Neurosurgery
CNS PUBLICATIONS

Proudly presents

RHOTON

CRANIAL ANATOMY & SURGICAL APPROACHES

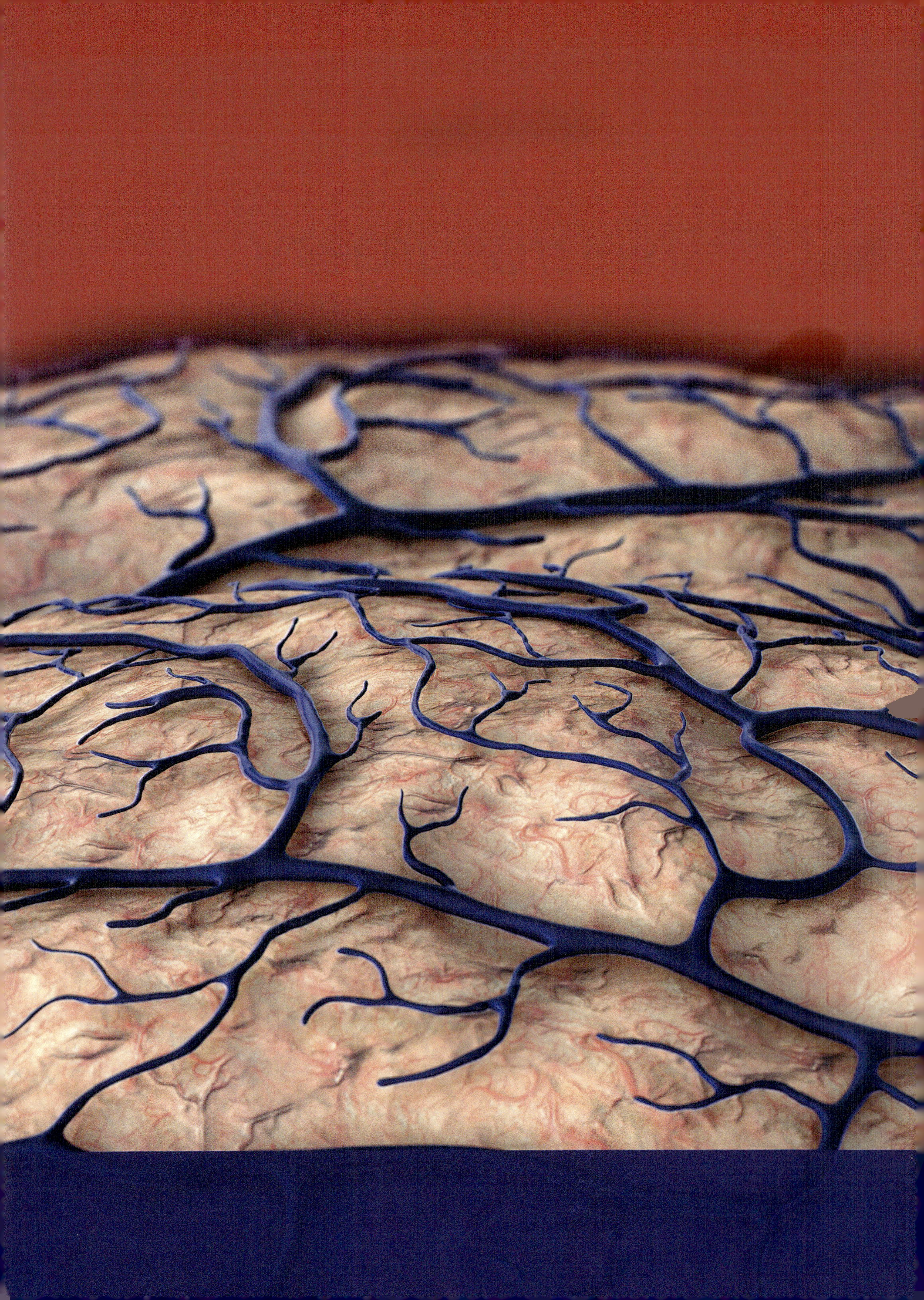

RHOTON

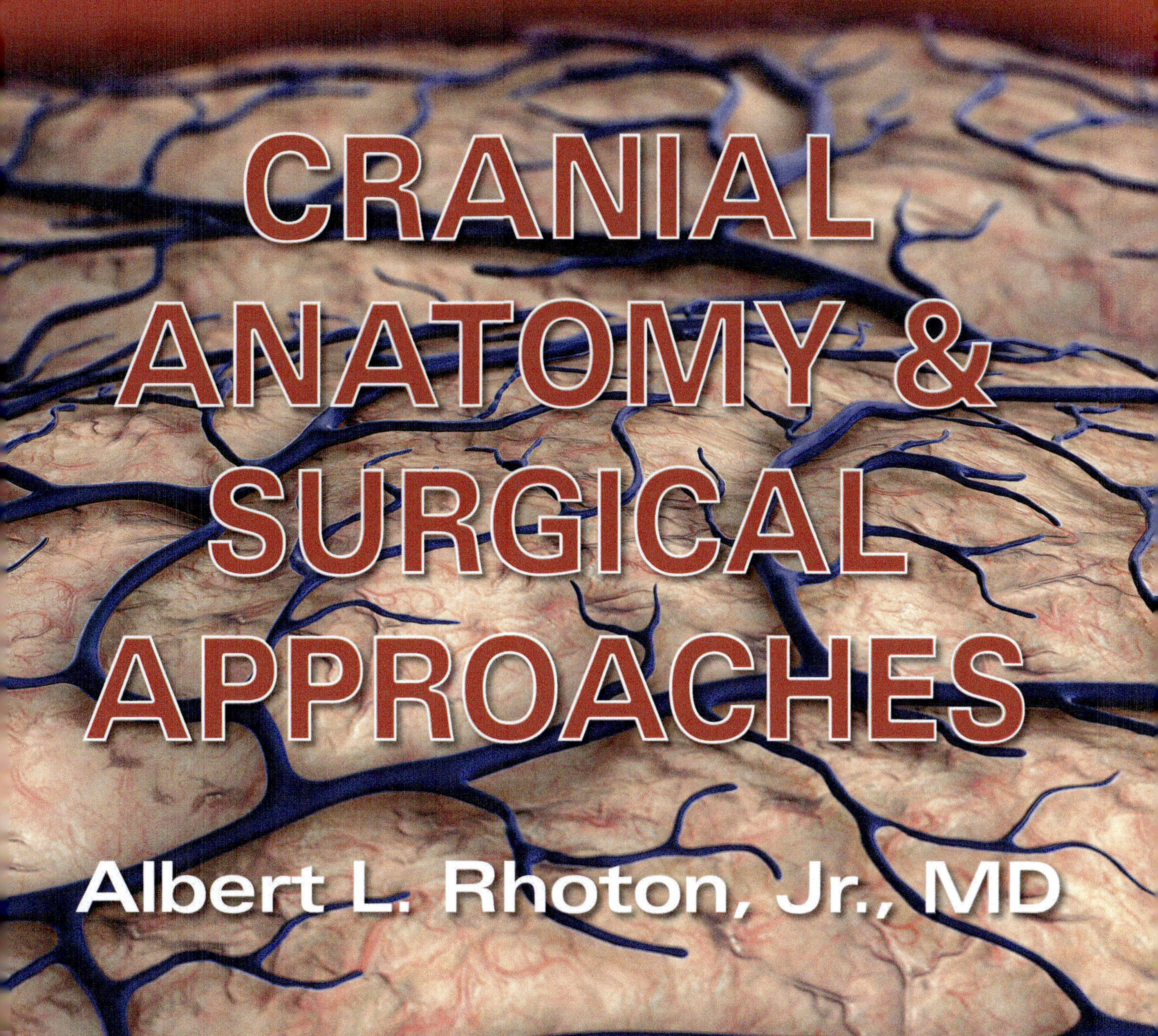

CRANIAL ANATOMY & SURGICAL APPROACHES

Albert L. Rhoton, Jr., MD

Wolters Kluwer
Philadelphia • Baltimore • New York • London
Buenos Aires • Hong Kong • Sydney • Tokyo

CONGRESS OF NEUROLOGICAL SURGEONS 1951 ERUDITIO OBSERVANTIA SOCIETAS CNS

Neurosurgery
CNS PUBLICATIONS

Acquisitions Editor: James Sherman
Senior Development Editor: Ariel S. Winter
Production Project Manager: Frances Gunning
Marketing Manager: Kirsten Watrud
Manager, Graphic Arts & Design: Stephen Druding
Manufacturing Coordinator: Lisa Bowling
Prepress Vendor: Aptara, Inc.

ISBN 978-1-9752-2687-9
ISSN 0148-397X

9 8 7 6 5 4 3 2
Printed in the United States of America

Library of Congress Cataloging-in-Publication Data available upon request.

shop.lww.com

MPP1125

Neurosurgery

CNS 1951

INFORMATION FOR SUBSCRIBERS

NEUROSURGERY (ISSN 0148-396X) is published monthly by Wolters Kluwer Health, Inc, at 1800 Dual Highway, Suite 201, Hagerstown, MD 21740-6636, for the Congress of Neurological Surgeons. Periodical postage paid at Hagerstown, MD, and additional mailing offices.

POSTMASTER: Send address changes to Neurosurgery, PO Box 1610, Hagerstown, MD 21740.

CNS MEMBERSHIP SERVICES
Congress of Neurological Surgeons
10 North Martingale Road, Suite 190
Schaumburg, IL 60173
TEL: 847/240-2500; FAX: 847/240-0804
TOLL-FREE: 877/517-1CNS
E-MAIL: info@cns.org

EDITORIAL CORRESPONDENCE
Brandon J. Fiedor, Director of Publications
Neurosurgery Publications
10 North Martingale Road, Suite 190
Schaumburg, IL 60173
TEL: 847/240-2500; FAX: 847/240-0804
TOLL-FREE: 877/517-1CNS
E-MAIL: neurosurgerypubs@cns.org

SUBSCRIPTION INFORMATION: All subscription inquiries: Customer Service, Wolters Kluwer Health, Inc., 1800 Dual Highway, Suite 201, Hagerstown, MD 21740-6636. Phone: 1-800-638-3030 (U.S., Canada, or Mexico). Outside North America call +1 (301) 223-2300. Email: customerservice@lww.com.

SUBSCRIPTION PRICE:
US subscriptions (NEUROSURGERY and OPERATIVE NEUROSURGERY package): Individuals: $1083.00. Institutions: $2250.00. International subscriptions (includes Canada and Mexico) in US dollars: Individuals: $1552.00. Institutions: $2940.00.

MEMBER SUBSCRIPTION INFORMATION: Congress of Neurological Surgeons member inquiries, change of address, back issues, claims, and membership renewal requests should be addressed to Congress of Neurological Surgeons, 10 North Martingale Road, Suite 190, Schaumberg, IL, 60173, Phone: 847-240-2500, Fax: 847-240-0804, Toll Free: 877-517-1CNS Web site: **www.cns.org;** Requests for replacement issues should be made within six months of the missing or damaged issue. Beyond six months and at the request of Congress of Neurological Surgeons, the publisher will supply replacement issues when losses have been sustained in transit and when the reserve stock permits.

ABSTRACTING AND INDEXING: The Journal is currently included by the following services in print and/or electronic format: PubMed, Index Medicus, Current Contents/Life Sciences, Clinical Medicine, and Science Citation Index.

INTERNATIONAL ADVISORY BOARD

NEUROSURGERY SPEAKS! OPERATIONS

COORDINATOR Jessica Striley — *Schaumburg, IL, USA*

ARABIC

Ahmed M. Alkhani — *King Abdulaziz Medical City, MNG-HA, Riyadh, Saudi Arabia*
Nasser El-Ghandour — *Faculty of Medicine, Cairo University, Cairo, Egypt*
Charbel Moussalem — *American University of Beirut Medical Center, Beirut, Lebanon*
Ibrahim Sbeih — *Farah Medical Campus, Amman, Jordan*

CHINESE

Zhuoying Du — *Huashan Hospital, Fudan University, Shanghai, China*
Xiaochun Jiang — *Yi Ji Shan Hospital (the First Affiliated Hospital), Wannan Medical College, Wuhu, China*
Hailiang Tang — *Huashan Hospital, Fudan University, Shanghai, China*
Junjie Wang — *Beijing Hospital, National Center of Gerontology, Beijing, China*
Kai Wang — *Weihai Central Hospital, Weihai, Shandong, China*
Xiang Zou — *Huashan Hospital, Shanghai Medical College, Fudan University, Shanghai, China*

ENGLISH

Ali Alaraj — *University of Illinois at Chicago, Chicago, IL, USA*
Fadi Al Saiegh — *Thomas Jefferson Hospital, Philadelphia, PA, USA*
Cargill H. Alleyne, Jr — *Piedmont Augusta, Augusta, GA, USA*
William Wallace Ashley — *Sinai Hospital and LifeBridge Health System, Baltimore, MD, USA*
Oluwakemi Aderonke Badejo — *University of Ibadan, College of Medicine, Ibadan, Nigeria*
Roberto Jose Diaz — *McGill University, Faculty of Medicine, Montreal, Quebec, Canada*
Mohamed Amin Soliman — *Cairo University, Faculty of Medicine, Cairo, Egypt*
Kunal Vakharia — *University of South Florida, Tampa, FL, USA*

FRENCH

Georges Abi Lahoud — *Institut de la Colonne Vertébrale et des NeuroSciences, Centre Médico-Chirurgical Bizet, Paris, France*
Michael Bruneau — *UZ Brussel, Vrije Universiteit Brussel (VUB), Brussels, Belgium*
Charbel Moussalem — *American University of Beirut Medical Center, Beirut, Lebanon*
Ulrick Sidney Kanmounye — *Geisinger Neuroscience Institute, Danville, PA, USA*

GREEK

Georgios A. Alexiou — *University Hospital of Ioannina, Ioannina, Greece*
George Georgoulis — *General Hospital of Athens "G. Gennimatas", Athens, Greece*
Stavros Matsoukas — *Mount Sinai Hospital, New York, NY, USA*
Themistoklis Papasilekas — *University of Athens Medical School, Athens, Greece*
Christos Tsitsipanis — *University Hospital of Heraklion, Heraklion, Greece*
Andreas Zigouris — *University Hospital of Ioannina, Ioannina, Greece*

ITALIAN

Francesco Acerbi — *Fondazione IRCCS Istituto Neurologico, C. Besta Milano, Milan, Italy*
Daniele Bongetta — *Ospedale Fatebenefratelli e Oftalmico, Milan, Italy*
Francesco Cardinale — *"Claudio Munari" Center for Epilepsy Surgery ASST GOM Niguarda, Milan, Italy*
Alfredo Conti — *Alma Mater Studiorum University of Bologna, and IRCCS Istituto delle Scienze Neurologiche di Bologna, Bologna, Italy*
Danilo De Paulis — *Hospital of the Sea, Naples, Italy*
Maurizio Iacoangeli — *Marche Polytechnic University, Umberto I General Hospital, Ancona, Italy*
Michele Rizzi — *Fondazione IRCCS Istituto Neurologico "Carlo Besta", Milan, Italy*
Andrea Ruggeri — *University of Rome "La Sapienza", Rome, Italy*

JAPANESE

Masaru Aoyagi — *Shioda Memorial Hospital, Nagara, Japan*
Kenichiro Asano — *Hirosaki University, Hirosaki, Japan*
Toshiki Endo — *Tohoku Medical and Pharmaceutical University, Sendai, Miyagi, Japan*
Toshiaki Hayashi — *Miyagi Children's Hospital, Sendai, Japan*
Yoshinori Higuchi — *Chiba University Graduate School of Medicine, Chiba City, Japan*
Tomoo Inoue — *Tohoku University Graduate School of Medicine, Sendai, Japan*
Hidehito Kimura — *Kobe University Graduate School of Medicine, Kobe, Japan*
Ryu Kurokawa — *Dokkyo Medical University Hospital, Tochigi, Japan*
Yoshikazu Matsuda — *Showa University, Tokyo, Japan*
Jun Muto — *Fujita Health University, Aichi, Japan*
Soichi Oya — *Saitama Medical Center/University, Saitama, Japan*

KOREAN

Tae Gon Kim — *Bundang CHA Medical Center, CHA University School of Medicine, Seongnam, Republic of Korea*
Sun Ha Paek — *Seoul National University, College of Medicine, Seoul, Republic of Korea*
Hye Ran Park — *Soonchunhyang University Seoul Hospital, Seoul, Republic of Korea*
Kawngwoo Park — *Gachon University Gil Medical Center, Incheon, Republic of Korea*

PORTUGUESE

Marcos Dellaretti — *Santa Casa de Belo Horizonte, Belo Horizonte, Brazil*
Hugo Leonardo Doria-Netto — *Universidade Federal de São Paulo - UNIFESP, and Hospital Beneficência Portuguesa de São Paulo, São Paulo, Brazil*
Eduardo Carvalhal Ribas — *Hospital das Clínicas, University of São Paulo Medicine School (HC-FMUSP), and Hospital Israelita Albert Einstein, São Paulo, Brazil*

RUSSIAN

Sergey Abeshaus — *Galilee Medical Center, Bar-Ilhan University, Nahariya, Israel*
Mikhail Gelfenbeyn — *University of Washington, Seattle, Washington*
Vsevolod Shurhkhay — *Burdenko Institute of Neurosurgery, Moscow, Russia*
Natalia Timchenko — *Sklifosovsky Research Institute of Emergency Medicine, Moscow, Russia*

SPANISH

Carlos Alarcon — *Department of Neurosurgery, Hospital Universitari Mutua de Terrassa, Barcelona, Spain*
Luis Ascanio-Cortez — *Icahn School of Medicine at Mount Sinai, Mount Sinai Health System, New York, NY, USA*
Juan Barges Coll — *University Hospital of Lausanne (CHUV), Lausanne, Switzerland*
Rodrigo Carrasco — *Hospital Universario Ramon y Cajal, Madrid, Spain*
Ricardo Diez Valle — *Quiron Group Hospitals, Madrid, Spain*
Alejandro Enriquez-Marulanda — *Beth Israel Deaconess Medical Center, Boston, MA, USA*
Ariel Kaen — *Hospital Virgen del Rocío, Sevilla, Spain*
Francisco Alberto Mannará — *Fernández Hospital, Buenos Aires City, Argentina*
Elizabeth Ogando-Rivas — *University of Florida, Gainesville, FL, USA*
Ramiro Antonio Pérez de la Torre — *Michigan Head and Spine Institute, Royal Oak, MI, USA*
Carlos Pérez-López — *University Hospital La Paz, Madrid, Spain*
Igor Paredes Sansinenea — *University Hospital "12 de Octubre", Madrid, Spain*

Neurosurgery

CNS PUBLICATIONS

First Published Rhoton's Anatomy October 2003 Volume 53 Pages 1-746

EDITOR'S LETTER:

THE TIMELESS VALUE OF RHOTON'S CRANIAL ANATOMY AND SURGICAL APPROACHES

Under Editor-in-Chief Michael L. J. Apuzzo, working with Professor Albert L. Rhoton, this book was created as a singular foundational document in neurosurgery. It remains an educational stalwart. The different printings, all desired by new practitioners of our craft, have allowed his work to reach more and more neurosurgeons across the world. The understanding of anatomy and the surgical principles upon which it is based, serve as our starting point in the understanding of disease, structure and function. The microneurosurgical era mandated the understanding of a "new' anatomy, and this then expanded to include the endoneurosurgical area, and other approaches whether with catheter, exoscope, or any other visualization tool. **Neurosurgery Publications** is proud to again present this essential work.

Douglas Kondziolka, MD, MSc
Editor-in-Chief, **Neurosurgery Publications**
New York, New York
2023

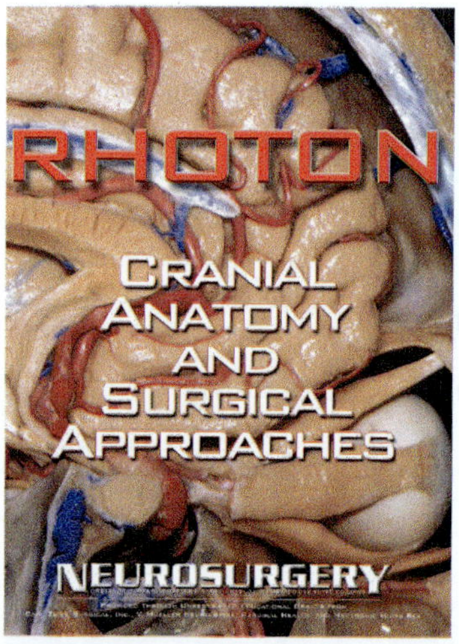

Lippincott Williams & Wilkins, 2007

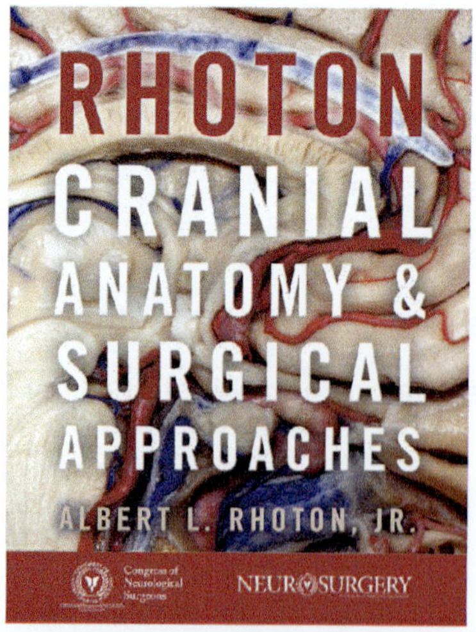

Oxford University Press, 2020

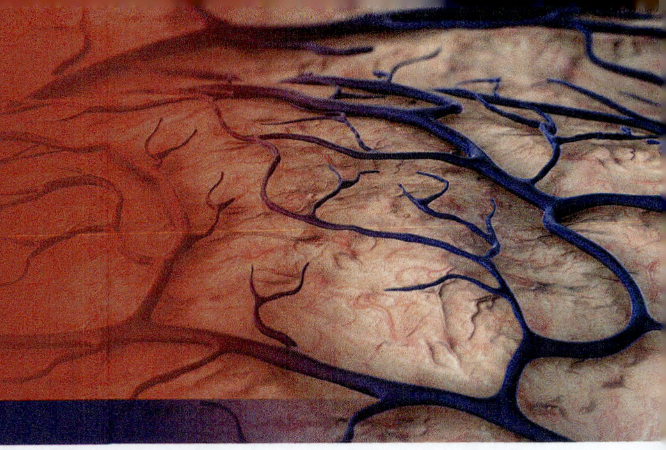

EDITOR'S LETTER

MIRABILE VISU

This volume stands as a tribute to the remarkable vision, diligence, and intelligence of Albert L. Rhoton, Jr. It is the concrete legacy of his character and persona. It serves as an example for all of us who would call ourselves neurosurgeons and represents the epitome of the term "contribution to the field" - a notion and goal that is the elusive "Holy Grail" for many of us.

In the progress of refinement of our surgical discipline over the centuries, the comprehension of anatomy, its quintessential building block, has been central to any surgical endeavor. All of our surgical ancestors, from Galen to Yasargil, have been aware of this truism. The challenge of the microneurosurgical era requires precise comprehension of the microsurgical anatomic substrate. In an effort spanning more than 40 years, Dr. Rhoton has developed and refined the field's comprehension of this critical foundation of our surgical enterprise. The work clearly stands alone as a remarkable contribution and accomplishment by an individual in this or any era. As a unique addition to the content of this volume, Dr. Rhoton's genius for instrument design and the practical craft of microneurosurgery is conveyed in generous detail.

NEUROSURGERY is proud to present the essential amalgam of the principal elements of this enterprise for our colleagues around the world, and we are particularly grateful to Dr. Rhoton for affording us the singular privilege of publishing this composite classic work. We are likewise indebted to Carl Zeiss Surgical, V. Mueller Neuro/Spine, Cardinal Health, and Medtronic Midas Rex for their generous and insightful support of this important project.

Michael L.J. Apuzzo
Editor-in-Chief Emeritus
Los Angeles, California

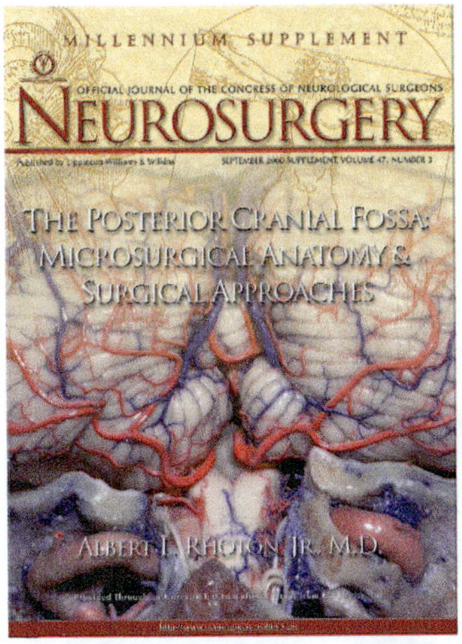

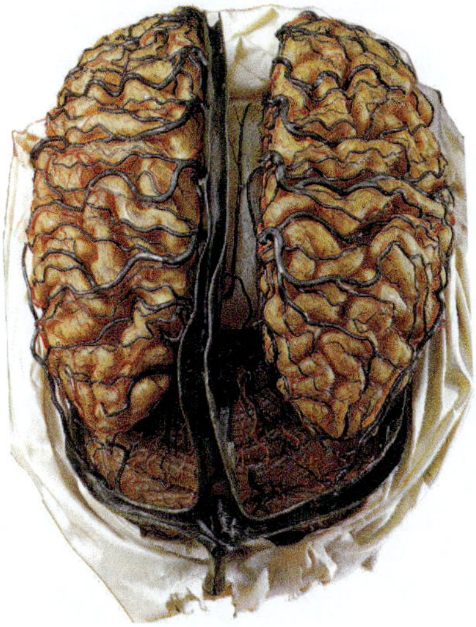

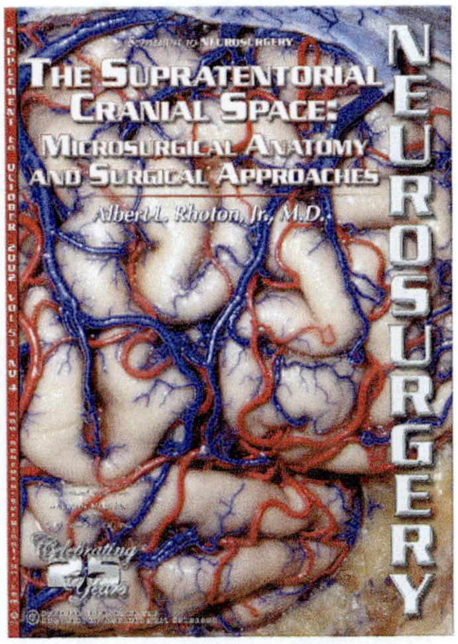

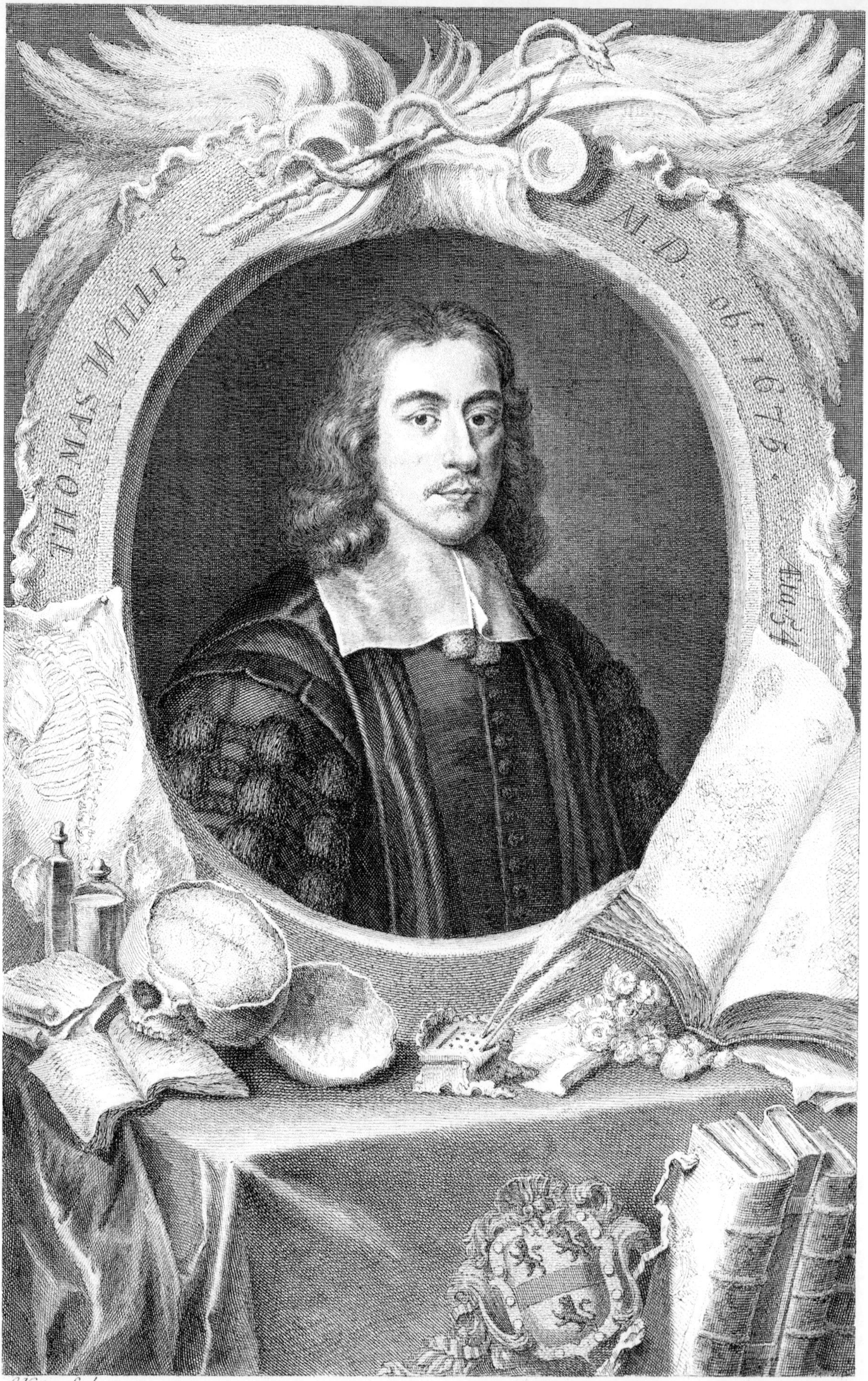

Portrait of Thomas Willis by Vertue, 1742, printed by Knapton. It is a copy of the earlier Laggan engraving done in 1666 when Willis was 45 years old.

FOREWORD

THE BRAIN AND CRANIAL BASE: MICROSURGICAL ANATOMY AND SURGICAL APPROACHES

I salute Cardinal Health V. Mueller, Carl Zeiss, Inc., and Medtronic Midas Rex on the occasion of the publication of this book and thank them for the grant that made it possible. Cardinal V. Mueller was added to the list of those whose grants made this second printing* possible. Cardinal V. Mueller has been producing microsurgical instruments for decades that allow us to take advantage of the anatomy displayed in this volume. It was my good fortune to begin work with Bill Merz of Cardinal V. Mueller nearly 40 years ago. Bill was among the best instrument makers in the world. Bill and V. Mueller have worked with the leading surgeons of the world and have produced instruments that have contributed greatly to the care of our patients. When I had a need for an instrument to make our work more accurate and safe, Bill Merz immediately sensed the possibilities. He derived great pride and joy from knowing he had met the need for an instrument that improved the outcome and lives of patients. In his later years, Mr. Merz established the William Merz Professorship in the Department of Neurosurgery at the University of Florida. I also salute Carl Zeiss and Medtronic on the occasion of the publication of this book and thank them for the grants that made this and the first printing possible. The increased safety and accuracy, and the improved results obtained with the Zeiss microscope are some of my greatest professional blessings and a great contributor to the quality of life of my patients. Medtronic Midas Rex, through the increased ease and delicacy of bone removal provided by their drills, has also made a worldwide contribution to the care of neurosurgical patients and allowed us to focus on dealing accurately and precisely with the delicate neural tissue that is the basis of our specialty. Midas Rex, Zeiss, and V. Mueller have continued to invest in modifying and upgrading their instruments by integrating them with modern technological advances in order to aid us in our work and provide new benefits to our patients. They have assisted with educational endeavors, like this book, that have improved neurosurgical care on every continent and have made the academic aspects of my career much more rewarding. I am grateful for their support of the publication of our studies on microsurgical anatomy and for partnering with neurosurgeons throughout the world to improve neurosurgical care (1). As stated in the Millennium and 25th Anniversary Issues of *Neurosurgery*, this work on microsurgical anatomy has grown out of my personal desire to improve the care of my patients (1, 2). It represents a 40 plus year attempt to gain an understanding of the anatomy and intricacies of the brain that would improve the safety, gentleness, and accuracy of my patients' surgery.

Before proceeding with some additional thoughts about the role of microsurgical anatomy in neurosurgery, I would like to share some thoughts about neurosurgery, some of which were included in my addresses as President of the AANS and CNS (1, 2). Neurosurgeons share a great professional gift; our lives have yielded an opportunity to help mankind in a unique and exciting way. In my early years, I never imagined that my life would hold as gratifying, exciting, and delicate a challenge as that of being a physician or a neurosurgeon. Neurosurgeons' work is performed in response to the idea that human life is sacred, that it makes sense to spend years of one's life in study to prepare to help others. Our training brings into harmony a knowledgeable mind, a skilled set of hands, and a well-trained eye, all of which are guided by a caring human being. The skills we use have been described as the most delicate, the most fateful, and, to the layperson, the most awesome of any profession. The Gallup Poll has reported that neurosurgeons are among the most prestigious and highly skilled members of American society. We share the opportunity to serve people in a unique way, dealing surgically with the most delicate of tissues.

Our ranking among the most highly skilled members of society tends to lead us to forget that our work and success are made possible by the benevolent order built into the universe around us. That people heal and survive after surgery provides us with our work and serves as a constant reminder of this benevolent protective order. We are surrounded by biological and physical forces that could overcome us, outstripping our finest medical and scientific achievements. The momentous process of injured tissues' knitting together is as essential to the work of the surgeon as the air people breathe is to their survival. The humanity survives and that neurosurgeons can play a role in the process of healing are examples of the compassion and love that surround us. A patient who writes a thank-you note or praises my efforts leads me to inwardly reflect that one of our greatest gifts is that we were created to help each other. I am grateful for the opportunity to be a participant in the miracle we call *neurosurgery*.

Another gift we share is a historical one based on the standards set by early physicians. Hippocrates taught that medicine is a difficult art that is inseparable from the highest morality and love of humanity. The noble values and loyal obedience of generations of physicians since Hippocrates have raised the calling to the highest of all professions. Many

*Printed in 2007

of us were attracted to neurosurgery by both the meticulousness of surgical craftsmanship and the intellectual challenge posed by modern clinical neurology and neurophysiology. All of us have submitted ourselves to the discipline of rigorous training, possibly the most demanding in modern society, and are capable of giving a great deal of ourselves.

Our work has grown out of the belief in absolute standards of value and worth in humanity. These values are reflected in the increasing importance of one man, one woman, or one child in American society and throughout the world. An example of the evolving importance of the individual is found in examining great human creations such as the Egyptian pyramids and the Great Wall of China. Through the decades and the centuries, humankind has evolved to the point where some of the pyramids of modern society are our modern medical centers. In them, society's most highly trained teams, using humankind's most advanced technology at great cost, are allowed to work for days trying to improve the lives of individual patients without regard to whether they are rich or poor. Issues related to the dignity and worth of a single man, woman, and child are clearer to us now than they were a century or two ago and provide the driving force behind our work. These values and standards, which are inseparable from the highest morality and love of humanity, are built into us just as the process of healing is built into our nature.

J. Lawrence Pool, who led the neurosurgery program at Columbia University, wrote, "As I look back on the pattern of my life I see how fortunate it was that I had chosen a career in neurosurgery, which I passionately loved despite its long hours and many grueling experiences." He concluded with a statement about his belief that the best surgeons have a strong sense of compassion. It is important that we grow in compassion just as we grow in competence. Competence is the possession of a required skill or knowledge. Compassion, on the other hand, does not require a skill or knowledge; it requires an innate feeling, commonly called love, toward someone else. Both competence and compassion need to be developed simultaneously, just as the giant oak develops its root system along with its leaves and branches. Competence without compassion is worthless. Compassion without competence is meaningless. It is a great challenge to guide patients competently and compassionately through neurosurgery. Death and darkness crowd near to our patients as we help them search for the correct path. Neurosurgical illness threatens not only their physical but also their financial security, because it is so expensive and the potential for disability is so great. No experience draws more frequently than the performance of neurosurgical procedures on the passage in Psalm 23, "though I walk through the valley of the shadow of death...." Neurosurgeons' competence should be reflected in our training, knowledge, and skill; our compassion should be reflected in our kindness, sincerity, and concern. The Saints and Buddhas taught that compassion and wisdom, which lead to competence, are one. Our patients are looking for help from someone who is knowledgeable, patient, and wise and who can provide clarity, wisdom, and enlightenment so that they can face life after surgery on the brain. That is the essence of integrating competence and compassion. Neurosurgeons have the responsibility to develop the dialogue in understandable terms to help the patient, the patient's family, and society understand the meaning of the patient's illness. One of my personal precepts is, "The best ally in the treatment of neurosurgical illness is a well-informed patient." Success requires more than advancing and applying medical knowledge. It also requires increased compassion so that we can respond sympathetically and with the best of our knowledge to all of our patients' questions and provide them with timely information that will help them understand their illness and plan their lives. There comes a time in our work when we can make as much of a difference in each other's lives by sitting for 30 minutes, for 1 hour, or longer to answer questions as we can by hours in surgery. There is no substitute for an honest, concerned, and sympathetic attitude. Success may not mean that every patient survives or is cured, because some problems are insolvable and some illnesses are incurable. Instead, success should mean giving every patient the feeling that he or she is cared about, no matter how desperate their situation, that their pain is felt, that their anger is understood, and that we care and will do our best. The greatest satisfaction in life comes from offering what you have to give. Devotion and giving to others gives purpose and meaning to life.

Another circumstance leading to the esteem that neurosurgeons enjoy is the magnificent tissue with which we work. The brain is the crown jewel of creation and evolution. It is a source of mystery and wonder. Of all the natural phenomena to which science can draw attention, none exceeds the fascination of the workings of the human brain. The brain holds our greatest unexplored biological frontiers. It is the only organ that is hidden and completely enclosed within a fortress of bone. The brain, although it does not move, is the most metabolically active of all organs, receiving 20% of cardiac output while representing only 3% of total body weight. It is the most frequent site of crippling, incurable disease. It is exquisitely sensitive to touch, anoxia, and derangements of its internal environment. Its status determines whether the humanity within us lives or dies. It yields all we know of the world. It controls both the patient and the surgeon.

Brain accounts for the mind, and through the mind, we are lifted from our immediate circumstances and are given an awareness of ourselves, our universe, our environment, and even the brain itself. Here, in two handsful of living tissue, we find an ordered complexity sufficient to preserve the record of a lifetime of the richest human experience and create computers that can store amounts of data that can be comprehended only by the mind. Perhaps the most significant achievement of this tissue is the ability, on the one hand, to conceive of a universe more than a billion light-years across and, on the other, to conceptualize a microcosmic world out of the reach of the senses and to model words completely separate from the reality that we can see, hear, smell, touch, and taste. Mind and brain are the source of happiness, knowledge, and wisdom. The brain is not the seat of the soul, but it is through the brain and mind that we become aware of our own souls.

In my early years, never in my wildest flights of imagination did I consider that life would yield such rewarding and challenging work as that of being a physician, and I was unaware that neurosurgery even existed. My early life was without exposure to physicians, hospitals, or other modern conveniences (Fig. 1). My birth was aided by a midwife in exchange for a bag of corn. As I entered college, the goal of being a physician seemed so unattainable that I had not considered that possibility. I first pursued chemistry, but the missing human element led me to major in social work. Social work also failed to satisfy me because it lacked the opportunity to touch and help others by working with the hands. That I might become a physician did not enter my mind until a psychology instructor invited me to see a brain operation performed in his laboratory. To my amazement, a tiny lesion improved the small animal's behavior, but without affecting its motor skills. That day, I sensed some of the amazement that must have been experienced in the 1870s when Broca presented his early observations regarding the cerebral localization of speech in his patient, Tan, and when Fritsch and Hitzig described their experiments on the cerebral motor cortex. Before their time, interest in the brain and its function centered on philosophical discussions of the brain as the seat of the mind and the soul and not as a site possessing the localizing features suitable for the application of a physician's or surgeon's skills. On that day in a psychology laboratory, I learned that surgery based on these concepts was possible, and I knew that I had found my calling. I know that many neurosurgeons have had a similar meaningful experience.

In medical school, I began to work in a neuroscience laboratory in my spare time. At the end of my residency, I completed a fellowship in neuroanatomy. It was during this fellowship that I realized the potential for greater knowledge of microneurosurgery and microneurosurgical anatomy to improve the care of my patients. I resolved early in my career to incorporate this new technique into my practice, because it seemed to increase the safety with which we could delve deep into and under the brain. One of my favorite personal goals has been to find images of a single operation performed perfectly, because the inner discipline of striving toward perfection leads to improvement. Such images are the essential building blocks for the improvement of operative techniques. During my training and thereafter, I lay awake many nights, as I know all neurosurgeons have, worrying about a patient who was facing a necessary, critical, high-risk operation the next day. With the use of this new technique, I found that difficult operations that carried significant risk were performed with greater accuracy and less postoperative morbidity. During my training, I did not see a facial nerve preserved during the surgical removal of an acoustic neuroma. Today, that goal is accomplished in a high percentage of microsurgical procedures on acoustic neuromas. In the past, in operating on patients with pituitary tumors, there was minimal discussion of preserving the normal pituitary gland; today, however, the combination of new diagnostic and surgical techniques has made tumor removal with the preservation of normal pituitary function a frequent achievement. The application of microsurgery in neurosurgery has yielded a whole new level of neurosurgical performance and competence, and microsurgical anatomy is the roadmap for applying microsurgical techniques.

As I began to work with microsurgical techniques, I realized that there was a need to train many neurosurgeons in their use. When I moved to the University of Florida, I began trying to develop a center for teaching neurosurgeons these techniques. Eventually, with the help of private contributions, my institution was able to purchase the necessary microscopes and equipment for a laboratory in which seven surgeons could learn at one time. The next task was to find seven individuals who were willing to come to the university for a course. Finally, after much solicitation, seven surgeons joined us for a 1-week course. I was quite apprehensive about that course, because I was not sure that we could keep seven surgeons busy learning microvascular skills for a whole week. It was comforting to learn that Harvey Cushing, early in his career, had developed a similar laboratory in which surgeons could practice and perfect their operative skills. I still remember and am grateful to each member of the initial group of neurosurgeons who were willing to invest 1 week of their valuable time in our first course, more than 25 years ago. During the first afternoon of that course, I walked into the laboratory and, to my amazement, found seven surgeons working quietly and diligently. Nothing was said for long periods of time. In the midst of their intense endeavor and amazing quietness, I realized that we had tapped into a great force: the desire of neurosurgeons to improve themselves. Each individual neurosurgeon can acquire new skills so that a new level of performance in the specialty is achieved. Over the years, more than 1000 neurosurgeons have attended courses in our microneurosurgery laboratories. Microtechniques are now being applied throughout the specialty, thus adding a new level of delicacy and gentleness to neurosurgery. The competence of the whole specialty has been improved and with this experience has come the realization that neurosurgeons, as a group, are constantly aspir-

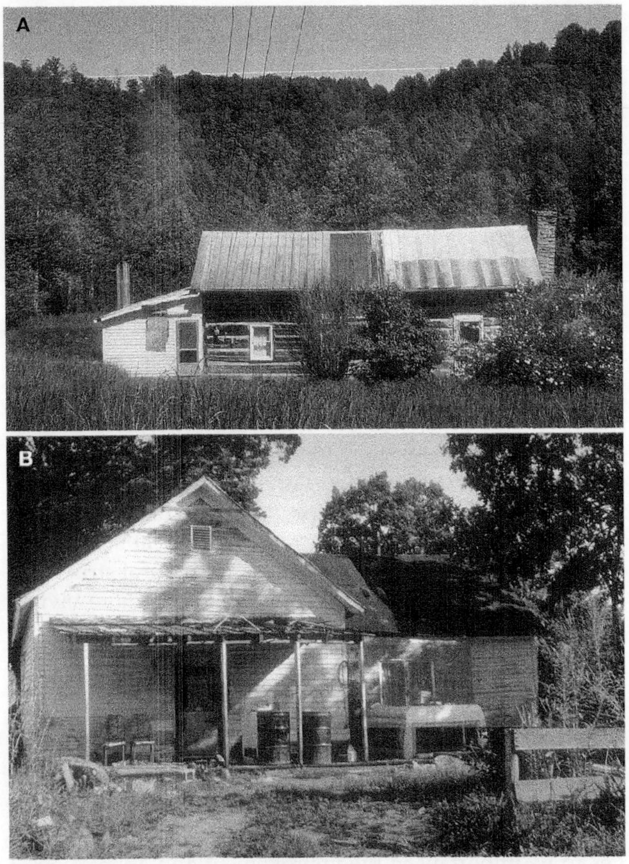

FIGURE 1. *Author's early home (A) and elementary school (B).*

ing to and achieving higher levels of performance that are not based on advances in diagnostic equipment and medication but are dependent on inspired individuals striving to improve their surgical skills to better serve their patients. Every year provides multiple examples of modifications in neurosurgery, based on the study and knowledge of microsurgical anatomy, that make operations more successful. It is amazing that, even after many years of study and practice, the insights gained from recent patients as well as continuing studies of microsurgical anatomy have lead to new and improved operative approaches. It is rewarding to see that most neurosurgery training programs now provide a laboratory for studying microsurgical anatomy and perfecting microsurgical techniques.

When we began our studies of anatomy more than 40 years ago, our dissections, even with microsurgical techniques, were crude by current standards. Photographs needed to be retouched to bring out the facets of anatomy important for achieving a satisfactory outcome at surgery. As we learned, over the years, to expose fine neural structures, the display of microsurgical anatomy became more vividly accurate and beautiful than we had imagined at the outset and has enhanced the accuracy and safety of our surgery. We hope that it will do the same for our readers.

Microsurgical anatomy will continue to be the science most fundamental to neurosurgery in the future. It will always occupy a major role in the training of neurosurgeons. The study and dissection of anatomic specimens improves surgical skill. The study of microsurgical anatomy continues to be important in the improvement and adaptation of old techniques to new situations. Its study will lead to numerous new and more accurate operative approaches and the application of new neurosurgical technologies in future. Microsurgical anatomy provides the basis for understanding the constantly improving imaging studies and provides an understanding of the safest and most effective surgical pathway for visualizing and treating neurosurgical pathology. Every year, there are advances in neurological technology that yield new therapeutic possibilities that must be evaluated and directed according to an enhanced understanding of anatomy.

The combination of the knowledge of microsurgical anatomy and the use of the operating microscope have improved the technical performance of many standard neurosurgical procedures (e.g., brain, spine, and cranial base tumor removal; aneurysm obliteration; neurorrhaphy; and even lumbar and cervical discectomy) and has opened new dimensions that were previously unattainable. The knowledge of microsurgical anatomy has improved operative results by permitting neural and vascular structures to be approached and delineated with greater accuracy, deep areas to be reached by safer routes with less brain retraction and smaller cortical incisions, bleeding to be controlled with less damage to adjacent neural and vascular structures, and nerves and perforating arteries to be preserved with greater frequency. The use of the microscope, when combined with the knowledge of microsurgical anatomy, has resulted in smaller wounds, less postoperative neural and vascular damage, better hemostasis, more accurate nerve and vascular repairs, and surgical treatment for some previously inoperable lesions. The microscopic study of anatomy has introduced a whole new era in surgical education by permitting the recording of minute anatomic detail not visible to the eye for later study and discussion.

Surgery with the operating microscope has led the neurosurgeon to the current limits of human dexterity, but in the future, robotically assisted microsurgery will open new frontiers of delicate surgery that will require additional microanatomic detail for optimization. The evolution of other technologies, such as endovascular surgery, will continue to require an accurate knowledge of microsurgical anatomy. In the endovascular treatment of aneurysms, an understanding of the variations in the anatomy of the parent vessel and the perforating arteries is as important as it is to microsurgical treatment. Microsurgical anatomy provided the basis for our entry into cranial base surgery and gave us a road map for reaching every site in the cranial base through carefully placed windows. The joint development of microsurgery in combination with image guidance has made it possible to work in long, narrow exposures to reach multiple deep sites within the brain. The study of microsurgical anatomy has led to the development of new approaches, such as the transchoroidal approaches to the third ventricle, the endonasal approach to pituitary tumor, and the telovelar approach to the fourth ventricle. In the future, there will be new, better, and safer procedures that will continue to evolve out of the continued study of microsurgical anatomy. It is hoped that the body of knowledge embodied in this volume will continue to be relevant to neurosurgical practice at the beginning of the next century and millennium.

Neurosurgery's 25th Anniversary issue (4) on the supratentorial area with 1000 color illustrations and the Millennium issue (3) on the posterior fossa with nearly 800 illustrations represent a distillation of more than 40 years of work and study in which 65 residents and fellows have participated, resulting in several hundred publications. For those wanting even greater detail than displayed in this volume, our prior works, published largely in *Neurosurgery* and the *Journal of Neurosurgery*, can be consulted. In this volume, we have attempted not only to display the brain and cranial base in the best views for understanding the anatomy but also to show the anatomy as exposed in the surgical routes to the supratentorial and infratemporal areas and cranial base. Areas examined include the cerebrum, the cerebellum, the lateral, third, and fourth ventricles, the cranial nerves, the cranial base, the orbit, the cavernous sinus, the temporal bone, the cerebellopontine angle, the foramen magnum, and numerous other structures. Our work is not complete in any area. Further study will yield new information that will improve the operative approach and operative results in dealing with pathology in each of the areas previously examined. There is no "finish line" for this effort. Future anatomic study will continue to yield new insights throughout the future of our specialty. Insights gained from the other medical sciences and new technologies, when combined with our increasing knowledge of microsurgical anatomy, will create new surgical possibilities, therapies, and cures.

It has been gratifying to view the role of our fellows and trainees in spreading this knowledge to other countries around the world and to see the benefits of neurosurgeons applying this knowledge to improve their patients' operations. Especially gratifying have been the relationships with Dr. Toshio Matsushima of Fukuoka, Japan, and Dr. Evandro de Oliveira of São Paulo, Brazil, whose studies of microsurgical anatomy have elevated the care of neurosurgical patients around the world. The following are the residents and fellows who have worked in the laboratory:

Hiroshi Abe, M.D., Japan
Hajime Arai, Japan
Allen S. Boyd, Jr., Tennessee
Robert Buza, Oregon
Alvaro Campero, Argentina
Alberto C. Cardoso, Brazil
Christopher C. Carver, California
Patrick Chaynes, France
Chanyoung Choi, Korea
Evandro de Oliveira, Brazil
Hatem El Khouly, Egypt
W. Frank Emmons, Washington
J. Paul Ferguson, Georgia
Andrew D. Fine, Florida
Brandon Fradd, Florida
Kiyotaka Fujii, Japan
Yutaka Fukushima, Japan
Adriano Scaff-Garcia, Brazil
Hirohiko Gibo, Japan
John L. Grant, Virginia
Kristinn Gudmundsson, Iceland
David G. Hardy, England
Frank S. Harris, Texas
Tsutomu Hitotsumatsu, Japan
Takuya Inoue, Japan
Tooru Inoue, Japan
Yukinari Kakizawa, Japan
Toshiro Katsuta, Japan
Masatou Kawashima, Japan
Chang Jin Kim, South Korea
Robert S. Knego, Florida
Shigeaki Kobayashi, Japan
Chae Heuck Lee, South Korea
Xiao-Yong Li, China
William Lineaweaver, California
J. Richard Lister, Illinois
Qing Liang Liu, China
Jack E. Maniscalco, Florida
Richard G. Martin, Alabama
Carolina Martins, Brazil
Haruo Matsuno, Japan
Toshio Matsushima, Japan
Juan C. Fernandez-Miranda, Spain
J. Robert Mozingo, deceased
Hiroshi Muratani, Japan
Antonio C.M. Mussi, Brazil
Shinji Nagata, Japan
Yoshihiro Natori, Japan
Kazunari Oka, Japan
Michio Ono, Japan
T. Glenn Pait, Arkansas
Wayne S. Paullus, Texas
David Perlmutter, Florida
Mark Renfro, Texas
Wade H. Renn, Georgia
Saran S. Rosner, New York
Pablo Rubino, Argentina
Naokatsu Saeki, Japan
Shuji Sakata, Japan
Eduardo R. Seoane, Argentina
Xiang-en Shi, China
Satoru Shimizu, Japan
Ryusui Tanaka, Japan
Necmettin Tanriover, Turkey
Helder Tedeschi, Brazil
Erdener Timurkaynak, Turkey
Xiaoguang Tong, China
Satoshi Tsutsumi, Japan
Arthur J. Ulm, Florida
Hung T. Wen, Brazil
C.J. Whang, South Korea
Isao Yamamoto, Japan
Alexandre Yasuda, Brazil
Nobutaka Yoshioka, Japan
Arnold A. Zeal, Florida

Special thanks go to our medical illustrators, David Peace and Robin Barry, who have worked with us for more than 2 decades. David and Robin's illustrations have graced hundreds of neurosurgical publications, including the covers of *Neurosurgery* and the *Journal of Neurosurgery*, for decades. I also extend special thanks to Ron Smith who has directed the microsurgery laboratory for many years, and to Laura Dickinson and Fran Johnson, who have labored over these and earlier manuscripts.

This work has been sustained by numerous private contributions to our department and the University of Florida. Most prominent among these has been that of the R.D. Keene family, who made the first $1 million gift to the University of Florida, a gift that has supported our work for many years. That gift was followed by additional endowments that have grown to nearly $20 million, which support many aspects of education and research in neurosurgery and the neurosciences at the University of Florida. These gifts have endowed the following chairs and professorships:

The R.D. Keene Family Chair
The C.M. and K.E. Overstreet Chair
The Mark Overstreet Chair
The Albert E. and Birdie W. Einstein Chair
The James and Newton Eblen Chair
The Dunspaugh-Dalton Chair
The Edward Shed Wells Chair
The Robert Z. and Nancy J. Greene Chair
The L.D. Hupp Chair
The William Merz Professorship
The Albert L. Rhoton, Jr. Chairman's Professorship

The most recent of these is the series of gifts and matching funds totaling nearly $5 million establishing the Albert L. Rhoton, Jr. Neurosurgery Professorship held by William A. Friedman, who followed me as chair of the Department of Neurosurgery. The efforts of the numerous clinicians and scientists recruited, as a result of the Endowed Chairs, contributed greatly to the founding the Evelyn F. and William L. McKnight Brain Institute of the University of Florida, where our studies of microsurgical anatomy are being completed. With this volume, we join our donors in their aspiration to improve the life of patients who undergo brain surgery throughout the world.

Before closing, I would like to thank my wife, Joyce, who has allowed microsurgical anatomy to become a hobby that has consumed much of my time away from the medical center. It is to Joyce that this volume is dedicated. In closing, I would also like to thank Editor Michael Apuzzo, not only from the bottom of my heart, but from the depths of my most valuable earthly possession, my brain, for allowing me to complete this work.

REFERENCES

1. Rhoton AL Jr: Presidential Address: Improving ourselves and our specialty. Clin Neurosurg 26:xiii-xix, 1979.
2. Rhoton AL Jr: Neurosurgery in the Decade of the Brain: The 1990 Presidential Address. J Neurosurg 73:487–495, 1990.
3. Rhoton AL Jr: The posterior cranial fossa: Microsurgical anatomy & surgical approaches. Neurosurgery 47[Suppl 1]:S1–S298, 2000.
4. Rhoton AL Jr: The supratentorial cranial space: Microsurgical anatomy and surgical approaches. Neurosurgery 51[Suppl 1]:S1-1–S1-410, 2002.

Albert L. Rhoton, Jr.
1932-2016
Gainesville, Florida

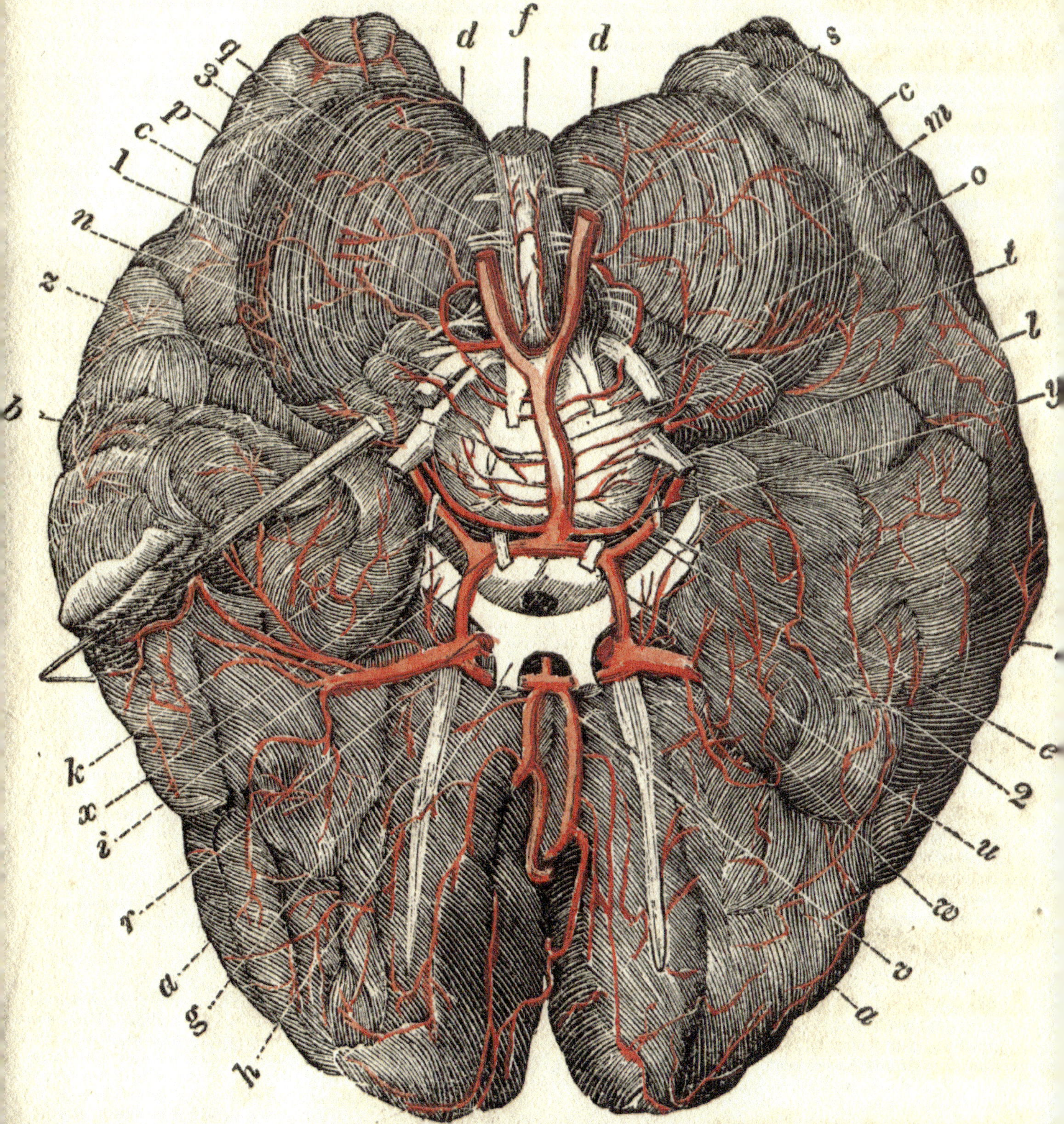

Basal view of human brain (from, Albrecht von Haller's Anatomical Description of the Arteries of the Human Body..., *Boston, Thomas B. Wait & Co., 1813), courtesy of Rare Book Room, Norris Medical Library, Keck School of Medicine, University of Southern California.*

Neurosurgery
CNS PUBLICATIONS

Proudly presents

RHOTON

CRANIAL ANATOMY & SURGICAL APPROACHES

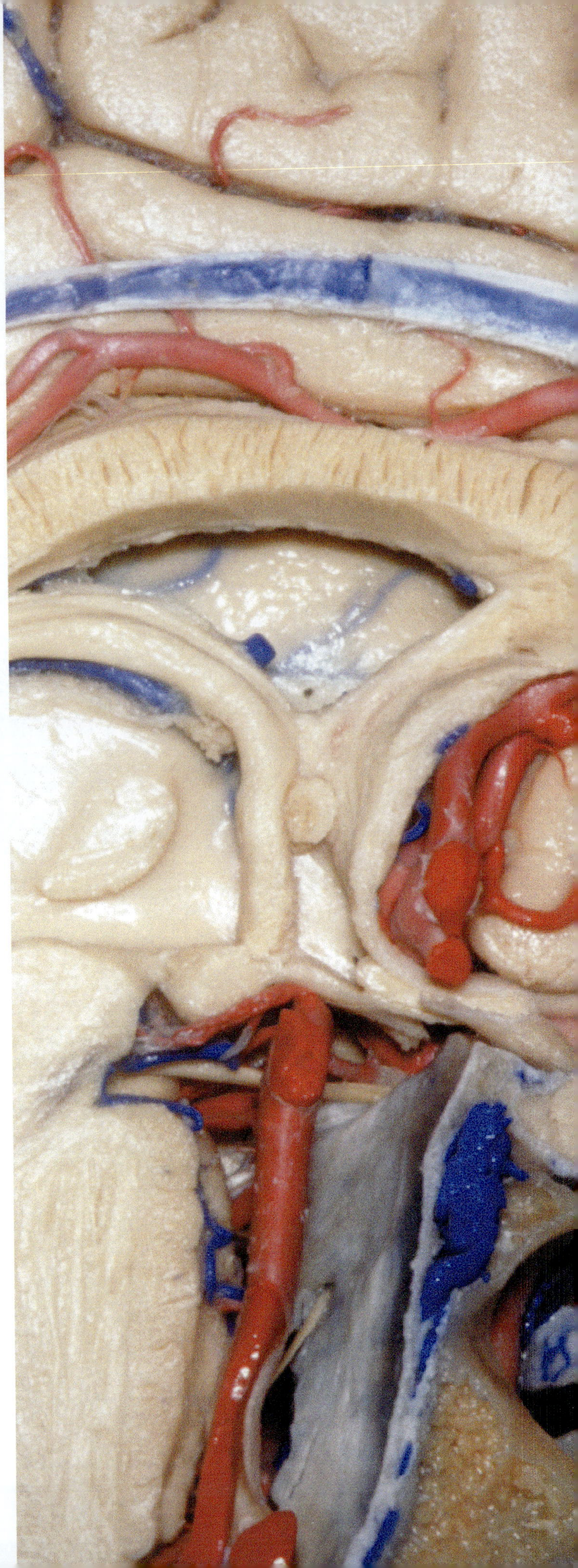

PART 1

Operative Techniques & Instrumentation for Neurosurgery

Operative Techniques and Instrumentation for Neurosurgery

Albert L. Rhoton, Jr., M.D.

Department of Neurological Surgery, University of Florida, Gainesville, Florida

Reprint requests:
Albert L. Rhoton, Jr., M.D., Department of Neurological Surgery, University of Florida McKnight Brain Institute, P.O. Box 100265, Gainesville, FL 32610-0265.
Email: rhoton@neurosurgery.ufl.edu

KEY WORDS: Cranial surgery, Craniotomy, Instrumentation, Microneurosurgery, Microsurgery, Operative techniques, Surgical instruments, Surgical microscope

The introduction of the operating microscope for neurosurgery brought about the greatest improvements in operative techniques that have occurred in the history of the specialty. The microscope has resulted in profound changes in the selection and use of instruments and in the way neurosurgical operations are completed. The advantages provided by the operating microscope in neurosurgery were first demonstrated during the removal of acoustic neuromas (4). The benefits of magnified stereoscopic vision and intense illumination provided by the microscope were quickly realized in other neurosurgical procedures. The operating microscope is now used for the intradural portion of nearly all operations involving the head and spine and for most extradural operations involving the spine and cranial base, converting almost all of neurosurgery into a microsurgical specialty.

Microsurgery has improved the technical performance of many standard neurosurgical procedures (e.g., brain tumor removal, aneurysm obliteration, neurorrhaphy, and lumbar and cervical discectomy) and has opened new, previously unattainable areas to the neurosurgeon. It has improved operative results by permitting neural and vascular structures to be delineated with greater visual accuracy, deep areas to be reached with less brain retraction and smaller cortical incisions, bleeding points to be coagulated with less damage to adjacent neural structures, nerves distorted by tumor to be preserved with greater frequency, and anastomosis and suturing of small vessels and nerves not previously possible to be performed. Its use has resulted in smaller wounds, less postoperative neural and vascular damage, better hemostasis, more accurate nerve and vessel repairs, and surgical treatment of some previously inoperable lesions. It has introduced a new era in surgical education, by permitting the observation and recording (for later study and discussion) of minute operative details not visible to the naked eye. Some general considerations are reviewed before discussion of instrument selection and operative techniques.

GENERAL CONSIDERATIONS

Achieving a satisfactory operative result depends not only on the surgeon's technical skill and dexterity but also on a host of details related to accurate diagnosis and careful preoperative planning. Essential to this plan is having a patient and family members who are well informed about the contemplated operation and who understand the associated side effects and risks. The surgeon's most important ally in achieving a satisfactory postoperative result is a well-informed patient.

Operating room scheduling should include information on the side and site of the pathological lesion and the position of the patient, so that the instruments and equipment can be properly positioned before the arrival of the patient (*Fig. 1.1*). Any unusual equipment required should be listed at the time of scheduling. There are definite advantages to having operating rooms dedicated to neurosurgery and to scheduling the same nurses, who know the equipment and procedures, for all neurosurgical cases.

Before induction, there should be an understanding between the surgeon and anesthesiologist regarding the need for administration of corticosteroids, hyperosmotic agents, anticonvulsants, antibiotics, and barbiturates, lumbar or ventricular drainage, and intraoperative evoked potential, electroencephalographic, or other specialized monitoring. Elastic or pneumatic stockings are placed on the patient's lower extremities, to prevent venous stagnation and postoperative phlebitis and emboli. A urinary catheter is inserted if the operation is expected to last more than 2 hours. If the patient is positioned so that the operative site is significantly higher than the right atrium, then a Doppler monitor is attached to the chest or inserted into the esophagus and a venous catheter is passed into the right atrium, so that venous air emboli can be detected and treated. At least two intravenous lines are established if significant bleeding is likely to occur.

Most intracranial procedures are performed with the patient in the supine, three-quarter prone (lateral oblique or park-bench), or fully prone position, with the surgeon sitting at the head of the table (*Fig. 1.1*). The supine position, with appropriate turning of the patient's head and neck and possibly elevation of one shoulder to rotate the upper torso, is selected for procedures in the frontal, temporal, and anterior parietal areas and for many cranial base approaches. The three-quarter prone position, with the table tilted to elevate the head, is used for exposure of the posterior parietal, occipital, and suboccipital areas (*Figs. 1.1–1.3*). Some sur-

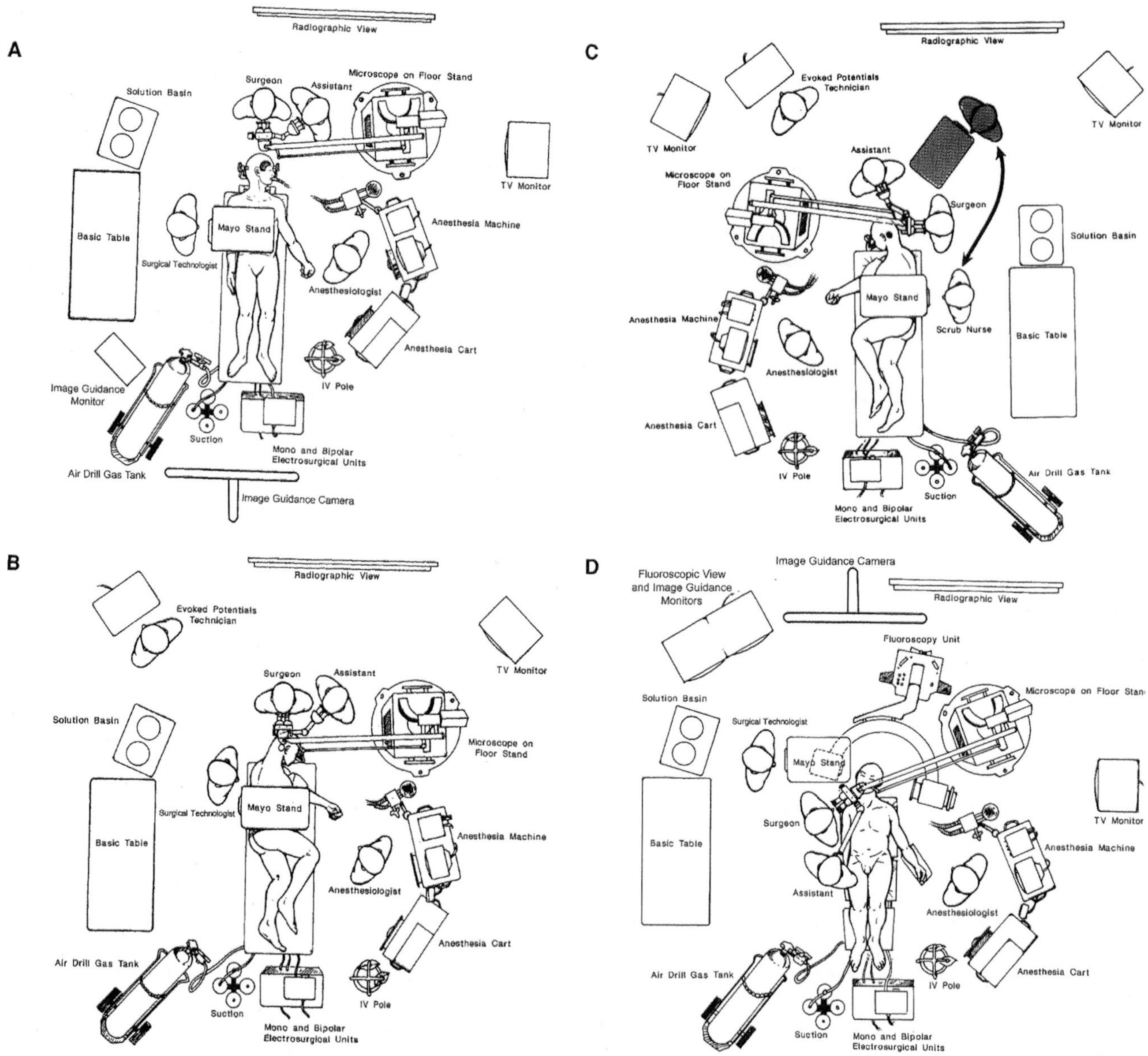

FIGURE 1.1. *Positioning of staff and equipment in the operating room.* A, *positioning for a right frontotemporal craniotomy. The anesthesiologist is positioned on the patient's left side, where the physician can have easy access to the airway, monitors on the chest, and the intravenous* (IV) *and intra-arterial lines. The microscope stand is positioned above the anesthesiologist. The scrub nurse, positioned on the right side of the patient, passes instruments to the surgeon's right hand. The position is reversed for a left frontotemporal craniotomy, with the anesthesiologist and microscope on the patient's right side and the nurse on the left side. Mayo stands have replaced the large heavy instrument tables positioned above the patient's trunk, which restricted access to the patient. The suction system, compressed air tanks for the drill, and electrosurgery units are positioned at the foot of the patient; the lines from these units are led up near the Mayo stand, so that the nurse can pass them to the surgeon as needed. A television* (TV) *monitor is positioned so that the nurse can anticipate the instrument needs of the surgeon. The infrared image guidance camera is positioned so that the surgeon, assistants, and equipment do not block the camera's view of the markers at the operative site.* B, *positioning for a right suboccipital craniotomy directed to the upper part of the posterior fossa, such as a decompression operation for treatment of trigeminal neuralgia. The surgeon is seated at the head of the patient. The anesthesiologist and microscope are positioned on the side the patient faces. The anesthesiologist and nurse shift sides for an operation on the left side.* C, *positioning for a left suboccipital craniotomy for removal of an acoustic neuroma. The surgeon is seated behind the head of the patient. For removal of a left acoustic tumor, the scrub nurse, with the Mayo stand, may move up to the* shaded area, *where instruments can be passed to the surgeon's right hand. For right suboccipital operations or for midline exposures, the positions are reversed, with the scrub nurse and Mayo stand being positioned above the body of the patient, which allows the nurse to pass instruments to the surgeon's right hand. In each case, the anesthesiologist is positioned on the side toward which the patient faces.* D, *positioning for transsphenoidal surgery. The surgeon is positioned on the right side of the patient and the anesthesiologist on the left side. The patient's head is rotated slightly to the right and tilted to the left, to provide the surgeon with a view directly up the patient's nose. The microscope stand is located just outside the C-arm on the fluoroscopy unit. The nurse and Mayo stand are positioned near the patient's head, above one arm of the fluoroscopy unit. The image guidance camera is positioned so that the surgeon does not block its view of the operative site.*

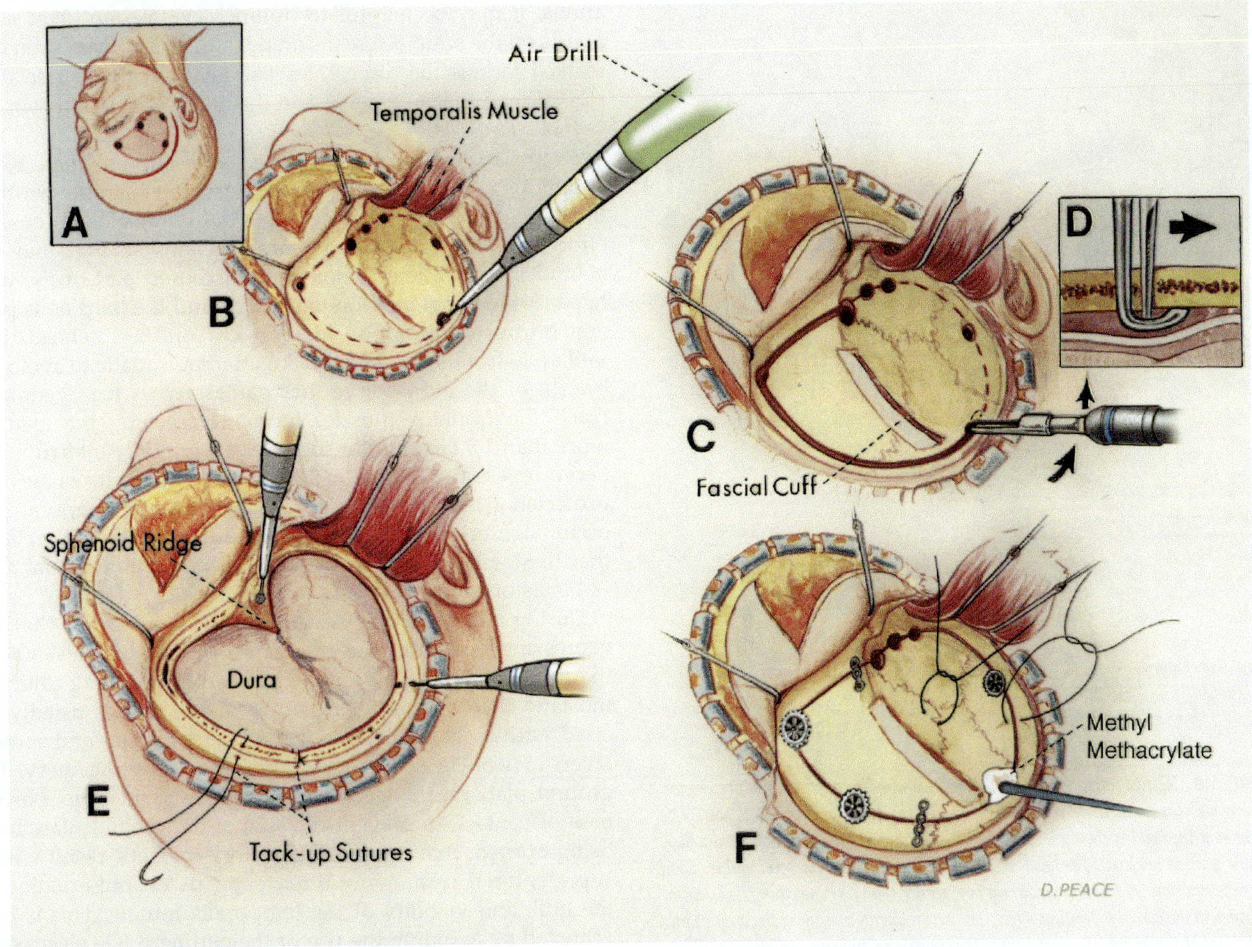

FIGURE 1.2. *Technique for craniotomy using a high-speed air or electric drill.* A, *right frontotemporal scalp and free bone flaps are outlined.* B, *the scalp flap has been reflected forward and the temporalis muscle downward. Elevation of the temporalis muscle with careful subperiosteal dissection with a periosteal elevator, rather than the cutting Bovie electrocautery, facilitates preservation of the muscle's neural and vascular supplies, which course in the periosteal attachments of the muscle to the bone. The high-speed drill prepares burr holes along the margins of the bone flap* (dashed line). C, *a narrow tool, with a foot plate to protect the dura, connects the holes.* D, *a cross sectional view of the cutting tool indicates how the foot plate strips the dura away from the bone.* E, *the high-speed drill removes the lateral part of the sphenoid ridge. A drill bit makes holes in the bone edge for tack-up sutures to hold the dura against the bony margin.* F, *after completion of the intradural part of the operation, the bone flap is held in place with plates and screws or burr hole covers that align the inner and outer tables of the bone flap and adjacent cranium. Silk sutures brought through drill holes in the margin of the bone flap may be used but do not prevent inward settling of the bone flap to the degree achieved with plating. Some methylmethacrylate may be molded into some burr holes or other openings in the bone, to provide firm cosmetic closure.*

geons still prefer to have the patient in the semi-sitting position for operations involving the posterior fossa and cervical region, because the improved venous drainage may reduce bleeding and because cerebrospinal fluid and blood do not collect in the depth of the exposure. Tilting the whole table to elevate the head of the patient in the lateral oblique position also reduces venous engorgement at the operative site. Extremes of turning of the head and neck, which may lead to obstruction of venous drainage from the head, should be avoided. Points of pressure or traction on the patient's body should be examined and protected.

Careful attention to the positioning of operating room personnel and equipment ensures greater efficiency and effectiveness. The anesthesiologist is positioned near the head and chest on the side toward which the head is turned, with easy access to the endotracheal tube and the intravenous and intra-arterial lines, rather than at the foot of the patient, where access to support systems is limited (*Fig. 1.1*). If the patient is treated in the supine or three-quarter prone position, then the anesthesiologist is positioned on the side toward which the face is turned and the scrub nurse is positioned on the other side, with the surgeon seated at the head of the patient (e.g., for a left frontal or frontotemporal approach, the anesthesiologist is positioned on the patient's right side and the scrub nurse is on the left side).

Greater ease in positioning the operating team around the patient is obtained when instruments are placed on Mayo stands, which can be moved around the patient. In the past, large, heavy, overhead stands with many instruments were positioned above the body of the patient. The use of Mayo stands, which are lighter and more easily moved, allows the scrub nurse and the instruments to be positioned and repositioned at the optimal site to

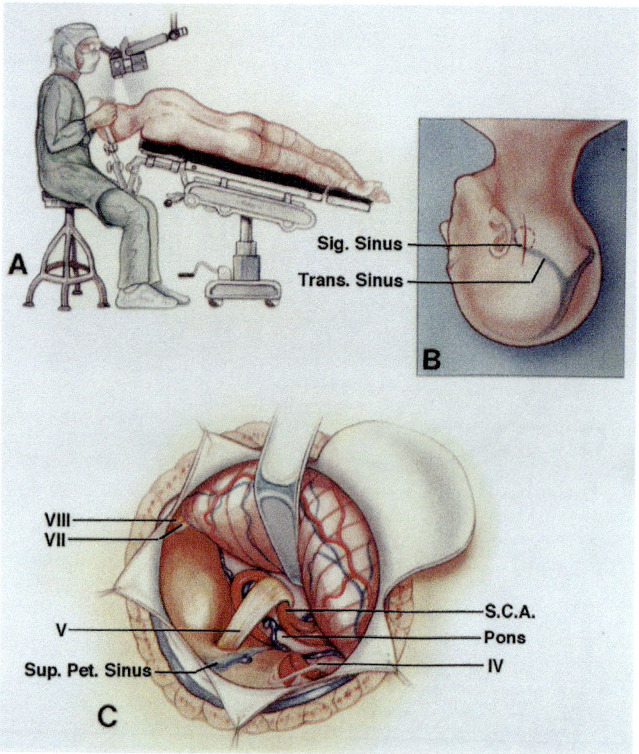

FIGURE 1.3. *Retrosigmoid approach to the trigeminal nerve for a decompression operation.* A, *the patient is positioned in the three-quarter prone position. The surgeon is at the head of the table. The patient's head is fixed in a pinion headholder. The table is tilted to elevate the head.* B, *the vertical paramedian suboccipital incision crosses the asterion. A small craniotomy flap, rather than a craniectomy, is used for approaches to the cerebellopontine angle. The superolateral margin of the craniotomy is positioned at the lower-edge junction of the transverse and sigmoid sinuses.* C, *the superolateral margin of the cerebellum is gently elevated with a tapered brain spatula, to expose the site at which the superior cerebellar artery loops down into the axilla of the trigeminal nerve. The brain spatula is advanced parallel to the superior petrosal sinus. The trochlear, facial, and vestibulocochlear nerves are in the exposure. The dura along the lateral margin of the exposure is tacked up to the adjacent muscles, to maximize the exposure. At the end of the procedure, the bone flap is held in place with magnetic resonance imaging-compatible plates.* Pet., *petrosal;* S.C.A., *superior cerebellar artery;* Sig., *sigmoid;* Sup., *superior;* Trans., *transverse* (from, *Rhoton AL Jr: Microsurgical anatomy of decompression operations on the trigeminal nerve, in Rovit RL (ed):* Trigeminal Neuralgia. *Baltimore, Williams & Wilkins, 1990, pp 165–200 [9]).*

assist the surgeon. It also provides the flexibility demanded by the more frequent use of intraoperative fluoroscopy, image guidance, and angiography. The control console for drills, suction, and coagulation is usually positioned at the foot of the operating table, and the tubes and lines are led upward to the operative site.

In the past, it was common to shave the entire head for most intracranial operations, but hair removal now commonly extends only 1.5 to 2 cm beyond the margin of the incision, with care being taken to shave and drape a wide enough area to allow extension of the incision if a larger operative field is needed and to allow drains to be led out through stab wounds. Some surgeons currently do not remove hair in preparation for a scalp incision and craniotomy. For supratentorial operations, it may be helpful to outline several important landmarks on the scalp before the drapes are applied. Sites commonly marked include the coronal, sagittal, and lambdoid sutures, the rolandic and sylvian fissures, and the pterion, inion, asterion, and keyhole (*Fig. 1.4*).

Scalp flaps should have a broad base and adequate blood supply (*Fig. 1.2*). A pedicle that is narrower than the width of the flap may result in the flap edges becoming gangrenous. An effort is made to position scalp incisions so that they are behind the hairline and not on the exposed part of the forehead. A bicoronal incision located behind the hairline is preferable to extension of an incision low on the forehead for a unilateral frontal craniotomy. An attempt is made to avoid the branch of the facial nerve that passes across the zygoma to reach the frontalis muscle. Incisions reaching the zygoma more than 1.5 cm anterior to the ear commonly interrupt this nerve unless the layers of the scalp in which it courses are protected ([14], see *Fig. 6.9*). The superficial temporal and occipital arteries should be preserved if there is the possibility that they will be needed for an extracranial-intracranial arterial anastomosis.

During elevation of a scalp flap, the pressure of the surgeon's and assistant's fingers against the skin on each side of the incision is usually sufficient to control bleeding until hemostatic clips or clamps are applied. The skin is usually incised with a sharp blade, but the deeper fascial and muscle layers may be incised with a cutting Bovie electrocautery. The ground plate on the electrocutting unit should have a broad base of contact, to prevent the skin at the ground plate from being burned. Achieving a satisfactory cosmetic result with a supratentorial craniotomy often depends on preservation of the bulk and viability of the temporalis muscle. This is best achieved by avoiding the use of the cutting Bovie electrocautery during elevation of the muscle from the bone. Both the vascular and neural supplies of the temporalis muscle course tightly along the fascial attachments of the muscle to the bone, where they could easily be damaged with a hot cutting instrument ([14], see *Fig. 6.9*). Optimal preservation of the muscle's bulk is best achieved by separation of the muscle from the bone via accurate dissection with a sharp periosteal elevator.

Bipolar coagulation is routinely used to control bleeding from the scalp margins, on the dura, and at intracranial sites. At sites where even gentle bipolar coagulation could result in neural damage, such as around the facial or optic nerves, an attempt is made to control bleeding with a gently applied hemostatic gelatinous sponge (Gelfoam; Upjohn Co., Kalamazoo, MI). Alternatives to gelatinous sponges include oxidized regenerated cellulose (Surgicel; Surigkos, New Brunswick, NJ), oxidized cellulose (Oxycell; Parke Davis, Morris Plains, NJ), and microfibrillar collagen hemostats (Avitene; Avicon, Inc., Fort Worth, TX). Venous bleeding can often be controlled with the light application of gelatinous sponges. Metallic clips, which were often used on the dura and vessels in the past, are now applied infrequently except on aneurysm necks, because they interfere with the quality of computed tomographic scans; if they are used, they should be composed of nonmagnetic alloys or titanium.

Use of a series of burr holes made with a manual or motor-driven trephine connected to a Gigli saw for elevating bone

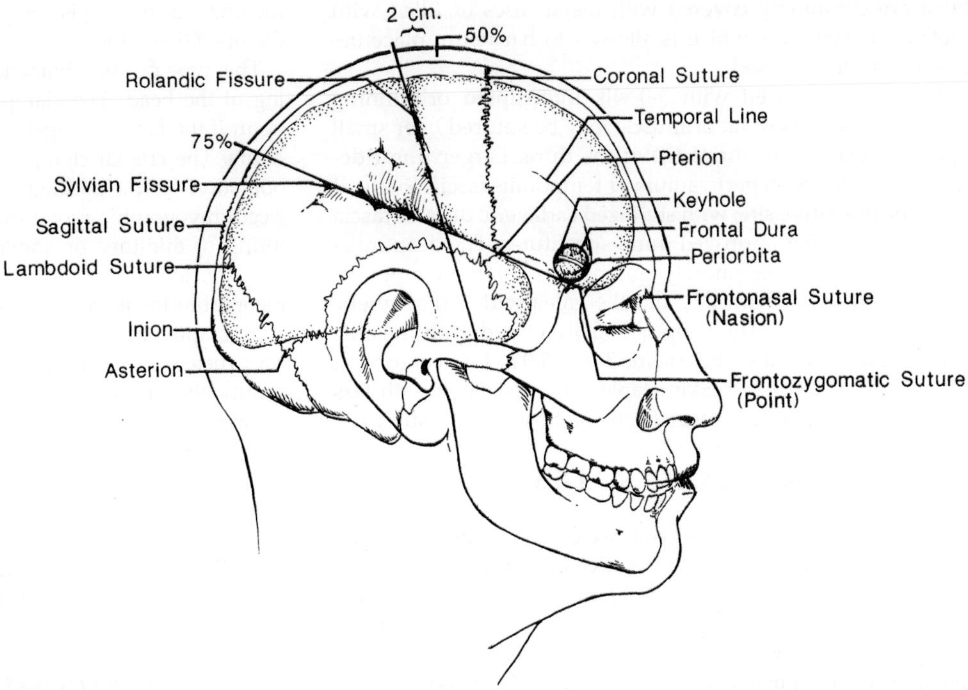

FIGURE 1.4. *Sites commonly marked on the scalp before application of the drapes, including the coronal, sagittal, and lambdoid sutures, the rolandic and sylvian fissures, and the pterion, inion, asterion, and keyhole. Approximation of the sites of the sylvian and rolandic fissures on the scalp begins with observation of the positions of the nasion, inion, and frontozygomatic point. The nasion is located in the midline, at the junction of the nasal and frontal bones. The inion is the site of a bony prominence that overlies the torcula. The frontozygomatic point is located on the orbital rim, 2.5 cm above the level at which the upper edge of the zygomatic arch joins the orbital rim and just below the junction of the lateral and superior margins of the orbital rim. The next steps are to construct a line along the sagittal suture and, with a flexible measuring tape, to determine the distance along this line from the nasion to the inion and to mark the midpoint and three-quarter point (50 and 75% points, respectively). The sylvian fissure is located along a line that extends backward from the frontozygomatic point, across the lateral surface of the head, to the three-quarter point. The pterion, i.e., the site on the temple approximating the lateral end of the sphenoid ridge, is located 3 cm behind the frontozygomatic point, on the sylvian fissure line. The rolandic fissure is located by identifying the upper and lower rolandic points. The upper rolandic point is located 2 cm behind the midpoint (50% plus 2 cm point), on the nasion-to-inion midsagittal line. The lower rolandic point is located where a line extending from the midpoint of the upper margin of the zygomatic arch to the upper rolandic point crosses the line defining the sylvian fissure. A line connecting the upper and lower rolandic points approximates the rolandic fissure. The lower rolandic point is located approximately 2.5 cm behind the pterion, on the sylvian fissure line. Another important point is the keyhole, the site of a burr hole that, if properly placed, has the frontal dura in the depths of its upper half and the periorbita in its lower half. It is approximately 3 cm anterior to the pterion, just above the lateral end of the superior orbital rim and under the most anterior point of attachment of the temporalis muscle and fascia to the temporal line* (from, *Rhoton AL Jr: The cerebrum.* ***Neurosurgery*** *51[Suppl 1]:S1-1–S1-51, 2002 [15]).*

flaps has given way to the use of high-speed drills for making burr holes and cutting the margins of bone flaps (*Fig. 1.2*). Commonly, a hole is prepared by using a cutting burr on a high-speed drill and a tool with a foot plate, to protect the dural cuts around the margins of the flap. Extremely long bone cuts should be avoided, especially if they extend across an internal bony prominence, such as the pterion, or across a major venous sinus. The risk of tearing the dura or injuring the brain is reduced by drilling several holes and making shorter cuts. A hole is placed on each side of a venous sinus and the dura is carefully stripped from the bone, after which the bone cut is completed, rather than the bone being cut above the sinus as part of a long cut around the whole margin of the flap. Bleeding from bone edges is stopped with the application of bone wax. Bone wax is also used to close small openings into the mastoid air cells and other sinuses, but larger openings in the sinuses are closed with other materials, such as fat, muscle, or pericranial grafts, sometimes in conjunction with a thin plate of methylmethacrylate or other bone substitute.

After elevation of the bone flap, it is common practice to tack the dura to the bony margin with a few 3-0 black silk sutures brought through the dura and then through small drill holes in the margin of the cranial opening (*Fig. 1.2*). If the bone flap is large, then the dura is also "snugged up" to the intracranial side of the bone flap with the use of a suture brought through drill holes in the central part of the flap. Care is taken to avoid placing drill holes for tack-up sutures that might extend into the frontal sinus or mastoid air cells. Tack-up sutures are more commonly used for dura over the cerebral hemispheres than for dura over the cerebellum. If the brain is pressed tightly against the dura, then the tack-up sutures are placed after treatment of the intradural pathological lesion, when the brain is relaxed and the sutures can be placed with direct observation of the deep surface of the dura. Tack-up sutures can also be led through adjacent muscles or pericranium, rather than a hole in the margin of the bone flap.

In the past, there was a tendency for bone flaps to be elevated and replaced over the cerebral hemispheres and for exposures in the suboccipital region to be performed as craniectomies, without replacement of the bone. Laterally placed suboccipital exposures are now commonly performed as craniotomies, with replacement of the bone flaps. Midline suboccipital operations are more commonly performed as craniectomies, especially if decompression at the foramen magnum is needed, because this area is protected by a greater thickness of overlying muscles.

Bone flaps are usually held in place with nonmagnetic plates and screws or small metal discs or burr hole covers that compress and align the inner and outer tables of the bone flap and the adjacent cranium (*Fig. 1.2F*). Remaining defects in the bone are commonly covered with metal discs or filled with methylmethacrylate, which is allowed to harden in place before the scalp is closed.

The dura is closed with 3-0 silk interrupted or running sutures. Small bits of fat or muscle may be sutured over small openings caused by shrinkage of the dura. Larger dural defects are closed with pericranium or temporalis fascia obtained from the operative site, with sterilized cadaveric dura or fascia lata, or with other approved dural substitutes. The deep muscles and fascia are commonly closed with 1-0, the temporalis muscle and fascia with 2-0, and the galea with 3-0 synthetic absorbable sutures. The scalp is usually closed with metallic staples, except at sites where some 3-0 or 5-0 nylon reenforcing sutures may be needed. Skin staples are associated with less tissue reaction than are other forms of closure with sutures.

HEAD FIXATION DEVICES

Precise maintenance of the firmly fixed cranium in the optimal position greatly facilitates the operative exposure (*Figs. 1.5* and *1.6*). Fixation is best achieved with a pinion headholder, in which the essential element is a clamp made to accommodate three relatively sharp pins. When the pins are placed, care should be taken to avoid a spinal fluid shunt, thin bones (such as those that overlie the frontal and mastoid sinuses), and the thick temporalis muscle (where the clamp, however tightly applied, tends to remain unstable). The pins should be applied well away from the eye and areas where they would hinder the incision. Shorter pediatric pins are available for thin crania. The pins should not be placed over the thin crania of some patients with a history of hydrocephalus. After the clamp has been secured on the head, the final positioning is completed and the headholder is fixed to the operating table.

This type of immobilization allows intraoperative repositioning of the head. The clamp avoids the skin damage that may occur if the face rests against a padded head support for several hours. The cranial clamps do not obscure the face during the operation (as do padded headrests), facilitating intraoperative electromyographic monitoring of the facial muscles and monitoring of auditory or somatosensory evoked potentials. Until recently, all head clamps were constructed from radiopaque metals, but the increasing use of intraoperative fluoroscopy and angiography has prompted the development of headholders constructed from radiolucent materials. The pinion headholder commonly serves as the site of attachment of the brain retractor system. The side arms of the head clamp should be shaped to accommodate the C-clamps securing the retractor system. The pinion headholder has a bolt that resembles a sunburst, for attachment to the operating table. Placement of three sunburst sites on the head clamp, rather than only one, allows greater flexibility in attachment of the head clamp to the operating table and provides extra sites for the attachment of retractor systems and components of the image guidance system.

INSTRUMENT SELECTION

Optimization of operative results requires the careful selection of instruments for the macrosurgical portion of the operation, performed with the naked eye, and the microsurgical part, performed with the eye aided by the operating microscope (10, 11). In the past, surgeons commonly used one set of instruments for conventional macrosurgery performed with

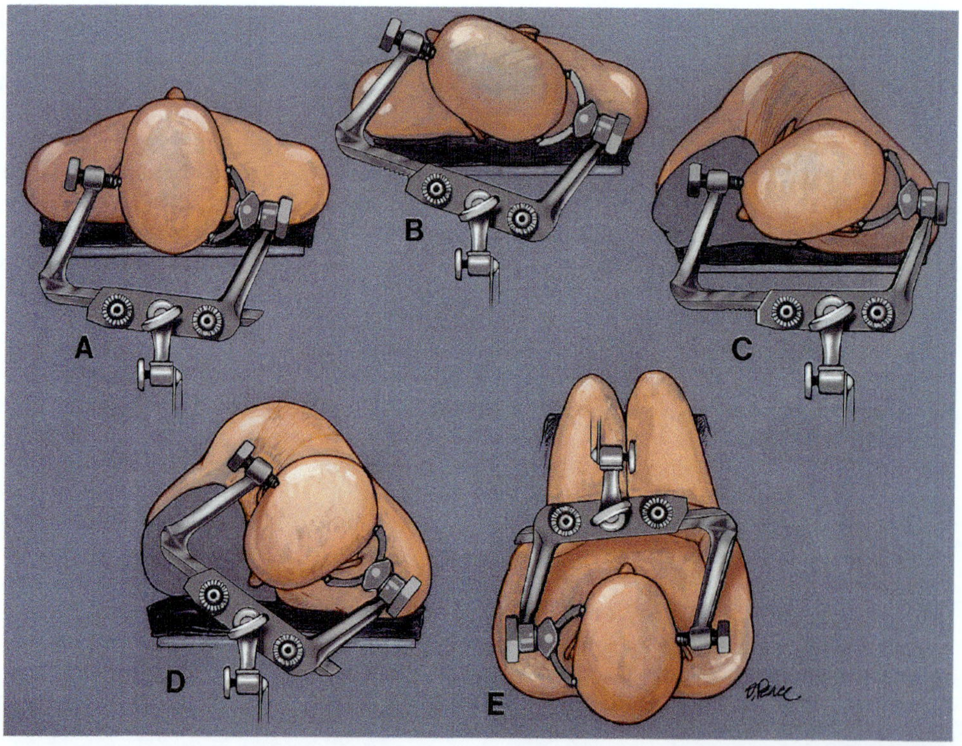

FIGURE 1.5. *Positioning of a pinion headholder for a craniotomy. Three pins penetrate the scalp and are firmly fixed to the outer table of the cranium.* A, *position of the headholder for a unilateral or bilateral frontal approach.* B, *position for a pterional or frontotemporal craniotomy.* C, *position for a retrosigmoid approach to the cerebellopontine angle.* D, *position for a midline suboccipital approach.* E, *position for a midline suboccipital approach with the patient in the semi-sitting position. The pins are positioned to avoid the thin bone over the frontal sinus and mastoid air cells and the temporalis muscle. The side arms of the head clamp should be shaped to accommodate the C-clamps holding the retractor system. The pinion headholder has a bolt that resembles a sunburst, for attachment to the operating table. Placement of three sunburst sites on the head clamp, rather than only one, allows greater flexibility in attaching the head clamp to the operating table and provides extra sites for the attachment of retractor systems and instruments for instrument guidance.*

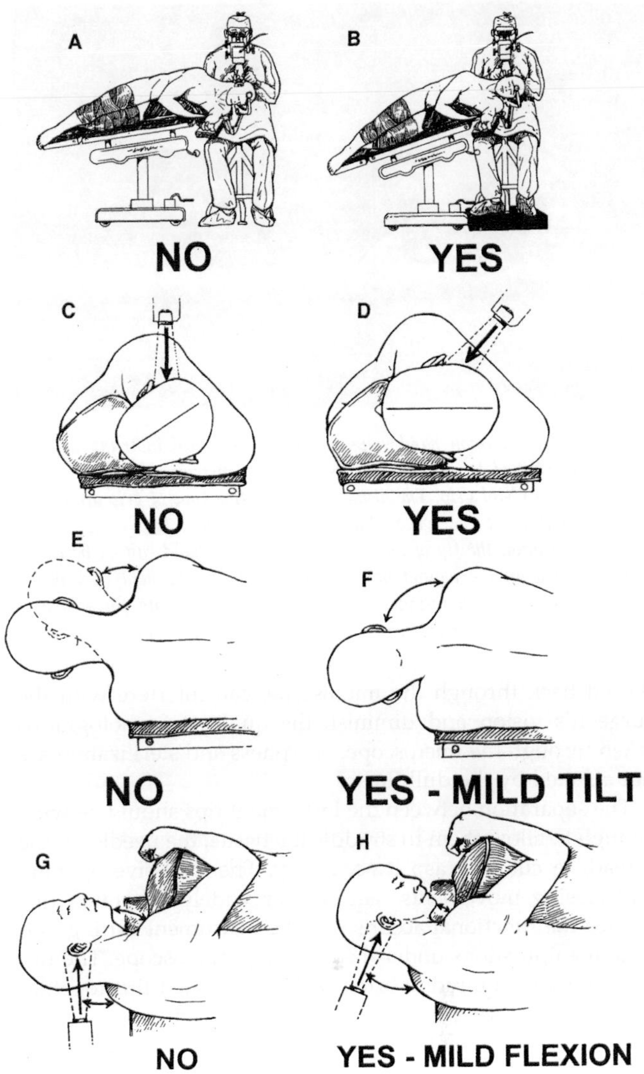

FIGURE 1.6. *Positioning of patients for acoustic neuroma removal and decompression for treatment of hemifacial spasm.* A *and* B, *the head of the table is elevated. In our initial use of the three-quarter prone position, the head of the operating table was tilted to elevate the head only slightly* (A). *It was later noted, however, that more marked tilting of the table significantly elevated the head and reduced the venous distension and intracranial pressure. I usually perform operations to treat acoustic neuromas and hemifacial spasm sitting on a stool positioned behind the head of the patient. In recent years, we have tilted the table to elevate the head to such a degree that the surgeon's stool must be placed on a platform* (B). *The patient should be positioned on the side of the table nearest the surgeon.* C *and* D, *the patient's head is rotated. There is a tendency to rotate the face toward the floor for acoustic neuroma removal* (C). *However, better operative access is obtained if the sagittal suture is placed parallel to the floor* (D). *Rotating the face toward the floor* (C) *places the direction of view through the operating microscope forward toward the shoulder, thus blocking or reducing the operative angle. Positioning the head so that the sagittal suture is parallel to the floor* (D) *allows the direction of view through the operating microscope to be rotated away from the shoulder and provides easier wider access to the operative field. The position shown in* D *is also used for decompression operations for treatment of hemifacial spasm. The position shown in* C *is used for decompression operations for treatment of trigeminal neuralgia, in which the surgeon is seated at the top of the patient's head, as shown in* Figure 1.3, *rather than behind the patient's head, as shown in* B. E *and* F, *it is better to gently tilt the head toward the contralateral shoulder than toward the ipsilateral shoulder. Tilting the vertex toward the floor, with the sagittal suture parallel to the floor, opens the angle between the shoulder and the head and increases operative access.* G *and* H, *extending the neck tends to shift the operative site toward the prominence of the shoulder and upper chest, whereas gentle flexion opens the angle between the upper chest and the operative site and broadens the range of access to the operative site.*

the naked eye and another set, with different handles and smaller tips, for microsurgery performed with the eye aided by the microscope. A trend is to select instruments with handles and tactile characteristics suitable for both macrosurgery and microsurgery and to change only the size of the instrument tip, depending on whether the use is to be macrosurgical or microsurgical. For example, forceps for macrosurgery have grasping tips as large as 2 to 3 mm and those for microsurgery commonly having tips measuring 0.3 to 1.0 mm.

If possible, the instruments should be held in a pencil grip between the thumb and the index finger, rather than in a pistol grip with the whole hand (*Fig. 1.7*). The pencil grip permits the instruments to be positioned with delicate movements of the fingers, but the pistol grip requires that the instruments be manipulated with the coarser movements of the wrist, elbow, and shoulder.

I prefer round-handle forceps, scissors, and needle-holders, because they allow finer movement. It is possible to rotate these instruments between the thumb and forefinger, rather than having to rotate the entire wrist (*Fig. 1.8*). I first used round-handle needle-holders and scissors to perform superficial temporal artery-middle cerebral artery anastomoses, and I later noted that the advantage of being able to rotate the instrument between the thumb and the fingers also improved the accuracy of other straight or bayonet instruments used for dissection, grasping, cutting, and coagulation (*Figs. 1.9* and *1.10*). Round-handle straight or bayonet forceps may be used for both macrosurgery and microsurgery.

The addition of round-handle straight forceps with teeth, called tissue forceps, increases the uses of instruments with round handles to include grasping of muscle, skin, and dura (*Fig. 1.11*). Tissue forceps with large teeth are used for the scalp and muscle, and ones with small teeth are used for the dura. The addition of round-handle forceps with fine serrations inside the tips, called dressing forceps, makes the set suitable for grasping arterial walls for endarterectomy and arterial suturing.

The instruments should have a dull finish, because the brilliant light from highly polished instruments, when re-

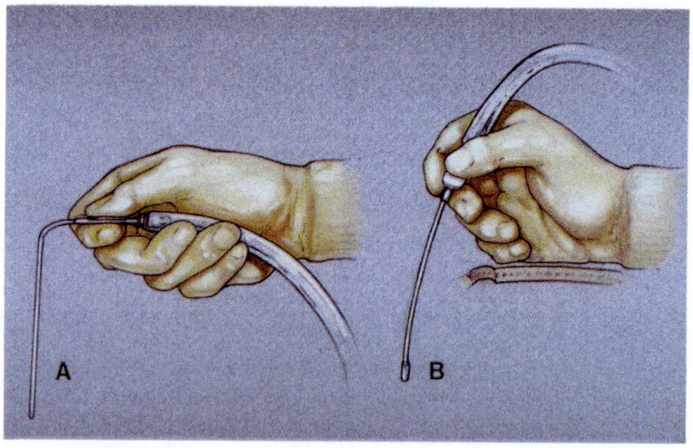

FIGURE 1.7. *Common hand grips for holding surgical instruments. The grip is determined largely by the design of the instrument. A, a suction tube held in a pistol grip. The disadvantages of this type of grip are that it uses movements of the wrist and elbow, rather than fine finger movements, to position the tip of the instrument and the hand cannot be rested and stabilized on the wound margin. B, a suction tube held in a pencil grip, which permits manipulation of the tip with delicate finger movements, while the hand rests comfortably on the wound margin.*

flected back through the microscope, can interfere with the surgeon's vision and diminish the quality of photographs taken through the microscope. Sharpness and sterilization are not affected by the dull finish.

The separation between the instrument tips should be wide enough to allow them to straddle the tissue, the needle, or the thread, to cut or grasp it accurately. The excessive opening and closing movements required for widely separated tips reduce the functional accuracy of the instrument during delicate manipulations under the operating microscope. The finger pressure required to bring widely separated tips together against firm spring tension often initiates a fine tremor and inaccurate movements. Microsurgical tissue forceps should have a tip separation of no more than 8 mm, microneedle-holder tips should open no more than 3 mm, and microscissors tips should open no less than 2 mm and no more than 5 mm, depending on the length of the blade and the use of the scissors.

The length of the instruments should be adequate for the particular task that is being contemplated (*Figs. 1.9* and *1.10*). Bayonet instruments (e.g., forceps, needle-holders, and scissors) should be available in at least the three lengths needed for the hand to be rested while the surgeon operates at superficial, deep, and extra-deep sites.

Bayonet Forceps

Bayonet forceps are standard neurosurgical instruments (*Figs. 1.9* and *1.10*). The bayonet forceps should be properly balanced so that, when its handle rests on the web between the thumb and index finger and across the radial side of the middle finger, the instrument remains there without falling forward when the grasp of the index finger and thumb is released. Poor balance prevents the delicate grasp required for microsurgical procedures.

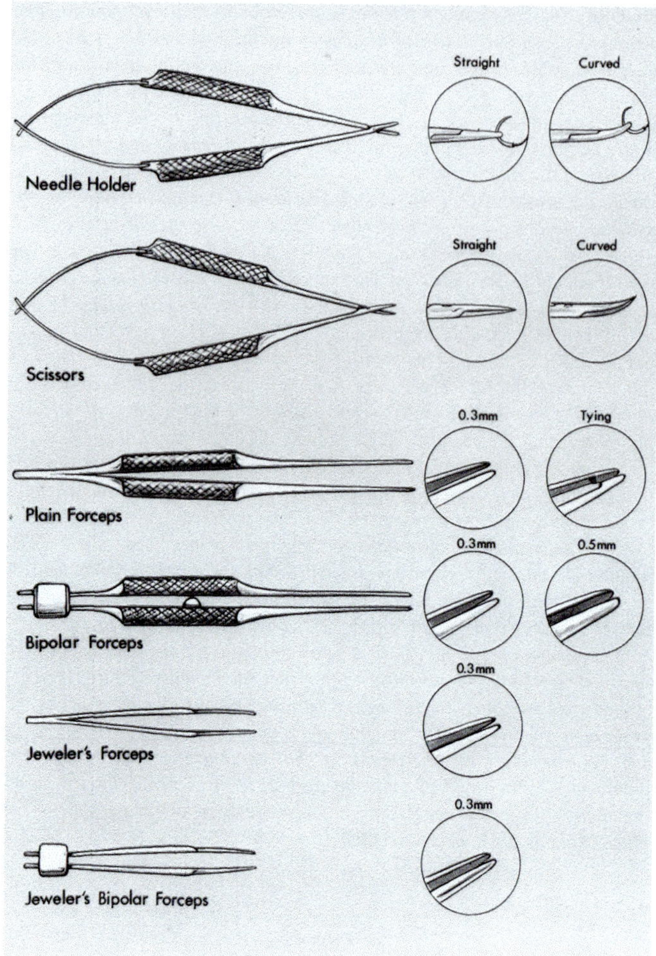

FIGURE 1.8. *Straight Rhoton instruments with round handles and fine tips, for use at the surface of the brain. These instruments are suitable for microsurgical procedures, such as extracranial-intracranial arterial anastomoses. The instruments include needle-holders with straight and curved tips, scissors with straight and curved tips, forceps with platforms for tying fine sutures, bipolar forceps with 0.3- and 0.5-mm tips, and plain and bipolar jeweler's forceps. Jeweler's forceps can be used as a needle-holder for placing sutures in fine microvascular anastomoses on the surface of the brain, but I prefer a round-handle straight needle-holder for that use.*

It is preferable to test forceps for tension and tactile qualities by holding them in the gloved hand, rather than the naked hand. Forceps resistance to closure that is perceived as adequate in the naked hand may become almost imperceptible in the gloved hand. The forceps may be used to develop tissue planes by inserting the closed forceps between the structures to be separated and releasing the tension so that the blades open and separate the structures. This form of dissection requires greater tension in the handles than is present in some delicate forceps.

In selecting bayonet forceps, the surgeon should consider the length of the blades needed to reach the operative site and the size of the tip needed for the specific task to be completed. Bayonet forceps with 8-, 9.5-, and 11-cm blades, with a variety

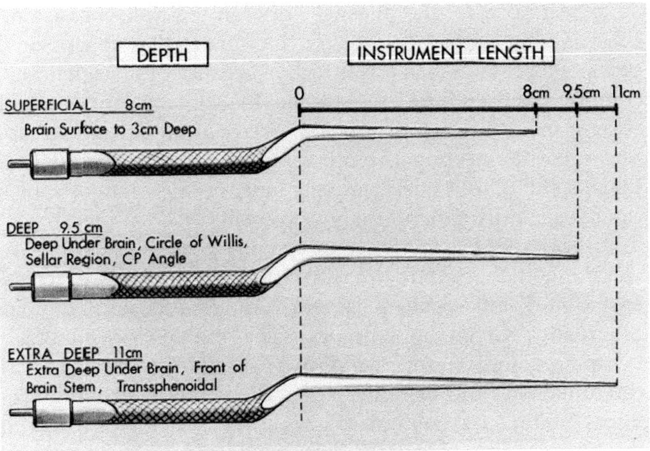

FIGURE 1.9. *Rhoton bayonet bipolar coagulation forceps for use at different depths. Bayonet forceps with 8-cm blades are suitable for coagulation on the surface of the brain and down to a depth of 3 cm. Bayonet forceps with 9.5-cm blades are needed for coagulation deep under the brain, in the region of the circle of Willis, the suprasellar area, or the cerebellopontine (CP) angle. Bayonet forceps with 11-cm blades are suitable for coagulation in extra-deep sites, such as in front of the brainstem or in transsphenoidal exposures. Some surgeons prefer that the forceps be coated, to ensure that the current is delivered to the tips, but the coating may obstruct the view at the tips during procedures performed under the microscope.*

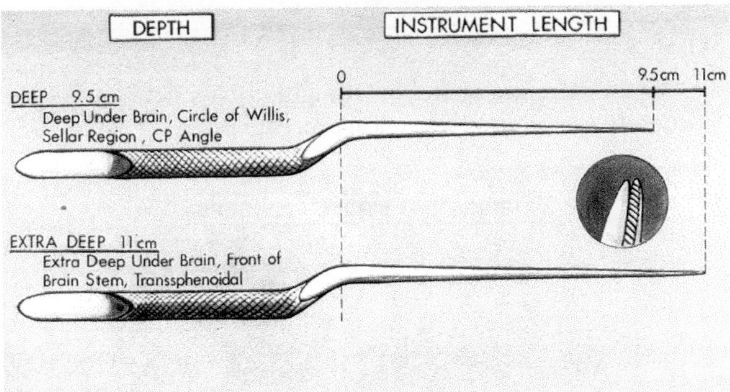

FIGURE 1.10. *Rhoton bayonet dissecting forceps with fine (0.5-cm) tips, for use at deep and extra-deep sites. Fine cross-serrations inside the tips (inset) facilitate grasping and manipulation of tissue. CP, cerebellopontine.*

of tip sizes (ranging from 0.5 to 2.0 cm), are needed (*Figs. 1.9, 1.10, and 1.12*). Bayonet forceps with 8-cm shafts are suitable for use on the brain surface and down to a depth of 2 cm below the surface. Bayonet forceps with blades of 9.5 cm are suitable for manipulating tissues deep under the brain, at the level of the circle of Willis (e.g., for treatment of an aneurysm), in the sellar region (e.g., for treatment of a pituitary tumor via a transcranial approach), and in the cerebellopontine angle (e.g., for removal of an acoustic neuroma or decompression of a cranial nerve). For dissection and coagulation in extra-deep sites, such as in front of the brainstem or in the depths of a transsphenoidal exposure, forceps with 11-cm blades are used. Some surgeons prefer that the forceps be coated with an insulating material except at the tips, to ensure that the current

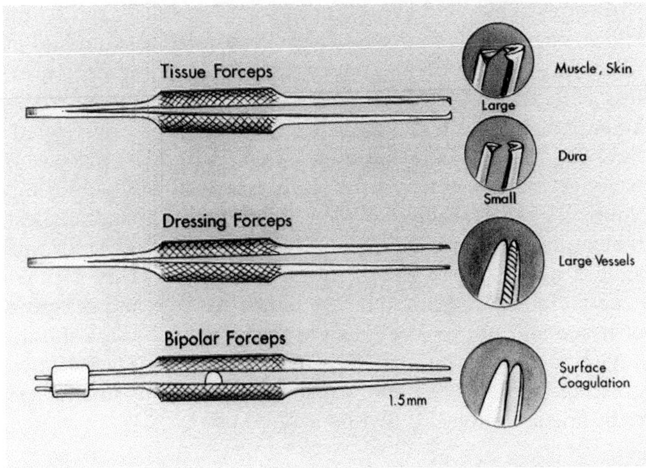

FIGURE 1.11. *Rhoton straight instruments with round handles needed to complete the set, so that the same type of handles can be used for macrosurgery performed with the naked eye and microsurgery performed with the eye aided by the microscope. Forceps with teeth, called tissue forceps, are needed to grasp dura, muscle, and skin. Small teeth are used for the dura, and large teeth are used for the skin and muscle. Forceps with cross-serrations, called dressing forceps, may be used during endarterectomies on larger arteries. Smooth-tip bipolar coagulation forceps with 1.5-mm tips are used for macrocoagulation of large vessels in the scalp, muscle, or dura.*

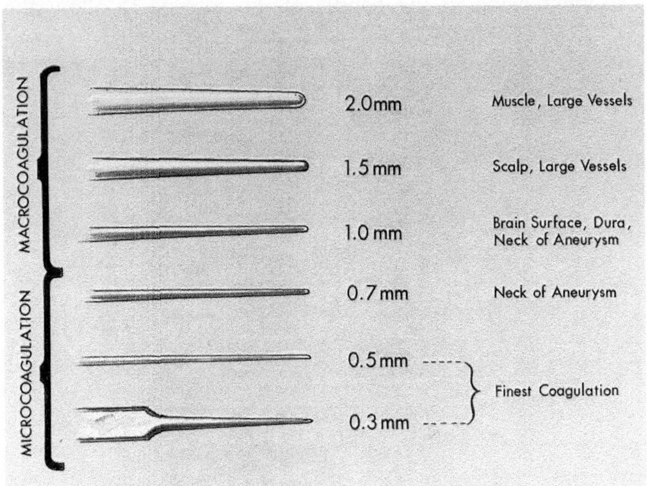

FIGURE 1.12. *Forceps tips needed for macro- and microcoagulation. Bipolar forceps with 1.5- and 2-mm tips are suitable for coagulation of large vessels and bleeding points in the scalp, muscle, and fascia. The 0.7- and 1-mm tips are suitable for coagulation on the dura and brain surface and for coagulation on tumor capsule surfaces. Fine coagulation at deep sites in the posterior fossa is performed with bayonet forceps with 0.5-mm tips. The 0.3-mm tip is suitable for use on short instruments such as jeweler's forceps. When tips as small as 0.3 mm are placed on bayonet forceps, the tips may scissor rather than oppose.*

is delivered to the tips, but the coating, if thick, may obstruct the view of the tissue being grasped during procedures performed under the microscope.

A series of bipolar bayonet forceps with tips of 0.3 to 2.0 mm allow coagulation of vessels of almost any size encountered in neurosurgery (*Fig. 1.12*). For coagulation of larger structures, tips with widths of 1.5 and 2 mm are needed. For microcoagulation, forceps with 1.0-, 0.7-, or 0.5-mm tips are selected. Fine 0.3-mm tips (like those on jeweler's forceps) placed on bayonet forceps may scissor, rather than firmly opposing, unless they are carefully aligned. A 0.5-mm tip is the smallest that is practical for use on many bayonet forceps. The forceps should have smooth tips if they are to be used for bipolar coagulation. If they are to be used for dissection and grasping of tissue and not for coagulation, then the inside tips should have fine cross-serrations (like dressing forceps) (*Fig. 1.10*). To grasp large pieces of tumor capsule, forceps with small rings with fine serrations at the tips may be used.

Bipolar Coagulation

The bipolar electrocoagulator has become fundamental to neurosurgery because it allows accurate fine coagulation of small vessels, minimizing the dangerous spread of current to adjacent neural and vascular structures (*Figs. 1.9, 1.12,* and *1.13*) (3, 5). It allows coagulation in areas where unipolar coagulation would be hazardous, such as near the cranial nerves, brainstem, cerebellar arteries, or fourth ventricle.

When the electrode tips touch each other, the current is short-circuited and no coagulation occurs. There should be enough tension in the handle of the forceps to allow the surgeon to control the distance between the tips, because no coagulation occurs if the tips touch or are too far apart. Some types of forceps, which are attractive because of their delicacy, compress with so little pressure that the surgeon cannot avoid closing them during coagulation, even with a delicate grasp. The cable connecting the bipolar unit and the coagulation forceps should not be excessively long, because longer cables can cause an irregular supply of current.

Surgeons with experience in conventional coagulation are conditioned to require maximal dryness at the surface of application, but some moistness is preferable with bipolar coagulation. Coagulation occurs even if the tips are immersed in saline solution, and keeping the tissue moist with local cerebrospinal fluid or saline irrigation during coagulation reduces heating and minimizes drying and sticking of tissue to the forceps. Fine irrigation units and forceps that dispense a small amount of fluid through a long tube in the shaft of the forceps to the tip with each coagulation step have been developed (*Fig. 1.14*). To avoid sticking after coagulation, the points of the forceps should be cleaned after each application to the tissue. If charred blood coats the tips, then it should be removed by wiping with a damp cloth rather than by scraping with a scalpel blade, because the blade may scratch the tips and make them more adherent to tissue during coagulation. The tips of the forceps should be polished if they become pitted and rough.

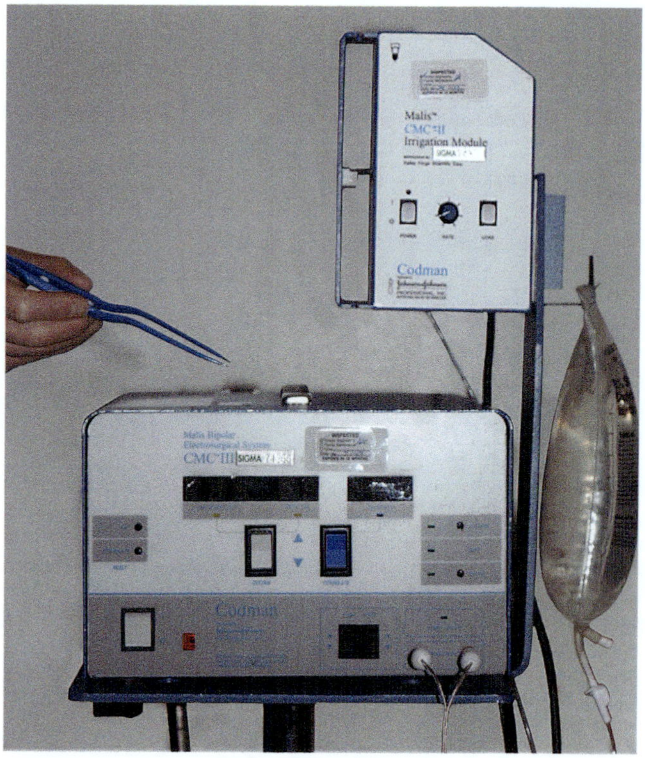

FIGURE 1.13. *Malis irrigation bipolar coagulation unit with coated Rhoton bayonet coagulation forceps. A small amount of fluid is dispensed at the tip of the forceps during each coagulation step.*

Scissors

Scissors with fine blades on straight or bayonet handles are frequently used for microsurgical procedures (*Figs. 1.8* and *1.15*).

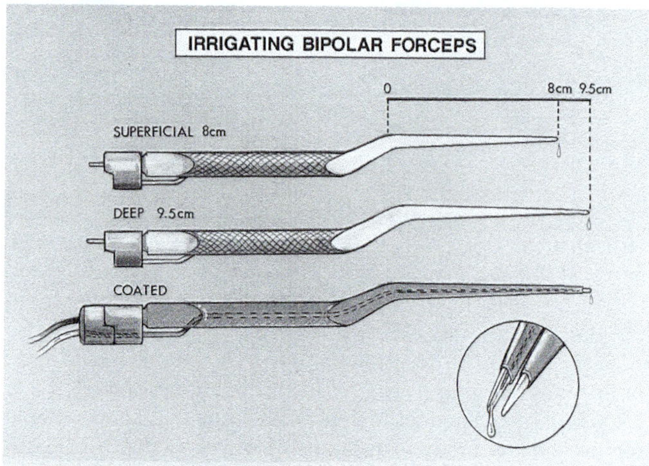

FIGURE 1.14. *Rhoton irrigating bipolar forceps. A small amount of fluid is dispensed at the tip of the forceps during each coagulation step. The small metal tube that carries the irrigating fluid is inlaid into the shaft of the instrument, so that it does not obstruct the view of the operative site when the surgeon is looking down the forceps into a deep narrow operative site. Irrigating forceps with 8-cm blades are suitable for coagulation at or near the surface of the brain. Bayonet forceps with 9.5-cm blades are used for coagulation deep under the brain. Some surgeons prefer that the forceps be coated, to ensure that the current is delivered to the tips, but the coating may obstruct the view at the tips during procedures performed under the microscope.*

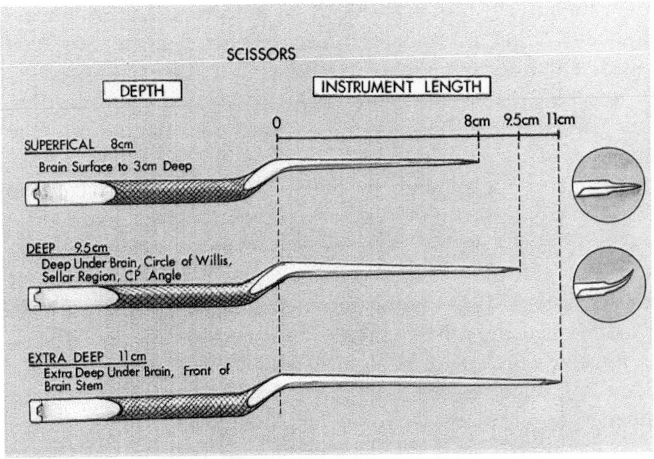

FIGURE 1.15. *Rhoton bayonet scissors with straight and curved blades. The bayonet scissors with 8-cm shafts are used at the surface of the brain and down to a depth of 3 cm. The scissors with 9.5-cm shafts are used deep under the brain, at the level of the circle of Willis, the suprasellar area, and the cerebellopontine (CP) angle. The scissors with 11-cm shafts are used at extra-deep sites, such as in front of the brainstem. The straight nonbayonet scissors shown in* Figure 8 *may also be used at the surface of the brain.*

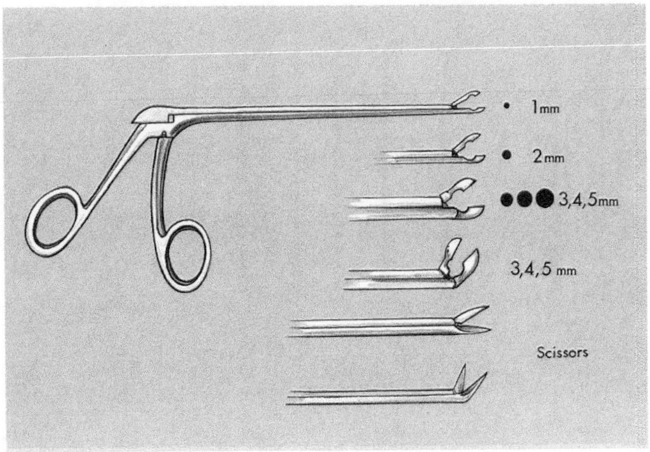

FIGURE 1.16. *Straight and angled alligator cup forceps and scissors. These fine cup forceps are used to grasp and remove tumors in deep narrow exposures. A 2-, 3-, or 4-mm cup is required for most microsurgical applications, but cup forceps as small as 1 mm or as large as 5 mm are occasionally needed. Straight and angled alligator scissors with the same mechanism of action as the cup forceps are required for deep narrow exposures, as in the depths of transsphenoidal approaches.*

Cutting should be performed with the distal half of the blade. If the scissors open too widely, then cutting ability and accuracy suffer. Delicate cutting near the surface, such as opening of the middle cerebral artery for anastomosis or embolectomy, should be performed with straight (not bayonet) scissors with fine blades that are approximately 5 mm long and open approximately 3 mm. Only delicate suture material and tissue should be cut with such small blades. Bayonet scissors with 8-cm shafts and curved or straight blades are selected for areas 3 to 4 cm below the cranial surface. Bayonet scissors with 9.5-cm shafts are selected for deep areas, such as the cerebellopontine angle or the suprasellar region. The blades should measure 14 mm in length and should open approximately 4 mm. For extra-deep sites, such as in front of the brainstem, the scissors should have 11-cm shafts. Scissors on an alligator-type shank with a long shaft are selected for deep narrow openings, as in transsphenoidal operations (*Fig. 1.16*).

Dissectors

The most widely used neurosurgical macrodissectors are of the Penfield or Freer types; however, the size and weight of these instruments make them unsuitable for microdissection around the cranial nerves, brainstem, and intracranial vessels. The smallest Penfield dissector, the no. 4, has a width of 3 mm. For microsurgery, dissectors with 1- and 2-mm tips are needed (*Fig. 1.17*). Straight, rather than bayonet, dissectors are preferred for most intracranial operations, because rotating the handle of a straight dissector does not alter the position of the tip but rotating the handle of a bayonet dissector causes the tip to move through a wide arc.

Round-tip dissectors, called canal knives, are used for separation of tumor from nerve (*Figs. 1.17–1.19*). An alternative method of fine dissection is to use the straight pointed instruments that I call needles (7). It may be difficult to grasp the margin of the tumor with forceps; however, a small needle dissector introduced into its margin may be helpful for retracting the tumor in the desired direction (*Figs. 1.18B* and *1.19A*). This type of pointed instrument can also be used to develop a cleavage plane between tumor and the arachnoid membrane, nerves, and brain. Spatula dissectors similar to, but smaller than, the no. 4 Penfield dissector are helpful in defining the neck of an aneurysm and separating it from adjacent perforating arteries. The 40-degree teardrop dissectors are especially helpful in defining the neck of an aneurysm and in separating arteries from nerves during vascular decompression operations, because the tip slides easily in and out of tight areas, without inadvertently avulsing perforating arteries or catching on delicate tissue (*Figs. 1.20* and *1.21*) (9, 13).

Any vessel located above the surface of an encapsulated tumor, such as an acoustic neuroma or meningioma, should be initially treated as if it were a brain vessel running over the tumor surface that could be preserved with accurate dissection. The surgeon should try to displace the vessel and adjacent tissue from the tumor capsule toward the adjacent neural tissues with a small dissector, after the tumor has been removed from within the capsule. Vessels that initially appear to be adhering to the capsule often prove to be neural vessels on the pial surface when dissected free of the capsule.

If the pia-arachnoid membrane is adhering to the tumor capsule or if a tumor mass is present within the capsule and prevents collapse of the capsule away from the brainstem and cranial nerves, then there is a tendency to apply traction to both layers and to tear neural vessels coursing on the pial surface. Before separating the pia-arachnoid membrane from the capsule, it is important to remove enough tumor so that the capsule is so thin it is almost transparent. If the surgeon is

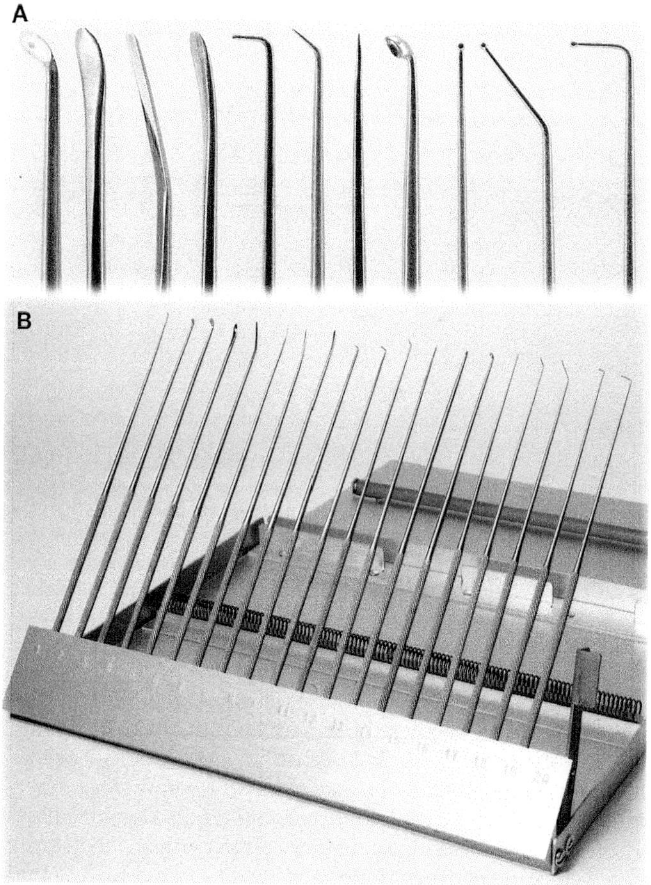

FIGURE 1.17. *Rhoton microdissectors for neurosurgery.* A, *the instruments shown (from* left to right) *are four types of dissectors (round, spatula, flat, and micro-Penfield), a right-angle nerve hook, angled and straight needle dissectors, a microcurette, and straight, 40-degree, and right-angle teardrop dissectors.* B, *a storage case permits easy access to the instruments and protects their delicate tips when they are not in use. The full set includes round and spatula dissectors in 1-, 2-, and 3-mm widths, straight and angled microcurettes, long and short teardrop dissectors in 40-degree and right-angle configurations, and one straight teardrop dissector.*

uncertain regarding the margin between the capsule and the pia-arachnoid membrane, then several gentle sweeps of a small dissector through the area can help clarify the appropriate plane for dissection.

For transsphenoidal operations, dissectors with bayonet handles are preferred because the handles help prevent the surgeon's hand from blocking the view down the long narrow exposure of the sella (*Fig. 1.22*) (8). Blunt ring curettes are frequently used during transsphenoidal operations, to remove small or large tumors of the pituitary gland and to explore the sella (*Figs. 1.23–1.26*).

Needles, Sutures, and Needle-holders

The operating room should have readily available microsutures ranging from 6-0 to 10-0, on a variety of needles (ranging in diameter from 50 to 130 μm) (*Table 1.1*) (18). For the most delicate suturing, as in extracranial-intracranial arterial anastomoses, nylon or Prolene sutures of 22-μm diameter (10-0) on needles of approximately 50- to 75-μm diameter are used.

Jeweler's forceps are commonly used to grasp microneedles, but they are too short for most intracranial operations. The handles of the microneedle-holders should be round, rather than flat or rectangular, so that rotating them between the fingers yields a smooth movement that drives the needle easily (*Figs. 1.8* and *1.27*). There should be no lock or holding catch on the microneedle. When such a lock is engaged or released, regardless of how delicately it is made, the tip jumps, possibly causing misdirection of the needle or tissue damage.

Jeweler's forceps or straight needle-holders are suitable for handling microneedles near the cortical surface (*Fig. 1.8*). For deeper applications, bayonet needle-holders with fine tips may be used (*Fig. 1.27*). Bayonet needle-holders with 8-cm shafts are suitable for use to a depth of 3 cm below the surface of the brain. Shafts measuring 9.5 cm are needed for suturing of vessels or nerves in deeper areas, such as in the suprasellar region, around the circle of Willis, or in the cerebellopontine angle. To tie microsutures, microneedle-holders, jeweler's forceps, or tying forceps may be used. Tying forceps have a platform in the tip to facilitate grasping of the suture; however, most surgeons prefer to tie sutures with jeweler's forceps or fine needle-holders.

Suction Tubes

Suction tubes with blunt rounded tips are preferred. Dandy designed and used blunt suction tubes, and his trainees have continued to use the Dandy type of tube (*Fig. 1.28*) (16). Yaşargil et al. (19) and Rhoton and Merz (16) reported the use of suction tubes with blunt rounded tips, which allowed the tubes to be used for the manipulation of tissue as well as for suction. The thickening and rounding of the tips reduce the problem of the small 3- and 5-French tubes becoming sharp when they are smoothly cut at right angles to the shaft. Some suction tubes, such as those of the curved Adson type, become somewhat pointed when prepared in sizes as small as 3 or 5 French, because the distal end of the tube is cut obliquely with respect to the long axis of the shaft, making the tubes less suitable for use near the thin walls of aneurysms.

Suction tubes should be designed to be held like a pencil, rather than like a pistol (*Fig. 1.7*). Frazier suction tubes are designed to be held like a pistol. The pencil grip design frees the ulnar side of the hand so that it can be rested comfortably on the wound margin, affording more precise, more delicate, and sturdier manipulation of the tip of the suction tube than is allowed with the unsupported pistol grip.

Selecting a tube of appropriate length is important because the arm tires during extended operations if the suction tube is too long to allow the hand to be rested (*Figs. 1.29* and *1.30*). Tubes with 8-cm shafts (i.e., the distance between the angle distal to the thumb piece and the tip) are used for suction at the level of the cranium or near the surface of the brain (*Fig. 1.31*). Tubes with 10-cm shafts allow the hand to rest along the wound margin during procedures performed in deep operative sites, such as in the cerebellopontine angle, suprasellar, or basilar

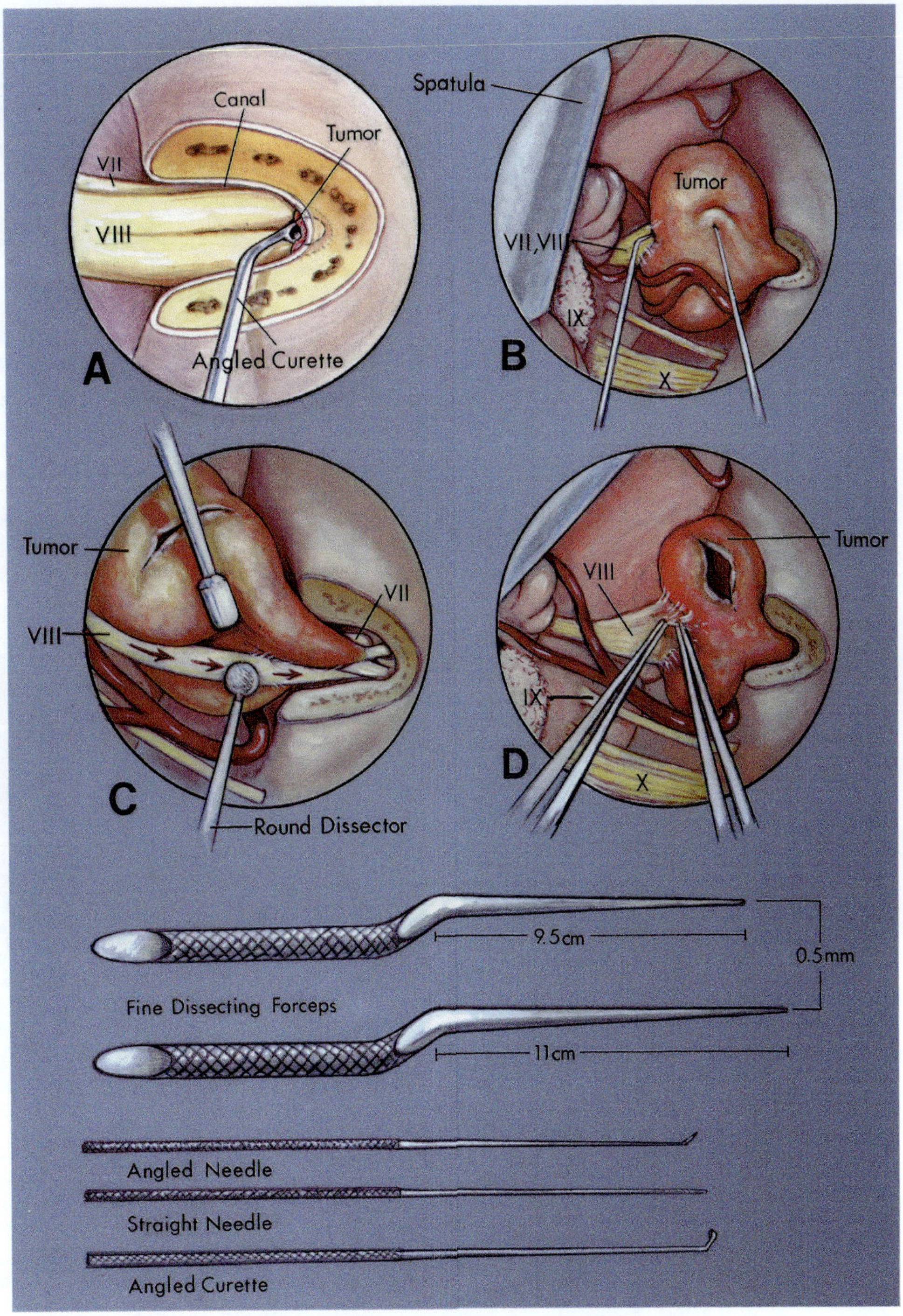

FIGURE 1.18. *Four methods of fine dissection for separation of the capsule of an acoustic neuroma from the nerves in the cerebellopontine angle.* A, *the posterior wall of the internal auditory canal has been removed and the entire tumor has been removed, except for a small fragment of the capsule in the lateral end of the canal, behind the vestibulocochlear and facial nerves. The angled curette is inserted in the meatal fundus behind the nerves and lifts the last fragment of capsule out of the lateral end of the meatus, after the tumor has been separated from the posterior surface of the nerves.* B, *a small acoustic neuroma is removed from the posterior surface of the vestibulocochlear nerve with angled and straight needles. The straight needle is used to retract the tumor capsule, and the angled needle separates the tumor capsule and nerve.* C, *the nerve and tumor capsule are separated with a round dissector. The strokes of the dissectors should be directed in the medial-to-lateral direction if there is a chance of preserving hearing. The facial nerve is exposed at the lateral end of the meatus.* D, *the capsule of a large tumor is removed from the posterior surface of the vestibulocochlear nerve with fine bayonet dissecting forceps with 0.5-mm tips, with small serrations on the inside edges of the tips to facilitate grasping of the tissue. Bayonet dissecting forceps with 9.5-cm shafts are used at deep sites, such as the cerebellopontine angle, and bayonet forceps with 11-cm shafts are used at extra-deep sites, such as in front of the brainstem. The glossopharyngeal and vagus nerves are below the tumor.*

apex regions or around the circle of Willis (*Fig. 1.32*). Suction tubes with 13-cm shafts may be used at extra-deep sites, such as in front of the brainstem, as well as for transsphenoidal operations. Suction tubes with 13-cm shafts, such as those used for transsphenoidal operations, have tips angled up and down (in addition to straight tips), for suction around the curves within tumor capsules or for treatment of asymmetrical tumor extensions (*Figs. 1.24* and *1.33*).

The suction tubes should encompass a range of diameters from 3 to 12 French, for use in macrosurgery and microsurgery (*Table 1.2*; *Fig. 1.30*). Conventional surgery performed with the naked eye uses 9-, 10-, or 12-French tubes. The French designation applies to the outer diameter. Three French units equal 1 mm; therefore, a 9-French tube has an outer diameter of 3 mm. The 10- and 12-French tubes are used during opening of the scalp, muscle, and bone and during heavy bleeding. The

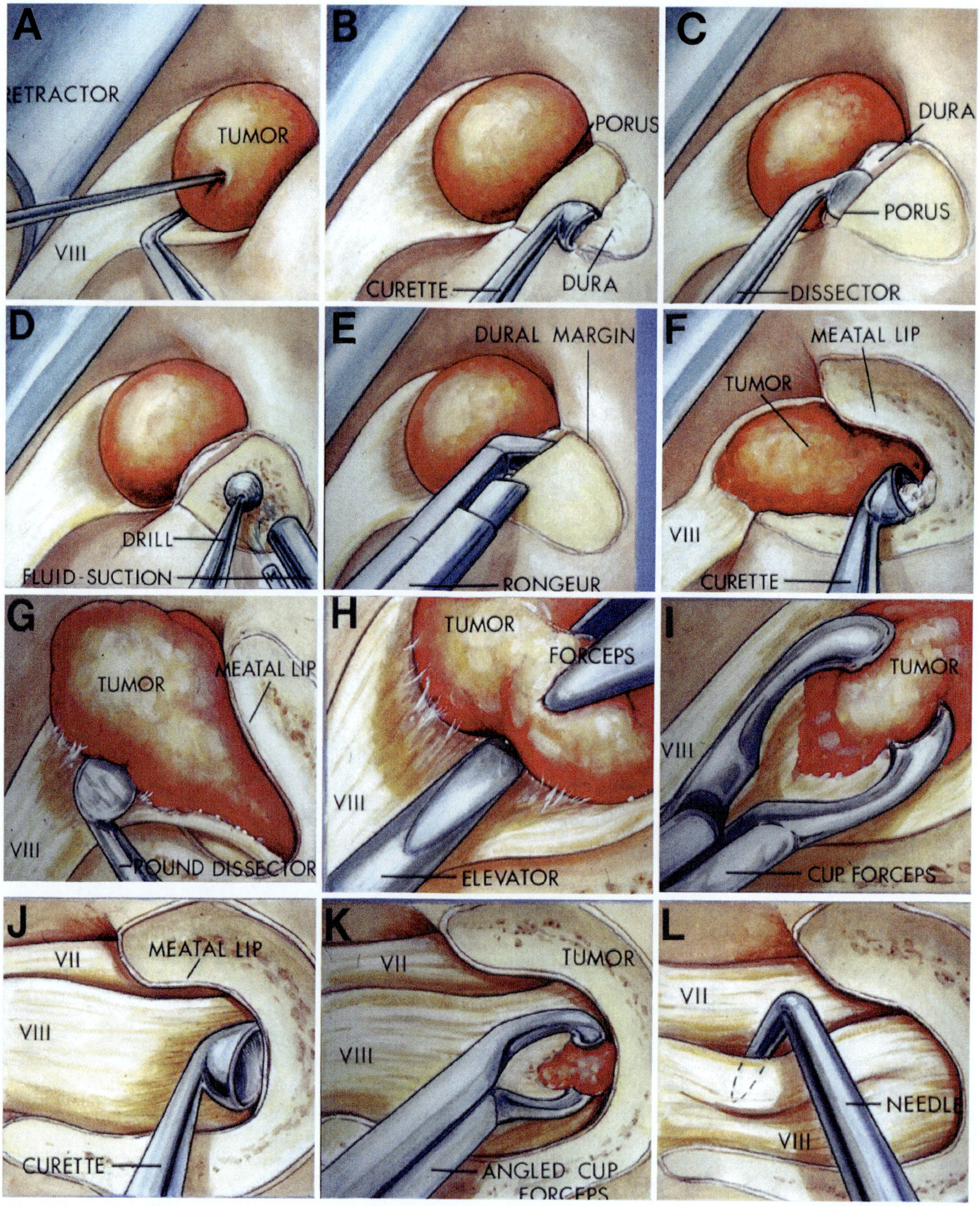

FIGURE 1.19. *Microinstruments used in the cerebellopontine angle. This illustration was prepared from 16-mm movie frames recorded at the time of removal of an acoustic neuroma in the right cerebellopontine angle. This operation resulted in preservation of the facial, acoustic, and vestibular nerves.* A,

most commonly used macrosuction tubes, the 9- and 10-French sizes, are too large for use after the dura has been opened. Stretched nerve fascicles or small vessels can easily become entrapped in such large tubes. Most microsurgical procedures require tube diameters of 5 and 7 French. The 3- and 5-French sizes are suitable for delicate applications, such as suction around the facial nerve during removal of an acoustic neuroma. The 5-French suction tube with a 10-cm shaft may be used as a suction-dissector in defining the neck of an aneurysm or as a suction-dissector in the cerebellopontine angle and near the cerebellar arteries and cranial nerves (*Fig. 1.32*). The 7-French tube is commonly used during intracapsular removal of an acoustic neuroma or meningioma of medium or large size. The 3-French tube is too small for most microsurgical procedures, but it is suitable for applications such as suction along the suture line of an extracranial-intracranial arterial bypass (*Fig. 1.31*).

The power of the suction is regulated by adjusting the degree to which the thumb occludes an air hole. The air holes should be large enough that the suction at the tip is markedly reduced when the thumb is not over the hole; however, the suction pressure may need to be adjusted at its source to avoid the risk of entrapping and damaging fine neural and vascular structures.

A continuous stream of irrigating fluid, which is often delivered through a tube fused to the suction tube, can be helpful during part of the operation (*Fig. 1.19D*). Irrigation discourages the formation of small blood clots and their adherence to the dissected surfaces; it also increases the effectiveness of bipolar coagulation forceps and reduces adhesion of the tips to tissue. Constant bathing with cerebrospinal fluid has the same effect.

Irrigation with physiological saline solution is also useful for cooling the drill, which may transmit heat to nearby neural structures, and for washing bone dust from the incision (*Fig. 1.19D*). The irrigation should be regulated so that the solution does not enter the operative field unless the surgeon's finger is removed from the suction release hole.

Brain Retractors

Self-retaining retraction systems are routinely used for most intracranial operations (2, 10, 19). They allow the surgeon to work in a relatively confined space unhindered by an assistant's hand. They are more dependable than the surgeon's or assistant's hand in maintaining constant gentle elevation of the brain. The retraction system should include tapered and rectangular brain spatulas that are applied to the protected surface of the brain, flexible arms that can support the brain spatulas in any position within the operating field, and a series of clamps and bars for attachment of the system to the pinion headholder or the operating table (*Fig. 1.34*). The most frequently used self-retaining retractor systems have flexible arms consisting of a series of ball-and-socket units (which resemble a string of pearls), with an internal cable that holds the arm in the desired position when tightened.

The stability of the system is increased if the flexible arms that hold the brain spatulas are constructed so that they are tapered, with the largest units near the bar to which the arm is attached and the smallest units at the end that holds the brain spatulas (*Fig. 1.34A*). Three lengths of flexible arms (20, 30, and 48 cm) allow the system to be used at diverse operative sites. Greater flexibility in positioning the flexible arms can be achieved if the arms are attached to the rigid bars with the use of a coupling that allows them to be rotated through a 360-degree arc (*Fig. 1.34A*). The flexible arms may be attached to a short bar that is fixed to the pinion headholder, or they may be attached to longer bars that are attached to the operating table or the headholder. The short handles used to tighten the flexible arms and joints in the system should be broad and flat, rather than narrow and round as in some systems (*Fig. 1.34A*). The broad flat handles increase the ease of adjustment of the arms and joints.

The clamps that attach the retractor system to the headholder or operating table should be firmly fixed in place before the flexible arms are attached to them. The clamps should be affixed to the headholder as close to the operative field as possible but should not decrease the ease with which the surgeon moves other instruments into the operative site. The retractor system should include straight and curved bars, a jointed bar, and clamps for attachment of the bars to the headholder or the operating table (*Fig. 1.34*). The retractor set may also include two hemi-rings, which can be positioned to create a circular halo around the operative site (*Fig. 1.34E*). It is helpful if the arms on the pinion headholder are shaped to accommodate the C-clamps that hold the bars to which the flexible arms are attached.

The flexible arms should be led into the operative site in such a way that they rest closely against the drapes around the

FIGURE 1.19. *Continued*
a brain spatula gently elevates the right cerebellum, to expose the tumor. Small pointed instruments called needles separate the tumor from the VIIIth cranial nerve. The straight needle retracts the tumor, and the 45-degree needle develops a cleavage plane between the tumor and the nerve. The facial nerve is hidden in front of the vestibulocochlear nerve. B, *a microcurette with a 1.5-mm cup strips the dura mater from the posterior wall of the meatus.* C, *a 1-mm round dissector separates the dura from the bone at the porus and within the meatus.* D, *a drill is used to remove the posterior wall of the meatus. Suction irrigation cools the area and removes bone dust.* E, *an alternative method involves removal of the posterior wall after it has been thinned by using a drill with a Kerrison rongeur, with a 1-mm-wide bite.* F, *the microcurette with a 1.5-mm cup removes the last bit of bone from the posterior meatal wall.* G, *the 1-mm round dissector separates tumor from the VIIIth cranial nerve.* H, *a flat dissector with a 1-mm tip separates tumor from the VIIIth cranial nerve.* I, *a microcup forceps with a 1-mm cup removes a tumor nodule from the nerve.* J, *a microcurette reaches into the meatus behind the VIIIth cranial nerve, to bring a tumor nodule into view. The facial nerve is anterior and superior to the vestibulocochlear nerve.* K, *the microcup forceps angled to the right removes the last remaining fragment of tumor from the lateral part of the meatus.* L, *the angled needle probes the area between the facial and vestibulocochlear nerves for residual tumor.*

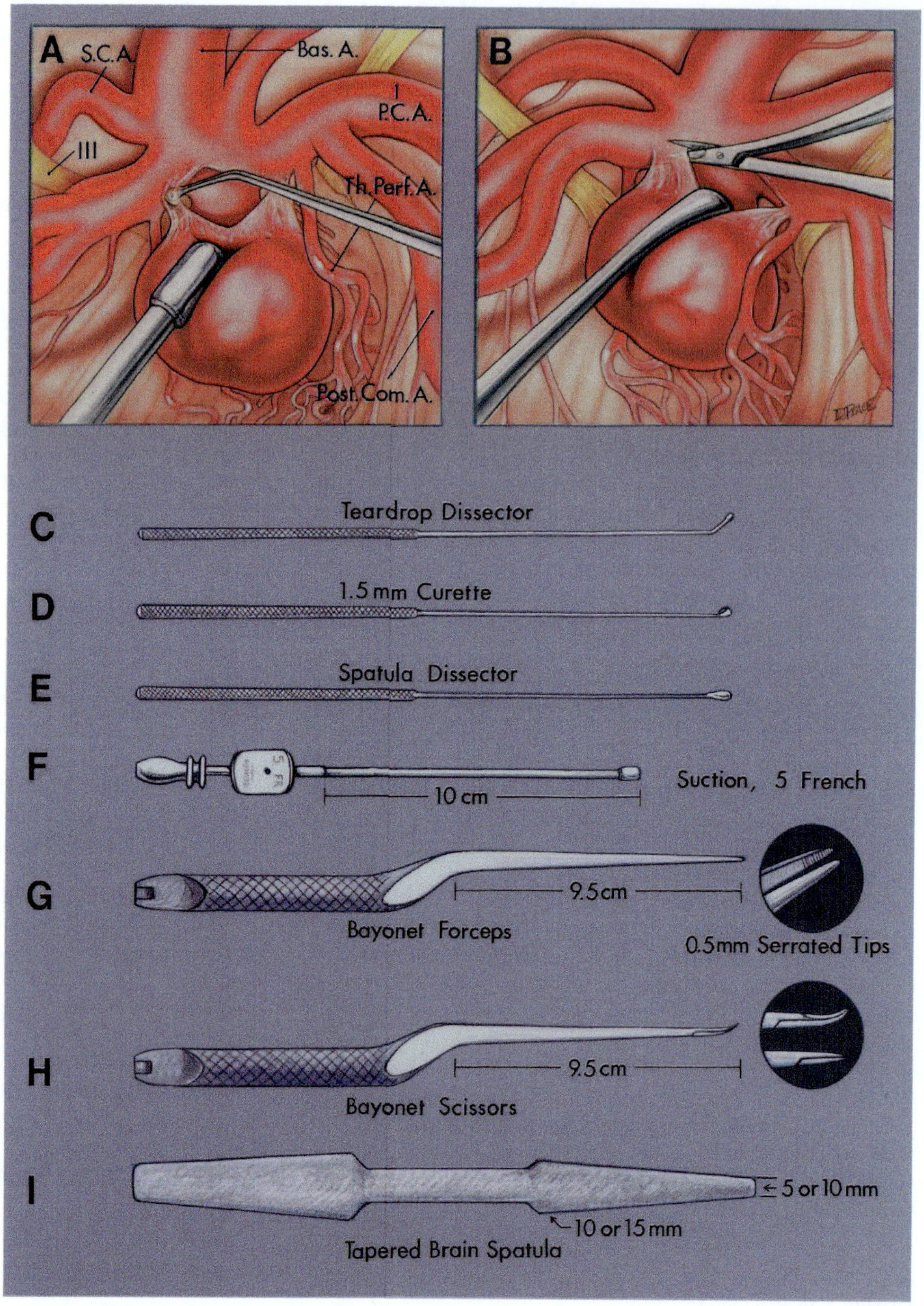

FIGURE 1.20. *Instruments for aneurysm dissection.* A, *a 40-degree teardrop dissector, separating perforating branches and arachnoidal bands from the neck of a basilar artery aneurysm. A blunt-tip, 5-French, suction tube provides suction and facilitates retraction of the aneurysm neck for dissection. Structures in the exposure include the superior cerebellar, posterior communicating, posterior cerebral, and posterior thalamoperforating arteries and the oculomotor nerve.* B, *the wall of an aneurysm being retracted with a spatula dissector, and tough arachnoidal bands around the neck being divided with microscissors.* C, *a 40-degree teardrop dissector, to define the neck and separate perforating vessels from the neck of an aneurysm.* D, *an angled microcurette with a 1.5-mm cup, which is useful for removing the dura from the anterior clinoid process.* E, *a spatula dissector, to define the neck and separate perforating vessels from the wall of an aneurysm.* F, *blunt-tip suction tube with a 10-cm shaft and a 5-French tip, for suction and dissection of an aneurysm. A 7- or 9-French blunt-tip suction tube may be needed if heavy bleeding occurs.* G, *bayonet forceps with 9.5-cm blades and 0.5-mm tips, with small serrations* (inset) *inside the tips for grasping arachnoidal and fibrous bands around an aneurysm.* H, *bayonet microscissors with 9.5-cm shafts and straight and curved blades* (inset) *for dividing adhesions around the neck of the aneurysm.* I, *brain spatulas most commonly used to elevate the brain during aneurysm surgery, tapered from 10 or 15 mm at the base to 5 or 10 mm at the tip.* A., *arteries;* Bas., *basilar;* Com., *communicating artery;* P.C.A., *posterior cerebral artery;* Post., *posterior;* S.C.A., *superior cerebellar artery;* Th.Perf., *thalamoperforating* (from, *Rhoton AL Jr: Aneurysms.* **Neurosurgery** *51[Suppl 1]:S1-121–S1-158, 2002 [13]).*

margin of the operative site. If the flexible arms are not positioned close to the drapes, then the suction tubing or the bipolar coagulator cable may become entangled with the arms and brain spatulas. Positioning near the drapes also reduces the chance that the nurse who is passing the instruments will bump the flexible arms. If the bar holding the flexible arms is positioned between the head of the patient and the surgeon, then the bar should be sufficiently close to the patient's head that the surgeon does not bump against it if he or she moves from one position to another around the head of the patient.

A series of tapered and rectangular brain spatulas should be available at the various operative sites (*Figs. 1.35–1.37*). Paired brain spatulas of the same size are frequently used for separation of the edges of the sylvian fissure or cortical incisions, and a single spatula is commonly used for elevation of the surface of the brain away from the cranial base, tentorium, or falx. A single spatula tapered from 15 to 25 mm at the base to 10 to 20 mm at the tip is commonly used for elevation of the frontal or temporal lobes or the cerebellum for tumor removal. A spatula with a 10-mm base that tapers to a 3-mm tip is

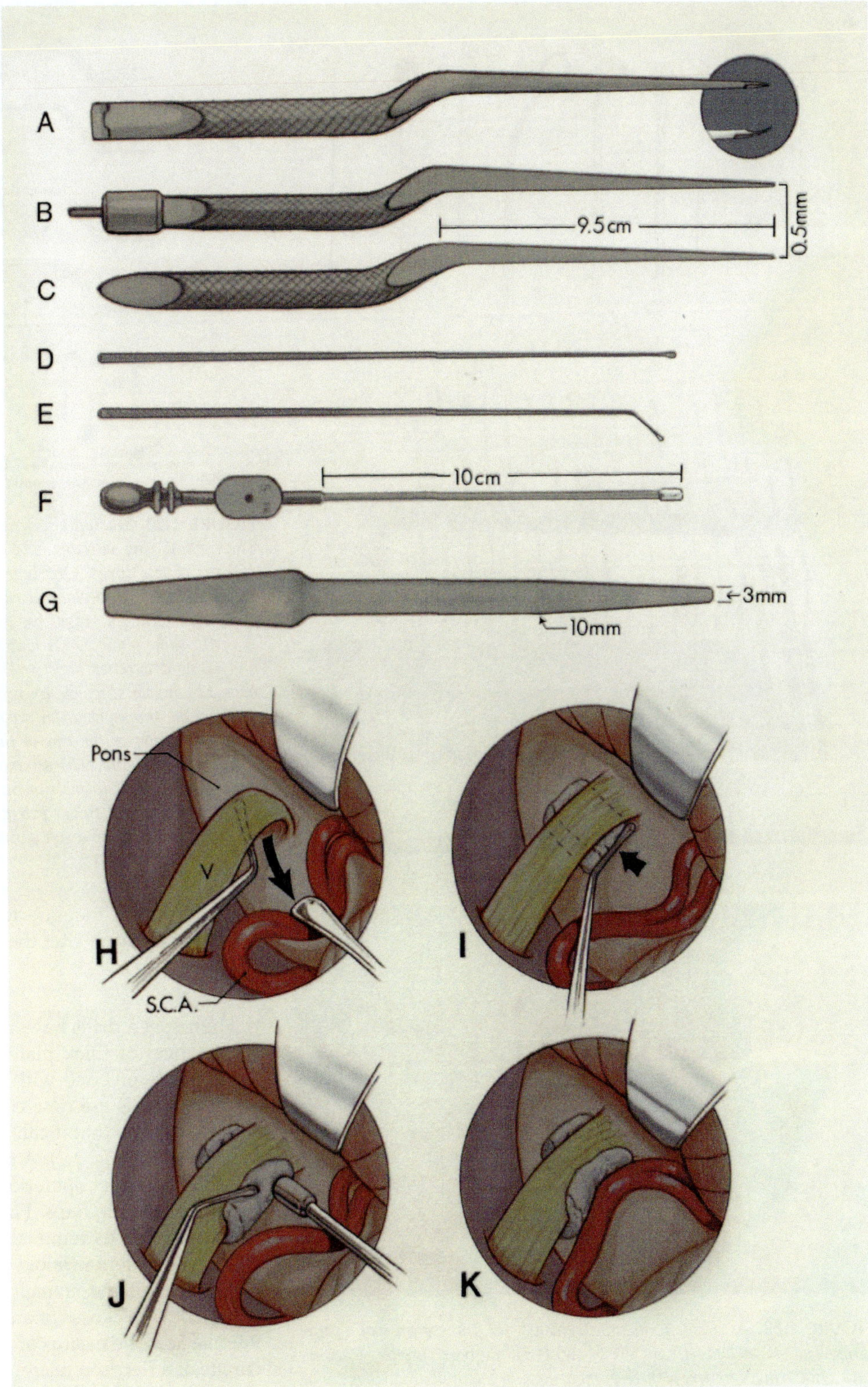

FIGURE 1.21. *Commonly used instruments for the microsurgical portion of a decompression operation for treatment of trigeminal neuralgia.* A, *bayonet scissors with 9.5-cm shafts and straight and curved blades are used for opening of the arachnoid membrane and cutting in the depths of the exposure.* B, *a bipolar bayonet forceps with 9.5-cm shafts and 0.5-cm tips is used for coagulation near the nerves or brainstem. A bipolar bayonet forceps with 0.7-mm tips is used for coagulation of large vessels in the superficial part of the exposure, and a forceps with 0.5-mm tips is used for deep coagulation.* C, *fine dissection around the arteries and nerves is performed with a plain bayonet forceps with 9.5-cm shafts and 0.5-cm tips.* D *and* E, *the two dissectors most commonly used around the trigeminal nerve are the small spatula microdissector* (D) *and a 40-degree teardrop dissector* (E). F, *suction around the nerve is performed with a blunt-tip suction tube with a 10-cm shaft and a 5-French tip.* G, *retraction is performed with a tapered brain spatula with a 10- or 15-mm width at the base and a 3- or 5-mm width at the tip. A self-retaining brain retractor system is used to hold the brain spatula in place.* H, *the orientation is the same as in* Figure 1.3C. *The right superior cerebellar artery is gently elevated away from the trigeminal nerve with the spatula dissector, and the area medial to the nerve is explored with the 40-degree teardrop dissector.* I, *a small foam pad is fit into the axilla of the nerve with the teardrop dissector.* J, *the separation between the superior surface of the nerve and the artery is maintained with a small foam prosthesis. A blunt-tip, 5-French, suction tube facilitates positioning of the small foam pad above the nerve.* K, *the small foam pad protects the medial and superior surfaces of the nerve* (from, *Rhoton AL Jr: Microsurgical anatomy of decompression operations on the trigeminal nerve, in Rovit RL (ed):* Trigeminal Neuralgia. *Baltimore, Williams & Wilkins, 1990, pp 165–200 [9]).*

commonly used during operations to treat trigeminal neuralgia or hemifacial spasm.

The surgeon should learn to manipulate the retractor while looking through the microscope. The retractor should not be applied so firmly that it blanches the vessels on the surface of the brain and causes infarction of the underlying brain tissue. Infarction occurs infrequently if blood pressure is normal; however, if induced hypotension is used intraoperatively, then inadequate

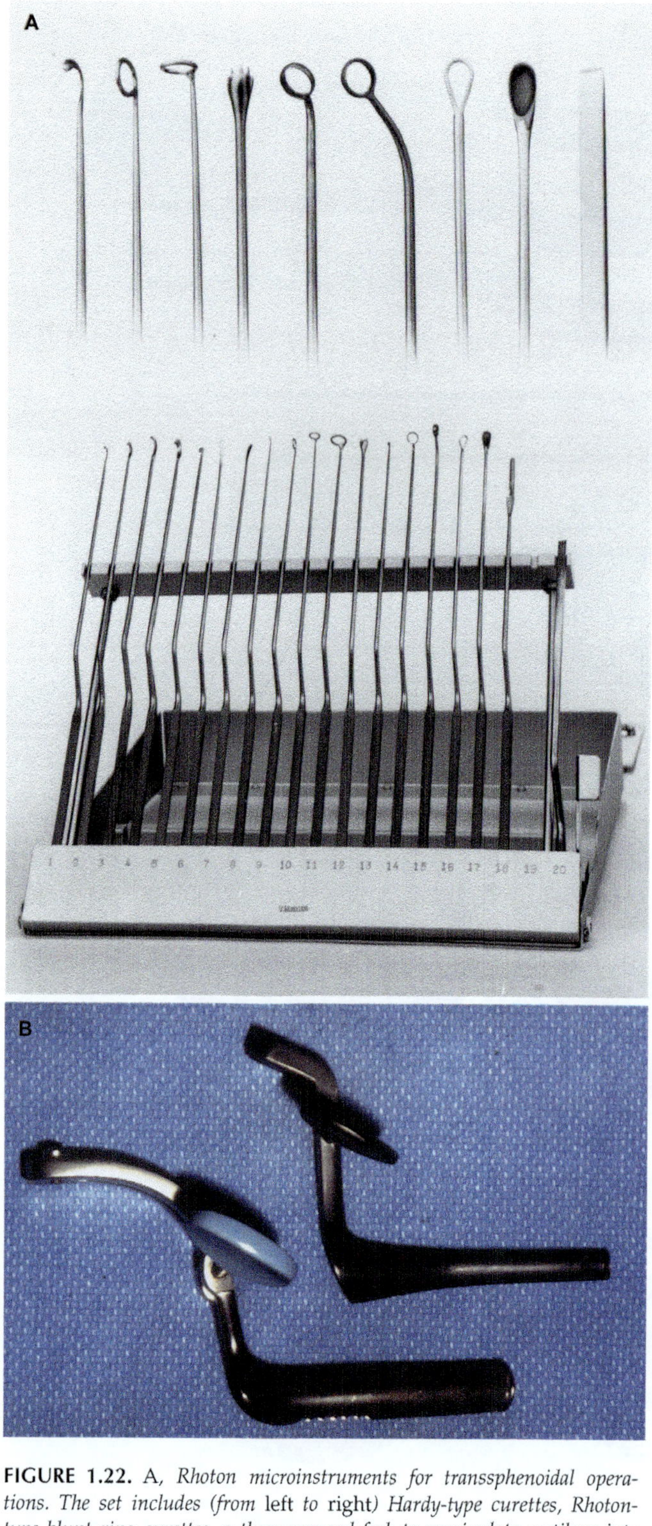

FIGURE 1.22. A, *Rhoton microinstruments for transsphenoidal operations. The set includes (from* left to right*) Hardy-type curettes, Rhoton-type blunt ring curettes, a three-pronged fork to manipulate cartilage into the sellar opening, Ray-type curettes, a malleable loop and spoon, and an osteotome to open the sellar wall.* B, *speculums for transsphenoidal surgery.* Right, *traditional transsphenoidal speculum, with thick wide blades.* Left, *Rhoton endonasal speculum, with smaller thinner blades, which is used for endonasal transsphenoidal tumor removal.*

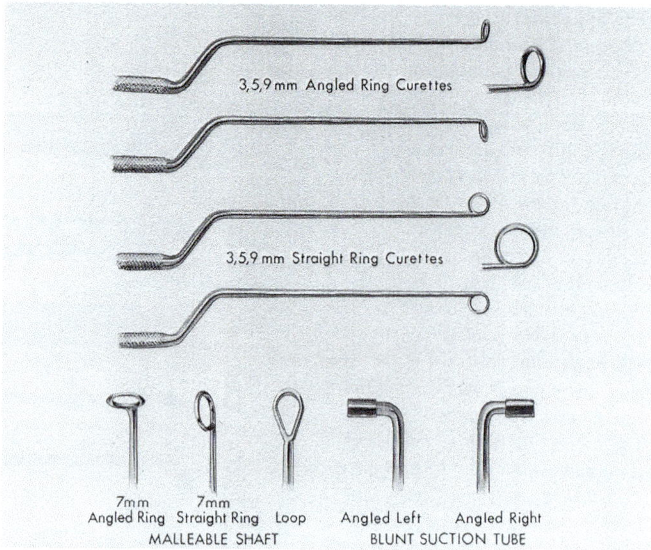

FIGURE 1.23. *Rhoton blunt ring curettes for transsphenoidal operations. These blunt ring curettes have small circular loops on the dissecting tip and are of two types. One type (angled rings) has a loop, the circumference of which is in a plane at right angles to the long axis of the shaft; the other type (straight rings) has a circular loop, the circumference of which is in the same plane as the long axis of the shaft. The rings on the angled and straight curettes have 3-, 5-, and 9-mm diameters. The instruments have 12-cm shafts, which are needed to reach the intracapsular/suprasellar area via the transsphenoidal exposure, and bayoneted handles, which facilitate observation of the tips of the instruments in the deep narrow transsphenoidal exposure. The set includes curettes with tips directed upward and downward. The instruments with malleable shafts can be bent for removal of unusual tumor extensions. The angled, blunt-tip, suction tubes are useful for removing soft parasellar and suprasellar tumor extensions.*

perfusion under the retractor may cause infarction, with subsequent hemorrhage after the retractor is removed.

Drills

High-speed drills have replaced the trephine and Gigli saw for removal of thick plates of bone. In the past, removal of thick plates of bone with rongeurs required great strength; however, drills are now commonly used to reduce the thickness of bone so that it can be gently removed without the use of great force (*Fig. 1.2*). A drill and its cutting attachments are used during most operations for placement of burr holes and elevation of bone flaps. Fine burrs are also available for delicate tasks such as removal of the wall of the internal acoustic meatus, the anterior clinoid process, part of the temporal bone, or protrusions of the cranial base (*Fig. 1.19D*). After a drill has reduced the thickness of an area such as the posterior lip of the internal acoustic meatus or the anterior clinoid process, a microcurette or a Kerrison microrongeur with a 1-mm lip may be used to remove the remaining thin layer of bone (*Fig. 1.19E*).

For delicate bone work, a drill that can reverse its direction may be preferable to one that cuts in only one direction. Most electric drills, but only a few air drills, are reversible. When reversible drills are used, the operation should be planned so that

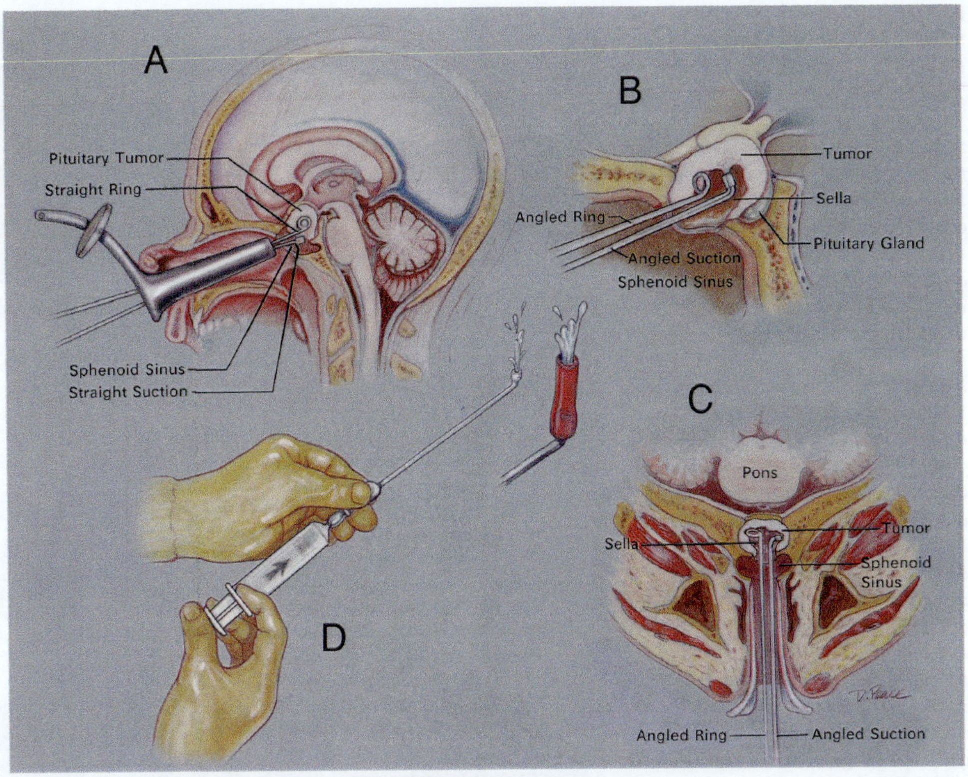

FIGURE 1.24. *Endonasal transsphenoidal removal of a large pituitary tumor with a suprasellar extension. A and B, midsagittal sections; C, oblique horizontal section through the plane along the transnasal route to the sphenoid sinus and sella turcica. A, the endonasal speculum has been advanced through the left nostril and along the side of the nasal septum to the sphenoid sinus. The straight ring curette breaks up the intracapsular contents of a suprasellar tumor, and the straight transsphenoidal suction tube aspirates tumor tissue from within the capsule. B, the angled ring curette and angled suction tube are directed upward for removal of the intracapsular contents of the suprasellar extension. C, the angled ring curette and suction tube remove tumor tissue extending into the parasellar region. D, placement of a syringe on the curved and straight tubes, with the thumb covering the thumb hole, allows the tube to be used for irrigation inside the tumor capsule, to soften, fragment, and remove tumor. A piece of red rubber catheter may be placed on the angled tubes, for suction and irrigation inside the capsule of large tumors.*

the burr rotates away from critical structures; if skidding occurs, it will be away from those areas. Diamond burrs are used near important structures. It is better for the surgeon to become skilled in the use of the drill in the laboratory before using it in a neurosurgical operation. Use of the drill can also be learned by assisting a surgeon who is experienced in its use and then practicing under the supervision of a skilled operator.

Drills that function at speeds from 10,000 to almost 100,000 rpm are available. At speeds of more than 25,000 rpm, the bone melts away so easily that the drill poorly transmits the tactile details of bony structure to the surgeon's hand. Slower speeds may be used for delicate procedures in which tactical control of the drill is important. A diamond bit is preferable for the most delicate bone removal.

The drill is held like a pen. Cutting is performed with the side rather than the end of the burr, except when making small calibrated holes for placement of sutures or screws at the margin of a bone flap. A large burr is used when possible. The greatest accuracy and control of the drill are obtained at higher speeds if a light brush action is used to remove the bone. Dangerous skidding may occur at lower speeds, because greater pressure is needed to cut the bone. The surgeon avoids running the burr across bone by using light intermittent pressure, rather than constant pressure of the burr at one spot. Overheating near nerves may damage them. Constant irrigation with physiological saline solution reduces heat transmission to the bone and nearby neural structures and prevents heat necrosis of the bone. Directing irrigating fluid toward the burr ensures optimal cleaning of the burr during irrigation of the operating field. The field may also be irrigated by using a suction-irrigation system. The teeth of the burr should be kept clean of bone dust. A coarse burr that clogs less easily is harder to control and skids across bone more easily, but this is reduced with irrigation. A burr should not be used to blindly make a long deep hole; instead, the hole should be beveled and as wide as possible. The surgeon should use a small curette to follow a small track, rather than pursuing it with a drill. Bone dust should be meticulously removed, because of its potent osteogenic properties.

Bone Curettes

Small curettes are frequently used for removal of the last shell of bone between a drill surface and neural or vascular structures. Straight and angled curettes are needed (*Figs. 1.17, 1.18A*, and *1.19, B, F*, and *J*). Curettes angled at 45 degrees are frequently used for special purposes, such as removal of the last thin shell of bone over the internal acoustic meatus or curettage of fragments of tumor from the lateral margin of the acoustic meatus or other cranial base areas. Curettes with tips as small as 1.5 mm are frequently needed. The curette is held so that the cutting edge is in full view. Cutting is performed with the side, rather than the tip, when possible. Pressure should be directed parallel to or away from important structures, rather than perpendicular to them. Properly sharpened curettes cut with less pressure and are safer than dull ones. The surgeon should try to use the largest curette possible.

Cup Forceps

A cup forceps, such as those used for intravertebral disc removal, is commonly used for removal of tumors (*Figs. 1.16* and *1.19, I* and

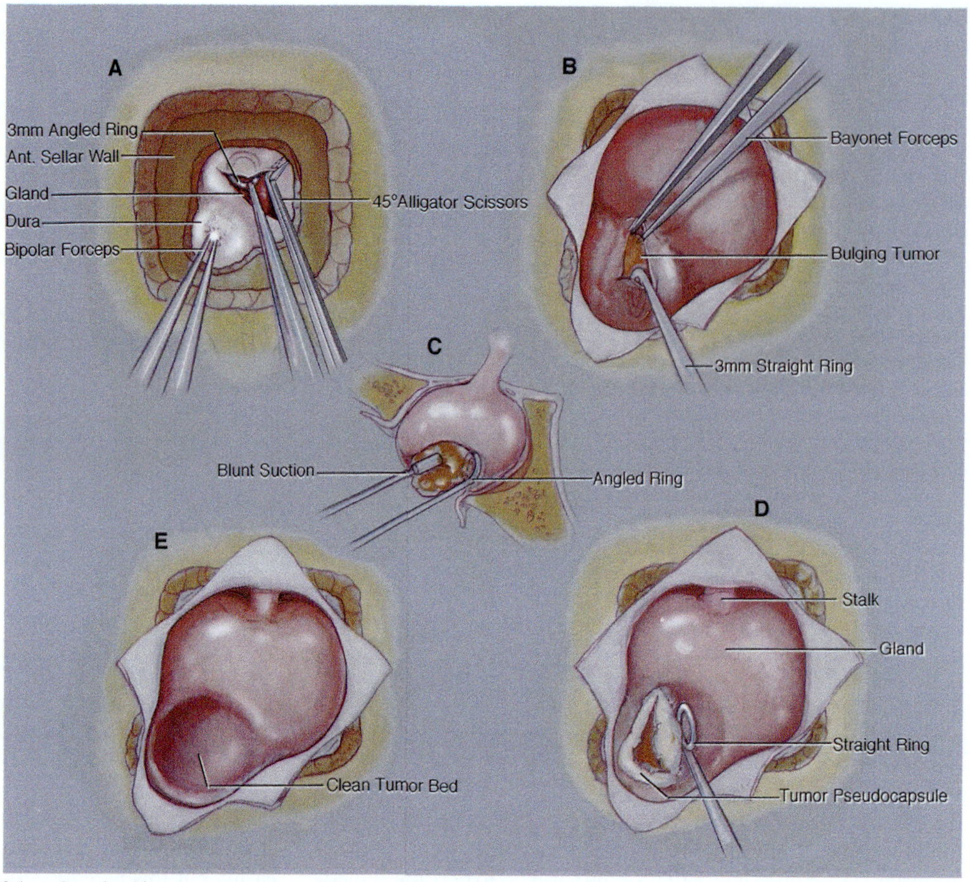

FIGURE 1.25. *Steps in the removal of a microadenoma. A, the sphenoid sinus and the anterior sellar wall have been opened. The thin bone and dura anterior to the tumor bulge in the inferior part of the right half of the sphenoid sinus. Bipolar forceps coagulate a vascular channel in the dura mater before the dura mater is opened. The dura is opened with a small vertical incision in the midline. A 3-mm, angled ring curette, inserted through the vertical incision, separates the dura from the anterior surface of the gland. Angled, 40-degree, alligator scissors, inserted through the vertical dural incision, open the dura from corner to corner. Incision of the dura in the corners and lateral margins of the sellar opening with a sharp pointed knife risks injury to the internal carotid arteries. B, the bulge at the site of the tumor is opened with the tips of a bayonet forceps or a small straight ring curette. The initial opening into the gland and the tumor is enlarged with the small straight ring curette. C, tumor tissue is removed from within the gland by using a blunt-tip suction tube and small angled ring curettes. The center of the tumor is often soft and gelatinous. D, the straight ring curette develops a cleavage plane between the firmer margin of tumor, which forms a pseudocapsule, and the gland. E, after removal of the tumor, the cavity within the gland is cleaned with irrigation. If the subarachnoid space was not opened during the procedure, then a small tumor bed can be cleaned of tumor cells by placing small pledgets of cottonoid immersed in absolute alcohol in the tumor bed.*

K). The most frequently used cup forceps have tips 3, 4, or 5 mm in width, suitable for intracapsular removal of large tumors. For removal of small tumors or small tumor fragments in critical locations, such as on the cranial nerves, in the acoustic meatus, or within the fourth ventricles, cup forceps with a diameter of 1 to 2 mm are used. To grasp small bits of tumor directly on or within the cranial nerves, the 1-mm cup forceps is used. The 2-, 3-, and 4-mm cups are suitable for intracapsular removal of small tumors. Angled microcup forceps enable the surgeon to reach around corners to grasp tissue or remove tumor. Cup forceps angled to the right are used to reach laterally to the right (e.g., to reach a right parasellar extension of a pituitary adenoma or to reach behind the facial and acoustic nerves in the right acoustic meatus), and cup forceps angled to the left are used on the left side (*Fig. 1.19K*). Angled cup forceps can also be used to reach on either side of a small capsular opening for intracapsular removal or to reach laterally into an intervertebral foramen for disc removal.

OPERATING MICROSCOPE

The use of the operating microscope and microsurgical techniques has disadvantages. Training in the use of the microscope is required, as is a shift from a tactile/manual technique using fingers to a vision-oriented technique (*Fig. 1.38*). The equipment is moderately expensive and requires additional space in the operating room, and its care places an additional burden on the nursing staff. It has been speculated that, by prolonging some procedures, microsurgical techniques may increase anesthesia-related risks and the risk of infection. However, by allowing operations to be performed through smaller openings and by permitting increased accuracy of dissection, microsurgical techniques may reduce the duration of procedures.

Performing operations with loupes (i.e., magnifying lenses attached to eyeglasses) is a form of microsurgery. Loupes represent an improvement over the naked eye but, even when combined with a headlight, they lack many of the advantages of the microscope. Most surgeons are unable to use loupes that provide more than two- to threefold magnification, the lower limit of resolution provided by the operating microscope. For craniotomies, many surgeons use loupes during the initial part of the operation and bring the microscope into the operative field just before or after opening of the dura mater.

Operations should be undertaken only after the surgeon has acquired proficiency in the use of the microscope. Clinical microtechniques should be applied first to procedures with which the surgeon is entirely familiar, such as excision of ruptured discs, before its use is expanded to new and technically more difficult procedures. Early in many surgeons' experience with the microscope, they tend to use it in less-

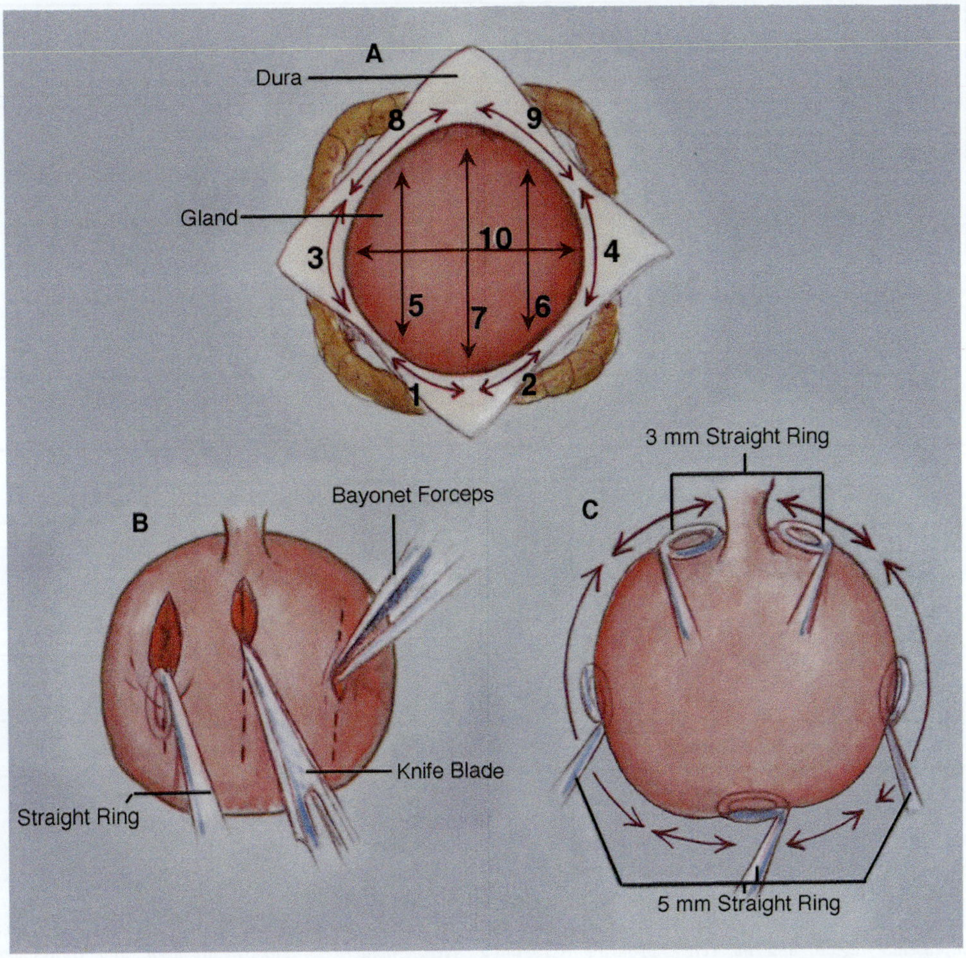

FIGURE 1.26. *Steps for exploration of the pituitary gland when a hypersecreting adenoma is known to be present but is not obvious after initial exposure of the gland. The order in which these steps are performed should be selected so that the fewest steps are required to locate the tumor. If equivocal or clear-cut radiological findings or results from petrosal sinus sampling suggest that the tumor is confined to a specific part of the sella, then exploration should begin in that area. Knowledge of the most common locations for each type of microadenoma is helpful for selection of the area in which to begin exploration. Tumors secreting growth hormone or prolactin commonly occur in the lateral aspect and corticotropin-secreting tumors occur in the central part of the gland.* A, *anterior view of the gland with the dura mater opened. Steps in the exploration of the gland are as follows: Step 1, separation of the inferior surface of the right half of the gland from the sellar floor; Step 2, separation of the inferior surface of the left half of the gland from the sellar floor; Step 3, separation of the right lateral surface of the gland from the medial wall of the cavernous sinus; Step 4, separation of the left lateral surface of the gland from the medial wall of the cavernous sinus; Step 5, vertical incision into the right half of the gland (the exploratory incisions into the gland are not carried through the superior, inferior, or lateral surfaces of the gland but are performed so as to preserve gland margins at both ends of the incision); Step 6, vertical incision into the left half of the gland; Step 7, vertical incision into the midportion of the gland; Step 8, separation of the superior surface of the right half of the gland from the diaphragm; Step 9, separation of the superior surface of the left half of the gland from the diaphragm; Step 10, transverse incision into the gland.* B, *methods of incision of the gland. The openings in the gland can be started by using a no. 11 knife blade or by introducing the closed tips of a pointed bayonet forceps into the surface of the gland and allowing the tips to open, splitting the gland. The incisions are enlarged with a 3-mm straight ring curette.* C, *direction (*arrows*) in which the straight ring curettes are slipped around the outer circumference of the gland to separate its surfaces from the sellar floor, the medial walls of the cavernous sinus, and the diaphragm. The 5-mm straight ring curette is used to separate the gland from the floor and medial walls of the cavernous sinus. The 3-mm straight ring curette is used to separate the superior surface of the gland from the diaphragm. Exploration of the superior surface of the gland is performed as a late step, to avoid entering the subarachnoid space and to reduce the risk of cerebrospinal fluid leakage and injury to the pituitary stalk. Most microadenomas can be removed without disturbing the superior surface of the gland and without making an opening into the subarachnoid space.*

demanding situations and to discontinue its use when they encounter hemorrhage or problems of unusual complexity. Increasing experience, however, makes it apparent that bleeding is more accurately and quickly controlled during operations in which magnification is used and that the hemorrhage that occurs during operations performed under the microscope tends to be of lesser magnitude than the hemorrhage that occurs during operations performed without magnification.

The surgeon should be knowledgeable about the basic optical and mechanical principles of the operating microscope, the common types of mechanical illumination, the types of electrical failure that affect illumination, and how to correct those failures, and the selection of lenses, eyepieces, binocular tubes, light sources, stands, and accessories for different operations (*Fig. 1.38*). The laboratory provides a setting in which the mental and physical adjustments required for performing microsurgery can be mastered. Training in the laboratory is essential before the surgeon undertakes microanastomotic procedures (e.g., superficial temporal artery-middle cerebral artery anastomoses) for patients. These techniques cannot be learned by watching others perform them; they must be perfected on specimens of cerebral vessels obtained at autopsy and on animals.

Microscope-assisted dissection of tissues obtained from cadavers may increase the surgeon's skill (*Fig. 1.39*). The performance of temporal bone dissection in the laboratory is an accepted component of microsurgical training for otological operations, and such exercises are of value to the neurosurgeon. The surgeon may gain skill in procedures in the cerebel-

TABLE 1.1. Recommended suture size in relation to vessel size[a]

Suture size	Vessel diameter (mm)	Example of blood vessel size	Suture diameter (μm)
6-0	5.0–6.0	Common carotid artery	
7-0	4.0–5.0	Internal carotid and vertebral arteries	
8-0	3.0–4.0	Basilar and middle cerebral arteries	45
9-0	2.0–3.0	Anterior and posterior cerebral arteries	35
10-0	0.8–1.5	Sylvian and cortical arteries	22
11-0			18

[a] From Yaşargil MG: Suturing techniques, in Yaşargil MG (ed): *Microsurgery Applied to Neurosurgery*. Stuttgart, Georg Thieme, 1969, pp 51–58 (18).

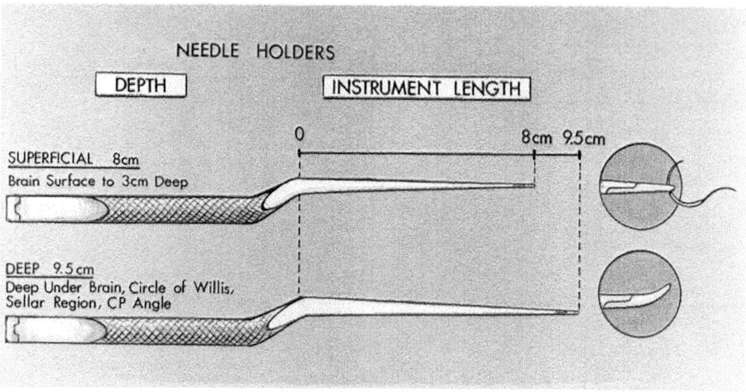

FIGURE 1.27. *Rhoton bayonet needle-holders with round handles. The bayonet needle-holders with 8-cm shafts are used at the surface of the brain and down to a depth of 3 cm. The needle-holders with 9.5-cm shafts are used deep under the brain, at the level of the circle of Willis, the suprasellar region, and the cerebellopontine (CP) angle. Needle-holders with straight and curved tips may be needed. The straight needle-holders shown in* Figure 1.8 *may also be used at the surface of the brain.*

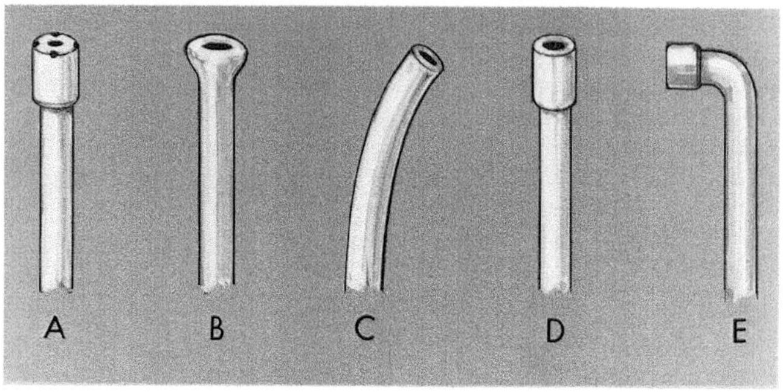

FIGURE 1.28. *Different types of suction tubes.* A, *Yankauer-type suction tube with a blunt tip. This tip is commonly used in general surgery.* B, *Dandy suction tube with a blunt tip.* C, *Adson suction tube with a curved tip. The distal tip of the Adson suction tube is oriented obliquely with respect to the long axis of the shaft.* D, *straight blunt tip for neurosurgery.* E, *angled blunt suction tubes for transsphenoidal surgery.*

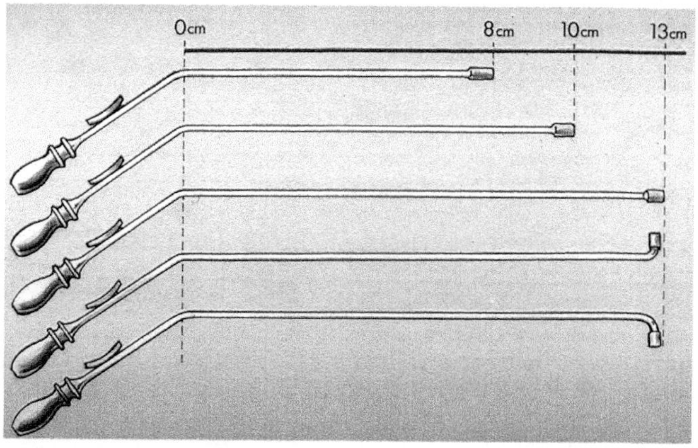

FIGURE 1.29. *Rhoton-Merz suction tubes of the three lengths needed for superficial, deep, and transsphenoidal or extra-deep neurosurgery. The 8-cm tube is used during opening of the cranium and at superficial intracranial sites. The 10-cm tube is used at deep intracranial sites, such as near the circle of Willis, in the suprasellar area, and in the cerebellopontine angle. The 13-cm tube is used at extra-deep sites, such as in front of the brainstem and in transsphenoidal operations. The transsphenoidal suction tubes have straight, angled-up, and angled-down tips in each of the 5-, 7-, and 10-French sizes.*

lopontine angle by dissecting temporal bone specimens and in transsphenoidal operations by dissecting sphenoid and sellar blocks (6, 17). Detailed microscopic exploration of the perforating branches of the circle of Willis and other common sites of aneurysm occurrence may improve the surgeon's technique for aneurysm treatment. As the need arises, other selected specimens may be used to increase the surgeon's acquaintance with other operative sites, such as the jugular foramen, cavernous sinus, pineal region, or ventricles.

The surgical nurse plays an especially important role in microneurosurgery (1). The nurse should make constant efforts to reduce the number of times the surgeon looks away from the microscope and to limit distractions. The scrub nurse may need to guide the surgeon's hands to the operative field. Communication between the nurse and the surgeon can be facilitated by a television system that allows the nurse to view the operative field on a nearby monitor and to place the proper instrument in the surgeon's hands, without the surgeon taking his or her eyes away from the microscope (*Fig. 1.1*). The nurse should be skilled in the operation and maintenance of the microscope, be able to balance and prepare it for par-

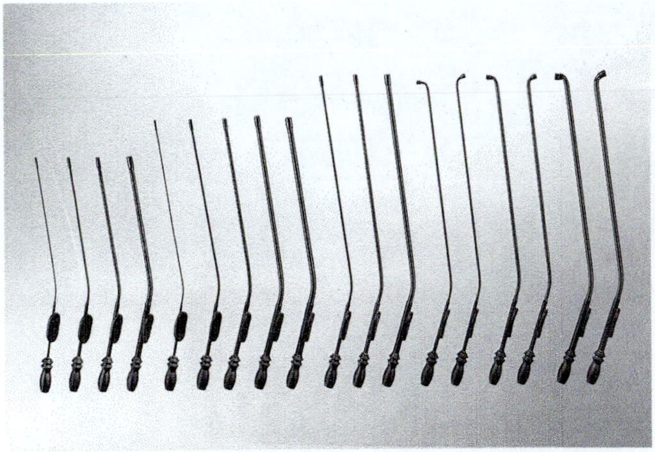

FIGURE 1.30. *Complete set of suction tubes for macroneurosurgery and microneurosurgery. The four short tubes (8-cm shafts)* (left) *have diameters of 3, 5, 7, and 10 French and are used at superficial sites. The five longer tubes (10-cm shafts)* (center) *have diameters of 3, 5, 7, 10, and 12 French and are used at deep sites. The nine longest tubes (13-cm shafts)* (right) *have three diameters (5, 7, and 10 French) and three tip configurations (straight, angled-up, and angled-down tips). They are used at extra-deep sites and for transsphenoidal operations. The angled tubes are used for transsphenoidal operations.*

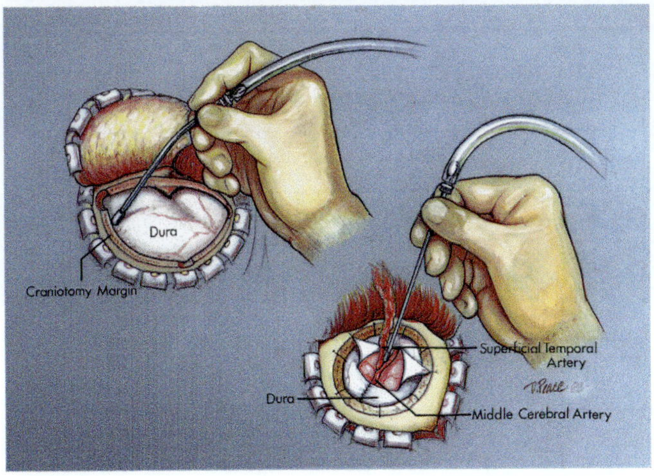

FIGURE 1.31. *Short tubes (8-cm shafts) used for suction during turning of bone flaps or during other operations near the surface of the brain. When held in a pencil grip for suction near the surface of the brain, the short tubes permit the hand to be rested on the wound margin and the tip to be manipulated with delicate finger movements. Use of a longer tube or a tube held in a pistol grip would not allow the hand to be rested on the wound margin. The short tube with a large diameter (10 French) is used for aspiration of bone dust and heavy bleeding during elevation of a craniotomy flap* (left)*. The short tube with the smallest diameter (3 French) is used for suction in the area of a superficial temporal artery-middle cerebral artery bypass* (right)*; a larger suction tube could injure the vessels or disrupt the suture line.*

ticular operations (with selection of the appropriate lenses), and be able to ready it for use with the patient in the supine, prone, or sitting position. The nursing staff should also be able to drape the microscope quickly and to address commonly encountered mechanical and electronic malfunctions. The circulating nurse must be immediately available to adjust the bipolar coagulator and suction system, rapidly change the microscope bulb or other light source, replace clouded or dirty objective lenses or eyepieces, and adjust all foot pedals and controls for the microscope. The nurse should record the surgeon's eyepiece settings, so that all replacement eyepieces are properly adjusted for use.

Developments in frameless stereotactic surgery permit the microscope to function as part of a stereotactic surgical system. An infrared localizing system for the microscope, when combined with digitization of the angle of view and the focal length, enables the surgeon to simultaneously view a reconstructed magnetic resonance imaging or computed tomographic scan matching the focal point of the image observed through the microscope. The surgeon knows exactly where the focal point of the image being viewed in the microscope is located in relation to the normal and pathological structures observed on computed tomographic and magnetic resonance imaging scans.

ULTRASONIC AND LASER DISSECTION

Ultrasonic and laser dissection units are alternatives to the use of cup forceps and suction for tumor removal. Such units are applied with the greatest degree of accuracy when guided by the magnified vision provided by the operating microscope. They are most commonly used to debulk tumors. Ultrasonic aspirators are preferred over laser dissection units because they can remove tumor tissue more rapidly. Tumor removal with a laser proceeds much more slowly. Neither instrument should be used to remove small tumor fragments on the surfaces of vessels or nerves. A special application of the laser is coagulation of tumor attachments to the cranial base but I think that the laser has no significant advantage, compared with carefully applied bipolar coagulation.

Ultrasonic Aspirators

Ultrasonic aspirators enjoy wider usage than lasers because of their ability to rapidly debulk large tumors but they must be used with extreme care, because they can quickly open through the surface of a tumor capsule and damage vessels and nerves adhering to the surface of the tumor. Aspirators are commonly used for the removal of large tumors. These vibrating suction devices fragment and aspirate tumor tissue. These units have a control console that regulates the amount of irrigation and suction at the hand piece and the vibration of the cutting tip. They are suitable for fragmenting firm tumors such as meningiomas, acoustic neuromas, and some gliomas. They can rapidly debulk the center of all except the most calcified tumors. They are commonly used to rapidly debulk neoplasms, after which the capsule is removed from nerves and vessels with fine dissecting instruments. These devices do not control bleeding, although some are designed to allow coagulation to be applied through the tip.

Laser Microsurgery

The fact that a laser beam can be focused to a fine point makes it an ideal tool to be directed by a magnified vision of the operating microscope (*Fig. 1.38*). The carbon dioxide laser,

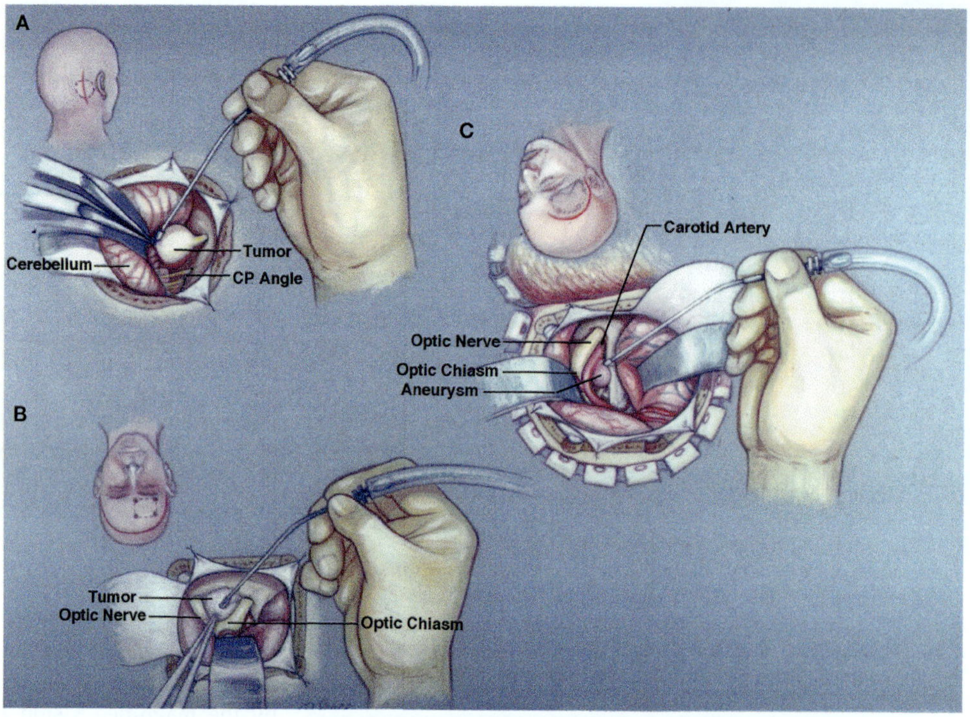

FIGURE 1.32. *Suction tubes with 10-cm shafts, used for deep intracranial operations in the cerebellopontine angle, in the suprasellar region, and around the circle of Willis. The* smaller drawings *show the scalp incisions (*solid line*) and the craniectomy or craniectomy sites (*dotted line*), and the* larger drawings *show the operative sites.* A, *the 10-cm suction tube facilitates exposure of a tumor in the right cerebellopontine (*CP*) angle.* B, *the 10-cm suction tube aspirates tumor from within the capsule of a suprasellar tumor.* C, *the 10-cm suction tube aspirates clot and facilitates dissection of the neck of an aneurysm arising on the internal carotid artery.*

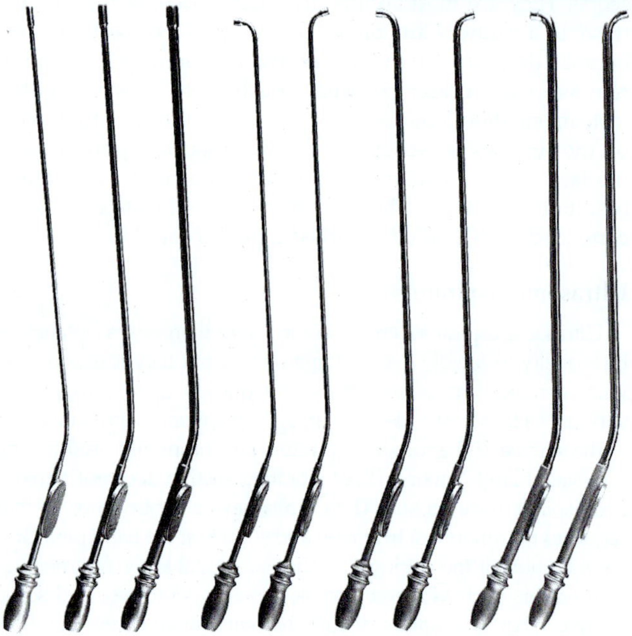

FIGURE 1.33. *Rhoton-Merz suction tubes for transsphenoidal operations. The transsphenoidal tubes have 13-cm shafts and are of three sizes (5, 7, and 10 French). Tubes of each of the three sizes have straight, angled-up, and angled-down tips.*

the type most commonly used in neurosurgery, can be used freehand but is more commonly linked to the operating microscope, by means of a direct mechanical or electromechanical manipulator. The beam from the carbon dioxide laser is invisible and must be identified with a coincident pilot helium-neon laser. The carbon dioxide and helium-neon beams must be absolutely coaxial; if they are not, then errors in the direction of the destructive carbon dioxide beam result. The carbon dioxide laser energy is immediately absorbed by and vaporizes tissues containing fluid. Because the beam cannot pass through fluid, its maximal effect is at the surface. The vaporized tissue is removed with a standard suction system.

TABLE 1.2. Uses for suction tubes

Diameter[a]	Use
3 French	Smallest nerves, vessel anastomosis
5 French	Aneurysm neck, pituitary gland, medium-size nerves
7 French	Microsurgical resection of larger tumors
10–12 French	Heavy bleeding, bone dust, flap elevation

[a] 3 French = 1-mm outer diameter.

The carbon dioxide laser is most commonly used for the removal of extra-axial tumors. The basic actions of incision, coagulation, and vaporization of tissue are functions of the amount of energy, measured in terms of watts applied to tissue. Lower wattages are used for coagulation, and higher wattages are used for incision and removal of tissue. The radiant energy is manipulated by altering the variables of power input, length of exposure, and surface area of the impact site. The beam is turned on by depressing a foot switch, and the power and length of exposure are determined by settings on the control console. The micromanipulator for

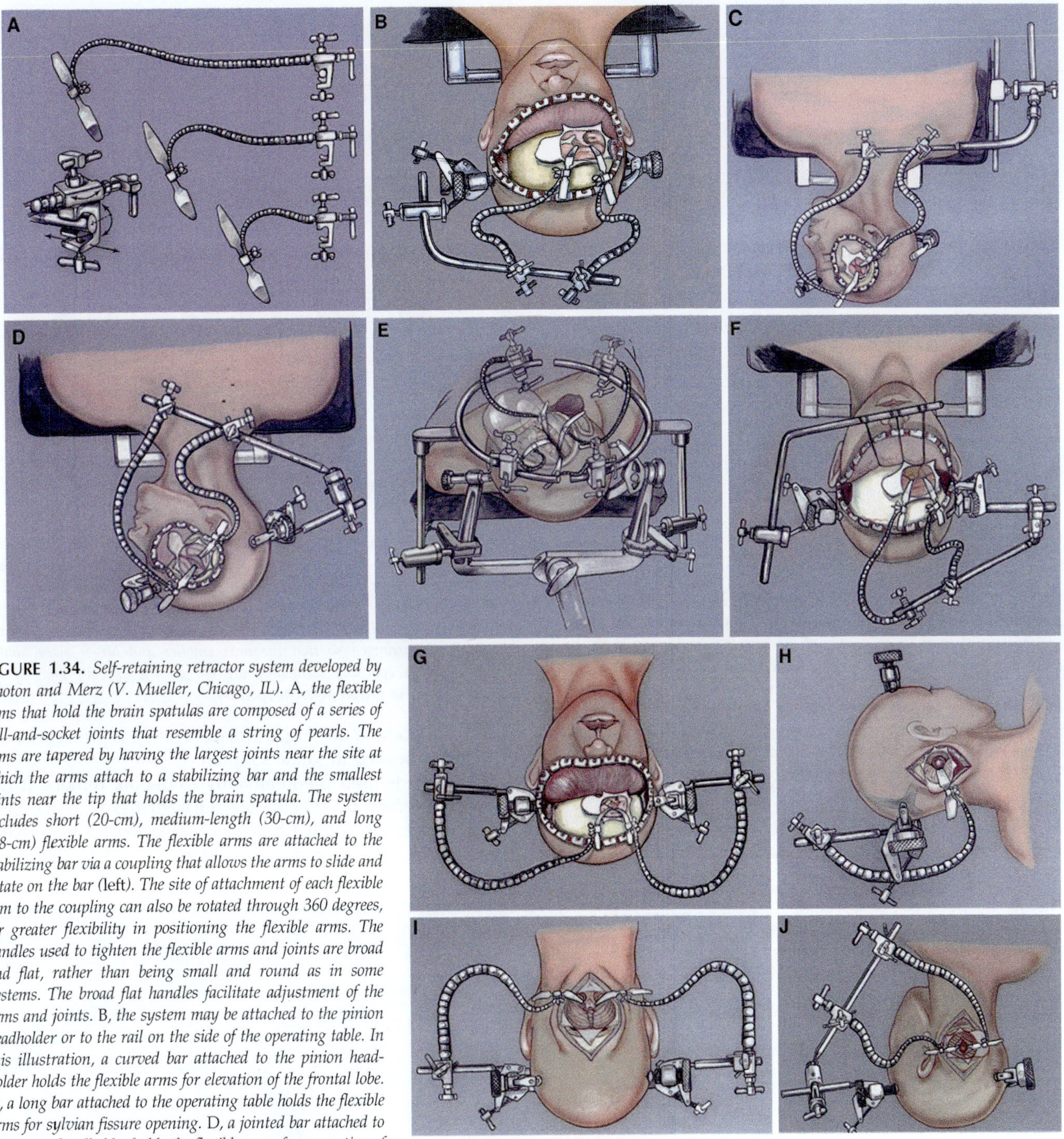

FIGURE 1.34. *Self-retaining retractor system developed by Rhoton and Merz (V. Mueller, Chicago, IL). A, the flexible arms that hold the brain spatulas are composed of a series of ball-and-socket joints that resemble a string of pearls. The arms are tapered by having the largest joints near the site at which the arms attach to a stabilizing bar and the smallest joints near the tip that holds the brain spatula. The system includes short (20-cm), medium-length (30-cm), and long (48-cm) flexible arms. The flexible arms are attached to the stabilizing bar via a coupling that allows the arms to slide and rotate on the bar (left). The site of attachment of each flexible arm to the coupling can also be rotated through 360 degrees, for greater flexibility in positioning the flexible arms. The handles used to tighten the flexible arms and joints are broad and flat, rather than being small and round as in some systems. The broad flat handles facilitate adjustment of the arms and joints. B, the system may be attached to the pinion headholder or to the rail on the side of the operating table. In this illustration, a curved bar attached to the pinion headholder holds the flexible arms for elevation of the frontal lobe. C, a long bar attached to the operating table holds the flexible arms for sylvian fissure opening. D, a jointed bar attached to the pinion headholder holds the flexible arms for separation of the margins of the sylvian fissure. E, two semicircular bars, attached by C-clamps to the pinion headholder, form a halo or ring around the craniotomy site that holds the flexible arms for splitting of the sylvian fissure. F, the jointed bar attached to the right side of the pinion headholder serves as the site of attachment of the flexible arms for elevation of the frontal lobe. A bar attached to the left side of the headholder serves as the site of attachment for the scalp retractors. G, the flexible arms are attached directly to the clamps on the pinion headholder for elevation of the frontal lobe. H, a flexible arm is attached to the clamp on the pinion headholder for removal of an acoustic neuroma. I, the flexible arms are attached to the clamp on the pinion headholder for separation of the cerebellar tonsils. J, the jointed bar holds the flexible arms for separation of the edges of an incision in the cerebellar hemisphere.*

direction of the site of impact of the beam is a straight lever situated near the objective lens of the microscope.

It is best to begin with low power and increase the power as appropriate. The cross sectional area of the impact zone is

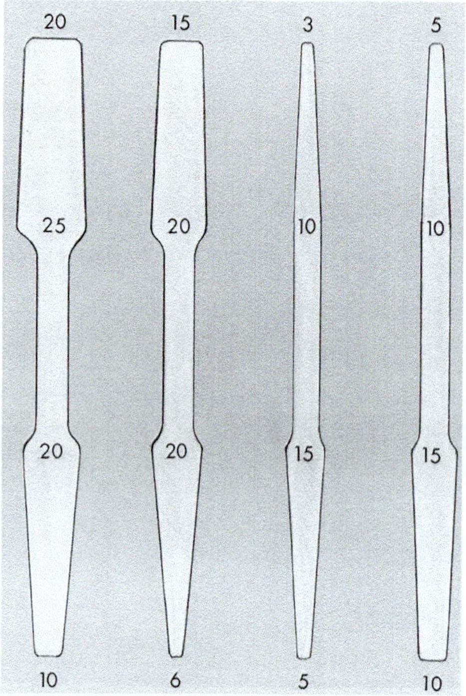

FIGURE 1.35. *Rhoton tapered brain spatulas of various widths. Spatulas of different widths may be needed, depending on the site and size of the lesion. A spatula tapered from 10 or 20 mm at the base to 5 to 15 mm at the tip is commonly selected for separation of the margins of the sylvian fissure, elevation of the frontal or temporal lobe, or exposure of lesions in the posterior fossa. A brain spatula tapered from 10 mm at the base to 3 or 5 mm at the tip is commonly selected for operations for treatment of trigeminal neuralgia or hemifacial spasm. A brain spatula with a 20- or 25-mm base and a 15- or 20-mm tip commonly serves for acoustic neuroma removal.*

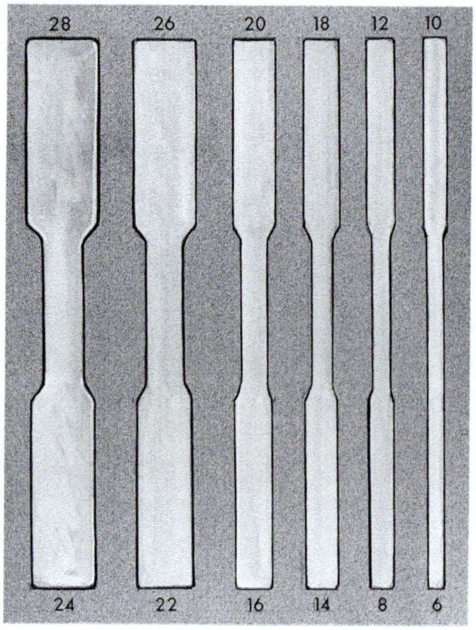

FIGURE 1.36. *Rhoton rectangular brain spatulas in a range of widths from 6 to 28 mm. Opposing brain spatulas of almost the same size are commonly used for opening of the sylvian fissure or fourth ventricle or exposure of lesions in the cerebral or cerebellar hemispheres. Each end of the brain spatulas has a different width. The widths of the two ends of the spatulas are arranged so that the next smaller and larger sizes, which could serve as opposing retractors, are not on the opposite ends of the same spatula but are on different spatulas.*

increased with beam defocusing. Shortening of exposure times tends to reduce the build-up of heat and thermal effects on tissues adjacent to the target. Adjacent tissue is protected with cottonoids soaked in saline solution.

The laser is used predominantly to debulk tumors. It decreases bleeding by coagulating adjacent tissue; however, I prefer accurately applied bipolar coagulation for hemostasis near critical neural structures. Accurate microdissection with

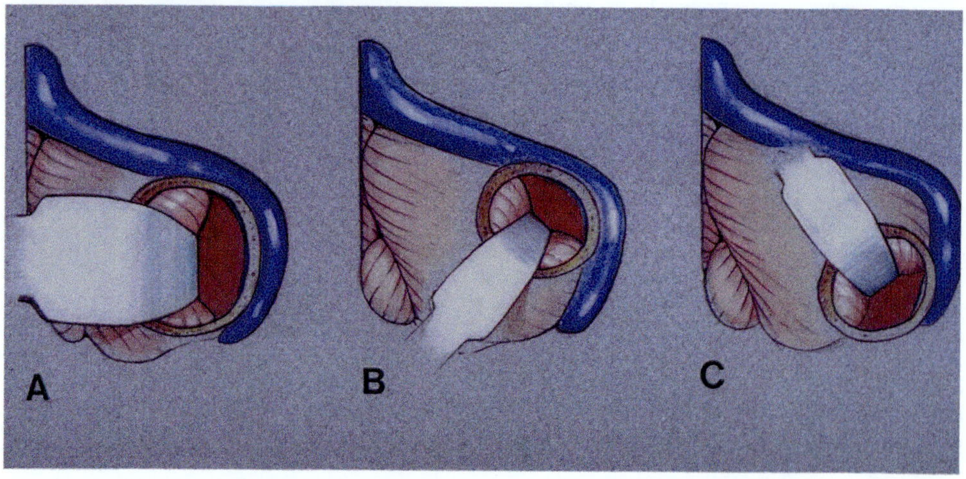

FIGURE 1.37. *Direction of application of brain spatulas for surgery in the various compartments of the cerebellopontine angle. A, retractor application for exposure of a lesion in the midportion of the cerebellopontine angle. The craniotomy is situated below the transverse sinus and medial to the sigmoid sinus. A brain spatula tapered from 20 or 25 mm at the base to 15 or 20 mm at the tip, depending on the size of the tumor, is commonly selected for elevation of the lateral surface of the cerebellum for acoustic neuroma removal. B, retractor application for exposure of the superolateral compartment of the posterior fossa for a vascular decompression operation for treatment of trigeminal neuralgia. A spatula tapered from 10 mm at the base to 3 mm at the tip is commonly selected. C, retractor application for exposure of the inferolateral compartment of the posterior fossa, such as for treatment of hemifacial spasm or glossopharyngeal neuralgia. A brain spatula tapered from 10 mm at the base to 3 mm at the tip is commonly used for operations for treatment of hemifacial spasm* (from, *Rhoton AL Jr: The cerebellopontine angle and posterior fossa cranial nerves by the retrosigmoid approach.* **Neurosurgery** *47[Suppl]:S93–S129, 2000 [12]).*

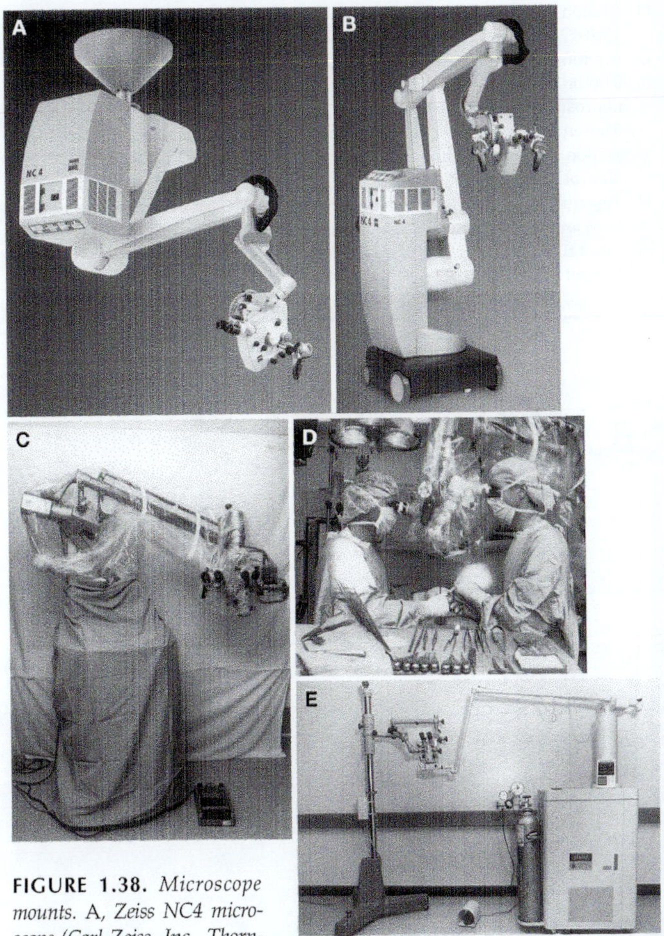

FIGURE 1.38. *Microscope mounts. A, Zeiss NC4 microscope (Carl Zeiss, Inc., Thornwood, NY) mounted on the ceiling. B, Zeiss motorized microscope on a floor stand. C, motorized zoom microscope draped for surgery. The motorized functions are controlled with foot switches on the floor or switches on the handles beside the microscope body. D, microscope being used for a spinal operation. The surgeon is on the left. The assistant, on the right, has a binocular viewing tube. E, carbon dioxide laser coupled to the operating microscope. The laser is activated with a foot switch. The power output and length of exposure are determined by settings on the control counsel. The site of impact of the beam is moved by using the straight lever to the left of the objective lens. The beam is delivered to the target via a series of deflecting mirrors located inside articulating tubular arms, which are mechanically coupled to the microscope.*

fine instruments is the preferred method for removing the final tumor fragments from neural and vascular structures.

Argon and neodymium:yttrium-aluminum-garnet lasers, although used less frequently than carbon dioxide lasers in neurosurgery, have some promise for the treatment of vascular tumors of the nervous system. The argon laser has found use in ophthalmology, because of the affinity of its wavelength for the melanin pigment in the retinal epithelium of the eye. The affinity of the neodymium:yttrium-aluminum-garnet laser for the red color of hemoglobin has led to its use for the treatment of lesions with high blood contents. Argon and neodymium:yttrium-aluminum-garnet laser beams can be delivered through optic fibers, but these fibers lead to an unacceptable loss of energy when used with a carbon dioxide laser.

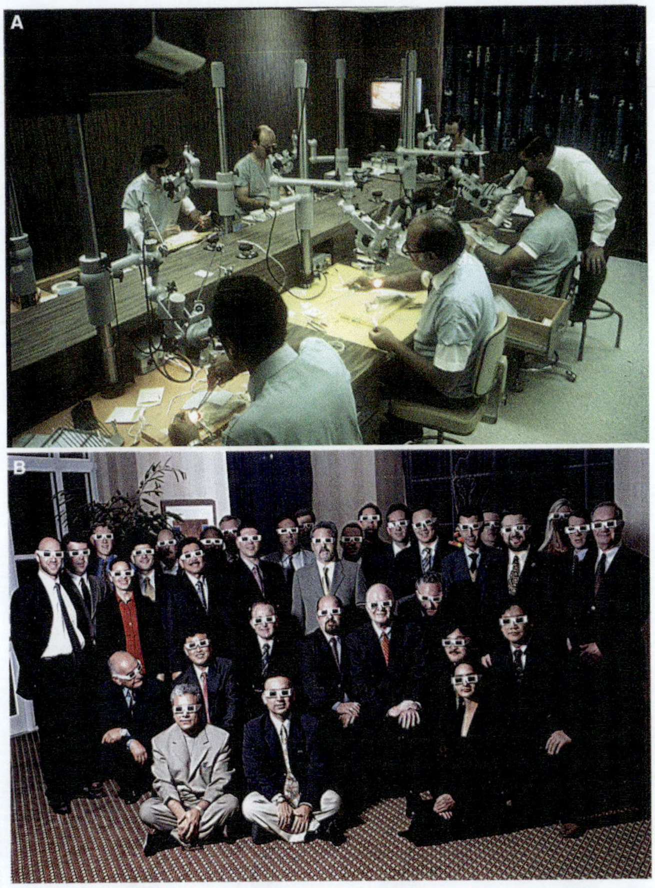

FIGURE 1.39. *A, participants working during the first microneurosurgery course held at the University of Florida, in 1975. B, participants in a recent course held at the McKnight Brain Institute at the University of Florida, in three-dimensional stereo glasses. Three-dimensional presentations have become an increasingly important part of the courses.*

The carbon dioxide beam is delivered to the target via a series of deflecting mirrors located inside articulating tubular arms that are mechanically coupled to the microscope. Individuals working around laser systems should wear protective lenses that are color-specific for the wavelength involved.

REFERENCES

1. Bader DC: Microtechnical nursing in neurosurgery. **J Neurosurg Nurs** 7:22–24, 1975.
2. Greenberg IM: Self-retaining retractor and handrest system for neurosurgery. **Neurosurgery** 8:205–208, 1981.
3. Greenwood J Jr: Two point coagulation: A new principle and instrument for applying coagulation current in neurosurgery. **Am J Surg** 50:267–270, 1940.
4. Kurze T: Microtechniques in neurological surgery. **Clin Neurosurg** 11:128–137, 1964.
5. Malis LL: Bipolar coagulation in microsurgery, in Yaşargil MG (ed): *Microsurgery Applied to Neurosurgery*. Stuttgart, Georg Thieme, 1969, pp 41–45.
6. Pait TG, Harris FS, Paullus WS, Rhoton AL Jr: Microsurgical anatomy and dissection of the temporal bone. **Surg Neurol** 8:363–391, 1971.
7. Rhoton AL Jr: Microsurgery of the internal acoustic meatus. **Surg Neurol** 2:311–318, 1974.
8. Rhoton AL Jr: Ring curettes for transsphenoidal pituitary operations. **Surg Neurol** 18:28–33, 1982.

9. Rhoton AL Jr: Microsurgical anatomy of decompression operations on the trigeminal nerve, in Rovit RL (ed): *Trigeminal Neuralgia*. Baltimore, Williams & Wilkins, 1990, pp 165–200.
10. Rhoton AL Jr: Instrumentation, in Apuzzo MJL (ed): *Brain Surgery: Complication Avoidance and Management*. New York, Churchill-Livingstone, 1993, vol 2, pp 1647–1670.
11. Rhoton AL Jr: General and micro-operative techniques, in Youmans JR (ed): *Neurological Surgery*. Philadelphia, W.B. Saunders Co., 1996, vol 1, pp 724–766.
12. Rhoton AL Jr: The cerebellopontine angle and posterior fossa cranial nerves by the retrosigmoid approach. **Neurosurgery** 47[Suppl 1]:S93–S129, 2000.
13. Rhoton AL Jr: Aneurysms. **Neurosurgery** 51[Suppl 1]:S1-121–S1-158, 2002.
14. Rhoton AL Jr: The anterior and middle cranial base. **Neurosurgery** 51[Suppl 1]:S1-273–S1-302, 2002.
15. Rhoton AL Jr: The cerebrum. **Neurosurgery** 51[Suppl 1]:S1-1–S1-51, 2002.
16. Rhoton AL Jr, Merz W: Suction tubes for conventional or microscopic neurosurgery. **Surg Neurol** 15:120–124, 1981.
17. Rhoton AL Jr, Hardy DG, Chambers SM: Microsurgical anatomy and dissection of the sphenoid bone, cavernous sinus and sellar region. **Surg Neurol** 12:63–104, 1979.
18. Yaşargil MG: Suturing techniques, in Yaşargil MG (ed): *Microsurgery Applied to Neurosurgery*. Stuttgart, Georg Thieme, 1969, pp 51–58.
19. Yaşargil MG, Vise WM, Bader DC: Technical adjuncts in neurosurgery. **Surg Neurol** 8:331–336, 1977.

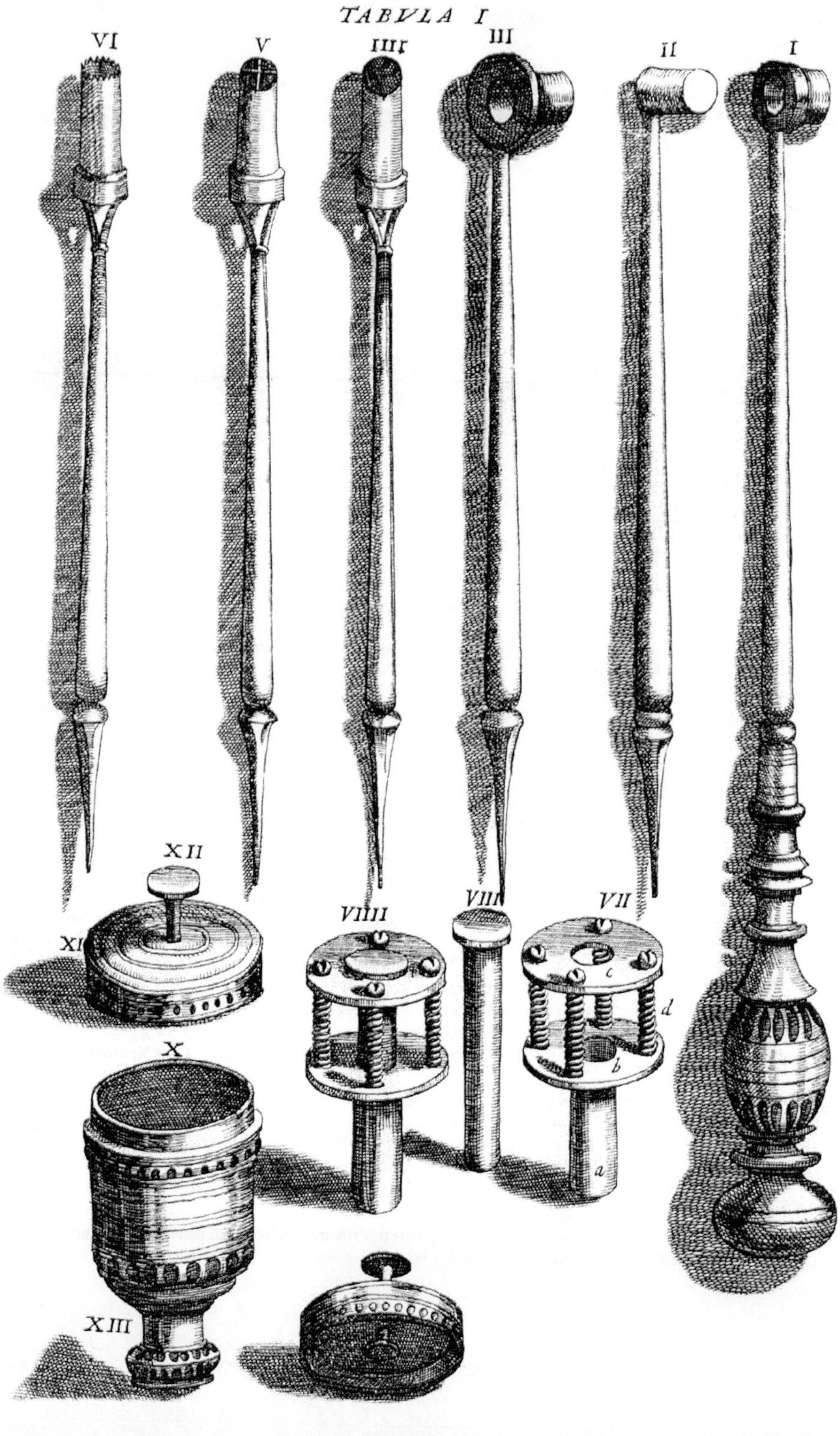

Surgical instruments as shown in Joannis Sculteti's Armamentarium Chirurgicum. . . . *This limited edition of 2500 copies was bound in half leather and Hahnemühle paper. From, Joannis Sculteti,* Armamentarium Chirurgicum XLII Tabulis Aeri Elegantissime Incisis. . . . *Ulm, B. Kühnen, 1655. Courtesy, Rare Book Room, Norris Medical Library, Keck School of Medicine, Los Angeles, California.*

PART 2

The Supratentorial Cranial Space: Microsurgical Anatomy & Surgical Approaches

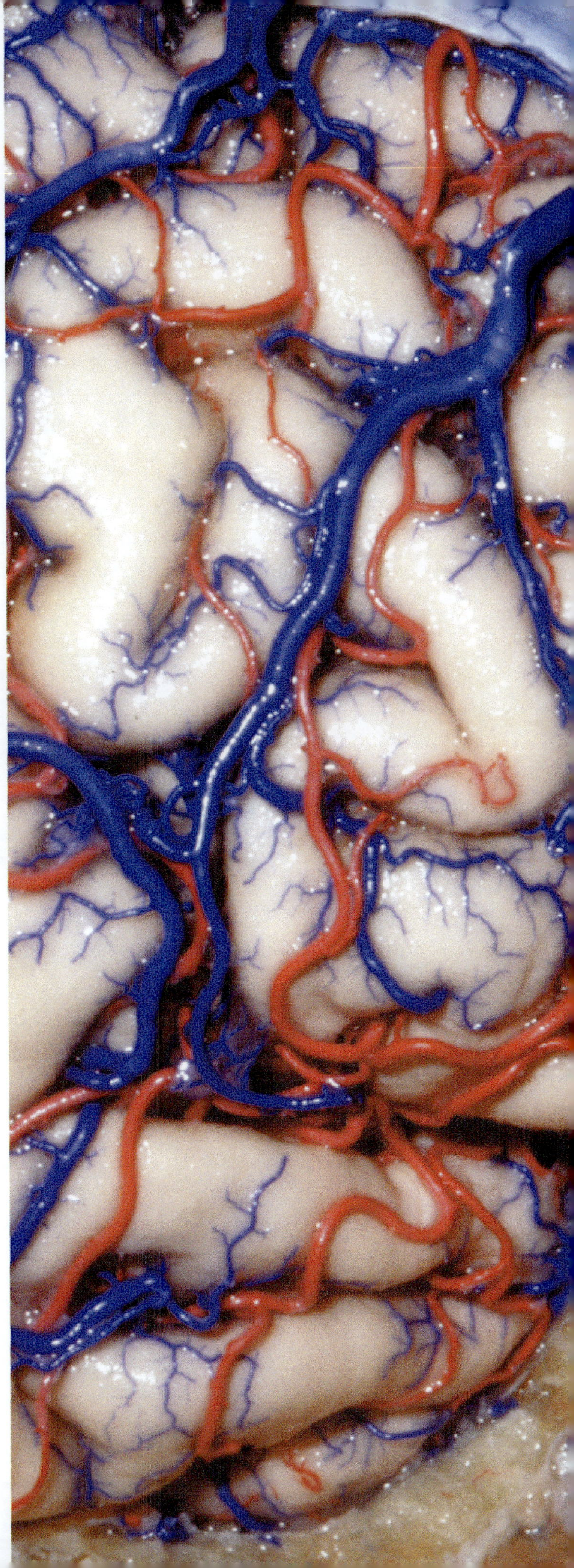

THE CEREBRUM

Albert L. Rhoton, Jr., M.D.
Department of Neurological Surgery, University of Florida, Gainesville, Florida

Correspondence:
Albert L. Rhoton, Jr., M.D., Department of Neurological Surgery, University of Florida, McKnight Brain Institute, P.O. Box 100265, 100 South Newell Drive, Building 59, L2-100, Gainesville, FL 32610-0265.
Email: rhoton@neurosurgery.ufl.edu

KEY WORDS: Basal ganglia, Cerebral hemispheres, Cerebrum, Craniotomy, Fiber dissections, Frontal lobe, Insula, Internal capsule, Lateral ventricles, Occipital lobe, Optic pathways, Parietal lobe, Sylvian fissure, Temporal lobe

The cerebrum is a remarkably beautiful and delicate structure (*Fig. 1.1*). The goal of the study of microsurgical anatomy is to perform gentle, precise, and accurate neurosurgery and to be able to navigate safely around and through the cerebrum and intracranial space. Essential to proceeding through the cranium and the brain's surface to the depths is an awareness of the site of the most valuable and vulnerable cortical and subcortical areas and the location of these eloquent areas in relation to the cranial and cerebral landmarks. This requires that the surgeon have a see-through x-ray-type microsurgical knowledge that visualizes deep structures in relation to the surface area exposed and weighs the value of tissue along each route to the targeted intracranial and intracerebral sites. The tentorium cerebelli, a dural projection, divides the intracranial space into supra- and infratentorial compartments. The posterior cranial fossa located below the tentorium in the infratentorial compartment was the subject of the Millennium issue of *Neurosurgery* (5). The supratentorial area and the anterior and middle cranial base are the focus of this issue.

In developing the concept of see-through x-ray-type knowledge of the supratentorial area, the location of selected deep structures are described in relation to the cranial and superficial cerebral landmarks. In numerous stepwise dissections, the author has tried not only to peel away and describe each layer, but also to clarify the relationships between structures in different layers (*Fig. 1.2*). One example is the relationship of the ventricles to the cerebral convexity. The frontal horn is located deep to the inferior frontal gyrus, the atrium is deep to the supramarginal gyrus, and the temporal horn is deep to the medial temporal gyrus. Another example is the relationship of the foramen of Monro to more superficial structures. At the cranial surface, the foramen of Monro is located deep to a point approximately 2 cm above the pterion, just behind the lower third of the coronal suture; at the cerebral surface, it is located deep to the central part of the pars opercularis of the inferior frontal gyrus; and at the insular level, it is located deep to the central part of the second short insular gyrus (*Fig. 1.2*). Many other relationships between superficial and deep structures are examined. In describing these relationships, the use of the terms superior, inferior, anterior, and posterior is the same as commonly applied in naming the cerebral gyri and sulci. The directional terms used are as follows: superior or above, situated toward the cranial vertex; inferior or below, situated toward the cranial base; anterior to or in front of, situated toward the frontal pole; and posterior or behind, situated toward the occipital pole.

THE HEMISPHERES

The paired cerebral hemispheres constitute the largest part of the brain. They are separated by the longitudinal fissure, interconnected by the corpus callosum, and merged with the diencephalon to establish continuity with the brainstem and the spinal cord. They encase the lateral and third ventricles. The cerebral hemispheres have three surfaces: lateral, medial, and basal; three margins: superior, inferior, and medial; three poles: frontal, temporal, and occipital; three types of white matter fibers: projection, commissural, and association; and five lobes: frontal, parietal, temporal, occipital, and the hidden insula. The most important landmarks for orienting surgery are the three borders, the three poles, the sylvian and interhemispheric fissures, and the central sulcus. The cerebral hemispheres have their greatest transverse diameter across the parietal lobes. The longitudinal fissure, the deep cleft separating the upper part of the paired hemispheres, contains a sickle-shaped process of dura called the falx cerebri that separates the anterior and posterior parts of the hemispheres (*Fig. 1.2*). The anterior portion of the falx cerebri is not as wide as its posterior part, leaving a wide space anteriorly between the free falx margin and the corpus callosum, where the medial surface of the hemispheres face each other and not the falx. Further posteriorly, the free margin slopes toward and becomes closely applied to the corpus callosum. The anterior part of the cingulate gyrus is below the free margin of the falx cerebri and is free to shift across the midline, whereas the middle and posterior parts have progressively less of the gyrus below and more above the free margin, where its displacement across the midline is limited by the rigidity of the falx (4). The shifts related to the tentorial incisura were reviewed in the Millennium issue of *Neurosurgery* (6).

Hemispheric Surfaces

The cerebral hemispheres have three surfaces: lateral, medial, and basal (*Fig. 1.3*). The lateral surface, referred to as the

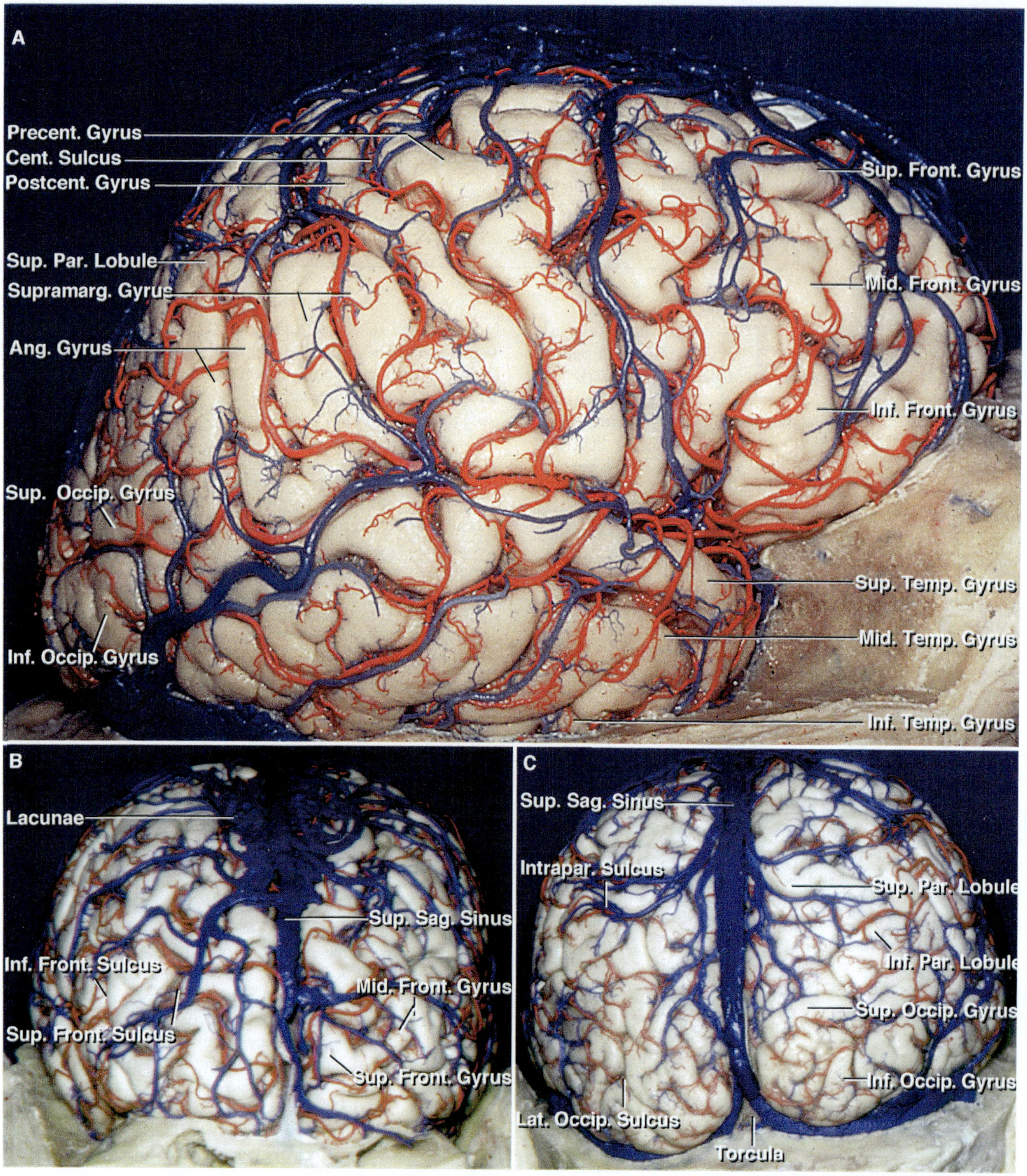

FIGURE 1.1. *Lateral view of the right cerebral hemisphere. A, the brain, when exposed carefully and accurately, is a remarkably beautiful structure. The arteries, veins, gyri, and sulci are organized in a complex array. The frontal convexity is made up of the superior, middle, and inferior frontal and precentral gyri. The parietal convexity is composed of the postcentral gyrus and the superior and inferior parietal lobules. The inferior parietal lobule is made up of the supramarginal and angular gyrus. The temporal convexity is composed of the superior, middle, and inferior temporal gyri. The occipital convexity is formed by the superior and inferior occipital gyri. B, anterior view. The superior and middle frontal gyri are separated by the superior frontal sulcus. The inferior frontal sulcus courses between the middle and inferior frontal gyri.*

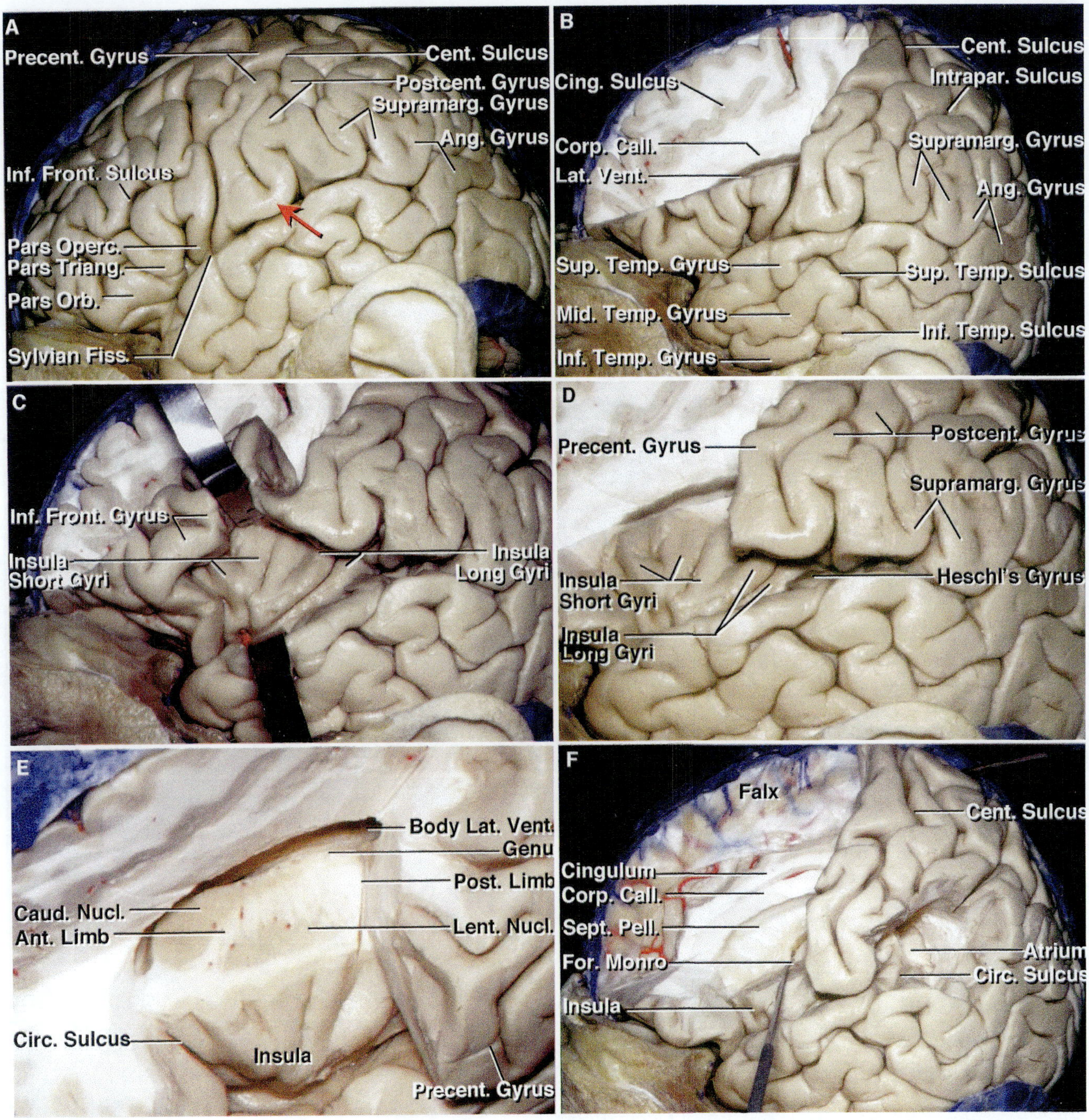

FIGURE 1.2. *Stepwise dissection of the left cerebral hemisphere. A, the inferior frontal gyrus is composed of the pars orbitalis, pars opercularis, and pars triangularis. The precentral gyrus borders the sylvian fissure behind the pars opercularis. The sylvian fissure extends* (Legend continues on next page.)

The veins from the anterior part of the hemisphere are directed backward to reach the superior sagittal sinus. A large venous lacunae extends over the superior margin of the frontal lobe adjacent to the superior sagittal sinus. C, posterior view of the hemisphere. The lateral occipital sulcus divides the lateral aspect of the occipital lobe into the superior and inferior occipital gyri. The veins from the occipital convexity are directed forward to enter the superior sagittal sinus. The posterior part of the parietal lobe is divided by the intraparietal sulcus into the superior and inferior parietal lobules. Ang., *angular;* Cent., *central;* Front., *frontal;* Inf., *inferior;* Intrapar., *intraparietal;* Lat., *lateral;* Mid., *middle;* Occip., *occipital;* Par., *parietal;* Postcent., *postcentral;* Precent., *precentral;* Sag., *sagittal;* Sup., *superior;* Supramarg., *supramarginal;* Temp., *temporal.*

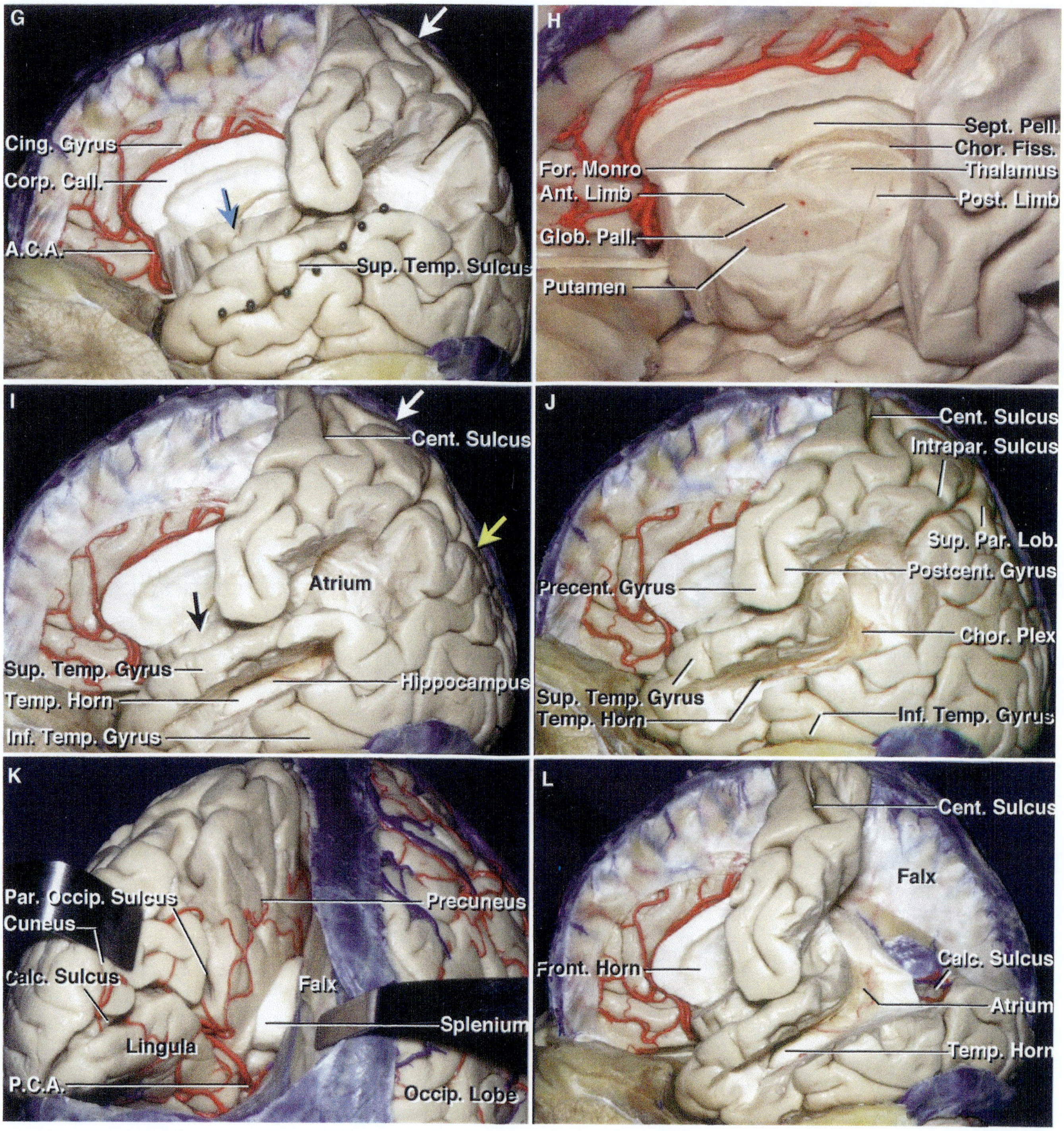

FIGURE 1.2. *Continued*
backward and turns up into the supramarginal gyrus at its posterior end. The lower part of the postcentral gyrus is positioned in front of the anterior bank of the supramarginal gyrus. The posterior bank of the supramarginal gyrus is continuous with the superior temporal gyrus. The central sulcus ascends between the pre- and postcentral gyri. There is commonly a gyral bridge (red arrow) connecting the pre- and postcentral gyri below the lower end of the central sulcus, so that the central sulcus does not open directly into the sylvian fissure. Often, with the limited craniotomy opening, the whole sylvian fissure is not exposed to aid in identification of the pre- and postcentral gyri and the central sulcus. The position of the lower end of the pre- and postcentral gyri can be approximated by identifying the pars opercularis just in front of the precentral gyrus and the anterior bank of the supramarginal gyrus just in back of the postcentral sulcus. The angular gyrus wraps around the upturned posterior end of the superior temporal sulcus. B, *the part of the frontal lobe above the inferior frontal gyrus and in front of the precentral sulcus has been removed while preserving a thin layer of the medial part of the hemisphere. The inferior frontal sulcus is located on the convexity at the deep level of the lower margin of the corpus callosum and roof of the frontal horn.*

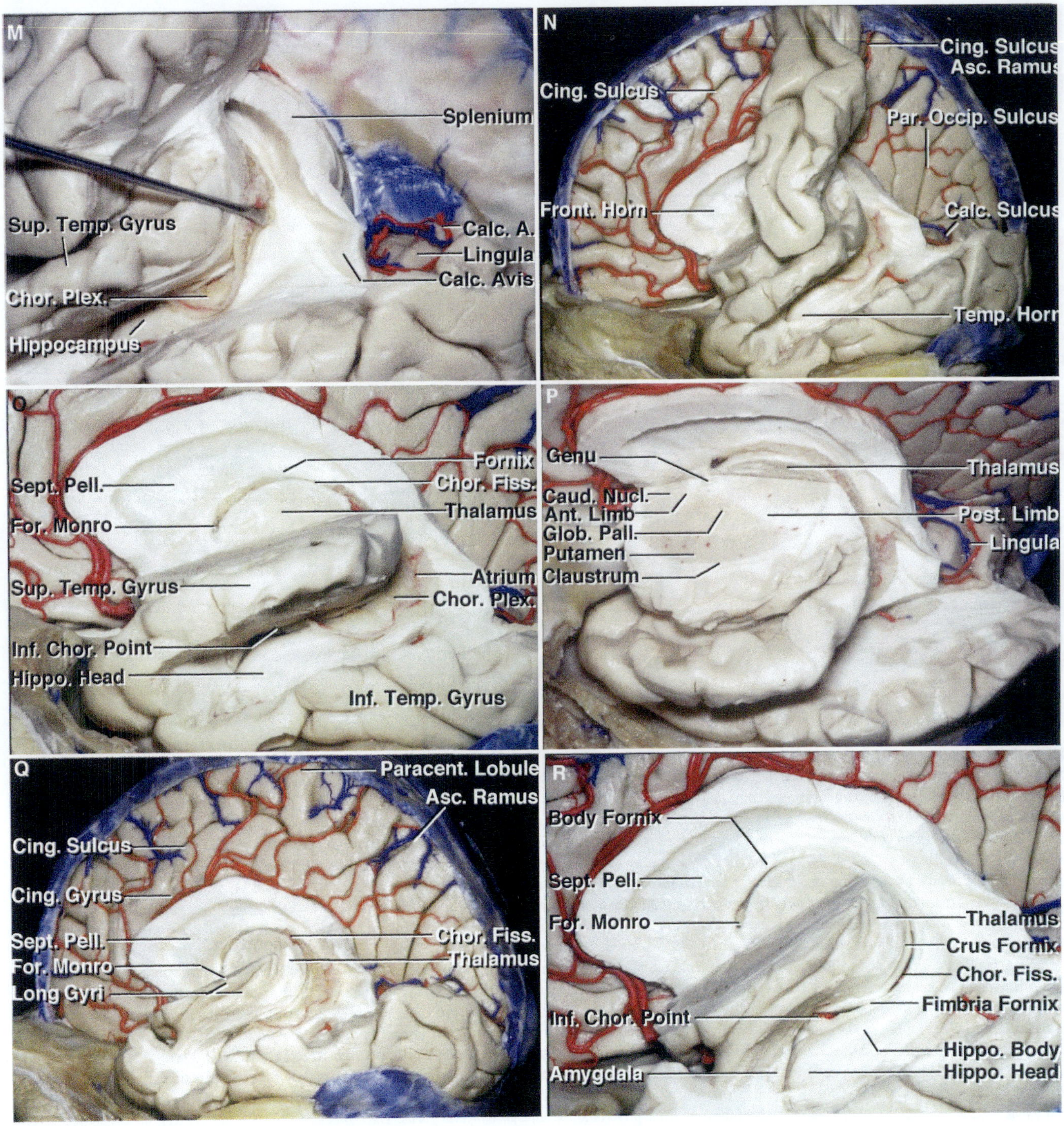

FIGURE 1.2. *Continued*

The gray matter of the cingulate sulcus is exposed above the corpus callosum. C, the opercular lips have been retracted to expose the insula, which is defined at its outer margin by the circular or limiting sulcus. The short gyri are located anteriorly and the long gyri posteriorly. D, enlarged view with the brain in front of the precentral gyrus removed. The insular gyri radiate upward and backward from the anteroinferior angle situated just lateral to the limen insulae. The short gyri are located deep to the pars triangularis and opercularis. Heschl's gyrus, the most anterior of the transverse temporal gyri, faces the lower end of the postcentral gyrus across the sylvian fissure. E, anterosuperior view of the central core of the hemisphere located deep to the insulae. The lentiform nucleus is exposed deep to the insula and is separated from the caudate nucleus by the anterior limb of the internal capsule. The circular sulcus surrounds the insula. F, the supramarginal gyrus has been removed to show its location superficial to the atrium. The posterior margins of the insula and circular sulcus are positioned superficial to the anterior edge of the atrium. The pre- and postcentral gyri are located lateral to the body of the ventricle and the splenium of the corpus callosum. The foramen of Monro is located deep to a point on the pars opercularis approximately 1 cm above the sylvian fissure and deep to the midlevel of the short gyri of the insula. *(Legend continues on next page.)*

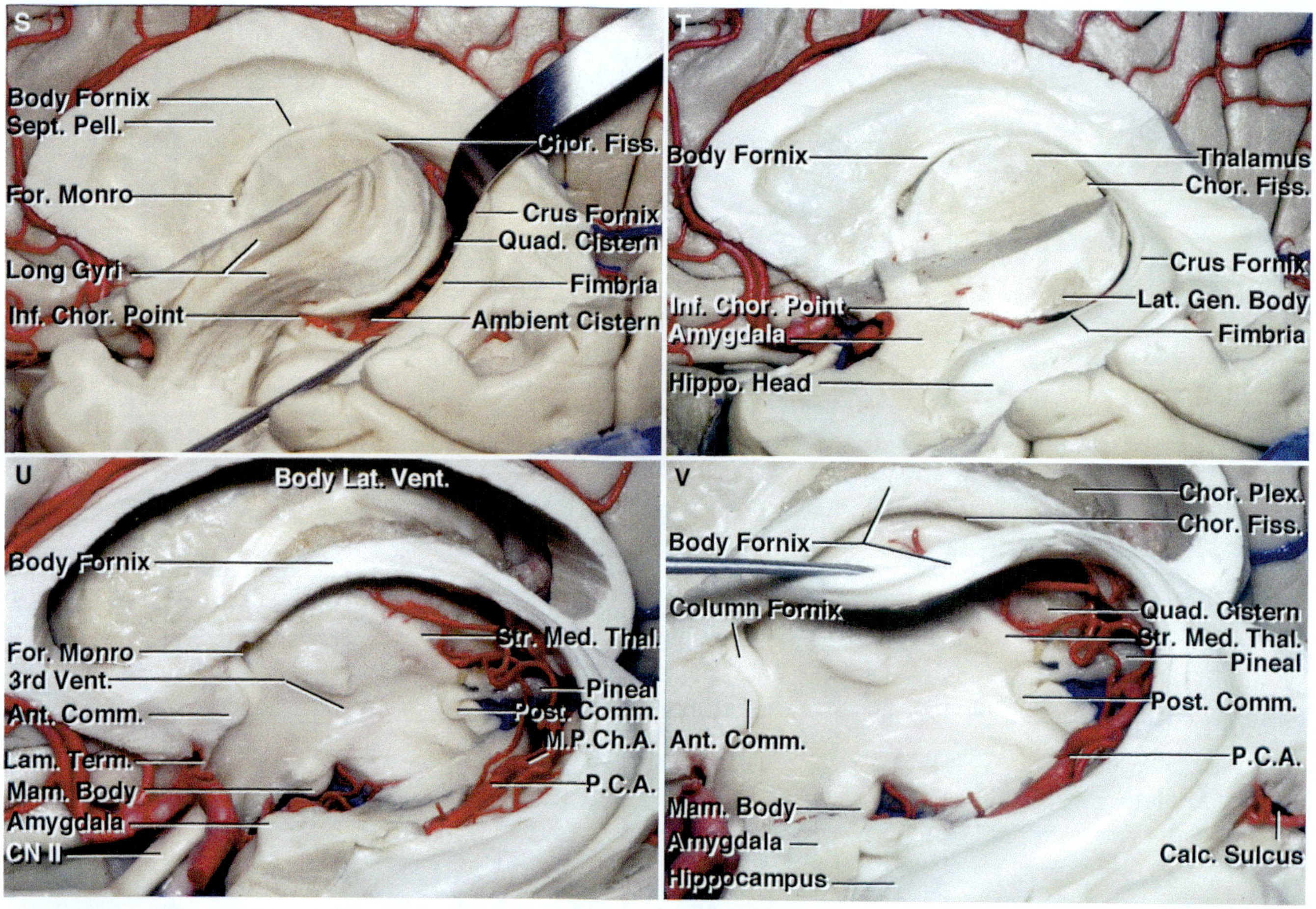

FIGURE 1.2. *Continued*

G, colored pins *have been placed along a line that corresponds to the lower margin of the insula, which is located deep to the superior temporal sulcus. A* blue arrow *has been placed on the foramen of Monro, which is located deep to the central part of the insula. The* white arrow *is located at the site where the upper end of the ascending ramus of the cingulate sulcus reaches the superior hemispheric border. The ascending ramus courses on the medial surface along the posterior margin of the paracentral lobule. H, the anterior limb of the internal capsule is located between the lentiform nucleus, formed by the putamen and globus pallidus, and the caudate nucleus. The posterior limb is located between the thalamus and lentiform nucleus. The genu of the internal capsule is located just lateral to the foramen of Monro. The choroidal fissure, along which the choroid plexus is attached, is situated between the fornix and thalamus. I, the temporal horn and hippocampus are located medial to the middle temporal gyrus, a segment of which has been removed. The hippocampus sits in the floor of the temporal horn. The atrium is deep to the supramarginal gyrus. The* black arrow *is on the foramen of Monro. The* white arrow *is located where the upper end of the ascending ramus of the cingulate sulcus reaches the superior hemispheric border. The* yellow arrow *is where the upper end of the parieto-occipital sulcus reaches the superior border. J, the remaining bridge of the superior temporal gyrus located superficial to the junction of the atrium and temporal horn has been removed. K, posterior view of the left hemisphere. The splenium is located deep in the interhemispheric fissure. The parieto-occipital and calcarine sulcus converge behind the splenium to give the medial surface a Y-shaped configuration. The parieto-occipital sulcus separates the precuneus and cuneus, and the calcarine sulcus separates the cuneus and lingula. L, the parietal lobe, above the level of the calcarine sulcus, has been removed. The upper lip of the calcarine sulcus, formed by the cuneus, has been removed to expose the lingula that forms the lower bank of the calcarine sulcus. The calcar avis is a prominence in the lower part of the medial atrial wall overlying the calcarine sulcus. M, the glomus of the choroid plexus has been reflected forward to expose the medial wall of the atrium. The lingula that forms the lower bank of the calcarine sulcus has been preserved. The calcar avis overlies the deep end of the calcarine sulcus. N, the falx has been removed to expose the medial part of the right hemisphere. The ascending ramus of the cingulate sulcus reaches the superior border of the hemisphere behind the paracentral lobule. O, the pre- and postcentral gyri have been removed while preserving the superior temporal gyrus. The choroidal fissure, the cleft between the thalamus and fornix, extends from the foramen of Monro through the body, atrium, and temporal horn to the inferior choroidal point located just behind the head of the hippocampus. P, superolateral view of the cross section of the central area of the hemisphere, positioned between the insula laterally and the ventricles medially. The central core of the hemisphere, the area between the insula laterally and the ventricles in the midline, includes the caudate and lentiform nucleus, thalamus, and anterior and posterior limbs and genu of the internal capsule. The claustrum is positioned between the insular cortex and the lentiform nucleus. Q, the superior temporal gyrus has been removed while preserving the long gyri of the insula. The ascending ramus of the cingulate sulcus marks the posterior edge of the paracentral lobule, the extension of the pre- and postcentral gyri onto the medial surface of the hemisphere. R, enlarged view of the choroidal fissure. The choroidal fissure extends from the foramen of Monro to the inferior choroidal point located behind the head of the hippocampus. The choroid plexus, which attaches along the choroidal fissure, has been removed. The outer edge of the choroidal fissure is formed by the body of the fornix in the body of the ventricle, the crus of the fornix in the atrium, and the fimbria of the fornix in the temporal horn. S, a* retractor *has been placed between the thalamus and the crus of the fornix to open the choroidal fissure. Opening the choroidal fissure in the body of the ventricle exposes the third ventricle.*

convexity, faces the cranial cap laterally. The medial surface of the frontal, parietal, and occipital lobes faces the falx cerebri medially, and the medial surface of the temporal lobe faces the lateral aspect of the midbrain. The basal surface faces the floor of the anterior and middle cranial fossae and the tentorium. The three borders separate the three cerebral surfaces. The superior border follows along the course of the superior sagittal sinus and upper edge of the interhemispheric fissure from the frontal to the occipital pole and separates the lateral convexity from the medial surface. The lateral border has anterior and posterior parts. The anterior part extends from the frontal pole along the lateral border of the basal surface of the frontal lobe to the sylvian fissure and separates the lateral and orbital surfaces of the frontal lobe. The posterior part of the lateral border has a gentle upward convexity that extends along and conforms with the lateral edge of the middle fossa floor and tentorium, and anteriorly turns upward around the temporal pole to reach the sylvian fissure. It separates the lateral surface of the temporal and occipital lobes from the basal surface that rests on the cranial base and tentorium. The medial border extends from the frontal to the occipital pole and has frontal and occipital parts. The frontal part extends in a straight line from the frontal pole to the lamina terminalis and separates the medial from the orbital surface of the frontal lobe. The occipital part of the medial border lies in the angle between the falx cerebri and tentorium cerebelli and extends parallel to the straight sinus from the occipital pole to just below the splenium of the corpus callosum, separating the medial and basal surfaces of the occipital lobe.

The frontal, occipital, and temporal lobes expand to all three cerebral surfaces (*Fig. 1.3*). The parietal lobe borders only two surfaces, the lateral and medial. The frontal lobe includes approximately a third of the hemispheric surface. It extends from the frontal pole to the central sulcus and is separated from the temporal lobe by the sylvian fissure. On the medial surface, the frontal lobe is separated from the corpus callosum by the callosal sulcus and from the parietal lobe by a line extending downward from the upper end of the central sulcus to the corpus callosum. The entire surface facing the orbital roof and referred to as the orbital surface belongs to the frontal lobe. The lateral surface of the parietal lobe is bounded anteriorly by the central sulcus, posteriorly by the upper half of the parietotemporal line that runs from the impression of the upper end of the parieto-occipital sulcus on the lateral surface to the preoccipital notch, and inferiorly by the posterior end of the sylvian fissure and the extended sylvian line that extends backward along the long axis of the sylvian fissure to the lateral parietotemporal line. On the medial surface, the boundary between the frontal and parietal lobes is a line extending downward from the upper end of the central sulcus to the corpus callosum. Between the parietal and occipital lobes is the parieto-occipital sulcus. The occipital lobe lies behind the parietotemporal line on the lateral surface and the parieto-occipital sulcus on the medial surface. On the basal surface, the occipital lobe is situated behind the lines extending from the junction of the calcarine and parieto-occipital sulci medially to the preoccipital notch laterally.

Boundaries and Surfaces of the Lobes

The frontal lobe presents four surfaces: three formed by a part of the lateral, medial, and basal cerebral surfaces, and a fourth sylvian surface facing the deep compartments of the sylvian fissure (*Fig. 1.3*). That latter surface, with the sylvian surface of the parietal lobe, forms the roof of the deep part of the sylvian fissure and faces the sylvian surface of the temporal lobe and the insula that form the floor and medial wall of the deep sylvian compartments. The temporal lobe also has four surfaces: larger lateral and basal surfaces, a smaller medial surface facing the brainstem, and a sylvian surface. The medial surface of the temporal lobe is formed by the part of the uncus, parahippocampal, and dentate gyri facing the midbrain. The upper surface of the temporal lobe forms the floor of the deep sylvian compartments and faces the sylvian surface of the frontal and parietal lobes and the insula. The parietal lobe has three surfaces: lateral, medial, and a sylvian surface that faces the sylvian surface of the temporal lobe and

Opening the choroidal fissure between the pulvinar and crus of the fornix exposes the quadrigeminal cistern, and opening the fissure between the lower surface of the thalamus and the fimbria of the fornix exposes the ambient cistern. T, the remaining insula has been removed to expose the thalamus forming the inner rim of the choroidal fissure. The lateral geniculate body is exposed at the lower margin of the thalamus. The optic radiations pass laterally above the hippocampus in the roof of the temporal horn and posteriorly around the lateral margin at the atrium to reach the calcarine sulcus. The anterior wall of the temporal horn is formed by the amygdala, which tilts backward above, but is separated from the hippocampal head by the temporal horn. U, the thalamus has been removed to expose the third ventricle. The body, crus, and fimbria of the fornix, forming the outer margin of the choroidal fissure, have been preserved. Opening the choroidal fissure in front of the crus of the fornix exposes the pineal region and quadrigeminal cistern. Opening the choroidal fissure adjacent to the body of the fornix exposes the third ventricle. Opening the choroidal fissure in the temporal horn exposes the ambient cistern and posterior cerebral arteries. The medial posterior choroidal arteries are exposed in the quadrigeminal cistern. The striae medullaris thalami marks the lower edge of the velum interpositum, in which the internal cerebral veins course. V, the left half of the body of the fornix has been folded downward to expose the right half of the body and medial aspect of the contralateral choroidal fissure located between the body of the fornix and the upper surface of the thalamus. The pineal gland and posterior commissure are exposed at the posterior margin and the anterior commissure and columns of the fornix are exposed at the anterior margin of the third ventricle. A., *artery;* A.C.A., *anterior cerebral artery;* Ang., *angular;* Ant., *anterior;* Asc., *ascending;* Calc., *calcar, calcarine;* Call., *callosum;* Caud., *caudate;* Cent., *central;* Chor., *choroid, choroidal;* Cing., *cingulate;* Circ., *circular;* CN, *cranial nerve;* Comm., *commissure;* Corp., *corpus;* Fiss., *fissure;* For., *foramen;* Front., *frontal;* Gen., *geniculate;* Glob., *globus;* Hippo., *hippocampal;* Inf., *inferior;* Intrapar., *intraparietal;* Lam., *lamina;* Lat., *lateral;* Lent., *lenticular, lentiform;* Lob., *lobule;* M.P.Ch.A., *medial posterior choroidal artery;* Mam., *mamillary;* Med., *medullaris;* Mid., *middle;* Nucl., *nucleus;* Occip., *occipital;* Operc., *opercularis;* Orb., *orbitalis;* P.C.A., *posterior cerebral artery;* Pall., *pallidus;* Par., *parietal;* Paracent., *paracentral;* Par. Occip., *parieto-occipital;* Pell., *pellucidum;* Plex., *plexus;* Post., *posterior;* Postcent., *postcentral;* Precent., *precentral;* Quad., *quadrigeminal;* Sept., *septum;* Str., *striae;* Sup., *superior;* Supramarg., *supramarginal;* Temp., *temporal;* Term., *terminalis;* Thal., *thalamic, thalamus;* Triang., *triangularis;* Vent., *ventricle.*

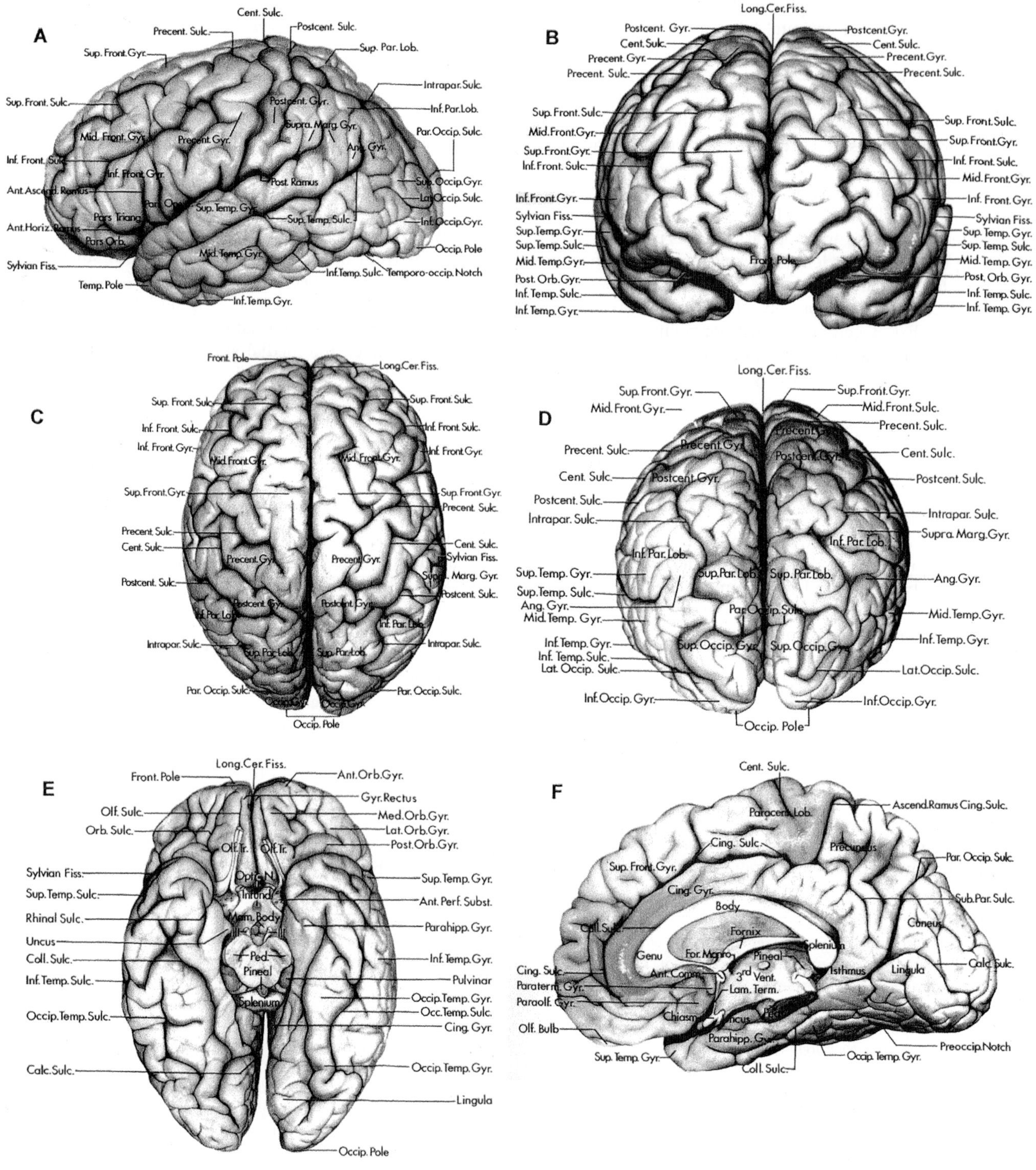

FIGURE 1.3. *Lateral, medial, and inferior surfaces of the cerebral hemispheres.* A–D, *lateral surface* (A, *lateral view;* B, *anterior view;* C, *superior view;* D, *posterior view).* E, *inferior surface.* F, *medial surface.* A–F, *the longitudinal cerebral fissure separates the cerebral hemispheres. The lateral surface of the frontal lobe extends from the frontal pole to the central sulcus and is demarcated inferiorly by the sylvian fissure. The precentral gyrus is situated between the central and precentral sulcus. The superior and inferior frontal sulci divide the part of the lateral surface in front of the precentral gyrus into the superior, middle, and inferior frontal gyri. The inferior frontal gyrus is divided by the anterior horizontal and the anterior ascending rami of the sylvian fissure into the pars orbitalis, pars triangularis, and pars opercularis. The parietal lobe is demarcated anteriorly by the central sulcus and posteriorly by a line extending from the superior limit of the parieto-occipital sulcus to the preoccipital notch. The anterior part of the parietal lobe is formed by the postcentral gyrus, which is situated between the central and postcentral sulci.*

the insula. The occipital lobe has three surfaces: lateral, medial, and basal, all formed by parts of the cerebral surfaces.

Sulci and Gyri

Although differences in the gyri and sulci can be identified between any two hemispheres, close inspection reveals a basic arrangement within which variations exist. The differences in the course and pattern of the sulci and gyri exist not only from person to person, but also between the hemispheres of the same brain. The greatest variability can be seen in the frontal and parieto-occipital regions (3). Commonly, the major sulci are discontinuous or have small side branches that create a significant variation in the shape and pattern of the gyri. Ono et al. (3) have classified the cerebral sulci into three groups based on their degree of continuity: the first group are those that are commonly continuous or uninterrupted; the second group are those that have low interruption rates; and the third group are those that are regularly interrupted. In our studies, the sulci that were uniformly continuous, not broken into several segments by gyral bridges crossing the sulcus, were the sylvian fissure and the callosal and parieto-occipital sulci. Another group that has a high, but not 100%, rate of continuity are the central, collateral, and calcarine sulci. Those sulci that are less commonly but still regularly interrupted are the postcentral, superior, and inferior frontal, superior temporal, cingulate, occipitotemporal, and the intraparietal sulci. Those that are usually interrupted by gyral bridges that break up their continuity are the precentral and inferior temporal sulci.

SYLVIAN FISSURE

The sylvian fissure and central sulcus are the most important landmarks on the lateral surface. The sylvian fissure is the most distinct and consistent landmark on the lateral surface. It is a complex fissure that carries the middle cerebral artery and its branches and provides a surgical gateway connecting the cerebral surface to the anterior part of the basal surface and cranial base (1).

The sylvian fissure is not a simple longitudinal cleft as its name implies (*Fig. 1.4*). It crosses both the basal and lateral cerebral surface and has a superficial and a deep part. The superficial part is visible on the surface of the brain and the deep part, often referred to as the sylvian cistern, is hidden below the basal surface. The superficial part has a stem and three rami; the stem begins medially at the anterior clinoid process and extends laterally along the sphenoid ridge between the junction of the frontal and temporal lobes to the pterion, where the stem divides into anterior horizontal, anterior ascending, and the posterior rami. The posterior ramus, the longest, represents the posterior continuation of the fissure. It is directed backward and upward, separating the frontal and parietal lobes above from the temporal lobe below. Its posterior end turns more sharply upward to terminate in the inferior parietal lobule, where the supramarginal gyrus wraps around its upturned posterior end.

The deep part of the sylvian fissure, hidden below the surface, is referred to as the sylvian cistern. It is more complex than the superficial part and is divided into sphenoidal and operculoinsular compartments. The sphenoidal compartment extends laterally from the cistern around the internal carotid artery, between the frontal and temporal lobes. The roof of the sphenoidal compartment is formed by the posterior part of the orbital surface of the frontal lobe and the anterior perforated substance. The caudate and lentiform nuclei and the anterior limb of the internal capsule are located above the roof. The floor is formed by the anterior part of the planum polare, an area free of gyri on the upper temporal pole, where a shallow cupped trench accommo-

The area behind the postcentral sulcus is divided by the intraparietal sulcus into the superior and inferior parietal lobules. The inferior parietal lobule includes the supramarginal gyrus, which surrounds the upturned end of the posterior ramus of the sylvian fissure, and the angular gyrus, which surrounds the upturned posterior end of the superior temporal sulcus. The lateral occipital sulcus divides the lateral aspect of the occipital lobe into the superior and inferior occipital gyri. The lateral surface of the temporal lobe behind the temporal pole is divided into the superior, middle, and inferior temporal gyri by the superior and inferior temporal sulci. The inferior surface of the frontal lobe is formed by the gyrus rectus and the orbital gyri. The olfactory tract courses in the olfactory sulcus, which separates the gyrus rectus from the orbital gyri. The orbital sulci divide the orbital surface of the frontal lobe into the anterior, medial, lateral, and posterior orbital gyri. The inferior surface of the temporal lobe, proceeding from medial to lateral, is formed by the parahippocampal, occipitotemporal, and inferior temporal gyri. The occipitotemporal sulcus separates the occipitotemporal and inferior temporal gyri. The collateral and rhinal sulci separate the parahippocampal and occipitotemporal gyri. A narrow strip of cortex at the posterior end of the parahippocampal gyrus, called the isthmus of the cingulate gyrus, wraps around the splenium of the corpus callosum and connects the posterior ends of the parahippocampal and cingulate gyri. On the medial surface of the hemisphere, the callosal sulcus separates the corpus callosum from the cingulate gyrus. The cingulate sulcus separates the cingulate gyrus from the superior frontal gyrus. The ascending ramus of the cingulate sulcus ascends along the posterior margin of the paracentral lobule. The subparietal sulcus separates the precuneus and the cingulate gyrus. The parieto-occipital sulcus separates the precuneus and the cuneus. The calcarine sulcus extends forward from the occipital pole and divides the medial surface of the occipital lobe between the cuneus and lingula. The paraterminal and paraolfactory gyri are situated below the corpus callosum in front of the lamina terminalis and anterior commissure. The inferior surface of the occipital lobe is formed by the lower part of the lingula and inferior occipital gyrus and the posterior part of the occipitotemporal gyrus. The mamillary bodies and infundibulum are in the floor of the third ventricle below the foramen of Monro. The oculomotor nerves arise on the medial surface of the cerebral peduncles. The optic nerves are situated at the medial ends of the sylvian fissures. Ang., *angular;* Ant., *anterior;* Ascend., *ascending;* Calc., *calcarine;* Cent., *central;* Cer., *cerebral;* Cing., *cingulate;* Coll., *collateral;* Comm., *commissure;* Fiss., *fissure;* For., *foramen;* Front., *frontal;* Gyr., *Gyrus;* Horiz., *horizontal;* Inf., *inferior;* Infund., *infundibulum;* Intrapar., *intraparietal;* Lam., *lamina;* Lat., *lateral;* Lob., *lobule;* Long., *longitudinal;* Mam., *mamillary;* Marg., *marginal;* Med., *medial;* Mid., *middle;* N., *nerve;* Occip., *occipital;* Olf., *olfactory;* Operc., *opercularis;* Orb., *orbital, orbitalis;* Par., *parietal;* Par. Occip., *parieto-occipital;* Paracent., *paracentral;* Parahipp., *parahippocampal;* Paraolf., *paraolfactory;* Paraterm., *paraterminal;* Ped., *peduncle;* Perf., *perforated;* Post., *posterior;* Postcent., *postcentral;* Precent., *precentral;* Preoccip., *preoccipital;* Sub. Par., *subparietal;* Subst., *substance;* Sulc., *sulcus;* Sup., *superior;* Supra. Marg., *supramarginal;* Temp., *temporal;* Temporo-occip., *temporo-occipital;* Term., *terminalis;* Tr., *tract;* Triang., *triangularis;* Vent., *ventricle.*

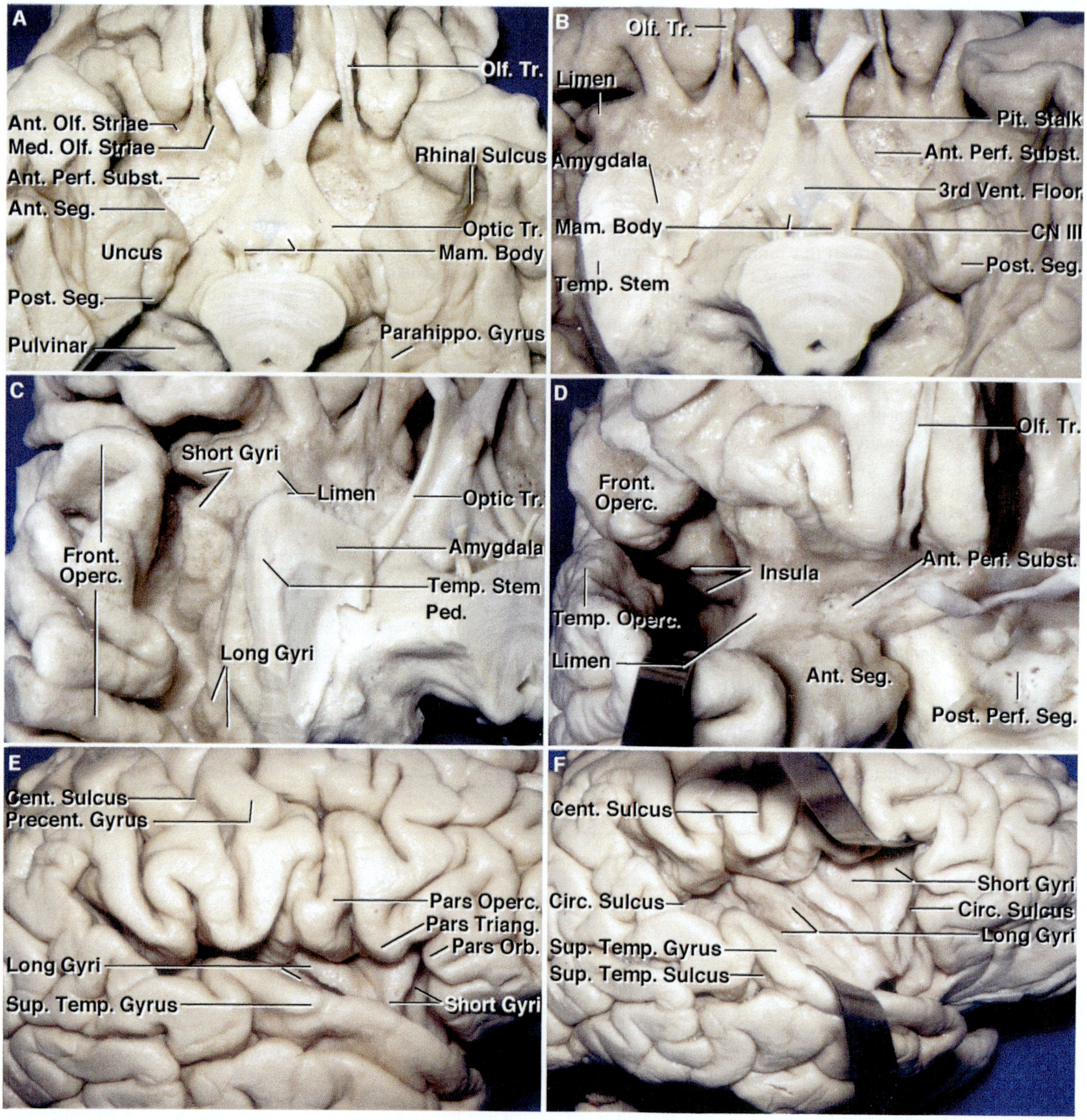

FIGURE 1.4. *Anterior perforated substance and sylvian fissure.* A, *inferior view. The anterior perforated substance forms of the roof of the sphenoidal compartment of the sylvian fissure. It extends from the olfactory striae anteriorly to the optic tract and stem of the temporal lobe posteriorly. On the medial side, it extends to the interhemispheric fissure and laterally to the limen insula. The anterior uncal segment faces the anterior perforated substance. The posterior segment faces the cerebral peduncle.* B, *the right temporal pole has been removed down to the level of the stem of the temporal lobe that forms the posterolateral margin of the anterior perforated substance. The limen insula is situated at the lateral margin of the anterior perforated substance anterior to the stem of the temporal lobe. On the left side, the lower part of the posterior uncal segment has been removed to expose the upper part formed largely by the hippocampal head. The anterior perforated substance has a salt-and-pepper appearance, created by small openings through which the perforating arteries and veins penetrate the hemisphere. The area where a third ventriculostomy is performed is located in front of the mamillary bodies.* C, *the view has been directed lateral to the limen to the insula and frontal operculum. The lower ends of the short and long gyri of the insula are exposed lateral to the stem of the temporal lobe and medial to the gyri on the frontal operculum.* D, *anterior view with the lips of the opening into the operculoinsular component of the sylvian fissure retracted. The sylvian fissure, lateral to the limen, extends backward and upward, and between the insula medially and the frontal and temporal opercula laterally.*

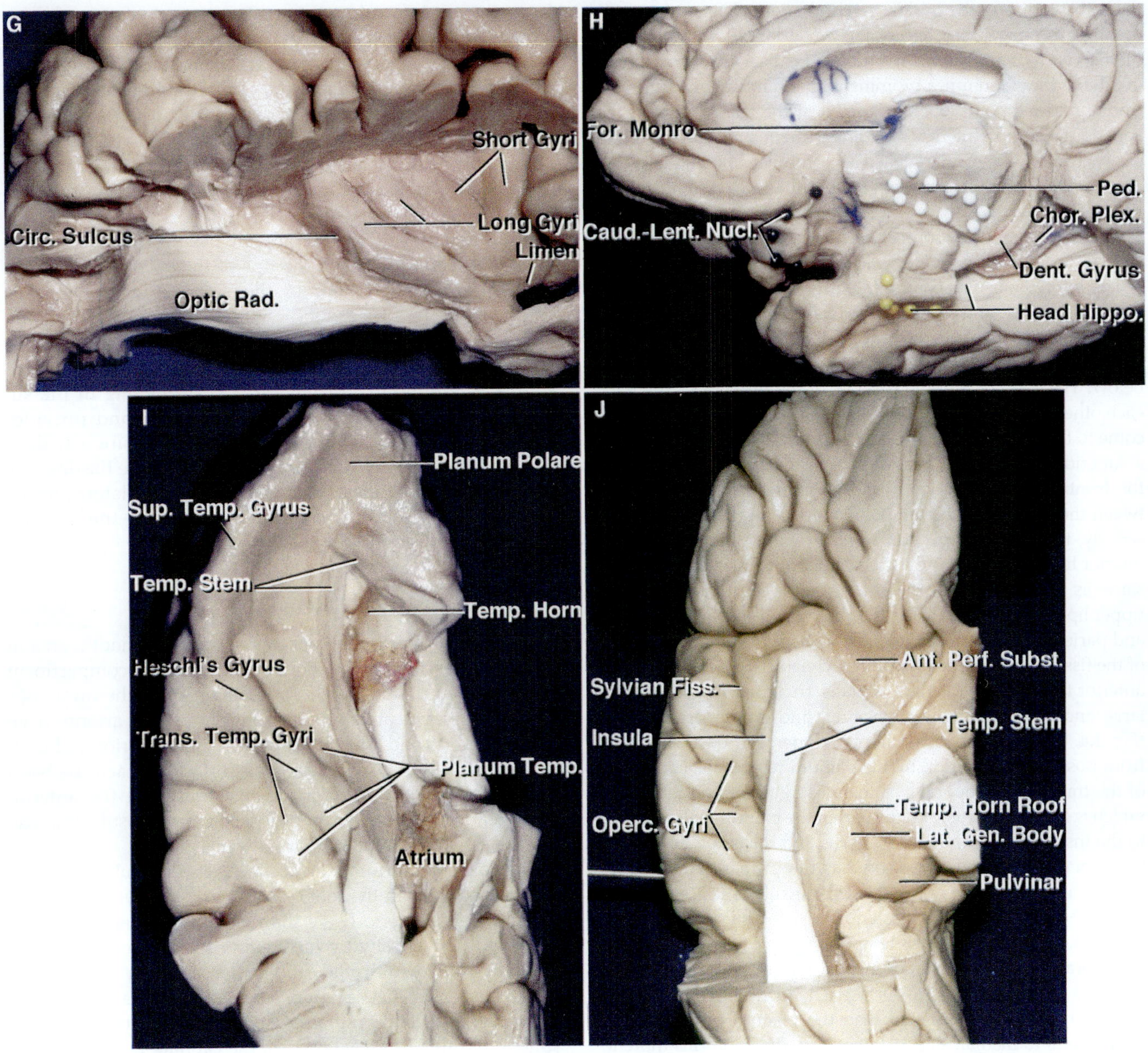

FIGURE 1.4. *Continued*

The posterior perforated substance is located between the cerebral peduncles. E, lateral view of the right hemisphere. In this hemisphere, the frontal and parietal opercula do not meet the temporal operculum, thus exposing the inferior part of the long and short gyri of the insula. F, the opercular lips have been retracted to expose the long and short gyri of the insula and the circular sulcus at the outer insular border. G, the temporal lobe has been removed and the optic radiations preserved. The lower margin of the insula is located superficially at approximately the deep level of the lateral geniculate body. The fibers of the optic radiation pass through the stem of the temporal lobe on their way back to the calcarine sulcus. H, inferomedial view of the basal frontal and medial temporal lobes. The white dots *outline the fibers descending to form the cerebral peduncle.* Black pins *outline the deep position of the caudate and lentiform nuclei above the anterior perforated substance and basal surface of the frontal lobe. The* yellow pins *outline the anterior margin of the head of the hippocampus. The posterior part of the head of the hippocampus has been exposed by removing the medial part of the parahippocampal gyrus. I, superior view of the upper surface of the temporal lobe that forms the floor of the sylvian fissure. The transverse temporal gyri, the most anterior of which is Heschl's auditory projection area, form the posterior part of the upper surface of the temporal lobe, called the planum temporale. The anterior part of the upper surface, called the planum polare, is free of gyri and has a shallow trough to accommodate the course of the middle cerebral artery. The lateral edge of the planum polare is formed by the superior temporal gyrus. The stem of the temporal lobe, the relatively thin layer of white and gray matter that connects the temporal lobe to the lower insula, is positioned above the lateral and anterior edge of the temporal horn. J, inferior view of the frontoparietal operculum. The gyri on the lateral surface extend around the lower border of the frontal and parietal lobes to form the upper lip of the sylvian fissure. The optic radiations pass laterally from the lateral geniculate body and course in the roof of the temporal horn along the temporal stem and lateral to the atrium to reach the calcarine sulcus on the medial aspect of the occipital lobe.* Ant., *anterior;* Caud., *caudate;* Cent., *(Legend continues on next page.)*

dates the course of the middle cerebral artery. The anterior segment of the uncus, the site of the amygdala, is located at the medial part of the floor. The limen insulae, the prominence overlying the cingulum, a prominent fiber bundle connecting the frontal and temporal lobes, is located at the lateral edge of the sphenoidal compartment. This compartment communicates medially through the sylvian vallecula, a tubular opening between the medial end of the opposing temporal and frontal lips of the fissure, through which the middle cerebral artery passes and provides a communication between the sylvian fissure and the cisterns around the optic nerve and carotid artery.

The operculoinsular compartment is formed by two narrow clefts: opercular and insular (*Fig. 1.4*). The opercular cleft is situated where the sylvian surfaces of the frontal lobe, and the parietal lobes above, face the sylvian surface of the temporal lobe below. The deep part of the surfaces of the three lobes that face each other across the opercular cleft are also oriented so that they come to face the lateral surface of the insula. The insular cleft has a superior limb, located between the insula and the opercula of the frontal and parietal lobes, and an inferior limb, located between the insula and the temporal operculum (*Fig. 1.4*) (1). Anteriorly, the superior limb has a greater vertical height than the inferior limb, but posteriorly, the height of the inferior limb is the same as or greater than the height of the superior limb. The upper lip of the opercular cleft is formed by the gyri of the frontal and parietal lobes that continue medially around the upper edge of the fissure to form the roof of the sylvian cistern and are, from anterior to posterior, the pars orbitalis, triangularis, and opercularis, and the precentral, postcentral, and supramarginal gyri (*Fig. 1.4, C* and *J*). The lower lip of the opercular cleft is formed, from posterior to anterior, by the planum temporale, composed of the transverse temporal gyri the most anterior and longest of which is Heschl's gyrus, and the part of the planum polare lateral to the insula (*Fig. 1.4I*). Heschl's gyrus and the adjoining part of the superior temporal gyrus serve as the primary auditory receiving area. The posterior edge of the insular surface approximates the position of the posterior edge of the pulvinar at a deeper level. The transverse temporal gyri seem to radiate anterolaterally from the posterior insular margin, widening as they progress toward the cortical surface. The plenum temporale has a more horizontal orientation than the plenum polare, which, from lateral to medial, slopes downward and conforms more to the convexly rounded insular surface.

The medially directed arterial apex, created by the most posterior middle cerebral artery branch turning sharply away from the insula, called the sylvian point, points medially toward the atrium, just as does the medial apex of the posterior convergence of the transverse temporal gyri. Each gyrus of the frontoparietal opercula faces and rests in close proximity to its counterpart on the temporal side. The supramarginal gyrus faces the gyri forming the posterior part of the planum temporale, the postcentral gyrus faces Heschl's gyrus, and the precentral gyrus and the pars opercularis, triangularis, and orbitalis are related to the lateral edge of the planum polare formed by the upper edge of the superior temporal gyrus. The site on the posterior ramus of the sylvian fissure, where the postcentral gyrus meets the Heschl's gyrus, is projected in the same coronal plane of the external acoustic meatus.

The medial wall of the sylvian fissure, formed by the insula, is seen only when the lips of the sylvian fissure are widely separated, except in the area below the inferior angle of the pars triangularis, which is often retracted upward to expose a small area of the insular surface (*Fig. 1.4*). The natural upward retraction of the apex of the pars triangularis commonly creates the largest opening in the superficial compartment of the sylvian fissure and provides an area on the convexity where the sylvian fissure is widest, and where it is often safest to begin opening the fissure. The apex of the pars triangularis is sited directly lateral to the anteroinferior part of the circular sulcus and the anterior limit of the basal ganglia.

Anterior Perforated Substance

The anterior perforated substance is a flat, smooth, area of gray matter located in the roof of the sphenoidal compartment of the sylvian fissure (*Fig. 1.4*). It is named for the numerous minute orifices created by numerous perforating arteries from the internal carotid, anterior choroidal, and anterior and middle cerebral arteries penetrating its surface to reach the basal ganglia, anterior portion of the thalamus, and the anterior limb, genu, and posterior limb of the internal capsule. It is also the exit site for the inferior striate veins.

The anterior perforated substance is a rhomboid-shaped area buried deep in the roof of the stem of the sylvian fissure. It is bounded anteriorly by the medial and lateral olfactory striae, posterolaterally by the stem of the temporal lobe, laterally by the limen insulae, and posteromedially by the optic tract. Medially, the anterior perforated substance extends above the optic chiasm to the anterior edge of the interhemispheric fissure. The frontal horn, the caudate head, the anterior part of the lentiform nucleus, and the anterior limb of the internal capsule are located above the anterior perforated substance. Just as the insula can be understood as the outer covering of the internal capsule, basal ganglia, and thalamus, the anterior perforated substance can be seen as the "floor" of the anterior half of the basal ganglia. The anterior perforated substance is where the basal ganglia reach the brain's surface.

FIGURE 1.4. *Continued*

central; Chor., *choroid, choroidal;* Circ., *circular;* CN, *cranial nerve;* Dent., *dentate;* Fiss., *fissure;* For., *foramen;* Front., *frontal;* Gen., *geniculate;* Hippo., *hippocampus;* Lat., *lateral;* Lent., *lentiform, lenticular;* Mam., *mamillary;* Med., *medial;* Nucl., *nucleus;* Olf., *olfactory;* Operc., *operculum, opercularis;* Orb., *orbitalis;* Parahippo., *parahippocampal;* Ped., *peduncle;* Perf., *perforated;* Pit., *pituitary;* Plex., *plexus;* Post., *posterior;* Precent., *precentral;* Rad., *radiations;* Seg., *segment;* Subst., *substance;* Sup., *superior;* Temp., *temporal, temporale;* Tr., *tract;* Trans., *transverse;* Triang., *triangularis;* Vent., *ventricle.*

Insula

The insula has a triangular shape with its apex directed anterior and inferiorly toward the limen insulae, a slightly raised area overlying the uncinate fasciculus, covered by a thin layer of gray matter, at the lateral border of the anterior perforated substance (*Figs. 1.2* and *1.4*). The limen is located at the junction of the sphenoidal and operculoinsular compartments of the sylvian fissure. The insula is encircled and separated from the frontal, parietal, and temporal opercula by a shallow limiting sulcus. The limiting sulcus, although roughly triangular in shape to conform to the shape of the insula, is commonly referred to as the circular sulcus because it encircles the insula. The sulcus has three borders: superior, inferior, and anterior; and three angles: anteroinferior, anterosuperior, and posterior where the borders join. The anterior border is located deep to the pars triangularis of the inferior frontal gyrus; the superior or upper border is nearly horizontal and separates the upper border of the insula and the sylvian surface of the frontal and parietal lobes; and the inferior or lower border is directed anteroinferiorly from the posterior apex and separates the insula from the sylvian surface of the temporal lobe. The anteroinferior angle, referred to as the insular apex, is located below the apex of the pars triangularis; the anterosuperior angle is located deep to the upper anterior edge of the pars triangularis; and the posterior angle is located deep to where the supramarginal gyrus wraps around the posterior end of the sylvian fissure. The anterosuperior angle is located directly lateral to the frontal horn and the posterior angle is located lateral to the atrium and corresponds to the sylvian point, the site at which the most posterior branch of the insular segment of the middle cerebral artery turns laterally between the opercular lips to reach the cortical surface, and the anteroinferior angle points to the lateral edge of the anterior perforated substance.

The sulci and gyri of the insula are directed superiorly and posteriorly in a radial manner from the apex at the limen insulae. The deepest sulcus, the central sulcus of insula, is a relatively constant sulcus that extends upward and backward across the insula, nearly parallel and deep to the central sulcus on the convexity. It divides the insula into a large anterior part that is divided by several shallow sulci into three to five short gyri, and a posterior part that is formed by the anterior and posterior long gyri. The insula covers the lateral surface of the central core of the hemispheric core formed by the extreme, external, and internal capsules, claustrum, lentiform (putamen plus globus pallidus), and caudate nuclei, and thalamus. It is approximately coextensive with the claustrum and putamen.

The upper margin of the insula is located superficial to the midlevel of the body and head of the caudate nucleus. The posterosuperior angle of the insula, the site of the sylvian point, is situated superficial to the anterior margin of the upper part of the atrium where the crus of the fornix wraps around the pulvinar. The majority of the atrium is located behind the level of the posterosuperior part of the circular sulcus. A surface landmark paralleling the lower border of the insula is the superior temporal sulcus, and a deep landmark paralleling the lower border is the optic tract coursing in the roof of the ambient cistern near the midline.

SULCI AND GYRI

Central Sulcus

The central sulcus, which separates the motor and sensory areas and the frontal and parietal lobes, follows in constancy after the sylvian fissure (*Figs. 1.1–1.3* and *1.5*). It begins at the superior border of the lateral surface extending onto the medial surface of the hemisphere in nearly 90% of cases. It intersects the upper hemispheric border approximately 2 cm behind the midpoint between the frontal and occipital poles. Below, it usually ends approximately 2.0 to 2.5 cm behind the anterior ascending ramus of the sylvian fissure without intersecting the sylvian fissure. From its upper end, it is directed laterally, inferiorly, and anteriorly, forming an angle of approximately 70 degrees with the anterior portion of the superior border of the hemisphere. It has two somewhat sinusoidal curves, the superior curve, or genu, has its convexity directed posteriorly, and an inferior curve, or genu, that is convex anteriorly, and together they resemble the shape of an inverted letter S (8). The upper genu is more well defined than the lower. The inferior end of the central sulcus often does not reach the sylvian fissure because a small gyral bridge frequently connects the lower ends of the precentral and postcentral gyri. Irregular limbs of the pre- and postcentral sulci may open into the central sulcus, in which case the pre- and postcentral gyri are divided into upper and lower or multiple segments.

The precentral gyrus, located between the central and precentral sulci, begins at the medial surface of the cerebrum, above the level of the splenium of the corpus callosum, and runs medially to laterally and posteriorly to anteriorly. It is positioned lateral to the following deep structures: body of the lateral ventricle, thalamus, posterior limb of the internal capsule, posterior part of the lentiform nucleus, and the midportion of the insula, to reach the sylvian fissure.

Lateral Convexity

The frontal, parietal, temporal, and occipital lobes contribute to the lateral convexity.

Frontal Lobe

The frontal lobe includes approximately a third of the hemispheric surface (*Figs. 1.3, 1.5,* and *1.6*). The lateral surface of the frontal lobe is bounded behind by the central sulcus and above by the superior hemispheric border. The lower border has an anterior part, the superciliary border, that faces the orbital roof, and a posterior part, the sylvian border, that faces the temporal lobe across the sylvian fissure. The lateral surface is traversed by three sulci, the precentral and the superior and inferior frontal sulci, that divide it into one vertical gyrus and three horizontal gyri. The precentral gyrus, the vertical gyrus, parallels the central sulcus and is bounded behind by the central sulcus and in front by the precentral sulcus. The sur-

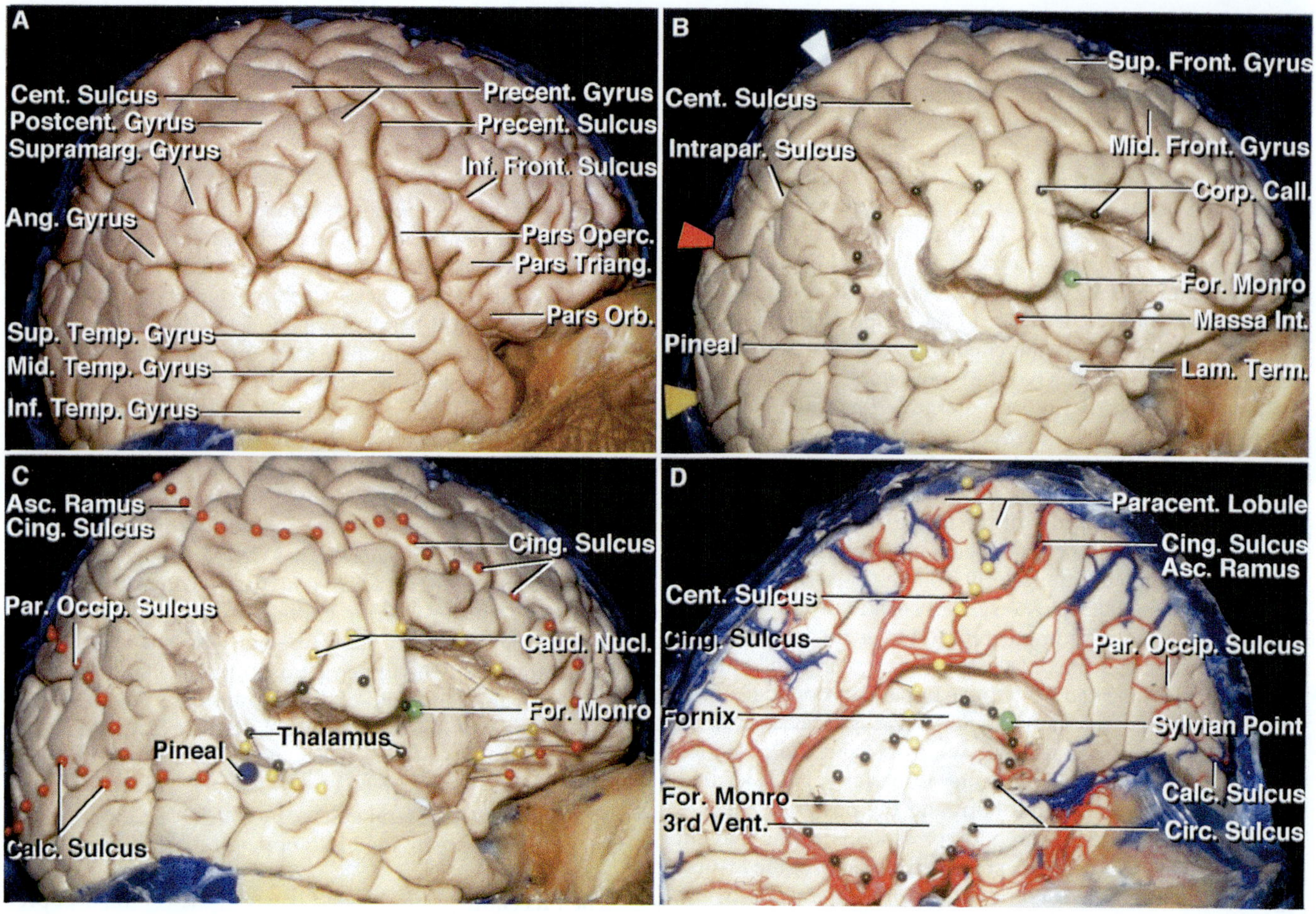

FIGURE 1.5. *Relationships between the medial and lateral surface. A, lateral view, right cerebrum. The inferior frontal gyrus is formed by the pars orbitalis, triangularis, and opercularis. The pre- and postcentral gyri are located between the pars opercularis anteriorly and supramarginal gyrus posteriorly. The precentral gyrus is broken into two gyral strips. B, the pars opercularis, triangularis, and orbitalis, and the superior temporal gyrus and part of the supramarginal gyrus have been removed to expose the insula. A number of pins have been placed on the cortical surface to identify the deep location of various structures: the* green pin *indicates the foramen of Monro; the* red pin, *the massa intermedia;* yellow pin, *the pineal gland;* white pin, *the lamina terminalis. The ovoid group of* dark pins *identifies the outer margin of the corpus callosum. The* arrows *along the posterior half of the superior margin identify the site at which sulci on the medial surface intersect the superior margin as follows:* white arrow, *the ascending (marginal) ramus of cingulate sulcus that marks the posterior edge of the paracentral lobule;* red arrow, *the parieto-occipital sulcus; and* yellow arrow, *the calcarine sulcus. C,* red pins *have been placed on the convexity directly lateral to the course of the calcarine and parieto-occipital sulci and the cingulate sulcus and its ascending ramus on the medial surface. The ascending ramus of the cingulate sulcus extends along the posterior edge of the paracentral lobule formed by the upper end of the pre- and postcentral gyrus overlapping onto the medial surface of the hemisphere. The parieto-occipital and calcarine sulci on the medial surface converge and join in a Y-shaped configuration.* Small black pins *outline the thalamus. The* yellow pins *outline the outer margin of the caudate nucleus. The* large blue pinhead *is located at the level of the pineal, and the* green pin *is located directly lateral to the foramen of Monro. D, medial surface of the same hemisphere. The* yellow pins *mark the location of the central sulcus. The lower end of the central sulcus is located just behind the foramen of Monro as is also shown in B and C. The* dark pins *outline the circular sulcus of the insula. The* green pin *is positioned at the sylvian point where the last branch of the middle cerebral artery turns laterally from the surface of the insula to reach the cortical surface.* Ang., *angular;* Asc., *ascending;* Calc., *calcarine;* Call., *callosum;* Caud., *caudate;* Cent., *central;* Cing., *cingulate;* Circ., *circular;* Corp., *corpus;* For., *foramen;* Front., *frontal;* Inf., *inferior;* Int., *intermedia;* Intrapar., *intraparietal;* Lam., *lamina;* Mid., *middle;* Nucl., *nucleus;* Operc., *opercularis;* Orb., *orbitalis;* Par. Occip., *parieto-occipital;* Paracent., *paracentral;* Postcent., *postcentral;* Precent., *precentral;* Sup., *superior;* Supramarg., *supramarginal;* Temp., *temporal;* Term., *terminalis;* Triang., *triangularis;* Vent., *ventricle.*

face in front of the precentral sulcus is divided by two sulci, the superior and inferior frontal sulci, that nearly parallel the superior border and divide the area into three roughly horizontal convolutions, the superior, middle, and inferior frontal gyri. The inferior frontal convolution, situated between the sylvian fissure and the inferior frontal gyrus, is divided, from anterior to posterior, into the pars orbitalis, pars triangularis, and pars opercularis by the anterior horizontal and anterior ascending rami of the sylvian fissure. The middle frontal gyrus is located between the inferior and superior frontal sulci, and the superior frontal gyrus is situated between the superior frontal sulcus and the superior margin of the hemi-

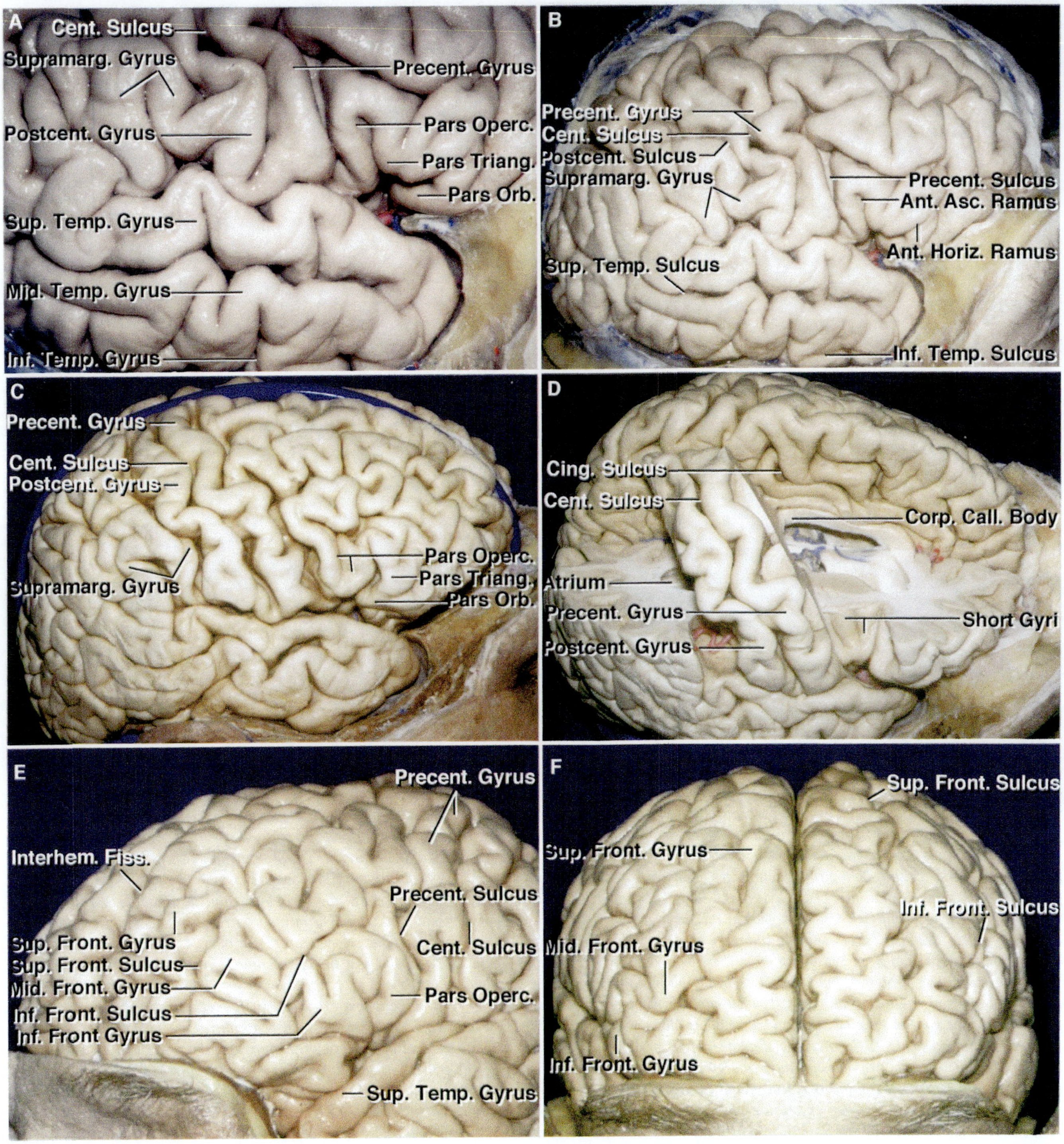

FIGURE 1.6. *Identification of the pre- and postcentral gyri and variations in the frontal and temporal lobe. A, right frontotemporal area adjoining the sylvian fissure. This is the area that would be exposed in a sizable frontotemporal craniotomy. The limited exposure may make it difficult to determine the site of the central sulcus and the precentral and postcentral gyri. Usually, the pre- and postcentral gyri can be located by examining the gyral pattern along the upper lip of the sylvian fissure. From anteriorly, the pars orbitalis, triangularis, and opercularis can be identified. The precentral gyrus is usually located at the posterior margin of the pars opercularis. The sylvian fissure also can be followed backward to its upturned posterior end that is capped by the supramarginal gyrus. Usually, the postcentral gyrus is the next gyrus along the sylvian fissure anterior to the supramarginal gyrus. B, overview of the right hemisphere shown in A. The central sulcus can be followed to the superior margin of the hemisphere. The precentral gyrus is broken up into several segments by crossing sulci. The relationships of the pars opercularis to the precentral gyrus and the supramarginal gyrus to the postcentral gyrus are quite consistent and are helpful in identifying the central sulcus and the pre- and postcentral gyri during the limited operative (Legend continues on next page.)*

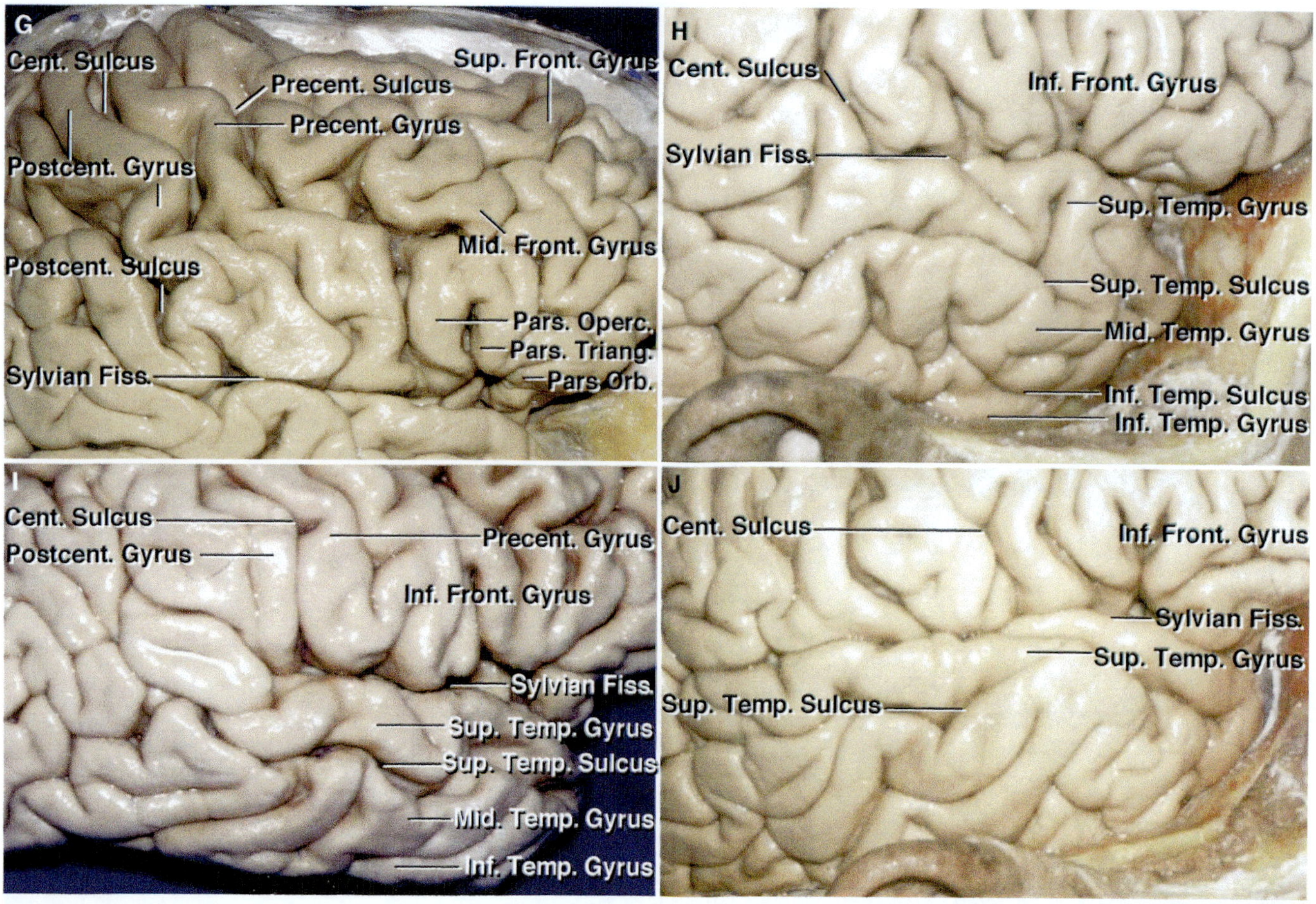

FIGURE 1.6. *Continued*
exposures along the sylvian fissure. The anterior horizontal ramus of the sylvian fissure separates the pars orbitalis and triangularis and the anterior ascending ramus separates the pars triangularis and opercularis. C, another right hemisphere. The lower end of the precentral gyrus is located behind a somewhat lobulated pars opercularis. The postcentral gyrus is located at the anterior edge of the supramar ginal gyrus, which wraps around the upturned posterior end of the sylvian fissure. D, the part of the right frontal and parietal lobes in front of and behind the pre- and postcentral gyri and central sulcus has been removed. The precentral gyrus is located lateral to the posterior part of the body of the ventricle. The postcentral gyrus is located lateral to the anterior part of the atrium. Both gyri adjoining the sylvian fissure are positioned lateral to the splenium of the corpus callosum. E–G, sulci and gyri of the frontal lobe. E, superolateral view of the left frontal lobe. The frontal lobe is often depicted as being split into three gyri, superior, middle, and inferior, by two sulci, superior and inferior. Often, as shown, the superior frontal gyrus is split into medial and lateral segments by irregular sulci and gyri. The middle frontal gyrus does not have a smooth, unbroken surface, but is broken up into multiple, tortuous segments. On the inferior frontal gyrus, formed by the pars orbitalis, triangularis, and opercularis, there can be multiple variations in the size and shape of the contributions from each part. The precentral gyrus, in this case, is broken up into several segments by limbs of the precentral sulcus. F, anterior view. A portion of the right superior frontal gyrus is broken into two longitudinal gyral strips. The left superior frontal gyrus is composed of multiple gyri that extend medially and laterally across the superior frontal area. The superior frontal sulci are continuous along both frontal lobes. The middle frontal gyri on both hemispheres are made up of numerous worm-like gyral segments. G, lateral view of another right frontal lobe. The pars triangularis and opercularis of the inferior frontal gyrus have a somewhat similar triangular appearance. Usually there is a gyral bridge at the lower margin of the central sulcus, but in this case the central sulcus opens into the sylvian fissure. The precentral gyrus is continuous from its lower to its upper margin and is not broken up into multiple segments as shown in B *and* E. *The middle frontal gyrus is made up of multiple irregular convolutions. H–J, variations in the sulcal and gyral patterns of the temporal lobe. H, right temporal lobe with a more typical pattern in which the three temporal gyri, superior, middle and inferior, are separated by two sulci, superior and inferior. The sulci have an irregular, tortuous course, but are largely continuous along the lateral temporal lobe from anterior to posterior. I, the superior temporal gyrus located above the superior temporal sulcus is easily identifiable. The part of the temporal lobe below the superior temporal sulcus is broken up into multiple obliquely oriented gyri that do not fit easily into a pattern of the expected middle and inferior gyri. J, the superior temporal gyrus is broken up into several segments but is fairly continuous. The middle and inferior temporal regions are formed by multiple obliquely oriented gyri and there is no clear inferior temporal sulcus.* Ant., *anterior;* Asc., *ascending;* Call., *callosum;* Cent., *central;* Cing., *cingulate;* Corp., *corpus;* Fiss., *fissure;* Front., *frontal;* Horiz., *horizontal;* Inf., *inferior;* Interhem., *interhemispheric;* Mid., *middle;* Operc., *opercularis;* Orb., *orbitalis;* Postcent., *postcentral;* Precent., *precentral;* Sup., *superior;* Supramarg., *supramarginal;* Temp., *temporal;* Triang., *triangularis.*

sphere. The superior frontal gyrus extends around the superior margin of the hemisphere to form the upper part of the medial surface of the lobe. It is frequently incompletely subdivided into an upper and lower part. The middle frontal gyrus may also be divided into upper and lower parts.

The middle frontal gyrus on the lateral surface is situated lateral to the cingulate gyrus on the medial surface, and the two are separated by the deep white matter forming the centrum semiovale. The inferior frontal sulcus is located at the level of the upper margin of the anterior part of the corpus callosum, and the posterior part of the inferior frontal gyrus is positioned lateral to the frontal horn, caudate head, and anterior part of the insula. The pars orbitalis is continuous medially with the orbital surface of the frontal lobe. The lower part of the pars opercularis may be connected by a gyral bridge to the lower part of the precentral gyrus. The pars opercularis and adjacent triangularis are frequently referred to as Broca's speech area. The apex of the pars triangularis is directed inferiorly toward the junction of the three rami–the anterior ascending, horizontal, and posterior rami–of the sylvian fissure; this junctional point coincides with the anterior part of the circular sulcus of the insula in the depth of the sylvian fissure. It also marks the anterior limit of the basal ganglia and the frontal horn of the lateral ventricle.

Parietal Lobe

The lateral surface of the parietal lobe is limited anteriorly by the central sulcus, superiorly by the interhemispheric fissure, inferolaterally by the sylvian fissure and a line, referred to as the extended sylvian line, extending posteriorly along the long axis of the sylvian fissure, and posteriorly by the line extending from the upper end of the parieto-occipital fissure to the preoccipital notch. Its two main sulci, the postcentral and intraparietal sulci, divide the lateral surface into three parts (*Figs. 1.1, 1.3,* and *1.5*). The postcentral sulcus divides the parietal lobe into an anterior convolution, the postcentral gyrus, situated behind and parallel to the central sulcus, and a large posterior part subdivided by the horizontal sulcus, the intraparietal sulcus, into superior and inferior parietal lobules. The postcentral sulcus is similar to the central sulcus in shape, but is frequently broken into several discontinuous parts by gyral bridges. The intraparietal sulcus is oriented anteroposteriorly, parallel, and 2 to 3 cm lateral to the superior border of the hemisphere. The depth of the intraparietal sulcus is directed toward the roof of the atrium and the occipital horn. The superior parietal lobule extends from the intraparietal sulcus to the superior margin of the hemisphere.

The inferior parietal lobule, the larger of the two lobules, is divided into an anterior part formed by the supramarginal gyrus, which arches over the upturned end of the posterior ramus of the sylvian fissure, and a posterior part formed by the angular gyrus, which arches over the upturned end of the superior temporal sulcus. The inferior parietal lobule blends posteriorly into the anterior part of the occipital lobe. The supramarginal gyrus arching over the upturned posterior end of the sylvian fissure forms the most posterior opercular lips of the sylvian fissure. The supramarginal gyrus is located lateral to the atrium of the lateral ventricle. The part of the supramarginal gyrus above the posterior end of the sylvian fissure is continuous in front with the lower end of the postcentral sulcus, and the part below the sylvian fissure is continuous with the superior temporal gyrus. The part of the angular gyrus above the superior temporal sulcus is continuous with the superior temporal gyrus, and below the superior temporal sulcus is continuous with the middle temporal gyrus.

Occipital Lobe

The occipital convexity is not separated from the temporal and parietal lobes by any clearly defined sulci (*Figs. 1.1* and *1.3*). It is composed of a number of irregular convolutions with considerable variability. The most consistent sulci, the lateral occipital sulcus, which is short and horizontal, divides the lobe into superior and inferior occipital gyri. The transverse occipital sulcus descends on the lateral surface behind the posterior part of the parieto-occipital arcus, a U-shaped gyrus that caps the short segment of the parieto-occipital sulcus that overlaps from the medial surface onto the lateral hemispheric surface. The anterior part of the arcus is parietal lobe and the posterior part is occipital lobe. The lambdoid suture joins the sagittal suture at approximately the parieto-occipital junction, but slopes downward across the occipital lobe behind the parieto-occipital junction. The calcarine sulcus, the most important sulcus on the occipital lobe, is located on the medial surface slightly below the midlevel of the lateral occipital surface at approximately the level of a line extending posteriorly along the long axis of the superior temporal sulcus.

Temporal Lobe

The lateral temporal surface, located below the sylvian fissure and the extended sylvian line and anterior to the line connecting the preoccipital notch and parieto-occipital sulci, is divided into three parallel gyri, the superior, middle, and inferior temporal gyri, by two sulci, the superior and inferior temporal sulci (*Figs. 1.1, 1.3,* and *1.6*). Both the gyri and sulci parallel the sylvian fissure. The superior temporal gyrus lies between the sylvian fissure and the superior temporal sulcus and is continuous around the lip of the fissure with the transverse temporal gyri, which extend obliquely backward and medially toward the posterosuperior angle of the insula to form the lower wall of the posterior part of the floor of the sylvian fissure. The middle temporal gyrus lies between the superior and inferior temporal sulci. The temporal horn and the ambient and the crural cisterns are located deep to the middle temporal gyrus. The inferior temporal gyrus lies below the inferior temporal sulcus and continues around the inferior border of the hemisphere to form the lateral part of the basal surface. The angular gyrus, a parietal lobe structure, caps the upturned posterior end of the superior temporal sulcus. One or more of the temporal gyri are frequently separated into two or three sections by sulcal bridges, giving the related gyri an irregular discontinuous appearance. The variation is greater with the middle and inferior temporal gyri than with the superior temporal gyrus. The inferior temporal gyrus is often composed

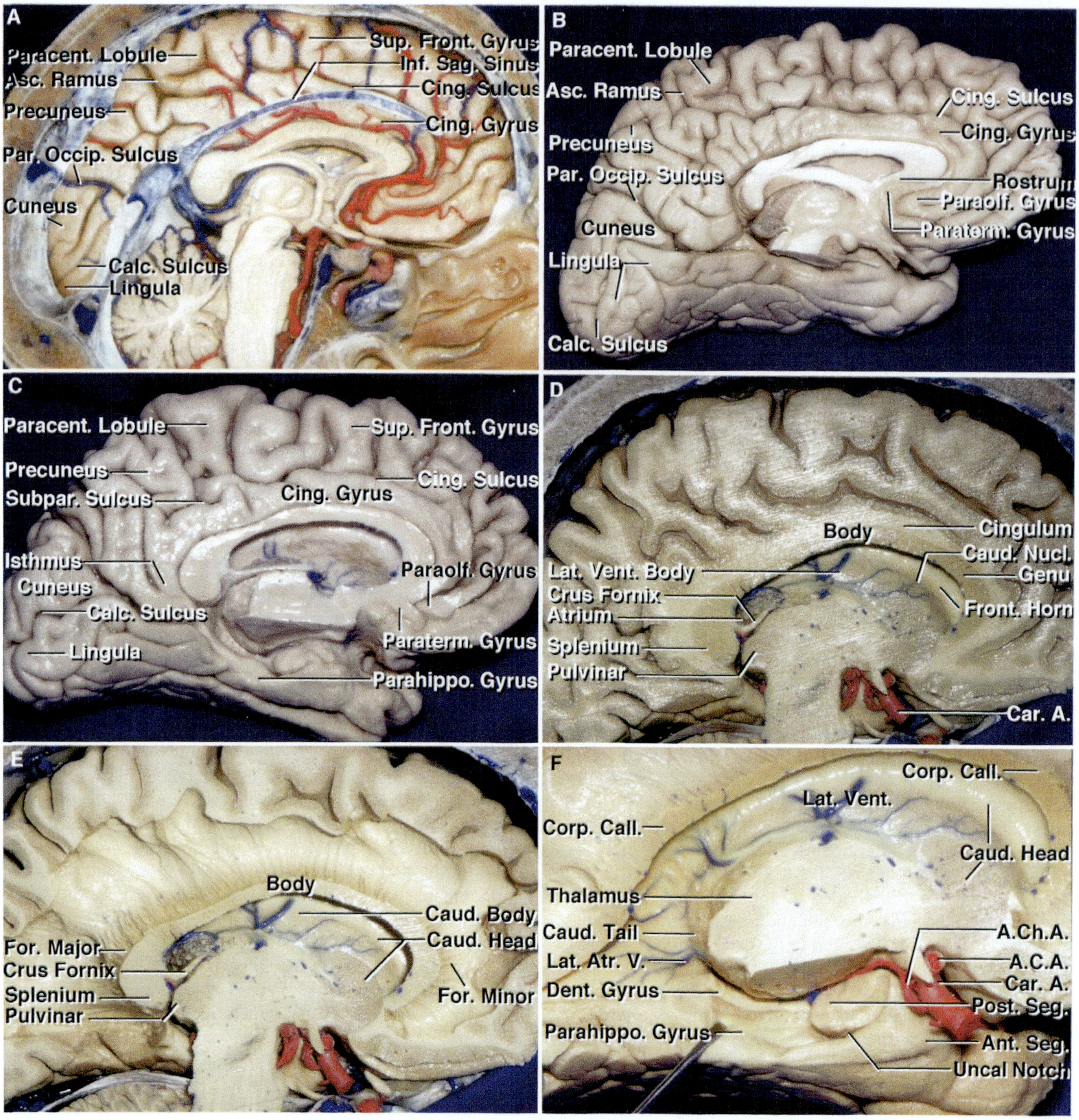

FIGURE 1.7. A–C, *medial surface of the right cerebral hemisphere.* A, *the falx, except for the inferior sagittal sinus, has been removed. The majority of the medial surface of the frontal lobe is formed by the cingulate and superior frontal gyri that are separated by the cingulate sulcus. The ascending ramus of the cingulate sulcus passes behind the paracentral lobule, the site of the extension of the pre- and postcentral gyri onto the medial surface of the hemisphere. The medial surface behind the paracentral lobule is formed by the precuneus, cuneus, and lingula and the posterior part of the cingulate sulcus. The precuneus is located between the paracentral lobule and parieto-occipital sulcus. The cuneus is located between the parieto-occipital and the calcarine sulci. The lingual gyrus (lingula) is located below the calcarine sulcus.* B, *medial surface of another hemisphere. The paraterminal and paraolfactory gyri are located below the rostrum of the corpus callosum. The precuneus is located between the ascending ramus of the cingulate sulcus, the parieto-occipital sulcus, and the subparietal sulcus, a posterior extension of the cingulate sulcus. The cuneus is located between the parieto-occipital and calcarine sulci, and the lingula is located below the calcarine sulcus. The parieto-occipital and calcarine sulci join to create a Y-shaped configuration. The parahippocampal gyrus forms the majority of the medial surface of the temporal lobe.* C, *another hemisphere. The medial surface is formed by the paraterminal, paraolfactory, superior frontal, and cingulate gyri and the paracentral lobule, precuneus, cuneus, lingula, and parahippocampal gyrus. The cingulate sulcus narrows*

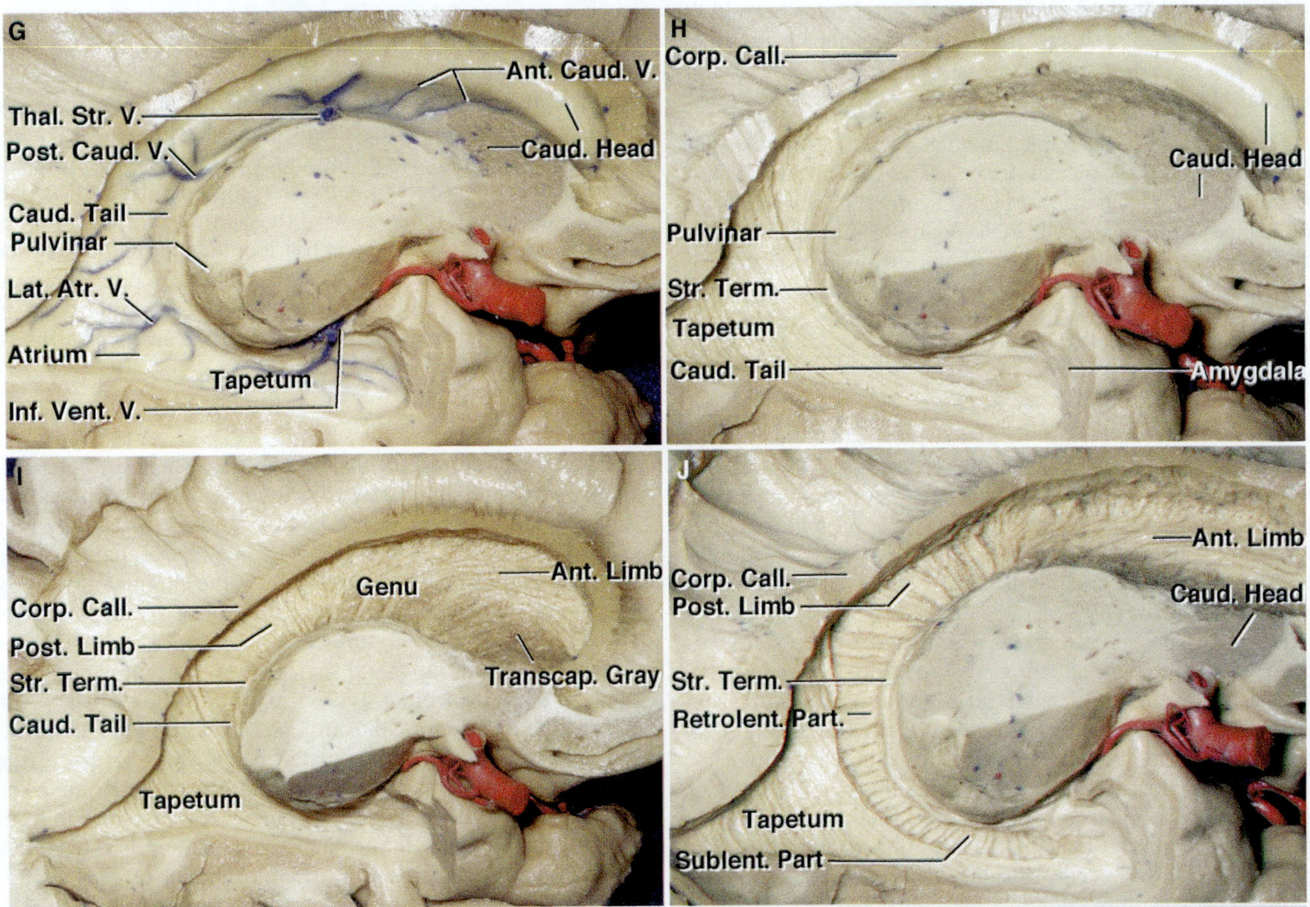

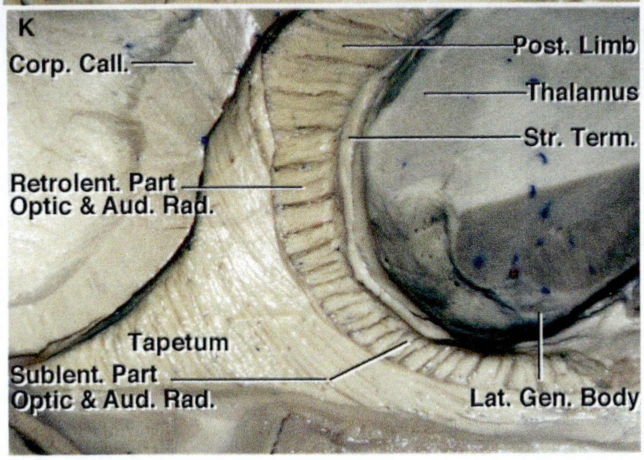

FIGURE 1.7. *Continued*
behind the splenium to form the isthmus of the cingulate sulcus that blends along the medial surface of the temporal lobe into the parahippocampal gyrus. D–K, fiber dissection of the medial surface of the hemisphere. D, the section extends through the medial part of the right hemisphere and thalamus. It crosses the medial part of the head of the caudate nucleus anteriorly and the pulvinar of the thalamus posteriorly. The genu of the corpus callosum wraps around the frontal horn. The body of the corpus callosum forms the roof of the body of the lateral ventricle and the splenium is located adjacent to the atrium. The caudate nucleus is exposed in the lateral wall of the frontal horn and the body of the ventricle. The cingulum, a bundle of association fibers, wraps around the outer border of the corpus callosum in the depths of the cingulate gyrus. E, the cingulum and gray matter of the cingulate gyrus have been removed to expose the fibers radiating laterally out of the corpus callosum. The cross section of the corpus callosum is the part nearest the reader and the fibers radiate away from the cut edge around the margins of the lateral ventricle. Fibers passing through the genu of the corpus callosum form the forceps minor and the anterior wall of the frontal horn and the large bundle passing posteriorly from the splenium forms the forceps major creating a prominence, the bulb of the corpus callosum, in the medial wall of the atrium. The crus of the fornix wraps around the pulvinar in the anterior wall of the atrium. F, the brainstem has been removed to expose the uncus, which has anterior and posterior segments. The anterior segment faces the internal carotid artery. The posterior segment, facing posteromedially, is divided into an upper and lower part by the uncal notch. Removing the brainstem also exposes the parahippocampal and dentate gyri. The crus of the fornix and splenium have been removed to expose the caudate tail extending around the pulvinar. G–K, fiber dissection of the medial surface of the hemisphere. G, the posterior segment of the uncus has been removed while preserving the anterior segment. The thalamostriate, anterior and posterior caudate, lateral atrial, and inferior ventricular veins cross the wall of the ventricle. The thalamostriate vein courses in the sulcus between the caudate nucleus and thalamus on the outer surface of the stria terminalis. The caudate tail extends around the pulvinar and into the roof of the temporal horn. H, the ependymal wall of the ventricle has been removed to expose the fibers in a subependymal area. The caudate tail is exposed below the pulvinar. The stria terminalis courses between the caudate and thalamus. The tapetum of the corpus callosum forms the roof and lateral wall of the atrium and temporal horn. The amygdala is located in the anterior segment of the uncus and forms the anterior wall of the temporal horn. (Legend continues on next page.)

of multiple fragmented gyri and may blend into the middle temporal gyrus without a clear sulcal demarcation.

Medial Hemispheric Surface

The frontal, parietal, occipital, and temporal lobes have medial surfaces (*Fig. 1.7*). The medial surfaces of the frontal, parietal, and occipital lobes are flattened vertically against the falx cerebri, are interconnected below the falx in the floor of the interhemispheric fissure by the corpus callosum, and are separated from the corpus callosum by the callosal sulcus. The medial surface of the temporal lobe is much more complex (9). It wraps around the cerebral peduncle and upper brainstem and forms the lateral wall of the cisterns above the tentorial incisura.

The general organization of the gyri of the frontal, parietal, and occipital lobes on the medial surface can be compared with that of a three-layer roll: the inner layer is represented by corpus callosum, the intermediate layer by cingulate gyrus, and the outer layer, from anterior to posterior, by the medial surface of the superior frontal gyrus, the paracentral lobule, precuneus, cuneus, and the lingula (8). The cingulate gyrus wraps around and is separated inferiorly from the corpus callosum by the callosal sulcus. The cingulate gyrus is separated on its outer margin from the remainder of the medial surface of the superior frontal gyrus and the paracentral lobule by the cingulate sulcus and from the precuneus and remainder of the parietal lobe by the subparietal sulcus, an indistinct posterior continuation of the cingulate sulcus behind the marginal ramus. The cingulate gyrus begins below the rostrum of the corpus callosum, curves around the genu and body of the corpus callosum, and turns downward behind the splenium, where it is connected by a narrow gyral bridge, the isthmus of the cingulate gyrus, to the parahippocampal gyrus. Several secondary rami, of which the paracentral and ascending rami are the most important, ascend from the cingulate sulcus to divide the outer layer into several sections. The paracentral ramus ascends from the cingulate sulcus at the level of the midportion of the corpus callosum to separate the superior frontal gyrus anteriorly from the paracentral lobule posteriorly. The marginal or ascending ramus ascends from the cingulate sulcus at the level of the posterior third of the corpus callosum and separates the paracentral lobule anteriorly from the precuneus posteriorly. The paracentral lobule, the extension of the pre- and postcentral gyri that wraps around the extension of the central sulcus onto the medial surface, is the site of the motor and sensory areas of the contralateral lower limb and perineal region and the voluntary control areas of defecation and micturition. The part of the paracentral lobule behind the central sulcus is a part of the parietal lobe. The paracentral lobule is located above the posterior half of the corpus callosum. The marginal ramus, present in almost all hemispheres, is an important aid in magnetic resonance imaging in locating the sensory or motor areas on the medial surface.

Frontal Lobe

The medial surface of the frontal lobe is formed predominantly by the medial surface of the superior frontal gyrus, the anterior half of the paracentral lobule, and the cingulate gyrus (*Figs. 1.3* and *1.7*). The superior frontal gyrus parallels the superior border and is separated from the cingulate gyrus by the cingulate sulcus. The cingulate sulcus parallels and is situated on the medial surface at the level of the superior frontal sulcus on the lateral surface. Anteriorly, the cingulate and the superior frontal gyri wrap around the genu and the rostrum of the corpus callosum and blend into the paraterminal and parolfactory gyri situated below the rostrum of the corpus callosum and in front of the lamina terminalis. The paraterminal gyrus is a narrow triangle of gray matter in front of the lateral edge of the lamina terminalis that is continuous with the indusium griseum, the thin lamina of gray matter that covers the upper surface of the corpus callosum. The paraterminal gyrus is separated at its anterior edge from the adjacent paraolfactory gyrus by the shallow posterior paraolfactory sulcus. The anterior paraolfactory sulcus, a short vertical sulcus, separates the paraolfactory gyrus from the anterior part of the frontal pole.

Parietal Lobe

The medial parietal surface is situated between the line from the upper end of the central sulcus to the corpus callo-

FIGURE 1.7. *Continued*
The anterior choroidal artery courses around the anterior and posterior segments of the uncus to reach the choroid plexus in the temporal horn. I, the caudate nucleus has been removed to expose the fibers constituting the internal capsule. The anterior thalamic peduncle and anterior limb of the internal capsule courses lateral to the caudate head. The anterior limb is crossed by bridges of transcapsular bridges gray matter interconnecting the caudate and lentiform nuclei that gives it a prominent striate appearance and a deeper color than the posterior part of the internal capsule. The superior thalamic peduncle and genu of the internal capsule are exposed above the thalamus. The posterior thalamic peduncle and posterior limb of the internal capsule are exposed behind the genu. The upper part of the optic radiations course behind the pulvinar in the retrolenticular part of the internal capsule. The tapetum sweeps downward to form the roof and lateral wall of the atrium and temporal horn. J, enlarged view. The stria terminalis wraps around the posterior margin of the thalamus and blends into the amygdala. The fibers forming the anterior and posterior limbs and the retro- and sublenticular parts of the internal capsule have been exposed. K, enlarged view. The sublenticular part of the optic and auditory radiations pass laterally and are separated from the temporal horn by only the tapetum. The retrolenticular part of the internal capsule contains some of the optic radiations. A., *artery;* A.C.A., *anterior cerebral artery;* A.Ch.A., *anterior choroidal artery;* Ant., *anterior;* Asc., *ascending;* Atr., *atrial;* Aud., *auditory;* Calc., *calcarine;* Call., *callosum;* Car., *carotid;* Caud., *caudate;* Cing., *cingulate;* Corp., *corpus;* Dent., *dentate;* For., *forceps;* Front., *frontal;* Gen., *geniculate;* Inf., *inferior;* Lat., *lateral;* Nucl., *nucleus;* Par. Occip., *parieto-occipital;* Paracent., *paracentral;* Parahippo., *parahippocampal;* Paraolf., *paraolfactory;* Paraterm., *paraterminal;* Post., *posterior;* Rad., *radiations;* Retrolent., *retrolenticular;* Sag., *sagittal;* Seg., *segment;* Str., *stria;* Sublent., *sublenticular;* Subpar., *subparietal;* Sup., *superior;* Term., *terminalis;* Thal. Str., *thalamostriate;* Transcap., *transcapsular;* V., *vein;* Vent., *ventricle, ventricular.*

sum anteriorly and the parieto-occipital sulcus posteriorly. It is formed by the precuneus and the posterior part of the cingulate gyrus and paracentral lobule (*Figs. 1.3, 1.5,* and *1.7*). The precuneus is a quadrilateral area bounded anteriorly by the ascending ramus of the cingulate sulcus, posteriorly by the parieto-occipital sulcus above the superior hemispheric border, and inferiorly from the cingulate gyrus by the subparietal sulcus. The posterior part of the cingulate gyrus wraps around the splenium and is separated from the precuneus by the subparietal sulcus and from the splenium by the callosal sulcus. The posterior part of the paracentral lobule is a medial extension of the postcentral gyrus, and the precuneus is the medial extension of the superior parietal lobule. The subparietal sulcus is located at approximately the level of the interparietal sulcus on the lateral surface.

Occipital Lobe

The medial surface of the occipital lobe is separated from the parietal lobe by the parieto-occipital sulcus (*Figs. 1.3, 1.5,* and *1.7*) (12). The calcarine fissure extends forward from the occipital pole toward the splenium and divides this surface into an upper part, the cuneus, and a lower part, the lingula. The cuneus is a wedge-shaped lobule, bounded in front by the parieto-occipital sulcus, below by the calcarine sulcus, and above by the superior border of the hemisphere. The lingula, a narrow convolution between the calcarine sulcus and the lower border of the medial surface, has, as its name suggests, a tongue-like appearance, with the tip of the tongue located at the occipital pole. The lingula blends anteriorly into the posterior part of the parahippocampal gyrus that extends backward from the temporal lobe.

The parieto-occipital sulcus is directed downward and forward from the superior border between the cuneus and precuneus at an angle of approximately 45 degrees. It descends to join the anterior part of the calcarine sulcus, giving the region a Y-shaped configuration. The parieto-occipital sulcus courses approximately parallel to the line on the convexity that connects the preoccipital notch and the upper end of the parieto-occipital sulcus.

The calcarine sulcus begins just above the occipital pole and courses forward with an upward convexity between the cuneus above and lingual below and joins the parieto-occipital sulcus. It continues anteriorly below the isthmus of the cingulate gyrus, where it may intersect the posterior part of the parahippocampal gyrus before terminating. The primary visual receiving area is located on the upper and lower banks and the depths of the posterior part of the calcarine sulcus. It may overlap for a short distance on the lateral aspect of the occipital pole, then continues anteriorly on the medial surface to intercept the isthmus of the cingulate gyrus. The portion of the calcarine sulcus anterior to the junction with the parieto-occipital sulcus extends so deeply into the medial surface of the hemisphere that it forms a prominence, the calcar avis, in the medial wall of the atrium. The part of the calcarine sulcus posterior to its junction with the parieto-occipital sulcus has the visual (striate) cortex on its upper and lower lips, and the part anterior to the junction with the parieto-occipital sulcus has visual cortex only on its lower lip (8). The basal surface of the occipital lobe slopes upward from its lateral edge, thus placing the calcarine sulcus higher relative to the convexity than it is on the medial surface. Although located low on the medial occipital surface, the anterior end of the calcarine sulcus is located deep to the posterior part of the superior temporal gyrus, and the posterior part is located deep to the midportion of the lateral occipital surface (*Fig. 1.5C*).

Temporal Lobe

The medial surface of the temporal lobe is the most complex of the medial cortical areas (*Figs. 1.8–1.10*) (10). It is formed predominantly by the rounded medial surfaces of the parahippocampal gyrus and uncus. This medial surface is composed of three longitudinal strips of neural tissue, one located above the other, which are interlocked with the hippocampal formation. The most inferior strip is formed by the rounded medial edge of the parahippocampal gyrus, the site of the subicular zones; the middle strip is formed by the dentate gyrus, a narrow serrated strip of gray matter located on the medial surface of the hippocampal formation; and the superior strip is formed by the fimbria of the fornix, a white band formed by the fibers emanating from the hippocampal formation and directed posteriorly into the crus of the fornix. The parahippocampal and dentate gyri are separated by the hippocampal sulcus, and the dentate gyrus and the fimbria are separated by the fimbriodentate sulcus. The amygdala and the hippocampal formation lie just beneath and are so intimately related to the mesial temporal cortex that they are considered in this section. The dentate gyrus blends posteriorly behind the splenium into the fasciolar gyrus, which is continuous with the indusium griseum.

The parahippocampal gyrus deviates medially at the site of the uncus that projects medially above the tentorial edge. The parahippocampal gyrus also extends around the lower border to form the medial part of the basal surface of the temporal lobe, where it is separated from the medially projecting uncus by the rhinal sulcus. Posteriorly, the part of the parahippocampal gyrus below the splenium of the corpus callosum is intersected by the anterior end of the calcarine sulcus, which divides the posterior portion of the parahippocampal gyrus into an upper part that is continuous above and posteriorly with the isthmus of the cingulate gyrus and continuous below and posteriorly with the lingual gyrus.

The uncus, the medially projecting anterior part of the parahippocampal gyrus, when viewed from above or below, has an angular shape with anterior and posterior segments that meet at a medially directed apex (*Figs. 1.8* and *1.9*). The anterior segment of the uncus faces anteromedial and the posterior segment faces posteromedial. The anterior segment has an undivided medial surface, but the posterior segment is divided into upper and lower parts by the uncal notch, a short sulcus that extends from posteriorly into the medial aspect of the posterior segment. The medial face of the anterior segment faces the proximal part of the sylvian, the carotid cistern, and the internal carotid and proximal middle cerebral arteries. The posterior segment faces the cerebral peduncle and, with the

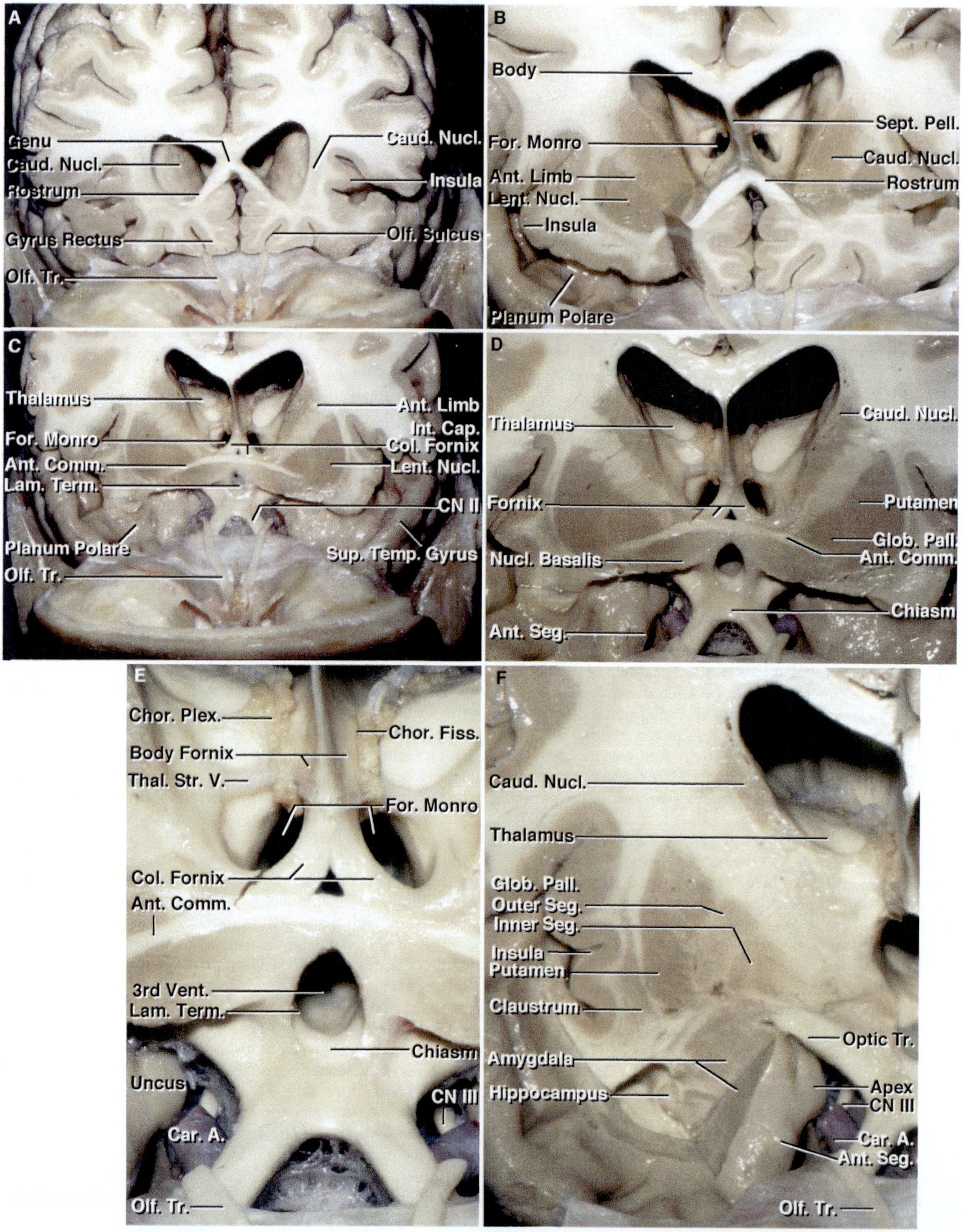

FIGURE 1.8. *(See legend beginning on page 52.)*

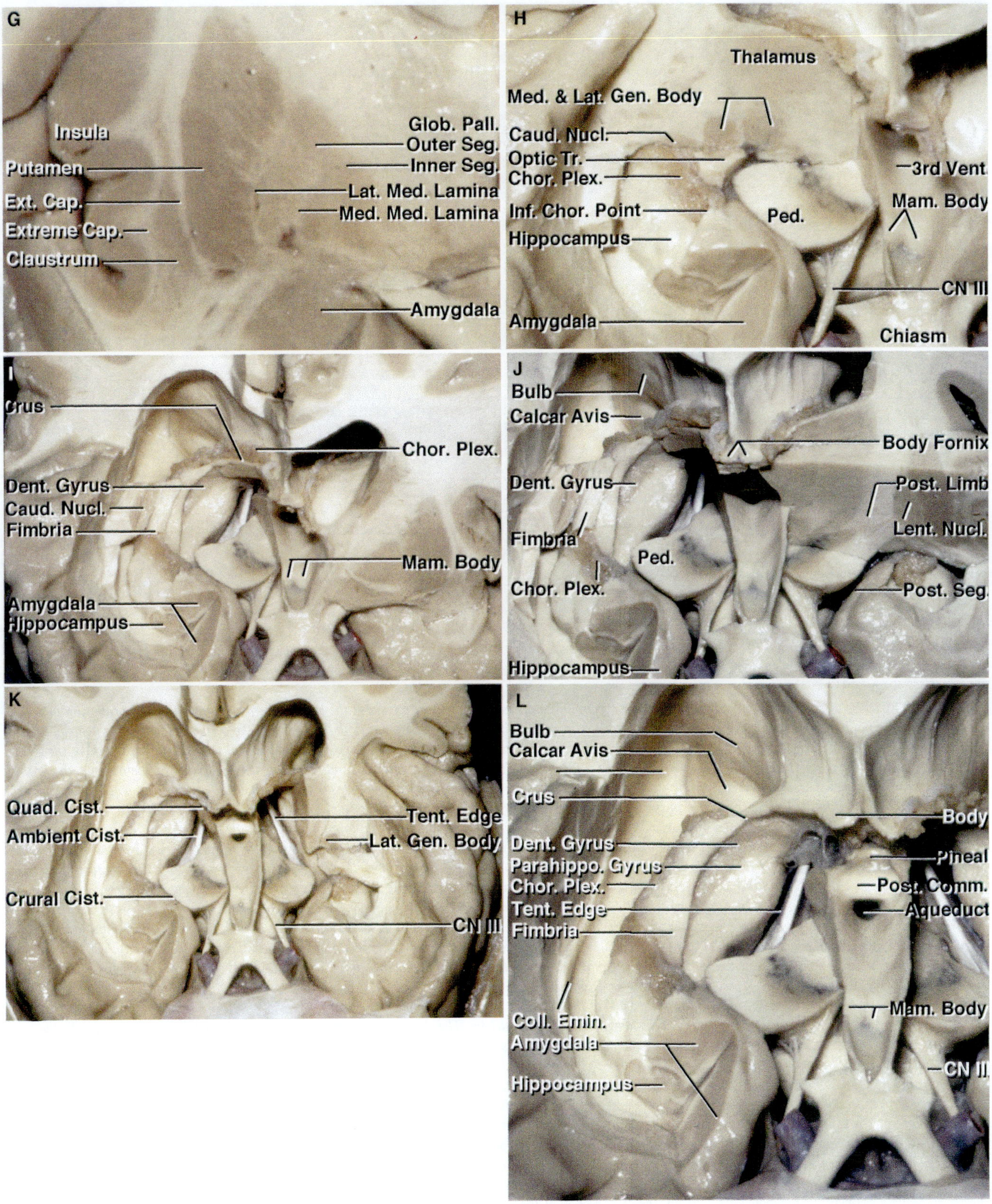

FIGURE 1.8. *(See legend beginning on page 52.)*

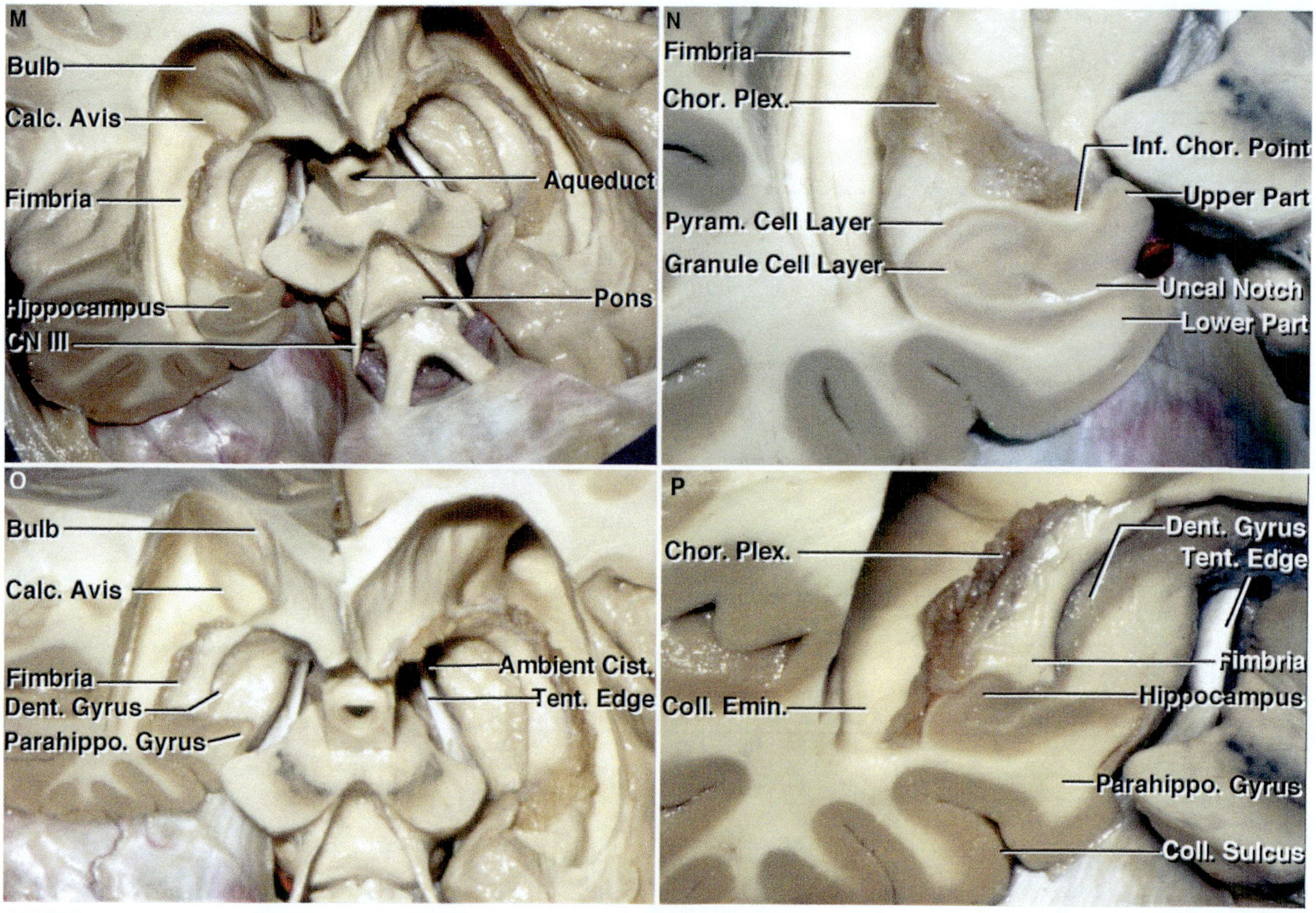

FIGURE 1.8. *Stepwise dissection of the cerebral hemispheres, beginning anteriorly.* A, *coronal section at the level of the rostrum of the corpus callosum and anterior part of the frontal horn. The anterior wall and adjacent part of the roof of the frontal horn are formed by the genu of the corpus callosum, the floor by the rostrum, and the lateral wall by the caudate nucleus. The insular surface is small at this level. The gyrus rectus is located medial to the olfactory tracts.* B, *the section has been extended to the midportion of the frontal horn. The roof is formed by the body of the corpus callosum, the lateral wall by the caudate nucleus, the floor by the rostrum, and the medial wall by the septum pellucidum. The anterior limb of the internal capsule passes between the caudate and the lentiform nuclei. The caudate nucleus blends into the lentiform nucleus in the area below the anterior limb of the internal capsule. The planum polare on the upper surface of the anterior part of the temporal lobe is devoid of gyri and has a shallow trough along which the middle cerebral artery courses.* C, *the cross section has been extended posteriorly to the level of the lamina terminalis and the anterior commissure. The columns of the fornix pass around the anterior and superior margin of the foramen of Monro and turn downward behind the lamina terminalis toward the mamillary bodies. At this level, the lentiform nucleus has taken on its characteristic triangular or lens shape in cross section.* D, *enlarged view. The lamina terminalis has been opened. The anterior limb of the internal capsule separates the caudate and lentiform nuclei. The lentiform nucleus is formed by the putamen and globus pallidus. The anteroinferior part of the caudate and lentiform nuclei blends without clear demarcation into the large mass of gray matter above the anterior perforated substance and adjacent part of the orbital surface of the frontal lobe that also includes the nucleus basalis and accumbens. The nucleus basalis is located below the anterior commissure and the accumbens is located anterior to the basalis without clear demarcation between these two nuclei or the adjacent part of the lentiform and caudate nuclei. The anterior segment of the uncus is exposed lateral to the carotid artery.* E, *enlarged view. The olfactory nerves pass posteriorly above the optic nerves. The choroidal fissure, the cleft between the thalamus and body of the fornix along which the choroid plexus is attached, begins at the posterior edge of the foramen of Monro. The thalamostriate vein courses through the posterior margin of the foramen of Monro and between the thalamus and caudate nucleus. The oculomotor nerves are exposed behind the carotid arteries.* F, *the cross section has been extended backward to the level of the foramen of Monro. At this level the caudate nucleus is considerably smaller than anteriorly. The globus pallidus has a clearly defined inner and outer segment. The anterior part of the roof of the temporal horn has been removed to expose the amygdala and anterior part of the hippocampus. The amygdala, at its upper margin, blends into the globus pallidus. The combination of the globus pallidus and amygdala seem to wrap around the lateral aspect of the optic tract. The apex of the uncus protrudes medially toward the oculomotor nerve. The anterior uncal segment is located lateral to the carotid artery. The claustrum is located between the insula and the lentiform nucleus. The amygdala fills most of the anterior segment of the uncus and forms the anterior wall of the temporal horn. The amygdala tilts backward above the anterior part of the hippocampal head and roof of the temporal horn.* G, *enlarged view of the lentiform nucleus and amygdala. The extreme capsule separates the claustrum and insula, and the external capsule separates the claustrum and lentiform nucleus. The lateral medullary lamina separates the putamen from the outer segment of the globus pallidus and the medial medullary lamina separates the medial and lateral segments of the globus pallidus.* H, *the cross section of the right hemisphere has been extended behind the cerebral peduncle and across the terminal part of the optic tract and the lateral and medial geniculate bodies. The section of the midbrain extends through the cerebral peduncle and substantia nigra.*

peduncle, forms the lateral and medial walls of the crural cistern through which the posterior cerebral, anterior choroidal, and medial posterior choroidal arteries pass. The optic tract passes above the medial edge of the posterior segment in the roof of the crural cistern. The amygdaloid nucleus forms almost all of the interior and comes to the medial surface of the upper part of the anterior segment. The upper part of the posterior segment is formed largely by the medial aspect of the head of the hippocampus. The apex, where the anterior and posterior segments meet, points medially toward the oculomotor nerve and posterior communicating artery. The head of the hippocampus reaches the medial surface in the upper part of the posterior segment at the anterior end of the dentate gyrus. Within the ventricle, a small medially projecting space, the uncal recess, situated between the ventricular surface of the amygdala and hippocampal head, is located lateral to the uncal apex.

The lower surface of the superior lip of the uncal notch is visible from below only after removing the lower lip formed by the parahippocampal gyrus (*Fig. 1.9*). The posterior segment is occupied by several small gyri that are continuations of the dentate gyri. The inferior choroidal point, the lower end of the choroidal fissure along which the choroid plexus is attached, is located just behind the upper edge of the posterior uncal segment, immediately behind the head of the hippocampus, at the site where the anterior choroidal artery passes through the choroidal fissure to enter the temporal horn. The anterior choroidal artery arises near the midlevel of the anterior segment and hugs its surface, sloping gently upward, unless extremely tortuous. It continues to ascend as it courses posteriorly around the uncal apex and reaches the upper part of the posterior segment, where it passes through the fissure at the inferior choroidal point. The dentate gyrus, named for its characteristic tooth-like elevations, extends posteriorly from the upper part of the posterior segment and has the most prominent denticulations anteriorly. The dentate gyrus is continuous posteriorly below and behind the splenium of the corpus callosum with the fasciolar gyrus, a smooth grayish band that blends above into the indusium griseum.

The amygdala can be considered as being entirely located within the boundaries of the uncus (*Figs. 1.8–1.10*). It forms the anterior wall of the temporal horn. Superiorly, the amygdala blends into the claustrum and globus pallidus without any clear demarcation. The upper posterior portion of the amygdala tilts back above the hippocampal head and the uncal recess to form the anterior portion of the roof of the temporal horn. Medially, it is related to the anterior and posterior segments of the uncus. In coronal cross section, the optic tract sits medial to the junction of the amygdala and globus pallidus. The amygdala gives rise to the stria terminalis, which courses between the thalamus and caudate nucleus deep to the thalamostriate vein.

The hippocampus, which blends into and forms the upper part of the posterior uncal segment, is a curved elevation, approximately 5 cm long, in the medial part of the entire length of the floor of the temporal horn (*Fig. 1.8*). It has the dentate gyrus along

The inferior choroidal point, the lower end of the choroidal fissure and attachment of the choroid plexus in the temporal horn, is located just behind the head of the hippocampus. The oculomotor nerve arises on the medial side of the cerebral peduncle. I, *the thalamus has been removed on the right side. The choroid plexus is attached along the choroidal fissure located between the fornix and thalamus. The tail of the caudate nucleus courses in the roof of the temporal horn above the hippocampus.* J, *the axial section on the left side has been extended through the midportion of the cerebral peduncle and the coronal section through the thalamus. The thalamus forms the floor of the body of the ventricle. At the midthalamic level, the lentiform nucleus is reduced markedly in size as compared with the more anterior levels where it forms a prominent part of the deep gray matter. As the cross section moves posteriorly, the thalamus forms a progressively greater part of the central core of the hemisphere located between the insula and ventricular surface. The temporal horn is located below the lentiform nucleus. The posterior segment of the uncus faces the cerebral peduncle. The bulb of the corpus callosum overlying the forceps major and the calcar avis overlying the calcarine sulcus are exposed in the medial wall of the atrium.* K, *all of the right thalamus and the medial part of the left thalamus have been removed to expose the crural, ambient, and quadrigeminal cisterns. The midbrain forms the medial wall and the parahippocampal and dentate gyri form the lateral wall of the ambient cistern. The crural cistern is located between the posterior uncus segment and the cerebral peduncle. The left lateral geniculate body has been preserved. The optic radiations arise in the lateral geniculate body and pass laterally above the temporal horn.* L, *enlarged view. The body of the fornix is in the lower medial part of the wall of the body of the lateral ventricles. The crus of the fornix forms part of the anterior wall of the atrium and the fimbria sits on the upper surface of the hippocampus in the floor of the temporal horn. The amygdala fills most of the anterior segment of the uncus and the hippocampal head extends into the posterior segment. The posterior commissure, aqueduct, and mamillary bodies are exposed in the walls of the third ventricle. The anterior part of the third ventricular floor between the mamillary bodies and the infundibular recess is quite thin and is the site frequently selected for a third ventriculostomy.* M, *oblique anterior view. The cross section of the right temporal lobe crosses the posterior uncal segment. The floor of the third ventricle has been removed back to the level of the aqueduct to expose the interpeduncular fossa located between the cerebral peduncles and above the pons. The posterior part of the floor of the third ventricle is formed by the midbrain.* N, *enlarged view of the medial part of the posterior segment of the uncus. The posterior uncal segment is divided by an uncal notch into upper and lower parts. The lower part is formed by the parahippocampal gyrus, which is the site of the subicular zones, and the upper part is formed predominantly by the hippocampal head. The inferior choroidal point, the lower end of the choroid plexus and choroidal fissure and the point where the anterior choroidal artery enters the temporal horn is located just behind the head of the hippocampus. The pyramidal and granule cell layers are organized to give the hippocampal formation its characteristic appearance.* O, *the cross section of the right temporal lobe has been extended back to the level of the midportion of the temporal horn. The ambient cistern is limited medially by the midbrain and laterally by the parahippocampal and dentate gyri.* P, *enlarged view. The collateral sulcus cuts deeply into the hemisphere and forms a prominence, the collateral eminence in the floor of the temporal horn on the lateral side of the hippocampus.* A., *artery;* Ant., *anterior;* Calc., *calcar;* Cap., *capsule;* Car., *carotid;* Caud., *caudate;* Chor., *choroid, choroidal;* Cist., *cistern;* CN, *cranial nerve;* Col., *column;* Coll., *collateral;* Comm., *commissure;* Dent., *dentate;* Emin., *eminence;* Ext., *external;* Fiss., *fissure;* For., *foramen;* Gen., *geniculate;* Glob., *globus;* Inf., *inferior;* Int., *internal;* Lam., *lamina;* Lat., *lateral;* Lent., *lentiform;* Mam., *mamillary;* Med., *medial, medullary;* Nucl., *nucleus;* Olf., *olfactory;* Pall., *pallidus;* Parahippo., *parahippocampal;* Ped., *peduncle;* Pell., *pellucidum;* Plex., *plexus;* Post., *posterior;* Pyram., *pyramidal;* Quad., *quadrigeminal;* Seg., *segment;* Sept., *septum;* Sup., *superior;* Temp., *temporal;* Tent., *tentorial;* Term., *terminalis;* Thal. Str., *thalamostriate;* Tr., *tract;* V., *vein;* Vent., *ventricle.*

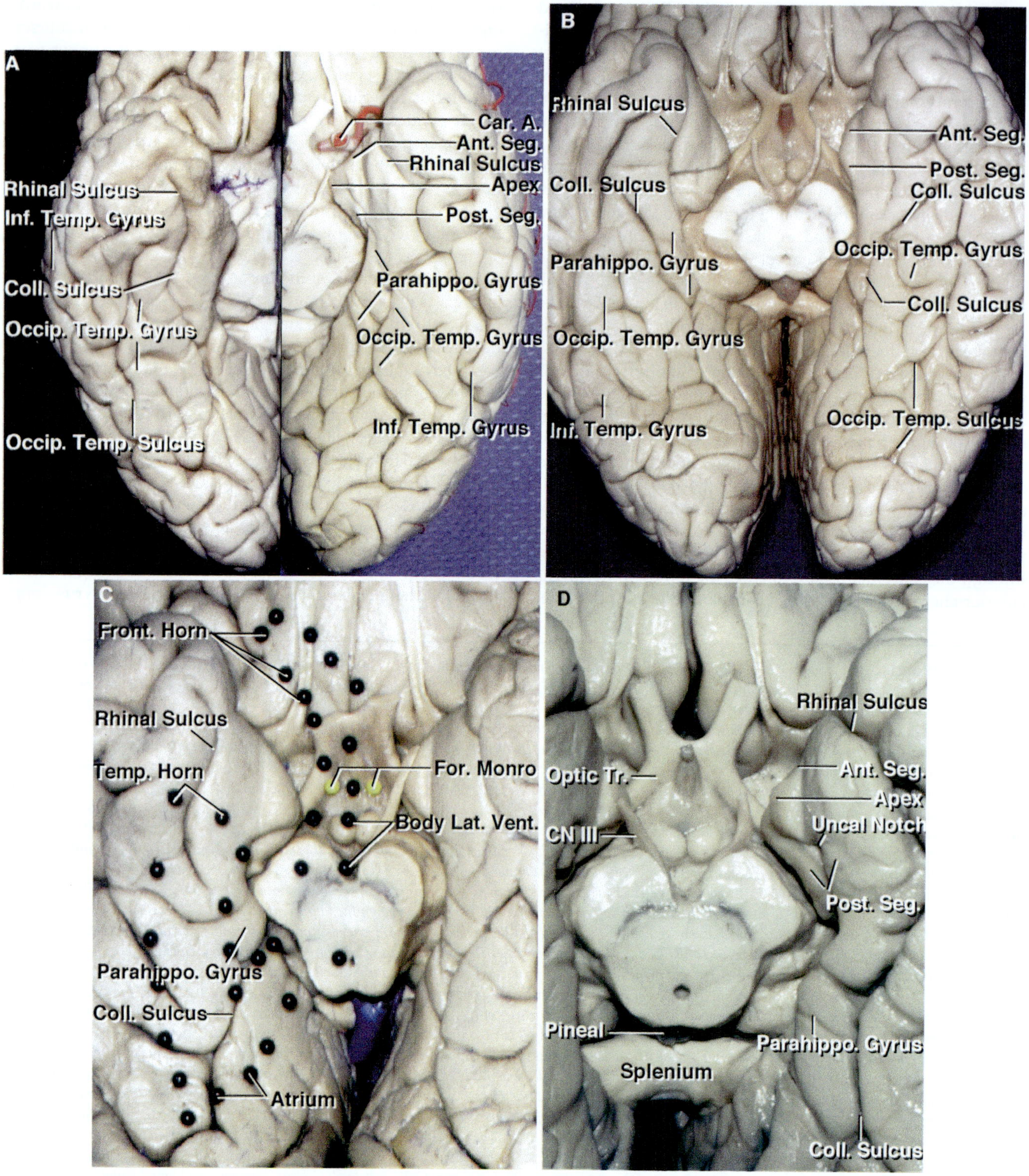

FIGURE 1.9. A, *basal surface of the temporal and occipital lobes from two different brains. The collateral sulcus separates the parahippocampal and occipitotemporal gyri and extends backward onto the occipital lobe. The parahippocampal gyrus is broken up into several segments on both hemispheres by sulci crossing it from medial to lateral. The occipitotemporal gyri that form the middle strip along the long axis of the basal surfaces are discontinuous, as are the inferior temporal gyri that fold from the convexity around the lower margin of the hemispheres. The rhinal sulci that extend along the lateral margin of the uncus are in continuity with the collateral sulci.* B, *another cerebrum. The rhinal sulcus on both sides extends along the lateral uncal margin, but is not continuous with the collateral sulcus as in* A.

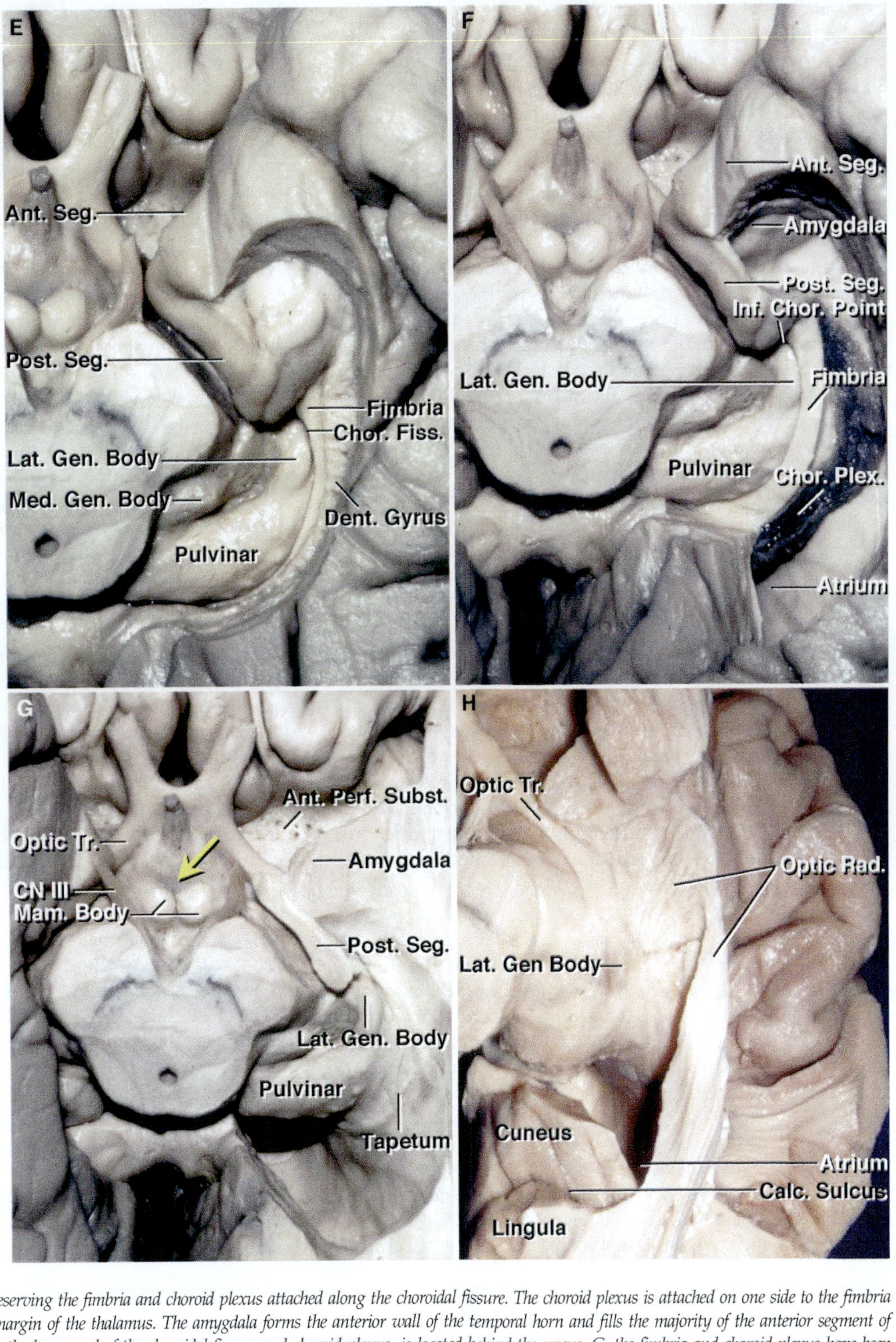

FIGURE 1.9. *Continued* *The parahippocampal, occipitotemporal, and the inferior temporal gyri are broken up into multiple segments. C, enlarged view.* Dark pins *outline the position of the lateral ventricle above the basal surface. The frontal horn is located above the posteromedial part of the basal surface of the frontal lobe. The body of the ventricle is located above the midbrain and thalamus. The temporal horn is located above the collateral sulcus and parahippocampal gyrus. There are prominences, the collateral eminence, in the floor of the temporal horn and the collateral trigone, in the floor of the atrium, that overlie the deep end of the collateral sulcus. D, basal surface of another temporal lobe. The uncus has an anterior segment that faces forward toward the carotid cistern and entrance into the sylvian cistern and a posterior segment that faces posteriorly toward the cerebral peduncle and crural cistern. The apex between the anterior and posterior segment is located lateral to the oculomotor nerve. The medial part of the parahippocampal gyrus faces the ambient cistern located between the lateral side of the midbrain and the parahippocampal gyrus. The rhinal sulcus courses along the lateral margin of the anterior part of the uncus and is continuous with the collateral sulcus. The posterior segment of the uncus is divided into an upper and lower part by the uncal notch. E, the part of the posterior uncal segment below the uncal notch and the medial part of the parahippocampal gyrus have been removed to expose the lower surface of the upper half of the posterior segment that blends posteriorly into the beaded dentate gyrus. The fimbria is exposed above the dentate gyrus. The head of the hippocampus folds into the posterior segment of the uncus. The choroidal fissure located between the thalamus and fimbria extends along the lateral margin of the lateral geniculate body. F, the hippocampus and dentate gyrus have been removed while preserving the fimbria and choroid plexus attached along the choroidal fissure. The choroid plexus is attached on one side to the fimbria and on the opposite side to the lower margin of the thalamus. The amygdala forms the anterior wall of the temporal horn and fills the majority of the anterior segment of the uncus. The inferior choroidal point, the lower end of the choroidal fissure and choroid plexus, is located behind the uncus. G, the fimbria and choroid plexus have been removed to expose the roof of the temporal horn. The lower part of the anterior uncal segment has been removed to expose the amygdala. A small portion of the posterior segment sitting below the optic tract has been preserved. The inferior choroidal point, the most anterior attachment of the choroid plexus in the temporal horn and the lower end of the choroidal fissure, is located behind the head of the hippocampus in front of the lateral geniculate body and at the posterior edge of the cerebral peduncle. The tapetum of the corpus callosum forms the roof and lateral wall of the atrium. (Legend continues on next page.)*

its medial edge and a curved collection of gray matter in its interior that is referred to as Ammon's horn. It sits above and is continuous below with the rounded medial surface of the parahippocampal gyrus referred to as the subicular surface. Ammon's horn is characterized in transverse sections of the hippocampal formation by its reversed C- or comma-shaped orientation and by its tightly packed pyramidal cell layer.

The hippocampus is divided into three parts: head, body, and tail (*Figs. 1.8* and *1.9*). The head of the hippocampus, the anterior and largest part, is directed anteriorly and medially, and forms the upper part of the posterior uncal segment. It is characterized by three or four shallow hippocampal digitations resembling that of a feline paw, giving it the name, pes hippocampus. The initial segment of the fimbria and the choroidal fissure are located at the posterior edge of the hippocampal head. Superiorly, the head of the hippocampus faces the posterior portion of the amygdala that is tilted backward above the hippocampal head to form the anterior part of the roof of the temporal horn. Anterior to the hippocampal head is the uncal recess, a cleft, located between the head of the hippocampus and the amygdala. The body of the hippocampus extends along the medial part of the floor of the temporal horn, narrowing into the tail that disappears as a ventricular structure at the anterior margin of the calcar avis, although histologically, the tail can be traced into a collection of gray matter that covers the inferior surface of the splenium.

The fimbria of the fornix arise on the ventricular surface of the hippocampus behind the head and just behind the choroidal fissure. The temporal horn extends into the medial part of the temporal lobe to just anterior to the hippocampal head and to just behind the amygdala. The temporal horn ends approximately 2.5 cm from the temporal pole. The inferior choroidal point, at the lower end of the choroidal fissure, is located just behind the head of the hippocampus and immediately lateral to the lateral geniculate body.

Basal Surface

The basal surface of the cerebrum has a smaller anterior part formed by the lower surface of the frontal lobe, which conforms to the orbital roof, and a larger posterior part formed by the lower surface of the temporal and occipital lobes, which conforms to the floor of the middle cranial fossa and the upper surface of the tentorium cerebelli.

Frontal Lobe

The entire inferior surface of the frontal lobe is concave from side to side and rests on the cribriform plate, orbital roof, and the lesser wing of the sphenoid bone (*Figs. 1.3* and *1.11*). The olfactory sulcus, which overlies the olfactory bulb and tract, divides the orbital surface into a medial strip of cortex, the gyrus rectus, and a larger lateral part, the orbital gyri, an irregular group of convolutions. The orbital gyri are divided by the roughly H-shaped orbital sulcus into the anterior, medial, posterior, and lateral orbital groups. The anterior orbital gyri are situated between the anterior pole and the transverse limb of the H. The posterior orbital gyri extend posteriorly from the transverse part of the H to the anterior margin of the anterior perforated substance. The lateral orbital gyri are positioned lateral to the lateral vertical limb of the H. The medial orbital gyri are situated between the medial vertical limb of the H and the olfactory sulcus. At a deep level, the anterior part of the genu of the corpus callosum and frontal horn extend forward above the orbital surface to approximately the level of the transverse part of the H-shaped orbital sulcus. The anterior limb of the internal capsule and the caudate and lentiform nuclei are positioned above the anterior perforated substance and the posterior orbital gyri. In the subfrontal approach to the suprasellar area, the exposure extends below the frontal horn and the caudate and lentiform nuclei, which blend below and anteriorly with clear borders into the nucleus basal and accumbens to form a massive gray matter complex above the posterior orbital gyri and anterior perforated substance.

Temporal and Occipital Lobes

The basal surfaces of the temporal and occipital lobes are formed by the same gyri that continue from anterior to posterior across their uninterrupted border (*Figs. 1.3* and *1.9*). They are traversed longitudinally by the longer collateral and occipitotemporal sulci and the shorter rhinal sulcus that divide the region from medial to lateral into the parahippocampal and occipitotemporal gyri and the lower surface of the inferior temporal gyrus. The basal surface of the parahippocampal gyrus forms the medial part of the inferior surface. It extends backward from the temporal pole to the posterior margin of the corpus callosum. Its anterior end projects medially to form the uncus. It is continuous anteriorly with the uncus without a limiting border and continues posteriorly to blend into the isthmus of the cingulate gyrus and lingula.

The collateral sulcus, one of the most constant cerebral sulci, begins near the occipital pole and extends anteriorly, parallel and lateral to the calcarine sulcus. Posteriorly, it separates the lingula and occipitotemporal gyrus, and anteriorly, it courses between the parahippocampal and the occipitotemporal gyri. The collateral sulcus may or may not be continuous anteriorly with the rhinal sulcus, the short sulcus extending along the lateral edge of the uncus. The collateral sulcus is located below the temporal horn and indents deeply into the basal surface producing a prominence, the collateral eminence, in the floor

FIGURE 1.9. *Continued*
H, the tapetum fibers have been removed to expose the fibers of the optic radiation arising from the lateral geniculate body and passing across the roof and around the lateral wall of the temporal horn and the lateral wall of the atrium. Only a thin layer of tapetal fibers separate the optic radiations from the temporal horn and atrium as they pass posteriorly to reach the calcarine sulcus. The cuneus forms the upper bank and the lingula forms the lower bank of the calcarine sulcus. A., *artery;* Ant., *anterior;* Calc., *calcarine;* Car., *carotid;* Chor., *choroid, choroidal;* CN, *cranial nerve;* Coll., *collateral;* Dent., *dentate;* Fiss., *fissure;* For., *foramen;* Front., *frontal;* Gen., *geniculate;* Inf., *inferior;* Lat., *lateral;* Mam., *mamillary;* Med., *medial;* Occip., *occipital;* Parahippo., *parahippocampal;* Perf., *perforated;* Plex., *plexus;* Post., *posterior;* Rad., *radiation;* Seg., *segment;* Subst., *substance;* Temp., *temporal;* Tr., *tract;* Vent., *ventricle.*

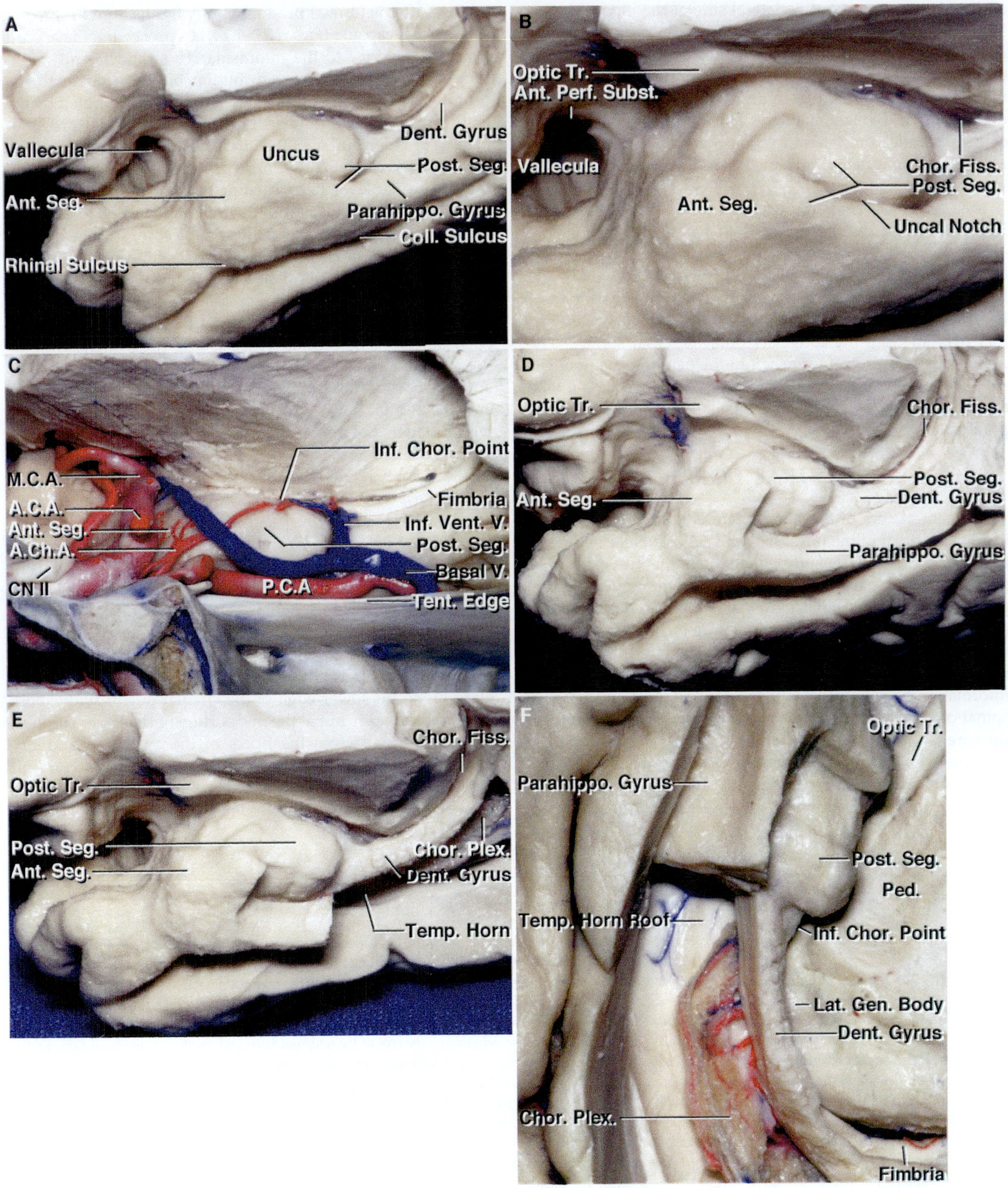

FIGURE 1.10. *Medial surface of the temporal lobe and uncus.* A, *the uncus, a medial projection at the anterior end of the parahippocampal gyrus, has an anterior and posterior segment. The sylvian vallecula is the site where the middle cerebral artery exits the carotid cistern to enter the sylvian cistern. The collateral sulcus extends along the lateral margin of the parahippocampal gyrus, and the rhinal sulcus extends along the lateral edge of the uncus.* *(Legend continues on next page.)*

of the temporal horn on the lateral side of the hippocampus. Posteriorly, in the area below the atrial floor, the collateral sulcus also indents deeply to produce a prominence in the triangular atrial floor called the collateral trigone. The temporal horn can be exposed from below by opening through the deep end of the collateral sulcus. The occipitotemporal sulcus courses parallel and lateral to the collateral sulcus and separates the occipitotemporal sulcus and basal surface of the inferior temporal gyrus.

The lower surface of the occipital lobe overlies the tentorium cerebelli (*Figs. 1.3* and *1.9*). It lies behind a line that extends laterally from the anterior end of the calcarine sulcus to the preoccipital notch. The inferior surface is formed by the lower part of the lingual gyrus or lingula, the posterior part of the occipitotemporal and the part of the lateral occipital gyri that overlap from the convexity onto the basal surface. The lingual gyrus blends anteriorly into the parahippocampal gyrus. The markings on the inferior surface of the occipital lobe are the posterior extension of the collateral and occipitotemporal sulci.

CENTRAL CORE

The central core of the hemisphere is located between the insula and the midline (*Figs. 1.12* and *1.13*). It is located deep to the pars triangularis and opercularis of the inferior frontal gyrus, the lower part of the pre- and postcentral gyri, anterior part of the supramarginal gyrus, and the superior temporal gyrus. The structures in the central core include the internal, external, and the extreme capsules, the caudate and lentiform nuclei, the claustrum and thalamus, and the fornix. All of the information passing between the cortex and the brainstem and spinal cord is relayed in or carried by fibers passing through the core.

In the core, medial to the anterior part of the insulae, the gray matter is formed predominantly by the caudate nucleus with a smaller contribution by the lentiform nucleus, and the white matter is formed predominantly by the anterior limb of the internal capsule (*Figs. 1.12–1.14*). In proceeding backward from the anterior to the midinsular level and lateral to the foramen of Monro, the contribution of the caudate to the central core is greatly diminished, and that contributed by the lentiform nucleus (putamen plus globus pallidus) predominates. The contribution of the internal capsule to the size of the core also increases greatly in proceeding from the anterior to the midinsular level. In proceeding backward from the middle to the posterior insular level, the thalamus begins to predominate as the dominant gray matter in the core, and the mass of white matter, representing the posterior limb of the internal capsule, is much greater than in the anterior part of the core.

The core is attached to the remainder of the hemisphere by the cerebral isthmus. The isthmus is located deep to the circular sulcus of the insula. There is a portion of the isthmus deep to the full circumference of the circular sulcus. The anterior part of the isthmus that separates the circular sulcus and the frontal horn is formed by a relatively thin layer of white matter. In cross section, the lateral edge of the frontal horn and circular sulcus seem to project toward each other, separated only by the isthmus (*Fig. 1.12, A–C*). It is the same at the posterior isthmus, where the circular sulcus and atrium are separated by only the relatively thin layer of white matter forming the isthmus. The transverse temporal gyri converge posteriorly and medially toward the lateral edge of the isthmus. The lower isthmus that connects the temporal lobe to the remainder of the hemisphere is also referred to as the stem of the temporal lobe. The lower isthmus is positioned between the circular sulcus and the roof of the temporal horn. Opening through the isthmus with an incision directed slightly downward along the lower edge of the circular sulcus will expose the temporal horn, but at the midportion of the lower isthmus, the incision will cross the fibers of the optic and auditory radiations just lateral to where they leave the lateral and medial geniculate bodies. The upper part of the isthmus separates the upper part of the circular sulcus and the body of the

FIGURE 1.10. *Continued*
The rhinal and collateral sulci are frequently not continuous, although they are in this case. B, *enlarged view. The posterior segment of the uncus is divided by the uncal notch into an upper and lower part. The lower part is formed by the parahippocampal gyrus and the upper part is formed predominantly by the hippocampal head. The dentate gyrus, at its anterior margin, blends into the upper part of the posterior segment.* C, *medial view of the uncus directed across the sella and tentorial edge. The carotid artery and middle cerebral artery face the anterior segment of the uncus. The posterior cerebral artery courses along the medial side of the posterior segment. The anterior choroidal artery ascends as it passes backward across the anterior segment to reach the upper part of the posterior segment. The anterior choroidal artery enters, and the inferior ventricular vein exits, the choroidal fissure by passing through the inferior choroidal point located just behind the head of the hippocampus and the posterior uncal segment. The inferior ventricular vein drains the roof of the temporal horn and empties in the basal vein.* D, *the medial part of the parahippocampal gyrus and the lower part of the posterior uncal segment have been removed to expose the dentate gyrus and the choroidal fissure. The beaded dentate gyrus blends into the posterior edge of the upper part of the posterior uncal segment and the medial side of the hippocampal head.* E, *additional parahippocampal gyrus has been removed while preserving the dentate gyrus to expose the choroid plexus in the temporal horn. The amygdala, partially enclosed in the anterior segment, forms the anterior wall of the temporal horn.* F, *inferior view of* E. *The part of the parahippocampal gyrus, lateral to the dentate gyrus, has been removed to expose the roof of the temporal horn, which is formed by the tapetum, the thin layer of fibers from the corpus callosum that separate the optic radiation from the wall of the temporal horn. The dentate gyrus and fimbria have been preserved. The choroid plexus is attached along the choroidal fissure located between the fimbria and lower margin of the thalamus. The inferior choroidal point at the lower end of the choroidal fissure is located behind the posterior uncal segment and the hippocampal head. The dentate gyrus and fimbria extend along the lateral edge of the lateral geniculate body.* A.C.A., *anterior cerebral artery;* A.Ch.A., *anterior choroidal artery;* Ant., *anterior;* Chor., *choroid, choroidal;* CN, *cranial nerve;* Coll., *collateral;* Dent., *dentate;* Fiss., *fissure;* Gen., *geniculate;* Inf., *inferior;* Lat., *lateral;* M.C.A., *medial cerebral artery;* P.C.A., *posterior cerebral artery;* Parahippo., *parahippocampal;* Ped., *peduncle;* Perf., *perforated;* Plex., *plexus;* Post., *posterior;* Seg., *segment;* Subst., *substance;* Temp., *temporal;* Tent., *tentorial;* Tr., *tract;* V., *vein;* Vent., *ventricular.*

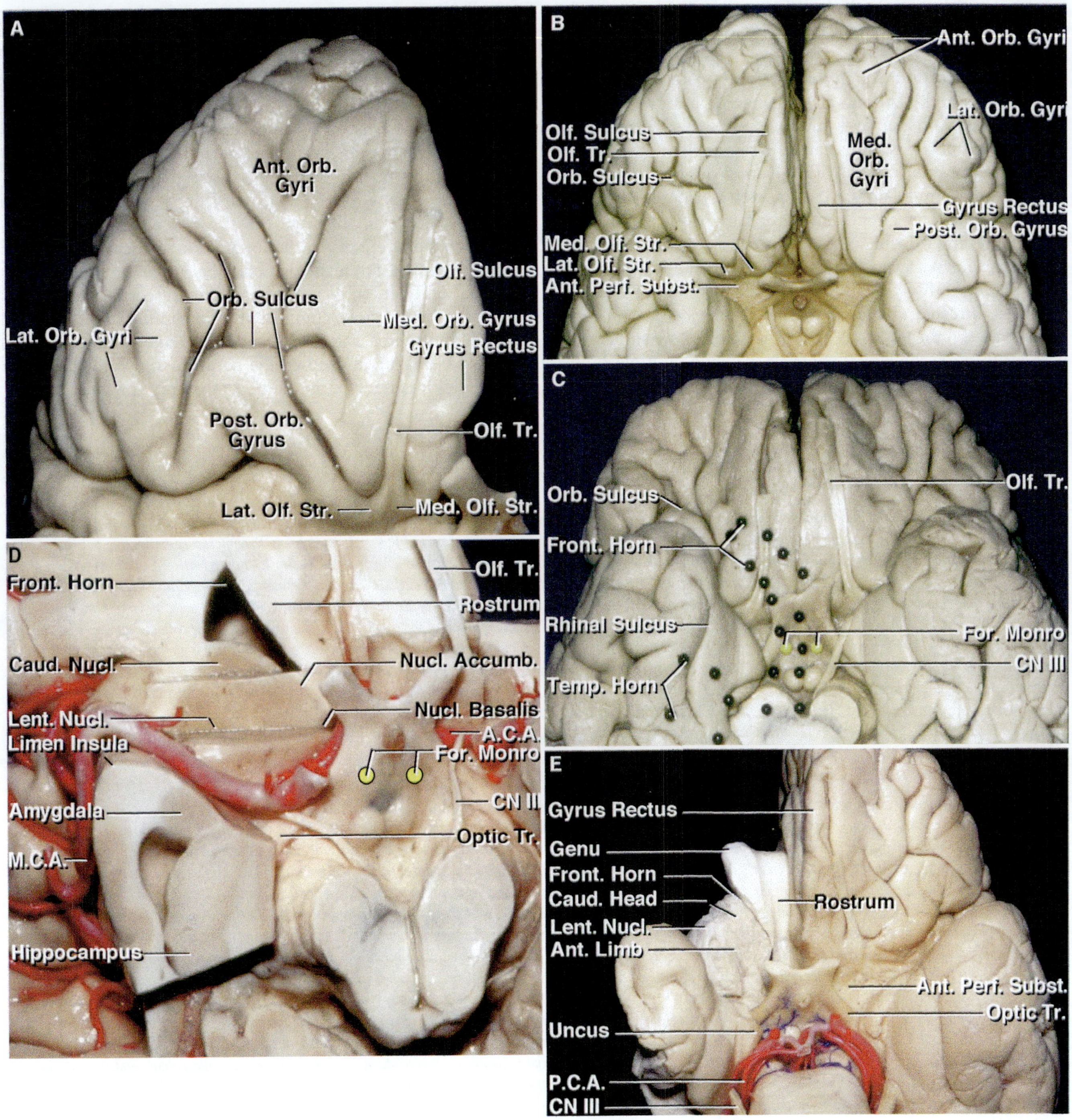

FIGURE 1.11. *Orbital surface of the frontal lobe. A, the olfactory tract extends along the olfactory sulcus on the lateral side of the gyrus rectus and divides at the edge of the anterior perforated substance into the medial and lateral olfactory striae. The orbital surface lateral to the gyrus rectus is divided by an H-shaped sulcus into anterior, posterior, medial, and lateral orbital gyri. B, another cerebrum. The olfactory sulci separate the gyrus rectus medially from the orbital gyri laterally. The orbital surface lateral to the gyrus rectus is divided by a number of sulci that tend to form an H-shaped configuration and divide the area into anterior, posterior, medial, and lateral orbital gyri. The most lateral of the lateral orbital gyri is continuous with the pars orbitalis of the inferior frontal gyrus. C, orbital surfaces of another hemisphere. The location of the frontal and temporal horns deep within the hemisphere has been outlined using colored* black pins. *The frontal horn extends forward in the frontal lobe to approximately the level of the transverse part of the H-shaped orbital sulcus. The deep site of the foramen of Monro, shown with* yellow pins, *in relationship to the basal surface is anterior to the mamillary bodies. D, the lower part of the right frontal lobe has been removed to expose the frontal horn. The caudate nucleus forms the lateral wall of the frontal horn and the rostrum of the corpus callosum forms the floor. At a more superior axial level, the caudate and lentiform nuclei are separated by the anterior limb of the internal capsule, but at this level below the anterior limb of the internal capsule, the nuclei form a solid, unbroken mass of gray (Legend continues on next page.)*

lateral ventricle and is thicker than at the other sites. The upper isthmus also contains the fibers forming the internal capsule.

Opening directly through the superior, posterior, and inferior margins of the isthmus risks damaging important motor, somatosensory, visual, and auditory pathways. Opening the anterior part of the isthmus carries less risk than opening the middle and posterior parts. Yaşargil and Wieser (11) reach the amygdala for amygdalohippocampectomy using a 1- to 2-cm incision through the circular sulcus and the lower isthmus just behind the limen insula. A number of operative routes that access various surfaces of the central core should be considered before transecting a part of the isthmus. These approaches, directed along the sylvian or interhemispheric fissures, between the basal surface of the hemisphere and cranial base, or through the lateral ventricle, provide multiple routes that access various surfaces and part of the central core. The routes to these deep areas are reviewed further below, in the discussion, and also in Chapter 5.

WHITE MATTER

The white matter of the cerebrum underlies the outer lamina of gray matter, intervenes between the cortical gray matter and the gray matter of the basal ganglia, and encases the ventricles (*Figs. 1.7, 1.15,* and *1.16*). In a horizontal section above the corpus callosum, the subcortical white matter in each hemisphere forms a semiovoid mass called the centrum semiovale. The white matter contains three types of fibers: association fibers interconnecting different cortical regions of the same hemisphere, commissural fibers interconnecting the two hemispheres across the median plane, and projection fibers passing up and down the neuraxis and connecting the cortex with caudal parts of the brain and spinal cord. The

FIGURE 1.11. *Continued*
matter located above the anterior perforated substance and adjoining part of the orbital surface. In addition, the lentiform and caudate nuclei blend medially without a clear border into the nucleus basalis and nucleus accumbens. The nucleus basalis is located in the medial part of this gray mass below the anterior commissure, and the nucleus accumbens is situated in front of the nucleus basalis. The amygdala is located below and blends into the lentiform nucleus at its upper border. E, *fiber dissection of the right hemisphere showing the relationship of the genu and rostrum of the corpus callosum to the orbital surface. The anterior margin of the genu of the corpus callosum is located above the midportion of the basal surface. The rostrum of the corpus callosum forms the floor of the frontal horn. The genu, along with its large fiber bundle, the forceps minor, forms the anterior wall of the frontal horn. The caudate nucleus forms the lateral wall of the frontal horn. The basal side of the caudate nucleus and the lentiform nucleus, formed by the putamen and globus pallidus, blend together in the area below the anterior limb of the frontal capsule to form a globular mass of gray matter that extends almost unbroken from the lower part of the frontal horn to the insula. At a more superior level, the anterior limb of the internal capsule cuts into the interval between the caudate and lentiform nuclei dividing them into separate nuclei.* A.C.A., *anterior cerebral artery;* Accumb., *accumbens;* Ant., *anterior;* Caud., *caudate;* CN, *cranial nerve;* For., *foramen;* Front., *frontal;* Lat., *lateral;* Lent., *lentiform;* M.C.A., *medial cerebral artery;* Med., *medial;* Nucl., *nucleus;* Olf., *olfactory;* Orb., *orbital;* P.C.A., *posterior cerebral artery;* Perf., *perforated;* Post., *posterior;* Str., *striae;* Subst., *substance;* Temp., *temporal;* Tr., *tract.*

FIGURE 1.12. *Central core of the hemisphere.* A, *superior view. The central core is the portion located between the insular surface laterally and the lateral and third ventricles medially. We refer to the narrow strip of white matter deep to the circular sulcus and connecting the central core to the remaining hemisphere as the cerebral isthmus. The isthmus, at the margin of the core, conveys all the fibers related to all of the motor and sensory pathways, including those that form the internal capsule and optic radiations. The anterior margin of the circular sulcus is separated from the frontal horn by the relatively thin anterior part of the isthmus, and the posterior margin of the circular sulcus is separated from the atrium by the narrow posterior part of the isthmus. The upper margin of the isthmus separating the upper margin of the circular sulcus and the lateral ventricle is somewhat thicker than the anterior or posterior margin of the isthmus. The transverse temporal gyri, the most anterior of which is Heschl's gyrus, are located lateral to the posterior margin of the insula on the planum temporale. An area without gyri anterior to the planum temporale on the anterior part of the upper surface of the temporal lobe, called the planum polare, faces the anterior part of the lateral surface of the insula. The transverse temporal gyri radiate forward and laterally from the posterior isthmus located lateral to the atrium. The sylvian point, the site at which the last insular branch of the middle cerebral artery turns laterally from the insula, is located lateral to the posterior isthmus and the posterior part of the circular sulcus.* B, *superior view of the central core and the anterior and posterior parts of the cerebral isthmus. The transverse temporal gyri seem to radiate laterally and forward from an apex situated lateral to the atrium, the posterior part of the circular sulcus, and the posterior isthmus. The section extends through the anterior and posterior limb and genu of the internal capsule, thalamus, and lentiform and caudate nuclei. The thalamus is located directly above the midbrain in the center of the tentorial incisura.* C, *superolateral view of the insula, circular sulcus, and the anterior and posterior isthmi. The circular sulcus extends completely around the margin of the insula and is located superficial to the white matter forming the cerebral isthmus. The isthmus is the thinnest area between the insular and ventricular surfaces.* D, *the upper surface of the left temporal lobe has been retracted to expose the lower part of the circular sulcus and isthmus located deep to the circular sulcus. An incision extending through the thin isthmus at the lower margin of the circular sulcus will expose the temporal horn, but will also cut across the optic and auditory radiations and the sublenticular part of the internal capsule, unless only a short segment of the anterior part of the lower isthmus is opened.* E, *lateral view of the central core. The cerebral hemisphere has been removed by dividing the isthmus, located deep to the circular sulcus and extending around the margin of the insula. The corpus callosum and fibers crossing the midline were also divided. Middle cerebral branches course along the insular surface. The lower margin of the circular sulcus is located deep to the superior temporal sulcus.* F, *all of the central core has been removed. It includes the caudate and lentiform nuclei, thalamus, and some of the corona radiata and internal capsule. The medial part of the core has been separated from the ventricular surface by opening the choroidal fissure, the natural cleft and cleavage plane between the thalamus and fornix. The body, crus, and fimbria of the fornix form the outer border of the choroidal fissure. The transverse temporal gyri, forming the planum temporale, radiate forward from the posterior edge of the circular sulcus located lateral to the atrium. The quadrigeminal cistern is located medial to the crus of the fornix.* A.C.A., *anterior cerebral artery;* Ant., *anterior;* Call., *callosum;* Cap., *capsule;* Caud., *caudate;* Circ., *circular;* Cist., *cistern;* Corp., *corpus;* Front., *frontal;* Int., *internal;* Lat., *lateral;* Lent., *lentiform;* M.C.A., *medial cerebral artery;* Nucl., *nucleus;* Post., *posterior;* Quad., *quadrigeminal;* Seg., *segment;* Str., *straight;* Temp., *temporal, temporale;* Tent., *tentorial;* Trans., *transverse;* Vent., *ventricle.*

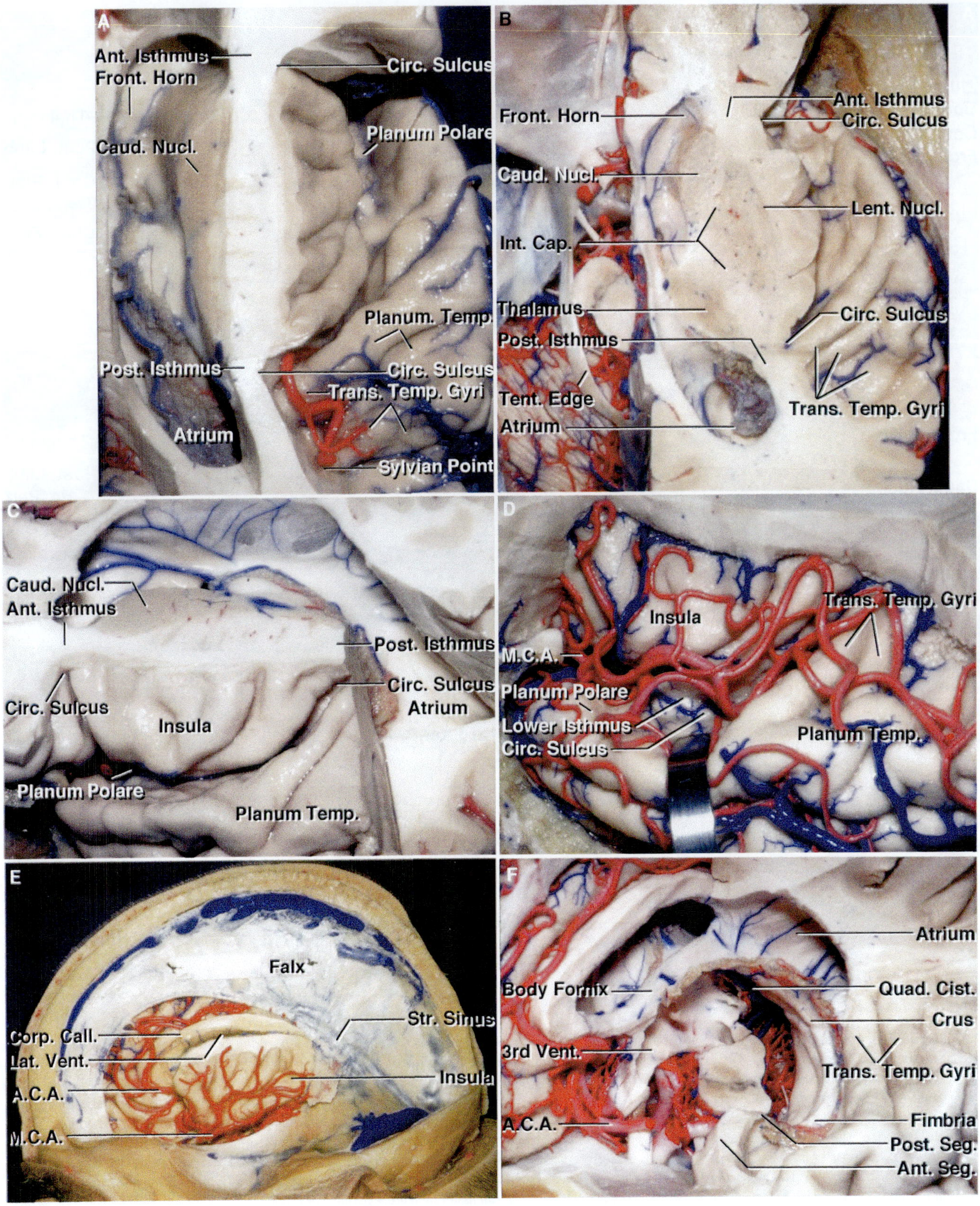
A
Ant. Isthmus
Front. Horn
Circ. Sulcus
Planum Polare
Caud. Nucl.
Planum. Temp.
Post. Isthmus
Circ. Sulcus
Trans. Temp. Gyri
Atrium
Sylvian Point
B
Ant. Isthmus
Front. Horn
Circ. Sulcus
Caud. Nucl.
Lent. Nucl.
Int. Cap.
Thalamus
Circ. Sulcus
Post. Isthmus
Tent. Edge
Trans. Temp. Gyri
Atrium
C
Caud. Nucl.
Ant. Isthmus
Post. Isthmus
Circ. Sulcus
Atrium
Circ. Sulcus
Insula
Planum Polare
Planum Temp.
D
Trans. Temp. Gyri
Insula
M.C.A.
Planum Polare
Lower Isthmus
Planum Temp.
Circ. Sulcus
E
Falx
Str. Sinus
Corp. Call.
Lat. Vent.
Insula
A.C.A.
M.C.A.
F
Atrium
Body Fornix
Quad. Cist.
Crus
3rd Vent.
Trans. Temp. Gyri
A.C.A.
Fimbria
Post. Seg.
Ant. Seg.

FIGURE 1.12.

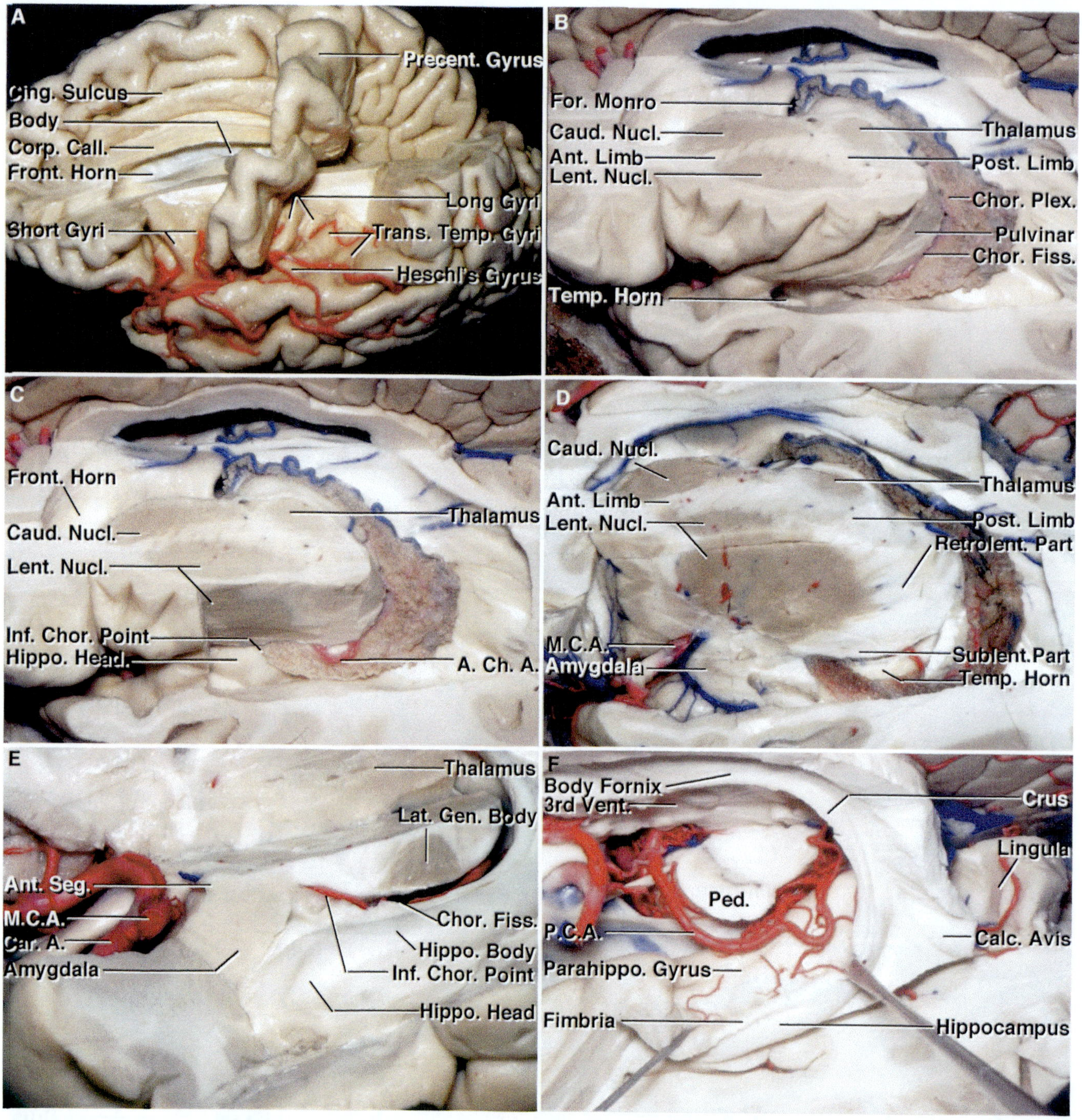

FIGURE 1.13. *Stepwise dissection of the central core of the hemisphere. A, superior view. The central core is the part of the cerebrum located between the insula and the third and lateral ventricles. The upper part of the left hemisphere, except the precentral gyrus, has been removed to expose the frontal horn and body of the ventricle. The precentral gyrus is located lateral to the posterior part of the body of the ventricle and lateral to the splenium of the corpus callosum. The postcentral gyrus, which has been removed, faces the most anterior of the transverse temporal gyri, called Heschl's gyrus. The short insular gyri are exposed anterior to and the long gyri behind the precentral gyrus. B, the axial section extending through the central core crosses the anterior and posterior limb and genu of the internal capsule, the thalamus, and the lentiform and caudate nuclei at the level of the foramen of Monro. The lateral wall of the atrium and the roof of the temporal horn have been removed by dividing the white matter along the circular sulcus of the insula. C, the posterior part of the lateral surface of the insula has been removed to expose the lateral surface of the lentiform nucleus. The choroid plexus is attached along the choroidal fissure that extends from the foramen of Monro to the inferior choroidal point located just behind the head of the hippocampus. D, the anterior part of the insular cortex has been removed to expose the lentiform nucleus in the area above and behind the sylvian fissure, and above the anterior perforated substance and temporal horn. The middle cerebral artery, in the stem of the sylvian fissure, passes below the anterior part of the caudate and lentiform nuclei. The sublenticular and retrolenticular parts of the internal capsule, including the optic and auditory radiations, pass below and behind the lentiform nucleus.*

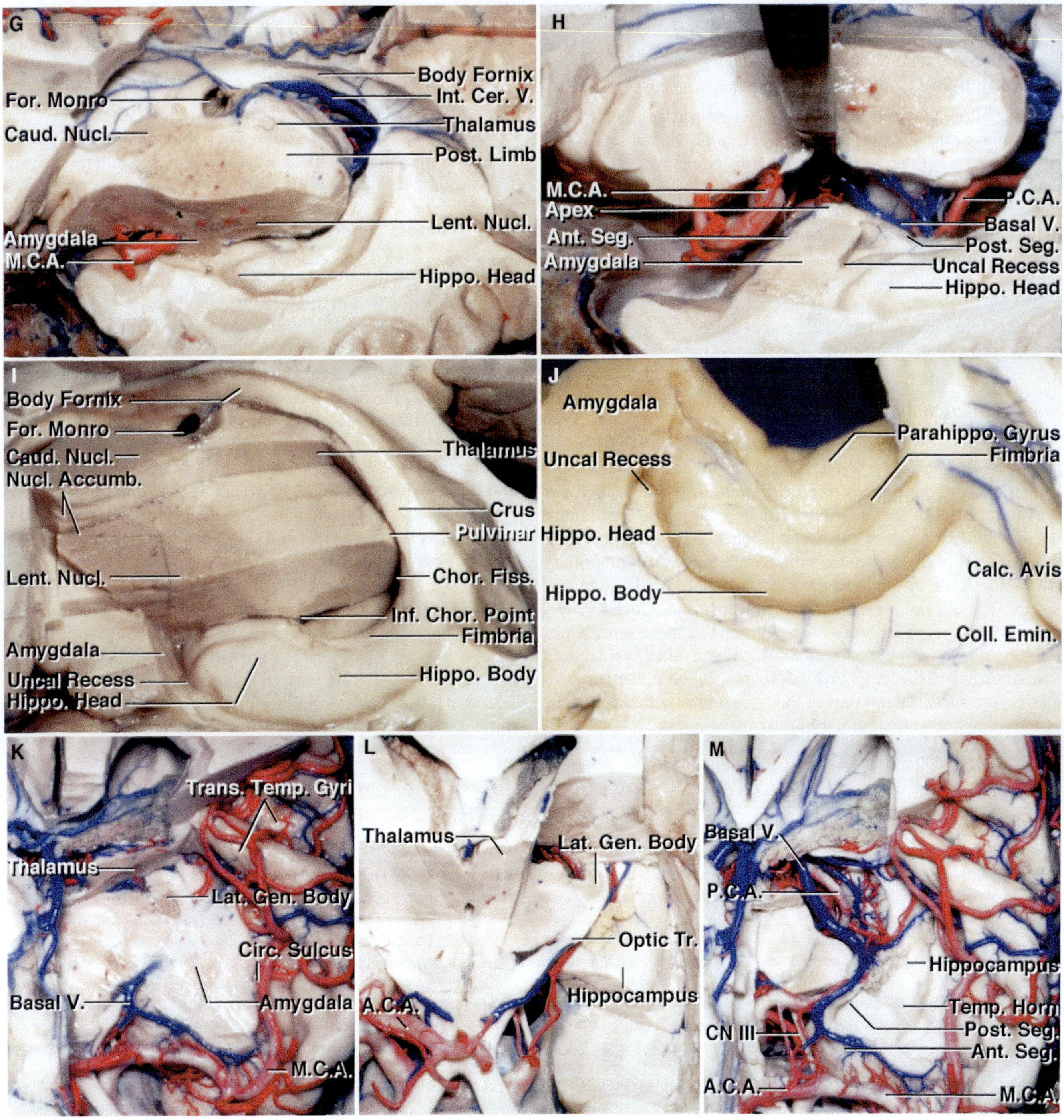

FIGURE 1.13. *Continued*

The anterior limb of the internal capsule is located between the caudate and lentiform nuclei, and the posterior limb is positioned between the lentiform nucleus and thalamus. E, *enlarged view of the lower margin of the thalamus and upper part of the uncus. The anterior segment of the uncus contains the amygdala and faces the carotid and middle cerebral arteries. The posterior segment of the uncus contains the head of the hippocampus and is located anterior to the lower end of the choroidal fissure. The lateral geniculate body is located just above the choroidal fissure and body of the hippocampus. The choroidal fissure, along which the choroid plexus is attached, is located between the fimbria and the thalamus. The inferior choroidal point, the lower end of the choroidal fissure, is located behind the hippocampal head.* F, *the thalamus has been removed and the fimbria of the fornix retracted laterally to expose the parahippocampal gyrus medial to the fimbria. The posterior cerebral artery courses through the crural and ambient cisterns on the medial side of the parahippocampal gyrus. The upper lip of the calcarine sulcus, formed by the cuneus, has been removed to expose the lower lip formed by the lingula. The deep end of the calcarine sulcus forms a prominence, the calcar avis, in the medial wall of the atrium.* G, *another hemisphere. (Legend continues on next page.)*

fornix, which contains both projection and commissural fibers, is considered below, under Commissural Fibers.

Association Fibers

Association fibers are of two types: short arcuate fibers that interconnect adjacent gyri and long arcuate fibers that interconnect widely separated gyri. The long arcuate fibers are situated deep to the short fibers and form several bundles. In our dissections of the white matter, the uncinate, cingulum, and superior longitudinal fasciculi have been the most distinct and identifiable (*Figs. 1.15* and *1.16*). Another association fiber bundle encountered in the ventricular margin is the stria terminalis (*Figs. 1.7* and *1.16M*). It arises in the amygdala and courses along the border between the caudate nucleus and the thalamus in the wall of the lateral ventricle deep to the thalamostriate vein.

Uncinate Fasciculus

The uncinate fasciculus is a hook-shaped bundle of fibers that curves around the stem of the sylvian fissure and connects the frontal and temporal lobes (*Figs. 1.15* and *1.16*). It is located at the lateral edge of the anterior perforated substance bordering the anteroinferior part of the insula. Its fibers course through the limen insulae and produce the prominence at the junction of the sphenoidal and operculoinsular compartments of the sylvian fissure. The uncinate fasciculus has an upper and a lower component. The lower part connects the gyri on the orbital surface of the frontal lobe with the parahippocampal and other gyri on the medial surface of the temporal lobe. The upper component unites gyri on the superolateral part of the frontal lobe with the cortex of the more lateral temporal gyri near the temporal pole.

Cingulum

The cingulum courses along the medial aspect of the cerebral hemisphere, following the curve of and forming much of the white matter within the cingulate gyrus (*Fig. 1.7*). It contains long- and short-association fibers that follow the curve of the cingulate gyrus and corpus callosum. It interconnects the subcallosal and paraolfactory areas located below the anterior part of the corpus callosum, the cingulate gyrus above the corpus callosum, and the isthmus of the cingulate sulcus and parahippocampal gyri located behind and below the corpus callosum.

Superior Longitudinal Fasciculus

The superior longitudinal fasciculus, the largest of the bundles, is located along the upper and lateral border of the lentiform nucleus and insula (*Figs. 1.15* and *1.16*). It arches backward from the frontal lobe lateral to the internal capsule and through the parietal to the occipital lobe, where it arches downward and forward to reach the temporal lobe. Less distinct fasciculi seen on our fiber dissections include the inferior longitudinal fasciculus that courses near but separated from the walls of the temporal and occipital horns by the optic radiations and the tapetum of the corpus callosum, and interconnects the occipital and temporal lobes. Other less distinctive and deeper bundles interconnect the frontal, occipital, and temporal lobes.

Projection Fibers

The projection fibers pass up and down the neural axis. Above the level of the thalamus, these projection fibers are arranged in a radiating pattern called the corona radiata (*Figs. 1.15* and *1.16*). The corona are continuous caudally with the more compact internal capsule whose fibers collect to form the

FIGURE 1.13. *Continued*
The choroid plexus has been removed to expose the choroidal fissure located between the thalamus and fornix. The lateral part of the body of the fornix has been removed to expose the internal cerebral veins in the roof of the third ventricle. The nuclear mass, formed by the caudate and lentiform nuclei, extends above the middle cerebral artery and the roof of the stem of the sylvian fissure, formed by the anterior perforated substance and posterior part of the orbital surface of the frontal lobe. The amygdala is positioned behind and below the middle cerebral artery. H, the incision has been extended forward from the inferior choroidal point through the amygdala. The amygdala occupies the anterior segment of the uncus and is crossed on its upper anterior surface by the middle cerebral artery. The head of the hippocampus blends into the posterior uncal segment. The middle cerebral artery courses above the anterior uncal segment and the posterior cerebral artery and basal vein course medial to the posterior segment. I, much of the thalamus has been removed to expose the body, crus, and fimbria of the fornix forming the outer margin of the choroidal fissure. The axial section extends through the area below the anterior limb of the internal capsule and anterior commissure where the caudate and lentiform nuclei and the nucleus accumbens and basalis blend together to form a massive collection of gray matter above the posterior part of the orbital surface of the frontal lobe and anterior perforated substance. J, axial sections through the temporal lobe and the anterior and posterior segments of the uncus. The amygdala fills the anterior segment and the head of the hippocampus fills the upper part of the posterior segment. The fimbria arises on the surface of the hippocampus. The parahippocampal gyrus extends medially below the hippocampus. The collateral eminence overlies the deep end of the collateral sulcus that runs along the basal surface on the lateral side of the parahippocampal gyrus. The hippocampus meets the calcar avis in the anterior part of the atrium. K, anterosuperior view. The axial section of the left hemisphere extends through the sylvian fissure, lateral geniculate body, amygdala, and the thin layer of white matter in the temporal stem below the lower edge of the circular sulcus. L, the cross sections extend along the optic tract and through the lower margin of the thalamus. The optic tract passes lateral to the lower margin of the thalamus to reach the lateral geniculate body. M, the optic tract and the thin layer of gray and white matter at the lower margin of the insula and circular sulcus that forms the stem of the temporal lobe have been removed to expose the temporal horn and the cisterns between the midbrain and parahippocampal gyrus. The anterior segment of the uncus faces the carotid and middle cerebral arteries. The apex faces the oculomotor nerve. The posterior segment faces the cerebral peduncle, crural cistern, posterior cerebral artery, and basal vein. A., *artery;* A.C.A., *anterior cerebral artery;* A.Ch.A., *anterior choroidal artery;* Accumb., *accumbens;* Ant., *anterior;* Calc., *calcar;* Call., *callosum;* Car., *carotid;* Caud., *caudate;* Cer., *cerebral;* Chor., *choroidal;* Cing., *cingulate;* Circ., *circular;* CN, *cranial nerve;* Coll., *collateral;* Corp., *corpus;* Emin., *eminence;* Fiss., *fissure;* For., *foramen;* Front., *frontal;* Gen., *geniculate;* Hippo., *hippocampal;* Inf., *inferior;* Int., *internal;* Lat., *lateral;* Lent., *lentiform;* M.C.A., *medial cerebral artery;* Nucl., *nucleus;* P.C.A., *posterior cerebral artery;* Parahippo., *parahippocampal;* Ped., *peduncle;* Plex., *plexus;* Post., *posterior;* Precent., *precentral;* Retrolent., *retrolenticular;* Seg., *segment;* Sublent., *sublenticular;* Temp., *temporal;* Tr., *tract;* Trans., *transverse;* V., *vein;* Vent., *ventricle.*

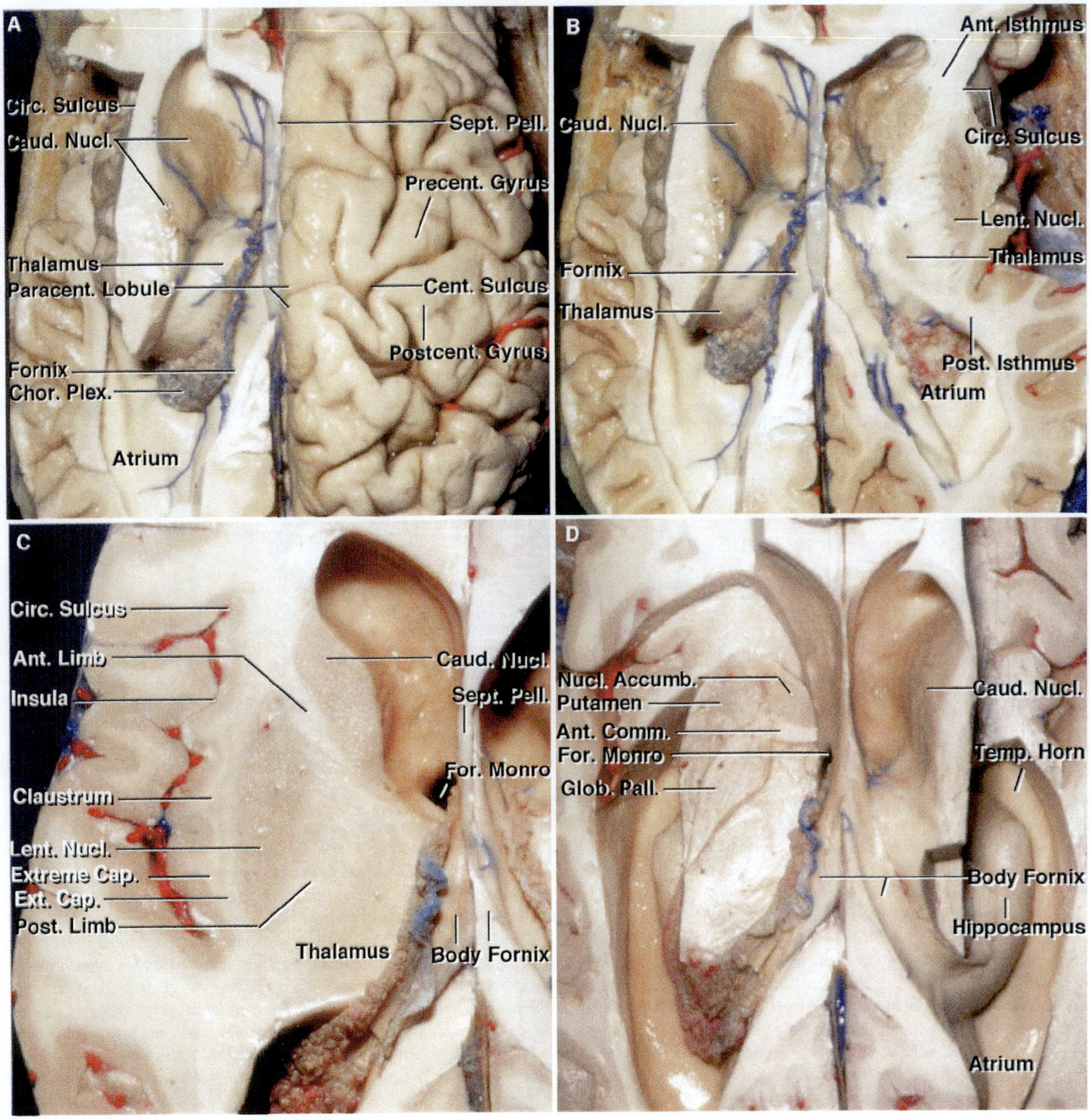

FIGURE 1.14. *Axial cross sections of the cerebral hemisphere and central core. A, superior view. The part of the left hemisphere above the upper edge of the insula and circular sulcus has been removed. The central sulcus ascends on the right hemisphere and intersects the superior margin of the hemisphere above the posterior part of the body of the lateral ventricle. The upper part of the body of the caudate that extends above the level of the upper margin of the circular sulcus has been removed. Anteriorly, the circular sulcus is located superficial to the anterior edge of the caudate head. The posterior edge of the circular sulcus is situated lateral to the anterior wall of the atrium. B, the section of the right hemisphere has been extended through the upper part of the lentiform nucleus, thalamus, and caudate head. On the left side, the axial section remains at the level of the upper edge of the circular sulcus. The anterior part of the cerebral isthmus is located between the frontal horn and anterior part of the circular sulcus and the posterior part is located between the posterior part of the circular sulcus and the anterior part of the atrium. C, the external and extreme capsule and the claustrum fill the interval between the insula and the lentiform nucleus. The axial section in the left hemisphere extends through the internal capsule just above and lateral to the foramen of Monro where the genu of the capsule reaches the ventricular surface. The anterior limb of the internal capsule is separated from the frontal horn by the caudate nucleus and the posterior limb is separated from the body of the ventricle by the thalamus, but the genu reaches the ventricular surface lateral to the foramen of Monro. D, the section through the left hemisphere has been extended downward below the frontal horn to the level of the anterior commissure. The anterior part of the section extends through the deep gray matter below the frontal horn anterior limb of the internal capsule. At higher levels, the lentiform* (Legend continues on next page.)

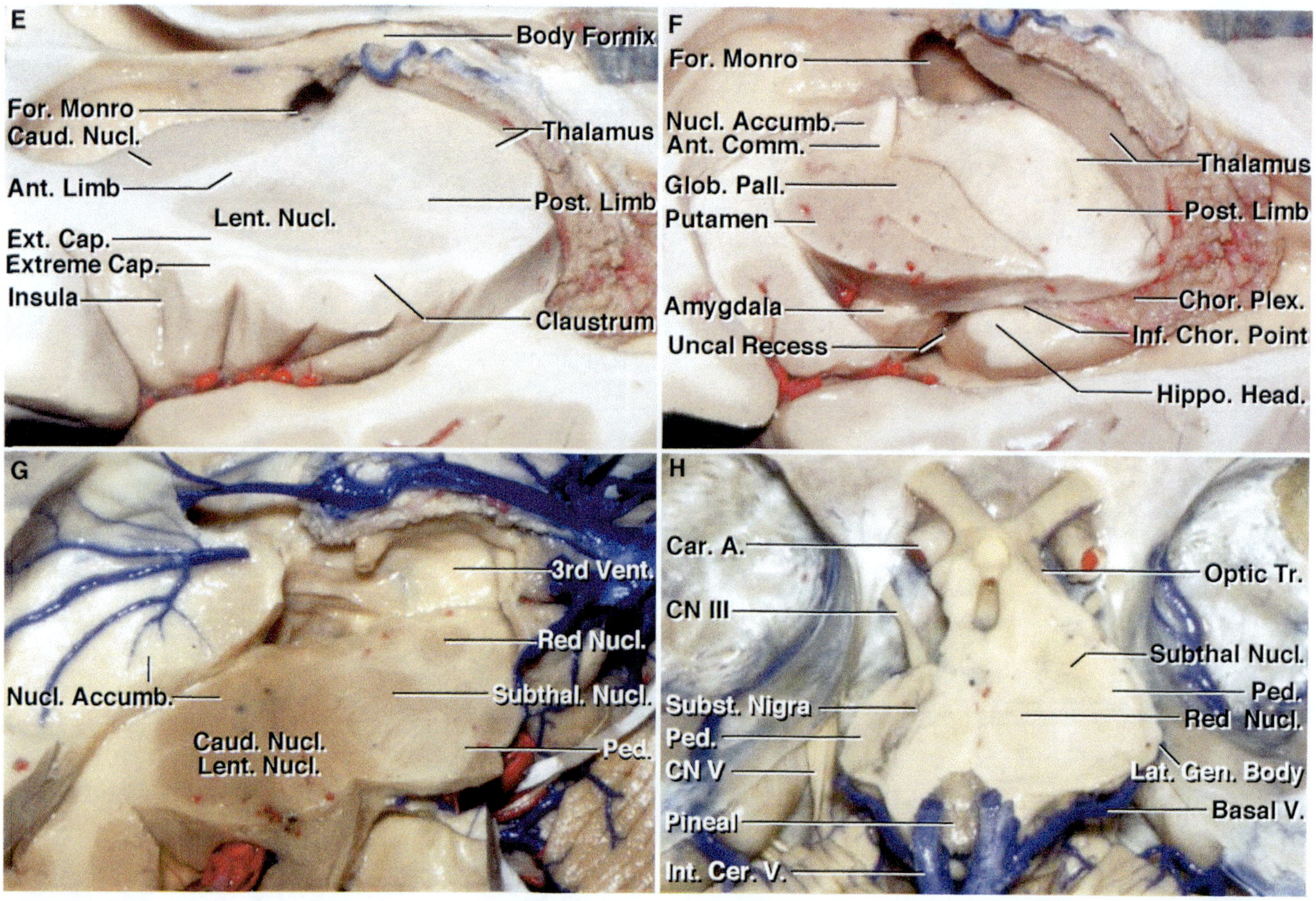

FIGURE 1.14. *Continued*

and caudate nuclei are separated by the anterior limb of the internal capsule, but at this level below the anterior limb of the internal capsule, the two nuclei blend into a mass of gray matter located above the anterior perforated substance and adjacent part of the orbital surface of the frontal lobe. The caudate and lentiform nuclei blend into the nucleus basalis located below the anterior commissure and the nucleus accumbens situated anterior to the nucleus basalis to form a massive collection of gray matter in the basal part of the hemisphere. E, *superolateral view at the foramen of Monro showing the genu of the capsule reaching the ventricular surface lateral to the foramen of Monro.* F, *superolateral view of the section at the level of the anterior commissure. At this level below the frontal horn and anterior limb of the internal capsule, and above the anterior perforated substance, the putamen, lentiform nucleus, globus pallidus, and caudate head blend into a large mass of gray matter. The posterior limb of the internal capsule, located between the lentiform nucleus and the thalamus, is still present in the cross section even though the anterior limb is absent. In coronal cross sections, the lentiform nucleus is typically lens-shaped, but in the axial cuts, as shown here, the lentiform nucleus, composed of the putamen and globus pallidus, has a tear-drop shape with a broad, rounded head anteriorly and a pointed tail posteriorly. The amygdala and head of the hippocampus, separated by the uncal recess, are exposed below the lentiform nucleus.* G, *superolateral view of a cross section extending below the frontal horn and through the red and subthalamic nuclei and upper part of the cerebral peduncle. At this level, just above the anterior perforated substance, the lentiform and caudate nuclei blend into the nucleus basalis and accumbens to create a large collection of gray matter. The red nucleus is located in the center of the midbrain. The right subthalamic nucleus is a lens-shaped nucleus situated in the interval between the cerebral peduncle and the midbrain.* H, *the part of the basal surface of the frontal lobe above the sylvian fissure has been removed to expose the upper edge of the cerebral peduncles and the red and subthalamic nuclei located just behind the peduncle. The optic tract passes laterally around the upper margin of the cerebellar peduncle. The left half of the brainstem has been sectioned obliquely to expose the substantia nigra located just below the subthalamic nucleus.* A., *artery;* Accumb., *accumbens;* Ant., *anterior;* Cap., *capsule;* Car., *carotid;* Caud., *caudate;* Cent., *central;* Cer., *cerebral;* Chor., *choroid, choroidal;* Circ., *circular;* CN, *cranial nerve;* Comm., *commissure;* Ext., *external;* For., *foramen;* Gen., *geniculate;* Glob., *globus;* Hippo., *hippocampal;* Inf., *inferior;* Int., *internal;* Lat., *lateral;* Lent., *lentiform;* Nucl., *nucleus;* Pall., *pallidus;* Paracent., *paracentral;* Ped., *peduncle;* Pell., *pellucidum;* Plex., *plexus;* Post., *posterior;* Postcent., *postcentral;* Precent., *precentral;* Sept., *septum;* Subst., *substantia;* Subthal., *subthalamic;* Temp., *temporal;* V., *vein;* Vent., *ventricle.*

cerebral peduncle. The internal capsule is a thick mass of white matter that is bounded laterally by the lentiform nucleus and medially by the caudate nucleus and the thalamus. The internal capsule has anterior and posterior limbs, a genu, and retro- and sublenticular parts. The internal capsule bends at a right angle around the medial margin of the pallidal part of the lentiform nucleus to form an anterior limb, located between the caudate nucleus medially and the lentiform nucleus laterally, and a posterior limb, interposed between the thalamus medially and the lentiform nucleus laterally. The two

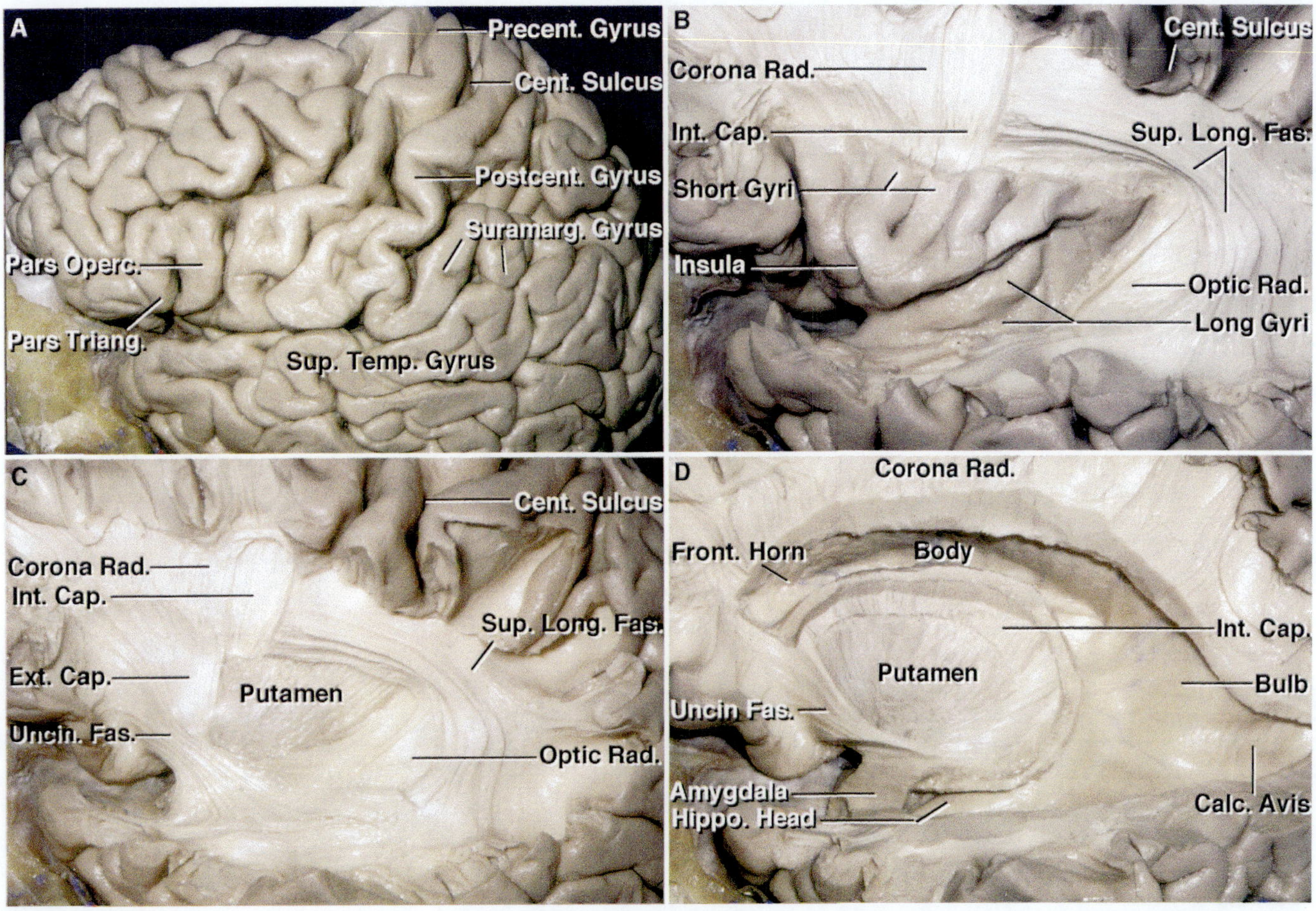

FIGURE 1.15. *Stepwise fiber dissection. A, left cerebral hemisphere. The pre- and postcentral gyri adjoin the central sulcus. The precentral gyrus is located behind the pars opercularis and the postcentral gyrus is located in front of the supramarginal gyrus. B, the frontal, parietal, and temporal operculi have been removed to expose the insula. The corona radiata and some of the fibers joining the internal capsule are exposed above the insula. The insular surface is composed of long and short gyri. The superior longitudinal fasciculus courses around the outer margin of the insula and lentiform nucleus. The retrolenticular part of the optic radiations are exposed behind the insula and deep to the superior longitudinal fasciculus. C, the claustrum and the posterior part of the external capsule have been removed to expose the putamen. The anterior part of the external capsule has been preserved. The uncinate fasciculus interconnects the frontal and temporal lobes. The retrolenticular part of the optic radiations is exposed behind the lentiform nucleus. The superior longitudinal fasciculus courses superficial to the optic radiations and deep to the extreme and external capsules. D, the frontal horn, body, atrium, and temporal horn of the lateral ventricle have been exposed. The fibers of the external capsule superficial to the putamen have been removed. The internal capsule courses medial to the lentiform nucleus, the outer segment of which is formed by the putamen. The lower part of the uncinate fasciculus has been removed to expose amygdala and the head of the hippocampus. The amygdala forms the anterior wall of the temporal horn. The calcar avis, overlying the deep end of the calcarine sulcus, and the bulb of the corpus callosum, overlying the fibers of the forceps major, are exposed in the medial wall of the atrium.* *(Legend continues on next page.)*

limbs join at the genu, where the fibers wrap around the medial apex of the globus pallidus. The medially directed apex is located lateral to the foramen of Monro, where the fibers in the genu reach the wall of the ventricle in the interval between the caudate nucleus and thalamus. The anterior limb is composed predominantly of fibers that connect the anterior and medial thalamus and the pontine nuclei to the frontal lobe. The genu of the internal capsule, in addition to the corticothalamic and thalamocortical fibers, contains corticobulbar fibers to the motor nuclei of the cranial nerves. The posterior limb, in addition to fibers interconnecting the thalamus and cortex, contains the corticospinal fibers to the motor nuclei of the upper and lower extremity and trunk. The fibers to the arm are nearer the genu than those coursing to the leg. The precentral gyrus is positioned superficial to the posterior limb.

Some fibers of the internal capsule curve around the posterior edge of the lentiform nucleus and are referred to as the retrolenticular fibers and others pass below the lentiform nucleus and are referred to as sublenticular fibers. The sublenticular part of the posterior limb contains the auditory radiation fibers directed from the medial geniculate body to the auditory area in the transverse temporal and adjacent parts of the superior temporal gyri and part of the optic radiations that course from the lateral geniculate to the walls of the calcarine sulcus. Some optic radiation fibers also pass through the re-

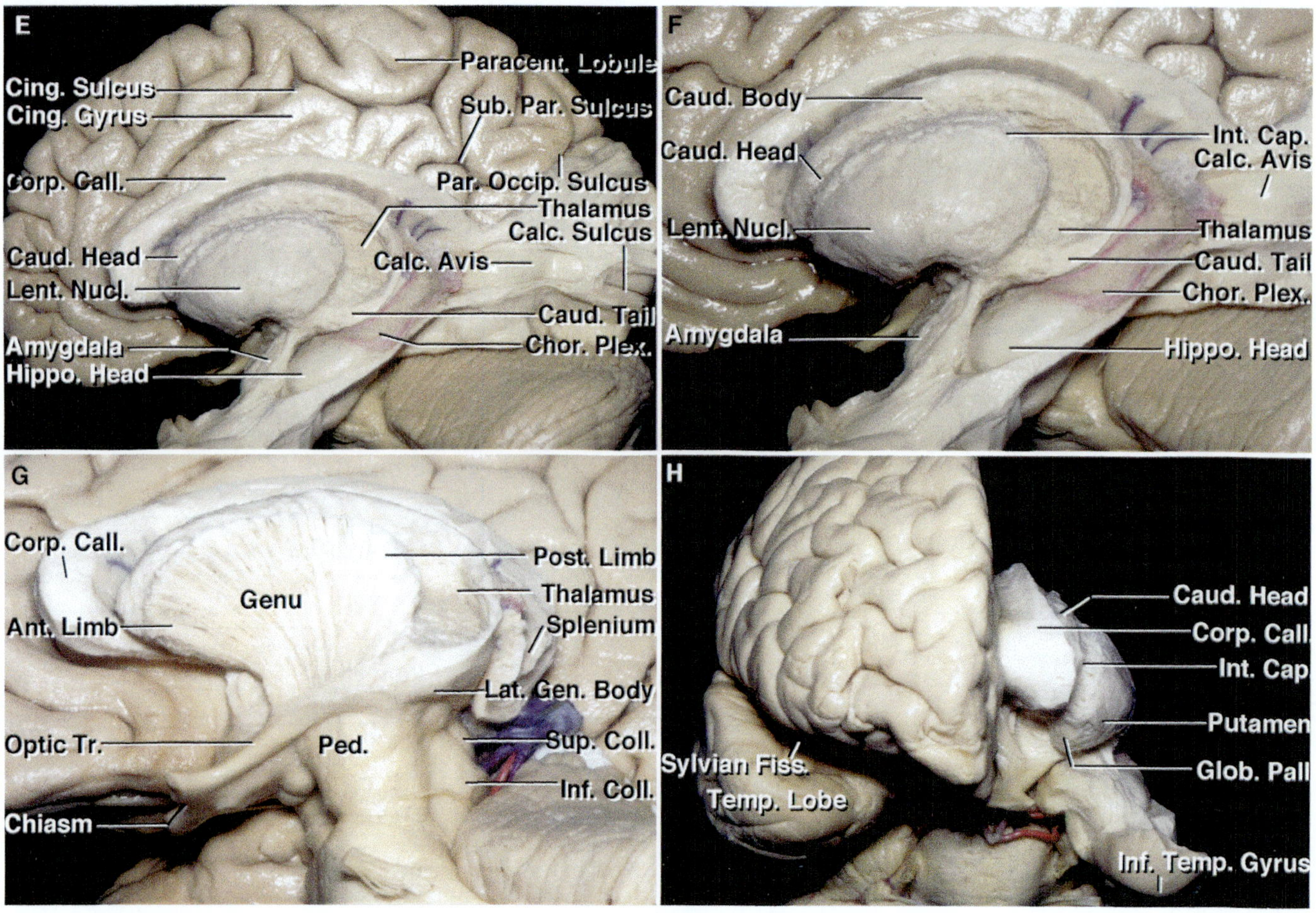

FIGURE 1.15. *Continued*

E, the fibers of the internal capsule that course between the posterior part of the lentiform nucleus and thalamus have been removed. The anterior limb of the internal capsule descends between the caudate head and lentiform nucleus and the posterior limb passes between the lentiform nucleus and thalamus. The head, body, and tail of the caudate nucleus are exposed in the wall of the ventricle. The tail of the caudate nucleus extends along the lateral edge of the thalamus. The head of the hippocampus is located in the floor of the temporal horn. The amygdala forms the anterior wall of the temporal horn. F, enlarged view. Some of the ependyma over the calcar avis has been removed. The choroid plexus is attached along the choroidal fissure. G, lateral view. The lentiform nucleus has been removed to expose the internal capsule. The anterior limb courses between the caudate nucleus and lentiform nucleus and has a darker color than the posterior limb because of the bridges of transcapsular gray matter extending across the internal capsule between the caudate and lentiform nuclei. The posterior limb of the internal capsule is located lateral to the thalamus. The optic tract passes backward to reach the lateral geniculate body. The fibers of the internal capsula descend to form the cerebral peduncle located medial to the optic tract. The superior and inferior colliculi are exposed in the quadrigeminal cistern. H, anterior view of dissection shown in G. The putamen and globus pallidus are positional on the lateral side of the internal capsule and the caudate nucleus is on the medial side. The anterior limb of the internal capsule descends between the caudate head and the lentiform nucleus. Ant., *anterior;* Calc., *calcar, calcarine;* Call., *callosum;* Cap., *capsule;* Caud., *caudate;* Cent., *central;* Chor., *choroid;* Cing., *cingulate;* Coll., *colliculi;* Corp., *corpus;* Ext., *external;* Fas., *fasciculus;* Fiss., *fissure;* Front., *frontal;* Gen., *geniculate;* Glob., *globus;* Hippo., *hippocampal;* Inf., *inferior;* Int., *internal;* Lat., *lateral;* Lent., *lentiform;* Long., *longitudinal;* Nucl., *nucleus;* Operc., *opercularis;* Pall., *pallidus;* Paracent., *paracentral;* Par. Occip., *parieto-occipital;* Ped., *peduncle;* Plex., *plexus;* Postcent., *postcentral;* Post., *posterior;* Precent., *precentral;* Rad., *radiata, radiations;* Sub. Par., *subparietal;* Sup., *superior;* Supramarg., *supramarginal;* Temp., *temporal;* Tr., *tract;* Triang., *triangularis;* Uncin., *uncinate.*

trolenticular part of the internal capsule, but most pass through the sublenticular part.

The optic radiations are separated from the roof and lateral wall of the temporal horn and the lateral atrial wall by only a thin layer of tapetal fibers. The fibers passing to the superior bank of the calcarine fissure leave the upper part of the lateral geniculate body and course almost directly posterior around the lateral aspect of the atrium to reach the striate visual cortex. Fibers from the lower part of the geniculate body destined for the inferior bank of the calcarine fissure initially loop forward and downward in the temporal lobe, forming Meyer's loop, before turning back to join the other fibers in the optic radiations.

The fibers of the optic radiation are divided into anterior, middle, and posterior groups (*Fig. 1.16H*). The anterior fibers, called Meyer's loop, subserve the upper half of the visual field.

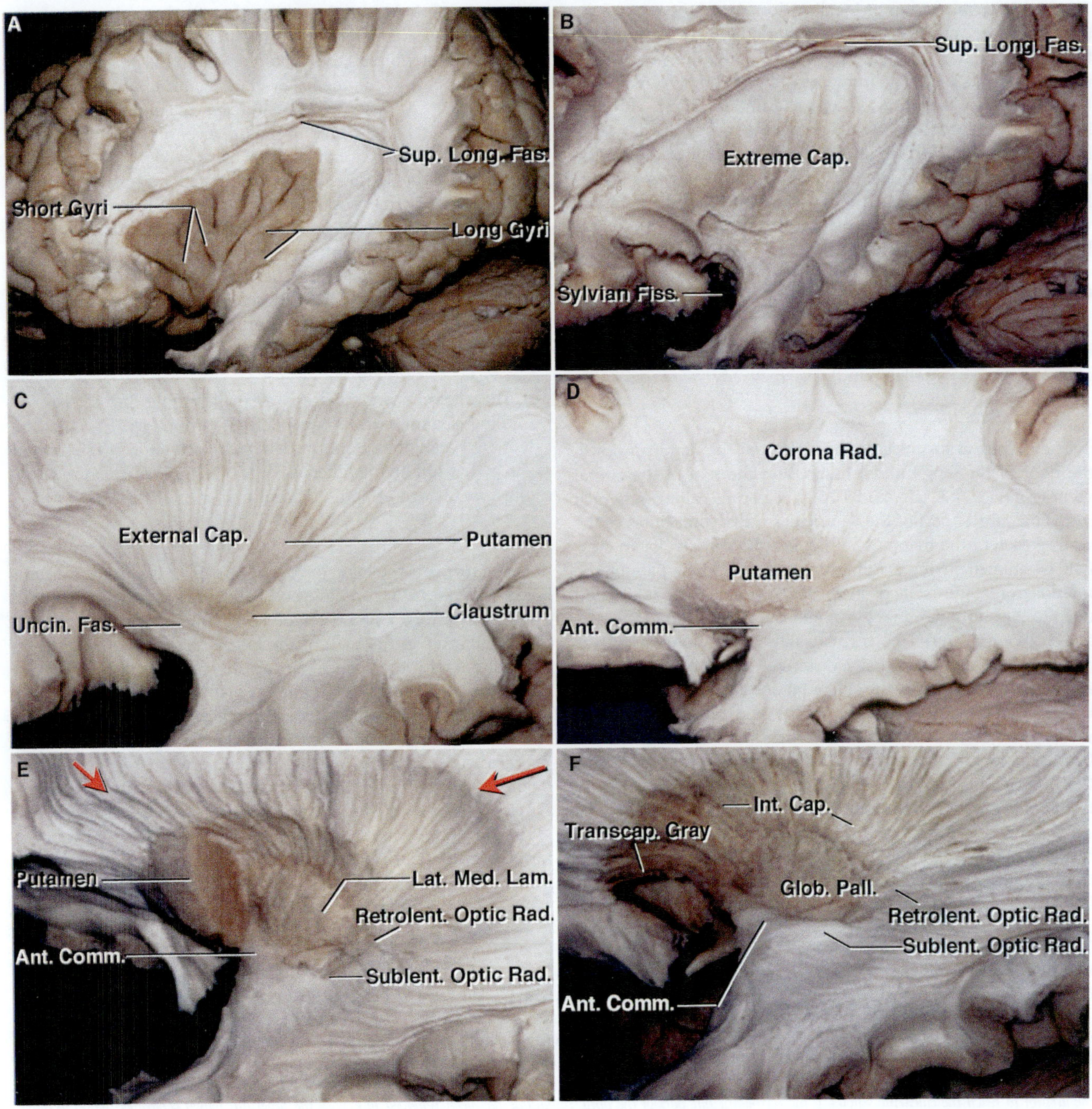

FIGURE 1.16. *Stepwise fiber dissection of the left cerebral hemisphere.* A, *the opercular lips of the sylvian fissure have been removed to expose the insula. The superior longitudinal fasciculus courses in the deep white matter around the outer edges of the insula and lentiform nucleus.* B, *the insular gray matter has been removed to expose the extreme capsule that separates the insular cortex from the claustrum. The superior longitudinal fasciculus arches around the outer margin of the insula and lentiform nucleus to interconnect the frontal, parietal, occipital, and temporal lobes.* C, *the extreme capsule has been removed. A small patch of the lower part of the claustrum remains. The external capsule, which separates the claustrum and lentiform nucleus, is exposed deep to the claustrum. Some of the fibers of the external capsule have been removed to expose the lateral surface of the putamen. The superior longitudinal fasciculus has also been removed. The uncinate fasciculus is located deep to the limen insula and interconnects the frontal and temporal lobes.* D, *the external capsule has been removed to expose the putamen. The anterior commissure, interconnecting the temporal and septal areas, is exposed below the putamen. The corona radiatus spreads out around the putamen.* E, *the posterior part of the putamen has been removed to expose the lateral medullary lamina that separates the putamen and globus pallidus. The white matter prominence* (red arrows) *around the putamen is created by the intersection of the fibers of the corpus callosum and the corona radiata. The optic radiations pass through the retrolenticular and sublenticular parts of the internal capsule to reach the visual cortex. Fibers of the anterior commissure spread laterally into the temporal lobe. (Legend continues on next page.)*

They initially take an anterior direction above the roof of the temporal horn, usually reaching as far anteriorly as the tip of the temporal horn, where they loop along the lateral and inferior aspects of the atrium and occipital horn to reach the lower lip of the calcarine fissure. The middle fibers, subserving the macula, course laterally above the roof of the temporal horn and turn posteriorly along the lateral wall of the atrium and the occipital horn. The posterior fibers responsible for the lower visual field course directly backward along the lateral wall of the atrium and the occipital horn to end in the upper lip of the calcarine fissure.

Commissural Fibers

The commisural fibers interconnect the paired cerebral hemispheres. The largest is the corpus callosum. The anterior commissure is a smaller bundle.

Corpus Callosum

The corpus callosum is located between the hemispheres in the floor of the longitudinal fissure and the roof of the lateral ventricles (*Figs. 1.7, 1.15,* and *1.16*). The corpus callosum, which forms the largest part of the ventricular walls, contributes to the wall of each of the five parts of the lateral ventricle. Its anterior half is situated in the midline deep to the upper part of the inferior frontal gyrus. Its posterior part, the splenium, is situated deep to the supramarginal gyrus and the lower third of the pre- and postcentral gyri. The corpus callosum has five parts: two anterior parts, the genu and rostrum; a central part, the body; and two posterior parts, the splenium and tapetum. The curved anterior part, the genu, wraps around and forms the anterior wall and adjacent part of the roof of the frontal horn. The genu blends below into the rostrum, a thin tapered portion that forms the floor of the frontal horn and is continuous downward, in front of the anterior commissure, with the lamina terminalis. The genu gives rise to a large fiber tract, the forceps minor, which forms the anterior wall of the frontal horn and interconnects the frontal lobes. The forceps minor sweeps obliquely forward and laterally, as does the anterior wall of the frontal horn. The genu blends posteriorly into the midportion, the body, located above the body of the lateral ventricle. The splenium, the thick, rounded posterior end, is situated dorsal to the pineal body and the upper part of the medial wall of the atrium. The splenium gives rise to a large tract, the forceps major, which forms a prominence called the bulb in the upper part of the medial wall of the atrium and occipital horn as it sweeps posteriorly to interconnect the occipital lobes. Another fiber tract, the tapetum, which arises in the posterior part of the body and splenium, sweeps laterally and inferiorly to form the roof and lateral wall of the atrium and the temporal and occipital horns. The tapetum separates the fibers of the optic radiations from the temporal horn and the atrium. The cingulate gyrus surrounds and is separated from the corpus callosum by the callosal sulcus.

Anterior Commissure

The anterior commissure is a small bundle that crosses the midline in front of the columns of the fornix (*Figs. 1.8* and *1.16*). It forms part of the anterior wall of the third ventricle. It is shaped somewhat like the handlebars of a bicycle. It interconnects the olfactory structures and temporal gyri on both sides.

Fornix

The fornix is the main efferent pathway from the hippocampal formation. It contains both commissural and projection fibers. The fornix is a C-shaped structure that wraps around the thalamus in the wall of the lateral ventricle and has relationships with the cortical surface that are similar to those at the outer edge of the thalamus (*Figs. 1.2, 1.8, 1.12,* and *1.13*). The fornix extends from the hippocampus to the mamillary bodies and has four parts: fimbria, crus, body, and columns. It arises in the floor of the temporal horn on the ventricular surface of the hippocampus from fibers that collect along the medial edge of the hippocampus and are directed backward. The fimbria is separated from the dentate gyrus by the fimbriodentate sulcus. The fimbria courses along the lateral edge of the lateral geniculate body and is separated from the geniculate body and optic and auditory radiations by the choroidal

FIGURE 1.16. *Continued*
F, all of the putamen has been removed to expose the lateral surface of the globus pallidus. The anterior commissure passes below the anterior part of the globus pallidus. Transcapsular bridges of gray matter extending between the lentiform and caudate nuclei cross the anterior part of the internal capsule to give it a dark appearance. G, *the posterior, but not the anterior, part of the globus pallidus has been removed. Transcapsular bridges of gray matter cross the anterior part of the internal capsule.* H, *the optic tract proceeds posteriorly toward the lateral geniculate body. Three bundles of the optic radiations are seen: an anterior one that is deeper and loops forward above the temporal horn before turning backward, the middle one passes laterally above the temporal horn, and the third bundle passes backward lateral to the atrium to reach the calcarine sulcus.* I, *the retrolenticular part of the optic radiations has been removed to expose the tapetum, which separates the optic radiations from the ventricular wall. The lateral ependymal wall of the atrium has been opened. The anterior commissure was transected and the lateral part removed. The middle part of the optic radiation has been elevated on a dissection.* J, *the optic radiations have been removed to expose the tail of the caudate blending into the amygdala. The optic tract has been exposed further posteriorly. The stria terminalis courses medial to the caudate tail and contains fibers passing from the amygdala to the septal area, thalamus, and mamillary body.* K, *the lateral ependymal wall of the lateral ventricle has been removed and some bundles of callosal fibers above the ventricle have been preserved. The calcar avis bulges into the medial wall of the atrium and occipital horn. The window in the white matter* (yellow arrow) *overlying the calcar avis exposes the cortical gray matter in the deep end of the calcarine sulcus. The* red pin *is positioned lateral to the deep site of the foramen of Monro. The genu of the internal capsule is located directly lateral to the foramen of Monro. The anterior limb of the capsule is located anterior to the* red dot *and lateral to the caudate head. The posterior limb is located posterior to the foramen of Monro. The internal capsule blends into the cerebral peduncle below the level of the optic tract.* L, *the head of the caudate has been folded downward to expose the foramen of Monro. The columns of the fornix pass superior and anterior to the foramen of Monro. The septum pellucidum is exposed above the rostrum of the corpus callosum. The amygdala is exposed below the optic tract.* M, *the tail of the caudate has been elevated to expose the stria terminalis, which arises within the amygdala. The collateral eminence overlies the deep end of the collateral sulcus. The tail of the caudate nucleus blends into the amygdala.* Ant., *anterior;* Calc., *Calcar;* Call.,

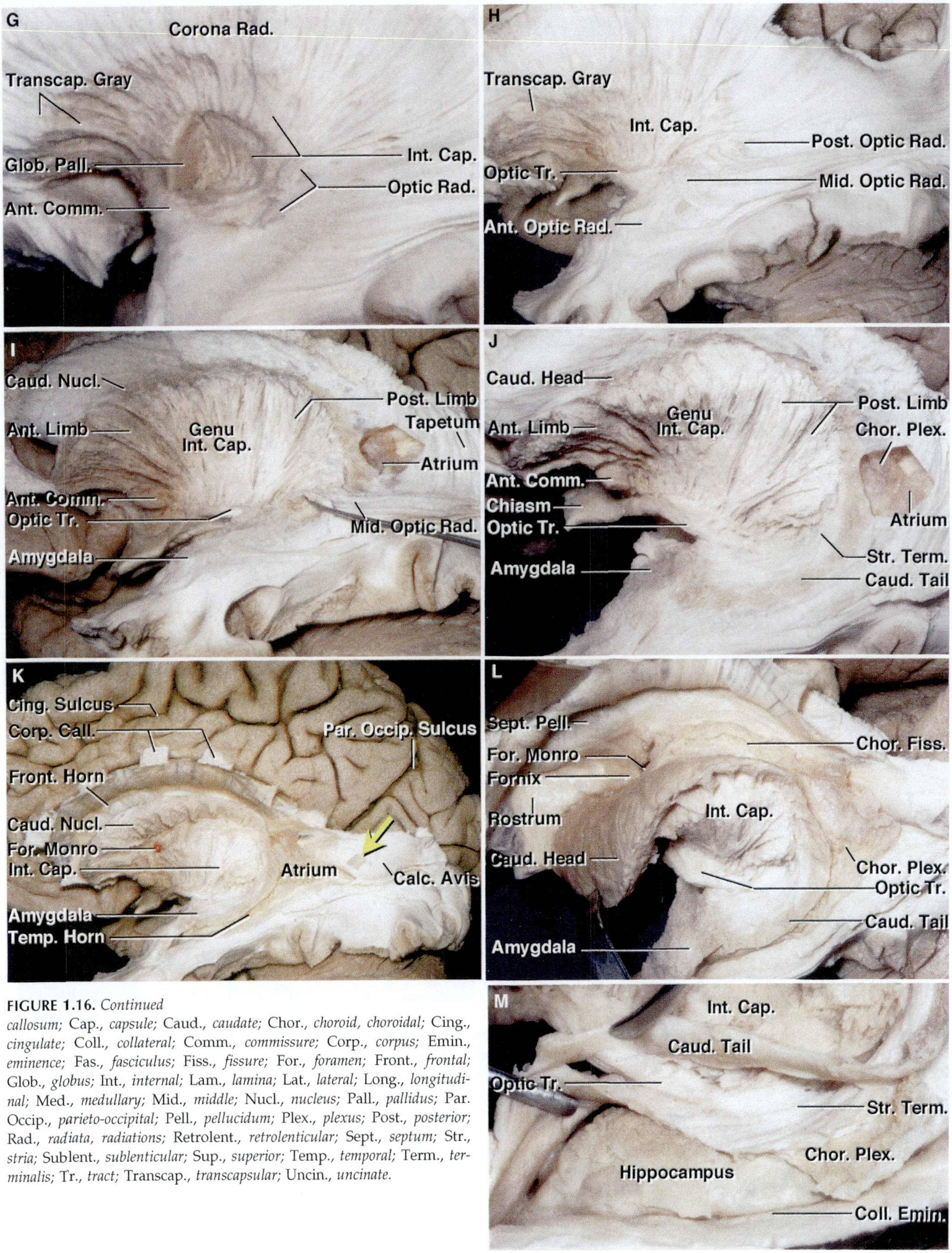

FIGURE 1.16. *Continued*
callosum; Cap., *capsule;* Caud., *caudate;* Chor., *choroid, choroidal;* Cing., *cingulate;* Coll., *collateral;* Comm., *commissure;* Corp., *corpus;* Emin., *eminence;* Fas., *fasciculus;* Fiss., *fissure;* For., *foramen;* Front., *frontal;* Glob., *globus;* Int., *internal;* Lam., *lamina;* Lat., *lateral;* Long., *longitudinal;* Med., *medullary;* Mid., *middle;* Nucl., *nucleus;* Pall., *pallidus;* Par. Occip., *parieto-occipital;* Pell., *pellucidum;* Plex., *plexus;* Post., *posterior;* Rad., *radiata, radiations;* Retrolent., *retrolenticular;* Sept., *septum;* Str., *stria;* Sublent., *sublenticular;* Sup., *superior;* Temp., *temporal;* Term., *terminalis;* Tr., *tract;* Transcap., *transcapsular;* Uncin., *uncinate.*

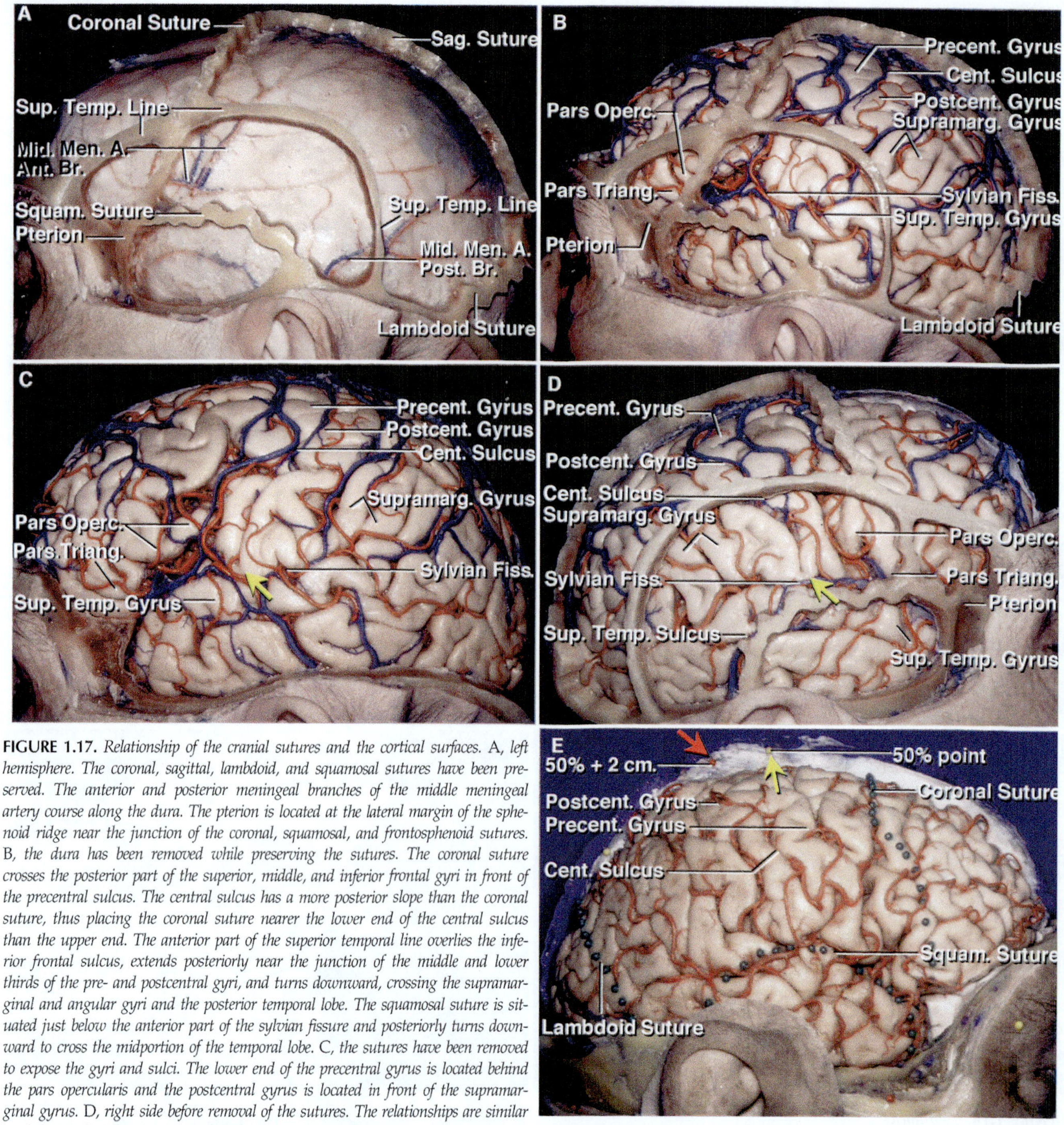

FIGURE 1.17. *Relationship of the cranial sutures and the cortical surfaces. A, left hemisphere. The coronal, sagittal, lambdoid, and squamosal sutures have been preserved. The anterior and posterior meningeal branches of the middle meningeal artery course along the dura. The pterion is located at the lateral margin of the sphenoid ridge near the junction of the coronal, squamosal, and frontosphenoid sutures. B, the dura has been removed while preserving the sutures. The coronal suture crosses the posterior part of the superior, middle, and inferior frontal gyri in front of the precentral sulcus. The central sulcus has a more posterior slope than the coronal suture, thus placing the coronal suture nearer the lower end of the central sulcus than the upper end. The anterior part of the superior temporal line overlies the inferior frontal sulcus, extends posteriorly near the junction of the middle and lower thirds of the pre- and postcentral gyri, and turns downward, crossing the supramarginal and angular gyri and the posterior temporal lobe. The squamosal suture is situated just below the anterior part of the sylvian fissure and posteriorly turns downward to cross the midportion of the temporal lobe. C, the sutures have been removed to expose the gyri and sulci. The lower end of the precentral gyrus is located behind the pars opercularis and the postcentral gyrus is located in front of the supramarginal gyrus. D, right side before removal of the sutures. The relationships are similar to those on the left side, except that the anterior part of the squamosal suture courses at the level of the anterior part of the sylvian fissure, rather than being positioned below the sylvian fissure as shown in B. The coronal suture has less slope from below to above than the central sulcus, thus placing the lower end of the central sulcus nearer the coronal suture than the upper end. In D there are relatively well-developed superior, middle, and inferior temporal gyri, but in C the temporal lobe is divided into a superior temporal gyrus, but there is no clear demarcation between the region of the middle and inferior temporal gyri that are broken into multiple segments by the oblique sulci. There is a gyral bridge* (yellow arrow) *below the central sulcus between the lower end of the pre- and postcentral gyri on both sides so that neither central sulcus reaches the sylvian fissure. The supramarginal gyrus wraps around the upturned posterior end of the superior temporal sulcus. E, another right hemisphere.* Green pinheads *have been placed along the site of the coronal, squamosal, and lambdoid sutures. The pterion is located at the junction of the squamosal and coronal sutures at the lateral end of the sphenoid ridge and stem of the sylvian fissure. A* yellow pin (yellow arrow) *has been placed along the edge of the superior sagittal sinus at the 50% point along the nasion-to-inion line. Another* red pin (red arrow) *has been placed 2 cm behind the 50% point, which is usually located at the upper end of the central sulcus. The central sulcus is usually placed 3.5 to 4.5 cm behind the coronal suture.* A., *artery;* Ant., *anterior;* Br., *branch;* Cent., *central;* Fiss., *fissure;* Men., *meningeal;* Mid., *middle;* Operc., *opercularis;* Post., *posterior;* Postcent., *postcentral;* Precent., *precentral;* Sag., *sagittal;* Squam., *squamosal;* Sup., *superior;* Supramarg., *supramarginal;* Temp., *temporal;* Triang., *triangularis.*

fissure. Posteriorly, the fimbria blends into the crus of the fornix that wraps around the posterior surface of the pulvinar in the medial part of the antrum and arches superomedial toward the lower surface of the splenium of the corpus callosum. At the junction between the atrium and the body of the lateral ventricle, the paired crura meet to form the body of the fornix, which passes above the thalamus and below the septum pellucidum in the lower part of the medial wall of the body of the lateral ventricle. At the anterior margin of the thalamus, the body of the fornix separates into two columns that arch along the superior and anterior margin of the foramen of Monro and blend into the walls of the third ventricle as they pass behind the anterior commissure and descend to reach the mamillary bodies. In the area below the splenium, a thin sheet of fiber, the hippocampal commissure, interconnects the medial edges of the crura of the fornix. The body and crus are located deep to the lower part of the pre- and postcentral gyri, and the fimbria is located deep to the lower part of the superior temporal gyrus. All of its parts are located deep to the posterior part of the insula. In the body of the lateral ventricle, the body of the fornix is in the lower part of the medial wall; in the atrium, the crus of the fornix is in the medial part of the anterior wall; and in the temporal horn, the fimbria of the fornix is in the medial part of the floor.

The inner border of the fornix forms the outer border of the choroidal fissure, the cleft between the thalamus and the fornix, along which the choroid plexus in the lateral ventricle attaches (2, 7). The choroidal fissure is a C-shaped arc that extends from the foramen of Monro through the body, atrium, and temporal horn of the lateral ventricle (*Figs. 1.2, 1.8,* and *1.13*) (2). The choroidal fissure is divided into three parts: the body part between the body of the fornix and the thalamus (9), the atrial part between the crus of the fornix and the pulvinar of the thalamus, and the temporal part between the fimbria of the fornix and the stria terminalis of the thalamus. The choroid plexus of the lateral ventricle is attached to the fornix and to the thalamus by an ependymal covering called taenia. The choroidal fissure is one of the most important landmarks in microneurosurgery involving the body and third ventricle and temporal lobe. In the body of the lateral ventricle, the fissure can be used as a route to the third ventricle. In the temporal region, it separates those structures located laterally that can be removed from those structures located medially that should be preserved during temporal lobectomy.

Septum Pellucidum

The septum pellucidum stretches across the interval between the anterior parts of the corpus callosum and the body of the fornix (*Figs. 1.8, 1.14,* and *1.16*). It is composed of paired laminae and separates the frontal horns and bodies of the lateral ventricles in the midline. In the frontal horn, the septum pellucidum is attached to the rostrum of the corpus callosum below, the genu anteriorly, and the body above. In the body of the lateral ventricle, the septum is attached to the body of the corpus callosum above and the body of the fornix below. The septum pellucidum disappears posteriorly where the body of the fornix meets the splenium. There may be a cavity, the cavum septum pellucidum, in the midline between the laminae of the septum pellucidum.

GRAY MATTER IN THE CENTRAL CORE

The central core of the hemisphere is the site of four large masses of gray matter located in the deep regions of the hemisphere (*Figs. 1.8* and *1.12–1.16*). These are the caudate nucleus putamen, globus pallidus, and thalamus. The putamen and globus pallidus combined have a lens shape in coronal cross sections and together are termed the lentiform nucleus. The thalamus is separated from the other nuclear masses by the internal capsule. The subcortical nuclear masses that include the caudate and lentiform nuclei plus the amygdala are referred to as the basal ganglia. The amygdala is located in the medial temporal lobe outside the central core. The amygdala is discussed above, with the medial surface of the temporal lobe. The superior and posterior parts of the caudate and lentiform nuclei are separated by the internal capsule, but anteroinferiorly, below the anterior limb of the internal capsule and above the anterior perforated substance, they fuse into a single nucleus mass. Further medially, below the anterior commissure and rostrum of the corpus callosum, they blend without clear demarcation into the nucleus basalis and accumbens. The tail of the caudate nucleus blends into the amygdala, and superiorly the amygdala blends into the lower surface of the globus pallidus. Two other nuclei that appear in axial sections of the basal gray matter, at the lower edge of the thalamus and medial to the cerebral peduncles, are the subthalamic and red nuclei (*Fig. 1.14*). This subthalamic nucleus is a biconvex lens-shaped structure located medial to the cerebral peduncle and above the substantia nigra. The substantia nigra is located below the subthalamic nucleus. The red nucleus is located in the center of the midbrain.

Caudate Nucleus

The caudate nucleus is an arched C-shaped structure that wraps around the lateral part of the thalamus (*Figs. 1.8, 1.13,* and *1.14*). It has a large head that tapers down to a smaller body and tail. The body extends backward from the head and is separated from the thalamus by the stria terminalis and thalamostriate vein. The head and body are so large that they produce a prominence in and form the lateral wall of the frontal horn and body of the lateral ventricle. The long slender tail arches downward in the atrial wall along the lateral edge of the pulvinar to form part of the lateral wall of the atrium. The tail reaches the roof of the temporal horn where it passes forward and blends into the junction between the amygdala and lower part of the lentiform nucleus. The tail is so slender that it does not produce a prominence in the wall of the atrium and temporal horn, as does the head in the horn and body. In the body of the lateral ventricle, the caudate nucleus is superolateral to the thalamus; in the atrium, it

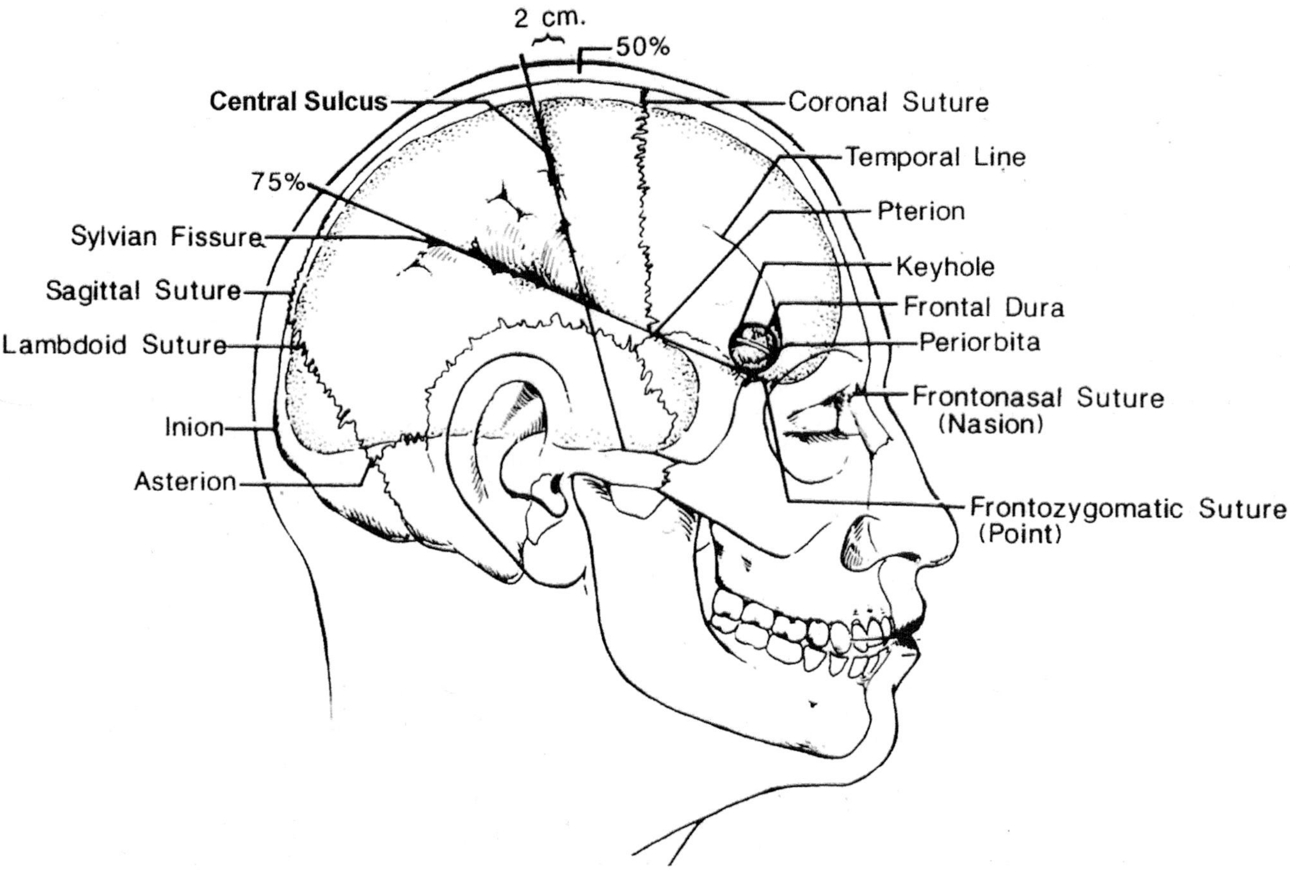

FIGURE 1.18. *Sites commonly marked on the scalp before applying the drapes include the coronal, sagittal, and lambdoid sutures; the central sulcus and sylvian fissures; and the pterion, inion, asterion, and keyhole. Approximating the site of the sylvian fissure and central sulcus on the scalp begins by noting the position of the nasion, inion, and frontozygomatic point. The nasion is located in the midline at the junction of the nasal and frontal bones. The inion is the site of a bony prominence that overlies the torcular herophili. The frontozygomatic point is located on the orbital rim 2.5 cm above the level where the upper edge of the zygomatic arch joins the orbital rim and just below the junction of the lateral and superior margins of the orbital rim. The next steps are to construct a line along the sagittal suture and, using a flexible measuring tape, to determine the distance along this line from the nasion to inion and mark the midpoint and three-quarter points (50% and 75% points). The sylvian fissure is located along a line that extends backward from the frontozygomatic point across the lateral surface of the head to the three-quarter point. The pterion, the site on the temple approximating the lateral end of the sphenoid ridge, is located 3 cm behind the frontozygomatic point on the sylvian fissure line. The central sulcus is located by identifying the upper and lower rolandic points. The upper rolandic point is located 2 cm behind the midpoint (50% plus 2 cm point) on the nasion-to-inion midsagittal line. The lower rolandic point is located where a line extending from the midpoint of the upper margin of the zygomatic arch to the upper rolandic point crosses the line defining the sylvian fissure. A line connecting the upper and lower rolandic points approximates the central sulcus. The lower rolandic point is located approximately 2.5 cm behind the pterion on the sylvian fissure line. Another important point is the keyhole, the site of a burr hole, which if properly placed, has the frontal dura in the depths of its upper half and the periorbita in its lower half. It is approximately 3 cm anterior to the pterion, just above the lateral end of the superior orbital rim and under the most anterior point of attachment of the temporalis muscle and fascia to the temporal line.*

is posterolateral to the thalamus; and, in the temporal horn, it is inferolateral to the thalamus.

Lentiform Nucleus

The lentiform nucleus is a wedge- or lens-shaped structure in cross section, located between the insula and the anterior and posterior limbs of the internal capsule (*Figs. 1.8* and *1.13–1.16*). Its lateral surface, all of which is medial to the insula, is slightly smaller than the insular surface area. Its anterior margin does not reach as far forward as the anterior part of the head of the caudate, which it faces across the anterior limb of the internal capsule. Its posterior margin does not reach as far posteriorly as the posterior part of the thalamus, which it faces across the posterior limb of the internal capsule. Its anterior edge is grooved by the anterior commissure. Its lower-anterior part blends into the lower part of the head of the caudate nucleus in the area below the anterior limb of the internal capsule and above the anterior perforated substance. It is divided by the lateral medullary lamina, a thin layer of white matter, into the larger, more laterally positioned putamen and the smaller medially placed globus pallidus. The putamen, the largest of the basal ganglia, forms a shell-like covering to the globus pallidus. The globus pallidus is subdivided into medial and lateral parts by the medial medullary lamina. The anterior limb of the internal capsule courses along the anterior margin of the lentiform nucleus and separates it from the caudate head. The posterior limb of the internal capsule courses along the posterior margin of the lentiform nucleus and separates the nucleus from the thalamus. The claustrum, a thin layer of gray matter interposed between the insular cortex and putamen, is separated from the putamen by a lamina of white matter, the external capsule, and from the outer gray cortex of the insula by another white matter layer, the extreme capsule.

Thalamus

The thalamus is located in the center of the lateral ventricle at the upper end of the brainstem. It is positioned deep to the posterior half of the insula and the lower part of the pre- and postcentral gyri and adjacent part of the superior temporal gyrus (*Figs. 1.2, 1.8,* and *1.13–1.15*). The anterior thalamic tubercle, the prominence overlying the anterior thalamic nucleus, forms the posterior edge of the foramen of Monro. The thalamus reaches the level of the posterior commissure posteriorly and the hypothalamus sulcus inferiorly. Its upper margin forms the floor of the lateral ventricle. The stria terminalis and thalamostriate veins are located dorsolaterally at the junction of the thalamus and caudate. Each lateral ventricle wraps around the superior, inferior, and posterior surfaces of the thalamus. The prominent posterior part, the pulvinar or buttock of the thalamus, presents in the wall of three different supratentorial compartments: the posterolateral part of the pulvinar forms the lateral half of the anterior wall of the atrium; the posteromedial part of the pulvinar is covered by the crus of the fornix and the part medial to the fornix forms part of the anterior wall of the quadrigeminal cistern; and the inferolateral part of the pulvinar in the region of the geniculate bodies forms part of the roof of the ambient cistern. The medial part of the thalamus forms the upper part of the lateral wall of the third ventricle.

DISCUSSION

Understanding the relationship of the sutures and other superficial landmarks to the cortical surfaces is helpful in positioning and directing operative approaches (*Fig. 1.17*). The pterion is located at the lateral end of the greater sphenoid wing and stem of the sylvian fissure near the junction of the squamosal, coronal, sphenoparietal, and frontosphenoid sutures. The lower end of the pars triangularis of the inferior frontal gyrus is located just behind the pterion. The coronal suture, as it descends from its junction with the sagittal suture, arches over the superior and middle frontal gyri in front of the precentral sulcus. The central sulcus is nearer the lower than the upper end of the coronal suture because the central sulcus, as it ascends, is directed more posteriorly than the coronal suture. The squamosal suture follows the anterior part of the posterior limb of the sylvian fissure before turning downward, at approximately the level of the postcentral gyrus, to cross the junction of the middle and posterior third of the temporal lobe. Another surface landmark is the superior temporal line that extends from the lateral frontal region in front of the pterion across the parietal and temporal region to the upper margin of the mastoid behind the ear. From its anterior end located lateral to the anterior margin of the pars orbitalis, it is directed obliquely upward, crossing the pars triangularis to reach the pars opercularis near the inferior frontal sulcus. Further posteriorly, it crosses superficial to the junction of the lower and middle thirds of the central sulcus, and turns downward and backward, crossing the posterosuperior margin of the supramarginal and angular gyri, finally reaching the parietomastoid suture. The lambdoid suture provides a rough estimate of the junction of the occipital lobe posteriorly with the parietal and temporal lobe anteriorly.

It may be helpful to outline several important landmarks on the scalp before applying the drapes (*Fig. 1.18*). Sites commonly marked include the coronal and sagittal sutures, the central sulcus and sylvian fissure, and the pterion, inion, and keyhole. Approximating the site of the sylvian fissure and central sulcus on the scalp begins with noting the position of the nasion, inion, and frontozygomatic point. The nasion is located in the midline at the junction of the nasal and frontal bones at the level of the upper rim of the orbit. The inion is the site of a bony prominence that overlies the torcular herophili and the attachment of the tentorium to the inner table of the cranium. The frontozygomatic point is the site of the frontozygomatic suture situated on the lateral orbital rim. It is positioned on the upper part of the lateral orbital rim just below where the frontal bone, which forms the upper margin of the orbital rim, joins the zygomatic bone, which forms the lateral margin of the orbital rim. The frontozygomatic point is situated on the orbital rim 2.5 cm above the level where the upper edge of the zygomatic arch joins the orbital rim.

The next step is to construct a line along the sagittal suture and, with the use of a flexible measuring tape, to determine the distance along the midsagittal line from the nasion to inion and to mark the midpoint and three-quarter point (the 50% and 75% points) along the line. The sylvian fissure is located along a line that extends backward from the frontozygomatic point across the lateral surface of the head to the three-quarter point on the nasion-to-inion midsagittal line. The pterion is located 3 cm behind the frontozygomatic point on the sylvian fissure line. The pterion approximates the lateral end of the sphenoid ridge, which extends along the stem of the sylvian fissure.

The central (rolandic) sulcus is located by identifying the upper and lower rolandic points that correspond to the upper and lower ends of the central sulcus. The upper rolandic point is located 2 cm behind the midpoint (50% plus 2 cm point) on the nasion-to-inion midsagittal line. The lower rolandic point is located where a line extending from the midpoint of the upper margin of the zygomatic arch to the upper rolandic point crosses the line defining the sylvian fissure. A line connecting the upper and lower rolandic points approximates the central sulcus. The lower rolandic point is located approximately 2.5 cm behind the pterion on the sylvian fissure line. The upper end of the central sulcus is usually located 3.5 to 4.5 cm behind the upper end of the central sulcus.

Another especially important point in approaches to the anterior part of the cerebrum is the keyhole, the site of a burr

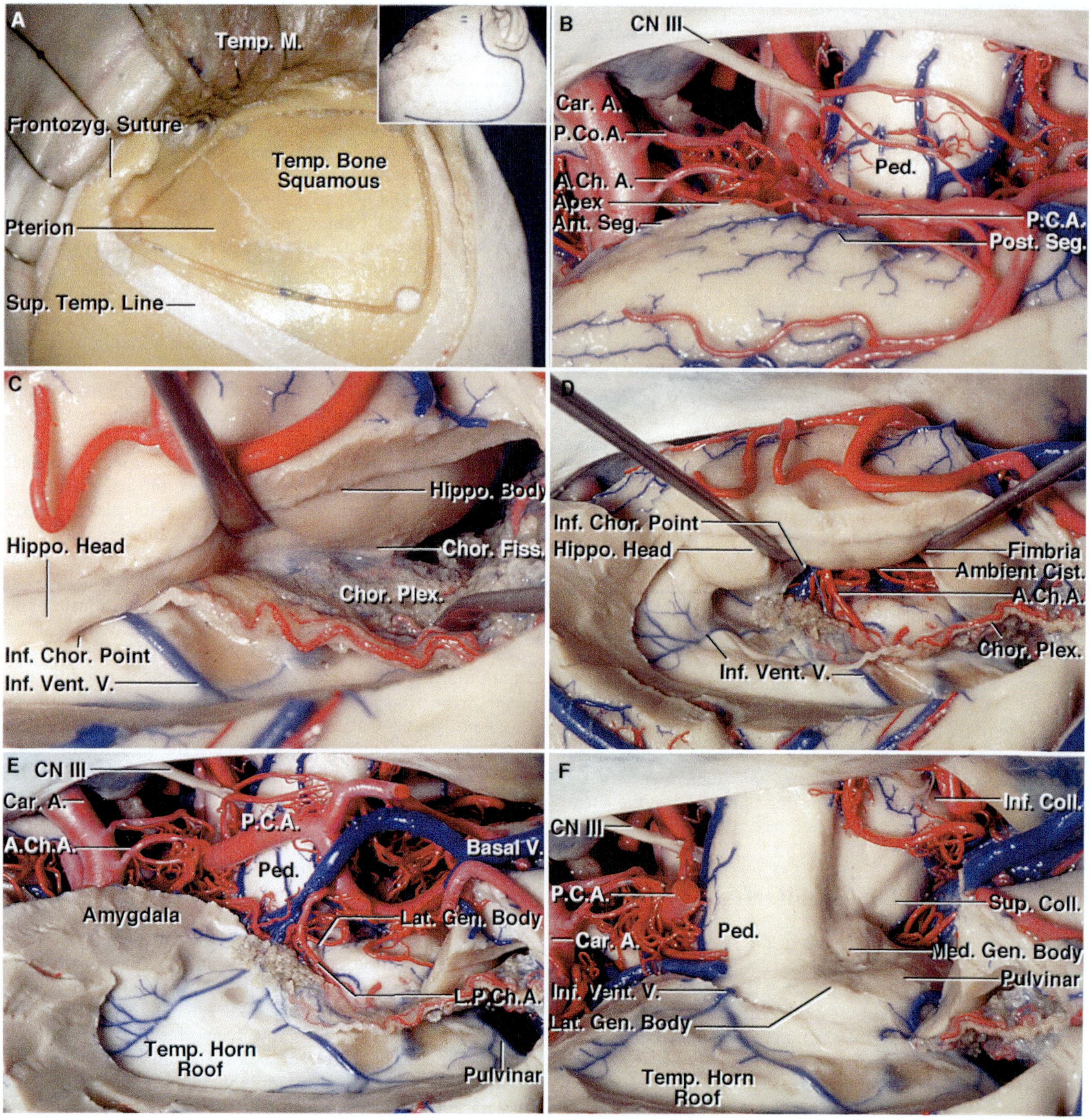

FIGURE 1.19. *Transchoroidal approach to the medial disconnection of the hippocampus during temporal lobectomy. A, the scalp incision is shown in the* inset *and the left frontotemporal bone flap has been outlined. A cuff of temporalis fascia is left along the superior temporal line for closure. B, the temporal lobe has been elevated to expose the anterior and posterior segment of the uncus. The anterior segment contains most of the amygdala and faces the internal carotid artery. The posterior segment contains the head of the hippocampus and faces the posterior cerebral artery and cerebral peduncle. The uncal apex is located lateral to the oculomotor nerve and posterior communicating artery. C, the temporal horn has been opened by incising through the collateral sulcus, and the inferior temporal and occipitotemporal gyri lateral to the collateral sulcus have been removed. The medial disconnection is performed by opening the choroidal fissure between the choroid plexus and fimbria. D, the taenia fimbria, which attaches the choroid plexus to the fimbria, has been divided and the choroid plexus elevated with the thalamus. Opening the choroidal fissure exposes the branches of the anterior choroidal artery entering the choroid plexus and the ambient cistern. The choroid plexus remains attached to the thalamus. E, the hippocampus and adjacent parahippocampal gyrus have been removed. The posterior cerebral artery courses through the crural and ambient cistern on the medial side of the uncus and parahippocampal gyrus. Some of the amygdala in the upper margin of the anterior uncal segment was not removed to avoid dissection and damage along the optic tract.*

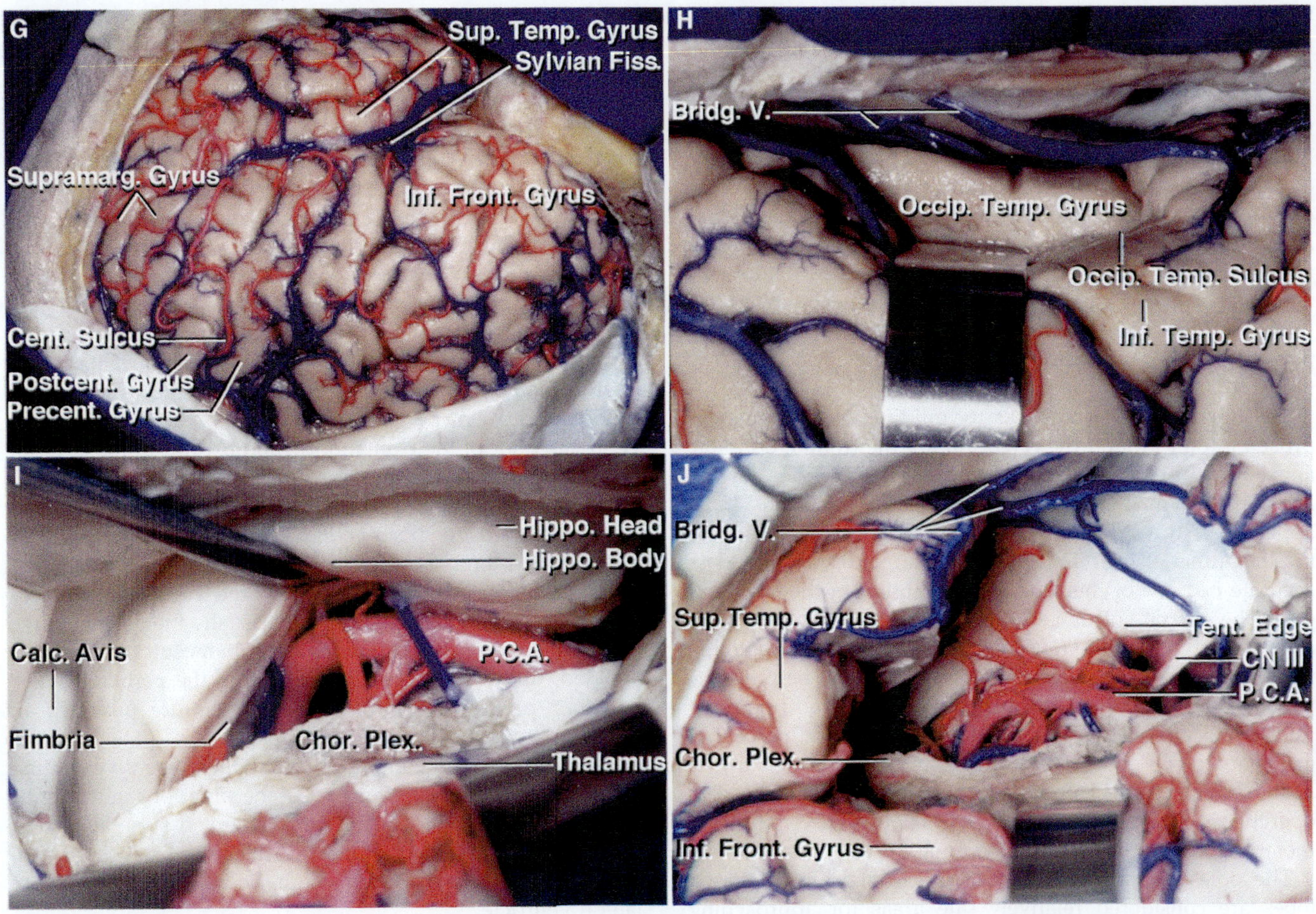

FIGURE 1.19. *Continued*
The lateral geniculate body is exposed medial to the choroidal fissure. The anterior and lateral posterior choroidal arteries enter the choroid plexus by passing through the choroidal fissure. F, *in this dissection, the posterior cerebral artery and basal vein were removed to expose the roof of the temporal horn and the lateral geniculate body. The inferior ventricular vein drains some of the central core of the hemisphere and passes medially across the roof of the temporal horn formed by the tapetum to the reach the basal vein.* G, *exposure for left temporal lobectomy. The exposure includes the frontal and temporal lobe, as might be used for extensive cortical recording and mapping. The exposure is greater than normally used for a standard temporal lobectomy.* H, *an approach that preserves more of the neocortical surface is to open through a sulcus like the occipitotemporal sulcus located between the inferior temporal and occipitotemporal gyri.* I, *the left temporal horn and hippocampal body and head have been exposed. The choroidal fissure has been opened by dividing the tenia fimbria that attaches the choroid plexus to the fimbria on the surface of the hippocampus. The choroid plexus remains attached to the thalamus.* J, *a temporal lobectomy has been completed. The third nerve, posterior cerebral artery, and tentorial edge are in the medial part of the exposure. A large bridging vein passes from the sylvian fissure below the temporal lobe to empty into a tentorial sinus. After disconnecting the hippocampus medially, the resection is extended across the head of the hippocampus behind the amygdala.* A., *artery;* A.Ch.A., *anterior choroidal artery;* Ant., *anterior;* Car., *carotid;* Cist., *cistern;* Chor., *choroid, choroidal;* CN, *cranial nerve;* Coll., *colliculus;* Fiss., *fissure;* Frontozyg., *frontozygomatic;* Gen., *geniculate;* Hippo., *hippocampal;* Inf., *inferior;* L.P.Ch.A., *lateral posterior choroidal artery;* Lat., *lateral;* M., *muscle;* Med., *medial;* P.C.A., *posterior cerebral artery;* P.Co.A., *posterior communicating artery;* Ped., *peduncle;* Plex., *plexus;* Post., *posterior;* Seg., *segment;* Sup., *superior;* Temp., *temporal;* V., *vein;* Vent., *ventricular.*

hole, which, if properly placed, has the frontal dura in the depths of its upper half and the periorbita in its lower half. The keyhole is located immediately above the frontozygomatic point. It is approximately 3 cm anterior to the pterion, just above the lateral end of the superior orbital rim and under the most anterior point of attachment of the temporalis muscle and fascia to the temporal line. Familiarity with these points and lines aids placement of a bone flap over the appropriate lobe and intracranial compartment.

A number of superficial cortical landmarks are helpful in estimating the position of the deep structures (*Figs. 1.2, 1.17,* and *1.18*). The temporal horn is located deep to the middle temporal gyrus, the atrium is located deep to the supramarginal gyrus, and the frontal horn is positioned deep to the inferior frontal gyrus. The splenium and posterior part of the body of the lateral ventricle are located deep to the pre- and postcentral gyri.

An understanding of the superficial relationships of a deep landmark, such as the foramen of Monro, is helpful in planning deep operative approaches. At the cranial surface, the foramen of Monro is located approximately 2 cm above the level of the pterion, just behind the lower third of the coronal suture. At the cerebral surface, it is located deep to the central part of the pars opercularis of the inferior frontal gyrus and, at the insular level, it is located deep to the central part of the second short insular gyrus (*Fig. 1.2*). The pineal is located at the level of the posterior part of the middle temporal gyrus. The thalamus sits at the center of the brain with the foramen of Monro positioned at one end and the pineal at the other end. Together the surface landmarks for the foramen of Monro and pineal approximate the deep position of both the thalamus and third ventricle. The foramen of Monro defines the anterosuperior thalamic margin and the pineal defines the posterior edge. The thalamus is positioned deep to the lower part of the pre- and postcentral gyri and the adjacent part of the superior temporal sulcus (*Fig. 1.2*).

The most reliable landmarks for guiding an operative approach into or around the cerebrum are the frontal, occipital, and temporal poles, the sylvian fissure, the superior, lateral, and medial hemispheric borders, and the central sulcus. If the approach is directed through the cortical surface distant to these landmarks, the orientation of the approach becomes less accurate because of their marked variability in the sulci and gyri. The central sulcus is the most reliable sulcal landmark after the sylvian fissure (*Figs. 1.2, 1.5,* and *1.6*). After opening the dura, its position adjoining the sylvian fissure between the pre- and postcentral gyri can usually be estimated by noting that it is located between the pars opercularis and precentral gyrus anteriorly and the postcentral and supramarginal gyri posteriorly. The precentral gyrus is located behind the pars opercularis, and the postcentral gyrus is positioned in front of the anterior bank of the supramarginal gyrus.

The poles and adjacent part of the frontal and temporal lobes are considered relatively safe areas for approaching deeper lesions, but opening the occipital pole carries significant risks to the visual pathways. If approaches to the midportions of the cerebrum are to be directed through the cortical surface and a lesion has not dissected a pathological pathway to the cortical surface, it is best to direct the approach through the middle and superior frontal gyri, superior parietal lobule, intraparietal sulcus, or the lower part of the lateral or basal surface of the temporal lobe. The deep end of the cerebral sulci are commonly directed toward the ventricular surface. Sulci suitable for approaching deep lesions, such as those in the lateral ventricles, include the superior frontal, inferior temporal, occipitotemporal, collateral, or the intraparietal sulci. The approaches to the lateral and third ventricle are reviewed in detail in Chapter 5.

Electrophysiological cortical mapping and studies of the sulci and gyri on magnetic resonance imaging also play a major role in directing an operative approach to the appropriate area. These more recent contributions, when combined with image guidance, have made intracerebral surgery much safer when applied with an accurate understanding of microsurgical anatomy.

The supratentorial area, fortunately, provides a number of natural pathways through which deep lesions can be approached. The sylvian fissure is a frequently used pathway for reaching all structures within and bordering the basal cisterns anterior to the quadrigeminal cistern. The neural and vascular structures within reach of transsylvian approaches include the insula, basal ganglia, uncus, orbit, anterior cranial fossa; the olfactory, optic, and oculomotor nerves; the chiasmatic, interpeduncular, carotid, lamina terminalis, and crural cisterns; the middle cerebral and proximal part of the anterior cerebral arteries; the internal carotid artery and its branches; the circle of Willis; and the upper part of the basilar artery. The major obstacles in working through the sylvian fissure are the trunks and perforating branches of the arteries that course through the cisterns. These are reviewed in Chapter 2.

The interhemispheric fissure provides another natural cleft for accessing deep areas of the brain. Approaches directed along the anterior part of the fissure access the subcallosal area in front of the lamina terminalis and rostrum of the corpus callosum and can be used as a route to the anterior third ventricle, floor of the frontal horn, and regions of the anterior communicating artery. Transcallosal approaches directed through the interhemispheric fissure just in front of the coronal suture access the portion of the corpus callosum above the foramen of Monro for dealing with colloid cysts and other lesions in the frontal horn and body of the lateral ventricle and the upper part of the third ventricle. Usually the portion of the interhemispheric fissure along the paracentral lobule is avoided, unless it is directly involved in the pathology. The posterior part of the interhemispheric fissure provides an excellent route to the quadrigeminal cistern, pineal region, and galenic venous complex because there are no bridging veins between the posterior part of the superior sagittal sinus and the occipital lobe. The interhemispheric fissure can also be used to access lesions that involve the corpus callosum, cingulate sulcus, and the frontal horn, body, and atrium of the lateral ventricle.

The area between the basal surface of the cerebrum and the cranial base also provides a route for reaching selected lesions. The approaches directed below the orbital surface of the frontal lobe provide access to the region of the cribriform plate, orbital roof, optic nerves, the chiasmatic and lamina terminalis cisterns, and the medial part of the sylvian fissure. The approach directed below the anterior part of the basal surface of the temporal lobe, called the anterior subtemporal approach, can be used to access lesions along the whole lateral margin of the tentorial incisura back to the junction of the ambient and quadrigeminal cisterns. Retracting the anterior part of the basal surface of the temporal lobe carries less risk than elevating the posterior part, because the bridging veins that drain the majority of the temporal lobe course below the posterior temporal lobe.

The central core of the hemisphere, although small relative to the surface cortical area, is the site of numerous vital structures and pathways that can be reached by a number of surgical routes. These approaches include the subfrontal approach, which accesses the area below the anterior perforated substance where the lentiform and caudate blend together below the anterior limb of the internal capsule in the roof of the sphenoidal part of the sylvian cistern; the anterior interhemispheric approach, with opening the lamina terminalis and rostrum of the corpus callosum, which accesses the lateral and third ventricle at the medial surface of the central core; the frontal and parietal transcallosal and transcortical approaches, which access the lateral ventricular surfaces of the core formed by the thalamus and caudate, and the medial thalamic surface facing the third ventricle; the transsylvian approach, which accesses the insular surface in the lateral aspect of the core and the caudate and lentiform nuclei facing the anterior perforated substance; and the subtemporal approach, which exposes the lower thalamic surface and the optic tract forming the roof of the ambient cistern in the lower part of the core.

Temporal Lobectomy and Amygdalohippocampectomy

The medial temporal lobe, one of the most complicated parts of the cerebrum, is the most common target for resections to treat convulsive disorders (*Figs. 1.2, 1.8–1.10, 1.12, 1.13,* and *1.19*) (10). Several important concepts aid in conceptualizing structures in the area. One is an understanding of the relationships of the anterior and posterior segments of the uncus to the amygdala and hippocampus and to the temporal horn. The amygdala forms the majority of the anterior segment of the uncus and the anterior wall and adjacent part of the roof of the temporal horn. The amygdala presents at the medial surface of the anterior segment just lateral to the internal carotid artery. The anterior segment and amygdala are crossed above by the middle cerebral artery. The anterior choroidal artery arises from the internal carotid artery medial to the anterior segment and ascends as it passes posteriorly along the medial surface of the anterior segment. The medially directed apex of the uncus is located lateral to the third nerve and posterior communicating artery. The posterior segment faces posteromedially toward the cerebral peduncle and is divided into an upper and lower part by the uncal notch, a short sulcus that extends into the posterior segment from its posterior edge (*Figs. 1.9* and *1.10*). The head of the hippocampus is located in the floor of the temporal horn and turns medially to form most of the upper half of the posterior uncal segment. The amygdala extends backward above the anterior part of the head of the hippocampus and roof of the temporal horn. Superiorly, the amygdala blends into the lower margin of the lentiform nucleus (*Fig. 1.8, F* and *G*). The uncal recess, a narrow medially projecting space between the hippocampal head and the ventricular surface of the amygdala, partially separates the two structures and is located lateral to the uncal apex (*Figs. 1.13J* and *1.14F*).

During a temporal lobectomy, the temporal horn, depending on the extent of the resection, can be entered through the middle or inferior temporal sulcus or through the basal surface on the medial side of the basal part of the inferior temporal or occipitotemporal gyri (*Fig. 1.19*). The temporal horn will be encountered approximately 2.5 cm from the temporal pole. There are several steps in completing the lobectomy. The first step is the lateral temporal or neocortical exposure and removal. The second step is the medial disconnection of the hippocampus, which can be achieved by opening the choroidal fissure. The third step is the anterior disconnection that includes separating the head of the hippocampus from the amygdala by using the uncal recess as a landmark for carrying the exposure through the medial aspect of the uncus. The next step is the posterior disconnection, which involves sectioning the hippocampus and parahippocampal gyrus as far posteriorly as indicated by electrophysiological and neuroradiological studies. The final step is removal of the remaining amygdala in front of the uncal recess. Usually, a small bit of amygdala is preserved superiorly where it is in close apposition to the optic tract, branches of the anterior choroidal and posterior cerebral arteries, and the lower surface of the lentiform nucleus.

Yaşargil and Wieser (11) approach the amygdala and hippocampus through the lower part of the sylvian fissure and circular sulcus, medial to the superior temporal gyrus and below the inferior trunk of the middle cerebral artery. The incision through the anteroinferior part of the circular sulcus exposes the amygdala in the anterior uncal segment (*Figs. 1.12* and *1.13*). The lower and lateral parts of the amygdala are removed, but the upper medial part adjacent the claustrum, optic tract, and lentiform nucleus is not removed. The anterior uncal area is removed using subpial suction, taking care to preserve the anterior choroidal and posterior communicating arteries, the oculomotor nerve, basal vein, and optic tract, which are visible through the pia arachnoid. The anterior portion of the temporal horn is then exposed and the choroidal fissure is opened in the area lateral to the cerebral peduncle while preserving the anterior choroidal artery, optic tract, and basal vein. The dissection is carried along the lateral side of the hippocampus to the rhinal and collateral sulcus, and the transverse section of the hippocampus and parahippocampal gyrus is carried out at the posterior edge of the cerebral peduncle, lateral to the level of the geniculate body and the ascension of the fimbria to form the crus of the fornix.

REFERENCES

1. Gibo H, Carver CC, Rhoton AL Jr, Lenkey C, Mitchell RJ: Microsurgical anatomy of the middle cerebral artery. **J Neurosurg** 54:151–169, 1981.
2. Nagata S, Rhoton AL Jr, Barry M: Microsurgical anatomy of the choroidal fissure. **Surg Neurol** 30:3–59, 1988.
3. Ono M, Kubik S, Abernathey CD: *Atlas of the Cerebral Sulci.* New York, Thieme Medical Publishers, 1990, pp 218.
4. Perlmutter D, Rhoton AL Jr: Microsurgical anatomy of the distal anterior cerebral artery. **J Neurosurg** 49:204–228, 1978.
5. Rhoton AL Jr: The posterior cranial fossa: Microsurgical anatomy and surgical approaches. **Neurosurgery** 47[Suppl 1]:S1–S297, 2000.
6. Rhoton AL Jr: Tentorial incisura. **Neurosurgery** 47[Suppl 1]:S131–S153, 2000.
7. Timurkaynak E, Rhoton AL Jr, Barry M: Microsurgical anatomy and operative approaches to the lateral ventricles. **Neurosurgery** 19:685–723, 1986.
8. Wen HT, Rhoton AL Jr: Basic neuroanatomy, in Layon AJ, Gabrielli A, Friedman WA (eds): *A Textbook of Neurointensive Care.* Philadelphia, W.B. Saunders Co. (in press).
9. Wen HT, Rhoton AL Jr, de Oliveira EP: Transchoroidal approach to the third ventricle: An anatomic study of the choroidal fissure and its clinical application. **Neurosurgery** 42:1205–1219, 1998.
10. Wen HT, Rhoton AL Jr, de Oliveira EP, Cardoso AC, Tedeschi H, Baccanelli M, Marino R Jr: Microsurgical anatomy of the temporal lobe: Part 1—Mesial temporal lobe anatomy and its vascular relationships as applied for amygdalohippocampectomy. **Neurosurgery** 45:549–592, 1999.
11. Yaşargil MG, Wieser HG: Selective amygdalohippocampectomy at the University Hospital, Zurich, in Engel J Jr (ed): *Surgical Treatment of the Epilepsies.* New York, Raven Press, 1987, pp 653–658.
12. Zeal AA, Rhoton AL Jr: Microsurgical anatomy of the posterior cerebral artery. **J Neurosurg** 48:534–559, 1978.

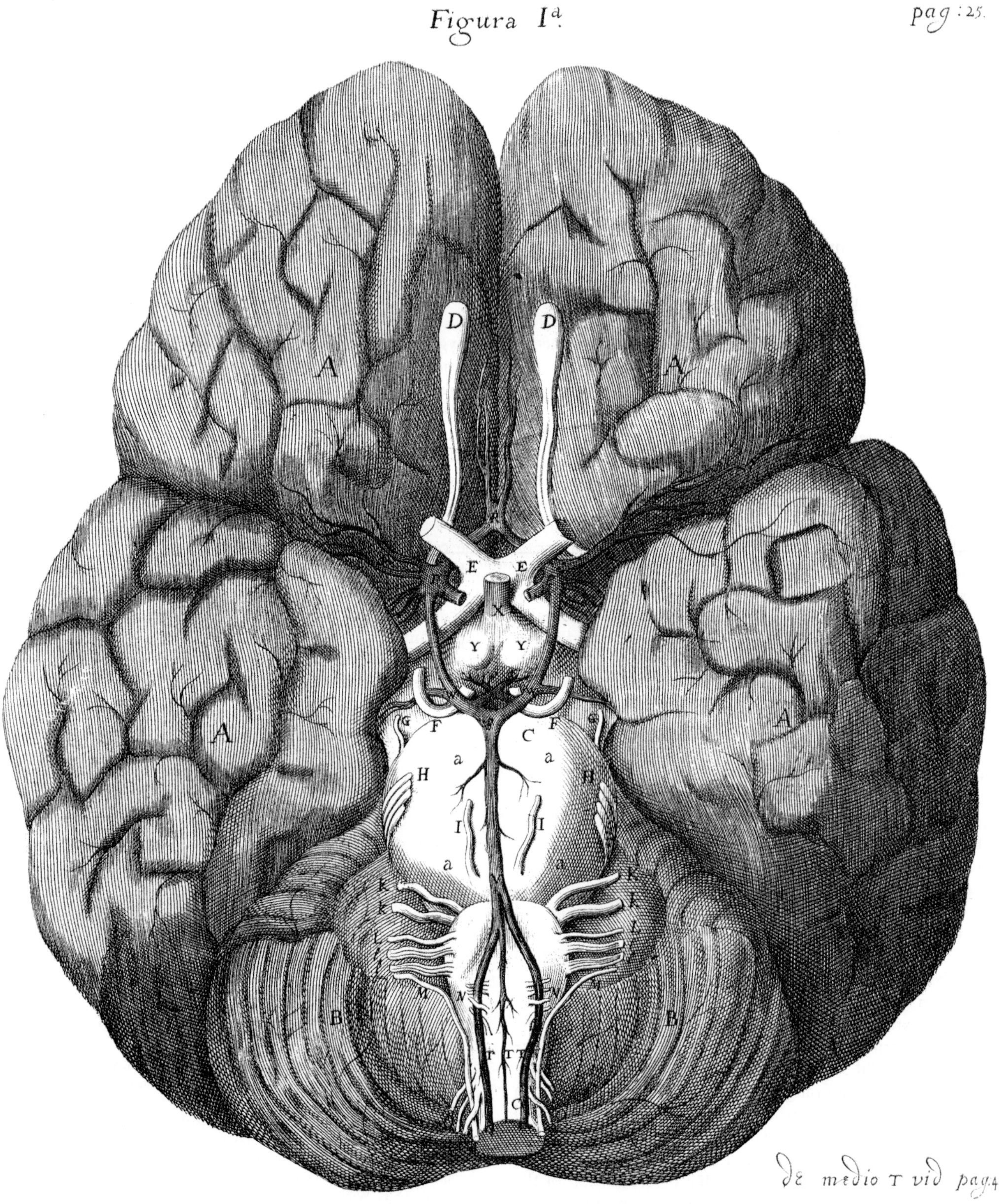

Image showing the inferior surface of the brain. From Thomas Willis' Cerebri Anatome. *London, 1664.*

The Supratentorial Arteries

Albert L. Rhoton, Jr., M.D.
Department of Neurological Surgery, University of Florida, Gainesville, Florida

Correspondence:
Albert L. Rhoton, Jr., M.D., Department of Neurological Surgery, University of Florida McKnight Brain Institute, P.O. Box 100265, 100 South Newell Drive, Building 59, L2-100, Gainesville, FL 32610-0265.
Email:
rhoton@neurosurgery.ufl.edu

KEY WORDS: Anterior cerebral artery, Anterior choroidal artery, Cerebral arteries, Cerebrovascular disease, Circle of Willis, Internal carotid artery, Intracranial aneurysms, Middle cerebral artery, Posterior cerebral artery, Supratentorial arteries

The supratentorial arteries include the supraclinoid portion of the internal carotid artery and its anterior and middle cerebral, ophthalmic, posterior communicating, and anterior choroidal branches, the components of the circle of Willis, which in the posterior midline includes the basilar apex, and finally, the posterior cerebral artery. The origin of all of these arteries is located deep under the center of the cerebrum and their proximal trunks are relatively inaccessible because they course in deep clefts like the sylvian or interhemispheric fissure or in the basal cisterns between the brainstem and temporal lobe (*Fig. 2.1*). Only the smaller terminal branches are accessible on lateral convexity and even there, these branches are often hidden in cortical sulci rather than coursing on the gyral surfaces. No single operative approach will access all of the branches of the three major cerebral arteries because of their long courses. Thus, each operative approach must be carefully tailored based on the relationships of the arterial segment involved. The relationship of these arteries to the common aneurysm sites and their operative exposure is reviewed in Chapter 3.

SUPRACLINOIDAL PORTION OF THE INTERNAL CAROTID ARTERY

The supraclinoidal portion of the internal carotid artery (ICA) is a common site of intracranial aneurysms, and its branches are frequently stretched, displaced, or encased by cranial base tumors. The ICA and its major and perforating branches are frequently exposed during operations on aneurysms of the circle of Willis and tumors of the sphenoid ridge, anterior and middle cranial fossae, and suprasellar region. Agenesis or aplasia of the internal carotid artery is rare.

Segments of the Internal Carotid Artery

The ICA is divided into four parts: the C1 or cervical portion extends from its junction with the common carotid artery to the external orifice of the carotid canal; the C2 or petrous portion courses within the carotid canal and ends where the artery enters the cavernous sinus; the C3 or cavernous portion courses within the cavernous sinus and ends where the artery passes through the dura mater forming the roof of the cavernous sinus; and the C4 or supraclinoid portion begins where the artery enters the subarachnoid space and terminates at the bifurcation into the anterior (ACA) and middle cerebral arteries (MCA) (*Fig. 2.2*) (25, 36).

The C4 begins where the artery emerges from the dura mater, forming the roof of the cavernous sinus. It enters the cranial cavity by passing along the medial side of the anterior clinoid process and below the optic nerve. It courses posterior, superior, and slightly lateral to reach the lateral side of the optic chiasm and bifurcates below the anterior perforated substance at the medial end of the sylvian fissure to give rise to the ACA and MCA. The C4 segment is defined as including the crotch from which the MCA and ACA arise, and the branches originating from the apex of the wall between the origin of the ACA and MCA are considered to be branches of the ICA, just as aneurysms arising at this apex are considered to be aneurysms of the bifurcation of the ICA. When viewed from laterally, the cavernous (C3) and intracranial (C4) portions have several curves that form an S-shape, and together these portions are called the carotid siphon. The lower half of the S, formed predominantly by the intracavernous portion, is convex anteriorly, and the upper half, formed by the supraclinoid portion, is convex posteriorly. The junction of the anteriorly and posteriorly convex segments passes along the medial side of the anterior clinoid process. The prebifurcation branches of the C4 are the ophthalmic, anterior choroidal (AChA), posterior communicating arteries (PComA), perforating, and superior hypophyseal arteries.

The intradural exposure of the C4 and the anterior portion of the circle of Willis is directed along the ipsilateral sphenoid ridge or orbital roof to the anterior clinoid process. In exposing the ICA, the approach is usually from proximal to distal, beginning with the ophthalmic segment and working distally toward the bifurcation. The ophthalmic artery is difficult to expose because of its short intradural length and its location under the optic nerve.

In exposing the C4 beyond the origin of the ophthalmic artery, the surgeon often sees the AChA before the PComA, although the AChA arises distal to the PComA (*Figs. 2.1* and *2.3*). This occurs because of three sets of anatomic circumstances. First, the C4 passes upward in a posterolateral direction, placing the origin of the AChA further lateral to the midline than the origin of the PComA. Second, the AChA

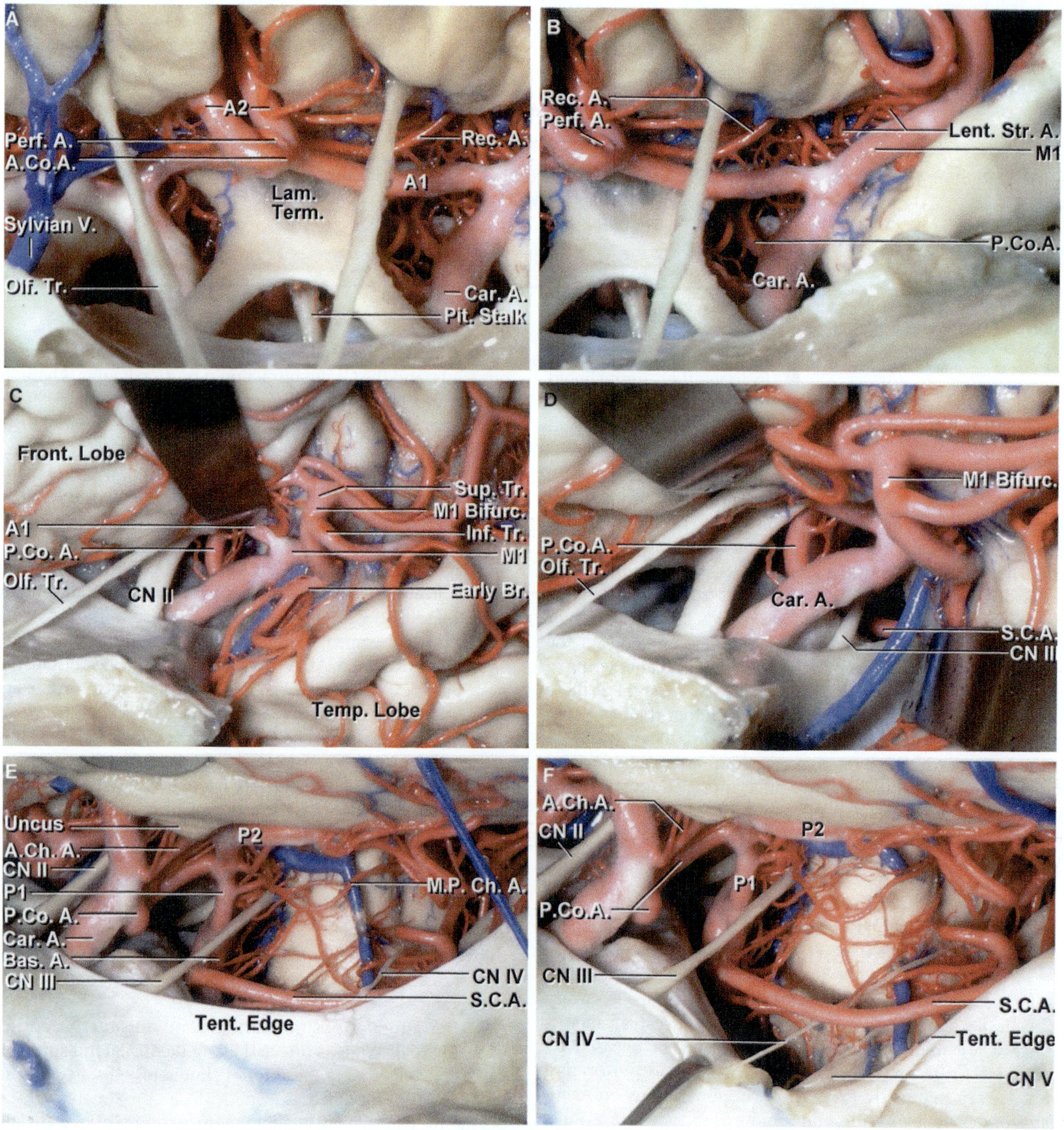

FIGURE 2.1. *Arteries in the basal cisterns.* A, *anterior view. A1s of nearly equal size cross the front of the lamina terminalis. The right A2 enters the interhemispheric fissure in front of the left A2. The left recurrent artery arises near the level of the anterior communicating artery (AComA) and passes laterally below the anterior perforated substance. A perforating artery arises from the AComA.* B, *the view has shifted laterally above the carotid bifurcation. The recurrent artery passes laterally above the A1 and intermingles with the lenticulostriate branches of the M1. The posterior communicating artery (PComA) is directed medially and is seen through the opticocarotid triangle located between the carotid artery, optic nerve, and the A1.* C, *anterolateral view. The PComA is seen through the opticocarotid triangle. The M1 bifurcates into superior and inferior trunks at the limen insula.* D, *the basal cisterns have been opened and the temporal pole retracted to expose the oculomotor nerve. The PComA is directed backward above and medial to the oculomotor nerve. The superior cerebellar artery courses below the oculomotor nerve.* E, *the temporal lobe has been elevated. The anterior choroidal artery (AChA) ascends on the medial side of the uncus. The PComA and the P1 join to form the P2, which continues backward on the medial side of the posterior part of the uncus. A medial posterior choroidal artery (MPChA) passes backward around the brainstem. The superior cerebellar artery passes below the oculomotor and trochlear nerves. The branches forming the P3 course through the quadrigeminal cistern. The P2 courses through the ambient and crural cisterns. A MPChA*

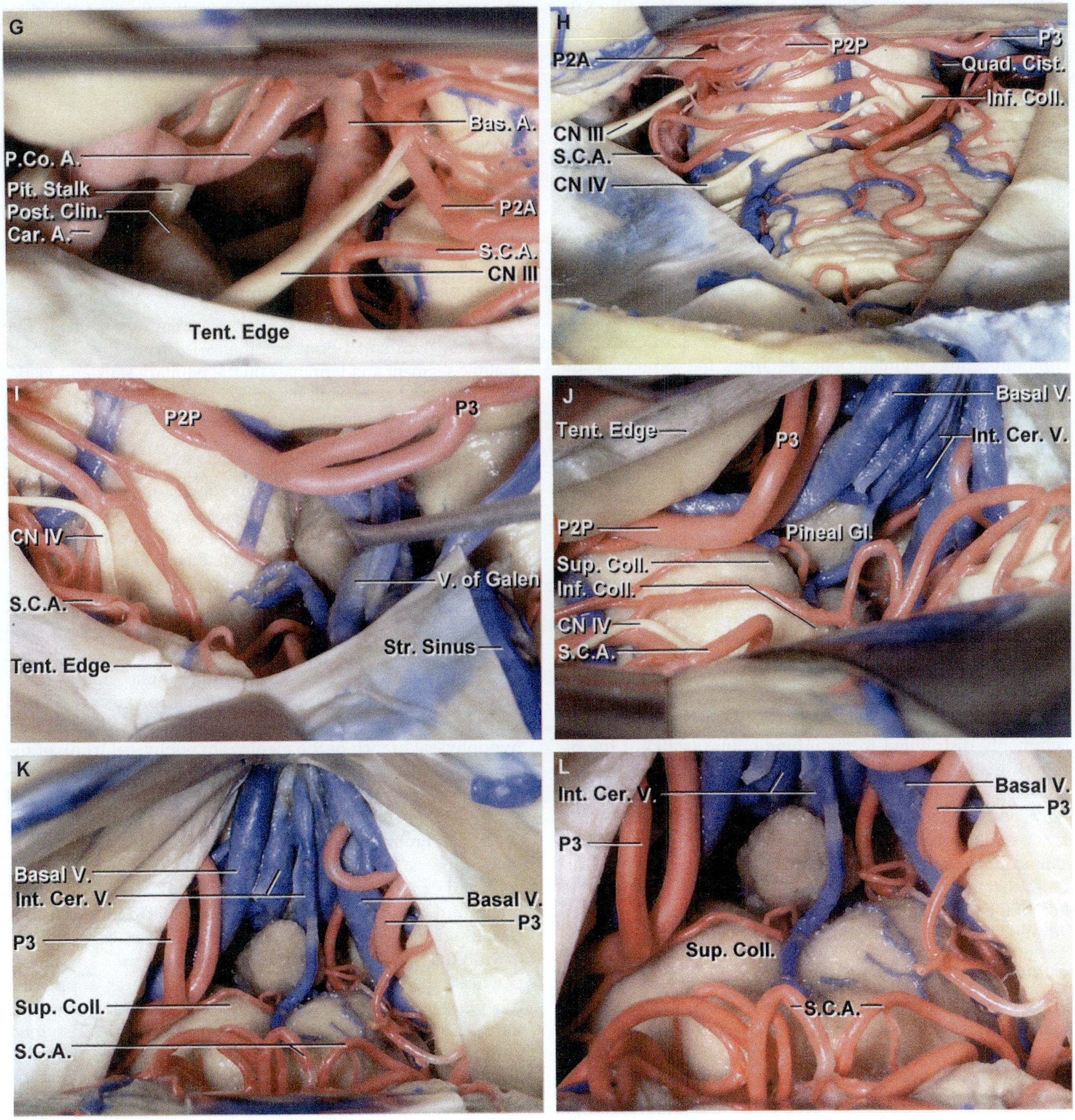

FIGURE 2.1. *Continued* *encircles the brainstem. F, the tentorium has been divided to expose the upper part of the basilar artery. The trigeminal nerve is exposed in the lateral margin of the tentorial opening. The posterior cerebral artery (PCA) courses above and the superior cerebellar artery courses below the oculomotor nerve. G, subtemporal exposure in another specimen. The PComA is larger than shown in D and E. The oculomotor nerve passes forward between the PCA and the superior cerebellar arteries. H, the exposure has been extended further posteriorly along the side of the brainstem to the quadrigeminal cistern. The tentorium has been divided to expose the upper part of the cerebellum. The PCA and superior cerebellar artery encircle the brainstem to reach the quadrigeminal cistern. The P2 is divided into a P2A that courses in the crural cistern between the uncus and cerebral peduncle, and a P2P that courses in the ambient cisterns between the parahippocampal gyrus on the midbrain. The P3 courses in the quadrigeminal cistern. The trochlear nerve arises below the inferior colliculus and crosses above the branches of the superior cerebellar artery. I, the exposure has been extended further posteriorly, above the tentorium to the left half of the quadrigeminal cistern. The tributaries of the vein of Galen have been retracted to expose the pineal. The PCA courses above the tentorium and the superior cerebellar* *(Legend continues on next page.)*

commonly arises further laterally on the posterior wall of the C4 portion than the PComA. The site of origin of the AChA from the posterior wall of the C4 portion is lateral to the site of origin of the PComA in 94% of hemispheres (33). Third, the AChA pursues a more lateral course than the PComA; the former passes laterally around the cerebral peduncle and into the temporal horn, whereas the latter is most commonly directed in its initial course in a posteromedial direction above the oculomotor nerve toward the interpeduncular fossa.

Segments of the C4

The C4 is divided into three segments based on the site of origin of the ophthalmic, PComA, and AChA. The ophthalmic segment extends from the roof of the cavernous sinus and the origin of the ophthalmic artery to the origin of the PComA; the communicating segment extends from the origin of the PComA to the origin of the AChA; and the choroidal segment extends from the origin of the AChA to the terminal bifurcation of the ICA. The ophthalmic segment is the longest, and the communicating segment is the shortest (15).

C4 Perforating Branches

Each of the three C4 segments gives off a series of perforating branches with a relatively constant site of termination. An average of 8 (range, 3–12) perforating arteries (excluding the ophthalmic, PComA, and AChA) arise from the C4 (*Figs. 2.4–2.6*).

Ophthalmic Segment

An average of four (range, one to seven) perforating arteries arise from the ophthalmic segment. Most arise from the posterior or medial aspect of the artery. These branches are most commonly distributed to the infundibulum (stalk) of the pituitary gland, the optic chiasm, and less commonly, in descending order of frequency, to the optic nerve, premamillary portion of the floor of the third ventricle, and the optic tract. A few vessels terminate in the dura mater covering the anterior clinoid process, sella turcica, and tuberculum sellae. The arteries that arise from this segment and pass to the infundibulum of the pituitary gland are called the superior hypophyseal arteries (13, 15).

Communicating Segment

No perforating branches arise from the communicating segment in more than half of hemispheres, and if present, only one to three are found. They arise from the posterior half of the wall and terminate, in descending order of frequency, in the optic tract, premamillary part of the floor of the third ventricle, the optic chiasm, and infundibulum, and infrequently, enter the anterior or posterior perforated substance. The branches are often stretched around the neck of posterior communicating aneurysms.

Choroidal Segment

An average of four (range, one to nine) branches arise from the choroidal segment. Most branches arise from the posterior half of the arterial wall and terminate, in descending order of frequency, in the anterior perforated substance, optic tract, and uncus.

Superior Hypophyseal and Infundibular Arteries

The superior hypophyseal arteries are a group of one to five (average, two) small branches that arise from the C4's ophthalmic segment and terminate on the pituitary stalk and gland, but also send branches to the optic nerves and chiasm and the floor of the third ventricle (*Figs. 2.4–2.6*). The largest of the branches is often referred to as the superior hypophyseal artery. Most branches arise from the posteromedial, medial, or the posterior aspects of the artery. The infundibular arteries are a group of arteries that originate from the PComA and are distributed to the infundibulum. There are fewer infundibular arteries than superior hypophyseal arteries. One-quarter of hemispheres have one or two infundibular arteries and the remainder have none.

The superior hypophyseal and infundibular arteries pass medially below the chiasm to reach the tuber cinereum. They intermingle and form a fine anastomotic plexus around the pituitary stalk called the circuminfundibular anastomosis. These arteries and the circuminfundibular plexus are distributed to the pituitary stalk and anterior lobe. The inferior hypophyseal branch of the meningohypophyseal trunk of the intracavernous carotid perfuses the posterior lobe. The capsular arteries also arise from the intracavernous carotid and supply the capsule of the pituitary gland (16).

This circuminfundibular plexus gives rise to ascending and descending arteries. The descending arteries include short-stalk and superficial arteries. The short-stalk arteries penetrate the infundibulum and form capillaries that lead into sinusoids running down the stalk. The superficial arteries course inferiorly on the outside of the stalk in the subarachnoid space and penetrate the anterior lobe. The ascending arteries supply the tuber cinereum, median eminence, and the inferior surface of the optic chiasm. The superior hypophyseal arteries also send branches to the chiasm and proximal portions of the optic nerves.

FIGURE 2.1. *Continued*
artery below. The trochlear nerve arises below the inferior colliculus and passes around the brainstem. J, the exposure has been directed below the tentorium. The internal cerebral veins exit the roof of the third ventricle and the basal veins exit the basal cisterns to join and form the vein of Galen. The P3 courses through the quadrigeminal cistern. K, midline infratentorial exposure. The pineal is exposed between the posterior cerebral arteries and basal veins and below the internal cerebral veins. The exposure into the fissure between the cerebellum and midbrain is not as great as can be achieved when the exposure is directed off to the side of the vermian apex in a paramedian location as shown in J. L, enlarged view of the midline infratentorial exposure. A., *artery, arteries;* A.Co.A., *anterior communicating artery;* Bas., *basilar;* Bifurc., *bifurcation;* Br., *branch;* Car., *carotid;* Cer., *cerebral;* Cist., *cistern;* Clin., *clinoid;* CN, *cranial nerve;* Coll., *colliculus;* Front., *frontal;* Gl., *gland;* Inf., *inferior;* Int., *internal;* Lam., *lamina;* Lent. Str., *lenticulostriate;* M.P.Ch.A., *medial posterior choroidal artery;* Olf., *olfactory;* P.Co.A., *posterior communicating artery;* Perf., *perforating;* Pit., *pituitary;* Post., *posterior;* Quad., *quadrigeminal;* Rec., *recurrent;* S.C.A., *superior cerebellar artery;* Str., *straight;* Sup., *superior;* Temp., *temporal;* Tent., *tentorial;* Term., *terminalis;* Tr., *tract, trunk;* V., *vein.*

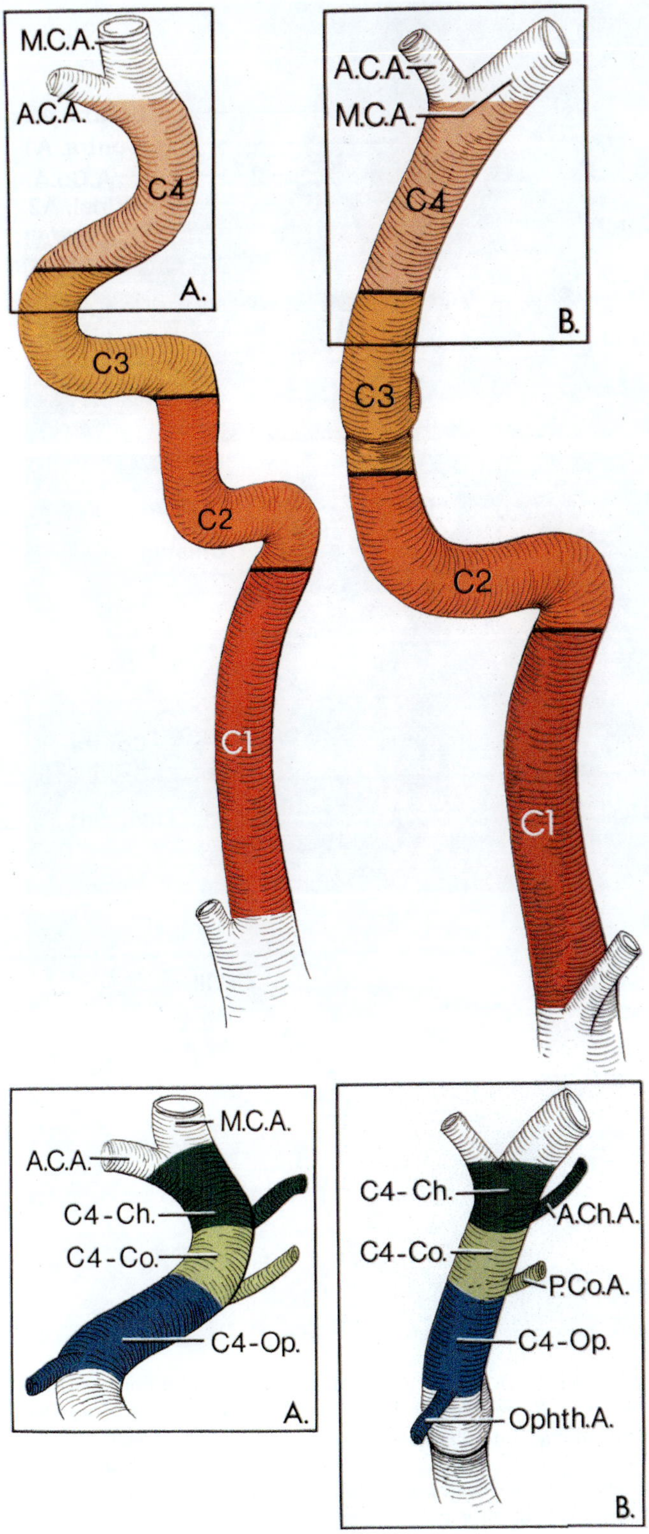

OPHTHALMIC ARTERY

The ophthalmic artery is the first branch of the C4. Most ophthalmic arteries arise below the optic nerve in the supraclinoid area above the dural roof of the cavernous sinus and pass anterolaterally below the optic nerve to enter the optic canal and orbit. The distal course is reviewed in Chapter 7. Eight percent of ophthalmic arteries originate within the cavernous sinus. The ophthalmic artery may rarely arise from the clinoid segment of the ICA located on the medial side of the anterior clinoid process or from the middle meningeal artery (16, 20, 29). It is rarely absent. The ophthalmic arteries uncommonly give rise to intracranial perforating branches and, if present, these branches run posteriorly and are distributed to the ventral aspect of the optic nerve and chiasm and the pituitary stalk.

The ophthalmic artery usually arises from the medial third of the superior surface of the C4 immediately distal to the cavernous sinus in the area below the optic nerve. In our earlier study, it arose above the medial third of the superior surface of the C4 in 78% of hemispheres and above the middle third of the superior surface in 22% of cases (15). None arise from the lateral third of the superior surface. It may kink laterally, infrequently presenting a short segment lateral to the optic nerve before entering the optic canal. The origin varies from as far as 5 mm anterior to 7 mm posterior to the tip of the anterior clinoid process and from 2 to 10 mm medial to the clinoid process (16). Most ophthalmic arteries arise anterior to the tip of the anterior clinoid process, approximately 5 mm medial to the anterior clinoid.

The intracranial segment of the ophthalmic artery is usually very short. In a previous study from this laboratory, 14% of the segments were found to exit the ICA and immediately enter the optic canal; in the remaining 86%, the maximum

FIGURE 2.2. *Lateral* (left) *and anterior views* (right) *of the left internal carotid artery (ICA) and* A *and* B, *segments of the supraclinoid (C4) portion.* A, *lateral view of the C4 portion.* B, *anterior view of the C4 portion. The ICA is divided into four parts. These parts, from proximal to distal, are the C1 through the C4 portions. The cervical portion (C1,* red*) extends from the origin of the ICA to the external orifice of the carotid canal in the petrous temporal bone. The petrous portion (C2,* orange*) extends from the external orifice of the carotid canal to where the artery exits the carotid canal to enter the cavernous sinus. The cavernous portion (C3,* yellow*) begins where the artery enters the cavernous sinus and terminates where it emerges from the dura mater on the medial side of the anterior clinoid process to enter the intracranial cavity. The intracranial (supraclinoid) portion (C4,* beige*) begins where the artery enters the cranial cavity medial to the anterior clinoid process and terminates below the anterior perforated substance where the artery bifurcates into the anterior and middle cerebral arteries. The ICA gives rise to the ophthalmic, posterior communicating, anterior choroidal, anterior cerebral, and the middle cerebral arteries. The supraclinoid portion of the ICA is divided into three segments based on the origin of these branches. The ophthalmic segment (C4-Op.,* dark blue*) extends from the origin of the ophthalmic artery to the origin of the PComA. The communicating segment (C4-Co.,* light green*) extends from the origin of the PComA to the origin of the anterior choroidal artery. The choroidal segment (C4-Ch.,* dark green*) extends from the origin of the anterior choroidal artery to the bifurcation of the internal carotid artery into the anterior and middle cerebral arteries.* A., *artery;* A.C.A., *anterior cerebral artery;* A.Ch.A., *anterior choroidal artery;* Ch., *choroidal;* Co., *communicating;* M.C.A., *middle cerebral artery;* Op., *ophthalmic;* Ophth., *ophthalmic;* P.Co.A., *posterior communicating artery.* (From, *Gibo H, Lenkey C, Rhoton AL Jr: Microsurgical anatomy of the supraclinoid portion of the internal carotid artery.* ***J Neurosurg*** *55:560–574, 1981 [15].)*

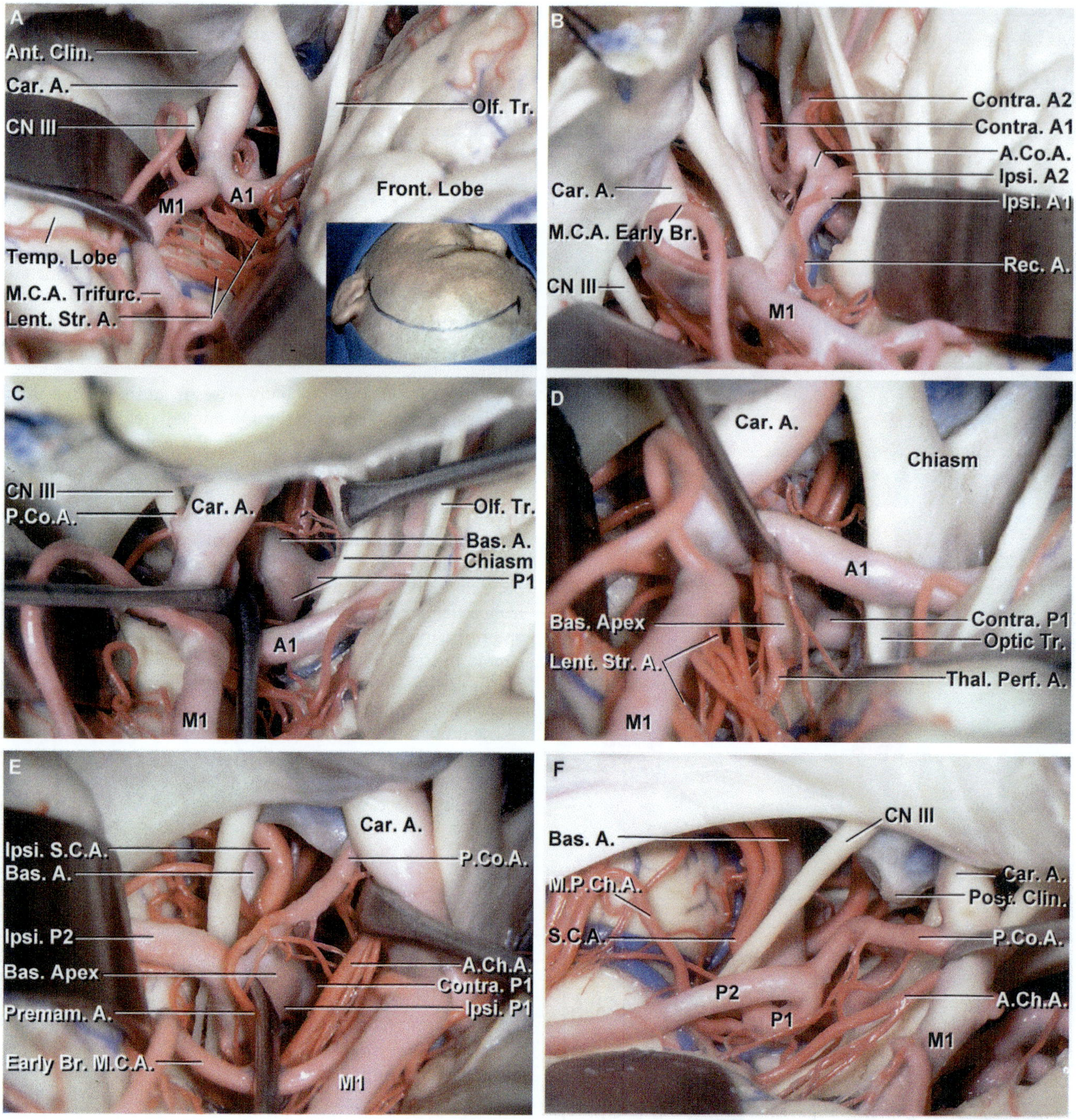

FIGURE 2.3. *Pterional exposure of the circle of Willis. A, a left frontotemporal bone flap has been elevated and the dura opened. The left frontal and temporal lobes have been retracted to expose the carotid artery entering the dura medial to the anterior clinoid process. The carotid bifurcation has been exposed. Lenticulostriate arteries arise from the M1. The M1 splits in a trifurcation pattern. B, the exposure has been extended between the chiasm and frontal lobe to the AComA and the contralateral A1 and A2s. A recurrent artery arising near the AComA passes laterally above the carotid bifurcation. C, the basilar bifurcation has been exposed through the opticocarotid triangle located between the internal carotid artery, A1, and optic nerve. D, the carotid bifurcation has been depressed to expose the basilar apex in the interval between the carotid bifurcation and the lower margin of the optic tract. Perforating branches crossing the area can make the approach hazardous. A thalamoperforating artery arises from the ipsilateral P1. E, the temporal pole has been retracted posteriorly for a pretemporal exposure. The carotid and anterior choroidal arteries have been elevated to expose the PComA, which gives rise to a large perforating branch referred to as a premamillary artery. The M1 gives rise to an early branch proximal to the trifurcation. The P2 extends above and the superior cerebellar artery (SCA) extends below the oculomotor nerve. F, anterior subtemporal view. The temporal pole and the carotid artery have been elevated to the expose the origin of the normal-sized PComA. The AChA passes backward along the medial edge of the uncus. A large MPChA arises from*

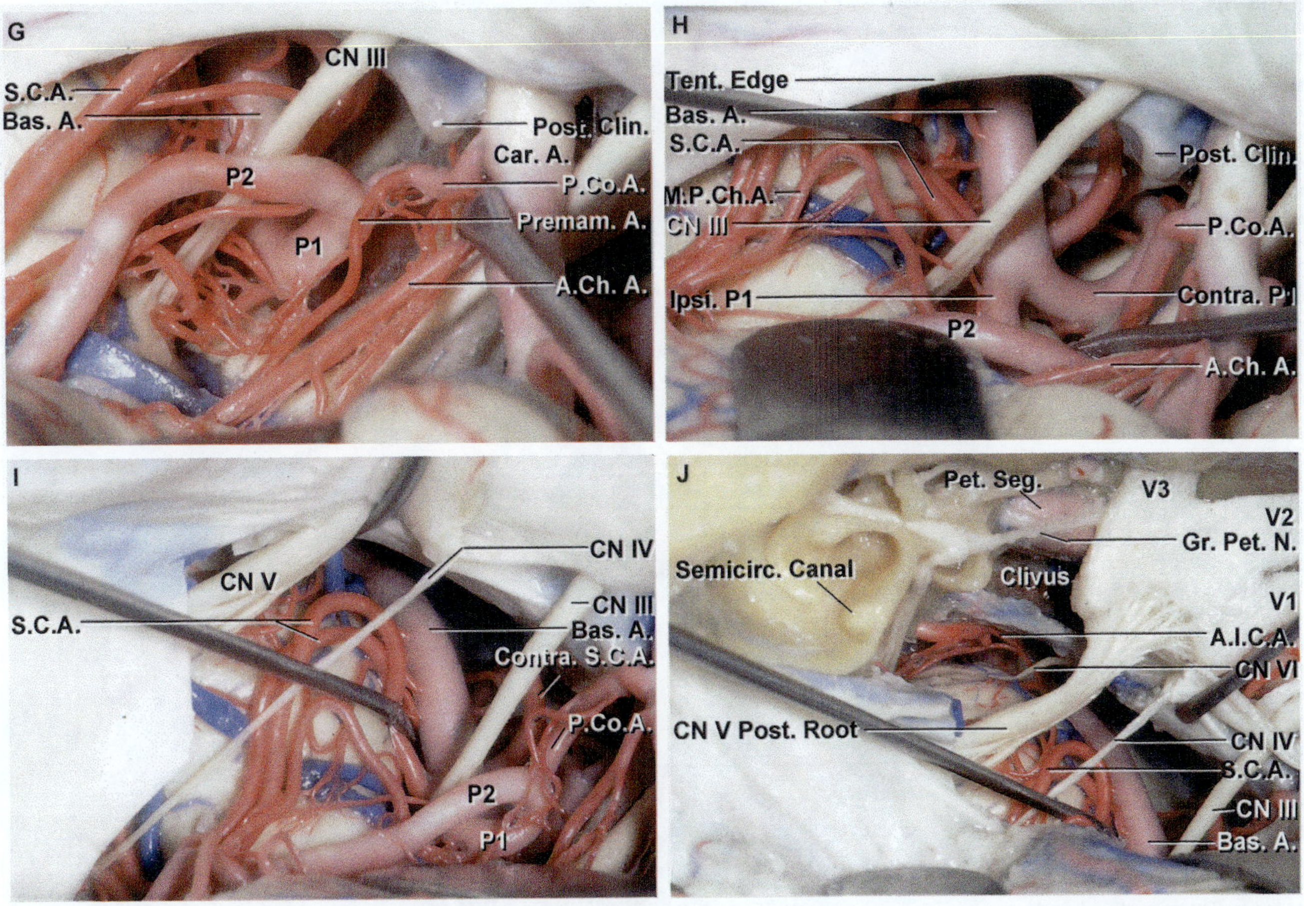

FIGURE 2.3. *Continued*
the P1 and loops downward as it passes to the quadrigeminal cistern. G, the AChA has been elevated to expose a large perforating branch of the PComA called a premamillary artery. H, the PComA has been elevated to provide an excellent exposure of the basilar apex and the P1s. The ipsilateral SCA arises as a duplicate artery. I, the tentorium has been divided behind where the trochlear nerve enters the edge. This increases the length of basilar artery exposed. The trunks of a duplicate superior cerebellar artery loop down toward the trigeminal nerve. J, the petrous apex has been removed to complete an anterior petrosectomy approach, which increases access to the front of the brainstem and the basilar artery. In this case, the labyrinth including the cochlea and semicircular canals, and the nerves in the internal acoustic meatus have been exposed to show the relationship of the drilling for the anterior petrosectomy in relationship to these structures. The drilling for an anterior petrosectomy is directed behind the petrous carotid artery medial to the labyrinth and proceeds medially to the inferior petrosal sinus and side of the clivus. The abducens nerve and the ICA are in the lower margin of the exposure. A., *arteries, artery;* A.Ch.A., *anterior choroidal artery;* A.Co.A., *anterior communicating artery;* A.I.C.A., *anteroinferior cerebellar artery;* Ant., *anterior;* Bas., *basilar;* Br., *branch;* Car., *carotid;* Clin., *clinoid;* CN, *cranial nerve;* Contra., *contralateral;* Front., *frontal;* Gr., *greater;* Ipsi., *ipsilateral;* Lent. Str., *lenticulostriate;* M.C.A., *middle cerebral artery;* M.P.Ch.A., *medial posterior choroidal artery;* N., *nerve;* Olf., *olfactory;* P.Co.A., *posterior communicating artery;* Pet., *petrosal;* Post., *posterior;* Premam., *premamillary;* Rec., *recurrent;* S.C.A., *superior cerebellar artery;* Seg., *segment;* Semicirc., *semicircular;* Temp., *temporal;* Tent., *tentorial;* Thal. Perf., *thalamoperforating;* Tr., *tract;* Trifurc., *trifurcation.*

length of the preforaminal segment was 7.0 mm, and the mean length was 3.0 mm (16). The intracranial segment usually arises from the medial third of the superior surface of the ophthalmic segment under the optic nerve and commonly enters the optic foramen within 1 to 2 mm of its origin. The exposure of the ophthalmic artery is facilitated by removing the anterior clinoid process and roof of the optic canal, and incising the falciform process, a thin fold of dura mater that extends medially from the anterior clinoid process and covers a 0.5- to 11-mm (average, 3.5 mm) segment of the optic nerve immediately proximal to the optic foramen (16).

POSTERIOR COMMUNICATING ARTERY

The PComA, which forms the lateral boundary of the circle of Willis, arises from the posteromedial surface of the C4 approximately midway between the origin of the ophthalmic artery and the terminal bifurcation (*Figs. 2.1, 2.3,* and *2.6–2.8*). It sweeps backward and medially below the tuber cinereum, above the sella turcica, and slightly above and medial to the oculomotor nerve to join the posterior cerebral artery (PCA). In the embryo, the PComA continues as the PCA, but in the adult, the latter artery is annexed by the basilar system. If the

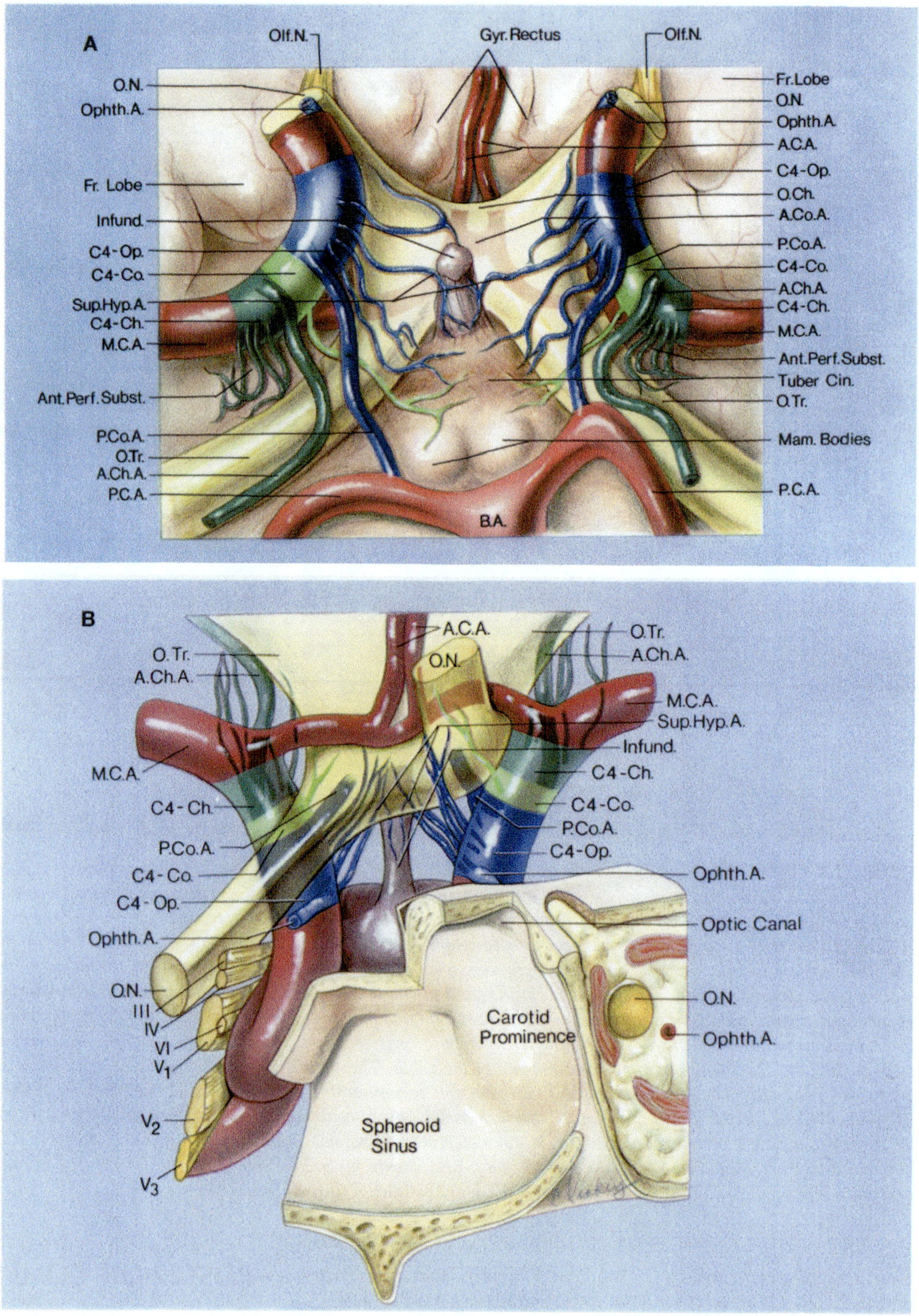

FIGURE 2.4. *Perforating branches of the ICA.* A, *inferior view. The internal carotid artery gives rise to the ophthalmic, posterior communicating, anterior choroidal, anterior cerebral, and the middle cerebral arteries. The supraclinoid portion of the ICA is divided into three segments based on the origin of these branches: an ophthalmic segment (C4-Op.,* blue*) that extends from the origin of the ophthalmic artery to the origin of the PComA; a communicating segment (C4-Co.,* light green*) that extends from the origin of the PComA to the origin of the AChA; and a choroidal segment (C4-Ch.,* dark green*) that extends from the origin of the AChA to the bifurcation of the ICA into the anterior and middle cerebral arteries. The perforating branches arising from the ophthalmic segment extend to the optic nerve, optic chiasm and the optic tracts, and the floor of the third ventricle around the infundibulum and tuber cinereum. The superior hypophyseal arteries arise from the ophthalmic segment and extend to the infundibulum of the pituitary gland. The branches arising from the communicating segment reach the optic tracts, floor of the third ventricle, and the area around the mamillary bodies. The perforating branches of the choroidal segment pass upward and enter the anterior perforated substance. The posterior cerebral arteries arise from the basilar artery and pass backward below the optic tracts. The ACA and AComA course above the optic chiasm and pass between the frontal lobes. The olfactory nerves are lateral to the gyrus rectus.* B, *anterior view. The left optic nerve has been divided near its entrance into the optic canal and elevated to give a clearer view of the perforating branches. The ophthalmic artery arises above the cavernous sinus. The carotid artery courses through the cavernous sinus and then laterally and produces a prominence in the wall of the sphenoid sinus before giving rise to the ophthalmic artery. The oculomotor, trochlear, abducens, and the ophthalmic, maxillary, and mandibular divisions of the trigeminal nerve pass lateral to the sphenoid sinus in the walls of the cavernous sinus. The superior hypophyseal arteries arise from the ophthalmic segment.*

PComA remains the major origin of the PCA, the configuration is termed fetal. If the PComA is of small or normal size, it courses posteromedially to join the PCA above and medial to the oculomotor nerve, but if it is of a fetal type, it courses further laterally above or lateral to the oculomotor nerve.

The PComA usually arises from the posteromedial or posterior aspect of the C4. The diameter at the carotid origin is slightly larger than at the junction with the PCA, but the difference is not usually more than 1 mm. Dilations of the origin of the PComA from the C4, known as functional dila-

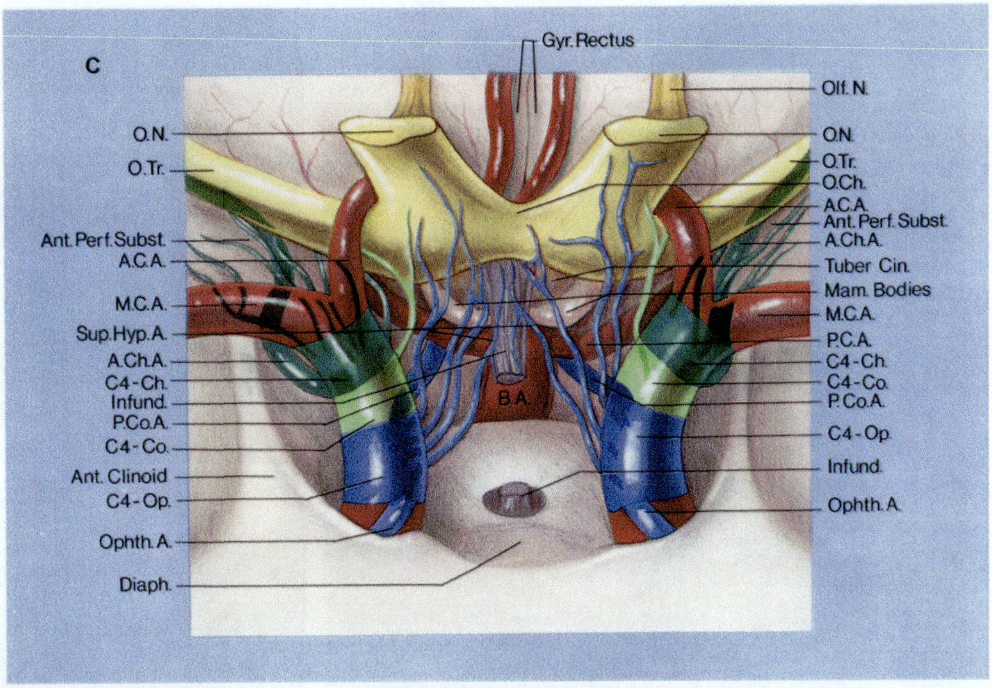

FIGURE 2.4. *Continued*
C, anterior view with both optic nerves divided and elevated to show the lower surface of the floor of the third ventricle and the perforating branches passing to it. The infundibulum has been divided above the diaphragma sellae. A., *artery;* A.C.A., *anterior cerebral artery;* A.Ch.A., *anterior choroidal artery;* A.Co.A., *anterior communicating artery;* Ant., *anterior;* Ch., *choroidal;* Cin., *cinereum;* Co., *communicating;* Diaph., *diaphragm;* Fr., *frontal;* Gyr., *gyrus;* Hyp., *hypophyseal;* Infund., *infundibulum;* M.C.A., *middle cerebral artery;* Mam., *mamillary;* N., *nerve;* O., *optic;* Olf., *olfactory;* Op., *ophthalmic;* Ophth., *ophthalmic;* P.C.A., *posterior cerebral artery;* P.Co.A., *posterior communicating artery;* Perf., *perforated;* Subst., *substance;* Sup., *superior;* Tr., *tract.* (From, *Gibo H, Lenkey C, Rhoton AL Jr: Microsurgical anatomy of the supraclinoid portion of the internal carotid artery.* **J Neurosurg** *55:560–574, 1981 [15].)*

tation or infundibular widening, are found in approximately 6% of hemispheres. Such dilation may be difficult to distinguish from an aneurysm. Some authors regard it as an early stage of aneurysm formation because the histological appearances are identical with those of aneurysms, but other authors, based on histological techniques, conclude that the junctional dilations are neither aneurysmal nor preaneurysmal (9, 17).

PComA Branches

An average of 8 (range, 4–14) perforating branches arise from the PComA, mostly from the superior and lateral surfaces, and course superiorly to penetrate, in decreasing order of frequency, the tuber cinereum and premamillary part of the floor of the third ventricle, the posterior perforated substance and interpeduncular fossa, the optic tract, the pituitary stalk, and the optic chiasm, to reach the thalamus, hypothalamus, subthalamus, and internal capsule (37). Branch origins are distributed relatively evenly along the course of the artery, with the anterior half having slightly more branches than the posterior half.

The premamillary artery is the largest branch that arises from the PComA. It enters the floor of the third ventricle in front of or beside the mamillary body between the mamillary body and optic tract (*Fig. 2.3*). There are commonly two or three branches terminating in the premamillary area, but only the largest branch is referred to as the premamillary artery. The premamillary artery has also been referred to as the anterior thalamoperforating artery. The premamillary artery most commonly originates on the middle third of the communicating artery, but can also arise on the anterior or posterior third. It supplies the posterior hypothalamus, anterior thalamus, posterior limb of the internal capsule, and subthalamus. The anterior group of PComA perforating branches supplies the hypothalamus, ventral thalamus, anterior third of the optic tract, and posterior limb of the internal capsule; the posterior group reaches the posterior perforated substance and subthalamic nucleus. Occlusion of the branches to the subthalamic nucleus leads to contralateral hemiballism.

ANTERIOR CHOROIDAL ARTERY

The AChA usually arises from the C4 as a single artery, with the majority arising nearer the origin of the PComA than to the carotid bifurcation (*Figs. 2.1, 2.9,* and *2.10*). It may infrequently arise from the C4 as two separate arteries or as a single artery that divides immediately into two trunks (47% of hemispheres) (33, 37). Infrequent origins, occurring in less than 1%, include the MCA and PComA. Its origin is similar in diameter to that of the ophthalmic artery, but smaller than those of the PComA, unless the PComA is small or hypoplastic. The origin of a fetal-type PComA may be more than twice the diameter of the AChA. The AChA is the first branch on the C4 distal to the PComA in two-thirds of hemispheres and the second, third, or even the fourth branch after one or more perforating branches, in descending order of frequency, in the remainder. The perforating branches arising between the PComA and AChA most commonly terminate in the optic tract, medial temporal lobe, and posterior perforated substance.

Course

The initial segment of the AChA is directed posteromedial behind the internal carotid artery. On the anteroposterior angiogram, the initial segment of the AChA is seen medial to the internal carotid artery. The origin of the artery is lateral to the optic tract, but the initial segment crosses from the lateral to the medial side of the optic tract in many hemispheres, only infrequently remaining lateral to the optic tract throughout its

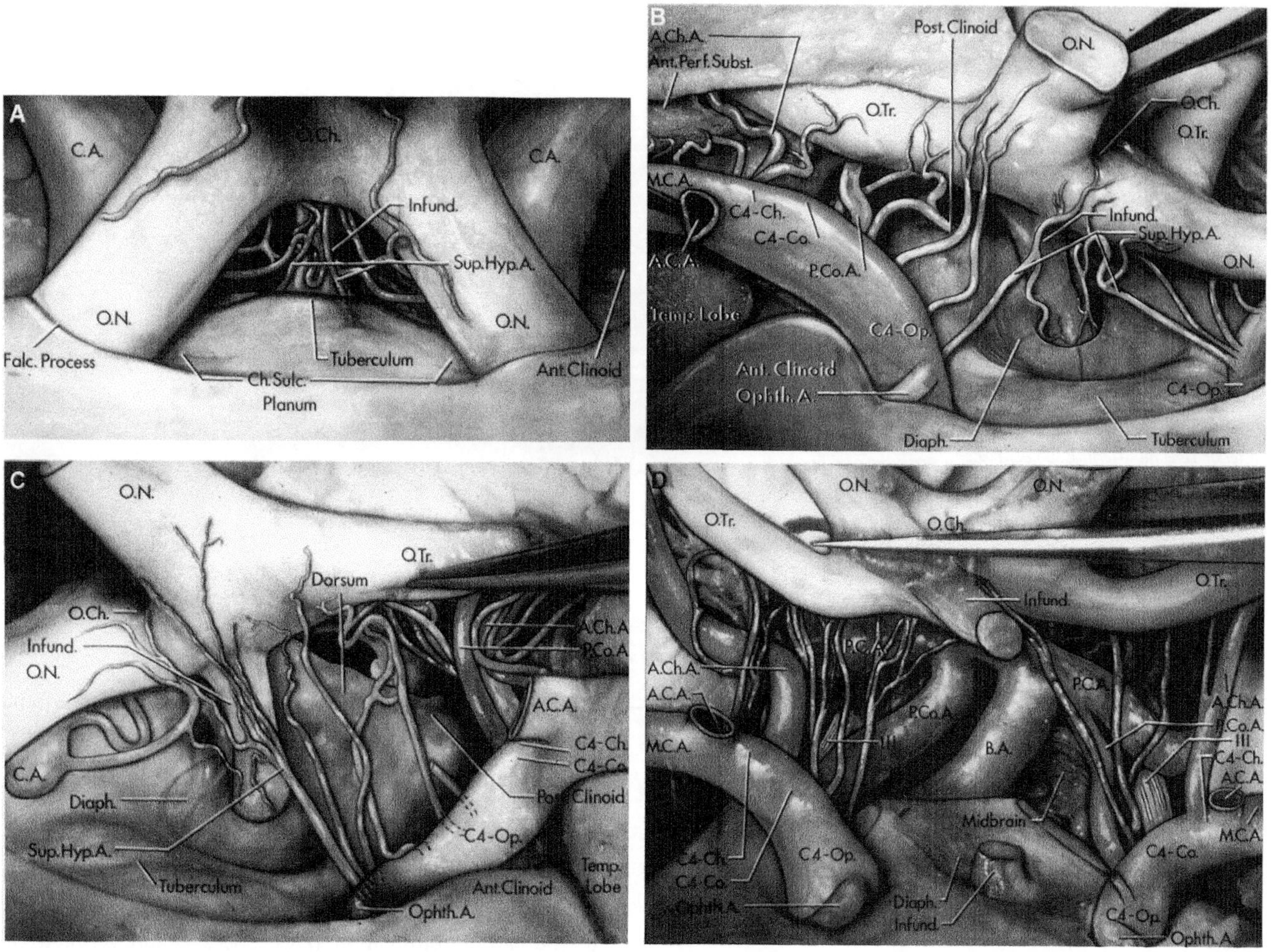

FIGURE 2.5. *Anterior and anteroinferior views of the supraclinoid portion of the internal carotid artery. A, anterior view. The optic nerves enter the optic canals medial to the anterior clinoid processes. The infundibulum passes inferiorly below the optic chiasm to the pituitary gland. The carotid arteries are posterior to the optic nerves. The planum sphenoidal is anterior to the chiasmatic sulcus and the tuberculum sellae. The perforating branches of the carotid artery pass medially in the subchiasmatic space. The superior hypophyseal arteries arise from the carotid artery and pass to the infundibulum. The falciform process is a fold of dura mater that passes above the optic nerve proximal to the optic foramen. B, the right optic nerve has been divided at the optic foramen and elevated to show the perforating branches of the supraclinoid portion of the carotid arteries. The right anterior cerebral artery was divided at its origin so that the optic nerve and chiasm could be elevated. The carotid artery gives rise to multiple perforating branches as well as the ophthalmic, posterior communicating, anterior choroidal, and the middle cerebral arteries. The supraclinoid portion of the ICA is divided into three segments based on the origin of its major branches: the ophthalmic segment (C4-Op.) extends from the origin of the ophthalmic artery to the origin of the PComA, the communicating segment (C4-Co.) extends from the origin of the PComA to the origin of the AChA, and the choroidal segment (C4-Ch.) extends from the origin of the AChA to the bifurcation of the carotid artery. The perforating branches arising from the ophthalmic segment pass to the optic nerve, chiasm, infundibulum, and the floor of the third ventricle. The perforating branches arising from the communicating segment pass to the optic tract and the floor of the third ventricle. The perforating branches arising from the choroidal segment pass upward and enter the brain through the anterior perforated substance. The diaphragma sellae surrounds the infundibulum above the pituitary gland. The temporal lobe is below the middle cerebral artery. C, the left optic nerve has been divided at the optic foramen and the anterior cerebral artery divided near its origin so that both optic nerves and the chiasm and tract could be elevated to show the perforating branches of the carotid artery. The Liliequist membrane is posterior to the infundibulum and hides the basilar artery, but not the posterior cerebral artery. The perforating branches of the ophthalmic segment pass upward to the infundibulum and the optic nerve, chiasm, and tract. D, both optic nerves and both ACAs and the infundibulum have been divided to permit the optic nerves and chiasm to be elevated with a forceps for this view under the optic chiasm and across the diaphragma sellae and dorsum to the upper part of the basilar artery and the oculomotor nerves. The oculomotor nerves pass forward below the PCAs. The perforating branches of the supraclinoid segment of the carotid artery pass upward to supply the infundibulum, the optic chiasm and tracts, and the floor of the third ventricle; some enter the brain through the anterior perforated substance. The right AChA is very large.* A., *artery;* A.C.A., *anterior cerebral artery;* A.Ch.A., *anterior choroidal artery;* Ant., *anterior;* B.A., *basilar artery;* C.A., *carotid artery;* Ch., *choroidal;* Ch., *chiasm, chiasmatic;* Co., *communicating;* Diaph., *diaphragm;* Falc., *falciform;* Hyp., *hypophyseal;* Infund., *infundibulum;* M.C.A., *middle cerebral artery;* N., *nerve;* O., *optic;* Op., Ophth., *ophthalmic;* P.C.A., *posterior cerebral artery;* P.Co.A., *posterior communicating artery;* Perf., *perforated;* Post., *posterior;* Subst., *substance;* Sulc., *sulcus;* Sup., *superior;* Temp., *temporal;* Tr., *tract.* (From, *Gibo H, Lenkey C, Rhoton AL Jr: Microsurgical anatomy of the supraclinoid portion of the internal carotid artery.* ***J Neurosurg*** *55:560–574, 1981 [15].)*

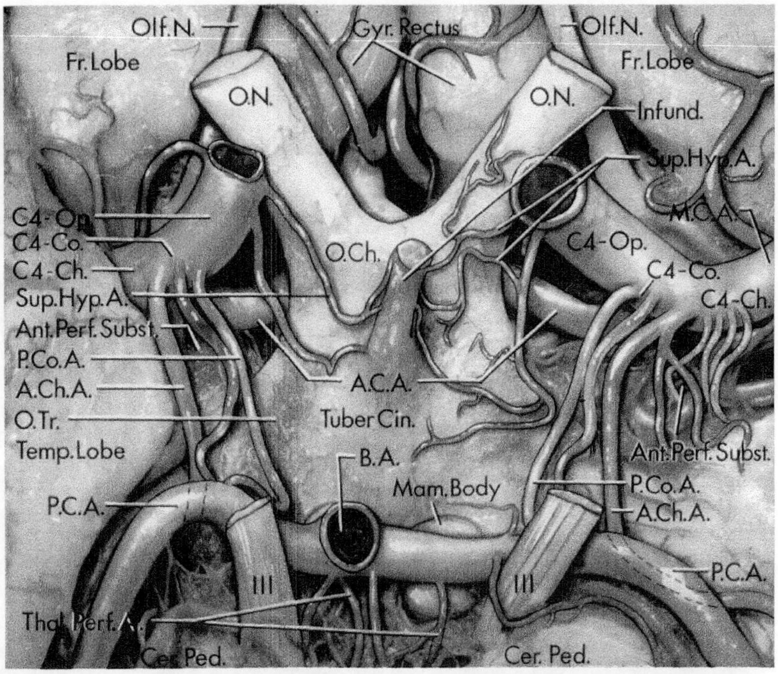

FIGURE 2.6. *Inferior view of the perforating branches of the supraclinoid portion of the internal carotid artery. The supraclinoid portion of the artery gives rise to the posterior communicating, anterior choroidal, middle cerebral, and anterior cerebral arteries. The supraclinoid portion of the artery is divided into three segments based on the site of origin of these branches: an ophthalmic segment (C4-Op.) that extends from the origin of the ophthalmic artery (not shown because the ICA was divided above the level of origin of the ophthalmic artery) to the origin of the PComA; a communicating segment (C4-Co.) that extends from the origin of the PComA to the origin of the AChA; and a choroidal segment (C4-Ch.) that extends from the origin of the AChA to the level of the bifurcation of the ICA into the anterior cerebral and middle cerebral arteries. The ophthalmic segment sends perforating branches to the optic nerves, optic chiasm, and the tuber cinereum. The superior hypophyseal arteries pass to the infundibulum of the hypophysis. The communicating segment sends one perforating branch on each side to the optic tracts and the region around the mamillary bodies. The perforating arteries are as large as the adjacent AChA and PComA. The choroidal segment sends its perforating branches into the anterior perforated substance. The posterior cerebral arteries arise from the basilar artery and pass laterally around the cerebral peduncles. The temporal lobe is lateral to the carotid artery. The frontal lobes, gyrus rectus, and olfactory nerves are above the optic nerves. The thalamoperforating arteries pass posteriorly between the oculomotor nerves.* A., *artery;* A.C.A., *anterior cerebral artery;* A.Ch.A., *anterior choroidal artery;* Ant., *anterior;* B.A., *basilar artery;* Cer.A., *cerebral artery;* Ch., *chiasm, choroidal;* Co., *communicating;* Fr., *frontal;* Gyr., *gyrus;* Hyp., *hypophyseal;* Infund., *infundibulum;* M.C.A., *middle cerebral artery;* Mam., *mamillary;* N., *nerve;* O., *optic;* Olf., *olfactory;* Op., *ophthalmic;* P.C.A., *posterior cerebral artery;* P.Co.A., *posterior communicating artery;* Ped., *peduncle;* Perf., *perforated;* Subst., *substance;* Sup., *superior;* Temp., *temporal;* Thal. Perf., *thalamoperforating;* Tr., *tract;* Tuber Cin., *tuber cinereum.* (From, *Gibo H, Lenkey C, Rhoton AL Jr: Microsurgical anatomy of the supraclinoid portion of the internal carotid artery.* **J Neurosurg** *55:560–574, 1981 [15].)*

course. It passes below or along the medial side of the optic tract to reach the lateral margin of the cerebral peduncle. The average length that the artery follows the optic tract is 12 mm (range, 5–25 mm) (33). At the anterior margin of the lateral geniculate body, the AChA again crosses the optic tract from medial to lateral and passes posterolateral through the crural cistern, located between the cerebral peduncle and uncus, to arrive superomedial to the uncus, where it passes through the choroidal fissure to enter the choroid plexus within the temporal horn. It courses along the medial border of the choroid plexus in close relation to the lateral posterior choroidal branches of the PCA. In some cases, it can pass dorsally along the medial border of the plexus, reaching the foramen of Monro.

Segments

The artery is divided into cisternal and plexal segments (33). The cisternal segment extends from the origin to the choroidal fissure and is divided at the anterior margin of the lateral geniculate body into a proximal and distal portion. The plexal segment is composed of one or more branches that pass through the choroidal fissure to branch and enter the choroid plexus of the temporal horn. The length from its origin to its passage through the choroidal fissure averages 2.4 cm (range, 20–34 mm). If there is a double artery, the distal branch usually terminates in the temporal lobe and the proximal branch nourishes the remaining anterior choroidal field.

Branches

The branches, which average 9 (range, 4–18), are divided on the basis of whether they arise from the cisternal or plexal segment. The branches from the cisternal segment penetrate, in decreasing order of frequency, the optic tract, uncus, cerebral peduncle, temporal horn, lateral geniculate body, hippocampus, dentate gyrus and fornix, and anterior perforated substance. These branches more commonly supply the optic tract, lateral part of the geniculate body, posterior two-thirds of the posterior limb of the internal capsule, most of the globus pallidus, the origin of the optic radiations, and the middle third of the cerebral peduncle. Less commonly supplied structures include part of the head of the caudate nucleus, pyriform cortex, the uncus, posteromedial part of the amygdaloid nucleus, substantia nigra, red nucleus, subthalamic nucleus, and the superficial aspect of the ventrolateral nucleus of the thalamus (1). None of these structures is always supplied by the artery, but, in approximately two-thirds of the hemispheres, it supplies the medial part of the globus pallidus, the posterior limb and retrolenticular part of the internal capsule, the optic tract and the lateral geniculate body. No structure other than the choroid plexus of the temporal horn received branches in every case. In approximately half of the hemispheres, it supplies the lateral part of the globus pallidus and the caudate tail; in one-third, it supplies the thalamus, hypothalamus, and subthalamus.

There is a marked interchangeability of the field of supply of the AChA and the nearby branches of the C4, PCA, PComA, and

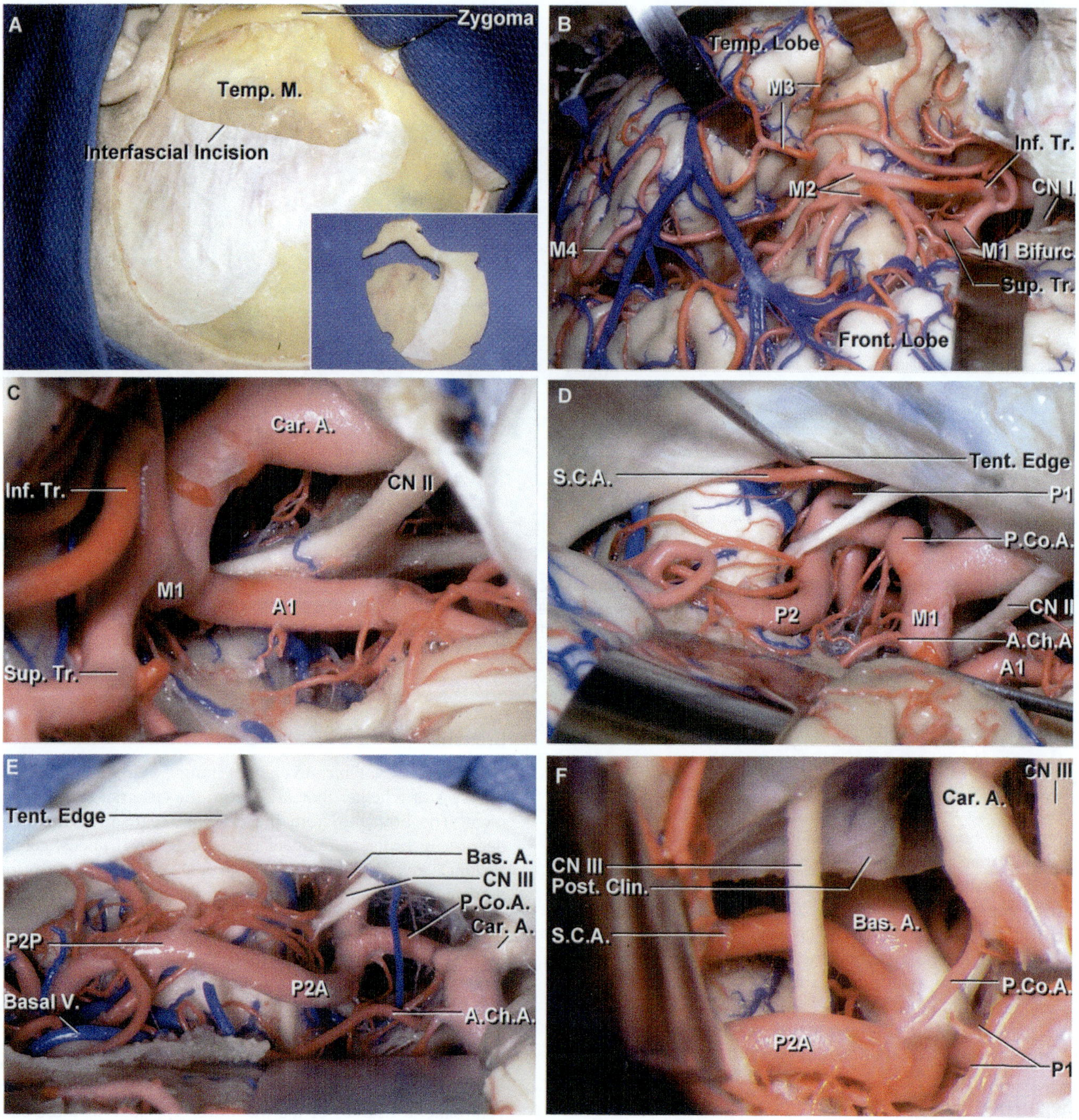

FIGURE 2.7. *Orbitozygomatic exposure of the arteries forming the circle of Willis including three variants (D, E, and F) in the size of the PComA. A, the scalp flap has been elevated and the interfascial incision has been completed so that the fat pad containing the branches of the facial nerve to the forehead can be folded downward with the scalp flap. The one-piece orbitozygomatic bone flap is shown in the* inset. *B, the sylvian fissure has been opened. The M1 bifurcates to form superior and inferior trunks of similar size. The branches forming the M2 begin at the limen insula and cross the insula. The branches forming the M3 loop over the opercular lips, and the M4 branches course on the lateral convexity. C, enlarged view of the carotid bifurcation. The M1 divides into superior and inferior trunks before reaching the limen insula, which is located at the lateral edge of the anterior perforated substance. A large A1 passes medially above the chiasm. D, the exposure has been directed under the temporal lobe. A large PComA of the fetal type provides the majority of flow to the P2 segment. As the PComA increases in size, it tends to shift laterally. The junction of the posterior communicating and P2 is situated medial to the oculomotor nerve. The tentorial edge has been depressed to expose the superior cerebellar artery. E, another subtemporal exposure showing a configuration in which the P1 and PComA are of approximately equal size. F, exposure oriented like C, showing a small PComA with the predominant P2 origin being from the P1. A., artery; A.Ch.A., anterior choroidal artery; Bas., basilar; Bifurc., bifurcation; Car., carotid; Clin., clinoid; CN, cranial nerve; Front., frontal; Inf., inferior; M., muscle; P.Co.A., posterior communicating artery; Post., posterior; S.C.A., superior cerebellar artery; Sup., superior; Temp., temporal, temporalis; Tent., tentorial; Tr., trunk; V., vein.*

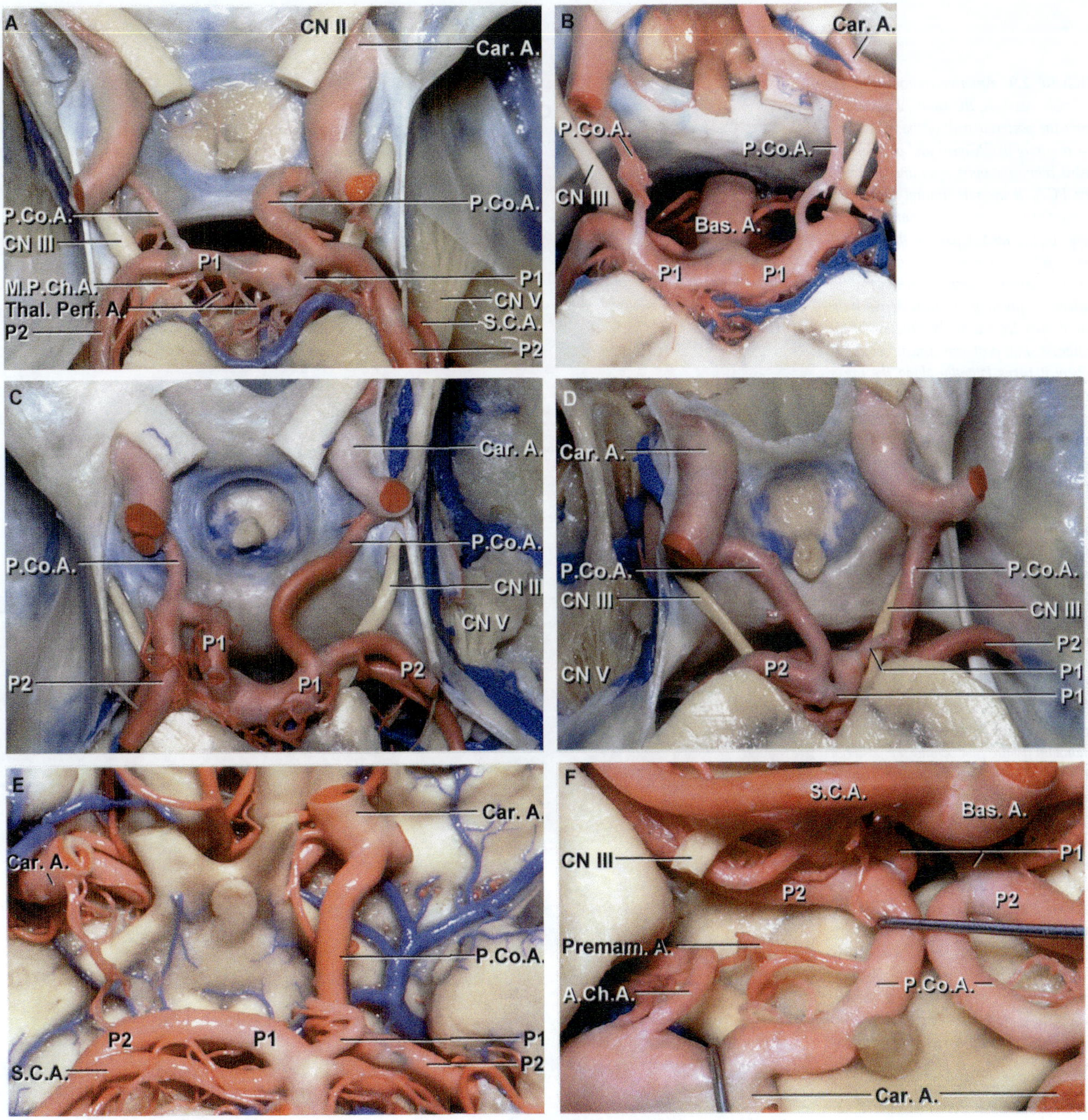

FIGURE 2.8. *Variations in the posterior circle of Willis include differing lengths and diameters of the PComAs or P1s.* A, *superior view. The left PComA is hypoplastic and the right is larger than its corresponding P1. The left PComA is straight and short and the right is long and convex medially. The right P2 segment is a direct continuation of the PComA. An MPChA courses medial to the left P2. Thalamoperforating branches arise at the basilar bifurcation.* B, *both P1s arise predominantly from the basilar artery. The hypoplastic PComAs course above and medial to the oculomotor nerves.* C, *the right PComA and P1 are of approximately equal size, and the junction of the PComA and the P2 is sharply angulated. The left P1 is directed anterior before joining the junction of the P2 and the PComA. The right PComA is much longer than the left.* D, *the right P1 arises predominantly from the PComA. The right P1 segment is small and short, being only long enough to reach above the oculomotor nerve. The left PComA and P1 are of approximately equal size, but the left P1 is short. The junction of the PComAs and the P2s are sharply angulated on both sides.* E, *inferior view. The left P1 is hypoplastic and the left P2 arises mainly from the PComA. The right PCA arises predominantly from the basilar artery.* F, *large tortuous PComAs almost touch in the midline. The P2s arise predominantly from the large PComAs, which are larger than the P1 segments. Premamillary perforating branches of the PComA arise on both sides.* A., *artery;* A.Ch.A., *anterior choroidal artery;* Bas., *basilar;* Car., *carotid;* CN, *cranial nerve;* M.P.Ch.A., *medial posterior choroidal artery;* P.Co.A., *posterior communicating artery;* Premam., *premamillary;* S.C.A., *superior cerebellar artery;* Thal. Perf., *thalamoperforating.*

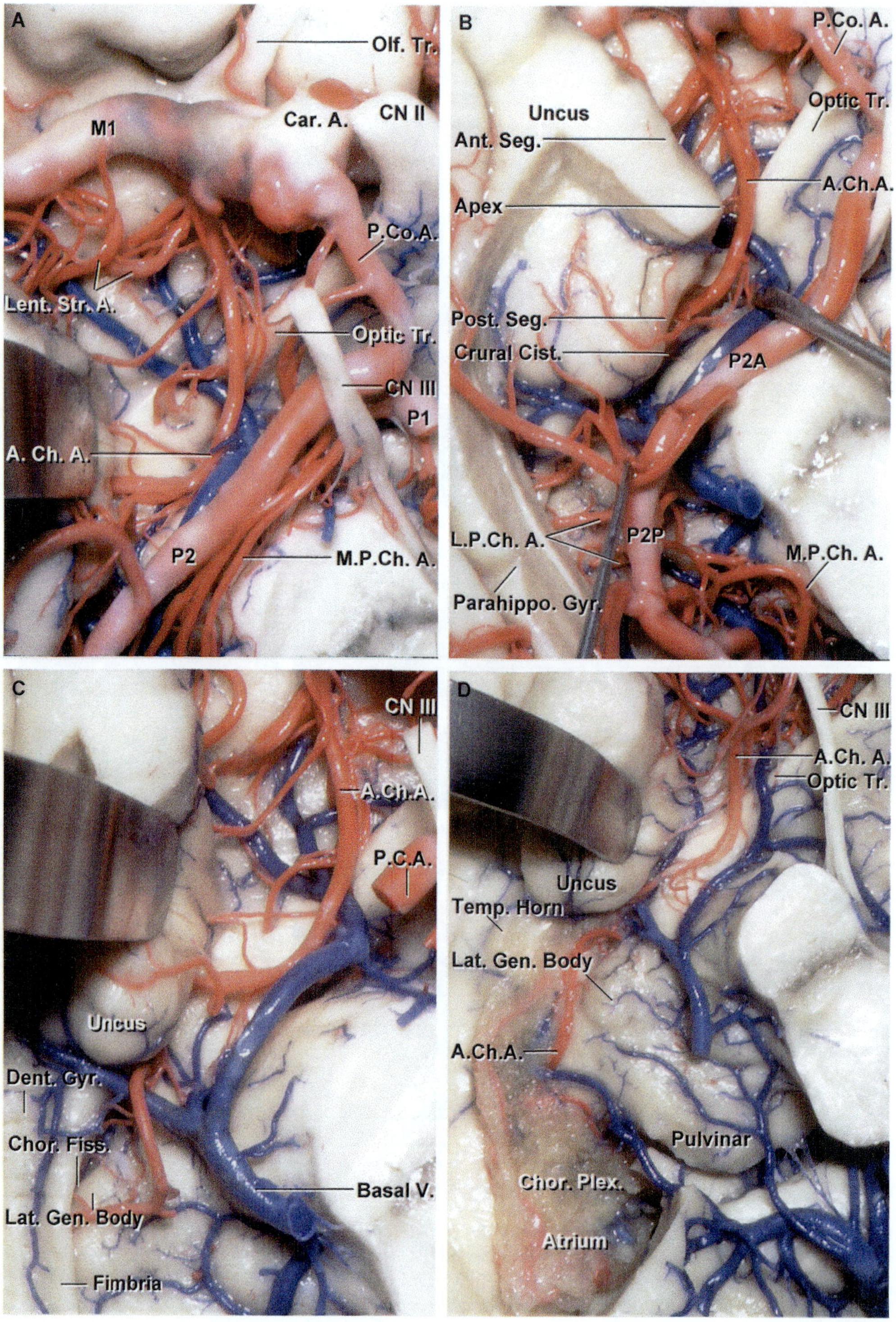

FIGURE 2.9. *Anterior choroidal artery. Inferior views.* A, *the right AChA arises from the posterior wall of the ICA above the origin of the PComA and passes backward below the optic tract and lateral to the PCA. It ascends around the medial surface of the uncus as it travels posteriorly.* B, *the medial part of the parahippocampal gyrus has been removed. The AChA courses backward medial to the anterior segment of the uncus to reach the uncal apex located at the junction of the anterior and posterior uncal segments where it turns laterally along the upper margin of the posterior uncal segment to reach the choroidal fissure.* C, *the posterior uncal segment has been retracted. The AChA passes above the posterior uncal segment and enters the temporal horn by passing through the choroidal fissure located between the thalamus above and fimbria of the fornix below. The lateral geniculate body forms the part of the thalamus above where the artery enters the choroidal fissure. The dentate gyrus is located at the lower edge of the fimbria.* D, *the floor of the temporal horn and the fimbria have been removed to expose the AChA entering the choroid plexus of the temporal horn by passing through the choroidal fissure just behind the posterior segment of the uncus. The lower end of the choroidal fissure and the site where the artery passes through the fissure are called the inferior choroidal point.* A., *arteries, artery;* A.Ch.A., *anterior choroidal artery;* Ant., *anterior;* Car., *carotid;* Chor., *choroid, choroidal;* Cist., *cistern;* CN, *cranial nerve;* Dent., *dentate;* Fiss., *fissure;* Gen., *geniculate;* Gyr., *gyrus;* L.P.Ch.A., *lateral posterior choroidal artery;* Lat., *lateral;* Lent. Str., *lenticulostriate;* M.P.Ch.A., *medial posterior choroidal artery;* Olf., *olfactory;* P.C.A., *posterior cerebral artery;* P.Co.A., *posterior communicating artery;* Parahippo., *parahippocampal;* Plex., *plexus;* Post., *posterior;* Seg., *segment;* Temp., *temporal;* Tr., *tract;* V., *vein.*

MCA. The C4 frequently gives rise to small arteries distributed to the areas commonly supplied by the proximal branches of the AChA. These arteries, as many as four, arising from the posterior wall of the carotid artery between the PComA and AChA, also frequently terminate, in decreasing order of frequency, in the optic tract, anterior perforated substance, uncus, hypothalamus, pituitary stalk, and cerebral peduncle (37).

Another example of the interchangeability of field occurs within the internal capsule. If the PComA is small, the anterior choroidal artery may take over its normal area of supply to the

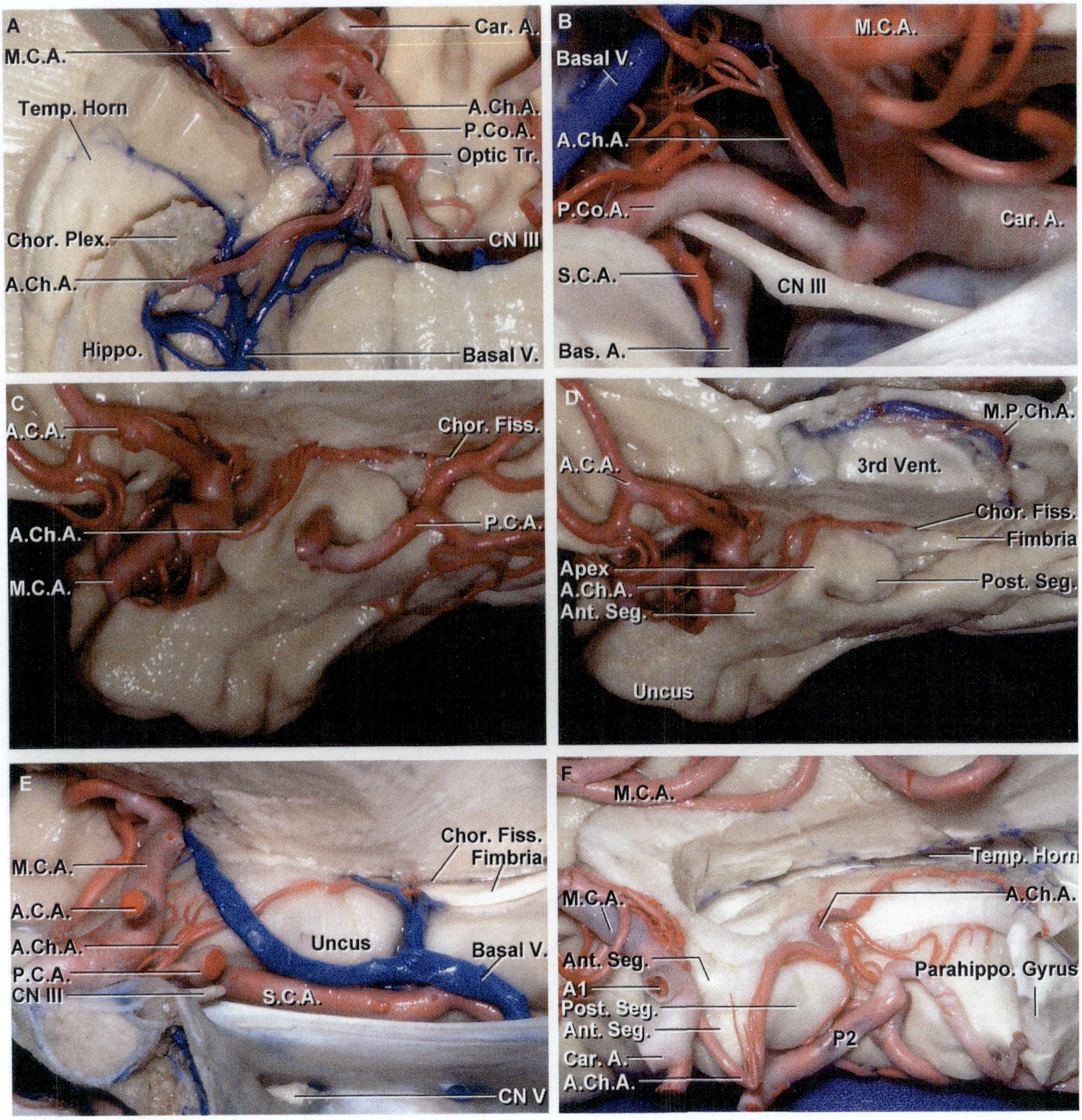

FIGURE 2.10. *Anterior choroidal artery. A, inferior view. The lower part of the right temporal pole has been removed to expose the AChA, which passes backward to reach the medial side of the optic tract where it turns laterally, passing again below the optic tract and around the uncus to enter the temporal horn. B, lateral view. The right AChA arises above the origin of the PComA and passes upward and backward around the uncus to reach the temporal horn. C, medial side of the right uncus. The AChA passes around the medial aspect of the uncus to reach the lower end of the choroidal fissure where it enters the temporal horn. The PCA courses along the posterior aspect of the uncus. D, the PCA has been removed. The AChA ascends along the anterior segment of the uncus to reach the uncal apex where it turns laterally above the posterior uncal segment to enter the inferior choroidal point at the lower end of the choroidal fissure located just behind the posterior uncal segment and the head of the hippocampus. The anterior uncal segment contains the amygdala and the posterior segment is formed predominantly by the head of the hippocampus. E, medial view of the right AChA in another specimen. The cross section extends through the midline of the sella. The view is directed laterally over the top of the sella to the medial aspect of the internal carotid artery, uncus, and the origin of the AChA. The AChA passes around the uncus to reach the lower end of the choroidal fissure. F, medial view of another temporal lobe. The AChA pursues an angulated course, descending along the anterior segment of the uncus, but at the uncal apex it turns sharply upward, reaching the upper part of the posterior uncal segment before entering the temporal horn.* A., *artery;* A.C.A., *anterior cerebral artery;* A.Ch.A., *anterior choroidal artery;* Ant., *anterior;* Bas., *basilar;* Car., *carotid;* Chor., *choroid, choroidal;* CN, *cranial nerve;* Fiss., *fissure;* Hippo., *hippocampus;* M.C.A., *middle cerebral artery;* M.P.Ch.A., *medial posterior choroidal artery;* P.C.A., *posterior cerebral artery;* P.Co.A., *posterior communicating artery;* Parahippo., *parahippocampal;* Plex., *plexus;* Post., *posterior;* S.C.A., *superior cerebellar artery;* Temp., *temporal;* seg., *segment;* Tr., *tract;* V., *vein;* Vent., *ventricle.*

genu and the anterior third of the internal capsule, or if the AChA is small, the field of supply of the PComA may enlarge to supply the greater part of the posterior limb of the internal capsule (1). Such inverse relationships, in which one artery's field of supply enlarges as the other's contracts, occur between the PCA and AChA in the supply to the cerebral peduncle, substantia nigra, red nucleus, subthalamic nucleus, optic tract, and lateral geniculate body. A large AChA is usually associated with a small PComA on that side.

The plexal segment, in most cases, originates as a single branch of the AChA, which passes through the choroidal fissure. Additional smaller branches to the choroid plexus may arise proximal to the choroidal fissure. These plexal branches divide and enter the medial border of the choroid plexus of the temporal horn to course in close relation to and frequently anastomose with branches of the lateral posterior choroidal arteries. Some branches of the AChA pass posteriorly into the choroid plexus in the atrium and then forward above the thalamus to supply the choroid plexus of the body as far forward as the foramen of Monro.

Nearly half of hemispheres have anastomoses between the PCA and AChA. The richest anastomoses are those located on the surface of the choroid plexus with the lateral posterior choroidal branches of the PCA. Anastomoses between the AChA and PCA are also found on the lateral surface of the lateral geniculate body and on the temporal lobe near the uncus. These complex and variable anastomoses make it difficult to predict the effects of occlusion of a single AChA, but explain some of the inconsistent results of AChA occlusion.

Clinical Features

The classic reported clinical features of occlusion of the AChA are contralateral hemiplegia, hemianesthesia, and hemianopsia (1, 11). The contralateral hemiplegia and hemianesthesia (to all sensory modalities) results from infarction in the posterior two-thirds of the posterior limb of the internal capsule and the middle third of the cerebral peduncle. The homonomous hemianopsia of varying degrees results from interruption of the supply to the origin of the optic radiations, the optic tract, and part of the lateral geniculate body. Infarction found in the globus pallidus seems to produce no symptoms.

Inconstant results, including absence of deficit, have followed surgical occlusion for the treatment of Parkinson's disease (5, 28). In 1952, while performing a pedunculotomy on a patient incapacitated with Parkinsonism, Coopers tore and had to clip the AChA (4, 5). The operation was terminated without cutting the peduncle. Postoperatively, there was disappearance of tremor and rigidity from the involved extremities, with preservation of voluntary motor function. This beneficial effect was presumed to be caused by ischemic necrosis of the globus pallidus. This represented a case of known occlusion of the AChA with none of the classic symptoms. The sparing of motor function was presumed to be caused by anastomosis over the lateral geniculate body and in the choroid plexus, which provided a collateral source for the capsular branches.

Surgical occlusions were then made by Cooper and his associates in 50 patients with Parkinsonism (4, 5). Each artery was clipped twice: once at its origin and once 1.5 cm from the origin, just distal to the pallidal branches. This distal clip was applied to prevent retrograde filling into the pallidal branches through the anastomosis in the choroid plexus. This was thought to isolate the pallidum and its efferent fiber tracts from their normal antegrade blood supply and from retrograde supply through anastomosis with the lateral posterior choroidal and other arteries. At the same time, it allowed the more distal structures, such as the internal capsule, the benefit of this retrograde collateral circulation. Cooper reported good relief of tremor and rigidity, a 20% morbidity, and 6% mortality in this group. Postoperative complications included a hemiplegia in three patients, a partial aphasia in one, and a homonymous quadrantanopsia in one. Twelve patients studied in detail had no visual defects. Several patients developed a memory loss and became confused, and it was not uncommon for the patients to remain somnolent for 1 to 10 days. Cooper assumed that collateral circulation spared the corticospinal fibers and the optic radiations, while failing to preserve the pallidum and / or its efferent fibers.

Rand et al. (28) later reported the results of occlusion of six arteries in five cases. Although finding no therapeutic value of AChA occlusion, these authors agreed that the artery could be occluded with little resultant damage. In four patients there was no effect on the Parkinsonism and no neurological deficit after the occlusion, but the fifth patient developed a contralateral hemiparesis after occlusion of the artery. A homonymous visual field defect occurred in two patients. In two cases, in which the brain became available for pathological examination, small and inconstant lesions were found within the areas supplied by the artery. The inconstant symptoms and infarction after AChA occlusion are attributed to collateral circulation through anastomoses with adjacent arteries and variations in the area of supply of the artery.

MIDDLE CEREBRAL ARTERY

The MCA is the largest and most complex of the cerebral arteries. Some of its branches are exposed in most operations in the supratentorial area, whether the approach is to the cerebral convexity, parasagittal region, or along the cranial base (*Figs. 2.1, 2.3, and 2.7*). In the past, surgical interest in the MCA has been directed at avoiding damage to its branches during operations within its territory, but micro-operative techniques have now made reconstruction of and bypass to the MCA an important method of preserving and restoring blood flow to the cerebrum.

The MCA arises as the larger of the two terminal branches of the internal carotid artery. The diameter of the MCA at its origin ranges from 2.4 to 4.6 mm (average, 3.9 mm), roughly twice that of the anterior cerebral artery. Its origin is at the medial end of the sylvian fissure, lateral to the optic chiasm, below the anterior perforated substance, and posterior to the division of the olfactory tract into the medial and lateral olfactory striae. From its origin, it courses laterally below the anterior perforated substance and parallel, but roughly 1 cm posterior, to the sphenoid ridge. As it passes below the anterior perforated substance, it gives rise to a series of perforating branches referred to as lenticulostriate arteries. It divides within the sylvian fissure and turns sharply posterosuperiorly at a curve, the genu, to reach the surface of the insula. At the periphery of the insula, the branches pass to the medial surface of the opercula of the frontal, temporal, and parietal lobes. Its branches pass around the opercula to reach the cortical surface and supply most of the lateral surface and some of the basal surface of the cerebral hemisphere.

Segments

The MCA is divided into four segments: Ml (sphenoidal), M2 (insular), M3 (opercular), and M4 (cortical) (*Figs. 2.11–2.14*). The M1 begins at the origin of the MCA and extends laterally within the depths of the sylvian fissure. It courses laterally, roughly parallel to and approximately 1 cm (range, 4.3–19.5 mm) posterior to the sphenoid ridge in the sphenoidal compartment of the sylvian fissure. This segment terminates at the site of a 90-degree turn, the genu, located at the junction of the sphenoidal and operculoinsular compartments of the sylvian fissure. The M1 is subdivided into a prebifurcation and postbifurcation part. The prebifurcation segment is composed of a single main trunk that extends from the origin to the bifurcation. The postbifurcation trunks of the M1 segment run in a nearly parallel course, diverging only minimally before reaching the genu. This bifurcation occurs proximal to the genu in nearly 90% of hemispheres (14). The small cortical branches arising from the main trunk proximal to the bifurcation are referred to as early branches.

The M2 segment includes the trunks that lie on and supply the insula (*Fig. 2.15*). This segment begins at the genu where the MCA trunks passes over the limen insulae and terminates at the circular sulcus of the insula. The greatest branching of the MCA occurs distal to the genu as these trunks cross the anterior part of the insula. The branches passing to the anterior cortical areas have a shorter path across the insula than those reaching the posterior cortical areas. The branches to the anterior frontal and anterior temporal areas cross only the anterior part of the insula, but the branches supplying the posterior cortical areas course in a nearly parallel but diverging path across the length of the insula. The frontal branches cross only the short gyri before leaving the insular surface, whereas the branches supplying the posterior parietal or angular regions pass across the short gyri, the central sulcus, and the long gyri of the insula before leaving the insular surface.

The M3 segment begins at the circular sulcus of the insula and ends at the surface of the sylvian fissure. The branches forming the M3 segment closely adhere to and course over the surface of the frontoparietal and temporal opercula to reach the superficial part of the sylvian fissure. The branches directed to the brain above the sylvian fissure undergo two 180-degree turns. The first turn is located at the circular sulcus, where the vessels coursing upward over the insular surface turn 180 degrees and pass downward over the medial surface of the frontoparietal operculum. The second 180-degree turn is located at the external surface of the sylvian fissure, where the branches complete their passage around the inferior margin of the frontoparietal operculum and turn in a superior direction on the lateral surface of the frontal and parietal lobes.

The arteries supplying the cortical areas below the sylvian fissure pursue a less tortuous course. These branches, on reaching the circular sulcus, run along its inferior circumference before turning upward and laterally on the medial surface of the temporal operculum, thus producing a less acute change in course at the inferior margin of the circular sulcus. On reaching the external surface of the sylvian fissure, these branches are directed downward and backward on the surface of the temporal lobe.

The M4 is composed of the branches to the lateral convexity. They begin at the surface of the sylvian fissure and extend over the cortical surface of the cerebral hemisphere. The more anterior branches turn sharply upward or downward after leaving the sylvian fissure. The intermediate branches follow a gradual posterior incline away from the fissure, and the posterior branches pass backward in nearly the same direction as the long axis of the fissure.

Perforating Branches

The perforating branches of the MCA enter the anterior perforated substance and are called the lenticulostriate arteries (*Fig. 2.16*). There is an average of 10 (range, 1–21) lenticulostriate arteries per hemisphere (36). Lenticulostriate branches arise from the prebifurcation part of the M1 in every case and from the postbifurcation part of the M1 segment in half of the hemispheres. Of the total number of lenticulostriate branches, approximately 80% arise from the prebifurcation part of the M1. Most of the remainder arise from the postbifurcation part of the M1, but a few arise from the proximal part of the M2 near the genu. The earlier the bifurcation, the greater the number of postbifurcation branches. No branches to the anterior perforated substance arise from the postbifurcation trunks if the bifurcation is 2.5 cm or more from the origin of the middle cerebral artery.

The lenticulostriate arteries are divided into medial, intermediate, and lateral groups, each of which has a unique origin, composition, morphology, and characteristic distribution in the anterior perforated substance. The medial group is the least constant of the three groups and is present in only half of the hemispheres (36). When present, it consists of one to five branches that arise on the medial prebifurcation part of the M1 segment near the carotid bifurcation or an early branch, and pursue a relatively direct course to enter the anterior perforated substance just lateral to the C4 branches. Most arise from the posterior or superior aspect of the main trunk. Branching before entering the anterior perforated substance is less common than in the intermediate or lateral groups.

The intermediate lenticulostriate arteries form a complex array of branches before entering the anterior perforated substance between the medial and lateral lenticulostriate arteries. They are present in more than 90% of hemispheres. The most distinctive feature of the intermediate group is that it possesses at least one major artery, which furnishes a complex arborizing array of as many as 30 branches to the anterior perforated substance. The fewer perforating branches in this group (average, three) and the division yielding a great number of total branches entering the anterior perforated sub-

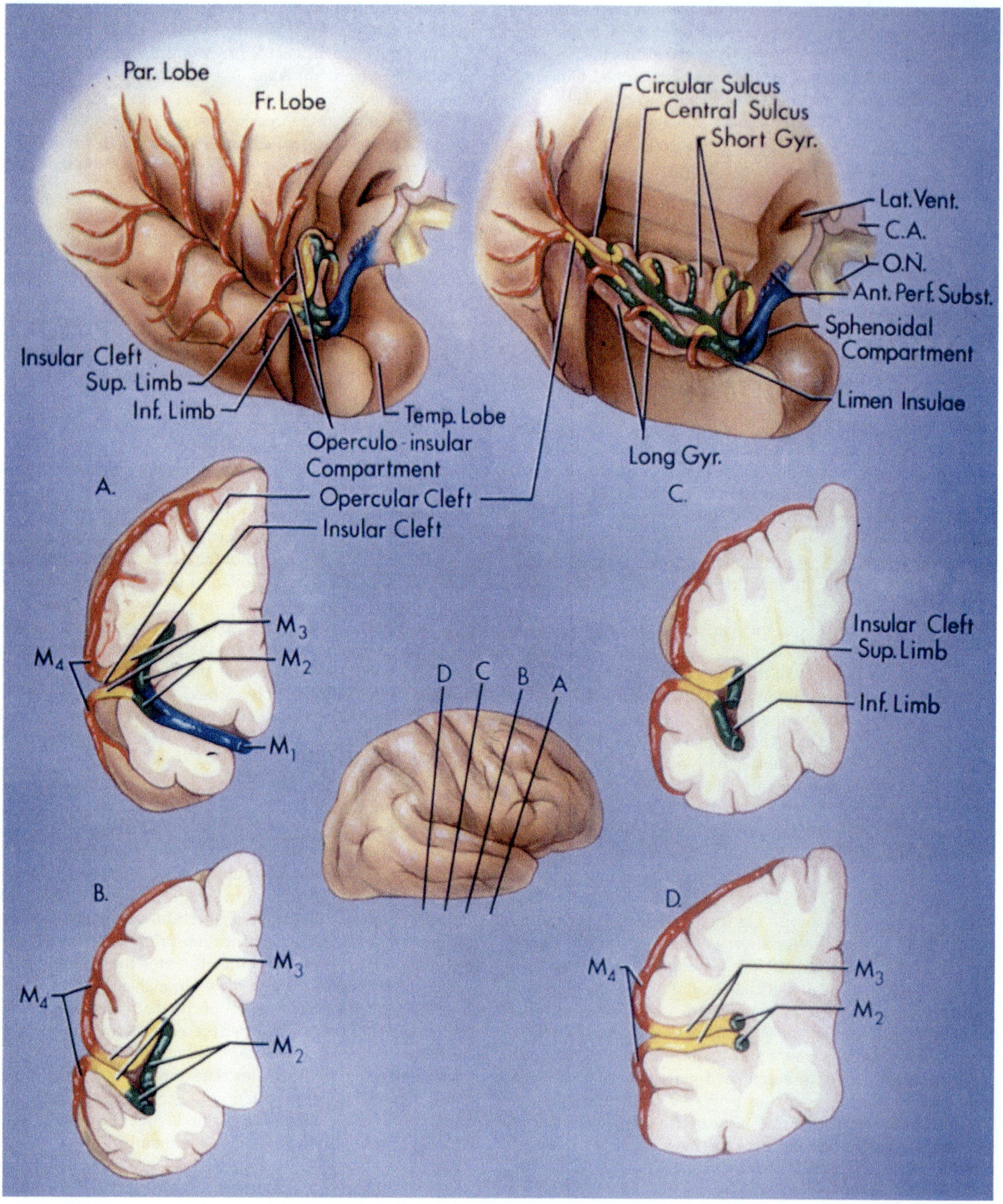

FIGURE 2.11. *Relationship of the M1* (blue), *M2* (green), *M3* (yellow), *and M4* (red) *segments of the middle cerebral arteries to the insula and sylvian fissure.* Upper left and right, *superolateral views of the right cerebral hemisphere with the anterior half of the frontal lobe and part of the frontoparietal and temporal opercula removed.* Upper left, *the removal exposes the anterior quarter of the insula.* Upper right, *the removal exposes the whole surface of*

stance is evidence of this distinctive morphology. The intermediate lenticulostriate arteries arise almost exclusively on the M1 or its early branches. Most arise from the posterior, posterosuperior, or superior aspect of the MCA. They arise predominantly from the main or prebifurcation part of the M1 or an early branch.

The lateral lenticulostriate arteries are present in almost all hemispheres. They originate predominantly on the lateral part of the M1, pursue an S-shaped course, and enter the posterolateral part of the anterior perforated substance. An average of five lateral lenticulostriate arteries per hemisphere divide to yield as many as 20 branches before they enter the anterior perforated substance. They may also arise from the early branches of the M1 or from the M2. They can arise from the pre- or postbifurcation trunks of the M1. More branches arise from postbifurcation branches if there is an early bifurcation; they could arise from either the superior or inferior trunk distal to the bifurcation, but there is a strong predilection for the inferior trunk. They arise from either the posterior, superior, or posterosuperior aspect of the parent trunks, travel medially with the parent trunks, then loop sharply posteriorly, laterally, and superiorly, and finally, turn posteromedially just before penetrating the anterior perforated substance. The branches with a more medial origin arise at a less acute angle to the parent vessel and pursue a more direct posterior, superior, and medial route to the anterior perforated substance.

The lateral and intermediate groups of lenticulostriate arteries pass through the putamen and arch medially and posteriorly to supply almost the entire anterior-to-posterior length of the upper part of the internal capsule and the body and head of the caudate nucleus. The medial lenticulostriate arteries irrigate the area medial to and below that supplied by the lateral and intermediate lenticulostriate arteries; this area includes the lateral part of the globus pallidus, the superior part of the anterior limb of the internal capsule, and the anterosuperior part of the head of the caudate nucleus.

The relationship of the lateral lenticulostriate arteries to the M1 bifurcation is important because the bifurcation is the site of most aneurysms arising from the middle cerebral artery. Nearly 30% of the lateral lenticulostriate arteries originate from the pre- or postbifurcation trunks 2.0 mm or less from the M1 bifurcation; and nearly 70% are positioned 5.0 mm or less from the bifurcation (36). Some branches arise directly on the bifurcation. Of the arteries originating near the bifurcation, there is a nearly even split between an origin on the pre- and postbifurcation trunks. The area of supply and clinical features are reviewed below, under the Anterior Perforating Arteries.

Cortical Distribution

The cortical territory supplied by the MCA includes the majority of the lateral surface of the hemisphere, all of the insular and opercular surfaces, the lateral part of the orbital surface of the frontal lobe, the temporal pole, and the lateral part of the inferior surface of the temporal lobe. The MCA territory does not reach the occipital or frontal poles or the upper margin of the hemisphere, but it does extend around the lower margin of the cerebral hemisphere onto the inferior surfaces of the frontal and temporal lobes (*Fig. 2.17*).

The narrow peripheral strip on the lateral surface of the cerebral hemisphere, supplied by the ACA and PCA rather than the MCA, extends along the entire length of the superior margin of the hemisphere from the frontal to the occipital pole. It is broadest in the superior frontal region and narrowest in the superior parietal area. This strip continues around the occipital pole and onto the posterior part of the lateral surface of the temporal lobe and narrows and disappears anteriorly on the temporal lobe where the branches of the MCA extend around the lower border of the hemisphere onto the inferior surface of the temporal lobe and the orbital surface of the frontal lobe.

The cortical area supplied by the MCA is divided into 12 areas (*Fig. 2.17*):

1. Orbitofrontal area. The orbital portion of the middle and inferior frontal gyri and the inferior part of the pars orbitalis.
2. Prefrontal area. The superior part of the pars orbitalis, the pars triangularis, the anterior part of the pars opercularis, and most of the middle frontal gyrus.
3. Precentral area. The posterior part of the pars opercularis and the middle frontal gyrus, and the inferior and middle portions of the precentral gyrus.
4. Central area. The superior part of the precentral gyrus and the inferior half of the postcentral gyrus.

the insula. The sylvian fissure is divided into sphenoidal and operculoinsular compartments. The sphenoidal compartment, in which the M1 segment courses, is located posterior to the sphenoid ridge. The M2 and M3 segments course in the operculoinsular compartment of the sylvian fissure. The operculoinsular compartment is divided into an insular and an opercular cleft. The opercular cleft is located between the frontoparietal and the temporal opercula. The insular cleft is located between the insula and the opercula. The insular cleft is divided into a superior limb, located medial to the frontoparietal operculum, and an inferior limb, located medial to the temporal operculum. The circular sulcus is located at the periphery of the insula. The short gyri of the insula are located above the central sulcus of the insula and the long gyri are located below. The carotid arteries and anterior perforated substance are at the medial end of the sylvian fissure. The lateral ventricles are above the optic nerves. A–D, *anterior views of coronal sections of the right cerebral hemisphere. The central diagram shows the level of the sections.* A, *coronal section at the level of the M1 segment. The M1 segment courses in the sphenoidal compartment, the M2 segment courses on the insulae, the M3 segment passes over the deep surface of the opercula, and the M4 segment courses on the cortical surface. At this anterior level, the frontal operculum covers more of the insula than the temporal operculum.* B, *coronal section at the midportion of the sylvian fissure where the frontal and temporal opercula are of nearly equal height.* C, *coronal section at a more posterior level where the temporal operculum covers more of the insula than does the frontoparietal operculum.* D, *coronal section from the posterior end of the sylvian fissure. Only the opercular cleft remains; the insular cleft has disappeared.* Ant., *anterior;* C.A., *carotid artery;* Fr., *frontal;* Gyr., *gyri;* Inf., *inferior;* Lat., *lateral;* N., *nerve;* O., *optic;* Par., *parietal;* Perf., *perforated;* Subst., *substance;* Sup., *superior;* Temp., *temporal;* Vent., *ventricle.* (From, *Gibo H, Carver CC, Rhoton AL Jr, Lenkey C, Mitchell RJ: Microsurgical anatomy of the middle cerebral artery.* ***J Neurosurg*** *54:151–169, 1981 [14].*)

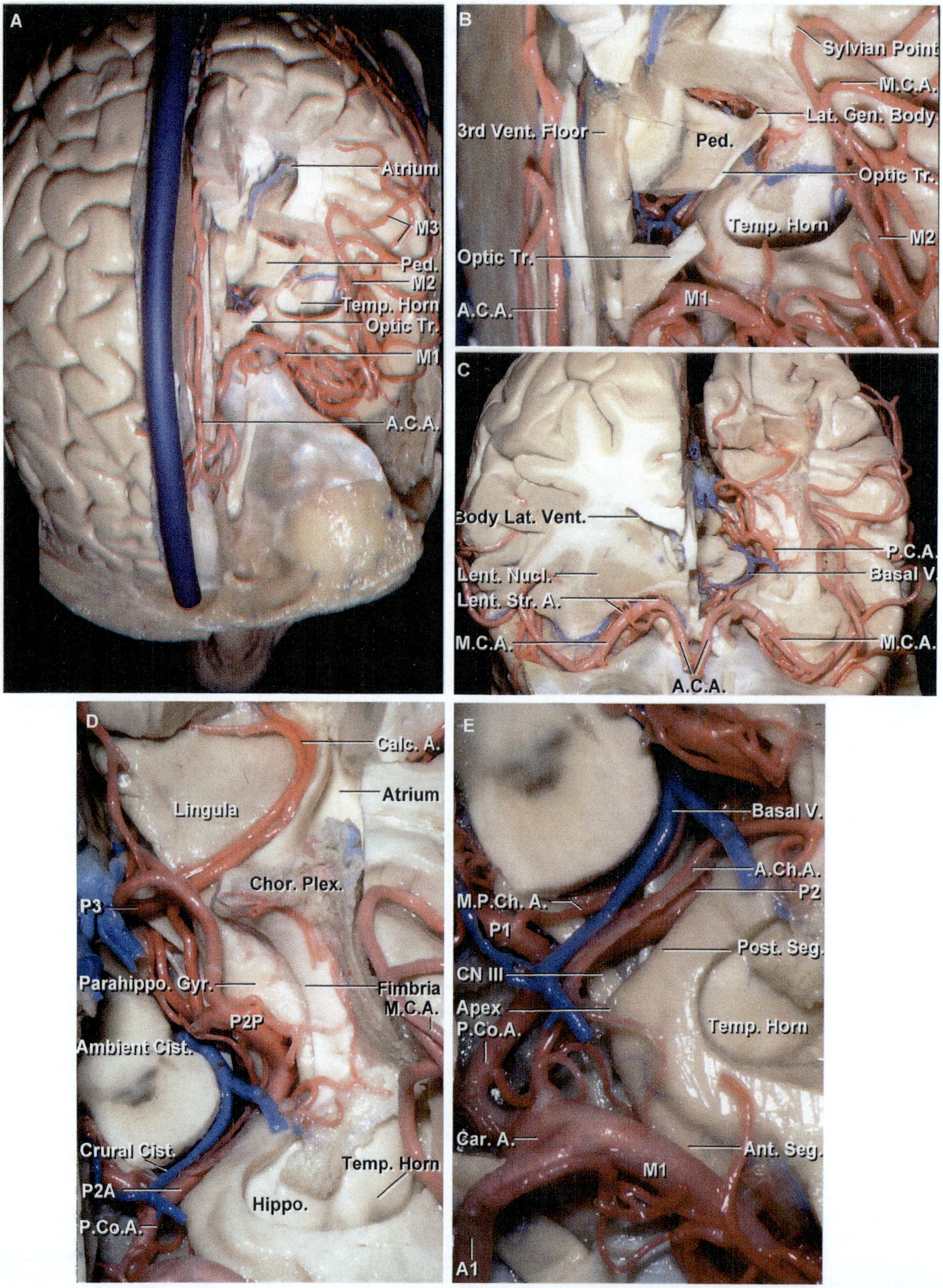

FIGURE 2.12. *Cerebral arteries, superior view. A, the upper part of the left hemisphere has been removed to expose the atrium and temporal horn. Part of the optic tract and cerebral peduncle has been preserved. The ACA crosses above the chiasm and along the medial surface of the hemisphere. The MCA*

5. Anterior parietal area. The superior part of the postcentral gyrus, and frequently, the upper part of the central sulcus, the anterior part of the inferior parietal lobule, and the anteroinferior part of the superior parietal lobule.
6. Posterior parietal area. The posterior part of the superior and inferior parietal lobules, including the supramarginal gyrus.
7. Angular area. The posterior part of the superior temporal gyrus, variable portions of the supramarginal and angular gyri, and the superior parts of the lateral occipital gyri (the artery to this area is considered the terminal branch of the MCA).
8. Temporo-occipital area. The posterior half of the superior temporal gyrus, the posterior extreme of the middle and inferior temporal gyri, and the inferior parts of the lateral occipital gyri.
9. Posterior temporal area. The middle and posterior part of the superior temporal gyrus, the posterior third of the middle temporal gyrus, and the posterior extreme of the inferior temporal gyrus.
10. Middle temporal area. The superior temporal gyrus near the level of the pars triangularis and pars opercularis, the middle part of the middle temporal gyrus, and the middle and posterior part of the inferior temporal gyrus.
11. Anterior temporal area. The anterior part of the superior, middle, and inferior temporal gyri.
12. Temporopolar area. The anterior pole of the superior, middle, and inferior temporal gyri.

Branching Pattern

The main trunk of the MCA divides in one of three ways: bifurcation into superior and inferior trunks; trifurcation into superior, middle, and inferior trunks; or division into multiple (four or more) trunks (*Figs. 2.18* and *2.19*). In our study, 78% of the MCAs divided in a bifurcation, 12% divided in a trifurcation, and 10% divided by giving rise to multiple trunks (14). The distal division of the MCA also generally occurs in a series of bifurcations. The small arteries that arise proximal to the bifurcation or trifurcation and are distributed to the frontal or temporal pole are referred to as early branches.

The MCAs that bifurcate are divided into three groups, designated equal bifurcation, superior trunk dominant, and inferior trunk dominant, based on the diameter and the size of the cortical area of supply of their superior and inferior trunks. The equal bifurcation (18% of hemispheres) yields two trunks with nearly equal diameters and size of cortical area. The inferior trunk supplies the temporal, temporo-occipital, and angular areas, and the superior trunk supplies the frontal and parietal regions. The superior trunk usually supplies the orbitofrontal to the posterior parietal areas, and the inferior trunk usually supplies the angular to the temporopolar areas. The inferior trunk dominant type of bifurcation (32% of hemispheres) yields a larger inferior trunk that supplies the temporal and parietal lobes and a smaller superior trunk that supplies all or part of the frontal lobe. The maximal area perfused by the inferior trunk includes all of the territory between and including the precentral and temporopolar areas. The superior trunk dominant type of bifurcation (28% of hemispheres) yields a larger superior trunk that supplies the frontal and parietal regions and a smaller inferior trunk that supplies only the temporal lobe. The maximal area supplied by the dominant superior trunk includes the orbitofrontal to the temporo-occipital areas.

Stem Arteries

The stem arteries arise from the trunks and give rise to the individual cortical branches (*Fig. 2.20*). They arise from the main trunk and the two or more trunks formed by a bifurcation, trifurcation, or division into multiple trunks. There is considerable variation in the number and size of the area supplied by the stem arteries. The most common pattern is made up of 8 stem arteries per hemisphere (range, 6 to 11) (14).

The individual stem arteries give rise to one to five cortical arteries. The most common pattern is for one of the 12 cortical areas to be supplied by a stem artery supplying one or two adjacent areas. The cortical areas most commonly receiving a stem artery serving only that area are the temporo-occipital, angular, and central areas. Stem arteries supplying four or five of the cortical areas are most commonly directed to the area below the sylvian fissure.

passes laterally below the anterior perforated substance and turns posteriorly in the depths of the sylvian fissure on the medial side of the opercular lips. The M1 segment courses below the anterior perforated substance and ends at the limen insula, the M2 segment crosses the insular, the M3 crosses the opercular lips, and the M4 branches course on the lateral convexity. B, *enlarged view. The initial segment of the optic tract has been preserved. The MCA courses laterally in the area above and anterior to the temporal pole and turns posteriorly in the sylvian fissure. The sylvian point, the site at which the last MCA turns away from the insula, coincides with the point where the most posterior of the transverse temporal gyri intersect the insula. The PCA is hidden below the optic tract and cerebral peduncle.* C, *the anterior part of the right hemisphere has been removed to show the symmetry of the MCAs. Lenticulostriate arteries are exposed below the lentiform nucleus. The upper part of the left cerebral peduncle and optic tract has been removed to expose the PCA and basal veins in the crural and ambient cisterns.* D, *enlarged view. The P2 arises at the level of the PComA and passes around the brainstem. The anterior part of the P2, the part that passes through the crural cistern, is designated the P2A, or crural segment, and the posterior part that courses in the ambient cistern is designated the P2P, or ambient segment. The P3 is located in the quadrigeminal cistern and the P4 segment consists of the cortical branches. The calcarine branch courses deeply within the calcarine sulcus, roofed above by the cuneus, which has been removed to exposed the floor of the calcarine sulcus formed by the lingula. The calcarine branch courses adjacent to the calcar avis, which is the prominence in the medial wall of the atrium formed by the deep end of the calcarine sulcus.* E, *enlarged view. The AChA courses around the anterior and posterior uncal segments and the uncal apex to reach the temporal horn just behind the posterior uncal segment. The PComA courses below and medial to the AChA and joins the P1 at the anterior edge of the crural cistern.* F, *another specimen in which the anterior portion of the hemisphere has been* *(Legend continues on next page.)*

FIGURE 2.12. *Continued* *removed to expose the temporal horn. The M1, M2, and M3 and the P2A, P2P, P3, and P4 have been exposed. The branches of the PCA pass back to the occipital pole. G, enlarged view. The anterior segment of the uncus faces the carotid, middle cerebral, anterior choroidal, and posterior communicating arteries. The posterior segment of the uncus, which forms the lateral margin of the crural cistern, faces the P2A, the basal terminal part of the AChA and the uncal apex is located lateral to the oculomotor nerve. The basal vein courses above the PCA. H, upper surface of the temporal and occipital lobes. The M1 courses along the stem of the sylvian fissure below the anterior perforated substance. The M2 begins at the limen insula and courses over the surface of the insula. The M3 courses over the opercular lips. The M4 is distributed to the cortical surface. The P2 has been preserved. It courses medial to the posterior segment of the uncus and parahippocampal gyrus and through the crural and ambient cisterns. The calcarine branch courses deep in the calcarine sulcus on the medial side of the atrium. I, inferior surface of the temporal lobe. The P2 branches are distributed to the inferior and the lower part of the lateral surfaces of the temporal and occipital lobes. The M1 courses above the anterior uncal segment.* A., *arteries, artery;* A.C.A., *anterior cerebral artery;* A.Ch.A., *anterior choroidal artery;* Ant., *anterior;* Calc., *calcarine;* Car., *carotid;* Chor., *choroid;* Cist., *cistern;* CN, *cranial nerve;* Gen., *geniculate;* Gyr., *gyrus;* Hippo., *hippocampal, hippocampus;* Lat., *lateral;* Lent., *lentiform;* Lent. Str., *lenticulostriate;* M.C.A., *middle cerebral artery;* M.P.Ch.A., *medial posterior choroidal artery;* Nucl., *nucleus;* P.C.A., *posterior cerebral artery;* P.Co.A., *posterior communicating artery;* Par. Occip., *parieto-occipital;* Parahippo., *parahippocampal;* Ped., *peduncle;* Plex., *plexus;* Post., *posterior;* Quad., *quadrigeminal;* Seg., *segment;* Temp., *temporal;* Tr., *tract;* Trans., *transverse;* V., *vein;* Vent., *ventricle.*

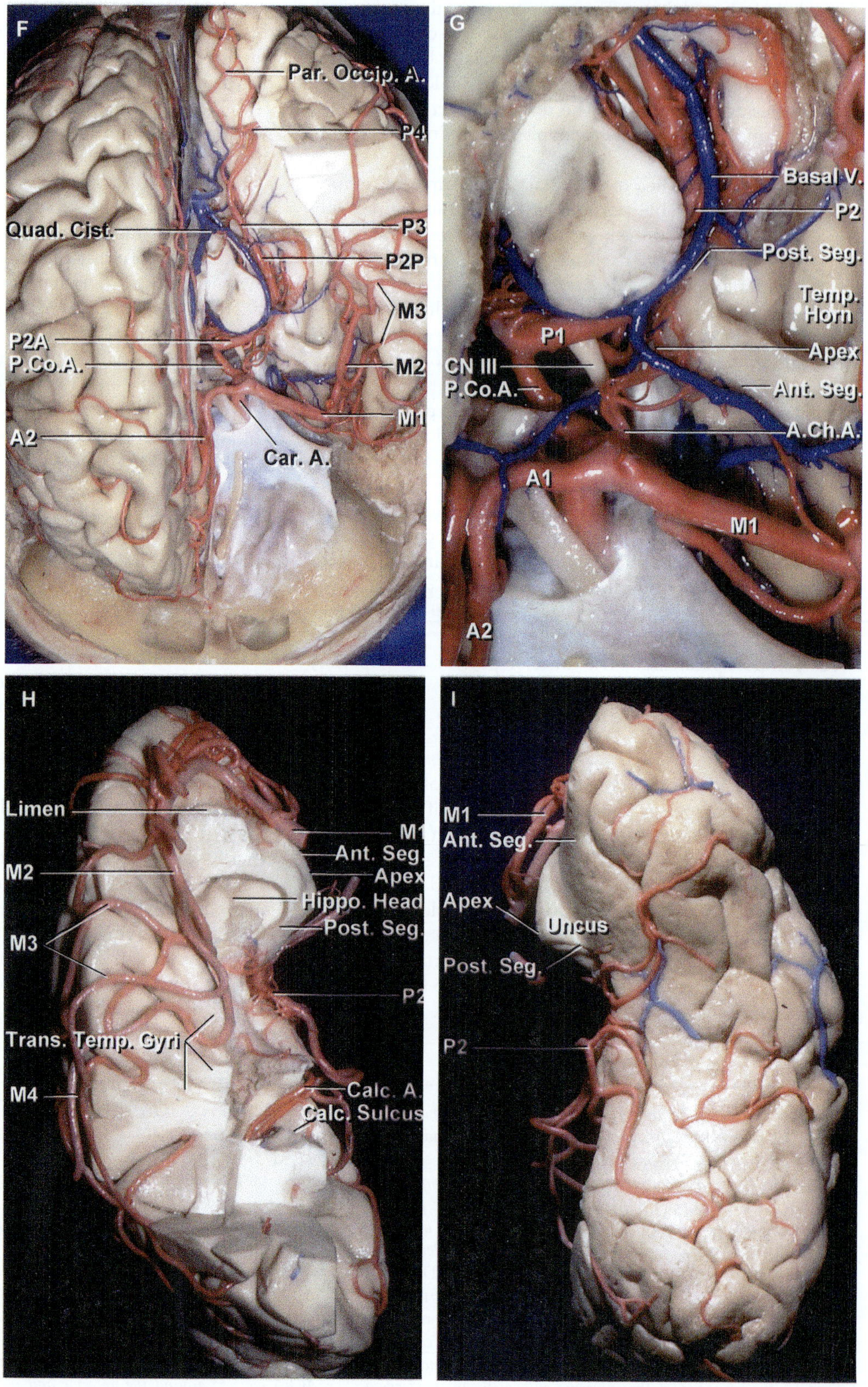

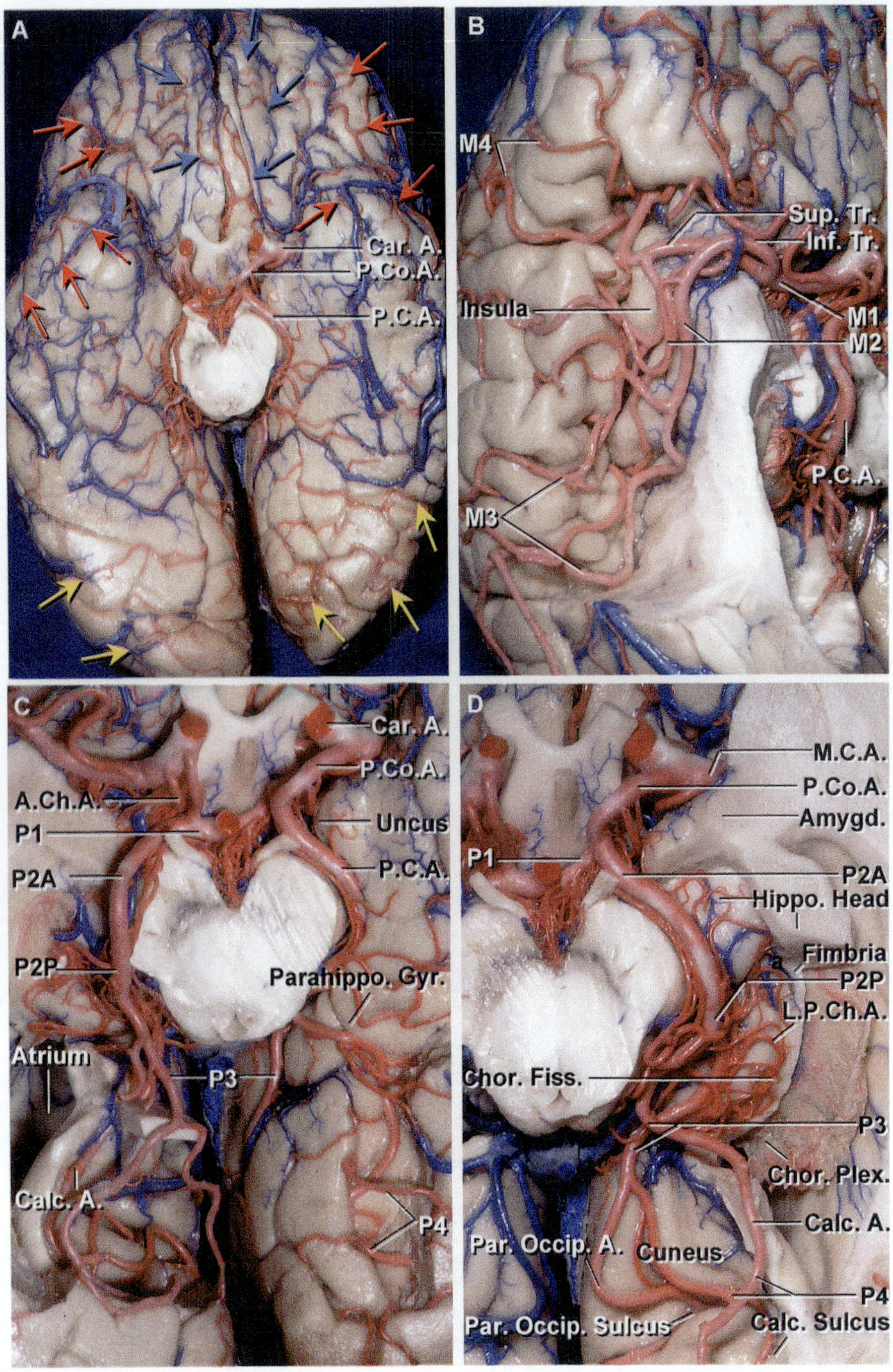

FIGURE 2.13. *Arteries of the basal surface.* A, *inferior view of the basal surface of the frontal, temporal, and occipital lobes. The orbital surface of the frontal lobe is supplied by the ACA and MCA. The branches of the ACA overlap from the interhemispheric fissure onto the adjacent part of the orbital surface of the frontal lobe* (blue arrows) *and the MCA branches overlap onto the lateral part of the orbital surface* (red arrows). *Most of the lower surface of the temporal and occipital lobes is supplied by the PCA; however, branches of the MCA overlap onto the basal surface of the temporal pole and adjacent part of the temporal lobe* (red arrows). *Branches of the PCA* (yellow arrows) *extend around the occipital pole lower hemispheric margin to reach the lateral surface of the temporal and occipital lobe* (yellow arrows). B, *the temporal lobe has been removed to expose the M1 bifurcating into superior and inferior trunks below the anterior perforated substance and passing across the insula and the frontoparietal operculi. The superior trunk supplies most of the lateral surface of the frontal lobe and the inferior trunk supplies most of the lateral surface of the parietal and temporal lobe. The M1 courses below the anterior perforated substance, the M2 courses on the insula, the M3 passes around the opercular lips, and the M4 is formed by the cortical branches.* C, *the PCAs arise in the interpeduncular cistern in front of the brainstem and pass through the crural cistern, located between the uncus and cerebral peduncle, and the ambient cistern, located between the midbrain and parahippocampal gyrus, to reach the quadrigeminal cisterns. The P2 segment courses in the crural and ambient cisterns, the P3 in the quadrigeminal cistern, and the P4 is the cortical segment. The P2 is divided into a P2A that courses in the crural cistern and a P2P that courses in the ambient cistern. The floor of the right atrium and the lower lip of the calcarine sulcus have been removed to expose the calcarine branches of the PCA coursing in the depths of the calcarine sulcus adjacent to the medial atrial wall. The PCA branches in the depths of the calcarine sulcus are separated from the medial wall of the atrium by only the thin layer of cortex and white matter that form the calcar avis, the prominence in the medial atrial wall overlying the deep end of the calcarine sulcus.* D, *the floor of the left temporal horn, except for some of the head of the hippocampus and the fimbria, has been removed. The head of the hippocampus folds into and constitutes most of the posterior segment of the uncus, which faces the P2A. The amygdala is located in the anterior uncal segment, which faces the carotid and PComAs. The lower lip of the calcarine sulcus, formed by the lingula, has been removed to expose the upper lip, formed by the cuneus, and the calcarine arteries coursing just outside the medial wall of the atrium. The calcarine branch courses deeply into the calcarine sulcus, and the parieto-occipital branch ascends in the parieto-occipital sulcus. The fimbria of the fornix has been preserved. The LPChAs arise below the thalamus and pass through the choroidal fissure, located between the thalamus and fimbria, to reach the choroid plexus in the temporal horn and atrium. The thalamogeniculate branches arise from the P2P and enter the roof of the ambient cistern by passing through the lower thalamus in the region of the geniculate bodies.* E, *inferior surface of* (Legend continues on next page.)

In our study, we also examined the stem arteries supplying each lobe (14). The frontal lobe is supplied by one to four stem arteries. The most common pattern, a two-stem pattern, had one stem giving rise to the orbitofrontal, prefrontal, and precentral arteries, and the other stem giving rise to the central artery. The parietal lobe and the adjoining part of the occipital lobe are supplied by one to three stem arteries. The most frequent pattern is for each of the three cortical areas to have its own stem. In the most frequent two-stem pattern, one stem gives rise to the anterior and posterior parietal arteries and the

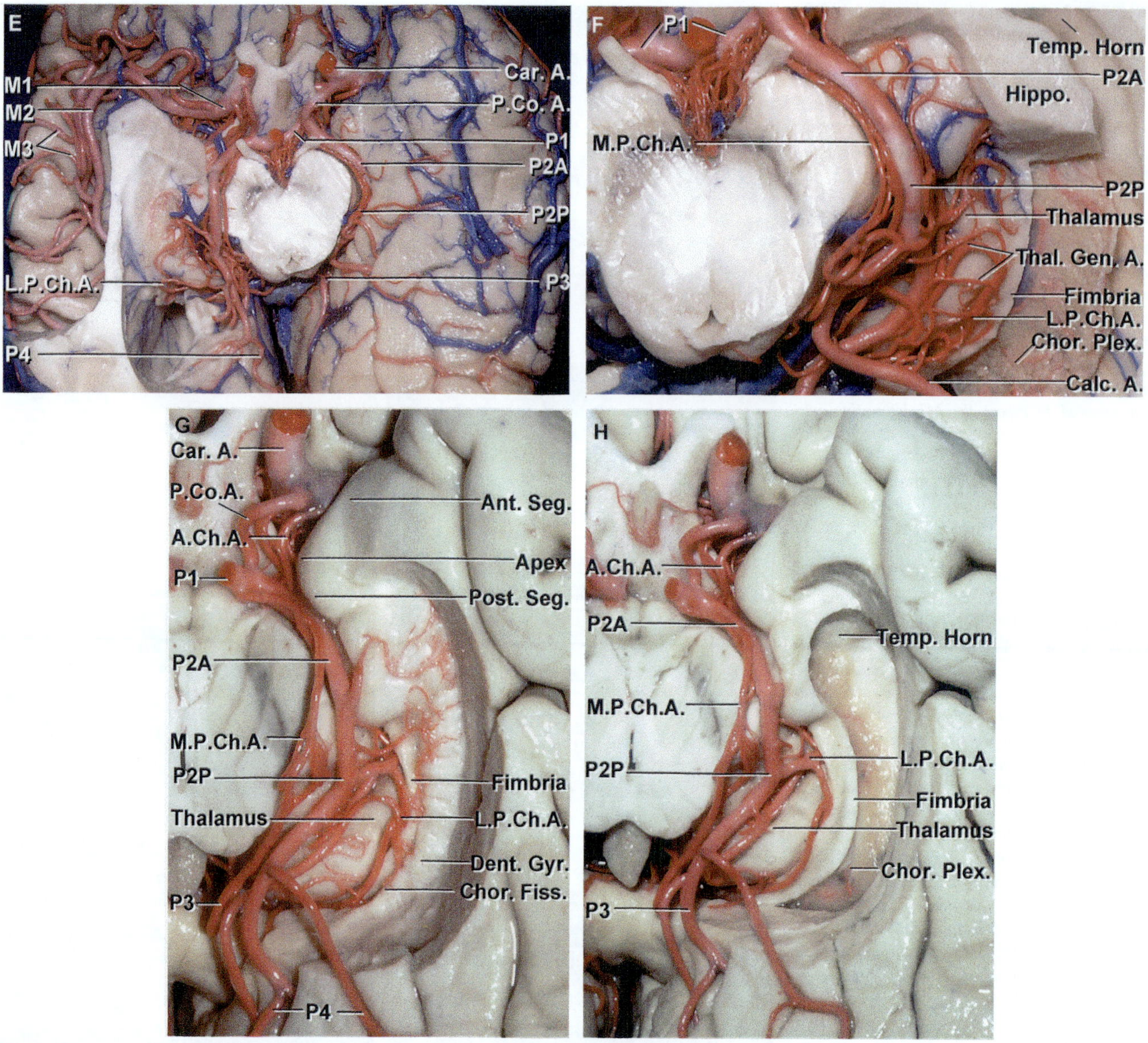

FIGURE 2.13. *Continued*
both cerebral hemispheres showing the MCA coursing along the sylvian cistern and the PCAs coursing through the crural, ambient, and quadrigeminal cisterns. F, enlarged view of the P2P coursing below the thalamus, which forms the roof of the ambient cistern. The left temporal horn has been opened by removing part of the floor. Some of the head of the hippocampus has been preserved. The P2P gives rise to a complex arborizing group of perforating arteries that enter the lower thalamus, some passing through the geniculate bodies, and constituting the thalamogeniculate arteries. G, inferior view of another cerebral hemisphere. The medial part of the parahippocampal gyrus has been removed to expose the PCA coursing through the crural, ambient, and quadrigeminal cisterns. The AChA courses around the uncus. The uncus has an anterior segment that faces the carotid, middle cerebral, anterior choroidal, and posterior communicating arteries, and a posterior segment that faces the posterior cerebral and the terminal segment of the AChA. The choroidal fissure is located between fimbria of the fornix and the lower surface of the thalamus and has its lower end just behind the posterior uncal segment. The LPChA pass laterally through the choroidal fissure located between the fimbria and the thalamus. The dentate gyrus is located below the fimbria. A MPChA courses medial to the PCA. H, the dentate gyrus and adjacent part of the parahippocampal gyrus has been removed to expose the choroid plexus in the temporal horn. The LPChAs pass laterally between the fimbria and the lower margin of the thalamus, formed in part by the lateral geniculate body and pulvinar, to reach the choroid plexus in the temporal horn and atrium. A., *artery;* A.Ch.A., *anterior choroidal artery;* Amygd., *amygdala;* Ant., *anterior;* Calc., *calcarine;* Car., *carotid;* Chor., *choroid, choroidal;* Dent., *dentate;* Fiss., *fissure;* Gyr., *gyrus;* Hippo., *hippocampal, hippocampus;* Inf., *inferior;* L.P.Ch.A., *lateral posterior choroidal artery;* M.C.A., *middle cerebral artery;* M.P.Ch.A., *medial posterior choroidal artery;* P.C.A., *posterior cerebral artery;* P.Co.A., *posterior communicating artery;* Par. Occip., *parieto-occipital;* Parahippo., *parahippocampal;* Plex., *plexus;* Post., *posterior;* Seg., *segment;* Sulc., *sulcus;* Sup., *superior;* Temp., *temporal;* Thal. Gen., *thalamogeniculate;* Tr., *trunk.*

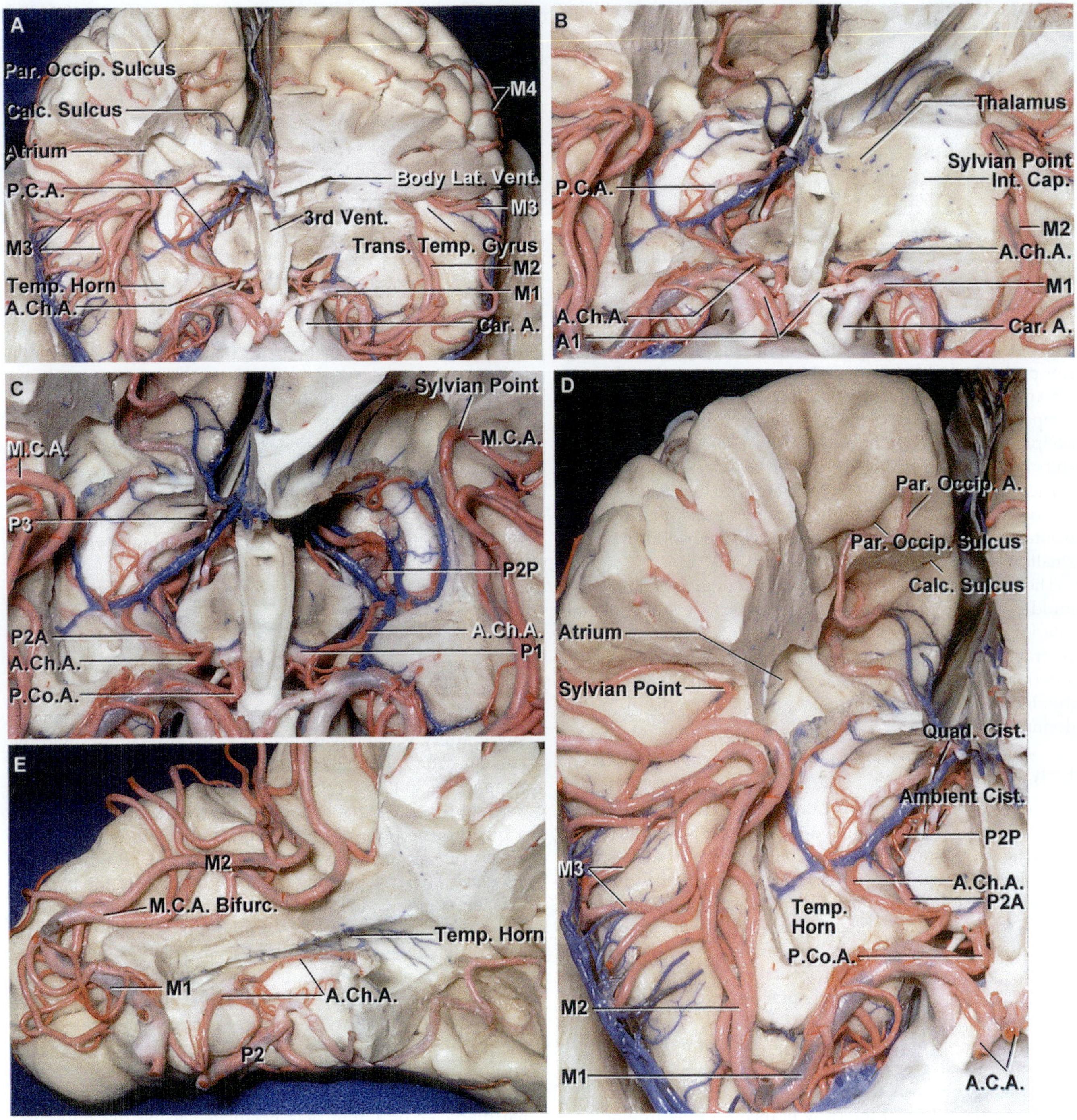

FIGURE 2.14. *Superior views of the cerebral arteries. A, the upper part of the right cerebral hemisphere has been removed to expose the temporal horn, atrium, and the basal cisterns. The part of the left hemisphere anterior to the midportion of the body of the lateral and above the sylvian fissure has been removed. The ICAs ascend on the lateral side of the optic nerves. The MCAs travel laterally in the sylvian fissures. The M1 crosses below the anterior perforated substance. The trunks of the M2 cross the insula and the M3 extends around the opercular lips. The M4 is formed by the cortical branches on the convexity. The PCAs pass posteriorly in the crural and ambient cisterns to reach the quadrigeminal cistern. The ACA passes above the optic chiasm. The floor of the third ventricle and the calcarine and parieto-occipital sulcus have been exposed. The upper lip of the parieto-occipital sulcus formed by the precuneus has been removed. The lower lip of the parieto-occipital sulcus is formed by the cuneus, which also forms the upper lip of the calcarine sulcus. B, enlarged view. The AChAs enter the choroid plexus in the temporal horn. The sylvian point is located where the most posterior branch of the M2 turns away from the insular surface and toward the lateral convexity. C, the anterior part of the left hemisphere has been removed down to the level of the temporal lobe and the midbrain. The AChAs pass around the upper medial part of the uncus to reach the temporal horn. The (Legend continues on next page.)*

other stem gives rise to the angular artery. The temporal lobe, along with the adjoining part of the occipital lobe, is supplied by one to five stem arteries; the most common pattern is to have four stem arteries. This lobe has more stem arteries than the other lobes supplied by the MCA.

Cortical Arteries

The cortical arteries arise from the stem arteries and supply the individual cortical areas. Generally, one, or less commonly, two cortical arteries (range, one to five) pass to each of the 12 cortical areas (*Figs. 2.17* and *2.20*). The smallest cortical arteries arise at the anterior end of the sylvian fissure and the largest arteries arise at the posterior limits of the fissure. The cortical branches to the frontal, anterior temporal, and anterior parietal areas are smaller than those supplying the posterior parietal, posterior temporal, temporo-occipital, and angular areas. The smallest arteries supply the orbitofrontal and temporopolar areas, and the largest ones supply the temporo-occipital and the angular areas. There is an inverse relationship between the size and number of arteries supplying a cortical area. The temporo-occipital area has the smallest number of arteries, but they are the largest in size, and the prefrontal area has the largest number of arteries, but they are smaller.

The temporopolar, temporo-occipital, angular, and anterior, middle, and posterior temporal arteries usually arise from the inferior trunk; the orbitofrontal, prefrontal, precentral, and central arteries usually arise from the superior trunk. The anterior and posterior parietal arteries have an origin evenly divided between the two trunks and usually arise from the dominant trunk.

Early Branches

The cortical arteries arising from the main trunk proximal to the bifurcation or trifurcation are called early branches (*Fig. 2.3*). The early branches are distributed to the frontal or temporal lobes. Nearly half of MCAs send early branches to the temporal lobe, but less than 10% give early branches to the frontal lobe (14). The temporal branches usually supply the temporopolar and anterior temporal areas. The frontal branches terminate in the orbitofrontal and prefrontal areas. A few MCAs will give rise to early branches to both the frontal and temporal areas.

There is most commonly only one early branch, but a few hemispheres will give rise to two early branches. In our study, the distance between the bifurcation or trifurcation of the MCA and the origin of the early branches to the frontal lobe was 5.5 mm (range, 5.0–6.0 mm) and 11.2 mm (range, 3.5–30.0 mm) for the temporal lobe (14).

Anomalies

Anomalies of the MCA, consisting of either a duplicate or an accessory MCA, are infrequent and occur less often than anomalies of the other intracranial arteries (14). A duplicated MCA is a second artery that arises from the internal carotid artery and an accessory MCA is one that arises from the anterior cerebral artery. Both the duplicate and accessory MCAs send branches to the cortical areas usually supplied by the MCA. The accessory MCAs usually arise from the anterior cerebral artery near the origin of the anterior communicating artery (AComA). The accessory MCA is differentiated from a recurrent artery of Heubner by the fact that the recurrent artery, although arising from the same part of the anterior cerebral artery as an accessory MCA, enters the anterior perforated substance, but the accessory MCA, although sending branches to the anterior perforated substance, also courses lateral to this area and sends branches to cortical areas normally supplied by the MCA (*Fig. 2.16H*).

MCA Branches for Extracranial-Intracranial Bypass

Important factors in selecting a cortical artery for a bypass procedure are its diameter and the length of artery available on the cortical surface. The largest cortical artery is the temporo-occipital artery (14). Nearly two-thirds are 1.5 mm or more in diameter, and 90% are 1 mm or more in diameter. The smallest cortical artery is the orbitofrontal artery; approximately one-quarter are 1 mm or more in diameter. The central sulcal artery is the largest branch to the frontal lobe, and the angular artery is the largest branch to the parietal lobe. The temporo-occipital and the posterior temporal arteries are the largest branches to the temporal lobe. The minimum length of a cortical artery needed to complete a bypass is 4 mm. The length of each of the cortical arteries on the cortical surface averages 11.8 mm or more. The angular, posterior parietal, and temporo-occipital arteries have the longest segments on the cortical surface, and the orbitofrontal and temporopolar arteries have the shortest cortical segment.

Chater et al. (3) undertook an analysis of the cortical branches of the MCA available in three circular cortical zones with a diameter of 4 cm. These three zones were centered over the convexity of the frontal lobe, the tip of the temporal lobe, and the region of the angular gyrus and were selected to be readily accessible by means of a small craniectomy. An external diameter of 1 mm was postulated to be the minimum

FIGURE 2.14. *Continued*
P2A courses medial to the uncus in the crural cistern, the P2P courses in the ambient cistern, and the P3 courses in the quadrigeminal cistern. D, *enlarged view. The M2 crosses the insula just above and lateral to the temporal horn. The artery forming the sylvian point often has its apex directed medially toward the atrium. The parieto-occipital branch of the PCA courses along the parieto-occipital sulcus. The calcarine branch is directed backward in the calcarine sulcus.* E, *the right temporal lobe has been removed while preserving the M1, M2, and M3. The P2 courses along the medial surface of the temporal lobe. The AChA arises from the carotid artery and takes a somewhat tortuous course to reach the choroid plexus and temporal horn.* A., *artery;* A.C.A., *anterior cerebral artery;* A.Ch.A., *anterior choroidal artery;* Bifurc., *bifurcation;* Calc., *calcarine;* Cap., *capsule;* Car., *carotid;* Cist., *cistern;* Int., *internal;* Lat., *lateral;* M.C.A., *middle cerebral artery;* P.C.A., *posterior cerebral artery;* P.Co.A., *posterior communicating artery;* Par. Occip., *parieto-occipital;* Quad., *quadrigeminal;* Temp., *temporal;* Trans., *transverse;* Vent., *ventricle.*

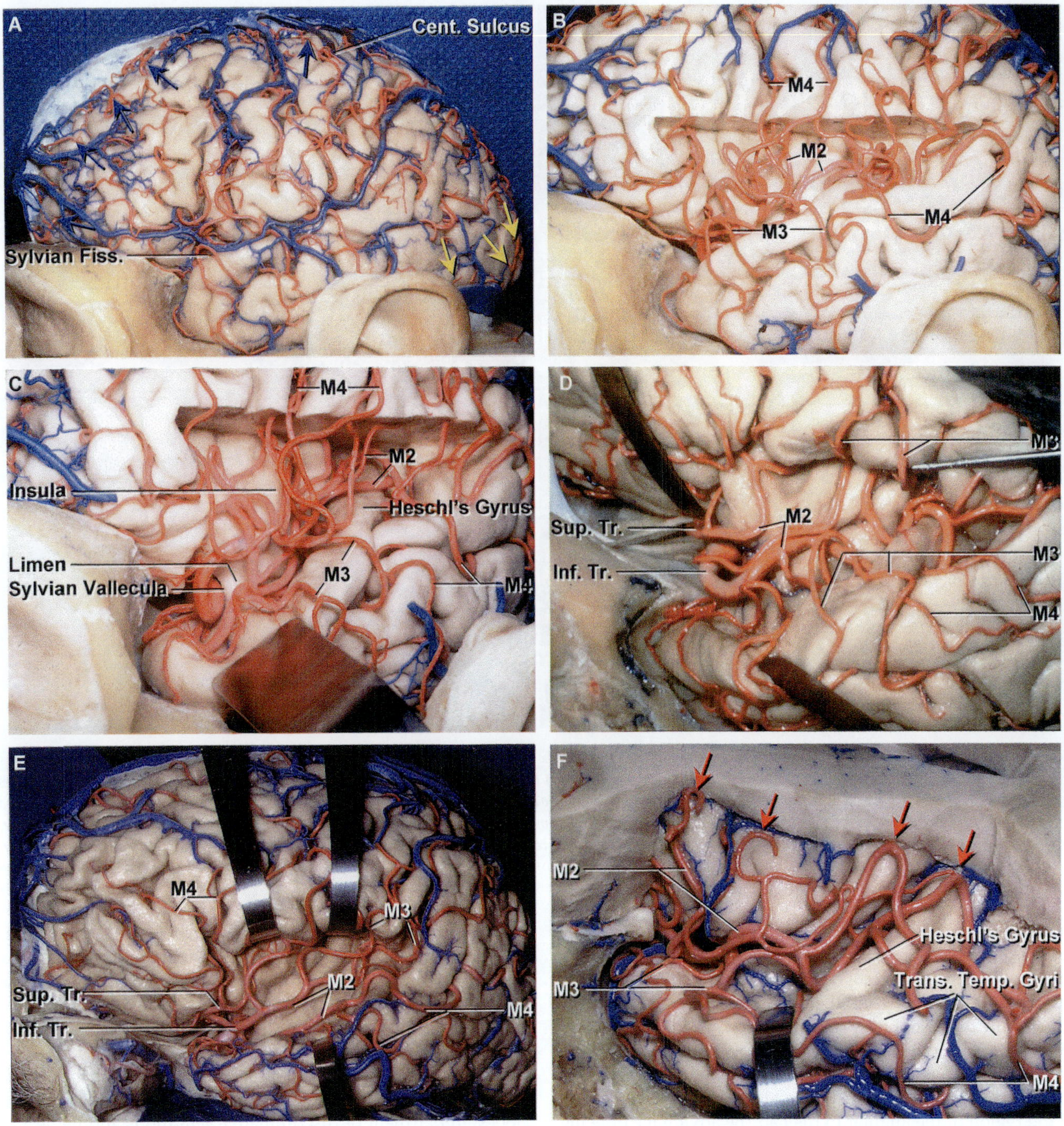

FIGURE 2.15. *The insula and middle cerebral arteries.* A, *left side. The cortical branches of the MCA, which form the M4, spread out from the sylvian fissure to supply the majority of the lateral convexity. Branches of the ACA* (yellow arrows) *spread over the superior hemispheric border to reach the lateral hemispheric surface, and branches of the PCA pass around the occipital pole and adjacent part of the temporal lobe to supply the adjacent part of the convexity* (red arrows). B, *the frontoparietal operculum that covers the upper part of the insula has been removed to show the M2 crossing the insula, the M3 curving around the opercular lips, and the M4 on the lateral cortical surface.* C, *enlarged view. The sylvian vallecula is the opening between the lips of the sylvian at the limen insula where the MCA turns posteriorly to form the M2 segment.* D, *another specimen with the lips of the sylvian fissure retracted. This shows a large dominant inferior trunk that gives rise to multiple branches that supply the majority of the lateral convexity.* E, *another hemisphere with the lips of the sylvian fissure retracted to expose the branches forming the M2, M3, and M4 crossing the insula and passing around the opercular lips to reach the cortical surface.* F, *the upper part of the hemisphere and the frontal and parietal operculum have been removed to expose the M2 branches crossing the insula. The posterior M3 branches cross the transverse temporal gyri, the most anterior of which forms Heschl's gyrus, to reach the cortical surface.* Cent., *central;* Fiss., *fissure;* Inf., *inferior;* Sup., *superior;* Temp., *temporal;* Tr., *trunk;* Trans., *transverse.*

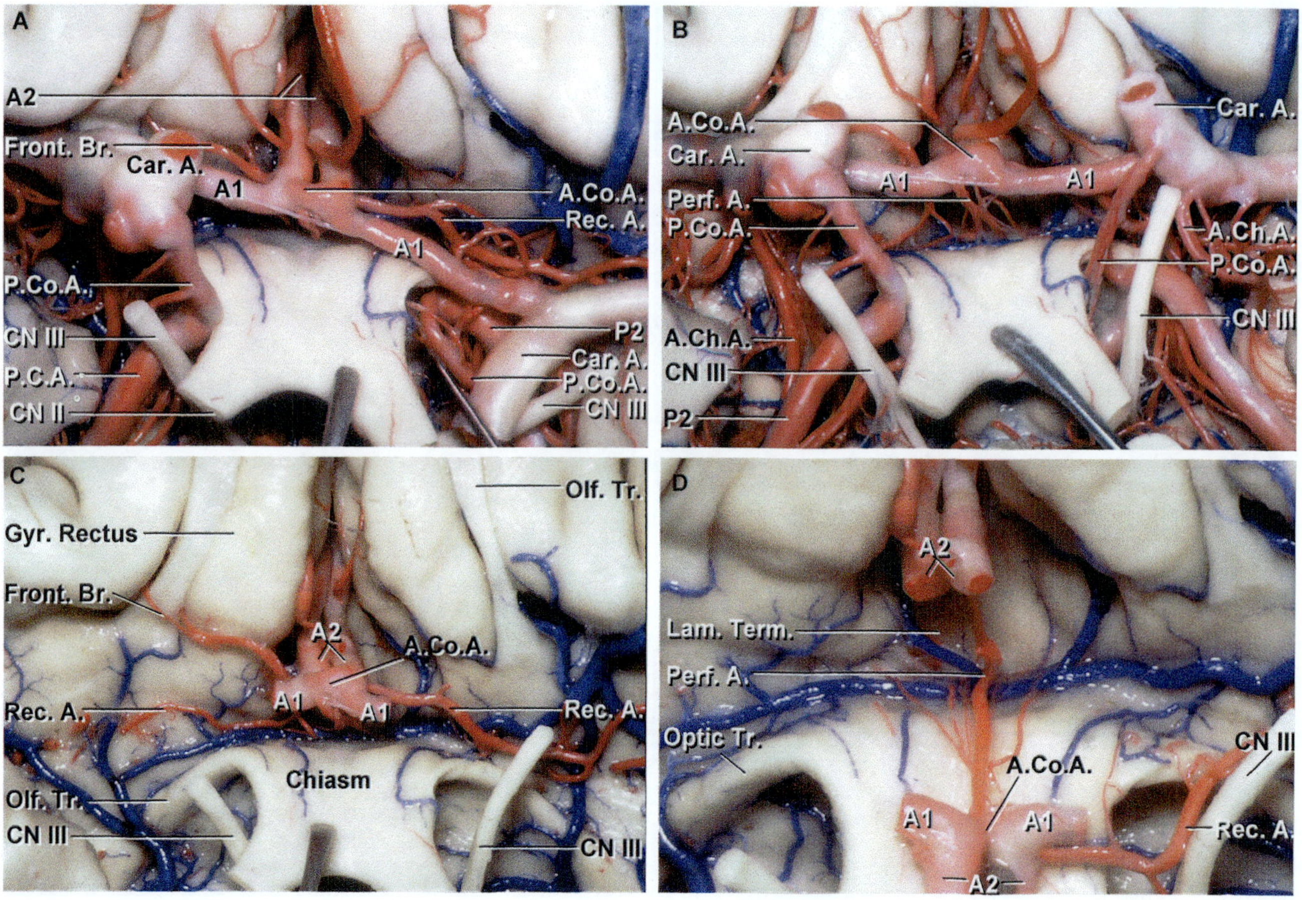

FIGURE 2.16. *Perforating branches of the anterior part of the circle of Willis.* A, *the A1, A2, and AComA are exposed above the optic chiasm. The left recurrent arteries arise from the ACA at the level of the AComA and travel laterally above the carotid bifurcation and below the anterior perforated substance. A small frontal branch arises at the same level on the right side. The stump of the right carotid artery has been folded upward and the left downward.* B, *the chiasm has been reflected downward and the ACA gently elevated to expose the perforating branches that arise from the AComA and pass backward to enter the diencephalon through the region of the lamina terminalis. The AChAs pass around the medial aspect of the uncus.* C, *the A1s have been removed to expose the recurrent arteries passing laterally below the anterior perorated substance. The left recurrent artery is larger than the right.* D, *the anterior communicating complex has been folded downward to expose the perforating branches that pass upward and enter the brain through the region of the lamina terminalis.*

required for long-term anastomosis patency. Chater et al. (3) found a cortical artery with a diameter of more than 1.4 mm in the angular zone in 100% of hemispheres. The arteries over the tip of the temporal lobe and the frontal lobe were considerably smaller. In the temporal zone, an artery with a diameter of more than 1.0 mm was present in 70% of hemispheres, and in the frontal zone, an arterial diameter of more than 1.0 mm was present in only 52%. These authors also noted that the vessels in the region of the angular gyrus had the advantage of being located so as to be accessible for anastomosis not only with the superficial temporal artery, but also with the occipital artery. They recommended that the craniotomy for exposing the cortical branches of the MCA be 4 cm in diameter, and that it be centered 6 cm above the external auditory canal.

Discussion

Occlusion of the individual cortical branches of the MCA, depending on the area supplied, may cause the following deficits: motor weakness caused by involvement of the corticospinal tract in the central gyrus; sucking and grasping reflex caused by involvement of the premotor area; motor aphasia resulting from involvement of the posteroinferior surface of the frontal cortex of the dominant hemisphere; changes in mentation and personality caused by involvement of the prefrontal area; visual field defects caused by a disturbance of the geniculocalcarine tract in the temporal, parietal, and occipital lobes; impairment of discriminative sensations and neglect of space and body parts resulting from involvement of the parietal lobes; finger agnosia, right-left disorientation, acalculia, and agraphia (Gerstmann's syndrome) caused by involvement of the functional area between the parietal and occipital lobes of the dominant hemisphere; or a receptive aphasia caused by disturbance of the dominant temporoparietal area.

Reports of specific clinical syndromes associated with occlusion of the individual cortical branches are rare. Occlusions of the individual cortical arteries are difficult to identify on angiograms, but, when detectable, they frequently correlate well with the

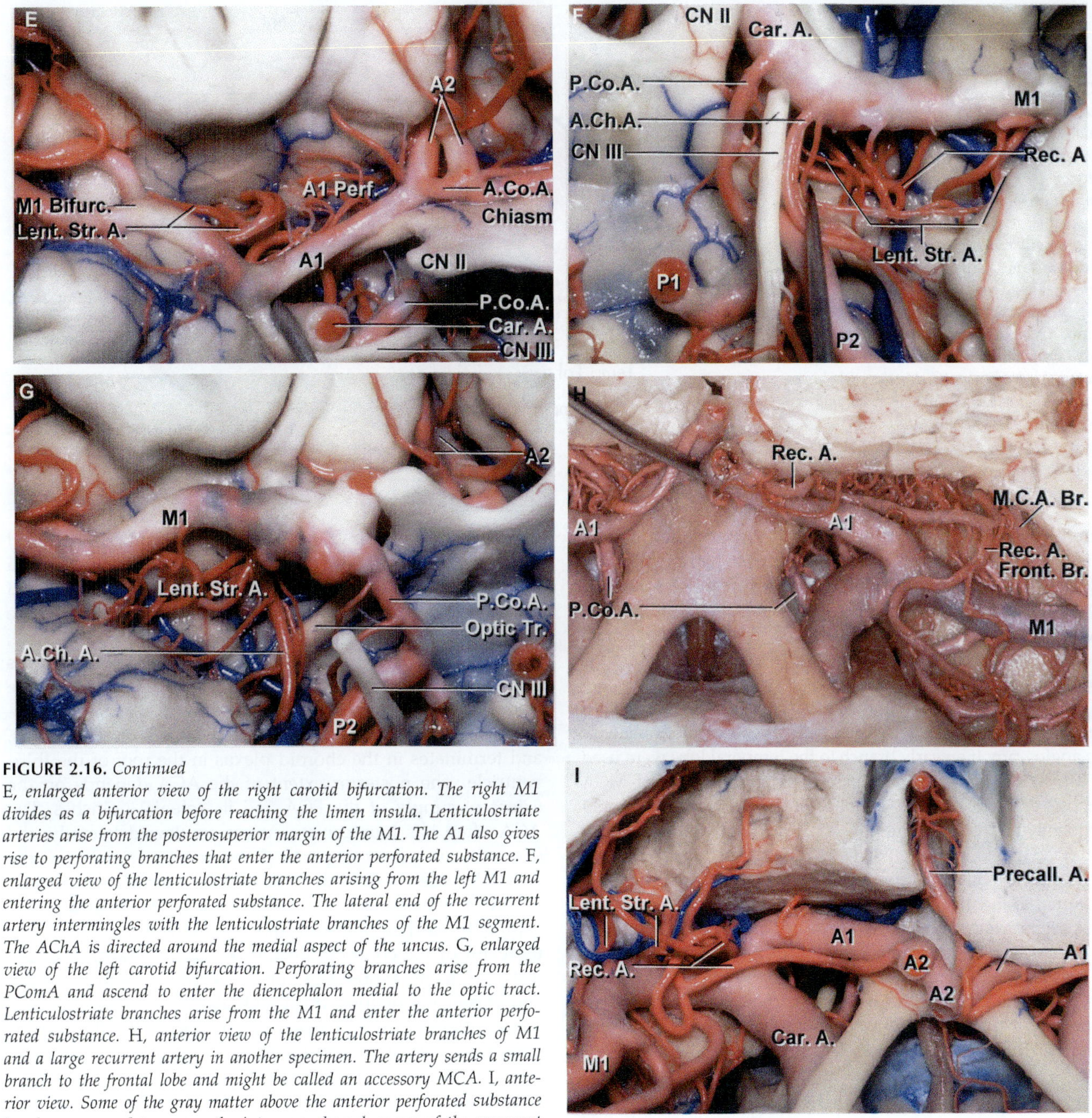

FIGURE 2.16. *Continued*
E, *enlarged anterior view of the right carotid bifurcation. The right M1 divides as a bifurcation before reaching the limen insula. Lenticulostriate arteries arise from the posterosuperior margin of the M1. The A1 also gives rise to perforating branches that enter the anterior perforated substance.* F, *enlarged view of the lenticulostriate branches arising from the left M1 and entering the anterior perforated substance. The lateral end of the recurrent artery intermingles with the lenticulostriate branches of the M1 segment. The AChA is directed around the medial aspect of the uncus.* G, *enlarged view of the left carotid bifurcation. Perforating branches arise from the PComA and ascend to enter the diencephalon medial to the optic tract. Lenticulostriate branches arise from the M1 and enter the anterior perforated substance.* H, *anterior view of the lenticulostriate branches of M1 and a large recurrent artery in another specimen. The artery sends a small branch to the frontal lobe and might be called an accessory MCA.* I, *anterior view. Some of the gray matter above the anterior perforated substance has been removed to expose the intraparenchymal course of the recurrent and lenticulostriate arteries.* A., *arteries, artery;* A.Ch.A., *anterior choroidal artery;* Bifurc., *bifurcation;* Br., *branch;* Car., *carotid;* CN, *cranial nerve;* Front., *frontal;* Gyr., *gyrus;* Lam., *lamina;* Lent. Str., *lenticulostriate;* M.C.A., *middle cerebral artery;* Olf., *olfactory;* P.C.A., *posterior cerebral artery;* P.Co.A., *posterior communicating artery;* Perf., *perforating;* Precall., *precallosal;* Rec., *recurrent;* Term., *terminalis;* Tr., *tract.*

neurological deficit (42). Embolism is a more frequent cause of occlusion of the MCA than thrombosis. In series of angiographically and autopsy-proven occlusions of the branches and trunks of the MCA, the ratio of embolic to thrombotic occlusions is approximately 13:1 to 16:1 (10).

Fisher (10) described the syndromes of obstructing the superior and inferior trunk of the MCA as follows: obstruction of the superior trunk causes a sensory-motor hemiplegia without receptive aphasia in the dominant hemisphere; obstruction of the inferior division causes a receptive aphasia in the absence of hemiplegia in the dominant side. Fisher's syndromes would apply if the trunks were nearly equal in size, with the superior trunk supplying the frontal and parietal regions and the inferior trunk supplying the temporal and occipital lobes. However, we

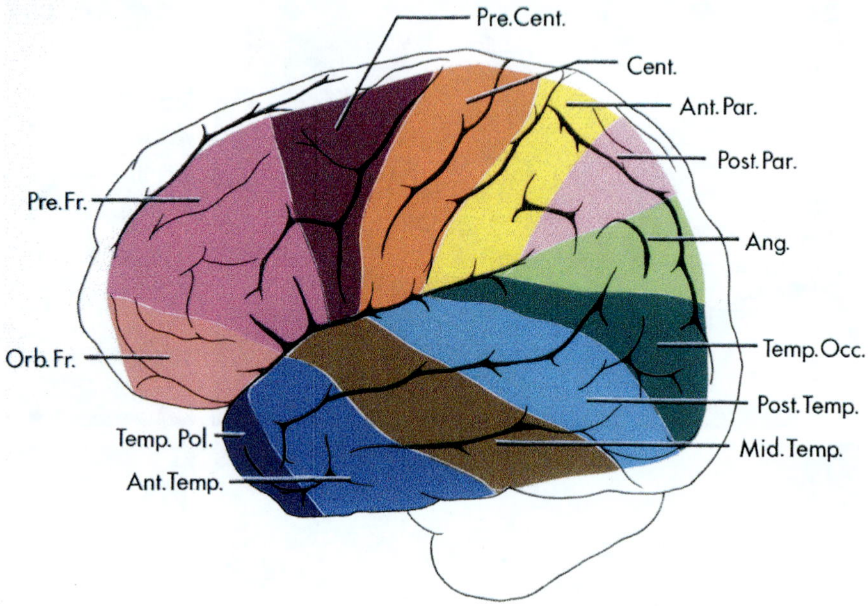

FIGURE 2.17. *Classification of the cortical areas used in this study The territory of the middle cerebral artery is divided into 12 areas: orbitofrontal, prefrontal, precentral, central, anterior parietal, posterior parietal, angular, temporo-occipital, posterior temporal, middle temporal, anterior temporal, and temporopolar.* Ang., *angular;* Ant., *anterior;* Cent., *central;* Mid., *middle;* Orb.Fr., *orbitofrontal;* Par., *parietal;* Post., *posterior;* Pre.Cent., *precentral;* Pre.Fr., *prefrontal;* Temp., *temporal;* Temp. Occ., *temporo-occipital;* Temp. Pol., *temporopolar.* (From, *Gibo H, Carver CC, Rhoton AL Jr, Lenkey C, Mitchell RJ: Microsurgical anatomy of the middle cerebral artery. J* **Neurosurg** *54:151–169, 1981 [14].)*

found marked variation in the size of the superior and inferior trunks and the area that they supply. In a few hemispheres, the inferior trunk supplied the temporal and parietal lobes and extended forward onto the precentral motor area, and, in another group of hemispheres, a large superior trunk supplied the frontal and parietal lobes and extended onto the speech centers on the posterior part of the temporal lobe.

The site of an MCA anastomosis for an MCA branch, trunk, or stem occlusion should be selected only after a careful review of the angiogram. If an early branch to the temporal lobe were used as a recipient vessel for a bypass operation, in cases of MCA stenosis or occlusion near the bifurcation, the new flow would frequently be channeled into the MCA proximal to the occlusion and none would have been delivered into the hypoperfused area distal to the occlusion. Some early branches, although arising proximal to the carotid bifurcation, may reach as far distally as the posterior temporal area. If one trunk of the MCA is stenotic or obstructed, an anastomosis to the other trunk will deliver blood to the proximal MCA and distally into the normal rather than into the ischemic area. Most surgeons use the angular, temporo-occipital, or posterior temporal branch of the MCA for a bypass, the three largest branches in this study (30).

ANTERIOR CEREBRAL ARTERY

The ACA, the smaller of the two terminal branches of the internal carotid artery, arises at the medial end of the sylvian fissure, lateral to the optic chiasm and below the anterior perforated substance (*Figs. 2.1* and *2.3*). It courses anteromedially above the optic nerve or chiasm and below the medial olfactory striate to enter the interhemispheric fissure. Near its entrance into the fissure, it is joined to the opposite ACA by the AComA, and ascends in front of the lamina terminalis to pass into the longitudinal fissure between the cerebral hemispheres.

The arteries from each side are typically not side by side as they enter the interhemispheric fissure and ascend in front of the lamina terminalis (*Figs. 2.1* and *2.21*). Rather, one distal ACA lies in the concavity of the other. Above the lamina terminalis, the arteries make a smooth curve around the genu of the corpus callosum and then pass backward above the corpus callosum in the pericallosal cistern. In their midcourse, one or both ACAs frequently turns away from the corpus callosum only to dip sharply back toward it. After giving rise to the cortical branches, the ACA continues around the splenium of the corpus callosum as a fine vessel, often tortuous, and terminates in the choroid plexus in the roof of the third ventricle. The posterior extent of the ACA depends on the extent of supply of the PCA and its splenial branches. The ACA often has four convex curves as viewed laterally: the convexity is posterosuperior between its origin and the AComA, anteroventral as it turns into the interhemispheric fissure, posterosuperior at the junction of the rostrum and genu of the corpus callosum, and anterior as it courses around the genu of the corpus callosum (*Fig. 2.22*). Branches of the distal ACA are exposed in surgical approaches to the sellar and chiasmatic regions, third and lateral ventricles, falx and parasagittal areas, and even in approaches to the medial parieto-occipital and pineal regions.

Segments

The ACA is divided at the AComA into two parts, proximal (precommunicating) and distal (post-communicating) (*Fig. 2.22*). The proximal part, extending from the origin to the AComA, constitutes the A1 segment. The distal part is formed by the A2 (infracallosal), A3 (precallosal), A4 (supracallosal), and A5 (posterocallosal) segments. The relationships of the four distal segments are reviewed below, under Distal Part.

A1 Segment and the Anterior Communicating Arteries

The A1 courses above the optic chiasm or nerves to join the AComA. The junction of the AComA with the right and left

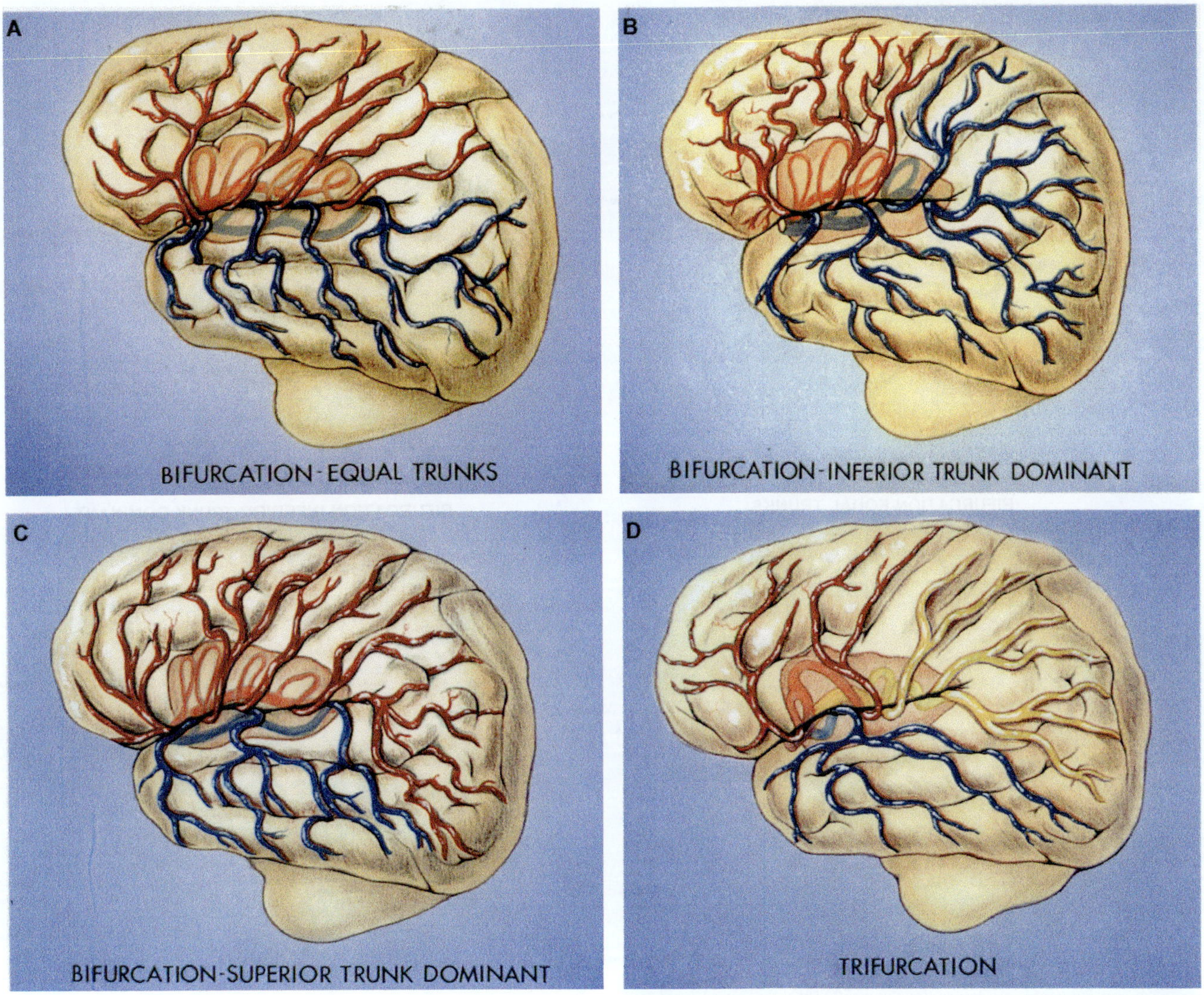

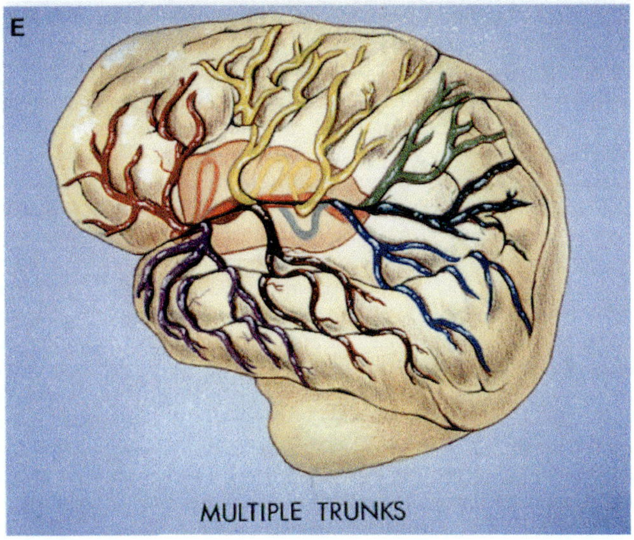

FIGURE 2.18. *Branching patterns of the middle cerebral artery. The main trunk divides in a bifurcation in 78% of hemispheres and in a trifurcation in 12%. In the remaining 10%, the main trunk divides into multiple (four or more) branches. A, bifurcation: equal trunk pattern (18% of hemispheres). The main trunk divides into superior* (red) *and inferior* (blue) *trunks that are of approximately the same diameter and supply cortical areas of similar size. The superior trunk supplies the frontal and parietal areas and the inferior trunk supplies the temporal and temporo-occipital areas. B, bifurcation: inferior trunk dominant (32% of hemispheres). The inferior trunk* (blue) *has a larger diameter and area of supply than the superior trunk* (red). *The inferior trunk supplies the temporal, occipital, and parietal areas, and the superior trunk supplies the frontal areas. C, bifurcation: superior trunk dominant (28% of hemispheres). The superior trunk* (red) *has the largest diameter and area of supply; it supplies the frontal, parietal, temporo-occipital, and posterior temporal areas, and the smaller inferior trunk* (blue) *supplies the temporopolar through the middle temporal areas. D, trifurcation pattern (12% of hemispheres). The main trunk of the middle cerebral artery divides into three trunks. The superior trunk* (red) *supplies the frontal areas, the middle trunk* (yellow) *supplies the areas around the posterior end of the sylvian fissure, and the inferior trunk* (blue) *supplies the temporal areas. E, multiple trunks (10% of hemispheres). The main trunk gives rise to multiple smaller trunks. Two trunks supply the frontal areas* (red and yellow), *two supply the parietal areas* (light green and dark green), *and three supply the temporal and occipital areas* (purple, brown, and blue). (From, *Gibo H, Carver CC, Rhoton AL Jr, Lenkey C, Mitchell RJ: Microsurgical anatomy of the middle cerebral artery.* ***J Neurosurg*** *54:151–169, 1981 [14].)*

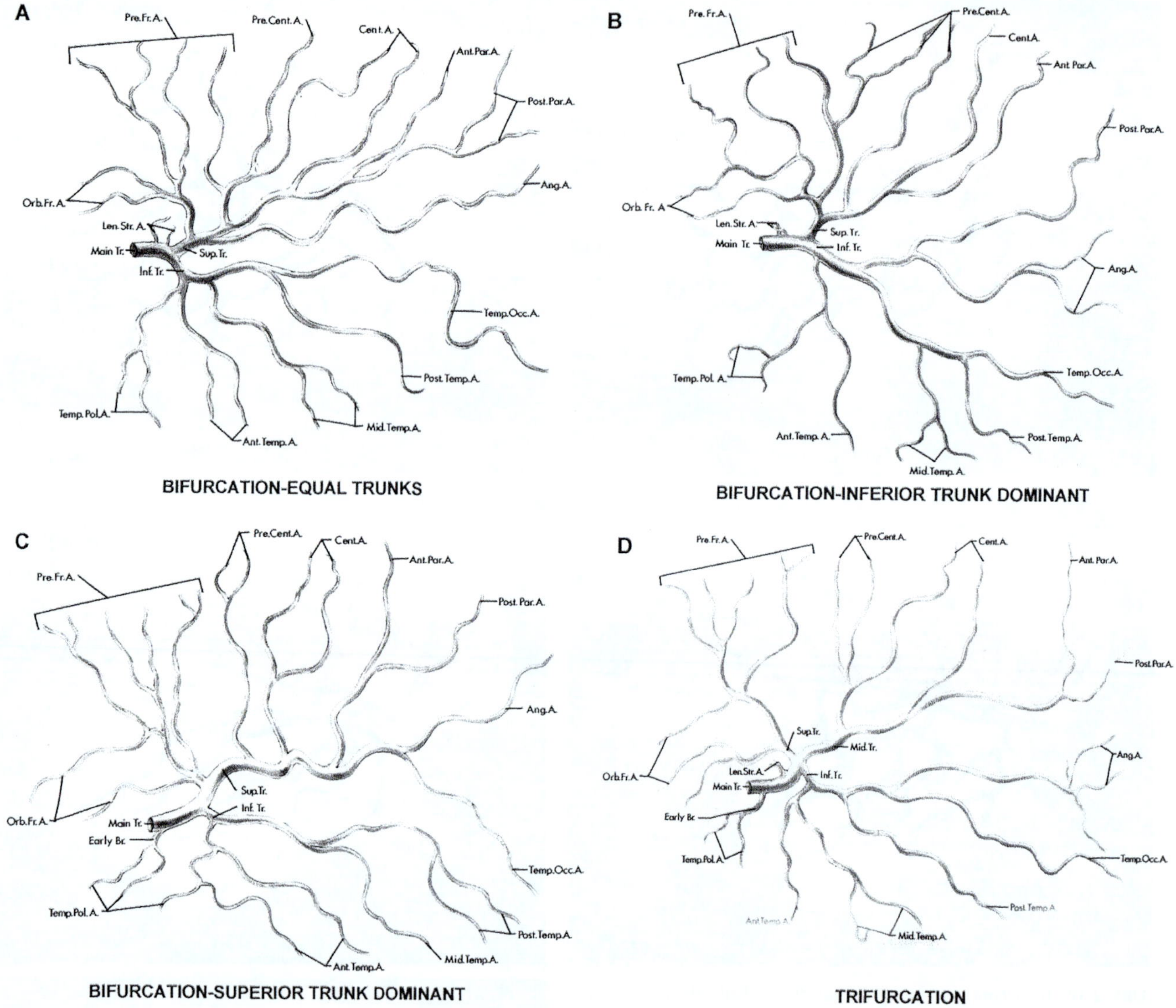

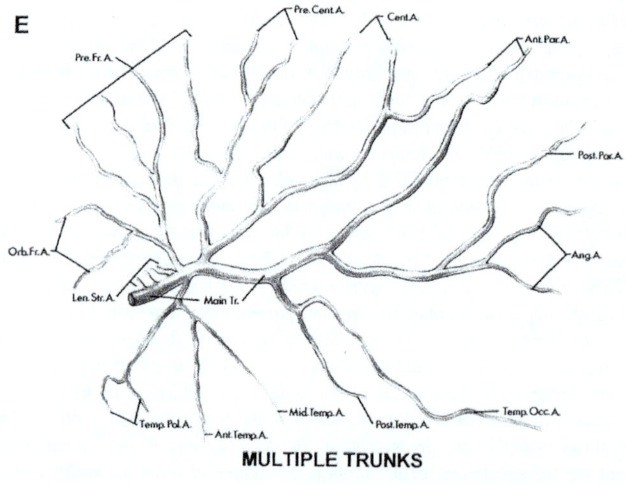

FIGURE 2.19. *Branching patterns of the middle cerebral artery. These drawings of MCAs dissected from five cerebral hemispheres show the different branching patterns of the main trunk. The main trunk divides in a bifurcation in 78% of hemispheres, in a trifurcation in 12%, and in a multiple branch pattern (four or more trunks) in 10%. The drawings show the main, superior, middle, and inferior trunks. These trunks give rise to the lenticulostriate, orbitofrontal, prefrontal, precentral, central, anterior parietal, posterior parietal, angular, temporo-occipital, posterior temporal, middle temporal, anterior temporal, and temporopolar arteries.* A, *bifurcation: equal trunks (18% of hemispheres). The main trunk divides into superior and inferior trunks that are of approximately the same diameter and supply cortical areas of similar size. The superior trunk gives rise to the orbitofrontal arteries through the angular arteries, and the inferior trunk gives rise to the temporopolar through the temporo-occipital arteries.* B, *bifurcation: inferior trunk dominant (32% of hemispheres). The inferior trunk has a larger diameter and area of supply than the superior trunk. The superior trunk supplies the orbitofrontal through the anterior parietal areas, and the inferior trunk supplies the posterior parietal through the temporopolar areas.* C, *bifurcation: superior trunk dominant (28% of hemispheres). The superior trunk has a larger diameter and area of supply than the inferior trunk. It supplies the orbitofrontal through the temporo-occipital areas, and the inferior trunk supplies the temporal areas except for the temporopolar area, which is supplied by an early branch* (Early Br.) *that arises from the main trunk.* D, *trifurcation pattern (12% of hemispheres). The main trunk of the MCA divides into three trunks. The superior trunk supplies the orbitofrontal and prefrontal areas, the middle trunk supplies the precentral through the posterior parietal areas,*

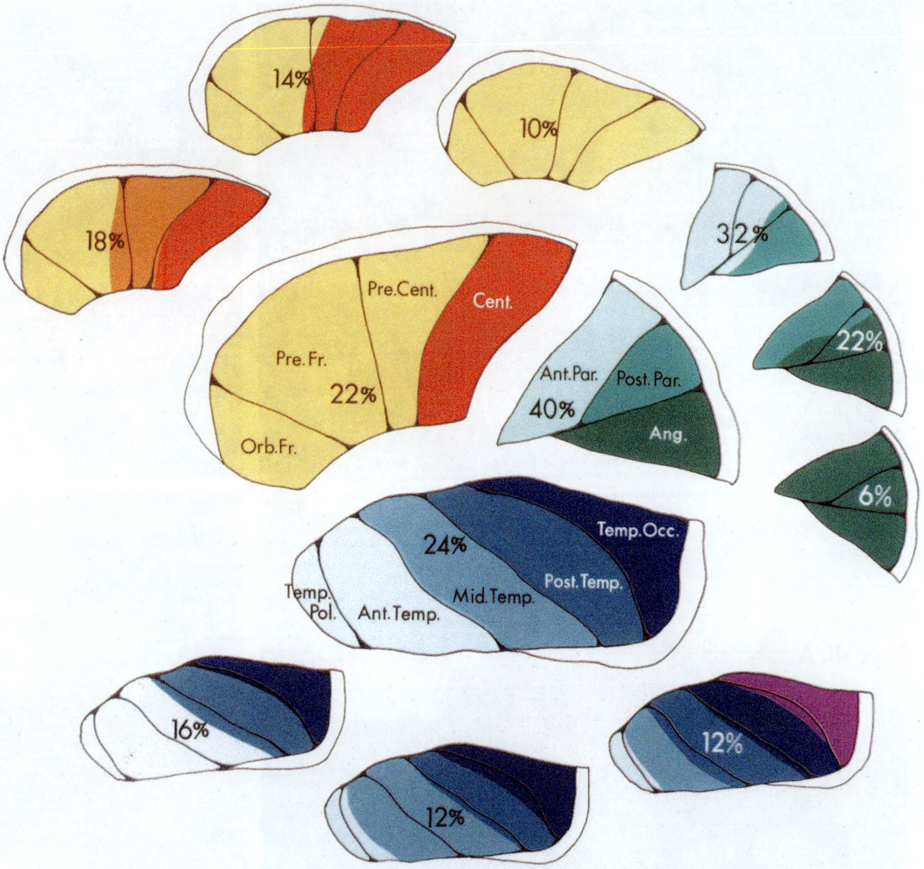

FIGURE 2.20. *Stem artery patterns. The stem arteries arise from the trunks and give rise to the cortical arteries. The central illustration shows the lateral surface of a left cerebral hemisphere with a space between the frontal, parietal, and temporal areas. The frontal lobe is formed by the orbitofrontal, prefrontal, precentral, and the central areas; the parietal lobe is composed of the anterior parietal, posterior parietal, and angular areas; the temporal and occipital lobes are formed by the temporopolar, anterior temporal, middle temporal, posterior temporal, and temporo-occipital areas. The posterior part of the central area, which is actually part of the parietal lobe, is included with the frontal lobe. The central diagram shows the most common stem pattern, and the peripheral diagrams show the next three most common patterns. Each color or shade of a color shows the area supplied by one stem artery. The percentage of hemispheres having the stem pattern shown is listed on each diagram. The most common frontal lobe pattern involves two stem arteries: one gives rise to the branches to the orbitofrontal, prefrontal, and precentral areas, and the other supplies the central area. The most common parietal lobe pattern involves three stem arteries, one each for the anterior and posterior parietal and the angular areas. The most common temporal and occipital lobe pattern involves four stem arteries: one stem artery supplies both the temporopolar and the anterior temporal areas, and there is one stem each for the middle temporal, posterior temporal, and temporo-occipital areas. The next three most common stem patterns for each lobe are shown on the peripheral diagrams. The four patterns shown for each lobe do not account for 100% of the hemispheres, but show only the four most common patterns for that lobe.* Ang., *angular;* Ant., *anterior;* Cent., *central;* Mid., *middle;* Orb. Fr., *orbitofrontal;* Par., *parietal;* Post., *posterior;* Pre. Cent., *precentral;* Pre. Fr., *prefrontal;* Temp., *temporal;* Temp. Occ., *temporo-occipital;* Temp. Pol., *temporopolar.* (From, *Gibo H, Carver CC, Rhoton AL Jr, Lenkey C, Mitchell RJ: Microsurgical anatomy of the middle cerebral artery.* ***J Neurosurg*** *54:151–169, 1981 [14].)*

A1 is usually above the chiasm (70% of brains) rather than above the optic nerves (30%) (*Figs.* 2.23 and 2.24) (26). Of those passing above the optic nerves, most journey above the nerve near the chiasm rather than distally. The shorter A1s are stretched tightly over the chiasm; the longer ones travel anteriorly over the optic nerves. The arteries with a more forward course are often tortuous and elongated, with some resting on the tuberculum sellae or planum sphenoidale. The A1 varies in length from 7.2 to 18.0 mm (average, 12.7 mm) (26). The length of the AComA is usually between 2 and 3 mm, but may vary from 0.3 to 7.0 mm (26). The longer AComAs are commonly curved, kinked, or tortuous.

A normal ACA-AComA complex is one in which an AComA connects A1s of nearly equal size, and both A1s and the AComA are of sufficient size to allow circulation between the two carotid arteries and through the anterior circle of Willis. The AComA diameter averages approximately 1 mm less than the average diameter of the A1. The AComA diameters are the same or larger than their smaller A1 in only 25% of the brains (26). Ten percent of the brains have an A1 of 1.5 mm or less in diameter and only 2% have an A1 with a diameter of 1.0 mm or less. The diameter of the AComA was 1.5 mm or smaller in 44% of brains and 1.0 mm or smaller in 16%.

and the inferior trunk supplies the angular through the anterior temporal areas. The temporopolar artery arises from the main trunk as an early branch. E, multiple trunks (10% of hemispheres). The main trunk gives rise to more than three trunks. There are five trunks in the specimen shown. A., arteries, artery; Ang., *angular;* Ant., *anterior;* Br., *branch;* Cent., *central;* Inf., *inferior;* Len. Str., *lenticulostriate;* Mid., *middle;* Orb.Fr., *orbitofrontal;* Par., *parietal;* Post., *posterior;* Pre. Cent., *precentral;* Pre. Fr., *prefrontal;* Sup., *superior;* Temp., *temporal;* Temp.Occ., *temporo-occipital;* Temp.Pol., *temporopolar;* Tr., *trunk.* (From, *Gibo H, Carver CC, Rhoton AL Jr, Lenkey C, Mitchell RJ: Microsurgical anatomy of the middle cerebral artery.* ***J Neurosurg*** *54:151–169, 1981 [14].)*

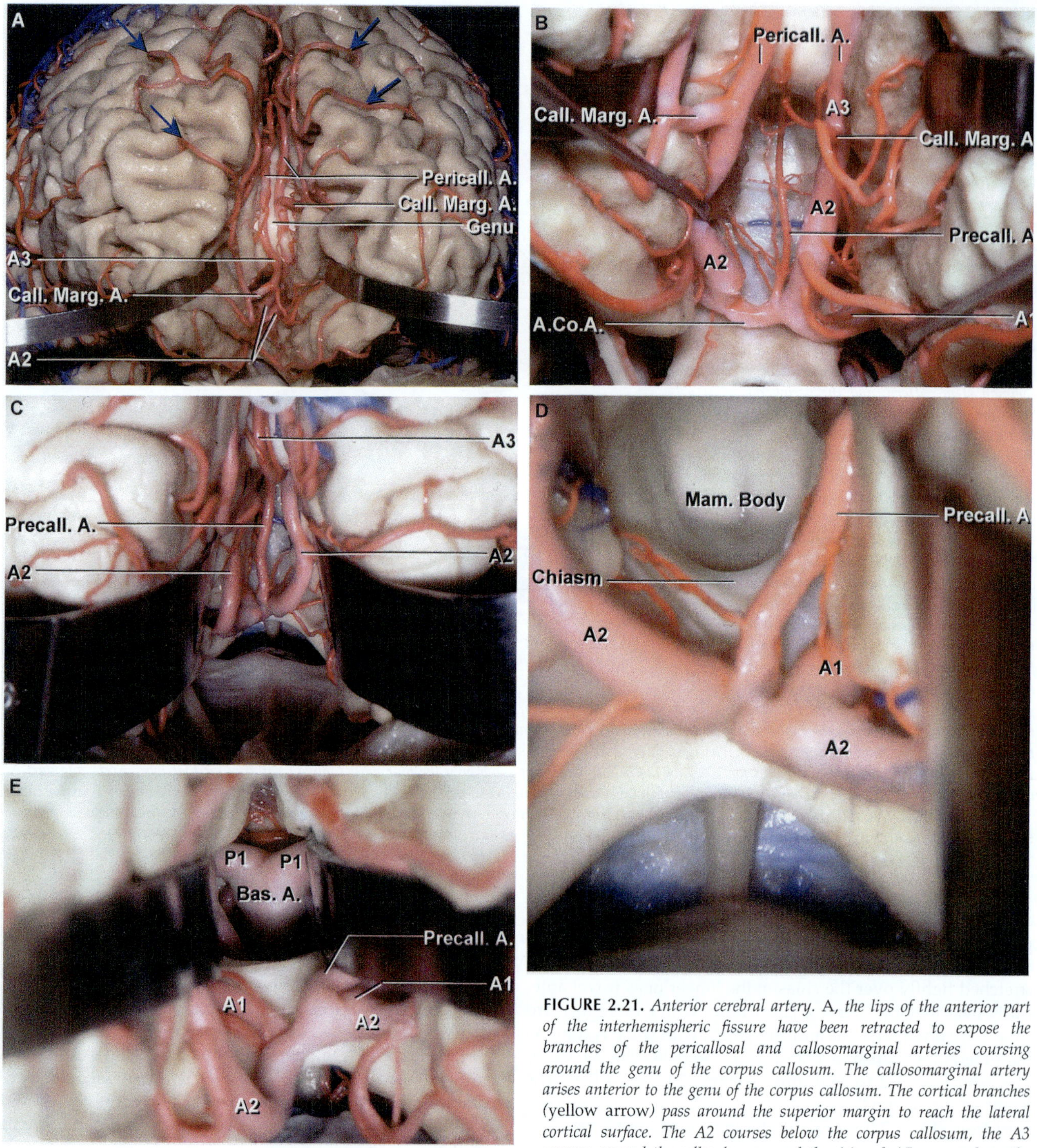

FIGURE 2.21. *Anterior cerebral artery.* A, *the lips of the anterior part of the interhemispheric fissure have been retracted to expose the branches of the pericallosal and callosomarginal arteries coursing around the genu of the corpus callosum. The callosomarginal artery arises anterior to the genu of the corpus callosum. The cortical branches* (yellow arrow) *pass around the superior margin to reach the lateral cortical surface. The A2 courses below the corpus callosum, the A3 courses around the callosal genu, and the A4 and A5 course above the corpus callosum.* B, *enlarged view. A precallosal artery arises from the AComA adjacent to the left ACA and passes upward in front of the lamina terminalis and rostrum of the corpus callosum, sending branches to the diencephalon and corpus callosum along its course.* C, *another specimen. The lips of the interhemispheric fissure have been retracted to expose a large precallosal artery that ascends around the genu to reach the upper callosal surface.* D, *the large precallosal artery has been retracted to the left and the lamina terminalis opened to expose the mamillary bodies in the floor of the third ventricle.* E, *the floor of the third ventricle has been opened to expose the apex of the basilar artery and origin of the P1s in the interpeduncular cistern at the posterior margin of the circle of Willis.* A., *artery;* A.Co.A., *anterior communicating artery;* Bas., *basilar;* Call. Marg., *callosomarginal;* Mam., *mamillary;* Pericall., *pericallosal;* Precall., *precallosal.*

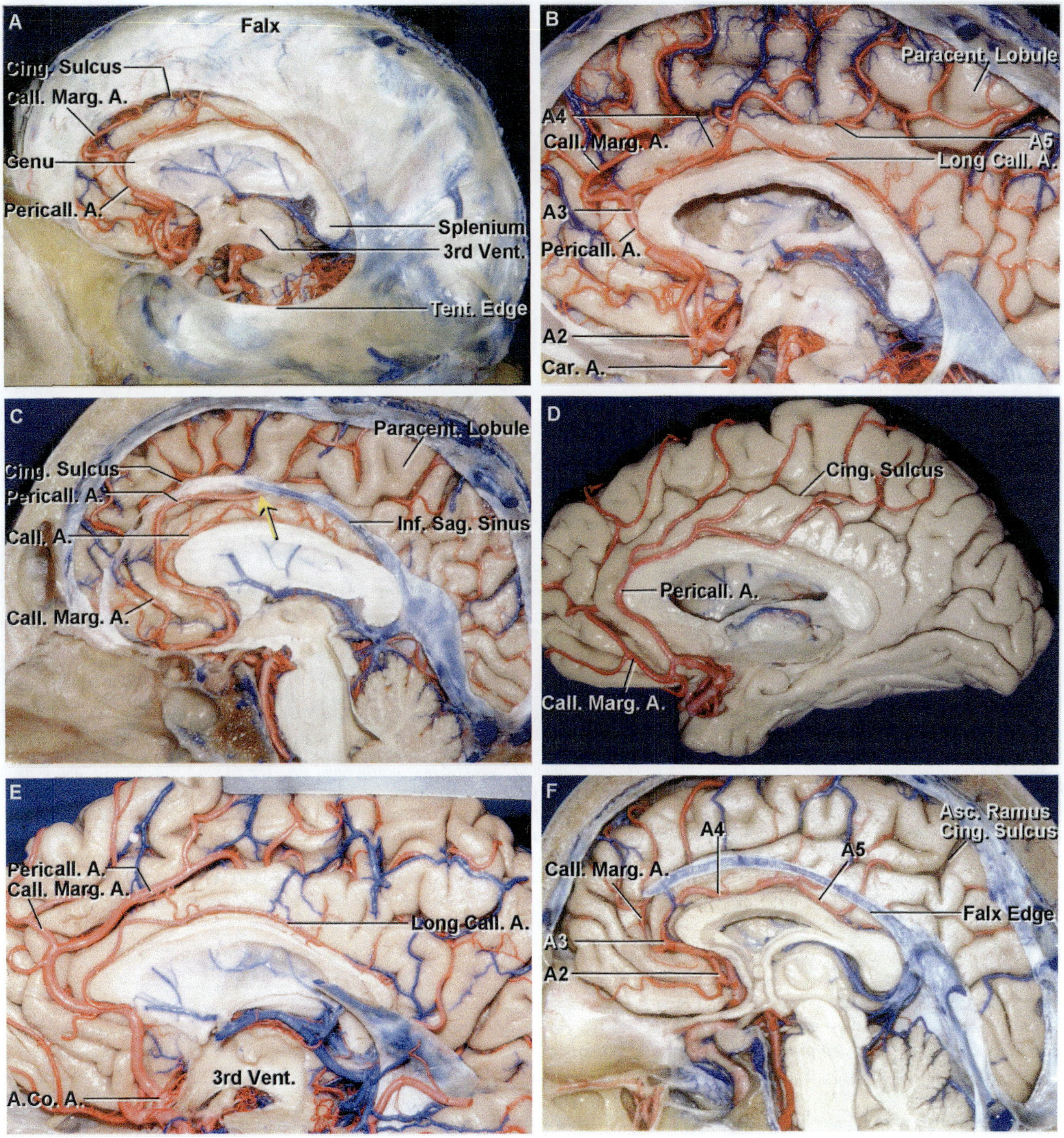

FIGURE 2.22. *Variations in the origin of the callosomarginal artery from the pericallosal artery. The pericallosal artery is defined as arising at the AComA and the callosomarginal is defined as the branch arising from the pericallosal to course along the cingulate sulcus and supply two or more cortical areas. The callosomarginal artery can arise from the pericallosal artery just distal to the AComA or at any site along the course of the pericallosal artery.* A *and* B *show the most common variation in which the callosomarginal artery arises as the pericallosal artery courses around the genu of the corpus callosum.* A, *the callosomarginal artery arises anterior to the genu of the corpus callosum. The distal part of the ACA, the part beginning at the AComA, is divided into four segments: The A2 extends from the AComA to the lower margin of the corpus callosum; the A3 courses around the anterior part of the corpus callosum; the A4 and A5 course above the anterior and posterior half of the corpus callosum, respectively. The anterior part of the falx cerebri is more widely separated from the corpus callosum than the posterior part. The inner edge of the anterior part of the falx is widely separated from the anterior part of the corpus callosum, but the space between the falx and callosal surface narrows as it proceeds posteriorly so that the posterior falx tightly hugs the splenium. The wide opening anteriorly between the falx and the corpus callosum permits the anterior part of the hemisphere and the more forward branches of the ACA to exhibit greater shift anteriorly than posteriorly.* B, *the falx has been removed. The distal* (Legend continues on next page.)

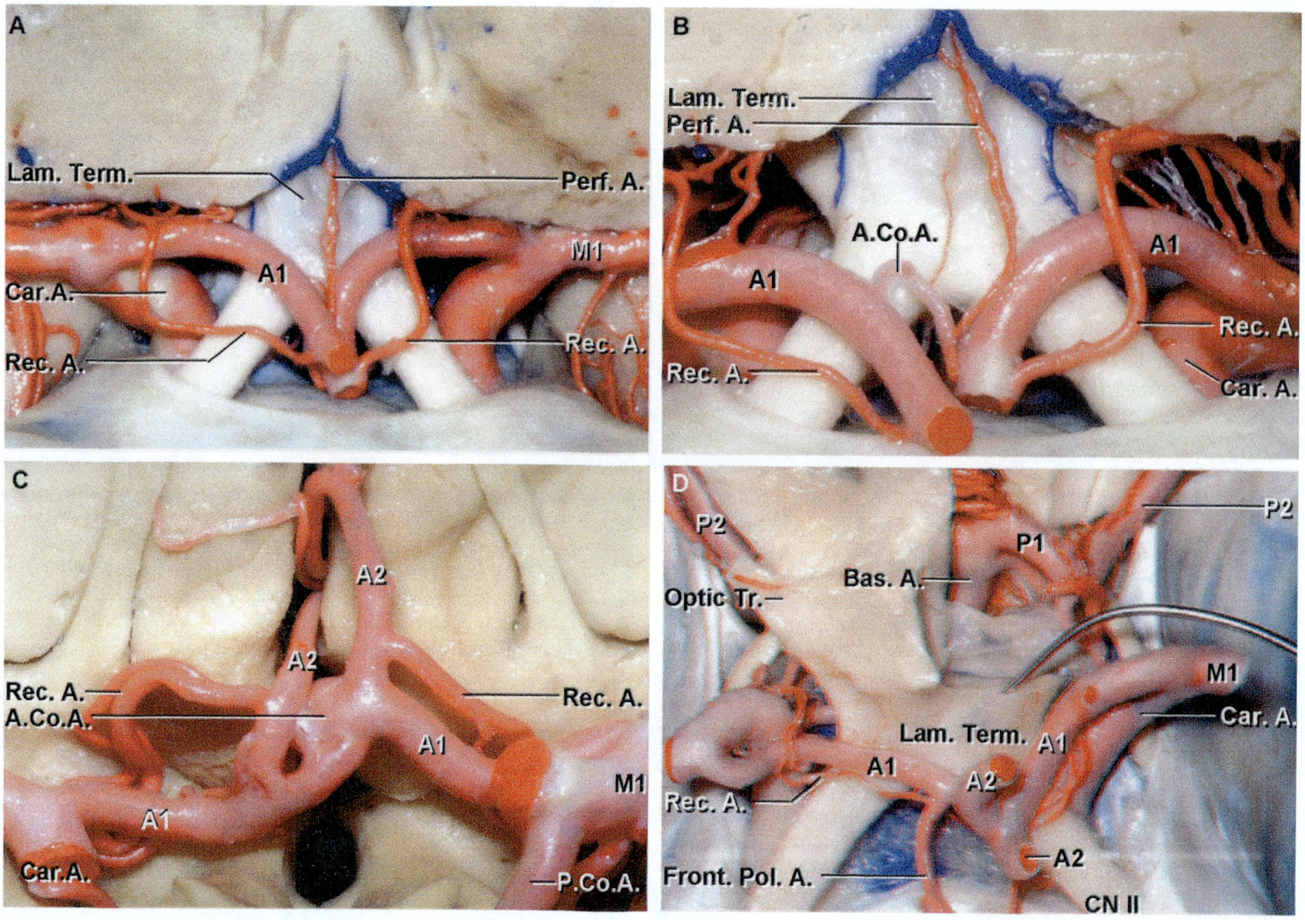

FIGURE 2.23. *Variations in the anterior part of the circle of Willis. A, anterior view of A1s of nearly equal size. The AComA is hypoplastic and is hidden between the ACAs. Recurrent arteries arise from the A2s at the same level on both sides. B, the A2s have been separated to expose the AComA, which is the site of a perforating branch that enters the brain through the region of the lamina terminalis. C, the A1s are of equal size and give rise to A2s of approximately the same size. The AComA is broad and somewhat dimpled and is expanding behind the right A2 in what may be the beginning of an aneurysm. Both recurrent arteries arise from the proximal A2. D, the left A1 is larger than the right A1. The right recurrent artery arises from a frontopolar artery and passes laterally toward the carotid bifurcation. The AComA is of approximately the same diameter as the left A1 and is the predominant source of flow to both A2s. The floor of the third ventricle has been opened to expose the basilar apex and the P1s. E, the left A1 gives rise to a frontopolar*

The A1 is the favorite site on the circle of Willis for hypoplasia. A1 hypoplasia has a high rate of association with aneurysms; it is found with 85% of AComA aneurysms (*Figs.* 2.23 and 2.24) (38). It is the only anatomic variant that correlates with the location of cerebral aneurysm. The importance of this variant in aneurysm formation is reviewed in more detail in Chapter 3.

There is a direct correlation between the difference in size of the right and left A1s and the size of the AComA. As the difference in diameter between the A1s increases, so does the

FIGURE 2.22. *Continued*
ACA branches extend around the margins of the hemisphere to reach the orbital surface of the frontal lobe and the anterior twothirds of the lateral convexity. The distal part of the pericallosal artery ascends to course along the cingulate sulcus to reach the paracentral lobule. C, the callosomarginal artery arises just distal to the AComA in the cistern of the lamina terminalis and ascends along the cingulate sulcus. The narrow band of the inner edge of the falx that contains the inferior sagittal sinus has been preserved to show the relationship of the branches of the pericallosal artery. The yellow arrow *shows the site at which the ACA would show a sharp angulation when shifted to the opposite side by a mass lesion. A callosal artery arises just below the genu of the corpus callosum and crosses the upper callosal surface toward the splenium.* D, *the pericallosal artery arises in the subcallosal area several millimeters distal to the AComA and sends branches across the superior margin of the hemisphere to supply the adjacent part of the lateral convexity.* E, *the pericallosal artery turns anteriorly at the level of the lower margin of the genu of the corpus callosum and courses along the cingulate sulcus, where it gives rise to the callosomarginal artery. The pericallosal artery gives rise to a long callosal artery that courses posteriorly to reach the splenium. F, the callosomarginal artery arises at the level of the lower margin of the callosal genu. The distal segments (A2 to A5) are shown. The ascending ramus of the cingulate sulcus marks the posterior border of the paracentral lobule formed by the central and precentral sulci overlapping onto the medical surface.* A., *artery;* A.Co.A., *anterior communicating artery;* Asc., *ascending;* Call., *callosal;* Call. Marg., *callosomarginal;* Car., *carotid;* Cing., *cingulate;* Inf., *inferior;* Sag., *sagittal;* Paracent., *paracentral;* Pericall., *pericallosal;* Tent., *tentorial;* Vent., *ventricle.*

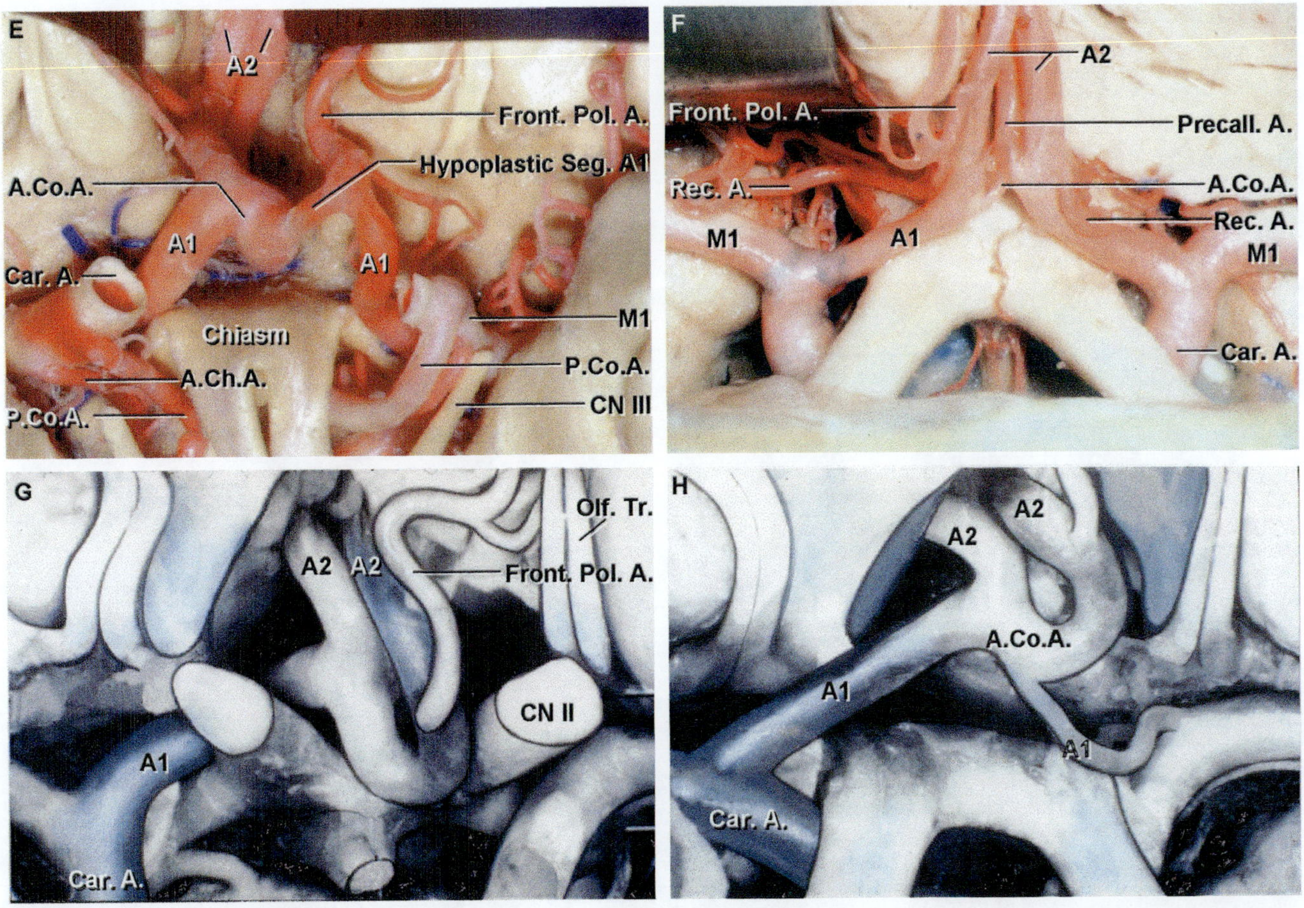

FIGURE 2.23. *Continued*
branch. The segment of the A1 between the origin of the frontopolar branch and the AComA is hypoplastic. The right A1 is dominant and provides the majority of the flow to both A2s. F, *anterior view. The left A1 is larger than the right. The AComA is short and small. A precallosal artery arises from the left A1-A2 junction near the AComA. The right recurrent artery arises from the frontopolar artery and passes laterally above the carotid bifurcation. The left recurrent artery arises at the level of the AComA.* G and H, *most common anatomic variant associated with an AComA aneurysm.* G, *the right A1 is dominant and gives rise to both A2s. The left A1 is hidden behind the optic nerve. The left A2 loops downward between the optic nerves.* H, *the anterior communicating complex has been elevated to show the hypoplastic left A1.* A., *artery;* A.Ch.A., *anterior choroidal artery;* Bas., *basilar;* Car., *carotid;* CN, *cranial nerve;* Front. Pol., *frontopolar;* Lam., *lamina;* Olf., *olfactory;* P.Co.A., *posterior communicating artery;* Perf., *perforating;* Precall., *precallosal;* Rec., *recurrent;* Seg., *segment;* Term., *terminalis;* Tr., *tract.*

size of the AComA. Thus, a large AComA is often associated with a significant difference in diameter between the right and left A1. This is understandable from a functional point of view because, with a small or hypoplastic A1, more collateral circulation flows across the AComA to make up the deficit. A difference in diameter of 0.5 mm or more between the right and left A1 is found in half of the brains and a difference of 1 mm or more in 12%. The average AComA diameter is 1.2 mm in the group of brains in which the difference in diameter between the right and left A1s is 0.5 mm or less and 2.5 mm if the difference is more than 0.5 mm. This correlation between the size of the A1s permits a rough estimate of the size of the AComA, even though the artery is not visualized, because it is the most difficult part of the circle of Willis to define on cerebral angiography.

Another difficulty in angiographically defining the AComA is that it is frequently not oriented in a strictly transverse plane. The length of the AComA is oriented in an oblique or straight anterior-posterior plane if one ACA passes between the hemispheres behind the other ACA. The ACAs are side by side as they pass between the cerebral hemispheres in approximately one in five hemispheres, and the left is anterior to the right more often than the right is anterior to the left. These variations may explain why angiography in the oblique position is often needed to define the AComA. The AComA usually has a round appearance, but it may seem flat because of a broad connection with both ACAs, or even triangular with a large base on one ACA and a threadlike connection on the other.

One AComA was present in 60%, two in 30%, and three in 10% of the brains we examined (*Fig. 2.24*) (26). Double AComAs can take a variety of forms; one is simply a hole in the middle of a broad or triangular artery separating arteries. The double or triple arteries can be approximately the same size or can vary markedly in diameter. A common pattern is for one to be large and the others relatively small. It is rare to find no

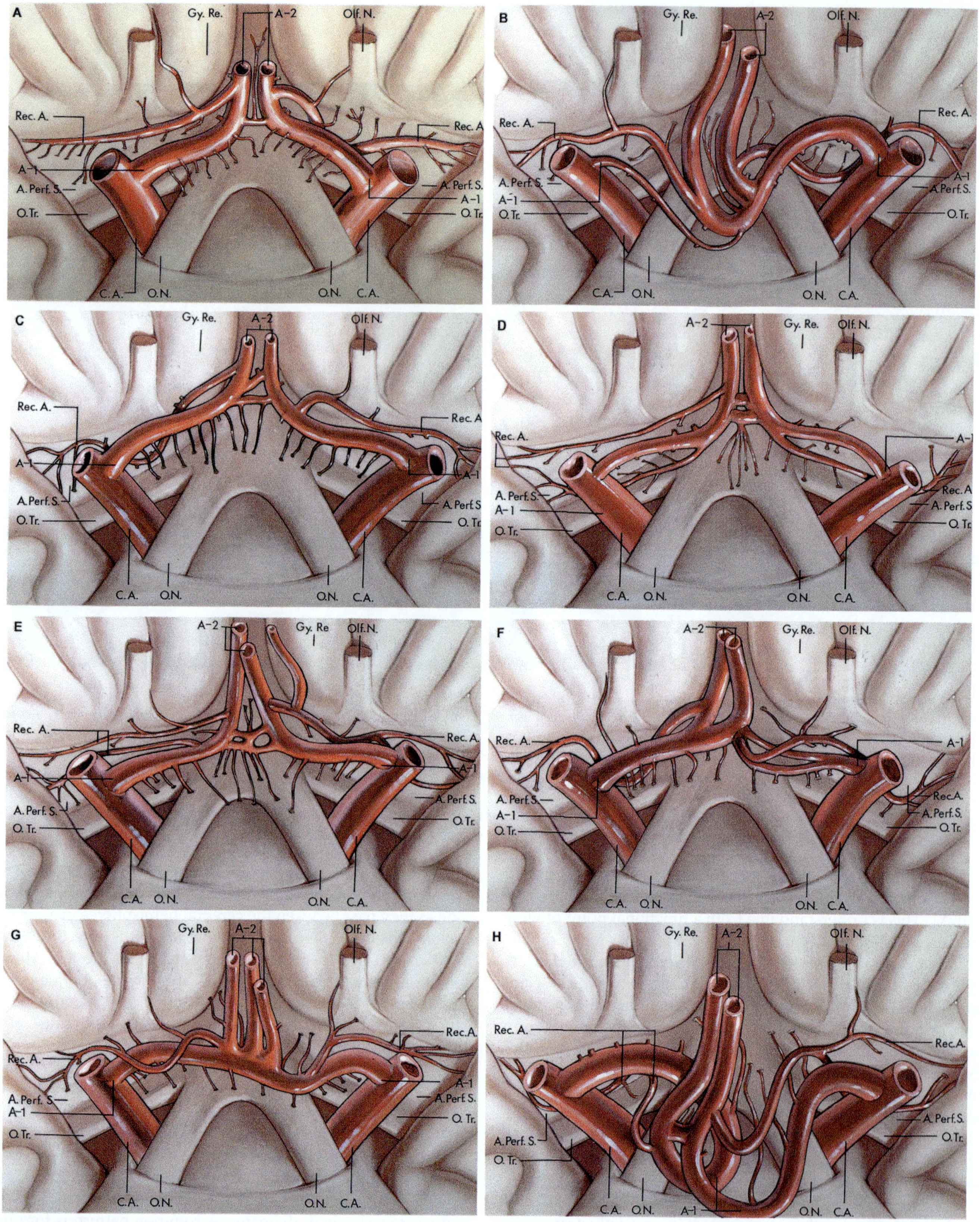
A
Gy. Re.
A-2
Olf. N.
Rec. A.
Rec. A
A-1
A. Perf. S.
O. Tr.
A. Perf. S.
A-1
O. Tr.
C.A.
O.N.
O.N.
C.A.
B
Gy. Re.
A-2
Olf. N.
Rec. A.
Rec. A.
A. Perf. S.
A-1
O. Tr.
A-1
A. Perf. S.
O. Tr.
C.A.
O.N.
O.N.
C.A.
C
Gy. Re.
A-2
Olf. N.
Rec. A.
Rec. A
A-1
A-1
A. Perf. S.
A. Perf. S
O. Tr.
O. Tr
C.A.
O.N.
O.N.
C.A.
D
A-2
Gy. Re.
Olf. N.
Rec. A.
A-1
Rec. A
A. Perf. S.
A. Perf. S
A-1
O. Tr.
O. Tr
C.A.
O.N.
O.N.
C.A.
E
A-2
Gy. Re
Olf. N.
Rec. A.
Rec. A.
A-1
A-1
A. Perf. S.
A. Perf. S.
O. Tr.
O. Tr.
C.A.
O.N.
O.N.
C.A.
F
A-2
Gy. Re.
Olf. N.
Rec. A.
A-1
A. Perf. S.
Rec. A.
A-1
A. Perf. S.
O. Tr.
O. Tr.
C.A.
O.N.
O.N.
C.A.
G
Gy. Re.
A-2
Olf. N.
Rec. A.
Rec. A.
A-1
A. Perf. S.
A. Perf. S.
A-1
O. Tr.
O. Tr.
C.A.
O.N.
O.N.
C.A.
H
Gy. Re.
A-2
Olf. N.
Rec. A.
Rec. A.
A. Perf. S.
O. Tr.
A. Perf. S.
O. Tr.
C.A.
O.N.
A-1
O.N.
C.A.

FIGURE 2.24.

connection between the two sides, but in some cases, the connection may be tiny—as small as 0.2 mm in diameter.

An infrequent finding is duplication of a portion of the A1. Another infrequent anomaly consists of a third or median ACA arising from the AComA. The median artery courses upward and backward above the corpus callosum. It frequently divides opposite the paracentral lobule and gives branches to the paracentral lobules of both sides. In such cases, the ACAs proper are usually small and supply the anteromedial surfaces of the hemispheres.

Recurrent Artery

The recurrent branch of the ACA, first described by Heubner in 1874, is unique among arteries in that it doubles back on its parent ACA and passes above the carotid bifurcation and MCA into the medial part of the sylvian fissure before entering the anterior perforated substance (*Figs. 2.16, 2.23,* and *2.24*) (18). It pursues a long, redundant path to the anterior perforated substance, sometimes looping forward on the gyrus rectus and inferior surface of the frontal lobe. In its journey to the anterior perforated substance, it is often closely applied to the superior or posterior aspect of the A1. It may seem, falsely, to be issuing from the A1 until further dissection clarifies its site of origin at the level of the AComA. The recurrent arteries arising proximally on the A1 follow a more direct path to the anterior perforated substance than those arising distally.

The recurrent branch is the largest artery arising from the A1 or the proximal 0.5 mm of the A2 in the majority of hemispheres (26). It may infrequently be absent on one side or arise as several branches. In our study, there was a single recurrent artery in 28% of the hemispheres, two in 48%, and three or four in 24% (26). If there were two or more recurrent arteries, both or at least one arose at the level of the junction of the A1 and A2 (36). Rarely does more than a single recurrent artery arise from the A1. If there are two recurrent arteries and one arises on the A1, the second usually arises at the junction of the A1 and A2. A large basal perforating artery may infrequently arise from the A1 between the AComA and the recurrent artery. The recurrent artery diameter is usually less than half that of the A1, but it may infrequently be as large as or exceed the A1 diameter if the A1 is hypoplastic.

The recurrent branch usually arises from the distal A1 or from the proximal part of the ACA segment just distal to the AComA, referred to as the A2; however, it may emerge at any point along the A1. It most commonly originates from the A2. In our study, it originated from the A2 in 78%, from the A1 in 14%, and at the A1–A2 junction at the level of the AComA in 8% (26). In 52%, it arose within 2 mm of the AComA, in 80% within 3 mm, and in 95% within 4 mm. The recurrent arteries arising near the AComA usually arise from the lateral side of the junction of the A1 and A2 at a right angle to the parent vessel. They may originate either in common with or give rise to the frontopolar artery.

Most recurrent arteries course anterior to the A1 and are seen on elevating the frontal lobe before visualizing the A1, but they may also course superior to the A1, between it and the anterior perforated substance, or may loop posterior to A1. It courses above the internal carotid bifurcation and the proximal middle cerebral artery in its lateral course.

The recurrent artery may enter the anterior perforated substance as a single stem or divide into many branches (average, four). Of the total branches, approximately 40% terminate in the anterior perforated substance medial to the origin of the ACA, and 40% terminate lateral to the ACA origin. The remaining branches pass to the inferior surface of the frontal lobe adjacent the anterior perforated substance. The recurrent artery supplies the anterior part of the caudate nucleus, anterior third of the putamen, anterior part of the outer segment of the globus pallidus, anteroinferior portion of the anterior limb of the internal capsule, and the uncinate fasciculus, and, less commonly, the anterior hypothalamus. The hypothalamic supply is less than from the A1. In the treatment of anterior communicating aneurysms, great care must be taken to avoid unnecessary manipulation or occlusion of Heubner's artery. Occlusion may cause hemiparesis with facial and brachial predominance because of compromise of that branch supplying the anterior limb of the internal capsule, and aphasia if the artery is on the dominant side.

FIGURE 2.24. *Anterior views of A1 and proximal A2 segments of the ACA, AComA, and recurrent arteries. Gyrus rectus, olfactory tract, and frontal lobe above; optic nerves and chiasm below. Arterioles to optic nerves, chiasm, and tracts, and lamina terminalis arise from the ACA and AComA.* A, *A1 segments of equal size and small communicating artery pass above the optic chiasm. Recurrent arteries arise from the lateral side of A2. Recurrent arteries pass anterosuperior to A1.* B, *both A2 segments arise from large left A1. The right A1 is small. A1 segments pass above the optic nerves. Recurrent arteries arise from A2 segments. Right recurrent artery is longer than the A1 segment. The left recurrent artery passes superior to the A1. Branches of the AComA supply the lamina terminalis above the optic chiasm.* C, *A1 segments are connected by a double communicating artery. The right recurrent artery arises from the A2 and courses above the A1. The left recurrent artery arises from and passes above the A1. Multiple arterioles pass to the optic chiasm and tract.* D, *A1 segments are connected by a double communicating artery. Two recurrent arteries arise on the right; one arises proximal and one distal to the communicating artery. The left recurrent artery arises from the posterior aspect of the A1. A spray of arterioles passes from the communicating artery to the optic chiasm.* E, *a multichanneled AComA gives rise to multiple arterioles to the optic nerves and chiasm and lamina terminalis. A double recurrent artery is on the right. The left recurrent artery gives rise to a large branch that passes below the gyrus rectus to the frontal tip.* F, *the left A1 segment is split into a double channel. Both A2 segments arise predominantly from the right A1. The left recurrent artery arises from one of the two A1 segments on the left. The right recurrent artery arises from the A2.* G, *triple A2 segments arise from the communicating artery area. The left recurrent artery arises from the A1 segment; right from the junction of the A1 and A2 segments.* H, *tortuous A1 segments loop forward to the area of the tuberculum sellae. The left recurrent artery arises from the A2 segment and the right recurrent artery arises from the A1 segment.* A., *anterior, artery;* C.A., *carotid artery;* Gy., *gyrus;* N., *nerve;* O., *optic;* Olf., *olfactory;* Perf., *perforated;* Re., *rectus;* Rec., *recurrent;* S., *substance;* Tr., *tract.* (From, *Perlmutter D, Rhoton AL Jr: Microsurgical anatomy of the anterior cerebral-anterior communicating-recurrent artery complex. **J Neurosurg** 45:259–272, 1976 [26].)*

Basal Perforating Branches

The A1 and A2 and the AComA give rise to numerous basal perforating arteries (*Figs. 2.16* and *2.24*). An average of 8 basal perforators (range, 2–15), exclusive of Heubner's artery, arise from each A1 (26, 27). The lateral half of A1 is a richer source of branches than the medial half. The A1 branches terminate, in descending order of frequency, in the anterior perforated substance, the dorsal surface of the optic chiasm or the suprachiasmatic portion of the hypothalamus, the optic tract, dorsal surface of the optic nerve, and the sylvian fissure between the cerebral hemispheres and the lower surface of the frontal lobe. The striking difference in the termination of A1 branches as compared with those from the recurrent artery is the lack of recurrent artery branches to the upper surface of the optic nerves and chiasm and the anterior hypothalamus and the greater number of recurrent branches entering the sylvian fissure. Approximately 40% of both A1 and recurrent artery branches terminate in the anterior perforated substance medial to the A1 origin, but almost no Heubner's branches enter the area around the optic chiasm and tract, although 40% of those from A1 terminated there. Approximately 40% of the recurrent artery branches enter the anterior perforated substance lateral to the carotid bifurcation.

The A1, excluding the recurrent artery and the A2, most consistently supplies the chiasm and anterior third ventricle and hypothalamic area, but only inconsistently supplies the caudate and globus pallidus. Heubner's artery, by contrast, provides a rich supply to the caudate and adjacent internal capsule, but much less to the hypothalamus than the A1. Involvement of the hypothalamic branches that arise mainly from A1, without implication of the recurrent artery, may result in emotional changes, personality disorders, and intellectual deficits, including anxiety and fear, weak spells, and symptoms referable to disordered mentation, such as dizziness, agitation, and hypokinesis without paralysis or alterations of the conscious or waking state (6, 26). The frequent inclusion of recurrent artery ischemia when the A1 branches are involved adds a hemiparesis with brachial predominance to the deficit. This contrasts with the crural weakness of distal ACA occlusion.

The AComA also frequently gives rise to perforating arteries that terminate in the superior surface of the optic chiasm and above the chiasm in the anterior hypothalamus (*Figs. 2.16, 2.23,* and *2.24*). The AComA is frequently the site of origin of one or two, but as many as four branches that terminate, in descending order of frequency, in the suprachiasmatic area, dorsal surface of the optic chiasm, anterior perforated substance, and frontal lobe, and perfuse the fornix, corpus callosum, septal region, and anterior cingulum (6, 8). Most arise from the superior or posterior surfaces of the AComA. The A2, to be discussed below, is also the site of origin of perforating branches terminating in the inferior frontal area, anterior perforated substance, dorsal optic chiasm, and the suprachiasmatic area.

Distal Part

The distal or postcommunicating part of the ACA begins at the AComA and extends around the corpus callosum to its termination (*Figs. 2.22* and *2.25*). The distal ACA is divided into four segments (A2 through A5). The A2 (infracallosal) segment begins at the AComA, passes anterior to the lamina terminalis, and terminates at the junction of the rostrum and genu of the corpus callosum. The A3 (precallosal) segment extends around the genu of the corpus callosum and terminates where the artery turns sharply posterior above the genu. The A4 (supracallosal) and A5 (postcallosal) segments are located above the corpus callosum and are separated into an anterior (A4) and posterior (A5) portion by a point bisected in the lateral view close behind the coronal suture. The A2 and A3 segments, together, and A4 and A5 have been referred to as the ascending and horizontal segments, respectively (27). In our discussion, the distal ACA is synonymous with the pre-callosal artery.

The Pericallosal Artery

The pericallosal artery is the portion of the ACA distal to the AComA around and on or near the corpus callosum (*Figs. 2.22, 2.25,* and *2.26*). Some authors reserve that term for the artery formed by the bifurcation near the genu of the corpus callosum into the pericallosal and callosomarginal arteries (27). We refer to the segment distal to the AComA as the pericallosal artery because both the AComA and pericallosal artery are consistently present, but the callosomarginal artery is inconsistent; it is quite variable with regard to its site of origin and is absent in nearly 20% of hemispheres (27). If one assumes the pericallosal artery begins at the callosomarginal origin, the variability of origin of the callosomarginal artery could place the origin of the pericallosal artery at any point from near the AComA to the genu of the corpus callosum, and, in addition, if the callosomarginal artery is absent, some arbitrary point must be selected as the origin of the pericallosal artery. Thus, the term pericallosal artery refers to the portion of the ACA beginning at the AComA, which includes the A2 to A5 segments.

The Callosomarginal Artery

The callosomarginal artery, the largest branch of the pericallosal artery, is defined as the artery that courses in or near the cingulate sulcus and gives rise to two or more major cortical branches (*Figs. 2.22, 2.25,* and *2.26*) (27). The callosomarginal artery is present in 80% of hemispheres. The callosomarginal artery cannot be defined in terms of a given group of vessels that arises from it because any of the usual branches of the callosomarginal artery may arise directly from the pericallosal artery. It follows a course roughly parallel to that of the pericallosal artery, coursing above the cingulate gyrus in or near the cingulate sulcus. Its origin varies from just distal to the AComA to the level of the genu of the corpus callosum. Its most frequent origin is from the A3, but it may also arise from the A2 or A4. Its branches ascend on the medial surface of the hemisphere and continue on to the lateral convexity for approximately 2 cm. Portions of the premotor, motor, and sensory areas are included in its area of perfusion.

The size of the pericallosal artery distal to the callosomarginal origin varies inversely with the size of the callosomarginal artery. Immediately past the origin of the callosomarginal artery, the

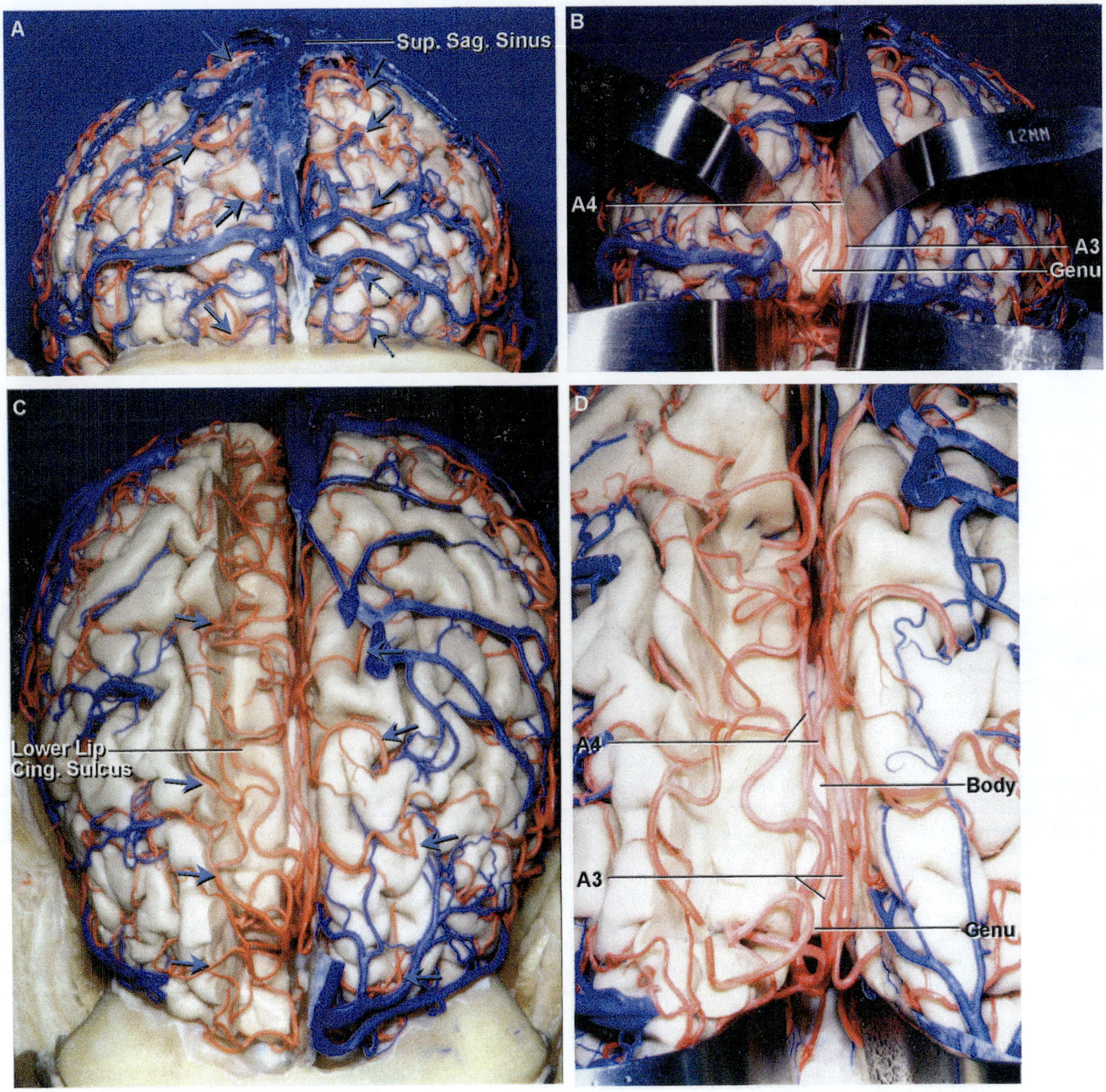

FIGURE 2.25. *Anterior cerebral artery. A, anterior view of the cerebral hemispheres. The branches of the ACA cross the superior and anterior margins of the hemisphere to supply the adjacent part of the lateral convexity* (arrows). *These ACA branches exiting the interhemispheric fissure course deep to the venous lacunae and the cortical veins entering the superior sagittal sinus. B, the falx and right frontal lobe have been retracted to expose the A3s passing around the genu of the corpus callosum deep in the interhemispheric fissure. The A4s course above the anterior part of the callosal body. C, the cortical strip above the right cingulate sulcus has been removed, while preserving the ACA branches looping deep within the sulci on the medial surface of the hemisphere. These branches often course within a sulci along the superior margin to reach the lateral surface. D, enlarged view of the branches of the ACA coursing deep within the cingulate sulcus. Some branches course deep within sulci along the superior margin of the hemisphere rather than looping over the upper edge of the superior margin to reach the lateral surface.* Cing., *cingulate;* Sag., *sagittal;* Sup., *superior.*

pericallosal and callosomarginal arteries are equal in diameter in only 20% of hemispheres; the pericallosal is larger in 50%; and the callosomarginal is larger in 30% (27). The callosomarginal artery should not be mistaken for the pericallosal artery in lateral angiography, because the mistaken wider curvature may be falsely interpreted as representing hydrocephalus.

The anterior portion of the falx cerebri is consistently narrower than its posterior part, with the free margin of its

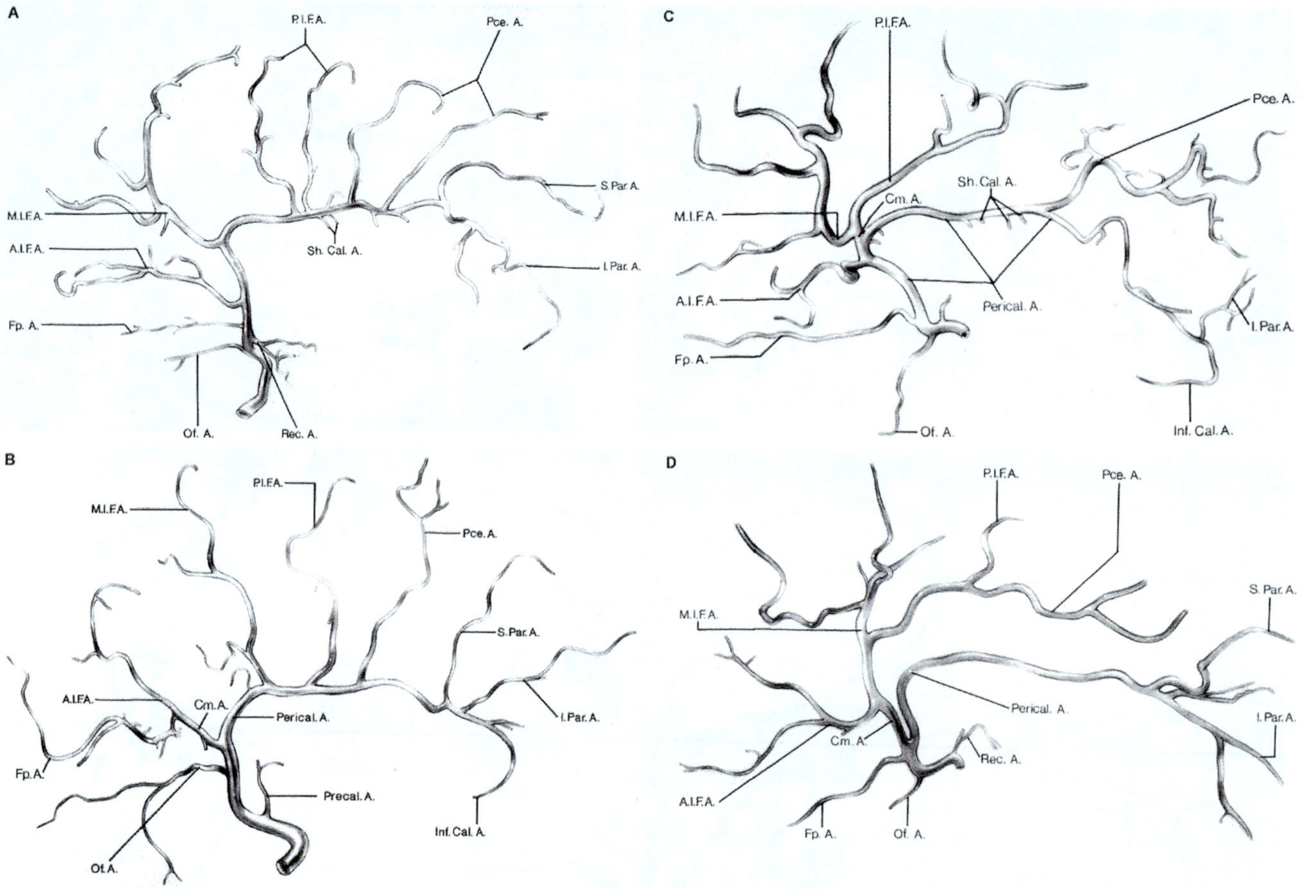

FIGURE 2.26. *Drawings of anterior cerebral arteries dissected from the cerebral hemispheres. The pericallosal, callosomarginal, orbitofrontal, frontopolar, anterior, middle and posterior internal frontal, paracentral, superior and inferior parietal, short callosal, inferior callosal, recurrent, and precallosal arteries are seen. A, there is no communicating artery and all the individual cortical branches of the ACA arise directly from the pericallosal artery. There are two posterior internal frontal and paracentral arteries. Short callosal branches arise from the pericallosal artery. B, the callosomarginal artery gives origin to two cortical branches: the frontopolar and anterior internal frontal arteries. The other cortical branches arise from the pericallosal artery. Precallosal and inferior callosal arteries are present. C, the callosomarginal artery gives origin to the middle internal frontal and posterior internal frontal arteries. Short and inferior callosal arteries are present. D, four cortical branches arise from the callosomarginal artery.* A., *artery;* A.I.F.A., *anterior internal frontal artery;* Cal., *callosal;* Cm., *callosomarginal;* Fp., *frontopolar;* I., *inferior;* Inf., *inferior;* M.I.F.A., *middle internal frontal artery;* Of., *orbitofrontal;* Par., *parietal;* Pce., *paracentral;* Perical., *pericallosal;* P.I.F.A., *posterior internal frontal artery;* Precal., *precallosal;* Rec., *recurrent;* S., *superior;* Sh., *short.* (From, *Perlmutter D, Rhoton AL Jr: Microsurgical anatomy of the distal anterior cerebral artery.* ***J Neurosurg*** *49:204–228, 1978 [27].)*

anterior portion lying well above the genu of the corpus callosum, whereas the free margin of its posterior portion is more closely applied to the splenium (*Fig. 2.22*). The entire course of the pericallosal artery, except for the posterior portion, is below the free margin of the falx cerebri and is free to shift across the midline. The callosomarginal artery, on the other hand, has only the most anterior portion below the free margin of the falx; the remainder lies above the free edge, and its displacement across the midline is limited by the rigidity of the falx (*Fig. 2.22, A–C*).

Distal ACA Branches

The distal ACA gives origin to two types of branches: 1) basal perforating branches to basal structures including the optic chiasm, suprachiasmatic area, lamina terminalis, and anterior hypothalamus, structures located below the rostrum of the corpus callosum; and 2) cerebral branches divided into cortical branches to the cortex and adjacent white matter and subcortical branches to the deep white and gray matter and the corpus callosum.

Basal Perforating Branches

The A2 segment typically gives rise to 4 or 5 (range, 0–10) basal perforating branches that supply the anterior hypothalamus, septum pellucidum, medial portion of the anterior commissure, pillars of the fornix, and anteroinferior part of the striatum (*Figs. 2.16, 2.23,* and *2.24*) (26, 27, 39). They commonly take a direct course from the A2 segment to the anterior diencephalon. In a few cases, the perforating branches may arise from a larger artery, referred to as the precallosal artery, that originates from A2 and passes upward between the A2 segment and the lamina terminalis toward the genu of the corpus callosum (*Figs. 2.21* and *2.23*). The recurrent artery may also arise from the A2, as described above.

Cortical Branches

The cortical branches supply the cortex and adjacent white matter of the medial surface from the frontal pole to the parietal lobe where they intermingle with branches of the PCA (*Figs. 2.25–2.27*). On the basal surface, the ACA supplies the medial part of the orbital gyri, the gyrus rectus, and the olfactory bulb and tract. On the lateral surface, the ACA supplies the area of the superior frontal gyrus and the superior parts of the precentral, central, and postcentral gyri. The band of lateral cortex supplied by the ACA is wider anteriorly, often extending beyond the superior frontal sulcus, and narrows progressively posteriorly. The distal ACA on one side sends branches to the contralateral hemisphere in nearly two-thirds of brains.

Eight cortical branches are typically encountered (*Figs. 2.26* and *2.27*). They are orbitofrontal, frontopolar, internal frontal, paracentral, and the parietal arteries; the internal frontal group is divided into the anterior, middle, and posterior frontal arteries, and the parietal group is divided into superior and inferior parietal arteries. The smallest cortical branch is the orbitofrontal artery, and the largest is the posterior internal frontal artery. The frontopolar and orbitofrontal arteries are present in nearly all hemispheres; the least frequent branch is the inferior parietal artery, present in approximately two-thirds of hemispheres. The most frequent ACA segment of origin of the cortical branches is as follows: orbitofrontal and frontopolar arteries, A2; the anterior and middle internal frontal and callosomarginal arteries, A3; the paracentral artery, A4; and the superior and inferior parietal arteries, A5. The posterior internal frontal artery arises with approximately equal frequency from A3, A4, and the callosomarginal artery. All of the cortical branches arise from the pericallosal artery more frequently than they do from the callosomarginal. Of the major cortical branches, one of the internal frontal arteries or the paracentral artery arises most frequently from the callosomarginal. The cortical branch that arises most frequently from the callosomarginal artery is the middle internal frontal artery. Of the callosomarginal arteries present in our study, 50% gave rise to two major cortical branches, 32% gave rise to three, 16% gave rise to four, and, in one hemisphere (2%), five of the eight major cortical branches arose from the callosomarginal artery (27).

1. Orbitofrontal Artery
   This artery, the first cortical branch of the distal ACA, is present in nearly all hemispheres. It commonly arises from the A2, but may also arise as a common trunk with the frontopolar artery. It may uncommonly arise from the A1

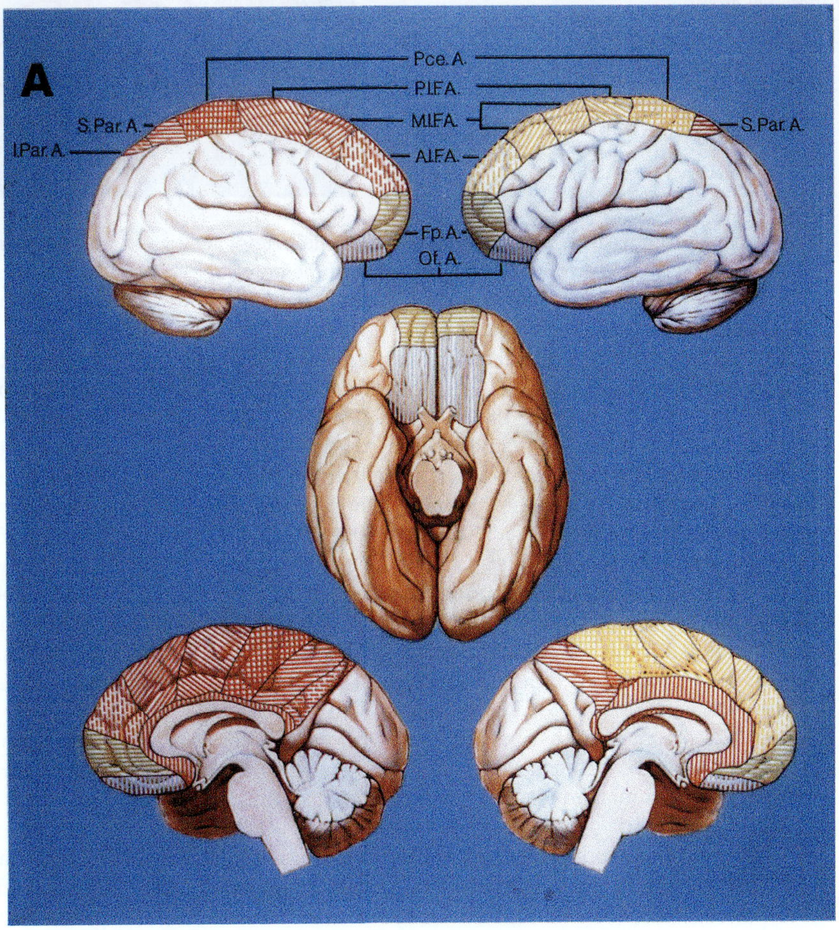

FIGURE 2.27. A–C, *area of supply of the distal anterior cerebral artery and its individual branches. The areas shown in* blue, green, and red *are supplied by branches arising directly from the pericallosal artery. Areas in* yellow *arise from branches of the callosomarginal artery. The orbitofrontal and frontopolar arteries are shown in* green *and* blue, *respectively. The anterior internal frontal artery shows as* vertical broken lines, *the middle internal frontal artery as* oblique lines passing upward to right; *the posterior internal frontal artery as* oblique lines passing downward to right; *the paracentral artery as* cross-hatched; *the superior parietal artery as* horizontal lines; *the inferior parietal artery as* horizontal broken lines; *and the pericallosal area supplied by short or terminal branches of the pericallosal artery as* vertical lines. A, *right cerebral hemisphere (*upper and lower left, *and* left half of basal view*). All cortical branches of the ACA arise directly from pericallosal artery and are shown in* blue, green, and red. *The callosomarginal artery is absent in 18% of hemispheres. Left hemisphere* (upper and lower right, and right half of basal view) *shows four of the major cortical branches arising from the callosomarginal artery* (yellow area). *The anterior internal frontal through the paracentral arteries arise from the callosomarginal artery. The maximum number of cortical branches that arise from the callosomarginal artery is five. The terminal branch of the pericallosal artery passes around the splenium of the corpus callosum toward the foramen of Monro. The inferior parietal artery is absent. (Legend continues on next page.)*

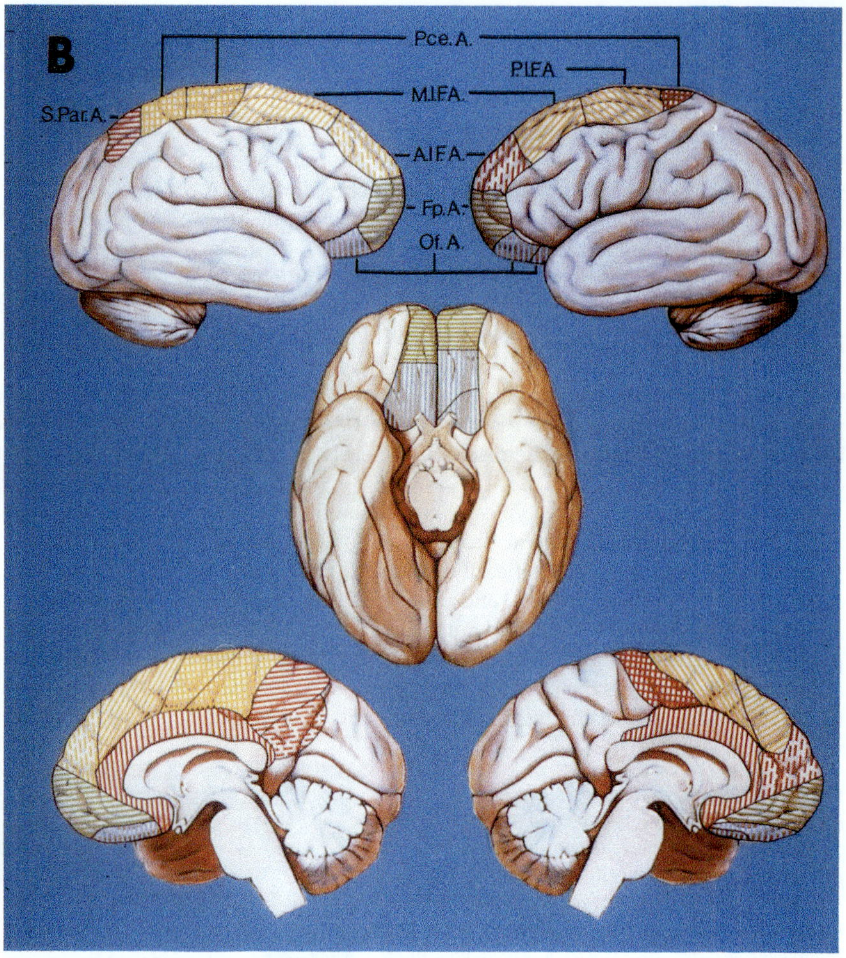

FIGURE 2.27. *Continued*
B, *the right hemisphere* (upper and lower left, and left half of basal view) *shows an unusually large area of supply of the ACA, extending beyond the parieto-occipital fissure to the cuneus. The posterior internal frontal artery is absent. The callosomarginal artery gives rise to the anterior and middle posterior frontal and the paracentral arteries* (yellow area). *The* black line *subdivides the* cross-hatched area *of the paracentral artery to show the two separate branches arising from the pericallosal artery to supply the area of the paracentral artery. The left hemisphere* (upper and lower right, and right half of basal view) *shows an unusually small area of supply of the ACA. The branches reach only the paracentral area. The callosomarginal artery gives origin to two cortical branches: the middle and posterior internal frontal arteries* (yellow area). *The superior and inferior parietal arteries are absent. The* black line *divides the orbitofrontal area* (blue lines) *to show that it was supplied by two separate branches of the pericallosal artery.*

segment just proximal to the AComA. From its origin, it passes down and forward toward the floor of the anterior cranial fossa to reach the level of the planum sphenoidale. It supplies the gyrus rectus, olfactory bulb, and tract, and the medial part of the orbital surface of the frontal lobe.

2. Frontopolar Artery
   The next cortical branch, the frontopolar artery, arises from the A2 segment of the pericallosal artery in 90% of hemispheres and from the callosomarginal artery in 10%. From its origin, it passes anteriorly along the medial surface of the hemisphere toward the frontal pole. It crosses the subfrontal sulcus and supplies portions of the medial and lateral surfaces of the frontal pole.
3. Internal Frontal Arteries
   The internal frontal arteries supply the medial and lateral surfaces of the superior frontal gyrus as far posteriorly as the paracentral lobule (6). They most commonly arise from the A3 segment of the pericallosal artery or from the callosomarginal artery. Combinations of origins in which one or two internal frontal arteries have separate origins from the pericallosal artery, but the remaining artery or arteries arise from the callosomarginal, are common.

   The anterior internal frontal artery usually arises as a separate branch of the A2 or A3, but may also arise from the callosomarginal artery; it supplies the anterior portion of the superior frontal gyrus. The origin, whether from the pericallosal or callosomarginal artery, is most often at or inferior to the level of the genu of the corpus callosum. The middle internal frontal artery arises with nearly equal frequency from the pericallosal and the callosomarginal arteries and courses posteriorly in the cingulate sulcus a short distance before turning vertically to cross over the superior cortical margin in the middle portion of the superior frontal gyrus. It supplies the middle portion of the medial and lateral surfaces of the superior frontal gyrus. It is the cortical branch that arises most frequently from the callosomarginal artery. The posterior internal frontal artery arises with nearly equal frequency from the A3 and A4 and the callosomarginal artery and courses upward to the cingulate sulcus, then backward for a short distance before turning superiorly to terminate in the uppermost limit of the precentral fissure. It supplies the posterior third of the superior frontal gyrus and part of the cingulate gyrus. Its branches frequently reach the anterior portion of the paracentral lobule.
4. Paracentral Artery
   This branch usually arises from the A4 or the callosomarginal artery approximately midway between the genu and

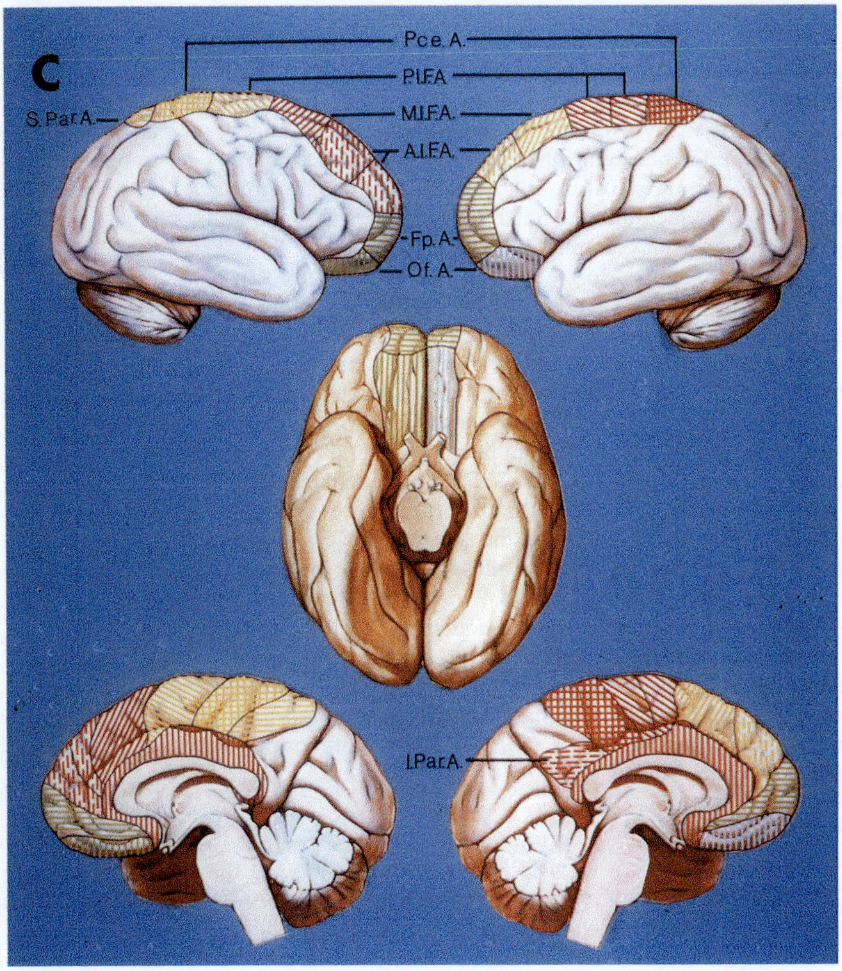

FIGURE 2.27. *Continued*
C, *the right hemisphere* (upper and lower left, and left half of basal view) *shows the orbitofrontal and frontopolar arteries arising from a common trunk* (both shown in green), *a relatively posterior area of supply of three branches arising from the callosomarginal artery* (yellow area), *and absence of the inferior parietal artery. The left hemisphere* (upper and lower right, and right half of basal view) *illustrates two cortical branches arising from the callosomarginal area* (yellow) *and absence of the superior and presence of the inferior parietal artery. The* black line *subdivides the area of posterior internal frontal artery to show that two separate branches arise from the pericallosal artery to supply this area.* A., *artery;* A.I.F.A., *anterior internal frontal artery;* Fp., *frontopolar;* I., *inferior;* M.I.F.A., *middle internal frontal artery;* Of., *orbitofrontal;* Par., *parietal;* Pce., *paracentral;* P.I.F.A., *posterior internal frontal artery;* S., *superior.* (From, *Perlmutter D, Rhoton AL Jr: Microsurgical anatomy of the distal anterior cerebral artery.* *J Neurosurg* *49:204–228, 1978 [27].)*

splenium or the corpus callosum. It usually courses anterior to the marginal limb of the cingulate sulcus or in the paracentral sulcus before turning vertically to the superior portion of the paracentral lobule, where it supplies a portion of the premotor, motor, and somatic sensory areas. It may represent the terminal portion of the ACA.

5. Parietal Arteries
   The parietal arteries, named the superior and inferior parietal arteries, supply the ACA distribution posterior to the paracentral lobule. The superior parietal artery arises from the A4 or A5 and from the callosomarginal artery and supplies the superior portion of the precuneus. It usually originates anterior to the splenium of the corpus callosum and courses in the marginal limb of the cingulate sulcus. If it courses posterior to the marginal limb, it often sends a branch to it. It is frequently the last cortical branch of the ACA. The inferior parietal artery most commonly arises from the A5 just before the latter courses around the splenium of the corpus callosum and supplies the posteroinferior part of the precuneus and adjacent portions of the cuneus. It is the least frequent cortical branch of the ACA (64% of hemispheres). An origin from the callosomarginal artery is uncommon.

Convexity Branches

There are large areas of the lateral cortical distribution of the ACA where there is a good chance of finding a vessel of sufficient diameter for a bypass anastomosis with a frontal branch of the superficial temporal artery. The area offering the best chance of finding an adequate ACA branch on the lateral surface was determined by drawing a circumferential line on the outer circumference of the hemisphere beginning at the sylvian fissure and continuing around the frontal pole and over the superior hemispheric margin toward the occipital pole. The minimum diameter needed for an anastomosis is usually considered to be 0.8 mm (27). An identical line was drawn 2 cm inside the circumferential line. The largest percentage of ACA branches crossing these lines was located on the anterior portion of the hemisphere between the 5-cm and 15-cm points on the circumferential line.

Callosal Branches

The ACA is the principal artery supplying the corpus callosum. The pericallosal artery sends branches into the rostrum, genu, body, and splenium and often passes inferiorly around the splenium. The terminal pericallosal branches are joined posteriorly by the splenial branches of the PCA. The corpus callosum is most commonly supplied by perforating branches, called short callosal arteries because they arise from the pericallosal artery and penetrate directly into the corpus callosum. As many as 20 short callosal branches (average, 7) may be found in one hemisphere (27). These branches not only supply the corpus callosum, but continue through it to supply the septum pellucidum, the anterior pillars of the fornix, and part of the anterior commissure.

In a few cases, well-formed longer branches, referred to as long callosal arteries, arise from the pericallosal artery and course parallel to the pericallosal artery, between it and the surface of the corpus callosum, to give origin to callosal perforating branches (*Fig. 2.22*). In addition to sending branches to the corpus callosum, they may supply adjacent cortex as well as the septal nuclei, septum pellucidum, and upper portions of the column of the fornix (27). The pericallosal artery frequently continues around the splenium of the corpus callosum, distal to the origin of the last cortical branch, and passes forward on the lower callosal surface, reaching the foramen of Monro in a few cases.

The precallosal artery, an infrequently occurring A2 or AComA branch, passes upward like a long callosal artery between the pericallosal artery and the lamina terminalis, sending branches into the anterior diencephalon and giving off multiple small branches to the rostrum and inferior part of the genu of the corpus callosum.

Anomalies

Anomalies of the distal ACA, including triplication of the postcommunical segment, failure of pairing of the distal ACA, and bihemispheric branches, are found in approximately 15% of brains (2). A bihemispheric branch is one that divides distal to the AComA and provides the major supply to the medial surface of both hemispheres. In the presence of such an anomaly, occlusion of one ACA distal to the AComA may produce bilateral cerebral injury similar to that produced by blocking both ACAs. The distal ACA on one side sends branches to the contralateral hemisphere in nearly two-thirds of brains (*Fig. 2.28*). However, most supply only a small area on the medial surface of the contralateral hemisphere. An infrequent anomaly is one in which the ACA distal to the A1 segment is unpaired and a single distal ACA divides to supply both hemispheres (26).

ANTERIOR PERFORATING ARTERIES

The anterior perforating arteries are the group of arteries that enter the brain through the anterior perforated substance (*Figs. 2.29–2.31*). The interrelationships between the anterior perforated arteries from the different sources and the vital tracts and nuclei they supply in the central part of the cerebrum make them deserving of special attention. These arteries have an intimate relationship to aneurysms of the internal carotid and the middle and anterior cerebral arteries, and to tumors arising deep under the brain (*Fig. 2.32*) (31, 35, 36).

The anterior perforated substance is a rhomboid-shaped area buried deep in the sylvian fissure, bounded anteriorly by the lateral and medial olfactory striae, posteriorly by the optic tract and the temporal lobe, laterally by the limen insulae; medially, it extends above the optic chiasm to the interhemispheric fissure (*Fig. 2.29*). The arteries passing below and sending branches into the anterior perforated substance are the ICA, MCA, and ACA, and the AChA. The perforating arteries from each parent artery enter a specific mediolateral and anteroposterior territory of the anterior perforated substance. The site of penetration in the mediolateral direction is described in relation to a line passing posteriorly along the olfactory tract. This line, dividing the anterior perforated substance into medial and lateral territories, crosses the anterior perforated substance near its greatest anterior-posterior dimension and transects the optic tract as it passes around the cerebral peduncle. The medial territory extends above the optic chiasm to the interhemispheric fissure, and the lateral

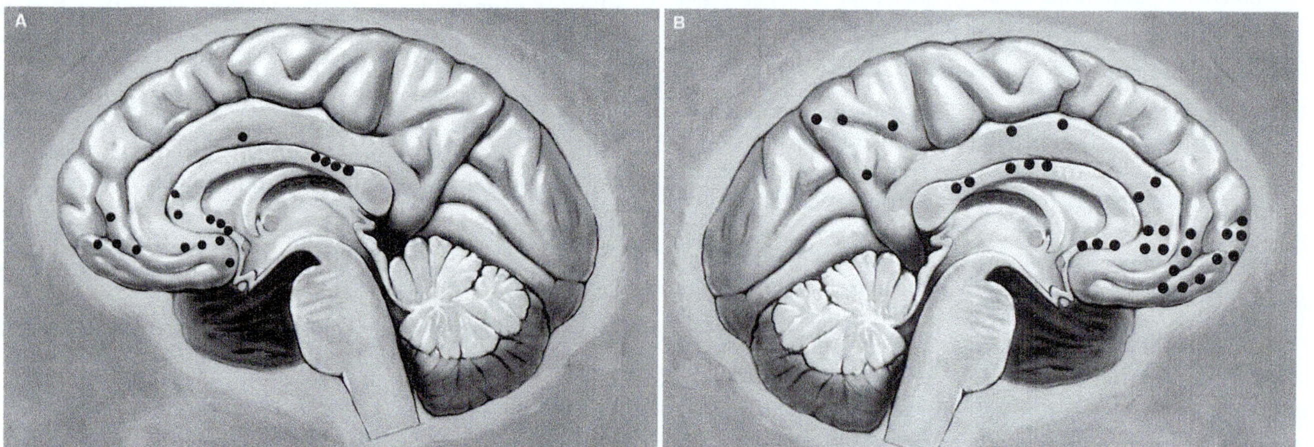

FIGURE 2.28. *Medial surface of cerebral hemispheres.* A, *right hemisphere;* B, *left hemisphere.* Black dots *indicate points where a branch from the opposite anterior cerebral artery arrives to supply the hemisphere shown. Based on the right and left hemispheres from 25 brains* (from, *Perlmutter D, Rhoton AL Jr: Microsurgical anatomy of the distal anterior cerebral artery.* ***J Neurosurg*** *49:204–228, 1978 [27]).*

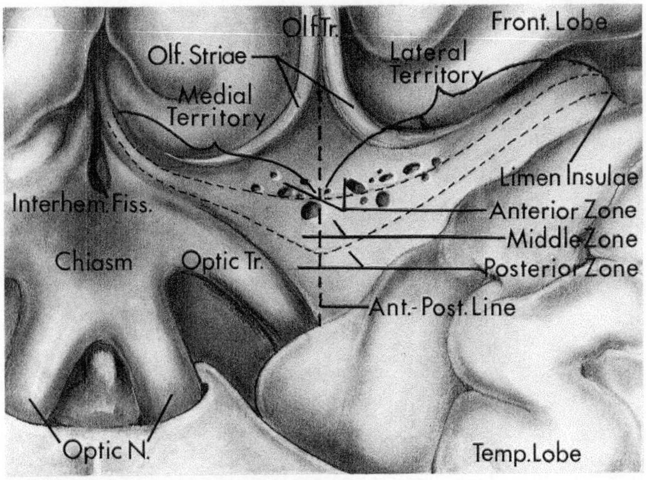

FIGURE 2.29. *Territories and zones within the anterior perforated substance. The anterior perforated substance lies between the frontal and temporal lobes. It is bounded anteriorly by the medial and lateral olfactory striae, and posteriorly by the temporal lobe and optic tract. The anterior perforated substance is divided into medial and lateral territories by a line drawn posteriorly along the olfactory tract. The medial territory extends above the optic nerve and chiasm to the interhemispheric fissure, and the lateral territory extends laterally in the sylvian fissure to the limen insulae. The anterior perforated substance is also divided into three transverse strips, the anterior, middle, and posterior zones, which extend from the interhemispheric fissure to the limen insulae, and correspond roughly to the anterior, middle, and posterior thirds of the anterior perforated substance. The point at which each artery penetrates these territories and zones is recorded. The medial and lateral olfactory striae are continuous anteriorly with the olfactory tract.* Ant., *anterior;* Interhem., *interhemispheric;* Fiss., *fissure;* Front., *frontal;* N., *nerve;* Olf., *olfactory;* Post., *posterior;* Temp., *temporal;* Tr., *tract.* (From, *Rosner SS, Rhoton AL Jr, Ono M, Barry M: Microsurgical anatomy of the anterior perforating arteries.* ***J Neurosurg*** *61:468–485, 1984 [36].)*

territory extends into the sylvian fissure to the limen insulae. The site of penetration of each group of arteries is also relatively constant in an anterior-posterior direction, based on subdivision of the anterior perforated substance into anterior, middle, and posterior zones extending across the full width of the anterior perforated substance, from the interhemispheric fissure to the limen insulae (*Figs. 2.29–2.31*).

Choroidal Segment of the C4

The C4 branches entering the anterior perforated substance arise from the choroidal segment (*Fig. 2.30, A* and *B*). The choroidal segment sends branches to the anterior perforated substance in nearly 100% of hemispheres (36). These branches tend to originate closer to the bifurcation than to the origin of the AChA. The branches arising at the bifurcation tend to be stouter than those arising below the bifurcation. Typically, these C4 branches follow a posterosuperior route to the posterior portion of the anterior perforated substance, near the optic tract. Approximately half of the branches penetrate the medial territory of the anterior perforated substance and half penetrate the lateral territory. Most enter the posterior or middle zones and very few enter the anterior zone.

Anterior Choroidal Artery

The AChA sends branches to the anterior perforated substance in 90% of hemispheres (13, 33, 36) (*Fig. 2.30, C–F*). The majority of the branches pursue a posterior, superior, and medial course, or a direct posterior and superior course to the anterior perforated substance. The branches arising at the origin of the AChA are somewhat stouter than those arising distally. These branches enter the posteromedial portion of the anterior perforated substance close to the optic tract and the line along the olfactory tract separating the medial and lateral territories. Approximately two-thirds of these branches enter the medial and one-third enter the lateral territory of the anterior perforated substance. Most enter the posterior zone or adjacent part of the middle zone of the anterior perforated substance.

Middle Cerebral Artery

The branches to the anterior perforated substance, called the lenticulostriate arteries, arise from the M1 and M2 and occasionally from the early branches (*Fig. 2.30, G–J*). They arise from the prebifurcation part of the M1 in every case and from the postbifurcation part of the M1 segment in half of the hemispheres. The lenticulostriate arteries are divided into medial, intermediate, and lateral groups. The medial group, present in half of the hemispheres, pursues a relatively direct course to enter the anterior perforated substance just lateral to the C4 branches. Ninety percent of the medial lenticulostriate arteries enter the lateral territory of the anterior perforated substance, whereas only 10% enter the medial territory (36). The predominant pattern is for them to enter the middle and posterior zones of the anterior perforated substance. In the hemispheres in which the medial group of lenticulostriate arteries are absent, their territory in the anterior perforated substance is occupied by branches from the C4 and the ACA, AChA, and the intermediate lenticulostriate arteries.

The intermediate lenticulostriate arteries entering the anterior perforated substance between the medial and lateral lenticulostriate arteries are present in more than 90% of hemispheres. They enjoy a generous area of distribution in the lateral territory of the anterior perforated substance. Nearly 90% enter the middle or posterior zones of the anterior perforated substance between the territory of the medial and lateral lenticulostriate arteries, lateral to the branches from the C4, and posterior to the branches of the recurrent artery.

The lateral lenticulostriate arteries, present in almost all hemispheres, originate predominantly on the lateral part of the M1, but may also arise from the early branches of the M1 or from the M2. They pursue an S-shaped course to enter the posterolateral part of the anterior perforated substance. All of the lateral lenticulostriate arteries enter the lateral territory of the anterior perforated substance near the limen insulae, and nearly all enter the posterior zone of the lateral part of the anterior perforated substance.

Anterior Cerebral Artery

The branches of the anterior cerebral artery to the anterior perforated substance arise from two sources. First, the A1

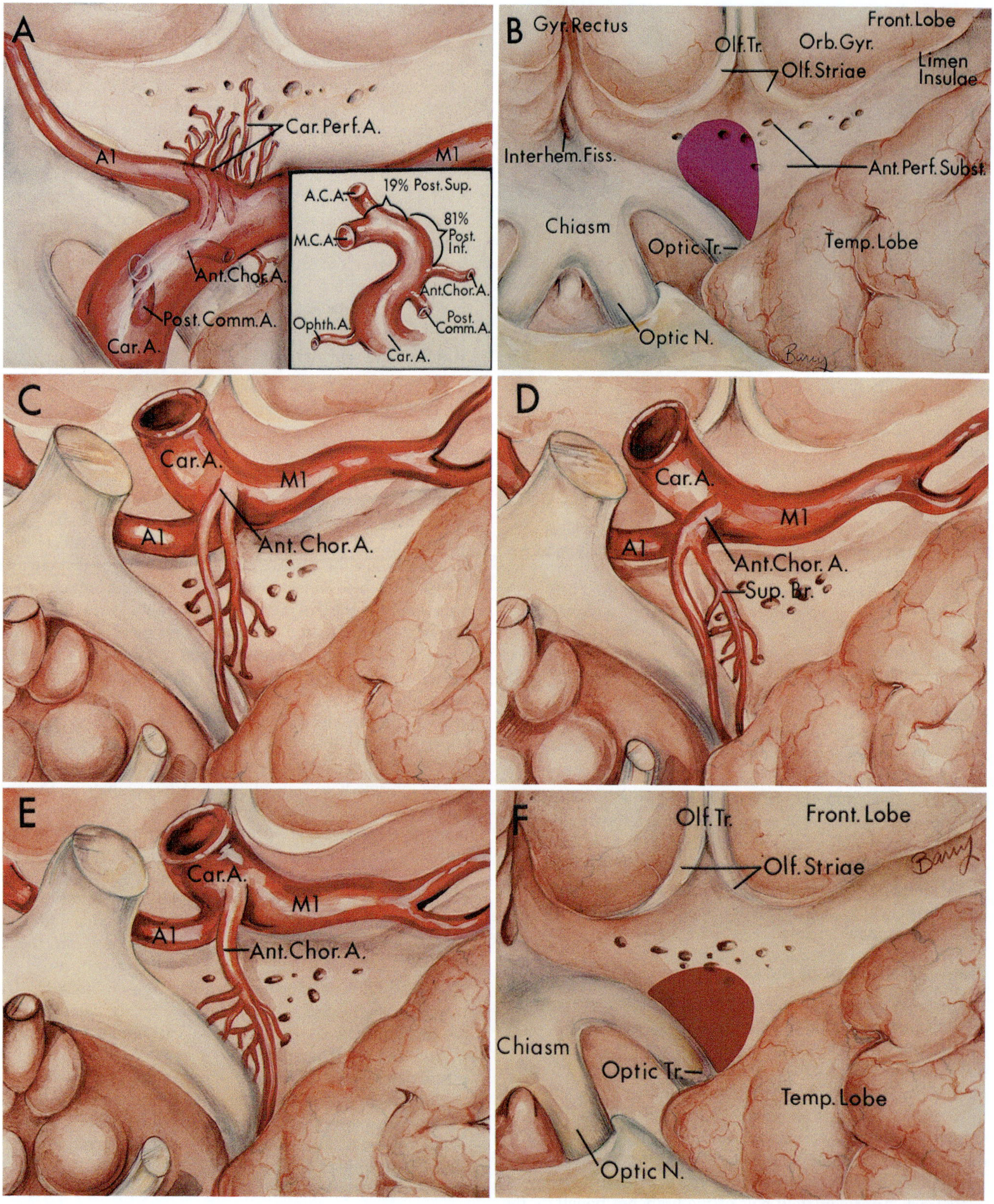

FIGURE 2.30. A–L, *arteries entering the anterior perforated substance. The internal carotid, anterior and middle cerebral, anterior choroidal, and recurrent arteries send branches to the anterior perforated substance. The carotid branches arise distal to the origin of the anterior choroidal artery, well above the origin of the ophthalmic and posterior communicating arteries. The middle cerebral branches arise from the M1 and M2 segments. The anterior cerebral branches, including the recurrent arteries, arise from the A1*

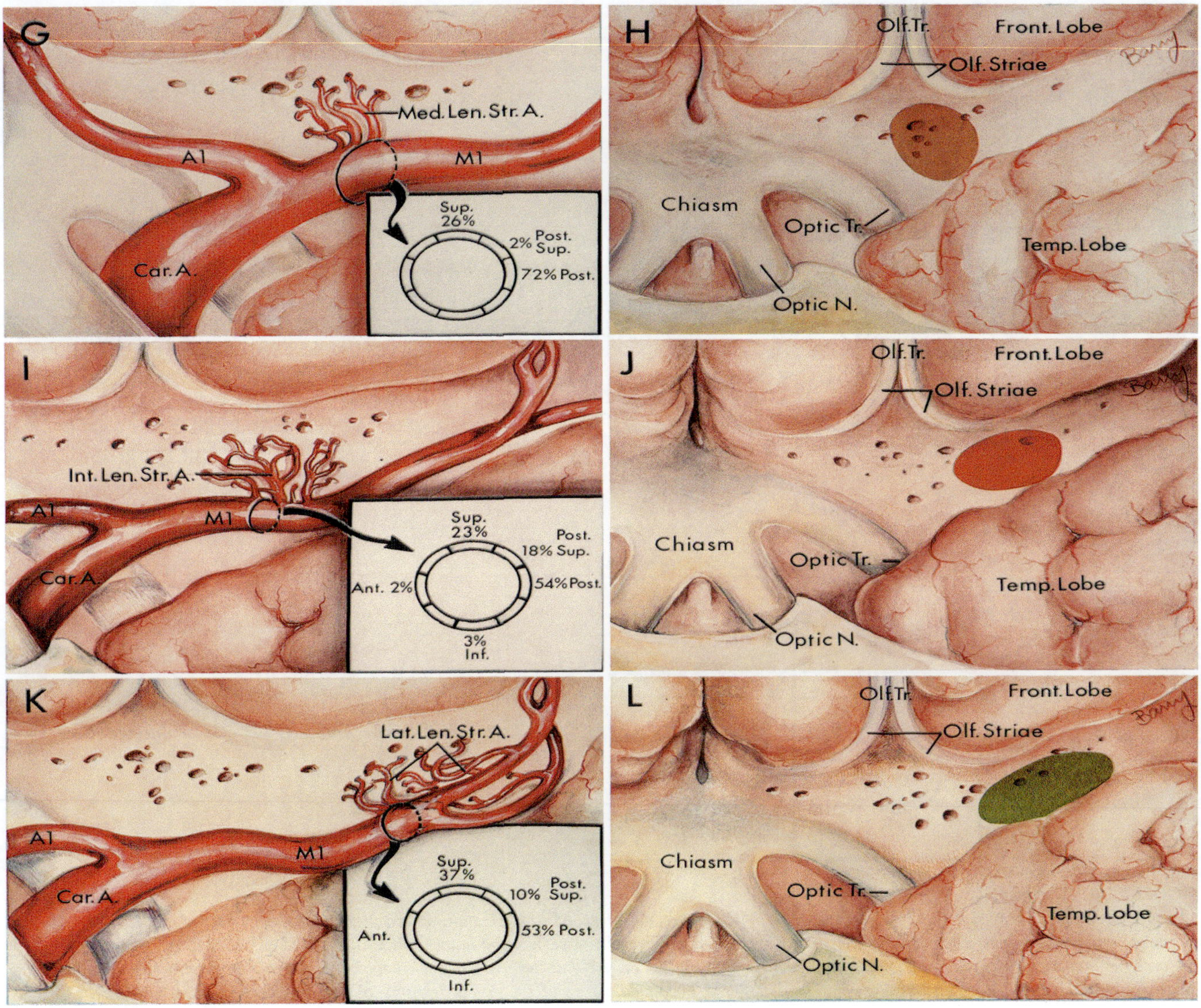

FIGURE 2.30. *Continued*
and A2 segments. The anterior perforated substance extends medially above the optic chiasm to the interhemispheric fissure, laterally to the limen insulae, anteriorly to the olfactory striae, and posteriorly to the optic tract and temporal lobe. The olfactory tract courses along the inferior surface of the frontal lobe at the junction of the gyrus rectus and the orbital gyri. A and B, *internal carotid artery.* A, *the branches from the internal carotid artery to the anterior perforated substance arise from the posterior wall above the anterior choroidal artery, and course upward behind the carotid bifurcation.* Inset: *lateral view of the carotid artery. Eighty-one percent of the branches to the anterior perforated substance arise from the posterior wall below the bifurcation and 18% arise from the posterosuperior surface of the wall, at or near the level of the bifurcation.* B, *internal carotid zone and territory in the anterior perforated substance. Most of the branches of the internal carotid artery enter the posterior and middle zones of the medial territory of the anterior perforated substance.* C–F, *anterior choroidal artery. Inferior views showing three patterns of origin* (C–E). C, *a branch to the anterior perforated substance arises in common with the origin of the anterior choroidal artery.* D, *the superior branch of the anterior choroidal artery gives rise to branches to the anterior perforated substance.* E, *the main trunk of the anterior choroidal artery gives off branches to the anterior perforated substance along its course to the choroid plexus in the temporal horn.* F, *the anterior choroidal branches enter the posterior and middle zones near the junction of the medial and lateral territories of the anterior perforated substance.* G–L, *lenticulostriate branches of the middle cerebral artery. The lenticulostriate branches are divided into medial, intermediate, and lateral groups.* G and H, *medial lenticulostriate arteries.* G, *the medial lenticulostriate arteries arise from the proximal part of the M1 segment.* Inset: *these arteries arise predominantly from the posterior and superior wall of the artery.* H, *they enter the middle and posterior zones of the medial part of the lateral territory of the anterior perforated substance.* I and J, *intermediate lenticulostriate arteries.* I, *these arteries arise from the M1 segment and, because of a complex branching, form a candelabra appearance as they approach the anterior perforated substance.* Inset: *they arise predominantly from the posterior, superior, and posterosuperior aspects of the wall.* J, *the arteries enter predominantly the middle and posterior zones of the central part of the lateral territory of the anterior perforated substance.* K and L, *lateral lenticulostriate arteries.* K, *these arteries arise in closer proximity to the bifurcation of the middle cerebral artery, from the M1 and M2 segments, and have an S-shaped course. First, they pass posterior, medial, and superior, then turn laterally, and finally complete an S-curve by turning medially just before entering the anterior perforated substance. Approximately half arise proximal and half arise distal to the bifurcation of the middle cerebral artery.* Inset: *site of origin. These arteries arise from the posterior, superior, or posterosuperior aspect of the parent trunk.* L, *the lateral lenticulostriate arteries enter predominantly the middle and posterior zones of the lateral territory of the anterior perforated substance.* *(Legend continues on next page.)*

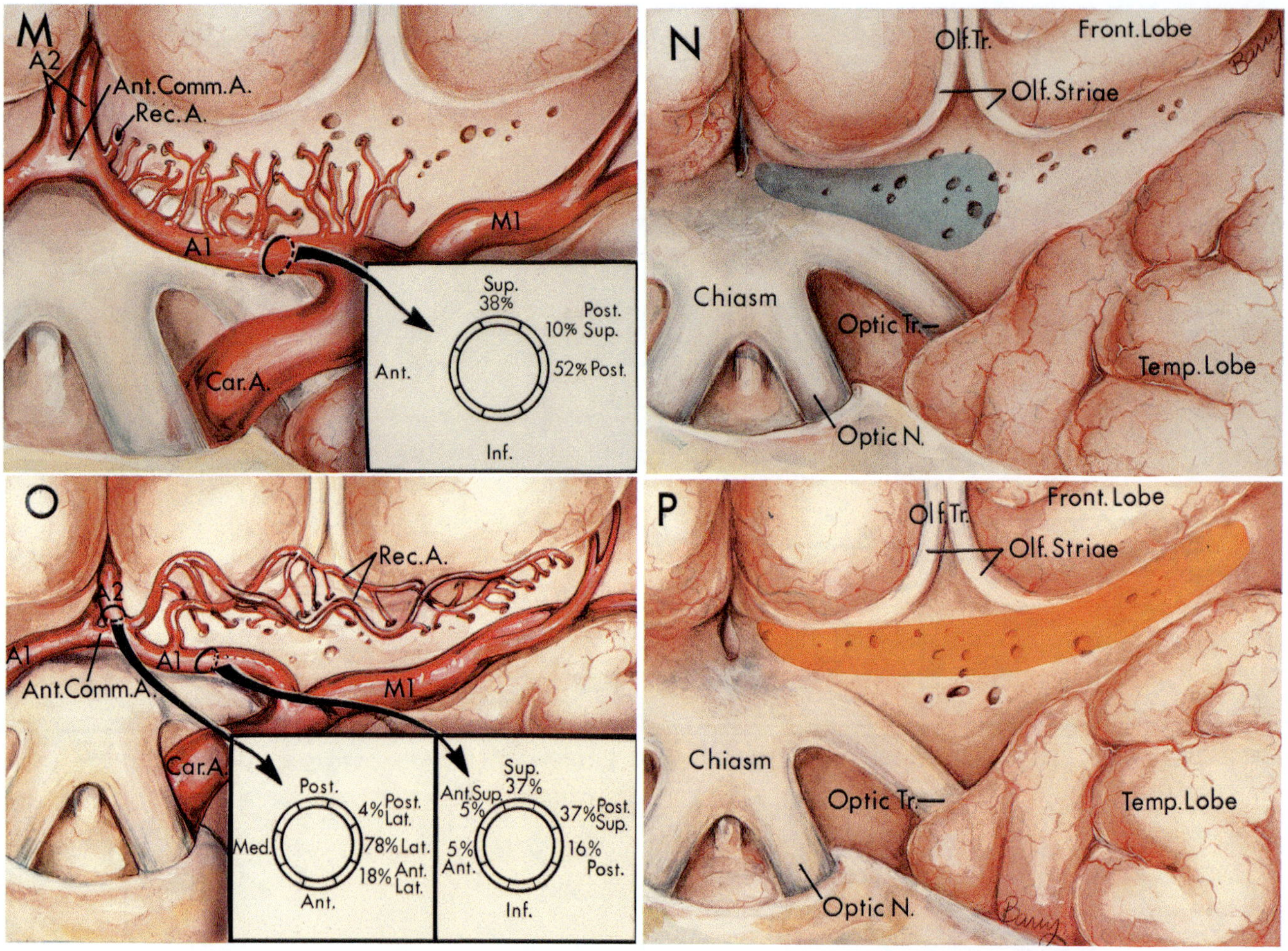

FIGURE 2.30. *Continued*
M and N, perforating branches of the A1 segment of the anterior cerebral artery. M, the A1 branches arise below the medial part of the anterior perforated substance and pass superior. The lateral half of the A1 segment is a richer site of perforating branches than the medial half. Inset: *the branches arise from the posterior, superior, or posterosuperior surface of the A1 segment. N, the A1 branches enter the narrow band of anterior perforated substance extending above the optic chiasm. They enter predominantly the posterior and middle zone of the medial territory of the anterior perforated substance. O and P, recurrent artery. O, as many as four recurrent arteries may arise from the anterior cerebral artery, either proximal to or near the level of the AComA. They pass laterally above the carotid bifurcation and give branches to the full mediolateral extent of the anterior perforated substance. They may wander forward on the posterior part of the orbital surface of the frontal lobe.* Inset (lower right)*: Site of origin of the recurrent arteries.* Left inset: *Recurrent artery origins near the junction of the A1 and A2 segments. The cross section of the artery at this level is oriented in a transverse plane. These branches arise predominantly from the lateral side of the vessel.* Right inset: *Site of origin of recurrent arteries arising from the A1 segments. The cross section of the artery at this level has an orientation in the sagittal plane. The branches arise predominantly from the superior or posterosuperior surface. P, the branches of the recurrent artery enter predominantly the anterior half of the anterior perforated substance along its full mediolateral extent, from the interhemispheric fissure to the limen insulae.* A., *arteries, artery;* A.C.A., *anterior cerebral artery;* Ant., *anterior;* Car., *carotid;* Chor., *choroidal;* Comm., *communicating;* Fiss., *fissure;* Front., *frontal;* Gyr., *gyrus;* Inf., *inferior;* Int., *intermediate;* Interhem., *interhemispheric;* Lat., *lateral;* Len. Str., *lenticulostriate;* M.C.A., *middle cerebral artery;* Med., *medial;* N., *nerve;* Olf., *olfactory;* Ophth., *ophthalmic;* Orb., *orbital;* Perf., *perforated, perforating;* Post., *posterior;* Subst., *substance;* Sup., *superior;* Tr., *tract, trunk;* Temp., *temporal.* (From, *Rosner SS, Rhoton AL Jr, Ono M, Barry M: Microsurgical anatomy of the anterior perforating arteries. **J Neurosurg** 61:468–485, 1984 [36].)*

gives rise to branches that pass directly to the anterior perforated substance. Second, the A1 and proximal part of the A2 give rise to the recurrent artery that sends branches to a broad extent of the anterior perforated substance (*Fig. 2.30, M–P*). Nearly all A1s send branches to the anterior perforated substance. Nearly 90% arise from the proximal half of the A1 and pursue a direct posterior and superior course to the anterior perforated substance. The ones with a more medial origin journey laterally to reach the anterior perforated substance. Most enter the medial territory of the anterior perforated substance near the optic chiasm and tract, and the remainder enter the lateral territory. Most enter the middle and posterior zones of the anterior perforated substance, predominantly posterior to the branches from the recurrent artery, anterome-

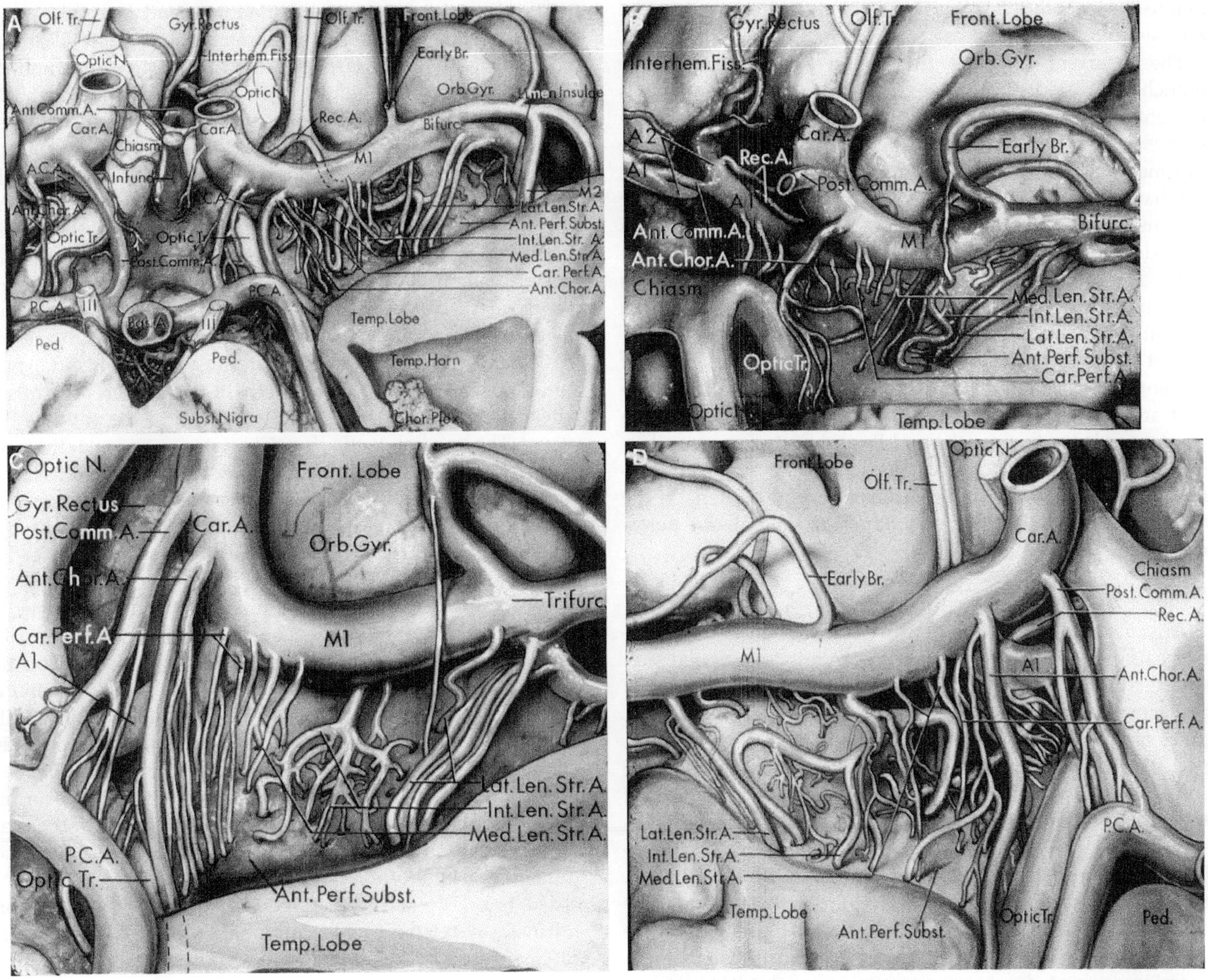

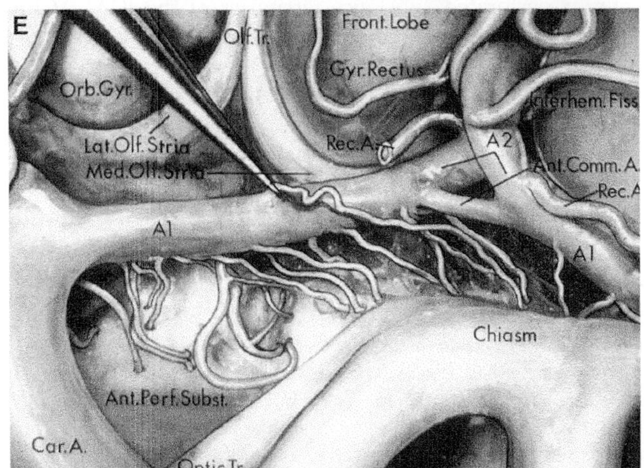

FIGURE 2.31. *Arteries entering the anterior perforated substance. A, inferior view. The anterior perforated substance on the left side extends anteriorly to the medial and lateral olfactory striae, posteriorly to the optic tract and temporal lobe, laterally to the limen insulae, and medially above the optic chiasm, to the interhemispheric fissure. The anterior part of the temporal lobe has been removed to expose the temporal horn. The internal carotid, anterior choroidal, and anterior and middle cerebral arteries (M1 and M2) give rise to branches to the anterior perforated substance. The PComA does not give branches to the anterior perforated substance. The middle cerebral branches, called the lenticulostriate arteries, are divided into medial, intermediate, and lateral lenticulostriate groups. The lateral lenticulostriate arteries arise laterally near the bifurcation of the M1 segment. The anterior choroidal and carotid branches enter the posterior part of the anterior perforated substance near the optic tract. The branches from the anterior cerebral artery enter the narrow strip of the anterior perforated substance above the optic chiasm. The recurrent artery arises from the anterior cerebral artery, near the level of the AComA, and passes laterally above the carotid bifurcation to enter the anterior perforated substance anterior to the branches from the other sources. The M1 segment gives rise to an early branch. B, another specimen. The optic nerve and chiasm have been reflected inferiorly. The branches from the left A1 segment enter the narrow medial sector of the anterior perforated substance extending above the optic chiasm to the interhemispheric fissure. A perforating artery arises from an early branch of the M1. Some of the lateral lenticulostriate arteries arise near the M1 bifurcation. The intermediate lenticulostriate arteries have a candelabra appearance. The anterior choroidal artery sends branches to the posterior half of the anterior perforated substance. Two recurrent arteries arise near the anterior communicating artery. C, another specimen. The anterior choroidal branches to the anterior perforated substance arise near the origin of the anterior choroidal artery. The lateral* *(Legend continues on next page.)*

dial to those from the internal carotid and anterior choroidal arteries, and medial to those from the middle cerebral artery.

The recurrent artery is the largest and longest of the branches directed to the anterior perforated substance. It is present, sending branches to the anterior perforated substance, in all hemispheres. The recurrent branches enter the full mediolateral extent of the anterior perforated substance, yet have a limited representation in the anterior-posterior dimension. The territory penetrated by recurrent branches extends into the narrow part of the medial territory above the optic chiasm and into the lateral territory as far as the inner margin of the limen insulae. Their anteroposterior distribution is limited in contrast to their rich mediolateral representation, in that they are confined predominantly to the anterior half of the anterior perforated substance. The branches from recurrent arteries with a more lateral origin from the A1 have a greater tendency to enter the middle and posterior zones than those arising at the junction of the A1 and A2. By virtue of its long mediolateral extent, the recurrent artery borders on the territory of all the other groups entering the anterior perforated substance.

Discussion

In summary, the ICA and AChA branches enter the posterior half of the central portion of the anterior perforated substance. The MCA enters the middle and posterior portions of the lateral half of the anterior perforated substance. The A1 gives rise to branches that enter the medial half of the anterior perforated substance above the optic nerve and chiasm. The recurrent artery sends branches into the anterior two-thirds of the full mediolateral extent of the anterior perforated substance. There are minimal anastomoses and limited overlap between the different groups at the level of the anterior perforated substance, making it most important that each of these groups be protected in operative approaches to the area. There is a reciprocal relationship between the intraparenchymal and anterior perforated substance territories of the ICA, AChA, ACA, and MCA such that the size of one artery's territory increases or decreases the other artery's territory in a reciprocal manner.

The deep cerebral structures located directly above the anterior perforated substance are the frontal horn and the anterior part of the caudate nucleus, putamen, and internal capsule (23). The anterior perforating arteries pass through the parts of the caudate nucleus, putamen, and internal capsule directly above the anterior perforated substance, and spread posteriorly to supply larger parts of these structures and the adjacent areas of the globus pallidus and thalamus (*Fig. 2.32*) (39, pp 30–33). The C4 branches penetrating the anterior perforated substance perfuse the genu of the internal capsule and the adjacent part of the globus pallidus, posterior limb of the internal capsule, and thalamus. The branches of the AChA entering the anterior perforated substance supply the medial two segments of the globus pallidus, the inferior part of the posterior limb of the internal capsule, and the anterior and ventrolateral nuclei of the thalamus. The lateral and intermediate groups of lenticulostriate arteries pass through the putamen and arch medially and posteriorly to supply almost the entire anterior-to-posterior length of the upper part of the internal capsule and the body and head of the caudate nucleus. The medial lenticulostriate arteries irrigate the area medial to and below that supplied by the lateral and intermediate lenticulostriate arteries; this area includes the lateral part of the globus pallidus, the superior part of the anterior limb of the internal capsule, and the anterosuperior part of the head of the caudate nucleus.

The A1 branches supply the area below the anteromedial part to the territory supplied by the lenticulostriate arteries. This region includes the area around the optic chiasm, the anterior commissure, the anterior hypothalamus, the genu of the internal capsule, and the anterior part of the globus pallidus. Its area of supply may less commonly extend to the contiguous part of the posterior limb of the internal capsule and to the anterior part of the thalamus (26). The recurrent artery supplies the most anterior and inferior parts of the head of the caudate nucleus and putamen, and the adjacent part of the anterior limb of the internal capsule (26).

The arteries entering the anterior perforated substance are intrinsically related to and commonly exposed in operations for aneurysms of the internal carotid, anterior communicating, and middle cerebral arteries. These relationships are reviewed in Chapter 3. The intradural exposure of the C4 and all of the arteries sending branches to the anterior perforated substance can be achieved using a small frontotemporal flap centered at the pterion. All of these aneurysms related to the anterior perforating arteries can be exposed by this approach along the ipsilateral sphenoid ridge, with opening of the sylvian fissure. Selected striatal arteriovenous malformations involving the

FIGURE 2.31. *Continued*
lenticulostriate arteries arise near the M1 trifurcation and have a roughly S-shaped course. The intermediate lenticulostriate arteries have a candelabra appearance. The medial lenticulostriate arteries pass near the perforating branches arising from the carotid artery and the medial half of the A1 segment. D, *inferior view, right side. The intermediate lenticulostriate arteries have a candelabra appearance. The A1 branches enter the anterior perforated substance medial to those from the internal carotid, anterior choroidal, and middle cerebral arteries. The recurrent artery arises above the optic chiasm, passes laterally above the carotid bifurcation, and gives rise to branches that enter the anterior perforated substance in front of those from other sources.* E, *perforating branches of the anterior cerebral artery, anterior view. The recurrent artery arises above the optic chiasm near the level of the AComA. The A1 segment arises from the carotid artery and its perforating branches to enter the medial half of the anterior perforated substance in the narrow sector extending above the optic chiasm.* A., *arteries, artery;* A.C.A., *anterior cerebral artery;* Ant., *anterior;* Bifurc., *bifurcation;* Car., *carotid;* Chor., *choroid, choroidal;* Comm., *communicating;* Br., *branch;* Fiss., *fissure;* Front., *frontal;* Gyr., *gyrus;* I.C.A., *internal cerebral artery;* Infund., *infundibulum;* Int., *intermediate;* Interhem., *interhemispheric;* Lat., *lateral;* Len. Str., *lenticulostriate;* Med., *medial;* N., *nerve;* Olf., *olfactory;* Orb., *orbital;* P.C.A., *posterior cerebral artery;* Ped., *peduncle;* Perf., *perforated, perforating;* Plex., *plexus;* Post., *posterior;* Rec., *recurrent;* Subst., *substance, substantia;* Temp., *temporal;* Tr., *tract;* Trifurc., *trifurcation.* (From, *Rosner SS, Rhoton AL Jr, Ono M, Barry M: Microsurgical anatomy of the anterior perforating arteries. **J Neurosurg** 61:468–485, 1984 [36].)*

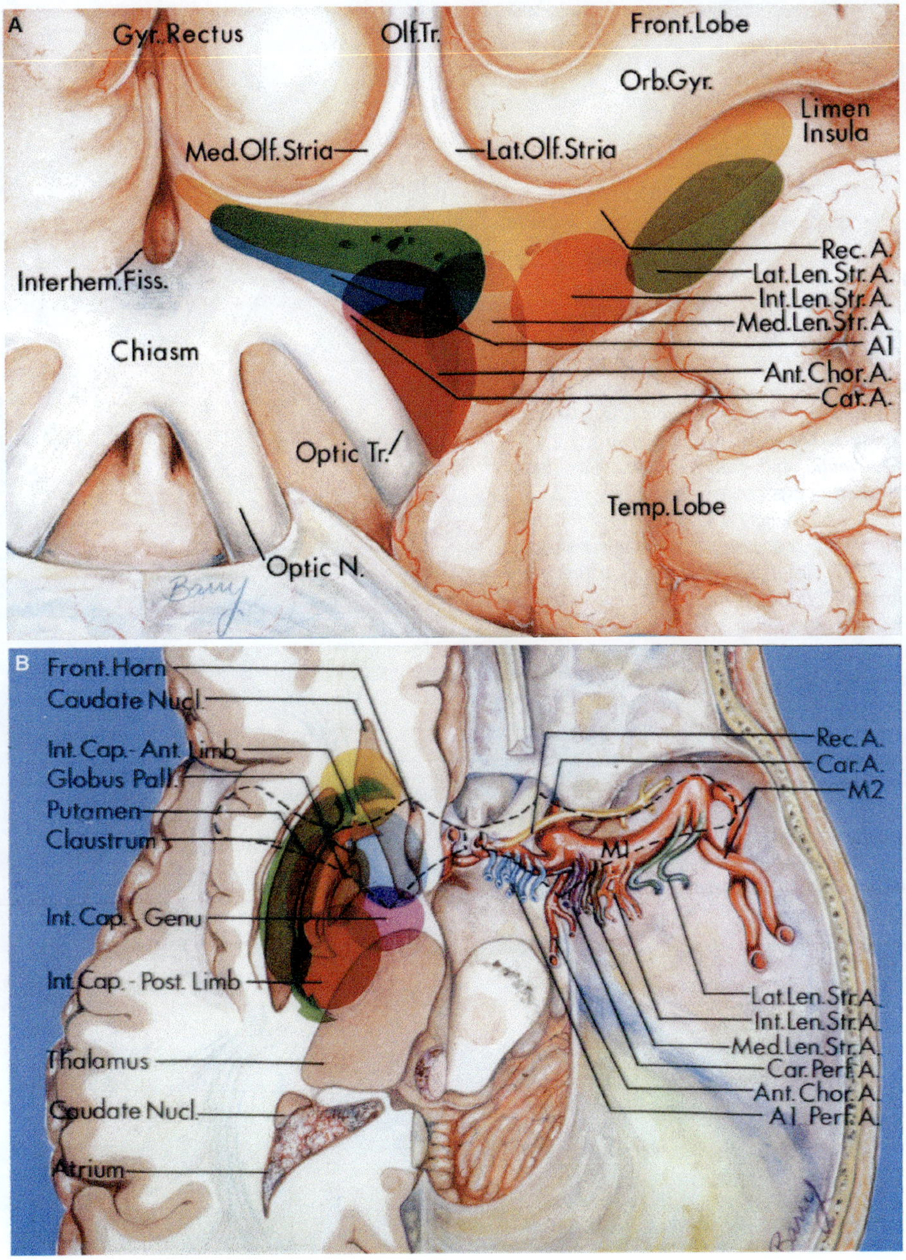

FIGURE 2.32. A, *site of entry of branches of the internal carotid, anterior choroidal, and anterior and middle cerebral arteries into the anterior perforated substance. The anterior perforated substance is located between the frontal and temporal lobes and is bordered anteriorly by the medial and lateral olfactory striae, laterally by the limen insulae, posteriorly by the optic tract and temporal lobe, and medially extends above the optic nerve and chiasm to the interhemispheric fissure. The A1 segment of the anterior cerebral artery gives rise to branches* (blue) *that enter the medial half of the anterior perforated substance above the optic nerve and chiasm. The internal carotid* (purple) *and anterior choroidal arteries* (red) *give rise to branches that enter the posterior part of the central portion of the anterior perforated substance. The middle cerebral artery gives rise to the medial* (brown)*, intermediate* (orange)*, and lateral lenticulostriate arteries* (green) *that enter the middle and posterior portions of the lateral half of the anterior perforated substance. The recurrent artery* (yellow) *sends branches into the anterior half of the full mediolateral extent of the anterior perforated substance. The olfactory tract divides the frontal lobe between the gyrus rectus and the orbital gyri.* B, *relationship of anterior perforating arteries to the deep cerebral structures. Superior view with all of the right cerebral hemisphere and the superior part of the left cerebral hemisphere removed. The site of the anterior perforated substance is shown on both sides by dotted lines. The deep neural structures above the anterior perforated substance are shown on the left side. The transverse section of the left cerebrum extends through the caudate nucleus, thalamus, globus pallidus, putamen, the anterior limb, genu, and posterior limb of the internal capsule, and the frontal horn and atrium of the lateral ventricle. The right side shows the site of origin of the perforating branches to the anterior perforated substance. The branches to the anterior perforated substance pass through the deep structures directly above the anterior perforated substance and spread posteriorly to supply larger parts of the caudate nucleus, putamen, internal capsule, and the adjacent parts of the globus pallidus and thalamus. The C4 branches* (purple) *perfuse the genu of the internal capsule, and the adjacent part of the globus pallidus, posterior limb of the internal capsule, and thalamus. The anterior choroidal branches* (red) *supply the medial two segments of the globus pallidus, the inferior part of the posterior limb of the internal capsule, and the anterior and ventrolateral nuclei of the thalamus. The lateral* (green) *and intermediate groups* (orange) *of lenticulostriate arteries pass through the putamen and the adjacent part of the globus pallidus and arch medially and posteriorly* (arrows) *to supply almost the entire anterior-to-posterior length of the upper part of the internal capsule and the body and head of the caudate nucleus. The medial lenticulostriate arteries* (brown) *irrigate the lateral part of the globus pallidus, the superior part of the anterior limb of the internal capsule, and the anterosuperior part of the head of the caudate nucleus. The A1 branches* (blue) *supply the genu of the internal capsule and the anterior part of the globus pallidus, and may extend to the adjacent part of the posterior limb of the internal capsule and, less commonly, to the thalamus. The recurrent artery* (yellow) *supplies the most anterior and inferior part of the head of the caudate nucleus and putamen, and the adjacent part of the anterior limb of the internal capsule.* (Legend continues on next page.)

arteries entering the anterior perforated substance have been treated by incision of the anterior perforated substance and occlusion of the feeding arteries without producing a deficit (*Fig. 2.16I*) (41). Operative treatment of these arteriovenous malformations is usually considered only if the lesion is located directly above the anterior perforated substance in the area anterior to the genu of the internal capsule, unless the genu and posterior limb of the internal capsule have already been damaged.

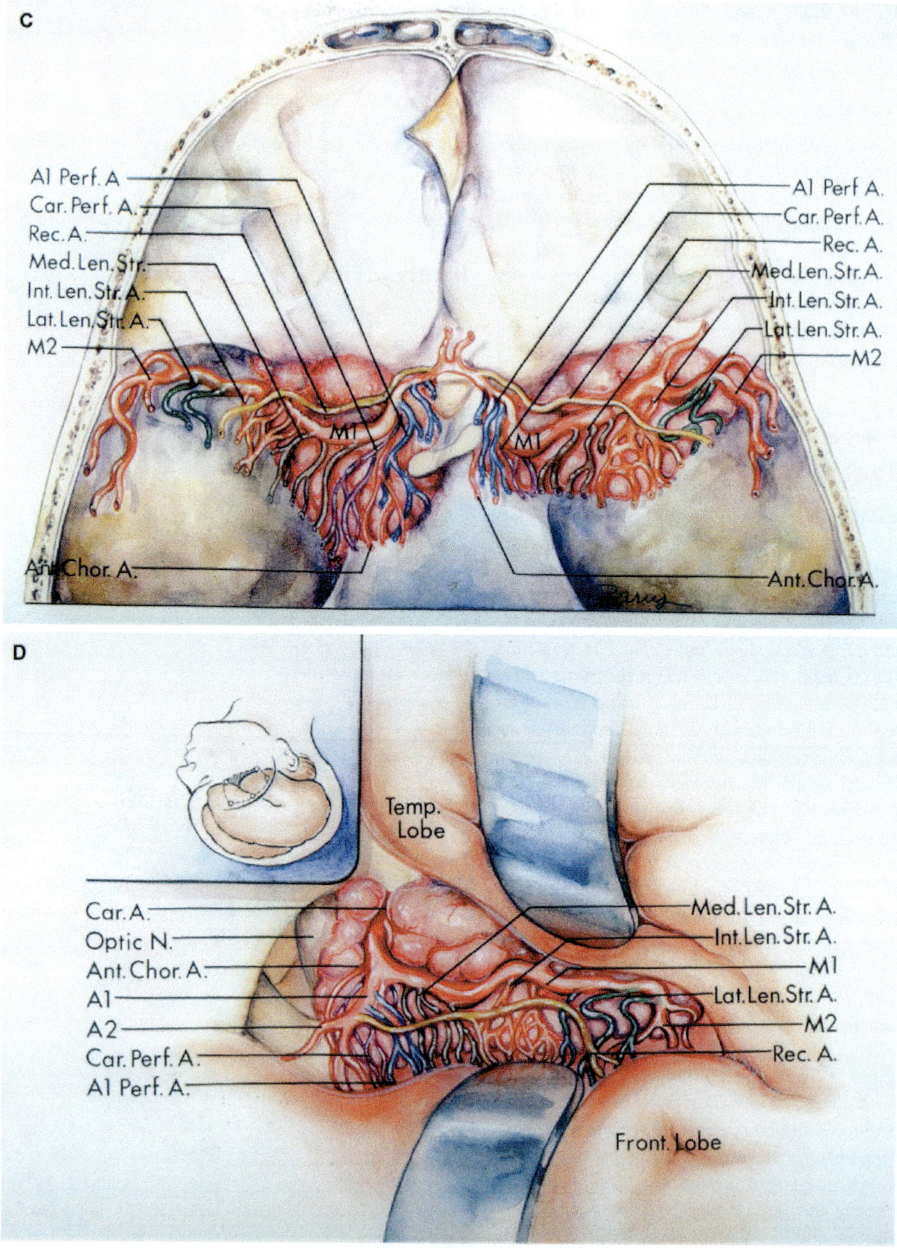

FIGURE 2.32. *Continued*
C–D, relationship of the anterior perforating arteries to tumors along the sphenoid ridge. C, superior view. The anterior perforating arteries are stretched across the upper surface of a sphenoid ridge meningioma. D, pterional exposure. The incision is shown in the inset. *The frontal and temporal lobes have been retracted to expose the carotid artery, which is encased by tumor. The anterior perforating arteries are stretched across the upper surface of the tumor. It is best to debulk a tumor of this type before separating the tumor capsule from the perforating arteries by using careful microtechnique.* A., *arteries, artery;* Ant., *anterior;* Cap., *capsule;* Car., *carotid;* Chor., *choroidal;* Fiss., *fissure;* Front., *frontal;* Gyr., *gyrus;* Int., *intermediate, internal;* Interhem., *interhemispheric;* Lat., *lateral;* Lent. Str., *lenticulostriate;* Med., *medial;* N., *nerve;* Nucl., *nucleus;* Olf., *olfactory;* Orb., *orbital;* Pall., *pallidus;* Perf., *perforating;* Post., *posterior;* Rec., *recurrent;* Temp., *temporal;* Tr., *tract.* *(From, Rosner SS, Rhoton AL Jr, Ono M, Barry M: Microsurgical anatomy of the anterior perforating arteries.* J Neurosurg *61:468–485, 1984 [36].)*

THE POSTERIOR PART OF THE CIRCLE OF WILLIS

The posterior part of the circle of Willis is formed by the proximal PCA and PComA and, together, in varying degrees, they provide the flow to the distal PCA (*Figs. 2.8, 2.33,* and *2.34*). The posterior circle is one of the most difficult sites to approach surgically because of its location in the midline below the third ventricle, the complex series of perforating vessels surrounding and arising from it, and its intimate relationship to the extraocular nerves and upper brainstem. Its branches are exposed in surgical approaches to the basilar apex, tentorial notch, lateral and third ventricles, inferior temporal and medial parieto-occipital areas, and the pineal region—all relatively inaccessible areas.

A normal posterior circle, in which the proximal PCAs have a diameter larger than their PComAs and are not hypoplastic, is present in approximately half of the brains (*Figs. 2.8* and *2.34*). The other half harbor anomalies of the posterior circle, including either a hypoplastic PComA or a fetal configuration in which the proximal PCA is small and the PComA provides the major supply to the PCA and is larger than the P1 (24).

A hypoplastic arterial segment is defined as one having a diameter of 1 mm or less. In our study, PComA hypoplasia was found unilaterally in 26% and bilaterally in 6%, and a fetal configuration, in which the PCA arises predominantly from

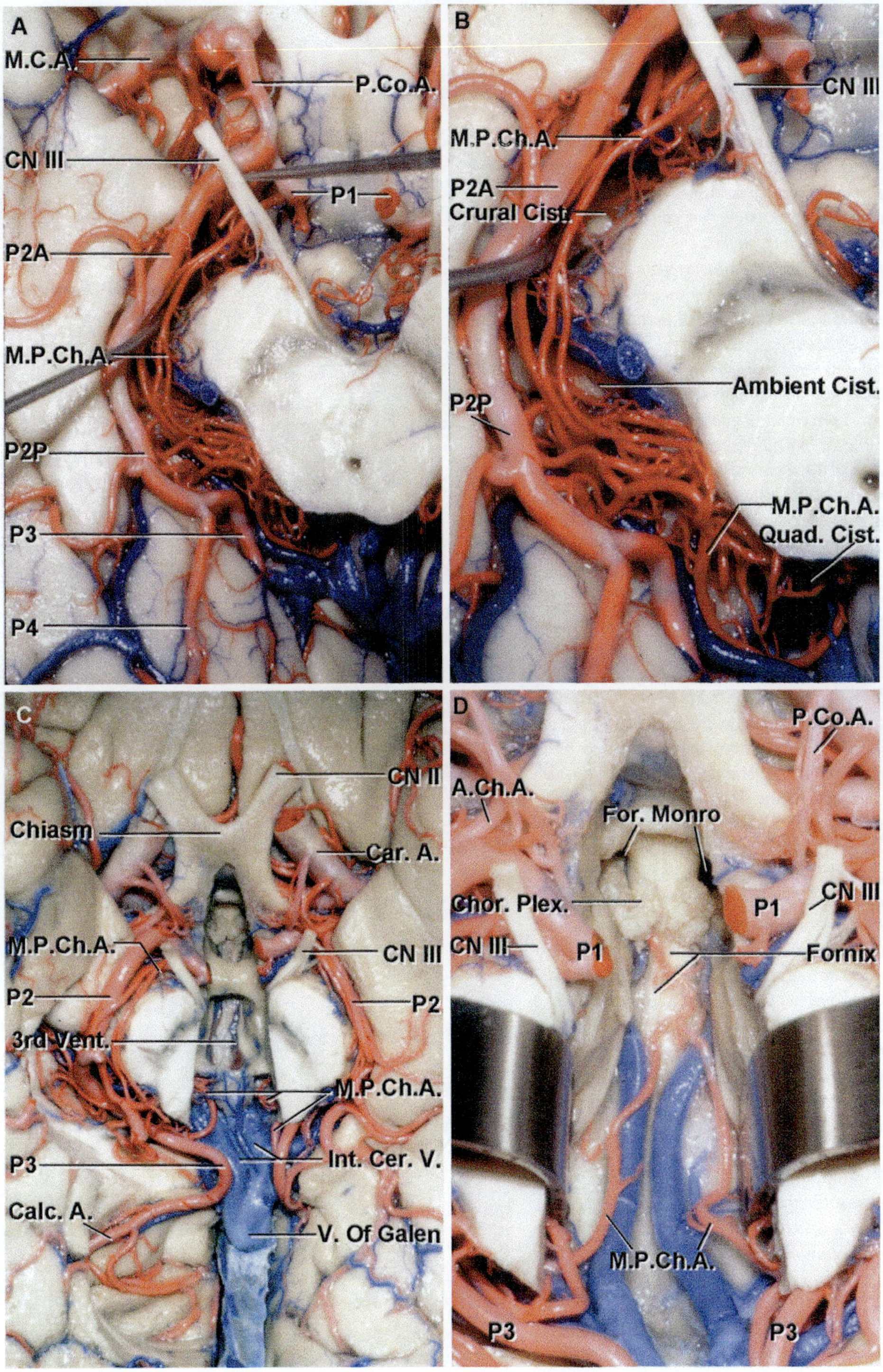

FIGURE 2.33. *Posterior choroidal arteries. A, inferior view of the posterior cerebral artery. The medial posterior choroidal artery arises from the P1 and encircles the brainstem on the medial side of the P2 and P3, giving off small branches to the brainstem along its course. The P3 is formed by the branches in the quadrigeminal cistern. B, enlarged view. The medial posterior choroidal artery encircles the brainstem in the crural, ambient, and quadrigeminal cisterns and turns forward beside the pineal in the quadrigeminal cistern to reach the roof of the third ventricle. C, inferior view of the posterior cerebral arteries in another specimen, with the floor of the third ventricle removed. The medial posterior arteries encircle the midbrain and turn forward in the quadrigeminal cistern to reach the roof of the third ventricle. Some of the medial part of the right parahippocampal gyrus has been removed to expose the branches arising from the P2. D, enlarged view. The lower layer of tela in the roof of the third ventricle has been opened to expose the medial posterior choroidal arteries coursing in the velum interpositum with the branches of the internal cerebral vein. The choroid plexus in the body of the lateral ventricle is continuous at the posterior margin of the foramen of Monro with the choroid plexus in the roof of the third ventricle, which has been removed. (Legend continues on next page.)*

the carotid artery, was found unilaterally in 20% and bilaterally in 2% (37). Eight percent had a hypoplastic communicating artery on one side and a fetal complex on the other side. Absence of either the communicating artery or a P1 segment is very uncommon. The PComA is described above.

The posterior portion of the circle of Willis sends a series of perforating arteries into the diencephalon and midbrain that may become stretched around suprasellar tumors or posterior circle aneurysms (*Figs. 2.33* and *2.34*). Some of the perforating branches arising from the upper part of the basilar artery overlap with some of those arising from the posterior circle. The risks of occlusion of these vital perforating vessels during tumor or aneurysm surgery include visual loss, somatesthetic disturbances, motor weakness, memory deficits, autonomic

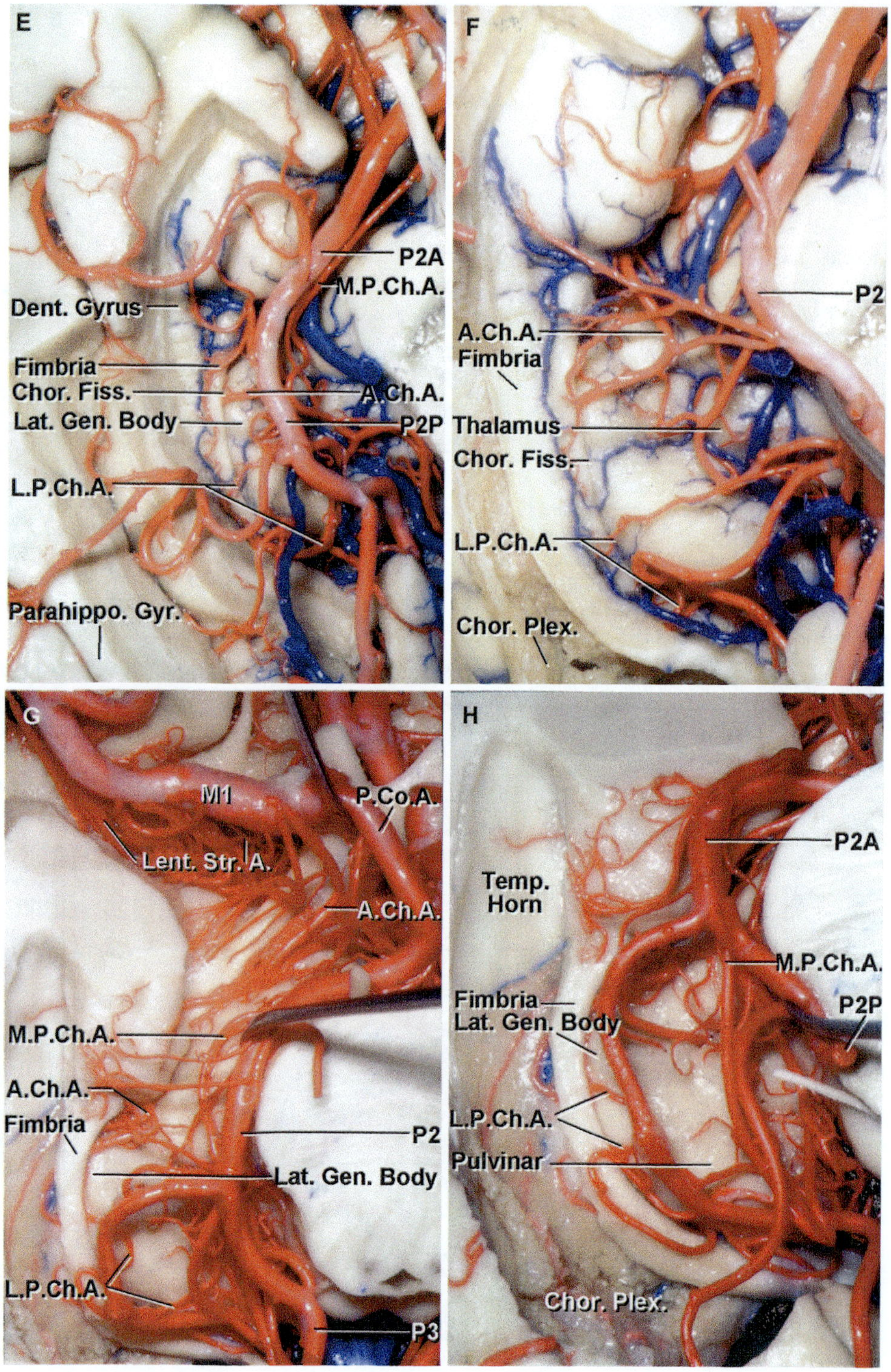

FIGURE 2.33. *Continued*
E, the medial part of the left parahippocampal gyrus has been removed to expose the lateral posterior choroidal arteries arising from the P2 and passing through the choroidal fissure located between the fimbria and thalamus to reach the choroid plexus in the temporal horn. Perforating branches like the thalamogeniculate arteries also arise from the P2 and ascend to penetrate the lower surface of the thalamus in the region of the geniculate bodies. F, enlarged view with the lower part of the hippocampal gyrus removed while preserving the fimbria. The P2 has been retracted medially to expose the lateral posterior choroidal arteries passing through the choroidal fissure located between the fimbria and thalamus to enter the choroid plexus in the temporal horn. The anterior choroidal artery is also seen passing through the fissure. G, another specimen. The M1 and P1 and P2 give rise to a series of perforating branches that enter the basal surface of the brain. The P2 has been retracted to expose the lateral posterior choroidal branches passing laterally through the choroidal fissure to reach the choroid plexus in the temporal horn and atrium. The parahippocampal gyrus has been removed. The fimbria and thalamus border the choroidal fissure. The lateral geniculate body protrudes from the lower margin of the thalamus. H, enlarged view. The lateral posterior choroidal artery passes laterally through the choroidal fissure to reach the choroid plexus. The medial posterior choroidal encircles the brainstem. A., *arteries, artery;* A.Ch.A., *anterior choroidal artery;* Calc., *calcarine;* Car., *carotid;* Cer., *cerebral;* Chor., *choroid, choroidal;* Cist., *cistern;* CN, *cranial nerve;* Dent., *dentate;* Fiss., *fissure;* For., *foramen;* Gen., *geniculate;* Gyr., *gyrus;* Int., *internal;* Lat., *lateral;* Lent. Str., *lenticulostriate;* L.P.Ch.A., *lateral posterior choroidal artery;* M.C.A., *middle cerebral artery;* M.P.Ch.A., *medial posterior choroidal artery;* Parahippo., *parahippocampal;* P.Co.A., *posterior communicating artery;* Plex., *plexus;* Quad., *quadrigeminal;* Temp., *temporal;* V., *vein;* Vent., *ventricle.*

imbalance, diplopia, alterations of consciousness, abnormal movements, and endocrine disturbances.

THE POSTERIOR CEREBRAL ARTERY

The PCA arises at the basilar bifurcation, is joined by the PComA at the lateral margin of the interpeduncular cistern, encircles the brainstem passing through the crural and ambient cisterns to reach the quadrigeminal cistern, and is distributed to the posterior part of the hemisphere (*Figs. 2.1, 2.3, 2.7–2.9, 2.12, 2.13, 2.33,* and *2.34*). The posterior cerebral artery supplies not only the posterior part of the cerebral hemispheres, as its name implies, but also sends critical branches to the thalamus, midbrain, and other deep structures, including the choroid plexus

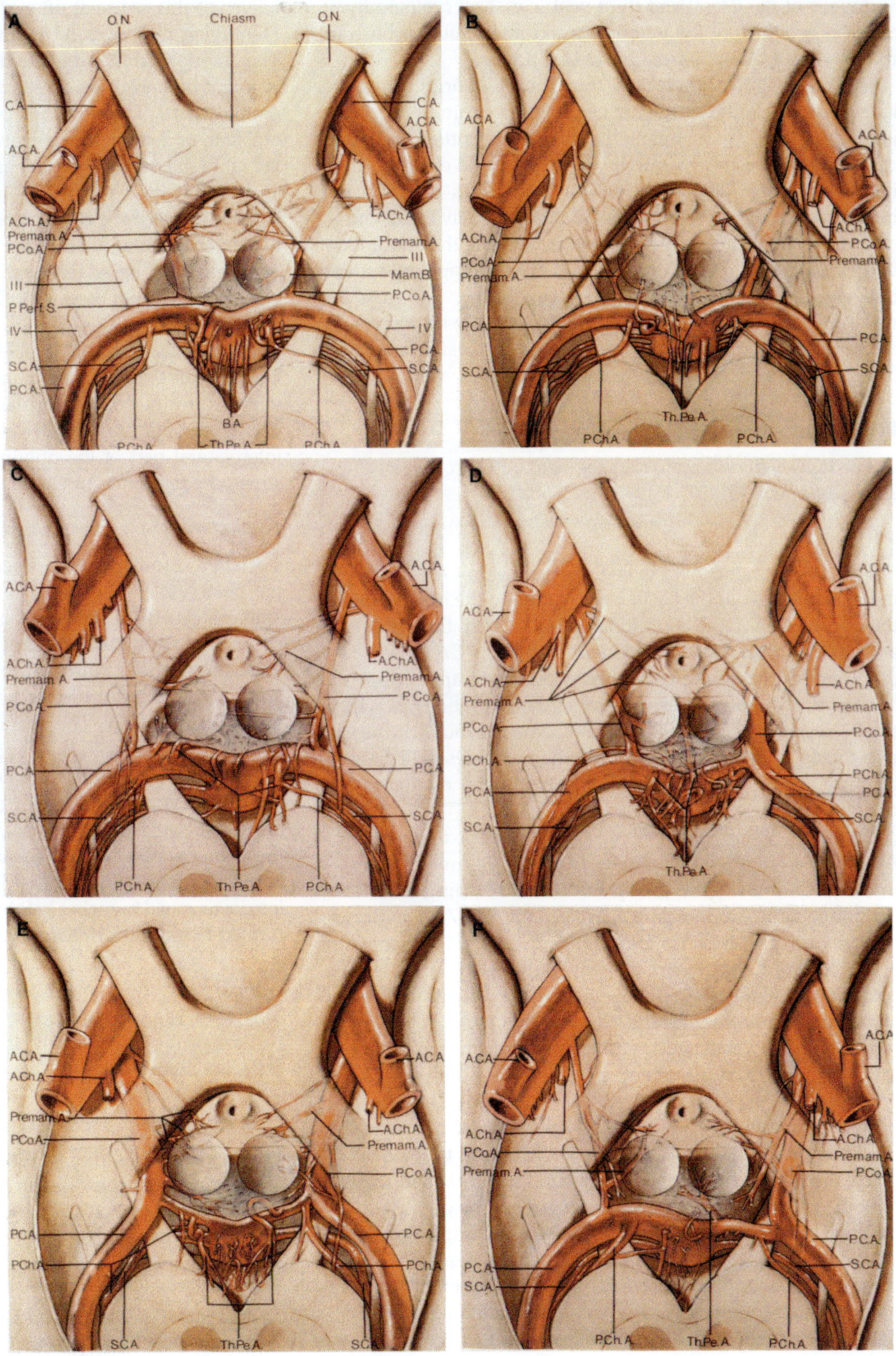

FIGURE 2.34. *Superior view of the basilar, superior cerebellar, P1, and distal segments of posterior cerebral, posterior communicating, internal carotid, and proximal anterior choroidal arteries. The arterial branches below the posterior perforating substance, mamillary bodies, optic tracts, chiasm, and nerves are shown in* half tone. *The third and fourth nerves course between the superior cerebellar and posterior cerebral arteries. Arterial branches to the upper pons, posterior mesencephalon, interpeduncular fossa, posterior perforating substance, mamillary bodies, tuber cinereum, optic tracts, and chiasm arise from the basilar, P1, posterior communicating, and internal carotid arteries.* A, *normal configuration of the posterior half of the circle of Willis; both P1s are larger than communicating arteries and the latter are not hypoplastic (diameter more than 1 mm). The right superior cerebellar artery is duplicated. The largest right P1 branch gives rise to both the thalamoperforating and the posterior choroidal arteries. Only two perforating arteries arise on the right P1. The left posterior choroidal arises on P2. Both premamillary arteries (largest communicating trunk to premamillary area) arise from the middle third of the PComAs. AChAs arise as a single trunk.* B, *hypoplastic left communicating artery. Thalamoperforating artery arises on P1 medial to the posterior choroidal arteries on both sides. The left premamillary artery arises from the posterior and the right from the anterior portion of the PComA. The superior cerebellar arteries are duplicated on both sides.* C, *PComAs are hypoplastic bilaterally. The largest right P1 branch gives rise to both the thalamoperforating and the PChAs. The thalamoperforating artery arises medial to the posterior choroidal artery on the left P1. The premamillary artery arises from the anterior third of the right PComA and from the middle third on the left. The left anterior choroidal arises from the carotid as two trunks.* D, *fetal origin of the right posterior cerebral artery. The thalamoperforating artery on the right arises near the basilar bifurcation. The right posterior choroidal artery arises on P2. The left posterior choroidal artery arises medial to the thalamoperforating artery. The right premamillary artery arises from the anterior portion of the communicating artery. The left premamillary area is supplied by a group of nearly equal-sized arteries. The anterior choroidal artery bifurcates immediately after origin on the left.* E, *bilateral fetal origin of the posterior cerebral artery. The right posterior choroidal artery arises lateral to the thalamoperforating artery. The largest left P1 branch gives rise to the thalamoperforating and choroidal arteries. The right premamillary artery arises from the middle portion of the communicating artery. A premamillary arterial complex is present on the left.* F, *fetal type of right posterior cerebral origin and hypoplastic left communicating artery. The right posterior choroidal artery arises lateral to the well-developed thalamoperforating artery. No thalamoperforating branches are present on the left. The right premamillary artery arises from the anterior and the left from the posterior portion of the communicating artery.* A., *artery;* A.C.A., *anterior cerebral artery;* A.Ch.A., *anterior choroidal artery;* B., *body;* B.A., *basilar artery;* C.A., *carotid artery;* Mam., *mamillary;* N., *nerve;* O., *optic;* P.C.A., *posterior cerebral artery;* P.Ch.A., *posterior choroid artery;* P.Co.A., *posterior communicating artery;* P.Perf.S., *posterior perforated substance;* Premam., *premamillary;* S.C.A., *superior cerebellar artery;* Th.Pe., *thalamoperforating.* (From, *Saeki N, Rhoton AL Jr: Microsurgical anatomy of the upper basilar artery and the posterior circle of Willis.* ***J Neurosurg*** *46:563–578, 1977 [37].)*

and walls of the lateral and third ventricles. Embryologically, it arises as a branch of the internal carotid artery, but by birth its most frequent origin is from the basilar artery.

The basilar bifurcation, and thus the PCA origin, may be located as far caudal as 1.3 mm below the pontomesencephalic junction and as far rostral as the mamillary bodies and adjacent floor of the third ventricle, which may be elevated by a high bifurcation. The artery usually bifurcates opposite the interpeduncular fossa, but some bifurcations may be as low as the upper pons or so high that they indent the mamillary bodies and floor of the third ventricle. The average separation between the basilar bifurcation and mamillary bodies is 8.1 mm (range, 0–14 mm). There is widening of the basilar artery at the bifurcation in 16% of cases, giving the basilar apex and bifurcation a cobra-like appearance (37, 43).

PCA Segments

The PCA is divided into four segments, P1 through P4 (*Figs. 2.12–2.14* and *2.33*) (37, 43).

P1 Segment

The P1 segment, also called the precommunicating segment, extends from the basilar bifurcation to the junction with the PComA. A fetal configuration, in which the P1 has a smaller diameter than the PComA and the PCA arises predominantly from the carotid artery, occurs in approximately one-third of hemispheres. A normal configuration, in which the P1 segment is larger than the PComA, is found in nearly two-thirds of hemispheres. A few hemispheres will have a PComA and P1 of the same diameter. A fetal configuration may be present on both sides.

P1 length varies, being longer if there is a fetal pattern. Average P1 length, which ranges from 3 to 14 mm, is approximately 9.0 mm in the group with a fetal configuration as compared with 7.0 mm in a normal pattern (37). The oculomotor nerve passes below and slightly lateral to the PComA if a normal configuration is present; but if a fetal pattern is present, P1 is longer and the nerve courses beneath or medial to the communicating artery.

The relatively constant branches arising from the P1 are 1) the thalamoperforating artery, which by definition enters the brain through the posterior perforated substance; 2) the medial posterior choroidal artery directed to the choroid plexus in the third ventricle and lateral ventricle; 3) the branch to the quadrigeminal plate; and 4) rami to the cerebral peduncle and mesencephalic tegmentum. The superior cerebellar artery (SCA) arises from the basilar artery at a level between the P1 origin and 7 mm below (average, 2.5 mm) (37). The SCA may infrequently have a common origin with the P1 or arise from P1. The initial segment gives rise to perforating vessels whose termination may overlap with those arising from the basilar apex and P1.

P2 Segment

The P2 segment begins at the PComA, lies within the crural and ambient cisterns, and terminates lateral to the posterior edge of the midbrain. The P2 is divided into an anterior and posterior part because the surgical approaches to the anterior and posterior halves of this segment often differ, and because it is helpful in identifying the origin of the many branches that arise from P2. The anterior part is designated the P2A or crural or peduncular segment because it courses around the cerebral peduncle in the crural cistern. The posterior part is designated the P2P or the ambient or lateral mesencephalic segment because it courses lateral to the midbrain in the ambient cistern. Both segments are approximately 25 mm long. The P2A begins at the PComA and courses between the cerebral peduncle and uncus that forms the medial and lateral walls of the crural cistern, and inferior to the optic tract and basal vein that crosses the roof of the cistern, to enter the proximal portion of the ambient cistern. The P2P commences at the posterior edge of the cerebral peduncle at the junction of the crural and ambient cisterns. It courses between the lateral midbrain and the parahippocampal and dentate gyri, which form the medial and lateral walls of the ambient cistern, below the optic tract, basal vein, and geniculate bodies and the inferolateral part of the pulvinar in the roof of the cistern, and superomedial to the trochlear nerve and tentorial edge.

P3 Segment

The P3 or quadrigeminal segment proceeds posteriorly from the posterior edge of the lateral surface of the midbrain and ambient cistern to reach the lateral part of the quadrigeminal cistern and ends at the anterior limit of the calcarine fissure. The PCA often divides into its major terminal branches, the calcarine and parieto-occipital arteries, before reaching the anterior limit of the calcarine fissure. The average length of the P3 segment is 2 cm. The P3s from both sides approach each other posterior to the colliculi. The point where the PCAs from each side are nearest is referred to as the collicular or quadrigeminal point. The separation averages 8.9 mm (range, 3.5–17 mm) (43). The artery forming the collicular point is the PCA trunk in approximately half of the hemispheres, and in the other half, in which the PCA bifurcates into its terminal branches before reaching the collicular point, it is formed by the calcarine artery.

P4 Segment

The P4 segment includes the branches distributed to the cortical surface. Posteriorly, it begins at the anterior end of the calcarine sulcus.

PCA Branches

The PCA gives rise to three types of branches: 1) central perforating branches to the diencephalon and midbrain; 2) ventricular branches to the choroid plexus and walls of the lateral and third ventricles and adjacent structures; and 3) cerebral branches to the cerebral cortex and splenium of the corpus callosum (*Fig. 2.33*). The central branches include the direct and circumflex perforating arteries, including the thalamoperforating, peduncular perforating, and thalamogeniculate arteries. The ventricular branches are the lateral and medial posterior choroidal arteries. The cerebral branches include the inferior temporal group of branches, which are divided into hippocampal and the anterior, middle, posterior, and common temporal branches, plus the parieto-occipital, calcarine, and splenial branches.

The long and short circumflex and thalamoperforating arteries arise predominantly from P1, and the other PCA branches most frequently arise from P2 or P3. The hippocampal, anterior temporal, peduncular perforating, and medial posterior choroidal arteries most frequently arise from P2A. The middle temporal, posterior temporal, common temporal, and lateral posterior choroidal arteries most frequently arise from P2P. The thalamogeniculate arteries arise only slightly more frequently from P2P than from P2A. The calcarine and parieto-occipital arteries most frequently arise from P3.

Perforating Branches

The central branches are divided into two groups: direct perforating and circumflex arteries (*Figs. 2.34* and *2.35*). The direct perforating branches pass directly from the parent trunk to the brainstem. This group includes the thalamoperforating arteries that arise from P1 and the thalamogeniculate and peduncular perforating arteries that arise from P2. The circumflex branches encircle the brainstem for a variable distance before entering the diencephalon and mesencephalon are divided into long and short groups, depending on how far they course around the brainstem.

An average of four, but as many as a dozen perforating branches, the largest of which may have a diameter of 1.5 mm, arise mainly from the superior and posterior surfaces of the P1, course superiorly and posteriorly, and divide into numerous branches that terminate in the interpeduncular fossa, posterior perforated substance, cerebral peduncle, mamillary bodies, and posterior midbrain. Perforating branches rarely arise from the anterior side of the basilar apex, but they arise from the anterior surface in a third of P1s, and terminate in the posterior perforated substance and mamillary bodies. The largest P1 branch is a thalamoperforating artery (42% of hemispheres), a posterior choroidal artery (40%), or a large trunk from which both arteries arise (18%) (37). The P1s with the larger branches tend to have few perforating branches. P1s having only one or two P1 perforators tend to have larger branches. If the largest P1 branch is relatively small, there will be more P1 branches. More perforating vessels arise on P1 lateral to the largest perforator than medial to it.

The posterior and lateral surfaces of the upper centimeter of the basilar artery is also a rich source of perforating arteries that overlap with those arising from the P1. An average of 8 (range, 3–18) branches arise from the upper centimeter; approximately

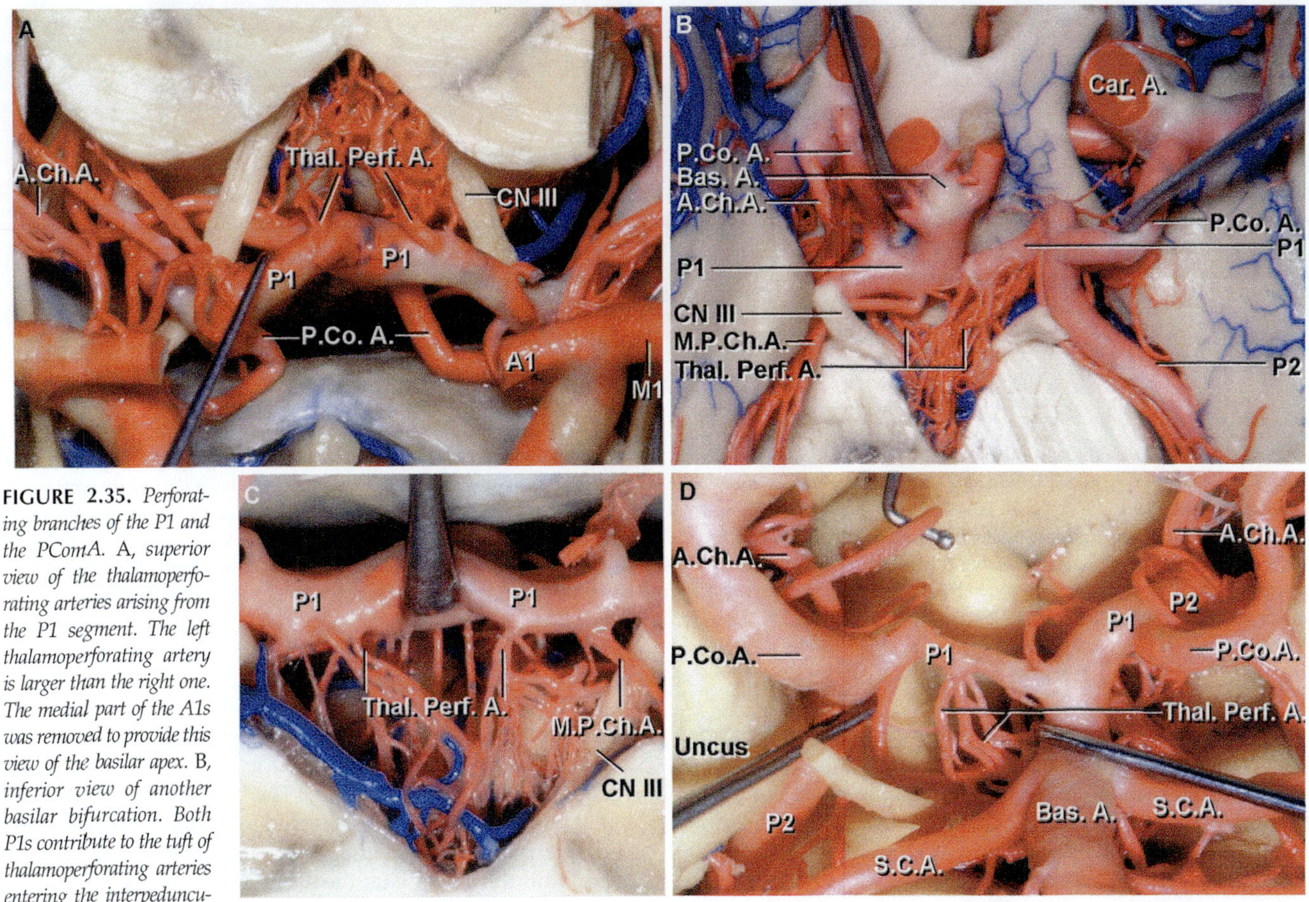

FIGURE 2.35. *Perforating branches of the P1 and the PComA. A, superior view of the thalamoperforating arteries arising from the P1 segment. The left thalamoperforating artery is larger than the right one. The medial part of the A1s was removed to provide this view of the basilar apex. B, inferior view of another basilar bifurcation. Both P1s contribute to the tuft of thalamoperforating arteries entering the interpeduncular fossa. The right AChA courses above and lateral to the PComA and turns laterally above the uncus. An MPChA arises from the right P1. C, superior view of the thalamoperforating arteries arising from P1. The basilar artery, below the P1 origins, also send perforating branches in the same area. D, inferior view. The right P1 is much smaller than the left P1, but the right P1 gives rise to a tuft of thalamoperforating arteries that pass upward to enter the interpeduncular fossa. A nerve hook holds up a premamillary branch of the PComA. (Legend continues on next page.)*

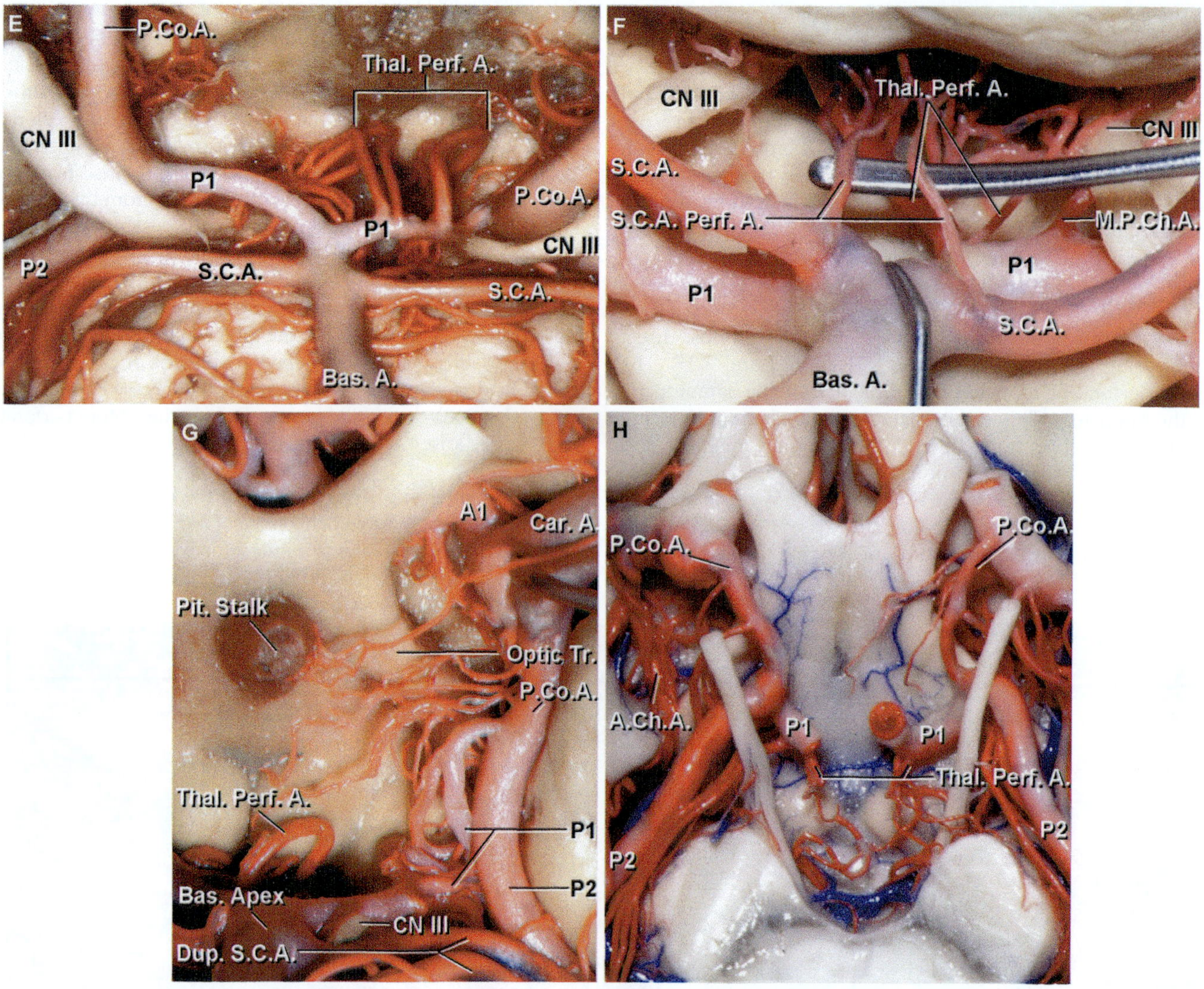

FIGURE 2.35. *Continued*
E, *both P1s are smaller than the PComAs, but both P1s give rise to thalamoperforating arteries. The smaller, or left, P1 gives rise to more and larger perforating arteries than the larger, right, P1.* F, *the dissector holds up two perforating branches that arise from the origin of the superior cerebellar artery and enter the brain through the same area as the thalamoperforating arteries.* G, *the left PCA has a fetal origin of the PComA. A series of perforating arteries arises from the PComA and enters the diencephalon medial to the optic tract in the region of the mamillary bodies and floor of the third ventricle. The P1 pursues a tortuous course to its junction with the P2.* H, *inferior view. The lateral parts of the P1s give rise to thalamoperforating arteries. Perforating branches also arise from the PComA.* A., *artery;* A.Ch.A., *anterior choroidal artery;* Bas., *basilar;* Car., *carotid;* CN, *cranial nerve;* Dup., *duplicate;* M.P.Ch.A., *medial posterior choroidal artery;* P.Co.A., *posterior communicating artery;* Perf., *perforating;* Pit., *pituitary;* S.C.A., *superior cerebellar artery;* Thal. Perf., *thalamoperforating;* Tr., *tract.*

half arise from the posterior surface and a quarter from each side (37). The more medial branches, called median or paramedian branches, enter the midbrain and pons near the midline, and the lateral ones, called transverse or circumferential branches, terminate in the lateral pons, peduncle, and posterior perforated substance.

Thalamoperforating Arteries

The thalamoperforating arteries arise on the P1 and enter the brain by passing through the posterior perforated substance and the medial part of the cerebral peduncles in the area behind the mamillary bodies in the upper part of the interpeduncular fossa (*Fig. 2.35*). The branches of the PComA that enter the same area are referred to as premamillary arteries. The majority of thalamoperforating arteries originate on the middle third of P1 as the P1 branch nearest the basilar bifurcation, but they may also arise on the medial or lateral third. If the first branch is not a thalamoperforating artery, it is a circumflex branch that terminates in the peduncle or posterior mesencephalic area. The thalamoperforating artery is the largest P1 branch in most cases (37). They almost always arise from the posterior or superior aspect of P1 and only infrequently from the anterior surface. A P1, even when of normal or large size, may infrequently not give rise to a thalamoperforating artery, in which case, the contralateral side will have well-developed thalamoperforating branches that supply the area normally perfused by the absent thalamoperforating artery. They supply the anterior and part of the posterior thalamus and hypothalamus, the subthalamus and the medial part of the upper midbrain, including the substantia nigra, red nucleus, oculomotor and trochlear nuclei, oculomotor nerve, mesencephalic reticular formation, pretectum, rostromedial floor of the fourth ventricle, and the posterior portion of the internal capsule (39, pp 96–99; 43).

Deficits related to the loss of these arteries include somatesthetic disturbances caused by involvement of the afferent pathways in the medial lemniscus or thalamus; motor weakness caused by involvement of the corticospinal tracts in the internal capsule or peduncle; memory deficits caused by involvement of hypothalamic pathways entering and exiting from the mamillary bodies; autonomic imbalance caused by disturbance of sympathetic and parasympathetic centers in the anterior and posterior diencephalon; diplopia caused by involvement of the extraocular nerves or nuclei in the midbrain; alterations of consciousness caused by ischemia of the midbrain reticular formation; abnormal movements caused by involvement of cerebellothalamic circuits in the midbrain and thalamus; and endocrine disturbances caused by involvement of the hypothalamic-pituitary axis. Occlusion of the thalamoperforating arteries, depending on the size of the area of ischemia, may produce a variety of more focal syndromes including contralateral hemiplegia, cerebellar ataxia, or a "rubral" tremor associated with ipsilateral oculomotor nerve paresis (Nothnagel's syndrome). If the lesion affects the subthalamus, it may produce contralateral hemiballismus, which abates into choreiform movements with time or treatment (43).

Peduncular Perforating Arteries

The peduncular perforating branches, usually two or three, but as many as six, arise from the P2 segment and pass directly from the PCA into the cerebral peduncle. They supply the corticospinal and corticobulbar pathways as well as the substantia nigra, red nucleus, and other structures of the tegmentum, and may send branches to the oculomotor nerve.

Circumflex Branches

The circumflex groups of arteries arise from the P1 and P2 and encircle the midbrain parallel and medial to the PCA. They are divided into a short and long circumflex group. The short circumflex branches reach only as far as the geniculate bodies. The long circumflex branches reach the colliculi. The short circumflex arteries course medial to the P2 and the medial posterior choroidal and the long circumflex arteries, and send branches to the cerebral peduncle as they proceed to their distal termination, which may range from the posterolateral border of the peduncle to the medial geniculate bodies. Those arising from P2 supply only the geniculate bodies and the midbrain tegmentum. The short circumflex arteries may send rami to the area of the interpeduncular fossa and posterior perforated substance, which are supplied predominantly by the thalamoperforating arteries (37).

The long circumflex arteries, referred to as the quadrigeminal arteries, are present in almost all hemispheres, pass around the brainstem to reach the quadrigeminal cistern, and supply the quadrigeminal bodies. They encircle the midbrain medial to the PCA and send small rami to the cerebral peduncle and geniculate bodies and occasionally to the tegmentum, pulvinar, and end at the quadrigeminal plate. They usually arise from the P1 or P2A. The terminal branches of the long circumflex form a rich arterial network over the colliculi, where they anastomose with branches from the superior cerebellar artery. The superior colliculus is supplied by the branches arising from the PCA and the inferior colliculus is supplied by branches of the superior cerebellar artery. Occlusion of the long circumflex (quadrigeminal) artery may result in defects of vertical gauge caused by infarction of the posterior commissure or of the nuclei of Darkschewitsch or Cajal (Parinaud's syndrome) (40).

Thalamogeniculate Arteries

The thalamogeniculate arteries arise directly from the P2 beneath the lateral thalamus and penetrate the part of the roof of the ambient cistern formed by the geniculate bodies and surrounding area. The PCA most commonly gives origin to two or three thalamogeniculate arteries, but there may be as many as seven. They arise near the junction of the crural (P2A) and ambient (P2P) segments, with a nearly equal number arising from each segment.

The thalamogeniculate arteries supply the posterior half of the lateral thalamus, posterior limb of the internal capsule, and the optic tract (39, pp 96–99). They meet the thalamoperforating branches of P1 near the middle of the thalamus and the thalamic branches of the PComA anteriorly in the lateral nucleus. The long and short circumflex and medial posterior choroidal arteries also send branches to this area as they encircle the brainstem, but the term thalamogeniculate arteries is reserved for those branches arising from the P2 and passing through the geniculate bodies and adjacent part of the roof of the ambient cistern.

Infarction of the area supplied by the thalamogeniculate arteries results in the thalamic syndrome of Dejerine and Roussy, consisting of a contralateral loss of superficial and particularly of deep sensation with an intense, intractable, hyperpathic pain on the affected side, with extreme hypersensitivity to mild touch, pain, and temperature stimuli, a contralateral hemiplegia, often transient and sometimes associated with choreoathetoid or dystonic movements of the paralyzed side, with possibly a homonymous hemianopsia (7, 22). There is usually a permanent disturbance of deep sensibility (position sense, heavy contact, and deep pressure) and, although the threshold to cutaneous stimuli is elevated, a threshold stimulus evokes a disagreeable burning, agonizing type of pain response, and there may be spontaneous pain. The limbs are affected more than the face.

In one such case reported in 1906, Dejerine and Roussy (7) found infarction in the posterior third of the lateral thalamic nucleus, part of the medial and centromedian nuclei and the pulvinar, the posterior limb of the internal capsule, and posterior part of the lentiform nucleus, but they did not find an occlusion of any PCA branch. The fact that the area is supplied not only by multiple thalamogeniculate arteries, but also by the circumflex and choroidal branches of the PCA, makes it unlikely that occlusion of a single thalamogeniculate artery would produce the complete syndrome. It would more likely be caused by a PCA occlusion proximal to the origin of all of these branches. Arterial occlusion is the most common cause of a typical thalamic syndrome, although vascular malformations or tumors of the thalamus may be a cause (43).

Ventricular and Choroid Plexus Branches

The posterior choroidal arteries, the branches of the PCA that enter the lateral and third ventricles to supply the choroid plexus and ventricular walls, are divided into medial and lateral groups referred to as the medial posterior (MPChA) and lateral posterior choroidal arteries (LPChA), depending on the origin and area of supply (*Figs. 2.12, 2.13,* and *2.33*) (13). The MPChAs most frequently arise from the posteromedial aspect of the proximal half of the PCA or one of its branches, encircle the midbrain medial to the main trunk of the PCA, turn forward at the lateral side of the pineal gland to enter the roof of the third ventricle between the thalami, and finally course through the choroidal fissure and foramen of Monro to enter the choroid plexus in the lateral ventricle. The MPChAs send branches along their course to the peduncle, tegmentum, geniculate bodies (medial and lateral, but primarily the former), the colliculi, pulvinar, pineal gland, and medial thalamus.

Most hemispheres have a single MPChA, but there may be as many as three (43). Most arise in the P2, but they may arise from the P3 or from the parieto-occipital and calcarine branches. Those MPChAs arising from the parieto-occipital and calcarine arteries and the distal PCA course in a retrograde fashion from their origin to enter the roof of the third ventricle.

The LPChAs arise from the PCA or its branches and pass laterally through the choroidal fissure to supply the choroid plexus of the lateral ventricle. The number of LPChAs in one hemisphere ranges from one to nine (average, four) (13). They most commonly arise directly from the P2P, but may also arise from the P2A or P3, or from some of the PCA branches. The largest LPChAs arise directly from the P2P in the ambient cistern, pass laterally through the choroidal fissure to the choroid plexus of the temporal horn and the glomus of the plexus in the atrium, and anastomose on the choroid plexus within the branches of the AChA and MPChA. The LPChAs may send branches to the cerebral peduncle, posterior commissure, part of the crura and body of the fornix, the lateral geniculate body, pulvinar, dorsomedial thalamic nucleus, and the body of the caudate nucleus (13, 43).

Cortical Branches

The cortical branches of the PCA are the inferior temporal, parieto-occipital, calcarine, and splenial branches (*Figs. 2.36* and *2.37*).

Inferior Temporal Arteries

The inferior temporal group of arteries arises from the PCA and the superior temporal arteries arise from the MCA. The inferior temporal arteries include the hippocampal and the anterior, middle, posterior, and common temporal arteries. These arteries supply the inferior parts of the temporal lobe. Branches of the inferior temporal arteries pass around the lower margin of the hemisphere to gain access to the lateral cerebral surface, reaching the middle temporal gyrus in 42% of hemispheres (43). They also give rise to some LPChAs.

The inferior temporal arteries are divided into five groups based on the branches present and the area they supply:

Group 1. All of the inferior temporal branches (hippocampal and anterior, middle, and posterior temporal arteries) are present (10% of hemispheres).

Group 2. A single large trunk, the common temporal artery, arises from the PCA and branches to supply the entire inferior temporal lobe (16%).

Group 3. Anterior, middle, and posterior temporal branches are present, but no hippocampal artery is present (20%).

Group 4. Anterior and posterior temporal branches are present, but no hippocampal or middle temporal arteries are present (10%).

Group 5. Hippocampal and anterior and posterior temporal branches are present, but no middle temporal artery is present. This is the most frequent pattern, present in 44% of hemispheres (43).

Hippocampal Arteries

The hippocampal artery, if present, arises in the crural or ambient cistern and is the first cortical branch of the PCA. It supplies the uncus, anterior parahippocampal gyrus, hippocampal formation, and the dentate gyrus. A small branch may extend to the lateral surface of the temporal lobe and forward to the temporal tip. If the first cortical branch supplies a significant portion of the inferior temporal lobe in addition to the hippocampal gyrus, the branch is classified as an anterior temporal artery. Bilateral occlusion of the vessels to the medial temporal area supplied by the hippocampal artery may cause a severe memory loss and a deficit resembling Korsakoff's syndrome (43).

Anterior Temporal Artery

The anterior temporal artery is usually the second cortical PCA branch. It is the first branch if there is no hippocampal artery. It usually arises in the proximal part of the ambient cistern and supplies the anteroinferior surface of the temporal lobe, occasionally reaching a portion of the temporal pole and the lateral cerebral surface in the region of the middle temporal sulcus and gyrus.

Middle Temporal Artery

This artery arises in the crural and ambient cisterns and supplies the inferior surface of the temporal lobe. It is the

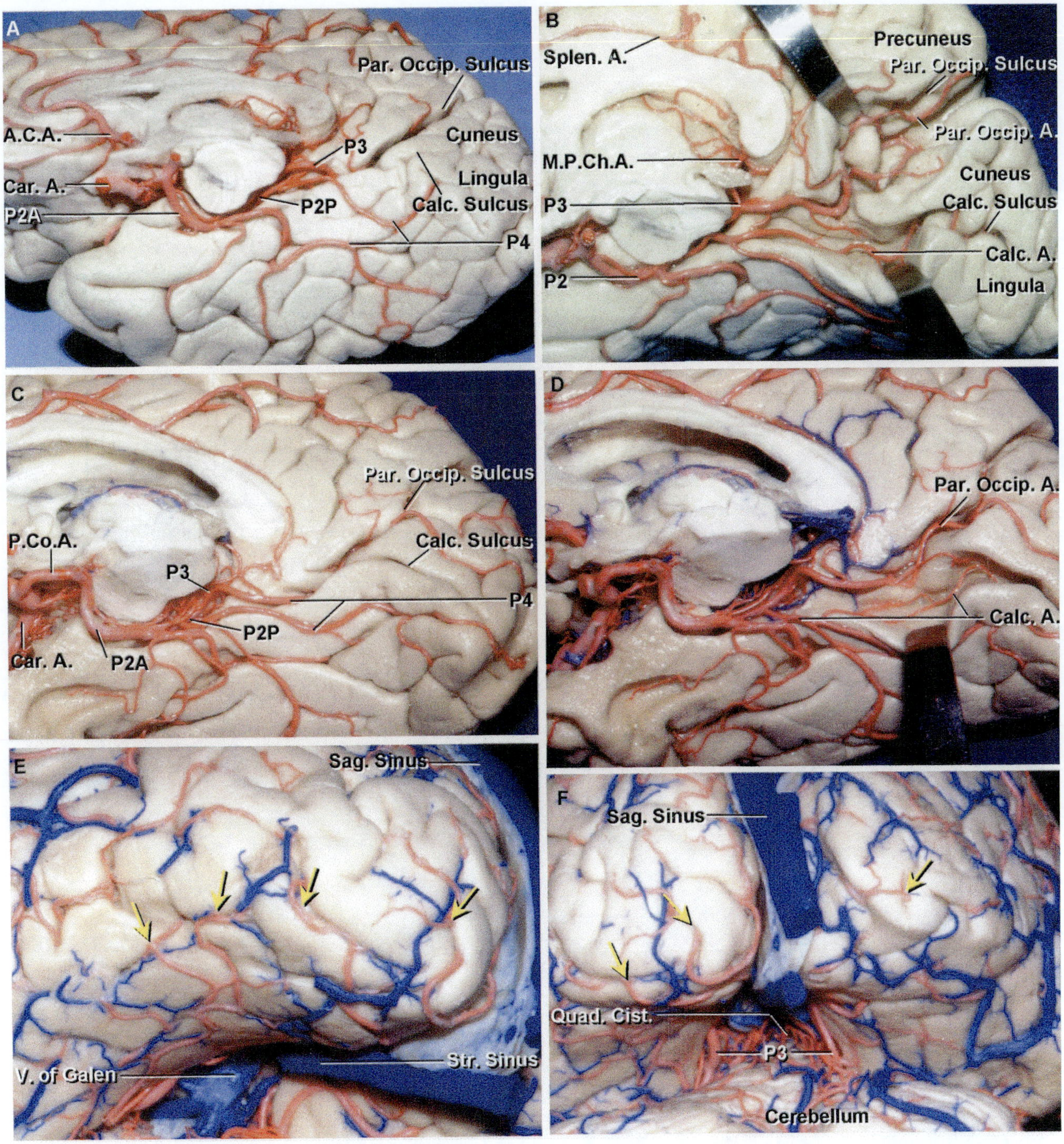

FIGURE 2.36. *Posterior cerebral arteries.* A, *the P2 divides into a P2A, which passes through the crural cistern located between the posterior segment of the uncus and the cerebral peduncle, and a P2P, which courses through the ambient cistern, located below the lateral midbrain and parahippocampal gyrus. The P3 passes through the quadrigeminal cistern where it gives rise to the P4 formed by the cortical branches, including the parieto-occipital and calcarine arteries that course in the parieto-occipital and calcarine sulci where they are commonly hidden between the sulcal lips.* B, *the lips of the parieto-occipital and calcarine sulci have been retracted to expose the parieto-occipital and calcarine branches coursing along the sulci. A MPChA encircles the brainstem to reach the third ventricular roof. The cuneus forms the upper lip and the lingula forms the lower lip of the calcarine sulcus. The precuneus forms the upper lip and the cuneus forms the lower lip of the parieto-occipital sulcus.* C, *another hemisphere. The terminal branches of the PCA pass posteriorly within the parieto-occipital and calcarine sulci. The* arrows *are on branches that pass around the occipital pole to reach the adjacent lateral surface.* D, *the lips of the parieto-occipital and calcarine sulci have been retracted. The parieto-occipital artery courses within its sulcus. The calcarine artery courses just below the calcarine sulcus and gives rise to several small branches that course along the depths of the sulcus.* E, *posteroinferior view of occipital pole showing the branches* (red arrow) *of the PCA coursing around the occipital pole to reach the adjacent part of the lateral convexity.* F, *posterior view of both occipital lobes. The P4 branches course around the posterior and lower border of the occipital lobe to reach the lateral cortical surface. The P3s course on the quadrigeminal cistern.* A., *artery;* A.C.A., *anterior cerebral artery;* Calc., *calcarine;* Car., *carotid;* Cist., *cistern;* M.P.Ch.A., *medial posterior choroidal artery;* P.Co.A., *posterior communicating artery;* Par. Occip., *parieto-occipital;* Quad., *quadrigeminal;* Sag., *sagittal;* Splen., *splenial;* Str., *straight;* V., *vein.*

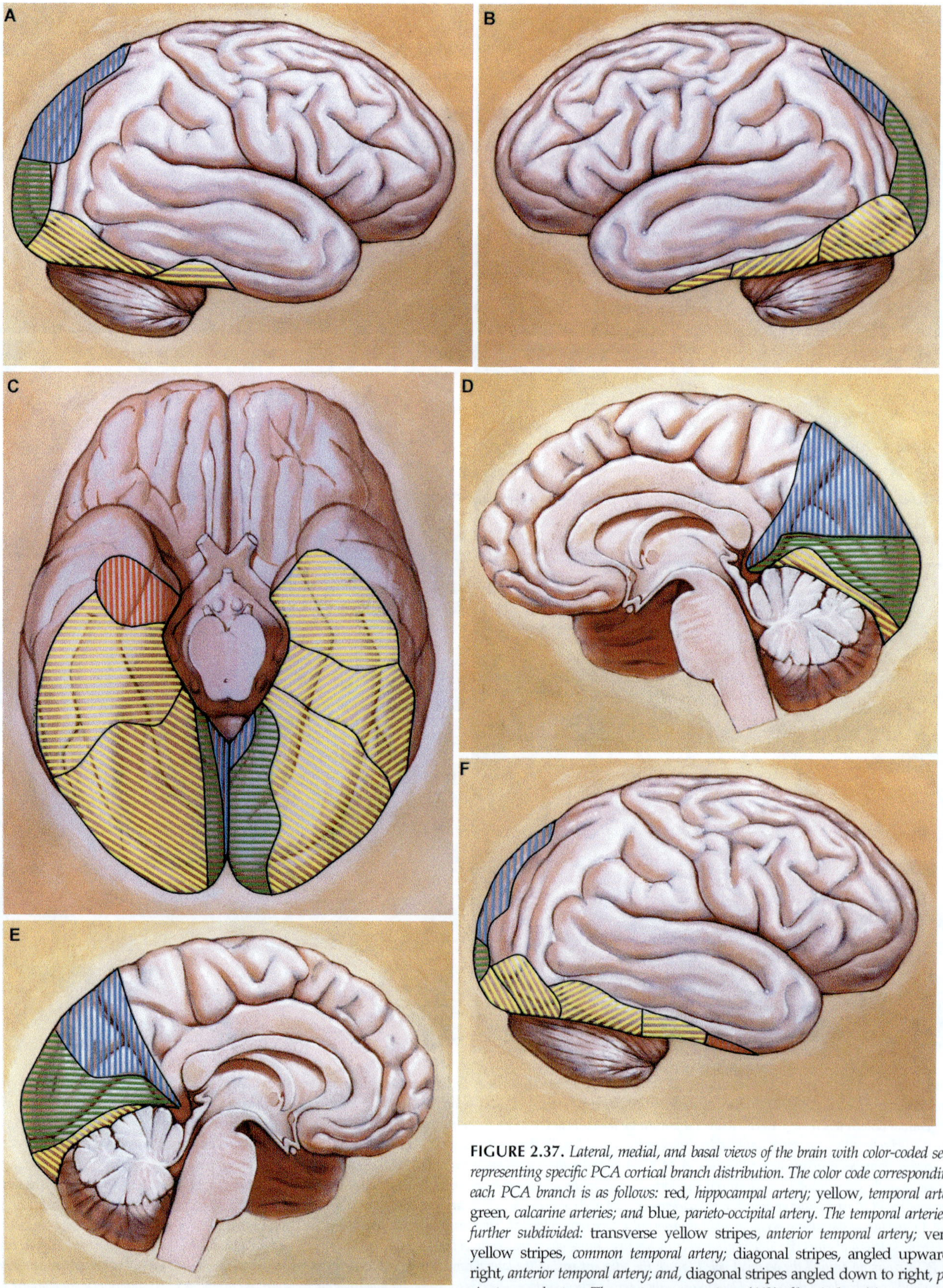

FIGURE 2.37. *Lateral, medial, and basal views of the brain with color-coded sectors representing specific PCA cortical branch distribution. The color code corresponding to each PCA branch is as follows:* red, *hippocampal artery;* yellow, *temporal arteries;* green, *calcarine arteries; and* blue, *parieto-occipital artery. The temporal arteries are further subdivided:* transverse yellow stripes, *anterior temporal artery;* vertical yellow stripes, *common temporal artery;* diagonal stripes, angled upward to right, *anterior temporal artery; and,* diagonal stripes angled down to right, *posterior temporal artery. The most common pattern (44% of hemispheres) is represented on the right cerebral hemisphere (*A and D, *and the left half of the basal view,* C*).*

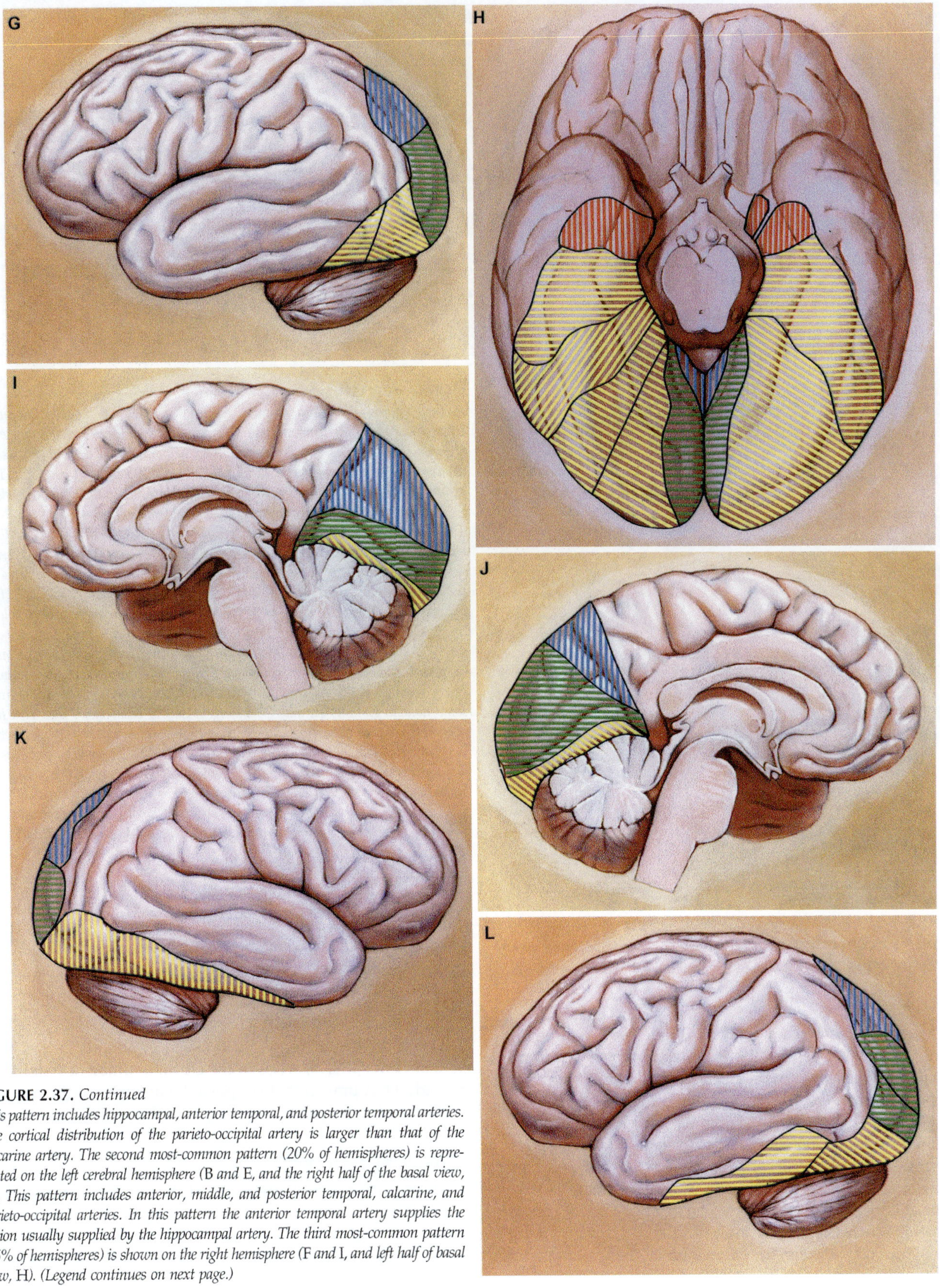

FIGURE 2.37. *Continued*
This pattern includes hippocampal, anterior temporal, and posterior temporal arteries. The cortical distribution of the parieto-occipital artery is larger than that of the calcarine artery. The second most-common pattern (20% of hemispheres) is represented on the left cerebral hemisphere (B and E, and the right half of the basal view, C). This pattern includes anterior, middle, and posterior temporal, calcarine, and parieto-occipital arteries. In this pattern the anterior temporal artery supplies the region usually supplied by the hippocampal artery. The third most-common pattern (16% of hemispheres) is shown on the right hemisphere (F and I, and left half of basal view, H). (Legend continues on next page.)

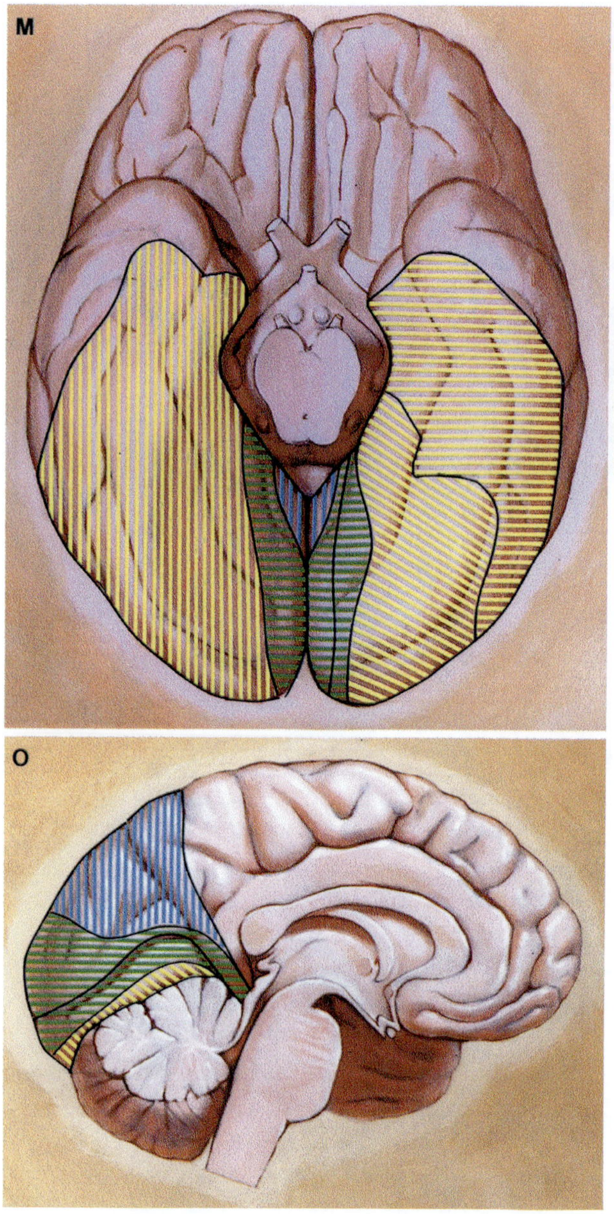

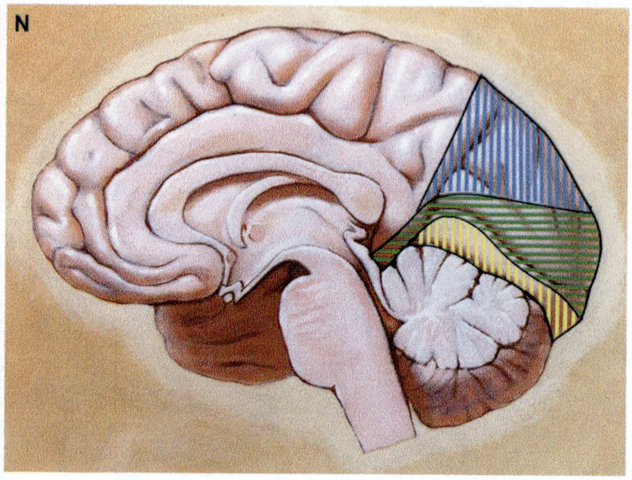

FIGURE 2.37. *Continued*
*In this pattern, there is a common temporal artery that supplies the entire inferior surface of the temporal lobe. The calcarine and parieto-occipital arteries are also present. The fourth most common pattern (10% of hemispheres) is depicted on the left hemisphere (*G *and* J, *and right half of basal view,* H*). This arrangement includes anterior and posterior temporal, calcarine, and parieto-occipital arteries, but no hippocampal or middle temporal branches of the PCA. The area of the calcarine artery is split into two sectors to illustrate that there were two calcarine arteries arising from the PCA, as occurs in 10% of hemispheres. The fifth most common pattern (10% of hemispheres) is illustrated on the right cerebral hemisphere (*K *and* N, *and left half of basal view,* M*). This pattern includes hippocampal, anterior, middle and posterior temporal, calcarine, and parieto-occipital arteries. The area supplied by the posterior temporal artery is split into two parts to show that two posterior temporal arteries arise from the PCA, as occurs in 6% of cerebral hemispheres. The parieto-occipital artery supplies the larger part of the medial surface. The last pattern illustrates some notable variants (*L *and* O, *and right half of basal view,* M*). Two hippocampal arteries arise from the PCA, a finding present in 12% of cerebral hemispheres. The anterior temporal artery supplies a smaller than usual amount of the anterior and lateral temporal surfaces, the remainder is supplied by the middle cerebral artery. The calcarine artery supplies an unusually large area on the medial surface.* (From, *Zeal AA, Rhoton AL Jr: Microsurgical anatomy of the posterior cerebral artery.* **J Neurosurg** *48:534–559, 1978 [43].)*

smallest, is frequently absent, and has the fewest branches of the inferior temporal arteries.

Posterior Temporal Artery

This artery, present in almost all hemispheres, arises from the inferior or lateral aspect of the PCA, most commonly in the ambient, but occasionally in the crural or quadrigeminal cisterns, and runs obliquely posterolateral toward the occipital pole to supply the inferior temporal and occipital surfaces, including the occipital pole and lingual gyrus. It has the largest trunk diameter and number of branches of any temporal artery except a common temporal artery from which all the temporal branches arise. Deficits after occlusions of the posterior temporal artery include dysphasia, which has usually been mild and transient, an amnestic syndrome, usually transient with homonymous hemianopsia, but without hemiparesis or sensory loss and inability to match colors to their names (21).

Common Temporal Artery

The common temporal artery, seen in slightly fewer than 20% of hemispheres, arises in the crural or ambient cisterns as a single PCA branch that supplies the majority of the inferior surface of the temporal and occipital lobes.

Parieto-occipital Artery

The parieto-occipital artery, one of the two terminal branches of the PCA, is present in almost all hemispheres. It consistently arises as a single branch and runs in the parieto-occipital fissure to supply the posterior parasagittal region, cuneus, precuneus, lateral occipital gyrus, and, rarely, the precentral and superior parietal lobules. It arises in the ambient or quadrigeminal cisterns. The arteries with a more proximal origin tend to be larger and donate branches to the midbrain, thalamus, pulvinar, and lateral geniculate bodies as they pass posteriorly within the hippocampal fissure. Those arteries with a proximal origin also send branches through the choroidal fissure to the choroid plexus in the lateral ventricle. This artery occasionally sends branches to the third ventricle in the area supplied by the MPChA or to the splenium of the corpus callosum.

Calcarine Artery

The calcarine artery, a terminal PCA branch, is present in all hemispheres. It courses within the calcarine fissure to reach the occipital pole, and has branches that fan out to the lingual gyrus and the inferior cuneus. It usually arises directly from the PCA in the ambient or quadrigeminal cisterns, but occasionally is a branch of the parieto-occipital artery.

The calcarine artery supplies the visual cortex, and the hallmark of an occlusion of this vessel is a homonymous visual field defect, usually with macular sparing. Occlusion may be associated with pain in the ipsilateral eye. Bilateral occipital lobe infarction may result in blindness with preserved pupillary reflexes or in Anton's syndrome, in which there is cortical blindness, confabulation, denial of blindness, and preservation of the pupillary reaction to light. The visual field may recover after ligation or occlusion of the calcarine artery (19).

Splenial Artery

The PCA, or its branches, gives rise to branches supplying the splenium of the corpus callosum in all hemispheres. They may arise from the following arteries: parieto-occipital, calcarine, medial posterior choroidal, posterior temporal, and lateral posterior choroidal. The splenial arteries anastomose with branches of the pericallosal artery a few centimeters anterior to the posterior tip of the splenium as previously noted. Retrograde filling of this artery through the pericallosal artery suggests occlusion of the PCA proximal to the origin of the splenial artery. Infarction of the dominant occipital pole (producing a hemianopsia) plus the splenium of the corpus callosum in the distribution of the splenial artery interrupts the fibers between the intact occipital pole and contralateral angular gyrus, resulting in the syndrome of dyslexia without dysgraphia (43).

Lateral Convexity Branches

All the cortical branches of the PCA may send branches to the lateral surface of the hemisphere, but of the seven cortical arteries, the posterior temporal artery is the most common site of origin of lateral cortical branches. The next most common source is the parieto-occipital artery. If a revascularization procedure using microvascular anastomoses between the superficial temporal or occipital arteries and a cortical branch of the PCA were undertaken, the area supplied by the posterior temporal artery would show the most promise of revealing a vessel of sufficient caliber to be used as a recipient, there being a higher than 75% chance of finding a vessel of sufficient size within this area (43). This corresponds with the region immediately anterior to the preoccipital notch. The majority of the cortical branches of the PCA are 0.4 to 0.6 mm in diameter when they pass around the margin to the lateral cerebral surface.

IIIrd and IVth Cranial Nerves

The relationship between the oculomotor and trochlear nerves and the PCA and SCA is constant (*Figs. 2.1* and *2.3*) (32). The oculomotor nerve consistently passes between the PCA and SCA near their origin, and the trochlear nerve passes between the two on the lateral margin of the brainstem. The relationship is unaltered even when the superior cerebellar origin is duplicated. When the SCA arises as duplicate trunks, the nerves pass between the superior trunk of the SCA and the PCA. The PCA consistently courses above the trochlear. A tortuous SCA may occasionally loop above a trochlear nerve.

Discussion

The PCA, more than any other intracranial vessel, subserves the function of vision. It supports a long list of ocular functions that include papillary reflexes, eye movement, visual memory, intrahemispheric transfer of visual information, binocular and visual spatial integration through its supply to the optic tracts, geniculate bodies, colliculi, extraocular nerves and their nuclei, the geniculocalcarine tracts, and the striate and peristriate cortex. The dysfunction caused by occlusion of the individual PCA branches has been reviewed in the subsection related to those branches. Occlusion of various branches may also lead to somesthetic disturbances caused by involvement of afferent pathways in the medial lemniscus or thalamus, motor weakness caused by involvement of the corticospinal tracts in the internal capsule or peduncle, memory deficits caused by involvement of the hypothalamic pathways entering and exiting the mamillary bodies, autonomic imbalance caused by disturbances of the sympathetic and parasympathetic pathways in the anterior and posterior diencephalon, alterations of consciousness caused by ischemia of the midbrain reticular formation, abnormal movements caused by involvement of cerebellothalamic circuits in the midbrain and thalamus, and endocrine disturbances caused by involvement of the hypothalamic pituitary axis.

Vascular complications in pituitary surgery result mainly from carotid artery injury and circulatory embarrassment after occlusion of the carotid artery. Occlusion of the perforating branches of the posterior circle is commonly neglected in discussions regarding complications in pituitary surgery. The arterial branches reviewed in this study, which would be stretched around the margin of suprasellar tumors, have the potential, when occluded, to cause personality disorders, memory disturbances, extraocular palsies, visual loss, and altered states of consciousness (12, 34). The branches stretched around pituitary tumors are discussed further in Chapter 8.

REFERENCES

1. Abbie AA: The clinical significance of the anterior choroidal artery. **Brain** 56:233–246, 1933.

2. Baptista AG: Studies on the arteries of the brain: Part II—The anterior cerebral artery: Some anatomic features and their clinical implications. **Neurology** 13:825–835, 1963.
3. Chater N, Spetzler RF, Tonnemacher K, Wilson CB: Microvascular bypass surgery: Part 1—Anatomical studies. **J Neurosurg** 44:712–714, 1976.
4. Cooper IS: Surgical alleviation of Parkinsonism: Effects of occlusion of the anterior choroidal artery. **J Am Geriatr Soc** 2:691–718, 1954.
5. Cooper IS: Surgical occlusion of the anterior choroidal artery in Parkinsonism. **Surg Gynecol Obstet** 99:207–219, 1954.
6. Critchley M: The anterior cerebral artery, and its syndromes. **Brain** 53:120–165, 1930.
7. Dejerine J, Roussy G: Le syndrome thalamique. **Rev Neurol** 14:521–532, 1906.
8. Dunker RO, Harris AB: Surgical anatomy of the proximal anterior cerebral artery. **J Neurosurg** 44:359–367, 1976.
9. Epstein F, Ransohoff J, Budzilovich GN: The clinical significance of junctional dilatation of the posterior communicating artery. **J Neurosurg** 33:529–531, 1970.
10. Fisher CM: Clinical syndromes in cerebral thrombosis, hypertensive hemorrhage, and ruptured saccular aneurysm. **Clin Neurosurg** 22:117–147, 1975.
11. Foix CH, Chavany JA, Hillemand P: Obliteration de l'artère choroidienne anterieure. Ramollissement cerebral hémiplégie, hémianesthesie et hémianopsie. **Soc d'Ophtal** May, 1925.
12. Fujii K, Chambers SM, Rhoton AL Jr: Neurovascular relationships of the sphenoid sinus: A microsurgical study. **J Neurosurg** 50:31–39, 1979.
13. Fujii, K, Lenkey C, Rhoton AL Jr: Microsurgical anatomy of the choroidal arteries: Lateral and third ventricles. **J Neurosurg** 52:165–188, 1980.
14. Gibo H, Carver CC, Rhoton AL Jr, Lenkey C, Mitchell RJ: Microsurgical anatomy of the middle cerebral artery. **J Neurosurg** 54:151–169, 1981.
15. Gibo H, Lenkey C, Rhoton AL Jr: Microsurgical anatomy of the supraclinoid portion of the internal carotid artery. **J Neurosurg** 55:560–574, 1981.
16. Harris FS, Rhoton AL Jr: Microsurgical anatomy of the cavernous sinus: A microsurgical study. **J Neurosurg** 45:169–180, 1976.
17. Hassler O, Saltzman GF: Angiographic and histologic changes in infundibular widening of the posterior communicating artery. **Acta Radiol** 1:321–327, 1963.
18. Heubner O: *Die luetische Erkrankung der Hirnarterien*. Leipzig, Vogel, 1874, p 183.
19. Hoyt WF, Newton TH: Angiographic changes with occlusion of arteries that supply the visual cortex. **N Z Med J** 72:310–317, 1970.
20. Liu Q, Rhoton AL Jr: Middle meningeal origin of the ophthalmic artery. **Neurosurgery** 49:401–407, 2001.
21. Mohr JP, Leicester J, Stoddard LT, Sidman M: Right hemianopia with memory and color deficits in circumscribed left posterior cerebral artery territory infarction. **Neurology** 21:1104–1113, 1971.
22. Newton TH, Hoyt WF, Margolis MT: Pathology of the posterior cerebral artery, in Newton TH, Potts PC (eds): *Radiology of the Skull and Brain*. St. Louis, C.V. Mosby, 1974, Vol II, Book 2, pp 1580–1627.
23. Ono M, Ono M, Rhoton AL Jr, Barry M: Microsurgical anatomy of the region of the tentorial incisura. **J Neurosurg** 60:365–399, 1984.
24. Padget DH: The development of the cranial arteries in the human embryo. **Contrib Embryol** 32:205–262, 1948.
25. Paullus WS, Pait TG, Rhoton AL Jr: Microsurgical exposure of the petrous portion of the carotid artery. **J Neurosurg** 47:713–726, 1977.
26. Perlmutter D, Rhoton AL Jr: Microsurgical anatomy of the anterior cerebral-anterior communicating-recurrent artery complex. **J Neurosurg** 45:259–272, 1976.
27. Perlmutter D, Rhoton AL Jr: Microsurgical anatomy of the distal anterior cerebral artery. **J Neurosurg** 49:204–228, 1978.
28. Rand RW, Brown WJ, Stern WE: Surgical occlusion of the anterior choroidal arteries in Parkinsonism. **Neurology** 6:390–401, 1956.
29. Renn WH, Rhoton AL Jr: Microsurgical anatomy of the sellar region. **J Neurosurg** 43:288–298, 1975.
30. Rhoton AL Jr: Microsurgical treatment of occlusive cerebrovascular disease. **Compr Ther** 5:39–47, 1979.
31. Rhoton AL Jr: Anatomy of saccular aneurysms. **Surg Neurol** 14:59–66, 1980.
32. Rhoton AL Jr: The cerebellar arteries. **Neurosurgery** 47[Suppl 1]:S29–S68, 2000.
33. Rhoton AL Jr, Fujii K, Fradd B: Microsurgical anatomy of the anterior choroidal artery. **Surg Neurol** 12:171–187, 1979.
34. Rhoton AL Jr, Hardy DG, Chambers SM: Microsurgical anatomy and dissection of the sphenoid bone, cavernous sinus and sellar region. **Surg Neurol** 12:63–104, 1979.
35. Rhoton AL Jr, Saeki N, Perlmutter D, Zeal A: Microsurgical anatomy of common aneurysm sites. **Clin Neurosurg** 26:248–306, 1979.
36. Rosner SS, Rhoton AL Jr, Ono M, Barry M: Microsurgical anatomy of the anterior perforating arteries. **J Neurosurg** 61:468–485, 1984.
37. Saeki N, Rhoton AL Jr: Microsurgical anatomy of the upper basilar artery and the posterior circle of Willis. **J Neurosurg** 46:563–578, 1977.
38. Stehbens WE: Aneurysms and anatomic variation of cerebral arteries. **Arch Pathol** 75:45–64, 1963.
39. Stephens RB, Stilwell DL: *Arteries and Veins of the Human Brain*. Springfield, Charles C Thomas, 1969, p 181.
40. Toole JF, Cole M: Ischemic cerebrovascular disease, in Baker AB, Baker LH (eds): *Clinical Neurology*. Hagerstown, Harper and Row, 1976, vol 1, pp 15–16.
41. Viale GL, Turtas S, Pau A: Surgical removal of striate arteriovenous malformations. **Surg Neurol** 14:321–324, 1980.
42. Waddington MM, Ring BA: Syndromes of occlusions of middle cerebral artery branches. **Brain** 91:685–696, 1968.
43. Zeal AA, Rhoton AL Jr: Microsurgical anatomy of the posterior cerebral artery. **J Neurosurg** 48:534–559, 1978.

Figure from D'Agoty Gautier's Essai d'anatomie, en tableaux imprimés. *Paris, 1748.*

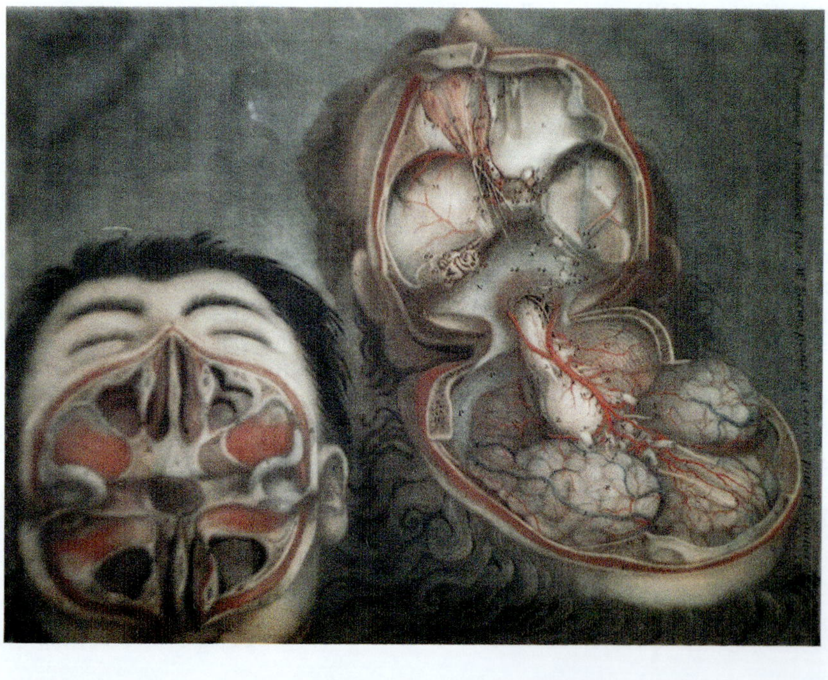

Aneurysms

Albert L. Rhoton, Jr., M.D.

Department of Neurological Surgery, University of Florida, Gainesville, Florida

Correspondence:
Albert L. Rhoton, Jr., M.D., Department of Neurological Surgery, University of Florida McKnight Brain Institute, P.O. Box 100265, 100 South Newell Drive, Building 59, L2-100, Gainesville, FL 32610-0265.
Email: rhoton@neurosurgery.ufl.edu

KEY WORDS: Aneurysms, Anterior cerebral artery, Basilar artery, Cerebrovascular disease, Craniotomy, Internal carotid artery, Microsurgery, Middle cerebral artery, Perforating arteries, Posterior cerebral artery, Subarachnoid hemorrhage, Vertebral artery, Vertebrobasilar system

In 1979, the author introduced three rules related to the anatomy of saccular aneurysms that should be considered when planning the operative approach to these lesions (18). These three aspects of anatomy are reviewed in this chapter in relation to each of the common aneurysm sites. First, these aneurysms arise at a branching site on the parent artery. This site may be formed either by the origin of a side branch from the parent artery, such as the origin of the posterior communicating artery from the internal carotid artery, or by subdivision of a main arterial trunk into two trunks, as occurs at the bifurcation of the middle cerebral or basilar arteries (*Figs. 3.1* and *3.2*). Second, saccular aneurysms arise at a turn or curve in the artery. These curves, by producing local alterations in intravascular hemodynamics, exert unusual stresses on apical regions that receive the greatest force of the pulse wave. Saccular aneurysms arise on the convex, not concave, side of the curve. Third, saccular aneurysms point in the direction that the blood would have gone if the curve at the aneurysm site were not present. The aneurysm dome or fundus points in the direction of the maximal hemodynamic thrust in the preaneurysmal segment of the parent artery. Since the original introduction of the three rules, our anatomic studies have revealed a fourth rule. The fourth rule is that there is a constantly occurring set of perforating arteries situated at each aneurysm site that need to be protected and preserved to achieve an optimal result (12, 13, 18).

Aneurysms are infrequently encountered on a straight, nonbranching segment of an intracranial artery. The aneurysms occurring on straight, nonbranching segments are more often found to have sacs that point longitudinally along the wall of the artery in the direction of blood flow and to project only minimally above the adventitial surface. Aneurysms having these characteristics are of a dissecting type, rather than of the congenital saccular type, and their development is heralded more frequently by the onset of ischemic neurological deficits than by the subarachnoid hemorrhage associated with congenital saccular aneurysms. It is rare to find an aneurysm on the concave side of an arterial curve or to find one that points in a direction opposite to that of the flow in the parent artery.

ANEURYSM SITES

Internal Carotid Artery Aneurysms

These four facets of anatomy, as they apply to aneurysm sites on the supraclinoid portion of the internal carotid artery, are considered first (*Figs. 3.1–3.4*). If all sites on the supraclinoid portion of the internal carotid artery (C4) are included, it is the most common site of intracranial aneurysms, accounting for approximately 35% of intracranial aneurysms (8). These aneurysms arise at five sites: the upper surface of the internal carotid artery at the origin of the ophthalmic artery, the medial wall at the origin of the superior hypophyseal artery, the posterior wall at the origin of the posterior communicating artery, the posterior wall at the origin of the anterior choroidal artery, and the apex of the carotid artery bifurcation into the anterior and middle cerebral arteries.

The intradural exposure of the supraclinoid carotid is along the sphenoid ridge or orbital roof to the anterior clinoid process and from proximal to distal (*Figs. 3.3* and *3.4*). Both the internal carotid artery and the optic nerve are medial to the anterior clinoid process. The artery exits the cavernous sinus on the medial side of the anterior clinoid process, beneath and slightly lateral to the optic nerve. It courses posterior, superior, and slightly lateral to reach the lateral side of the optic chiasm, where it turns forward to complete the upper half of the S-shaped curve of the carotid siphon. It bifurcates in the area below the anterior perforated substances to give rise to the anterior and middle cerebral arteries.

The supraclinoid portion of the internal carotid artery is divided into three segments on the basis of the site of origin of the ophthalmic, posterior communicating, and anterior choroidal arteries (*Figs. 2.4* and *3.5*). The ophthalmic segment extends from the origin of the ophthalmic artery at the roof of the cavernous sinus to the origin of the posterior communicating artery; the communicating segment extends from the origin of the posterior communicating artery to the origin of the anterior choroidal artery; and the choroidal segment extends from the origin of the anterior choroidal artery to the terminal bifurcation of the internal carotid artery. The ophthalmic segment is the longest and the communicating segment the shortest. Each internal carotid artery gives off from 3 to 16 (average, 8.2) perforating branches with a relatively constant origin and termination (3). The relationships of the perforating branches to each of the common aneurysm sites are reviewed below.

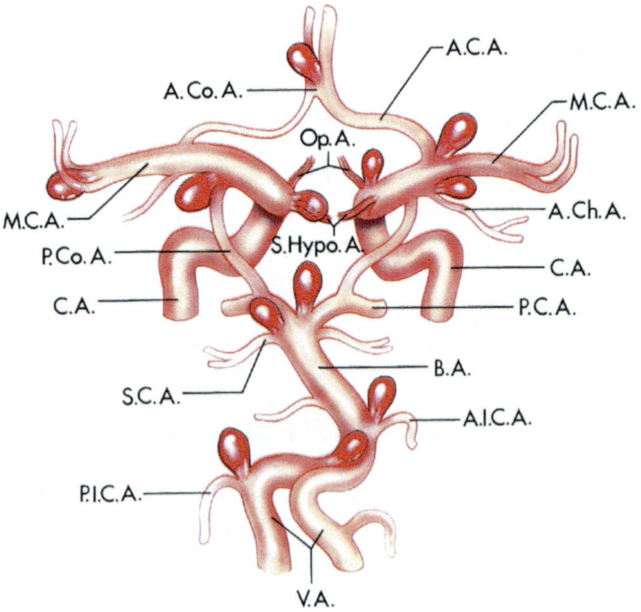

FIGURE 3.1. *Most-common sites of saccular aneurysms. Each aneurysm arises from the branching site of a large artery. Most are located on or near the circle of Willis. More than 90% are located at one of the following five sites: (a) the internal carotid artery at the level of the posterior communicating artery; (b) the junction of the anterior cerebral and anterior communicating arteries; (c) the proximal bifurcation of the middle cerebral artery; (d) the junction of the posterior cerebral and basilar arteries, and (e) the bifurcation of the carotid artery into the anterior cerebral and middle cerebral arteries. Other aneurysm sites on the carotid artery are at the origins of the ophthalmic, superior hypophyseal, and anterior choroidal arteries. Other sites on the vertebral and basilar arteries include the sites of origin of the anteroinferior cerebellar, posteroinferior cerebellar, and the superior cerebellar arteries and the junction of the basilar and vertebral arteries.* A.C.A., *anterior cerebral artery;* A.Ch.A., *anterior choroidal artery;* A.Co.A., *anterior communicating artery;* A.I.C.A., *anteroinferior cerebellar artery;* B.A., *basilar artery;* C.A., *internal carotid artery;* M.C.A., *middle cerebral artery;* Op.A., *ophthalmic artery;* P.C.A., *posterior cerebral artery;* P.Co.A., *posterior communicating artery;* P.I.C.A., *posteroinferior cerebellar artery;* S.C.A., *superior cerebellar artery;* S.Hypo.A., *superior hypophyseal artery;* V.A., *vertebral artery.*

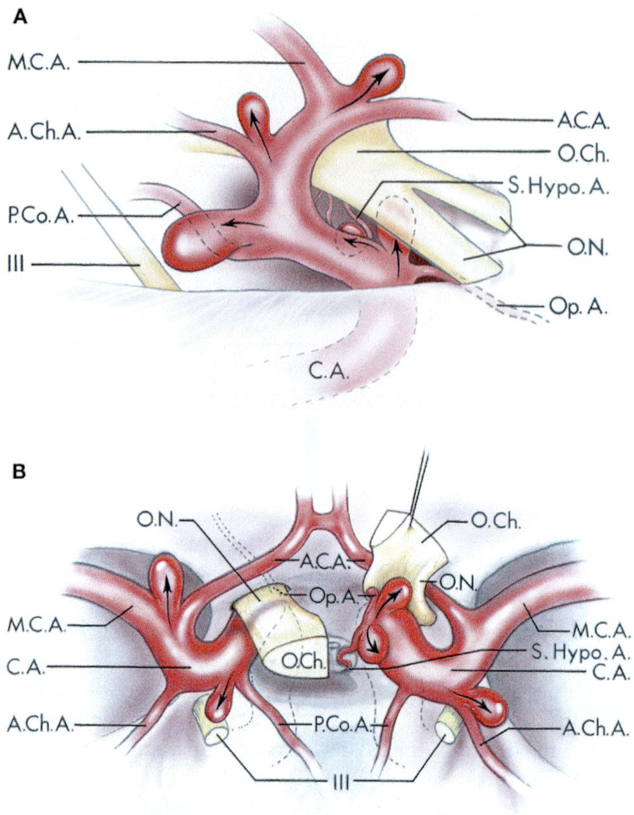

FIGURE 3.2. *Lateral* (A) *and superior* (B) *views of common aneurysm sites on the supraclinoid portion of the internal carotid artery.* A, *lateral view of the right internal carotid artery.* B, *superior view of the internal carotid arteries, with the right optic nerve and right half of the optic chiasm reflected forward to expose the origin of the ophthalmic artery. The intracavernous portion of both carotid arteries and the course of the left ophthalmic artery are shown by* dotted lines. *The aneurysms arise on curves in the artery at the site of origin of its branches. The aneurysms point in the direction* (arrows) *of the maximal hemodynamic force immediately proximal to the aneurysm site and in the direction the blood would have gone if there were no curve at the aneurysm site. The aneurysm sites on the internal carotid artery are usually located immediately distal to the origins of its branches. Aneurysms arising at the origin of the ophthalmic artery point upward into the optic nerve. Aneurysms arising at the origin of the superior hypophyseal artery point medially under the optic chiasm. Aneurysms arising near the origin of the posterior communicating artery point posteriorly toward the oculomotor nerve and are usually located superolateral to the posterior communicating artery. Aneurysms arising near the origin of the anterior choroidal artery point posterolaterally and are usually located immediately superior to the origin of the anterior choroidal artery. Aneurysms arising at the carotid bifurcation into the anterior and middle cerebral arteries point upward lateral to the optic chiasm toward the anterior perforated substance.* A.C.A., *anterior cerebral artery;* A.Ch.A., *anterior choroidal artery;* C.A., *internal carotid artery;* M.C.A., *middle cerebral artery;* O.Ch., *optic chiasm;* O.N., *optic nerve;* Op.A., *ophthalmic artery;* P.Co.A., *posterior communicating artery;* S.Hypo.A., *superior hypophyseal artery.*

Carotid-Ophthalmic Aneurysms

Aneurysms arising at the carotid-ophthalmic artery junction commonly arise from the superior wall of the carotid artery at the distal edge of the origin of the ophthalmic artery at or above the roof of the cavernous sinus, where the superiorly directed intracavernous segment turns posteriorly (*Figs. 3.2, 3.3, 3.5,* and *3.6*). At this turn, the maximal hemodynamic thrust is directed toward the superior wall of the carotid artery just distal to the ophthalmic artery, and the aneurysm projects upward toward the optic nerve.

The origin of the ophthalmic artery is difficult to expose because of its short intradural length and its location under the optic nerve (*Fig. 3.6*). It arises from the carotid artery below the optic nerve and reaches the orbit by one of three routes. It usually passes through the optic canal to enter the orbit. In a few cases it will arise in the cavernous sinus and enter the orbit through the superior orbital fissure (5). The least common course is for it to penetrate a foramen in the

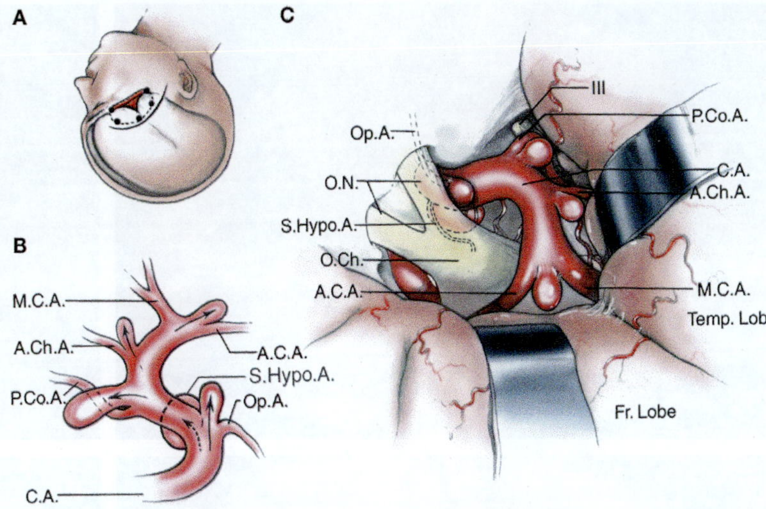

FIGURE 3.3. *Operative view of aneurysm sites on the internal carotid artery.* A, *scalp incision* (solid line), *bone flap* (dotted line), *and craniectomy* (red area) *for approaching internal carotid artery aneurysms.* B, *lateral view of the right internal carotid artery showing aneurysm sites.* C, *operative view provided by a right frontotemporal craniotomy with brain spatulas on the frontal and temporal lobes. These aneurysms point in the direction* (arrows in B) *of the maximal hemodynamic force proximal to the aneurysm site and in the direction the blood would have gone if there were no curve in the parent artery at the aneurysm site. The aneurysm sites on the internal carotid artery are located immediately distal to the origin of its branches. Aneurysms arising at the origin of the ophthalmic artery point upward into the optic nerve. Aneurysms arising at the origin of the superior hypophyseal artery point medially under the optic chiasm. Aneurysms arising near the origin of the posterior communicating artery point posteriorly toward the oculomotor nerve and are usually located superolateral to the posterior communicating artery. Aneurysms arising near the origin of the anterior choroidal artery point posterolaterally and are usually located immediately superior to the origin of the anterior choroidal artery. Aneurysms arising at the carotid bifurcation into the anterior and middle cerebral arteries point upward lateral to the optic chiasm toward the anterior perforated substance. Each of the aneurysms can be approached through a frontotemporal craniotomy.* A.C.A., *anterior cerebral artery;* A.Ch.A., *anterior choroidal artery;* C.A., *internal carotid artery;* Fr., *frontal;* M.C.A., *middle cerebral artery;* O.Ch., *optic chiasm;* O.N., *optic nerve;* Op.A., *ophthalmic artery;* P.Co.A., *posterior communicating artery;* S.Hypo.A., *superior hypophyseal artery;* Temp., *temporal.*

bony strut that separates the optic foramen and the superior orbital fissure, or to arise from the middle meningeal artery (7).

Aneurysms arising in the region of the origin of the ophthalmic artery and the anterior clinoid process are among the most complicated aneurysms because of the variable origin and course of the ophthalmic artery and the involvement of the dural folds in the region of the optic foramen and clinoid process (*Fig. 3.6, A–C*). Ophthalmic aneurysms are relatively uncomplicated if they arise above the cranial base; however, their complexity increases as they get closer to and involve the segment of the internal carotid artery, referred to as the clinoid segment, exposed by removing the anterior clinoid process (*Figs. 3.4* and *3.7*) (5). The clinoid segment and its exposure is discussed in Chapter 9 of this issue. The clinoid segment is located at the junction of the intracavernous and subarachnoid segments of the artery, between the dural folds coming off the upper and lower margins of the anterior clinoid process. The dura that extends medially from the top of the anterior clinoid process forms the upper dural ring around the carotid artery. The dura that extends medially from the lower margin of the anterior clinoid surrounds the artery to form the lower dural ring, which marks the lower margin of the clinoid segment. The layer that extends medially to form the lower dural ring separates the lower margin of the clinoid process from the upper surface of the oculomotor nerve. The upper ring forms a tight collar around the artery, but inspection under the operating microscope reveals that there is often a narrow depression in the dura at the site at which the ring hugs the anteromedial aspect of the artery, called the carotid cave. The cave, the short downward pouching, extends a variable distance below the level of the upper dural ring (*Fig. 3.6, A* and *B*) and is most prominent on the anteromedial side of the artery, where it may extend down to near the lower ring. The cave seems to become less prominent as the arteries elongate with advancing age. Carotid cave aneurysms are distinct from clinoid segment aneurysms, which arise from the clinoid segment of the internal carotid artery located between the upper and lower dural ring. Aneurysms that arise from the clinoid segment of the internal carotid artery have been referred to as clinoid segment aneurysms, and those located above the upper ring, but extending into the cave adjacent the upper ring, are referred to as carotid cave aneurysms.

The anatomy of ophthalmic aneurysms varies depending on the site of origin and course of the ophthalmic artery and whether the aneurysm involves the clinoid segment or the carotid cave. If the aneurysm arises on the upper surface of the carotid artery above the upper ring, it will project upward into the optic nerve and involve neither the cave nor the clinoid segment (*Fig. 3.6, D* and *E*). If the ophthalmic artery has an even longer subarachnoid segment and arises distal to the upper ring along the superomedial side of the carotid artery, the aneurysm may project medially under the optic nerve in the anterior presellar area and mimic an anteriorly situated superior hypophyseal aneurysm, although it arises at the origin of the ophthalmic artery (*Fig. 3.6, F* and *G*). If the aneurysm arises in the carotid cave, the fundus will extend upward out of the carotid cave on the anteromedial aspect of the carotid artery (*Fig. 3.6, H* and *I*). The ophthalmic artery also may arise further proximally on the carotid artery and pass through an anomalous foramen in the optic strut, the bridge of bone that separates the lateral margin of the optic canal from the medial edge of the superior orbital fissure, to reach the orbit, rather than passing through the optic canal (*Fig. 3.6, J* and *K*). This anomalous foramen in the optic strut is called the ophthalmic foramen (*Fig. 7.3L*). Aneurysms arising at the origin of an ophthalmic artery that passes through the optic strut have their neck along the anterior or lateral part of the clinoid

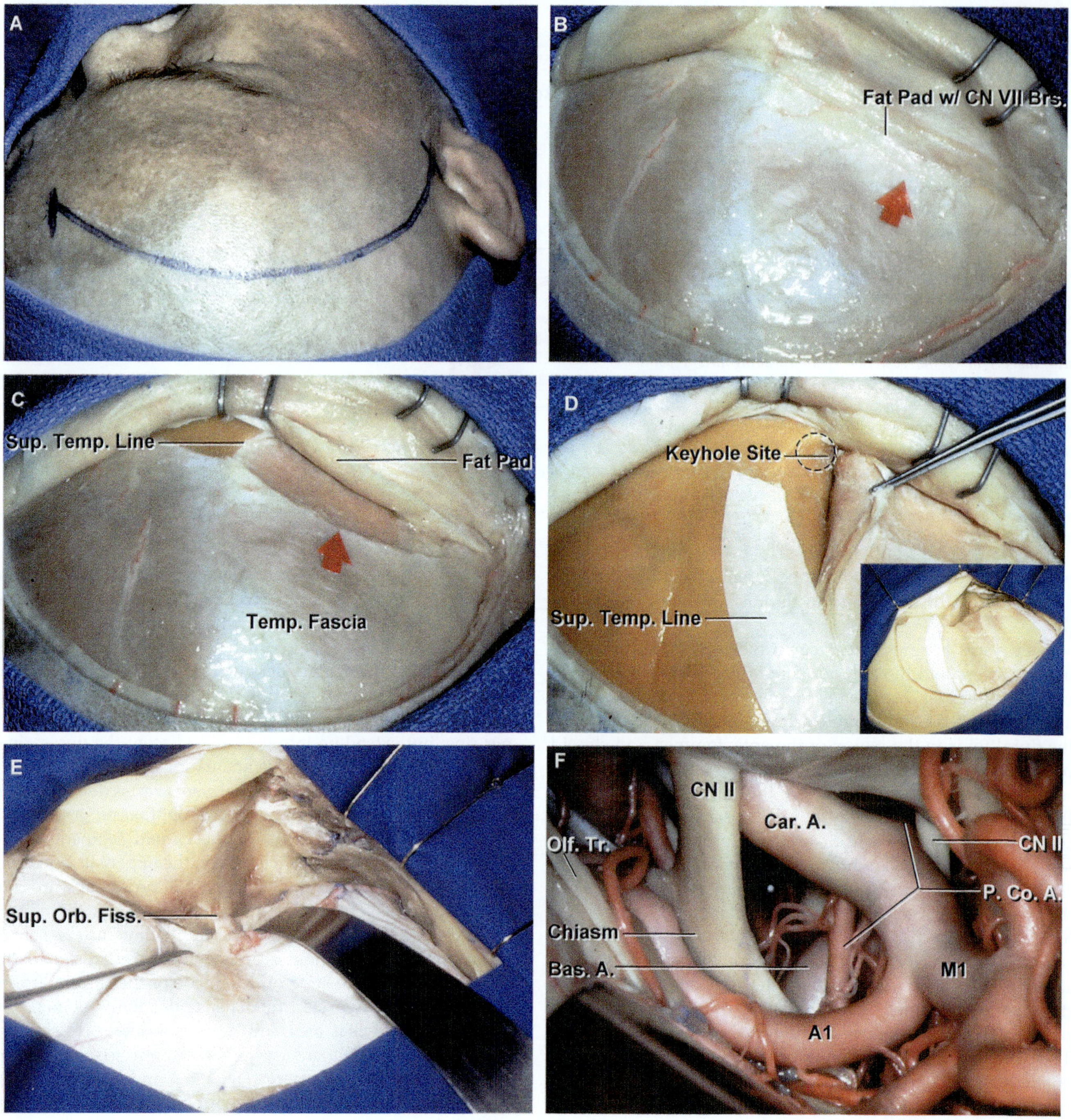

FIGURE 3.4. *Frontotemporal (pterional) craniotomy used to expose aneurysms on the circle of Willis. A, the anterior end of the scalp incision is located near the midline behind the hairline. The posterior end is located at the zygomatic arch near the tragus. B, the scalp flap has been reflected downward using a subgaleal dissection. The fat pad, in which the facial nerve branches course, is exposed at the lower margin of the exposure. C, an incision through the superficial temporal fascia covering the lower part of the temporalis muscle allows the superficial fascia, with the fat pad that encloses the facial nerve branches, to be folded downward with the scalp flap. D, the keyhole, the site of a burr hole, which is located behind the anterior part of the superior temporal line, is outlined. The keyhole has the anterior fossa dura in its upper margin and the periorbita in its lower margin. The inset shows the burr holes and bone flap. E, the sphenoid ridge has been removed leaving a thin shell of bone over the roof and lateral wall of the orbit. The bone removal is extended downward to increase access to the middle fossa floor. F, the dura and sylvian fissure have been opened to expose the supra- and parasellar areas. The olfactory tract and the optic and oculomotor nerves are exposed. The posterior communicating and basilar arteries are seen through the opticocarotid triangle located between the optic nerve and carotid and anterior cerebral arteries. The posterior communicating artery courses medial to the oculomotor nerve in the suprasellar area.*

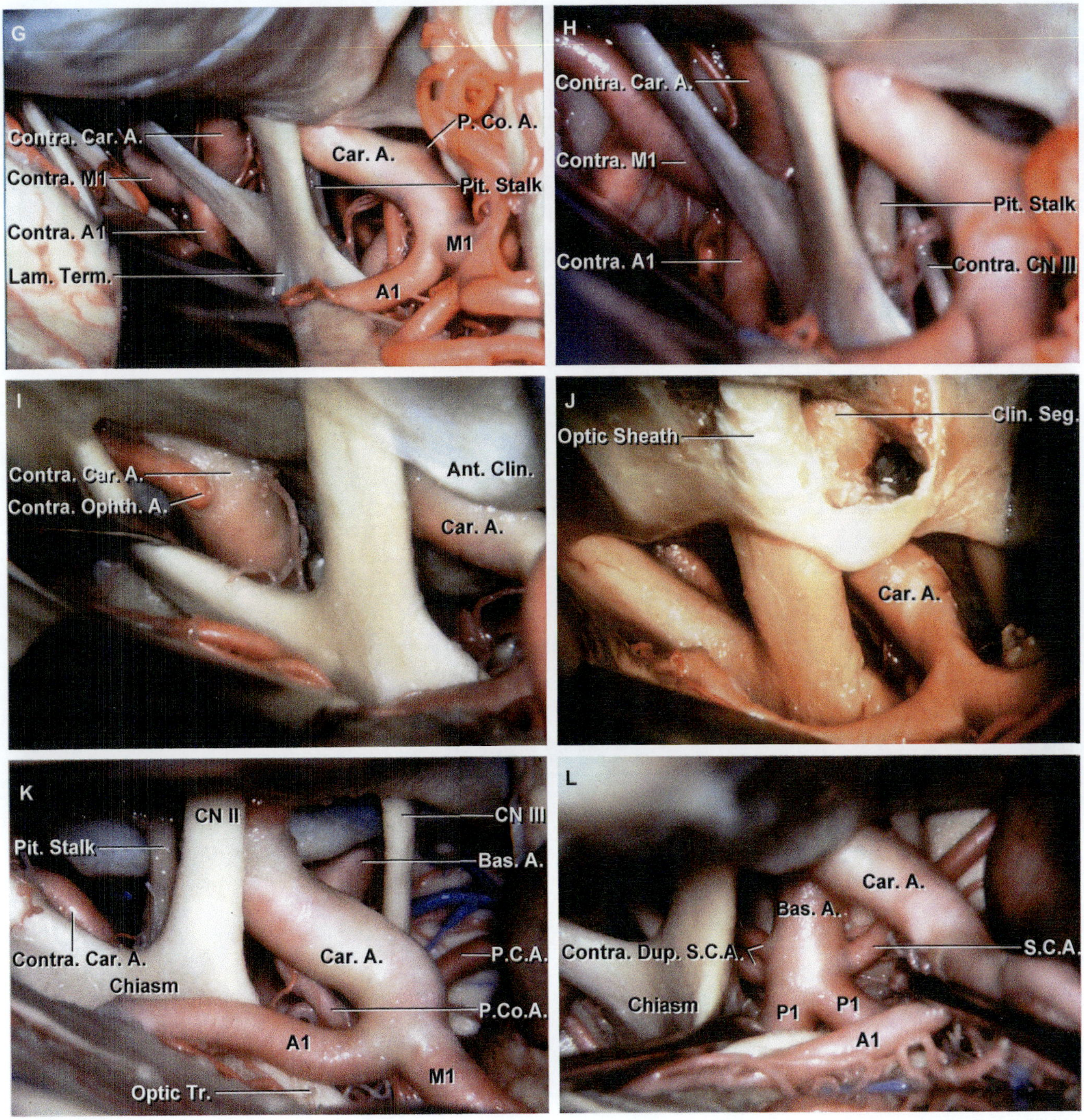

FIGURE 3.4. *Continued*
G, the exposure has been extended to the opposite side by further elevation of the frontal lobe. The exposure includes both optic nerves and the ipsilateral and contralateral carotid and middle cerebral arteries. The lamina terminalis extends upward from the optic chiasm. The pituitary stalk is exposed below the optic chiasm. H, further elevation of the frontal lobes exposes the opposite sylvian fissure to the level of the bifurcation of the contralateral middle cerebral artery. The pituitary stalk and contralateral oculomotor nerve are seen through the opticocarotid triangle. I, the left optic nerve has been elevated to expose the contralateral ophthalmic artery. J, the anterior clinoid process has been removed to expose the clinoid segment of the internal carotid artery. K–P, examines four routes to the apex of the basilar apex that can be accessed through a frontotemporal (pterional) craniotomy. These routes are: 1) through the opticocarotid triangle located between the internal carotid artery, optic nerve, and anterior cerebral artery; 2) through the carotid bifurcation-optic tract interval located between the bifurcation of the internal carotid artery and the optic tract; 3) through the carotid-oculomotor interval located between the carotid artery and the oculomotor nerve and above the posterior communicating artery; and 4) through the carotid-oculomotor interval and below the posterior communicating artery. K and L, exposure directed through the opticocarotid triangle. K, pterional exposure of supra- and parasellar area in another specimen. The pituitary stalk and contralateral internal carotid artery are seen below the optic chiasm. L, (Legend continues on next page.)

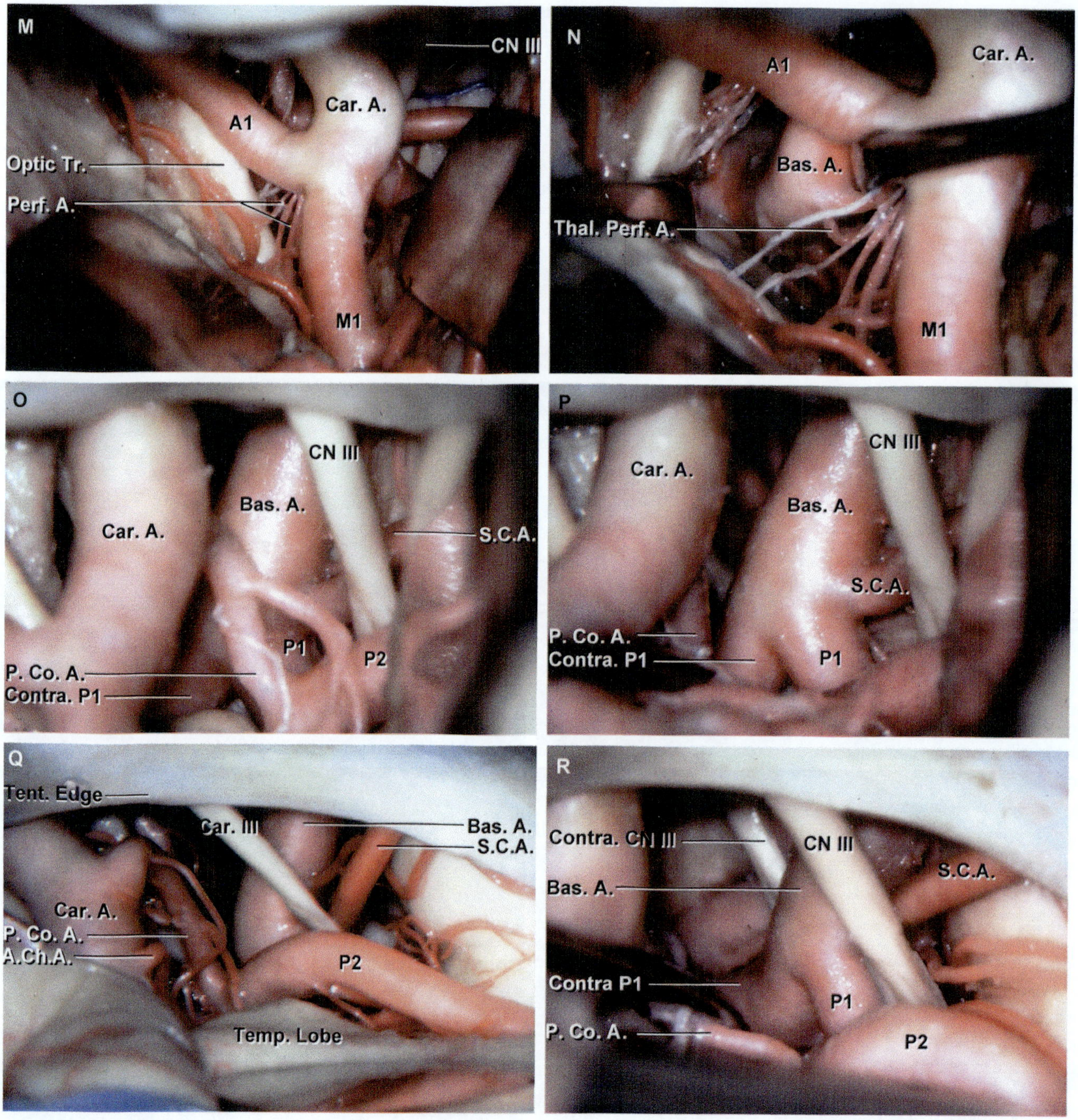

FIGURE 3.4. *Continued*
the opticocarotid triangle has been opened by gently elevating the optic chiasm and displacing the carotid artery laterally to access the bifurcation of the basilar artery and the origin of both superior cerebellar and posterior cerebral arteries. The contralateral superior cerebellar artery arises as a duplicate artery. This exposure is adequate if the opticocarotid triangle is large, as occurs if both the internal carotid and anterior cerebral arteries are long, but is inadequate if the internal carotid and anterior cerebral arteries are short and the internal carotid artery courses tightly beside the optic nerve and chiasm. The basilar bifurcation cannot be exposed by this route if the bifurcation is especially high or is located below the dorsum sellae. M *and* N, *exposure directed through the carotid bifurcation optic tract interval* M, *the exposure is redirected to the area above the carotid bifurcation.* N, *the carotid bifurcation has been depressed and the optic tract elevated to expose the basilar bifurcation. A thalamoperforating artery arises from the basilar bifurcation.* O *and* P, *exposure directed through the carotid-oculomotor interval located between the carotid artery and the oculomotor nerve.* O, *the posterior communicating artery passes in front of the basilar bifurcation. Gently depressing or elevating the posterior communicating artery, which crosses in front of the basilar artery, will increase access to the basilar apex.* P, *the posterior communicating artery has been elevated to expose the origin of the superior cerebellar arteries and the basilar bifurcation.* Q *and* R, *anterior subtemporal exposure obtained through the frontotemporal craniotomy by elevating the anterior part of the temporal lobe.* Q, *this oculomotor nerve arises from the medial surface of the cerebral peduncle and passes between the posterior cerebral and superior cerebellar artery to enter the roof of the cavernous sinus.* R, *the posterior communicating artery has been elevated to expose the basilar apex, both oculomotor nerves, and the junction of the right posterior communicating artery with the right posterior cerebral artery.*

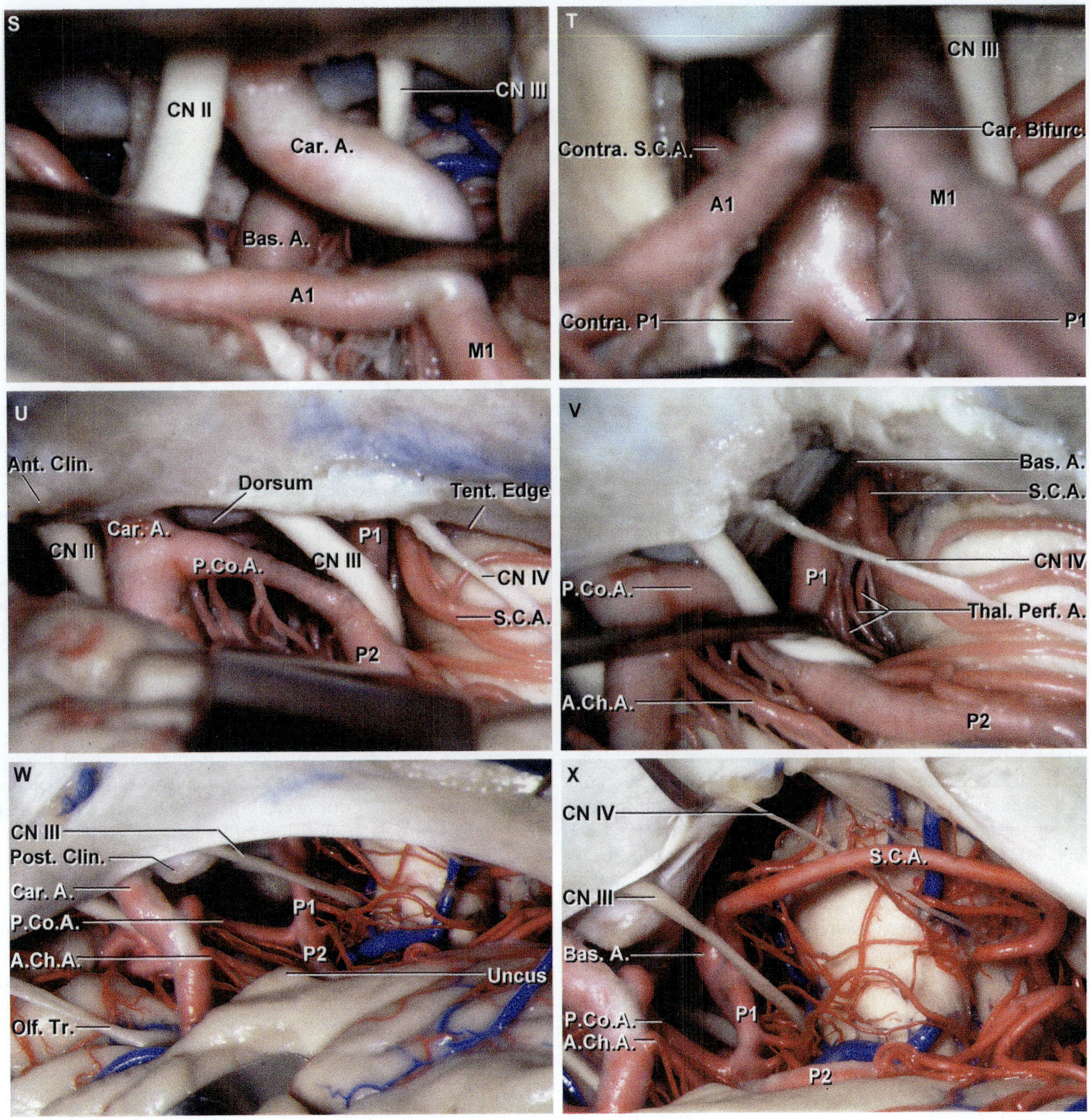

FIGURE 3.4. *Continued*
S and T, exposure of a high basilar bifurcation through a frontotemporal craniotomy S, the basilar artery can be seen through the opticocarotid triangle, but the basilar bifurcation is so high that it cannot be seen. T, the optic tract has been gently elevated and the carotid bifurcation depressed to expose the basilar apex. U–X, subtemporal transtentorial exposure of low basilar bifurcation. U, the right temporal lobe has been elevated to expose the optic, oculomotor, and trochlear nerves above the tentorial edge. The posterior communicating artery passes backward superomedial to the oculomotor nerve. The basilar bifurcation is located behind the dorsum sellae, just below the tentorial edge. V, the tentorial edge has been divided just behind where the trochlear nerve joins the tentorium to expose the basilar bifurcation located in back of the dorsum sellae. Elevating the posterior cerebral artery exposes the thalamoperforating arteries. W, another exposure. The bifurcation is located behind the dorsum. The P1 extends upward on the medial side of the oculomotor nerve. X, the tentorium has been divided while preserving the trochlear nerve to expose the upper part of the basilar artery and the bifurcation. The posterior cerebral artery passes above and the superior cerebellar artery below the oculomotor nerve. A., *artery;* A.Ch.A., *anterior choroidal artery;* Ant., *anterior;* Bas., *basilar;* Bifurc., *bifurcation;* Brs., *branches;* Car., *carotid;* Clin., *clinoid;* CN, *cranial nerve;* Contra., *contralateral;* Dup., *duplicate;* Fiss., *fissure;* Lam., *lamina;* Olf., *olfactory;* Ophth., *ophthalmic;* Orb., *orbital;* P.C.A., *posterior cerebral artery;* P.Co.A., *posterior communicating artery;* Perf., *perforating;* Pit., *pituitary;* Post., *posterior;* S.C.A., *superior cerebellar artery;* Seg., *segment;* Sup., *superior;* Temp., *temporal, temporalis;* Tent., *tentorial;* Term., *terminalis;* Thal. Perf., *thalamoperforating;* Tr., *tract.*

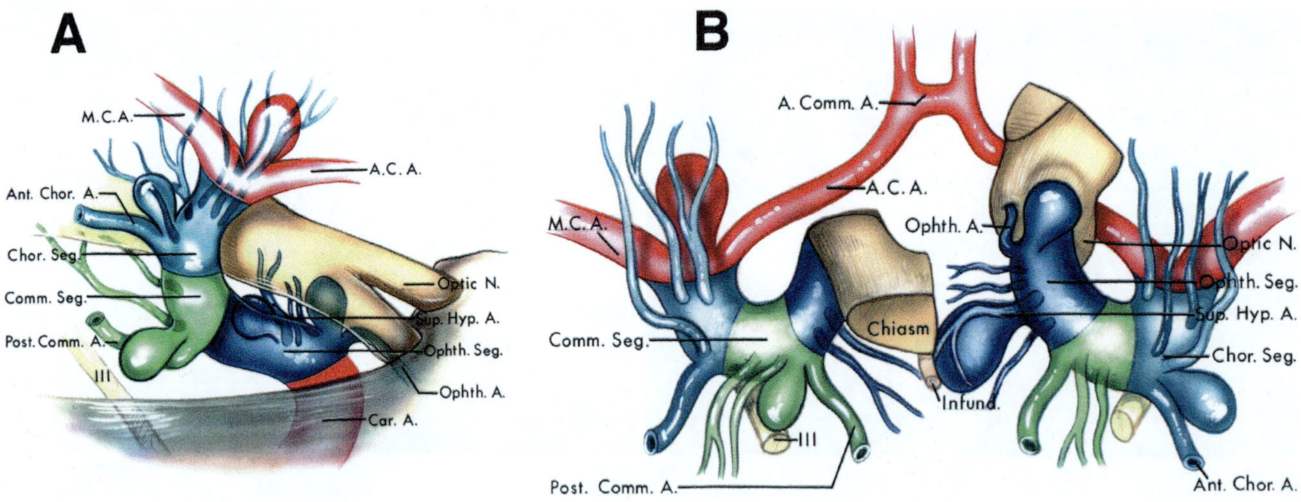

FIGURE 3.5. *Perforating arteries at the common aneurysm sites on the supraclinoid portion of the internal carotid artery.* A, *lateral view.* B, *superior view, with the right optic nerve and right half of the optic chiasm reflected forward to expose the origin of the ophthalmic artery.* A and B, *ophthalmic aneurysms arise at the origin of the ophthalmic artery from the ophthalmic segment and point upward into the optic nerve. The perforating branches arising from the ophthalmic segment are on the medial side of this aneurysm. Posterior communicating aneurysms arise at the origin of the posterior communicating artery from the communicating segment and point posteriorly toward the oculomotor nerve. The perforating branches arising from the communicating segment are often stretched around the neck of posterior communicating aneurysms. Anterior choroidal aneurysms arise at the origin of the anterior choroidal artery from the choroidal segment and point posterolaterally. They are usually located superior or superolateral to the origin of the anterior choroidal artery. Aneurysms arising at the bifurcation into the anterior and middle cerebral arteries point upward lateral to the optic chiasm and tract toward the anterior perforated substance. The perforating branches arising from the choroidal segment are usually stretched along the posterior wall of the aneurysm arising at the bifurcation.* A., *artery;* Ant., *anterior;* Comm., *communicating;* A.C.A., *anterior cerebral artery;* Chor., *choroidal;* Car., *carotid;* Hyp., *hypophyseal;* Infund., *infundibulum;* M.C.A., *middle cerebral arteries;* N., *nerve;* Ophth., *ophthalmic;* Post., *posterior;* Seg., *segment;* Sup., *superior.*

segment or carotid cave and project upward out of the cave into the subarachnoid space. The fifth variant of the ophthalmic aneurysm is one that is associated with an ophthalmic artery that arises within the cavernous sinus and passes through the superior orbital fissure to reach the orbit (*Fig. 3.6, L* and *M*). This aneurysm will point upward, but almost immediately encounters the lower margin of the anterior clinoid process and cannot break into the subarachnoid space.

The ophthalmic artery usually arises from the medial third of the superior surface of the carotid in the area below the optic nerve (*Figs. 3.4* and *3.6C*). Gentle elevation of the optic nerve away from the internal carotid artery is often required to see the preforaminal segment. The ophthalmic artery, after exiting the carotid, may immediately enter the optic canal, but in most cases, there is a 2- to 5-mm preforaminal segment. Exposure of the neck of this aneurysm may be facilitated by the removal of the anterior clinoid process and adjacent part of the lesser sphenoid wing, by removing the roof of the optic foramen and adjacent part of the orbital roof to allow some mobilization of the optic nerve, and by incision of the falciform process, a thin fold of dura mater that extends medially from the anterior clinoid process to the tuberculum sellae and covers the segment of the optic nerve immediately proximal to the optic foramen. It is helpful to divide the upper and sometimes the lower dural ring to mobilize the carotid artery for clipping aneurysms. Most ophthalmic arteries arise anterior to the tip of the anterior clinoid process, approximately 5 mm medial to the clinoid process (3).

The perforating arteries arising from the ophthalmic segment take origin from posterior or medial aspects of the internal carotid artery and are distributed to the stalk of the pituitary gland, the optic nerve, chiasm, and tracts and floor of the third ventricle around the infundibulum (*Fig. 3.5*). Ophthalmic aneurysms typically arise on the upper anterior wall of the carotid artery, not on the side from which the perforating arteries arise, and point upward away from the perforating branches arising from the ophthalmic segment. The risk of damaging the adjacent perforating branches is less in clipping an ophthalmic aneurysm than at other sites on the internal carotid artery because ophthalmic aneurysms typically point upward, away from these perforating branches.

Carotid-Superior Hypophyseal Aneurysms

The segment of the carotid artery just distal to the origin of the ophthalmic artery, and from which the superior hypophyseal artery arises, has a medially convex curve in the area lateral to the pituitary stalk (*Figs. 3.2, 3.3, 3.5,* and *3.6N*). It is on this medially convex curve that the superior hypophyseal aneurysm arises. The aneurysm arises at the distal edge of the origin of the superior hypophyseal artery and points medially into the area between the lower surface of the optic chiasm and the diaphragma sellae. The aneurysms are often confused, on lateral angiograms, with intracavernous aneurysms, because they frequently project below the level of the anterior clinoid process, although they are located in the subarachnoid

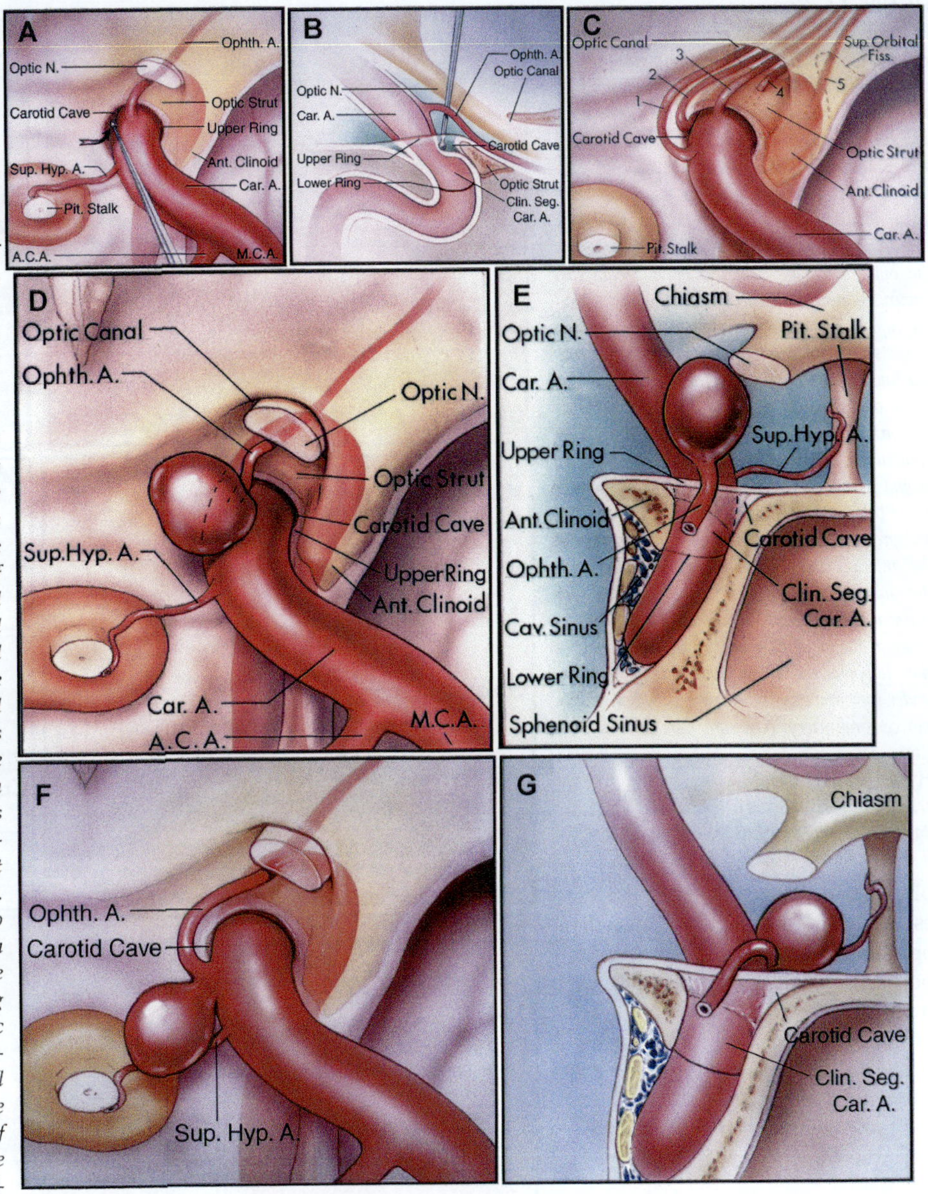

FIGURE 3.6. *Relationship of ophthalmic and superior hypophyseal aneurysms to the clinoid segment of the carotid artery and the carotid cave.* A, *the clinoid segment of the carotid artery is the segment situated medial to the anterior clinoid process. The upper dural ring, which surrounds the upper edge of the clinoid segment, is formed by the dura that extends medially from the upper margin of the anterior clinoid process. The lower dural ring extends medially from the lower margin of the anterior clinoid process. The ophthalmic artery arises from the superior surface of the initial supraclinoid segment of the carotid artery and passes forward under the optic nerve to enter the optic foramen. The upper ring often seems to be adherent to and forms a collar around the carotid artery. However, in many cases there is a space between this ring and the anteromedial aspect of the artery that extends downward to form a cave around the artery, referred to as the carotid cave. The cave is most prominent on the anteromedial side of the carotid artery at the roof of the cavernous sinus. If the ophthalmic artery arises within the carotid cave, the neck of the aneurysm will also be located in the cave, and the aneurysm will extend upward out of the cave into the subarachnoid space. The superior hypophyseal artery arises from the medial wall of the internal carotid artery and courses toward the pituitary stalk. The optic strut is the bridge of bone that separates the optic foramen from the superior orbital fissure. This strut extends from the lower surface of the anterior clinoid process to the body of the sphenoid bone. The strut forms the inferolateral margin of the optic foramen. The anterior and middle cerebral arteries are also in the exposure.* B, *sagittal cross section through the clinoid segment and carotid cave. The cave extends downward between the upper dural ring and the wall of the carotid artery. The ophthalmic artery usually arises from the carotid artery immediately above the carotid cave and upper dural ring. A probe is inserted in the carotid cave, the space between the upper dural ring and the wall of the carotid artery. This clinoid segment of the carotid artery is situated medial to the anterior clinoid process.* C, *various patterns* (1–5 *in* C) *of the origin and passage of the ophthalmic artery that determine the degree of involvement by an aneurysm of the clinoid segment and carotid cave.* 1, *the ophthalmic artery arises from the superomedial wall of the artery well above the carotid cave. An aneurysm arising at the origin of this ophthalmic artery will mimic a superior hypophyseal aneurysm.* 2, *the ophthalmic artery arises in the carotid cave.* 3, *the artery arises just above the carotid cave.* 4, *the artery arises in the carotid cave and passes through the optic strut to enter the optic canal.* 5, *the artery arises in the cavernous sinus and passes through the superior orbital fissure.* D *and* E, *superior and anterior views of the most common ophthalmic aneurysm. This aneurysm arises above the clinoid segment and the carotid cave from the medial part of the superior wall of the carotid artery and projects upward into the optic nerve. The cavernous sinus is located below the anterior clinoid process in the anterior view.* F *and* G, *superior and anterior view of an ophthalmic aneurysm that mimics a superior hypophyseal aneurysm. The ophthalmic artery has a relatively long course to the optic foramen. This aneurysm projects medially below the optic chiasm and mimics the superior hypophyseal aneurysm, although it arises at the origin of the ophthalmic artery. The neck of the aneurysm is proximal to the origin of the superior hypophyseal artery. This aneurysm, on lateral angiography, may be seen medial to and below the upper margin of the anterior clinoid process.* *(Legend continues on next page.)*

space below the optic chiasm. The superior hypophyseal artery and the ophthalmic segment perforating branches described above are stretched around the neck of this aneurysm.

The superior hypophyseal arteries are small branches, usually two, that arise from the medial or posterior aspect of the ophthalmic segment (*Figs. 2.4, 3.2.* and *3.5*, and *8.1*) (3). One branch often predominates. These arteries pass medially to reach the floor of the third ventricle, optic nerves, and the chiasm and pituitary stalk. The perforating arteries and the hypophyseal vascular supply may be compromised if the aneurysm expands medially. Diabetes insipidus and amenorrhea may result from occlusion of these branches. Removing the anterior clinoid process and adjacent part of the roof of the optic canal and orbital roof is often helpful in exposing the neck of the superior hypo-

FIGURE 3.6. *Continued*
H and I, superior and anterior views of an aneurysm arising below the upper dural ring, within the carotid cave. This aneurysm projects upward out of the carotid cave toward the optic nerve and has the upper dural ring around its base. J and K, superior and anterior views of an ophthalmic aneurysm that arises in association with an ophthalmic artery, having its origin in the carotid cave and passing through a foramen in the optic strut to reach the optic canal. This aneurysm neck is located further laterally than the typical ophthalmic aneurysm. The aneurysm projects upward out of the cave into the subarachnoid space. L and M, superior and anterior views of an aneurysm that arises at the ophthalmic artery origin in the cavernous sinus. This ophthalmic artery passes through the superior orbital fissure to reach the orbit. This aneurysm arises below the clinoid segment and carotid cave and projects upward against the lower margin of the anterior clinoid process and does not reach the subarachnoid space. N, superior view of superior hypophyseal aneurysm. The aneurysm arises at the distal edge of the origin of the superior hypophyseal artery and points medially under the optic chiasm. A., artery; A.C.A., anterior cerebral artery; Ant., anterior; Car., carotid; Cav., cavernous; Clin., clinoid; Fiss., fissure; Hyp., hypophyseal; M.C.A., middle cerebral artery; N., nerve; Ophth., ophthalmic; Pit., pituitary; Seg., segment; Sup., superior.

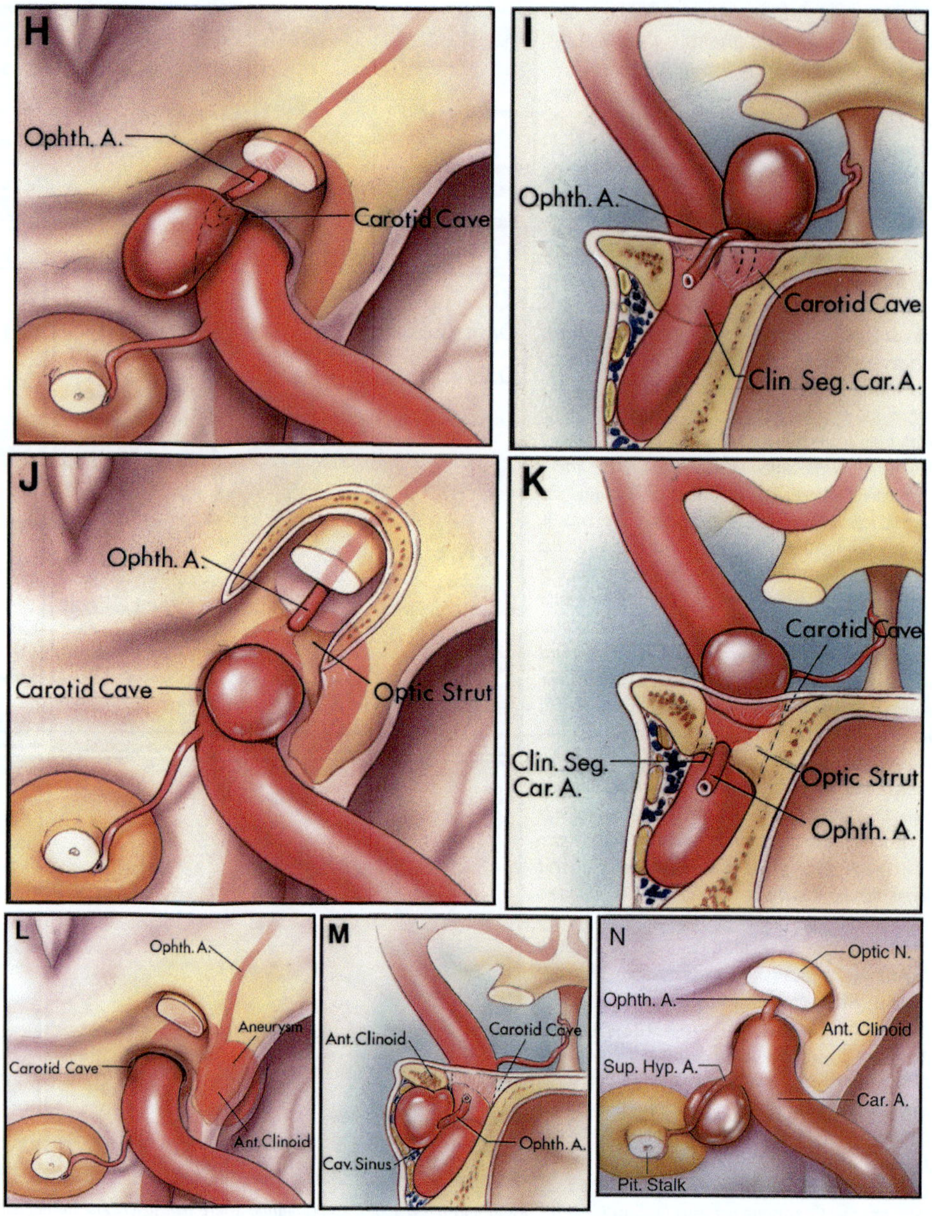

physeal aneurysms. In some cases, especially in older individuals, the ophthalmic artery and supraclinoid portion of the internal carotid artery may elongate, thus placing the neck of the ophthalmic aneurysm further posteriorly so that it mimics the position and medial projection under the optic chiasm of the superior hypophyseal aneurysm.

Carotid-Posterior Communicating Aneurysms

The initial segment of the supraclinoid carotid is directed posteriorly, but the segment after the origin of the superior hypophyseal artery turns upward toward the anterior perforated substance to form a curve that is convex posteriorly (*Figs. 3.2, 3.3, 3.5,* and *3.8*). The posterior communicating and anterior choroidal arteries arise from the posterior wall on this convex curve as the carotid artery passes upward toward its bifurcation. The most common carotid aneurysm arises at the carotid-posterior communicating artery junction. These aneurysms arise from the posterior wall of the carotid artery near the apex of this turn, immediately above the distal edge of the origin of the posterior communicating artery. Another important relationship in this area is that of the oculomotor nerve to the internal carotid artery. The oculomotor nerve enters the dura lateral to the posterior clinoid process and medial to the dural band passing from the tentorium cerebelli toward the anterior clinoid process. The oculomotor nerve pierces the dura between 2 and 7 mm (average, 5 mm) posterior to the initial supraclinoid segment. Aneurysms arising at the origin of the posterior communicating artery point downward and backward and may compress the oculomotor nerve at its entrance into the dural roof of the cavernous sinus when they reach 4 to 5 mm in diameter.

The posterior communicating artery is usually found inferomedial and the anterior choroidal artery superior or superolateral to the neck of the aneurysm (*Figs. 3.4, 3.7,* and *3.8*). In exposing the carotid artery beyond the origin of the ophthalmic artery, the surgeon often sees the anterior choroidal artery before

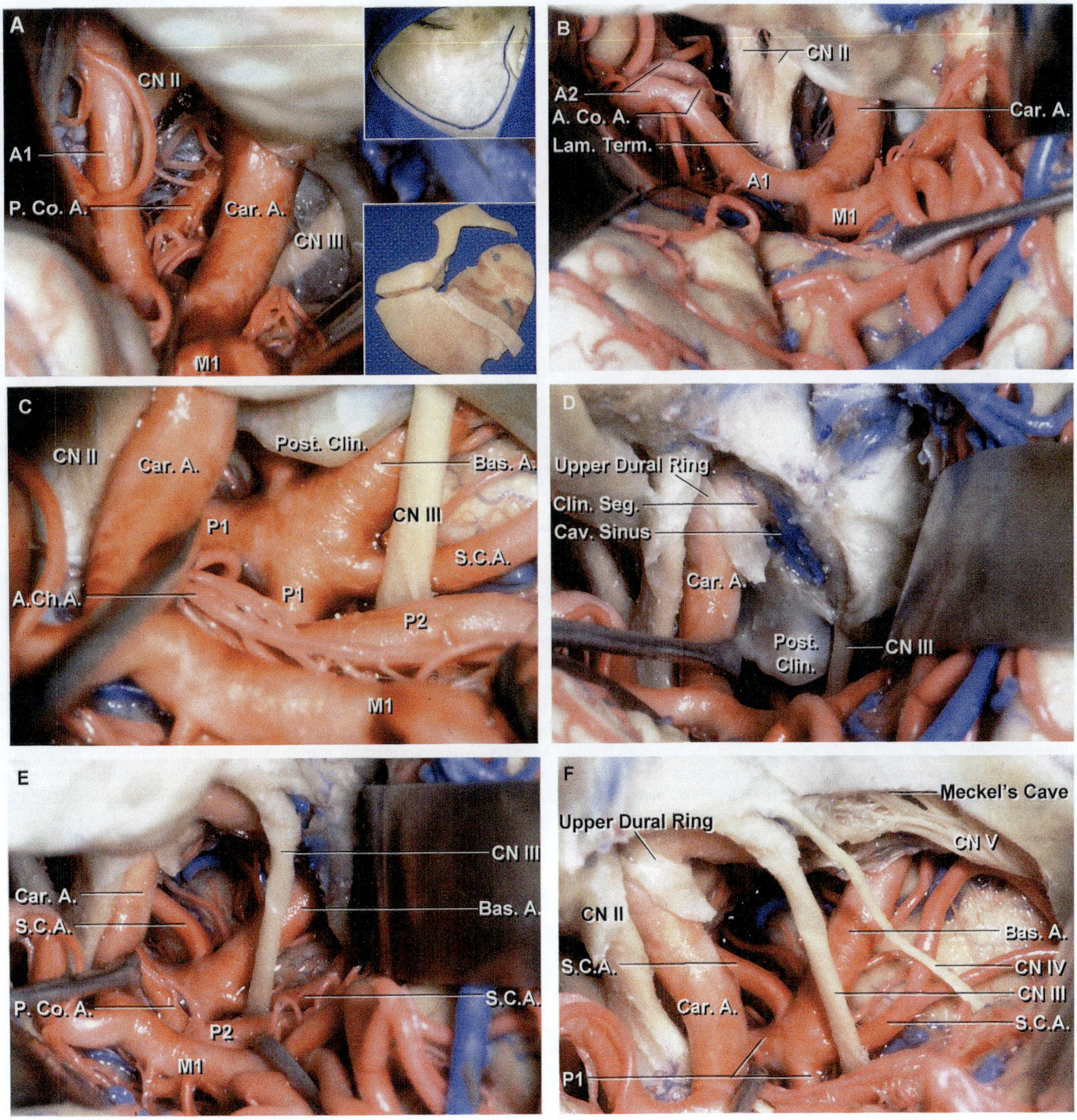

FIGURE 3.7. A, *orbitozygomatic craniotomy and transcavernous approach to basilar apex.* A, *the* inset (upper right) *shows the scalp incision and the* inset (lower right) *shows the two-piece orbitozygomatic craniotomy. The frontal and temporal lobes have been retracted to expose the optic and oculomotor nerves and the anterior and middle cerebral and posterior communicating arteries.* B, *the exposure has been directed medially above the optic chiasm to the region of the anterior communicating artery.* C, *the carotid artery has been elevated to expose the basilar artery apex through the interval between the carotid artery and oculomotor nerve. The posterior clinoid process blocks access to the basilar artery.* D, *the anterior clinoid process and the roof of the cavernous sinus have been removed to provide access to the clinoid segment of the internal carotid artery and the posterior clinoid process. The upper dural ring extends medially from the upper margin of the anterior clinoid process.* E, *the posterior clinoid process has been removed to increase access to the upper portion of the basilar artery.* F, *the anterior part of the tentorial edge has been removed to expose the upper margin of the posterior trigeminal root in Meckel's cave and to provide increased access to the upper part of the basilar artery. The trochlear nerve was preserved in opening the anterior part of the tentorial edge. Note the difference in the length of basilar arteries exposed in* C *and* F. A., *artery;* A.Ch.A., *anterior choroidal artery;* A.Co.A., *anterior communicating artery;* Bas., *basilar;* Car., *carotid;* Cav., *cavernous;* Clin., *clinoid;* CN, *cranial nerve;* Lam., *lamina;* P.Co.A., *posterior communicating artery;* Post., *posterior;* S.C.A., *superior cerebellar artery;* Seg., *segment;* Term., *terminalis.*

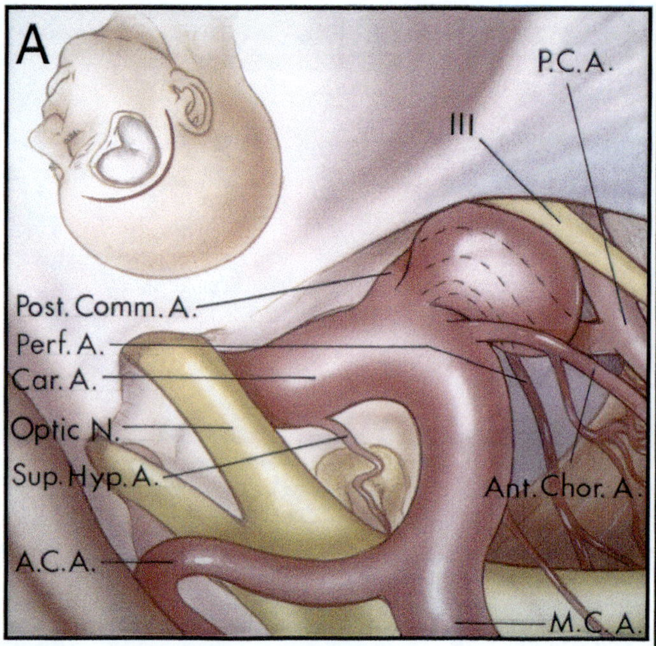

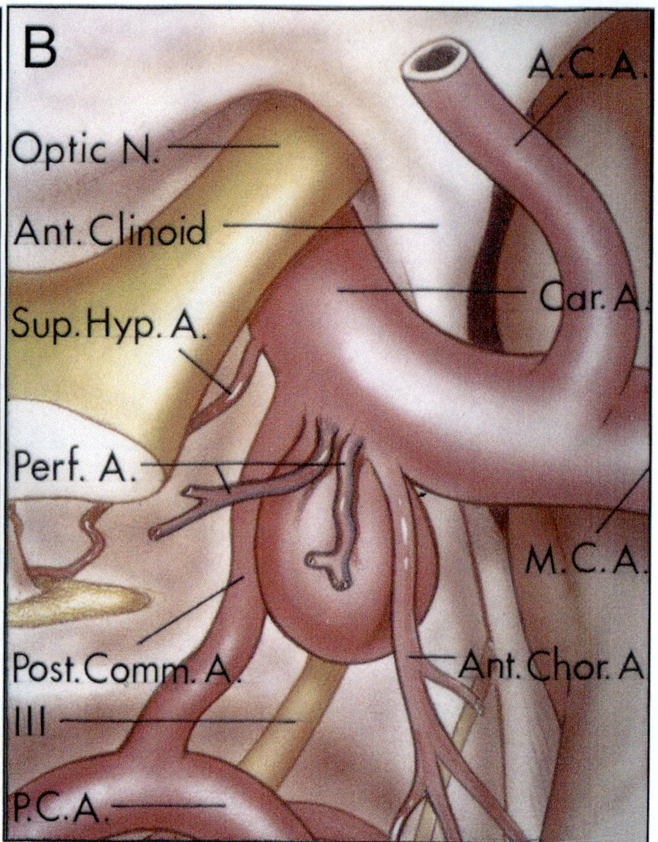

FIGURE 3.8. *Carotid-posterior communicating aneurysm. A, lateral operative view. The* inset (upper left) *shows the site of the right frontotemporal craniotomy. The aneurysm arises from the carotid artery at the distal edge of the origin of the posterior communicating artery and projects backward toward the oculomotor nerve. The posterior communicating artery is on the inferomedial margin of the neck and the anterior choroidal artery is on the superolateral margin. Perforating arteries that may be as large as either the posterior communicating or the anterior choroidal artery arise around the neck of the aneurysms. Other structures in the exposure include the optic nerves and the anterior, middle, and posterior cerebral and superior hypophyseal arteries.* B, *superior view. The posterior communicating artery is on the inferomedial edge of the neck of the aneurysm and the anterior choroidal artery is on the superolateral margin, with perforating branches arising along the neck of the aneurysm. The anterior clinoid process is lateral to the carotid artery.* A., *artery;* A.C.A., *anterior cerebral artery;* Ant., *anterior;* Car., *carotid;* Chor., *choroidal;* Comm., *communicating;* Hyp., *hypophyseal;* M.C.A., *middle cerebral artery;* N., *nerve;* P.C.A., *posterior cerebral artery;* Perf., *perforating;* Post., *posterior;* Sup., *superior.*

the posterior communicating artery, although the anterior choroidal artery arises distal to the posterior communicating artery. This occurs because of three sets of anatomic circumstances. First, the supraclinoidal segment of the internal carotid artery passes upward in a posterolateral direction, placing the origin of the more distally arising branch, the anterior choroidal artery, further lateral to the midline than the origin of the posterior communicating artery, which arises more proximally. Second, the anterior choroidal artery arises further laterally on the posterior wall of the carotid than the posterior communicating artery. Third, the anterior choroidal artery pursues a more lateral course than the posterior communicating artery; the former passes laterally below the optic tract, around the cerebral peduncle, and into the temporal horn, whereas the latter is directed in a posteromedial direction above and medial to the oculomotor nerve toward the interpeduncular fossa. Care should be taken to preserve both the posterior communicating artery and the anterior choroidal artery at the time of obliteration of internal carotid artery aneurysms. Occlusion of either of these arteries may cause a hemiplegia, homonymous hemianopsia, and reduced levels of consciousness.

The posterior communicating artery, which forms the lateral boundary of the circle of Willis, arises from the posteromedial surface of the internal carotid artery and sweeps backward above the sella turcica and above and medial to the oculomotor nerve to join the posterior cerebral artery (*Figs. 3.4, 3.7,* and *3.8*). If the posterior communicating artery remains the major origin of the posterior cerebral artery, the configuration is termed fetal. If the posterior communicating artery is of small or normal size, it courses posteromedially to join the posterior cerebral artery medial to the oculomotor nerve, but if it is of a fetal type, it courses posterolaterally above or above and lateral to the oculomotor nerve.

Fewer perforating branches arise from the communicating segment of the carotid artery than from the ophthalmic or choroidal segments (*Fig. 3.5*) (3). However, they are of critical importance because some of them may be larger than either the anterior choroidal or the posterior communicating arteries, especially if the latter artery is hypoplastic. These branches arise from the posterior half of the arterial wall at the same site as the neck of the aneurysm and are often stretched around the neck of the aneurysm. These branches terminate in the optic

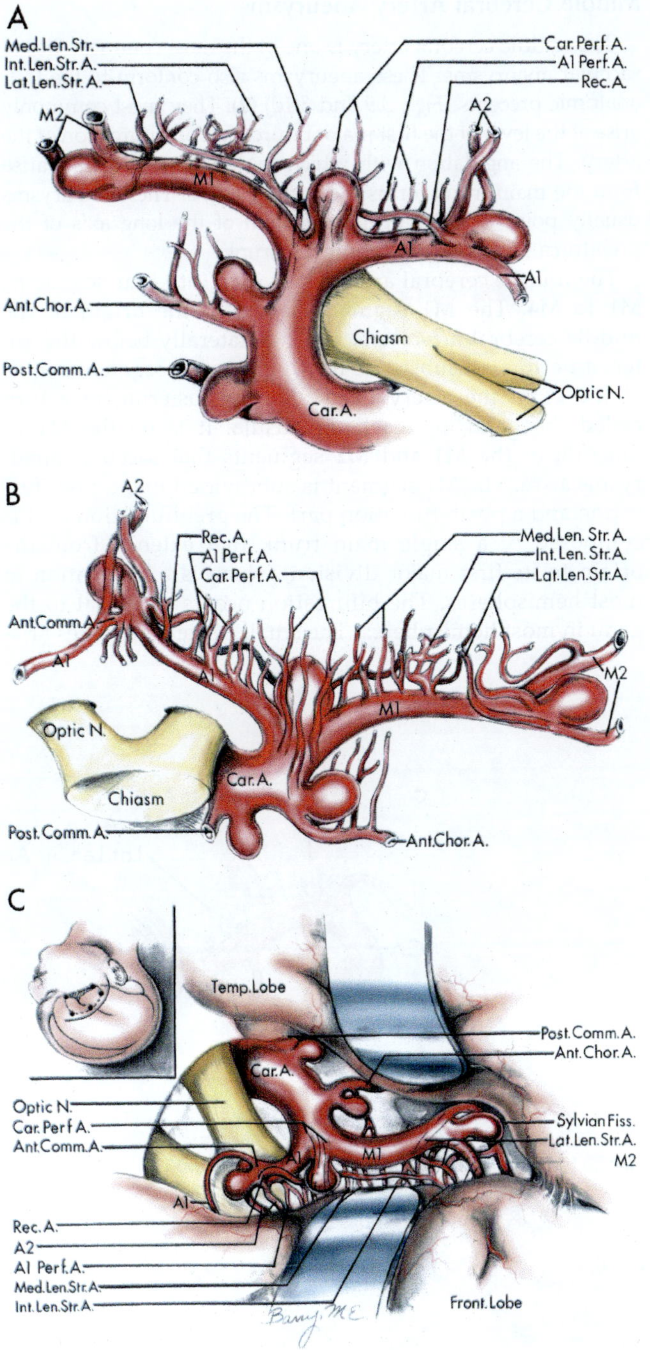

chiasm and tract, floor of the third ventricle, infundibulum, the posterior perforated substance, and medial temporal lobe.

Carotid-Anterior Choroidal Aneurysms

The apex of the posteriorly convex curve of the supraclinoid carotid may also be located at the level of the origin of the anterior choroidal artery, which shifts the hemodynamic force distally from the level of origin of the posterior communicating artery to that of the anterior choroidal artery (*Figs. 3.2, 3.3, and 3.5*). An aneurysm arising at the level of the anterior choroidal artery is usually located just distal, superior, or superolateral to the origin of the anterior choroidal artery. They point posteriorly or posterolaterally, usually well above the oculomotor nerve. In opening the sylvian fissure, the origin and proximal portion of the anterior choroidal artery is often exposed before the posterior communicating artery, because of its more lateral origin and course.

The anterior choroidal artery arises from the posterolateral aspect of the carotid artery (*Figs. 3.4, 3.7, and 3.8*) (19). It may arise as two or duplicate arteries. Perforating branches arising in this area may be as large as the anterior choroidal artery. From its origin, it courses posteriorly below the optic tract and terminates by joining the choroid plexus in the temporal horn. Occlusion causes a variable deficit that includes contralateral hemiplegia, hemianesthesia, and hemianopsia.

Aneurysms arising from the choroidal segment commonly have more perforating branches stretched around their neck than those arising from the communicating or ophthalmic segment because the choroidal segment has a greater number of perforating branches arising from it and the majority arise from the posterior wall, where the neck of the aneurysm is situated (*Figs. 3.5 and 3.9*). On average, four, but as many as

FIGURE 3.9. *Relationship of the arteries entering the anterior perforated substance to common aneurysm sites. A, lateral view and B, superior view. The aneurysms involving these perforating arteries arise at four sites: (a) the internal carotid artery at the origin of the anterior choroidal artery; (b) the terminal bifurcation of the internal carotid artery into the anterior and middle cerebral arteries; (c) the bifurcation of the middle cerebral artery; and (d) the region of the anterior communicating artery. The aneurysms arising from the internal carotid artery at the level of the posterior communicating artery do not involve the branches to the anterior perforated substance, unless they become very large. The aneurysms arising from the internal carotid artery at the level of, or just distal to, the anterior choroidal artery, point posteriorly and posterolaterally and may have branches to the anterior perforated substance from both the internal carotid and anterior choroidal arteries near the neck, and from the anterior choroidal artery on the inferior or inferomedial margin. Aneurysms arising at the carotid bifurcation have the carotid perforating branches passing upward behind the neck to enter the anterior perforated substance adjacent to where the medial lenticulostriate arteries and the proximal perforating branches of the A1 enter the anterior perforated substance. The recurrent artery passes above the carotid bifurcation and may be incorporated into the arachnoidal bands around the neck and fundus of this aneurysm. Aneurysms arising at the bifurcation of the middle cerebral artery commonly have the origin of some of the lateral lenticulostriate arteries near their neck. If the prebifurcation segment of the M1 is very short, the intermediate lenticulostriate arteries will arise near the neck. The aneurysm arising at the level of the anterior communicating artery is located above the optic nerve and chiasm at the junction of the A1 and A2 segments of the anterior cerebral artery. This aneurysm usually arises in the setting where one A1 segment is dominant and the opposite A1 segment is hypoplastic. The A1 perforating branches and the recurrent artery arise near the neck of the aneurysm. C, operative exposure through a frontotemporal craniotomy. The sylvian fissure has been opened between the frontal and temporal lobes. The* inset (upper left) *shows the skin incision* (solid line)*, the site of the craniotomy* (dotted line)*, and the craniectomy* (hatched area)*.* A., *arteries, artery;* Ant., *anterior;* Car., *carotid;* Chor., *choroidal;* Comm., *communicating;* Fiss., *fissure;* Front., *frontal;* Int., *intermediate;* Lat., *lateral;* Len. Str., *lenticulostriate;* Med., *medial;* N., *nerve;* Perf., *perforating;* Post., *posterior;* Rec., *recurrent;* Temp., *temporal.* (From, *Rosner SS, Rhoton AL Jr, Ono M, Barry M: Microsurgical anatomy of the anterior perforating arteries.* ***J Neurosurg*** *61:468–485, 1984 [19].)*

nine, perforating branches arise from the posterior wall of this segment. These branches pass superiorly behind the choroidal segment and the bifurcation of the internal carotid artery to enter the anterior perforated substance with the perforating branches of the anterior cerebral, recurrent, middle cerebral, and anterior choroidal arteries and ascend to the internal capsule (3, 19). An oculomotor nerve deficit, as frequently occurs with a carotid-posterior communicating artery aneurysm, is uncommon and rarely occurs before rupture.

Carotid Bifurcation Aneurysms

The fifth aneurysm site on the internal carotid artery is at its bifurcation. These aneurysms most easily fit the four principles described above (*Figs. 3.2, 3.3, 3.5,* and *3.9*). These aneurysms arise at the apex of the T-shaped bifurcation. They point upward in the direction of the long axis of the prebifurcation segment of the artery toward the anterior perforated substance. The perforating branches arising from the choroidal segment of the internal carotid and the proximal part of the anterior and middle cerebral arteries are stretched around the back side of the neck and wall of the aneurysm and should be dissected free of the aneurysm (*Figs. 3.4, 3.5, 3.7,* and *3.9*).

Middle Cerebral Artery Aneurysms

The middle cerebral artery is one of the most common sites of saccular aneurysms. These aneurysms also conform to the four anatomic precepts (*Figs. 3.9* and *3.10*) (2). They most commonly arise at the level of the first major bifurcation or trifurcation of the artery. The angulation with which the bifurcating trunks arise from the main trunk forms the turn or curve. These aneurysms usually point laterally in the direction of the long axis of the prebifurcation segment of the main trunk.

The middle cerebral artery is divided into four segments, M1 to M4. The M1 segment begins at the origin of the middle cerebral artery and extends laterally below the anterior perforated substance to where the M2 segment begins at the point the artery turns sharply posterior, at a turn called the genu, to reach the insula. It is on the M1 or junction of the M1 and M2 segments that saccular aneurysms arise. The M1 segment is subdivided into a prebifurcation and a postbifurcation part. The prebifurcation part is composed of a single main trunk that extends from the origin to its first major division, which is a bifurcation in most hemispheres. The bifurcation occurs proximal to the genu in most hemispheres. The small cortical branches aris-

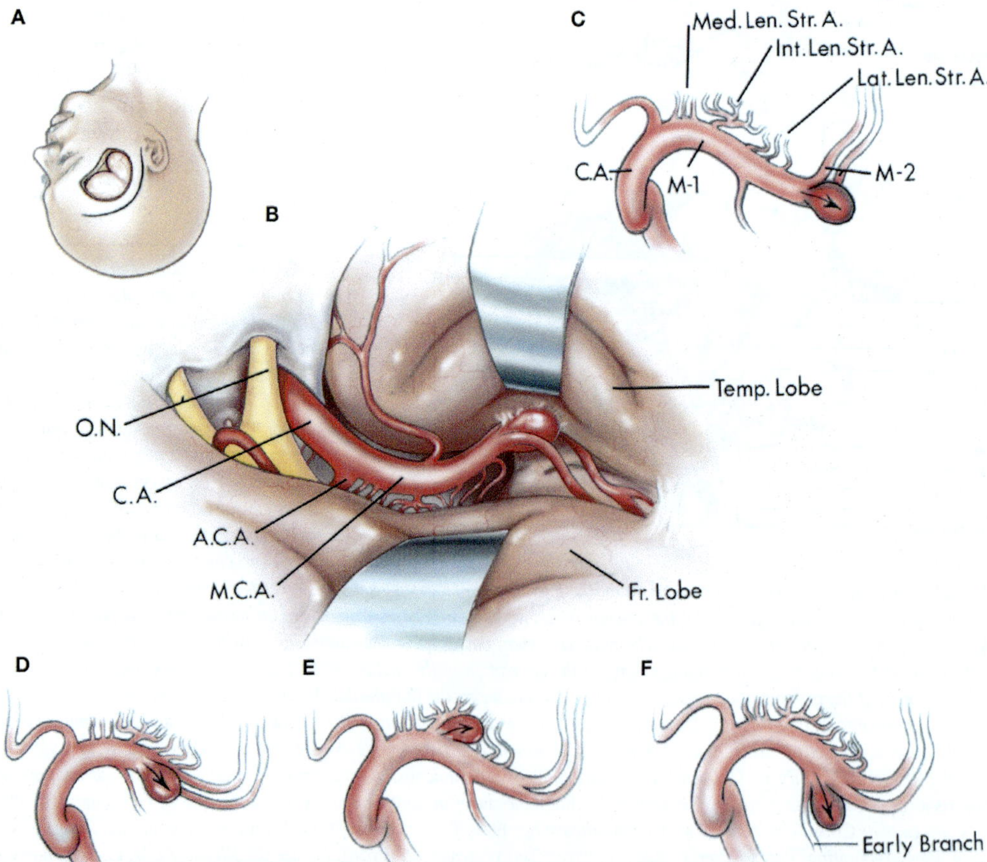

FIGURE 3.10. *Middle cerebral aneurysms.* A, *scalp incision and craniotomy for approaching aneurysms arising on the middle cerebral artery.* B, *operative view provided by a right frontotemporal craniotomy. The right sylvian fissure has been split to provide this view of the optic nerves and the carotid and middle and anterior cerebral arteries. Brain spatulas are on the temporal and frontal lobes.* C, *middle cerebral aneurysms are usually located at the bifurcation near the genu of the artery. The arrows show the direction of hemodynamic force at the aneurysm site. The medial, intermediate, and lateral lenticulostriate arteries arise from the middle cerebral artery.* D, *aneurysm arising on an early bifurcation.* E, *aneurysm arising at a large lenticulostriate branch.* F, *aneurysm arising at an early branch.* A., *arteries, artery;* A.C.A., *anterior cerebral artery;* C.A., *internal cerebral artery;* Fr., *frontal;* Int., *intermediate;* Lat., *lateral;* Len.Str., *lenticulostriate;* M.C.A., *middle cerebral artery;* Med., *medial;* O.N., *optic nerve;* Temp., *temporal.*

ing from the M1 segment proximal to the bifurcation, called early branches, may be the site of origin of aneurysms arising proximal to the bifurcation. The early branches are directed to the frontal and temporal lobes.

The middle cerebral artery branches to the anterior perforated substance are called the lenticulostriate arteries (*Figs. 2.30, 2.31, 3.9,* and *3.10*). On average, there are 10 (range, 1–20) lenticulostriate arteries per hemisphere (19). Eighty percent of lenticulostriate arteries arise from the prebifurcation part of the M1 segment, 17% arise from the postbifurcation part of the M1 segment, and 3% arise from the proximal part of the M2 segment near the genu. The earlier the bifurcation, the greater the number of branches arising distal to the bifurcation. An aneurysm may infrequently arise at the origin of a large lenticulostriate branch. The lenticulostriate arteries are divided into medial, intermediate, and lateral groups (*Figs. 2.30* and *3.9*) (19). Each group has a unique origin, composition, and characteristic distribution in the anterior perforated substance. The distinct morphology of each group has led to the medial group being referred to as straight because they pursue a straight course, the intermediate group as candelabra because of their complex branching as they approach the anterior perforated substance, and the lateral group as S-shaped, describing their curved course. All three groups are encountered in splitting the sylvian fissure and following the artery medially. The number and type of perforating branches stretched around the neck of the aneurysm is dependent on the level of the bifurcation (*Figs. 3.9* and *3.10*). If the prebifurcation segment is very short, the neck of the aneurysm may have the straight or candelabra branches stretched around the neck, whereas an aneurysm arising at the apex of a long prebifurcation segment may involve the area of the S-shaped lenticulostriate branches.

Instruments helpful in dissecting the neck and in separating the perforating arteries from the wall of the aneurysm include the 40-degree-angled teardrop dissectors and the 1-, 2-, or 3-mm wide spatula dissectors (*Fig. 3.11*) (14, 15). A small angled curette with a 1.5-mm cup is useful in removing the dura over the clinoid process. A 5-French suction, 10-cm long provides a useful suction dissector. Bayonet scissors with 9.5-cm shafts are the appropriate length to divide arachnoidal bands. For grasping and separating arachnoidal adhesions, bayonet tissue forceps with fine serrations on the inside of the tips of the forceps are needed. Brain spatulas tapered from 10 or 15 mm at the base to 5 or 10 mm at the tip are suitable for elevating the brain at most aneurysm sites.

Anterior Communicating Aneurysms

The most common aneurysm site on the anterior cerebral artery is at the level of the anterior communicating artery (*Fig. 3.12*). These aneurysms are made complex by the frequently associated variants of anatomy and the difficulties in fully visualizing the major arterial trunks and perforating arteries in the area (12). The segment of the anterior cerebral artery between the internal carotid and anterior communicating arteries is referred to as the A1 segment, and the segment between the anterior communicating artery and the rostrum of the corpus callosum is referred to as A2 segment. Aneurysms usually occur in the setting where one A1 segment is hypoplastic and the dominant A1 gives rise to both A2s (*Fig. 3.12*). The aneurysm arises at the point where the dominant A1 segment bifurcates at the level of the anterior communicating artery to give rise to both the left and right A2 segments. These aneurysms usually point away from the dominant segment toward the opposite side. They may also project in other directions. The direction in which the fundus points is determined by the course of the anterior cerebral arteries proximal to their junction with the anterior communicating artery. Tortuosity of the arteries may create a situation in which the hemodynamic thrust varies, so that these aneurysms may project not only to the opposite side, but also in the anterior, posterior, or inferior direction (*Fig. 3.12*).

The anterior cerebral artery gives rise to numerous perforating branches (*Figs. 2.16, 2.24, 3.9,* and *3.13*). The branches arise from two sources. First, the A1 segment gives rise to branches that pass directly to the anterior perforated substance; and second, the A1 and the proximal part of the A2 segments give rise to the recurrent artery. The recurrent branch of the anterior cerebral artery is the largest and longest of the branches directed to the anterior perforated substance. It may be the first artery seen on elevating the frontal lobe to approach the anterior communicating aneurysm (*Fig. 3.13*). It is unique among arteries in that it doubles back on its parent vessel, passing above the carotid bifurcation, and accompanying the middle cerebral artery into the sylvian fissure before entering the anterior perforated substance. If the A1 segment is hypoplastic, the recurrent artery on that side may be as large as the hypoplastic A1 segment and might even be confused with it, since both will be passing along the area between the carotid bifurcation and interhemispheric fissure (*Figs. 2.24* and *3.13*). The recurrent artery may lie in any direction from the A1 segment. Its origin may adhere to the wall of the anterior communicating aneurysms. The inverting adventitia of A1 may so obscure the recurrent artery that inadvertent occlusion by a clip may easily occur, even under the operating microscope. The recurrent artery pursues a long, redundant path, looping forward on the gyrus rectus or the posterior part of the orbital surface of the frontal lobe where it could be damaged and occluded in removing the posterior 1 or 2 cm of the gyrus rectus, as is common practice in exposing anterior communicating aneurysms (*Fig. 3.9*). It may arise from a common stem with the frontopolar artery (*Fig. 3.13*). Ischemia in the area supplied by Heubner's artery may cause hemiparesis with facial and brachial predominance, because of compromise of the branch supplying the anterior limb of the internal capsule, and may cause aphasia if the artery is on the dominant side (19).

The anterior communicating artery is the site of origin of as many as four perforating branches to the dorsal surface of the optic chiasm and suprachiasmatic area (*Figs. 2.16* and *2.24*) (11). These perforating branches perfuse the fornix, corpus callosum, and septal region. Their occlusion results in personality and memory disturbances.

Pericallosal Aneurysms

The next most common aneurysm site on the distal anterior cerebral artery is at the level of origin of the callosomarginal

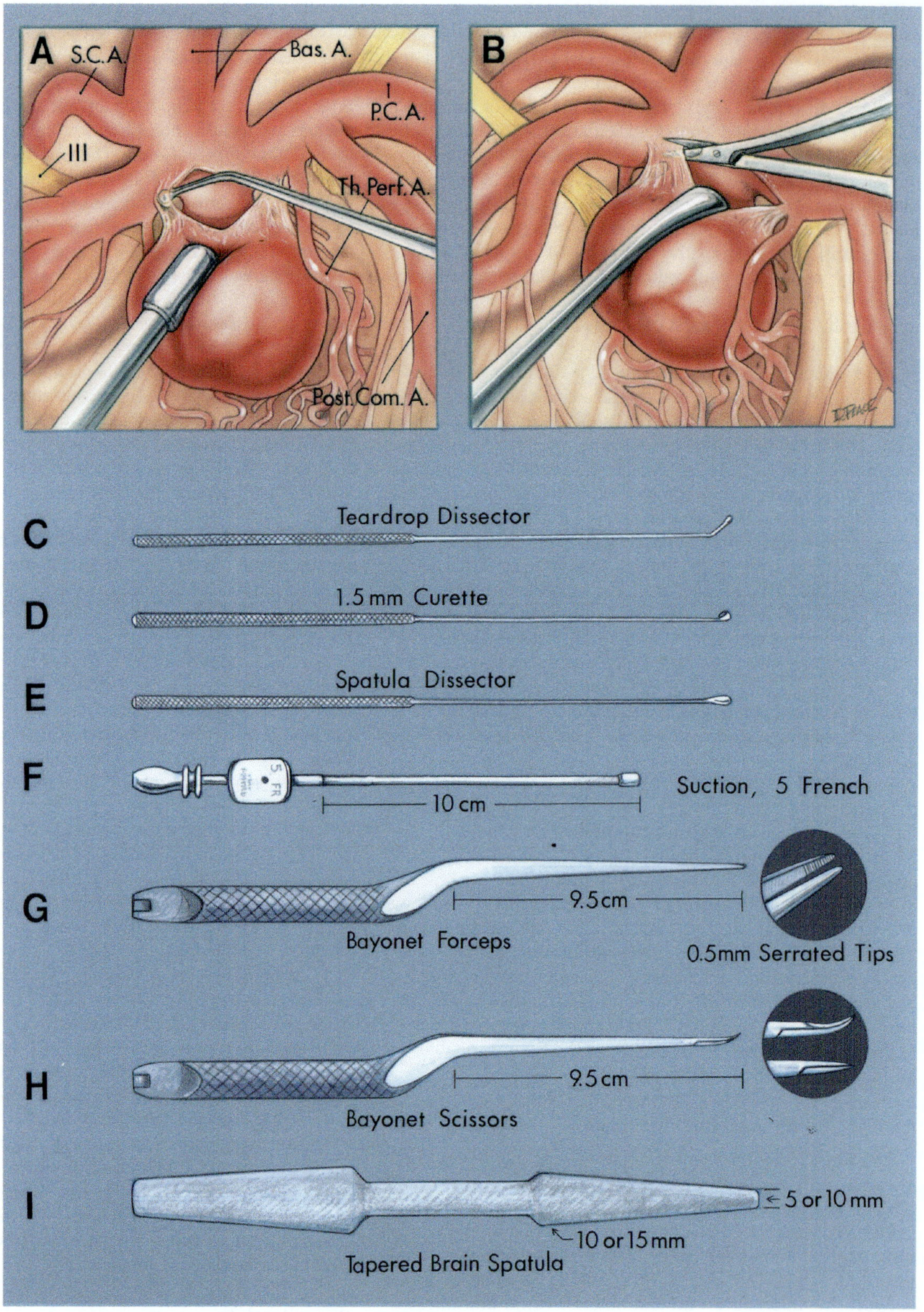

FIGURE 3.11. *Instruments for aneurysm dissection. A, the 40-degree-angled teardrop dissector separates perforating branches and arachnoidal bands from the neck of an aneurysm of the basilar artery. The blunt tip suction of a 5-French size provides suction and aids in the retraction of the aneurysm neck for dissection. Structures in the exposure include the superior cerebellar, posterior communicating, posterior cerebral, and thalamoperforating arteries and the oculomotor nerve. B, the wall of the aneurysm is being retracted with a spatula dissector, and tough arachnoidal bands around the neck are being divided with a microscissors. C, 40-degree-angled teardrop dissector for defining the neck and separating perforating vessels from the neck of the aneurysm. D, angled microcurette with 1.5-mm cup, useful in removing the dura from the anterior clinoid process. E, spatula dissector for defining the neck and separating perforating vessels from the wall of an aneurysm. F, blunt tip suction of 5-French size for suction and dissection of an aneurysm. A 7- or 9-French blunt tip suction may be needed if heavy bleeding should occur. G, bayonet forceps with 9.5-cm blades and 0.5-mm tips with small serrations (inset) inside tips for grasping arachnoidal and fibrous bands around an aneurysm. H, bayonet microscissors with 9.5-cm shafts and straight and curved blades (inset) for dividing adhesions around the neck of the aneurysm. I, the brain spatulas most commonly used to elevate the brain in aneurysm surgery are tapered from 10 or 15 mm at the base to 5 or 10 mm at the tip. A., arteries, artery; Bas., basilar;* Com., *communicating;* P.C.A., *posterior cerebral artery;* Post., *posterior;* S.C.A., *superior cerebellar artery;* Th.Perf., *thalamoperforating.*

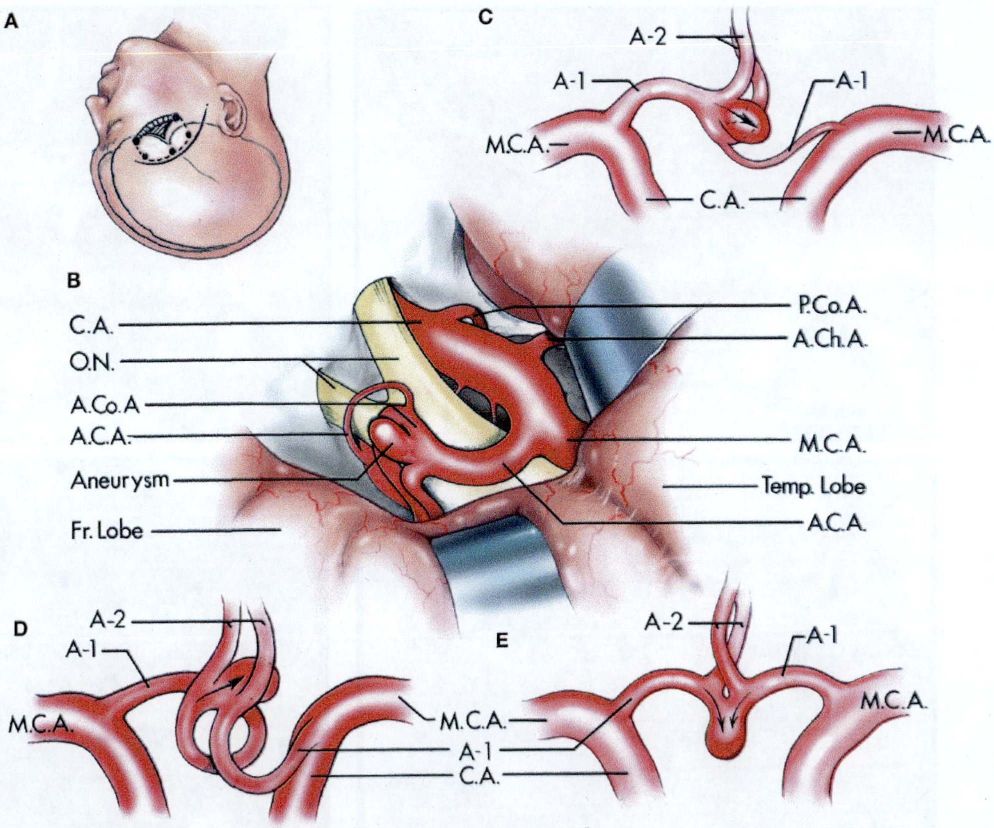

FIGURE 3.12. *Anterior communicating artery aneurysms.* A, *scalp incision (solid line), bone flap (dotted line), and craniectomy (hatched area).* B, *operative view of the most common anterior communicating artery aneurysm. The aneurysm points downward and forward away from the dominant anterior cerebral artery. Structures in the exposure include the carotid, anterior cerebral, middle cerebral, anterior communicating, posterior communicating, and anterior choroidal arteries, optic nerves, and the frontal and temporal lobes.* C, D, *and* E, *anterior views showing three different aneurysm configurations created by the different hemodynamic forces (arrows) associated with the various sizes and shapes of proximal and distal segments of the anterior cerebral arteries. The most common aneurysm* (C) *is associated with a hypoplastic A1 segment. Less common projections of these aneurysms are posterior* (D) *or straight forward* (E). *The direction in which the fundus points is determined by the course of the artery proximal to its junction with the anterior communicating artery.* A.C.A., *anterior cerebral artery;* A.Ch.A., *anterior choroidal artery;* A.Co.A., *anterior communicating artery;* C.A., *internal carotid artery;* Fr., *frontal;* M.C.A., *middle cerebral artery;* O.N., *optic nerve;* P.Co.A., *posterior communicating artery;* Temp., *temporal.*

artery from the pericallosal artery, usually in close proximity to the anterior part of the corpus callosum, near the point of greatest angulation of the artery at the genu (*Figs. 2.22* and *3.14*). The curve is formed by the angulation of the branching and the artery's passage around the rostrum of the corpus callosum. The aneurysm points distally into the interval between the junction of the pericallosal and callosomarginal arteries. Unusual variants, such as a connection between the two pericallosal arteries at their major bifurcation, may cause aneurysms by producing alterations in hemodynamics.

Vertebral and Basilar Artery Aneurysms

Approximately 15% of saccular aneurysms occur in the vertebrobasilar system, the majority of which (63%) occur at the basilar bifurcation. The incidence of anomalies consisting of either a hypoplastic communicating or a fetal posterior cerebral origin is more common with aneurysms than in normal groups. Aneurysms arising on the branches of the vertebral and basilar arteries also share the same four facets of anatomy described above. They arise at an apical branching site on a curve, point in the direction the blood would have followed if the curve were not present, and are surrounded by a constantly occurring set of perforating branches (*Fig. 3.15*). The basilar apex aneurysm arises at the branching of the posterior cerebral arteries from the basilar artery and points upward in the direction of the long axis of the basilar artery (*Figs. 3.15* and *3.16, A* and *B*). Because of these variations, posterior cerebral artery aneurysms may be visualized on carotid as well as on vertebral angiography, especially when the P1 segment is hypoplastic (fetal type).

Aneurysms arising from the basilar artery at the level of origin of the superior cerebellar or anteroinferior cerebellar artery, or from the vertebral artery at the level of origin of the posteroinferior cerebellar artery, initially seem to conform poorly to the first three facets of anatomy applicable to the other aneurysms because the basilar and vertebral arteries are often pictured as straight arteries, with the cerebellar arteries arising at right angles from them (*Fig. 3.15*) (18). However, most of the arteries harboring aneurysms are tortuous, and the change in direction of flow associated with the curves creates hemodynamic stress on the wall of the basilar or vertebral arteries near the origins of the cerebellar arteries. These aneurysms point in the direction the blood would have gone had there not been a curve at the level of origin of the involved branch.

Basilar Apex Aneurysms

The majority of the 15% of aneurysms occurring in the vertebral-basilar system are located on the posterior part of the circle of Willis at the bifurcation of the basilar artery (*Figs. 3.4, 3.15,* and *3.16, A* and *B*). The basilar apex aneurysm arises at the branching of the posterior cerebral arteries from the basilar artery. The curve at the aneurysm site is related to the change from the vertical direction of the basilar artery to a lateral direction of the posterior cerebral arteries. These aneu-

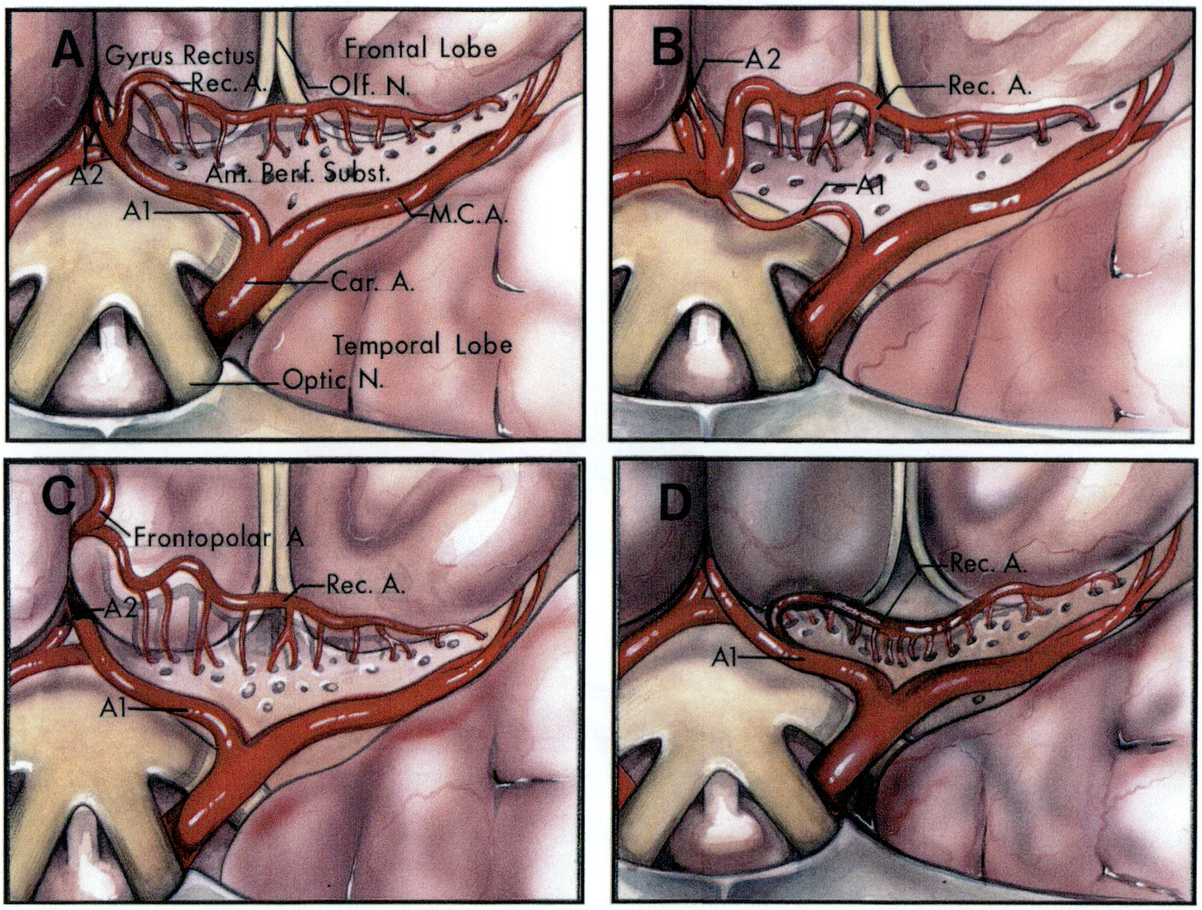

FIGURE 3.13. *Variants in the origin and course of the recurrent artery.* A, *the recurrent artery arises at the junction of the A1 and A2 segments and passes laterally above the bifurcation of the carotid artery to be distributed to a long strip of the anterior perforating substance. It commonly loops forward on the gyrus rectus, where it could be injured in removing a small area of the gyrus for exposure of an anterior communicating aneurysm.* B, *the recurrent artery may be as large or larger than the hypoplastic A1 segment in the area between the carotid bifurcation and the interhemispheric fissure. It may be the first artery seen on elevating the frontal lobe as one dissects medially from the carotid bifurcation to the region of the anterior communicating artery. It often loops forward on the gyrus rectus and could easily be damaged as the posterior centimeter of the gyrus rectus is removed to expose the junction of the A1 and A2 segments.* C, *the recurrent artery arises as a common trunk with the frontopolar artery and passes laterally across the gyrus rectus.* D, *the recurrent artery arises from the A1 segment.* A., *artery;* Ant., *anterior;* Car., *carotid;* M.C.A., *middle cerebral artery;* N., *nerve;* Olf., *olfactory;* Perf., *perforated;* Rec., *recurrent;* Subst., *substance.*

rysms project upward in the direction of the long axis of the basilar artery. The basilar bifurcation is most commonly situated opposite the interpeduncular fossa, but it may be located as far as 1.3 mm below the pontomesencephalic junction in front of the pons, or as far rostral as the mamillary bodies (20). High bifurcations may indent and push the mamillary bodies and floor of the third ventricle upward. High or low bifurcations are best approached by the subtemporal rather than the pterional route.

In the subtemporal approach for basilar aneurysm, the neck of the aneurysm at the bifurcation is best found by following the inferior side of the posterior cerebral artery medially as it curves around the peduncle, because the inferior surface is the most infrequent site of origin for perforating branches, thus making it the safest approach to the P1 and basilar bifurcation (*Figs. 3.17* and *3.18*).

The region of the basilar bifurcation may be the site of multiple anomalies (20, 22). The segment of the posterior cerebral artery between the basilar bifurcation and the posterior communicating artery is referred to as P1 and the segment just distal to the communicating as P2. A normal posterior circle, defined as one in which both P1 segments have a diameter larger than their posterior communicating arteries—and the latter are not hypoplastic—is found in approximately half of cases. In the remainder, anomalies are found consisting of either a hypoplastic posterior communicating artery or a fetal arrangement in which the P1 segment is hypoplastic and the posterior communicating artery provides the major supply to the posterior cerebral artery.

A hypoplastic posterior communicating artery, or a fetal configuration in which the posterior cerebral artery arises predominantly from the carotid artery, may be found on one

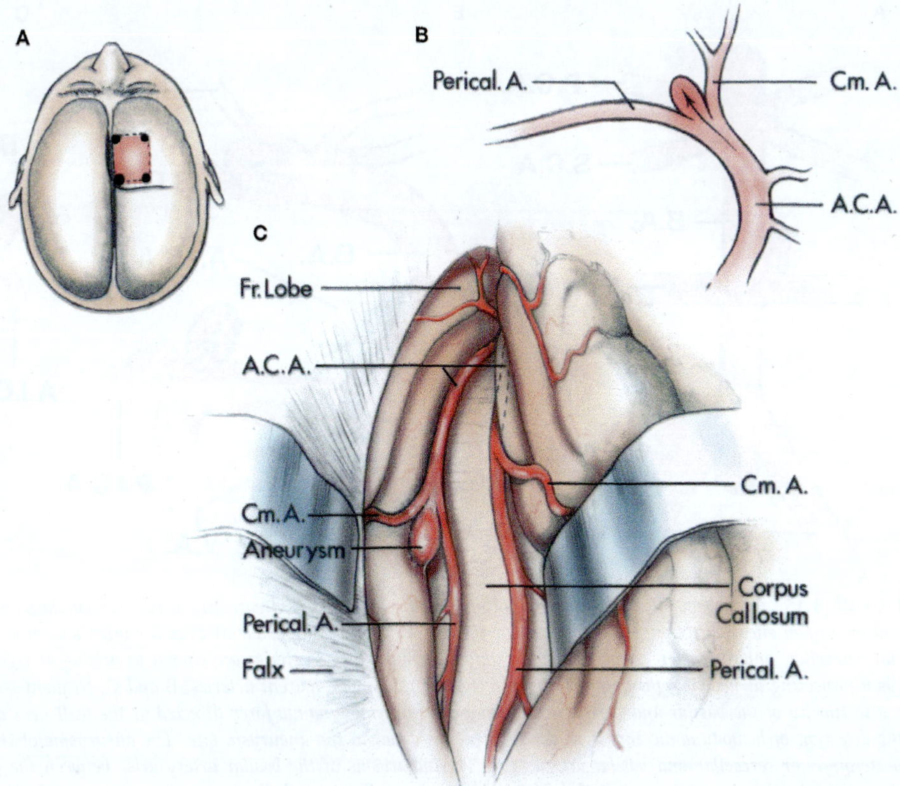

FIGURE 3.14. *Lateral and operative views of the most common aneurysm site on the distal part of the anterior cerebral artery. A, scalp incision* (solid line) *and bone flap* (dotted line). *B, medial surface of the right anterior cerebral artery. The aneurysm arises on the medial surface of the frontal lobe at the anterior margin of the corpus callosum. The hemodynamic thrust* (arrow) *and the aneurysm are directed distally in the interval between the pericallosal and callosomarginal arteries. C, the right frontal lobe is retracted to expose the anterior cerebral arteries, the falx, and the aneurysm arising above the corpus callosum at the origin of the callosomarginal and pericallosal arteries. The exposure may be centered lower on the forehead if the origin of the callosomarginal artery and the aneurysm are located below the corpus callosum. A., artery;* A.C.A., *anterior cerebral artery;* Cm., *callosomarginal;* Fr., *frontal;* Perical., *pericallosal.*

or both sides (*Figs. 2.8* and *2.34*). Transection of a hypoplastic posterior communicating artery or P1 segment has been recommended to gain access to basilar bifurcation aneurysms on the assumption that they have fewer branches. However, the number and diameter of perforating branches is relatively constant, regardless of trunk size; therefore, a hypoplastic segment supplies the same perforating area as a larger vessel, despite its smaller size (20).

The posterior portion of the circle of Willis sends a series of perforating arteries into the diencephalon and midbrain that may become stretched around basilar apex aneurysms. The most important and largest of these are the thalamoperforating arteries, which arise from the P1 in the region of the basilar apex aneurysm (*Figs. 3.18* and *3.19*) (20, 22). They originate from P1 and enter the brain behind the maxillary bodies through the posterior perforated substance in the interpeduncular fossa and medial cerebral peduncles. They are both the largest branches of the P1 and the branch nearest the bifurcation in most cases. One P1 may not give rise to a thalamoperforating artery, in which case a well-developed or dominant thalamoperforating branch on the contralateral side will supply the area normally perfused by the branches of both P1s. The risks from occlusion of these vital perforating vessels include visual loss, paralysis, somesthetic disturbances, weakness, memory deficits, autonomic and endocrine imbalance, abnormal movements, diplopia, and depression of consciousness.

The posterior and lateral surfaces of the upper centimeter of the basilar artery is also a rich source of perforating arteries. An average of 8 (range, 3–18) branches arise from the upper centimeter (*Figs. 2.34* and *2.35*) (20, 22). Approximately half arise from the posterior surface and a quarter arise from each side. Perforating branches rarely arise from the anterior surface of the basilar artery. The patient with basilar bifurcation aneurysms has been viewed more gravely than the patient with aneurysms in other areas because of the greater tendency of vital perforators to be involved in aneurysm dissection and clipping. In basilar bifurcation aneurysms, the more posterior the aneurysm, the poorer the prognosis, because the tendency for vital perforators to be involved becomes greater as the aneurysm projects more posteriorly (1). The anterior surface of the basilar bifurcation is infrequently the site of perforators, thus surgical results are better with anteriorly projecting aneurysms. The rich plexus on the posterior basilar surface, 2 to 3 mm below the bifurcation, entering the interpeduncular fossa and terminating in the medial midbrain makes this the most dangerous site. The basilar apex is intermediate in risk because the thalamoperforating artery is easier to identify at surgery, and there are fewer perforators than on the posterior aspect of the bifurcation.

An aneurysm of the posterior cerebral artery distal to the origin is uncommon. The most common site is at the origin of the first major branch, as the posterior cerebral artery winds around the midbrain either on the P1 or P2 in the crural or ambient cisterns. Distal posterior cerebral artery aneurysms tend to become larger than other aneurysms before their identification, often mimicking neoplasms in the region. The most frequent neurological deficit with posterior cerebral aneurysms is a partial or complete oculomotor nerve deficit.

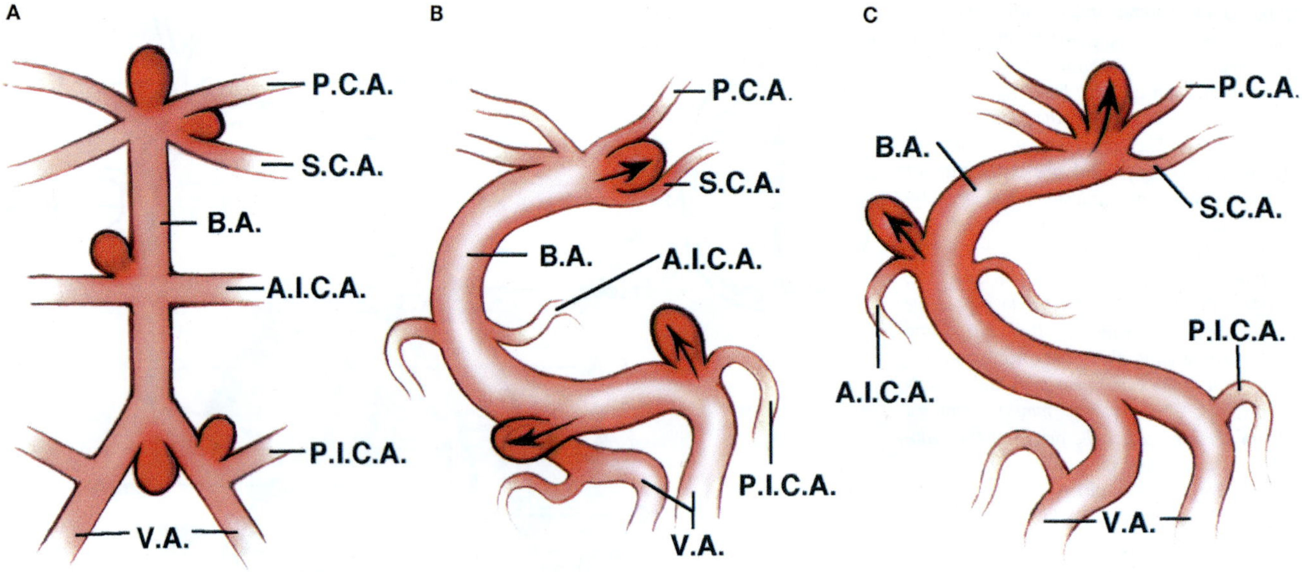

FIGURE 3.15. *Aneurysm sites on the vertebral and basilar arteries.* A, *frequently used diagrammatic representation of the vertebral and basilar arteries and aneurysm sites that often proves to be incorrect. The vertebral and basilar arteries are often shown as straight vessels, and the posterior cerebral, superior cerebellar, anteroinferior cerebellar, and posteroinferior cerebellar arteries are shown as arising at right angles from the parent arteries, with the aneurysm projecting at nearly right angles to the direction of flow in the parent arteries.* B and C, *frequent configurations associated with aneurysms in which the tortuosity of the basilar and vertebral arteries creates a hemodynamic force directed at the wall near a branching site, with the aneurysms pointing in the direction of hemodynamic thrust in the segment proximal to the aneurysm site. The aneurysms of the vertebral artery arise at its junctions with the posteroinferior cerebellar and basilar arteries* (B)*. The aneurysms of the basilar artery arise between the posterior cerebral and superior cerebellar arteries* (B)*, at the basilar apex* (C)*, and at the origin of the anteroinferior cerebellar artery* (C)*. All point in the direction of the long axis of the preaneurysmal segment of the artery and in the direction of maximal hemodynamic thrust* (arrows) *at the aneurysm site.* A.I.C.A., *anteroinferior cerebellar artery;* B.A., *basilar artery;* P.C.A., *posterior cerebral artery;* P.I.C.A., *posteroinferior cerebellar artery;* S.C.A., *superior cerebellar artery;* V.A., *vertebral artery.*

Basilar Trunk Aneurysms

The basilar aneurysm at the level of the superior cerebellar artery often arises where there is a curvature and tilt of the upper basilar artery, so that the hemodynamic thrust created by flow along the basilar artery is just above the origin of the superior cerebellar artery rather than at the basilar apex (*Figs. 3.15* and *3.16C*) (4). The aneurysm located at the origin of the anteroinferior cerebellar artery commonly arises from the convex side of the curve in the basilar artery and points in the direction of the long axis of the basilar segment immediately proximal to the aneurysm (*Fig. 3.16D*) (10).

The most common aneurysm site on the vertebral artery is at the level of origin of the posteroinferior cerebellar artery. The vertebral artery is often depicted as being straight; however, if an aneurysm is present, the vertebral artery is usually found to have a convex upward curve with an apex where the posteroinferior cerebellar artery arises (*Figs. 3.15* and *3.16F*) (6). The aneurysm arises from the apex of this curve at the origin of the posteroinferior cerebellar artery and points upward.

Aneurysms arising infrequently at the junction of the two vertebral arteries with the basilar artery may initially seem difficult to fit into these precepts. When examined in multiple angiographic projections, however, they are often found to conform to these same anatomic principles applied in predicting the site and direction of projection of the more common saccular aneurysms. These aneurysms often arise on the convex side of a tortuous curve formed at the vertebrobasilar junction (*Figs. 3.15* and *3.16E*). One vertebral artery is often dominant and the smaller vertebral artery acts as the branch site. If this tortuous configuration is not present, it is likely that the aneurysm is associated with a fenestration in the lower part of the basilar artery.

ANATOMIC PRINCIPLES DIRECTING SURGERY

The following basic surgical principles are helpful in directing the attack on intracranial aneurysms.

1. The parent artery should be exposed proximal to the aneurysm. This allows control of flow to the aneurysm if it ruptures during dissection. Exposure of the internal carotid artery above the cavernous sinus will give proximal control for aneurysms arising at the level of the posterior communicating or anterior choroidal artery. Exposure of the internal carotid artery at the level of the ophthalmic and superior hypophyseal arteries is commonly achieved by removing the anterior clinoid process, the adjacent part of the roof of the optic canal, and the posterior part of the orbital roof to gain access to the clinoid segment of the internal carotid artery. An operative plan that permits cervical internal carotid occlusion

FIGURE 3.16. A–E, *common aneurysm sites in the posterior cranial fossa. Diagrams on the* upper right *show the basilar, vertebral, posterior cerebral, superior cerebellar, posteroinferior cerebellar, and anteroinferior cerebellar arteries; the site of the aneurysm; and the direction of hemodynamic force* (arrow) *at the aneurysm site. Diagrams on the* upper left *show the scalp incision* (dotted lines) *and bone flap* (solid lines) *or craniectomy* (hatched area) *used to expose the aneurysm.* A, *a basilar apex aneurysm is shown arising at the origin of the posterior cerebral arteries, as exposed by a right anterior subtemporal craniotomy. Note scalp incision and bone flap or craniectomy. The retractor is on the temporal lobe, and the tentorium cerebelli has been divided to expose the basilar, posterior cerebral, superior cerebellar, posterior communicating, and internal carotid arteries and the oculomotor, trochlear, and trigeminal nerves.* B, *a basilar apex aneurysm is exposed by a frontotemporal approach. The sylvian fissure has been split and the frontal and temporal lobes are retracted to expose the aneurysm. The middle cerebral, anterior cerebral, and anterior choroidal arteries and the optic nerves are also exposed. The carotid artery is retracted with a spatula dissector to expose the aneurysm. (Legend continues on next page.)*

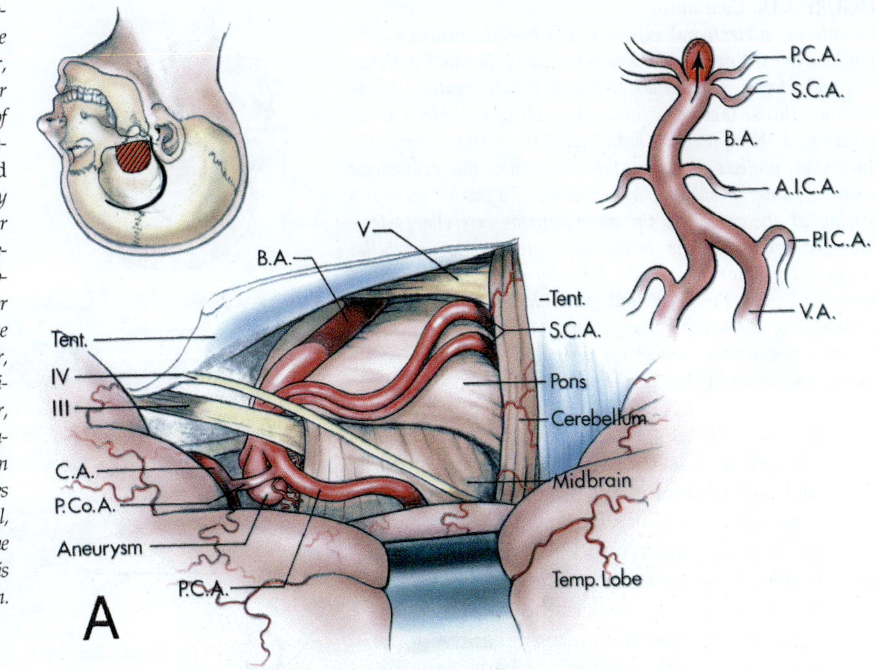

in the neck, either by balloon catheter or by direct exposure, should be considered if anterior clinoid removal and proximal supraclinoid exposure is unlikely to yield adequate proximal control. The supraclinoid carotid or the preaneurysmal trunks of the middle cerebral or anterior cerebral arteries should also be exposed initially to obtain proximal control of middle cerebral and anterior cerebral artery aneurysms. The exposure can be directed laterally from the internal carotid artery for middle cerebral aneurysms and medially over the optic nerves and chiasm for anterior communicating aneurysms. For basilar apex aneurysms, control of the basilar artery proximal to the aneurysm can be obtained by following the inferior surface of the posterior cerebral artery or the superior surface of the superior cerebellar artery to the basilar artery and then working up the side of the basilar artery to the neck of the aneurysm. An operative plan that includes proximal balloon may also be considered. There are several operative routes, discussed below, under Operative Approaches, that increase the length of basilar artery below the apex that can be exposed.

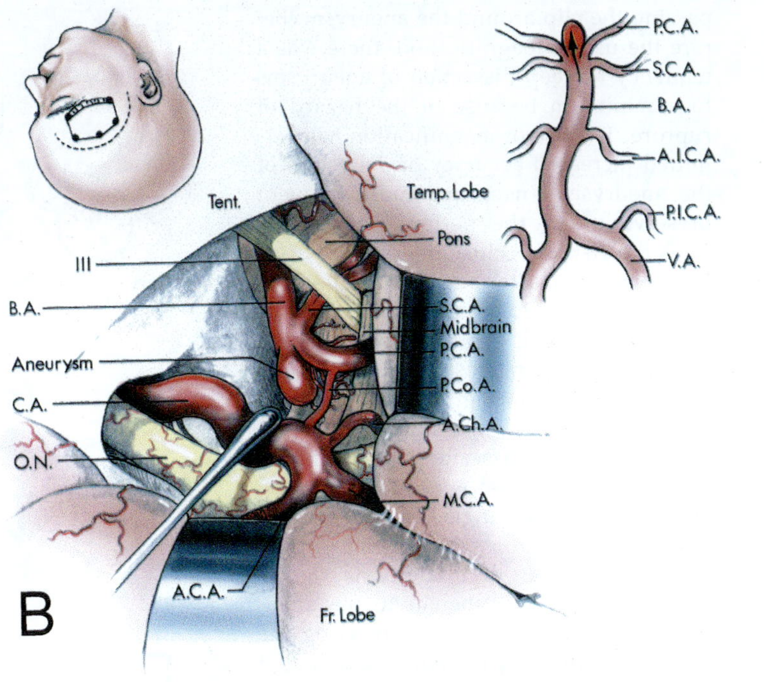

2. If possible, the side of the parent vessel away from or opposite to the site on which the aneurysm arises should be exposed before dissecting the neck of the aneurysm. The dissection can then be carried around the wall of the parent vessel to the origin of the aneurysm.
3. The aneurysmal neck should be dissected before the fundus. The neck is the area that can tolerate the greatest manipulation, has the least tendency to rupture, and is to be clipped. Unfortunately, it is the portion of the aneurysm that is most likely to incorporate the origin of a

FIGURE 3.16. *Continued*
C, anterior subtemporal exposure of a basilar aneurysm arising between the origin of the superior cerebellar and posterior cerebral arteries. The basilar artery curvature creates a hemodynamic thrust (arrow) *against the wall of the artery at the junction of the upper two branches of the basilar artery. The aneurysm projects laterally below or into the oculomotor nerve.* D, *anterior subtemporal exposure of a basilar aneurysm arising at the origin of the anteroinferior cerebellar artery. The abducens nerve is below the anteroinferior cerebellar artery. The tentorium is split laterally above the trigeminal nerve to expose the facial and vestibulocochlear nerves. The curvature of the basilar artery creates a hemodynamic thrust* (arrow) *against the wall of the artery at the junction of the basilar and anteroinferior cerebellar arteries.*

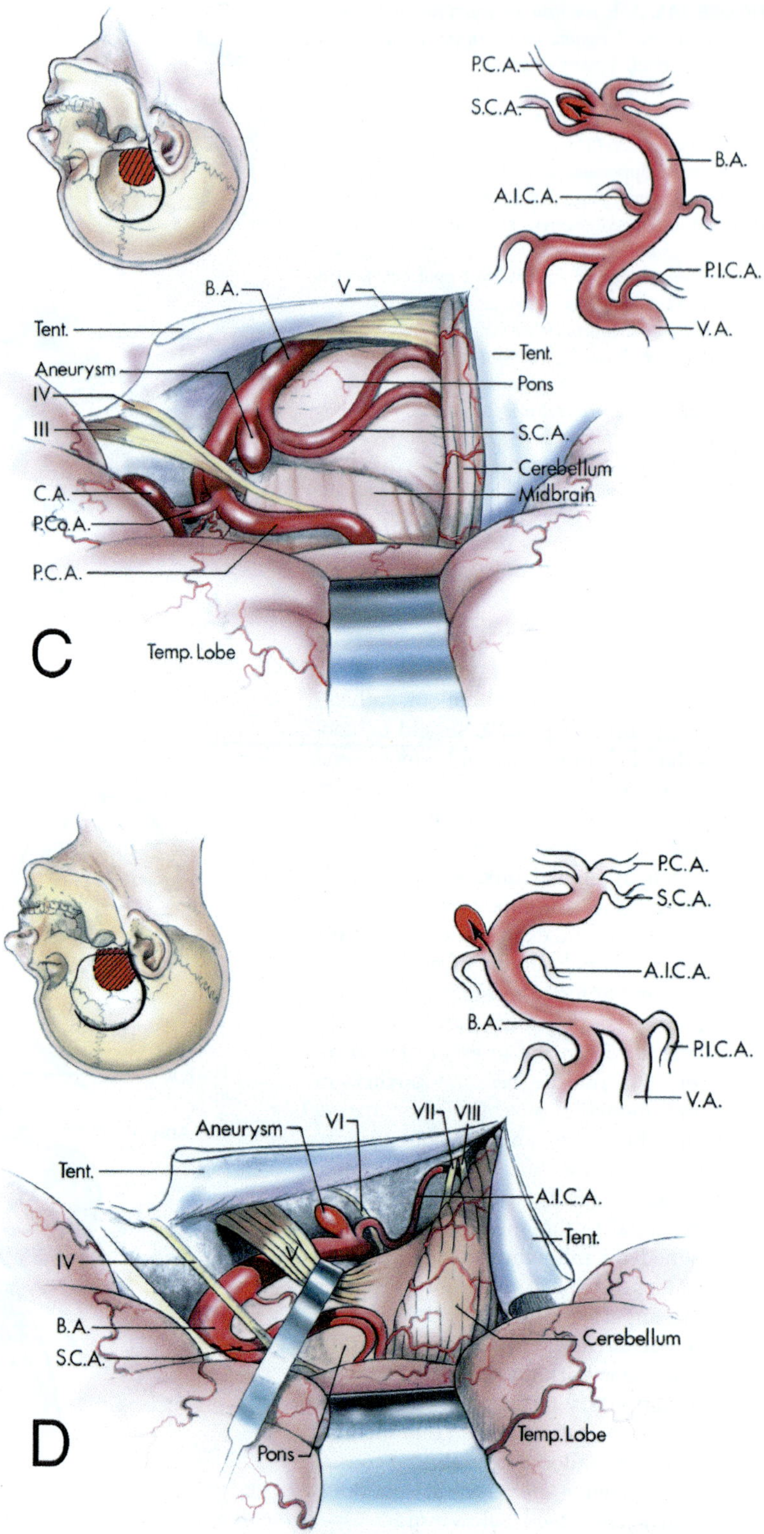

parent arterial trunk or perforating vessel. Therefore, dissection of the neck and proximal part of the fundus should be performed carefully, with full visualization, to prevent passage of a clip around the parental arterial trunk or significant perforating branches that arise near the neck of the aneurysm. The dissection should not be started at the dome, because this is the area most likely to rupture before or during surgery.

4. All perforating arterial branches should be separated from the aneurysmal neck before passing the clip around the aneurysm. Before the use of magnification, there was a tendency to keep dissection of aneurysms to a minimum because of the hazard of rupture. The use of magnification has permitted increased accuracy of dissection of the aneurysmal neck and more frequent preservation of the perforating arteries. Thus the risk of occlusion of perianeurysmal perforating arterioles that results from placement of a clip on an inadequately exposed aneurysm is greater than the hazard of rupture with microsurgical dissection. Separating perforating arteries from the neck of an aneurysm requires appropriately sized microdissectors. Small spatula dissectors 1- or 2-mm wide (Rhoton No. 6 or 7) or 40-degree-angle teardrop dissectors are suitable.

Separating the perforators, if tightly packed against or adherent to the aneurysm, may be facilitated by lowering the blood pressure or by temporary clipping of the parent artery. In other cases, where the middle portion of the body, but not the neck of the aneurysm can be separated from the perforating arteries, placing a clip around the middle portion will sometimes reduce the width of the aneurysm neck so that the perforators can be separated from the neck before moving the clip to the aneurysm neck. Perforators may also be placed in the open area of a fenestrated clip in some cases where one cannot separate the perforator from the neck. An endoscopic view of the neck with

FIGURE 3.16. *Continued*
E, suboccipital exposure of an aneurysm arising at the junction of the vertebral and basilar arteries. Although shown here in the upright position, the operation shown in E and F is performed in the three-quarter prone position. The right half of the cerebellum is elevated to expose the facial, vestibulocochlear, glossopharyngeal, vagus, and spinal accessory nerves and the internal acoustic meatus. One of the vertebral arteries often joins the other in a configuration resembling the branching seen at other aneurysm sites or is associated with a fenestration in the lower basilar artery. Angiographic views in multiple projections reveal the aneurysm pointing in the direction of flow in the preaneurysmal segment of the larger vertebral artery. F, suboccipital exposure of an aneurysm arising at the origin of the right vertebral and posteroinferior cerebellar arteries. The angulation of the vertebral artery creates a hemodynamic thrust (arrow) *in the direction in which the aneurysm points. The flocculus and choroid plexus protrude into the cerebellopontine angle.* A.C.A., *anterior cerebral artery;* A.Ch.A., *anterior choroidal artery;* A.I.C.A., *anteroinferior cerebellar artery;* B.A., *basilar artery;* C.A., *internal carotid artery;* Ch., *choroid;* Fr., *frontal;* M.C.A., *middle cerebral artery;* O.N., *optic nerve;* P.C.A., *posterior cerebral artery;* P.Co.A., *posterior communicating artery;* P.I.C.A., *posteroinferior cerebellar artery;* Pl., *plexus;* S.C.A., *superior cerebellar artery;* Temp., *temporal;* Tent., *tentorium;* V.A., *vertebral artery.*

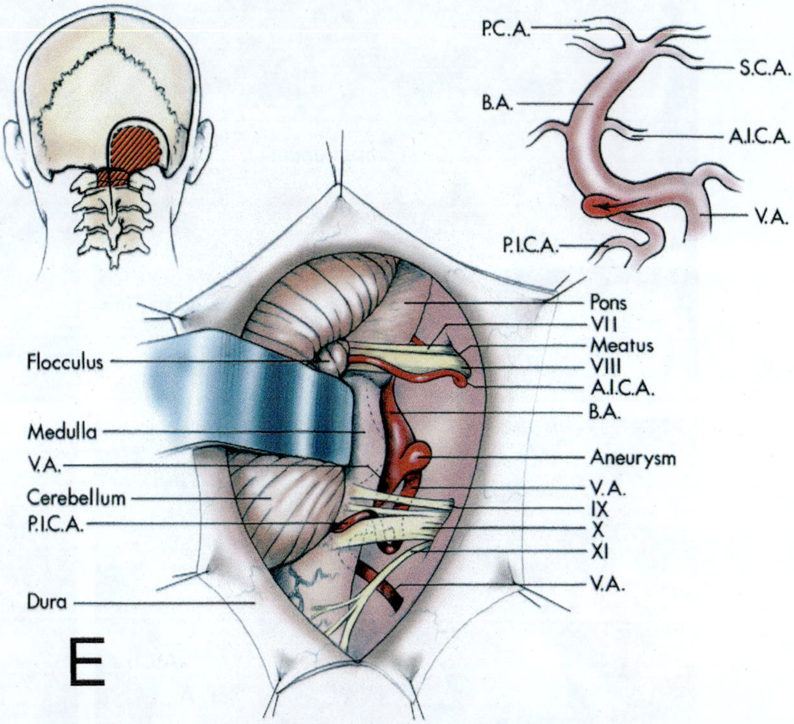

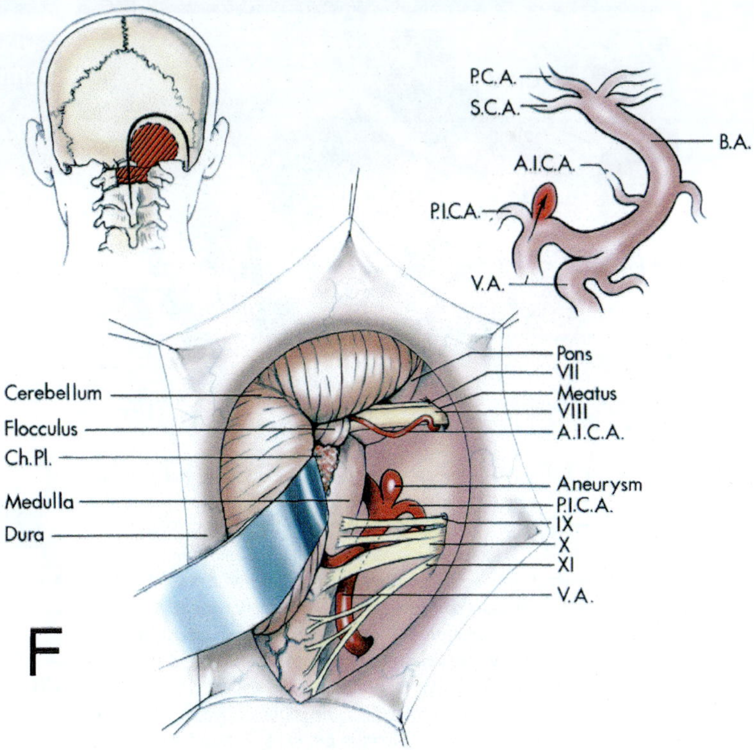

angled endoscopes may aid by revealing the position of perforating branches not seen in the view provided by the surgical microscope.

5. If rupture occurs during microdissection, bleeding should be controlled by applying a small cotton pledget to the bleeding point and concomitantly reducing mean arterial pressure. If this technique does not stop the hemorrhage, temporary occlusion with a clip or occluding balloon can be applied to the proximal blood supply, but only for a brief time.
6. The bone flap should be placed as low as possible to minimize the need for retraction of the brain in reaching the area (*Figs. 3.4, 3.7, 3.17, 3.20,* and *3.21*). Most aneurysms are located on or near the circle of Willis under the central portion of the brain. Cranial-base resection, such as is performed in the orbitozygomatic, anterior petrosectomy, presigmoid, or far lateral approaches, should be used if it will minimize brain retraction, improve vascular exposure, and broaden the operative angle available for attacking the aneurysm.
7. A clip with a spring mechanism that allows it to be removed, repositioned, and reapplied should be used.
8. After the clip is applied, the area should always be inspected, sometimes with intraoperative angiography, to make certain the clip does not kink or obstruct a major vessel and that no perforating branches are included in it.

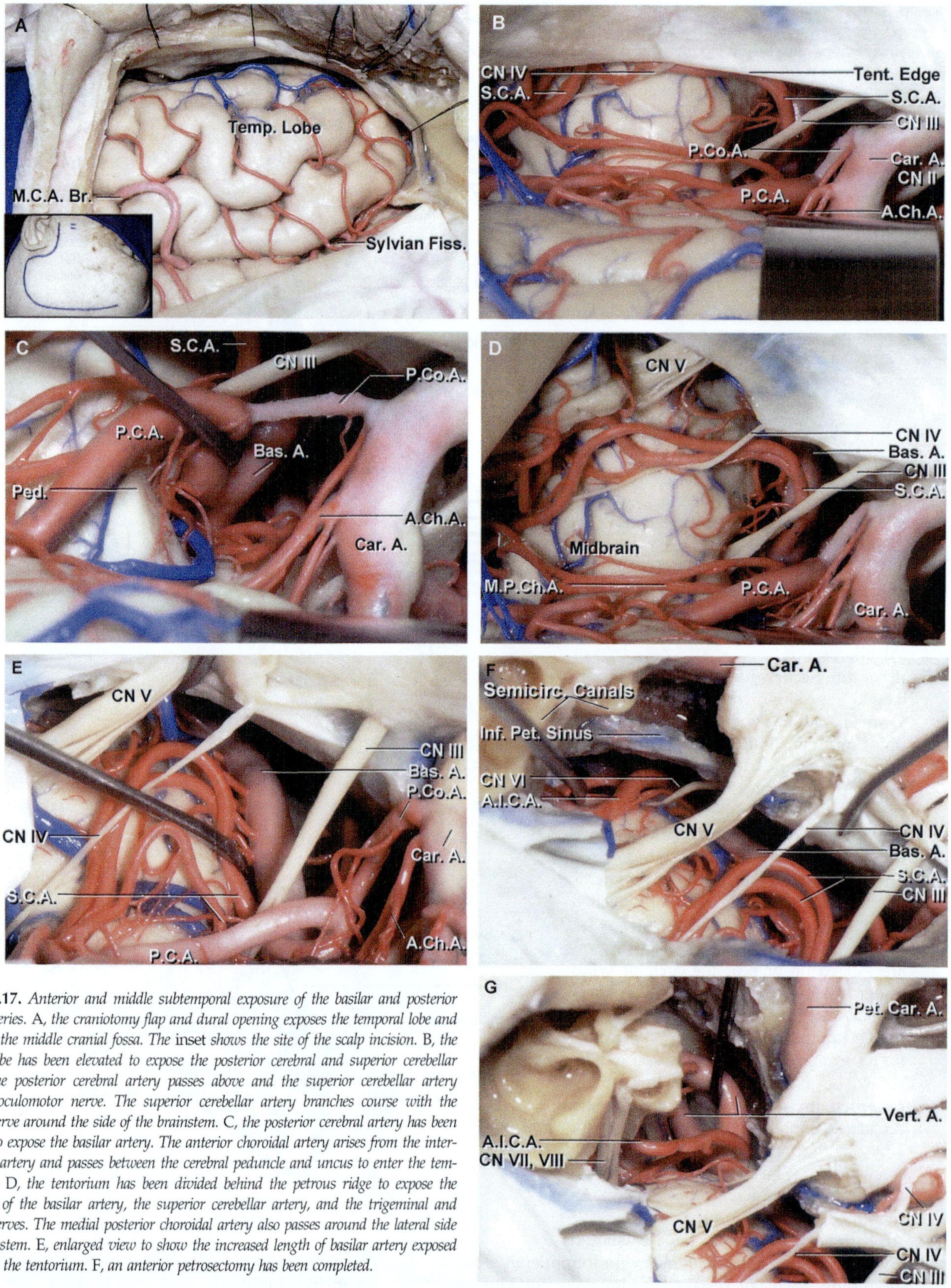

FIGURE 3.17. *Anterior and middle subtemporal exposure of the basilar and posterior cerebral arteries. A, the craniotomy flap and dural opening exposes the temporal lobe and the floor of the middle cranial fossa. The inset shows the site of the scalp incision. B, the temporal lobe has been elevated to expose the posterior cerebral and superior cerebellar arteries. The posterior cerebral artery passes above and the superior cerebellar artery below the oculomotor nerve. The superior cerebellar artery branches course with the trochlear nerve around the side of the brainstem. C, the posterior cerebral artery has been depressed to expose the basilar artery. The anterior choroidal artery arises from the internal carotid artery and passes between the cerebral peduncle and uncus to enter the temporal horn. D, the tentorium has been divided behind the petrous ridge to expose the upper part of the basilar artery, the superior cerebellar artery, and the trigeminal and trochlear nerves. The medial posterior choroidal artery also passes around the lateral side of the brainstem. E, enlarged view to show the increased length of basilar artery exposed by dividing the tentorium. F, an anterior petrosectomy has been completed.*

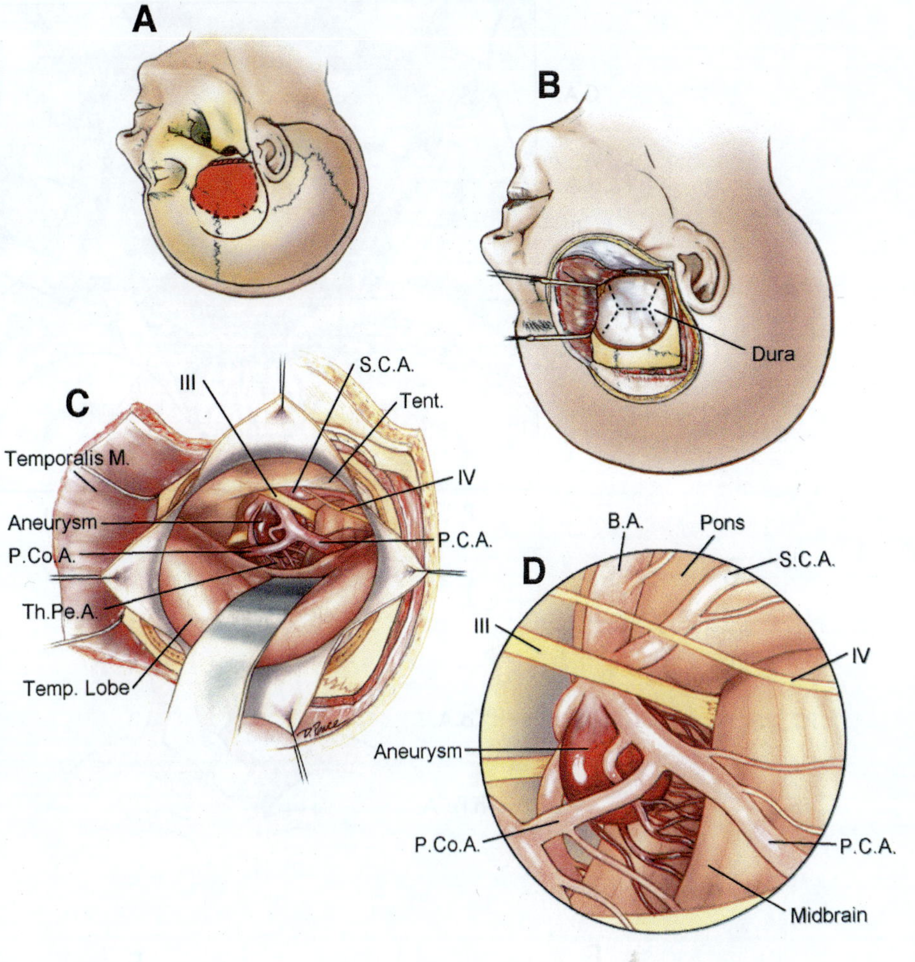

FIGURE 3.18. *Anterior subtemporal exposure for aneurysms of the upper part of the basilar artery. A, the scalp incision* (solid line) *in the shape of a question mark and the bone flap are located above the zygoma. The upper edge of the zygoma* (hatched area) *is removed with a drill if it blocks access to a low exposure along the floor of the middle fossa.* B, *the bone flap has been elevated to expose the site of the dural opening* (broken line). *The temporalis muscle is reflected forward. A small craniectomy at the lower margin of the bone flap combined with removal of the upper part of the zygoma may be needed to bring the line of vision down to the floor of the middle cranial fossa.* C, *the temporal lobe has been elevated to expose the basilar, thalamoperforating, posterior cerebral, posterior communicating, and superior cerebellar arteries, the trochlear and oculomotor nerves, and tentorium. The temporalis muscle is reflected forward.* D, *enlarged view. The thalamoperforating arteries course along the posterolateral margin of the neck of the aneurysm.* A., *arteries;* B.A., *basilar artery;* M., *muscle;* P.C.A., *posterior cerebral artery;* P.Co.A., *posterior communicating artery;* S.C.A., *superior cerebellar artery;* Temp., *temporal;* Tent., *tentorium;* Th.Pe., *thalamoperforating.*

9. If an aneurysm has a broad-based neck that will not easily accept the clip, the neck may be reduced by bipolar coagulation. Nearby perforating arteries are protected with a cottonoid sponge during coagulation. The tips of the bipolar coagulation forceps are inserted between adjacent vessels and the neck of the aneurysm, and are gently squeezed during coagulation. Short bursts of low current are used, and the tips of the forceps are relaxed and opened between applications of current to prevent them from adhering to the aneurysm, and to evaluate the degree of shrinkage.

OPERATIVE APPROACHES

Ninety-five percent of aneurysms are found at one of five sites, all of which are located in close proximity to the circle of Willis (*Fig. 3.1*). These sites are 1) the internal carotid artery between the posterior communicating and the anterior choroidal arteries; 2) the anterior communicating artery area; 3) the initial bifurcation or trifurcation of the middle cerebral artery; 4) the internal carotid bifurcation; and 5) the basilar bifurcation. The frontotemporal craniotomy with slight modifications is commonly selected for approaching all of these aneurysms

The petrous apex in the area behind the internal carotid artery and medial to the semicircular canals has been removed. The dural opening has been extended downward to expose the lateral edge of the clivus and the inferior petrosal sinus coursing along the petroclival fissure. The abducens nerve and the anteroinferior cerebellar artery are in the lower margin of the exposure. G, the angle of view has been changed to show the vertebral arteries in the lower margin of the exposure. The facial and vestibular nerves and the labyrinth and semicircular canals, which are to be avoided in the anterior petrosectomy approach, have been exposed to show their relationship to the approach. A., *artery;* A.Ch.A., *anterior choroidal artery;* A.I.C.A., *anteroinferior cerebellar artery;* Bas., *basilar;* Br., *branch;* Car., *carotid;* CN, *cranial nerve;* Fiss., *fissure;* Inf., *inferior;* M.C.A., *middle cerebral artery;* M.P.Ch.A., *middle posterior choroidal artery;* P.C.A., *posterior cerebral artery;* P.Co.A., *posterior communicating artery;* Ped., *peduncle;* Pet., *petrosal, petrous;* S.C.A., *superior cerebellar artery;* Semicirc., *semicircular;* Temp., *temporal;* Tent., *tentorial;* Vert., *vertebral.*

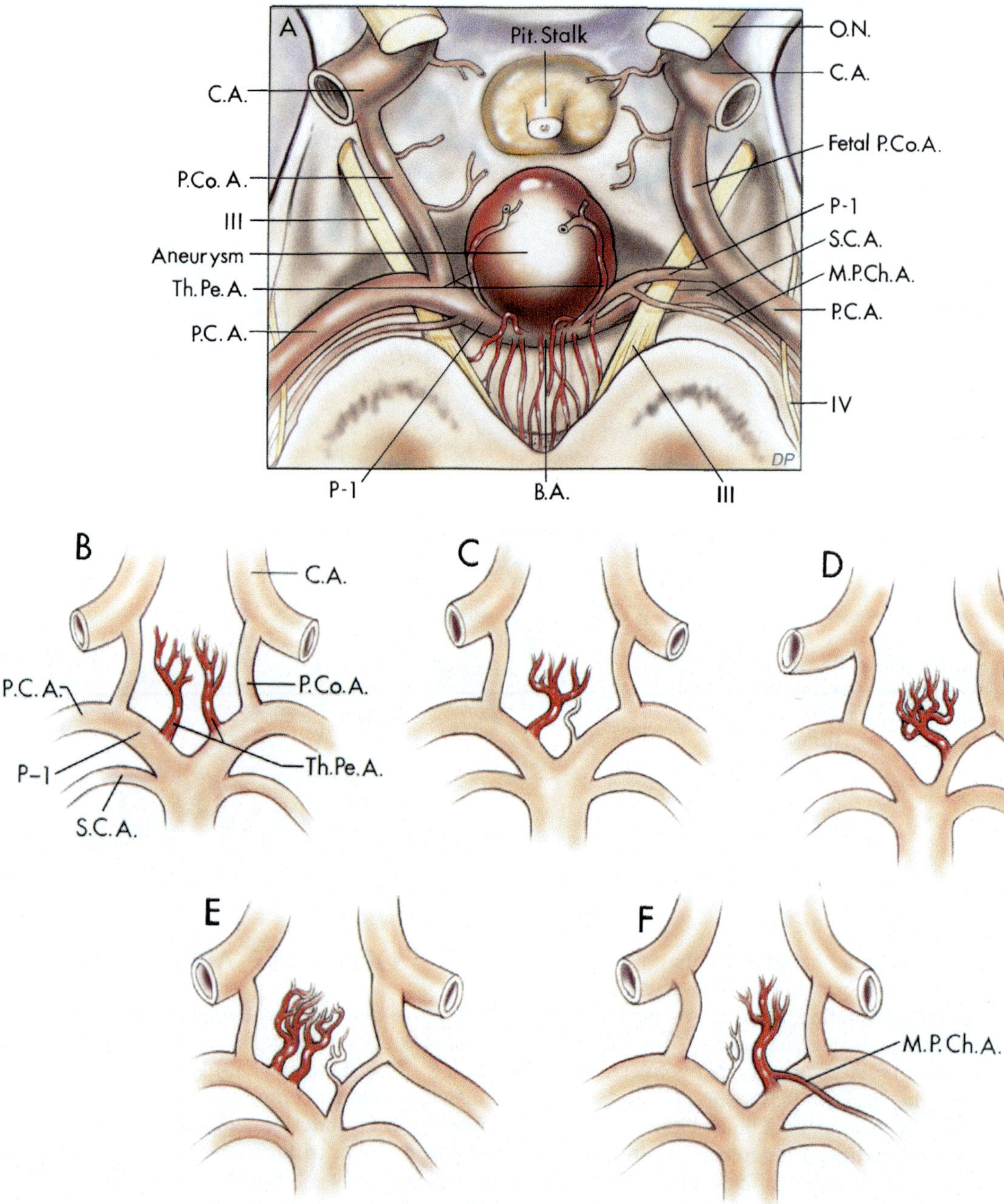

FIGURE 3.19. *Basilar apex aneurysm.* A, *superior view. The aneurysm points upward from the apex of the basilar artery and has the thalamoperforating arteries stretched around the posterior margins of the wall. The communicating artery on the left is of normal size, being neither hypoplastic nor fetal type. The right posterior cerebral artery is a fetal type arising predominately from the internal carotid artery. The right P1 is hypoplastic and the left P1 is of normal size. Other structures in the exposure include the oculomotor and optic nerves, pituitary stalk, and superior cerebellar and medial posterior choroidal arteries.* B–F, *patterns of origin of the thalamoperforating arteries. They are the most important perforating branches in the region of a basilar apex aneurysm.* B, *most common pattern of origin. The thalamoperforating arteries are paired and arise from P1 segments, which are not hypoplastic.* C, *the perforating artery on the left is much larger than the one on the right.* D, *a single or dominant thalamoperforating artery arises from the hypoplastic right P1. The right posterior cerebral artery has a fetal configuration, arising predominately from the carotid artery.* E, *there are two thalamoperforating arteries on the left and a smaller one arising from the hypoplastic right P1.* F, *paired thalamoperforating arteries. The right one arises from a common trunk with the medial posterior choroidal artery.* A., *arteries;* B.A., *basilar artery;* C.A., *internal carotid artery;* M.P.Ch.A., *medial posterior choroidal artery;* O.N., *optic nerve;* P.C.A., *posterior cerebral artery;* P.Co.A., *posterior communicating artery;* Pit., *pituitary;* S.C.A., *superior cerebellar artery;* Th.Pe., *thalamoperforating.*

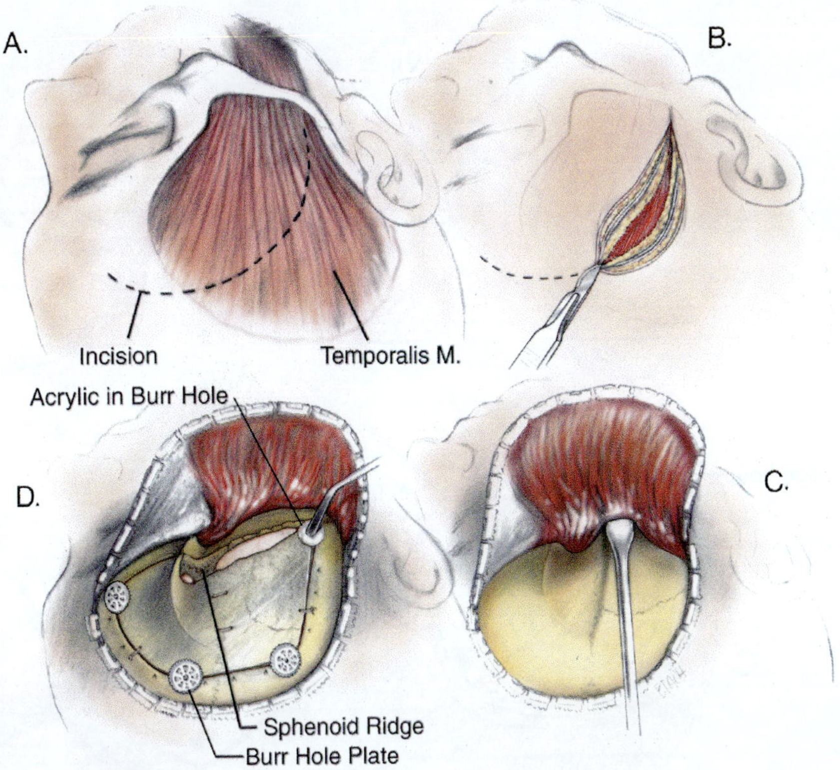

FIGURE 3.20. *Frontotemporal craniotomy used to expose aneurysms on the anterior part of the circle of Willis at or above the level of the posterior communicating artery.* A–C, *the scalp and temporalis muscle and fascia are elevated as a single layer.* D, *as the craniotomy flap is closed, soft acrylic may be molded into the burr holes and allowed to harden under direct vision to minimize the cosmetic deformity if the plating system does not cover the burr holes.* M., *muscle.*

arising from the anterior circle of Willis, and for some originating from the upper basilar artery (21). A frontotemporal flap centered at the pterion (pterional craniotomy) may be used for internal carotid artery aneurysms (*Figs. 3.4, 3.20,* and *3.21*). The flap may be enlarged posterosuperiorly for reaching aneurysms of the middle cerebral artery and of the internal carotid artery bifurcation, forward for approaches to the anterior communicating area, and posteriorly to provide a pterional-pretemporal or anterior subtemporal approach for an aneurysm of the basilar apex.

The scalp incision for this flap begins above the zygoma and extends across the temporal region and forward to the frontal region behind the hairline. The method of opening the scalp for the frontotemporal exposure varies, depending on the site of the aneurysm (*Figs. 3.20* and *3.21*). If the aneurysm is located at the level of or above the posterior communicating artery, the skin, galea, pericranium, and temporalis muscle and fascia are reflected as a single layer. If the aneurysm is located at the level of the ophthalmic or superior hypophyseal artery, the skin and galea are elevated in one layer and the temporalis muscle and fascia are elevated in a second layer. The two-layer scalp opening provides a lower exposure and better access for removing the anterior clinoid process and adjacent part of the orbital roof than the single-layer flap.

A small, free bone-flap, having the center of its base below the pterion, is elevated. The opening in the cranium is extended inferiorly and medially by removing the sphenoid ridge and reducing the thickness of the orbital roof and lateral wall to a thin shell of bone. The time required to prepare this flap, in which all of the soft tissue layers are reflected together, is less than that required to separate and reflect each layer individually. The incidence of weakness of the frontalis muscle is reduced with the single-layer exposure because the layers superficial to the temporalis fascia, in which the facial nerve branches to the frontalis muscle, are not disturbed. Decreased dissection around the temporalis muscle diminishes the incidence of contractures that limit opening of the mouth and reduces cosmetic deformities caused by scarring and atrophy of the temporalis muscle. Any burr holes or craniectomy site that would heal with a cosmetic deformity are closed with cranioplasty material or nonmagnetic plates. The cranioplasty material is molded into position and allowed to harden under direct vision to ensure that the hardened material fits the natural contour of the area.

The frontotemporal scalp flap is modified so that the scalp and galea are elevated as one layer and the temporalis muscle and fascia are elevated as a second layer if the aneurysm is located at the origin of the superior hypophyseal or ophthalmic artery or if a basilar apex aneurysm is to be reached by this approach (*Fig. 3.21*). This allows the temporalis muscle to be reflected into the posteroinferior part of the exposure and provides a lower exposure for removal of the anterior clinoid process, roof of the optic canal, and adjacent part of the roof of the orbit, which are commonly needed to manage aneurysms that arise proximal to the posterior communicating artery.

Cranial-base approaches, such as orbitozygomatic osteotomy, anterior petrosectomy, and various modifications of the presigmoid and far lateral approaches, have been used with increasing frequency in dealing with aneurysms because they reduce the need for brain retraction, increase the width of the operative route, and broaden the angle for dissection and clip application. The orbitozygomatic craniotomy, with elevation of the superior and lateral orbital rim and the zygomatic arch, may facilitate the exposure of all aneurysms on the supraclinoid carotid and circle of Willis, but the benefits are greatest with ophthalmic and superior hypophyseal aneurysms (*Figs. 3.7* and *3.22*). The orbitozygomatic craniotomy may be combined with any of the following: anterior clinoidectomy and removal of the roof of the optic canal and orbital apex for ophthalmic and superior hypophyseal aneurysms; anterior clinoidectomy opening of the roof of the cavernous sinus; and

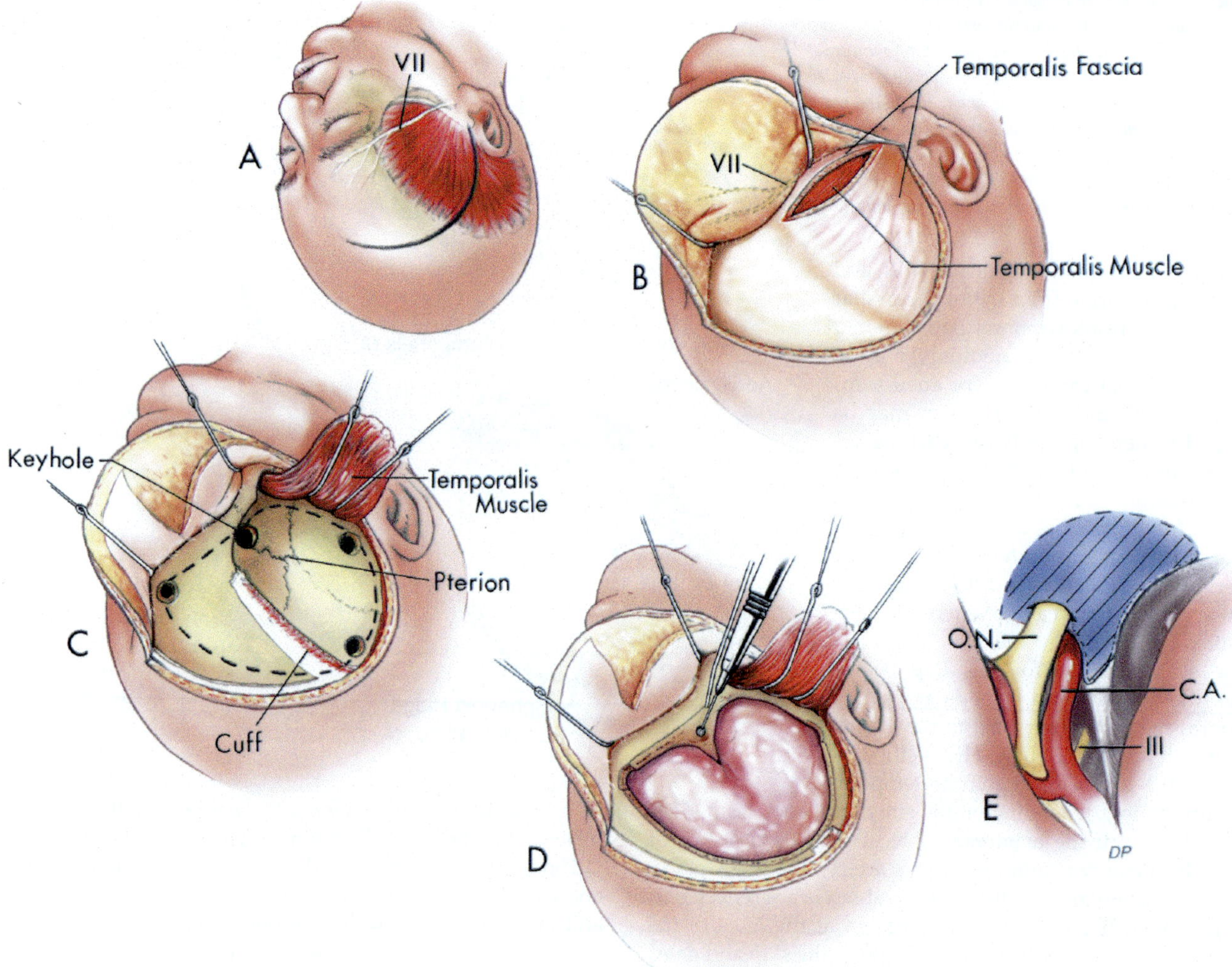

FIGURE 3.21. *Modification of the frontotemporal craniotomy for exposing aneurysms arising at the origin of the ophthalmic and superior hypophyseal arteries. This two-layer scalp opening provides a lower exposure and easier access for removal of the anterior clinoid process and the adjacent part of the orbital roof than when the scalp flap is turned as a single layer, as shown in Fig. 3.20. Site of scalp incision* (solid line) *and bone flap* (broken line). A, *the branches of the facial nerve pass across the zygoma to reach the muscles of the forehead.* B, *the scalp, including the galea, is reflected downward by opening the plane between the pericranium and the galea. An incision is made in the temporalis fascia (but not the temporalis muscle), just above the fat pad containing the branches of the facial nerve to the forehead so that the fat pad and facial branches can be reflected downward with the scalp flap, thus reducing the possibility of damaging these branches of the facial nerve.* C, *the scalp flap and temporalis muscle have been reflected to expose the keyhole and pterion. A cuff of pericranium and temporalis fascia is preserved along the anterior part of the temporal line to facilitate closure of the temporalis muscle and fascia.* D, *the frontotemporal bone flap has been elevated and the lateral part of the sphenoid ridge is being removed. The temporalis muscle and fascia are reflected into the posteroinferior margin of the exposure.* E, *the anterior clinoid process, roof of the optic canal, and adjacent part of the orbital roof and lesser wing of the sphenoid are commonly removed* (hatched area) *to access the internal carotid artery proximal to ophthalmic and superior hypophyseal aneurysms.* C.A., *internal carotid artery;* O.N., *optic nerve.*

posterior clinoidectomy (transcavernous approach) or anterior petrosectomy for reaching a low-lying basilar apex or basilar trunk aneurysm (*Figs. 3.7, 3.17, 3.22,* and *3.23*). The far lateral approaches that expose the vertebral artery as it courses behind the atlanto-occipital joint are used with increasing frequency for vertebral, vertebrobasilar, and lower basilar trunk aneurysms (*Figs. 3.24* and *3.25*). The presigmoid approaches with varying degrees of temporal bone resection may be considered for aneurysms located in the central part of the posterior fossa, although many of these aneurysms may be reached with the various modifications of the orbitozygomatic, anterior petrosectomy, or far lateral approaches (*Figs. 3.26* and *3.27*). The various modifications of the orbitozygomatic approach are reviewed in Chapter 9 of this issue and the far lateral and presigmoid approaches were reviewed in the Millennium issue of *Neurosurgery* (16, 17).

After the pterional or orbitozygomatic bone flap is elevated and the dura opened, the arachnoid is opened, usually beginning below the pars triangularis of the inferior frontal gyrus. The frontal lobe adjoining the anterior part of the sylvian

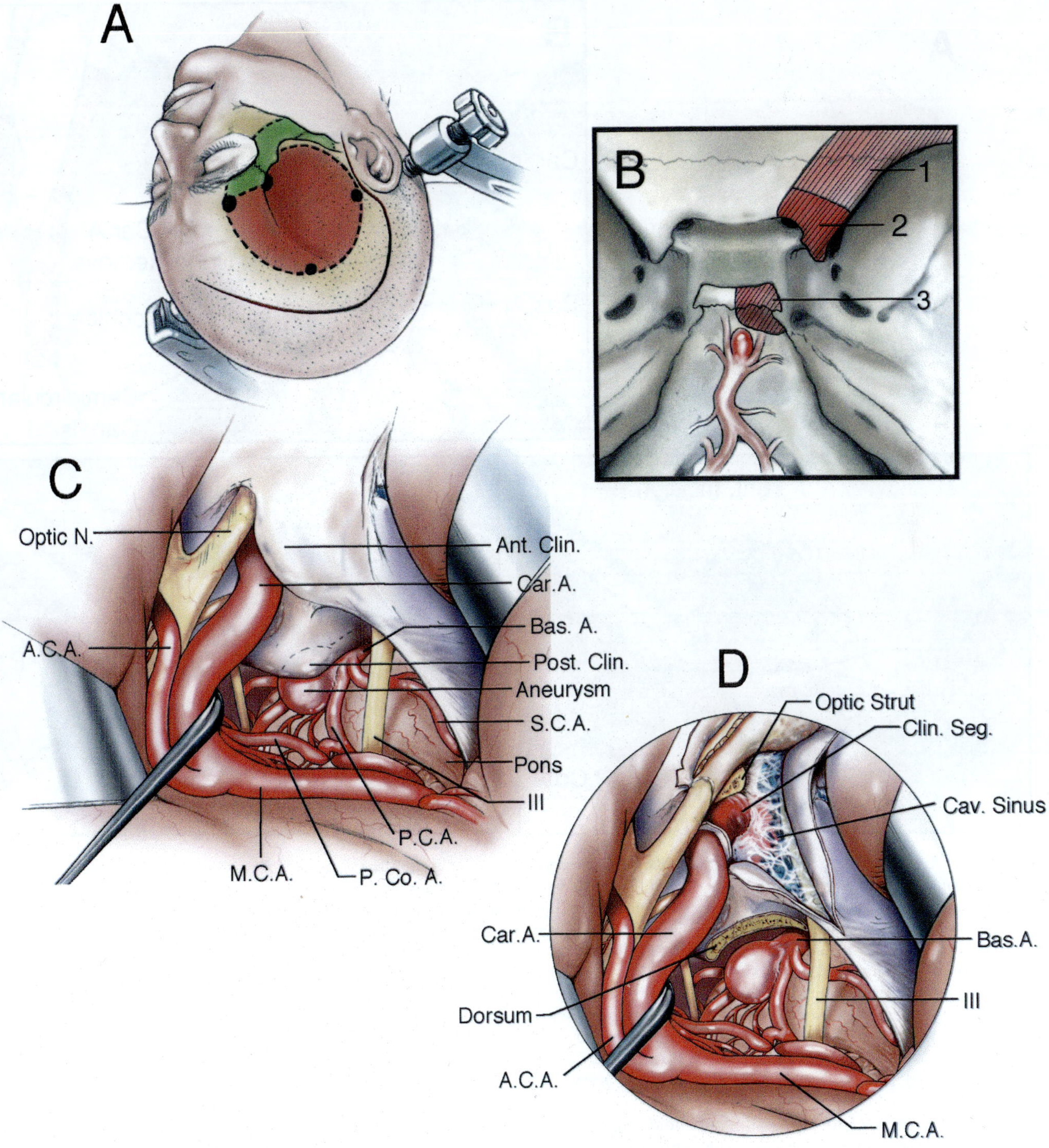

FIGURE 3.22. *Orbitozygomatic transcavernous approach to a basilar apex aneurysm.* A, *head position and site of cranio-orbitozygomatic osteotomies. A pterional bone flap* (red) *is elevated as the first piece, and the orbitozygomatic osteotomy* (green) *is elevated as the second piece. The two-piece approach allows more of the orbital roof to be preserved than when the bone, included in the two osteotomies, is elevated as one piece.* B, *the bone removal* (red hatched area) *may include the sphenoid ridge* (1), *and anterior* (2) *and posterior clinoid processes and adjacent dorsum sellae* (3). C, *operative exposure of low basilar apex aneurysm. The exposure is directed between the carotid artery and oculomotor nerve. The posterior communicating artery has been elevated. The neck of the aneurysm is located behind the dorsum sellae and posterior clinoid process.* D, *the anterior clinoid process has been removed to expose the clinoid segment of the internal carotid artery and the roof of the cavernous sinus. The dura of the roof has been opened back to the level of the posterior clinoid process, and the posterior clinoid and adjacent part of the dorsum have been removed to expose the basilar artery below the neck of the aneurysm.* A., *artery;* A.C.A., *anterior cerebral artery;* Ant., *anterior;* Bas., *basilar;* Car., *carotid;* Cav., *cavernous;* Clin., *clinoid;* M.C.A., *middle cerebral artery;* N., *nerve;* P.C.A., *posterior cerebral artery;* P.Co.A., *posterior communicating artery;* Post., *posterior;* S.C.A., *superior cerebellar artery;* Seg., *segment.*

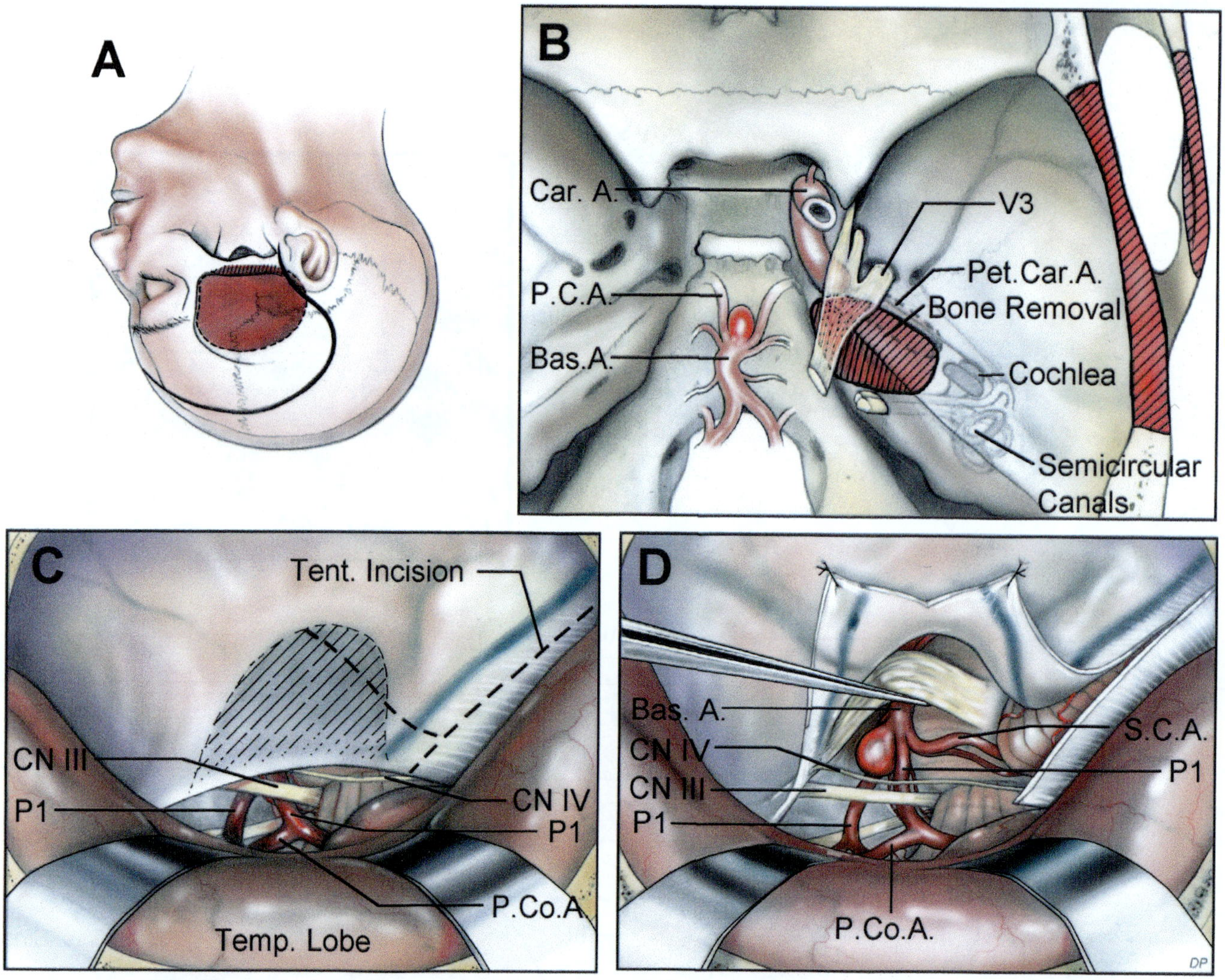

FIGURE 3.23. *Anterior petrosectomy for low basilar bifurcation aneurysms.* A, *a question-mark-shaped scalp flap* (solid line) *is elevated. A bone flap extending down to the floor of the middle fossa is elevated* (shaded area inside the broken line). *Some bone is removed at the lower margin of the flap and possibly at the upper margin of the zygomatic arch* (hatched area) *to increase access along the floor of the middle fossa.* B, *diagrammatic representation of the low basilar bifurcation aneurysm and the site of the bone removal for the anterior petrosectomy. The anterior part of the petrous apex behind the petrous segment of the internal carotid artery in front of the internal acoustic meatus and medial to the cochlea is removed. Bone is removed at the lower edge of the bone flap, including the upper part of the zygomatic arch* (hatched area) *to increase access to the floor of the middle fossa.* C, *the temporal lobe has been elevated. The tentorial incision extends through the medial edge behind the entrance of the trochlear nerve into the tentorial edge* (broken line). *The dural incision extends forward into the area of the anterior petrosectomy. The P1s and posterior communicating artery and the oculomotor and trochlear nerves are exposed at the medial margin of the tentorial edge.* D, *the dura has been opened and the trigeminal nerve has been depressed to expose an aneurysm on the low basilar bifurcation.* A., *artery;* Bas., *basilar;* Car., *carotid;* CN, *cranial nerve;* P.C.A., *posterior cerebral artery;* P.Co.A., *posterior communicating artery;* Pet., *petrous;* S.C.A., *superior cerebellar artery;* Temp., *temporal;* Tent., *tentorial.*

fissure may be elevated to expose the sphenoid ridge to the depth of the anterior clinoid process. The sylvian veins emptying into the anterior part of the cavernous sinus are usually preserved (*Fig. 4.12*). The arachnoid walls of the cistern around the optic nerve and carotid artery are opened. The surgeon is at the desired location if the aneurysm arises from the internal carotid artery (*Figs. 3.3, 3.4,* and *3.7*). Exposure of the neck of ophthalmic and superior hypophyseal aneurysms is facilitated by the removal of the anterior clinoid process, unroofing the optic canal and adjacent part of the orbital roof, and incision of the falciform process of the dura extending above the optic nerve to allow mobilization of the optic nerve. The anterior clinoid removal for exposure of an aneurysm is usually performed intra- rather than extradurally.

In approaching posterior communicating aneurysms, the anterior or anterolateral surface of the supraclinoid carotid is exposed initially before exposing the wall on the posterior or posteromedial side from which the aneurysm arises (*Fig. 3.8*). It has been suggested that the posterior communicating artery can be clipped with the neck of the aneurysm, especially if the

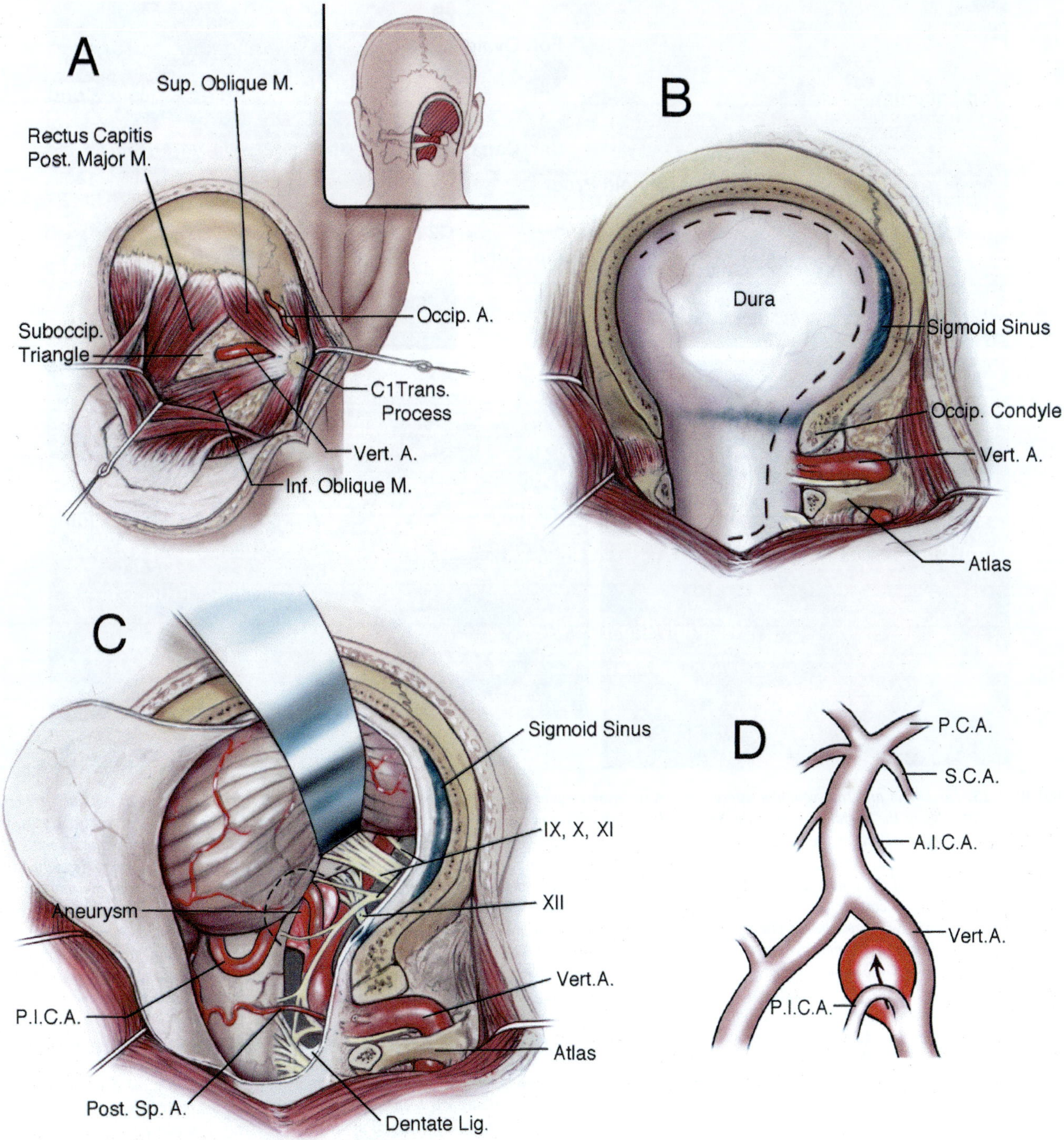

FIGURE 3.24. *Far lateral approach.* A, *the procedure is shown in the upright position; however, the operation is usually performed in the three-quarter prone position. The* inset *shows the site of the scalp incision* (solid line) *and the bony opening* (shaded area). *All of the suboccipital muscles, except those bordering the suboccipital triangle, are folded downward in one layer with a scalp flap. The vertebral artery courses behind the atlanto-occipital joint in the depths of the suboccipital triangle, located between the superior and inferior oblique and rectus capitis posterior major muscles.* B, *the posterior part of the occipital condyle has been removed. The dura is opened as shown.* C, *the vertebral artery and the low origin of the posteroinferior cerebellar artery from the vertebral artery are shown. The aneurysm projects between the posteroinferior cerebellar artery and the vertebral artery and in front of the brainstem. The glossopharyngeal, vagus, accessory, and hypophyseal nerves are in the exposure.* D, *posteroinferior cerebellar artery vertebral aneurysm for which a far lateral approach would be considered.* A., *artery;* A.I.C.A., *anteroinferior cerebellar artery;* B.A., *basilar artery;* Lig., *ligament;* Inf., *inferior;* M., *muscle;* Occip., *occipital;* P.C.A., *posterior cerebral artery;* P.I.C.A., *posteroinferior cerebellar artery;* Post., *posterior;* S.C.A., *superior cerebellar artery;* Sp., *spinal;* Suboccip., *suboccipital;* Sup., *superior;* Trans., *transverse;* Vert., *vertebral.*

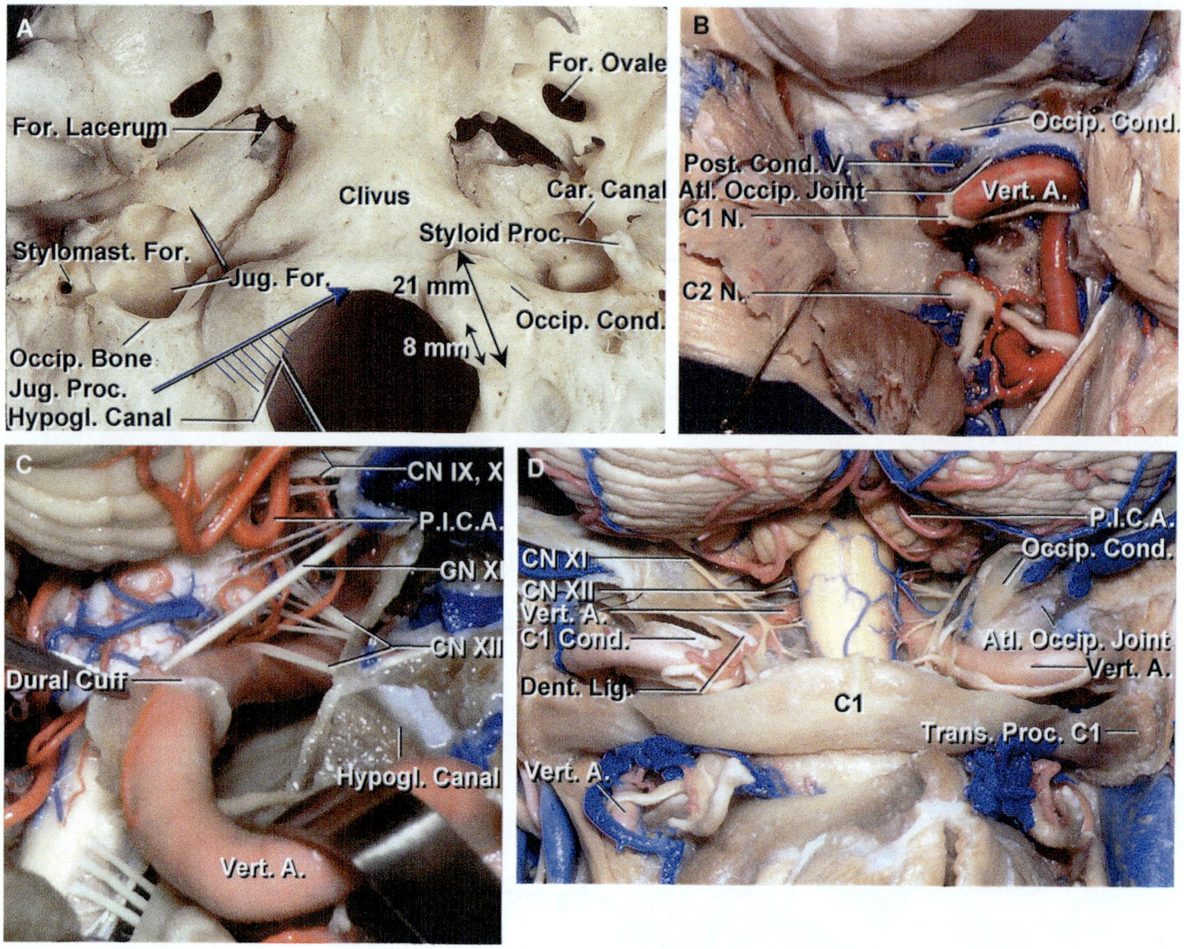

FIGURE 3.25. *Far lateral and transcondylar approaches. A, inferior view of the occipital condyles and foramen magnum. The occipital condyles are ovoid structures located along the lateral margin of the anterior half of the foramen magnum. The hypoglossal canal, through which the probe has been passed, is located above the middle third of the occipital condyle and is directed from posterior to anterior and from medial to lateral. The intracranial end of the hypoglossal canal is located approximately 5 mm above the junction of the posterior and middle third of the occipital condyle, and approximately 8 mm from the posterior edge of the condyle. The extracranial end of the canal is located approximately 5 mm above the junction of the anterior and middle third of the condyle. The far lateral approach is directed through the area behind the condyle, and the transcondylar approach involves removal of some of the condyle. The* large arrow *shows the direction of the transcondylar approach and the* hatched area *shows the portion of the occipital condyle that can be removed without exposing the hypoglossal nerve in the hypoglossal canal. B, right side. A suboccipital craniectomy has been completed and the right half of the posterior arch and the posterior root of the transverse foramen of the atlas have been removed. The vertebral artery passes medially behind the atlanto-occipital joint. A posterior condylar vein passes through the occipital condyle. C, the drilling in the supracondylar area exposes the hypoglossal nerve in the hypoglossal canal and can be extended extradurally to the level of the jugular tubercle to increase access to the front of the brainstem. The dura has been opened. The dural incision completely encircles the vertebral artery, leaving a narrow dural cuff on the artery so that the artery can be mobilized. D, comparison of the exposure with the far lateral and transcondylar approaches. On the right side, the far lateral exposure has been extended to the posterior margins of the atlantal and occipital condyles and the atlanto-occipital joint. The prominence of the condyles limits the exposure along the anterolateral margin of the foramen magnum. On the left side, a transcondylar exposure has been completed by removing the posterior part of the condyles. The dura can be reflected further laterally with the transcondylar approach than with the far lateral approach. The condylar drilling provides an increased angle of view and room for exposure and dissection. The dentate ligament and accessory nerve ascend from the region of the foramen magnum.* A., *artery;* Atl.Occip., *atlanto-occipital;* Car., *carotid;* CN, *cranial nerve;* Cond., *condylar, condyle;* Dent., *dentate;* For., *foramen;* Hypogl., *hypoglossal;* Jug., *jugular;* Lig., *ligament;* N., *nerve;* Occip., *occipital;* P.I.C.A., *posteroinferior cerebellar artery;* Post., *posterior;* Proc., *process;* Stylomast., *stylomastoid;* Trans., *transverse;* V., *vein;* Vert., *vertebral.*

artery is hypoplastic (9). However, hypoplastic segments of the circle of Willis give rise to the same number and size of perforating branches as do normal or large segments.

In approaching internal carotid aneurysms along the sylvian fissure, the origin and proximal portion of the anterior choroidal artery is often exposed before the posterior communicating artery because of its more lateral origin and course. The anterior choroidal aneurysm usually projects posterolaterally above and medial to the anterior choroidal artery, thus providing an angle of separation for safe application of a clip.

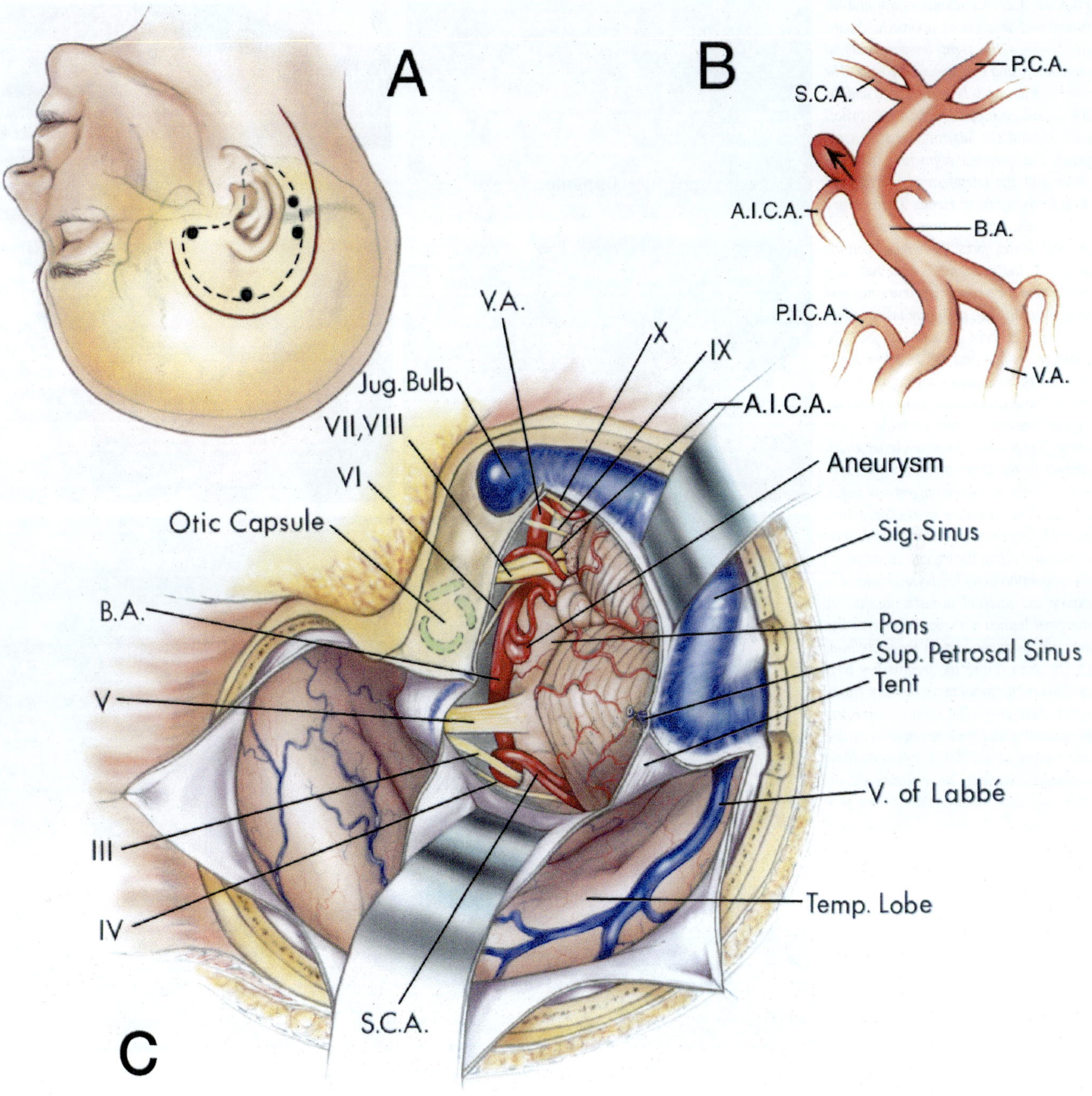

FIGURE 3.26. *Combined supra- and infratentorial presigmoid approach to the basilar artery. A, site of the scalp incision (solid line) and bone removal (broken lines). B, type of aneurysm for which this approach might be considered. C, the supra- and infratemporal areas have been exposed. A mastoidectomy has been completed with care taken to preserve the otic capsule and bone over the semicircular canals. The dura is opened in front of the sigmoid sinus. The dural incision is carried across the superior petrosal sinus and tentorial edge with care taken to preserve the trochlear nerve. This provides access to the upper part of the vertebral artery and the full length of the basilar artery. This approach may be used for aneurysms arising from the basilar artery at the origin of the anteroinferior cerebellar artery or at the junction of the vertebral arteries with the basilar artery. This approach may also be selected for vertebral aneurysms arising at the origin of the posteroinferior cerebellar artery if the aneurysm is located high and deep in the posterior fossa. The jugular bulb may block access to the lower part of the intracranial part of the vertebral artery. Care is taken to preserve the vein of Labbé as the temporal lobe is elevated. Other structures in the exposure include the oculomotor, trigeminal, abducens, facial, vestibulocochlear, glossopharyngeal, and vagus nerves and the superior cerebellar artery.* A.I.C.A., *anteroinferior cerebellar artery;* B.A., *basilar artery;* Jug., *jugular;* P.C.A., *posterior cerebral artery;* P.I.C.A., *posteroinferior cerebellar artery;* S.C.A., *superior cerebellar artery;* Sig., *sigmoid;* Sup., *superior;* Temp., *temporal;* Tent., *tentorium;* V., *vein;* V.A., *vertebral artery.*

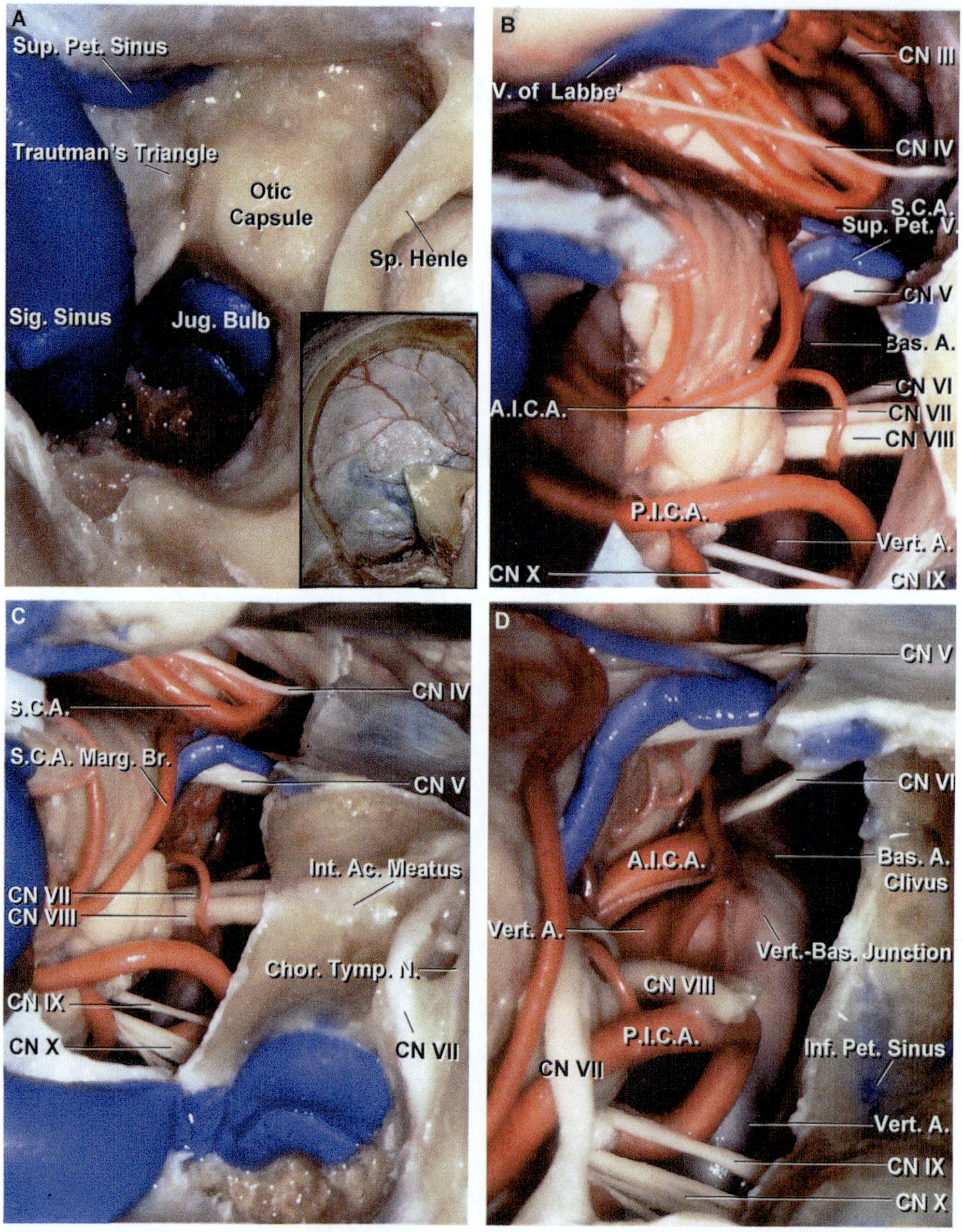

FIGURE 3.27. *Combined supra- and infratentorial presigmoid approach.* A, *the inset shows the right temporo-occipital craniotomy and the mastoid exposure. The mastoidectomy has been completed and the otic capsule, composed of the dense cortical bone around the labyrinth, has been exposed. The tympanic segment of the facial nerve and the lateral canal are situated deep to the spine of Henle. Trautmann's triangle, the patch of dura in front of the sigmoid sinus, faces the cerebellopontine angle.* B, *the presigmoid dura has been opened and the superior petrosal sinus and tentorium divided, with care taken to preserve both the vein of Labbé that joins the transverse sinus and the trochlear nerve that enters the anterior edge of the tentorium. The abducens and facial nerves are exposed medially to the vestibulocochlear nerve. The posteroinferior cerebellar artery courses in the lower margin of the exposure with the glossopharyngeal and vagus nerves. The superior cerebellar artery passes below the oculomotor and trochlear nerves and above the trigeminal nerve.* C, *the labyrinthectomy has been completed to expose the internal acoustic meatus. A marginal branch of the superior cerebellar artery loops downward on the cerebellum.* D, *the dura lining the meatus has been opened and the facial nerve has been transposed posteriorly. The cochlear nerve has been divided and bone removed to expose and remove the cochlea. The transcochlear exposure, completed by removing the cochlea and surrounding petrous apex, provides access to the front of the brainstem and vertebrobasilar junction, but at the cost of loss of hearing caused by the labyrinthectomy and almost certain temporary or permanent facial weakness associated with the transposition of the facial nerve.* A., *artery;* Ac., *acoustic;* A.I.C.A., *anteroinferior cerebellar artery;* Bas., *basilar;* Br., *branch;* Chor., *chorda;* CN, *cranial nerve;* Inf., *inferior;* Int., *internal;* Jug., *jugular;* Marg., *marginal;* N., *nerve;* P.I.C.A., *posteroinferior cerebellar artery;* Pet., *petrosal;* S.C.A., *superior cerebellar artery;* Sig., *sigmoid;* Sp., *spine;* Sup., *superior;* Tymp., *tympani;* V., *vein;* Vert., *vertebral;* Vert.-Bas., *vertebrobasilar.*

The neck is inferior, medial, or inferior and medial. The aneurysm may also arise within a multivessel origin of the anterior choroidal artery and displace its branches both laterally and medially. It may be helpful to work over the carotid bifurcation to expose a portion of the neck.

The anterior communicating area is most commonly approached by the pterional route and less frequently by a subfrontal, bifrontal, or anterior interhemispheric approach. For anterior communicating artery aneurysms, the dissection in the pterional approach is directed superiorly to the bifurcation of the internal carotid artery and over the optic nerve and chiasm along the anterior cerebral artery to the neck of the aneurysm (*Figs. 3.4* and *3.12*). The majority of the aneurysms point anteriorly, inferiorly, and toward the side opposite the dominant A1. An approach along the pterion facilitates exposure of the base before the fundus. Some surgeons approach all anterior communicating aneurysms from the right side. The author has selected the left side if a left frontal hematoma is present, if the fundus of the aneurysm projects toward the right, or if the left anterior cerebral artery is dominant and the right is hypoplastic. It is important to have control of the dominant anterior cerebral artery, because the majority of these aneurysms occur in association with dominance of one A1 and hypoplasia of the other. Gyrus rectus removal is not necessary if the aneurysm is exposed in the subarachnoid cistern above the chiasm. If resection is required to visualize both A1s and proximal A2s and the recurrent and anterior communicating arteries, it should be kept to a minimum.

The recurrent artery of Heubner is frequently exposed before the A1 segment in defining the neck on anterior cerebral aneurysms because it commonly courses anterior to A1 (*Figs. 3.9* and *3.13*). The first artery seen on frontal lobe elevation may be the recurrent artery. If A1 is hypoplastic, the recurrent artery on that side may be nearly as large as the A1 segment and might even be confused with it because it may have the same course as the A1. The recurrent artery may lie in any direction from the A1 segment, but if followed, usually joins the A2 segment just distal to the anterior communicating artery. The recurrent artery may be adherent to the wall of aneurysms. It may loop forward or cross the gyrus rectus where it could be occluded in removing the posterior part of the gyrus rectus, as performed in the gyrus rectus approach. The investing adventitia of A1 may so obscure Heubner's artery that inadvertent occlusion by a clip may easily occur, even under the microscope. Hypoplastic A1s should be preserved because they may give rise to perforating branches even when very small. Temporary clips should be placed on the A1 at a site that avoids the perforating branches, the majority of which arise from the lateral half of the A1 segment. Placement of a clip on an inadequately exposed aneurysm risks occlusion of perianeurysmal perforating arterioles, and is to be avoided.

Aneurysms of the distal anterior cerebral artery are located in or near the midline. They should be approached from the nondominant right side through a unilateral frontal craniotomy anterior to the coronal suture and extending up to the midline as needed to obtain exposure along the falx without undue retraction (*Fig. 3.14*). The craniotomy is preferably placed far enough forward that the proximal part of the pericallosal artery can be exposed and temporarily occluded if bleeding should occur during exposure. The craniotomy may be modified so that a second aneurysm, which occurs more frequently than with aneurysms in other sites, can also be approached at the same operation. The distal portion of the anterior cerebral artery is difficult to expose because of its location deep in the interhemispheric fissure. At no other location do the main trunks of two major cerebral arteries run side by side as do the distal anterior cerebral arteries and because of cross-over of branches from one side to the other, injuries to one anterior cerebral artery may cause infarction in the contralateral cerebral hemisphere. A less satisfactory, more difficult approach, suitable only for lesions of the proximal A2, is through a pterional or subfrontal craniotomy with elevation of the frontal lobe and following the anterior cerebral artery distally from near the carotid origin. Before retracting the medial surface of the frontal lobe, it may be necessary to sacrifice a bridging vein passing from the superior margin of the hemisphere to the sagittal sinus. Most frequently, only one vein must be sacrificed. From this point, the surgery is often tedious because of the limited exposure provided by the interhemispheric fissure, the frequent attachment of the aneurysm to the falx, and because aneurysms at this site are more prone to rupture during exposure than other supratentorial aneurysms.

Intracerebral hemorrhage occurs after rupture slightly more frequently with aneurysms of the distal anterior cerebral artery than with aneurysms in other locations, because of the absence of a subarachnoid cistern into which to bleed and the closely applied cerebral surfaces. The hemorrhage may be into the hemisphere opposite the anterior cerebral artery harboring the aneurysm. A significant hematoma may dictate that the approach be on the side of the hematoma.

The pericallosal and callosomarginal arteries and variants of normal anatomy should be identified before dissecting the aneurysm (*Fig. 2.22*). Connections between the two anterior cerebral arteries may occur proximal or distal to the area of the aneurysm, or the aneurysm may occur at the apex of a single pericallosal artery created by a fusion of the pericallosal arteries from both sides to form a single artery. The necks of distal anterior cerebral artery aneurysms are often wide and atherosclerotic.

Middle cerebral artery aneurysms are exposed by splitting the sylvian fissure (*Figs. 3.4, 3.9,* and *3.10*). Usually, opening the sylvian fissure and working in the superior part of the exposure below the frontal lobe will allow the proximal M1 segment and its postbifurcation trunks to be exposed before encountering the neck and fundus of the aneurysm. These aneurysms usually arise distal to the lenticulostriate arteries near the genu at the M1 bifurcation or trifurcation, but they may also arise at the origin of an early branch of the M1 segment to the frontal or temporal lobes. Aneurysms arising at an early branch site arise from the same part of the M1 segment from which the lenticulostriate arteries arise. An aneurysm may also arise at the origin of a large lenticulostriate artery. These aneurysms arising at the genu, the most common site, point downward, forward, and laterally and may be attached to the sphenoid ridge, in which case the operative approach may need to be modified to avoid avulsing the fundus of the aneurysm at the sphenoid ridge.

There are several approaches to basilar apex aneurysms. They may be exposed through a pterional, pretemporal, anterior subtemporal, or subtemporal approach. The four routes to the apex of the basilar apex that can be accessed through a frontotemporal (pterional) craniotomy are: 1) through the opticocarotid triangle, located between the internal carotid artery, optic nerve, and anterior cerebral artery; 2) between the bifurcation of the internal carotid artery below and the optic tract above; 3) through the interval between the carotid artery and the oculomotor nerve and above the posterior communicating artery; and 4) between the internal carotid artery and oculomotor nerve and below the posterior communicating artery (*Figs. 3.4* and *3.28*).

Some basilar apex aneurysms may be exposed through the opticocarotid triangle if the interval between the optic nerve, carotid artery, and A1 is sufficiently wide and the aneurysm projects superiorly or anteriorly (*Figs. 3.4* and *3.28*). The triangle

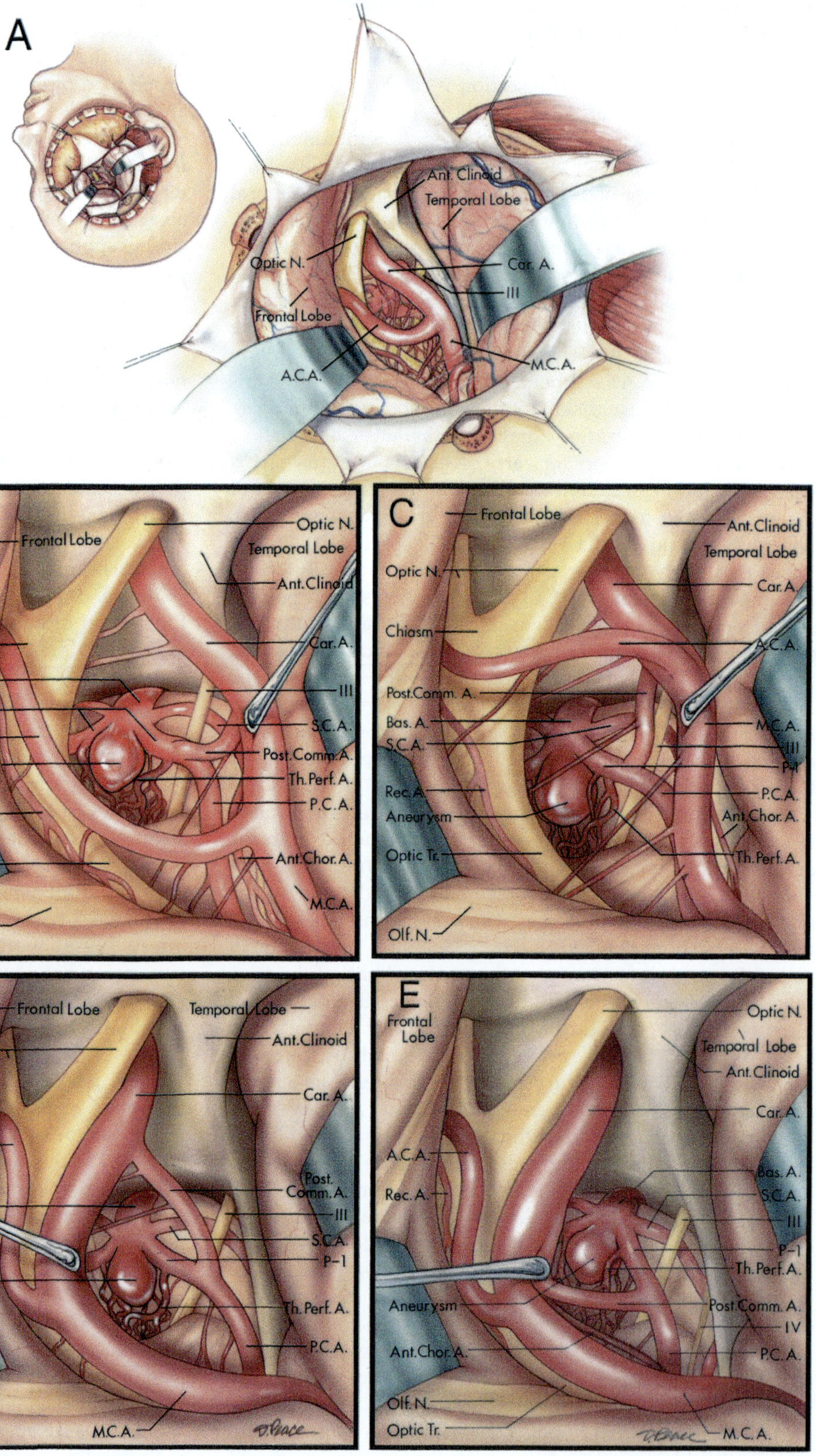

FIGURE 3.28. *Four operative routes directed through a frontotemporal craniotomy to a basilar apex aneurysm.* A, *site of the frontotemporal craniotomy* (upper left). *The sylvian fissure has been split to expose the carotid and anterior and middle cerebral arteries, the optic and oculomotor nerves, and the anterior clinoid process* (lower right). B, *the basilar apex is exposed through the opticocarotid triangle, located between the carotid artery, optic nerve, and anterior cerebral artery. This approach may be used if the internal carotid artery and the initial segment of the anterior cerebral arteries are long, thus providing a wide opening through this triangular space. Other structures exposed include the basilar, posterior cerebral, posterior communicating, thalamoperforating, superior cerebellar, recurrent arteries, and the olfactory and optic tract. The P1 extends from the basilar artery to the junction with the posterior communicating artery. Perforating branches of the carotid and posterior communicating arteries may provide an obstacle and should be preserved in each of the four approaches.* C, *approach through the interval between the carotid bifurcation and the optic tract. This approach may be used if the carotid artery is short, thus providing an opening between the bifurcation and the optic tract. The perforating branches arising in the region of the bifurcation of the carotid artery may limit access through this area.* D, *approach directed behind the carotid artery and above the posterior communicating artery, through the interval between the carotid artery and oculomotor nerve. The perforating branches of the posterior communicating artery may need to be separated to reach the basilar apex.* E, *approach directed below the posterior communicating artery, through the interval between the carotid artery and oculomotor nerve. The posterior communicating artery has been elevated with a small dissector.* A., *arteries, artery;* A.C.A., *anterior cerebral artery;* Ant., *anterior;* Bas., *basilar;* Car., *carotid;* Chor., *choroidal;* Comm., *communicating;* M.C.A., *middle cerebral artery;* N., *nerve;* Olf., *olfactory;* P.C.A., *posterior cerebral artery;* Post., *posterior;* Rec., *recurrent;* S.C.A., *superior cerebellar artery;* Th.Perf., *thalamoperforating;* Tr., *tract.*

is widened if the supraclinoid carotid and A1 are elongated, and is small if these arteries are short. If this approach is used, care should be taken to preserve the vital perforating branches that arise on the internal carotid artery and cross this space to supply the optic nerve and tract and diencephalon. Aneurysms arising on a high basilar bifurcation may also be exposed through the interval between the bifurcation of the internal carotid artery below and the optic tract above, usually by depressing the bifurcation, but again, the perforating arteries crossing this interval must be protected (*Figs. 3.4* and *3.28*). The approach may be applicable if the supraclinoid carotid is short so that there is a wide space between the carotid bifurcation, lower surface of the optic tract, and anterior perforated substances. In the pterional route, the aneurysm is more commonly approached through the space between the internal carotid artery and the oculomotor nerve (*Figs. 3.4* and *3.28*). This exposure is facilitated by elevating the carotid artery and proximal M1 segment. After exposing the area between the carotid artery and the oculomotor nerve, a decision must be made regarding whether to expose the aneurysm by operating above or below the posterior communicating artery. If a basilar aneurysm arises from the posterior aspect of the upper basilar artery, it is best to elevate the temporal lobe and approach the area along the floor of the middle fossa (*Figs. 3.4, 3.17,* and *3.18*).

Most basilar artery aneurysms are approached through an anterior subtemporal approach (*Figs. 3.17* and *3.18*). The anterior subtemporal and subtemporal approaches are facilitated if the pterional scalp incision and bone flap are extended backward in a question-mark incision above the anterior part of the ear and downward onto the zygomatic arch near the tragus to facilitate exposure along the floor of the middle fossa. Turning the temporalis muscle and fascia as a separate layer from the scalp and folding the temporalis muscle downward and forward facilitates the exposure along the middle fossa floor. Elevating the anterior part of the temporal lobe provides an anterior subtemporal exposure with visualization of the oculomotor nerve as it arises from the medial surface of the cerebral peduncle and passes between the posterior cerebral and superior cerebellar arteries to enter the roof of the cavernous sinus. Elevating the posterior communicating artery and temporal lobe exposes the basilar apex, both oculomotor nerves, and the junction of the right posterior communicating artery with the right posterior cerebral artery. The subtemporal approach, when combined with sectioning of the tentorium cerebelli posterior to the junction of the trochlear nerve with the tentorial edge, accesses aneurysms arising on a low basilar bifurcation or at the origin of the superior cerebellar artery. Aneurysms arising at the origin of the anteroinferior cerebellar arteries may also be approached by this route if the origin is high on the upper basilar artery (*Fig. 3.17*).

In the subtemporal approaches, the neck of the aneurysm at the basilar bifurcation is best found by following the inferior side of the posterior cerebral artery medial as it curves around the peduncle. The inferior surface of the P1 is the most infrequent site of origin for perforating branches, thus making it the safest approach to the proximal part of the posterior cerebral artery and the basilar bifurcation (*Figs. 3.17* and *3.18*). The approach under the anterior temporal lobe in front of the vein of Labbé gives better exposure of the perforating arteries that commonly arise from the posterior aspect of the basilar artery than does the pterional approach along the sphenoid ridge. These perforating branches are especially important because they supply diencephalic areas controlling consciousness. Transection of a hypoplastic posterior communicating artery or P1 may be considered to gain access to basilar bifurcation aneurysms and some tumors on the assumption that they have fewer branches and the brain is less dependent on them. However, the number and diameter of perforating branches are relatively constant, regardless of trunk size. If a hypoplastic segment is divided, care should be taken not to sacrifice any small perforating branches (20). In ligating or placing clips on the posterior cerebral artery, the small circumferential arteries on its medial surface that may not be visible from the lateral subtemporal route must be avoided. These small circumferential arteries are often incorporated into the same arachnoid bundle with the posterior cerebral artery trunk and can be preserved only by dissecting them away from the main trunk.

Cranial-base approaches have been used with increasing frequency in dealing with basilar apex aneurysms. An orbitozygomatic craniotomy, in which the orbital roof and lateral wall and the zygomatic arch are removed, increases the angle of exposure, whether the approach be transsylvian, pretemporal, anterior subtemporal, or midsubtemporal (*Figs. 3.7* and *3.22*). Two other modifications that have been used to reach the low basilar bifurcation are the orbitozygomatic craniotomy combined with a transcavernous approach, in which the anterior and posterior clinoid processes and the roof of the cavernous sinus are removed (*Figs. 3.7* and *3.22*). An alternative to the transcavernous approach is the anterior petrosectomy approach, in which the part of the petrous apex behind the petrous carotid artery and under the trigeminal nerve is removed extradurally before opening the dura, either through a frontotemporal or orbitozygomatic craniotomy (*Figs. 3.17* and *3.23*). After the drilling is complete, the dura is opened and the tentorium divided. The exposure allows the trigeminal nerve to be depressed, thus significantly increasing the length of basilar artery that can be exposed as compared with that seen with tentorial section without petrosectomy.

Aneurysms arising at the vertebrobasilar junction are approached through a subtemporal transtentorial exposure if the aneurysm and junction are high in the posterior fossa, through a combined supra- and infratentorial presigmoid exposure if the junction is deep in the middle part of the posterior fossa, or through a lateral suboccipital or far lateral approach if the vertebrobasilar junction is low (*Figs. 3.16E* and *3.24–3.27*). Vertebral aneurysms arising at the origin of the posteroinferior cerebellar artery are approached through lateral suboccipital craniectomy or far lateral approach if they are located low in the posterior fossa, and through a combined supra and infratentorial presigmoid exposure if they are deep in the middle portion of the posterior fossa (*Figs. 3.16F* and *3.24–3.27*). If the far lateral suboccipital approach is selected, the ipsilateral half of the posterior C1 arch may be removed to provide adequate exposure of the segment of the vertebral artery proximal to the aneurysm. The side for the suboccipital approach should be selected only after carefully reviewing the angiogram, because aneurysms of one vertebral artery may lie on the side of the brainstem opposite the side of the vertebral artery from which it fills because of extreme tortuosity of these arteries.

REFERENCES

1. Drake CG: Bleeding aneurysms of the basilar artery: Direct surgical management in four cases. **J Neurosurg** 18:230–238, 1961.
2. Gibo H, Carver CC, Rhoton AL Jr, Lenkey C, Mitchell RJ: Microsurgical anatomy of the middle cerebral artery. **J Neurosurg** 54:151–169, 1981.
3. Gibo H, Lenkey C, Rhoton AL Jr: Microsurgical anatomy of the supraclinoid portion of the internal carotid artery. **J Neurosurg** 55:560–574, 1981.
4. Hardy DG, Peace DA, Rhoton AL Jr: Microsurgical anatomy of the superior cerebellar artery. **Neurosurgery** 6:10–28, 1980.
5. Inoue T, Rhoton AL Jr, Theele D, Barry ME: Surgical approaches to the cavernous sinus: A microsurgical study. **Neurosurgery** 26:903–932, 1990.
6. Lister JR, Rhoton AL Jr, Matsushima T, Peace DA: Microsurgical anatomy of the posterior inferior cerebellar artery. **Neurosurgery** 10:170–199, 1982.
7. Liu QL, Rhoton AL Jr: Middle meningeal origin of the ophthalmic artery. **Neurosurgery** 49:401–407, 2001.
8. Locksley HB: Natural history of subarachnoid hemorrhage, intracranial aneurysms and arteriovenous malformations: Based on 6368 cases in the cooperative study. **J Neurosurg** 25:219–239, 1966.
9. Lougheed WM, Marshall BM: Management of aneurysms of the anterior circulation by intracranial procedures, in Youmans JR (ed): *Neurological Surgery*. Philadelphia, W.B. Saunders Co., 1973, vol 2, pp 731–767.
10. Martin RG, Grant JL, Peace D, Theiss C, Rhoton AL Jr: Microsurgical relationships of the anterior inferior cerebellar artery and the facial-vestibulocochlear nerve complex. **Neurosurgery** 6:483–507, 1980.
11. Perlmutter D, Rhoton AL Jr: Microsurgical anatomy of the anterior cerebral-anterior communicating-recurrent artery complex. **J Neurosurg** 45:259–272, 1976.
12. Rhoton AL Jr: Anatomy of saccular aneurysms. **Surg Neurol** 14:59–66, 1980.
13. Rhoton AL Jr: Microsurgical anatomy of saccular aneurysms, in Wilkins RH, Rengachary SS (eds): *Neurosurgery*. New York, McGraw-Hill, 1985, vol 2, pp 1330–1340.
14. Rhoton AL Jr: Micro-operative techniques, in Youmans JR (ed): *Neurological Surgery*. Philadelphia, W.B. Saunders Co., 1990, vol 2, ed 3, pp 941–991.
15. Rhoton AL Jr: Instrumentation, in Apuzzo MLJ (ed): *Brain Surgery: Complication Avoidance and Management*. New York, Churchill-Livingstone, 1993, vol 2, pp 1647–1670.
16. Rhoton AL Jr: Far lateral approach and its transcondylar, supracondylar, and paracondylar extensions. **Neurosurgery** 47[Suppl 1]:S195–S209, 2000.
17. Rhoton AL Jr: Temporal bone and transtemporal approaches. **Neurosurgery** 47[Suppl 1]:S211–S265, 2000.
18. Rhoton AL Jr, Saeki N, Perlmutter D, Zeal A: Microsurgical anatomy of common aneurysm sites. **Clin Neurosurg** 26:248–306, 1979.
19. Rosner SS, Rhoton AL Jr, Ono M, Barry M: Microsurgical anatomy of the anterior perforating arteries. **J Neurosurg** 61:468–485, 1984.
20. Saeki N, Rhoton AL Jr: Microsurgical anatomy of the upper basilar artery and the posterior circle of Willis. **J Neurosurg** 46:563–578, 1977.
21. Yaşargil MG, Fox JL: The microsurgical approach to intracranial aneurysms. **Surg Neurol** 3:7–14, 1975.
22. Zeal AA, Rhoton AL Jr: Microsurgical anatomy of the posterior cerebral artery. **J Neurosurg** 48:534–559, 1978.

Figure from D'Agoty Gautier's Essai d'anatomie, en tableaux imprimés. *Paris, 1748.*

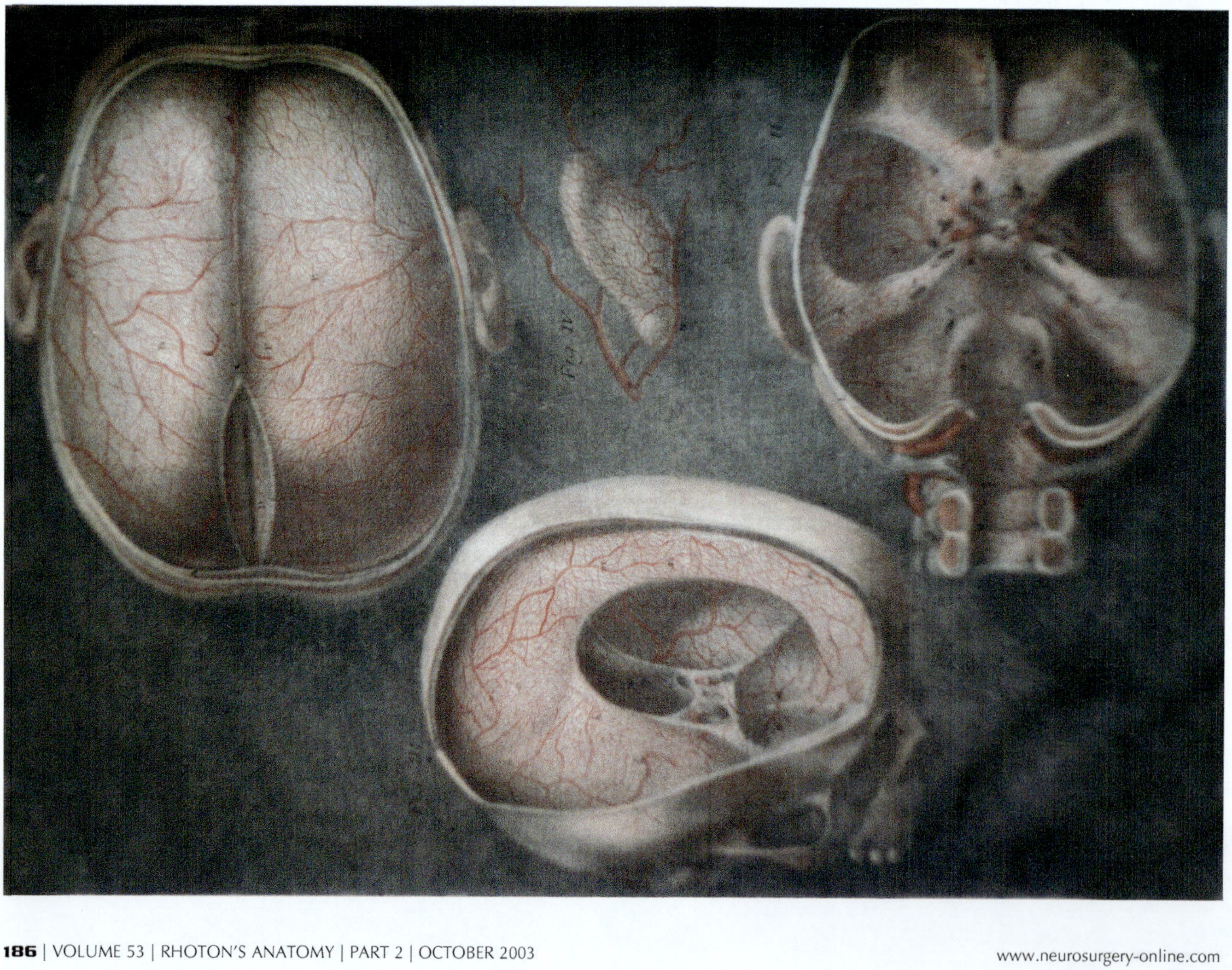

THE CEREBRAL VEINS

Albert L. Rhoton, Jr., M.D.

Department of Neurological Surgery, University of Florida, Gainesville, Florida

Correspondence:
Albert L. Rhoton, Jr., M.D., Department of Neurological Surgery, University of Florida McKnight Brain Institute, P.O. Box 100265, 100 South Newell Drive, Building 59, L2-100, Gainesville, FL 32610-0265.
Email: rhoton@neurosurgery.ufl.edu

KEY WORDS: Basal vein, Brain, Cerebral hemisphere, Cortical vein, Deep venous system, Dural venous sinus, Great vein, Internal cerebral vein, Microsurgical anatomy, Superficial cerebral vein

There are several reasons that the veins of the cerebrum have received little attention in the neurosurgical literature. Earlier studies of these veins have focused predominantly on the lateral surface of the cerebrum and lacked the detail needed for operations on the medial and basal surfaces. Frequent variations in the size and connections of these veins have made it difficult to define a normal pattern, and the nomenclature used to describe the veins has infrequently been applicable to the operative situation. The fact that sacrifice of the major trunks of the deep venous system only infrequently leads to venous infarction with mass effect and neurological deficit is attributed to the diffuse anastomoses between the veins. On the other hand, injury to this complicated venous network may cause severe deficits, including hemiplegia, coma, and death. The cerebral veins may pose a major obstacle to operative approaches to deep-seated lesions, especially in the pineal region under the temporal lobe and along the central part of the superior sagittal sinus. At numerous sites, the displacement of the veins may provide more accurate localizing information on neuroradiological studies than the arteries, because the veins are often more adherent to the brain than the arteries, which are not tightly adherent to the cortical surface as they pass through the cisterns, fissures, and sulci. The ventricular veins also provide larger and more valuable landmarks in the lateral ventricle than the arteries, especially if hydrocephalus—a common result of ventricular tumors—is present, because the borders between the neural structures in the ventricular walls become less distinct as the ventricles dilate.

The cerebral veins are divided into a superficial group and a deep group. The superficial group drains the cortical surfaces. The deep group drains the deep white and gray matter and collects into channels that course through the walls of the ventricles and basal cisterns to drain into the internal cerebral, basal, and great veins.

THE SUPERFICIAL VEINS

Drainage Groups

The superficial veins drain the cortical surfaces. They collect into four groups of bridging veins: a superior sagittal group that drains into the superior sagittal sinus; a sphenoidal group that drains into the sphenoparietal or cavernous sinus; a tentorial group that converges on the sinuses in the tentorium; and a falcine group that empties into the inferior sagittal or straight sinus, or their tributaries (*Fig. 4.1*). The latter group includes the cortical veins that reach the straight sinus by emptying into the internal cerebral, basal, and great veins. The superior sagittal, sphenoidal, or tentorial group may drain the majority of the hemisphere if its tributaries are large.

Superior Sagittal Group

The superior sagittal group is composed of the veins that drain into the superior sagittal sinus (*Figs. 4.1–4.3*). It includes the veins from the superior part of the medial and lateral surfaces of the frontal, parietal, and occipital lobes and from the anterior part of the orbital surface of the frontal lobe. There is usually a free segment of vein, 1 to 2 cm in length, in the subdural space between the vein's exit from its bed in the pia-arachnoid and its entrance into the sinus. These veins may empty directly into the superior sagittal sinus or may join a meningeal sinus in the dura mater en route to the superior sagittal sinus.

Sphenoidal Group

The sphenoidal group is formed by the bridging veins that empty into the sinuses that course on the inner surface of the sphenoid bone (*Fig. 4.1*). This group, formed by the terminal ends of the superficial sylvian and occasionally the deep sylvian veins, drains the part of the frontal, temporal, and parietal lobes adjoining the sylvian fissure. These veins drain into the sphenoparietal or cavernous sinus and, less commonly, into the sphenobasal or sphenopetrosal sinuses.

Tentorial Group

The tentorial group of bridging veins drains into the sinuses coursing in the tentorium, called the tentorial sinuses, or into the transverse and superior petrosal sinuses in the tentorial margins (*Figs. 4.4* and *4.5*). This group is composed of the veins draining the lateral surface of the temporal lobe and the basal surface of the temporal and occipital lobes. This group includes the temporobasal and occipitobasal veins and the descending veins, including the vein of Labbé, from the lateral surface of the temporal lobe. These veins converge on the preoccipital notch and, although they may enter the transverse sinus, most of them, except the vein of Labbé, usually course

A

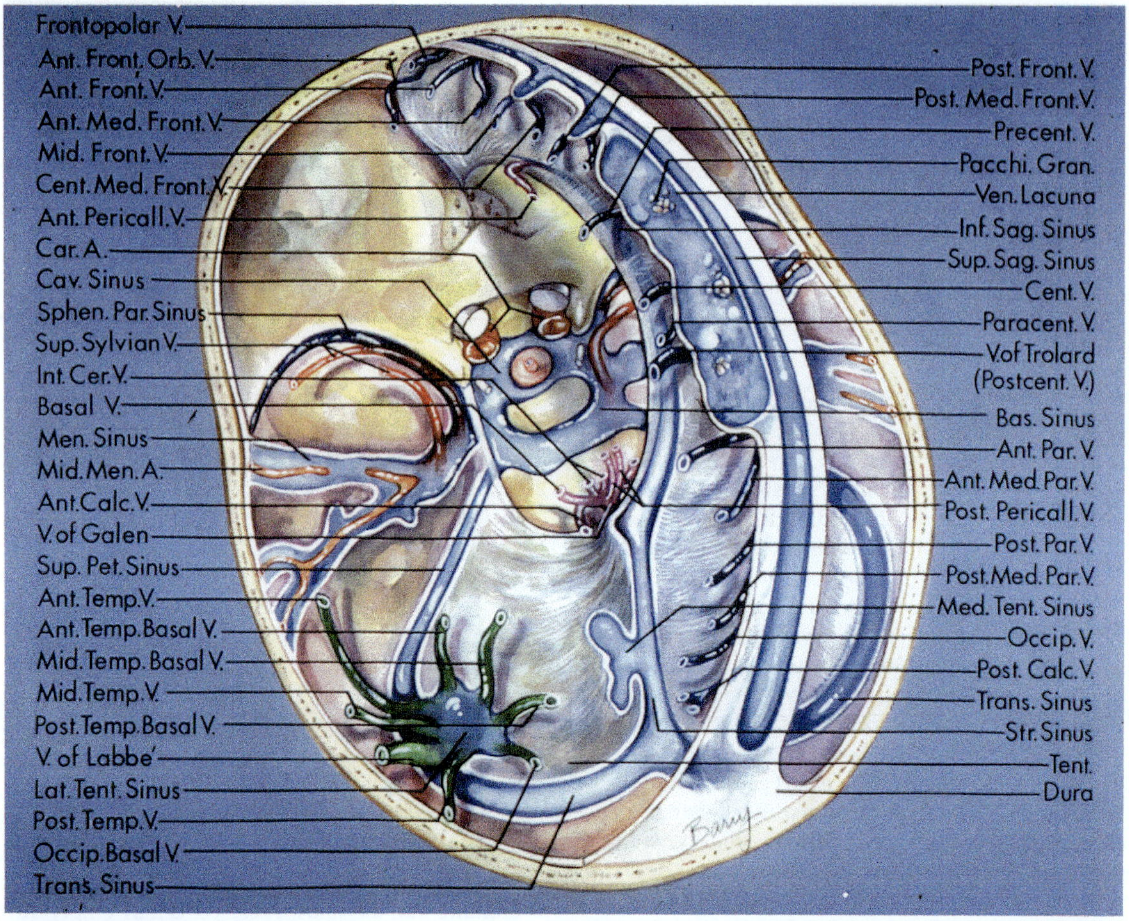
Frontopolar V.
Ant. Front. Orb. V.
Ant. Front. V.
Ant. Med. Front. V.
Mid. Front. V.
Cent. Med. Front. V.
Ant. Pericall. V.
Car. A.
Cav. Sinus
Sphen. Par. Sinus
Sup. Sylvian V.
Int. Cer. V.
Basal V.
Men. Sinus
Mid. Men. A.
Ant. Calc. V.
V. of Galen
Sup. Pet. Sinus
Ant. Temp. V.
Ant. Temp. Basal V.
Mid. Temp. Basal V.
Mid. Temp. V.
Post. Temp. Basal V.
V. of Labbe'
Lat. Tent. Sinus
Post. Temp. V.
Occip. Basal V.
Trans. Sinus
Post. Front. V.
Post. Med. Front. V.
Precent. V.
Pacchi. Gran.
Ven. Lacuna
Inf. Sag. Sinus
Sup. Sag. Sinus
Cent. V.
Paracent. V.
V. of Trolard
(Postcent. V.)
Bas. Sinus
Ant. Par. V.
Ant. Med. Par. V.
Post. Pericall. V.
Post. Par. V.
Post. Med. Par. V.
Med. Tent. Sinus
Occip. V.
Post. Calc. V.
Trans. Sinus
Str. Sinus
Tent.
Dura

B

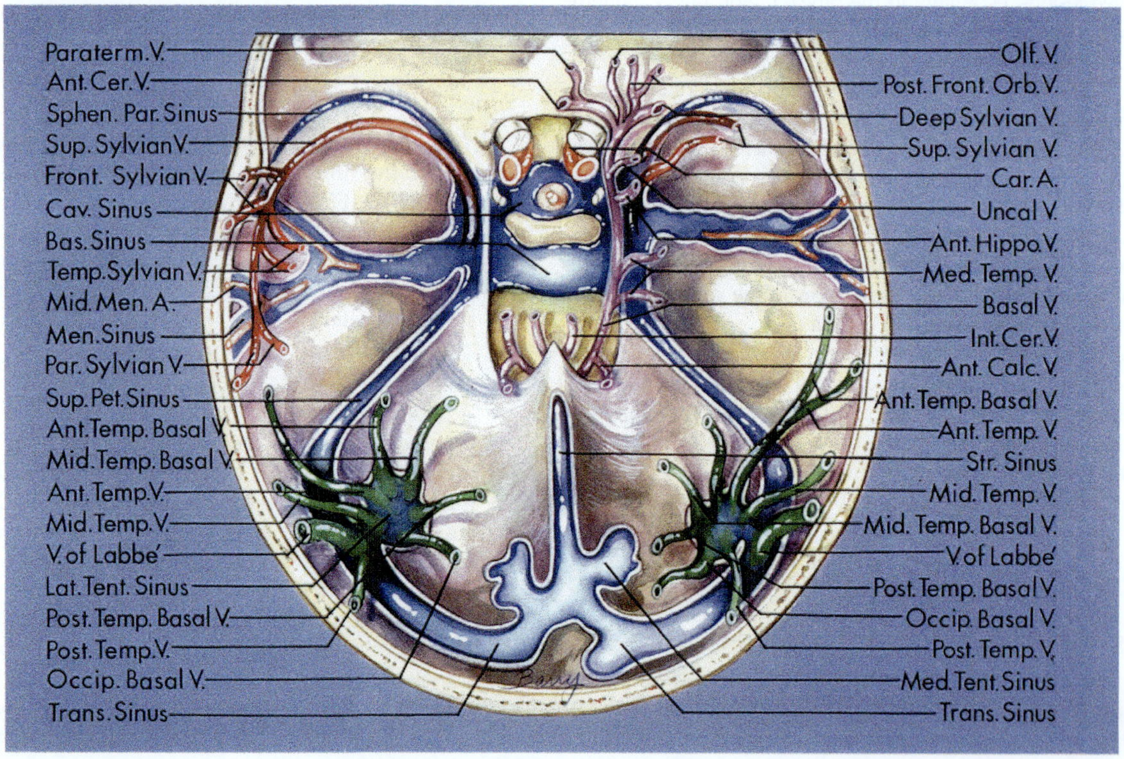
Paraterm. V.
Ant. Cer. V.
Sphen. Par. Sinus
Sup. Sylvian V.
Front. Sylvian V.
Cav. Sinus
Bas. Sinus
Temp. Sylvian V.
Mid. Men. A.
Men. Sinus
Par. Sylvian V.
Sup. Pet. Sinus
Ant. Temp. Basal V.
Mid. Temp. Basal V.
Ant. Temp. V.
Mid. Temp. V.
V. of Labbe'
Lat. Tent. Sinus
Post. Temp. Basal V.
Post. Temp. V.
Occip. Basal V.
Trans. Sinus
Olf. V.
Post. Front. Orb. V.
Deep Sylvian V.
Sup. Sylvian V.
Car. A.
Uncal V.
Ant. Hippo. V.
Med. Temp. V.
Basal V.
Int. Cer. V.
Ant. Calc. V.
Ant. Temp. Basal V.
Ant. Temp. V.
Str. Sinus
Mid. Temp. V.
Mid. Temp. Basal V.
V. of Labbe'
Post. Temp. Basal V.
Occip. Basal V.
Post. Temp. V.
Med. Tent. Sinus
Trans. Sinus

FIGURE 4.1.

around the inferior margin of the hemisphere to reach the lateral tentorial sinus. The vein of Labbé usually enters the transverse sinus. The bridging veins from the basal surface frequently adhere to the dura mater covering the middle fossa or the tentorium surface before joining the venous sinuses.

Falcine Group

The falcine group is formed by the veins that empty into the inferior sagittal or straight sinus, either directly or through the internal cerebral, basal, and great veins (*Figs. 4.1* and *4.6*). The cortical area drained by the falcine group corresponds roughly to the limbic lobe, a group of convolutions that form a continuous cortical strip that wraps around the corpus callosum and upper brainstem. The largest cortical areas are the parahippocampal and cingulate gyri, but the area also includes the paraterminal, paraolfactory gyri, and the uncus. The veins on the paraterminal and paraolfactory gyri drain posteriorly toward the anterior cerebral vein, which empties into the anterior end of the basal vein. The anterior parts of the cingulate gyrus and corpus callosum are drained by the anterior pericallosal veins, which may join the inferior sagittal sinus or the anterior cerebral vein. The posterior part of the cingulate gyrus is drained by the posterior pericallosal vein, which drains into the great or internal cerebral veins in the quadrigeminal cistern. The area adjoining the isthmus of the cingulate gyrus and the area surrounding the anterior part of the calcarine fissure is drained by anterior calcarine veins, which cross the quadrigeminal cistern to reach the great vein or its tributaries. The medial part of the parahippocampal gyrus and uncus are drained by the uncal, anterior hippocampal, and medial temporal veins, which pass medially to empty into the basal vein in the crural and ambient cisterns.

Dural Sinuses and Veins

The dural sinuses into which the cortical veins empty are the superior and inferior sagittal, straight, transverse, tentorial, cavernous, sphenoparietal, sphenobasal, and sphenopetrosal sinuses. These sinuses form the terminal part of the superficial cortical venous system. The small sinuses that accompany the meningeal arteries, referred to as the meningeal veins, are also reviewed in this section.

Superior Sagittal Sinus and Venous Lacunae

The superior sagittal sinus courses in the midline beginning just behind the frontal sinuses and grows larger as it continues posteriorly in the shallow groove on the inner table of the cranium (*Figs. 4.1–4.3*). It may communicate through the foramen cecum with the veins of the nasal cavity. It drains into the transverse sinus at the internal occipital protuberance through a plexiform confluent venous complex, called the torcular herophili, that connects the superior sagittal, transverse, straight, and occipital sinuses. Although the superior sagittal sinus may drain equally to the right and left transverse sinuses or predominantly or wholly to either side, it is usually the right transverse sinus that receives the majority of its drainage. The superior sagittal sinus drains the anterior part of the inferior surface of the frontal lobe and the superior portions of the lateral and medial surfaces of the frontal, parietal, and occipital lobes.

The veins from each cortical area join the superior sagittal sinus in a characteristic configuration (*Figs. 4.2, 4.3,* and *4.7*). The veins arising near the frontal pole are directed posteriorly, in the usual direction of flow within the sinus, at their junction with the sinus. The veins arising from the posterior part of the frontal lobe are directed forward as they join the sinus, in a

FIGURE 4.1. *Dural sinuses and bridging veins.* A, *oblique superior view;* B, *direct superior view with the falx and superior sagittal sinus removed.* A *and* B, *the veins are divided into four groups based on their site of termination: a superior sagittal group* (dark blue*), which drains into the superior sagittal sinus; a tentorial group* (green*), which drains into the transverse or lateral tentorial sinus; a sphenoidal group* (red*), which drains into the sphenoparietal or cavernous sinus; and a falcine group* (purple*), which drains into the straight or inferior sagittal sinus either directly or through the basal, great, or internal cerebral veins. The veins emptying into the superior sagittal sinus* (blue*) drain the upper part of the medial or lateral surfaces of the frontal, parietal, and occipital lobes and the anterior part of the orbital surface of the frontal lobe. The veins from the lateral surface that terminate in the superior sagittal sinus are the frontopolar, anterior frontal, middle frontal, posterior frontal, precentral, central, anterior parietal, posterior parietal, and occipital veins and the vein of Trolard, which, in this case, is a large postcentral vein. The veins from the medial surface that drain into the superior sagittal sinus* (blue*) are the anteromedial frontal, centromedial frontal, posteromedial frontal, paracentral, anteromedial parietal, posteromedial parietal, and posterior calcarine veins. The veins from the orbital surface that drain into the superior sagittal sinus are the anterior orbitofrontal veins. The veins emptying into the sinuses in the tentorium* (green*) drain the lateral and basal surfaces of the temporal lobe and the basal surface of the occipital lobe. The veins from the lateral surface that drain into the sinuses in the tentorium are the anterior temporal, middle temporal, and posterior temporal veins and the vein of Labbé. The veins from the inferior surface that drain into the sinuses in the tentorium are the anterior temporobasal, middle temporobasal, posterior temporobasal, and occipitobasal veins. The veins that empty into the cavernous or sphenoparietal sinus* (red*) course along the sylvian fissure and drain the parts of the frontal, parietal, and temporal lobes adjoining the sylvian fissure. These branches are the superficial sylvian vein and its tributaries, the frontosylvian, parietosylvian, and temporosylvian veins. The veins emptying into the straight sinus* (purple*) or its tributaries drain the part of the frontal and parietal lobes surrounding the corpus callosum and the medial part of the temporal lobe. The area drained by this group corresponds roughly to the limbic lobe of the brain. The veins in this group are the paraterminal, posterior fronto-orbital, olfactory, anterior pericallosal, posterior pericallosal, uncal, anterior hippocampal, medial temporal, and anterior calcarine veins. The right superficial sylvian veins are directed toward the sphenoparietal sinus and the anterior part of the cavernous sinus, and the left superficial sylvian veins are directed further posteriorly toward a lateral extension of the cavernous sinus. The deep sylvian and anterior cerebral veins also empty into the anterior end of the basal vein. The carotid arteries pass through the cavernous sinuses. The meningeal sinuses in the floor of the middle cranial fossae course with the middle meningeal arteries. The medial tentorial sinuses receive tributaries from the cerebellum and join the straight sinus. The basilar sinus sits on the clivus. Pacchionian granulations protrude into the venous lacuane.* A., *artery;* Ant., *anterior;* Ant.Med., *anteromedial;* Bas., *basilar;* Calc., *calcarine;* Car., *carotid;* Cav., *cavernous;* Cent., *central;* Cer., *cerebral;* Front., *frontal;* Front.Orb., *fronto-orbital;* Hippo., *hippocampal;* Inf., *inferior;* Int., *internal;* Lat., *lateral;* Med., *medial;* Men., *meningeal;* Mid., *middle;* Occip., *occipital;* Olf., *olfactory;* Pacci. Gran., *Pacchionian granulations;* Par., *parietal;* Paracent., *paracentral;* Paraterm., *paraterminal;* Pericall., *pericallosal;* Pet., *petrosal;* Post., *posterior;* Post.Med., *posteromedial;* Precent., *precentral;* Sag., *sagittal;* Sphen.Par., *sphenoparietal;* Str., *straight;* Sup., *superior;* Temp., *temporal;* Tent., *tentorial, tentorium;* Trans., *transverse;* V., *vein;* Ven., *venous.*

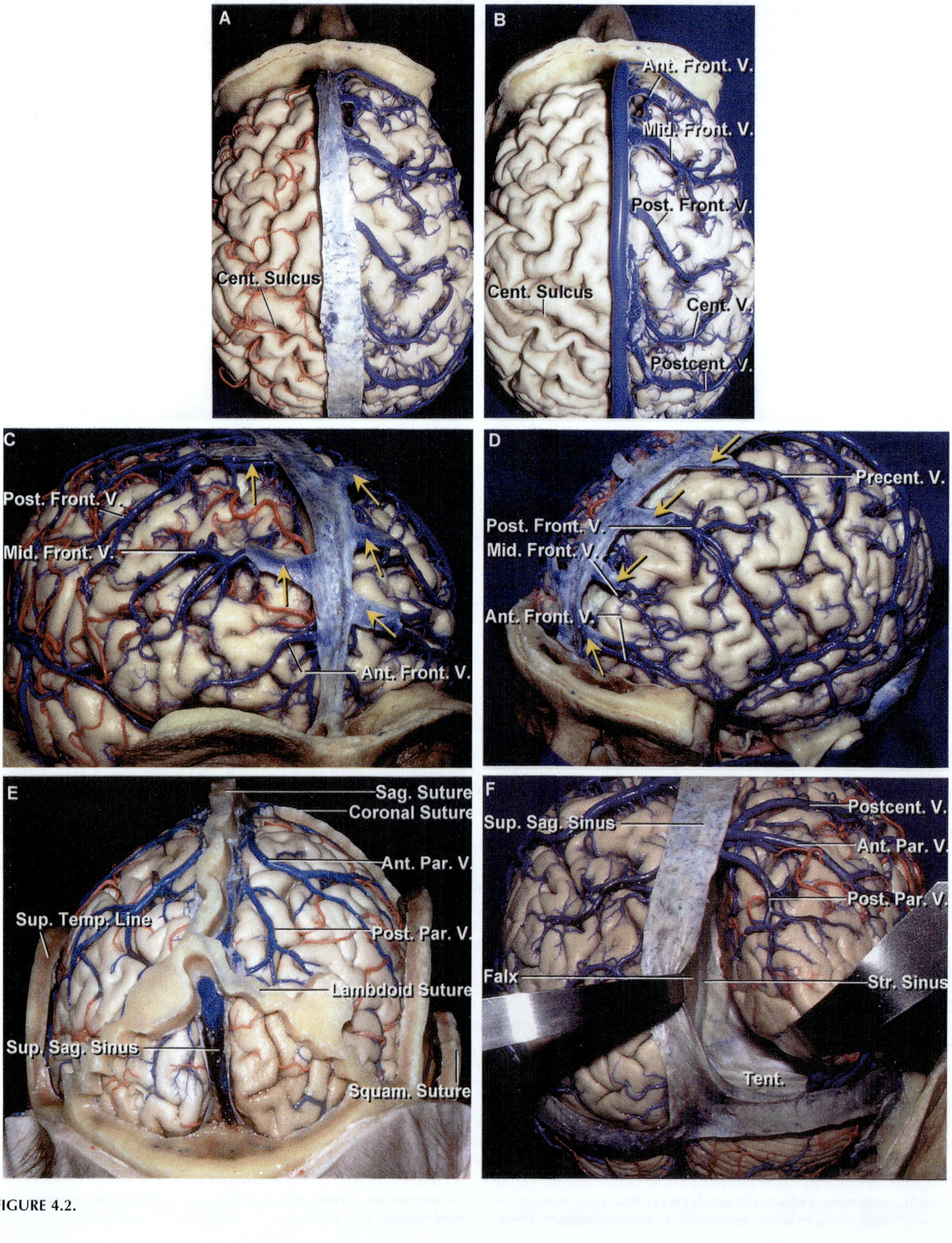
A
Cent. Sulcus
B
Ant. Front. V.
Mid. Front. V.
Post. Front. V.
Cent. Sulcus
Cent. V.
Postcent. V.
C
Post. Front. V.
Mid. Front. V.
Ant. Front. V.
D
Precent. V.
Post. Front. V.
Mid. Front. V.
Ant. Front. V.
E
Sag. Suture
Coronal Suture
Ant. Par. V.
Sup. Temp. Line
Post. Par. V.
Lambdoid Suture
Sup. Sag. Sinus
Squam. Suture
F
Postcent. V.
Sup. Sag. Sinus
Ant. Par. V.
Post. Par. V.
Falx
Str. Sinus
Tent.

FIGURE 4.2.

direction opposed to the direction of flow within the sinus, and those from the intermediate frontal areas join the sinus at approximately a right angle. The terminal ends of the parietal and occipital veins are directed forward and enter the superior sagittal sinus at an angle opposed to the direction of flow. The more posterior veins course anteriorly and slightly inferiorly to enter the lower margin of the sinus. They may adhere to the lateral wall of the sinus before joining it. The length of the veins adherent to the sinus wall varies and is greatest with the most posterior veins, which may have as much as 8 cm of vein adherent to the sinus wall (17).

Enlarged venous spaces, called lacunae, are contained in the dura mater adjoining the superior sagittal sinus (*Figs. 4.2, 4.3,* and *4.8*). The lacunae are largest and most constant in the parietal and posterior frontal regions. Smaller lacunae are found in the occipital and anterior frontal regions. In some cases, the separate lacunae are replaced by a single lacuna on each side of the sinus (17). The lacunae receive predominantly the drainage of the meningeal veins, which accompany the meningeal arteries in the dura mater. Some investigators have recorded that the lacunae do not receive the drainage of the cortical veins; however, we did find sites of communication between the cortical veins and the lacunae (17, 29). The cortical veins that empty into the superior sagittal sinus characteristically pass beneath rather than emptying directly into the lacunae to reach the sinus. The majority of the veins that pass beneath the lacunae open into the sinus separately from the lacunae, but some may share a common opening into the sinus with the lacunae. Very few cortical veins empty directly into the lacunae.

Arachnoid granulations, finger-like outpouchings of clumps of arachnoid cells, project into the floor and walls of the lacunae (9). The arachnoid granulations infrequently project into the superior sagittal sinus. In the granulations, the arachnoid cells rest against the endothelium lining the venous spaces. The increase in size of the lacunae with advancing age is thought to accompany the increase in size of the arachnoid granulations with age (9). O'Connell (17) emphasized the fact that, although a few granulations are found projecting into the venous sinuses, the vast majority project into the lacunae, which in the adult are carpeted with granulations. The arachnoid granulations are also found in proximity to the transverse, cavernous, superior petrosal, sphenoparietal, and straight sinuses (16).

The superior sagittal sinus is triangular in cross section and has right and left lateral angles at its junction with the dura mater covering the convexities and an inferior angle at its junction with the falx. The cortical veins may pass directly to the superior sagittal sinus, or they may join the meningeal sinuses, which empty into the superior sagittal sinus. The cortical veins passing directly to the superior sagittal sinus may join the lateral angles, lateral walls, or inferior angle of the sinus. Other cortical veins join the meningeal sinuses in the dura mater over the convexity 0.5 to 3.0 cm lateral to the superior sagittal sinus. These meningeal sinuses course medially to join the lateral angle of the superior sagittal sinus (*Figs. 4.2* and *4.8*). Several cortical veins may join a single meningeal sinus. Two or three meningeal sinuses may join to form a vestibule just before reaching the superior sagittal sinus. There is a tendency for the veins draining the lateral surface of the anterior frontal and posterior parietal regions to join the meningeal sinus in the dura mater lateral to the superior sagittal sinus. The veins from the posterior frontal and parietal region most commonly dip beneath the venous lacunae and pass directly to the superior sagittal sinus.

The veins from the medial surface of the hemisphere enter the inferior border of the sinus or turn laterally onto the superior margin of the hemisphere to join the veins from the lateral surface before entering the sinus. The segment of the superior sagittal sinus in the frontal region above the genu of the corpus callosum receives fewer bridging veins than any other area except the 4 to 6 cm proximal to the torcular herophili, where bridging veins infrequently enter the superior sagittal sinus.

Inferior Sagittal Sinus

The inferior sagittal sinus courses in the inferior edge of the falx (*Figs. 4.1* and *4.6*). It originates above the anterior portion of the corpus callosum and enlarges as it courses posteriorly to

FIGURE 4.2. A, *superior view. The dura covering the cerebrum has been removed to expose the cortical veins entering the superior sagittal sinus. The branches of the left anterior and middle cerebral arteries have been preserved. The veins entering the most anterior part of the sagittal sinus are directed slightly posteriorly. Those from the midportion of the frontal lobe enter the sagittal sinus at a right angle and, proceeding posteriorly, the veins entering the sinus are progressively angulated further forward. The central sulcus reaches the superior hemispheric border.* B, *the arteries on the left side have been removed. The veins entering the posterior part of the sagittal sinus are directed forward. Anterior, middle, and posterior frontal, and central and postcentral veins ascend to the superior sagittal sinus. The posterior frontal vein drains the area normally drained by precentral and posterior frontal veins.* C, *right anterolateral view. The right middle and posterior frontal veins join sinuses in the dura that empty medially into the superior sagittal sinus. The right anterior frontal vein empties directly into the superior sagittal sinus.* Yellow arrows *are on two dural sinuses on the right and three on the left side.* D, *left anterolateral view. The left anterior, middle, and posterior frontal and precentral veins do not pass directly to the superior sagittal sinus, but empty into dural sinuses that cross the upper border of the frontal lobe to reach the superior sagittal sinus.* Yellow arrows *are on four left dural sinuses.* E, *posterior view. The veins on the occipital lobe are directed forward so that the area below the lambdoid suture is often completely devoid of bridging veins to the superior sagittal sinus. This often allows the occipital lobe to be retracted away from the sagittal sinus without sacrificing any bridging veins. There is an intrasutural bone in each lambdoid suture.* F, *another specimen. The lambdoid suture has been removed to show the absence of bridging veins entering the posterior part of the superior sagittal sinus. Right postcentral and anterior and posterior parietal veins empty into the superior sagittal sinus. The right occipital lobe has been retracted to expose the tentorium, falx, and straight sinus. There are no bridging veins between the occipital pole and the superior sagittal or straight sinus.* Ant., *anterior;* Cent., *central;* Front., *frontal;* Mid., *middle;* Par., *parietal;* Post., *posterior;* Postcent., *postcentral;* Precent., *precentral;* Sag., *sagittal;* Squam., *squamosal;* Str., *straight;* Sup., *superior;* Temp., *temporal;* Tent., *tentorium;* V., *vein.*

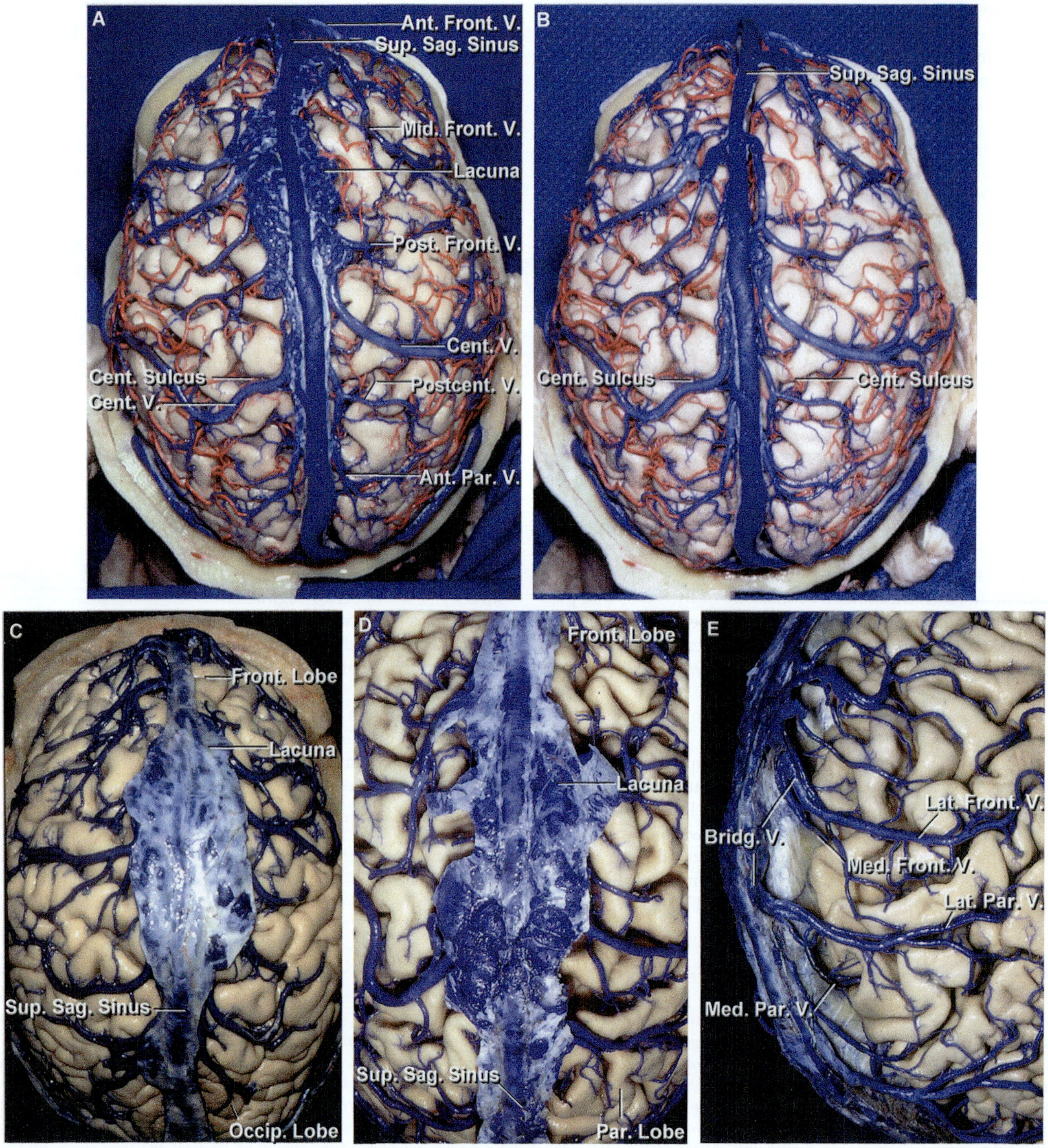

FIGURE 4.3. *Venous lacunae and bridging veins to the superior sagittal sinus. A, superior view. A large venous lacunae adjoining the sagittal sinus extends above the bridging veins emptying into the superior sagittal sinus. The veins from the right hemisphere emptying into the superior sagittal sinus are the anterior, middle, and posterior frontal, central, postcentral, and anterior parietal veins. The precentral and central areas are drained by the large central vein. The veins draining the posterior part of the hemisphere are directed forward. B, the large venous lacunae have been removed to show the veins passing below the lacunae to enter the superior sagittal sinus. The left central vein joins the superior sagittal sinus at the upper end of the central sulcus. The right central vein passes forward across the precentral gyrus to join the superior sagittal sinus. C, the frontal lobe is above and the occipital lobe is below. A large venous lacunae covers the central part of the cerebral vertex. D, some of the dura covering the upper surface of another venous lacunae have been removed. Most of the veins draining into the sagittal sinus proceed medially below the lacunae to reach the sinus. E, right lateral view of the sagittal sinus after removal of the lacunae shown in D. The veins entering the sagittal sinus pass below the large venous lacunae. The medial and lateral, frontal and parietal veins often join to form a common stem before emptying into the sagittal sinus.* Ant., *anterior;* Bridg., *bridging;* Cent., *central;* Front., *frontal;* Lat., *lateral;* Med., *medial;* Mid., *middle;* Occip., *occipital;* Par., *parietal;* Postcent., *postcentral;* Sag., *sagittal;* Sup., *superior;* V., *vein.*

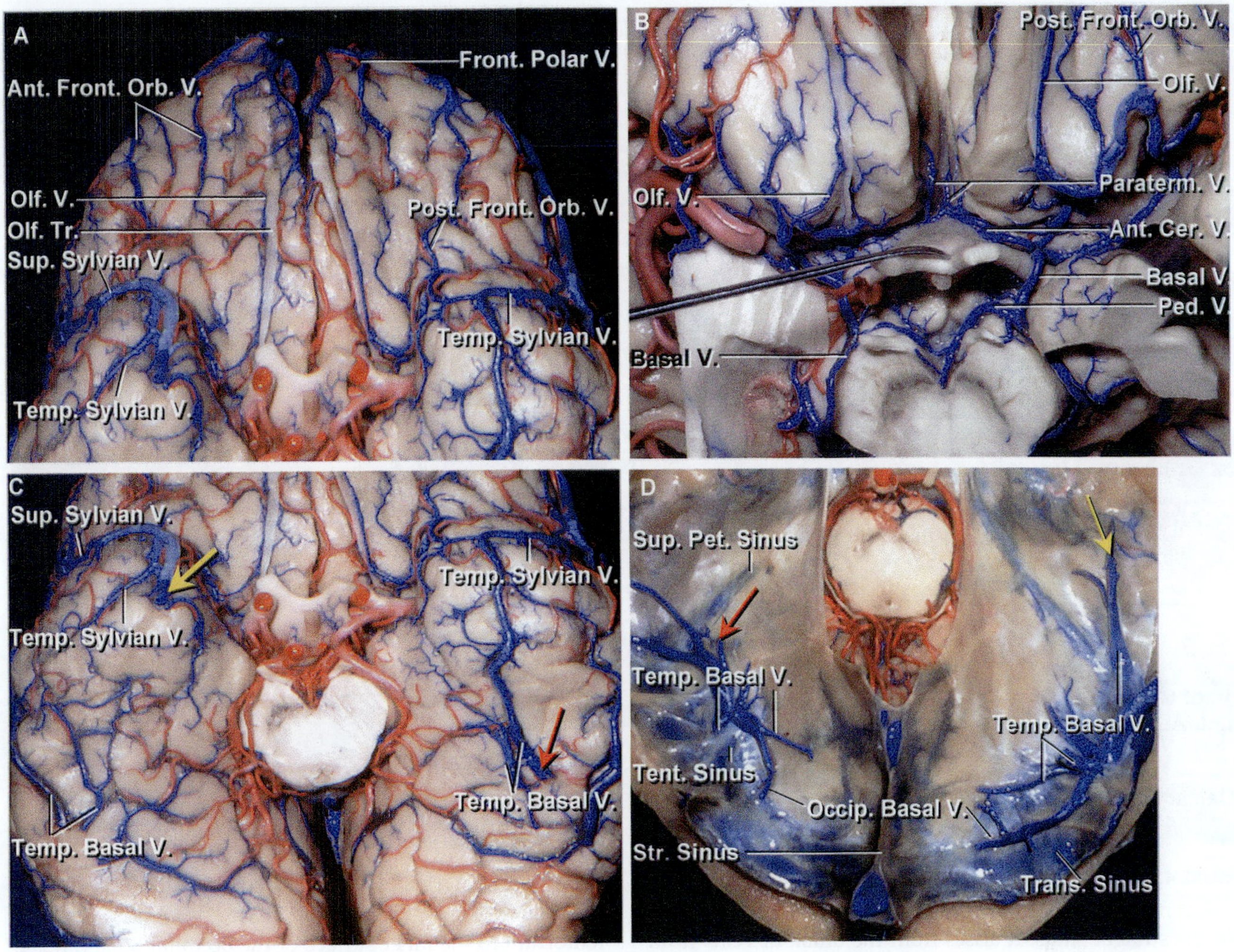

FIGURE 4.4. *Veins of the basal surface. A, the basal surface of the frontal lobe is drained by the frontopolar, anterior and posterior fronto-orbital veins, and the olfactory veins. The anterior fronto-orbital veins empty into the anterior part of the superior sagittal sinus or its tributaries. The posterior fronto-orbital veins empty into the veins below the anterior perforated substance that converge on the anterior end of the basal vein. B, enlarged view. The optic chiasm has been reflected downward to expose the anterior cerebral veins passing above the optic chiasm and being joined by the paraterminal veins that course along the medial surface of the hemisphere below the genu of the corpus callosum. The olfactory, paraterminal, anterior cerebral, and posterior fronto-orbital veins converge on the anterior end of the basal vein. C, basal surface of the temporal lobe. The anterior part of the basal surface of the temporal lobe is drained by the temporosylvian veins that empty into the veins along the sylvian fissure. The right temporobasal veins empty into a tentorial sinus located just medial to the transverse sinus. The area normally drained by the left anterior and middle temporobasal veins is drained predominantly by a long trunk that passes along the long axis of the basal surface and empties at a tentorial sinus. The* yellow *and* red arrows *are on the terminal end of veins that empty into the right and left tentorial sinuses shown in D. D, superior view of the tentorial sinuses into which the temporobasal veins shown in C empty. The long vein on the left basal surface empties into the tributary of the left tentorial sinus shown by the* red arrow. *The temporobasal veins on the right side empty into the right tentorial sinus with multiple tributaries. The vein shown with the* yellow arrow *in C empties into the tributary of right tentorial sinus shown with a* yellow arrow *in D. E, enlarged view of the area below the left anterior perforated substance. The olfactory, anterior cerebral, posterior fronto-orbital, and deep sylvian veins join to form the basal vein. The inferior ventricular vein joins the basal vein at the posterior edge of the cerebral peduncle. F, inferior view of the cerebral hemispheres with the parahippocampal gyri removed to expose the temporal horns and atria. The left fimbria and posterior cerebral artery have been preserved. The left inferior ventricular vein passes above the choroid plexus and through the choroidal fissure located between the fimbria and thalamus. The lateral atrial veins also pass through the choroidal fissure. The lower lip of the calcarine sulcus has been removed on both sides to expose the anterior calcarine veins and calcarine artery and the upper lip of the fissure formed by the cuneus. G, the left fimbria, posterior cerebral artery, and choroid plexus have been removed to expose the inferior ventricular vein crossing the roof of the temporal horn. The anterior calcarine veins, which empty into the vein of Galen, are exposed below the cuneus. H, the floor of the third ventricle has been removed to expose the fornix coursing above the foramen of Monro. The massa intermedia and posterior commissure are exposed. The basal veins pass around the midbrain to join the vein of Galen. Small hypothalamic veins join the anterior end of the basal vein.* Ant., *anterior;* Atr., *atrial;* Calc., *calcarine;* Cer., *cerebral;* CN, *cranial nerve;* Comm., *commissure;* For., *foramen;* Front., *frontal;* Front.Orb., *fronto-orbital;* Inf., *inferior;* Int., *intermedia;* Lat., *lateral;* Occip., *occipital;* Olf., *olfactory;* Paraterm., *paraterminal;* P.C.A., *posterior cerebral artery;* Ped., *peduncular;* Pet., *petrosal;* Post., *posterior;* Str., *straight;* Sup., *superior;* Temp., *temporal;* Tent., *tentorial;* Tr., *tract;* Trans., *transverse;* V., *vein;* Vent., *ventral. (Figure continues on next page.)*

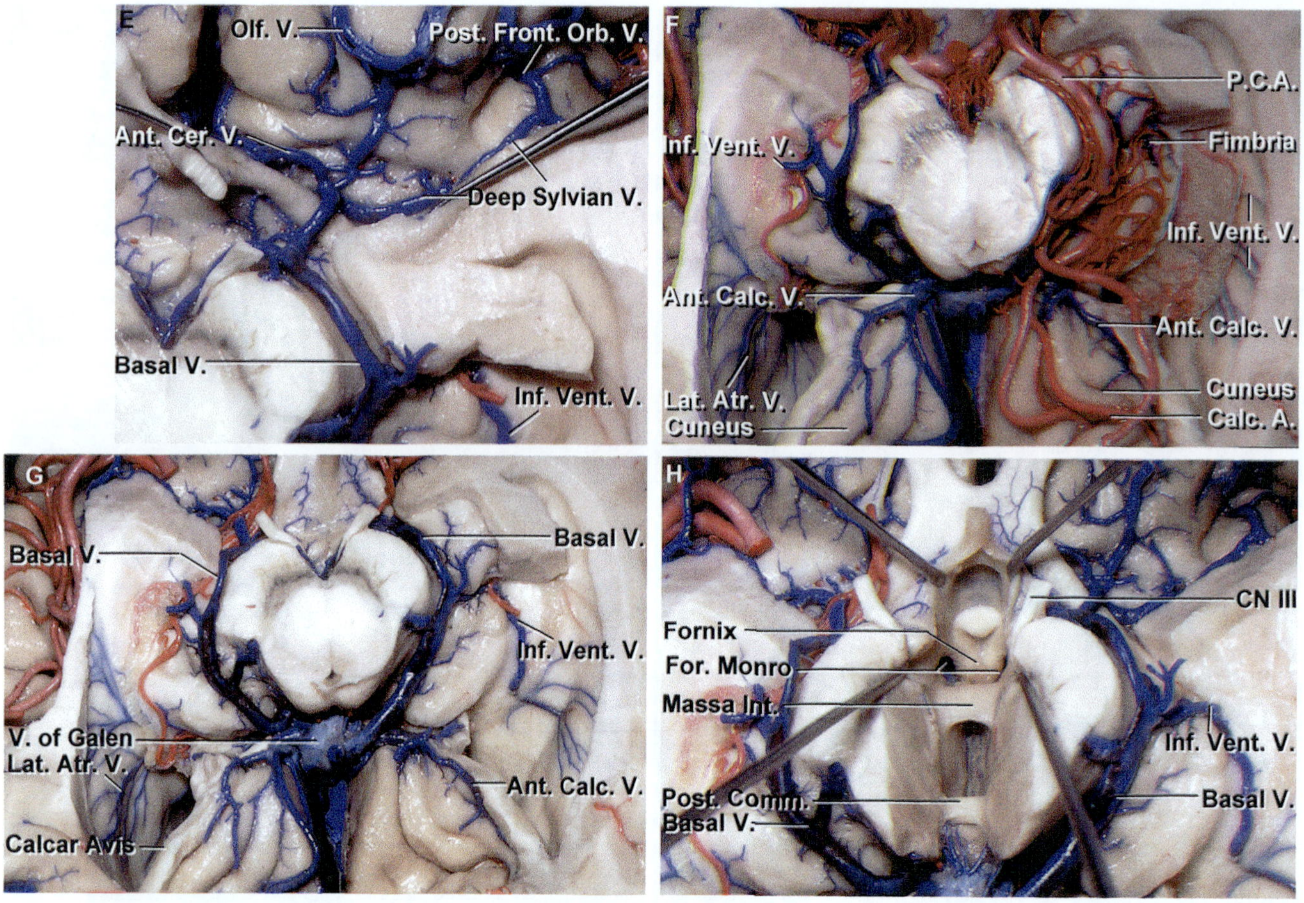

FIGURE 4.4. *Continued*

join the straight sinus. It arises from the union of veins from the adjacent part of the falx, corpus callosum, and cingulate gyrus. The junction of the veins from the cingulate gyrus and corpus callosum with the sinus often forms an acute hook-like bend, with the apex directed forward. The largest tributaries of the inferior sagittal sinus are the anterior pericallosal veins. The superior sagittal sinus may communicate through a venous channel in the falx with the inferior sagittal sinus. This connection may infrequently be so large that the superior sagittal sinus drains predominantly into the inferior sagittal and straight sinuses (26).

Straight Sinus

The straight sinus originates behind the selenium of the corpus callosum at the union of the inferior sagittal sinus and the great vein (*Figs. 4.1, 4.2, 4.4,* and *4.5*). It continues posteriorly and downward in the junction of the tentorium and falx. It may drain into either transverse sinus, but most commonly drains predominantly into the left transverse sinus.

Transverse Sinus

The right and left transverse sinuses originate at the torcular herophili and course laterally from the internal occipital protuberance in a shallow groove between the attachments of the tentorium to the inner surface of the occipital bone (*Figs. 4.1, 4.4, 4.5,* and *4.9*). The transverse sinus exits the tentorial attachments to become the sigmoid sinus at the site just behind the petrous ridge, where the transverse and superior petrosal sinuses meet. Although the superior sagittal sinus may drain equally to the left and right transverse sinus or predominantly or wholly to either side, it is the right transverse sinus that is usually larger and receives the majority of the drainage from the superior sagittal sinus. The left transverse sinus is usually smaller and receives predominantly the drainage of the straight sinus. Thus, the right transverse sinus, right sigmoid sinus, and right jugular vein contain blood from the superficial parts of the brain, and the left transverse sinus, left sigmoid sinus, and left internal jugular vein contain blood mainly from the deep parts of the brain drained by the internal cerebral, basal, and great veins. The difference in symptoms caused by blockage of the venous drainage on one side or the other and the differences in Queckenstedt's sign with compression of the jugular veins on either the left or right side have been explained by the differences in drainage on each side.

The cortical veins from the lateral surface of the temporal lobe may drain into the transverse sinus, but before entering it, they commonly pass medially below the hemisphere to join a short sinus in the tentorium, which courses within the tento-

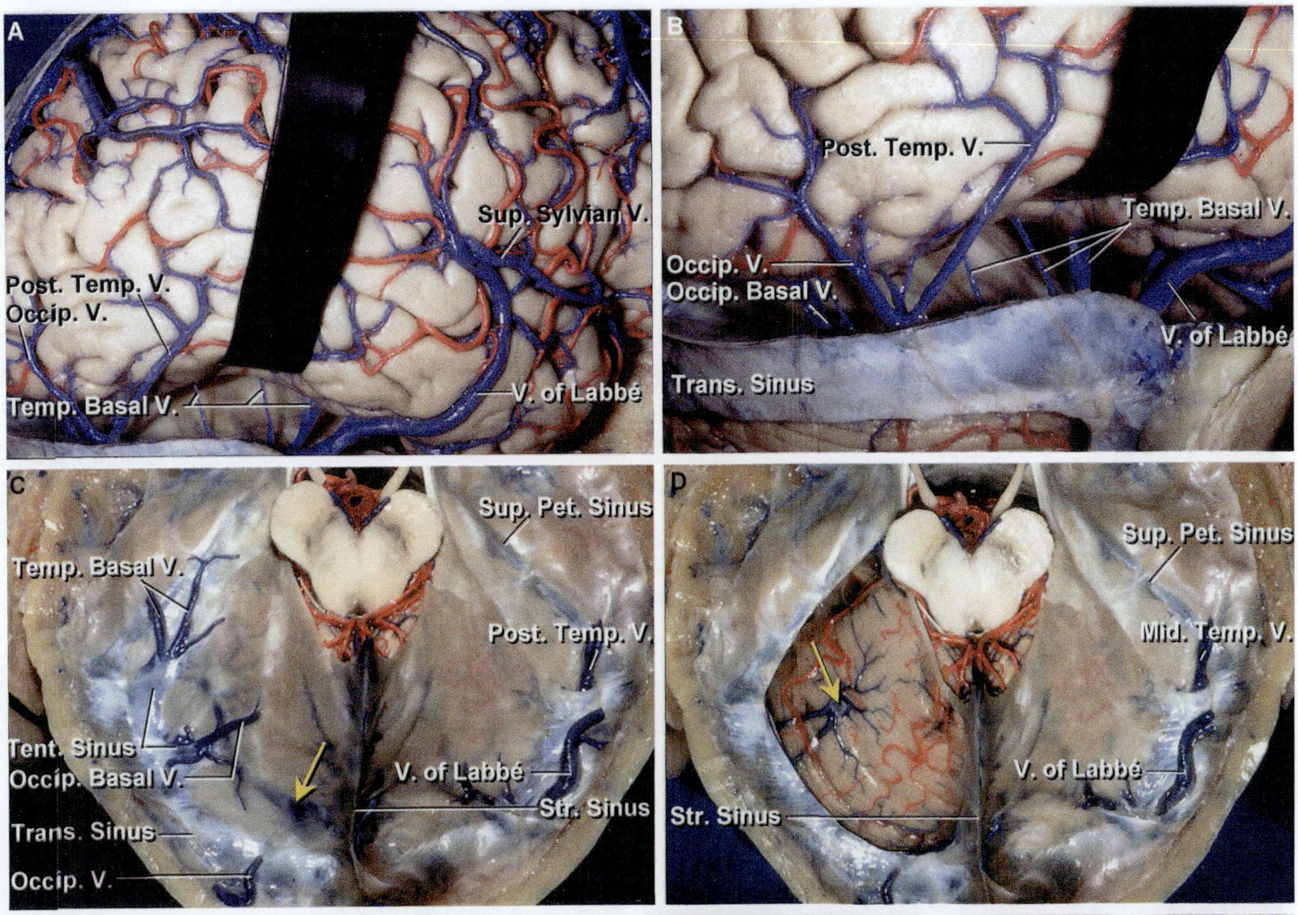

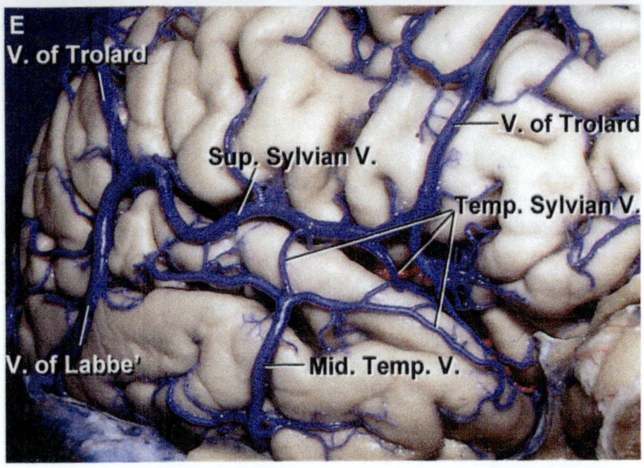

FIGURE 4.5. *Tributaries of the transverse and tentorial sinuses. A, posterolateral view. The posterior temporal lobe has been elevated to expose the vein of Labbé and the posterior temporal and occipital veins from the lateral surface joining the transverse sinus and the temporobasal veins from the basal surface of the temporal lobe emptying into the tentorial sinuses. Some veins from the lateral surface of the temporal and occipital convexity do not pass directly to the transverse sinus, but turn medially under the basal surface to empty into sinuses in the tentorium. B, enlarged view. The vein of Labbé is exposed anteriorly. Reaching the tentorial incisura by the posterior subtemporal route may require the sacrifice of multiple temporobasal and occipitobasal veins draining into the tentorial sinuses in addition to the vein of Labbé and other veins from the lateral surface of the temporal and occipital lobes. C, superior view of the tentorium. On the left side, the temporobasal and occipitobasal veins converge on two short tentorial sinuses located just medial to the transverse sinus. On the right side, the vein of Labbé and a posterior temporal vein drain directly into the transverse sinus. Another sinus within the left tentorium* (yellow arrow) *receives drainage from the cerebellum and passes medially across the tentorium to empty into the torcular herophili. D, the left half of the tentorium has been removed. The bridging cerebellar vein, shown in D with a* yellow arrow, *empties into the tentorial sinus shown in C with the* yellow arrow. *E, lateral surface of the right temporal lobe and sylvian fissure in another specimen. The anterior part of the superficial sylvian vein is small and the posterior part that empties into the vein of Labbé is larger. A middle temporal vein that courses along the superior temporal sulcus forms a bridging vein that passes around the lower margin of the hemisphere to empty into a tentorial sinus. The sylvian vein also has connections with the superior sagittal sinus through two anastomotic veins of Trolard: one crosses the frontal lobe and the other crosses the parietal lobe. The temporosylvian veins drain the superior temporal gyrus and empty into the superficial sylvian and middle temporal veins.* Mid., *middle;* Occip., *occipital;* Pet., *petrosal;* Post., *posterior;* Str., *straight;* Sup., *superior;* Temp., *temporal;* Tent., *tentorial;* Trans., *transverse;* V., *vein.*

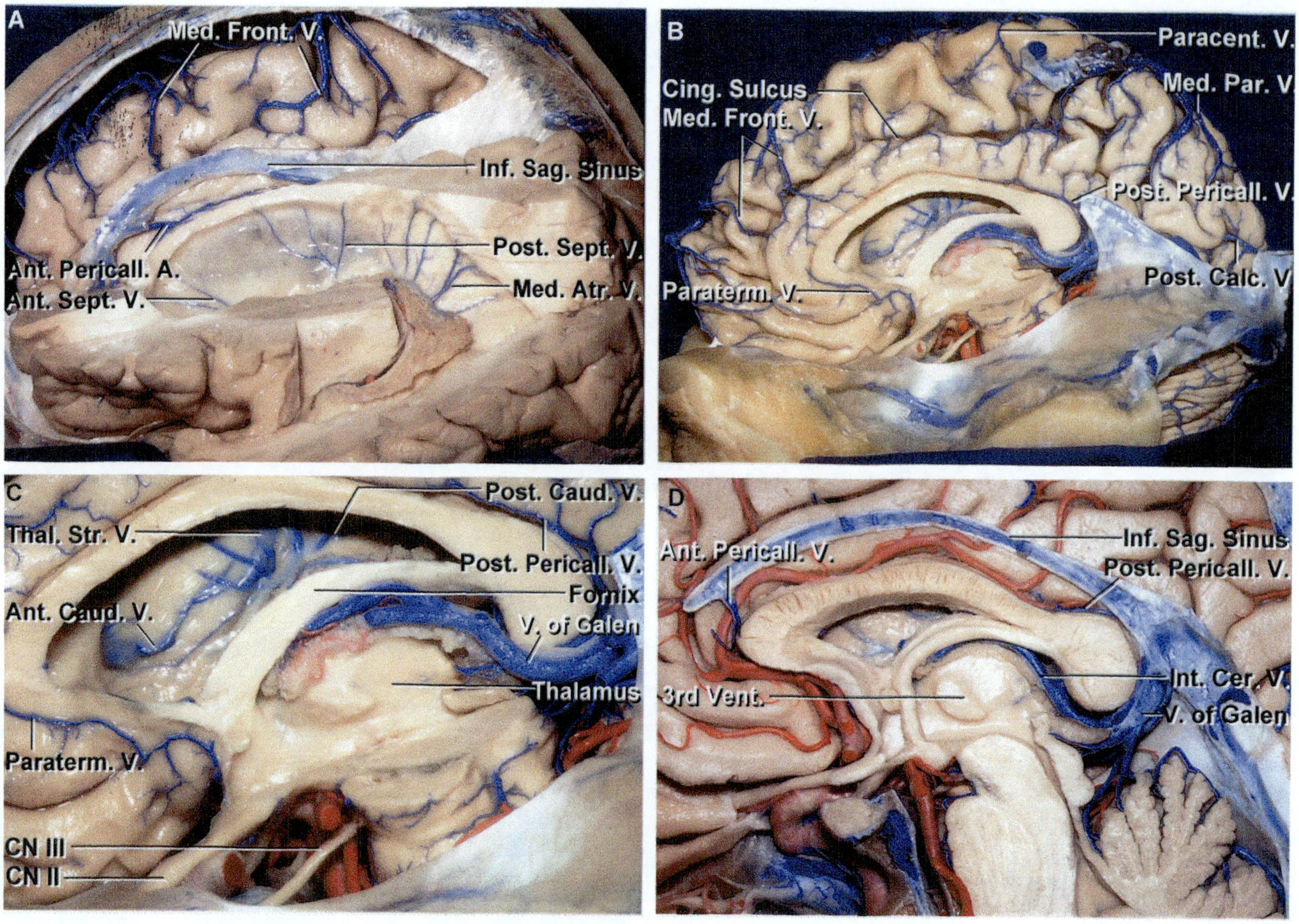

FIGURE 4.6. *Veins of the medial surface. A, the upper part of the left cerebral hemisphere has been removed to expose the medial surface of the right hemisphere. An anterior pericallosal vein empties into the inferior sagittal sinus. The medial frontal veins draining the area above the cingulate sulcus empty into the superior sagittal sinus. The veins from the medial surface often join the veins from the lateral surface to form a common stem before emptying into the superior sagittal sinus. The veins from the part of the cingulate sulcus bordering the corpus callosum commonly empty into the paraterminal veins or the pericallosal veins. The anterior and posterior septal and medial atrial veins cross the medial wall of the frontal horn, body, and atrium. The anterior pericallosal vein empties into the anterior end of the inferior sagittal sinus. B, the remainder of the left hemisphere has been removed. The medial frontal and parietal veins draining the outer strip of the medial surface empty into the superior sagittal sinus. The veins draining the part of the cingulate sulcus facing the corpus callosum empty into the anterior and posterior pericallosal, paraterminal, and great veins. The posterior calcarine vein drains the posterior part of the calcarine sulcus and commonly empties into the veins on the lateral surface. C, enlarged view. The anterior and posterior caudate and thalamostriate veins in the lateral wall of the frontal horn and body pass through the choroidal fissure between the fornix and thalamus to empty into the internal cerebral veins. The paraterminal vein courses downward in front of the lamina terminalis to empty into the anterior cerebral vein. A posterior pericallosal (splenial) vein passes around the splenium of the corpus callosum and empties into the vein of Galen. D, enlarged view of the inferior sagittal sinus coursing in the lower edge of the falx. An anterior pericallosal vein empties into the anterior end of the inferior sagittal sinus. A small posterior pericallosal vein empties into the vein of Galen.* A., *artery;* Ant., *anterior;* Atr., *atrial;* Calc., *calcarine;* Caud., *caudal;* Cer., *cerebral;* Cing., *cingulate;* CN, *cranial nerve;* Front., *frontal;* Inf., *inferior;* Int., *internal;* Med., *medial;* Par., *parietal;* Paracent., *paracentral;* Paraterm., *paraterminal;* Pericall., *pericallosal;* Pet., *petrosal;* Post., *posterior;* Sag., *sagittal;* Sept., *septal;* Thal. Str., *thalamostriate;* V., *vein;* Vent., *ventricle.*

rium for approximately 1 cm before draining into the terminal part of the transverse sinus (*Figs. 4.1, 4.4,* and *4.5*). The cortical veins from the basal surface of the temporal and occipital lobes usually join the lateral tentorial sinus. The vein of Labbé commonly ends in the transverse sinus, but may curve around the inferior margin of the hemisphere to join the lateral tentorial sinus. The transverse sinus may communicate through emissary veins in the occipital bone with the extracranial veins.

Tentorial Sinuses

Each half of the tentorium has two constant but rarely symmetrical venous channels, the medial and lateral tentorial sinuses (*Figs. 4.1, 4.4,* and *4.5*) (3). The medial tentorial sinuses are formed by the convergence of veins from the superior surface of the cerebellum, and the lateral tentorial sinuses are formed by the convergence of veins from the basal and lateral surfaces of the temporal and occipital lobes. The lateral tento-

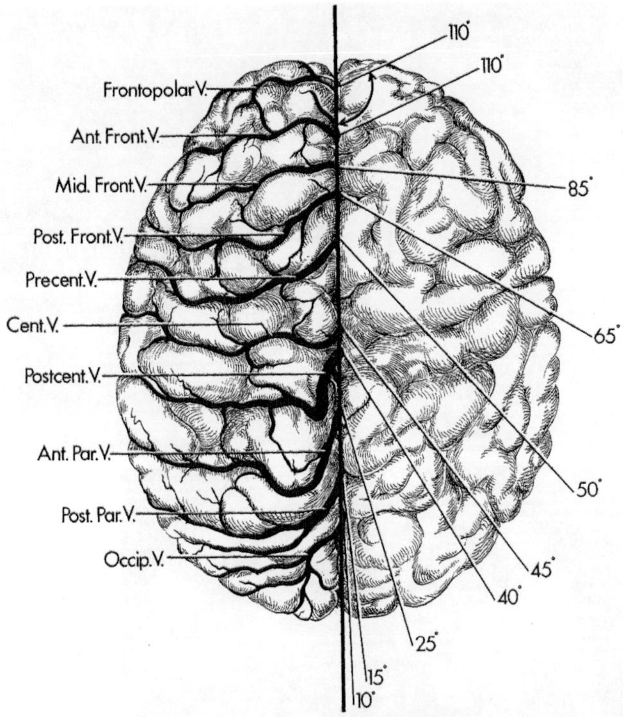

FIGURE 4.7. *Superior view of the cerebral hemispheres showing the veins from the lateral surface of the cerebrum entering the superior sagittal sinus. The veins entering the superior sagittal sinus are shown on the* left *and the average angles at which the veins enter the sinus are shown on the* right. *From anterior to posterior, the angles at which the veins join the sinus decrease. The average angles between the individual veins and the sinuses are as follows: frontopolar and anterior frontal veins, 110 degrees; middle frontal vein, 85 degrees; posterior frontal vein, 65 degrees; precentral vein, 50 degrees; central vein, 45 degrees; postcentral vein, 40 degrees; anterior parietal vein, 25 degrees; posterior parietal vein, 15 degrees; occipital vein, 10 degrees.* Ant., *anterior;* Cent., *central;* Front., *frontal;* Mid., *middle;* Occip., *occipital;* Par., *parietal;* Post., *posterior;* Precent., *precentral;* V., *vein.* (From, *Oka K, Rhoton AL Jr, Barry M, Rodriguez R: Microsurgical anatomy of the superficial veins of the cerebrum.* **Neurosurgery** *17:711–748, 1985 [18].)*

rial sinuses arise within the lateral part of the tentorium and course laterally to drain into the terminal portion of the transverse sinus. The medial tentorial sinuses course medially to empty into the straight sinus or the junction of the straight and transverse sinuses.

Cavernous Sinus

The paired cavernous sinuses are situated on each side of the sella turcica and are connected across the midline by the anterior and posterior intercavernous sinuses, which course in the junction of the diaphragma sellae with the dura lining the sella (*Fig. 4.1*). Anteriorly, each cavernous sinus communicates with the sphenoparietal sinus and the ophthalmic veins. Its middle portion communicates through a lateral extension on the inner surface of the greater sphenoid wing with the pterygoid plexus via small veins that pass through the foramina spinosum and ovale. Posteriorly, the cavernous sinus opens directly into the basilar sinus, which sits on the clivus. It communicates through the superior petrosal sinus with the junction of the transverse and sigmoid sinuses and through the inferior petrosal sinus with the sigmoid sinus. Our studies of the cavernous sinus are reported in Chapter 9 in this issue, and other publications (23, 24).

Superior Petrosal Sinus

The superior petrosal sinus courses within the attachment of the tentorium to the petrous ridge (*Figs. 4.1, 4.4,* and *4.5*). Its medial end connects with the posterior end of the cavernous sinus, and its lateral end joins the junction of the transverse and sigmoid sinuses. The bridging veins that join it usually arise from the cerebellum and brainstem, not the cerebrum. The sinus may course over, under, or around the posterior root of the trigeminal nerve. The superficial sylvian veins may empty into an infrequent tributary of the superior petrosal sinus called the sphenopetrosal sinus.

Sphenoparietal, Sphenobasal, and Sphenopetrosal Sinuses

The sphenoparietal sinus is the largest of the meningeal channels coursing with the meningeal arteries (*Fig. 4.1*). It accompanies the anterior branch of the middle meningeal artery above the level of the pterion. Below this level, it deviates from the artery and courses in the dura mater just below the sphenoid ridge to empty into the anterior part of the cavernous sinus. Its upper end communicates through the meningeal veins with the superior sagittal sinus. The sinus coursing along the sphenoid ridge may turn inferiorly to reach the floor of the middle cranial fossa rather than emptying into the anterior part of the cavernous sinus. From here, it courses posteriorly to empty into a lateral extension of the cavernous sinus on the greater sphenoid wing or joins the sphenoidal emissary veins, which pass through the floor of the middle fossa to reach the pterygoid plexus. It also may pass further posteriorly to join the superior petrosal or lateral sinuses. The variant in which the sinus exits the cranium by joining the sphenoidal emissary veins and the pterygoid plexus is referred to as the sphenobasal sinus, and the variant in which the sinus courses further posteriorly along the floor of the middle fossa and drains into the superior petrosal or lateral sinus is called the sphenopetrosal sinus. The superficial sylvian veins commonly empty into the sphenoparietal sinus. If the sphenoparietal sinus is absent or poorly developed, the sylvian veins may drain directly into the cavernous sinus or they may turn inferiorly around the anterior pole and inferior surface of the temporal lobe to empty into the sphenobasal or sphenopetrosal sinuses.

Anastomotic Veins

The largest veins on the lateral surface are the veins of Trolard and Labbé and the superficial sylvian veins (*Figs. 4.10–4.12*). The vein of Trolard is the largest anastomotic vein joining the superior sagittal sinus with the veins along the

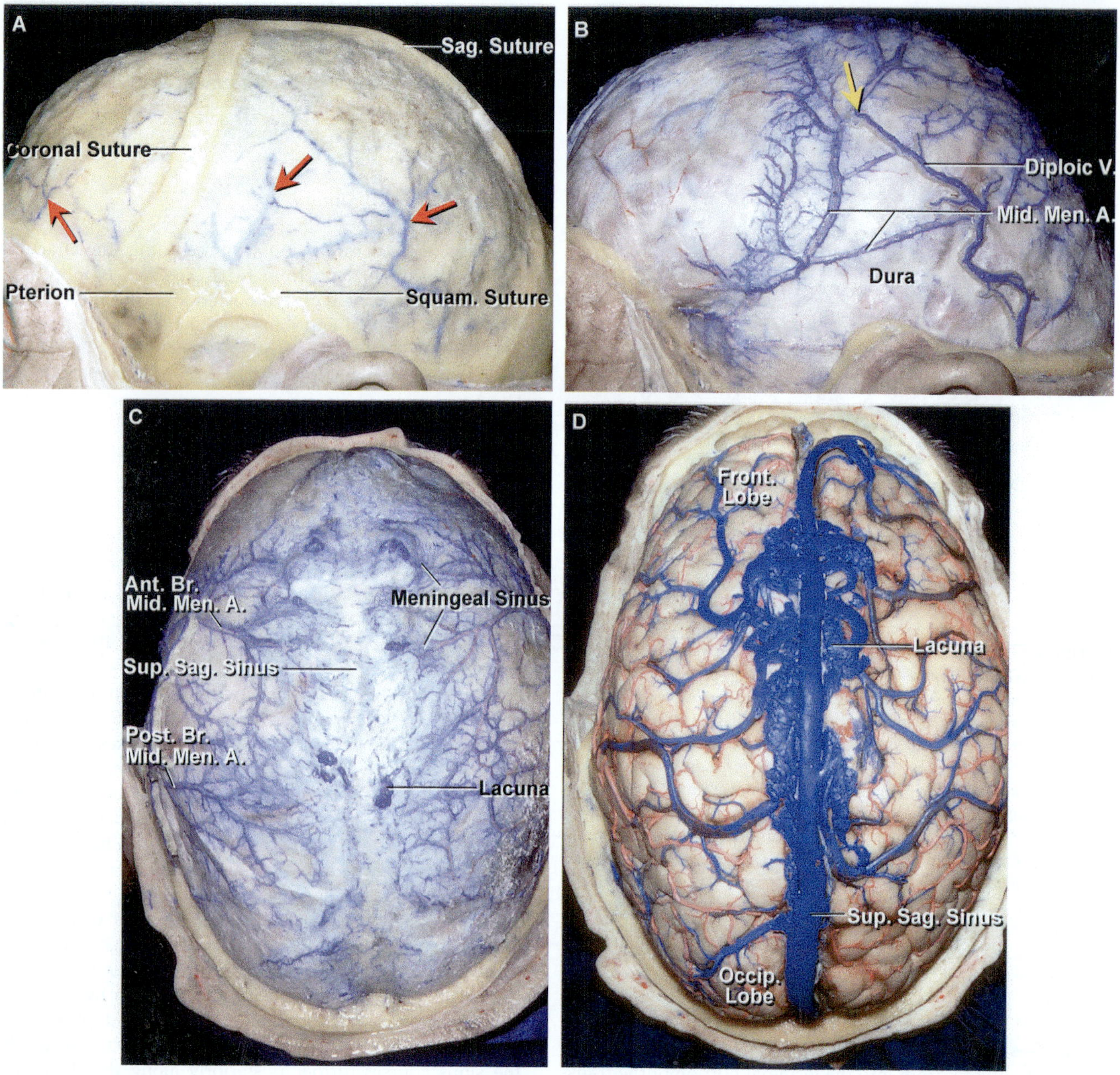

FIGURE 4.8. A, *the outer table of the cranium has been removed, while preserving the sutures, to expose the diploic veins* (red arrows) *coursing between the inner and outer table.* B, *the inner table has been removed to expose the meningeal sinuses coursing along the middle meningeal artery, while preserving the large posterior diploic vein in the bone. The upper end of the diploic vein joins the venous sinuses around the middle meningeal artery at the* yellow arrow. C, *superior view. The dura covering the cerebral hemispheres contains a plexus of small meningeal sinus veins that follow the branches of the meningeal arteries. The largest meningeal sinuses course along the anterior and posterior branches of the middle meningeal artery and extend up to the superior sagittal sinus and the region of the venous lacunae.* D, *the dura has been opened and the venous lacunae preserved. The veins from the posterior part of the hemisphere are directed forward.* A., *artery;* Ant., *anterior;* Br., *branch;* Men., *meningeal;* Mid., *middle;* Occip., *occipital;* Post., *posterior;* Sag., *sagittal;* Squam., *squamosal;* Sup., *superior;* V., *vein.*

sylvian fissure. The vein of Labbé is the largest vein connecting the veins along the sylvian fissure with the transverse sinus (6, 7). The superficial sylvian vein courses along the surface of the sylvian fissure and drains predominantly into the dural sinuses along the sphenoid ridge. Although the veins of Trolard and Labbé and the superficial sylvian vein may be of nearly equal size, it is more common for one or two of them to predominate and the other to be small or absent. Usually, there is asymmetry between the right and left hemispheres in the size of these channels.

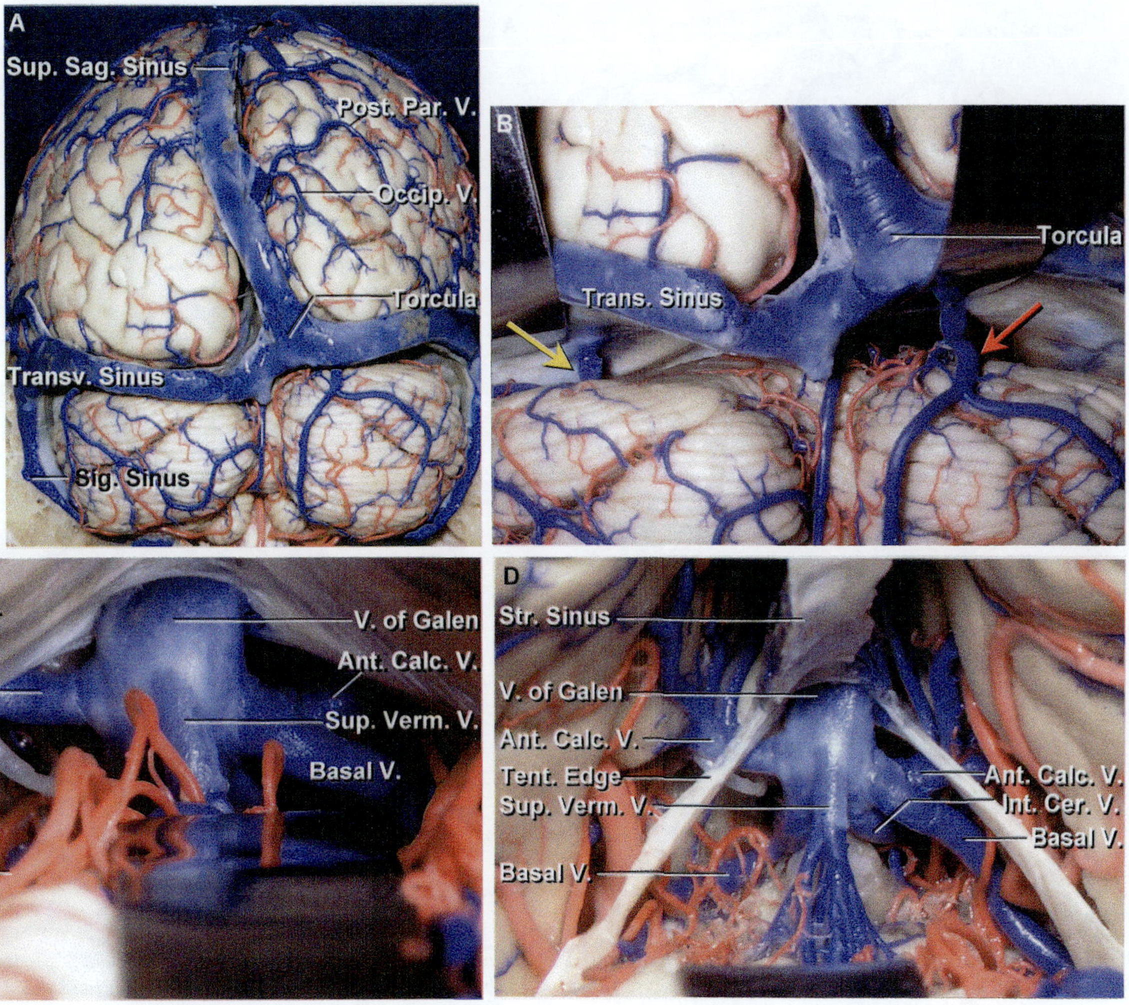

FIGURE 4.9. *Posterior view of the cerebral and cerebellar hemispheres.* A, *the superior sagittal sinus is connected through the torcular herophili with the transverse sinuses. The right transverse sinus is slightly larger than the left. The veins arising along the posterior part of the hemisphere are directed forward and join the superior sagittal sinus well above the torcular herophili, leaving a void along the medial occipital lobe where there are no bridging veins emptying into the sinus.* B, *the tentorium has been elevated to show the veins from the cerebellum forming bridging veins that enter the sinuses in the lower margin of the tentorium. On the left side, a large vein* (yellow arrow) *passes from the superior surface of the cerebellar hemisphere to enter a tentorial sinus. On the right side, a large bridging vein from the suboccipital cerebellar surface* (red arrow) *turns forward on the superior surface and empties into a tentorial sinus in front of the torcular herophili.* C, *view below the tentorium. The vein of Galen empties into the straight sinus. A large superior vermian vein empties into the vein of Galen. The right basal and the right and left anterior calcarine veins are exposed. The left basal vein is hidden in front of the left superior cerebellar artery.* D, *the tentorium has been removed, while preserving the straight sinus and the tentorial edge. The vein of Galen and its tributaries are exposed in the quadrigeminal cistern. Both basal veins are exposed. Large anterior calcarine veins drain the calcarine sulcus and adjacent part of the atrium. The branches of the posterior cerebral artery course in the upper part of the quadrigeminal cistern and the branches of the superior cerebellar artery course in the lower part.* Ant., *anterior;* Calc., *calcarine;* Cer., *cerebral;* Int., *internal;* Occip., *occipital;* Par., *parietal;* P.C.A., *posterior cerebral artery;* Post., *posterior;* Sag., *sagittal;* S.C.A., *superior cerebellar artery;* Sig., *sigmoid;* Str., *straight;* Sup., *superior;* Tent., *tentorium, tentorial;* Trans., Transv., *transverse;* V., *vein;* Verm., *vermian.*

Vein of Trolard

The vein of Trolard, also called the superior anastomotic vein, is the largest anastomotic vein crossing the cortical surface of the frontal and parietal lobes between the superior sagittal sinus and the sylvian fissure (*Figs. 4.10* and *4.11*). In 15 of the 20 hemispheres examined in this study, the vein of Trolard was located at a site that would correspond to the precentral, central, or postcentral vein. It was most commonly located at the level of the postcentral vein. The most anterior vein of Trolard was situated at the level of the anterior frontal veins and connected the anterior part of the sagittal sinus with the anterior part of the superficial sylvian vein. The most posterior vein of Trolard was located at the level of the anterior parietal veins. The vein of Trolard usually joins the superior sagittal sinus as a single channel that is directed forward against the direction of flow as it joins the sinus. It is com-

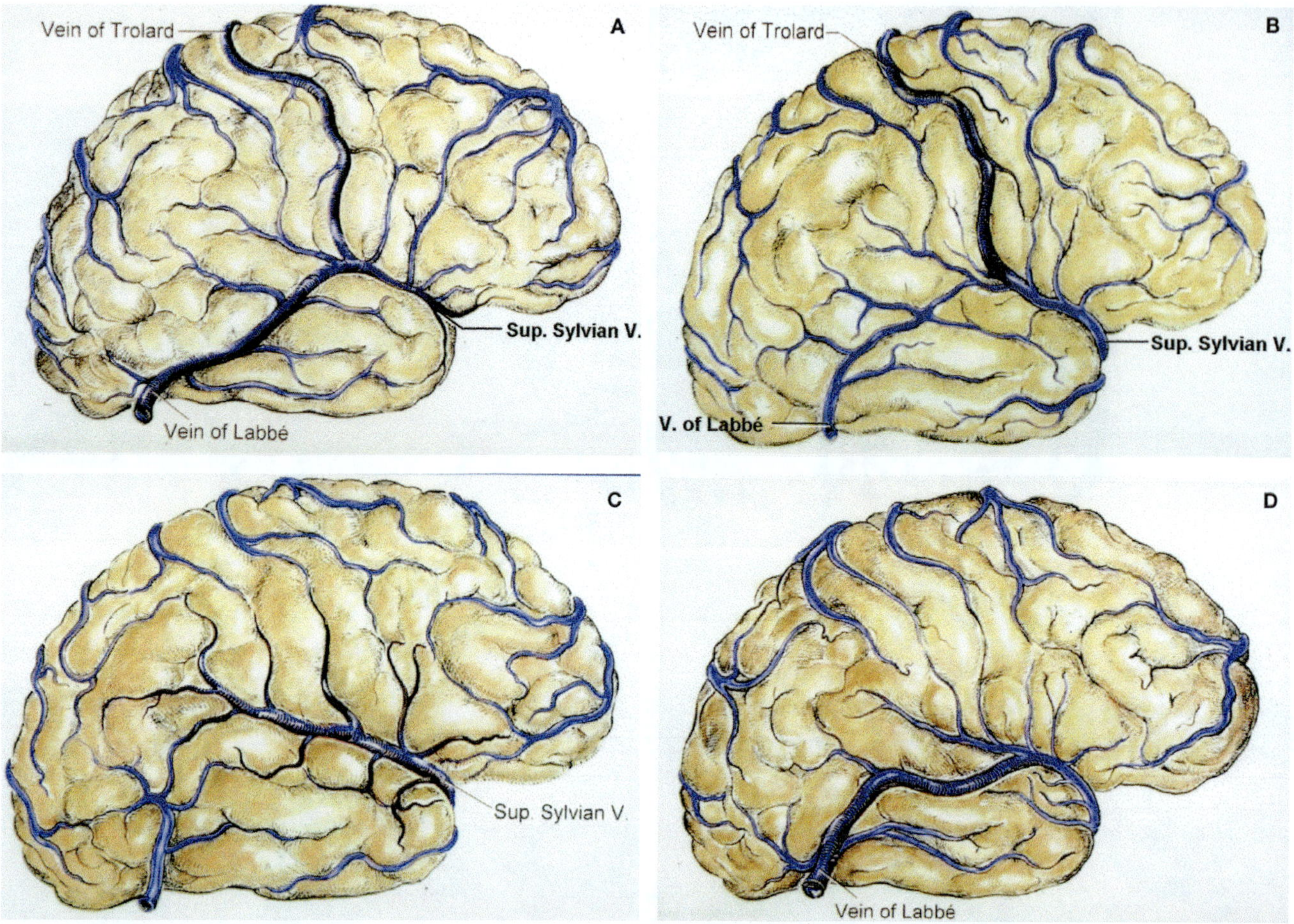

FIGURE 4.10. *Major anastomotic veins. A–D, different patterns. The dominant vein is darkly shaded. The vein of Trolard is the largest vein connecting the superficial sylvian vein with the superior sagittal sinus. The vein of Labbé is the largest vein connecting the superficial sylvian vein with the transverse sinus. The superficial sylvian vein drains the areas along the sylvian fissure and empties into the sinuses along the sphenoid ridge. A, all three anastomotic veins are present, but the veins of Labbé and Trolard are dominant. B, dominant superficial sylvian and vein of Trolard. C, dominant superficial sylvian vein. D, dominant vein of Labbé.* Sup., *superficial;* V., *vein.*

monly joined by other veins immediately proximal to the sinus. Its lower end is usually a single channel that anastomoses with the veins along the sylvian fissure, but it may split on the lower part of the frontal and parietal convexity into multiple channels that join the superficial sylvian vein. There may be duplicate veins of Trolard, in which case two large veins of similar size cross the interval between the sylvian fissure and the superior sagittal sinus.

Vein of Labbé

The vein of Labbé, also called the inferior anastomotic vein, is the largest anastomotic channel that crosses the temporal lobe between the sylvian fissure and the transverse sinus (*Figs. 4.5, 4.10,* and *4.11*). It usually arises from the middle portion of the sylvian fissure and is directed posteriorly and inferiorly toward the anterior part of the transverse sinus. It may cross the temporal lobe as far back as the posterior limit of the lobe or as far forward as the anterior third of the lateral surface. In the 20 hemispheres examined in this study, the vein of Labbé was located at the level of the middle temporal vein in 12, the posterior temporal vein in 6, and the anterior temporal vein in 2. There may be double veins of Labbé, in which case the posterior vein is usually larger (18).

Superficial Sylvian Vein

The superficial sylvian vein usually arises at the posterior end of the sylvian fissure and courses anteriorly and inferiorly along the lips of the fissure (*Figs. 4.5* and *4.10–4.12*). It may arise as two trunks, but these usually merge into a single channel before emptying into the venous sinuses along the sphenoid ridge. The superficial sylvian vein receives the frontosylvian, parietosylvian, and temporosylvian veins and commonly anastomoses with the veins of Trolard and Labbé. It penetrates the arachnoid covering the anterior end of the sylvian fissure and joins the sphenoparietal sinus as it courses just below the medial part of the sphenoid ridge, or it may pass directly to the cavernous sinus. It may also leave the sylvian fissure and course around the temporal pole to reach

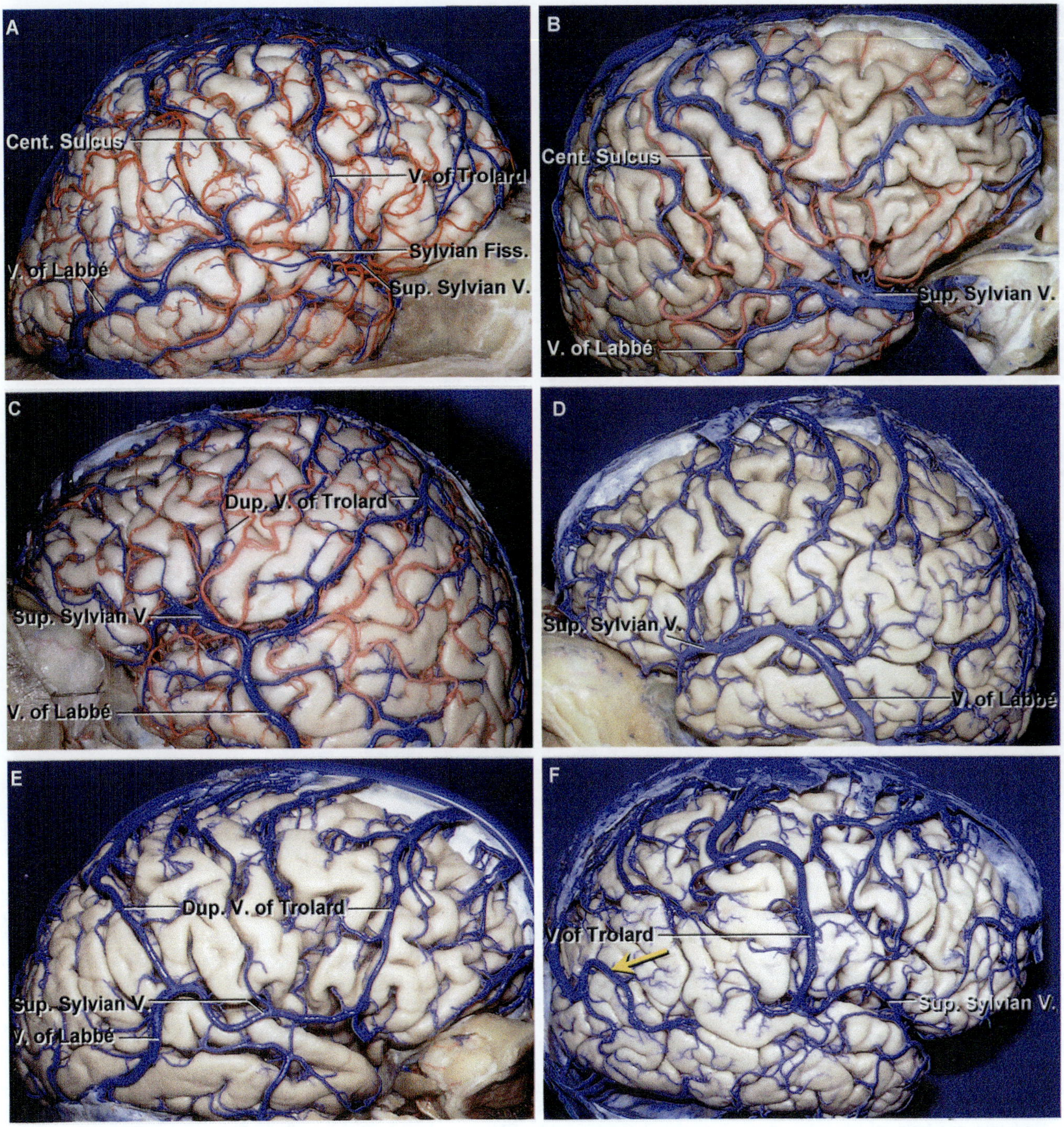

FIGURE 4.11. *Comparison of the drainage pattern of different cerebral hemispheres. A, right lateral view. The veins draining this cerebral hemisphere are directed to the superior sagittal and transverse sinuses. The superficial sylvian vein is small. One small anastomotic vein of Trolard links the superior sagittal sinus and sylvian fissure. B, another right hemisphere. The superficial sylvian vein is large. There is minimal anastomosis between the superficial sylvian vein and the veins draining into the superior sagittal sinus, but there is a connection between the superficial sylvian vein and the vein of Labbé. In opening the sylvian fissure by the pterional approach, the drainage pattern for the whole hemisphere is not seen. Sacrificing the superficial sylvian vein shown in A would probably not affect the hemisphere, but sacrificing the large superficial sylvian vein shown in B could lead to venous drainage problems along the frontal and temporal lobes adjoining the sylvian fissure. C, left hemisphere. A superficial sylvian vein has a large connection with the vein of Labbé. In addition, two small or duplicate veins of Trolard connect the superior sagittal sinus and the sylvian vein. The posterior one joins the superficial sylvian vein near the junction with the vein of Labbé. D, left hemisphere. There are no significant connections between the veins in the sylvian fissure and the superior sagittal sinus, but there is a large anastomosis between the superficial sylvian vein and the vein of Labbé. E, right hemisphere. Duplicate veins of Trolard connect the superior sagittal sinus to the superficial sylvian veins; one crosses the frontal lobe and one crosses the parietal lobe. The superficial sylvian vein also has a large anastomosis with the vein of Labbé. F, right hemisphere. A single large vein of Trolard coursing in the region of the central sulcus connects the superficial sylvian vein and the superior sagittal sinus. This is no well-developed vein of Labbé, but a large vein from the posterior parietal and temporal areas* (yellow arrow) *empties into the superior sagittal sinus.* Cent., *central;* Dup., *duplicate;* Fiss., *fissure;* Sup., *superior;* V., *vein.*

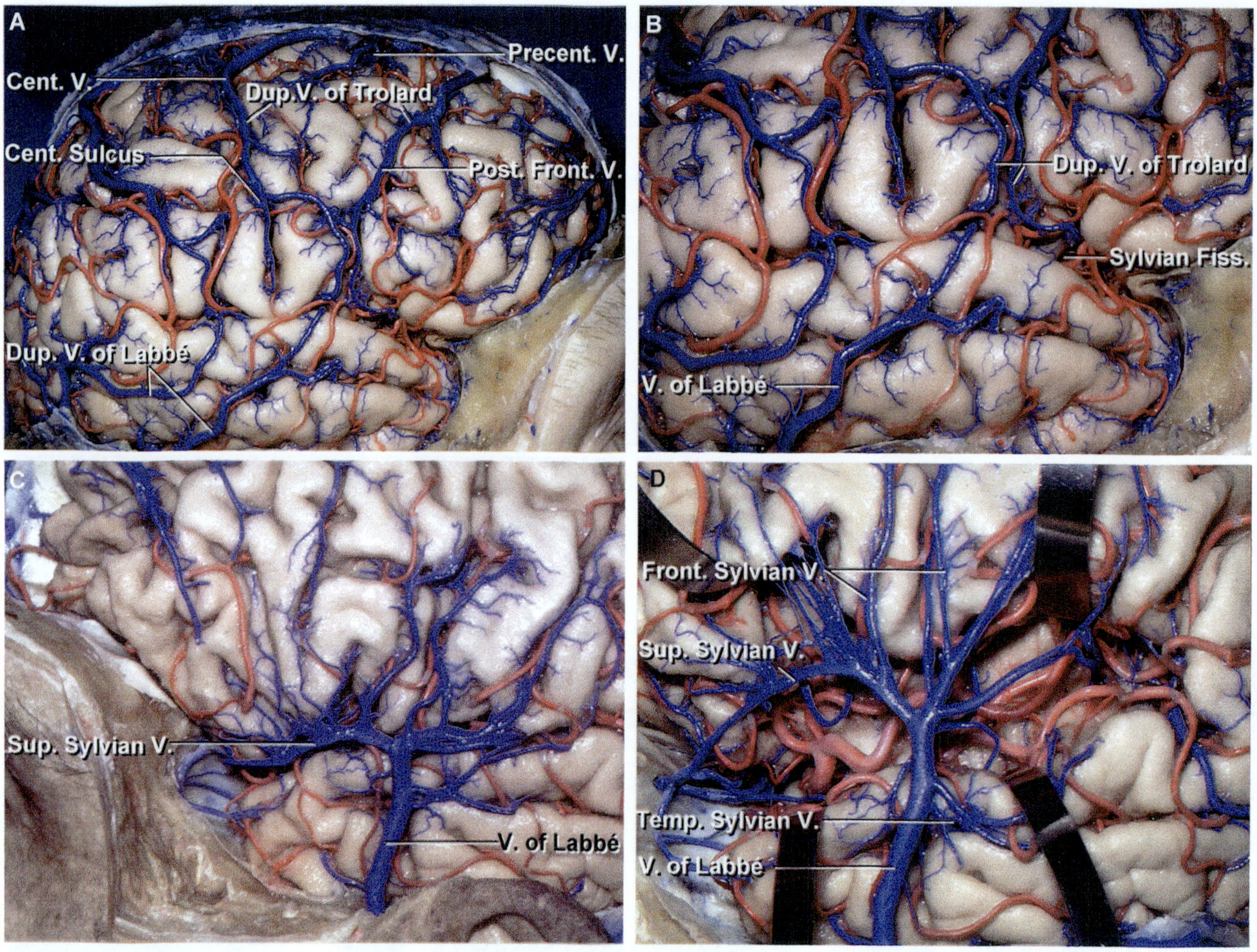

FIGURE 4.12. *Lateral view. Comparison of drainage pattern along the sylvian fissure on the right side (*A *and* B*) and left side (*C *and* D*) of the same brain.* A, *right lateral view. There is no significant superficial sylvian vein. The veins draining the frontal and parietal areas are relatively evenly dispersed over the frontal and parietal lobes and drain predominantly into the superior sagittal sinus. There are two, or duplicate, veins of nearly equal size that cross from the sylvian fissure to the transverse sinus and fit the description of a vein of Labbé. Central and posterior frontal veins of approximately the same size connect the sylvian fissure and superior sagittal sinus, and together constitute a duplicate vein of Trolard. The lower part of the central vein passes along the central sulcus.* B, *enlarged view of sylvian fissure. Duplicate veins of Labbé and Trolard drain much of the area along the sylvian fissure.* C, *left side. There is a large superficial sylvian vein that has minimal connections with the superior sagittal sinus; however, a significant part of the drainage from this area is directed through a vein of Labbé that crosses the midtemporal area.* D, *the sylvian fissure has been opened below the superficial sylvian vein that empties anteriorly into the sphenoparietal sinus coursing below the sphenoid ridge and posteriorly into a large vein of Labbé.* E, *right orbitozygomatic craniotomy. The temporalis muscle has been reflected downward, the bone flap elevated, and the dural incision* (solid line) *outlined. The inset shows the one-piece orbitozygomatic bone flap.* F, *the dura has been opened to expose a large superficial sylvian vein that empties into the dural sinuses along the sphenoid ridge.* G, *the sylvian fissure has been opened and the large superficial sylvian vein retracted to expose the internal carotid and middle cerebral artery.* H, *another orbitozygomatic exposure. In this case, the anterior segment of the superficial sylvian vein is absent and the veins draining the posterior part of the sylvian fissure empty into veins crossing the frontal and temporal lobes.* A., *artery;* Car., *carotid;* Cent., *central;* CN, *cranial nerve;* Dup., *duplicate;* Fiss., *fissure;* Front., *frontal;* M., *muscle;* M.C.A., *middle cerebral artery;* Olf., *olfactory;* Post., *posterior;* Precent., *precentral;* Sup., *superior;* Temp., *temporal, temporalis;* Tr., *tract;* V., *vein. (Figure continues on next page.)*

the dural sinuses in the floor of the middle fossa, which empty into the superior petrosal sinus or exit the intracranial cavity through the foramina in the sphenoid bone to reach the pterygoid plexus. The deep sylvian veins, which drain the insula and adjacent walls of the sylvian fissure, were reviewed in our studies on the deep venous system of the brain (20).

If the superficial sylvian vein is small or absent, the adjacent veins will take over its drainage area (*Figs. 4.5* and *4.10–4.12*). The veins arising on the upper lip of the sylvian fissure will ascend to join the veins that empty into the superior sagittal sinus, and those arising on the lower lip will be directed posteroinferiorly to join the veins entering the sinuses below

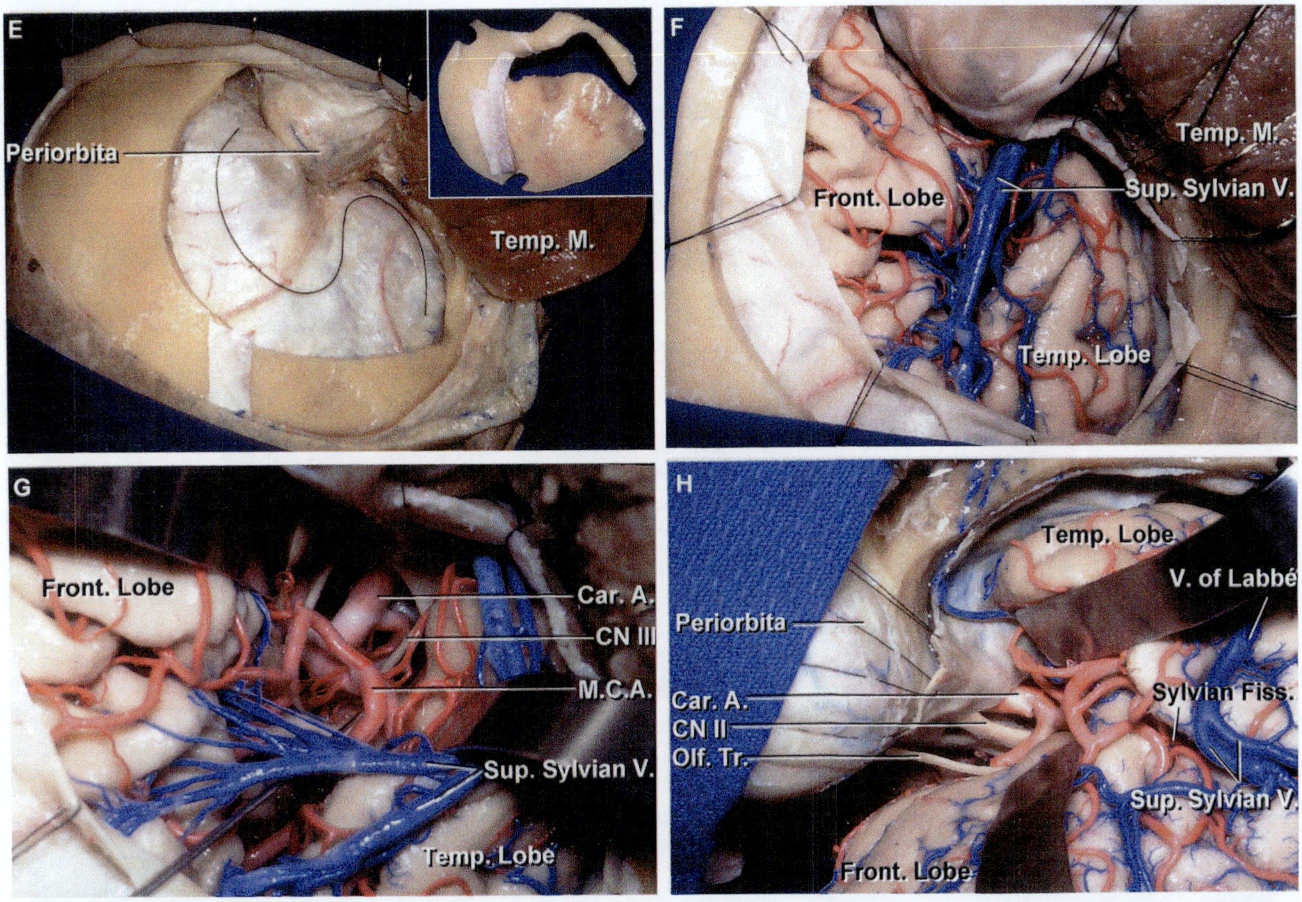

FIGURE 4.12. *Continued*

the temporal lobe. If the central segment of the vein is absent, the anterior segment will join the sinuses along the sphenoid ridge and the posterior segment will join the anastomotic veins of Trolard and Labbé that drain into the superior sagittal and transverse sinuses.

Cortical Veins

The superficial cortical veins are divided into three groups based on whether they drain the lateral, medial, or inferior surface of the hemisphere (*Fig. 4.13*). The cortical veins on the three surfaces are further subdivided on the basis of the lobe and cortical area that they drain. The largest group of cortical veins terminate by exiting the subarachnoid space to become bridging veins that cross the subdural space and empty into the venous sinuses in the dura mater. A smaller group of cortical veins terminate by joining the deep venous system of the brain (20).

Most of the individual veins outlined are formed by a single channel with multiple tributaries; however, two or more channels may infrequently pass from the individual cortical areas to the adjacent dural sinuses. There is a reciprocal relationship between the veins from adjacent areas so that, as the territory of one vein increases, the territory of the adjacent vein decreases. There is a similar reciprocal relationship between the major venous groups draining a surface or lobe.

The individual cortical veins from adjoining areas may join to form a single bridging vein before their termination in a dural sinus (*Fig. 4.14*). In addition, the veins draining the adjacent areas on the medial, lateral, and inferior surfaces may join along the margins of the hemisphere to form a single bridging vein before emptying into one of the sinuses. The ascending veins from the medial and lateral surfaces frequently join along the superior margin of the hemisphere before emptying into the superior sagittal sinus, and the descending veins from the lateral surface and the laterally directed veins from the inferior surface often join along the inferior margin of the hemisphere before draining into the sinuses along the cranial base. The individual veins from each of the lobes are considered next.

Frontal Lobe

The veins of the frontal lobe are divided into groups that drain the lateral, medial, and basal surfaces of the lobe (*Figs. 4.1–4.4, 4.6,* and *4.11–4.14*). The lateral frontal veins are divided into an ascending group, which empties into the superior sagittal sinus, and a descending group, which courses

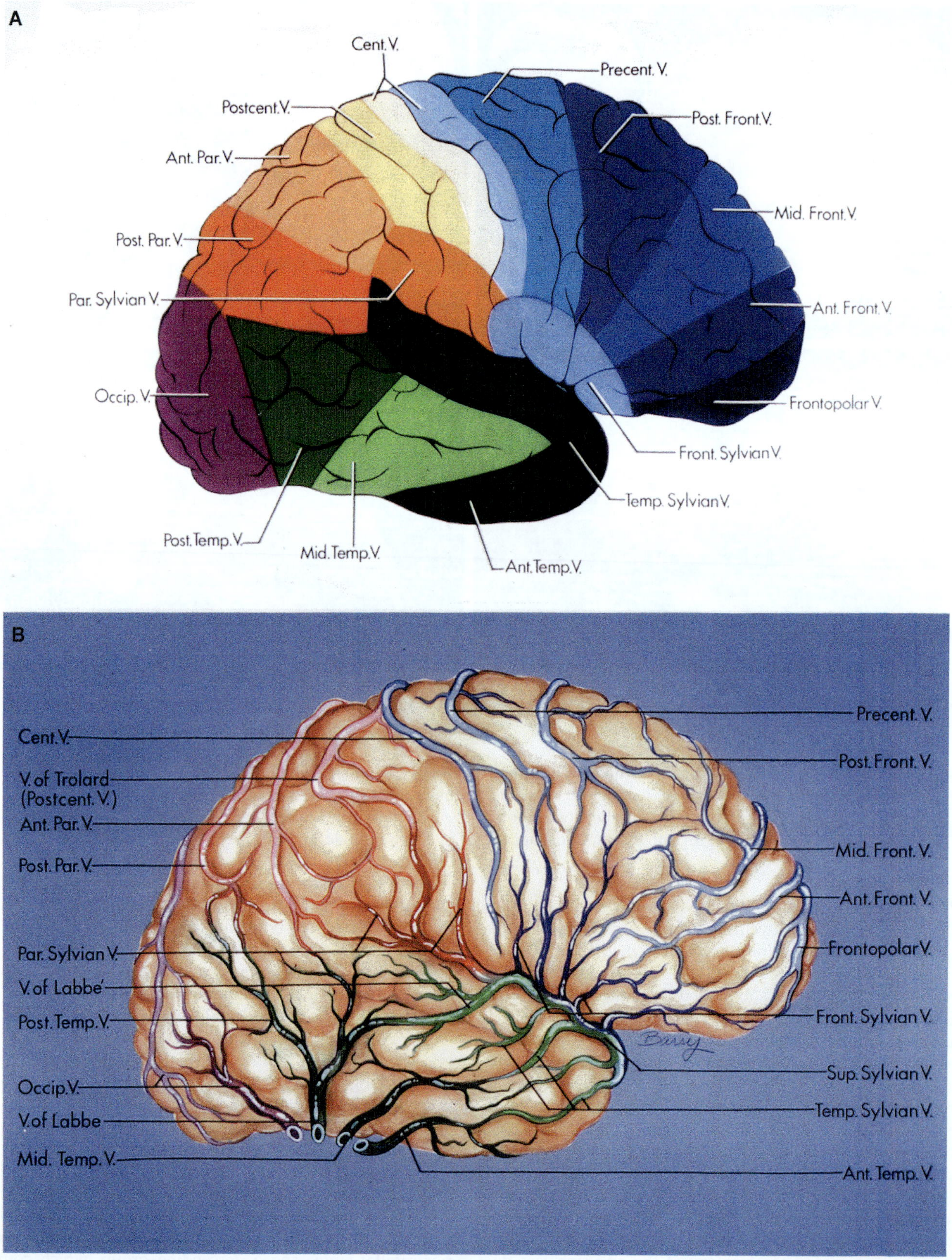

FIGURE 4.13. *(Legend is on page 206.)*

C

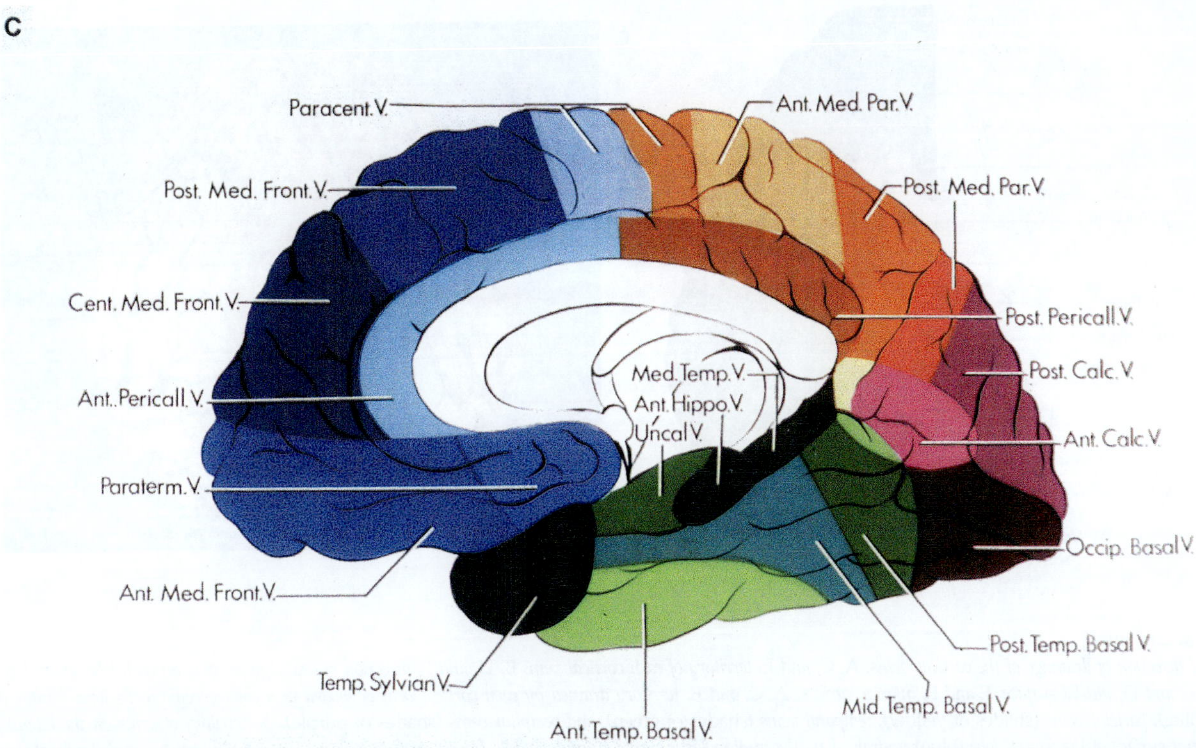

D

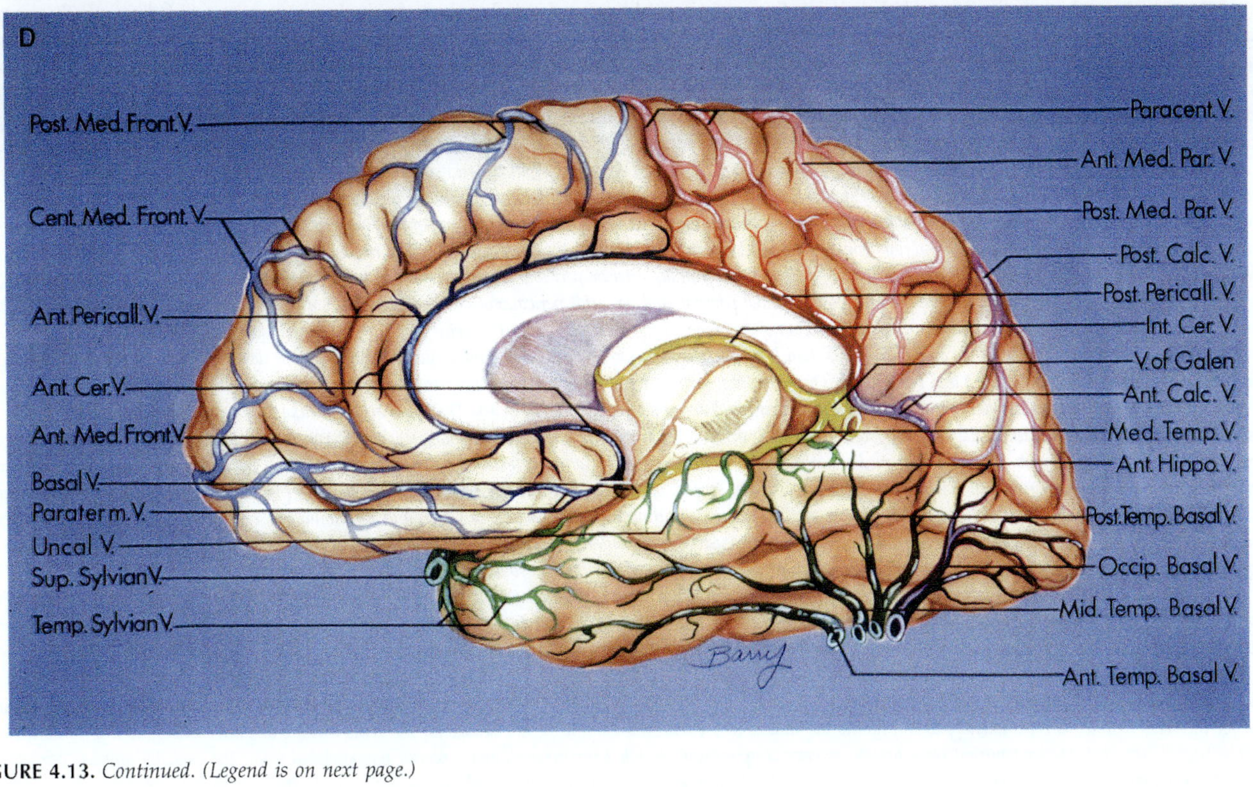

FIGURE 4.13. *Continued. (Legend is on next page.)*

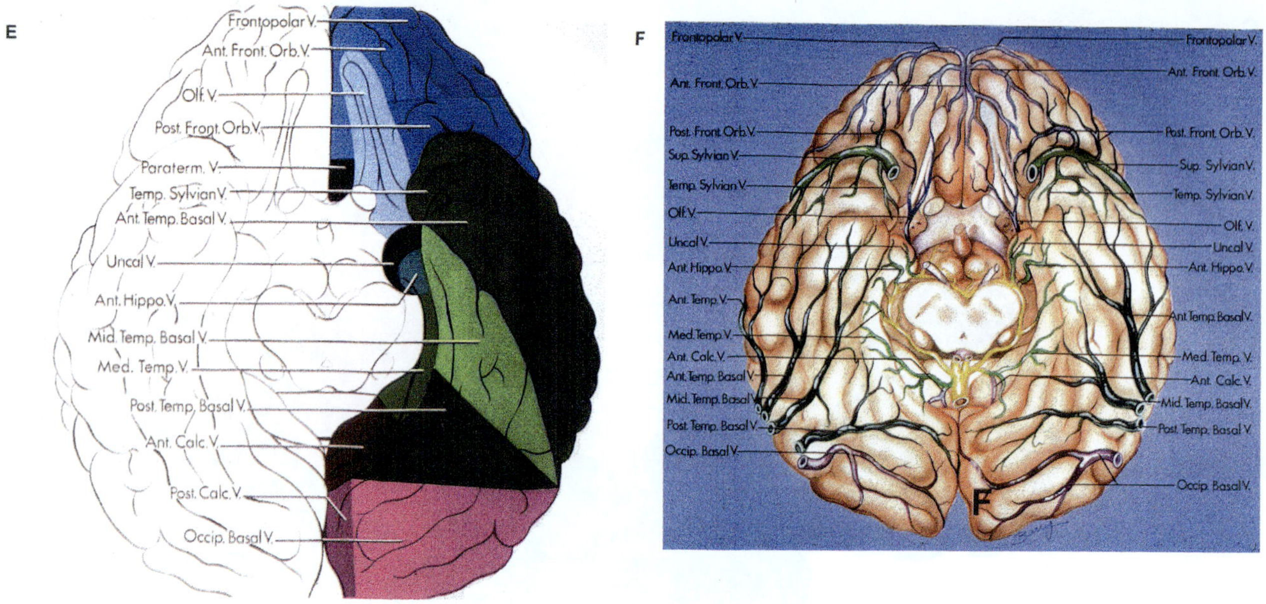

FIGURE 4.13. *Continued*

Territory and direction of drainage of the cortical veins. A, C, *and* E, *territory of each cortical vein.* B, D, *and* F, *direction of drainage of veins on each lobe.* A *and* B, *lateral surface.* C *and* D, *medial surface.* E *and* F, *inferior surface.* A, C, *and* E, *territory drained by each cortical vein is shaded in a color specific to its lobe: frontal veins* (shades of blue), *parietal veins* (shades of yellow), *temporal veins* (shades of green), *and occipital veins* (shades of purple). A, *territory of veins on the lateral surface. The lateral surface of the frontal lobe* (blue) *is drained by the frontopolar, anterior frontal, middle frontal, posterior frontal, precentral, central, and the frontosylvian veins. The lateral surface of the parietal lobe* (yellow) *is drained by the central, postcentral, anterior parietal, posterior parietal, and parietosylvian veins. The lateral surface of the occipital lobe* (purple) *is drained by the occipital veins. The lateral surface of the temporal lobe* (green) *is drained by the anterior temporal, middle temporal, posterior temporal, and temporosylvian veins.* B, *direction of drainage on the lateral surface. The veins draining the lateral surface of the frontal lobe are shown in two shades of* blue: *a* lighter shade *for the ascending veins, which drain into the superior sagittal sinus, and a* darker shade *for the descending veins, which drain into the superficial sylvian vein. The ascending frontal veins are the frontopolar; anterior frontal, middle frontal, and posterior frontal veins; and precentral and central veins. The descending lateral frontal veins are the frontosylvian veins. The veins draining the lateral surface of the parietal lobe are shown in two shades of* red: *a* light shade *for the ascending veins, which drain into the superior sagittal sinus, and a* darker shade *for the descending veins, which drain into the superficial sylvian vein. The ascending lateral parietal veins are the central, postcentral, anterior parietal, and posterior parietal veins. The vein of Trolard corresponds to a large postcentral vein. The descending lateral parietal veins are the parietosylvian veins. The veins draining the lateral surface of the occipital lobe are shown in* purple: *they are predominantly ascending veins called occipital veins, which ascend to join the superior sagittal sinus. A few occipital veins may descend to join the transverse sinus or tentorial sinus. The veins draining the lateral surface of the temporal lobe are shown in two shades of* green: *a* light shade *for the veins that ascend to empty into the superficial sylvian vein and a* darker shade *for the veins that descend to reach the sinuses in the tentorium. The ascending lateral temporal veins are the temporosylvian veins. The descending lateral temporal veins are the anterior temporal, middle temporal, and posterior temporal veins.* C, *territory of veins on the medial surface. The medial surface of the frontal lobe* (blue) *is drained by the paraterminal, anteromedial frontal, centromedial frontal, posteromedial frontal, anterior pericallosal, and paracentral veins. The medial surface of the parietal lobe* (yellow) *is drained by the paracentral, anteromedial parietal, posteromedial parietal, and posterior pericallosal veins. The medial surface of the occipital lobe* (purple) *is drained by the anterior calcarine and posterior calcarine veins.* D, *direction of drainage on the medial surface. The veins draining the medial surface of the frontal lobe are shown in two shades of* blue: *a* lighter shade *for the ascending veins, which pass to the superior sagittal sinus, and a* darker shade *for the descending veins, which drain into the inferior sagittal sinus and anterior cerebral and basal veins. The ascending medial frontal veins are the anteromedial frontal, centromedial frontal, posteromedial frontal, and paracentral veins. The descending medial frontal veins are the paraterminal and anterior pericallosal veins. The veins on the medial surface of the parietal lobe are shown as two shades of* red: *a* lighter shade *for the ascending veins, which drain into the superior sagittal sinus, and a* darker shade *for the descending veins, which drain into the vein of Galen and its tributaries. The ascending medial parietal veins are the paracentral, anteromedial parietal, and posteromedial parietal veins. The descending medial parietal veins are the posterior pericallosal veins. The veins on the medial surface of the occipital lobe are shown in two shades of* purple: *a* lighter color *for the ascending veins draining into the superior sagittal sinus and a* darker shade *for the veins draining into the vein of Galen and its tributaries. The ascending medial occipital vein is the posterior calcarine vein, and the vein draining into the deep venous system is the anterior calcarine vein.* E, *territory of veins on the inferior surface. The inferior surface of the frontal lobe* (blue) *is drained by the frontopolar, anterior fronto-orbital, posterior fronto-orbital, olfactory, and paraterminal veins. The inferior surface of the temporal lobe* (green) *is drained by the anterior temporobasal, middle temporobasal, posterior temporobasal, anterior hippocampal, uncal, medial temporal, and temporosylvian veins. The interior surface of the occipital lobe* (purple) *is drained by the occipitobasal vein.* F, *direction of drainage on the inferior surface. The veins on the inferior surface of the frontal lobe are shown in two shades of* blue: *a* lighter shade *for the anterior veins, which drain into the superior sagittal sinus, and a* darker color *for the posterior veins, which empty into the anterior end of the basal vein. The anterior group of the inferior frontal veins are the anterior fronto-orbital veins. The posterior group of inferior frontal veins are the posterior fronto-orbital and olfactory veins. The veins on the inferior surface of the temporal lobe are shown in two shades of* green: *a* darker shade *for the veins that are directed laterally to empty into the sinuses in the tentorium and a* lighter shade *for the veins that are directed medially to drain into the basal vein. The laterally directed inferior temporal veins are the anterior temporobasal, middle temporobasal, and posterior temporobasal veins; the medially directed veins are the uncal, anterior hippocampal, and medial temporal veins. The veins on the inferior surface of the occipital lobe are shown as* one shade of purple, *because there is only one group, the occipitobasal veins, that empty into the sinuses in the tentorium. The internal cerebral vein joins the vein of Galen.* Ant., *anterior;* Calc., *calcarine;* Cent., *central;* Front., *frontal;* Front.Orb., *fronto-orbital;* Hippo., *hippocampal;* Med., *medial;* Mid., *middle;* Occip., *occipital;* Olf., *olfactory;* Orb., *orbital;* Par., *parietal;* Paracent., *paracentral;* Paraterm., *paraterminal;* Pericall., *pericallosal;* Post., *posterior;* Postcent., *postcentral;* Post.Med., *posteromedial;* Precent., *precentral;* Temp., *temporal;* V., *vein.*

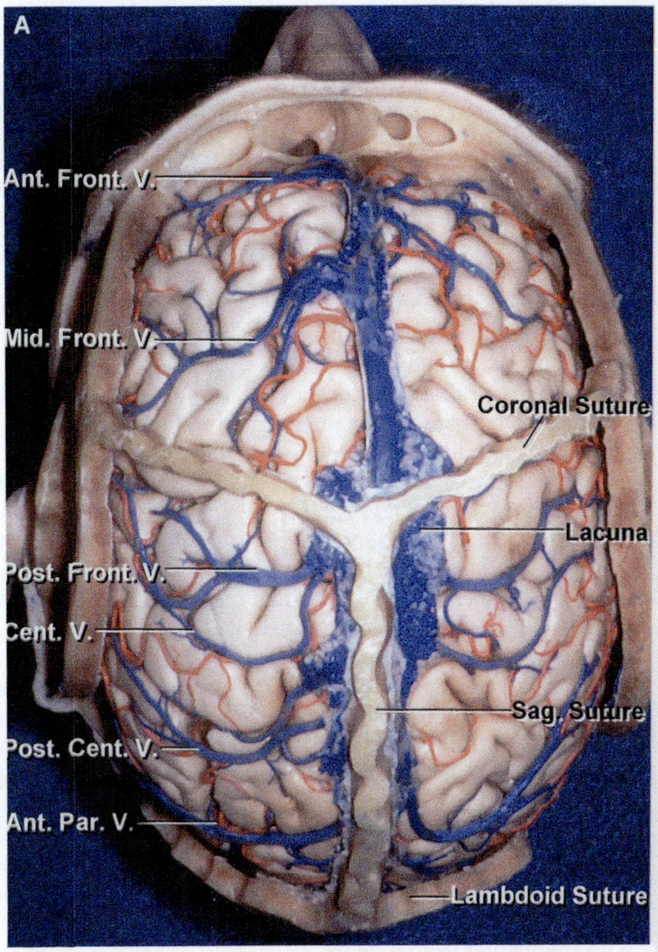

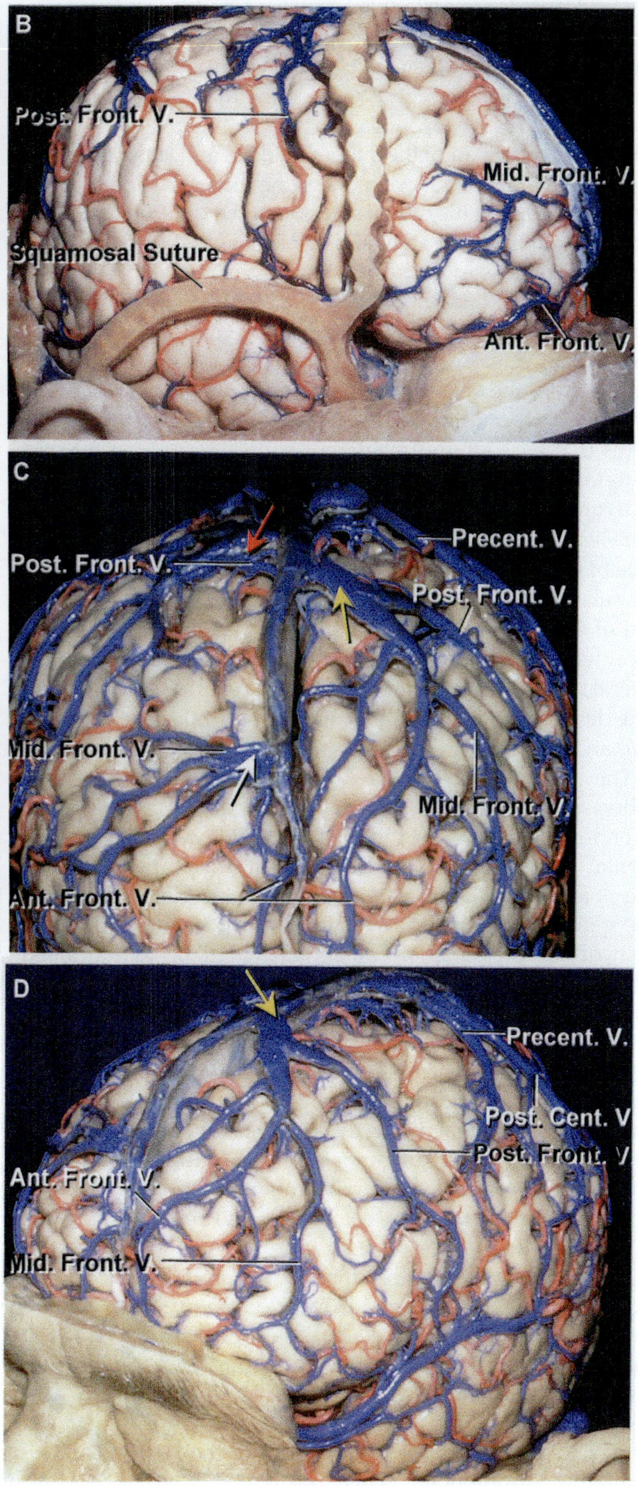

FIGURE 4.14. A, *cerebrum with the coronal and sagittal sutures preserved, superior view. There is commonly an area devoid of bridging veins entering the superior sagittal sinus just in front of the coronal suture, as shown, that would be a suitable site for a transcallosal approach. The author places the flap for a transcallosal approach exposure one-third behind and two-thirds in front of the coronal suture.* B, *lateral view, right hemisphere. The area in front of the coronal sutures is devoid of bridging veins emptying into the superior sagittal sinus.* C and D, *anterior and left anterolateral views of another cerebrum.* C, *anterior view. On the left side, a large bridging vein* (yellow arrow)*, into which the anterior, middle, and posterior frontal veins empty, drains almost all of the left frontal lobe. On the right side, two large bridging veins* (red and white arrows) *drain most of the frontal lobe.* D, *anterolateral view of the left hemisphere. A large part of the left frontal lobe is drained by a single large bridging vein* (yellow arrow). *In the limited exposures used for surgical approaches, it is difficult to know how significant the anastomotic channels are. Sacrificing the large bridging vein on the left frontal lobe is more likely to produce a disturbance of venous drainage than sacrificing the smaller frontal bridging veins on the right side.* Ant., *anterior;* Cent., *central;* Front., *frontal;* Mid., *middle;* Par., *parietal;* Post., *posterior;* Precent., *precentral;* Sag., *sagittal;* V., *vein.*

toward the sylvian fissure and joins the superficial sylvian veins. The ascending veins are the frontopolar; anterior, middle, and posterior frontal; precentral; and central veins. The vein may join the veins from the adjoining parts of the basal and medial surfaces before emptying into the sinus. The descending group is composed of the frontosylvian veins. The area drained by the ascending group is larger than the area drained by the descending group.

The lateral frontal veins and the areas they drain are as follows: the frontopolar vein drains the anterior part of the inferior, middle, and superior frontal gyri; the anterior, middle, and posterior frontal veins drain the anterior, middle, and posterior part of the frontal convexity, in the area between the frontopolar and precentral veins; the precentral vein drains the lower part of the precentral gyrus, the opercular part of the inferior frontal gyrus, and the adjacent part of the inferior, middle, and superior frontal gyri; the central rolandic vein drains the precentral and postcentral gyri bordering the central sulcus; and the frontosylvian veins drain the inferior and adjoining part of the middle frontal gyri and the inferior part of the precentral gyrus.

The medial surface of the frontal lobe is divided by the curved cingulate sulcus into inner and outer zones. The medial frontal veins are divided into an ascending group, which drains into the superior sagittal sinus, and a descending group, which empties into the inferior sagittal sinus or into the veins that pass around the corpus callosum to drain into the anterior end of the basal vein. The ascending veins are the anteromedial, centromedial, and posteromedial frontal and paracentral veins. They drain the majority of the medial surface of the superior frontal gyrus and the adjoining part of the cingulate gyrus. They commonly curve over the superior margin of the hemisphere onto the upper part of the lateral surface, where they join the terminal end of the veins from the lateral surface before emptying into the superior sagittal sinus. The descending veins are the anterior pericallosal, paraterminal, and anterior cerebral veins.

The medial frontal veins and the areas they drain are as follows: the anteromedial frontal vein drains the cingulate and superior frontal gyri behind the frontal pole; the centromedial frontal vein drains the medial surface of the superior frontal gyrus and the adjacent part of the cingulate gyrus in front of the genu of the corpus callosum; the posteromedial frontal vein drains the superior frontal and cingulate gyri situated above the genu of the corpus callosum; the paracentral vein drains the cingulate gyrus above the body of the corpus callosum and adjacent paracentral lobule; the anterior pericallosal veins—paired veins—drain the genu and rostrum of the corpus callosum and adjacent part of the cingulate gyri; the anterior cerebral vein drains the area below the rostrum of the corpus callosum near the upper margin of the optic chiasm; and the paraterminal vein drains the paraterminal and paraolfactory gyri in the area below the rostrum of the corpus callosum.

The inferior frontal veins, draining the orbital surface of the frontal lobe, are divided into an anterior group, which courses toward the frontal pole and empties into the superior sagittal sinus, and a posterior group, which drains backward to join the veins at the medial part of the sylvian fissure, that converge on the anterior perforated substance to form the basal vein. The anterior group is composed of the anterior orbitofrontal and frontopolar veins. The posterior group is composed of the olfactory and the posterior orbitofrontal veins.

The inferior frontal veins and the areas they drain are as follows: the anterior orbitofrontal vein drains the anterior part of the gyrus rectus and the anteromedial part of the orbital gyri; the posterior orbitofrontal veins drain the posterior portion of the orbital surface of the frontal lobe; and the olfactory vein drains the olfactory sulcus and the adjacent part of the gyrus rectus and medial orbital gyri.

Parietal Lobe

The veins of the parietal lobe are divided on the basis of whether they drain the lateral or medial surfaces of the lobe (*Fig. 4.1–4.3, 4.6,* and *4.13*). The veins draining the lateral surface are divided into an ascending group, which empties into the superior sagittal sinus, and a descending group, which drains into the veins along the sylvian fissure. The ascending veins are the central and postcentral veins and the anterior and posterior parietal veins. The descending group is formed by the parietosylvian veins.

The veins and the areas they drain are as follows: the postcentral vein drains the anterior part of the supramarginal gyrus and superior parietal lobule and the posterior part of the postcentral gyrus; the anterior parietal vein drains the supramarginal and angular gyri; the posterior parietal vein drains the posterior part of the inferior parietal lobule and the adjacent part of the occipital lobe; and the parietosylvian veins drain the postcentral gyrus and the inferior parietal lobule.

The medial parietal veins are divided into an ascending group, which drains into the superior sagittal sinus, and a descending group, which courses around the splenium of the corpus callosum to empty into the vein of Galen or its tributaries. The ascending veins are the paracentral and the anteromedial and posteromedial parietal veins. The descending veins are the posterior pericallosal veins. The ascending veins from the medial and lateral surfaces commonly join along the superior margin of the hemisphere before emptying into the superior sagittal sinus. The paracentral veins, which drain the adjacent parts of the frontal and parietal lobes, are described with the medial frontal veins.

The medial parietal veins and the areas they drain are as follows: the anteromedial parietal vein drains the upper edge of the cingulate gyrus and the anterior part of the precuneus; the posteromedial parietal vein drains the posterior part of the precuneus and the adjacent part of the occipital lobe; and the posterior pericallosal veins—paired veins—drain the posterior part of the corpus callosum, cingulate gyrus, and the precuneus.

Temporal Lobe

The veins of the temporal lobe are divided into a lateral group, which drains the convexity, and an inferior group, which drains the basal surface of the lobe (*Figs. 4.1, 4.4, 4.5,* and *4.11–4.13*). The lateral temporal veins are divided into an ascending group, which courses toward the sylvian fissure, and a descending group, which empties into the venous sinuses below the temporal lobe. The ascending group is formed by the temporosylvian veins. The descending group is formed by the anterior, middle, and posterior temporal veins.

The lateral group of veins and the areas they drain are as follows: the anterior temporal vein drains the anterior third of the lateral surface, with the exception of the superior temporal gyrus; the middle temporal vein drains the midportion of the temporal convexity; the posterior temporal vein drains the posterior third of the temporal convexity and occasionally the angular gyrus and the anterior part of the occipital lobe; and the temporosylvian veins drain the superior temporal gyrus from the temporal pole to the posterior end of the sylvian fissure.

The inferior temporal veins are divided into a lateral group, which drains into the sinuses in the anterolateral part of the tentorium, and a medial group, which empties into the basal vein as it courses along the medial edge of the temporal lobe. The lateral group is composed of the anterior, middle, and posterior temporobasal veins. The temporobasal veins seem to radiate from the preoccipital notch across the inferior surface of the temporal lobe. The medial group is formed by the uncal, anterior hippocampal, and medial temporal veins. The part of the basal surface adjoining the temporal pole is commonly drained by the temporosylvian veins.

The inferior temporal veins and the areas they drain are as follows: the anterior temporobasal vein drains the anterior third of the inferior temporal and occipitotemporal gyri and the adjacent part of the parahippocampal gyrus; the middle temporobasal vein drains the middle third of the inferior surface of the lobe; the posterior temporobasal vein drains the basal surface of the temporal lobe and the anterior part of the occipital lobe; the uncal veins drain the uncus and the adjacent part of the parahippocampal gyrus; the anterior hippocampal vein drains the posterior portion of the uncus and the adjacent part of the parahippocampal gyrus; and the medial temporal veins drain the parahippocampal gyri bordering the basal cisterns beside the upper midbrain.

Occipital Lobe

The veins draining the occipital lobe are divided into groups that drain the lateral, medial, or inferior surfaces of the lobe (*Figs. 4.1, 4.2, 4.5,* and *4.13*). The veins draining the posterior part of the temporal and parietal lobes may drain the anterior part of the occipital lobe. The fact that the lateral occipital veins are directed forward rather than backward means that no large veins enter the superior sagittal sinus for a distance of 4 to 5 cm proximal to the torcular herophili, or directly medial to the posterior part of the occipital lobe.

The medial surface of the occipital lobe is drained by the anterior and posterior calcarine veins. The anterior calcarine vein (also referred to as the internal occipital vein) drains the anterior portion of the cuneus and lingula, and the posterior calcarine vein drains the area bordering the posterior part of the calcarine fissure.

The inferior surface of the occipital lobe is drained by the occipitobasal vein. The occipitobasal vein arises from tributaries that drain the inferolateral part of the lingula and the adjacent part of the occipitotemporal and inferior temporal gyri. It courses anterolaterally toward the preoccipital notch and frequently joins the posterior temporobasal vein before emptying into the lateral tentorial sinus. This vein may infrequently course anteromedial to join the basal vein.

Meningeal Veins

The small venous channels that drain the dura mater covering the cerebrum are called the meningeal veins (*Fig. 4.8*). They are actually small sinuses that usually accompany the meningeal arteries. The meningeal veins accompanying the meningeal arteries course between the arteries and the overlying bone. The fact that the artery presses into the veins gives them the appearance of parallel channels on each side of their respective arteries. The largest meningeal veins accompany the middle meningeal artery. The meningeal veins drain into the large dural sinuses along the cranial base at their lower margin and into the venous lacunae and superior sagittal sinus at their upper margin. The veins accompanying the anterior branch of the middle meningeal artery join the sphenoparietal or cavernous sinus or the sphenoidal emissary veins, and those accompanying the posterior branch of the middle meningeal artery join the lateral sinus. The meningeal veins may course through a superficial tunnel on the inner surface of the bone so that they have both an intradiploic and an intradural course. The meningeal veins receive diploid veins from the calvarium.

THE DEEP VEINS

The deep venous system collects into channels that course through the walls of the ventricles and basal cisterns and converge on the internal cerebral, basal, and great veins (*Figs. 4.15–4.17*). During operations on the lateral ventricles, the deep veins more commonly provide orienting landmarks than the arteries because the arteries in the ventricular walls are small and poorly seen and the veins are larger and are easily visible through the ependyma. These venous landmarks are especially helpful in the presence of hydrocephalus, in which the normal angles between the neural structures disappear. The deep veins in the basal cisterns pose a major obstacle in operative approaches to deep-seated tumors, especially in the pineal region where multiple veins converge on the vein of Galen. On cerebral angiograms, these veins may provide a more accurate estimation of the site and size of a lesion than the arteries, because they are more closely adherent to the pial and ependymal surfaces of the brain than the arteries.

The deep venous system of the brain consists of the internal cerebral, basal, and great veins and their tributaries. These veins drain the deep white and gray matter surrounding the lateral and third ventricles and the basal cisterns. The deep veins are divided into a ventricular group, composed of the veins draining the walls of the lateral ventricles, and a cisternal group, which includes the veins draining the walls of the basal cisterns. The internal cerebral vein is discussed with the ventricular group, because it is predominantly related to the ventricles. The basal and great veins, although they receive some ventricular veins, are discussed with the cisternal group, because they course through the basal cisterns. The choroidal veins are included with the ventricular veins, because they arise on the choroid plexus in the ventricles. The thalamic veins are discussed in both the ventricular and the cisternal groups, because some course on the ventricular surface and others course in the basal cisterns. There are frequent anastomosis with veins from adjacent areas and it is common for veins from adjacent areas to form common stems before terminating in the larger draining veins.

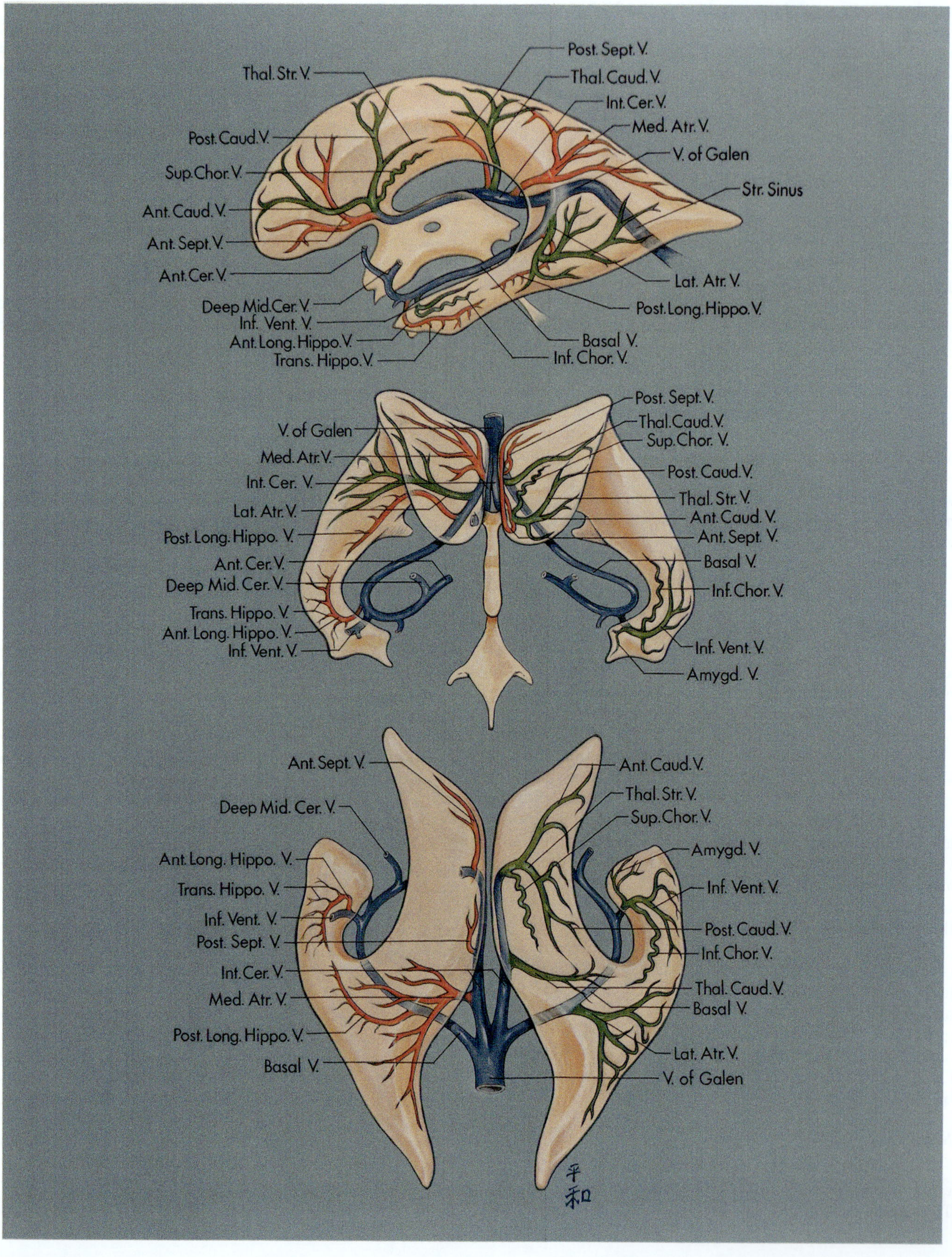
Post. Sept. V.
Thal. Str. V.
Thal. Caud. V.
Int. Cer. V.
Post. Caud. V.
Med. Atr. V.
V. of Galen
Sup. Chor. V.
Str. Sinus
Ant. Caud. V.
Ant. Sept. V.
Ant. Cer. V.
Lat. Atr. V.
Deep Mid. Cer. V.
Post. Long. Hippo. V.
Inf. Vent. V.
Ant. Long. Hippo. V.
Basal V.
Trans. Hippo. V.
Inf. Chor. V.
Post. Sept. V.
V. of Galen
Thal. Caud. V.
Sup. Chor. V.
Med. Atr. V.
Post. Caud. V.
Int. Cer. V.
Thal. Str. V.
Lat. Atr. V.
Ant. Caud. V.
Post. Long. Hippo. V.
Ant. Sept. V.
Ant. Cer. V.
Basal V.
Deep Mid. Cer. V.
Inf. Chor. V.
Trans. Hippo. V.
Ant. Long. Hippo. V.
Inf. Vent. V.
Inf. Vent. V.
Amygd. V.
Ant. Sept. V.
Ant. Caud. V.
Thal. Str. V.
Deep Mid. Cer. V.
Sup. Chor. V.
Amygd. V.
Ant. Long. Hippo. V.
Inf. Vent. V.
Trans. Hippo. V.
Inf. Vent. V.
Post. Caud. V.
Post. Sept. V.
Inf. Chor. V.
Int. Cer. V.
Thal. Caud. V.
Med. Atr. V.
Basal V.
Post. Long. Hippo. V.
Lat. Atr. V.
Basal V.
V. of Galen
平
和

FIGURE 4.15.

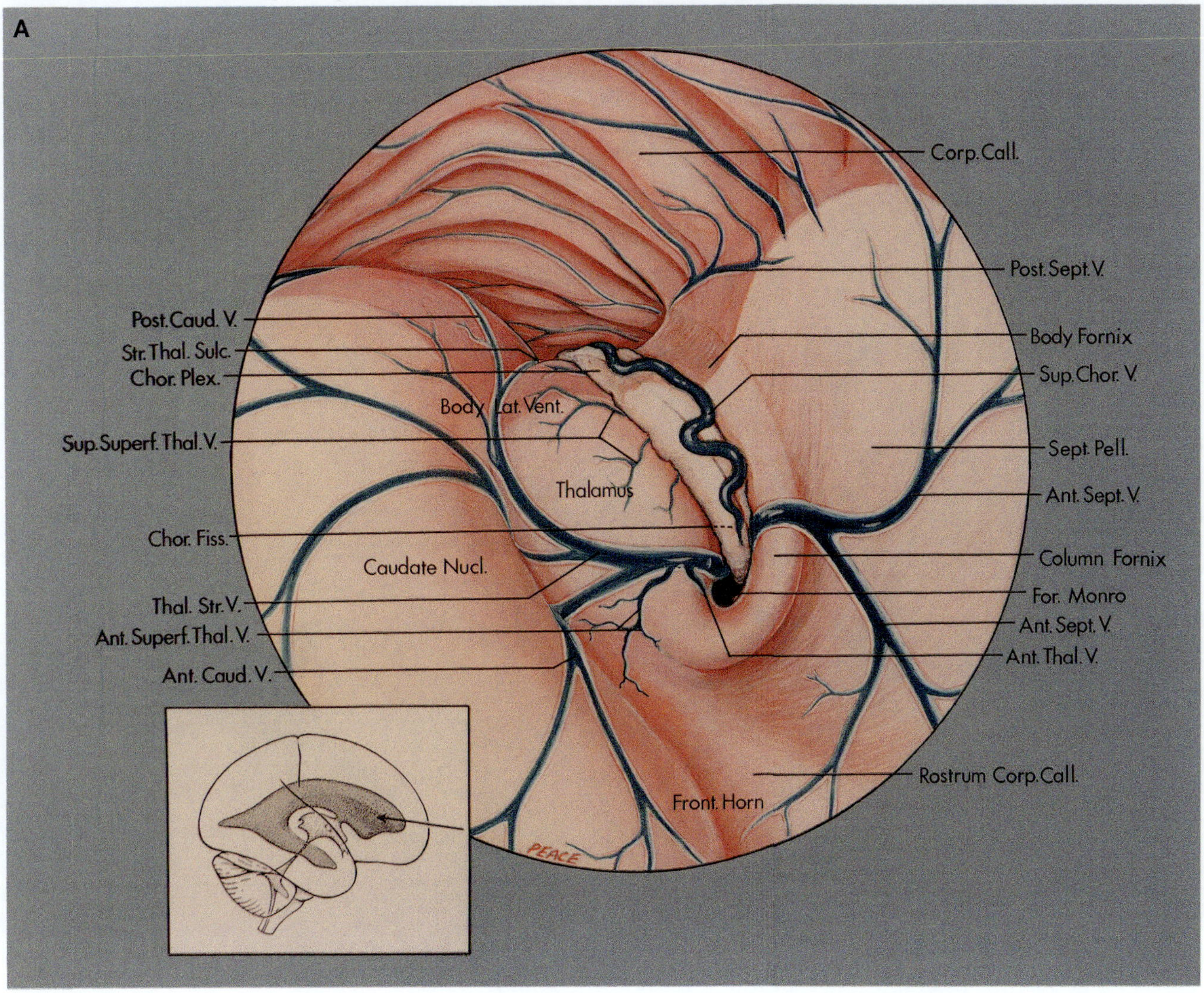

FIGURE 4.16. *Ventricular veins.* A, *anterior view* (along the arrow in the inset) *into the frontal horn and body of the lateral ventricle. The frontal horn is located anterior to the foramen of Monro and has the septum pellucidum in the medial wall, the genu and body of the corpus callosum in the roof, the caudate nucleus in the lateral wall, the genu of the corpus callosum in the anterior wall, and the rostrum of the corpus callosum in the floor. The body of the lateral ventricle has the thalamus in its floor, the caudate nucleus in the lateral wall, the body of the fornix and septum pellucidum in the medial wall, and the corpus callosum in the roof. The choroid plexus is attached along the choroidal fissure, the cleft between the fornix and thalamus. The anterior septal veins cross the roof and medial wall of the frontal horn and pass posteriorly toward the foramen of Monro, where they join the anterior end of the internal cerebral veins. The anterior caudate veins cross the lateral wall of the frontal horn and join the thalamostriate vein, which passes through the foramen of Monro. The superior choroidal vein courses on the choroid plexus in the body. The posterior septal veins cross the roof and medial wall of the body and pass through the margin of the choroidal fissure. The posterior caudate veins cross the lateral wall of the body and join the thalamostriate vein, which courses along the striothalamic sulcus. Anterior and superior superficial thalamic veins cross the surface of the thalamus. The anterior thalamic vein drains the nuclei in the anterosuperior part of the thalamus.* *(Legend continues on next page.)*

FIGURE 4.15. *Schematic drawing of the ventricular veins. Lateral* (top), *anterior* (middle), *and superior* (lower) *views. The ventricular veins are divided into a medial* (orange) *and a lateral* (green) *group. The ventricular veins drain into the internal cerebral, basal, and great veins. The lateral group consists of the anterior caudate vein in the frontal horn; the thalamostriate in the frontal horn; the thalamostriate, posterior caudate, and thalamocaudate veins in the body; the lateral atrial vein in the atrium; and the inferior ventricular vein and amygdalar veins in the temporal horn. The medial group is formed by the anterior septal vein in the frontal horn, the posterior septal veins in the body, the medial atrial vein in the atrium, and the transverse hippocampal veins in the temporal horn. The transverse hippocampal veins drain into the anterior and posterior longitudinal hippocampal veins. The superior choroidal veins drain into the thalamostriate and internal cerebral veins, and the inferior choroidal vein drains into the inferior ventricular vein. The vein of Galen drains into the straight sinus. The anterior and deep middle cerebral veins join to form the basal vein.* Amygd., *amygdala;* Ant., *anterior;* Atr., *atrial;* Caud., *caudate;* Cer., *cerebral;* Chor., *choroidal;* Hippo., *hippocampal;* Inf., *inferior;* Int., *internal;* Lat., *lateral;* Long., *longus;* Med., *medial;* Mid., *middle;* Post., *posterior;* Sept., *septal;* Str., *straight;* Sup., *superior;* Thal.Caud., *thalamocaudate;* Thal.Str., *thalamostriate;* Trans., *transverse;* V., *vein;* Vent., *ventricular.* (From, *Ono M, Rhoton AL Jr, Peace D, Rodriguez R: Microsurgical anatomy of the deep venous system of the brain.* **Neurosurgery** *15:621–657, 1984 [20].)*

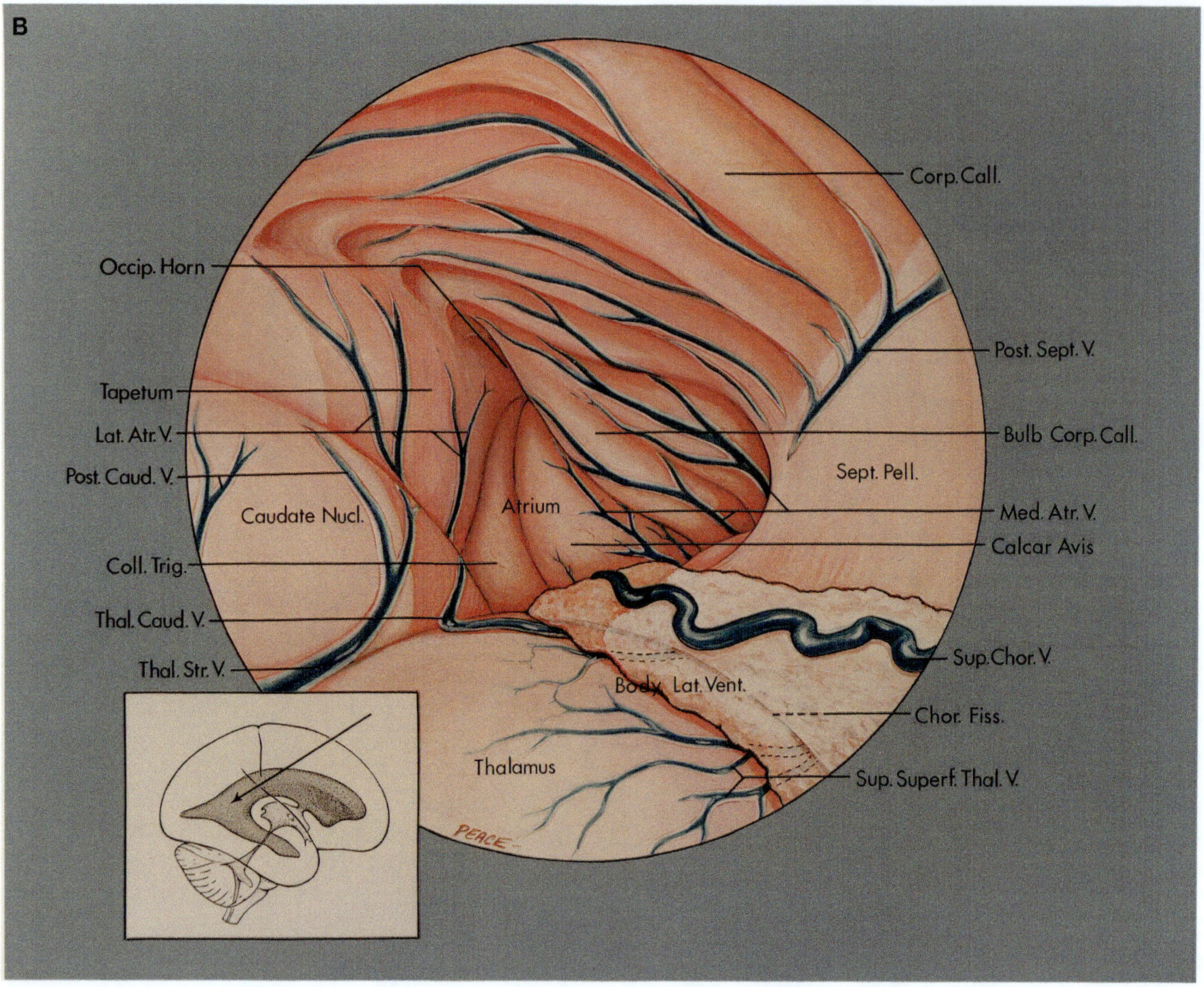

FIGURE 4.16. *Continued*

B, *anterosuperior view* (along the arrow in the inset) *into the body, atrium, and occipital horn of the lateral ventricle. The calcar avis and bulb of the corpus callosum form the medial wall of the atrium and occipital horn. The floor of the atrium is formed by the collateral trigone. The roof and posterior part of the lateral walls are formed by the tapetum of the corpus callosum. The caudate nucleus is in the anterior part of the lateral wall of the atrium. The medial and lateral atrial veins pass forward on the medial and lateral walls of the atrium toward the choroidal fissure. A thalamocaudate vein crosses the lateral wall posterior to the thalamostriate vein. The superior choroidal vein courses toward the foramen of Monro.*

VENTRICULAR GROUP

Neural Relationships

Each lateral ventricle is a C-shaped cavity that wraps around the thalamus and is situated deep within the cerebrum (*Figs. 4.15* and *4.16*). Each ventricle has five parts: the frontal, temporal, and occipital horns and the body and atrium. Each of these five parts has medial and lateral walls, a roof, and a floor. In addition, the frontal and temporal horns and the atrium have anterior walls. These walls are formed predominantly by the thalamus, septum pellucidum, deep cerebral white matter, corpus callosum, and two C-shaped structures, the caudate nucleus and fornix, that wrap around the thalamus. These neural relationships of the ventricles are reviewed in detail in Chapter 5.

Choroid Plexus and Choroidal Fissure

The choroid plexus in the lateral ventricle has a C-shaped configuration that parallels the fornix (*Figs. 4.15, 4.16,* and *4.18–4.20*) (8). It is attached along the choroidal fissure, a narrow cleft between the fornix and the thalamus, in the medial part of the body, atrium, and temporal horn. The choroid plexus extends through the foramen of Monro into the roof of the third ventricle. In the atrium, the choroid plexus has a prominent triangular tuft called the glomus. The edges of the thalamus and fornix bordering this fissure have small ridges, the teniae, along which the tela choroidea, the membrane in which the choroid plexus arises, is attached. The choroidal fissure extends from the foramen of Monro along the medial wall of the body, atrium, and temporal horn to its

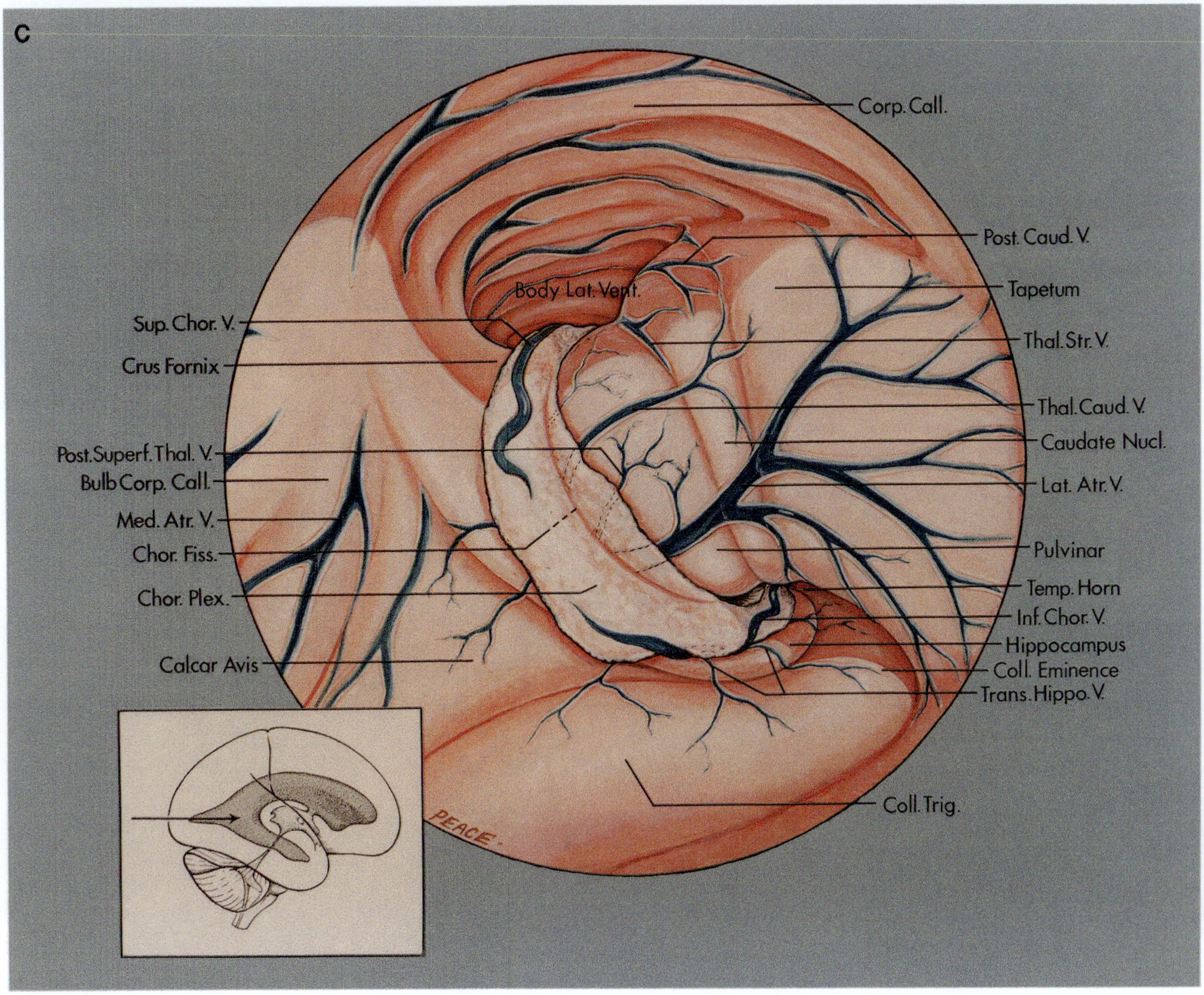

FIGURE 4.16. *Continued*
C, posterior view (along the arrow in the inset) *into the atrium and temporal horn. The inferior choroidal vein courses on the choroid plexus in the temporal horn. The lateral atrial veins arise on the lateral wall and cross the tail of the caudate nucleus and the pulvinar to pass through the choroidal fissure. The medial atrial veins pass forward and penetrate the crus of the fornix near the choroidal fissure to reach the quadrigeminal cistern. Some of the medial atrial veins also drain the roof and floor. Transverse hippocampal veins cross the floor of the atrium and temporal horn. Posterior superficial thalamic veins cross the atrial surface of the thalamus. (Legend continues on next page.)*

inferior termination, the inferior choroidal point, located just behind the uncus and hippocampal head. The veins coursing in the walls of the lateral ventricles exit the ventricles by passing, in a subependymal location, through the margin of this fissure to reach the internal cerebral, basal, or great veins.

Velum Interpositum

The velum interpositum, on which many of the ventricular veins converge to reach the internal cerebral veins, is located in the roof of the third ventricle below the fornix and between the superomedial surfaces of the thalami (*Figs. 4.17* and *4.18*). The velum interpositum is usually a closed space. It is widest posteriorly where it extends from the lower margin of the splenium to the upper margin of the pineal and tapers to a narrow apex just behind the foramen of Monro. It may infrequently have an opening situated between the splenium and the pineal body that communicates with the quadrigeminal cistern to form the cisterna velum interpositum. The upper and lower walls of the velum interpositum are formed by the two membranous layers of tela choroidea in the roof of the third ventricle. The upper wall is formed by the layer that is attached to the lower surface of the fornix and the hippocampal commissure. The lower wall is attached to the striae medullaris thalami, habenular commissure, and pineal. The internal cerebral veins arise in the anterior part of the velum interpositum, just behind the foramen of Monro, and they exit the velum interpositum above the pineal body to enter the quadrigeminal cistern and join the great vein.

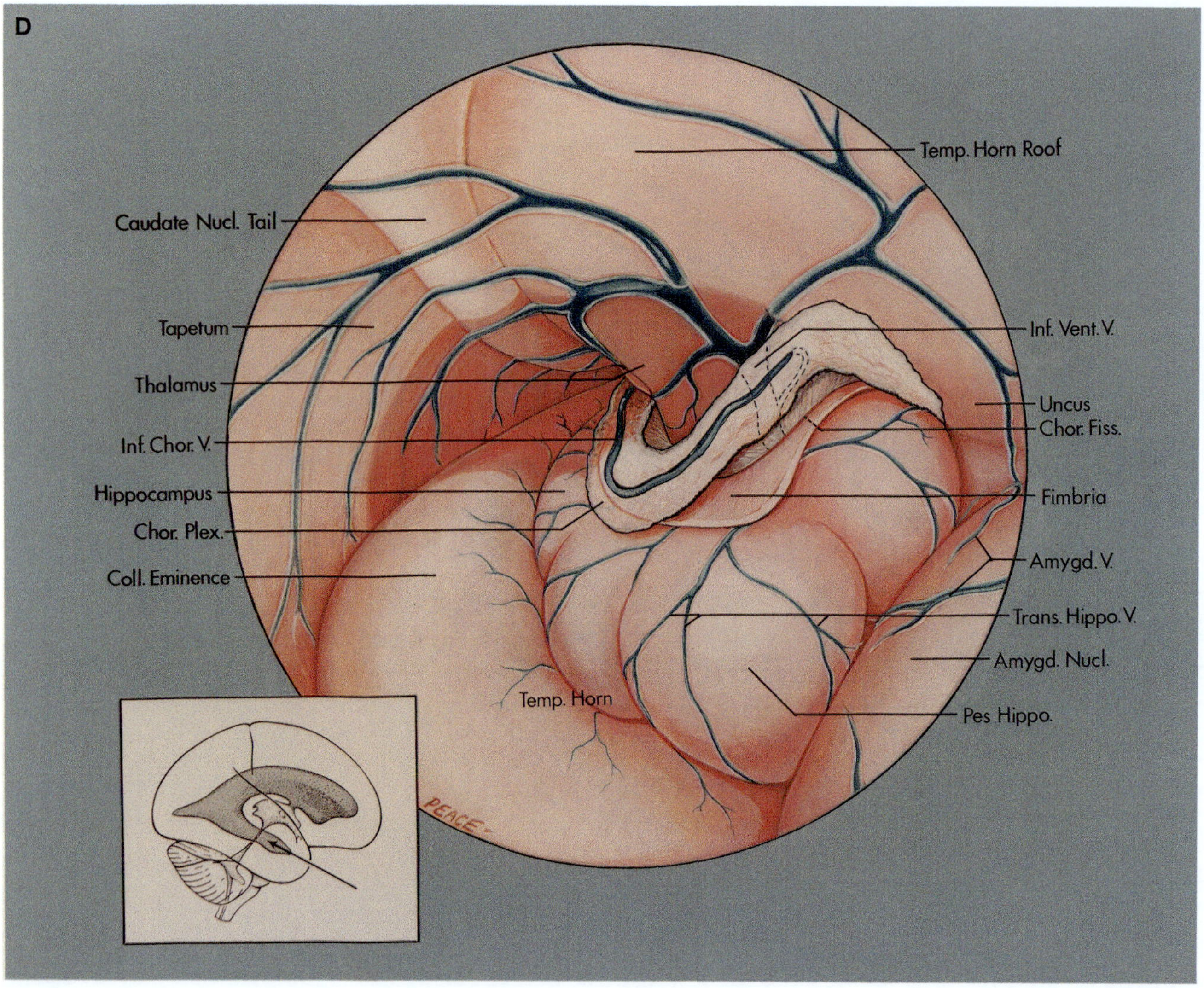

FIGURE 4.16. *Continued*
D, anterior view (along the arrow in the inset) *into the temporal horn. The floor of the temporal horn is formed by the collateral eminence and the hippocampal formation. The roof and lateral wall are formed, from medial to lateral, by the thalamus, the tail of the caudate nucleus, and the tapetum of the corpus callosum. The medial wall is little more than the cleft between the inferior surface of the thalamus and the fimbria. The amygdaloid nucleus bulges into the anteromedial part of the temporal horn. The pes hippocampus, the bulbous digitated anterior end of the hippocampal formation, is in the anterior part of the floor. The fimbria of the fornix arises on the surface of the hippocampal formation and passes posteriorly to become the crus of the fornix. The choroid plexus is attached along the choroidal fissure. The inferior ventricular vein drains the roof of the temporal horn and receives the amygdalar vein from the ventricular surface of the amygdaloid nucleus. The inferior choroidal vein joins the inferior ventricular vein. The transverse hippocampal veins draining the floor of the temporal horn pass medially through the choroidal fissure to enter the basal vein or its tributaries.* Amygd., *amygdaloid;* Ant., *anterior;* Atr., *atrial;* Call., *callosum;* Caud., *caudate;* Chor., *choroid, choroidal;* Coll., *collateral;* Corp., *corpus;* Fiss., *fissure;* For., *foramen;* Front., *frontal;* Hippo., *hippocampal;* Inf., *inferior;* Lat., *lateral;* Med., *medial;* Nucl., *nucleus;* Occip., *occipital;* Pell., *pellucidum;* Plex., *plexus;* Post., *posterior;* Sept., *septal, septum;* Str., *straight;* Sulc., *sulcus;* Sup., *superior;* Superf., *superficial;* Temp., *temporal;* Thal., *thalamic;* Thal.Caud., *thalamocaudate;* Thal.Str., *thalamostriate;* Trans., *transverse;* Trig., *trigone;* V., *vein;* Vent., *ventricle.* (From, *Ono M, Rhoton AL Jr, Peace D, Rodriguez R: Microsurgical anatomy of the deep venous system of the brain.* **Neurosurgery** *15:621–657, 1984 [20].)*

Ventricular Veins

The ventricular veins arise from tributaries that drain the basal ganglia, thalamus, internal capsule, corpus callosum, septum pellucidum, fornix, and deep white matter (*Figs. 4.15, 4.16,* and *4.18–4.20*). These tributaries converge on the lateral edge of the lateral ventricles, where they split into medial and lateral groups based on whether they course through the thalamic or the forniceal side of the choroidal fissure. The lateral group passes through the thalamic or inner side of the fissure, and the medial group passes through the outer or forniceal circumference of the fissure. Both groups course along the walls of the ventricle in a subependymal location

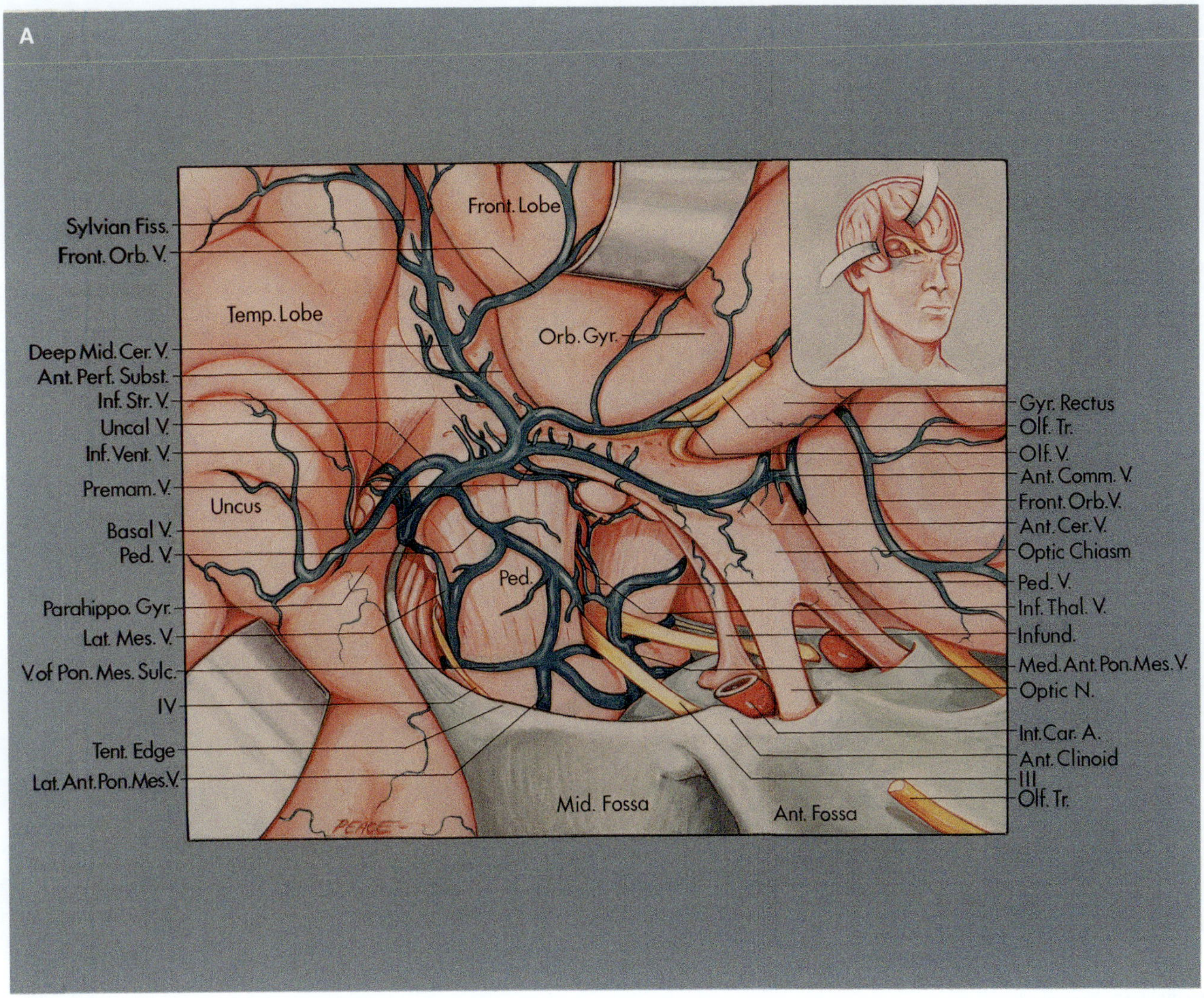

FIGURE 4.17. *Cisternal veins. A, anterolateral view. The inset shows the direction of view. The frontal and temporal lobes have been retracted away from the floor of the anterior and middle cranial fossae. The veins converging on the anterior end of the basal vein below the anterior perforated substance are the deep middle cerebral veins from the sylvian fissure; the olfactory vein, which drains posteriorly along the olfactory tract near the gyrus rectus; the orbitofrontal veins, which drain the orbital gyri; the inferior striate veins, which exit the anterior perforated substance; and the anterior cerebral veins, which are joined above the optic chiasm by the anterior communicating vein. The peduncular vein passes around the cerebral peduncle above the oculomotor nerve and joins the median anterior pontomesencephalic vein in the midline and the basal vein laterally. The infundibulum passes inferiorly behind the anterior clinoid process, optic nerve, and internal carotid artery. The lateral anterior pontomesencephalic vein joins the vein of the pontomesencephalic sulcus below and the basal vein above. The inferior thalamic veins arise behind and the premamillary veins arise in front of the mamillary bodies. The inferior ventricular vein exits the temporal horn above the parahippocampal gyrus and enters the basal vein. An uncal vein passes medially from the uncus. The trochlear nerve courses near the tentorial edge. (Legend continues on next page.)*

toward the choroidal fissure. The lateral group drains the lateral wall and passes along the inner or thalamic side of the ventricle. This group drains the lateral wall and the floor of the frontal horn, body, atrium, and occipital horn, and the roof of the temporal horn. The veins in this group pass, in a subependymal location, through the thalamic side of the choroidal fissure to terminate in the internal cerebral, basal, and great vein. The medial group drains the medial wall plus the ventricular wall opposite the thalamus. This group drains the medial wall and the roof of the frontal horn, body, atrium, and occipital horn and the floor of the temporal horn. After reaching the medial part of the ventricle near the choroidal fissure, the veins in the medial group exit the ventricle by piercing the fornix to join the internal cerebral, basal, or great vein.

The veins of the medial and lateral groups frequently join near the choroidal fissure to form a common stem before terminating in the large veins in the velum interpositum and basal cisterns. In general, the veins draining the frontal horn and the body of the lateral ventricle drain into the internal cerebral vein as it courses through the velum interpositum, those draining the temporal

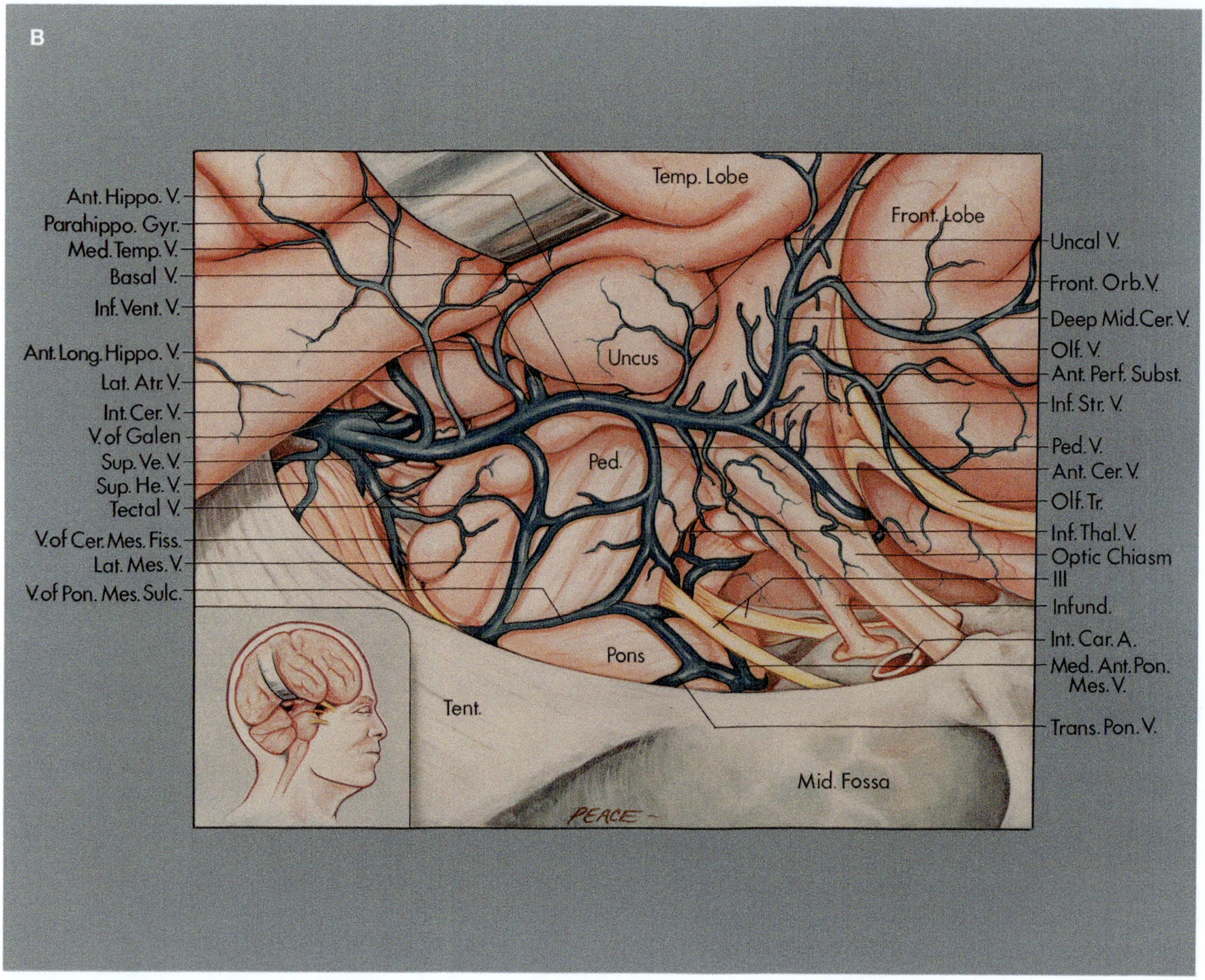

FIGURE 4.17. *Continued*
B, lateral view, right side. The temporal lobe has been elevated, as shown in the inset. The tentorium extends along the side of the brainstem. The basal vein passes around the brainstem and joins the vein of Galen. The tributaries of the basal veins lateral to the brainstem include the lateral mesencephalic vein, which courses in the lateral mesencephalic sulcus; the inferior ventricular vein, which drains the roof of the temporal horn; the anterior hippocampal vein, which courses along the sulcus between the uncus and the parahippocampal gyrus; the anterior longitudinal hippocampal vein, which courses along the dentate gyrus; and the medial temporal veins from the inferomedial surface of the temporal lobe. In the pineal region, the basal vein receives the lateral atrial vein from the lateral wall of the atrium. The internal cerebral veins pass above the pineal body. The superior vermian and superior hemispheric veins from the cerebellum and the vein of the cerebellomesencephalic fissure from the fissure between the midbrain and cerebellum ascend to join the vein of Galen. Tectal veins drain the colliculi. A transverse pontine vein crosses the pons.

horn drain into the segment of the basal vein coursing through the ambient and crural cisterns, and the veins from the atrium drain into the segments of the basal, internal cerebral, and great veins coursing through the quadrigeminal cistern. The internal cerebral veins, as they course through the velum interpositum, receive tributaries from the thalamus, the fornix, and the walls of the third ventricle, in addition to tributaries from the walls of the lateral ventricle.

Frontal Horn

The frontal horn, the part of the lateral ventricle located anterior to the foramen of Monro, has a medial wall formed by the septum pellucidum, an anterior wall formed by the genu of the corpus callosum, a lateral wall composed of the head of the caudate nucleus, and a narrow floor formed by the rostrum of the corpus callosum. The columns of the fornix, as they pass anterior to the foramen of Monro, are in the posteroinferior part of the medial wall.

The medial group of veins in the frontal horn consists of the anterior septal veins, and the lateral group consists of the anterior caudate veins (*Figs. 4.15, 4.16,* and *4.18*). The anterior septal veins are formed by tributaries from the deep white matter near the frontal pole. They course medially across the roof and anterior wall to reach the septum pellucidum, where

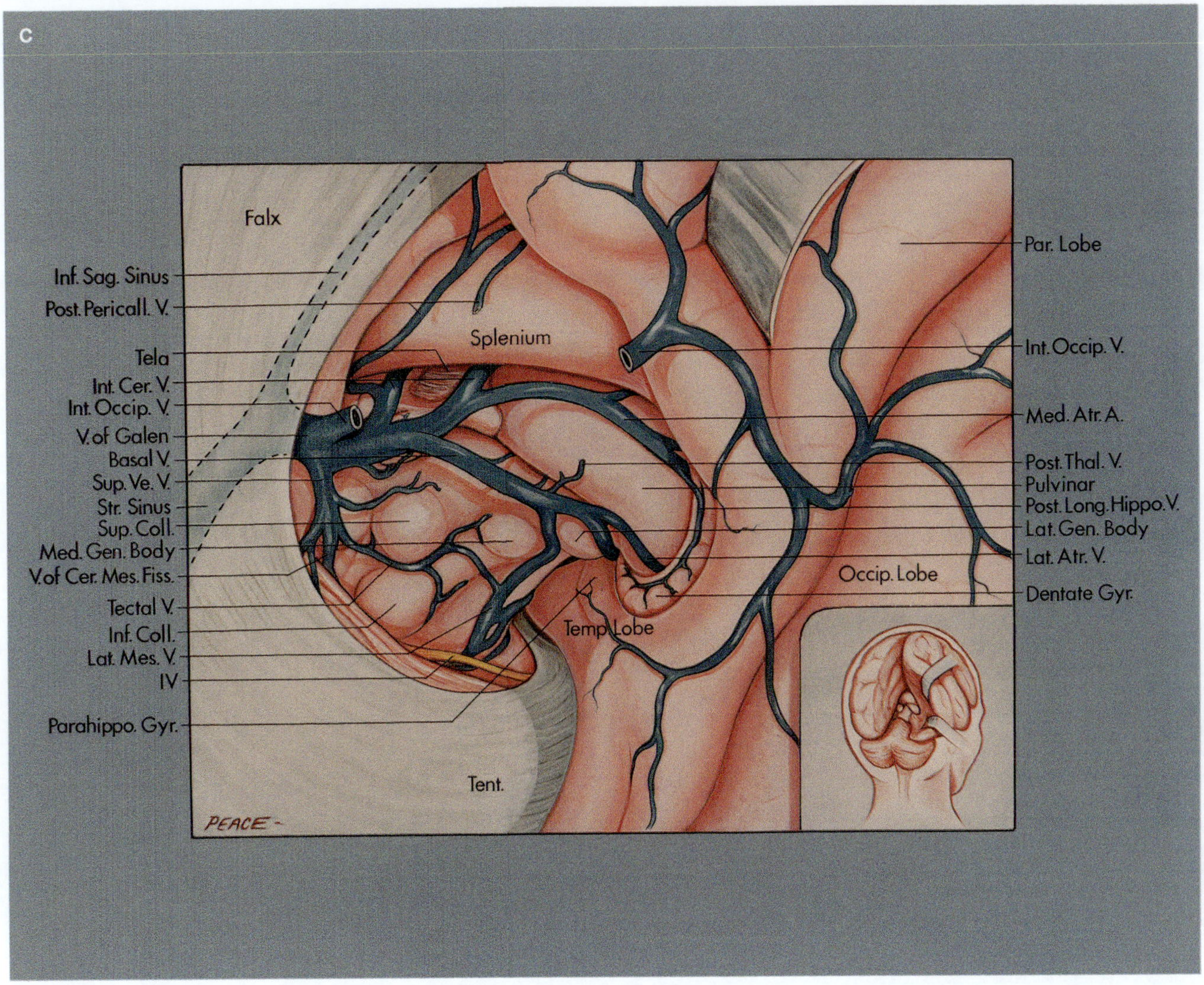

FIGURE 4.17. *Continued*
C, posterior view. The inset *shows the direction of view. The occipital and parietal lobes have been retracted to expose the termination of the internal cerebral and basal veins in the vein of Galen. The internal occipital and posterior pericallosal veins join the internal cerebral vein. The posterior longitudinal hippocampal vein passes along the dentate gyrus and joins the medial atrial vein. The lateral mesencephalic, posterior thalamic, and inferior ventricular veins join the basal vein. Tectal veins pass from the superior and inferior colliculi. The medial and lateral geniculate bodies are below the pulvinar. The inferior sagittal sinus and the vein of Galen join the straight sinus. (Legend continues on next page.)*

they turn posteriorly toward the foramen of Monro, pass around the column of the fornix just above the foramen of Monro to enter the velum interpositum, and terminate in the internal cerebral vein. The anterior caudate veins are formed from small tributaries at the anterolateral and superolateral to the frontal horn, course on the ventricular surface of the head of the caudate nucleus, and terminate near the foramen of Monro in the thalamostriate or thalamocaudate veins. They may also empty directly into the internal cerebral vein.

Body of the Lateral Ventricle

The body of the lateral ventricle extends from the posterior edge of the foramen of Monro to the point where the septum pellucidum disappears and the corpus callosum and fornix meet. The roof is formed by the body of the corpus callosum, the medial wall by the septum pellucidum above and the body of the fornix below, the lateral wall is formed by the body of the caudate nucleus, and the floor is formed by the thalamus. The medial group of veins in the body is formed by the posterior septal veins, and the lateral group consists of the thalamostriate, thalamocaudate, and posterior caudate veins.

The thalamostriate is the best known of the subependymal veins because it is the one most frequently seen on angiography (*Figs. 4.15, 4.16,* and *4.18*). In our study, it was present in 18 of the 20 hemispheres examined (20). The thalamostriate arises from tributaries that converge on the striothalamic sul-

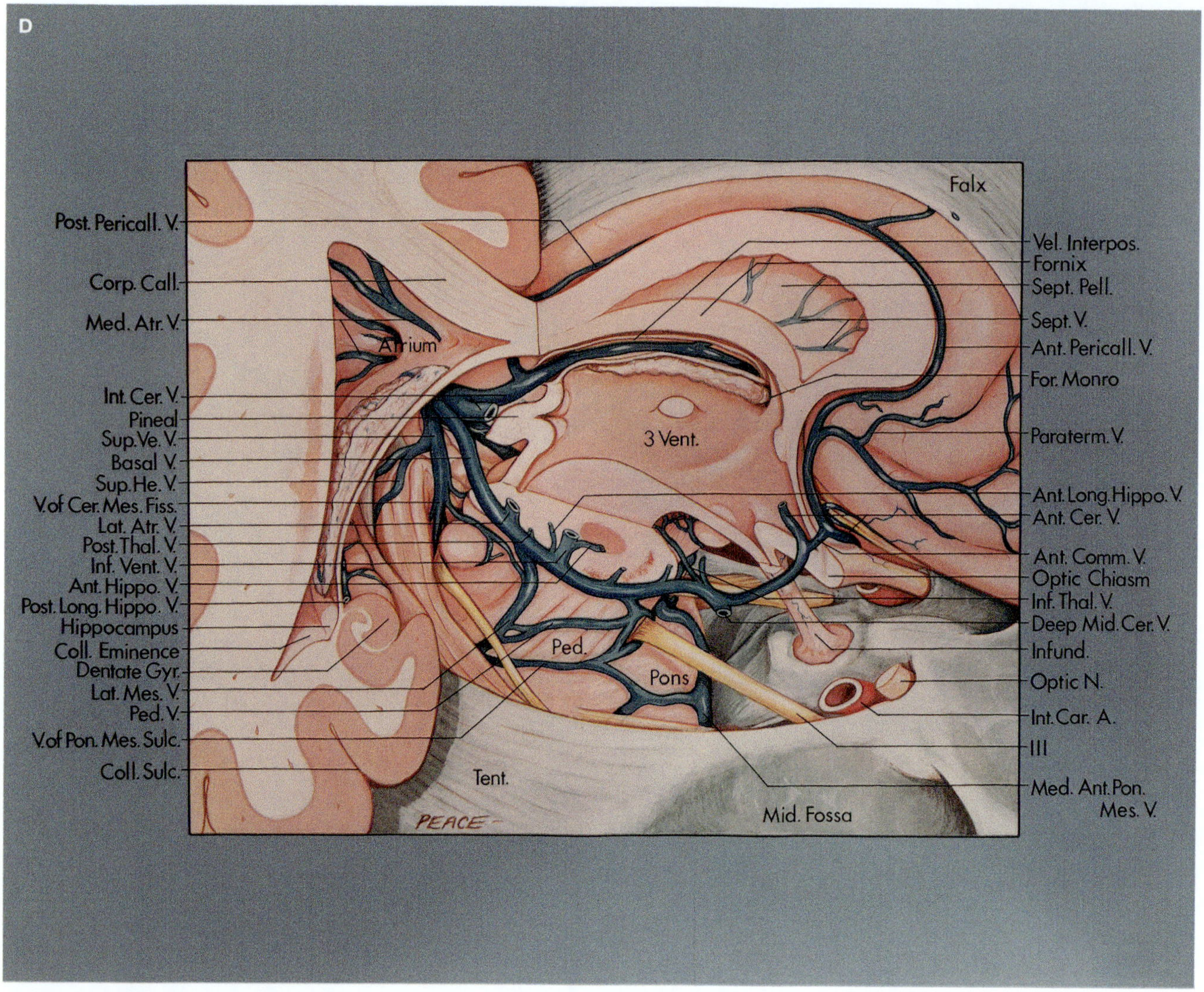

FIGURE 4.17. *Continued*

D, right anterolateral view with the anterior portion of the right cerebral hemisphere removed to expose the upper brainstem and the third ventricle in the midline. The brainstem was sectioned at the level of the cerebral peduncle. The anterior cerebral veins join the deep middle cerebral vein to form the basal vein. The basal vein encircles the brainstem and along its course receives the peduncular, inferior ventricular, anterior hippocampal, anterior longitudinal hippocampal, posterior thalamic, lateral atrial, lateral anterior pontomesencephalic, and lateral mesencephalic veins. The superior vermian vein receives the superior hemispheric and tectal veins and the vein of the cerebellomesencephalic fissure. The paraterminal and anterior pericallosal veins join the anterior cerebral vein. The internal cerebral vein courses in the velum interpositum in the roof of the third ventricle. The collateral eminence sits above the collateral sulcus in the floor of the temporal horn. Septal veins cross the septum pellucidum. The choroid plexus passes through the foramen of Monro to reach the roof of the third ventricle. A., *artery;* Ant., *anterior;* Atr., *atrial;* Call., *callosum;* Car., *carotid;* Cer., *cerebral;* Cer.Mes., *cerebellomesencephalic;* Coll., *collateral;* Comm., *communicating;* Corp., *corpus;* Fiss., *fissure;* For., *foramen;* Front., *frontal;* Front.Orb., *orbitofrontal;* Gen., *geniculate;* Gyr., *gyrus;* He., *hemispheric;* Hippo., *hippocampal, hippocampus;* Inf., *inferior;* Infund., *infundibulum;* Int., *internal;* Interpos., *interpositum;* Lat., *lateral;* Long., *longus;* Med., *medial;* Mes., *mesencephalic;* Mid., *middle;* N., *nerve;* Occip., *occipital;* Olf., *olfactory;* Orb., *orbital;* Par., *parietal;* Parahippo., *parahippocampal;* Paraterm., *paraterminal;* Ped., *peduncle, peduncular;* Pell., *pellucidum;* Perf., *perforated;* Pericall., *pericallosal;* Pon., *pontine;* Pon.Mes., *pontomesencephalic;* Premam., *premamillary;* Sag., *sagittal;* Sept., *septal, septum;* Str., *straight;* Subst., *substance;* Sulc., *sulcus;* Sup., *superior;* Temp., *temporal;* Tent., *tentorial, tentorium;* Thal., *thalamic;* Tr., *tract;* Trans., *transverse;* V., *vein;* Ve., *vermian;* Vel., *velum;* Vent., *ventricle, ventricular.* (From, *Ono M, Rhoton AL Jr, Peace D, Rodriguez R: Microsurgical anatomy of the deep venous system of the brain.* ***Neurosurgery*** *15:621–657, 1984 [20].)*

cus located between the caudate nucleus and thalamus and passes toward the foramen of Monro, where it turns sharply posteriorly through the posterior margin of the foramen of Monro or the adjacent part of the choroidal fissure and enters the velum interpositum to join the internal cerebral vein. The angle formed by the junction of the thalamostriate and the internal cerebral veins at the thalamic tubercle, the venous angle, as seen on the lateral view of the cerebral angiogram, approximates the site of the foramen of Monro. In our study, the venous angle was situated 0 to 6.0 mm (average, 1.5 mm) from the posterior edge of the foramen of Monro (20). If the thalamostriate vein is absent, as occurred in two cases in our study, or is small, the thalamocaudate vein, which courses directly medial across the caudate nucleus and thalamus toward the choroidal fissure, drains the same area. In some cases, there are double thalamostriate veins, called the anterior and posterior thalamostriate veins, that course forward near the striothalamic sulcus and converge on the internal cerebral vein near the foramen of Monro.

The thalamocaudate vein courses medially across the caudate nucleus and thalamus behind the posterior extension of the thalamostriate vein and terminates in the internal cerebral vein (*Figs. 4.15* and *4.16*). The size of the thalamocaudate vein is inversely proportional to the size of the thalamostriate vein. If the thalamostriate vein is large and extends backward to the posterior part of the body, the thalamocaudate vein will be absent or small, and if the thalamostriate vein is absent, the thalamocaudate vein will be large. The thalamocaudate vein is not directed anteriorly along the striothalamic sulcus, as is the thalamostriate vein, but is directed medially or posteriorly across the lateral wall and floor of the body. It passes through the margin of the choroidal fissure well behind the foramen of Monro and ends in the internal cerebral, medial atrial, or posterior septal veins. The thalamocaudate vein was larger and the thalamostriate vein was absent in 4 of 20 hemispheres in our study (20).

The posterior caudate veins originate at the superolateral angle of the body and course inferomedial across the caudate nucleus toward the striothalamic sulcus, where they terminate in the thalamostriate or thalamocaudate veins. The posterior septal veins consist of one or two veins that originate along the roof of the body, course across the septum pellucidum, and terminate by penetrating the junction of the fornix and the septum pellucidum to enter the velum interpositum, where they join the internal cerebral vein.

Atrium and Occipital Horn

The atrium and occipital horn together form a roughly triangular cavity, with the apex posteriorly in the occipital lobe and the base anteriorly on the pulvinar (*Figs. 4.15* and *4.16*). The lateral wall has an anterior part formed by the caudate nucleus and a posterior part formed by the fibers of the tapetum of the corpus callosum. The anterior wall has a medial part composed of the crus of the fornix and a lateral part formed by the pulvinar. The floor has a medial part composed of the hippocampus and a lateral part formed by the collateral trigone, the triangular prominence deep to the posterior end of the collateral sulcus. The occipital horn extends posteriorly into the occipital lobe from the atrium. Its size varies widely, from absence to extension far posteriorly in the occipital lobe, and its size may differ from one hemisphere to the other.

The medial group of veins in the atrium and occipital horn consists of the medial atrial veins, and the lateral group is composed of the lateral atrial veins (*Figs. 4.4, 4.15, 4.16, 4.18–4.21*). The medial atrial veins drain forward on the medial wall of the atrium and occipital horn toward the choroidal fissure. They may also drain the adjacent part of the roof or floor. They pass through the choroidal fissure or crus of the fornix and terminate within the velum interpositum or quadrigeminal cistern in the internal cerebral or basal veins or their tributaries. The lateral atrial veins drain the anterior and lateral walls of the atrium and occipital horn and the adjacent part of the roof and floor. These veins course forward on the lateral wall across the tail of the caudate nucleus to reach the anterior wall, where they turn medially on the posterior surface of the pulvinar and pass through the choroidal fissure to reach the ambient or quadrigeminal cisterns. There they join the internal cerebral, basal, or great vein. The medial and lateral atrial veins may join near the choroidal fissure to form a common trunk called the common atrial vein.

The transverse hippocampal veins course medially across the collateral trigone and hippocampus on the floor of the temporal horn and penetrate the fimbria. They enter the ambient cistern by passing between the fimbria and dentate gyrus to terminate on the dentate gyrus in the posterior longitudinal hippocampal veins.

Temporal Horn

The temporal horn extends forward from the atrium below the pulvinar into the medial part of the temporal lobe and ends blindly in the anterior wall situated immediately behind the amygdaloid nucleus (*Fig. 4.16*). The floor is formed by the hippocampus and collateral eminence, the roof by the thalamus and caudate tail, the lateral wall by the tapetum, and the medial wall by the choroid fissure. The medial group of veins courses on the roof, and the lateral group of veins courses on the floor. The roof is drained predominantly by the inferior ventricular vein, with a lesser contribution from the amygdalar vein, and the floor is drained by the transverse hippocampal veins. The veins from the temporal horn join the basal vein or its tributaries. The posterior part of the roof and floor may be drained by the veins coursing in the walls of the atrium.

The inferior ventricular vein is in the posterolateral part of the roof of the temporal horn and courses obliquely anteromedial near the tail of the caudate nucleus (*Figs. 4.4, 4.15, 4.16,* and *4.19–4.21*). It exits the temporal horn just behind the inferior choroidal point to join the basal vein near the lateral geniculate body at the junction of the crural and ambient cisterns. The amygdalar vein courses medially across the anterior wall on or near the ventricular surface of the amygdaloid nucleus. It terminates in the inferior ventricular, basal, or anterior longitudinal hippocampal vein near the inferior choroid point, either before or after it has passed through the choroidal fissure to enter the crural cistern. The amygdalar vein may receive the inferior choroidal veins and drain the adjacent part of the roof. The transverse hippocampal veins are a group of very fine veins that course medially across the hippocampal formation and collateral eminence. They penetrate the attachment of the fimbria to the hippocampus to enter the ambient cistern through the fimbriodentate sulcus to drain into the anterior and posterior longitudinal hippocampal veins.

Choroidal Veins

The superior and inferior choroidal veins are the most consistent veins on the choroid plexus (*Figs. 4.15, 4.16,* and *4.18*). The superior choroidal vein, the largest of the choroidal

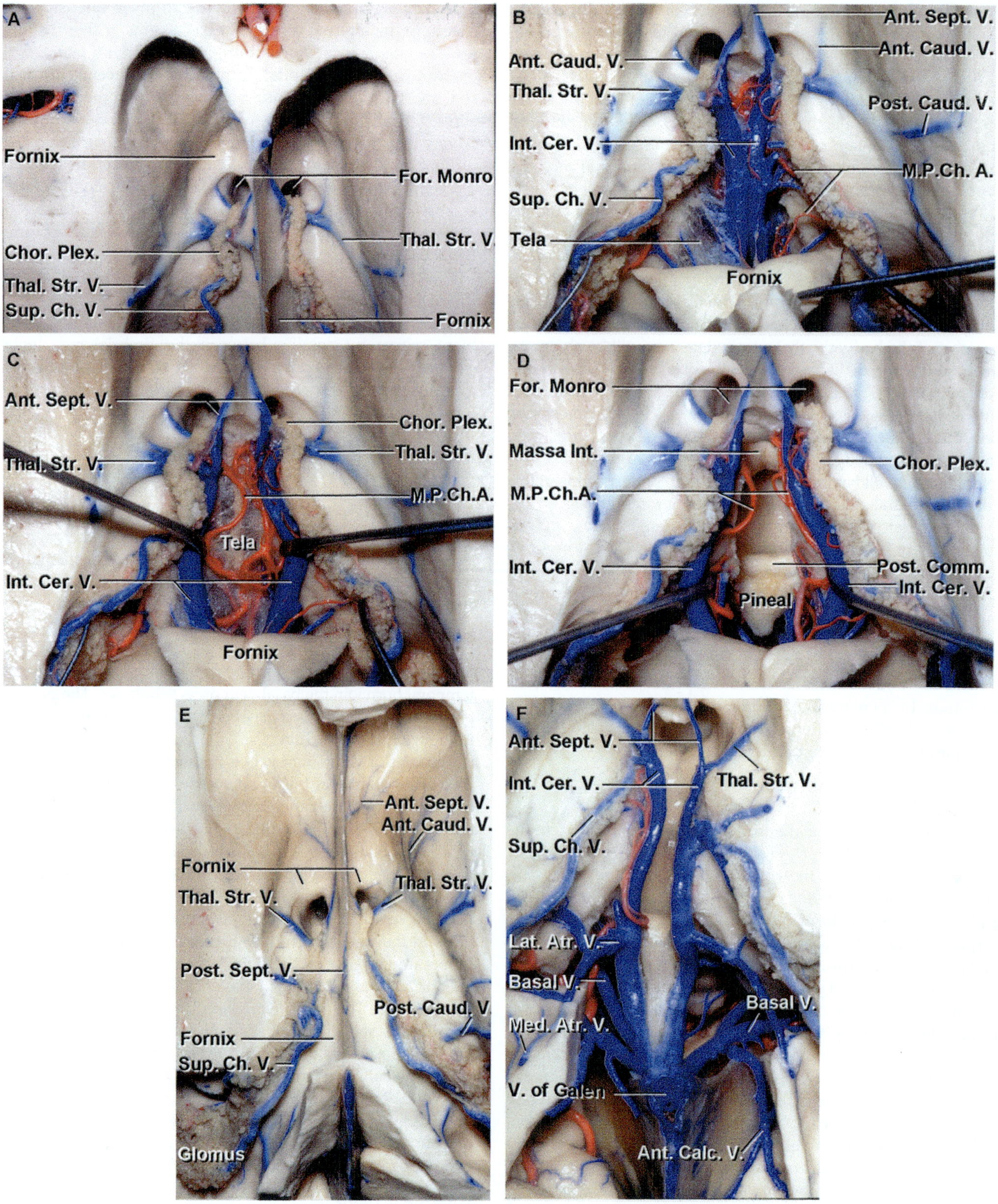
A
Fornix
For. Monro
Chor. Plex.
Thal. Str. V.
Thal. Str. V.
Sup. Ch. V.
Fornix
B
Ant. Sept. V.
Ant. Caud. V.
Ant. Caud. V.
Thal. Str. V.
Post. Caud. V.
Int. Cer. V.
M.P.Ch. A.
Sup. Ch. V.
Tela
Fornix
C
Ant. Sept. V.
Chor. Plex.
Thal. Str. V.
Thal. Str. V.
M.P.Ch.A.
Tela
Int. Cer. V.
Fornix
D
For. Monro
Massa Int.
Chor. Plex.
M.P.Ch.A.
Int. Cer. V.
Post. Comm.
Int. Cer. V.
Pineal
E
Ant. Sept. V.
Ant. Caud. V.
Fornix
Thal. Str. V.
Thal. Str. V.
Post. Sept. V.
Post. Caud. V.
Fornix
Sup. Ch. V.
Glomus
F
Ant. Sept. V.
Int. Cer. V.
Thal. Str. V.
Sup. Ch. V.
Lat. Atr. V.
Basal V.
Basal V.
Med. Atr. V.
V. of Galen
Ant. Calc. V.

FIGURE 4.18.

veins, runs forward on the choroid plexus in the body of the lateral ventricle and terminates near the foramen of Monro in the thalamostriate or internal cerebral veins or their tributaries. The inferior choroidal vein, the next most consistent choroidal vein, courses anteriorly in the temporal horn along the inferior end of the choroid plexus. It terminates by joining the inferior ventricular and amygdaloid vein or by passing through the choroidal fissure near the inferior choroidal point to reach the basal cisterns, where it terminates in the basal vein or its tributaries. The superior and inferior choroidal veins frequently anastomose through the veins draining the glomus of the choroid plexus.

Internal Cerebral Veins

The paired internal cerebral veins originate just behind the foramen of Monro and course posteriorly within the velum interpositum (*Figs. 4.6, 4.15, 4.17–4.19,* and *4.22*). Initially, they follow the gentle convex upward curve of the striae medullaris thalami and, further distally, as they course along the superolateral surface of the pineal body, they follow the concave upward curve of the inferior surface of the splenium. The union of the paired veins to form the great vein may be located above or posterior to the pineal body and inferior or posterior to the splenium. The length of the internal cerebral vein varies from 19 to 35 mm (average, 30.2) (20).

The veins from the frontal horn, body, and part of the atrium terminate in the internal cerebral veins as they course through the velum interpositum. The tributaries of the internal cerebral vein from the lateral and third ventricles include the anterior septal, anterior caudate, posterior septal, posterior caudate, thalamostriate, thalamocaudate, anterior thalamic, anterior superficial thalamic, superior choroidal, superior thalamic, and superior superficial thalamic veins and the veins draining the striae medullaris thalami. The internal cerebral veins also receive numerous fine tributaries from the fornix, hippocampal commissure, choroid plexus of the third ventricle, and the thalamic surfaces forming the lateral walls of the third ventricle. Other veins that may join the internal cerebral, basal, or great veins include the medial and lateral atrial, posterior longitudinal hippocampal, internal occipital, and posterior pericallosal veins.

CISTERNAL GROUP

The cisternal group of deep veins drains the area beginning anteriorly in front of the third ventricle and extending laterally into the sylvian fissure and backward to include the walls of the chiasmatic, interpeduncular, crural, ambient, and quadrigeminal cisterns (*Figs. 4.17,* and *4.19–4.22*). The veins draining the structures anterior to the quadrigeminal cistern drain into the basal vein, and those in the region of the quadrigeminal cistern drain into the basal, internal cerebral, or great veins.

The area drained by the cisternal group of veins is divided into three regions depending on their relationship to the brainstem and tentorial incisura: an anterior incisural region located in front of the brainstem, a middle incisural region situated lateral to the brainstem, and a posterior incisural space located behind the brainstem (19). The incisural spaces are reviewed in detail in Chapter 5 of the Millennium issue of *Neurosurgery* (21). The major veins in the cisternal group are the basal and great veins.

The basal vein is formed below the anterior perforated substance by the union of veins draining the walls of the anterior incisural space. It proceeds posteriorly between the midbrain and the temporal lobe to drain the walls of the middle incisural space, and terminates within the posterior incisural space by joining the internal cerebral or great vein (*Figs. 4.4* and *4.20–4.22*). The basal vein is divided into anterior, middle, and posterior segments that correspond to the parts of the vein coursing within the anterior, middle, and posterior incisural regions. The anterior and middle incisural regions are drained, almost totally, by tributaries of the basal vein. The veins in the posterior incisural region join the internal cerebral and great veins, as well as the basal vein.

FIGURE 4.18. *Internal cerebral veins in the roof of the third ventricle. A, superior view of the frontal horn and body. The thalamostriate and superior choroidal veins converge on the posterior edge of the foramen of Monro. The superior and anterior margin of the foramen of Monro is formed by the fornix. B, the fornix has been folded backward to expose the tela choroidea and the internal cerebral veins in the roof of the third ventricle. A thin layer of ependyma extends above and partially hides the thalamostriate veins coursing along the sulcus between the thalamus and caudate nucleus. The anterior caudate and anterior septal veins cross the lateral and medial wall of the frontal horn. The posterior caudate veins cross the lateral wall of the body of the ventricle. Only a small part of the upper layer of tela located between the fornix and internal cerebral veins remains. C, the internal cerebral veins have been separated to expose the branches of the medial posterior choroidal artery and the lower layer of tela choroidea that forms the floor of the velum interpositum in the roof of the third ventricle. The lower wall of the velum interpositum, in which the internal cerebral veins and medial posterior choroidal arteries course, is formed by the layer of tela attached along the medial side of the thalamus to the striae medullaris thalami. D, the lower layer of tela has been opened and the internal cerebral veins and the medial posterior choroidal arteries have been retracted to expose the posterior commissure, pineal gland, and massa intermedia. E, another hemisphere. The upper part of the hemisphere has been removed to expose the frontal horn, body and atrium of the lateral ventricle. The choroid plexus is attached along the choroidal fissure. The anterior and posterior caudate veins cross the lateral wall and the anterior and posterior septal veins cross the medial wall of the frontal horn and body of the lateral ventricle. The superior choroidal veins course along the choroid plexus. The thalamostriate veins pass through the posterior margin of the foramen of Monro. The choroid plexus in the atrium expands to a large tuft called the glomus. F, the body of the fornix has been removed to expose the internal cerebral veins coursing in the roof the third ventricle. The medial and lateral atrial and anterior calcarine veins join the posterior end of the internal cerebral veins. The basal veins are exposed below and lateral to the internal cerebral veins.* Ant., *anterior;* Atr., *atrial;* Calc., *calcarine;* Caud., *caudate;* Cer., *cerebral;* Ch., *choroidal;* Chor., *choroid;* Comm., *communicating;* For., *foramen;* Int., *intermedia, internal;* Lat., *lateral;* Med., *medial;* Plex., *plexus;* M.P.Ch.A., *medial posterior choroidal artery;* Post., *posterior;* Sept., *septal;* Sup., *superior;* Thal.Str., *thalamostriate;* V., *vein.*

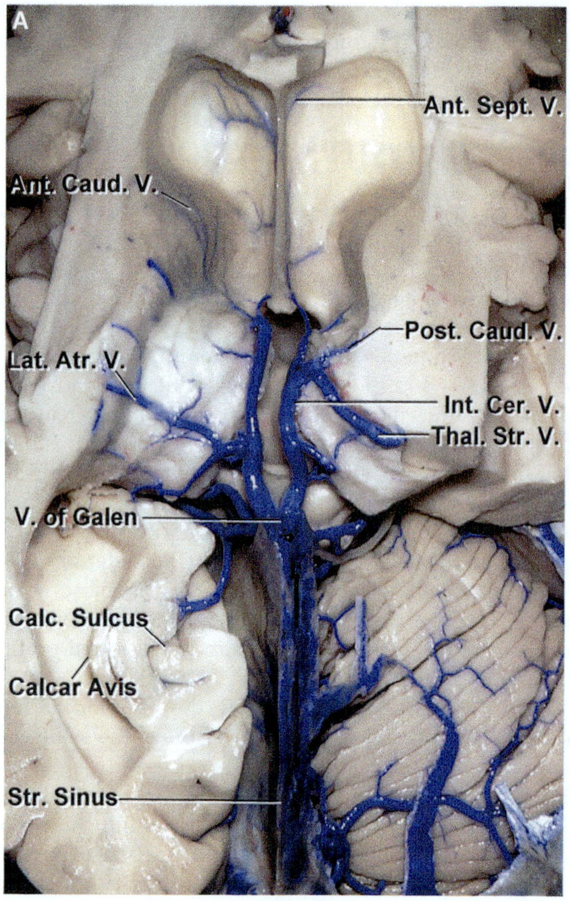

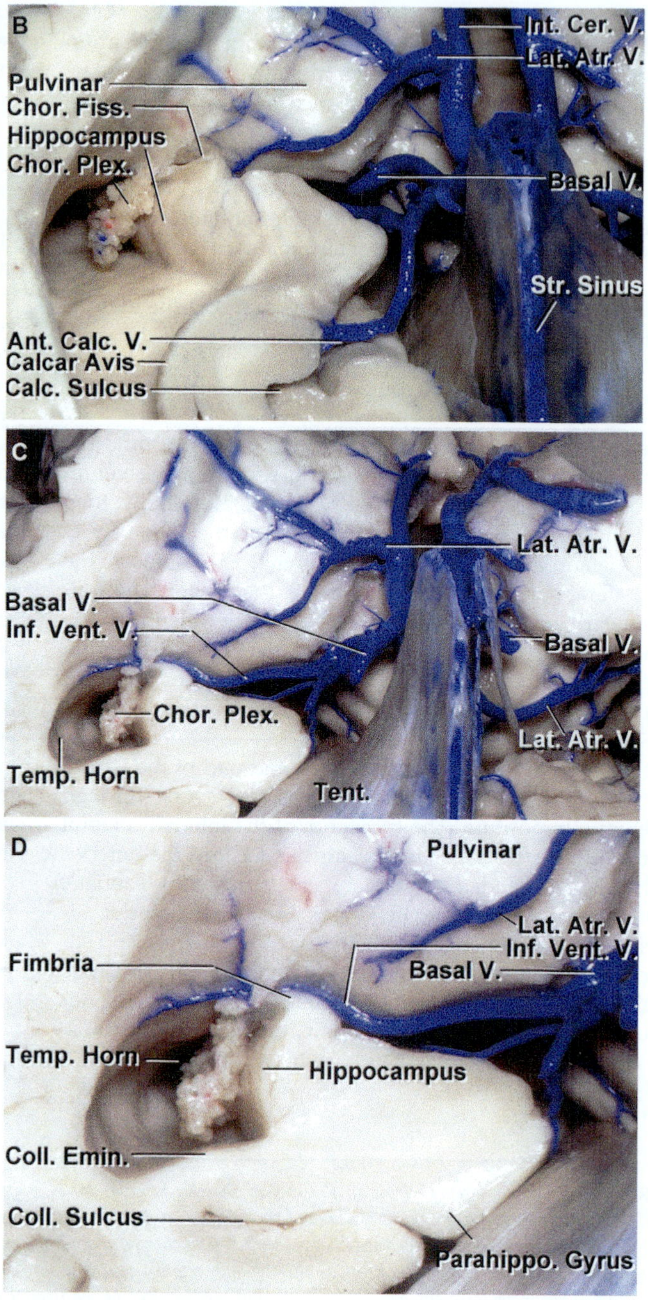

FIGURE 4.19. A, *posterosuperior view of the ventricles with the upper part of the cerebral hemisphere removed. The right occipital lobe and the adjacent tentorium have been removed to expose the upper surface of the cerebellum. Anterior caudate and anterior septal veins drain the walls of the frontal horn and empty into the anterior end of the internal cerebral vein. The posterior caudate veins drain the lateral wall of the body of the ventricle.* B, *enlarged view. The internal cerebral and basal veins converge on the vein of Galen. The lateral atrial vein crosses the pulvinar and empties into the internal cerebral vein. The anterior calcarine vein drains the depths of the calcarine sulcus and joins the vein of Galen near its junction with the basal vein. The calcarine sulcus forms a prominence, the calcar avis, in the medial wall of the atrium. The posterior end of the hippocampus is located at the anterior edge of the calcar avis. The veins exiting the ventricle pass through the margins of the choroidal fissure located between the fornix and thalamus.* C, *the section of the left cerebrum has been extended forward into the temporal horn and hippocampus. The inferior ventricular vein drains the roof of the temporal horn and passes through the choroidal fissure to empty into the basal vein. The lateral atrial vein crosses the posterior surface of the pulvinar to empty into the internal cerebral vein. Only the stump of the basal vein remains.* D, *enlarged view of the inferior ventricular vein passing through the choroidal fissure located between the fimbria and lower surface of the pulvinar, to join the basal vein. The deep end of the collateral sulcus, located on the lateral margin of the parahippocampal gyrus, forms a prominence, the collateral eminence, in the floor of the temporal horn lateral to the hippocampus.* Ant., *anterior;* Atr., *atrial;* Calc., *calcarine;* Caud., *caudate;* Cer., *cerebral;* Chor., *choroid, choroidal;* Coll., *collateral;* Emin., *eminence;* Fiss., *fissure;* Inf., *inferior;* Int., *internal;* Lat., *lateral;* Parahippo., *parahippocampal;* Plex., *plexus;* Post., *posterior;* Sept., *septal;* Str., *straight;* Temp., *temporal;* Tent., *tentorium;* Thal. Str., *thalamostriate;* V., *vein;* Vent., *ventricular.*

Anterior Incisural Region

The anterior incisural region is located anterior to the brainstem and extends upward around the optic chiasm to the subcallosal area and laterally below the anterior perforated substance into the sylvian fissure and over the surface of the insula (*Figs. 4.4, 4.17,* and *4.21*). This region includes the walls of the subcallosal, chiasmatic, interpeduncular, and sylvian cisterns. The anterior perforated substance, on which numer-

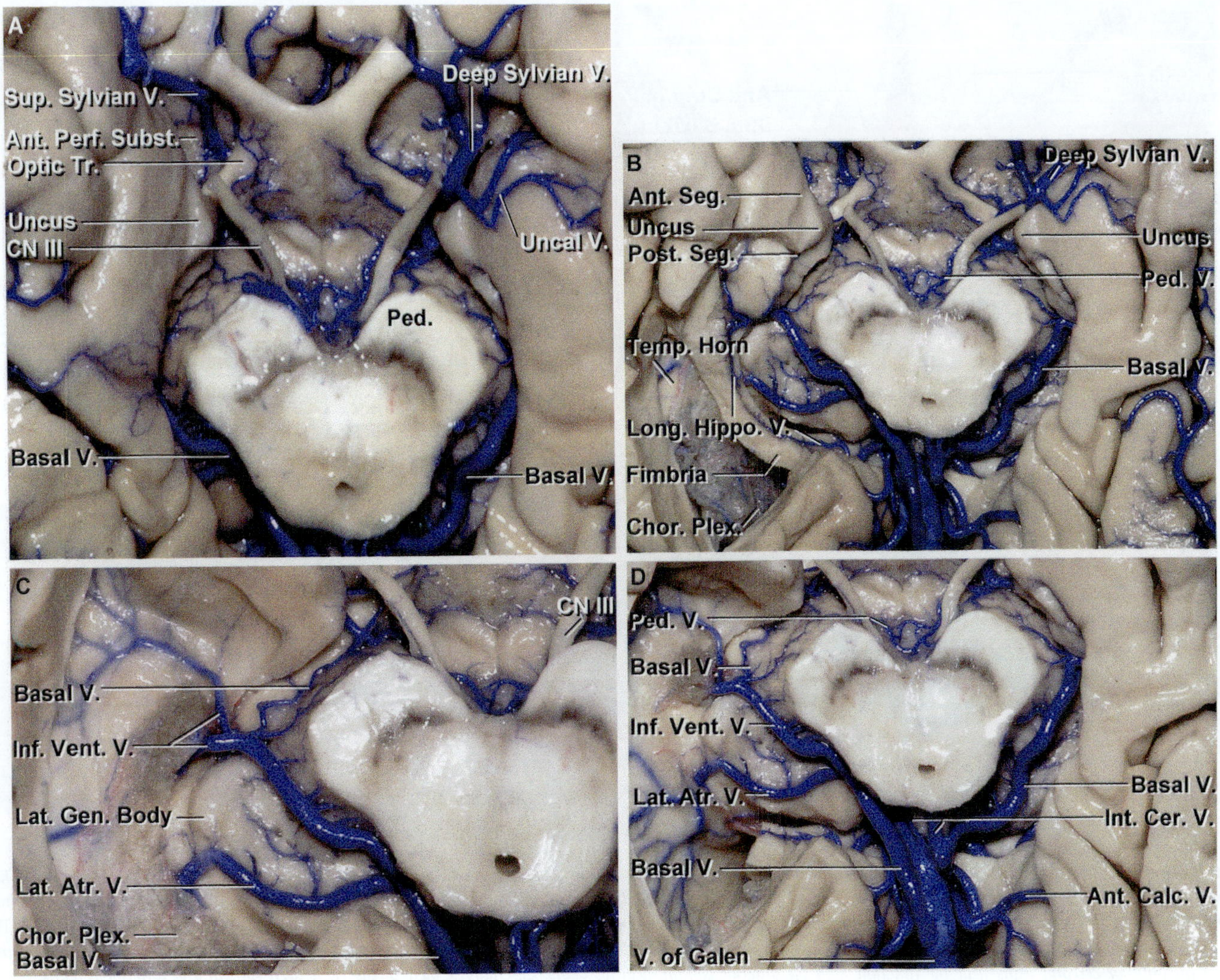

FIGURE 4.20. *Inferior view of the basal cisterns.* A, *the basal veins are formed below the anterior perforated substance by the union of the posterior orbitofrontal, superficial and deep sylvian, and uncal veins and course posteriorly across the optic tracts. Only the anterior and posterior segments of the basal vein are exposed because the middle part is hidden above the uncus and parahippocampal gyrus.* B, *the uncus has an anterior and posterior segment. The lower part of the posterior segment of the right uncus and adjacent part of the parahippocampal gyrus has been removed, while preserving the fimbria of the fornix, to expose the inferior ventricular and lateral atrial veins. The segment of the right basal veins coursing lateral to the cerebral peduncle is very small. The inferior ventricular and lateral atrial veins pass through the choroidal fissure, situated between the thalamus and fimbria, to empty into the basal vein. The longitudinal hippocampal veins course along the fimbria. The peduncular veins, in this case, are quite small. The lateral atrial veins, which drain the lateral atrial wall and the posterior part of the roof of the temporal horn, pass below the pulvinar to reach the basal vein.* C, *enlarged view after removal of the fimbria. The large veins draining the roof of the temporal horn and lateral atrial wall and crossing the lower and posterior surface of the thalamus, are analogous to the thalamostriate vein that crosses the upper surface of the thalamus. All three veins drain a portion of the central core of the hemisphere and pass through the choroidal fissure between the thalamus and choroid plexus.* D, *the choroid plexus has been removed.* Ant., *anterior;* Atr., *atrial;* Calc., *calcarine;* Chor., *choroid;* CN, *cranial nerve;* Gen., *geniculate;* Hippo., *hippocampal;* Inf., *inferior;* Lat., *lateral;* Long., *longus;* Ped., *peduncle, peduncular;* Perf., *perforated;* Plex., *plexus;* Post., *posterior;* Seg., *segment;* Subst., *substance;* Sup., *superior;* Temp., *temporal;* Tr., *tract;* V., *vein;* Vent., *ventricular.*

ous veins converge to form the basal vein, is in the central part of the roof of the anterior incisural space.

The cortical areas bordering the anterior incisural region, which may also be drained by the basal vein, include the insula and the orbital surface of the frontal lobe. The insular veins, one of the major contributing groups to the first part of the basal vein, are named for their relationship to the insular sulci and gyri.

The major venous structure in the anterior incisural space is the anterior segment of the basal vein (*Figs. 4.4, 4.17,* and *4.21*). This segment begins at the union of the deep middle cerebral and anterior cerebral veins, below the anterior perforated substance, and passes posteriorly to end where the peduncular vein joins the basal vein at the anterolateral part of the cerebral peduncle. The tributaries of this segment are the deep middle cerebral, anterior cerebral, insular, orbitofrontal, olfac-

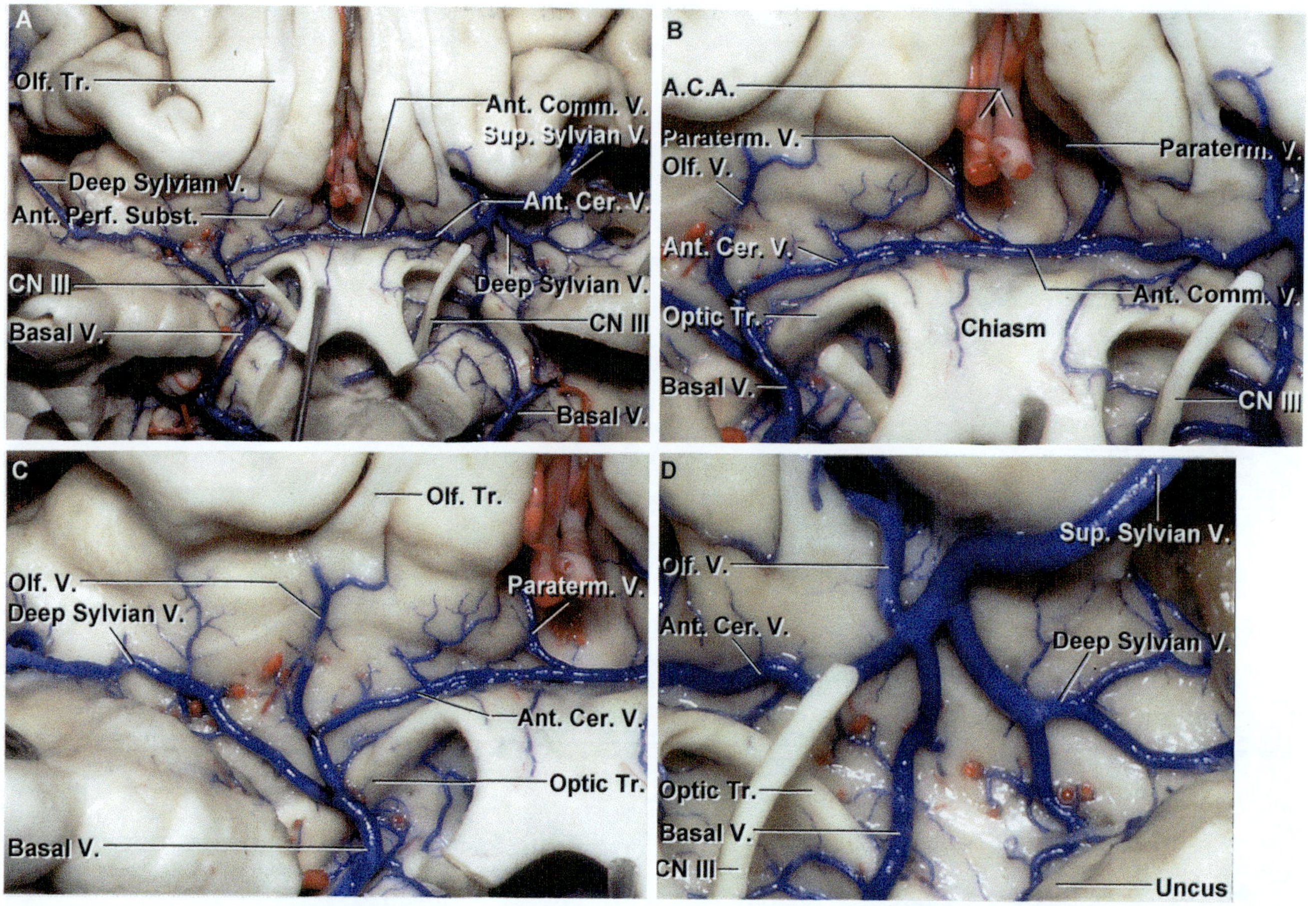

FIGURE 4.21. *Territory of the basal vein. A, inferior view of the frontal lobe and anterior perforated substance with the optic chiasm reflected downward. The anterior cerebral veins pass above the optic chiasm and are joined across the midline by an anterior communicating vein. The anterior cerebral veins join the veins draining the posterior part of the orbital surface of the frontal lobe and the superficial and deep sylvian veins to constitute the anterior end of the basal vein. B, enlarged view of the anterior cerebral and anterior communicating veins. Paraterminal veins, draining the cortical areas below the genu of the corpus callosum, join the anterior cerebral veins near the junction with the anterior communicating veins. C, enlarged view of the right deep sylvian and anterior cerebral veins joining below the anterior perforated substance to form the anterior end of the basal vein. D, enlarged view of the large left superficial sylvian and smaller deep sylvian veins joining the anterior cerebral and olfactory veins to empty into the anterior end of the basal vein. E, inferior view of the basal cisterns in the same cerebrum. The medial part of the right parahippocampal gyrus has been removed to expose the temporal horn while preserving the uncus and the fimbria of the fornix. The left posterior cerebral artery and the medial temporal structures have been preserved. The lower lip of the right calcarine sulcus has been removed to expose the cuneus and anterior calcarine veins. The basal vein courses posteriorly around the cerebral peduncle and below the thalamus. The right anterior choroidal artery passes between the lateral geniculate body and the fimbria to reach the choroid plexus in the temporal horn. The left basal vein courses above the posterior cerebral artery. F, the left posterior cerebral artery has been removed to expose the basal vein. The anterior part of the left basal vein is hidden deep to the uncus. The right anterior and posterior longitudinal hippocampal veins course along the fimbria. G, the lower part of the posterior segment of the left uncus plus the parahippocampal gyrus and fimbria have been removed to expose the roof of the left temporal horn. The posterior segment of the left basal vein is missing, because the anterior part drained into a sinus in the tentorial that has been removed instead of draining into the vein of Galen. Uncal veins converge on the basal vein, as does the peduncular vein. The lateral atrial and thalamic veins converge on the calcarine vein. H, overview. The sylvian veins join the anterior cerebral veins to form the anterior end of the basal vein. The anterior cerebral veins are connected above the optic chiasm by the anterior communicating veins. The anterior segment of the right basal vein is larger than the left. The left atrial veins join the anterior calcarine vein before emptying into the vein of Galen.* A., *artery;* A.C.A., *anterior cerebral artery;* A.Ch.A., *anterior choroidal artery;* Ant., *anterior;* Atr., *atrial;* Calc., *calcarine;* Car., *carotid;* Cer., *cerebral;* Chor., *choroid;* CN, *cranial nerve;* Comm., *communicating;* Hippo., *hippocampal;* Inf., *inferior;* Lat., *lateral;* Long., *longus;* Olf., *olfactory;* Paraterm., *paraterminal;* P.C.A., *posterior cerebral artery;* Ped., *peduncle;* Perf., *perforated;* Plex., *plexus;* Post., *posterior;* Subst., *substance;* Sup., *superior;* Temp., *temporal;* Tr., *tract;* V., *vein;* Vent., *ventricular.*

tory, uncal, peduncular, and inferior striate veins. In our study, two hemispheres lacked an anterior segment of the basal vein (20). A number of these veins may join before emptying into the basal vein.

The deep middle cerebral vein is formed by the union of the insular veins near the limen insula. It passes medially across the anterior perforated substance, where it unites with the anterior cerebral vein to form the basal vein. The deep middle

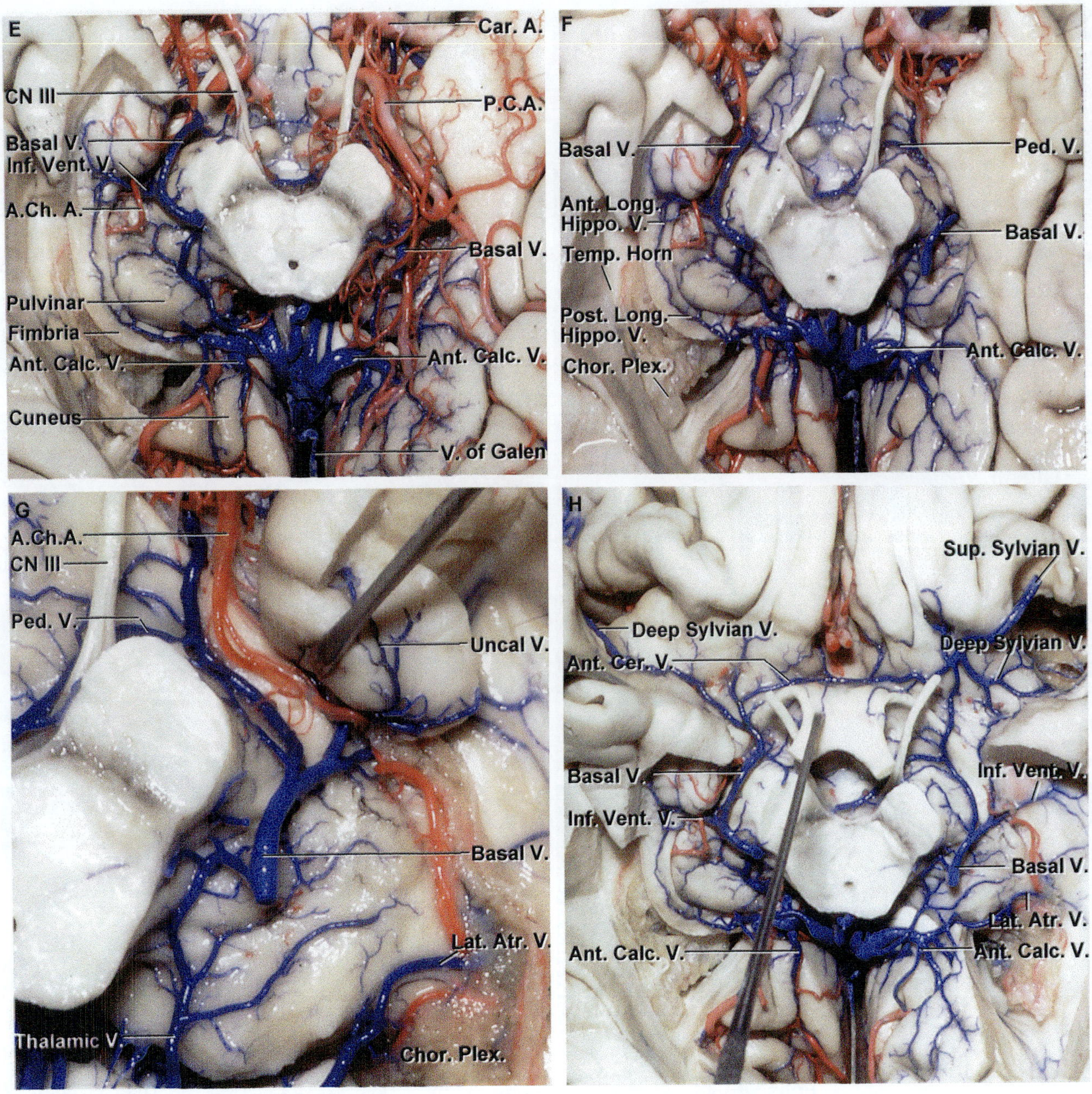

FIGURE 4.21. *Continued*

cerebral vein, the anterior segment of the basal vein, or their tributaries may be connected by a bridging vein to the sphenoparietal or cavernous sinus.

The veins draining the insula empty predominantly through the deep middle cerebral vein into the basal vein, but some may terminate in the superficial cortical veins bordering the sylvian fissure (*Fig. 4.23*). The anterior cerebral veins originate near the upper margin of the optic chiasm and are often joined across the midline by the anterior communicating vein. They course along the superolateral boundary of the optic chiasm and tract, and terminate, most commonly, by joining the deep middle cerebral vein. The orbitofrontal veins consist of one or more veins that drain the orbital surface of the frontal lobe and empty into the anterior end of the basal vein or its tributaries. The olfactory vein courses on the inferior surface of the frontal lobe, near the olfactory sulcus, and terminates in the tributaries of the basal vein.

The inferior striate veins exit the anterior perforated substance and join the deep middle cerebral and basal veins. They drain a large area above the anterior perforated substance that includes the putamen, caudate nucleus, and internal capsule. In the lateral view of the cerebral venogram, they have a fan-shaped appear-

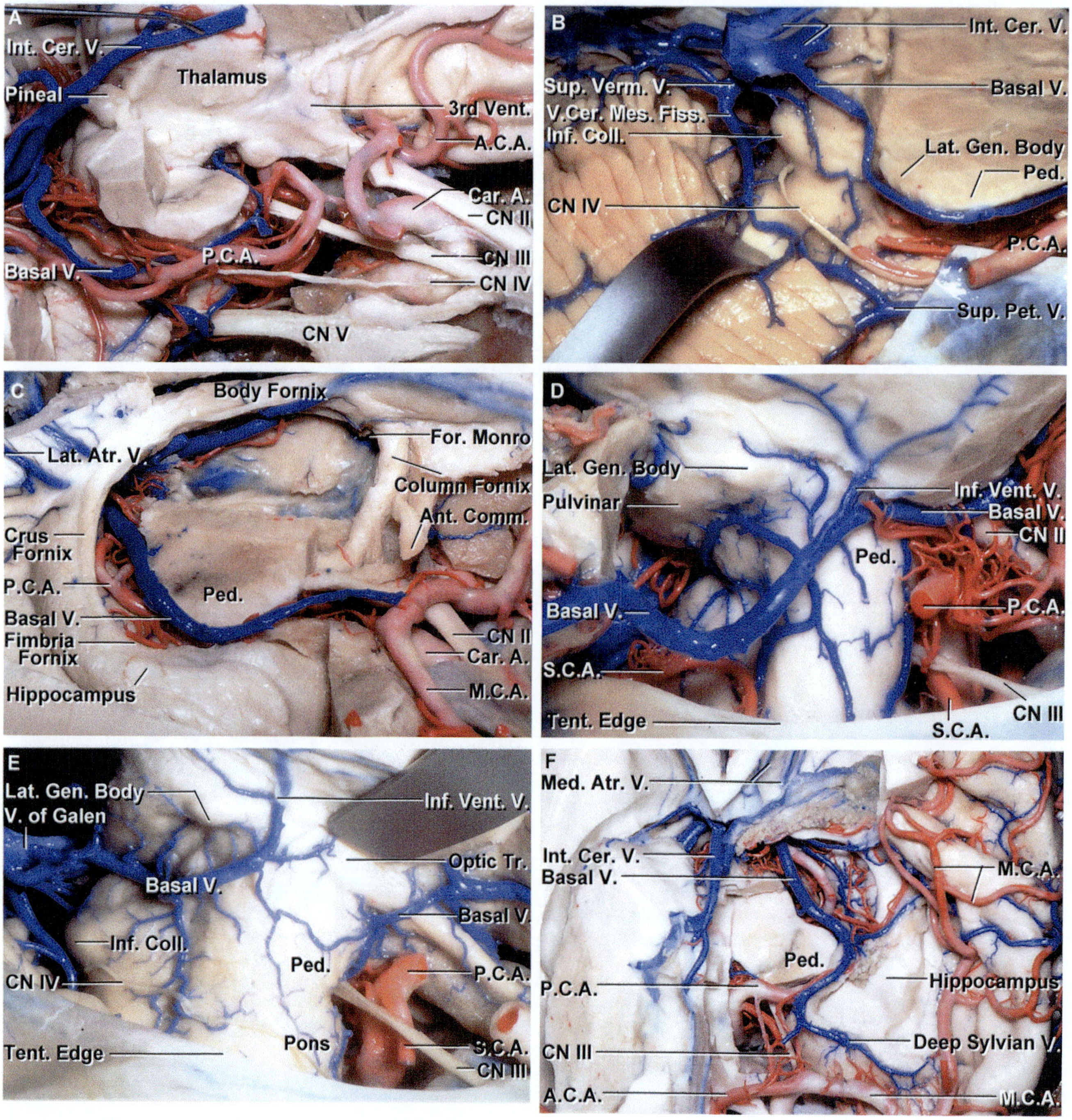

FIGURE 4.22. *Basal vein. A, lateral view with the right hemisphere removed. The internal cerebral veins course between the upper parts of the thalami. The basal vein courses posteriorly above the posterior cerebral artery. The nerves in the wall of the cavernous sinus have been exposed. B, superolateral view of the quadrigeminal cistern. The section of the brainstem extends through the cerebral peduncle and lateral geniculate body. The basal vein passes posteriorly above the posterior cerebral artery to join the internal cerebral vein in the quadrigeminal cistern. A vein courses parallel and below the basal vein connecting the veins in the quadrigeminal cistern and cerebellomesencephalic fissure with the superior petrosal veins emptying into the superior petrosal sinus. The trochlear nerve arises below the inferior colliculus. C, the right hemisphere including the thalamus has been removed to expose the basal vein coursing through the crural, ambient, and quadrigeminal cisterns and the internal cerebral veins coursing in the roof of the third ventricle. The hippocampus and fimbria have been preserved. The internal cerebral and basal veins course in close relationship to the fornix. The internal cerebral vein courses below the body of the fornix. The basal vein courses medial to the fimbria and the basal and internal cerebral veins join to form the vein of Galen in the area medial to the crus of the fornix. A column of the fornix and the anterior commissure are at the anterior margin of the exposure. D, the right temporal lobe, including the hippocampus and the choroid plexus, has been removed to expose the right basal vein passing through the ambient and quadri-*

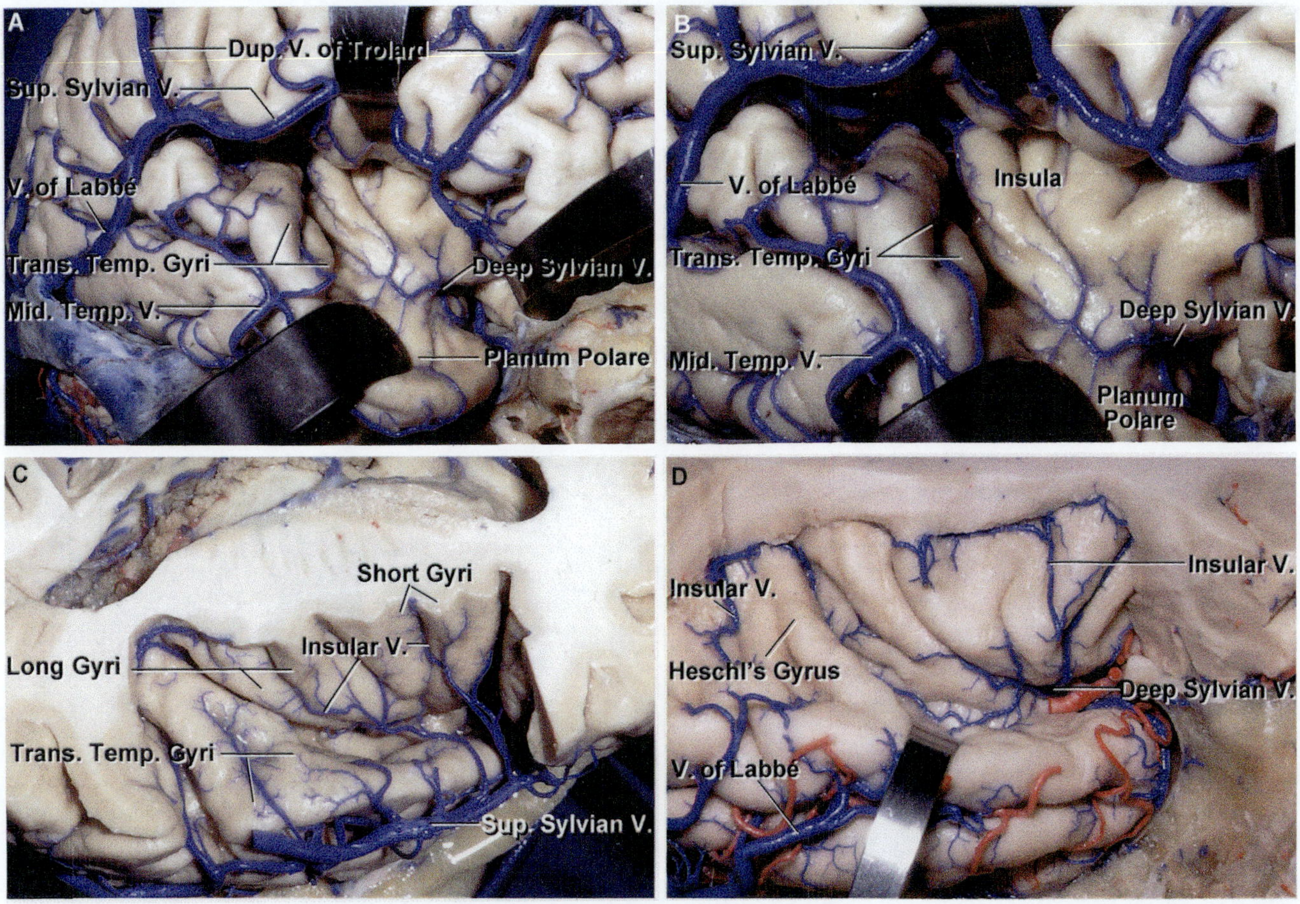

FIGURE 4.23. A, *sylvian and insular veins. Lateral view of the sylvian fissure. The posterior two-thirds of the superficial sylvian vein is larger than the anterior third, which is very small. The large posterior segment of this superficial sylvian vein joins the vein of Labbé and the anterior end joins an anastomotic vein crossing the frontal lobe. Duplicate anastomotic veins fitting the criteria for a vein of Trolard connect the sagittal sinus to the sylvian veins: one crosses the frontal lobe and the other crosses the parietal lobe. The lip of the sylvian fissure has been retracted to expose a small deep sylvian vein, which crosses the insula and passes medially below the anterior perforated substance to join the basal vein. The lower retractor is on the planum polare, an area free of gyri on the upper surface of the temporal lobe. Further posteriorly on the upper surface of the temporal lobe are the transverse temporal gyri that form the planum temporale.* B, *enlarged view of another specimen. The lower opercular lip has been retracted to expose the deep sylvian veins passing around the lumen insula to course below the anterior perforated substance and join the anterior end of the basal vein.* C, *the frontoparietal operculum has been removed. The veins draining the opercular lips and insula pass predominantly to the large superficial sylvian vein rather than forming a large deep sylvian vein.* D, *another specimen showing the veins on the insula converging to form a deep sylvian vein that passes above the middle cerebral artery and below the anterior perforated substance to join the anterior end of the basal vein. The most anterior of the transverse temporal gyri is Heschl's gyrus.* Dup., *duplicate;* Mid., *middle;* Sup., *superior;* Temp., *temporal;* Trans., *transverse;* V., *vein.*

◄

geminal cistern. The roof of the temporal horn formed by the thalamus and tapetum of the corpus callosum is drained by the inferior ventricular vein that joins the basal vein by passing through the choroidal fissure. This basal vein in this case does not empty into the vein of Galen, but passes laterally below the temporal lobe to empty into a tentorial sinus. E, *lateral view of another basal vein. The middle segment of this basal vein is hypoplastic. The posterior segment of the basal vein receives the inferior ventricular vein and passes around the midbrain to empty into the vein of Galen. The anterior part of the territory normally drained by the basal vein empties into the sylvian veins, leaving a hypoplastic midsegment lateral to the peduncle.* F, *anterosuperior view of the left basal vein coursing through the crural, ambient, and quadrigeminal cisterns. The basal vein arises at the union of the sylvian and anterior cerebral veins and passes posteriorly above the posterior cerebral artery in the crural cistern, located between the peduncle and uncus. It exits the crural cistern to enter the ambient cistern, located between the midbrain and parahippocampal gyrus, and terminates in the quadrigeminal cistern. The third nerve passes below the posterior cerebral artery. Medial atrial veins cross the medial atrial wall and empty into the veins in the quadrigeminal cistern. The internal cerebral vein courses in the roof of the third ventricle.* A., *artery;* A.C.A., *anterior cerebral artery;* Ant., *anterior;* Atr., *atrial;* Car., *carotid;* Cer., *cerebral;* Cer.Mes., *cerebellomesencephalic;* CN, *cranial nerve;* Coll., *collateral;* Fiss., *fissure;* For., *foramen;* Gen., *geniculate;* Inf., *inferior;* Int., *internal;* Lat., *lateral;* M.C.A., *medial cerebral artery;* Med., *medial;* P.C.A., *posterior cerebral artery;* Ped., *peduncle;* Pet., *petrosal;* S.C.A., *superior cerebellar artery;* Sup., *superior;* Tent., *tentorial;* Tr., *tract;* V., *vein;* Vent., *ventricle, ventricular;* Verm., *vermian.*

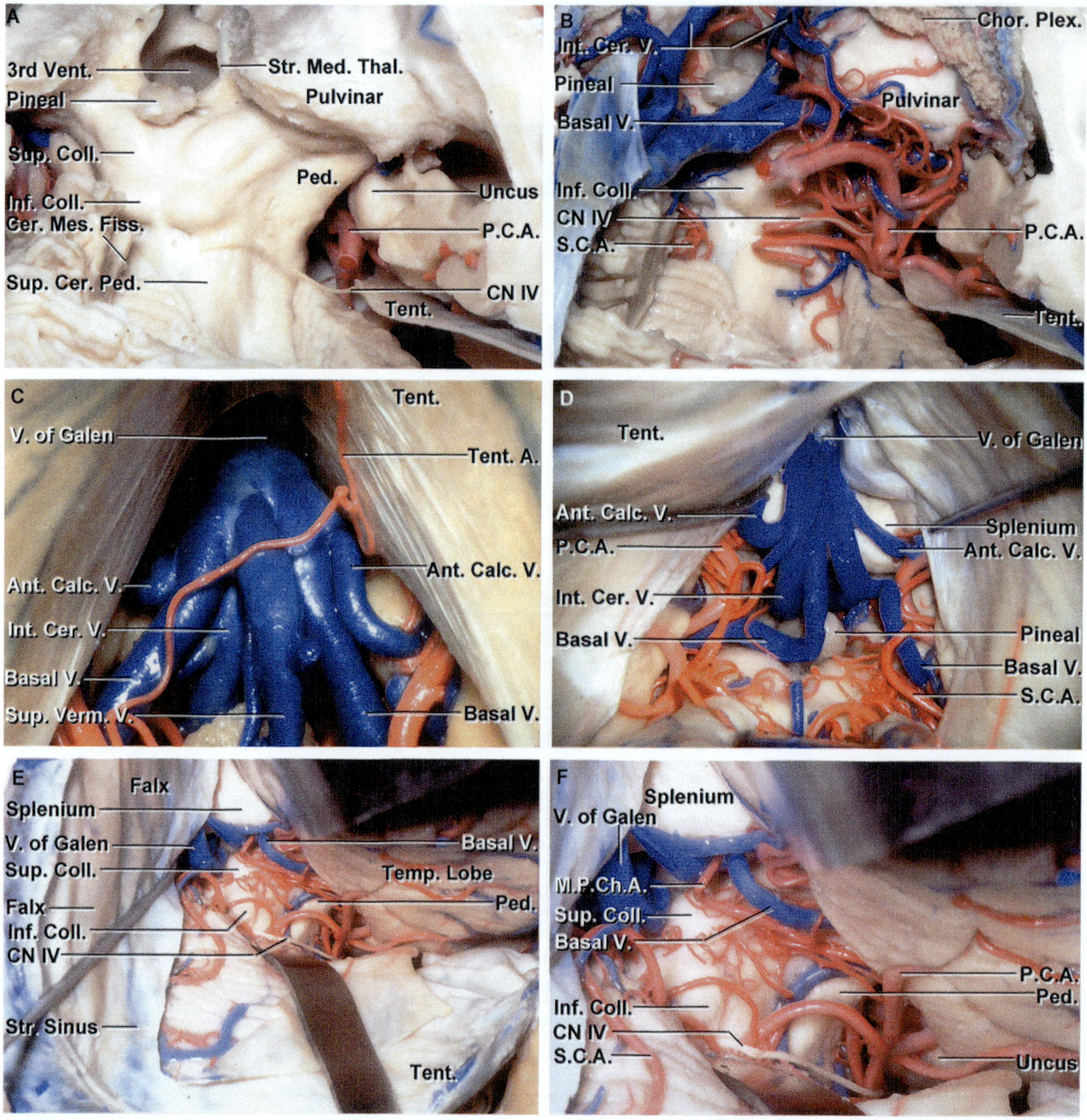

FIGURE 4.24. *Venous relationships in the quadrigeminal cistern. A, neural structures in the quadrigeminal cistern. The anterior wall of the quadrigeminal cistern is formed by the pulvinar, superior, and inferior colliculi and the superior cerebellar peduncles. The cistern extends downward between the cerebellum and midbrain into the cerebellomesencephalic fissure. The roof of the third ventricle, anterior to the pineal, has been opened. The striae medullaris thalami extend forward along the lateral wall of the third ventricle, beginning posteriorly at the habenular commissure. The right temporal horn, uncus, and cerebral peduncle have been exposed. B, the internal cerebral and basal veins join in the quadrigeminal cistern to form the vein of Galen. The posterior cerebral arteries enter the upper part of the quadrigeminal cistern and the superior cerebellar arteries enter the lower part. The trochlear nerve courses between the superior cerebellar and posterior cerebral arteries. C, infratentorial exposure of the venous complex in the supracerebellar area. The basal, internal cerebral, anterior calcarine, and superior vermian veins converge on the vein of Galen. The left posterior cerebral artery gives rise to a branch that enters the lower surface of the tentorium. D, another specimen. The internal cerebral, basal, and anterior calcarine veins converge on the vein of Galen. E and F, occipital transtentorial exposure. E, the occipital lobe has been retracted and the tentorium divided adjoining the straight sinus to expose the quadrigeminal cistern. F, enlarged view. The exposure extends forward to the margin of the cerebral peduncle, uncus, and the crural cistern. The basal vein*

ance and converge to an apex at the anterior perforated substance. The peduncular vein originates on the posterior perforated substance, courses laterally around the cerebral peduncle, and usually joins the basal vein at the junction of the anterior and middle cerebral incisural spaces. Small veins from the anterior part of the medial surface of the uncus cross the anterior incisural space and terminate in the deep middle cerebral vein or the anterior part of the basal vein.

Middle Incisural Space

The middle incisural region, which is drained by the middle segment of the basal vein, is located between the midbrain and the temporal lobe (*Figs. 4.4, 4.17,* and *4.20–4.22*). Its anterior part contains the crural cistern, and its posterior part contains the ambient cistern. The venous relationships in the middle incisural space are relatively simple. The major venous trunk in this space is the middle segment of the basal vein, which courses along the upper part of the cerebral peduncle and below the pulvinar to reach the posterior incisural space. The basal vein may infrequently terminate in a tentorial sinus in the free edge at this level. The tributaries of this segment of the basal vein are from the temporal horn and medial temporal surface, including the uncus and lateral midbrain.

The veins in this area are as follows: the inferior ventricular vein, which drains the roof of the temporal horn; the anterior longitudinal hippocampal vein, which courses anteriorly along the dentate gyrus toward the inferior choroidal point; the anterior hippocampal vein, which originates on the uncus and the posterior portion of the amygdaloid nucleus and proceeds posteriorly along the anterior hippocampal sulcus to form a common stem with the inferior ventricular or anterior longitudinal hippocampal vein; the lateral mesencephalic vein, which courses along the lateral mesencephalon; the temporal cortical veins from the posterior two-thirds of the uncus; and the medial temporal veins from the adjacent part of the parahippocampal and occipitotemporal gyri.

Posterior Incisural Region

The posterior incisural space is situated posterior to the midbrain and corresponds to the pineal region (*Figs. 4.9, 4.17, 4.19, 4.22,* and *4.24*). This space is occupied by the quadrigeminal cistern. The venous relationships in the posterior incisural region are the most complex in the cranium because the internal cerebral, basal, and great veins and many of their tributaries converge on this area. The internal cerebral veins exit the velum interpositum to reach the posterior incisural space, where they join to form the vein of Galen. The posterior segment of the basal vein begins at the posterior margin of the ambient cistern, where the vein passes to the posterior margin of the midbrain to reach the quadrigeminal cistern, and it terminates in the internal cerebral or great veins. If the posterior segment of the basal vein is absent, the middle segment drains into a sinus in the tentorial edge. The great vein passes below the splenium to enter the straight sinus at the tentorial apex. The junction of the vein of Galen with the straight sinus varies from being nearly flat if the tentorial apex is located below the splenium to forming an acute angle if the tentorial apex is located above the level of the splenium, so that the great vein must turn sharply upward to reach the straight sinus at the tentorial apex.

The tributaries of the internal cerebral, basal, and great veins in the quadrigeminal cistern are as follows: the atrial veins, which are described above, under Ventricular Veins; the posterior longitudinal hippocampal vein, which courses along the posterior portion of the dentate gyrus; the posterior pericallosal vein, which courses around the posterior surface of the splenium; the superior vermian vein, the largest vein from the infratentorial part of the posterior incisural space, which arises on the vermic surface forming the floor of the posterior incisural space and receives the superior hemispheric veins from the adjacent cerebellar surface and the vein of the cerebellomesencephalic fissure and empties into the great vein; the tectal veins originating on or near the superior and inferior colliculi; the epithalamic veins, which emerge from the posterior part of the third ventricle in the region of the pineal body and drain the posteromedial part of the thalamus and adjacent epithalamic areas, including the pineal body, posterior and habenular commissures, and neighboring portions of the thalamus—the most posterior of the medial temporal veins draining the posterior part of the parahippocampal and occipitotemporal gyri; the medial occipitotemporal veins, which arise on the lingula and the occipitotemporal gyri; the internal occipital veins, which originate in the area of the calcarine and parietooccipital sulci; and the thalamic veins from the superior and medial portions of the thalamus that drain into the internal cerebral or great veins, and these form the inferior and lateral portions of the thalamus, which drain into the basal vein or its tributaries. The term, thalamostriate vein, implies a relationship with the thalamus but, despite its course along the lateral margin of the thalamus, none of the thalamic veins join it.

The deep thalamic veins are divided into anterior, superior, inferior, and posterior thalamic veins. The anterior thalamic vein drains the anterior portion of the thalamus and terminates in the adjacent part of the internal cerebral, anterior septal, thalamostriate, or anterior caudate vein, or other

passes around the brainstem on the medial side of the temporal lobe to reach the quadrigeminal cistern. The internal cerebral veins exit the roof of the third ventricle and empty into the vein of Galen. A combined supra- and infratentorial exposure can be obtained by dividing the transverse sinus and tentorium, but should only be considered if there is a nondominant transverse sinus on the side of the exposure. Ant., *anterior;* Calc., *calcarine;* Cer., *cerebellar;* Cer.Mes., *cerebellomesencephalic;* Chor., *choroid;* CN, *cranial nerve;* Coll., *collateral;* Fiss., *fissure;* Inf., *inferior;* Int., *internal;* Med., *medial;* M.P.Ch.A., *medial posterior choroidal artery;* P.C.A., *posterior cerebral artery;* Ped., *peduncle;* Plex., *plexus;* S.C.A., *superior cerebellar artery;* Str., *straight;* Sup., *superior;* Temp., *temporal;* Tent., *tentorial, tentorium;* Thal., *thalamus;* V., *vein;* Vent., *ventricle;* Verm., *vermian.*

smaller veins in the region. The superior thalamic vein is the largest of the thalamic veins. It arises in the central superior part of the thalamus, runs medially to emerge from the mesial surface of the thalamus near the striae medullaris thalami, runs posteriorly below the internal cerebral vein in the velum interpositum, and ends in the internal cerebral or the great vein. The inferior thalamic veins arise in the anteroinferior part of the thalamus and traverse the posterior perforated substance to drain into the posterior communicating or peduncular vein.

The posterior thalamic veins drain the posterior inferolateral portion of the thalamus and empty into the posterior part of the basal vein or the veins coursing on the posterolateral surface of the midbrain. The superficial thalamic veins course along the ventricular surface of the thalamus in a subependymal location and drain into the adjacent veins in the ventricle, velum interpositum, or basal cisterns.

DISCUSSION AND OPERATIVE APPROACHES

The distribution of the superficial cortical veins is not as irregular and variable as is generally supposed, and their examination during the venous phase of the cerebral angiogram may prove helpful in localizing expanding lesions by revealing poor filling and displacement and alteration in the direction of flow. Although the majority of the superficial cortical veins do not course along the sulci, some may be helpful in locating the sulci. The veins that most commonly approximate the position of a sulcus (and their respective sulci) are the superficial sylvian veins and the sylvian fissure, the precentral vein and the precentral sulcus, the central vein and the central sulcus, the postcentral vein and the postcentral sulcus, the anteromedial parietal vein and the ascending ramus of the cingulate sulcus, the posteromedial parietal vein and the parieto-occipital sulcus, and the anterior and posterior pericallosal veins and the anterior and posterior parts of the callosal sulcus. The tendency of these veins to approximate the position of a sulcus becomes less prominent as the veins approach the sinuses.

There is considerable variation in the size of the individual cortical veins, not only in different brains, but also from side to side in the same brain. The veins on the lateral surface are larger than those on the medial and inferior surfaces. The largest veins on the lateral surface are usually in the region of the central sulcus. The veins on the lateral surface are arranged like the spokes of a wheel; they radiate outward from the stem of the sylvian fissure. The three largest pathways of cortical drainage on the lateral surface are through the veins of Trolard and Labbé and the superficial sylvian veins (*Figs. 4.10* and *4.11*). According to DiChiro (7), the vein of Labbé predominates in the dominant hemisphere nearly twice as often as it predominates in the nondominant hemisphere, and the vein of Trolard predominates in the nondominant hemisphere with approximately the same frequency.

The fact that sacrifice of the individual cortical veins only infrequently leads to venous infarction, hemorrhage, swelling, and neurological deficit is attributed to the diffuse anastomoses between the veins. There are abundant anastomoses between the individual cortical veins draining adjacent cortical areas and between the superficial cortical veins and the deep ventricular and cisternal veins. There are also anastomoses along the borders of the hemisphere between the veins draining the adjacent parts of the lateral, medial, and basal surfaces. The latter anastomoses are located at the terminal ends of the veins just proximal to where the bridging veins enter the dural sinuses.

Obliteration of the superficial and deep bridging veins, including the great, basal, and internal cerebral veins, is inescapable in some operative approaches; however, the number of these veins and their branches to be sacrificed should be kept to a minimum because of the possible undesirable sequelae, which, although usually transient, may be permanent. Before sacrificing these veins, the surgeon should try to work around them, displacing them out of the operative route, or placing them under moderate or even severe stretch, accepting the fact that they may be torn, if this will yield some possibility of their being saved. Another option is to divide only a few of their small tributaries, which may allow the displacement of the main trunk out of the operative field. The natural reluctance to sacrifice a bridging vein should be increased if the vein in the operative exposure seems larger than normal (*Fig. 4.12*). The increase in size usually signifies that the vein drains a larger area than normal and increases the likelihood of ill effect if it is sacrificed. In some cases, a large vein of Trolard or Labbé or a large superficial sylvian vein may drain the majority of the lateral surface of a hemisphere. Occlusion of the bridging veins formed by the terminal end of several cortical veins causes more difficulty than sacrifice of a bridging vein formed by the terminal end of one vein or obliteration of the individual vein on the cortical surface.

In opening the dura mater adjoining the superior sagittal sinus, one should attempt to preserve the meningeal sinuses, which may arise as far as 2.5 cm lateral to the superior sagittal sinus (*Fig. 4.2, C* and *D*). These sinuses may receive the terminal end of numerous cortical veins. In removing a parasagittal tumor deep to these sinuses, the dura is opened along the edges of the sinus while preserving the sinus' proximal junction with the cortical veins and its distal junction with the superior sagittal sinus. The tumor is then separated from the lower margin of the meningeal sinus without sacrificing the sinus.

The lacunae may present a significant obstacle in operative approaches to the parasagittal region, where they spread out over the upper extent of the precentral, central, and postcentral gyri (*Fig. 4.3*). The lacunae are reported to be absent in the fetus and increase in size with advancing age (17). The increase in the size of the lacunae is accompanied by an increase in the size of the pacchionian granulations that project into the lacunae. The lacunae may extend along the medial extent of the hemisphere adjacent to the falx and as far as 3 cm laterally over the convexity. Entering or occluding a lacuna at operation does not necessarily result in occlusion of the cortical veins or the superior sagittal sinus because most of the veins course deep to the lacunae and usually empty into the sinus separately from the lacunae. The lacunae, even when large, do not have a diffuse communication with the superior sagittal sinus, but open into it through smaller apertures, which may be occluded without loss of patency of the sinus. Parasagittal meningiomas usually arise from the arachnoid granulations in the lacunae and do not necessarily occlude the adjacent cortical veins, which frequently course under rather than through the lacunae to reach the superior sagittal sinus. These veins should be carefully separated from the deep margin of the tumor by micro-operative techniques, rather than obliterating them when they are exposed along the margin of the tumor.

The operative approach directed along the falx toward the anterior part of the corpus callosum may require the sacrifice of a bridging vein to the superior sagittal sinus. Occasionally, the corpus callosum may be reached in the area between the anterior and posterior frontal veins without sacrificing any bridging veins because there is frequently a several-centimeter segment of the superior sagittal sinus between the anterior and middle frontal veins or between the middle and posterior frontal veins where no tributaries join the superior sagittal sinus (*Fig. 4.14*). Obliteration of the bridging veins to the superior sagittal sinus in the region of the precentral, central, or postcentral gyri frequently causes a contralateral hemiparesis that is more prominent in the lower than the upper extremity and is usually transient. Spontaneous occlusion of the veins in this region causes a hemiparesis that is commonly accompanied by headache and seizures (12, 14). The bridging veins joining the inferior sagittal sinus, which arise from the upper end of the anterior pericallosal vein, are infrequently mentioned in discussing the transcallosal operative approaches. These veins vary in size from a tiny tuft that drains a small cortical area to several large veins that drain both the upper portion of the corpus callosum and most of the adjacent part of the medial surface of the frontal lobes.

In the subfrontal approach, bridging veins are rarely encountered in the area between the frontal lobe and the orbital roof. The anterior end of the basal vein may be seen below the anterior perforated substance (*Figs. 4.4* and *4.21*). The veins most commonly sacrificed in this approach are those along the medial part of the exposure, which drain into the anterior end of the superior sagittal sinus, and those on the lateral side of the exposure, which empty into the sphenoparietal and cavernous sinuses adjacent to the sphenoid ridge. The posterior part of the orbital surface of the frontal lobe can usually be retracted away from the upper surface of the sphenoid ridge without sacrificing any veins because most of the tributaries along the sphenoid ridge join the sphenoparietal sinus below the edge of the ridge.

Reaching lesions in the basal cisterns by the frontotemporal (pterional) and subtemporal approaches may require the sacrifice of one or more bridging veins entering the dual sinuses adjacent to the sphenoid ridge, which courses toward the cavernous sinus (*Figs. 4.5* and *4.12*). It is often necessary to sacrifice one or more of the veins entering the sphenoparietal, sphenobasal, or cavernous sinus to retract the temporal pole away from the adjacent part of the sphenoid ridge. It may be possible to preserve the bridging veins entering the sinuses along the sphenoid ridge if the frontotemporal approach is entirely above the sphenoid ridge or if the subtemporal approach is entirely below the temporal pole. It is usually necessary to sacrifice some of the superficial or deep sylvian bridging veins if both the posterior frontal area and the temporal tip are retracted away from the sphenoid ridge. Obliteration of the superficial or deep sylvian veins along the sphenoid ridge may cause seizures and a facial palsy plus aphasia if the occlusion is on the left side (2, 13).

Many bridging veins are encountered further posteriorly under the temporal lobe (*Fig. 4.5*). These veins include the temporal, occipital, temporobasal, and occipitobasal veins and the vein of Labbé. Sacrifice of these veins, which pass from the lower part of the hemisphere to the transverse and tentorial sinuses, frequently causes some degree of venous infarction and edema of the temporal lobe. A contralateral hemiparesis, more marked in the face and arm than the leg, with an aphasia if the dominant hemisphere is affected, may follow occlusion of these veins (4). The reason for the frequent difficulties encountered after retraction of the temporal lobe away from the area above the junction of the transverse and superior petrosal sinuses is that the veins from most of the lateral and basal surfaces of the temporal lobe converge on this area. These sequelae, encountered after the subtemporal operative approaches, are frequently ascribed to occlusion of the vein of Labbé; however, it is infrequent that only the vein of Labbé is sacrificed in these approaches, because there are numerous other bridging veins in the region that must also be sacrificed if the subtemporal operative exposure extends medial under the temporal lobe to the tentorial incisura.

In the occipital transtentorial operative approach, the occipital pole can usually be retracted from the straight sinus and the junction of the falx and the tentorium without sacrificing any veins to the superior sagittal or transverse sinuses (*Fig. 4.2*). The superior sagittal sinus is commonly devoid of bridging veins in the area just in front of the torcular herophili, but bridging veins are encountered if the exposure is directed further forward along the superior sagittal sinus in the posterior parietal area. The posterior calcarine vein, which empties into the veins on the lateral surface and into the superior sagittal sinus 4 to 9 cm proximal to the torcular herophili, is infrequently encountered in the occipital transtentorial approaches. However, the anterior calcarine (internal occipital) vein, which crosses at a much deeper level, frequently blocks access to the quadrigeminal cistern as it passes from the anterior end of the calcarine fissure to the great vein, thus making its obliteration unavoidable in reaching some tumor in the pineal region (*Figs. 4.9* and *4.24*). Sacrificing the anterior calcarine vein may cause a homonymous hemianopsia. No bridging veins pass directly from the occipital lobe to the straight sinus.

The medial and lateral tentorial sinuses may be encountered in the operative approaches in which the tentorium is divided (*Figs. 4.4* and *4.5*). The medial tentorial sinus would be encountered in incising the tentorium from anterior to posterior adjacent to the straight sinus, as might be conducted in an occipital transtentorial or infratentorial supracerebellar approach. The lateral tentorial sinus would be encountered in the lateral part of an incision in the tentorium extending from the free edge toward the transverse sinus in the area just behind the petrous ridge, as would be conducted in a subtemporal approach to the front of the brainstem. The veins that arise on the brainstem and cerebellum and drain into the superior petrosal sinus are also encountered in sectioning the anteromedial edge of the tentorium through a subtemporal craniectomy to expose the trigeminal nerve. The temporobasal bridging veins, which have relatively strong adhesions to the dura mater of the middle fossa and the superior surface of the tentorium, could be injured proximal to their termination during elevation of the temporal lobe in the course of a subtemporal operative approach to the basal cisterns.

The deep cerebral veins may pose a major obstacle to operative approaches to deep-seated lesions, especially in the pineal region, where multiple veins converge on the great vein (*Figs. 4.9, 4.17,* and *4.24*) (25, 31). The fact that sacrifice of the major trunks of the deep venous system only infrequently leads to venous infarction with mass effect and neurological deficit is attributed to the diffuse anastomoses between the veins. Dandy (5) noted that, not infrequently, one internal cerebral vein has been sacrificed without effect and, on a few occasions, both veins and even the great vein have been ligated with recovery without any apparent disturbance of function. On the other hand, injury to this complicated venous network has caused diencephalic edema, mental symptoms, coma, hyperpyrexia, tachycardia, tachypnea, miosis, rigidity of limbs, and exaggeration of deep tendon reflexes (2, 15, 27, 28). Occlusion of the thalamostriate and other veins at the foramen of Monro may cause drowsiness, hemiplegia, mutism, and hemorrhagic infarction of the basal ganglia (11).

The ventricular veins provide valuable landmarks in directing the surgeon to the foramen of Monro and the choroidal fissure during operations on the ventricles (*Figs. 4.18* and *4.19*). This is especially true if hydrocephalus, a common result of ventricular tumors, is present, because the borders between the neural structures in the ventricular walls become less distinct as the ventricles dilate. The thalamostriate vein is helpful in delimiting the junction of the caudate nucleus and the thalamus because it usually courses along the sulcus separating these structures.

The fact that the ventricular veins converge on the choroidal fissure assists in identifying this fissure, which is situated on the periphery of the thalamus and through which operative procedures may be directed to the third ventricle, pineal region, and crural, ambient, and quadrigeminal cisterns (*Figs. 4.16* and *4.18–4.21*). Opening through the choroidal fissure in the body of the ventricle will expose the velum interpositum and the roof of the third ventricle; opening through the fissure in the atrium will expose the quadrigeminal cistern and the pineal region; and opening through the fissure in the temporal horn will expose the crural and ambient cisterns. The venous drainage of arteriovenous malformations and tumors fed by the choroidal arteries will drain through the margin of the choroidal fissure to reach the major deep venous trunks. The arterial supply of these malformations also commonly passes through the choroidal fissure (8, 10, 22).

In the anterior transcortical or transcallosal approach through the anterior part of the corpus callosum, the veins in the frontal horn are seen to drain posteriorly toward the foramen of Monro, because the choroidal fissure does not extend into this area. The anterior caudate, anterior septal, superior choroidal, and thalamostriate veins usually join the internal cerebral veins at or near the foramen of Monro. However, these veins may pass through the choroidal fissure behind the foramen of Monro to enter the velum interpositum and course adjacent to the internal cerebral vein for a considerable distance before joining the internal cerebral vein. The junction of the thalamostriate vein with the internal cerebral vein, as seen on the lateral angiogram, usually forms an acute angle at the posterior margin of the foramen of Monro; however, the thalamostriate vein may pass through the choroidal fissure and join the internal cerebral vein posterior to the foramen of Monro, thus suggesting on the angiogram that the foramen of Monro is shifted posteriorly when it is not.

The internal cerebral vein is not seen on opening into the frontal horn because it courses in the roof of the third ventricle below the body of the fornix (*Fig. 4.18*). The anterior part of the internal cerebral vein can be exposed only by opening through or displacing the structures forming the roof of the third ventricle. One method of increasing the exposure of the roof of the third ventricle is to section a column of the fornix anterosuperior to the foramen on one side, but this will permit the exposure of no more than a short anterior segment of the internal cerebral vein. To prevent the complications associated with sectioning the fornix, Hirsch et al. (11) sectioned the thalamostriate vein at the posterior margin of the foramen of Monro, rather than damaging the fornix to enlarge the opening in the roof of the third ventricle. They stressed that interruption of this vein was harmless; however, some of their patients developed drowsiness, hemiplegia, and mutism, and occlusion of the veins at the foramen of Monro has caused hemorrhagic infarction of the basal ganglia. Other routes to the anterior part of the internal cerebral vein are by the interforniceal approach, in which the body of the fornix is split in the midline and the tela choroidea below the fornix is opened to expose the internal cerebral veins, or by the transchoroidal approach, in which the choroidal fissure is opened between the fornix and thalamus, thus allowing the fornix to be pushed to the opposite side to expose the structures in the roof of the third ventricle (1, 30). The transchoroidal and interforniceal approaches have the advantage of giving access to the central portion of the third ventricle by displacing, rather than dividing, the fibers in the fornix. These approaches are reviewed in detail in Chapter 5.

In the transcortical approach to the posterior part of the body and atrium of the lateral ventricle, the medial and lateral atrial, posterior septal, posterior caudate, and thalamocaudate veins will be seen to converge on the choroidal fissure, which, in this area, is located between the crus of the fornix and the pulvinar. These veins join the posterior end of the internal cerebral vein in the velum interpositum or the basal, internal cerebral, or great vein in the quadrigeminal cistern. To reach these veins by the transventricular approaches, the surgeon must open through the choroidal fissure or the crus of the fornix.

In these approaches through the temporal horn, the inferior ventricular vein in the roof of the temporal horn and the smaller transverse hippocampal veins in the floor of the temporal horn will be seen to converge on the choroidal fissure (*Figs. 4.16* and *4.19–4.21*). After entering the temporal horn, the choroidal fissure is opened to expose the crural and ambient cisterns and the basal peduncular, lateral mesencephalic, basal hippocampal, and inferior ventricular veins.

Lesions medial to the atrium in the quadrigeminal cistern may be reached from above the tentorium along the inferomedial surface of the occipital lobe using an occipital-transtentorial approach, through the posterior part of the lateral ventricle using a posterior transventricular approach, through the corpus callosum using a posterior interhemispheric-transcallosal approach, or from below the tentorium through the supracerebellar space using an infratentorial-supracerebellar approach. The infratentorial-supracerebellar approach is selected for many lesions because the deep venous system that caps the dorsal aspect of pineal tumors does not obstruct access to the tumor. The occipital-transtentorial approach is preferred for lesions centered at or above the tentorial edge and above the vein of Galen. The posterior transcallosal approach, in which the splenium is divided, would be used only if the lesion seems to arise in the splenium above the vein of Galen. The posterior transventricular approach through the superior parietal lobule may provide the optimal approach to a tumor involving the quadrigeminal cistern if the tumor extends into the pulvinar or involves the atrium or glomus of the choroid plexus. The approaches to the ventricle are reviewed in detail in Chapter 5.

REFERENCES

1. Apuzzo MLJ, Chikovani OK, Gott PS, Teng EL, Zee C, Giannotta SL, Weiss MH: Transcallosal, interfornicial approaches for lesions affecting the third ventricle: Surgical considerations and consequences. **Neurosurgery** 10:547–554, 1982.
2. Bailey P: Peculiarities of the intracranial venous system and their clinical significance. **Arch Neurol Psychiatry** 32:1105, 1934.
3. Braun JP, Tournade A, Panisset JL, Straub P: Anatomical and neuroradiological study of the veins of the tentorium and the floor of the middle cranial fossa, and their drainage to dural sinuses. **J Neuroradiol** 5:113–132, 1978.
4. Cambria S: Thrombosis of the vein of Labbé with hemorrhagic cerebral infarction. **Rev Neurol (Paris)** 136:321–326, 1980.
5. Dandy WE: Operative experience in cases of pineal tumor. **Arch Surg** 33:19–46, 1936.
6. Delmas A, Pertuiset B, Bertrand G: Les veines du lobe temporal. **Rev Otoneuroophtalmol** 23:224–230, 1951.
7. DiChiro G: Angiographic patterns of cerebral convexity veins and superficial dural sinuses. **AJR Am J Roentgenol** 87:308–321, 1962.
8. Fujii K, Lenkey C, Rhoton AL Jr: Microsurgical anatomy of choroidal arteries: Lateral and third ventricles. **J Neurosurg** 52:165–188, 1980.
9. Grossman CB, Potts DG: Arachnoid granulations: Radiology and anatomy. **Radiology** 113:95–100, 1974.
10. Heros RC: Arteriovenous malformations of the medial temporal lobe: Surgical approach and neuroradiologic characterization. **J Neurosurg** 56:44–52, 1982.
11. Hirsch JF, Zouaoui A, Renier D, Pierre-Kahn A: A new surgical approach to the third ventricle with interruption of the striothalamic vein. **Acta Neurochir (Wien)** 47:135–147, 1979.
12. Kalberg RM: Cerebral venous thrombosis, in Kapp JD, Schmidek HH (eds): *The Cerebral Venous System and Its Disorders*. Orlando, Grune & Stratton, 1984, pp 505–536.
13. Kaplan HA: Results of obliteration of specific cerebral veins and dural sinuses: Animal and human studies, in Kapp JD, Schmidek HH (eds): *The Cerebral Venous System and Its Disorders*. Orlando, Grune & Stratton, 1984, pp 275–281.
14. Krayenbühl H: Cerebral venous and sinus thrombosis. **Clin Neurosurg** 14:1–24, 1967.
15. Kunicki A: Operative experiences in eight cases of pineal tumor. **J Neurosurg** 17:815–823, 1960.
16. Le GrosClark WE: On the pacchionian bodies. **J Anat** 55:40–48, 1920.
17. O'Connell EA: Some observation of the cerebral veins. **Brain** 57:484–503, 1934.
18. Oka K, Rhoton AL Jr, Barry M, Rodriguez R: Microsurgical anatomy of the superficial veins of the cerebrum. **Neurosurgery** 17:711–748, 1985.
19. Ono M, Ono M, Rhoton AL Jr, Barry M: Microsurgical anatomy of the region of the tentorial incisura. **J Neurosurg** 60:365–399, 1984.
20. Ono M, Rhoton AL Jr, Peace D, Rodriguez RJ: Microsurgical anatomy of the deep venous system of the brain. **Neurosurgery** 15:621–657, 1984.
21. Rhoton AL Jr: Tentorial incisura. **Neurosurgery** 47[Suppl 1]:S131–S153, 2000.
22. Rhoton AL Jr, Fujii K, Fradd B: Microsurgical anatomy of the anterior choroidal artery. **Surg Neurol** 12:171–187, 1979.
23. Rhoton AL Jr, Hardy DG, Chambers SM: Microsurgical anatomy and dissection of the sphenoid bone, cavernous sinus and sellar region. **Surg Neurol** 12:63–104, 1979.
24. Rhoton AL Jr, Harris FS, Fujii K: Anatomy of the cavernous sinus, in Kapp JP, Schmidek HH (eds): *The Cerebral Venous System and Its Disorders*. Orlando, Grune & Stratton, 1984, pp 61–91.
25. Rhoton AL Jr, Yamamoto I, Peace DA: Microsurgery of the third ventricle: Part 2—Operative approaches. **Neurosurgery** 8:357–373, 1981.
26. Stephens RB, Stilwell DL: *Arteries and Veins of the Human Brain*. Springfield, Charles C Thomas, 1969.
27. Stern WE, Batzdorf U, Rich JR: Challenges of surgical excision of tumors in the pineal region. **Bull Los Angeles Neurol Soc** 36:105–118, 1971.
28. Suzuki J, Iwabuchi T: Surgical removal of pineal tumors (pinealomas and teratomas): Experience in a series of 19 cases. **J Neurosurg** 23:565–571, 1965.
29. Symington J: On the valvular arrangement in connection with the cranial venous circulation. **Br Med J** 2:1037, 1882.
30. Viale GL, Turtas S: The subchoroid approach to the third ventricle. **Surg Neurol** 14:71–74, 1980.
31. Yamamoto I, Rhoton AL Jr, Peace DA: Microsurgery of the third ventricle: Part 1—Microsurgical anatomy. **Neurosurgery** 8:334–356, 1981.

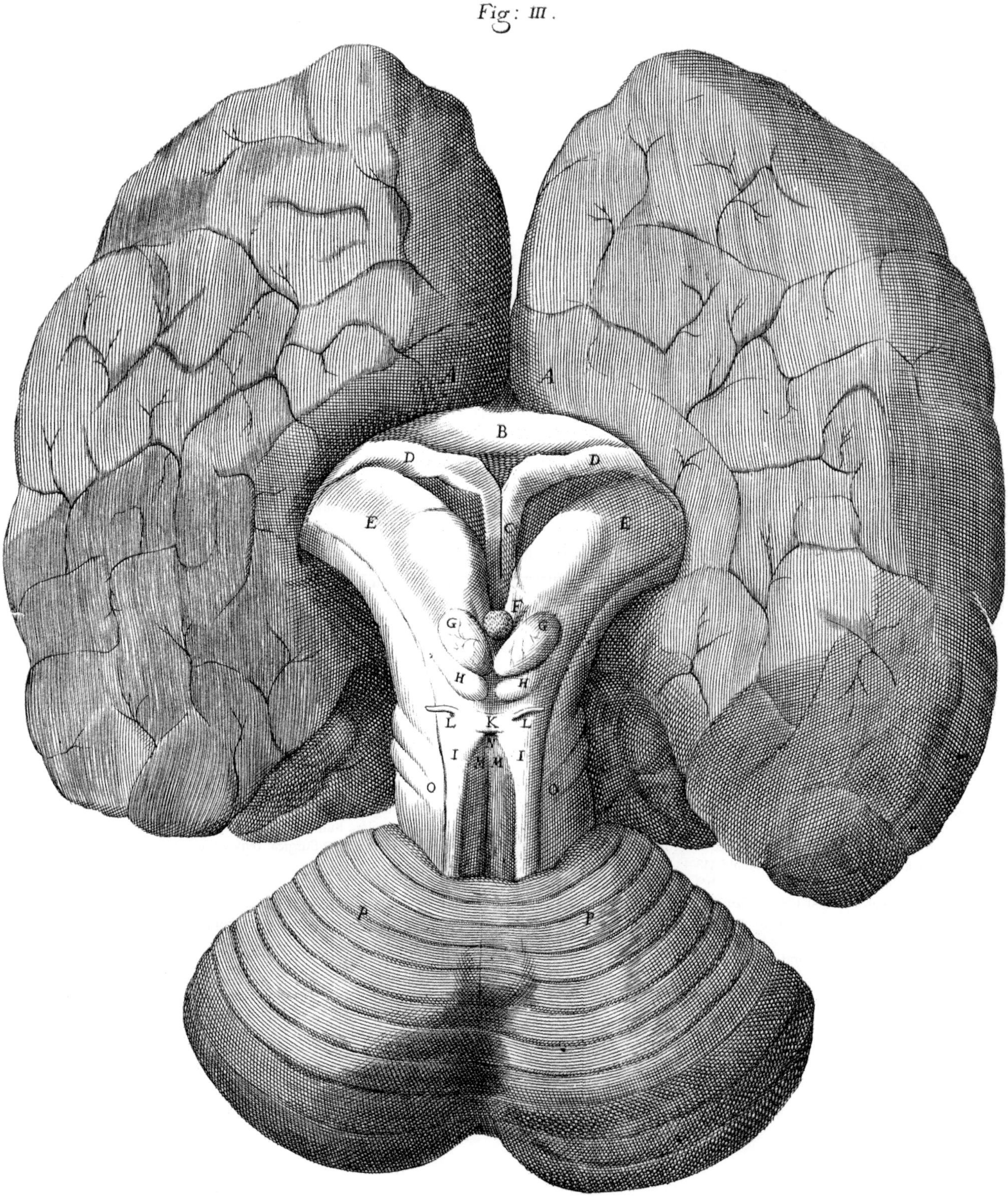

Image from Thomas Willis' Cerebri Anatome. *London, 1664, showing the outmost or superior surfaces of the human brain.*

The Lateral and Third Ventricles

Albert L. Rhoton, Jr., M.D.

Department of Neurological Surgery, University of Florida, Gainesville, Florida

Correspondence:
Albert L. Rhoton, Jr., M.D., Department of Neurological Surgery, University of Florida McKnight Brain Institute, P.O. Box 100265, 100 South Newell Drive, Building 59, L2-100, Gainesville, FL 32610-0265.
Email:
rhoton@neurosurgery.ufl.edu

KEY WORDS: Cerebral arteries, Cerebral veins, Cerebrum, Choroid plexus, Choroidal fissure, Colloid cyst, Intraventricular tumors, Lateral ventricle, Microsurgical anatomy, Operative approaches, Third ventricle

Operative approaches to the lateral and third ventricles are made challenging by their deep position near the center of intracranial space, complete encasement in neural tissue, curved shape within the cerebrum, variable shape and size in the different lobes, narrow communicating orifices making them susceptible to obstruction, expansile nature allowing them to act as mass lesions, and walls containing important motor, sensory, and visual pathways and vital autonomic and endocrine centers. The lateral ventricles provide deep cavities through which the third ventricle and basal cisterns may be approached. In this chapter, the neural and vascular relationships that provide the basis for optimizing the results obtained with intraventricular operations are reviewed before the individual operative approaches are described. Many of the structures that form part of the walls of the lateral ventricle are also seen in the third ventricle. Both the lateral and third ventricles are intimately related to the deep venous system, and numerous arteries supply the walls of both the lateral and third ventricles.

LATERAL VENTRICLE

Neural Relationships

Each lateral ventricle is a C-shaped cavity that wraps around the thalamus and is situated deep within the cerebrum (*Fig. 5.1*). Each lateral ventricle has five parts: the frontal, temporal, and occipital horns, the body, and the atrium. Each of these five parts has medial and lateral walls, a roof, and a floor. In addition, the frontal and temporal horns and the atrium have anterior walls. These walls are formed predominantly by the thalamus, septum pellucidum, deep cerebral white matter, corpus callosum, and two C-shaped structures, the caudate nucleus and the fornix, that wrap around the thalamus.

Thalamus

The thalamus is located in the center of the lateral ventricle. Each lateral ventricle wraps around the superior, inferior, and posterior surfaces of the thalamus (*Fig. 5.1A*). The body of the lateral ventricle is above the thalamus, the atrium and occipital horn are posterior to the thalamus, and the temporal horn is inferolateral to the thalamus. The superior surface of the thalamus forms the floor of the body, the posterior surface of the pulvinar of the thalamus forms the anterior wall of the atrium, and the inferior surface of the thalamus is situated at the medial edge of the roof of the temporal horn.

Caudate Nucleus

The caudate nucleus is an arched, C-shaped, cellular mass that wraps around the thalamus and constitutes an important part of the wall of the lateral ventricle (*Fig. 5.1B*). It has a head, body, and tail. The head bulges into the lateral wall of the frontal horn and body of the lateral ventricle. The body forms part of the lateral wall of the atrium, and the tail extends from the atrium into the roof of the temporal horn and is continuous with the amygdaloid nucleus near the anterior tip of the temporal horn. In the body of the lateral ventricle, the caudate nucleus is superolateral to the thalamus; in the atrium, it is posterolateral to the thalamus; and in the temporal horn, it is inferolateral to the thalamus. The stria terminalis, a fiber tract that runs parallel and deep to the thalamostriate vein, arises in the amygdaloid nucleus and courses along the border between the caudate nucleus and the thalamus in the wall of the ventricle from the temporal horn to the body.

Fornix

The fornix is another C-shaped structure that wraps around the thalamus in the wall of the ventricle (*Fig. 5.1A*). The fornix consists mainly of hippocampomamillary tract fibers that originate from the hippocampus, subiculum, and dentate gyrus of the temporal lobe. The fimbria arises in the floor of the temporal horn on the ventricular surface of the hippocampal formation and passes posteriorly to become the crus of the fornix. The crus wraps around the posterior surface of the pulvinar of the thalamus and arches superomedially toward the lower surface of the splenium of the corpus callosum. At the junction of the atrium and the body of the lateral ventricle, the paired crura meet to form the body of the fornix, which runs forward along the superomedial border of the thalami in the medial wall of the body of the lateral ventricle. The body of the fornix separates the roof of the third ventricle from the floor of the bodies of the lateral ventricles. At the anterior margin of the thalamus, the body of the fornix separates into two columns that arch along the superior and anterior margins of the foramen of Monro in their course toward the mamillary bodies. In the area below the

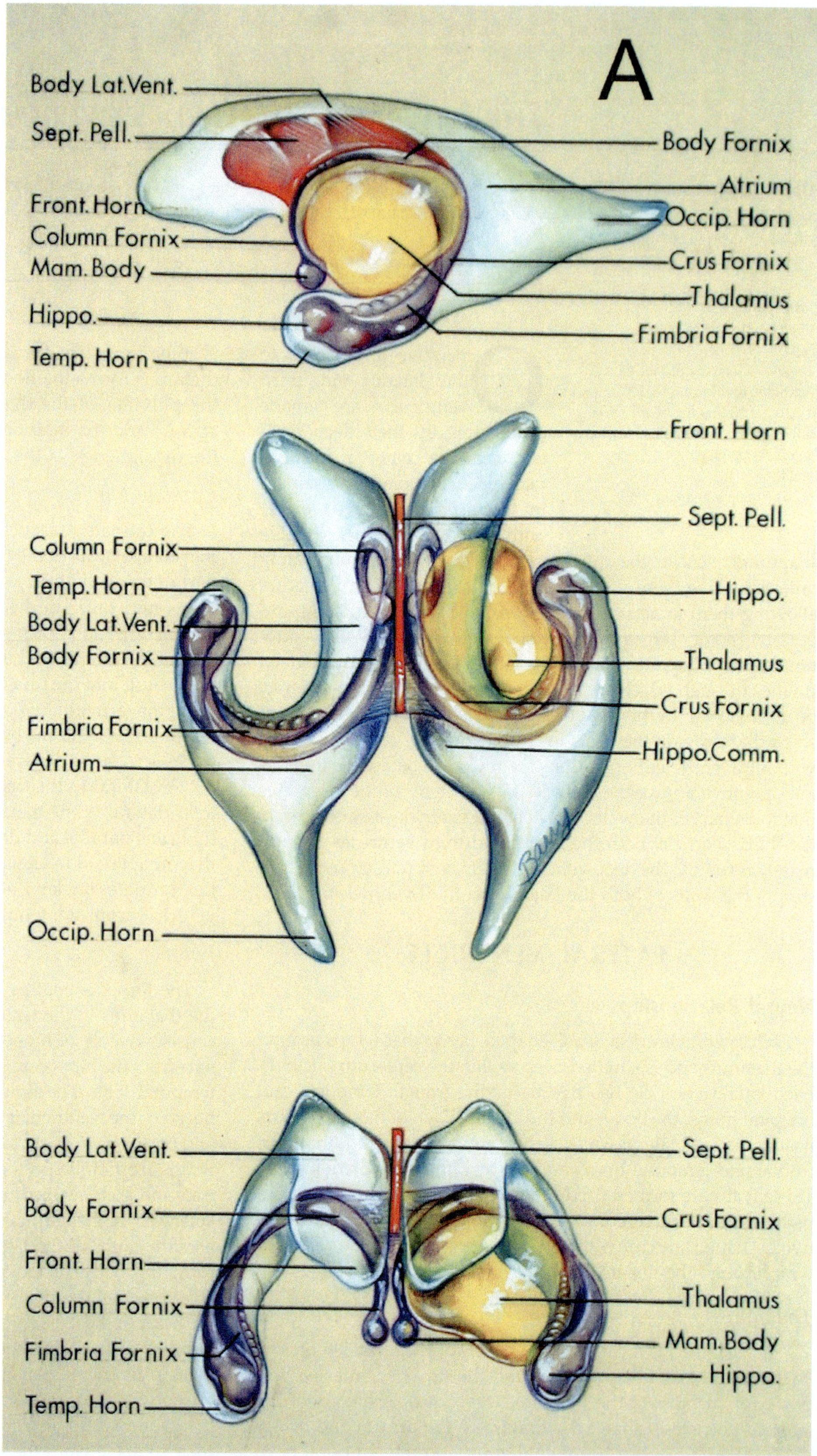

FIGURE 5.1. *Neural relationships.* A, *relationship of the septum pellucidum* (orange), *thalamus* (yellow), *and hippocampal formation and fornix* (purple) *to the lateral ventricles.* Top, *lateral view;* middle, *superior view;* bottom, *anterior view. Each lateral ventricle wraps around the thalamus. The frontal horn is anterior to the thalamus, the body is above the thalamus, the atrium and occipital horn are behind the thalamus, and the temporal horn is below and lateral to the thalamus. The septum pellucidum is in the medial wall of the frontal horn and body of the lateral ventricle. The hippocampal formation is in the floor of the temporal horn. The fornix arises in the hippocampal formation and wraps around the thalamus in the medial part of the temporal horn, atrium, and body. The fimbria of the fornix arises on the surface of the hippocampal formation in the temporal horn. The crus of the fornix is posterior to the thalamus in the wall of the atrium. The body of the fornix passes above the thalamus in the lower part of the medial wall of the body. The columns of the fornix are formed at the level of the foramen of Monro and pass inferior to the mamillary bodies. The crura of the fornix are connected across the midline in the roof of the third ventricle by the hippocampal commissure. The septum pellucidum, which separates the frontal horns in the midline, does not extend to the anterior tip of the frontal horn in the lateral view because the frontal horn is directed forward and laterally from the anterior margin of the septum pellucidum.*

FIGURE 5.1. *Continued*
B, *relationship of the corpus callosum* (red), *caudate nucleus* (green), *and fornix and hippocampal formation* (purple) *to the lateral ventricles.* Top, *view through medial surface of the hemisphere;* middle, *view through inferior surface of the hemisphere;* bottom, *view through the anterior surface of the hemisphere. The head and body of the caudate nucleus form the lateral wall of the frontal horn and body of the lateral ventricle. The tail of the caudate nucleus extends into the anterior part of the lateral wall of the atrium and into the medial part of the roof of the temporal horn to the level of the amygdaloid nucleus, which is in the anterior wall of the temporal horn. The corpus callosum is made up of the rostrum (which is in the floor of the frontal horn), the genu (which forms the anterior wall and roof of the frontal horn), the body (which forms the roof of the body of the lateral ventricle), and the splenium (which gives rise to the fiber bundles making up the forceps major, which forms a prominence in the medial wall of the atrium called the bulb of the corpus callosum). The genu of the corpus callosum gives rise to a fiber bundle called the forceps minor, which forms the anterior wall of the frontal horn. The body and splenium give rise to a fiber bundle called the tapetum, which sweeps downward to form the roof and lateral wall of the atrium and temporal horn. The relationship of the hippocampal formation, fornix, and mamillary bodies to these structures is shown in the* middle *figure. A prominence in the medial wall of the atrium, called the calcar avis, overlies the calcarine sulcus.* Amygd., *amygdaloid;* Calc., *calcarine;* Comm., *commissure;* Corp., *corpus;* Front., *frontal;* Hippo., *hippocampal, hippocampus;* Lat., *lateral;* Mam., *mamillary;* Nucl., *nucleus;* Occip., *occipital;* Pell., *pellucidum;* Sept., *septum;* Sulc., *sulcus;* Temp., *temporal;* Vent., *ventricle.*

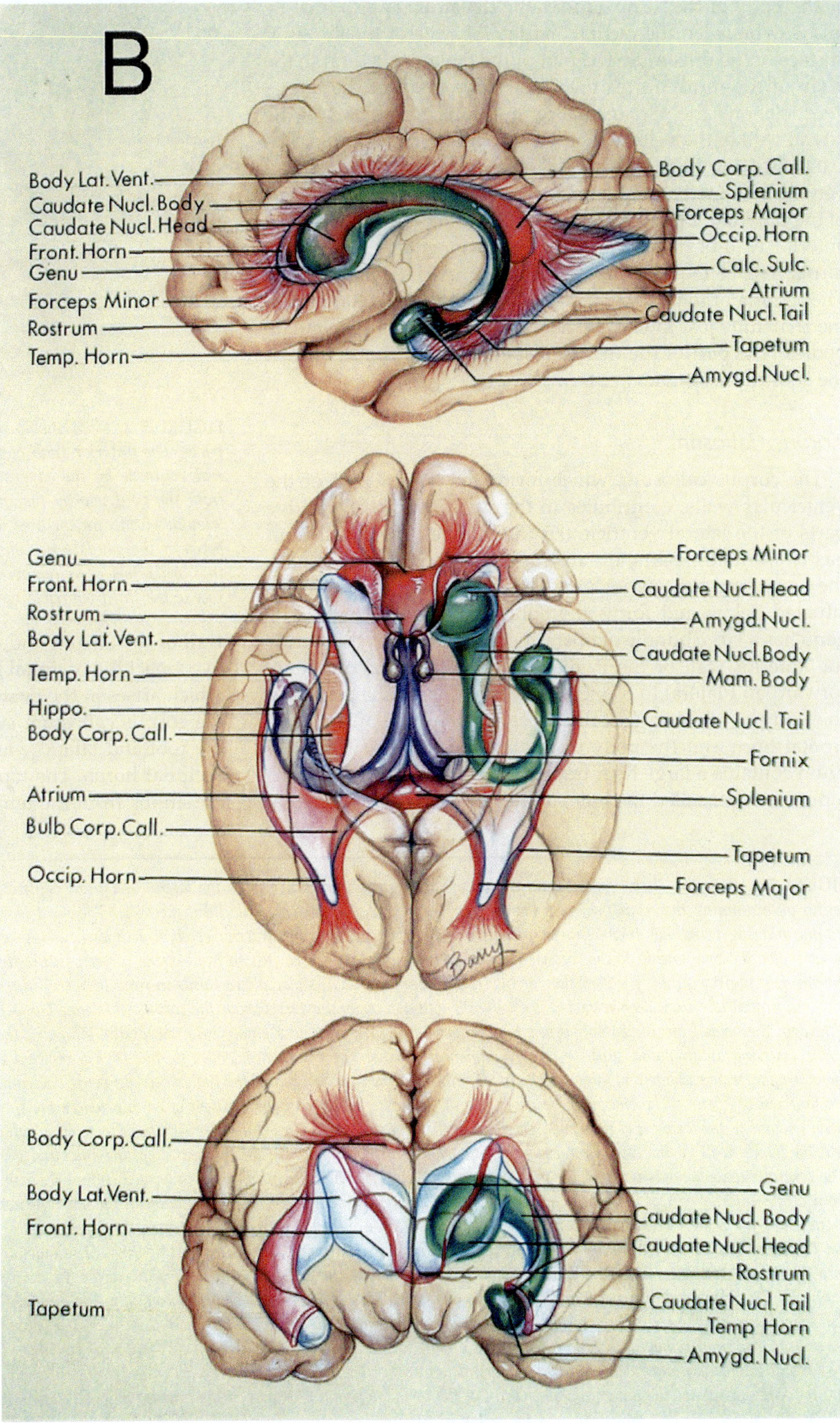

splenium, a thin sheet of fibers interconnects the medial margins of the crura to form the hippocampal commissure. In the body of the lateral ventricle, the body of the fornix is in the lower part of the medial wall; in the atrium, the crus of the fornix is in the medial part of the anterior wall; and in the temporal horn, the fimbria of the fornix is in the medial part of the floor.

The body of the fornix crosses the thalamus approximately midway between the medial and lateral edge of the superior surface of the thalamus. The part of the thalamus lateral to the body of the fornix forms the floor of the body of the lateral ventricle, and the part medial to the fornix forms part of the lateral wall of the velum interpositum and third ventricle. The crus of the fornix crosses the pulvinar approximately midway between the medial and lateral edge of the pulvinar. The part of the pulvinar lateral to the crus of the fornix forms part of the anterior wall of the atrium, and the part medial to the fornix forms part of the anterior wall of the quadrigeminal cistern. The fimbria of the fornix passes below the inferolateral part of the thalamus just lateral to the medial and lateral geniculate bodies. The part of the thalamus medial to the fimbria forms the roof of the ambient cistern.

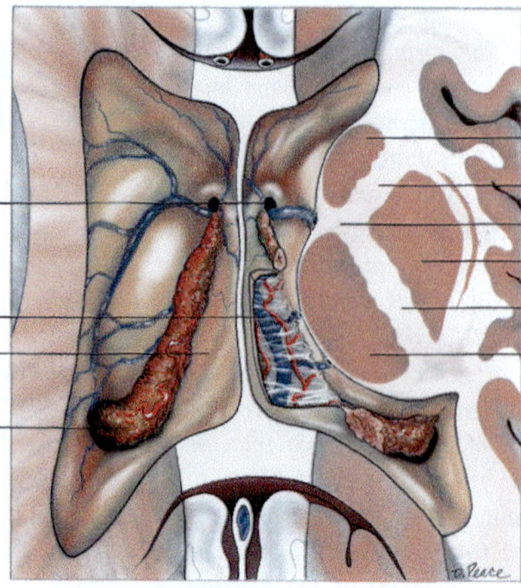

FIGURE 5.2. *Relationship of the internal capsule to the right lateral ventricle. The anterior limb of the internal capsule is separated from the lateral ventricle by the caudate nucleus, and the posterior limb is separated from the ventricle by the thalamus. The genu comes directly to the ventricular surface in the area lateral to the foramen of Monro in the interval between the caudate nucleus and thalamus. The right half of the body of the fornix has been removed to expose the internal cerebral veins in the roof of the third ventricle.*

Corpus Callosum

The corpus callosum, which forms the largest part of the ventricular walls, contributes to the wall of each of the five parts of the lateral ventricle (*Fig. 5.1B*). The corpus callosum has two anterior parts, the rostrum and genu, a central part, the body, and a posterior part, the splenium. The rostrum is situated below and forms the floor of the frontal horn. The genu has a large bundle of fibers, the forceps minor, that forms the anterior wall of the frontal horn as it sweeps obliquely forward and lateral to connect the frontal lobes. The genu and the body of the corpus callosum form the roof of both the frontal horn and the body of the lateral ventricle. The splenium contains a large fiber tract, the forceps major, that forms a prominence, called the bulb, in the upper part of the medial wall of the atrium and occipital horn as it sweeps posteriorly to connect the occipital lobes. Another fiber tract, the tapetum, which arises in the posterior part of the body and splenium of the corpus callosum, sweeps laterally and inferiorly to form the roof and lateral wall of the atrium and the temporal and occipital horns. The tapetum separates the fibers of the optic radiations from the temporal horn.

FIGURE 5.3. *Stepwise dissection used during our microsurgery courses to expose the lateral and third ventricles and the choroidal fissure. A, the dissection is begun by examining the relationships in the anterior transcallosal approach to the third ventricle. The right frontal lobe, between the large middle and posterior frontal bridging veins, has been retracted away from the falx to expose the anterior cerebral arteries coursing on the upper surface of the corpus callosum. The inset shows the relationship to the coronal suture. There is usually an area just in front of the coronal suture that is relatively devoid of bridging veins entering the superior sagittal sinus. The bone flap for the transcallosal approach is placed two-thirds in front and one-third behind the coronal suture. B, enlarged view. The falx and frontal lobe have been retracted to expose the anterior cerebral arteries above the corpus callosum. The veins draining the medial surface of the hemisphere often join the veins from the lateral surface to form large bridging veins that empty into the sagittal sinus. C, the corpus callosum has been opened to expose the fornix coursing anterior and superior to the foramen of Monro. The transcallosal opening has been completed without sacrificing a bridging vein. D, enlarged view. The anterior caudate and superior choroidal veins join the anterior end of the thalamostriate vein. The column of the fornix passes anterior and superior to the foramen of Monro. The choroidal fissure begins at the posterior edge of the foramen of Monro where the choroid plexus is attached by the tenia fimbria and tenia thalami to the fornix and thalamus. The floor of the frontal horn is formed by the rostrum of the corpus callosum, the medial wall by the septum pellucidum, and the lateral wall by the caudate nucleus. E, lateral view of the hemisphere. In the next step, the sulci and gyri on the lateral surface are examined (Fig. 1.1). The central sulcus ascends between the pre- and postcentral gyri. The precentral gyrus is located behind the pars opercularis. The postcentral gyrus is located in front of the anterior part of the supramarginal gyrus. To expose the ventricles for the dissection in the laboratory, an axial cut through the hemisphere is completed 1 cm above the posterior end of the long axis of the sylvian fissure (broken line). F, the same hemisphere after removal of the arteries and veins. The site of the cut (broken line) to expose the ventricles crosses the inferior frontal gyrus, the lower part of the central sulcus, and the supramarginal gyrus. G, superior view into the lateral ventricles. The caudate nucleus forms the lateral wall and the septum pellucidum forms the medial wall of the frontal horn and body of the lateral ventricle. The rostrum of the corpus callosum forms the floor of the frontal horn. The thalamus is in the floor of the body of the lateral ventricle. The third ventricle is located below the body of the fornix. The choroid plexus is attached along the choroidal fissure located between the fornix and thalamus. H, the frontoparietal operculum has been removed to expose the insula lateral to the frontal horn and body of the lateral ventricle. Branches of the middle cerebral artery cross the insula and the plana temporale and polare. I, superolateral view. The middle cerebral artery enters the operculoinsular compartment of the sylvian fissure by crossing the limen insula at the anteroinferior margin of the insula. The anterior part of the circular sulcus is separated from the frontal horn by the anterior isthmus of the central core of the hemisphere, and the posterior part of the circular sulcus is separated from the atrium by the posterior isthmus. J, enlarged view of the middle cerebral branches coursing along the insula. The upper temporal surface is formed posteriorly by the planum temporale where the transverse temporal gyri are located and anteriorly by the planum polare, an area free of gyri, which contains a shallow trough along which the middle cerebral artery courses. The lower part of the circular sulcus is located medial to the planum polare and temporale above the roof of the temporal horn.* (Legend continues on page 243.)

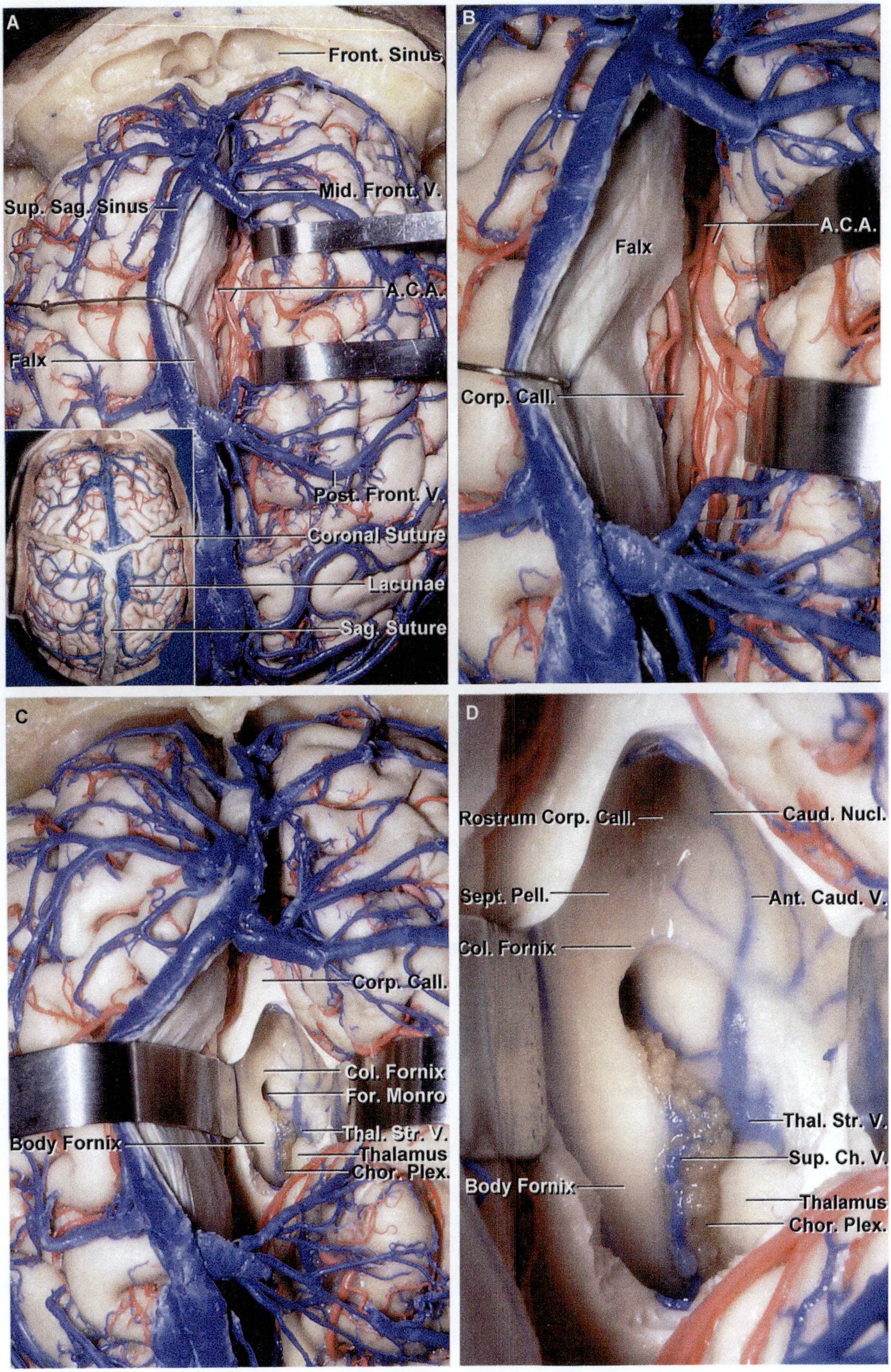
A
Front. Sinus
Mid. Front. V.
Sup. Sag. Sinus
A.C.A.
Falx
Post. Front. V.
Coronal Suture
Lacunae
Sag. Suture
B
Falx
A.C.A.
Corp. Call.
C
Corp. Call.
Col. Fornix
For. Monro
Thal. Str. V.
Body Fornix
Thalamus
Chor. Plex.
D
Rostrum Corp. Call.
Caud. Nucl.
Sept. Pell.
Ant. Caud. V.
Col. Fornix
Thal. Str. V.
Sup. Ch. V.
Body Fornix
Thalamus
Chor. Plex.

FIGURE 5.3.

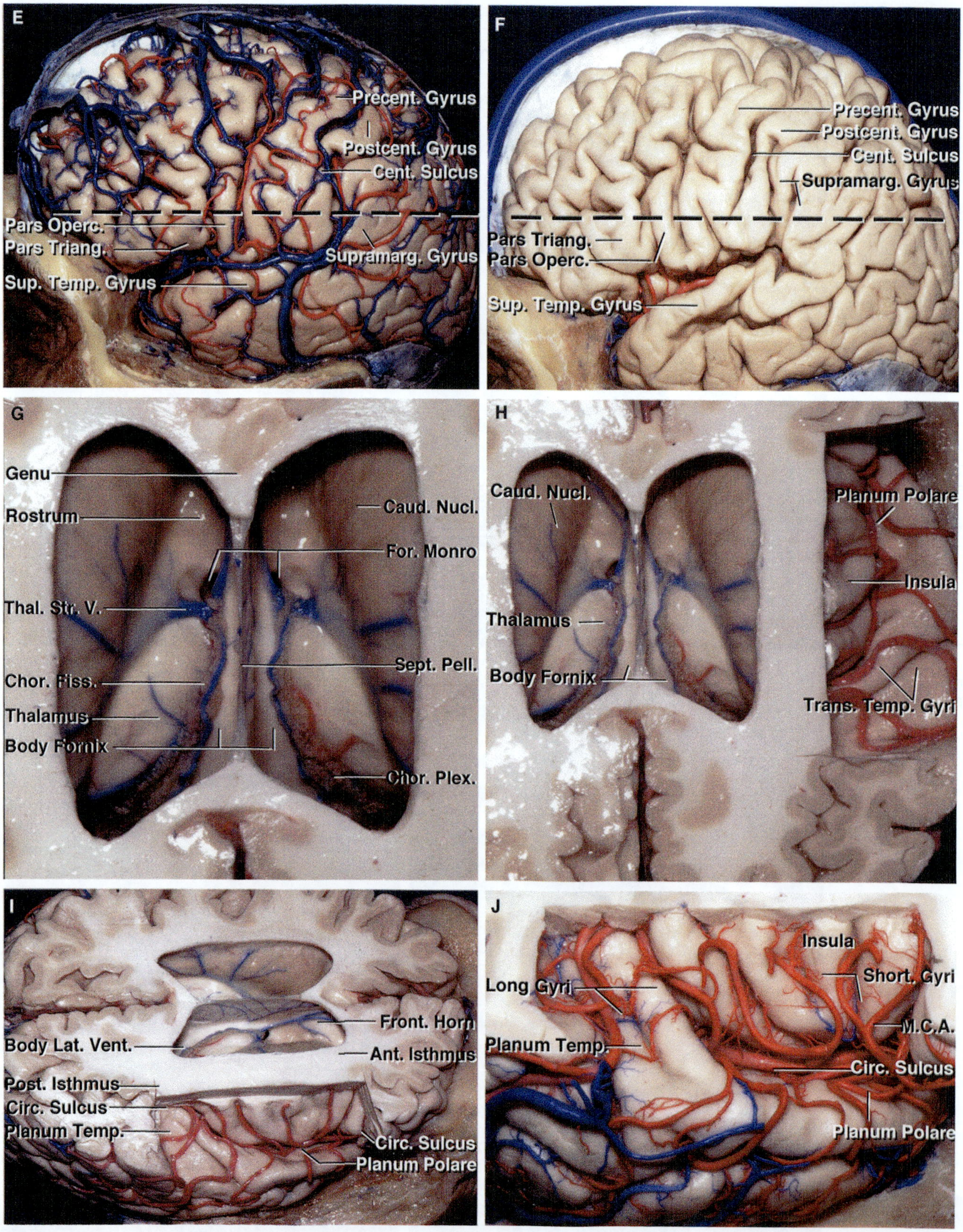

FIGURE 5.3. *Continued*

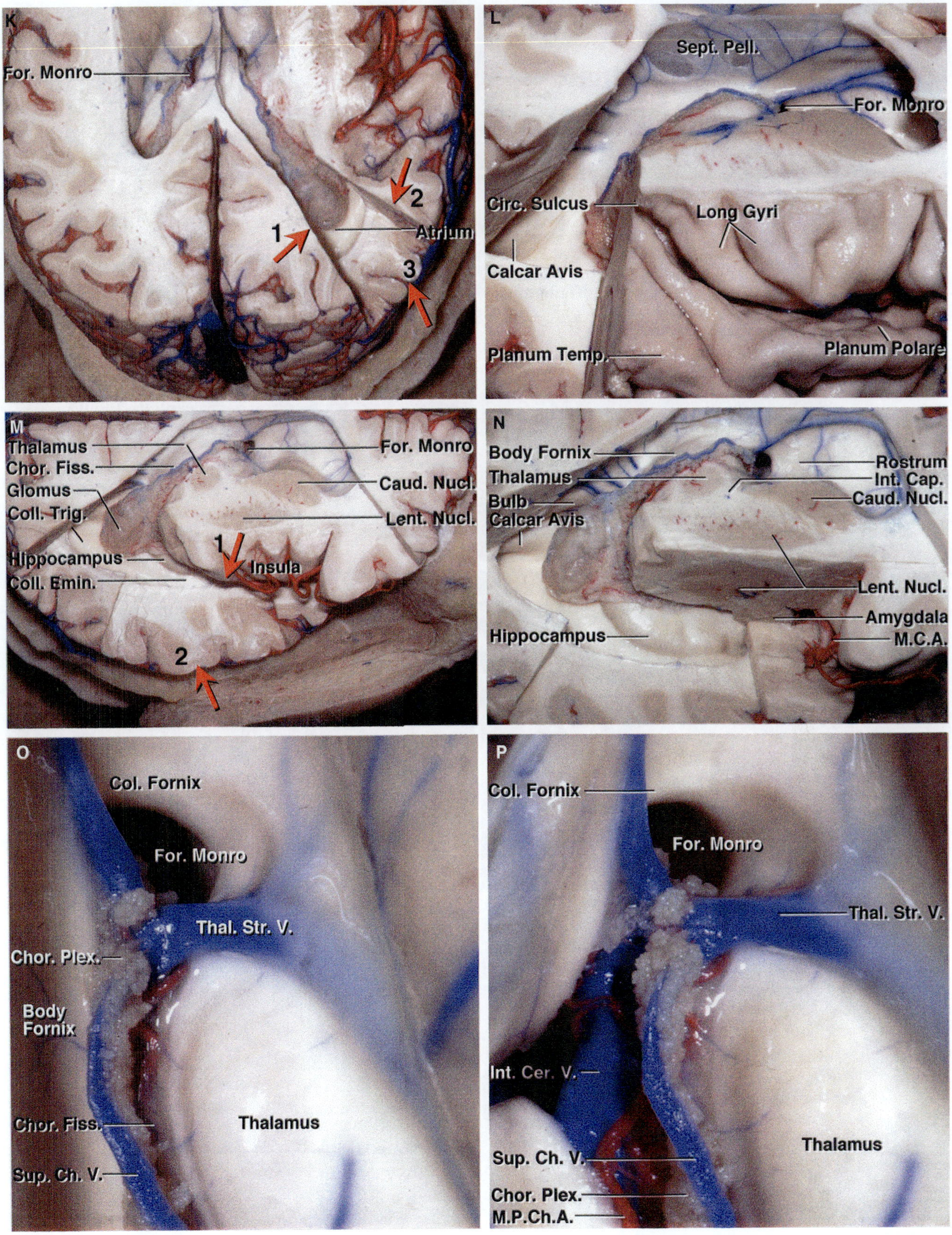

FIGURE 5.3. *Continued*

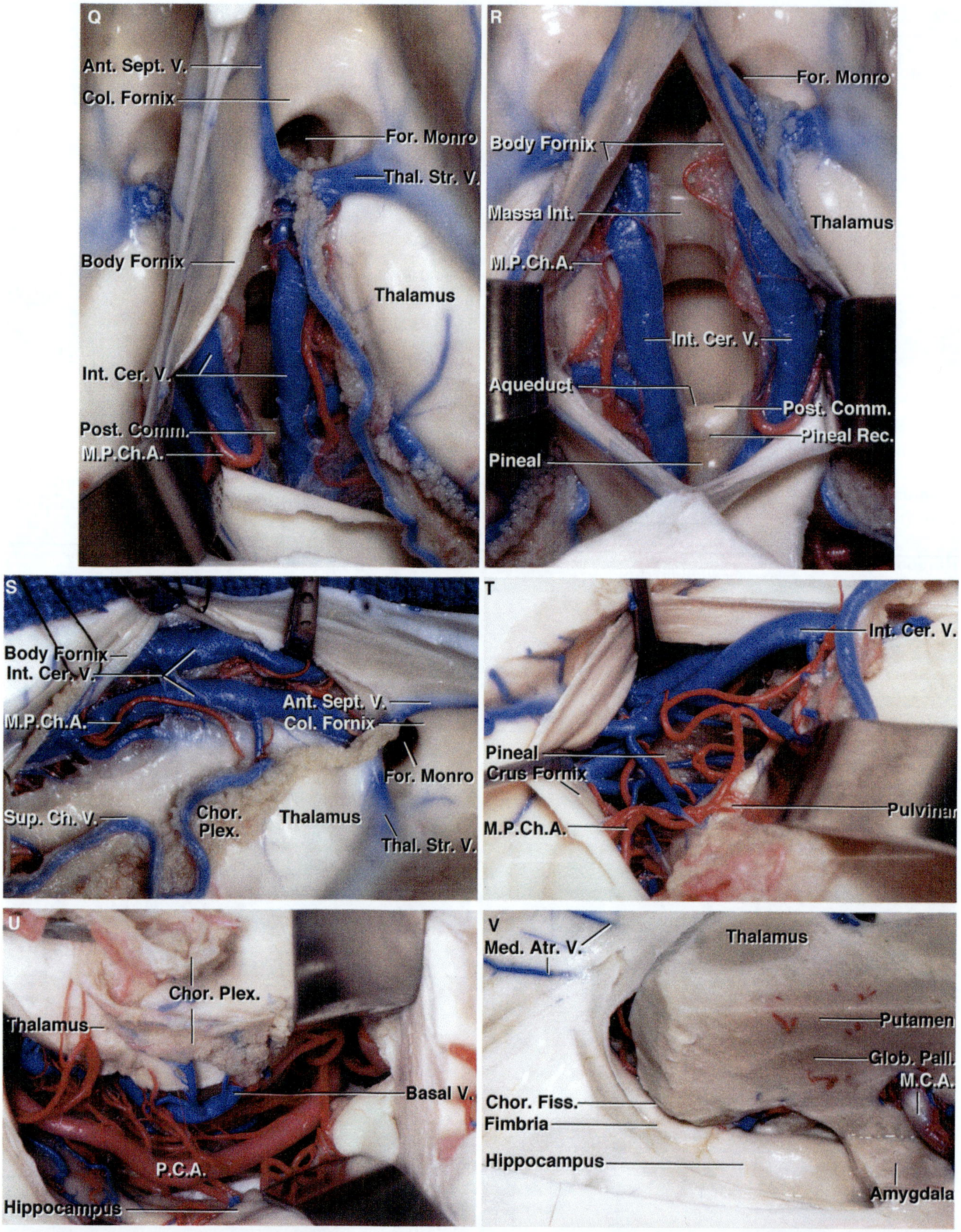

FIGURE 5.3. *Continued*

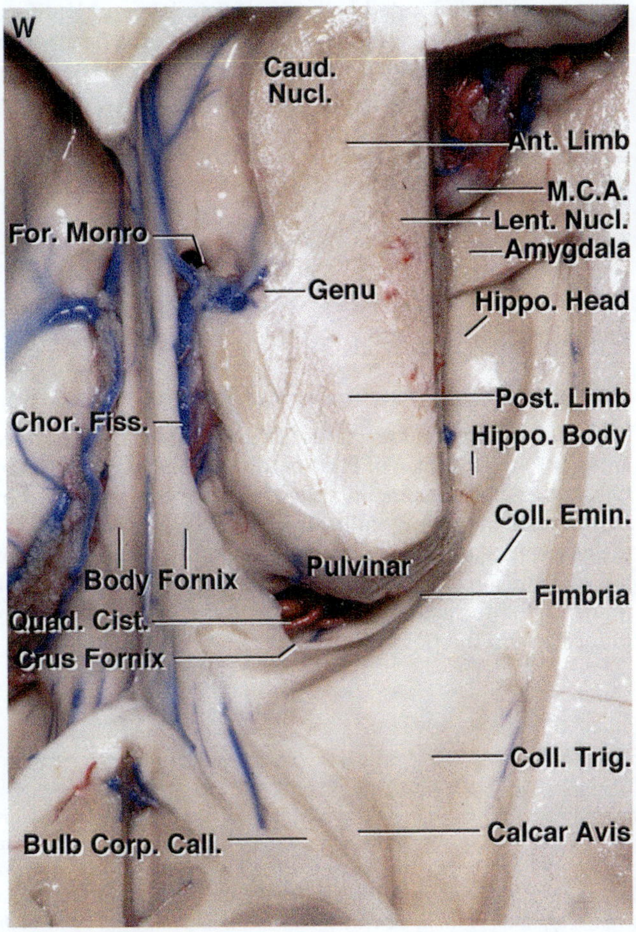

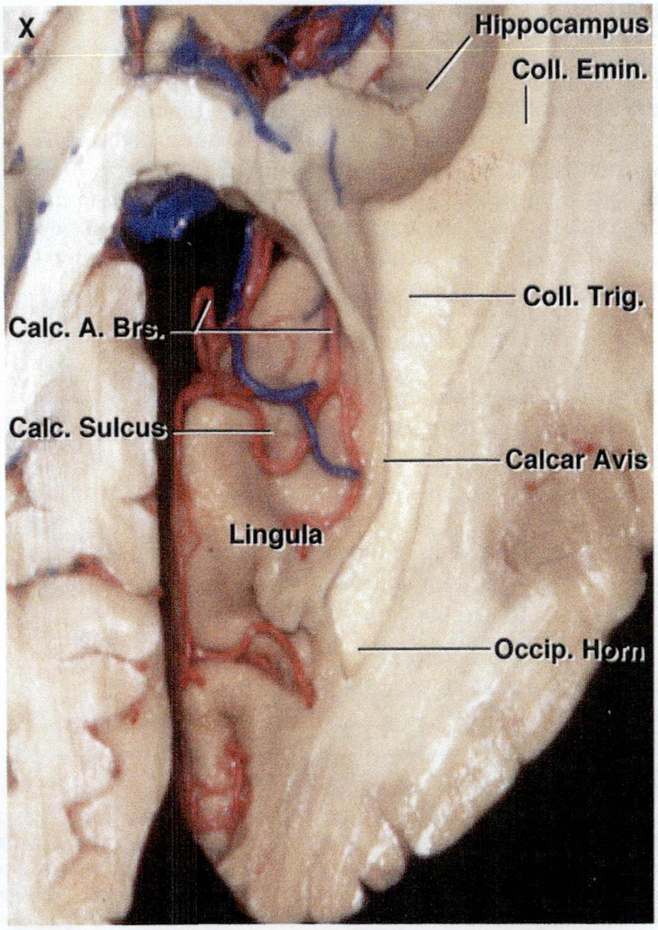

FIGURE 5.3. *Continued*
K, the initial cut through the hemisphere exposes the frontal horns and bodies of the lateral ventricles. Three cuts, two coronal cuts and one horizontal, are then completed to expose the atrium and posterior part of the temporal horn. The posterior coronal cut (No. 1) is directed obliquely forward along the medial wall of the atrium. The second coronal cut (No. 2) crosses the hemisphere at the anterior part of the atrium just behind the pulvinar. The horizontal cut (No. 3) is located at the level of the floor of the atrium. The three cuts expose the atrium from the pulvinar back to the medial wall. L, superolateral view obtained with cuts shown in K. M, the temporal horn is exposed using two cuts. One (No. 1) is directed through the lower margin of the circular sulcus to the temporal horn, and the second is a transverse cut (No. 2) located at the level of the floor of the temporal horn. Removing the block of tissue between the two cuts exposes the temporal horn. The collateral eminence overlying the deep end of the collateral sulcus is well seen, but it is difficult to see the hippocampus because it is located further medially below the insula and lentiform nucleus. N, a sagittal cut medial to the insula exposes the lentiform nucleus. The incision extends through the lentiform nucleus and amygdala. The full length of the choroidal fissure from the foramen of Monro to the inferior choroidal point, located behind the head of the hippocampus, is exposed. The bulb of the corpus callosum overlying the forceps major and the calcar avis overlying the deep end of the calcarine sulcus are exposed in the medial wall of the atrium. O, enlarged view of the foramen of Monro. The columns of the fornix pass around the superior and anterior margins of the foramen of Monro. The anterior nucleus of the thalamus sits in the posterior margin of the foramen of Monro. The thalamostriate vein passes forward between the caudate nucleus and thalamus and through the posterior margin of the foramen of Monro. The choroidal fissure in the body of the lateral ventricle is located between the body of the fornix and the thalamus. A superior choroidal vein passes along the choroid plexus. *(Legend continues on next page.)*

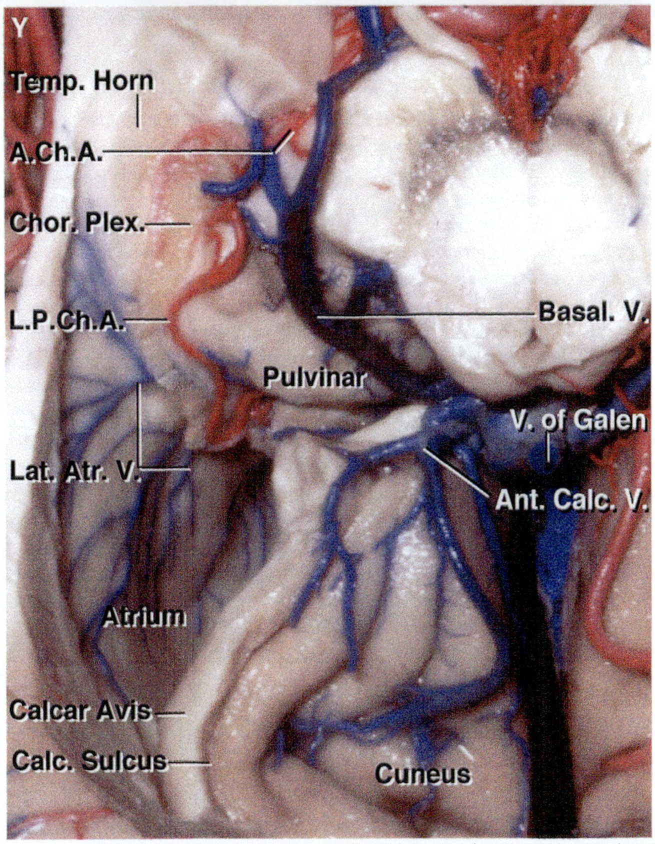

Septum Pellucidum

The septum pellucidum, which is composed of paired laminae, separates the frontal horns and bodies of the lateral ventricles in the midline (*Fig. 5.1A*). In the frontal horn, the septum pellucidum is attached to the rostrum of the corpus callosum below, the genu anteriorly, and the body above. In the body of the lateral ventricle, the septum is attached to the body of the corpus callosum above and the body of the fornix below. The septum pellucidum is tallest anteriorly and shortest posteriorly, disappearing near the junction of the body and crura of the fornix where the crura and hippocampal commissure fuse with the lower surface of the corpus callosum. The anterior-posterior length of the septum pellucidum varies from 28 to 50 mm. There may be a cavity, the cavum septum pellucidum, in the midline between the laminae of the septum pellucidum.

Internal Capsule

The close relationship of the internal capsule to the lateral wall of the frontal horn and body of the lateral ventricle is often forgotten in planning operative approaches to the ventricles (*Figs.* 5.2 and 5.3). The anterior limb of the internal capsule, which is located between the caudate and lentiform nuclei, is separated from the frontal horn by the head of the caudate nucleus, and the posterior limb, which is situated between the thalamus and the lentiform nucleus, is separated from the body of the lateral ventricle by the thalamus and body of the caudate nucleus. However, the genu of the internal capsule comes directly to the ventricular surface and touches the wall of the lateral ventricle immediately lateral to the foramen of Monro, in the interval between the caudate nucleus and the thalamus.

Lateral Ventricular Walls

Frontal Horn

The frontal horn, the part of the lateral ventricle located anterior to the foramen of Monro, has a medial wall formed by the septum pellucidum, an anterior wall and roof formed by the genu of the corpus callosum, a lateral wall composed of the head of the caudate nucleus, and a narrow floor formed by the rostrum of the corpus callosum (*Figs. 5.3–5.5*). The columns of the fornix, as they pass anterior to the foramen of Monro, are in the posteroinferior part of the medial wall.

FIGURE 5.3. *Continued*

P, the opening in the choroidal fissure is begun by dividing the tenia fornix, the delicate membrane that attaches the lateral margin of the fornix to the choroid plexus. Opening the tenia on the thalamic side, by opening the tenia thalami, carries greater risk of damaging the thalamostriate vein than opening the forniceal side of the fissure. The internal cerebral vein and medial posterior choroidal arteries are exposed in the roof of the third ventricle. Q, the opening in the choroidal fissure has been extended back to the area above the posterior commissure by dividing the tenia fornix. The choroid plexus is not disturbed on the thalamic side of the choroidal fissure. Branches of the medial posterior choroidal artery course with the internal cerebral veins. R, an interforniceal approach, in which the body of the fornix is divided longitudinally in the midline, has been completed. The massa intermedia, aqueduct, posterior commissure, pineal recess, and pineal are exposed. S, superolateral view of the dissection. The velum interpositum, located between the upper and lower layers of tela and in which the internal cerebral veins and medial posterior choroidal arteries course, has been exposed. The lower layer of tela attached to the striae medullaris thalami has not been opened. Both internal cerebral veins are exposed posterior to the foramen of Monro. If a vein at the foramen of Monro is to be sacrificed, it is preferable to sacrifice the anterior septal rather than the thalamostriate vein. T, the exposure has been extended back to the atrium where the choroid fissure has been opened by dividing the tenia fornix along the edge of the crus of the fornix. The medial posterior choroidal arteries pass along the side of the pineal and through the quadrigeminal cistern to reach the roof of the third ventricle. U, the opening in the choroidal fissure has been extended to the temporal horn. The choroidal fissure has been opened by dividing the tenia on the edge of the fimbria of the fornix to expose the posterior cerebral artery and basal veins. The choroid plexus remains attached to the thalamus. V, the choroid plexus in the right lateral ventricle has been removed. The medial atrial vein drains into the internal cerebral veins. The amygdala is exposed below the globus pallidus and just behind the middle cerebral artery coursing in the sylvian fissure. The amygdala forms the anterior wall and anterior part of the roof of the temporal horn and superiorly blends into the lower margin of the lentiform nucleus. The middle cerebral artery courses above the amygdala in the medial part of the sylvian fissure. W, superior view. The choroid plexus in the right lateral ventricle has been removed after opening the choroidal fissure from the foramen of Monro to the inferior choroidal point located just behind the head of the hippocampus. The axial section through the right hemisphere extends through the internal capsule. The genu of the internal capsule comes directly to the ventricular surface in the area lateral to the foramen of Monro. The lateral part of the floor of the temporal horn is formed by the collateral eminence, and the floor of the atrium is formed by the collateral triangle. Both the collateral eminence and trigone overlie the deep end of the collateral sulcus, which courses along the basal surface of the hemisphere between the parahippocampal and occipitotemporal gyri. The calcar avis, overlying the deep end of the calcarine sulcus, and the bulb, overlying the forceps major, are exposed in the medial wall of the atrium. X, superior view of the temporal and occipital horns with the upper part of the hemisphere removed. The section extends through the depths of the calcarine sulcus. The cuneus, forming the upper lip of the calcarine sulcus, has been removed to expose the lingula, forming the lower lip of the fissure. The calcarine sulcus extends so deeply into the medial part of the hemisphere that it produces a prominence, the calcar avis, in the medial wall of the atrium and occipital horn. Y, inferior view of the calcar avis. The lingula, forming the lower lip of the calcarine sulcus, has been removed to expose the cuneus, forming the upper lip of the sulcus. The calcarine sulcus cuts so deeply into the hemisphere that it produces a prominence in the medial wall of the atrium. The lateral atrial veins cross the lateral atrial wall. The lower part of the temporal lobe has been removed to expose the roof of the temporal lobe. The choroid plexus is attached to the lower surface of the thalamus. The anterior and lateral posterior choroidal arteries course along the medial edge of the choroid plexus. The anterior calcarine vein drains the depths of the calcarine sulcus. A.C.A., *anterior cerebral artery;* A.Ch.A., *anterior choroidal artery;* Ant., *anterior;* Atr., *atrial;* Calc., *calcarine;* Call., *callosum;* Cap., *capsule;* Caud., *caudate;* Cent., *central;* Cer., *cerebral;* Ch., *choroidal;* Chor., *choroid, choroidal;* Circ., *circular;* Cist., *cistern;* Col., *column;* Coll., *collateral;* Corp., *corpus;* Emin., *eminence;* Fiss., *fissure;* For., *foramen;* Front., *frontal;* Glob., *globus;* Hippo., *hippocampal;* Int., *intermedia, internal;* Lat., *lateral;* Lent., *lenticular;* M.C.A., *middle cerebral artery;* Med., *medial;* Mid., *middle;* M.P.Ch.A., *medial posterior choroidal artery;* Nucl., *nucleus;* Operc., *opercularis;* Pall., *pallidus;* P.C.A., *posterior cerebral artery;* Pell., *pellucidum;* Plex., *plexus;* Post., *posterior;* Postcent., *postcentral;* Precent., *precentral;* Quad., *quadrigeminal;* Rec., *recess;* Sag., *sagittal;* Sept., *septal, septum;* Sup., *superior;* Supramarg., *supramarginal;* Temp., *temporal, temporale;* Thal. Str., *thalamostriate;* Triang., *triangularis;* Trig., *trigone;* V., *vein.*

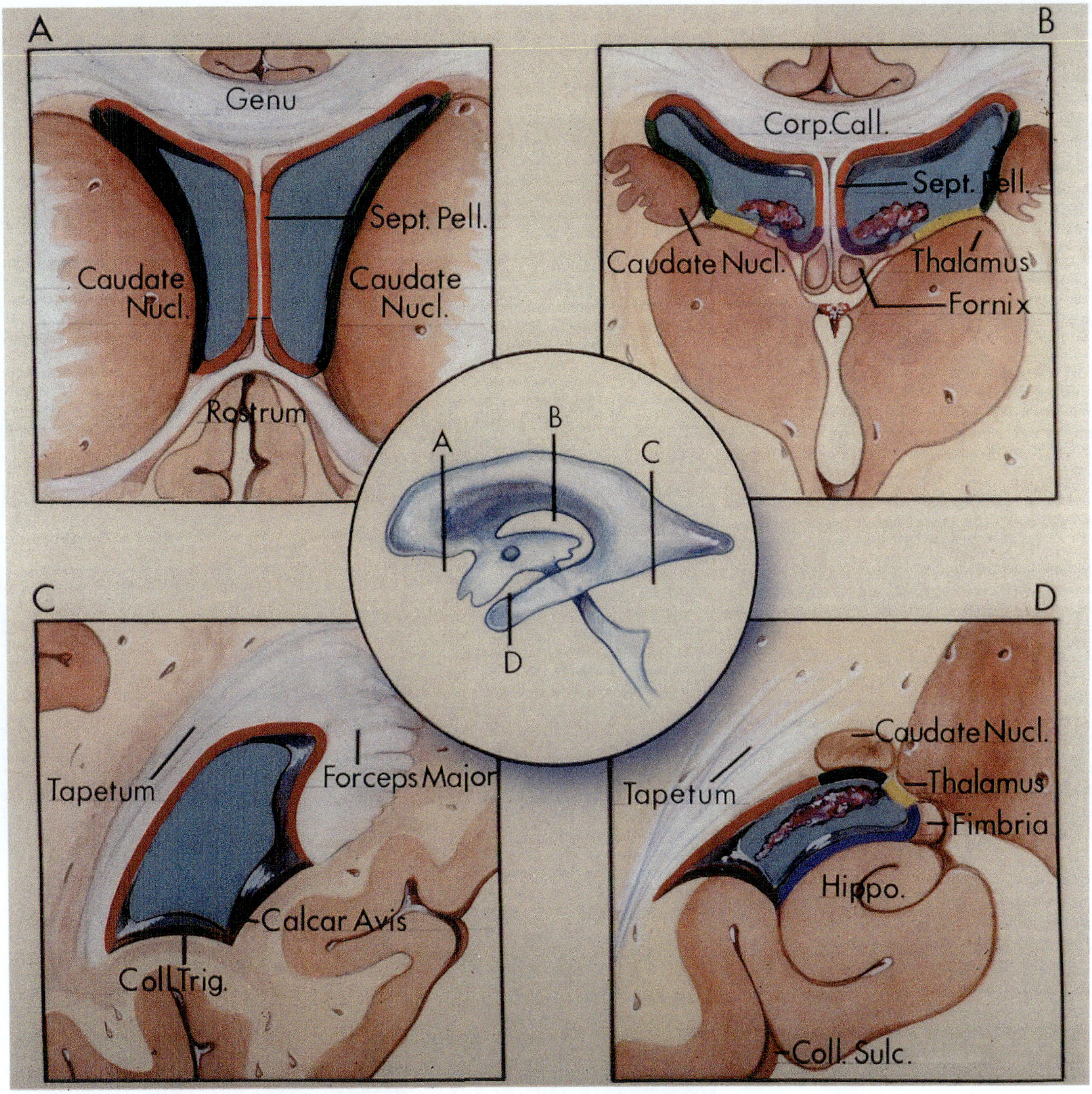

FIGURE 5.4. *Structures in the walls of the lateral ventricles. The* central *diagram shows the level of the cross sections through the frontal horn* (A), *body* (B), *atrium* (C), *and temporal horn* (D). *The ventricular surfaces formed by the various structures are shown in different colors: corpus callosum,* red; *thalamus,* yellow; *fornix and hippocampal formation,* purple; *caudate nucleus,* green; *septum pellucidum,* orange; *and the prominences overlying the collateral and calcarine sulci,* brown. A, *frontal horn. The genu of the corpus callosum is in the roof, the caudate nucleus is in the lateral wall, the rostrum of the corpus callosum is in the floor, and the septum pellucidum is in the medial wall.* B, *body of the lateral ventricle. The body of the corpus callosum is in the roof, the caudate nucleus is in the lateral wall, the thalamus is in the floor, and the septum pellucidum and fornix are in the medial wall. The choroidal fissure, the site of the attachment of the choroid plexus in the lateral ventricle, is situated between the fornix and the thalamus.* C, *atrium. The lateral wall and roof are formed by the tapetum of the corpus callosum, and the floor is formed by the collateral trigone, which overlies the collateral sulcus. The inferior part of the medial wall is formed by the calcar avis, the prominence that overlies the deep end of the calcarine sulcus, and the superior part of the medial wall is formed by the bulb of the corpus callosum, which overlies the forceps major.* D, *temporal horn. The medial part of the floor of the temporal horn is formed by the prominence overlying the hippocampal formation, and the lateral part of the floor is formed by the prominence called the collateral eminence, which overlies the deep end of the collateral sulcus. The roof is formed by the caudate nucleus and the tapetum of the corpus callosum, the lateral wall is formed by the tapetum of the corpus callosum, and the medial wall of the temporal horn is little more than the cleft between the fimbria of the fornix and the inferolateral aspect of the thalamus.* Call., *callosum;* Coll., *collateral;* Corp., *corpus;* Hippo., *hippocampus;* Nucl., *nucleus;* Pell., *pellucidum;* Sept., *septum;* Sulc., *sulcus;* Trig., *trigone.*

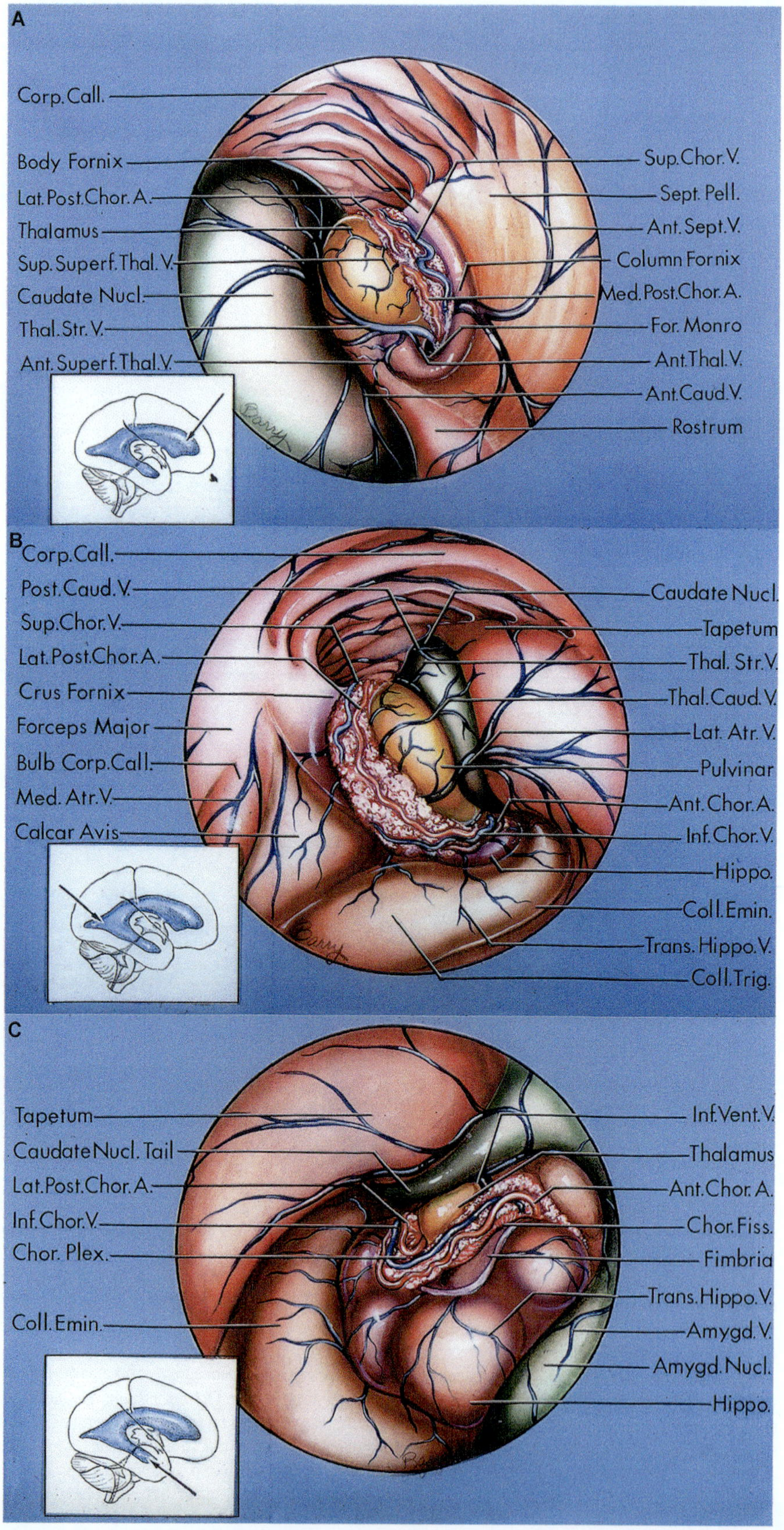

FIGURE 5.5. *Views into the lateral ventricles. The structures in the walls of the ventricle are shown in different colors: thalamus,* yellow; *caudate and amygdaloid nucleus,* green; *corpus callosum,* red; *fornix and hippocampal formation,* purple; *septum pellucidum,* orange; *and the prominences over the calcarine and collateral sulci,* brown. A, *anterior view, along the* arrow in the inset, *into the frontal horn and body of the lateral ventricle. The frontal horn is located anterior to the foramen of Monro and has the septum pellucidum in the medial wall, the genu and the body of the corpus callosum in the roof, the caudate nucleus in the lateral wall, the genu of the corpus callosum in the anterior wall, and the rostrum of the corpus callosum in the floor. The body of the lateral ventricle has the thalamus in its floor, the caudate nucleus in the lateral wall, the body of the fornix and septum pellucidum in the medial wall, and the corpus callosum in the roof. The choroid plexus is attached along the choroidal fissure, the cleft between the fornix and thalamus. The superior choroidal vein and branches of the lateral and medial posterior choroidal arteries course on the surface of the choroid plexus. The anterior and posterior septal veins cross the roof and the medial wall of the frontal horn and body. The anterior and posterior caudate veins cross the lateral wall of the frontal horn and body and join the thalamostriate vein, which passes through the foramen of Monro. A superior superficial thalamic vein courses on the thalamus.* B, *posterior view, along the* arrow in the inset, *into the atrium. The atrium has the tapetum of the corpus callosum in the roof, the bulb of the corpus callosum and the calcar avis in its medial wall, the collateral trigone in the floor, the caudate nucleus and tapetum in the lateral wall, and the crus of the fornix, pulvinar, and choroid plexus in the anterior wall. The temporal horn has the hippocampal formation and collateral eminence in the floor and the thalamus, tail of the caudate nucleus, and tapetum in the roof and the lateral wall. Branches of the anterior and lateral posterior choroidal arteries course on the surface of the choroid plexus. A thalamocaudate vein drains the part of the lateral wall of the body behind the area drained by the thalamostriate vein. The inferior choroidal vein courses on the choroid plexus in the temporal horn. The lateral and medial atrial veins cross the medial and lateral walls of the atrium. Transverse hippocampal veins cross the floor of the atrium and temporal horn.* C, *anterior view, along the* arrow in the inset, *into the temporal horn. The floor of the temporal horn is formed by the collateral eminence and the hippocampal formation. The roof and lateral wall are formed, from medial to lateral, by the thalamus, the tail of the caudate nucleus, and the tapetum of the corpus callosum. The medial wall is little more than the cleft between the thalamus and the fimbria, called the choroidal fissure, along which the choroid plexus is attached. The amygdaloid nucleus bulges into the anteromedial part of the temporal horn. The fimbria of the fornix arises on the surface of the hippocampal formation. Branches of the anterior and lateral posterior choroidal arteries course on the surface of the choroid plexus. The inferior ventricular vein drains the roof of the temporal horn and receives the amygdalar vein from the ventricular surface of the amygdaloid nucleus. The inferior choroidal vein joins the inferior ventricular vein. The transverse hippocampal veins drain the floor of the temporal horn.* A., *artery;* Amygd., *amygdaloid;* Ant., *anterior;* Atr., *atrial;* Call., *callosum;* Caud., *caudate;* Chor., *choroid, choroidal;* Coll., *collateral;* Corp., *corpus;* Emin., *eminence;* For., *foramen;* Hippo., *hippocampal, hippocampus;* Inf., *inferior;* Lat., *lateral;* Med., *medial;* Nucl., *nucleus;* Pell., *pellucidum;* Plex., *plexus;* Post., *posterior;* Sept., *septal, septum;* Sup., *superior;* Superf., *superficial;* Thal., *thalamic;* Thal.Str., *thalamostriate;* Trans., *transverse;* Trig., *trigone;* V., *vein.*

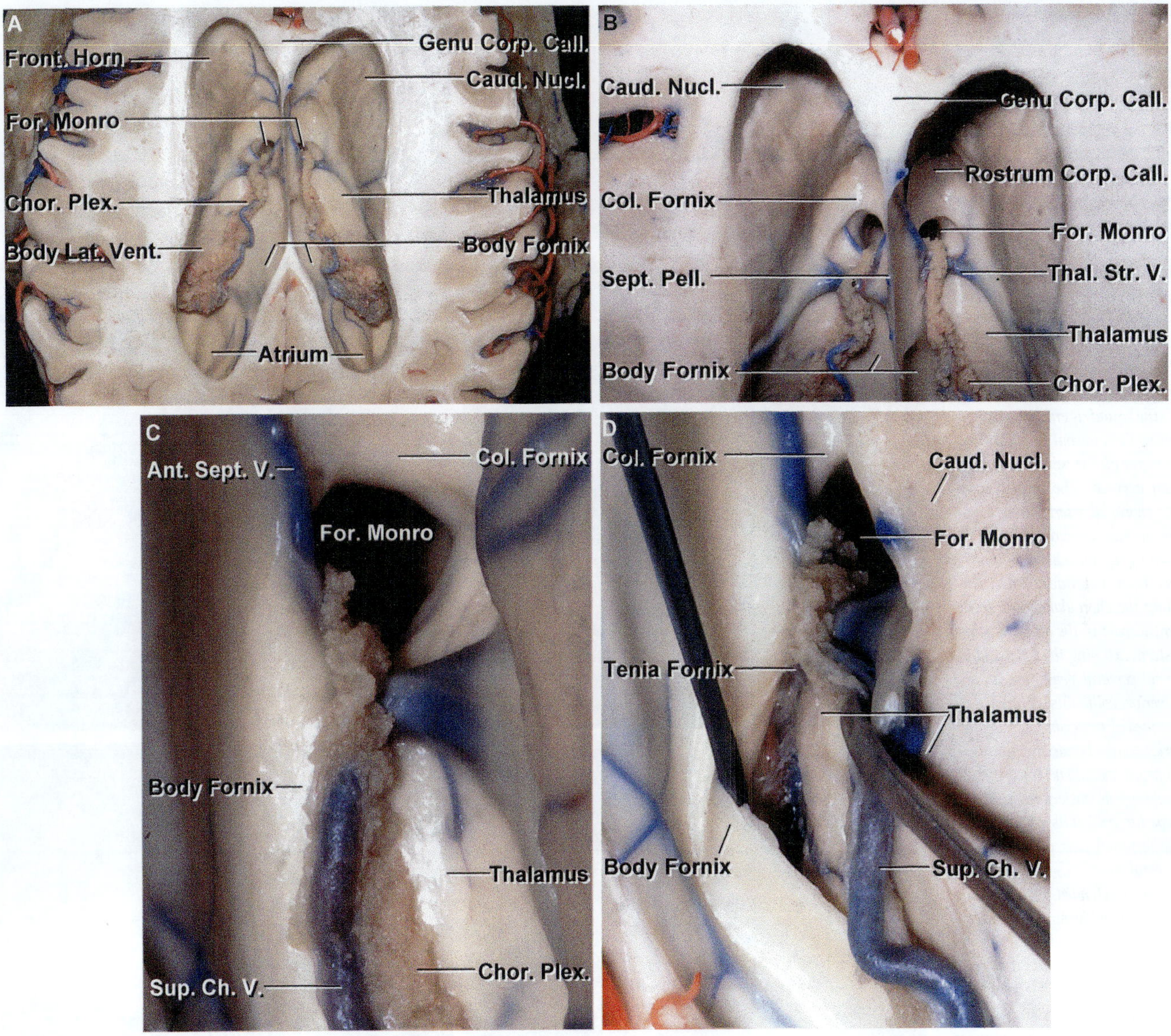

FIGURE 5.6. *Stepwise dissection of the choroidal fissure.* A, *superior view of the lateral ventricles. The choroidal fissure is the cleft between the fornix and the thalamus along which the choroid plexus is attached. The frontal horn is located anterior and the ventricular body behind the foramen of Monro. The thalamus forms the floor of the body of the lateral ventricle and the anterior wall of the atrium.* B, *enlarged view. The columns of the fornix form the anterior and superior margins of the foramen of Monro. The choroid plexus in the body extends through the posterior margin of the foramen of Monro and is continuous with the choroid plexus in the roof of the third ventricle. The right thalamostriate vein passes through the posterior edge of the foramen of Monro and the left thalamostriate vein passes through the choroidal fissure behind the foramen. The floor of the frontal horn is formed by the rostrum, and the anterior wall is formed by the genu of the corpus callosum. The lateral wall is formed by the caudate nucleus. The septum pellucidum is attached to the upper edge of the body of the fornix.* C, *enlarged view of the foramen of Monro. The columns of the fornix form the anterior and superior margins of the foramen. An anterior septal vein passes backward along the septum pellucidum and crosses the column of the fornix. The thalamostriate vein passes forward between the caudate nucleus and thalamus and turns medially to pass through the posterior margin of the foramen of Monro to empty into the internal cerebral vein. The choroid plexus is attached medially by the tenia fornix to the body of the fornix and laterally by the tenia thalami to the thalamus.* D, *the transchoroidal exposure is begun by dividing the tenia fornix that attaches the choroid plexus to the margin of the fornix. The tenia thalami that attaches the choroid plexus to the thalamus is not opened.* E, *the opening of the choroidal fissure has been extended backward from the foramen of Monro to expose both internal cerebral veins and the medial posterior choroidal arteries coursing in the velum interpositum. The anterior septal vein crosses the septum pellucidum. The lower layer of tela choroidea, attached to the striae medullaris thalami deep to the internal cerebral veins, is intact.* F, *the lower layer of tela choroidea that forms the floor of the velum interpositum has been opened, exposing the massa intermedia and posterior commissure within the third ventricle.* G, *the internal cerebral veins have been separated to expose the anteroinferior part of the third ventricle. The upper end of the midbrain forms the posterior part of the floor of the third ventricle. The mamillary bodies are situated in the midportion of the floor. The floor anterior to the mamillary bodies and behind the infundibular recess in very thin and is the site commonly opened in a third ventriculostomy. The chiasmatic recess extends forward above the posterior edge of the optic chiasm and below the anterior commissure.* *(Legend continues on next page.)*

FIGURE 5.6. *Continued* *H, enlarged view of the inner surface of the anterior wall of the third ventricle. The columns of the fornix extend downward behind the anterior commissure toward the mamillary bodies. The lamina terminalis, chiasmatic recess, posterior edge of the chiasm, and the infundibular recess are located along the anterior and lower wall of the third ventricle. I, the opening along the choroidal fissure has been extended posteriorly by opening the tenia fornix along the edge of the body and crus of the fornix. The upper part of the quadrigeminal cistern, where the internal cerebral veins converge on the vein of Galen, has been exposed. The medial posterior choroidal arteries course with the internal cerebral veins. J, the opening of the choroidal fissure has been extended downward along the choroidal fissure to the central part of the quadrigeminal cistern, exposing the basal and internal cerebral veins, pineal, and superior colliculus. Branches of the medial posterior choroidal arteries course beside the pineal. K, enlarged view. The tip of the pineal projects posteriorly above the superior colliculus and between the terminal part of the internal cerebral veins. L, the dissection has been extended forward along the choroidal fissure toward the temporal horn by dividing the tenia on the edge of the fimbria of the fornix to expose the basal vein, posterior cerebral arteries, and trochlear nerve in the posterior part of the ambient cistern below the thalamus. M, the choroidal fissure in the temporal horn has been opened by dividing the tenia fimbria. The choroid plexus attachment to the thalamus has not been disturbed. The posterior cerebral artery and basal vein course through the ambient cistern on the medial side of the temporal portion of the choroidal fissure.*

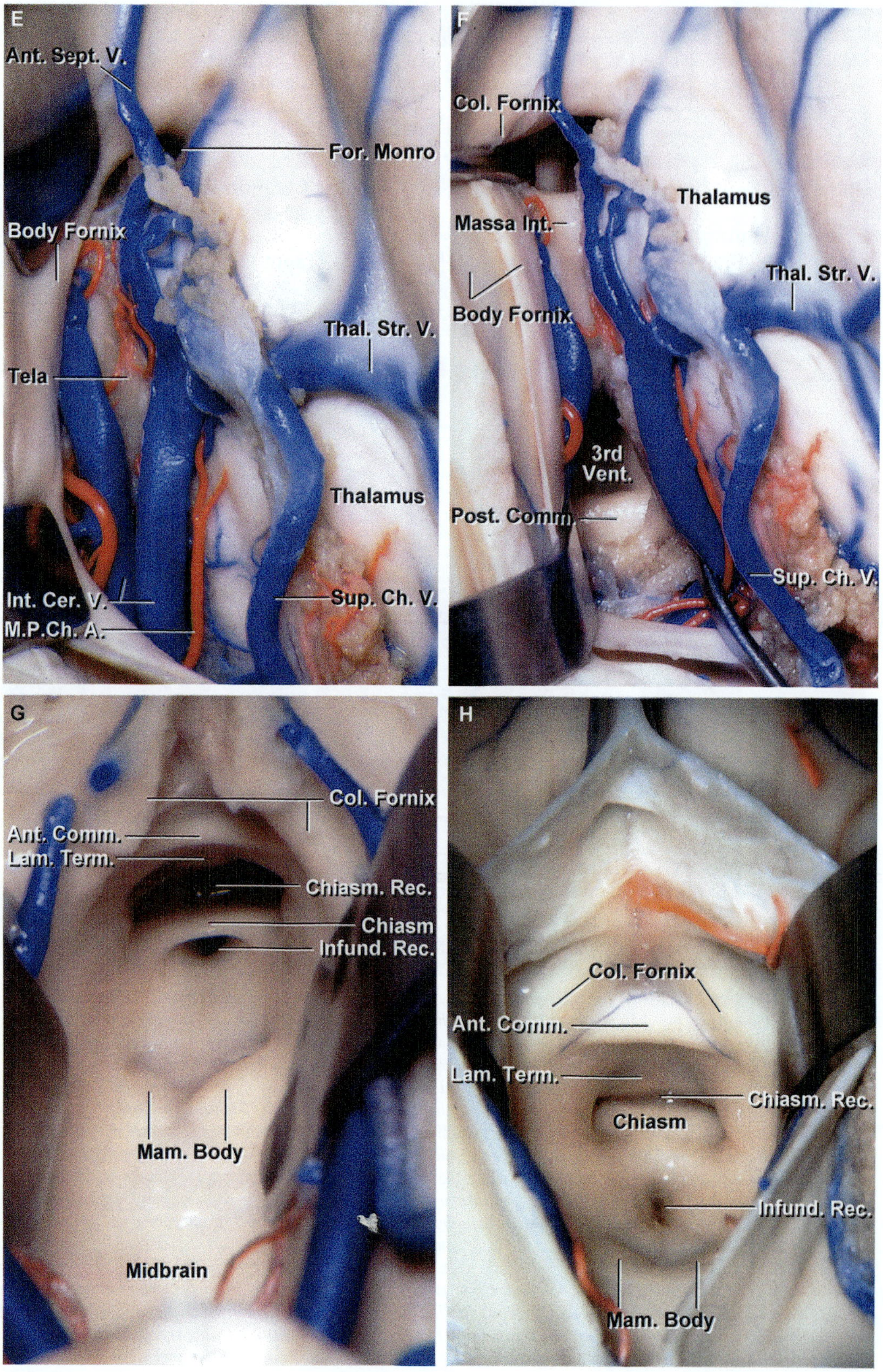

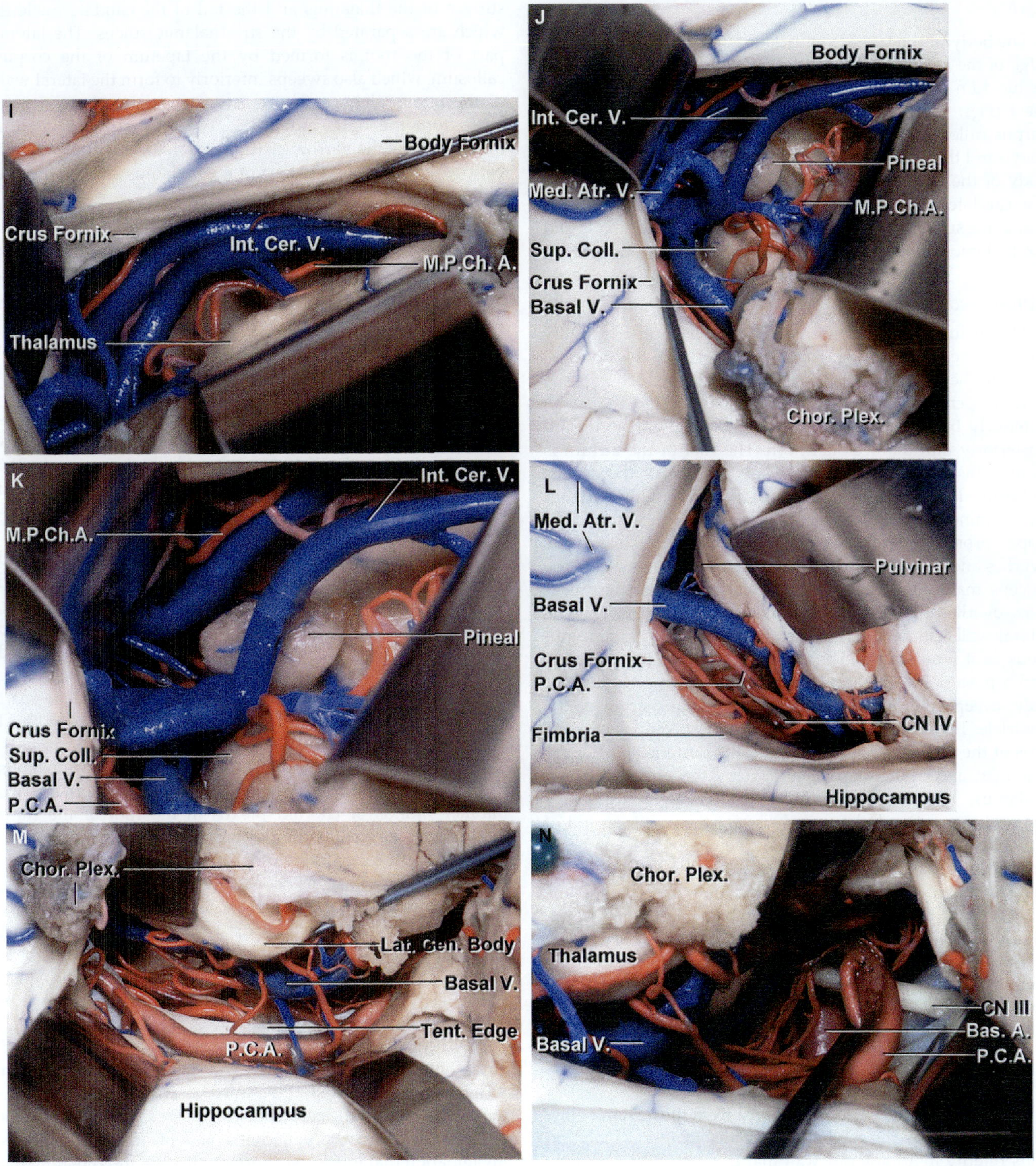

FIGURE 5.6. *Continued*

N, *the exposure has been extended through the amygdala anterior to the choroidal fissure to expose the oculomotor nerve and origin of the posterior cerebral artery. The posterior cerebral artery passes above the oculomotor nerve.* A., *artery;* Ant., *anterior;* Bas., *basilar;* Call., *callosum;* Caud., *caudate;* Cer., *cerebral;* Ch., *choroidal;* Chiasm., *chiasmatic;* Chor., *choroid;* Col., *column;* Coll., *colliculus;* Comm., *commissure;* Corp., *corpus;* CN, *cranial nerve;* For., *foramen;* Front., *frontal;* Gen., *geniculate;* Infund., *infundibular;* Int., *intermedia, internal;* Lam., *lamina;* Lat., *lateral;* Mam., *mamillary;* M.P.Ch.A., *medial posterior choroidal artery;* Nucl., *nucleus;* P.C.A., *posterior cerebral artery;* Pell., *pellucidum;* Plex., *plexus;* Rec., *recess;* Sept., *septal, septum;* Tent., *tentorial;* Term., *terminalis;* Thal. Str., *thalamostriate;* V., *vein;* Vent., *ventricle.*

Body

The body of the lateral ventricle extends from the posterior edge of the foramen of Monro to the point where the septum pellucidum disappears and the corpus callosum and fornix meet (*Figs. 5.3–5.5*). The roof is formed by the body of the corpus callosum, the medial wall by the septum pellucidum above and the body of the fornix below, the lateral wall by the body of the caudate nucleus, and the floor by the thalamus. The caudate nucleus and thalamus are separated by the striothalamic sulcus, the groove in which the stria terminalis and the thalamostriate vein course.

Atrium and Occipital Horn

The atrium and occipital horn together form a roughly triangular cavity, with the apex posteriorly in the occipital lobe and the base anteriorly on the pulvinar (*Figs. 5.3–5.5*). The atrium opens anteriorly above the thalamus into the body, anteriorly below the thalamus into the temporal horn, and posteriorly into the occipital horn. The roof of the atrium is formed by the body, splenium, and tapetum of the corpus callosum. The medial wall is formed by two roughly horizontal prominences that are located one above the other. The upper prominence, called the bulb of the corpus callosum, overlies and is formed by the large bundle of fibers called the forceps major, and the lower prominence, called the calcar avis, overlies the deepest part of the calcarine sulcus. The lateral wall has an anterior part, formed by the caudate nucleus as it wraps around the lateral margin of the pulvinar, and a posterior part, formed by the fibers of the tapetum as they sweep anteroinferiorly along the lateral margin of the ventricle. The anterior wall has a medial part composed of the crus of the fornix as it wraps around the posterior part of the pulvinar, and a lateral part, formed by the pulvinar of the thalamus. The floor is formed by the collateral trigone, a triangular area that bulges upward over the posterior end of the collateral sulcus. In the atrium, the choroid plexus has a prominent tuft called the glomus.

The occipital horn extends posteriorly into the occipital lobe from the atrium. It varies in size from being absent to extending far posteriorly in the occipital lobe, and it may vary in size from side to side. Its medial wall is formed by the bulb of the corpus callosum and the calcar avis, the roof and lateral wall are formed by the tapetum, and the floor is formed by the collateral trigone.

Temporal Horn

The temporal horn extends forward from the atrium below the pulvinar into the medial part of the temporal lobe and ends blindly in an anterior wall that is situated immediately behind the amygdaloid nucleus (*Figs. 5.3–5.5*). The floor of the temporal horn is formed medially by the hippocampus, the smooth prominence overlying the hippocampal formation, and laterally by the collateral eminence, the prominence overlying the collateral sulcus that separates the parahippocampal and occipitotemporal gyri on the inferior surface of the temporal lobe. The medial part of the roof is formed by the inferior surface of the thalamus and the tail of the caudate nucleus, which are separated by the striothalamic sulcus. The lateral part of the roof is formed by the tapetum of the corpus callosum, which also sweeps inferiorly to form the lateral wall of the temporal horn. The tapetum separates the temporal horn from the optic radiations. The only structure in the medial wall is the narrow cleft, the choroidal fissure, situated between the inferolateral part of the thalamus and the fimbria of the fornix.

Choroidal Fissure and Choroid Plexus

The choroidal fissure is the narrow C-shaped cleft between the fornix and the thalamus along which the choroid plexus is attached (*Figs. 5.3–5.6*). When the choroid plexus of the lateral ventricle is torn away, the fissure is seen as a narrow cleft situated in the medial part of the body, atrium, and temporal horn. The fornix forms the outer margin of the fissure, and the thalamus forms the inner margin. The choroidal fissure is limited in the body of the ventricle by the body of the fornix superiorly and by the thalamus inferiorly, in the atrium by the crus of the fornix posteriorly and the pulvinar anteriorly, and in the temporal horn by the fimbria of the fornix below and the stria terminalis and thalamus above. The choroidal fissure extends in a C-shaped arc from the foramen of Monro around the superior, inferior, and posterior surfaces of the thalamus to its inferior termination, called the inferior choroidal point, which is located just behind the head of the hippocampus and lateral to the lateral geniculate body. The thalamus is situated so that the part of its surface lateral to the choroidal fissure forms part of the wall of the lateral ventricle, and the part medial to the fissure forms part of the wall of the third ventricle or basal cisterns.

The choroid plexus from each lateral ventricle extends through the foramen of Monro and is continuous with the two parallel strands of choroid plexus in the roof of the third ventricle. In the atrium, the choroid plexus forms a prominent triangular tuft called the glomus. The edges of the thalamus and fornix bordering this choroidal fissure have small ridges, called the teniae, along which the tela choroidea, the membrane in which the choroid plexus arises, is attached. The tenia on the thalamic side is called the tenia thalami or tenia choroidea. The tenia on the forniceal side of the fissure is called the tenia fornicis, except in the temporal horn where it is referred to as the tenia fimbriae.

The choroidal fissure is formed at approximately 8 weeks of embryonic development when the vascular pia mater that forms the epithelial roof of the third ventricle invaginates into the medial wall of the cerebral hemisphere. No nervous tissue develops between the ependyma and pia mater along this invagination that forms the choroidal fissure, thus creating the thinnest site in the wall of the lateral ventricle. The choroidal arteries, which supply the choroid plexus, arise from the internal carotid and posterior cerebral arteries and enter the ventricles through the choroidal fissure. In addition, the veins coursing in the walls of the ventricles exit the ventricles by passing through the margin of the choroidal fissure in the subependymal location to reach the internal cerebral, basal, or great veins. Opening through the fissure from the lateral ventricle during intracranial operations provides access to several structures that are difficult or impossible to expose through the extracerebral route.

The choroidal fissure is divided into body, atrial, and temporal parts. The body portion is situated in the body of the lateral ventricle between the body of the fornix and the superior surface of the thalamus (*Figs. 5.5* and *5.7*). The velum interpositum, through which the internal cerebral veins course, is located on the medial side of the body portion of the fissure in the roof of the third ventricle. Opening through the choroidal fissure from the body of the ventricle will expose the velum interpositum and the roof of the third ventricle. The choroidal fissure and choroid plexus do not extend into the frontal horn; however, some operative approaches to the superior part of the choroidal fissure are directed through the frontal horn and adjacent part of the body. The atrial part is located in the atrium of the lateral ventricle between the crus of the fornix and the pulvinar (*Figs. 5.5* and *5.8*). The fissure does not extend into the occipital horn. The quadrigeminal cistern, the pineal region, and the posterior portion of the ambient cistern can be exposed by opening through the fissure from the atrium. The temporal part is situated in the temporal horn between the fimbria of the fornix and the inferolateral surface of the thalamus (*Figs. 5.5* and *5.9*). Opening through the choroidal fissure in the temporal horn exposes the structures in the ambient and posterior part of the crural cisterns. The cisternal side of the temporal portion of the fissure is situated in the superolateral edge of the ambient cistern. The fissure is the thinnest site in the wall of the lateral ventricle bordering the basal cisterns and the roof of the third ventricle.

THIRD VENTRICLE

The third ventricle is located in the center of the head, below the corpus callosum and the body of the lateral ventricle, above the sella turcica, pituitary gland, and midbrain, and between the cerebral hemispheres, the two halves of the thalamus, and the two halves of the hypothalamus (*Figs. 5.10* and *5.11*). It is intimately related to the circle of Willis and its branches and the great vein of Galen and its tributaries. Tumors in the region of the third ventricle are among the most difficult to expose and remove.

Manipulation of the walls of the third ventricle may cause hypothalamic dysfunction, as manifested by disturbances of consciousness, temperature control, respiration, and hypophyseal

FIGURE 5.7. *Transchoroidal approach directed through the body portion of the choroidal fissure using an opening through the corpus callosum. The site of the scalp incision and bone flap are shown in the inset. A, operative exposure of the frontal horn and body of the right lateral ventricle. The choroidal fissure lies deep to the choroid plexus. Structures in the wall of the lateral ventricle include the thalamus, caudate nucleus fornix, foramen of Monro, septum pellucidum, and the rostrum of the corpus callosum. Vascular structures that converge on the choroidal fissure include the medial and lateral posterior choroidal arteries and the anterior and posterior septal, anterior and posterior caudate, superior choroidal, and thalamostriate veins. B, the choroidal fissure has been opened by incising along the tenia fornicis. The layers of tela choroidea in the roof of the third ventricle have been opened and the massa intermedia and interior and floor of the third ventricle have been exposed by separating the internal cerebral veins. The medial posterior choroidal arteries course around the internal cerebral veins.* A., *artery;* Ant., *anterior;* Call., *callosum;* Caud., *caudate;* Cer., *cerebral;* Chor., *choroid, choroidal;* Fiss., *fissure;* For., *foramen;* Front., *frontal;* Int., *intermedia, internal;* Lat., *lateral;* Med., *medial;* Nucl., *nucleus;* Pell., *pellucidum;* Plex., *plexus;* Post., *posterior;* Sept., *septal, septum;* Sup., *superior;* Thal. Str., *thalamostriate;* V., *vein;* Vent., *ventricle. (From, Nagata S, Rhoton AL Jr, Barry M: Microsurgical anatomy of the choroidal fissure.* ***Surg Neurol*** *30:3–59, 1988 [15].)*

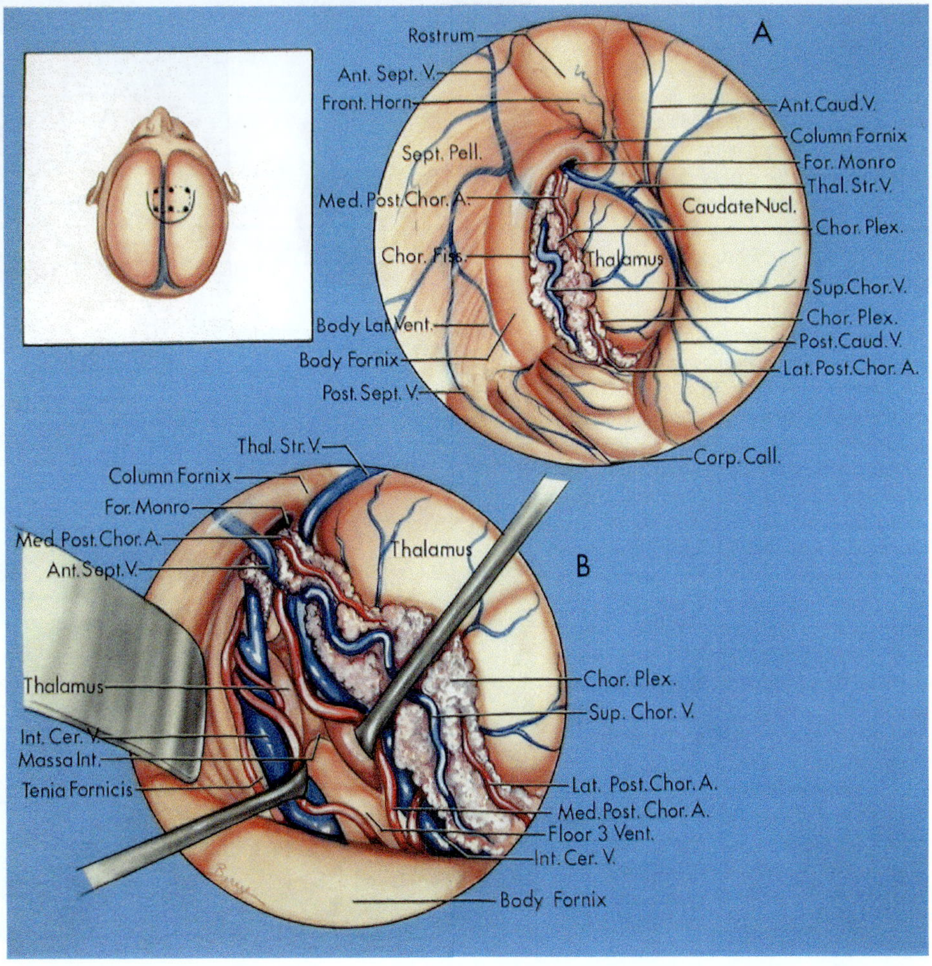

secretion, visual loss due to damage of the optic chiasm and tracts, and memory loss due to injury to the columns of the fornix in the walls of the third ventricle (24, 28, 37).

Neural Relationships

The third ventricle is a narrow, funnel-shaped, unilocular, midline cavity. It communicates at its anterosuperior margin with each lateral ventricle through the foramen of Monro and posteriorly with the fourth ventricle through the aqueduct of sylvius. It has a roof, a floor, and an anterior, posterior, and two lateral walls.

Roof

The roof of the third ventricle forms a gentle upward arch, extending from the foramen of Monro anteriorly to the suprapineal recess posteriorly (*Figs. 5.10–5.13*). The roof has four layers: one neural layer formed by the fornix, two thin membranous layers of tela choroidea, and a layer of blood vessels between the sheets of tela choroidea. The choroidal fissure is located in the lateral margin of the roof. The upper layer of the anterior part of the roof of the third ventricle is formed by the body of the fornix, and the posterior part of the roof is formed by the crura and the hippocampal commissure. The septum pellucidum is attached to the upper surface of the body of the fornix.

The tela choroidea forms two of the three layers in the roof below the layer formed by the fornix. The tela choroidea consists of two thin, semiopaque membranes derived from the pia mater, which are interconnected by loosely organized trabeculae. The final layer in the roof is a vascular layer located between the two layers of tela choroidea. The vascular layer consists of the medial posterior choroidal arteries and their branches and the internal cerebral veins and their tributaries. Parallel strands of choroid plexus project downward on each side of the midline from the inferior layer of tela choroidea into the superior part of the third ventricle.

The velum interpositum is the space between the two layers of tela choroidea in the roof of the third ventricle. It is located on the medial side of the body portion of the choroidal fissure in the roof of the third ventricle below the body of the fornix and between the superomedial surfaces of the thalami. The upper layer of the tela choroidea is attached to the lower surface of the fornix and the hippocampal commissure. The lower wall has an anterior part that is attached to the small ridges on the free edge of the fiber tracts, called the striae medullaris thalami, that extend along the superomedial bor-

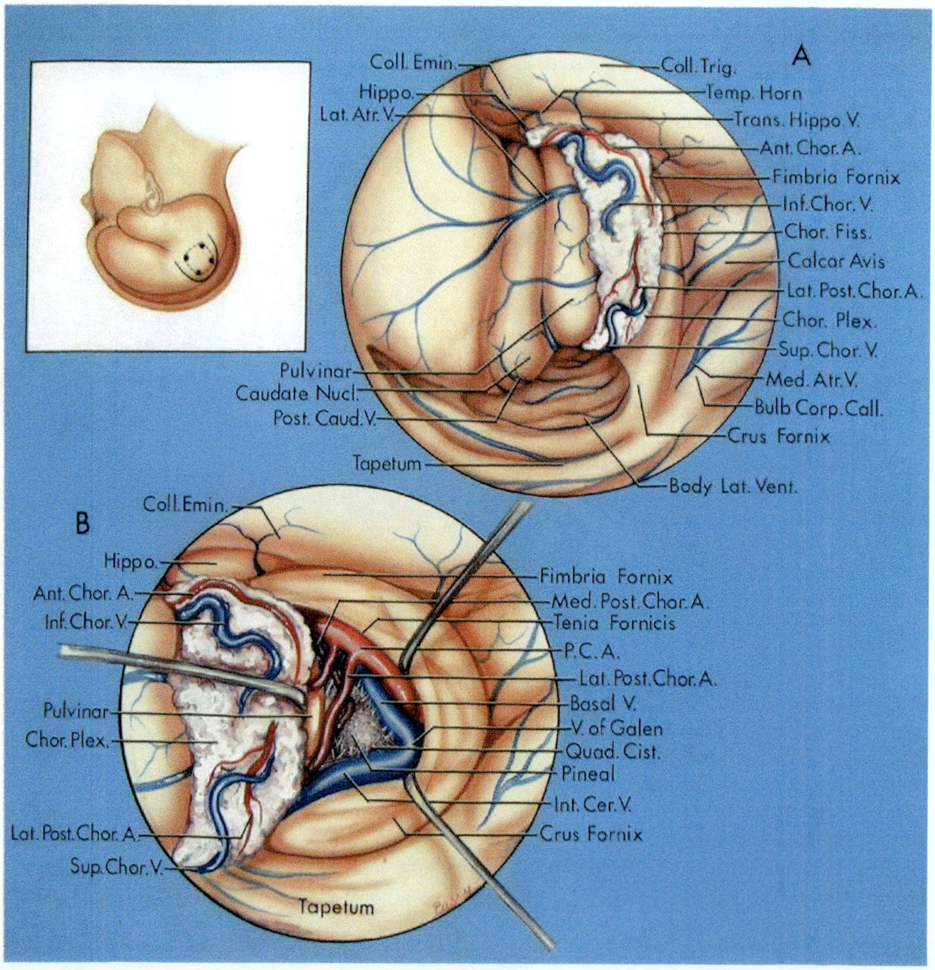

FIGURE 5.8. *Transchoroidal approach directed through the atrial portion of the choroidal fissure using a cortical incision in the superior parietal lobule. The site of the scalp incision, bone flap, and cortical incision are shown in the* inset. A, *the choroid plexus is attached along the choroidal fissure. The atrial portion of the choroidal fissure is situated between the crus of the fornix and the pulvinar. Structures in the wall of the atrium, body, and temporal horn of the lateral ventricle include the pulvinar, fornix, caudate nucleus, tapetum and bulb of the corpus callosum, calcar avis, hippocampal formation, and the collateral eminence and trigone. Vascular structures that converge on the choroidal fissure include the anterior and lateral posterior choroidal arteries and the lateral and medial atrial, posterior caudate, superior and inferior choroidal, and transverse hippocampal veins.* B, *the choroidal fissure has been opened by incising the tenia fornicis and retracting the crus of the fornix posteriorly to expose the quadrigeminal cistern, posterior cerebral and medial posterior choroidal arteries, pineal body, and internal cerebral, basal, and great veins.* A., *artery;* Ant., *anterior;* Atr., *atrial;* Call., *callosum;* Caud., *caudate;* Cer., *cerebral;* Chor., *choroid, choroidal;* Cist., *cistern;* Coll., *collateral;* Corp., *corpus;* Emin., *eminence;* Fiss., *fissure;* Hippo., *hippocampal, hippocampus;* Inf., *inferior;* Int., *internal;* Lat., *lateral;* Med., *medial;* Nucl., *nucleus;* P.C.A., *posterior cerebral artery;* Plex., *plexus;* Post., *posterior;* Quad., *quadrigeminal;* Sup., *superior;* Temp., *temporal;* Trans., *transverse;* Trig., *trigone;* V., *vein;* Vent., *ventricle.* (From, *Nagata S, Rhoton AL Jr, Barry M: Microsurgical anatomy of the choroidal fissure.* **Surg Neurol** *30:3–59, 1988 [15].)*

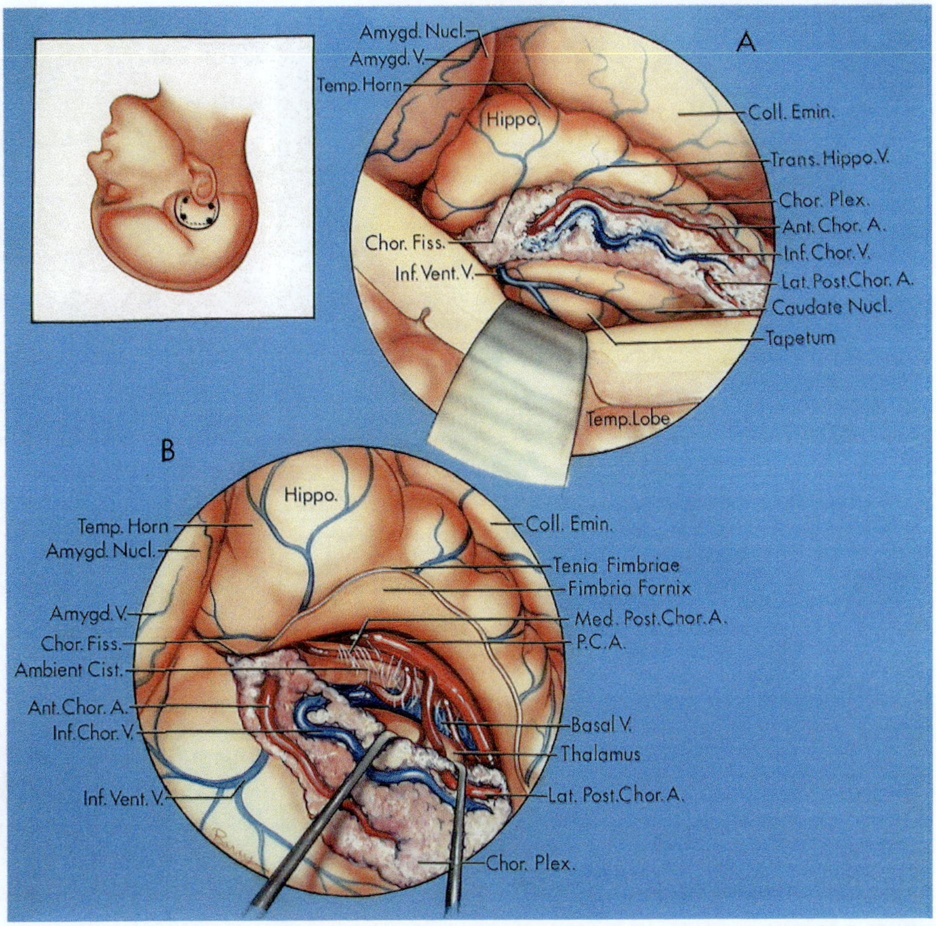

FIGURE 5.9. *Transchoroidal approach directed through the temporal portion of the choroidal fissure. The inset shows the site of the scalp incision and bone flap. A, the inferior surface of the temporal lobe has been opened to expose the temporal horn. The choroid plexus is attached along the choroidal fissure. Structures in the wall of the temporal horn include the hippocampal formation, collateral eminence, amygdaloid and caudate nuclei, and the tapetum of the corpus callosum. Vascular structures that pass through the choroidal fissure include the anterior and lateral posterior choroidal arteries and the transverse hippocampal, amygdalar, inferior choroidal, and inferior ventricular veins. B, the choroidal fissure has been opened by incising along the tenia fimbriae and retracting the choroid plexus upward. This exposes the ambient cistern, branches of the posterior cerebral artery, and tributaries of the basal vein. The medial posterior choroidal artery courses medial to the posterior cerebral artery.* A., *artery;* Amygd., *amygdalar, amygdaloid;* Ant., *anterior;* Caud., *caudate;* Chor., *choroid, choroidal;* Cist., *cistern;* Coll., *collateral;* Emin., *eminence;* Fiss., *fissure;* Hippo., *hippocampal, hippocampus;* Inf., *inferior;* Lat., *lateral;* Med., *medial;* Nucl., *nucleus;* P.C.A., *posterior cerebral artery;* Plex., *plexus;* Post., *posterior;* Temp., *temporal;* Trans., *transverse;* V., *vein;* Vent., *ventricle.* (From, *Nagata S, Rhoton AL Jr, Barry M: Microsurgical anatomy of the choroidal fissure.* **Surg Neurol** *30:3–59, 1988 [15].)*

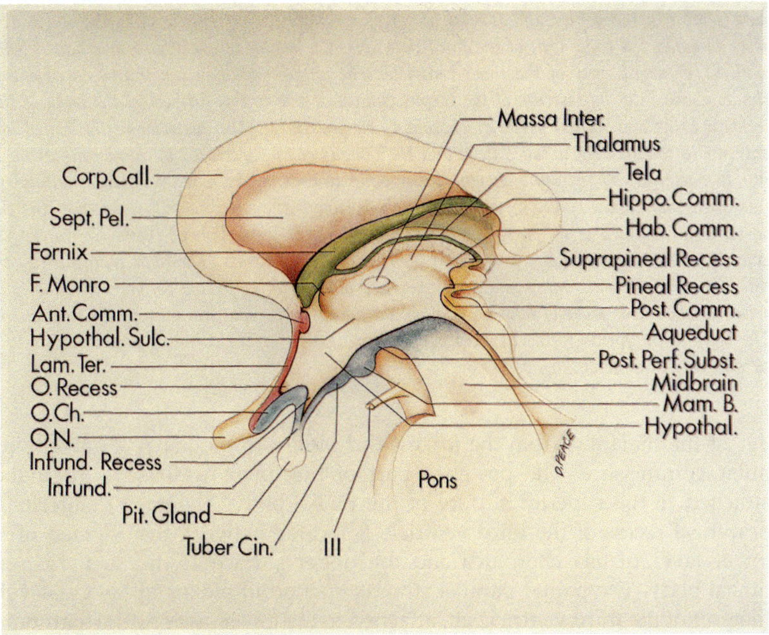

FIGURE 5.10. *Midsagittal section of the third ventricle. The floor* (blue) *extends from the optic chiasm to the aqueduct of sylvius and includes the lower surface of the optic chiasm, the infundibulum, the infundibular recess, the pituitary gland, the tuber cinereum, the mamillary bodies, the posterior perforated substance, and the part of the midbrain anterior to the aqueduct. The anterior wall* (red) *extends from the optic chiasm to the foramen of Monro and includes the upper surface of the optic chiasm, the optic recess, the lamina terminalis, the anterior commissure, and the foramen of Monro. The roof* (green) *extends from the foramen of Monro to the suprapineal recess and is formed by the fornix and the layers of tela choroidea, between which course the internal cerebral vein and the medial posterior choroidal artery. The hippocampal commissure, corpus callosum, and septum pellucidum are above the roof. The posterior wall extends from the suprapineal recess to the aqueduct and includes the habenular commissure, pineal gland, pineal recess, and posterior commissure. The oculomotor nerve exits from the midbrain. The hypothalamic sulcus forms a groove between the thalamic and hypothalamic surfaces of the third ventricle.* Ant., *anterior;* B., *body;* Call., *callosum;* Ch., *chiasm;* Cin., *cinereum;* Comm., *commissure;* Corp., *corpus;* For., *foramen;* Hab., *habenular;* Hippo., *hippocampal;* Hypothal., *hypothalamic, hypothalamus;* Infund., *infundibular, infundibulum;* Inter., *intermedia;* Lam., *lamina;* Mam., *mamillary;* N., *nerve;* O., *optic;* Pel., *pellucidum;* Perf., *perforated;* Pit., *pituitary;* Post., *posterior;* Sept., *septum;* Subst., *substance;* Sulc., *sulcus;* Ter., *terminalis.*

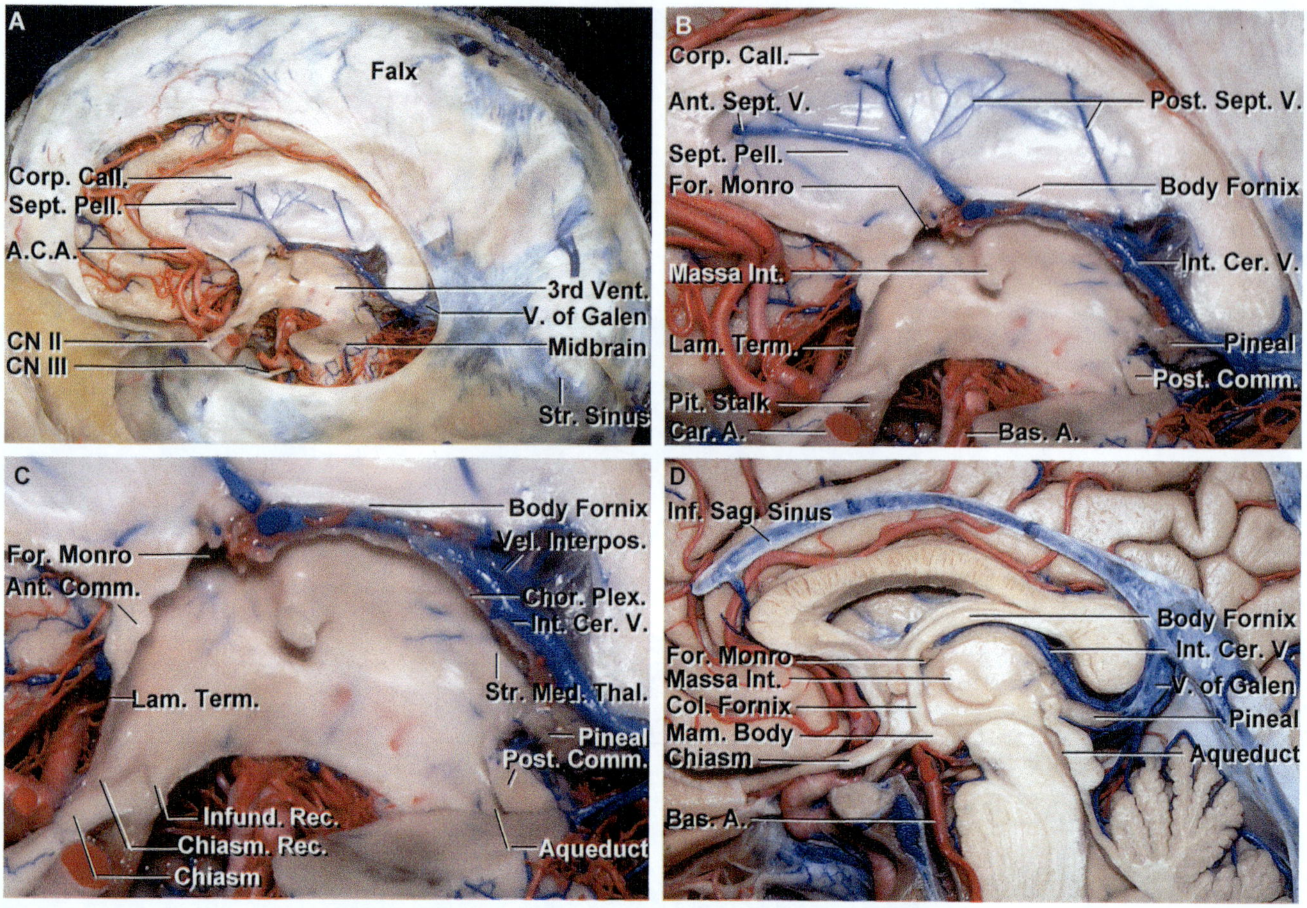

FIGURE 5.11. *Midsagittal views of the third ventricle.* A, *the third ventricle sits in the center of the cranium below the corpus callosum, body of the lateral ventricles, and septum pellucidum, above the midbrain and interpeduncular fossa, anterior to the quadrigeminal cistern and vein of Galen, and posterior to the anterior cerebral arteries. The interhemispheric fissure, along the side of the falx, offers one avenue to the third ventricle. The posterior part of the third ventricle can also be approached along the junction of the falx and tentorium, adjacent the straight sinus.* B, *enlarged view. The septum pellucidum separates the bodies and frontal horns of the lateral ventricles and is crossed by anterior and posterior septal veins. The anterior cerebral artery ascends along the front wall of the third ventricle, the basilar bifurcation is positioned below the floor, and the vein of Galen blocks access to the posterior wall.* C, *enlarged view of the third ventricle. The anterior wall of the third ventricle is formed by the lamina terminalis and anterior commissure and blends above into the rostrum of the corpus callosum. The roof is formed by the body of the fornix and the velum interpositum through which the internal cerebral veins and medial posterior choroidal arteries course. The posterior wall, formed by the pineal and habenular and posterior commissures, is located anterior to the quadrigeminal cistern and the venous complex created by numerous veins converging on the vein of Galen. The floor is formed, from anterior to posterior, by the optic chiasm, tuber cinereum above the pituitary stalk, mamillary bodies, and upper midbrain. The section extends to the lateral side of the mamillary bodies. The velum interpositum is the space within the roof of the third ventricle along which the internal cerebral veins and medial posterior choroidal arteries pass. The body of the fornix is located above the velum interpositum. The upper wall of the velum interpositum is formed by the layer of tela choroidea attached to the lower margin of the fornix. The floor is formed by the layer of tela attached along the striae medullaris thalami. The internal cerebral veins and medial posterior choroidal arteries course between the two layers of tela. The choroid plexus in the roof of the third ventricle arises in the lower layer of tela.* D, *another third ventricle. This section extends just to the left of the midline through the column and body of the fornix. The body of the fornix forms the roof of the third ventricle. The columns pass anterior to the foramen of Monro and descend behind the anterior commissure to reach the mamillary bodies.*

der of the thalamus from the foramen of Monro to the habenular commissure. The posterior part of the lower wall is attached to the superior surface of the pineal body. The suprapineal recess of the third ventricle is located between the lower layer of tela choroidea and the upper surface of the pineal body. The paired parallel strands of choroid plexus in the roof of the third ventricle are attached to the lower layer of tela choroidea. Many of the veins draining the frontal horn and body converge on the velum interpositum to form the internal cerebral veins. The internal cerebral veins arise in the anterior part of the velum interpositum, just behind the foramen of Monro, and they exit the velum interpositum above the pineal body to enter the quadrigeminal cistern and join the great vein. The velum interpositum is usually a closed space that tapers to a narrow apex just behind the foramen of Monro, but it may infrequently have an opening situated

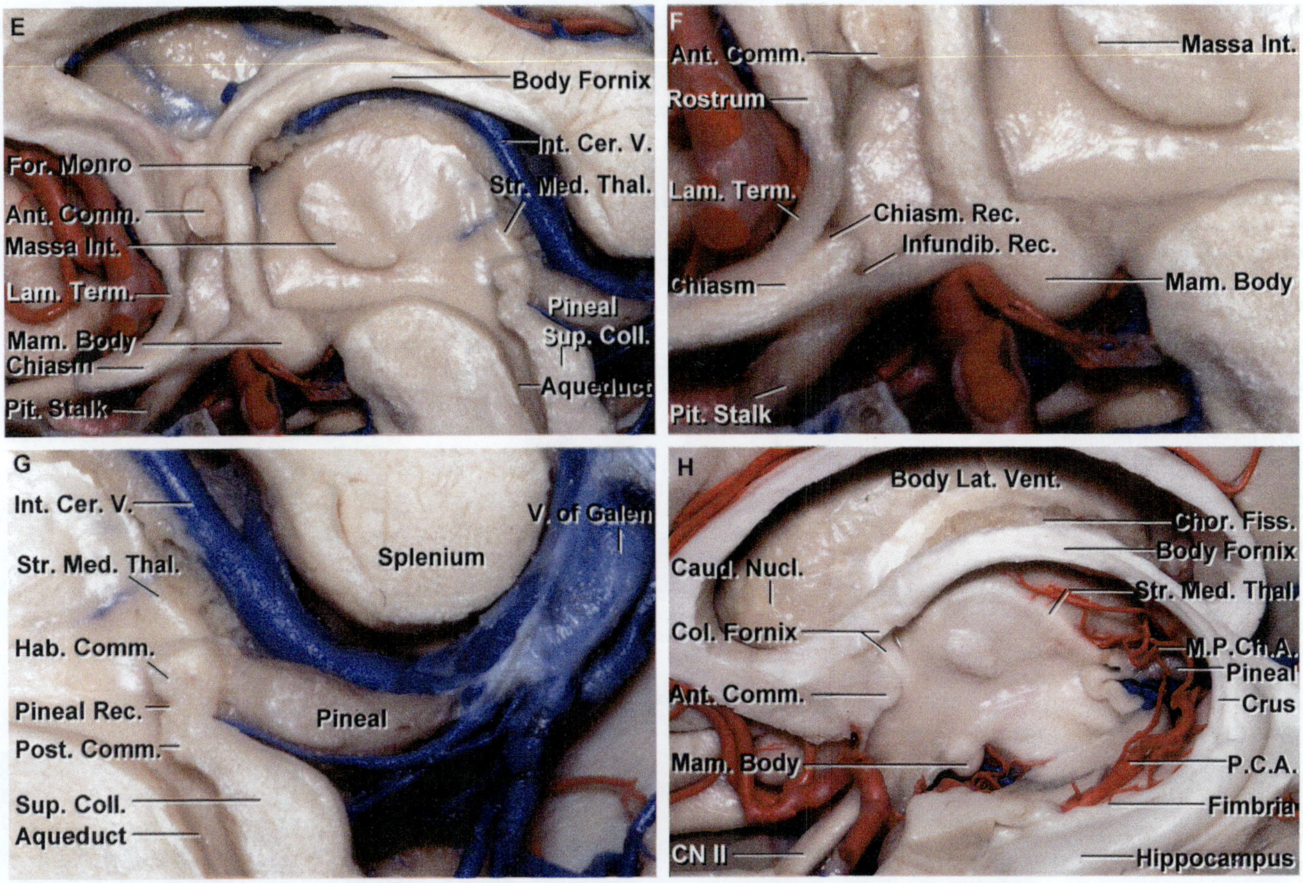

FIGURE 5.11. *Continued*
E, enlarged view. The anterior wall is made up of the lamina terminalis and the anterior commissure. The optic chiasm, mamillary bodies, and midbrain are in the floor. F, enlarged view. The chiasmatic recess is located above the optic chiasm and behind the lamina terminalis. The infundibular recess is located below and behind the optic chiasm. The lamina terminalis blends into the rostrum of the corpus callosum. The anterior commissure is positioned between the rostrum of the corpus callosum and the columns of the fornix. The thalamus and hypothalamus form the lateral wall of the third ventricle. G, enlarged view of the posterior part of the third ventricle. The posterior wall of the third ventricle is formed by the aqueduct, pineal, and habenular and posterior commissures. The pineal recess extends into the base of the pineal in the interval between the habenular and posterior commissures. H, lateral view of the third ventricle with the hippocampus and fornix preserved. The body of the fornix forms the roof of the third ventricle. The velum interpositum, through which the internal cerebral veins course, is located between the body of the fornix and the striae medullaris thalami. The quadrigeminal cistern and pineal region are located anteromedial to the crus of the fornix, and the ambient cistern and posterior cerebral artery are located medial to the temporal horn and the fimbria. Opening the choroidal fissure adjacent to the body of the fornix exposes the third ventricle. The medial posterior choroidal arteries turn forward beside the pineal to reach the velum interpositum. A., *artery;* A.C.A., *anterior cerebral artery;* Ant., *anterior;* Bas., *basilar;* Call., *callosum;* Car., *carotid;* Caud., *caudate;* Cer., *cerebral;* Chiasm., *chiasmatic;* Chor., *choroid;* CN, *cranial nerve;* Col., *column;* Coll., *colliculus;* Comm., *commissure;* Corp., *corpus;* For., *foramen;* Hab., *habenular;* Infund., *infundibular;* Int., *intermedia, internal;* Interpos., *interpositum;* Lam., *lamina;* Lat., *lateral;* Mam., *mamillary;* Med., *medial;* M.P.Ch.A., *medial posterior choroidal artery;* Nucl., *nucleus;* P.C.A., *posterior cerebral artery;* Pell., *pellucidum;* Pit., *pituitary;* Plex., *plexus;* Post., *posterior;* Rec., *recess;* Sag., *sagittal;* Sept., *septal, septum;* Str., *straight;* Sup., *superior;* Term., *terminalis;* Thal., *thalami;* V., *vein;* Vel., *velum;* Vent., *ventricle.*

between the splenium and pineal body that communicates with the quadrigeminal cistern to form the cisterna velum interpositum. There also may be a space above the velum interpositum between the hippocampal commissure and splenium called the cavum vergae.

Floor

The floor extends from the optic chiasm anteriorly to the orifice of the aqueduct of sylvius posteriorly (*Figs. 5.10, 5.13,* and *5.14*). The anterior half of the floor is formed by diencephalic structures, and the posterior half is formed by mesencephalic structures. When viewed from inferiorly, the structures forming the floor include, from anterior to posterior, the optic chiasm, the infundibulum of the hypothalamus, the tuber cinereum, the mamillary bodies, the posterior perforated substance, and (most posteriorly) the part of the tegmentum of the midbrain located above the medial aspect of the cerebral peduncles. The optic chiasm is located at the junction of the floor and the anterior wall of the third ventricle. The chiasm slopes posteriorly and superiorly from its junction with the optic nerves. The inferior surface

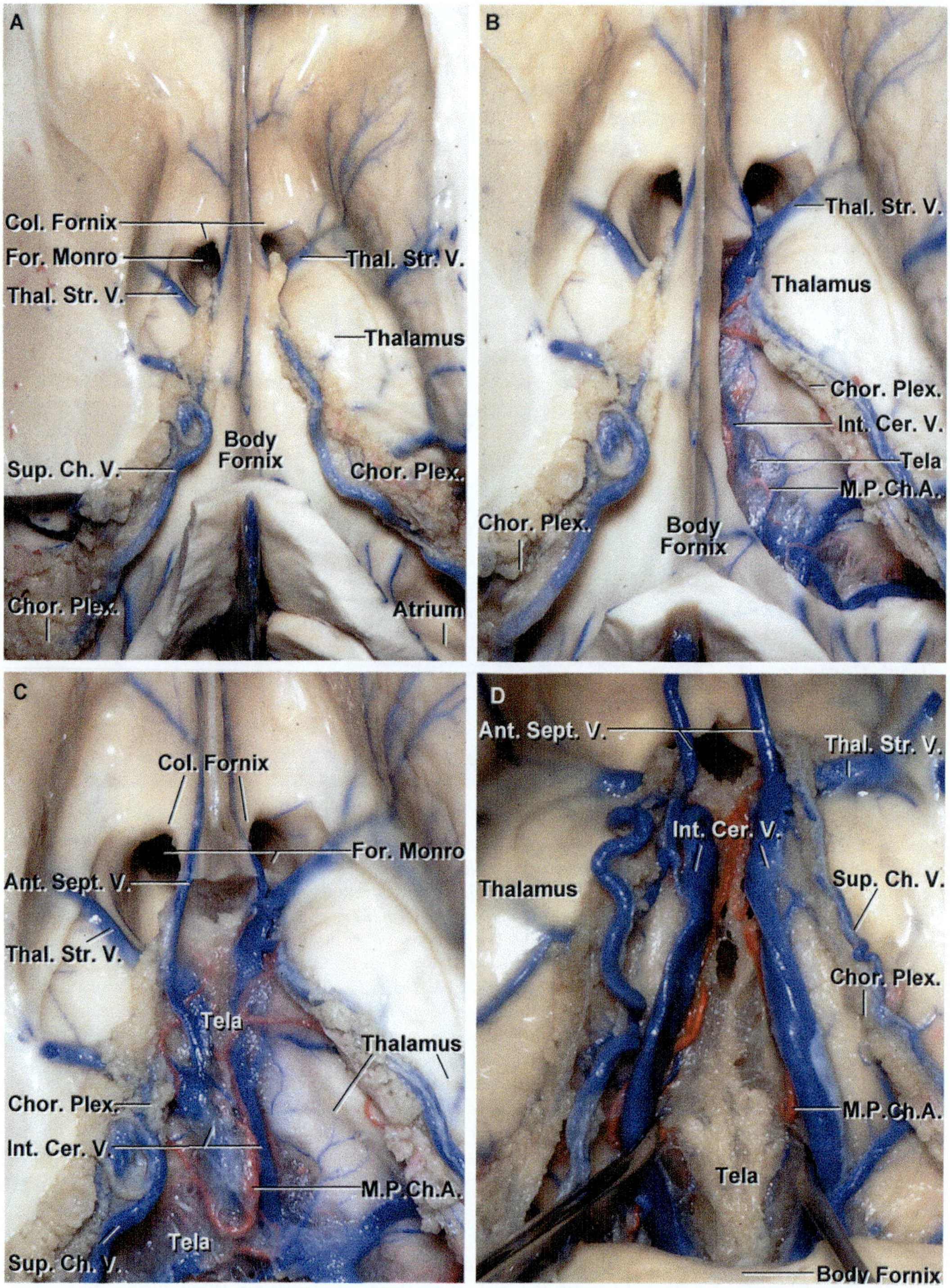

FIGURE 5.12. *Roof of the third ventricle. Superior views.* A, *the upper part of the hemispheres has been removed to expose the frontal horn and body of the lateral ventricle. The choroid plexus is attached along the choroidal fissure located between the body of the fornix and the thalamus. The superior choroidal veins course along the choroid plexus. The thalamostriate veins pass through the posterior margins of the foramen of Monro. The columns of the fornix pass anterior and superior to the foramen of Monro. The body of the fornix forms the upper part of the roof of the third ventricle.* B, *the right lateral edge of the fornix has been removed to expose the upper layer of tela choroidea that spans the interval below the body of the fornix and forms the upper wall of the velum interpositum in the roof of the third ventricle. The velum is positioned between an upper layer of tela attached to the lower surface of the body of the fornix and a lower layer of tela attached below the internal cerebral veins to the striae medullaris thalami. The internal cerebral veins and medial posterior choroidal arteries course in the velum interpositum.* C, *the body of the fornix has been folded backward. The upper layer of tela that rests against the lower surface of the body of the fornix has been preserved. The tela is a thin, arachnoid-like membrane, through which the internal cerebral veins and the medial posterior choroidal arteries can be seen. The anterior septal veins pass above the foramen of Monro.* D, *the upper layer of tela has been removed to expose the internal cerebral veins and medial posterior choroidal arteries. The internal cerebral veins have been retracted laterally. The anterior septal veins course along the septum and join the internal cerebral veins near the foramen of Monro.* E, *the tela has been opened to expose the massa intermedia, mamillary bodies, and posterior commissure.* F, *the exposure has been directed to the posterior part of the third ventricle. The aqueduct is positioned below the posterior and habenular commissures. The pineal recess extends posteriorly between the habenular and posterior commissures into the base of the pineal.* Ant., *anterior;* Cer., *cerebral;* Ch., *choroidal;* Chor., *choroid;* Col., *column;* Comm., *commissure;* For., *foramen;* Hab., *habenular;* Int., *intermedia, internal;* Mam., *mamillary;* M.P.Ch.A., *medial posterior choroidal artery;* Plex., *plexus;* Post., *posterior;* Rec., *recess;* Sept., *septal;* Sup., *superior;* Thal.Str., *thalamostriate;* V., *vein.*

of the chiasm forms the anterior part of the floor, and the superior surface forms the lower part of the anterior wall. The optic tracts arise from the posterolateral margin of the chiasm and course obliquely away from the floor toward the lateral margin of the midbrain. The infundibulum, tuber cinereum, mamillary bodies, and posterior perforated substance are located in the

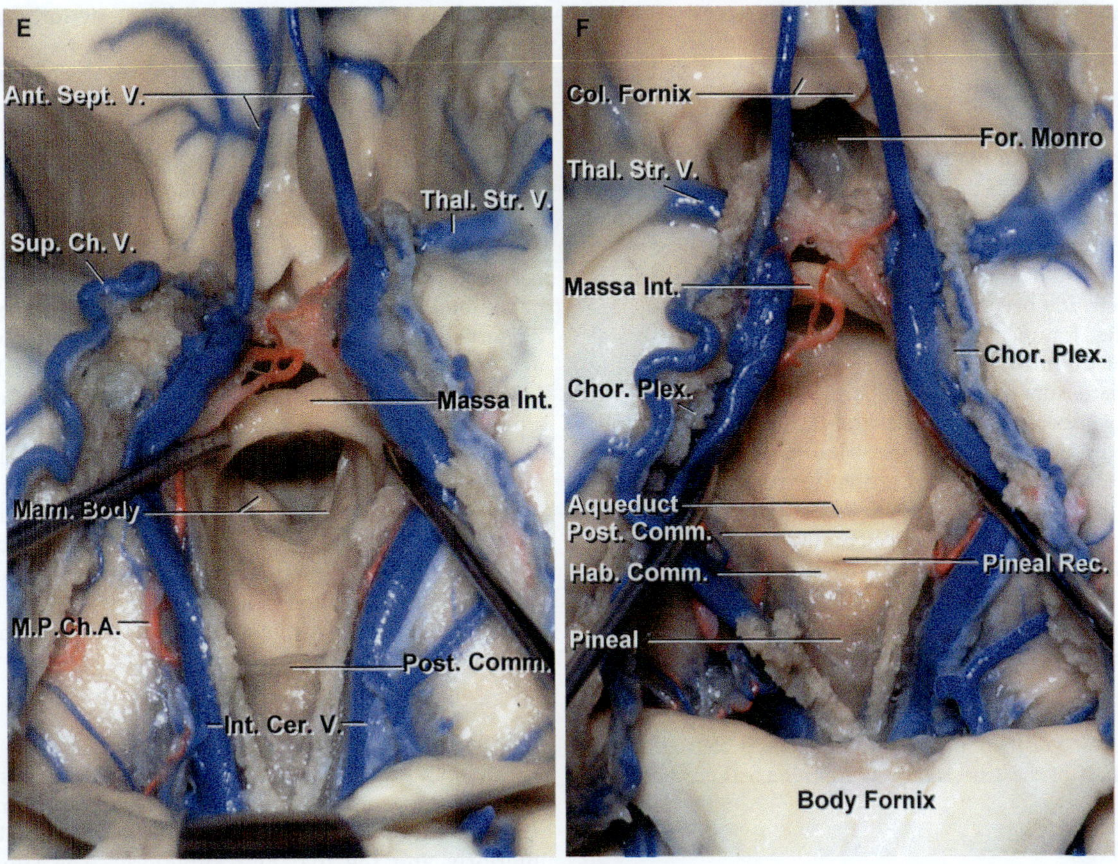

FIGURE 5.12. *Continued*

space limited anteriorly and laterally by the optic chiasm and tracts and posteriorly by the cerebral peduncles.

The infundibulum of the hypothalamus is a hollow, funnel-shaped structure located between the optic chiasm and the tuber cinereum. The pituitary gland (hypophysis) is attached to the infundibulum, and the axons in the infundibulum extend to the posterior lobe of the hypophysis. The tuber cinereum is a prominent mass of hypothalamic gray matter located anterior to the mamillary bodies. The tuber cinereum merges anteriorly into the infundibulum. The tuber cinereum around the base of the infundibulum is raised to form a prominence called the median eminence. The mamillary bodies form paired, round prominences posterior to the tuber cinereum. The posterior perforated substance is a depressed, punctuated area of gray matter located in the interval between the mamillary bodies anteriorly and the medial surface of the cerebral peduncles posteriorly. The posterior part of the floor extends posterior and superior to the medial part of the cerebral peduncles and superior to the tegmentum of the midbrain.

When viewed from above and inside the third ventricle, the optic chiasm forms a prominence at the anterior margin of the floor. The infundibular recess extends into the infundibulum behind the optic chiasm. The mamillary bodies form paired prominences on the inner surface of the floor posterior to the infundibular recess. The part of the floor between the mamillary bodies and the aqueduct of sylvius has a smooth surface that is concave from side to side. This smooth surface lies above the posterior perforated substance anteriorly and the medial part of the cerebral peduncles and the tegmentum of the midbrain posteriorly.

Anterior Wall

The anterior margin of the third ventricle extends from the foramina of Monro above to the optic chiasm below (*Figs. 5.10, 5.11,* and *5.15*). Only the lower two-thirds of the anterior surface is seen on the external surface of the brain; the upper third is hidden posterior to the rostrum of the corpus callosum. The part of the anterior wall visible on the surface is formed by the optic chiasm and the lamina terminalis. The lamina terminalis is a thin sheet of gray matter and pia mater that attaches to the upper surface of the chiasm and stretches upward to fill the interval between the optic chiasm and the rostrum of the corpus callosum.

When viewed from within, the boundaries of the anterior wall are formed, from superior to inferior, by the columns of the fornix, foramina of Monro, anterior commissure, lamina terminalis, optic recess, and optic chiasm. The foramen of Monro on each side is located at the junction of the roof and the anterior wall. The foramen is a ductlike canal that opens between the fornix and the thalamus into the lateral ventricle and extends inferiorly below the fornix into the third ventricle as a single channel. The foramen of Monro is bounded anteriorly by the junction of the body and the columns of the fornix and posteriorly by the anterior pole of the thalamus. The size and shape of the foramina of Monro depend on the size of the ventricles: if the ventricles are small, each foramen is a crescent-shaped opening bounded anteriorly by the concave curve of the fornix and posteriorly by the convex anterior tubercle of the thalamus. As the ventricles enlarge, the foramen on each side becomes rounder. The structures that pass through the foramen are the choroid plexus, the distal branches of the medial posterior choroidal arteries, and the thalamostriate, superior choroidal, and septal veins.

The anterior commissure is a compact bundle of fibers that crosses the midline in front of the columns of the fornix. The anterior-posterior diameter of the anterior commissure varies from 1.5 to 6.0 mm (37). In our specimens, the distance from the posterior end of the anterior commissure to the anterior border of the foramen of Monro ranged from 1.0 to 3.5 mm (average, 2.2 mm), and the distance from the upper edge of the optic chiasm to the anterior border of the anterior commissure ranged from 8 to 12 mm (average, 10 mm). The lamina terminalis fills the interval between the anterior commissure and the optic chiasm. The lamina attaches to the midportion of the superior surface of the chiasm, leaving a small cleft between the upper half of the chiasm and the lamina, called the optic recess.

Posterior Wall

The posterior wall of the third ventricle extends from the suprapineal recess above to the aqueduct of sylvius below (*Figs. 5.10* and *5.11*). When viewed from anteriorly and within the third ventricle, it consists, from above to below, of the suprapineal recess, the habenular commissure, the pineal body and its recess, the posterior commissure, and the aqueduct of sylvius. The suprapineal recess projects posteriorly between the upper surface of the pineal gland and the lower layer of tela choroidea in the roof. The pineal gland extends posteriorly into the quadrigeminal cistern from its stalk. The stalk of the pineal gland has an upper and a lower lamina. The habenular commissure, which interconnects the habenulae, crosses the midline in the upper lamina, and the posterior commissure crosses in the lower lamina. The pineal recess projects posteriorly into the pineal body between the two laminae. The shape of the orifice of the aqueduct of sylvius is triangular; the base of the triangle is on the posterior commissure and the other two limbs are formed by the central gray matter of the midbrain.

When viewed from posteriorly, the only structure in the posterior wall is the pineal body. The pineal gland projects posteriorly into the quadrigeminal cisterns and is concealed by the splenium of the corpus callosum above, the thalamus laterally, and the quadrigeminal plate and the vermis of the cerebellum inferiorly.

Lateral Wall

The lateral walls are not visible on the external surface of the brain, but are hidden between the cerebral hemispheres (*Figs. 5.10* and *5.11*). They are formed by the hypothalamus inferiorly and the thalamus superiorly. The lateral walls have an outline like the lateral silhouette of a bird's head with an open beak. The head is formed by the oval medial

FIGURE 5.13. *Floor and roof of the third ventricle.* A, *the floor of the third ventricle is located medial to the uncus and anterior perforated substance and above the midbrain. From anterior to posterior, the floor includes the lower margin of the optic chiasm, the pituitary stalk surrounded by the tuber cinereum, mamillary bodies, and the midbrain. The interpeduncular fossa is located below the posterior part of the floor. The anterior part of the optic tract extends along the lateral margin of the floor, but further posteriorly, the tracts deviate laterally away from the floor to pass around the upper margin of the cerebral peduncle.* B, *enlarged view. The tuber cinereum is situated around the pituitary stalk. The infundibular recess extends into the base of the stalk. A third ventriculostomy is commonly performed by opening through the thin area* (yellow arrow) *in the floor just in front of the mamillary bodies. The oculomotor nerves arise behind the mamillary bodies below the posterior part of the floor of the third ventricle.* C, *another specimen showing the thin area in front of the mamillary bodies* (yellow arrow) *through which a third ventriculostomy is completed. The anterior perforated substance and optic tracts are positioned lateral to the anterior part of the floor of the third ventricle. The mamillary bodies and upper midbrain are positioned below the posterior part of the floor.* D, *view of another third ventricle from below with the vascular structure preserved. The internal carotid, posterior communicating, anterior choroidal, and posterior cerebral arteries all give rise to branches that reach the walls of the lateral and third ventricles. The thalamoperforating branches of the posterior cerebral artery supply some of the posterior part of the floor of the third ventricle.* E, *inferior view with the floor of the third ventricle removed to expose the roof. The pituitary stalk has been reflected forward to expose the ventricular side of the infundibular recess and lamina terminalis. The lamina terminalis slopes upward from the upper edge of the chiasm to the area in front of the anterior commissure where it blends into the rostrum of the corpus callosum. The columns of the fornix cross above and anterior to the foramen of Monro and descend toward the mamillary bodies. The massa intermedia crosses the midportion of the third ventricle. The velum interpositum, in which the internal cerebral veins and medial posterior choroidal arteries course, is positioned between the thalami in the roof of the third ventricle. The posterior commissure is exposed below the pineal gland. The vein of Galen, into which the basal veins empty, is located just behind the third ventricle.* F, *enlarged view. The infundibular recess is located below the optic chiasm in the base of the pituitary stalk, and the chiasmatic recess is located above the optic chiasm. The lamina terminalis forms the anterior wall of the chiasmatic recess. The anterior commissure crosses the anterior wall in front of the columns of the fornix. The foramina of Monro open upward into both lateral ventricles. The lower wall of the velum interpositum is formed by the layer of tela choroidea, in which the choroid plexus in the roof of the third ventricle arises, and which is attached laterally to the striae medullaris thalami. The internal cerebral veins can be seen through the layer of tela forming the lower wall of the velum interpositum.* G, *another specimen with the floor of the third ventricle removed. The posterior cerebral arteries, from which the lateral and medial posterior choroidal arteries arise, passes around the midbrain. The lamina terminalis is exposed above the optic chiasm and slopes upward toward the anterior commissure. The columns of the fornix pass along the anterior and superior margins of the foramen of Monro and behind the anterior commissure. The lower layer of tela choroidea in the velum interpositum has been removed to expose the vascular layer in the roof of the third ventricle formed by the internal cerebral veins and medial posterior choroidal arteries. Another layer of tela, which spans the interval above the internal cerebral veins and below the body of the fornix, separates the vascular layer from the body of the fornix.*

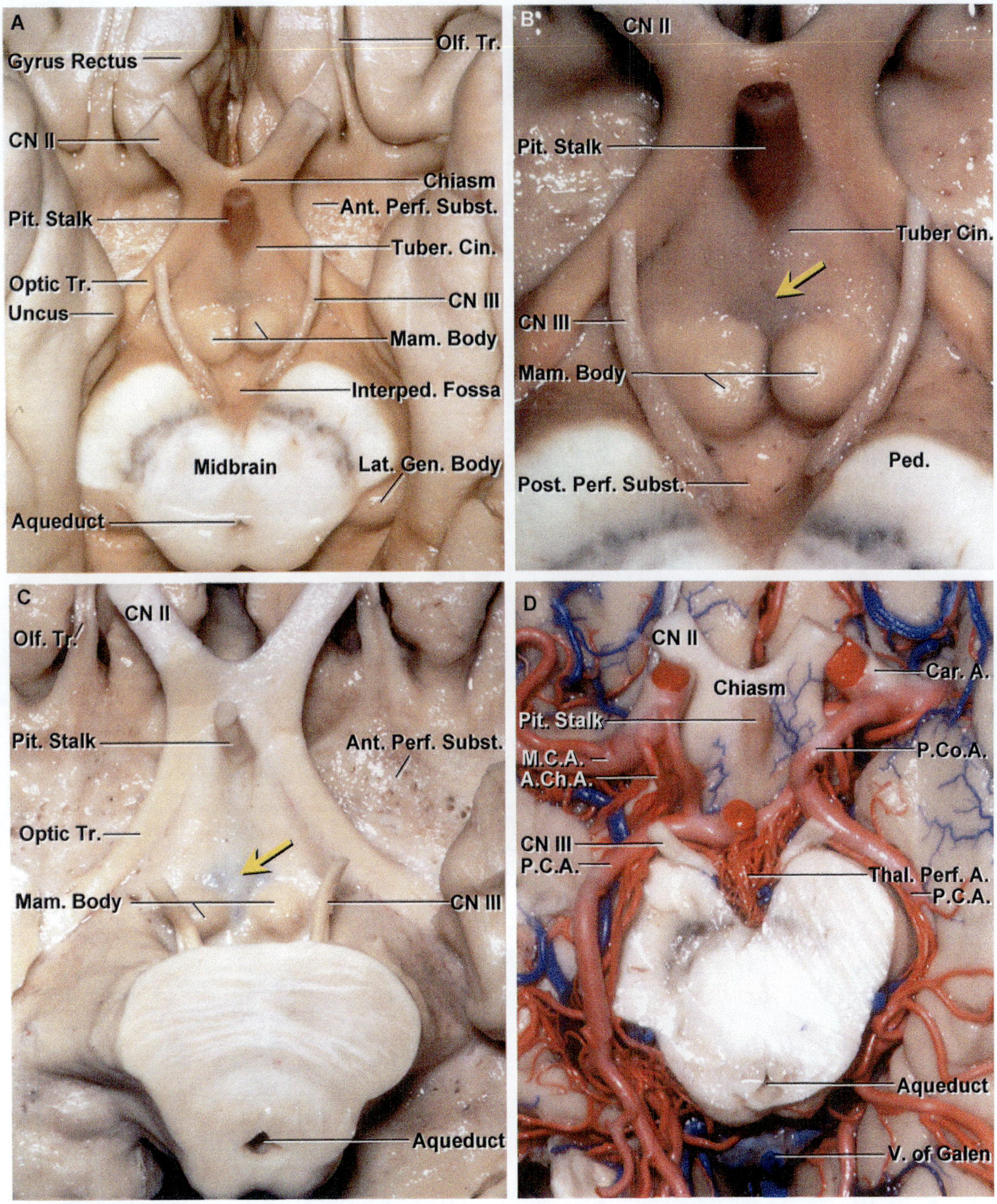

FIGURE 5.13. *Continued*
H, enlarged view. The upper layer of tela choroidea that spans the interval below the body of the fornix has been removed. The body of the fornix, exposed by removing the upper layer of tela, blends anteriorly into the columns of the fornix that pass along the anterior and superior margin of the foramen of Monro. The lamina terminalis has been opened in the interval between the optic chiasm and anterior commissure to expose the perforating branches of the anterior cerebral artery. A., *artery;* A.C.A., *anterior cerebral artery;* A.Ch.A., *anterior choroidal artery;* Ant., *anterior;* Calc., *calcarine;* Car., *carotid;* Cin., *cinereum;* CN, *cranial nerve;* Col., *column;* Comm., *commissure;* For., *foramen;* Gen., *geniculate;* Infund., *infundibular;* Int., *intermedia, internal;* Interped., *interpeduncular;* Interpos., *interpositum;* Lam., *lamina;* Lat., *lateral;* Mam., *mamillary;* M.C.A., *middle cerebral artery;* M.P.Ch.A., *medial posterior choroidal artery;* Olf., *olfactory;* P.C.A., *posterior cerebral artery;* P.Co.A., *posterior communicating artery;* Ped., *peduncle;* Perf., *perforated;* Pit., *pituitary;* Post., *posterior;* Rec., *recess;* Subst., *substance;* Term., *terminalis;* Thal.Perf., *thalamoperforating;* Tr., *tract;* V., *vein;* Vel., *velum. (Figure continues on next page.)*

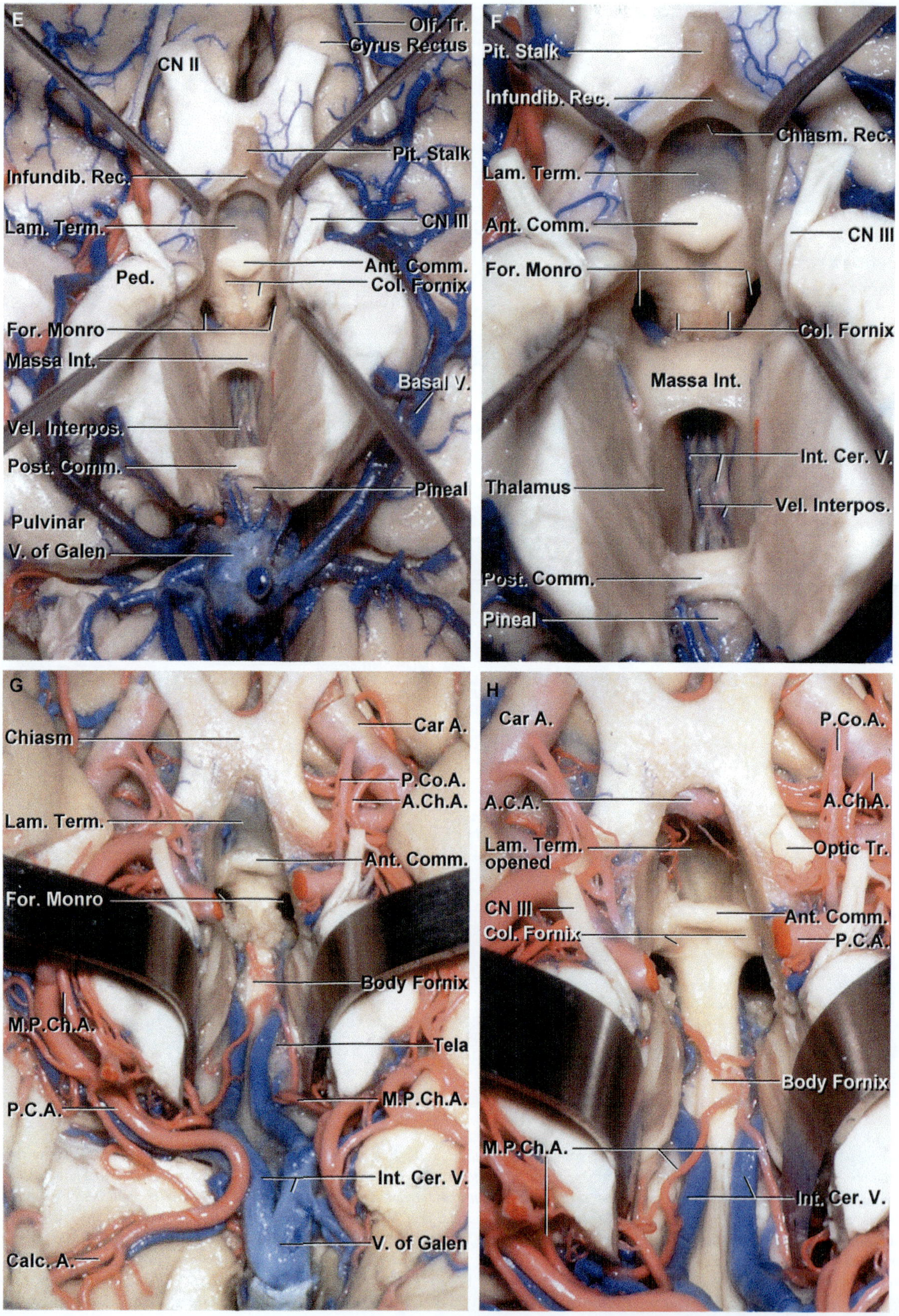

FIGURE 5.13. *Continued*

surface of the thalamus; the open beak, which projects anteriorly and inferiorly, is represented by the recesses in the hypothalamus: the pointed upper beak is formed by the optic recess and the lower beak is formed by the infundibular recess. The hypothalamic and thalamic surfaces are separated by the hypothalamic sulcus, a groove that is often ill-defined and extends from the foramen of Monro to the aqueduct of sylvius. The superior limit of the thalamic surfaces of the third ventricle is marked by narrow, raised ridges, known as the striae medullaris thalami. These striae extend forward from the habenulae along the superomedial surface of the thalamus near the attachment of the lower layer of the tela choroidea. The habenulae are small eminences on the dorsomedial surfaces of the thalamus just in front of the pineal gland. The habenulae are connected across the midline in the rostral stalk of the pineal gland by the habenular commissure.

The massa intermedia projects into the upper half of the third ventricle and often connects the opposing surfaces of the thalamus. It is present in approximately 75% of brains, being located 2.5 to 6.0 mm (average, 3.9 mm) posterior to the foramen of Monro. The columns of the fornix form distinct prominences in the lateral walls of the third ventricle just below the foramina of Monro, but inferiorly they sink below the surface.

Tentorial Incisura

The lateral and third ventricles are situated above the tentorial incisura, the triangular space situated between the free edges of the tentorium and the dorsum sellae (*Fig. 5.16*) (18, 23, 27). The apex of the incisura is dorsal to the midbrain in the area posterior to the pineal body, and the base is on the dorsum sellae. The midbrain is situated in the center of the incisura. The area between the midbrain and the free edges is divided into (a) an anterior incisural space located in front of the brainstem; (b) paired middle incisural spaces situated lateral to the midbrain; and (c) a posterior incisural space located behind the midbrain. The frontal horns are located above the anterior incisural space; the bodies of the lateral ventricles are located directly above the central part of the incisura, where they sit on and are separated from the central part of the incisura by the thalamus; the atria are located above the posterior incisural space; and the temporal horns are situated superolateral to the middle incisural space. The three incisural spaces contain some of the basal cisterns and are so intimately related to the lateral ventricles that some operative approaches to the basal cisterns situated within the incisura are directed through the lateral ventricles and choroidal fissure.

The anterior incisural space, which is situated anterior to the midbrain, extends obliquely upward around the optic chiasm along the anterior wall of the third ventricle to the area below the rostrum of the corpus callosum and the floor of the frontal horn. This space contains the interpeduncular cistern, which is situated between the cerebral peduncles, and the chiasmatic cistern, which is located below the optic chiasm. The chiasmatic cistern communicates around the optic chiasm with the cisternal laminae terminalis, which lies anterior to the lamina terminalis in the area below the floor of the frontal horn.

The middle incisural space, which is located between the temporal lobe and the midbrain, is so intimately related to the temporal horn and temporal part of the choroidal fissure that some operative approaches to this space are directed through the temporal horn. The temporal horn extends into the medial part of the temporal lobe lateral to the middle incisural space and ends approximately 3 cm from the anterior pole of the temporal lobe. This space is the site of the crural and ambient cisterns. The crural cistern, located between the cerebral peduncle and uncus and roofed by the optic tract, opens posteriorly into the ambient cistern.

The ambient cistern is a narrow communicating channel demarcated medially by the midbrain, above by the pulvinar, and laterally by the parahippocampal and dentate gyri and the fimbria of the fornix. The cisternal side of the temporal portion of the choroidal fissure is located in the superolateral part of the ambient cistern between the fimbria and the lower thalamic surface. The crural cistern cannot be reached through the choroidal fissure because the fissure ends just behind the uncus and the cistern at the inferior choroidal point. The crural cistern can be exposed from the temporal horn by an incision extending forward from the inferior choroidal point through the amygdala.

The posterior incisural space, the site of the quadrigeminal cistern, is located medial to the atrium. This cistern encloses a space that corresponds to the pineal region and has a roof, floor, and anterior and lateral walls. The choroid fissure lies at the junction of the anterior and lateral walls of the quadrigeminal cistern. The lateral walls of the quadrigeminal cistern separate the cistern from the atria. Each lateral wall has anterior and posterior parts: the anterior part is formed by the crus of the fornix and the posterior part is formed by the part of the medial surface of the occipital lobe situated below the splenium.

The anterior wall of the cistern has medial and lateral parts. The medial part of the anterior wall is formed by the quadrigeminal plate and pineal body. The suprapineal recess of the third ventricle bulges into the cistern above the pineal body. The lateral part of the anterior wall of the cistern is formed by the part of the pulvinar that lies medial to the crus of the fornix. Below the colliculi, the cistern extends into the cleft between the midbrain and cerebellum called the cerebellomesencephalic fissure. This fissure cannot be reached through the choroidal fissure. The trochlear nerves arise below the inferior colliculi and course laterally around the midbrain and below the pulvinars to enter the ambient cisterns.

The roof of the cistern is formed by the lower surface of the splenium and the broad membranous envelope that surrounds the great vein and its tributaries. This broad envelope of arachnoid tissue is applied to the lower surface of the splenium and is continuous anteriorly with the velum interpositum. It is within this envelope, in the superomedial part of the cistern, that the venous structures are found in the greatest density. The superomedial location of the major veins in the cistern contrasts with the location of the large arteries that are found in the inferolateral part of the cistern.

The quadrigeminal cistern opens anteriorly below the pulvinars into the ambient cisterns. The quadrigeminal cistern may communicate with the velum interpositum. Another potential

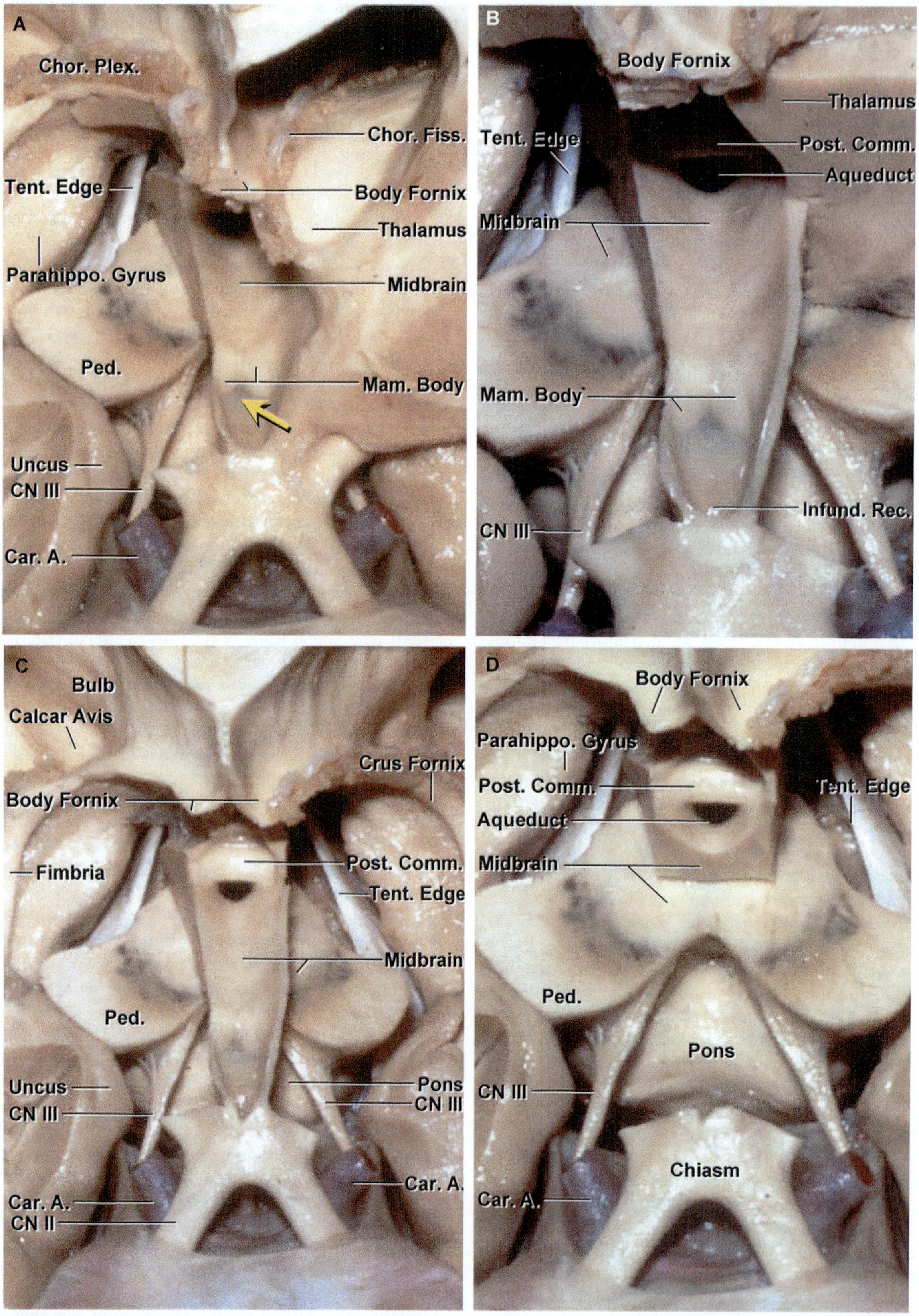
A
Chor. Plex.
Chor. Fiss.
Tent. Edge
Body Fornix
Thalamus
Parahippo. Gyrus
Midbrain
Ped.
Mam. Body
Uncus
CN III
Car. A.
B
Body Fornix
Thalamus
Tent. Edge
Post. Comm.
Aqueduct
Midbrain
Mam. Body
Infund. Rec.
CN III
C
Bulb
Calcar Avis
Crus Fornix
Body Fornix
Fimbria
Post. Comm.
Tent. Edge
Midbrain
Ped.
Uncus
Pons
CN III
CN III
Car. A.
Car. A.
CN II
D
Body Fornix
Parahippo. Gyrus
Post. Comm.
Tent. Edge
Aqueduct
Midbrain
Ped.
Pons
CN III
Chiasm
Car. A.

FIGURE 5.14.

cavity that may communicate with the quadrigeminal cistern is the cavum vergae, which is located immediately above the velum interpositum between the hippocampal commissure and the splenium. The cavum vergae is infrequently present because the hippocampal commissure commonly fuses to the lower surface of the splenium.

ARTERIAL RELATIONSHIPS

Each part of the lateral and third ventricles has surgically important arterial relationships. All of the arterial components of the circle of Willis are located in the anterior incisural space below the frontal horns and bodies of the lateral ventricles. The internal carotid arteries bifurcate into the anterior and middle cerebral arteries in the area below the frontal horns and give rise to the anterior choroidal arteries, which send branches through the choroidal fissures to the choroid plexus. The posterior part of the circle of Willis and the apex of the basilar artery are situated below the thalami, bodies of the lateral ventricles, floor of the third ventricle, and between the temporal horns. The anterior cerebral arteries pass around the anterior wall of the third ventricle and the floor and anterior wall of the frontal horns to reach the roof of the frontal horns and bodies. The posterior cerebral arteries pass medial to the temporal horns and atria and give rise to the posterior choroidal arteries, which pass through the choroidal fissure to supply the choroid plexus in the temporal horns, atria, and bodies. The posterior cerebral, pericallosal, superior cerebellar, and choroidal arteries pass adjacent to the posterior wall. Both the anterior and posterior cerebral arteries send branches into the roof, and the middle cerebral arteries pass below the frontal horns to reach the sylvian fissures and then course over the insulae, where they are lateral to the bodies of the lateral ventricle. The internal carotid, anterior choroidal, anterior and posterior cerebral and the anterior and posterior communicating arteries give rise to perforating branches that reach structures in or near the walls of the lateral and third ventricles (*Figs. 5.17* and *5.18*) (8, 9, 20, 21, 29, 30). The relationships between these arteries and the ventricles are reviewed in greater detail below.

Choroidal Arteries

The arteries most intimately related to the lateral ventricles and choroidal fissures are the choroidal arteries that supply the choroid plexus in the lateral and third ventricles. They arise from the internal carotid and posterior cerebral arteries in the basal cisterns and reach the choroid plexus by passing through the choroidal fissures (*Figs. 2.9, 2.10, 2.33,* and *5.19; Tables 5.1–5.3*).

The choroid plexus of the lateral ventricles is supplied by the anterior and posterior choroidal arteries (7, 26). The posterior choroidal arteries are divided into lateral and medial groups called the lateral and medial posterior choroidal arteries. Illustrations and text related to the course of each of these arteries is reviewed in Chapter 2. Each of the choroidal arteries gives off branches to the neural structures along its course. The most common pattern is for the anterior choroidal arteries to supply a portion of the choroid plexus in the temporal horn and atrium; the lateral posterior choroidal arteries to supply a portion of the choroid plexus in the atrium, body, and posterior part of the temporal horn; and the medial posterior choroidal arteries to supply the choroid plexus in the roof of the third ventricle and part of that in the body of the lateral ventricle. The size of the plexal areas supplied by the anterior and posterior choroidal arteries is inversely related: as the area supplied by one artery enlarges, the area supplied by the other decreases. The same inverse relationship occurs between the areas supplied by the lateral and medial posterior choroidal arteries. The lateral and medial posterior choroidal arteries arising on one side may infrequently send branches to the choroid plexus in the opposite lateral ventricle.

The anterior choroidal artery arises from the internal carotid artery in the anterior incisural space and courses posteriorly to reach the middle incisural space, where it passes through the choroidal fissure near the inferior choroidal point and courses along the medial border of the choroid plexus in close relation to the lateral posterior choroidal arteries. It passes posteriorly and dorsally along the plexus, reaching the foramen of Monro in a few hemispheres. There are frequent anastomoses between the branches of the anterior and lateral posterior choroidal arteries on the surface of the choroid plexus.

The lateral posterior choroidal arteries are a group that arise in the ambient and quadrigeminal cisterns from the posterior cerebral artery or its cortical branches. These branches enter the ventricle behind the branches of the anterior choroidal artery. They pass laterally around the pulvinar and through the choroidal fissure at the level of the fimbria, crus, and body of the fornix to reach the choroid plexus in the temporal horn, atrium, and

FIGURE 5.14. *Anterior view of the floor and lower part of the third ventricle.* A, *the right thalamus has been removed. The posterior part of the floor of the third ventricle is formed by the upper surface of the midbrain located behind the mamillary bodies. The tentorial edges join at the tentorial apex located in the quadrigeminal cistern behind the aqueduct. The choroidal fissure in the body of the ventricle is located between the body of the fornix and the upper surface of the thalamus. The floor between the optic chiasm and mamillary bodies is located above the chiasmatic cistern. The most common site for a third ventriculostomy is located just in front of the mamillary bodies.* B, *the anterior part of the left thalamus has been removed to expose the cerebral peduncles and upper midbrain on both sides of the third ventricle. The oculomotor nerves arise below the posterior part of the floor of the third ventricle. The infundibular recess is located behind the optic chiasm. The pons is exposed below the mamillary bodies and infundibular recess.* C, *both thalami have been removed. The third ventricular floor extends from the optic chiasm to the aqueduct. The choroidal fissure in the body of the ventricle is located between the body of the fornix and the thalamus, in the atrium it is between the crus of the fornix and the pulvinar, and in the temporal horn it is between the fimbria and lower surface of the thalamus.* D, *enlarged view. The upper midbrain and pons are located below the floor of the third ventricle. The oculomotor nerves exit the midbrain below the floor. The aqueduct and posterior commissure are positioned in the posterior wall of the third ventricle in front of the tentorial apex and quadrigeminal cistern.* A., *artery;* Car., *carotid;* Chor., *choroid;* CN, *cranial nerve;* Comm., *commissure;* Infund., *infundibular;* Mam., *mamillary;* Parahippo., *parahippocampal;* Ped., *peduncle;* Plex., *plexus;* Post., *posterior;* Rec., *recess;* Tent., *tentorial.*

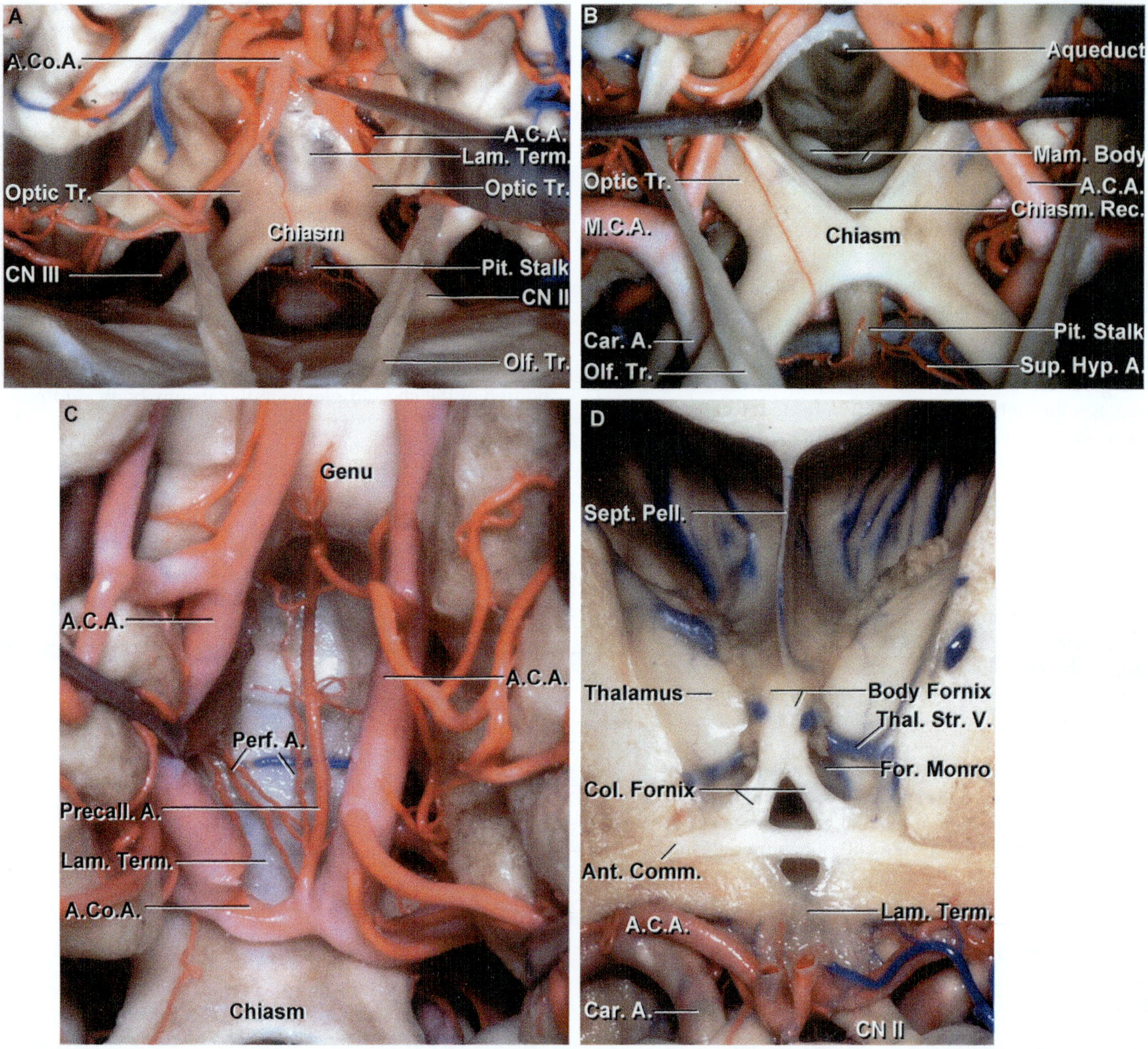

FIGURE 5.15. *Anterior wall of the third ventricle.* A, *the frontal lobe and the anterior carotid arteries have been elevated to expose the optic chiasm and lamina terminalis. The pituitary stalk extends downward from the floor of the third ventricle. The optic tracts pass along the lateral margin of the floor of the third ventricle. The lamina terminalis blends above into the rostrum of the corpus callosum. The olfactory tracts pass backward above the optic nerves.* B, *the lamina terminalis has been opened to expose the chiasmatic recess, mamillary bodies, and aqueduct. The pituitary stalk is exposed below the infundibular recess located behind the optic chiasm and in front of the mamillary bodies. Superior hypophyseal arteries pass medially from the carotid artery.* C, *another third ventricle. The anterior communicating artery commonly passes in front of the lamina terminalis. Perforating arteries arise from a precallosal branch of the anterior communicating artery and penetrate the anterior wall of the third ventricle to reach the columns of the fornix.* D, *anterior view of a cross section through the anterior part of the third ventricle and body of the lateral ventricle. The lamina terminalis, which has been opened, extends upward in front of the anterior commissure and blends into the rostrum of the corpus callosum. The anterior cerebral arteries have been folded forward. The choroid plexus extends through the foramen of Monro into the roof of the third ventricle below and the body of the lateral ventricle above.* E, *the cross section of another third ventricle extends through the anterior commissure. The body of the fornix sits in the floor of the body of the ventricle. The columns of the fornix pass around the superior and anterior margins of the foramen of Monro and behind the anterior commissure. The lamina terminalis extends upward from the chiasm.*

body. If the anterior choroidal artery supplies the choroid plexus in the temporal horn and atrium, the lateral posterior choroidal arteries will course outside the ventricle along the medial edge of the temporal and atrial parts of the choroidal fissure and reach the choroid plexus by passing through the body portion of the choroidal fissure. The lateral posterior choroidal arteries may

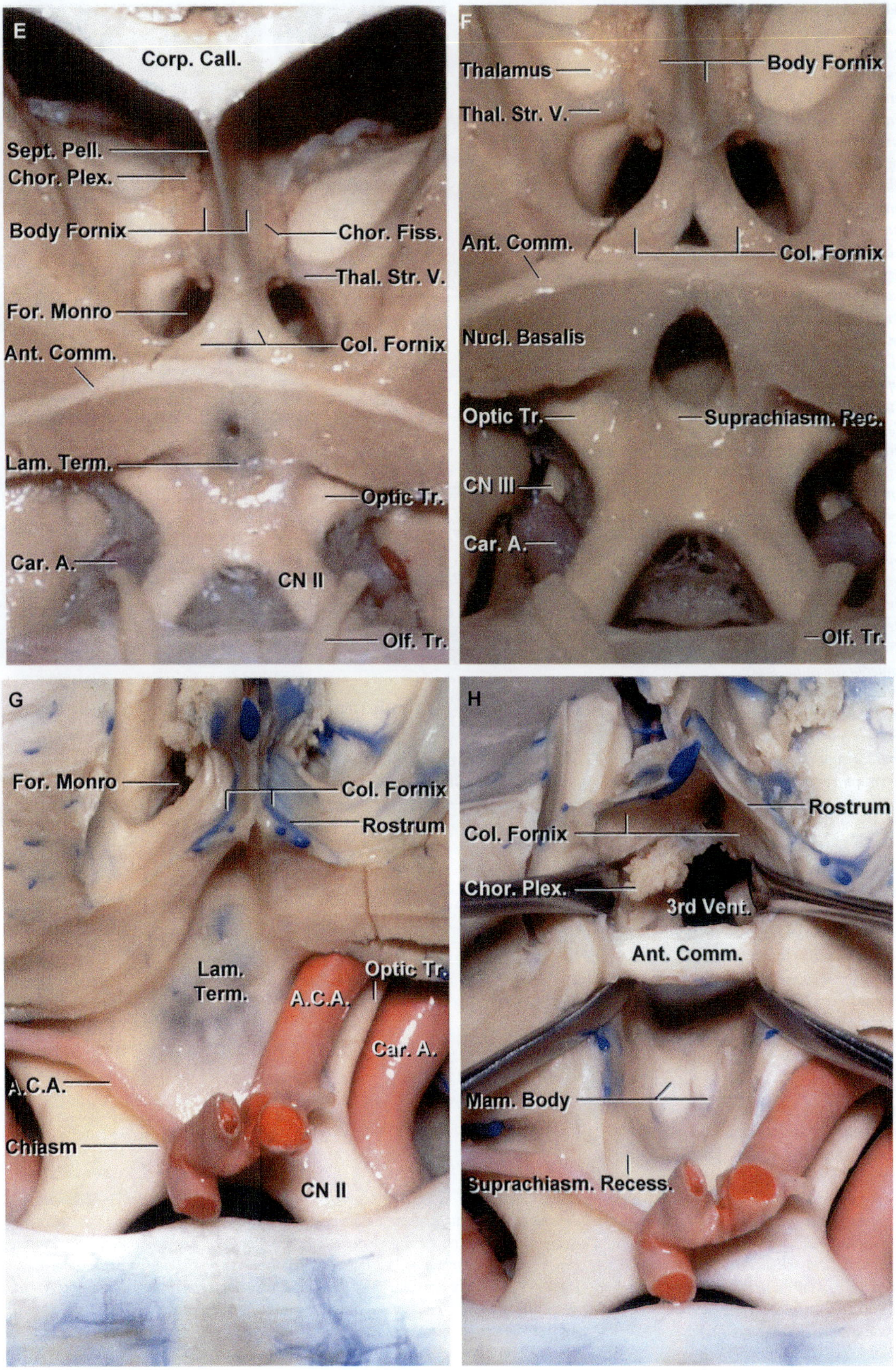

FIGURE 5.15. *Continued* F, *enlarged view. The lamina terminalis has been opened. The chiasmatic recess is located between the lower part of the lamina terminalis and the posterior part of the optic chiasm. The nucleus basalis is located below the lateral part of the anterior commissure.* G, *another third ventricle. The lamina terminalis extends upward from the optic chiasm and blends into the rostrum of the corpus callosum.* H, *the lamina terminalis has been opened. The posterior margin of the chiasm is exposed behind the anterior communicating artery. The anterior commissure is exposed behind the upper edge of the lamina terminalis. The incision has been extended upward through the rostrum of the corpus callosum between the columns of the fornix. This exposes the roof of the third ventricle above the anterior commissure. The choroid plexus hangs down from the tela into the roof of the third ventricle. The mamillary bodies are exposed in the floor.* A., *artery;* A.C.A., *anterior cerebral artery;* A.Co.A., *anterior communicating artery;* Ant., *anterior;* Car., *carotid;* Chiasm., *chiasmatic;* Chor., *choroid;* CN, *cranial nerve;* Col., *column;* Fiss., *fissure;* For., *foramen;* Hyp., *hypophyseal;* Lam., *lamina;* Mam., *mamillary;* M.C.A., *middle cerebral artery;* Nucl., *nucleus;* Olf., *olfactory;* Pell., *pellucidum;* Perf., *perforating;* Pit., *pituitary;* Plex., *plexus;* Precall., *precallosal;* Rec., *recess;* Sept., *septum;* Sup., *superior;* Suprachiasm., *suprachiasmatic;* Term., *terminalis;* Thal. Str., *thalamostriate;* Tr., *tract;* V., *vein;* Vent., *ventricle.*

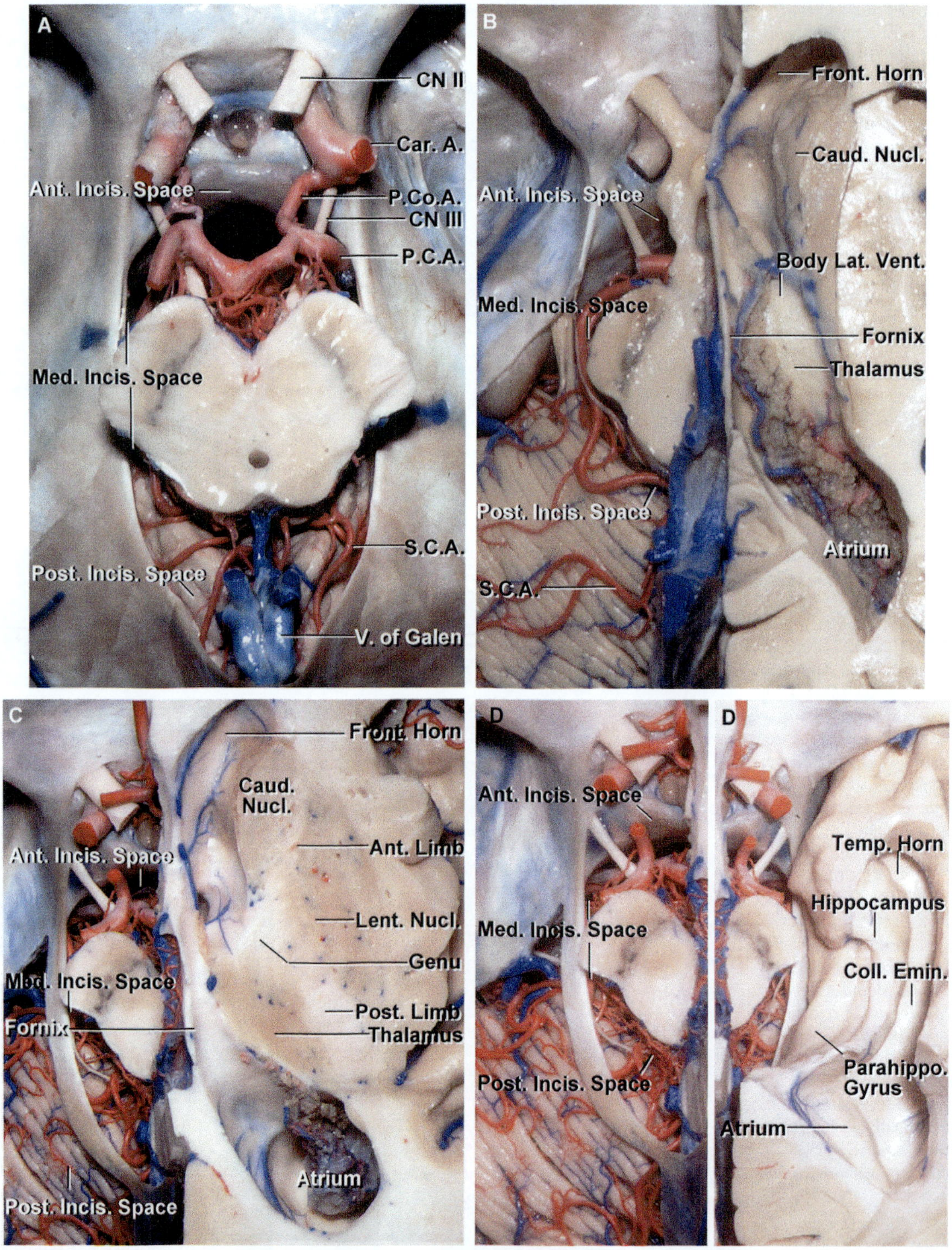

FIGURE 5.16. *Superior views showing the relationships of the lateral ventricles to the tentorial incisura. A, the tentorial incisura is divided into an anterior incisural space located anterior to the brainstem, a middle incisural space located between the midbrain and tentorial edge, and a posterior incisural space located between the tentorial apex and posterior surface of the midbrain. The anterior incisural space contains the chiasmatic and interpeduncular cisterns. The middle incisural space communicates with the ambient and crural cistern. The posterior incisural space contains the quadrigeminal cistern. B, superior view with the left cerebrum and left half of the tentorium removed. The frontal horn sits above the anterior incisural space. The thalamus sits directly above the midbrain in the center of the tentorial incisura. The middle incisural space is located between the midbrain and tentorial edge. The atrium faces the posterior incisural space and quadrigeminal cistern. C, another specimen. The axial section of the right hemisphere extends through the internal capsule. The frontal horn is located above the anterior incisural space. The thalamus is located above the midbrain in the center of the incisura and above the middle incisural spaces. The medial wall of the atrium forms the lateral wall of the quadrigeminal cistern and posterior incisural space. The internal capsule is situated above the lateral edge of the three incisural spaces. D, comparison of the relationships in the tentorial incisura (*D-left*) and temporal horn (*D-right*). The neural structures on the right have been removed except the temporal horn. The temporal lobe on the left was removed to expose the tentorial incisura. The choroidal fissure opens between the fimbria and the thalamus into the middle incisural space located lateral to the midbrain. The temporal horn is positioned lateral to the middle incisural space. The lower part of the medial wall of the atrium faces the posterior incisural space. A., artery;* Ant., *anterior;* Car., *carotid;* Caud., *caudate;* CN, *cranial nerve;* Coll., *collateral;* Front., *frontal;* Incis., *incisural;* Lat., *lateral;* Lent., *lenticular;* Med., *medial;* Nucl., *nucleus;* Parahippo., *parahippocampal;* P.C.A., *posterior cerebral artery;* P.Co.A., *posterior communicating artery;* Post., *posterior;* S.C.A., *superior cerebellar artery;* Temp., *temporal;* V., *vein;* Vent., *ventricle.*

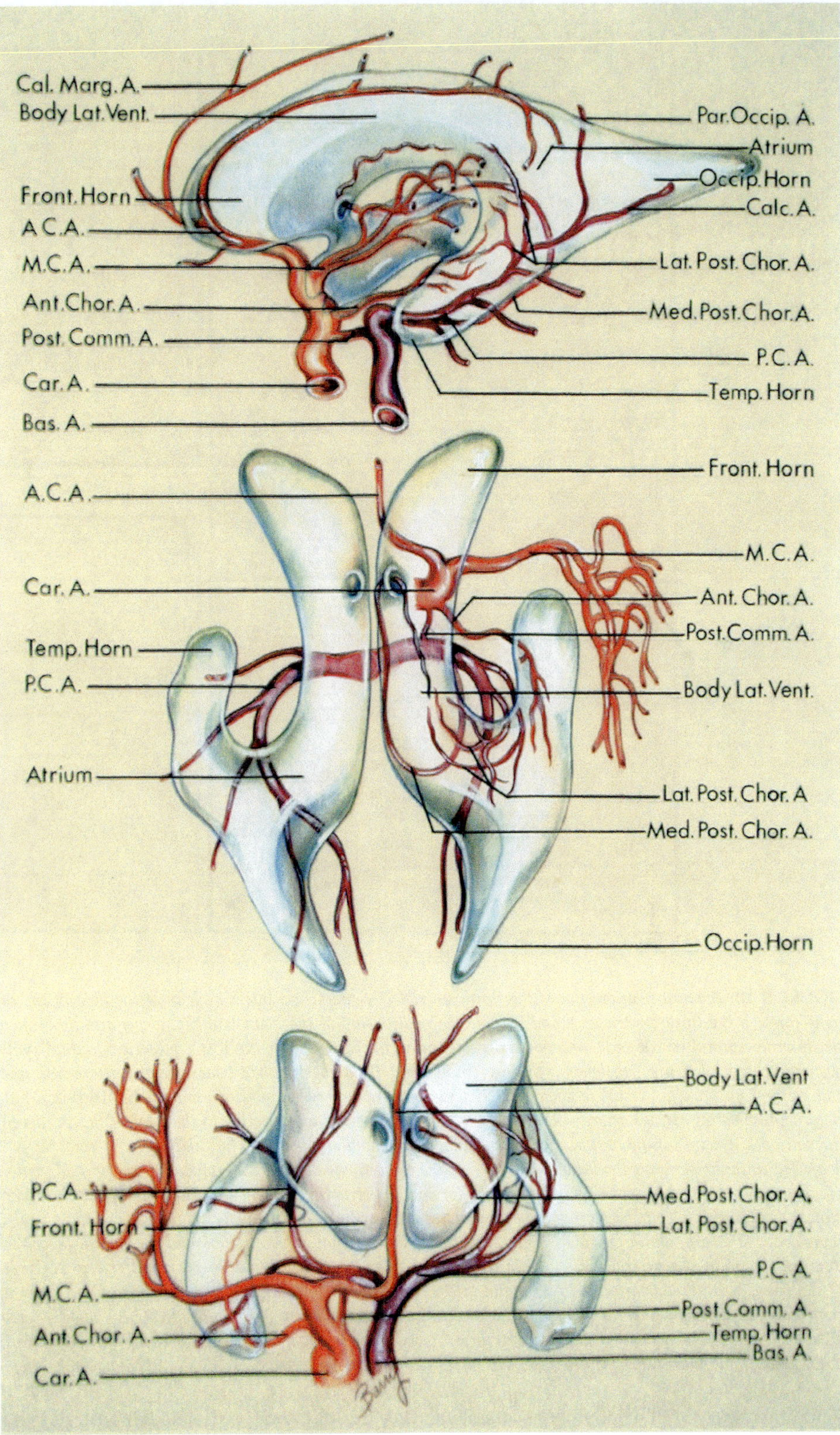

FIGURE 5.17. *Arterial relationships of the lateral ventricles. Lateral (top), superior (middle), and anterior (bottom) views. The internal carotid artery and its branches are shown in orange, and the basilar artery and its branches are shown in red. The internal carotid, basilar, anterior, middle, posterior cerebral, and anterior, lateral, and medial posterior choroidal arteries all have important relationships to the frontal, temporal, and occipital horns and the atria and bodies of the lateral ventricles. The carotid arteries bifurcate into their anterior and middle cerebral branches in the area below the posterior part of the frontal horns. The origins of the middle cerebral arteries are situated below the frontal horns. The anterior cerebral arteries pass anteromedially below the frontal horns and give rise to the pericallosal and callosomarginal branches, which curve around the anterior wall and roof of the frontal horn. The anterior choroidal arteries enter the anterior part of the temporal horns. The posterior communicating arteries are situated below the thalami and bodies of the lateral ventricles. The basilar artery bifurcates below the bodies of the lateral ventricles into the posterior cerebral arteries, which course below the thalami near the medial aspect of the temporal horns and atria. The medial posterior choroidal arteries arise from the proximal part of the posterior cerebral arteries, encircle the brainstem below the thalami, and pass forward in the roof of the third ventricle, where they give branches to the choroid plexus in the roof of the third ventricle and the bodies of the lateral ventricles. The lateral posterior choroidal branches of the posterior cerebral arteries pass laterally through the choroidal fissures to enter the temporal horns and atria of the lateral ventricles. The middle cerebral arteries course on the insulae in the area above the temporal horns and lateral to the bodies of the lateral ventricles. The posterior cerebral arteries bifurcate into the calcarine and parieto-occipital arteries in the area medial to the atria.* A., *artery;* A.C.A., *anterior cerebral artery;* Ant., *anterior;* Bas., *basilar;* Cal. Marg., *callosomarginal;* Calc., *calcarine;* Car., *carotid;* Chor., *choroidal;* Comm., *communicating;* Front., *frontal;* Lat., *lateral;* M.C.A., *middle cerebral artery;* Occip., *occipital;* Par. Occip., *parieto-occipital;* P.C.A., *posterior cerebral artery;* Post., *posterior;* Temp., *temporal;* Vent., *ventricle.*

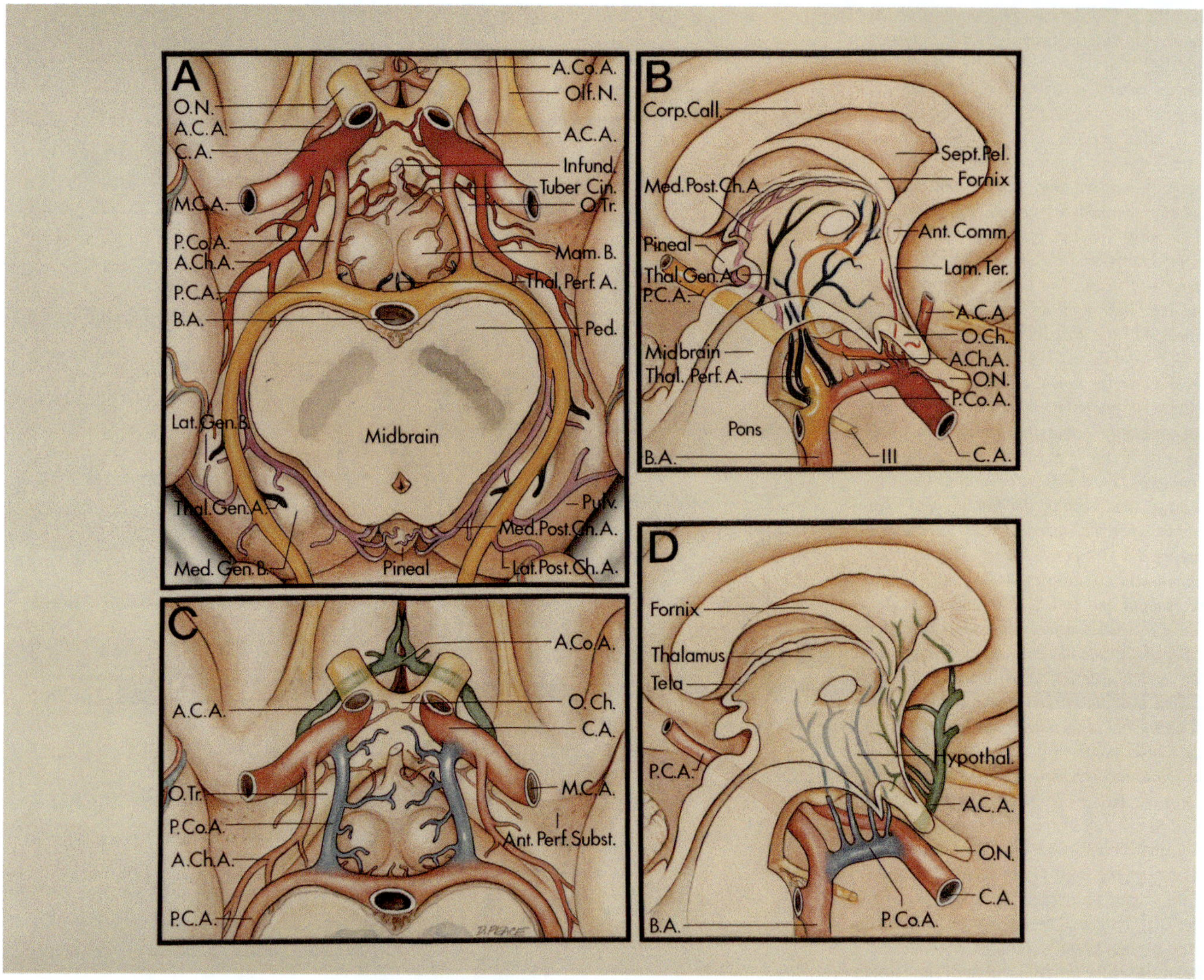

FIGURE 5.18. *Arterial relationships of the third ventricle.* A *and* C *are inferior views of the floor of the third ventricle and* B *and* D *are midsagittal sections through the third ventricle.* A *and* B *show the relationship of the main trunks and perforating branches of the following arteries to the third ventricle: internal carotid* (dark red), *anterior choroidal* (orange), *basilar apex* (yellow), *posterior cerebral* (yellow), *medial posterior choroidal* (pink), *lateral posterior choroidal* (pink), *thalamoperforating* (blue), *and thalamogeniculate* (dark green) *arteries.* C *and* D *show the relationships of the main trunks and perforating branches of the following arteries to the third ventricle: anterior cerebral* (light green), *anterior communicating* (light green), *and posterior communicating* (blue) *arteries. The olfactory and optic nerves are anterior to the floor of the third ventricle. The structures in the floor are the optic chiasm, optic tracts, infundibulum, tuber cinereum, and mamillary bodies. The midbrain and cerebral peduncles are inferior to the posterior half of the floor. The anterior perforated substance is lateral to the optic tracts. The lateral geniculate and medial geniculate bodies are attached to the lower margin of the thalamus near the pulvinar, lateral to the midbrain. The structures in the anterior wall of the third ventricle are the anterior commissure, lamina terminalis, and optic chiasm. The corpus callosum and septum pellucidum are above the roof of the third ventricle. The roof is formed of the two layers of tela choroidea, the fornix, and a vascular layer composed of the internal cerebral veins and the medial posterior choroidal arteries. The oculomotor nerve exits from the midbrain.* A., *artery;* A.C.A., *anterior cerebral artery;* A.Ch.A., *anterior choroidal artery;* A.Co.A., *anterior communicating artery;* Ant., *anterior;* B., *body;* B.A., *basilar artery;* C.A., *carotid artery;* Call., *callosum;* Ch., *chiasm, choroidal;* Cin., *cinereum;* Comm., *commissure;* Corp., *corpus;* Gen., *geniculate;* Hypothal., *hypothalamus;* Lam., *lamina;* Lat., *lateral;* Mam., *mamillary;* M.C.A., *middle cerebral artery;* Med., *medial;* N., *nerve;* O., *optic;* Olf., *olfactory;* P.C.A., *posterior cerebral artery;* P.Co.A., *posterior communicating artery;* Ped., *peduncle;* Pell., *pellucidum;* Perf., *perforated;* Post., *posterior;* Pulv., *pulvinar;* Sept., *septum;* Subst., *substance;* Term., *terminalis;* Thal.Gen., *thalamogeniculate;* Thal.Perf., *thalamoperforating;* Tr., *tract.*

send branches from the body of one lateral ventricle through the foramen of Monro, or between the fornix and thalamus to the choroid plexus in the third ventricle, or through the foramen of Monro to the choroid plexus in the body of the contralateral lateral ventricle. These branches intermingle with the branches of the medial posterior choroidal artery in the body of the ventricle and at the foramen of Monro.

The medial posterior choroidal arteries most frequently arise as one to three branches from the posteromedial aspect of the proximal part of the posterior cerebral artery in the interpedun-

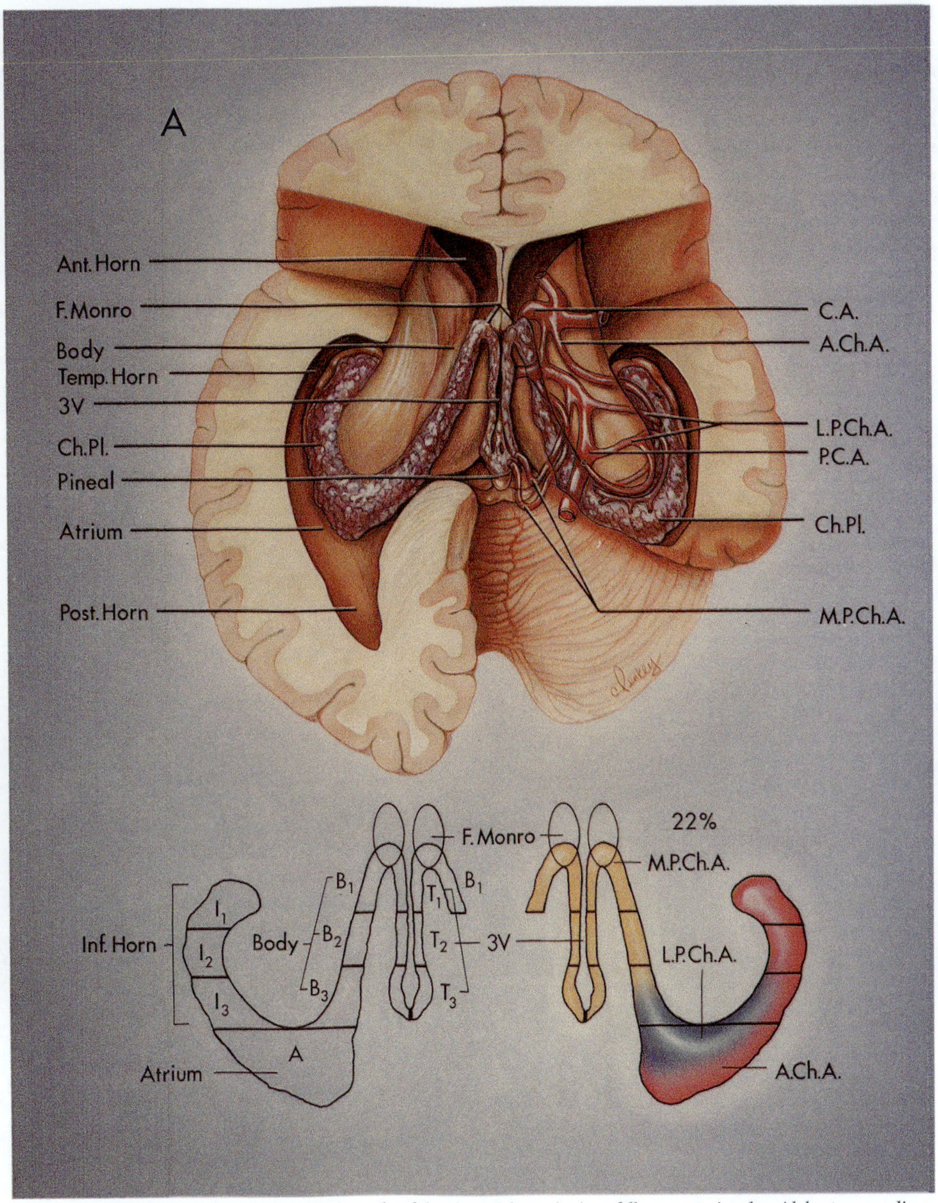

FIGURE 5.19. A. Upper: *Superior view with part of the cerebral hemispheres, corpus callosum, and the fornix removed to show the relationship between the lateral and third ventricle and the choroid plexus. The left hemisphere shows the relationship of the ventricles to the choroid plexus. The choroid plexus of the lateral ventricle extends from the temporal horn into the atrium and body of the lateral ventricle. It does not extend backward into the posterior horn or forward into the anterior (frontal) horn, but passes through the foramen of Monro and continues posteriorly in the roof of the third ventricle to the suprapineal recess above the pineal body. The right hemisphere shows the relationships between the choroidal arteries and the choroid plexus. The anterior choroidal artery arises from the carotid artery and supplies the plexus of the temporal horn and atrium. The lateral posterior choroidal arteries arise from the posterior cerebral artery or its branches and supply the plexus in the posterior part of the temporal horn, atrium, and body of the lateral ventricle. The medial posterior choroidal arteries arise from the posterior cerebral artery and supply the plexus in the third and, in many cases, the body of the lateral ventricle.* Lower left: *Classification of the choroid plexus. The portion of the choroid plexus within the temporal horn and body of the lateral ventricle and the third ventricle is subdivided into an anterior, middle, and posterior third. The subdivisions within the lateral and third ventricles are designated as follows: inferior (temporal) horn of the lateral ventricle—anterior third I_1, middle third I_2, and posterior third I_3; atrium of the lateral ventricle—A; body—anterior third B_1, middle third B_2, and posterior third B_3; and third ventricle—anterior third T_1, middle third T_2, and posterior third T_3. The criteria used to divide the area of supply of each artery into small, medium, and large groups are listed in* Table 5.1. Lower right: *Schematic illustration of the choroid plexus showing the most common pattern of supply (22% of hemispheres). The anterior choroidal artery is shown in* red, *the lateral posterior choroidal artery in* blue, *the medial posterior choroidal artery in* yellow, *and the contralateral lateral posterior choroidal artery in* green. *The area of the field of supply of the choroidal arteries is as follows: anterior choroidal artery, medium; lateral posterior choroidal artery, small; and medial posterior choroidal artery, large. The medial posterior choroidal arteries are shown together in both hemispheres. (Legend continues on next page.)*

cular and crural cisterns. These branches encircle the midbrain medial to the main trunk of the posterior cerebral artery, turn forward at the side of the pineal gland to enter the roof of the third ventricle, and course in the velum interpositum, between the thalami, adjacent to the internal cerebral veins and the opposite medial posterior choroidal arteries. A few medial posterior choroidal arteries may arise from the distal parts of the posterior cerebral artery or its cortical branches and run in an anterior or retrograde course from their origin to reach the roof of the third ventricle. The medial posterior choroidal arteries supply the choroid plexus in the roof of the third ventricle and sometimes pass through the ipsilateral foramen of Monro or choroidal fissure to supply the choroid plexus in the lateral ventricle. They occasionally send branches through the contralateral foramen of Monro and choroidal fissure to supply the choroid plexus in the contralateral lateral ventricle. They may send tiny branches along their course to the cerebral peduncle, geniculate bodies, tegmentum, colliculi, pulvinar, pineal body, posterior commissure, habenula, striae medullaris thalami, occipital cortex, and thalamus.

Internal Carotid Artery

The internal carotid artery exits the cavernous sinus along the medial surface of the anterior clinoid process and bifurcates below the frontal horn (*Figs. 5.15–5.18*) (9, 29). The branches arising from the ophthalmic and communicating segments pass to the optic nerves, chiasm, and tract, and the

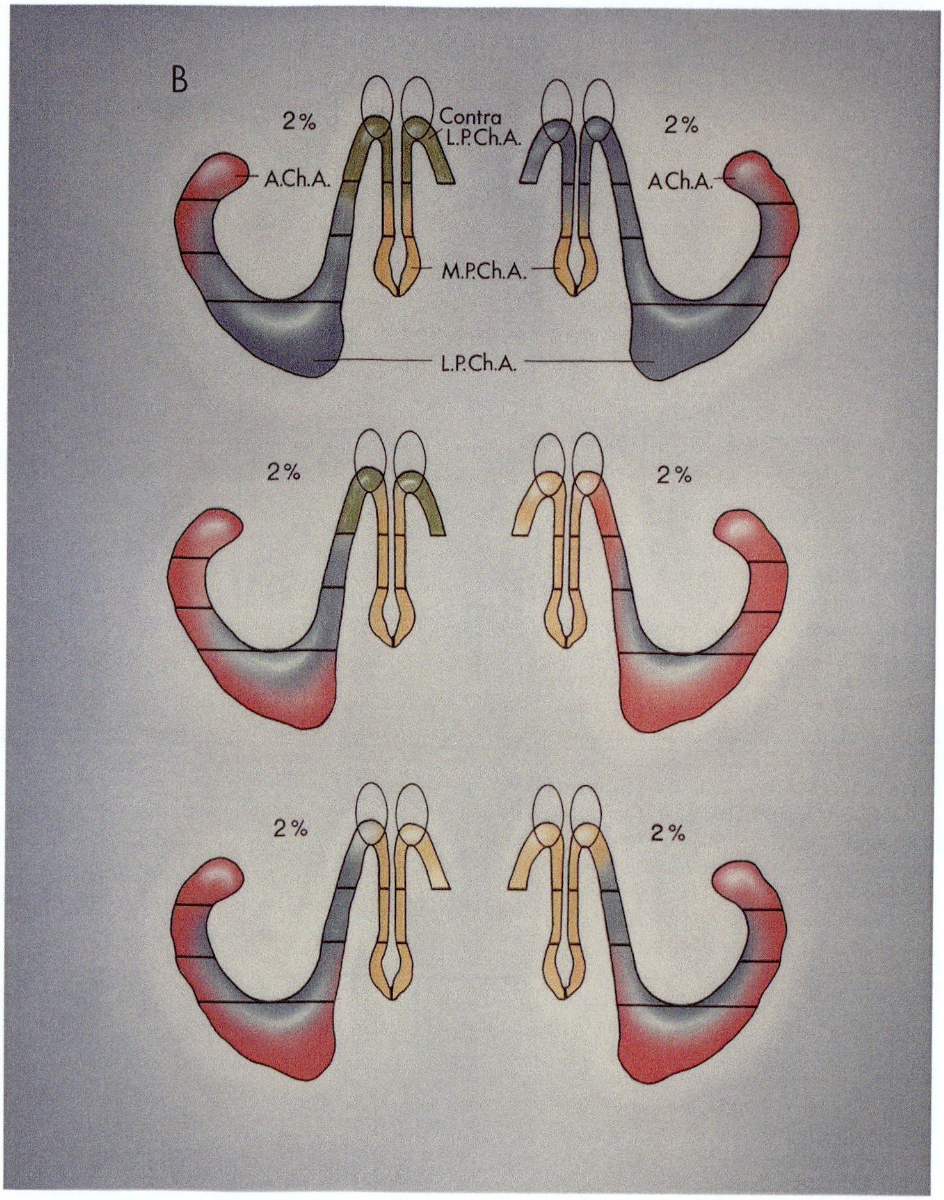

FIGURE 5.19. *Continued*
B, schematic illustration of the choroid plexus showing size of the area supplied by the choroidal arteries. The criteria used to divide the area of supply of each artery into small, medium, and large groups are listed in Table 5.1. *The second to seventh most common patterns are listed in* Table 5.2.

floor of the third ventricle, but the branches arising from the choroidal segment are directed upward through the anterior perforated substance to supply structures in or near the walls of the lateral and third ventricles, which include the genu and posterior limb of the internal capsule, the adjacent part of the globus pallidus, and the thalamus. The internal carotid artery also gives off the superior hypophyseal artery, which runs medially below the floor of the third ventricle, to reach the tuber cinereum and join its mate of the opposite side to form a vascular ring around the infundibulum.

Posterior Communicating Artery

The posterior communicating artery arises from the posterior wall of the internal carotid artery below the frontal horn in the anterior incisural space and courses posteromedially below the optic tracts and the floor of the third ventricle to join the posterior cerebral artery (*Figs. 2.8, 5.17,* and *5.18*). Its branches penetrate the floor of the third ventricle between the optic chiasm and carotid peduncle to reach the hypothalamus, thalamus, subthalamus, and internal capsule in the area below the body of the lateral ventricle.

Anterior Cerebral and Anterior Communicating Arteries

The anterior cerebral artery ascends in front of the lamina terminalis and anterior wall of the third ventricle to reach the area below the floor of the frontal horn (*Figs. 5.11, 5.15, 5.17,* and *5.18*) (20, 21). It then passes below the rostrum and around the genu of the corpus callosum in close proximity to the floor, anterior wall, and roof of the frontal horn and the roof of the body of the lateral ventricle. The tightness of the curve around the frontal horn is a good indicator of

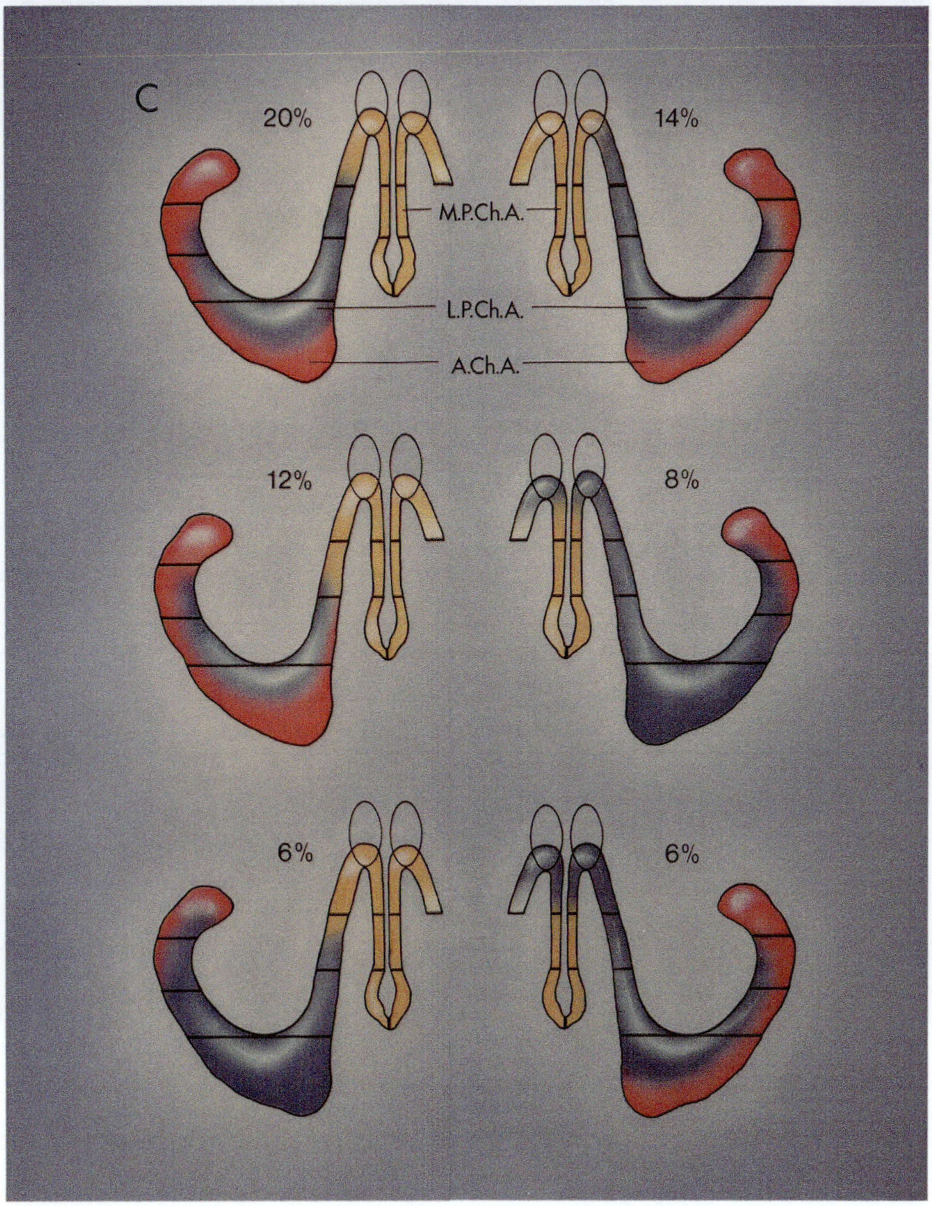

FIGURE 5.19. *Continued*
C, schematic illustration of the choroid plexus showing the size of area supplied by the choroidal arteries. The criteria used to divide the area of supply into small, medium, and large groups are listed in Table 5.1. *The least common patterns are listed in* Table 5.3. A.Ch.A., *anterior choroidal artery;* Ant., *anterior;* C.A., *carotid artery;* Ch., *choroid;* F., *foramen;* Inf., *inferior;* L.P.Ch.A., *lateral posterior choroidal artery;* M.P.Ch.A., *medial posterior choroidal artery;* P.C.A., *posterior cerebral artery;* Pl., *plexus;* Post., *posterior;* Temp., *temporal;* V, *ventricle.*

the size of the lateral ventricles. The distal part of the anterior cerebral artery may be exposed not only above, but also below the corpus callosum, because the terminal branch of the pericallosal artery may pass around the splenium and course forward in the roof of the third ventricle, reaching as far anterior as the foramen of Monro. The pericallosal branches that penetrate the corpus callosum reach the septum pellucidum and the fornix in the medial wall of the frontal horn and body.

The anterior cerebral and anterior communicating arteries give rise to perforating branches that terminate in the whole anterior wall of the third ventricle and reach the adjacent parts of the hypothalamus, fornix, septum pellucidum, and striatum. A precallosal artery may originate from the anterior cerebral or the anterior communicating artery, run upward across the lamina terminalis, and send branches into the anterior wall.

The recurrent branch of the anterior cerebral artery is frequently encountered in approaches below the anterior part of the third ventricle and frontal horn. It and the segment of the anterior cerebral artery proximal to the anterior communicating artery send branches into the area near the lateral wall of the frontal horn and body. These branches supply part of the genu and anterior limb of the internal capsule, globus pallidus, and less commonly, the thalamus.

Middle Cerebral Artery

The middle cerebral artery arises below the frontal horn (*Figs. 5.17* and *5.18*) (8). The penetrating branches of the mid-

TABLE 5.1. Criteria for classification of area supplied by the choroidal arteries by size[a]

Artery and size of field supply	Plexal area supplied	Percentage of hemispheres
Anterior choroidal		
Small	Only I_1, I_2, I_3	18
Medium	I_1, I_2, I_3, A	64
Large	I_{1-3}, A, and extends into body	18
Lateral posterior choroidal		
Small	Only I_3, A, B_3	38
Medium	I_2, I_3, A, B_3, B_2, and infrequently B_1	46
Large	I_1, I_2–B_1, and the plexus in third ventricle and/ or contralateral ventricle	16
Medial posterior choroidal		
Small	Only T_3, T_2	10
Medium	T_3, T_2, T_1	28
Large	T_3, T_2, T_1, and the plexus in lateral ventricle	62

[a] A, atrium of the lateral ventricle; B, body of the lateral ventricle: B_1 anterior third, B_2 middle third, B_3 posterior third; I, inferior (temporal) horn of the lateral ventricle: I_1 anterior third, I_2 middle third, and I_3 posterior third; and T, third ventricle: T_1 anterior third, T_2 middle third, and T_3 posterior third.

TABLE 5.2. Most common patterns of supply by the choroidal arteries[a]

Hemispheres present	% present	AChA (red)	LPChA (blue)	MPChA (yellow)
Upper				
Left	20%	Medium	Medium	Large
Right	14%	Medium	Medium	Medium
Middle				
Left	12%	Large	Small	Large
Right	8%	Small	Large	Medium
Lower				
Left	6%	Small	Medium	Large
Right	6%	Medium	Large	Small

[a] AChA, anterior choroidal artery; LPChA, lateral posterior choroidal artery; MPChA, medial posterior choroidal artery.

dle cerebral artery that supply structures in the area lateral to the frontal horn and body of the lateral ventricle are called the lenticulostriate arteries. They enter the deep structures lateral to the frontal horn and body of the lateral ventricle, including the lentiform nucleus, the entire anterior-posterior length of the internal capsule, and the body and head of the caudate nucleus.

Posterior Cerebral Artery

The bifurcation of the basilar artery into the posterior cerebral arteries is located below the posterior half of the floor of the third ventricle and below the bodies of the lateral ventricles (*Figs. 5.13, 5.17,* and *5.18*) (30, 38). A high basilar bifurcation may indent the floor. Its branches reach the walls of the temporal horn, atrium, and body of the lateral ventricle, and the floor, roof, and posterior and lateral walls of the third ventricle.

The thalamogeniculate and the thalamoperforating arteries are two of the larger perforating branches of the posterior cerebral artery. The thalamoperforating arteries enter the brain through the posterior perforated substance to supply structures in the floor and lateral walls of the third ventricle, including the anterior two-thirds of the thalamus in the area below the floor of the body of the lateral ventricle. They also send branches into the cerebral peduncle, hypothalamus, midbrain, and internal capsule. The thalamogeniculate arteries arise in the ambient and enter the brain in the region of the geniculate bodies and send branches into the posterolateral part of the thalamus, including the geniculate bodies and the adjacent part of the internal capsule.

Superior Cerebellar Artery

This artery arises from the basilar artery, encircles the midbrain below the posterior cerebral artery, and passes through

TABLE 5.3. Least common patterns of supply by the choroidal arteries[a]

Hemispheres present	% present	AChA (red)	LPChA (blue)	MPChA (yellow)
Upper				
Left	2%[b]	Small	Medium	Small
Right	2%	Small	Large	Small
Middle				
Left	2%[b]	Medium	Small	Medium
Right	2%	Large	Small	Medium
Lower				
Left	2%	Large	Medium	Medium
Right	2%	Large	Medium	Large

[a] AChA, anterior choroidal artery; LPChA, lateral posterior choroidal artery; MPChA, medial posterior choroidal artery.
[b] Partially supplied by the large contralateral lateral posterior choroidal artery (green).

the quadrigeminal cistern to reach the superior surface of the cerebellum (10). The segment of the artery in the quadrigeminal cistern is exposed in the supra- and infratentorial operative approaches to the posterior part of the third ventricle, and its cortical branches are exposed in the infratentorial approaches. The perforating branches of the posterior cerebral and superior cerebellar arteries supply the walls of the cistern. The posterior cerebral arteries supply the structures above the level of the sulcus, between the superior and inferior colliculi, and the superior cerebellar arteries supply the structures below this level.

VENOUS RELATIONSHIPS

The deep cerebral venous system is intimately related to the walls of the lateral and third ventricles and the basal cisterns. Illustrations and more extensive text related to these veins is provided under Deep Veins in Chapter 4 (*Figs. 4.16, 4.17,* and *5.20*). These veins represent a formidable obstacle to the operative approaches directed from the lateral ventricle to the third ventricle, and in the region of the posterior wall, atrium, pineal region, and quadrigeminal cistern, where the internal cerebral vein and the basal vein of Rosenthal on each side converge on the great vein of Galen.

The deep venous system of the brain collects into channels that course in a subependymal location through the walls of the lateral and third ventricles as they converge on the internal cerebral, basal, and great veins (*Figs. 5.3, 5.6, 5.11, 5.12,* and *5.20*) (14, 17, 19). The veins from the frontal horn, the body of the lateral ventricle, and the surrounding gray and white matter drain into the internal cerebral vein; the veins from the temporal horn and the adjacent periventricular structures drain into the basal veins; and those draining the atrium and adjacent parts of the brain drain into the basal, internal cerebral, or great vein. The veins collecting blood from the periventricular white and gray matter join to form subependymal channels in the walls of the lateral ventricles.

During operations on the lateral ventricles, the veins provide orienting landmarks more commonly than the arteries because the arteries in the ventricular walls are small and poorly seen, but the veins are larger and are easily visible through the ependyma. These venous landmarks are especially helpful in the presence of hydrocephalus, when the normal angles between the neural structures disappear. On cerebral angiograms, these veins may provide a more accurate estimate of the site and size of a lesion than the arteries, because they are more closely adherent to the ependymal and pial surfaces of the brain than the arteries.

The ventricular veins arise from tributaries that drain the basal ganglia, thalamus, internal capsule, corpus callosum, septum pellucidum, fornix, and deep white matter and course along the walls of the ventricle in a subependymal location toward the choroidal fissure. The ventricular veins are divided into medial and lateral groups based on whether they course through the thalamic or forniceal side of the choroidal fissure: the lateral group passes through the thalamic or inner side of the fissure, and the medial group passes through the outer or forniceal circumference of the fissure.

The lateral group drains the lateral wall of the frontal, temporal, and occipital horns, the body, and the atrium, the floor of the body, the anterior wall of the atrium, and the roof of the temporal horn. The medial group drains the medial wall and roof of the frontal and occipital horns, body, and atrium and the floor of the temporal horn. The veins comprising the medial and lateral groups frequently join near the choroidal fissure to form a common stem before terminating in the large veins in the velum interpositum and basal cisterns.

The medial group of veins in the frontal horn consists of the anterior septal veins, and the lateral group consists of the anterior caudate veins. The medial group of veins in the body is formed by the posterior septal veins, and the lateral group consists of the thalamostriate, thalamocaudate, and posterior caudate veins. The medial group of veins in the atrium and occipital horn consists of the medial atrial veins, and the

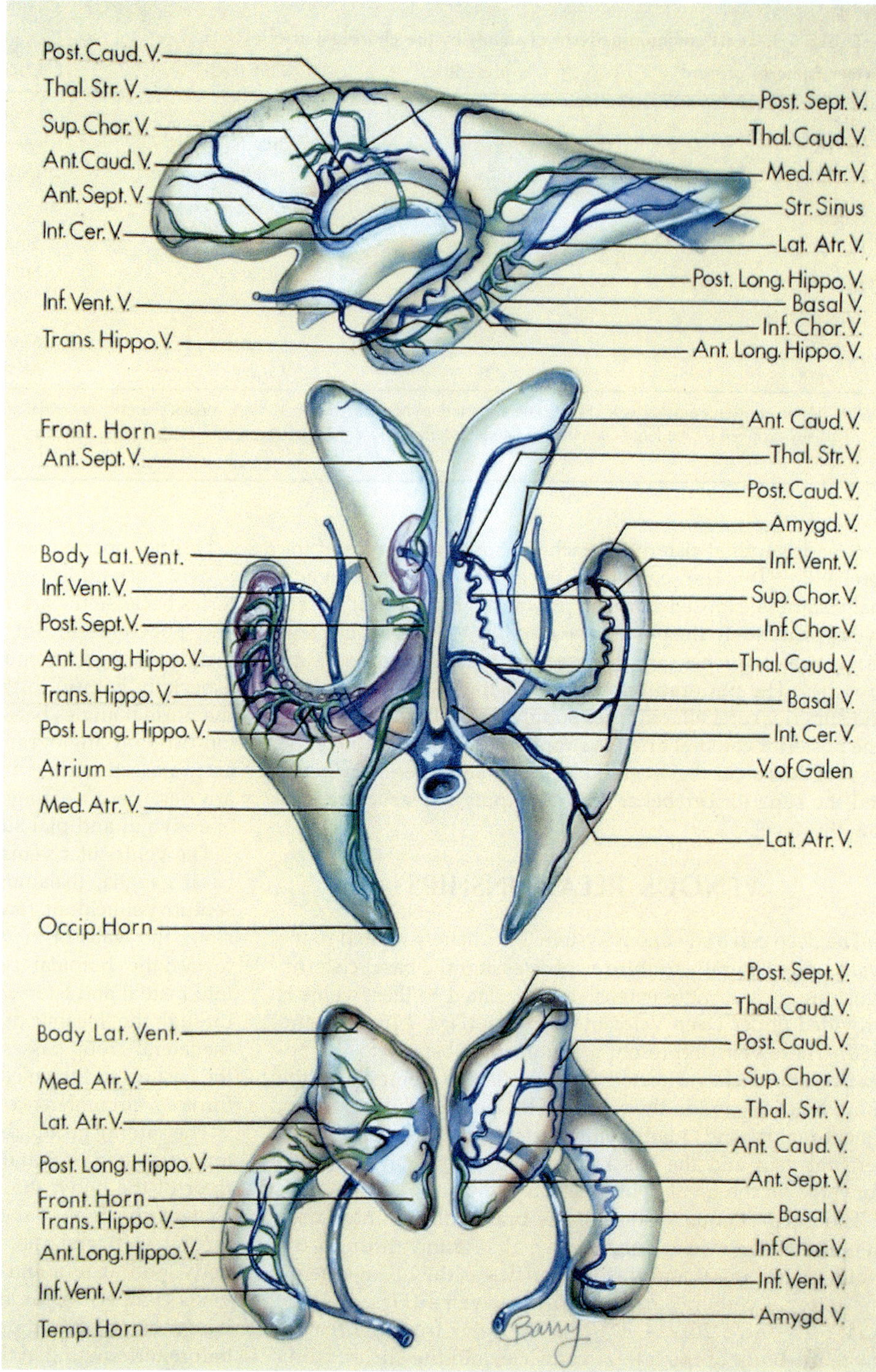

FIGURE 5.20. *Venous relationships of the lateral ventricles. Lateral* (top), *anterior* (middle), *and superior* (lower) *views. The ventricular veins are divided into medial and lateral groups. The ventricular veins drain into the internal cerebral, basal, and great veins. The lateral group consists of the anterior caudate vein in the frontal horn; the thalamostriate, posterior caudate, and thalamocaudate veins in the body; the lateral atrial veins in the atrium and occipital horn; and the inferior ventricular and amygdalar veins in the temporal horn. The medial group is formed by the anterior septal vein in the frontal horn; the posterior septal veins in the body; the medial atrial veins in the atrium; and the transverse hippocampal veins in the temporal horn. The transverse hippocampal veins drain into the anterior and posterior longitudinal hippocampal veins. The superior choroidal veins drain into the thalamostriate and internal cerebral veins, and the inferior choroidal vein drains into the inferior ventricular vein. The great vein drains into the straight sinus.* Amygd., *amygdalar;* Ant., *anterior;* Atr., *atrial;* Caud., *caudate;* Cer., *cerebral;* Chor., *choroidal;* Front., *frontal;* Hippo., *hippocampal;* Inf., *inferior;* Int., *internal;* Lat., *lateral;* Long., *longitudinal;* Med., *medial;* Occip., *occipital;* Post., *posterior;* Sept., *septal;* Str., *straight;* Sup., *superior;* Temp., *temporal;* Thal.Caud., *thalamocaudate;* Thal.Str., *thalamostriate;* Trans., *transverse;* V., *vein;* Vent., *ventricular, ventricle.*

lateral group is composed of the lateral atrial veins. The medial group of veins courses on the floor of the temporal horn, and the lateral group courses on the roof. The roof and lateral wall are drained predominantly by the inferior ventricular vein and the floor is drained by the transverse hippocampal veins.

Choroidal Veins

The superior and inferior choroidal veins are the largest veins on the choroid plexus (*Figs. 5.3, 5.6,* and *5.12*) (19). The superior choroidal vein, the largest of the choroidal veins, runs forward on the choroid plexus in the body of lateral ventricle and terminates near the foramen of Monro in the thalamostri-

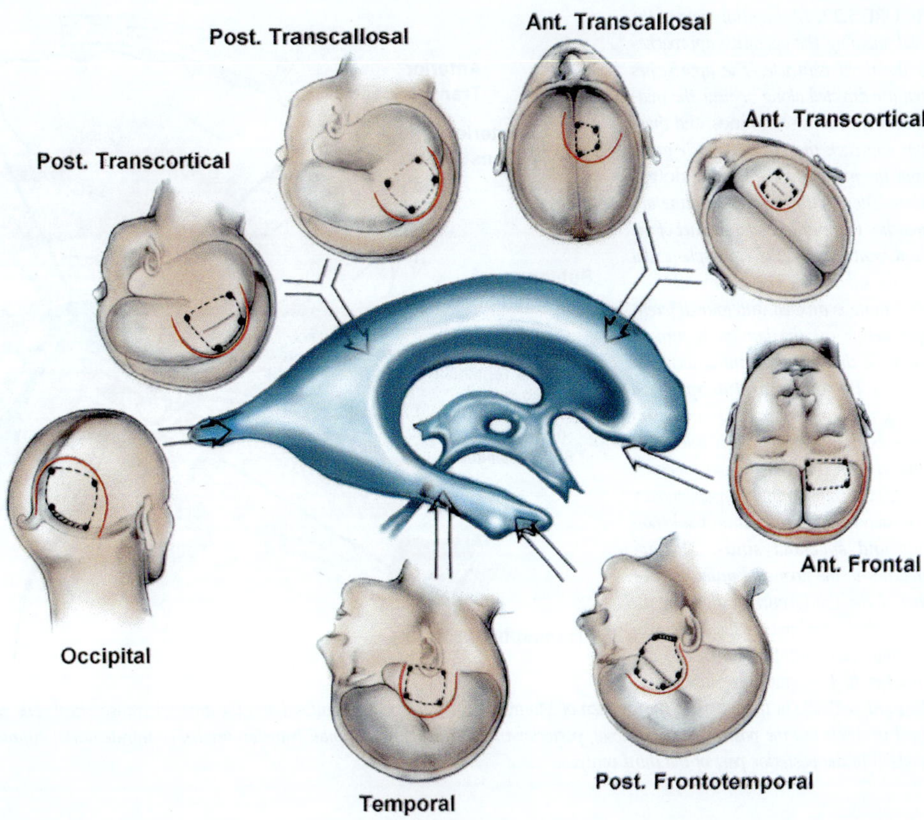

FIGURE 5.21. *Surgical approaches to the lateral ventricles. The site of the skin incision* (solid line) *and the bone flap* (broken line) *are shown for each approach. The anterior part of the lateral ventricle may be reached by the anterior transcallosal, anterior transcortical, and the frontal approaches. The posterior routes to the lateral ventricle are the posterior transcallosal, posterior transcortical, and occipital approaches. The inferior part of the lateral ventricle are reached using the frontotemporal and temporal approaches.* Ant., *anterior;* Post., *posterior.*

ate or internal cerebral veins or their tributaries. The inferior choroidal vein drains the choroid plexus in the temporal horn and atrium.

Internal Cerebral, Basal, and Great Veins

The venous relationships in the quadrigeminal cistern medial to the atrium are the most complex in the cranium because the internal cerebral, basal, and great veins and many of their tributaries converge on this area (*Figs. 5.3, 5.6, 5.11, 5.12,* and *5.20*). The internal cerebral veins exit the velum interpositum and the basal veins exit the ambient cisterns to reach the quadrigeminal cistern, where they join to form the vein of Galen.

The internal cerebral vein originates from multiple tributaries at the foramen of Monro and courses posteriorly in the roof of the third ventricle above the striae medullaris thalami between the two layers of the tela choroidea. Its anterior portion courses adjacent to the midline beside its mate from the opposite side. It diverges from the midline along the superolateral surface of the pineal. Further posteriorly, beneath the splenium of the corpus callosum, it converges on the midline and unites with its mate from the opposite side to form the vein of Galen.

The basal vein originates on the surface of the anterior perforated substance by the union of multiple veins and passes through the crural and ambient cisterns. It courses posteromedially above the uncus to reach the anterior portion of the cerebral peduncle. At the most medial point of the basal vein anterior to the peduncle, it turns posterolaterally to reach the lateral most point of the cerebral peduncle and then turns posteromedially around the inferior and posterior aspects of the pulvinar to join the vein of Galen or the internal cerebral vein in the quadrigeminal cistern.

SURGICAL CONSIDERATIONS

The lateral and third ventricles are among the most surgically inaccessible areas in the brain. Numerous operative approaches to the ventricles have been described since the pioneer work of Dandy (*Figs. 5.21* and *5.22*) (3–5). The routes through which the lateral and third ventricles can be reached are (a) from above, through the corpus callosum or the cerebral cortex; (b) from anterior, through the anterior interhemispheric fissure, corpus callosum, and lamina terminalis; (c) from below, through the basal cisterns, suprasellar region, or through or below the temporal lobe; and (d) from posterior, through the interhemispheric fissure, quadrigeminal cisterns, corpus callosum, and cerebral cortex. The selection of the best operative approach is determined by the relationship of the lesion to the lateral and third ventricles, the size of the ventricles and the structures involved, including the foramen of Monro, aqueduct of sylvius, optic nerves and chiasm, pineal gland, sella turcica, pituitary gland, fornix, midbrain, thalamus, corpus callosum, interhemispheric fissure, and basal cisterns. Before considering the specific operative approaches, some general principles are reviewed. These principles apply to all of the operative approaches discussed in this issue of *Neurosurgery*.

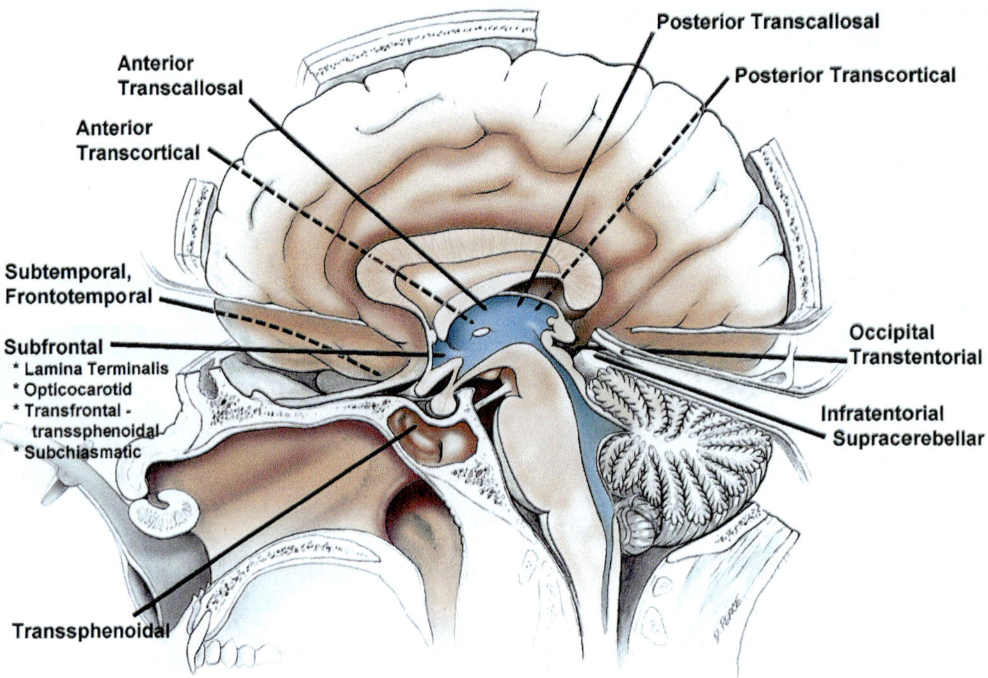

FIGURE 5.22. *Midsagittal view of the head showing the operative approaches to the third ventricle. The approaches that are directed along or near the midline are shown as* solid lines, *and those that approach the third ventricle away from the midline are shown as* dotted lines. *The midline or near-midline approaches to the anteroinferior part of the third ventricle are the transsphenoidal and the subfrontal. The subfrontal operative route is divided into four different approaches: (a) the lamina terminalis approach through the lamina terminalis; (b) the opticocarotid approach through the opticocarotid triangle; (c) the subchiasmatic approach below the optic chiasm between the optic nerves; and (d) the transfrontal-transsphenoidal approach through the planum sphenoidale and sphenoid sinus. The approaches to the floor and anteroinferior part of the third ventricle that are directed off the midline are the subtemporal and the frontotemporal. The approaches to the anterosuperior part of the third ventricle in the region of the foramen of Monro are the anterior transcallosal and the anterior transcortical. The supratentorial approaches to the posterior part of the third ventricle are the posterior transcallosal, posterior transcortical, and occipital transtentorial. The infratentorial supracerebellar approach is directed below the tentorium cerebelli to the posterior part of the third ventricle.*

Craniotomy Placement

The craniotomy flap should be placed so as to minimize the need for brain retraction. The sites of retraction used to reach the walls of the lateral and third ventricles include the orbital surface of the frontal lobe to reach the chiasmatic area; the frontal and parietal parasagittal cortex for the transcallosal approaches; the inferior and medial surfaces of the frontal lobe for the anterior frontal approach; the inferior surface of the frontal lobe and the anterior and inferior parts of the temporal lobe for the frontotemporal approaches; the inferior surface of the temporal lobe for the subtemporal approach; the inferior and medial surface of the occipital lobe for the occipital approach; and the superior surface of the cerebellum for the infratentorial approaches. To minimize the need for brain retraction, the surgeon should place the craniotomy as follows. For the parasagittal approaches, the flaps should extend to or across the midline. For the occipital approach, the flap should reach the margins of the sagittal and transverse sinuses and the torcular herophili. For the anterior frontal approach, the flap should have its medial margin on the midline and, if needed, its anterior margin on the floor of the anterior fossa. For the subfrontal, subtemporal, and frontotemporal approaches, the flap should have its lower border on the floor of the anterior and / or middle fossa. For the posterior frontotemporal approach, the flap should be based on the floor of the frontal and temporal fossae and the lateral half of the sphenoid ridge should be removed. For the infratentorial approaches the opening should reach the margin of the transverse sinus and torcular herophili.

Self-retaining, rather than hand-held, retractors are used. The extracerebral space is increased and the need for retraction is further reduced by draining cerebrospinal fluid through a ventriculostomy if hydrocephalus is present, through a basal cistern if hydrocephalous is not significant and a cistern in accessible in the exposure, or through a lumbar spinal drain if there is no ventricular obstruction.

Neural Incisions

It is impossible to reach the lateral and third ventricles without opening some neural structures. The surgical approaches to the lateral and third ventricles may require cortical incisions in the frontal, parietal, or temporal lobes and the anterior or posterior part of the corpus callosum, displacement or division of the fornix, and opening of the lamina terminales, choroidal fissure, septum pellucidum, floor of the third ventricle, and dissection and separation of the tumor from the quadrigeminal plate, the optic nerves, chiasm, and tracts, the pituitary gland and its stalk, and the cerebral peduncle. The brain may be retracted to expose an external wall of the third or lateral ventricle, such as the corpus callosum or lamina terminalis, but then the wall must be incised to reach the ventricle. After reaching the lateral ventricles, opening of the choroidal fissure or another neural incision through a site such as the fornix is needed to expose those lesions that extend into the third ventricle or the basal cisterns. Opening through the choroidal fissure in the body of the ventricle will expose the velum interpositum and the roof of the third ventricle, opening through the fissure in the atrium will expose the quadrigeminal cistern and the pineal region, and opening through it in the temporal horn will expose the ambient cistern. When opening the choroidal fissure, it is better to open through the tenia fornicis than through the tenia choroidea, because fewer arteries and veins pass through the tenia fornicis (*Figs. 5.3, 5.6–5.9,* and *5.23*).

The incision and retraction of neural structures to reach the lateral and third ventricles, such as the olfactory and oculomotor nerves, the optic pathways, and the quadrigeminal plate, causes deficits that are well defined and that correspond to the area injured. The sacrifice of other neural structures has produced variable results: in some cases there was no deficit, and in others the deficit was transient or permanent or resulted in the loss of life. Structures sacrificed with variable results include the anterior and posterior parts of the corpus callosum and various parts of the fornix. Callosal incisions have resulted in disorders of the interhemispheric transfer of information, visuospatial transfer, the learning of bimanual motor tasks, and memory and have also resulted in such deficits as alexia, apraxia, and astereognosis (15, 24, 28, 33). Division of the fornix on both sides may cause a memory loss. The cerebral retraction needed for the anterior and posterior transcallosal approaches and the cortical incisions for the transventricular surgical approaches have caused convulsions, hemiplegia, mutism, impairment of consciousness, and visual field loss. Manipulation of lesions extending into the walls of the third ventricle may cause hypothalamic dysfunction as manifested by disturbances of temperature control, respiration, consciousness, and hypophyseal secretion; visual loss due to damage of the optic chiasm and tracts; and memory loss due to injury to the body and columns of the fornix. Dissection medial to the atrium in the area of the quadrigeminal plate may cause disorders of eye movement, edematous closure of the aqueduct of sylvius, blindness from edema in the colliculi or geniculate bodies, and extraocular palsies due to edema of the nuclei of the nerves or the central pathways in the brainstem (5).

Opening the choroidal fissure carries the risk of damaging the fornix. However, unilateral damage to the fornix produces no deficit, and damage to the forniceal fibers from both hemispheres does not usually produce a permanent memory loss (15, 24, 28, 33). Opening the temporal part of the choroidal fissure risks damaging the fimbria and hippocampal formation. There is abundant experimental and clinical evidence that massive bilateral damage of the hippocampal formation, causes impairment of recent memory. However, unilateral damage of the hippocampal formation produces no deficit. The stria terminalis that borders the temporal portion of the choroidal fissure is the most prominent efferent pathway from the amygdaloid nuclear complex to the nuclei of the stria terminalis. However, there is no evidence that unilateral lesions of the stria terminalis or amygdaloid nucleus cause emotional disturbances. Bilateral lesions of the amygdaloid complex may produce a reduction in emotional excitability.

Arterial Considerations

Intraventricular tumors and arteriovenous malformations are commonly supplied by the choroidal arteries (*Fig. 5.19; Tables 5.1–5.3*). The fact that the choroidal arteries converge on and pass through the choroidal fissure assists in identifying this fissure situated on the periphery of the thalamus through which operative procedures may be directed to the third ventricle, pineal region, and ambient and quadrigeminal cisterns. Opening through the fissure will expose these arteries proximal to a ventricular lesion; opening through the fissure in the body of ventricle will expose the medial posterior choroidal arteries in the velum interpositum and the roof of the third ventricle; opening through the fissure in the atrium will expose the medial and lateral posterior choroidal arteries in the quadrigeminal cistern and the pineal region; and opening through it in the temporal horn will expose the anterior, medial, and lateral posterior choroidal arteries in the ambient cistern.

Other arteries that may also be exposed in removing tumors of the lateral and third ventricles are the anterior cerebral and anterior communicating arteries in the region of the anterior wall of the third ventricle and the frontal horns and bodies of the lateral ventricle; the posterior part of the circle of Willis, the apex of the basilar artery, and the proximal part of the posterior cerebral arteries in the area below the third ventricular floor and medial to the temporal horns; the distal part of the posterior cerebral arteries in the area of the posterior third ventricle and medial to the atria; the posterior cerebral, pericallosal, superior cerebellar, and choroidal arteries adjacent to the posterior wall of the third ventricle and medial to the atria; and both the anterior and posterior cerebral arteries that send branches into the roof of the lateral ventricle. In addition, the internal carotid artery, anterior, middle, and posterior cerebral arteries, and anterior and posterior communicating arteries give rise to perforating branches that reach the walls of the lateral and third ventricles. Only infrequently should any of these be sacrificed. Occlusion of the perforating branches of these arteries at the anterior part of the circle of Willis is likely to result in disturbances in memory and personality, and occlusion of those at the posterior part of the circle of Willis is more likely to result in disorders of the level of consciousness and are frequently combined with disorders of extraocular motion. Sacrifice of the perforating branches of the posterior communicating artery in the subtemporal approaches has resulted in infarction in the basal ganglia (32). Obliteration of the thalamoperforating arteries in the cisterns medial to the temporal horn may cause coma and death. Injuries to the superior cerebellar artery in approaches to the posterior part of the third ventricle may cause a cerebellar deficit.

Venous Considerations

The ventricular veins provide valuable landmarks in directing the surgeon to the foramen of Monro and choroidal fissure during operations on the ventricles (*Figs. 5.3, 5.6, 5.11, 5.12, 5.20,* and *5.23*). This is especially true if hydrocephalus is present, as commonly occurs with ventricular tumors, because the borders between the neural structures in the ventricular walls become less distinct as the ventricles dilate. The thalamostriate vein is helpful in delimiting the junction of the caudate nucleus and thalamus, because it usually courses along the sulcus separating these structures.

The number of veins sacrificed in approaching a ventricular lesion should be kept to a minimum because of the undesir-

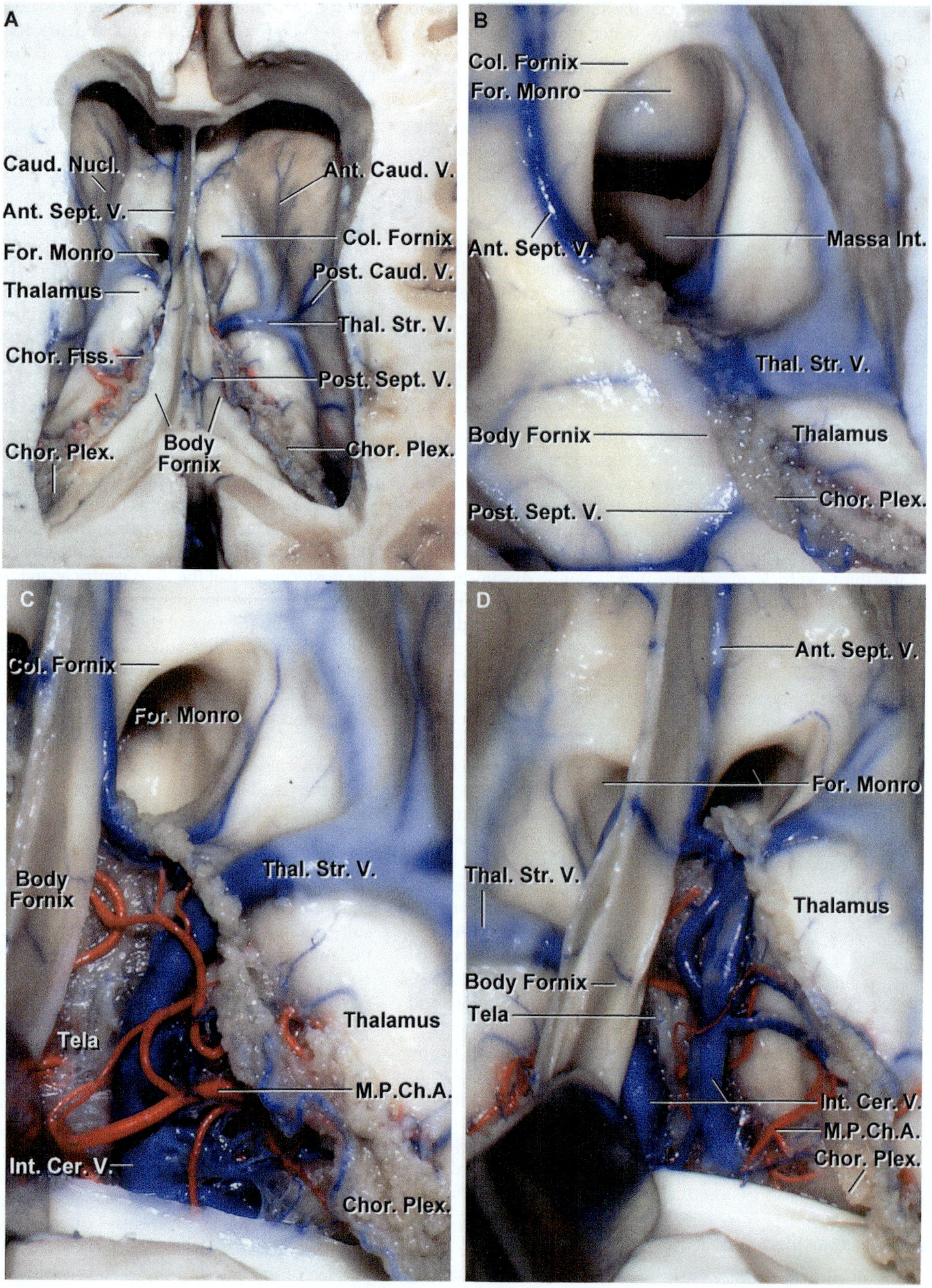

FIGURE 5.23. *Transchoroidal approach to the third ventricle directed along the forniceal side of the choroidal fissure. A, superior view of the frontal horn and body of the lateral ventricle. The body of the fornix forms the upper part of the roof of the third ventricle. The left thalamostriate vein passes through the posterior margin of the foramen of Monro and the right thalamostriate vein passes through the choroidal fissure a few millimeters behind the foramen. Anterior septal and anterior caudate veins cross the wall of the frontal horn. Posterior septal and posterior caudate veins cross the wall of the body of the lateral ventricle. The thalamus sits in the floor of the body. The choroidal fissure, located between the thalamus and fornix, is opened by dividing the tenia fornix that attaches the choroid plexus to the lateral edge of the fornix, leaving the attachment of the choroid plexus to the thalamus undisturbed. B, enlarged view. The columns of the fornix form the anterior and superior wall of the foramen of Monro. The massa intermedia is seen through the foramen. Anterior and posterior septal veins cross the septum pellucidum and fornix. C, the tenia fornix, which attaches the choroid plexus to the fornix, has been divided and the body of the fornix retracted medially to expose the internal cerebral vein and medial posterior choroidal arteries. The lower layer of tela, which attaches to the striae medullaris thalami and forms the floor of the velum interpositum, is intact. D, the separation of the fornix and choroid plexus has been extended posteriorly to the junction of the atrium and body of the ventricle. The lower layer of tela remains intact. E, the lower layer of tela has been opened to expose the massa intermedia, posterior commissure, and the floor of the third ventricle. The ependyma covering the anterior septal vein has been opened so that a short segment of the vein can be mobilized. The possibility of damaging the thalamostriate vein is reduced by allowing the choroid plexus to remain attached to the thalamus and the upper surface of the vein.*

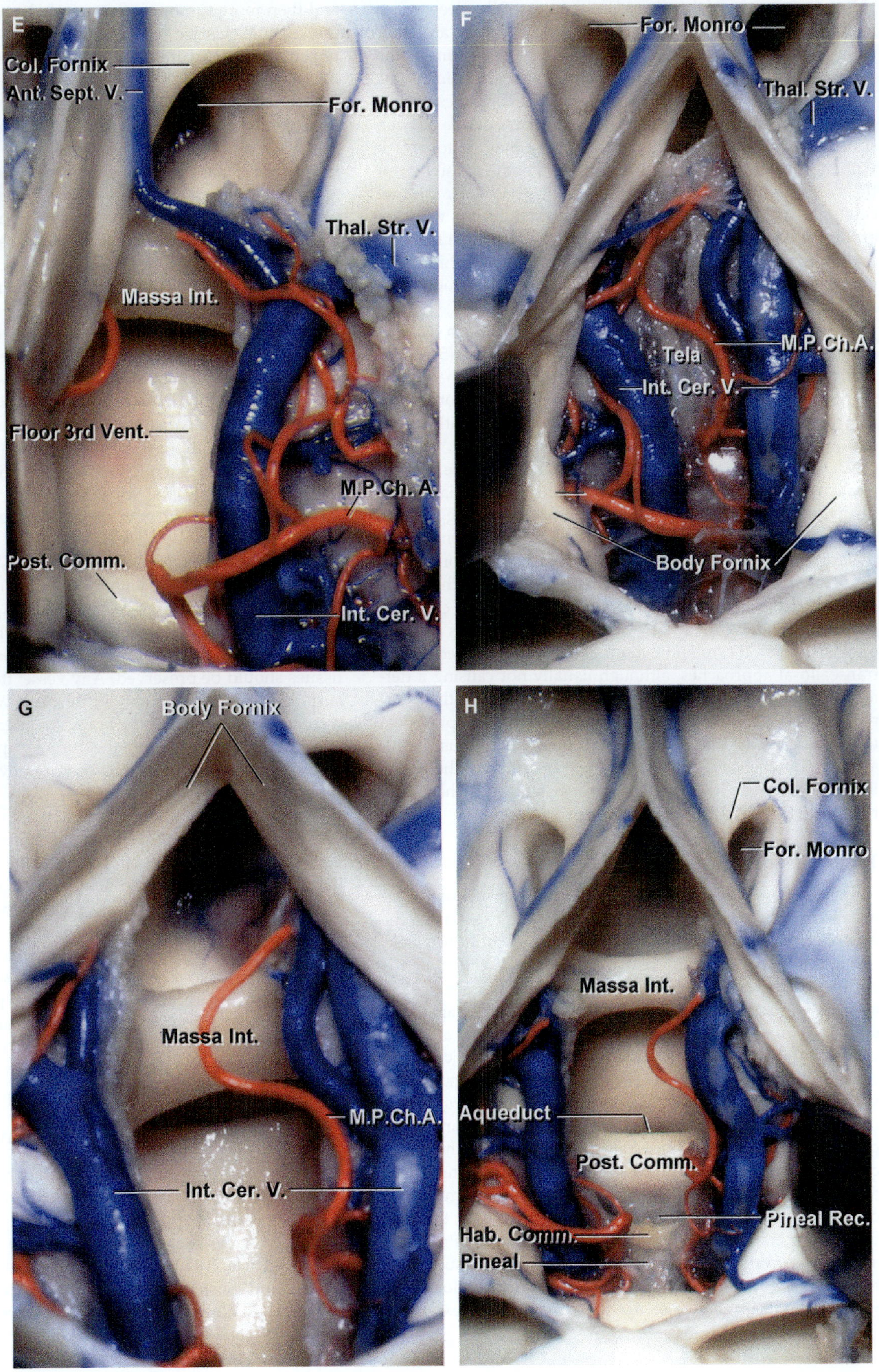

FIGURE 5.23.
Continued
F–H, *interforniceal approach.* F, *the interforniceal approach is completed by incising the fornix longitudinally in the midline. Each half of the body of the fornix has been retracted laterally to expose the internal cerebral veins, medial posterior choroidal arteries, and the layer of tela choroidea that attaches to the striae medullaris thalami.* G, *the tela has been opened to expose the floor of the third ventricle and the massa intermedia.* H, *the view has been directed posteriorly toward the aqueduct and the posterior and habenular commissures. The pineal recess extends into the base of the pineal between the habenular and posterior commissures. The pineal gland extends backward from the pineal recess.* Ant., *anterior;* Caud., *caudate;* Cer., *cerebral;* Chor., *choroid;* Col., *column;* Comm., *commissure;* Fiss., *fissure;* For., *foramen;* Hab., *habenular;* Int., *intermedia, internal;* M.P.Ch.A., *medial posterior choroidal artery;* Nucl., *nucleus;* Plex., *plexus;* Post., *posterior;* Rec., *recess;* Sept., *septal;* Thal.Str., *thalamostriate;* V., *vein;* Vent., *ventricle.*

able consequences of their loss. Obliteration of the deep veins, including the great, basal, and internal cerebral veins and their tributaries, and the bridging veins from the cerebrum to the dural sinuses is inescapable in reaching and removing some tumors in or near the ventricles. Before sacrificing these veins, the surgeon should try placing them under moderate or even severe stretch (accepting the fact that they may be torn) if it will allow satisfactory exposure and yield some possibility of the veins being saved. Before sacrificing the basal, internal cerebral, and great veins, the surgeon should try working around them or displacing them out of the operative route or try dividing only a few of their small branches, which may allow displacement of the main trunk out of the operative field.

Sacrificing branches of the superficial and deep venous systems has produced inconstant deficits. Dandy (5) noted that, not infrequently, one internal cerebral vein had been sacrificed without effect, and on a few occasions both veins and even the great vein of Galen had been ligated with recovery without any apparent disturbance of function. On the other hand, injury to this venous network may cause diencephalic edema, mental symptoms, coma, hyperpyrexia, tachycardia, tachypnea, miosis, rigidity of limbs, and exaggeration of deep tendon reflexes (15, 24, 28, 33). Occlusion of the thalamostriate and other veins at the foramen of Monro may cause drowsiness, hemiplegia, mutism, and hemorrhagic infarction of the basal ganglia. Obliteration of veins coursing between the cerebrum and the superior sagittal sinus anterior or posterior to the rolandic vein, as may be required in the transcallosal approaches, although usually not causing a deficit, may be accompanied by hemiplegia. Sacrificing the internal occipital vein or the bridging veins from the occipital pole to the superior sagittal or transverse sinuses may cause hemianopsia. Cerebellar swelling after the transection of the bridging vein between the cerebellum and tentorium has been reported (15, 24, 28, 33).

Tumor Removal

Tissue should be removed from within the capsule of an encapsulated ventricular tumor before trying to separate the capsule from adjacent structures. If the tumor could be cystic, the initial step is aspiration with a needle. If the tumor is encapsulated, the capsule is opened, the tumor is biopsied, and an intracapsular removal is completed. The capsule is separated from the neural and vascular structures after the contents of the capsule have been removed. The most common cause of tumor appearing to be tightly adherent is not adhesions between the capsule and surrounding structures; rather, it is residual tumor within the capsule wedging the tumor into position. As the intracapsular contents are removed, the tumor collapses, thus making it possible to remove more tumor through the small exposure. Tumors are not commonly so densely adherent that they defy easy removal after their intracapsular contents are removed. If the tumor does not separate easily from the neural tissue after the intracapsular contents have been removed, a brief wait often allows the pulsation of the brain to dislodge the tumor into the exposure, and then more tumor can frequently be removed from within the capsule. Under magnification, individual adhesions between vital structures and the tumor can be divided with microinstruments. This technique has been especially helpful in removing craniopharyngiomas. It is frequently possible to remove the capsule of craniopharyngiomas and epidermoid tumors involving the third ventricle, but not that of chromophobe adenomas. The capsule of the chromophobe adenoma is the dura mater of the cranial base, which has been stretched upward over the tumor. The stretched dura over the dome of the chromophobe adenoma may be excised, but an attempt to pull this pseudocapsule of dura mater from its attachment to the cranial base may cause severe vascular and neural injury. A remnant of the tumor capsule may be left if it is attached firmly to vital structures such as the optic nerves or chiasm, colliculi, thalamus, or hypothalamus. The response of craniopharyngiomas, chromophobe adenomas, pinealomas, and some gliomas to radiation therapy is sufficiently good that it may be relied on to deal with residual neoplasm. The removal is limited frequently to biopsy only or an internal decompression if the tumor is malignant or infiltrative.

A colloid cyst is first aspirated with a needle through the foramen of Monro. It is often possible to perform the entire operation through the foramen of Monro, especially if it is enlarged. Grumous material within the cyst is then removed using a microsuction, perhaps with the addition of forceps extraction. In the case of a very large colloid cyst, an approach through the choroidal fissure is preferable to dividing the fornix.

The arteries that pass over the tumor capsule to neural tissues should be preserved. Any vessel that stands above the surface of the capsule should be dealt with initially as if it were a vessel supplying the brain. An attempt should be made to displace the vessel off the tumor capsule using a small dissector after the tumor has been removed from within the capsule.

A shunt may be needed if obstruction to the flow of cerebrospinal fluid at the foramen of Monro, aqueduct of sylvius, third ventricle, or tentorial incisura persists at the end of the operation. If the initial operation creates an opening from the third ventricle through the lamina terminalis, floor of the third ventricle, or pineal region into the subarachnoid space, this may suffice. The floor of the third ventricle in front of the mamillary body may be opened using endoscopic techniques. If a suboccipital exposure has been used to approach a tumor of the pineal region, a tube may be led from the lateral ventricle or from an opening in the posterior part of the third ventricle to the cisterna magna, thus creating a Torkildsen shunt.

OPERATIVE APPROACHES

The operative approaches to the lateral ventricles are divided into anterior, posterior, and inferior approaches (*Fig. 5.21*). The anterior approaches are directed to the frontal horn and body of the lateral ventricle and the anterior part of the third ventricle. The posterior approaches are directed to the atrium and posterior third ventricle, and the inferior approaches are directed to the temporal horn and basal cisterns.

The anterior approaches are the anterior transcallosal, anterior transcortical, and anterior frontal. The posterior approaches are the posterior transcallosal, posterior transventricular, occipital transtentorial, and infratentorial supracerebellar. The lateral approaches are the pterional, posterior frontotemporal, and subtemporal. The transsphenoidal and subfrontal approaches may also be used for selected lesions involving the anterior wall and floor of the third ventricle; however, these approaches are most commonly used for lesions involving the sella and are reviewed in Chapter 8.

Anterior Approaches

Anterior Transcallosal Approach

This approach, directed through the corpus callosum, is suitable for reaching lesions located within the frontal horn and body of the lateral ventricle and the anterosuperior part of the third ventricle (*Fig. 5.24*). The alternative to the anterior transcallosal approach is the anterior transcortical approach directed through the middle frontal gyrus. It is easier to expose the opening of the foramen of Monro into both lateral ventricles through this approach than through the anterior transcortical approach. The transcallosal approach is easier to perform than the transventricular approach if the ventricles are of a normal size or are minimally enlarged.

The patient is positioned supine with the sagittal suture in the vertical plane and the head elevated 20 to 30 degrees. An alternative position is the lateral position with the right side down, so that gravity will assist the retraction of the medial surface of the right cerebral hemisphere away from the right side of the falx. A right frontal horseshoe, bicoronal, or S-shaped skin incision is used. The right frontal bone flap extending to the lateral edge of or across the sagittal sinus is located two-thirds in front and one-third behind the coronal suture. The dura mater is opened with the base on the sagittal sinus. The area in front of the coronal suture is often relatively devoid of bridging veins entering the superior sagittal sinus; some, usually no more than one, may have to be divided to allow retraction of the medial surface of the right frontal lobe away from the falx (*Fig. 5.3*). The arachnoid membrane, encountered deep to the free edge of the falx, is opened to expose the corpus callosum and the anterior cerebral arteries. Smaller veins from the corpus callosum and adjacent part of the frontal lobe that empty into the anterior end of the inferior sagittal sinus may have to be sacrificed. Opening the arachnoid below the falx exposes the branches of the anterior cerebral arteries, which may cross the midline above the corpus callosum. The right and left cingulate gyri, which face each other, are separated to expose the corpus callosum and the pericallosal arteries. The approach is best directed between the pericallosal arteries, although some of their branches may cross the midline above the corpus callosum. If both pericallosal arteries are retracted to one side, it may be necessary to divide some of the branches that run laterally from the pericallosal arteries to the corpus callosum and the cingulate gyrus to reach the corpus callosum.

The part of the corpus callosum above the foramen of Monro is split in the midline. An incision 2 cm in length provides satisfactory access to both lateral ventricles. Image guidance will aid in selecting the site to open the corpus callosum. After the ventricle is opened by either the transcallosal or transventricular approach, the foramen of Monro is found by following the choroid plexus and the thalamostriate vein anteriorly to where they converge on the foramen. The choroid plexus is attached along the choroidal fissure between the fornix and thalamus, and the thalamostriate vein courses in a more lateral position in the groove between the thalamus and caudate nucleus. The veins in the frontal horn are seen to drain posteriorly toward the foramen of Monro because the choroidal fissure through which they pass to reach the internal cerebral vein does not extend into the frontal horn.

The close relationship of the genu of the internal capsule to the foramen of Monro should be kept in mind when retracting the walls of the lateral ventricle (*Figs. 5.2* and *5.3*). The genu of the internal capsule touches the wall of the ventricle in the area lateral to the foramen of Monro near the anterior pole of the thalamus. Care should be exercised in retracting this area because a thin brain spatula could easily cut into the ventricular wall in this critical region resulting in hemiplegia.

The callosal opening may expose the frontal horn and body on the same or opposite side of the cranial exposure, but the anatomy makes this obvious. A simple rule for determining whether the left or right lateral ventricle has been exposed is to determine whether the thalamostriate vein is to the left or right side of the choroid plexus; the left lateral ventricle has been opened if the thalamostriate vein is further to the patient's left side than the choroid plexus; the right lateral ventricle has been entered if the thalamostriate vein is further to the patient's right side than the choroid plexus. Entry into a cavum between the leaves of the septum pellucidum may be confusing until the surgeon realizes that no intraventricular structures are present. Opening the septum pellucidum will provide access to the opposite lateral ventricle and the opening of the foramen of Monro into both lateral ventricles.

There are several methods of enlarging the opening at the foramen of Monro if needed to explore a deeper portion of the third ventricle (*Fig. 5.24B*). One is to incise the ipsilateral column of the fornix at the anterosuperior edge of the foramen of Monro. A preferable alternative to incising the fornix is the transchoroidal approach in which the choroidal fissure, located between the fornix and thalamus, is opened, thus allowing the fornix to be pushed to the opposite side to expose the structures in the roof of the third ventricle (*Figs. 5.23* and *5.24*). The fissure is the thinnest site in the wall of the lateral ventricle bordering the roof of the third ventricle. Another alternative is the interforniceal approach, in which the body of the fornix is split in the midline, in the direction of its fibers, to expose the velum interpositum (2, 13, 35). The transchoroidal and interforniceal approaches have the advantage of giving access to the central portion of the third ventricle behind the foramen of Monro by displacing, rather than transecting, the fibers in the fornix (15, 36). Both approaches provide a satisfactory view into the third ventricle with the transcallosal approach. Sectioning the thalamostriate vein at the posterior

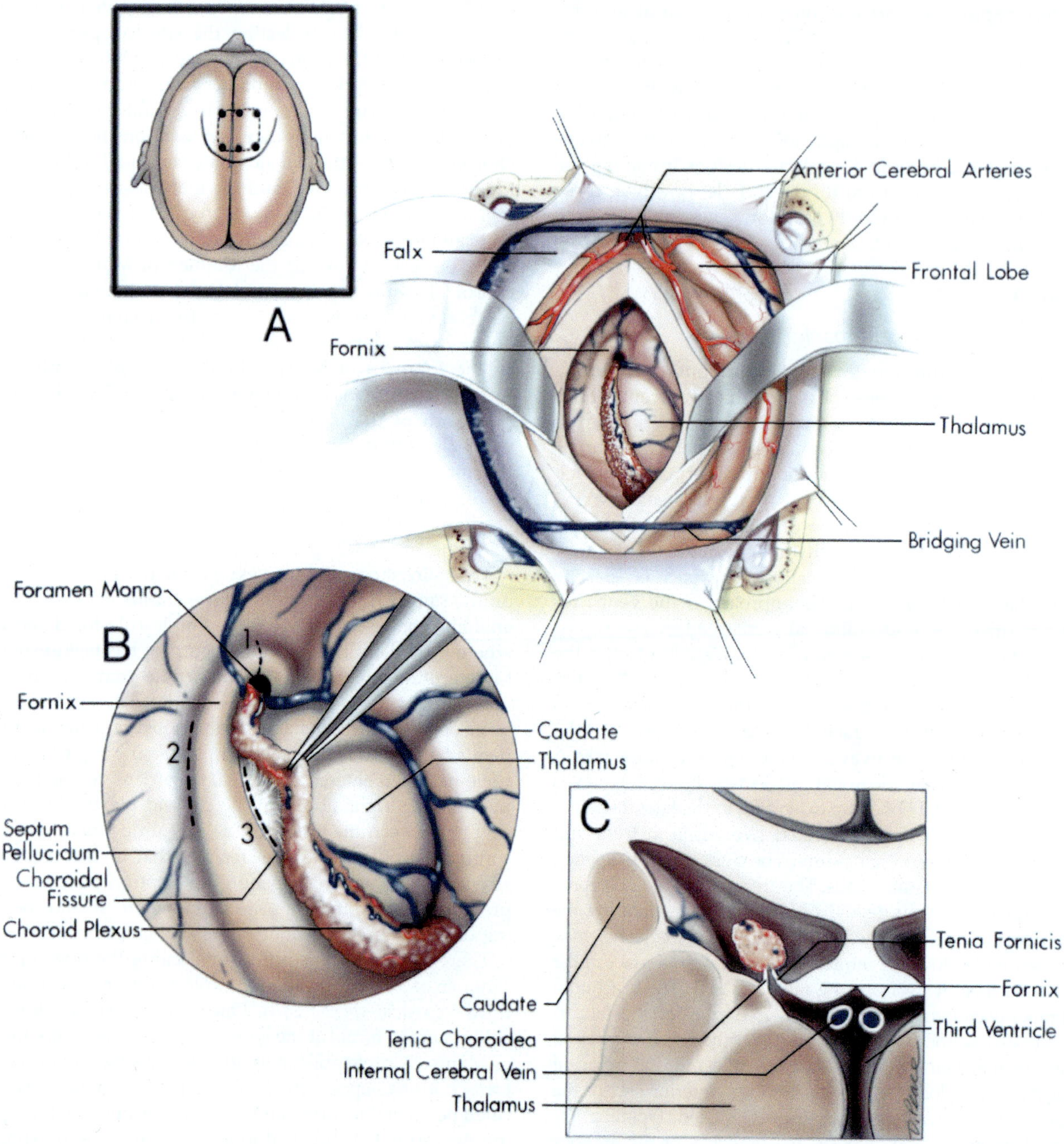

FIGURE 5.24. *Transcallosal approach to the lateral and third ventricles. A–C, normal ventricular anatomy. A, the body and frontal horn of the right lateral ventricle have been exposed through an incision in the anterior part of the corpus callosum. The inset on the upper left shows the head position, scalp incision* (solid line) *and bone flap* (broken line). *The bone flap extends across the superior sagittal sinus. An alternative would be to use a Souttar incision and to have the bone flap extend only to the lateral edge of the superior sagittal sinus. B, sites of incisions used to reach lesions in the third ventricle:* (No. 1) *the foramen of Monro may be enlarged by incising the ipsilateral column of the fornix, at the anterosuperior margin of the foramen of Monro;* (No. 2) *the transforniceal approach is completed using an incision along the body of the fornix in the midline; and* (No. 3) *the transchoroidal approach is completed by opening the choroidal fissure by incising along the tenia fornicis. C, the transchoroidal approach is completed by incision along the tenia fornicis rather than the tenia choroidea, also referred to as the tenia thalami, because more veins and arteries pass through the tenia choroidea than the tenia fornicis. The internal cerebral veins course in the roof of the third ventricle. D and F, removal of a large colloid cyst by the transchoroidal approach.*

margin of the foramen of Monro has also been advocated as an alternative to incising the fornix for enlarging the opening into the third ventricle; however, this may cause drowsiness, hemiplegia, and mutism, and occlusion of the veins of the foramen of Monro has caused hemorrhagic infarction of the basal ganglia.

In the transchoroidal approach, the third ventricle is exposed by opening the choroidal fissure along the tenia fornicis

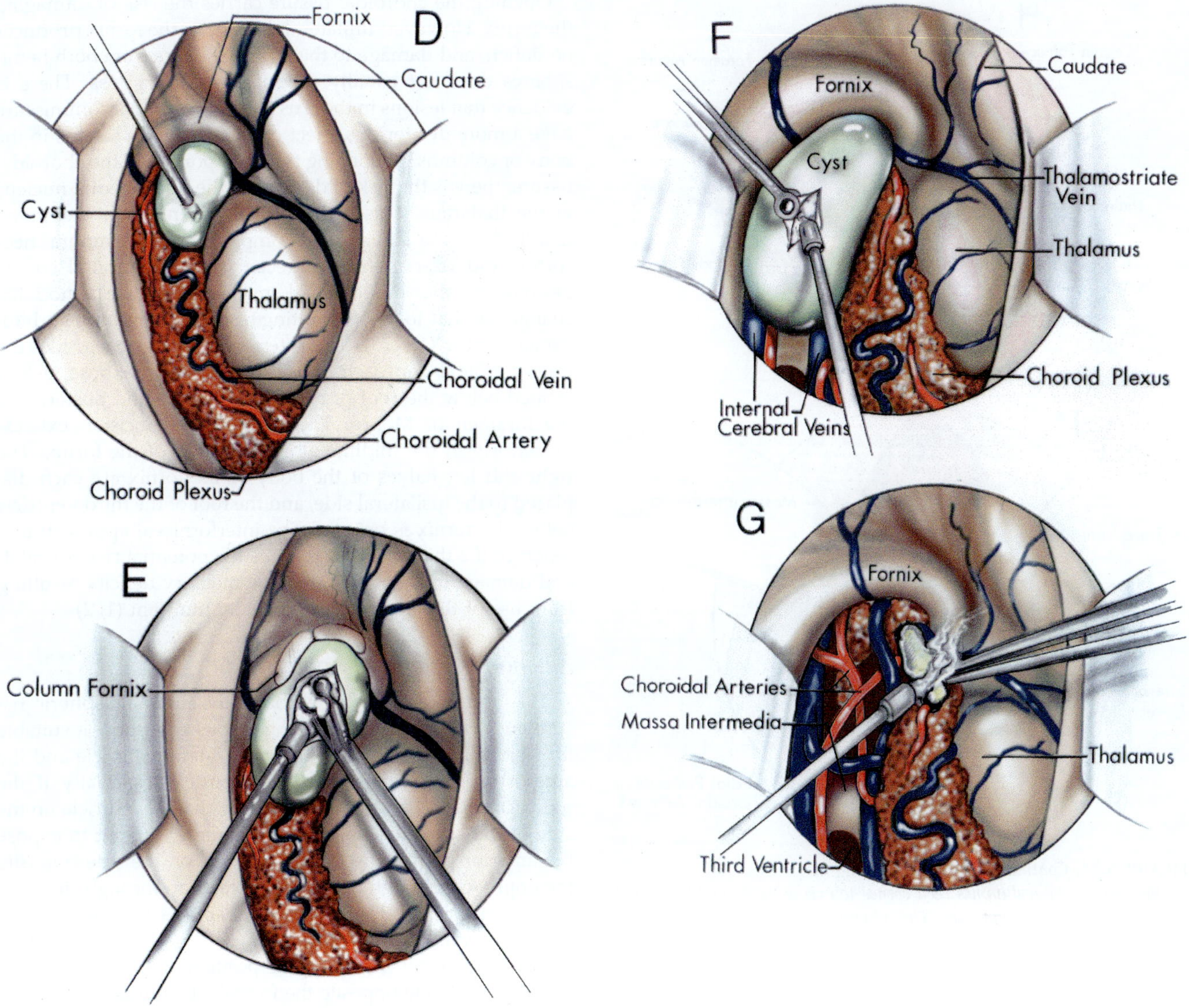

FIGURE 5.24. *Continued*
D, a colloid cyst that obstructs the foramen of Monro is being aspirated with a needle. E, a colloid cyst that obstructs the foramen of Monro has been exposed by opening the choroidal fissure along the attachment of the choroid plexus to the fornix. The internal cerebral veins and medial posterior choroidal arteries are exposed behind the foramen of Monro. The cyst's contents are being removed with a suction. F, the final remnant of the attachment of the cyst to the choroid plexus is being coagulated. G, the column of the fornix has been divided to enlarge the foramen of Monro and the semigelatinous material within the cyst is being removed using a cup forceps and suction. (Legend continues on next page.)

beginning at the posterior edge of the foramen of Monro and displacing the fornix to the opposite side, after which the roof of the third ventricle is entered by opening the layers of tela choroidea (*Figs. 5.23* and *5.24*). Opening 1 cm of the choroidal fissure beginning at the posterior edge of the foramen of Monro usually provides a view of the ventricular floor back to the aqueduct. It is safer to direct the transchoroidal approach through the tenia fornicis than through the tenia thalami because the large veins, like the thalamostriate vein that drains the internal capsule and central part of the hemisphere and the choroidal arteries, pass through the tenia thalami rather than through the tenia fornicis. The transchoroidal approach is especially well suited to lesions that are fed by the terminal branches of the choroidal arteries.

The roof of the third ventricle can commonly be entered without sacrificing any branches of the internal cerebral veins if the approach is directed between the veins; however, it is often necessary to sacrifice some of the branches of the internal cerebral vein if the third ventricle is entered on the lateral side of the internal cerebral vein between the vein and thalamus

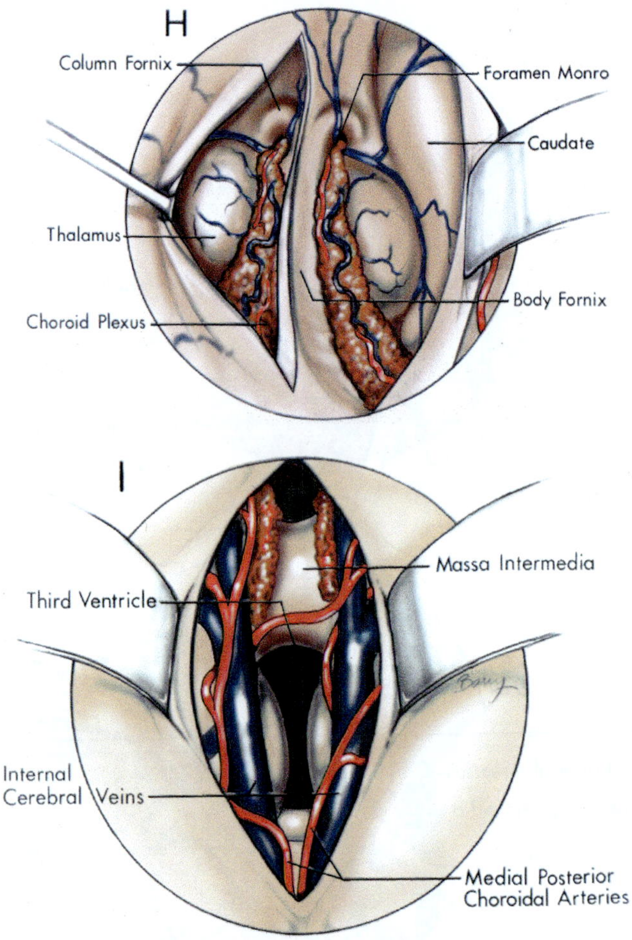

FIGURE 5.24. *Continued*
H, the septum pellucidum has been opened to expose the frontal horns and bodies of both lateral ventricles. The columns of the fornix arch anterior and superior to the openings of the foramen of Monro into both lateral ventricles. The body of the fornix forms part of the roof of the third ventricle. I, the body of the fornix has been split in the midline to expose the third ventricle. The internal cerebral veins and medial posterior choroidal arteries course in the roof of the third ventricle. This transforniceal approach is suitable for exposing lesions located in the third ventricle behind the foramen of Monro.

(*Figs.* 5.12 and 5.23). The tiny branches of the medial and lateral posterior choroidal arteries may cross the midline in the velum interpositum, but the risk of sacrificing these fine branches is minimal. After opening the lower layer of tela choroidea, the choroid plexus in the roof of the third ventricle, massa intermedia, and the floor of the third ventricle are encountered.

In earlier reports, the choroidal fissure was opened by incising the tenia thalami. This approach, referred to as the subchoroidal approach, risks damaging the thalamus and the vessels that pass through the thalamic side of the fissure by penetrating the tenia choroidea (6, 11, 13). We refer to the approach directed through the tenia fornix as the transchoroidal or suprachoroidal approach to distinguish it from the subchoroidal approach.

Opening the choroidal fissure carries the risk of damaging the fornix. However, unilateral damage to the fornix produces no deficit, and damage to the forniceal fibers from both hemispheres does not usually produce a memory loss. There is evidence that lesions in the crus and hippocampal commissure have a more deleterious effect on memory than lesions in the body or columns. In opening the body portion of the choroidal fissure, there is the risk of damage to the dorsomedial nucleus of the thalamus. This nucleus has afferent fibers stemming mainly from the amygdaloid complex and the temporal neocortex, and efferent fibers directed to the prefrontal cortex. Lesions in the dorsomedial nucleus produce emotional changes similar to those resulting from ablations of the orbitofrontal cortex (15, 28). The interforniceal approach, like the transchoroidal approach, can also be used to expose lesions located below the roof of the third ventricle and posterior to the foramen of Monro. The interforniceal incision extends posteriorly in the midline along the body of the fornix. The right and left halves of the body of the fornix are each displaced to the ipsilateral side, and the roof of the third ventricle below the fornix is opened. The interforniceal approach to a lesion of the third ventricle carries the potential risk for bilateral damage to the fornix, but the memory deficits resulting from use of this approach are usually transient (1, 2).

Anterior Transcortical Approach

This approach, directed through the interhemispheric fissure and the anterior part of the corpus callosum, is suitable for lesions in the anterior part of the lateral ventricle and the anterosuperior part of the third ventricle, especially if the tumor is situated predominantly in the lateral ventricle on the side of the approach (*Fig. 5.25*). It is more difficult to expose the anterior part of the lateral ventricle on the side opposite the approach through the transcortical than through the transcallosal approach. The transcortical approach is facilitated if the lateral ventricles are enlarged.

With the patient in the supine position, the head is rotated slightly to the side opposite the frontal lobe through which the ventricle is to be approached. The scalp and bone flaps are positioned over the central part of the middle frontal gyrus of the nondominant hemisphere. The dominant hemisphere is selected only if there is a major extension of the tumor into the lateral ventricle of the dominant hemisphere. If the approach is through the dominant hemisphere, care is taken to place the cortical incision above and anterior to the expressive speech centers on the inferior frontal gyrus and anterior to the precentral motor strip. The dilated frontal horn is reached through a small cortical incision located in the long axis of the middle frontal gyrus. The landmarks within the ventricle are described in the section on the transcallosal approach. It may be necessary to enlarge the opening into the third ventricle by opening the choroidal fissure. The transchoroidal opening provides a better view into the roof of the third ventricle than the interforniceal opening with the transcortical approach. For most lesions, opening the choroidal fissure is preferable to the interforniceal approach or sectioning the ipsilateral column of the fornix. Opening the septum pellucidum will provide access to both frontal horns and bodies.

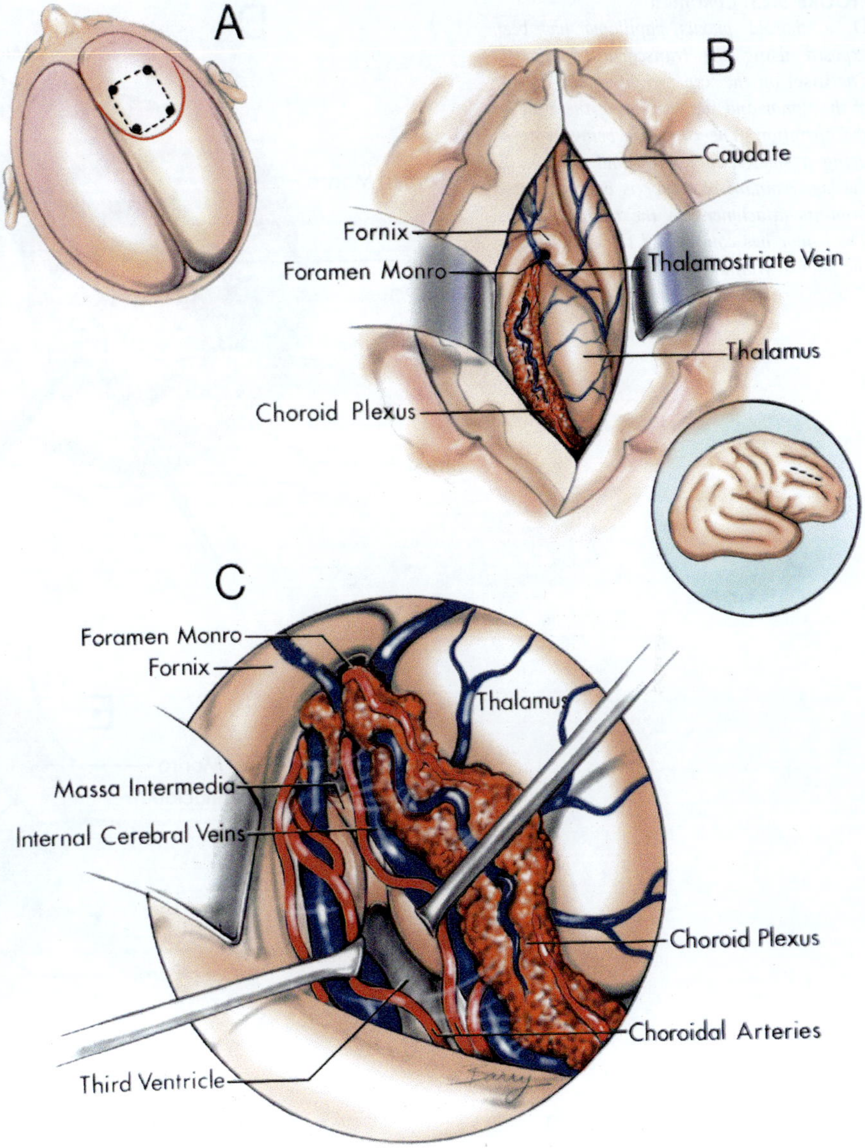

FIGURE 5.25. *Transcortical approach to the lateral and third ventricles.* A, *the scalp incision* (solid line) *and bone flap* (dotted line) *are centered over the middle frontal gyrus.* B *and* C, *normal ventricular anatomy.* B, *The cortical opening exposes the right lateral ventricle. The* inset *on the lower right shows the site of the cortical incision. The opening into the right lateral ventricle exposes the caudate nucleus, fornix, foramen of Monro, thalamus, and thalamostriate vein.* C, *the third ventricle has been exposed by opening the choroidal fissure along the site of the attachment of the choroid plexus to the fornix. This exposes the internal cerebral veins and medial posterior choroidal arteries in the roof of the third ventricle. (Legend continues on next page.)*

Anterior Frontal Approach

The anterior frontal approach may infrequently be considered for a lesion involving the structures forming the anteroinferior wall of the frontal horn and the adjacent part of the third ventricle (*Figs. 5.15* and *5.26*) (28). This approach would be adequate to expose lesions involving the floor and lower part of the anterior wall of the frontal horn or lesions that extend from the rostrum of the corpus callosum into the third ventricle behind the lamina terminalis. This approach is not suitable for reaching a lesion in the region of the posterior part of the frontal horn near the foramen of Monro, in the floor of the body of the lateral ventricle, or in the superior part of the third ventricle behind the foramen of Monro.

The patient is positioned supine with the face looking directly upward. A Souttar scalp incision is used. A unilateral bone flap extending up to the edge of the superior sagittal sinus is elevated on the side of the lesion. The bone flap is positioned in the interval between the supraorbital ridge and the coronal suture, depending on the site of the lesion. The lower margin of the flap will border the supraorbital ridge if the lesion is in the region of the rostrum and the adjacent part of the lamina terminalis, but will be placed higher on the forehead if the lesion is centered in the lower part of the genu of the corpus callosum. The dura mater is opened with the base on the superior sagittal sinus. Elevating the orbital surface of the frontal lobe will allow the arachnoid in front of the optic chiasm and along the medial part of the sylvian fissure to be opened to expose the supraclinoid portion of the internal carotid artery, the initial segments of the anterior and middle cerebral arteries, and the anterior communicating and recurrent arteries. One olfactory nerve may need to be divided above the cribriform plate to expose the area above the optic chiasm. Further retraction will expose the lamina terminalis above the optic chiasm and possibly the lower part of the

FIGURE 5.25. *Continued*
D, a choroid plexus papilloma has been exposed using the transcortical approach. The inset on the upper right shows the site of the tumor and the position of the head for the operation. The tumor is being removed using a small cup forceps and suction. E, the last remnant of tumor is being removed from its attachment to the choroid plexus. The tumor has compressed the structures in the floor at frontal horn.

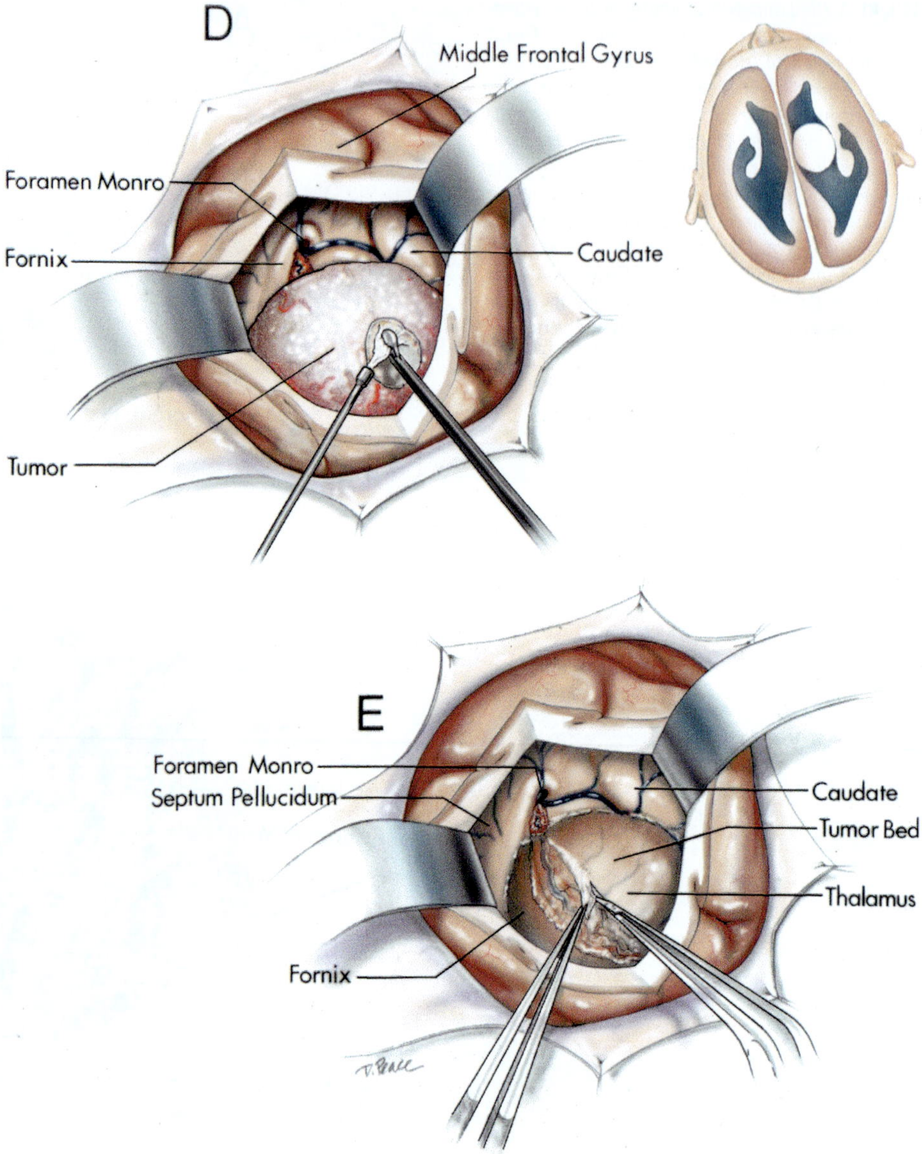

rostrum. The medial surface of the frontal lobe is retracted away from the anterior part of the falx to expose the anterior part of the interhemispheric fissure in the region of the rostrum and genu of the corpus callosum. One or two small cortical veins entering the lateral margin of the superior sagittal sinus may need to be sacrificed to retract the frontal pole away from the falx. Small veins entering the anterior end of the inferior sagittal sinus may need to be obliterated and divided before the arachnoid in the depths of the interhemispheric fissure is opened. Opening the arachnoid will expose the A2 segments of the anterior cerebral arteries and their bifurcation into the pericallosal and callosomarginal arteries. The surgeon may need to push the anterior cerebral arteries toward their respective hemispheres or to one side to reach the rostrum part of the corpus callosum. Care should be taken to avoid occluding the perforating branches of the anterior communicating artery, which extend into the walls of the third ventricle to supply columns of the fornix. A vertical incision beginning in the lamina terminalis and extending upward into the rostrum of the corpus callosum will expose a lesion in the floor of the frontal horn formed by the anteroinferior part of the corpus callosum and straddling the lateral and third ventricular sides of the foramen of Monro.

Posterior Approaches

The approaches suitable for lesions in the posterior part of the lateral and third ventricles are the posterior transcortical, posterior transcallosal, occipital transtentorial, and infratentorial supracerebellar (*Figs. 5.21* and *5.22*). The posterior transcortical and transcallosal approaches are best suited to atrial lesions, but may be used for selected lesions that involve

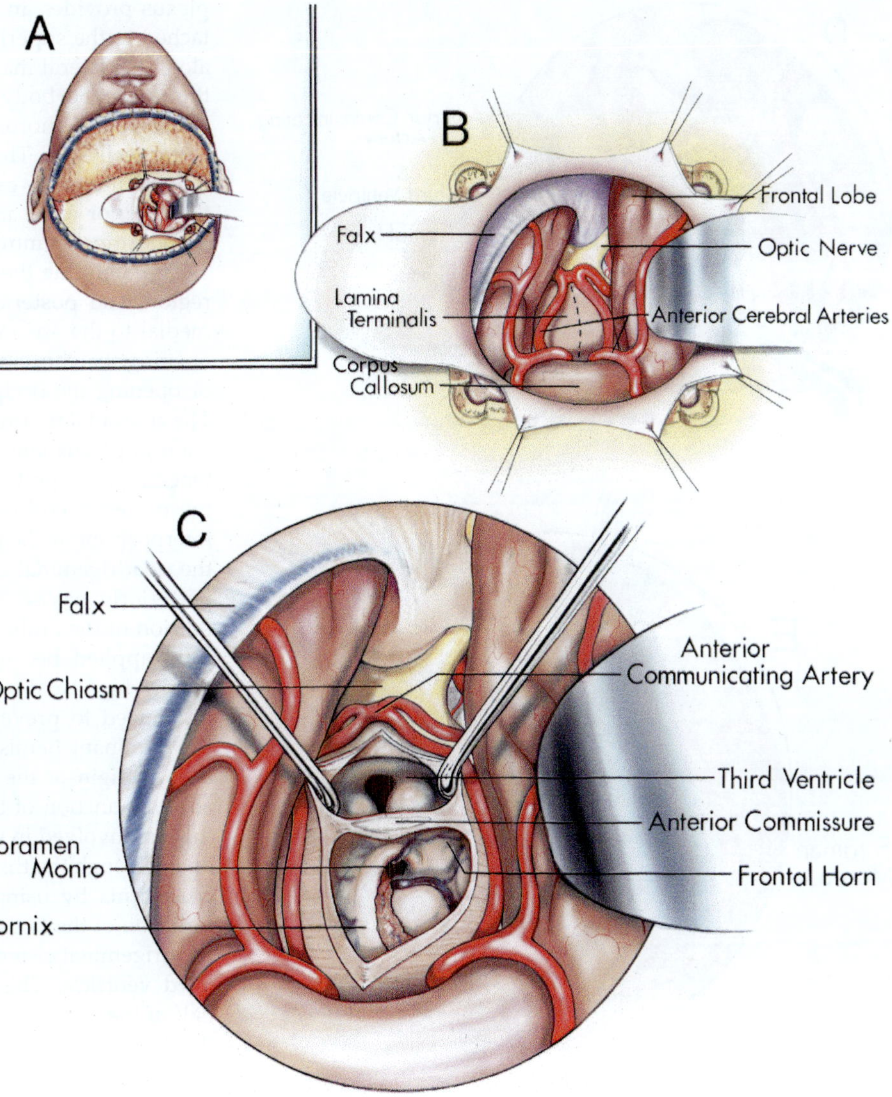

FIGURE 5.26. *Transfrontal approach to the anterior part of the lateral and third ventricles.* A, *site of scalp and bone flaps.* B, *the right frontal lobe has been retracted away from the falx to expose the optic nerves, lamina terminalis, rostrum of the corpus callosum, and the anterior cerebral arteries.* C, *normal ventricular anatomy. The lamina terminalis and rostrum of the corpus callosum have been opened to expose the third ventricle and the frontal horn. The anterior commissure and columns of the fornix have been preserved. (Legend continues on next page.)*

the medial wall of the atrium and extend into the quadrigeminal cistern and posterior third ventricle. The occipital transtentorial and infratentorial supracerebellar approaches are best suited to lesions in the posterior third ventricle and quadrigeminal cistern.

Lesions situated entirely within the atrium and posterior part of the body of the lateral ventricle are best exposed using the posterior transcortical approach. Selected lesions may be exposed by the posterior transcallosal or occipital interhemispheric approaches. The transcallosal approach is considered if the lesion involves the splenium of the corpus callosum and extends into the lateral ventricle from the roof or the upper part of the medial wall of the atrium. The occipital approach directed along the occipital pole and interhemispheric fissure would be used if a lesion involving the medial wall of the atrium extended into the third ventricle and medial wall of the quadrigeminal cistern.

Pineal tumors have been removed by a posterior transcortical approach directed through the medial wall of the atrium. However, this area is very narrow and is heavily vascularized, making it difficult to approach pineal tumors by this route. The occipital-transtentorial approach and the infratentorial-supracerebellar approaches are most commonly used for exposing pineal tumors.

Posterior Transcortical Approach

This approach, directed through a cortical incision in the superior parietal lobule, exposes the interior of the atrium and the posterior part of the body and may be the preferred approach for a lesion situated entirely within the atrium, or arising in the glomus of the choroid plexus or a lesion that involves the atrium, posterior third ventricle, and quadrigeminal cistern (*Fig. 5.27*).

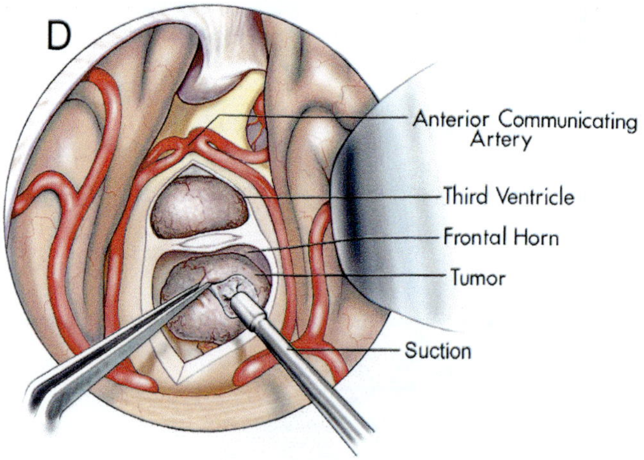

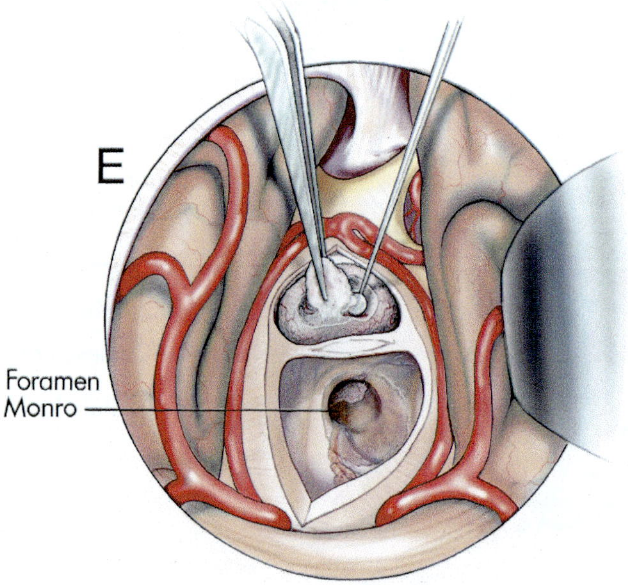

FIGURE 5.26. *Continued*
D, a tumor that straddles the foramen of Monro and extends into both the frontal horn and third ventricle has been exposed. The portion of the tumor within the frontal horn is being removed using a suction and forceps. E, the part of the tumor within the third ventricle is being removed using a fine dissector.

The patient is positioned in the three-quarter prone position with the face turned toward the floor so as to place the parietal area to be operated uppermost. A high posterior parietal bone flap, centered behind the postcentral gyrus over the superior parietal lobule, is elevated. The cortex is incised in the long axis of the superior parietal lobule in the region behind the postcentral gyrus, preferably in a sulcus crossing the lobule. This cortical incision avoids the visual pathways traversing the parietal lobe and the speech areas at the junction of the parietal and temporal lobes. The lateral ventricle is entered above the junction of the body and atrium and above the body and crus of the fornix (*Figs. 5.3, 5.6,* and *5.8*). The choroid plexus provides an orienting landmark. It forms a fringe attached to the superior and posterior surfaces of the thalamus along the lateral margin of the body and crus of the fornix. In this area, the body and crus of the fornix fill the interval between the choroid plexus and the lower surface of the corpus callosum. This approach will expose the calcar avis and bulb of the corpus callosum in the medial wall, the pulvinar in the anterior wall, and the collateral trigone in the floor. The hippocampal commissure is medial to the crus of the fornix.

After entering the atrium, the quadrigeminal cistern, pineal region, and posterior part of the third ventricle, which are medial to the atrium, can be reached by one of three routes: opening the choroidal fissure, opening along the crus fornix, or opening the occipital lobe forming the medial atrial wall. The choroidal fissure is opened by retracting the glomus of the choroid plexus laterally and opening along the tenia fornicis. Opening through the crus or the choroidal fissure will expose the posterior end of the internal cerebral vein in the velum interpositum or the basal, internal cerebral, and great veins in the quadrigeminal cistern. Retracting the crus medially and posteriorly exposes the quadrigeminal cistern and the caudal portion of the ambient cistern. The retraction should be carefully applied because it may damage the calcar avis and underlying visual cortex. Retraction of the pulvinar should be minimized to prevent language and speech disturbances in the dominant hemisphere, because the pulvinar is the main site of origin of the thalamic fibers to the association cortex and the junction of the parietal, temporal, and occipital lobes that are involved in speech and vision. An alternate route is to open through the thin medial wall of the atrium formed by the crus fornix by using an arcuate incision directed along the direction of the fibers in the crus. This incision opens into the quadrigeminal cisterns and provides a route to the roof of the third ventricle. This incision should spare the contralateral half of the fornix. However, avoiding the contralateral half of the fornix is easier in the atrium than in the body of the ventricle because the crura are more widely separated at the level of the atrium. If the pulvinar bulges too far posteriorly a supplemental horizontal incision in the medial wall of the atrium behind the crus may be needed to avoid retraction of the pulvinar. However, extending this incision posteriorly into the calcar avis will cause a visual field deficit, which increases in severity as the incision is increased further posteriorly. The internal cerebral and great veins and the medial posterior choroidal arteries commonly block the exposure. These vascular structures should be gently displaced after dividing only those branches required to expose and remove the tumor, rather than sacrificing their main trunks.

The lower part of the atrium may also be approached through cortical incisions in the superior and middle temporal gyri and the temporoparietal junction, although the preferred route is through the superior parietal lobule. The atrium was first approached through a parieto-occipital bone flap and a cortical incision extending from the posterior end of the superior temporal gyrus into the inferior part of the parietal lobe (34). Exposing the atrium through the temporoparietal junction may cause a homonymous visual field deficit due to the

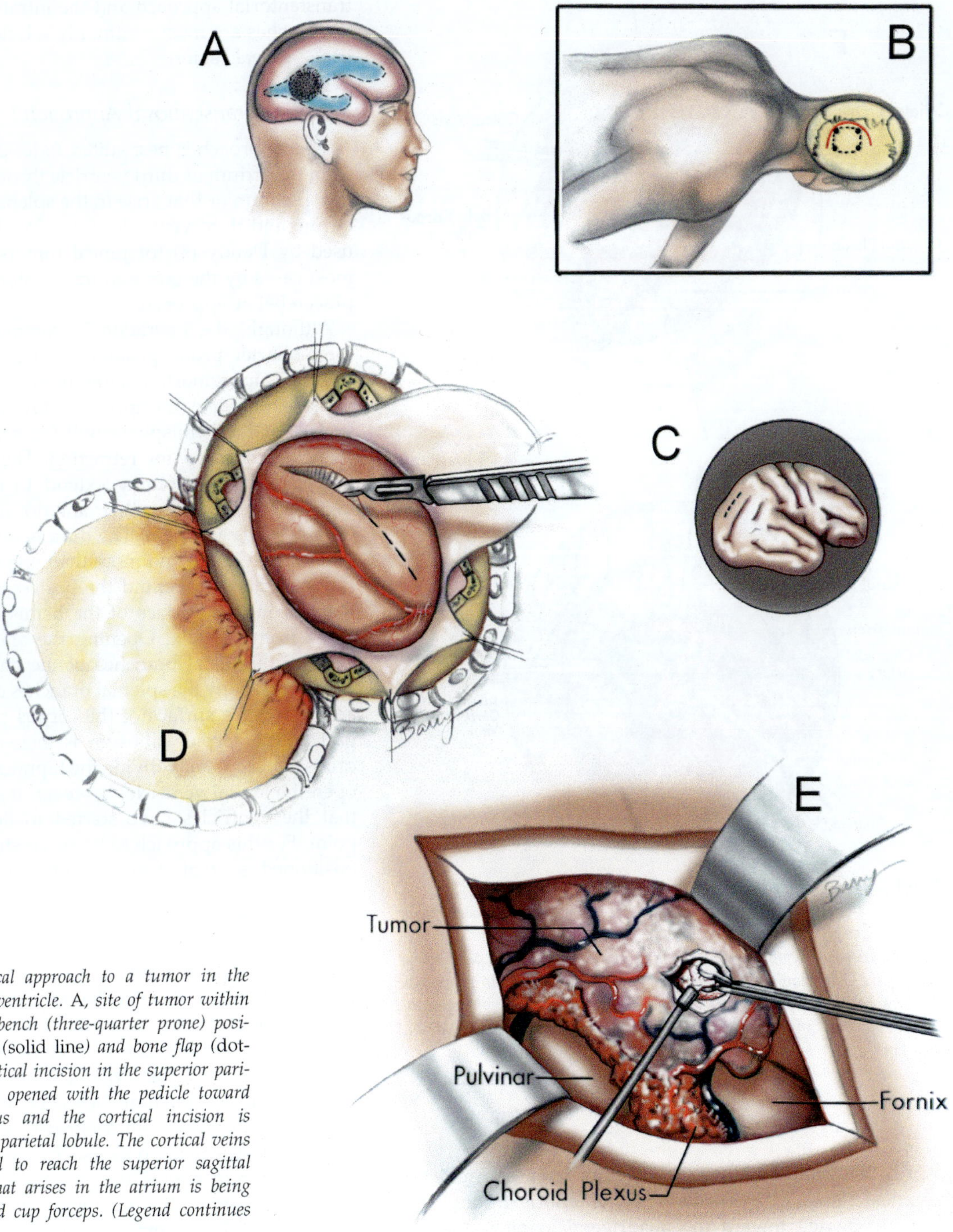

FIGURE 5.27. *Transcortical approach to a tumor in the atrium of the right lateral ventricle.* A, *site of tumor within the right atrium.* B, *park bench (three-quarter prone) position. Site of scalp incision* (solid line) *and bone flap* (dotted line). C, *site of the cortical incision in the superior parietal lobule.* D, *the dura is opened with the pedicle toward the superior sagittal sinus and the cortical incision is directed along the superior parietal lobule. The cortical veins pass forward at this level to reach the superior sagittal sinus.* E, *a meningioma that arises in the atrium is being debulked using suction and cup forceps. (Legend continues on next page.)*

interruption of the optic radiations in either hemisphere, disturbances of visuospatial function in the nondominant hemisphere, and aphasia and agnostic disorders in the dominant hemisphere (15, 24, 28, 33). Opening through the middle temporal gyrus might be considered for a lesion in the dominant hemisphere. However, cortical mapping during surgery has revealed an occasional extension of the speech representative into the middle temporal gyrus (16). The lower the approach, the more readily accessible is the anterior choroidal supply to tumors arising in the trigonal region. It is possible to slip beneath such tumors as meningiomas in the trigone by this route, after partially debulking them, to pick up the medial blood supply from the lateral posterior choroidal vessels.

The transcortical-transventricular exposures are more difficult to perform if the ventricles are not dilated. These approaches through the atrium do not provide satisfactory ex-

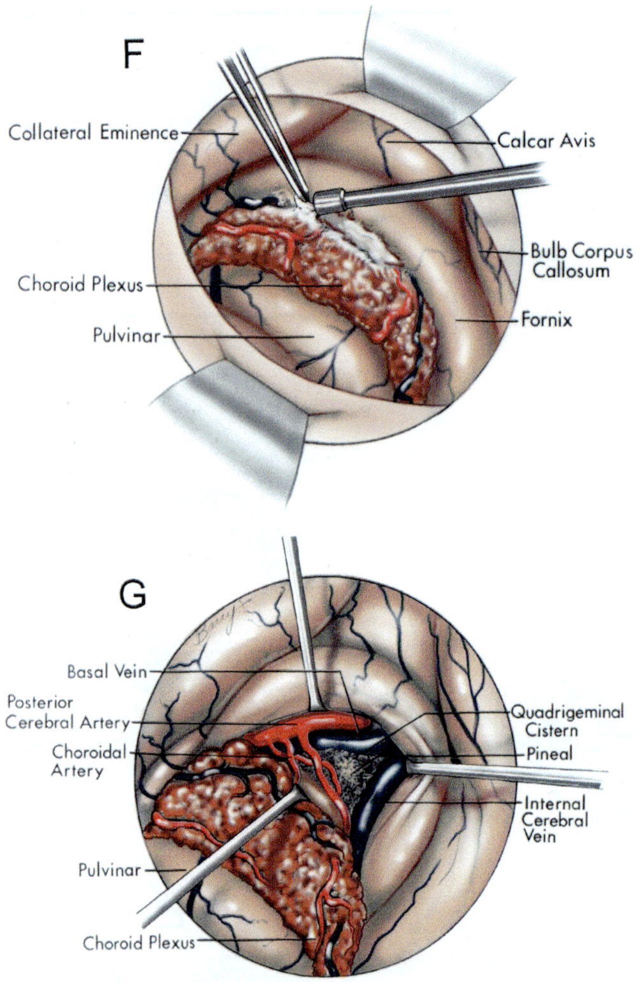

FIGURE 5.27. *Continued*
F, the last remnant of tumor has been removed and its attachment to the choroid plexus is being coagulated. G, the choroidal fissure has been opened by incising along the attachment of the choroid plexus to the crus of the fornix. The choroid plexus has been retracted forward to expose the structures in the quadrigeminal cistern, which include the pineal body, posterior cerebral and choroidal arteries, and the internal cerebral and basal veins.

posure of the typical midline pineal tumor and are unsuited to the pineal tumor that extends posteroinferiorly through the tentorial opening toward the quadrigeminal plate and the cerebellum. The posterior transcortical approach directed through the choroidal fissure is most commonly used for arteriovenous malformations or vascular tumors that are located behind the pulvinar and are fed and drained by vessels passing through the choroidal fissure. Pineal tumors have been removed by a transventricular approach directed through the medial wall of the atrium; however, the narrowness and heavy vascularization of the pineal area make it difficult to approach pineal tumors by this route. The occipital transtentorial approach and the infratentorial supracerebellar approaches are most commonly selected for exposing tumors in the pineal region.

Posterior Transcallosal Approach

This approach is best suited to lesions that extend upward from the atrium or third ventricle through the posterior part of the splenium or that arise in the splenium and extend into the atrium and third ventricle (*Fig. 5.28*). The approach, although used by Dandy (5) for pineal tumors, has been replaced in most cases by the occipital transtentorial or infratentorial supracerebellar approach.

Although, the operation is commonly performed in the three-quarter prone position with the parietal region to be operated uppermost, a better alternative with some lesions is to place the side of the approach downward so that the medial surface of the hemisphere will fall away from the falx, thus reducing the need for retraction. The parieto-occipital scalp flap and the craniotomy extend to or across the superior sagittal sinus and have their anterior margin behind the postcentral gyrus and vein. The dura is reflected toward the sagittal sinus. Usually, no more than one vein entering the superior sagittal sinus behind the postcentral gyrus is divided so that the medial surface of the hemisphere may be retracted away from the falx. Opening the arachnoid below the falx exposes the distal branches of the anterior cerebral arteries and occasionally the splenial branches of the posterior cerebral arteries on the surface of the corpus callosum. The posterior part of the corpus callosum is incised in the midline. This callosal incision may divide the hippocampal commissure and open the lateral ventricle; however, it should be remembered that the ventricles have started to deviate laterally at this point. For this approach to be successful, the lesion should be positioned so that it comes into view as the splenium is exposed and opened. The junction of the internal cerebral veins with the great vein comes into view below the splenium and above the pineal gland. These veins may separate easily from the dorsal surface of a tumor lying within the third ventricle, but they also may be frequently so embedded within the upper surface of a tumor that their sacrifice is inescapable. Dandy (5), in some cases, resected the great and internal cerebral veins and the straight sinus in this region without neurological dysfunction; however, every effort should be made to spare these venous structures, because their obliteration may cause major deficits. The medial posterior choroidal and other branches of the posterior cerebral and superior cerebellar arteries, the trochlear nerves, the quadrigeminal plate, and the basal veins come into view in the depths of this exposure. The roof of the third ventricle will be encountered anterior to the pineal body. Opening the layers of tela choroidea in the roof of the third ventricle will expose the cavity of the third ventricle and the choroid plexus in the roof. The most dangerous dissection is in the area of the quadrigeminal plate, because some tumors are adherent to or embedded in this area. The tentorium may be divided longitudinally beside the straight sinus, and the falx may be split vertically to facilitate the exposure posteriorly and to the opposite side.

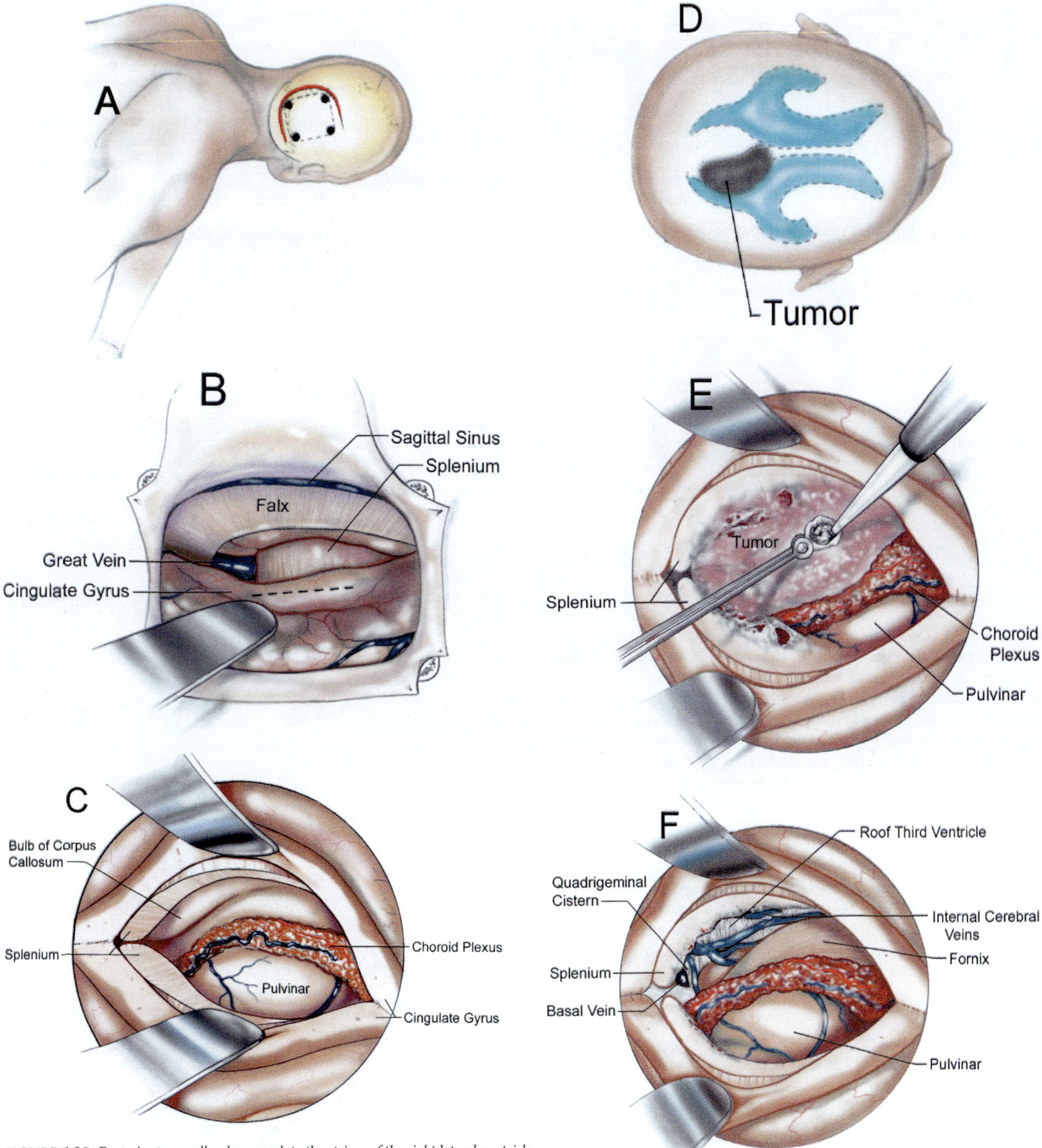

FIGURE 5.28. *Posterior transcallosal approach to the atrium of the right lateral ventricle.*
A, *three-quarter prone position. The side of the tumor is placed downward to facilitate the exposure along the interhemispheric fissure. The scalp incision* (solid line) *and the bone flap* (broken line) *extends up to or across the midline.* B, *the dura is open with the pedicle toward the superior sagittal sinus. The medial surface of the right parietal lobe has been retracted away from the falx. The cortical incision extends through the posterior part of the cingulate gyrus. The corpus callosum is opened to the right of the midline to expose the right atrium.* C, *normal ventricular anatomy. The opening through the cingulate gyrus encounters the lateral part of the splenium. Opening through the splenium in the midline would expose the roof of the third ventricle. The opening through the lateral part of the splenium into the atrium exposes the crus of the fornix, bulb of the corpus callosum, pulvinar, and choroid plexus.* D, *the glial tumor is situated in the forceps major and the bulb of the corpus callosum.* E, *the tumor is being removed with an ultrasonic aspirator. The choroid plexus and pulvinar are pushed forward by the tumor.* F, *the tumor has been removed. Removing the bulb of the corpus callosum exposes the internal cerebral veins in the roof of the third ventricle and the quadrigeminal cistern. Residual tumor is present in the corpus callosum.*

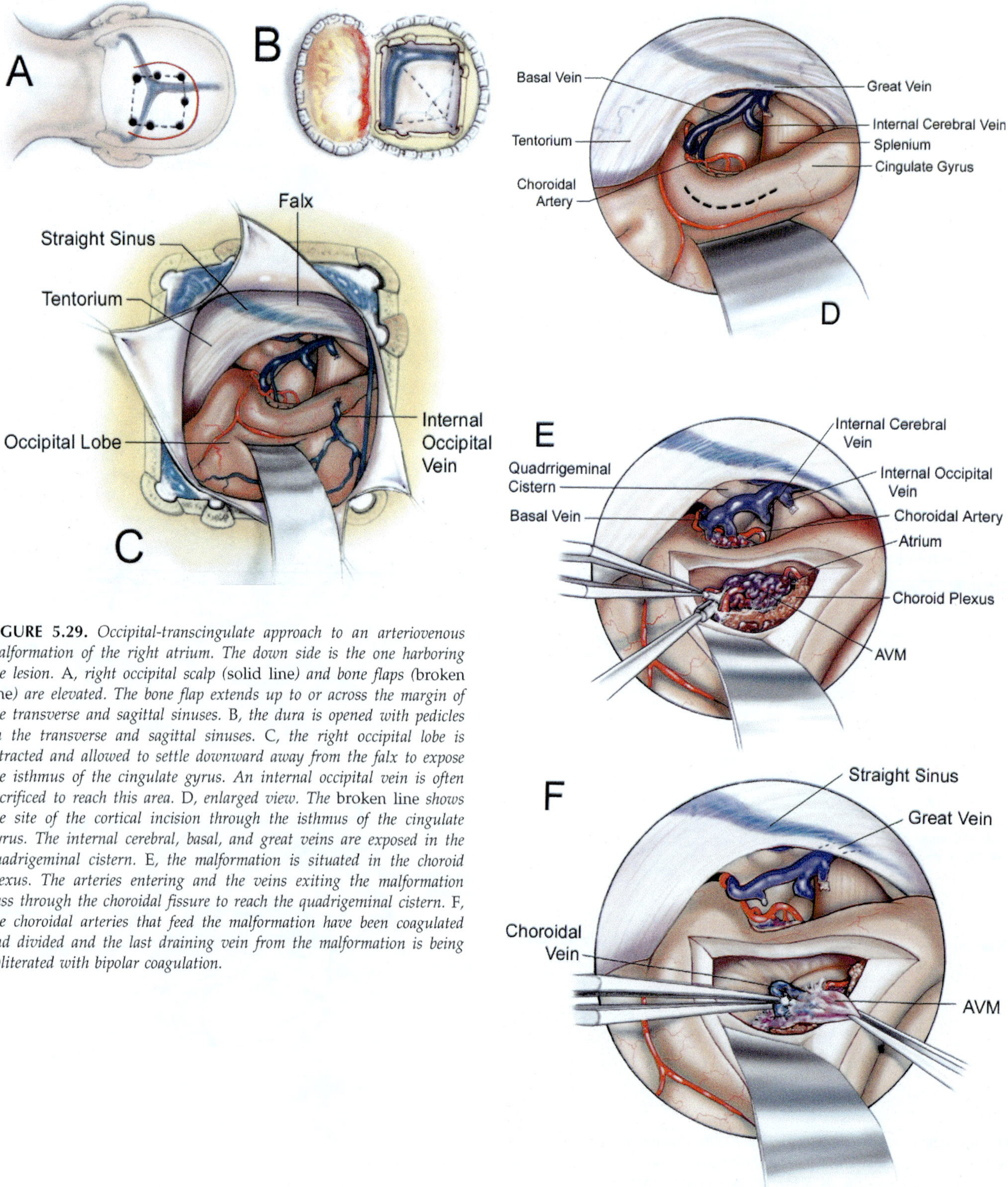

FIGURE 5.29. *Occipital-transcingulate approach to an arteriovenous malformation of the right atrium. The down side is the one harboring the lesion. A, right occipital scalp* (solid line) *and bone flaps* (broken line) *are elevated. The bone flap extends up to or across the margin of the transverse and sagittal sinuses. B, the dura is opened with pedicles on the transverse and sagittal sinuses. C, the right occipital lobe is retracted and allowed to settle downward away from the falx to expose the isthmus of the cingulate gyrus. An internal occipital vein is often sacrificed to reach this area. D, enlarged view. The* broken line *shows the site of the cortical incision through the isthmus of the cingulate gyrus. The internal cerebral, basal, and great veins are exposed in the quadrigeminal cistern. E, the malformation is situated in the choroid plexus. The arteries entering and the veins exiting the malformation pass through the choroidal fissure to reach the quadrigeminal cistern. F, the choroidal arteries that feed the malformation have been coagulated and divided and the last draining vein from the malformation is being obliterated with bipolar coagulation.*

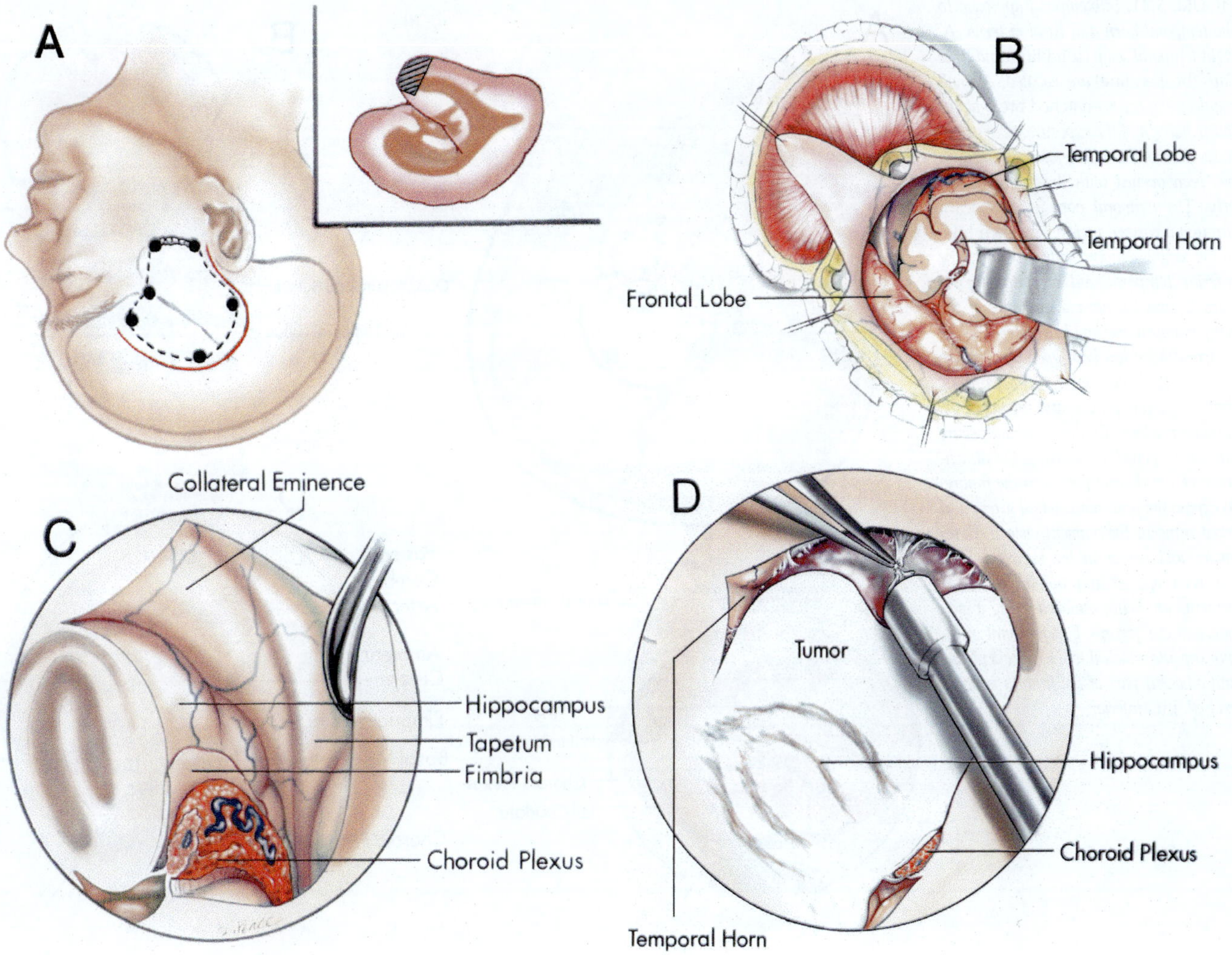

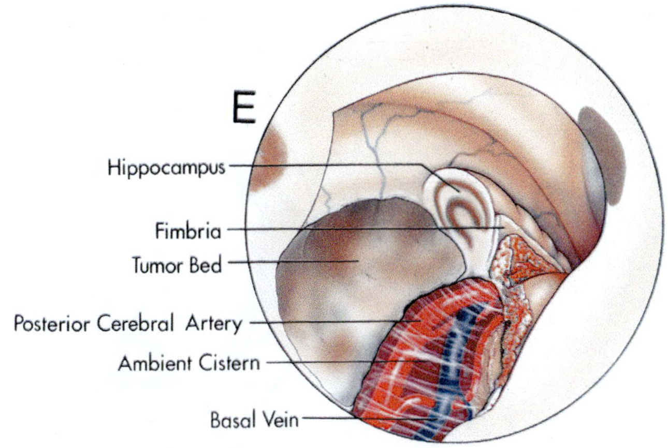

FIGURE 5.30. *Right frontotemporal craniotomy and approach to temporal horn through a temporal lobectomy.* A, *right frontotemporal scalp* (solid line) *and bone flaps* (broken line) *are elevated. The* inset *shows the extent of the temporal lobectomy.* B *and* C, *normal ventricular anatomy.* B, *the lobectomy extends across the anterior part of the temporal horn.* C, *structures exposed in the wall of temporal horn include the hippocampal formation, fimbria, choroid plexus, collateral eminence, and the tapetum of the corpus callosum.* D, *a glial tumor that arises in the hippocampus is being removed with bipolar coagulation and fine suction.* E, *removal of the tumor and the anterior part of the hippocampus exposes the posterior cerebral artery and basal vein in the ambient cistern. The normal hippocampus is exposed behind the tumor.*

For the approach to the atrium, an incision is made in the cingulate gyrus behind the posterosuperior part of the corpus callosum. This cortical incision is directed obliquely forward through the lateral part of the splenium to enter the atrium just above the bulb of the corpus callosum. The landmarks within the ventricle are described above, under the posterior transcortical approach.

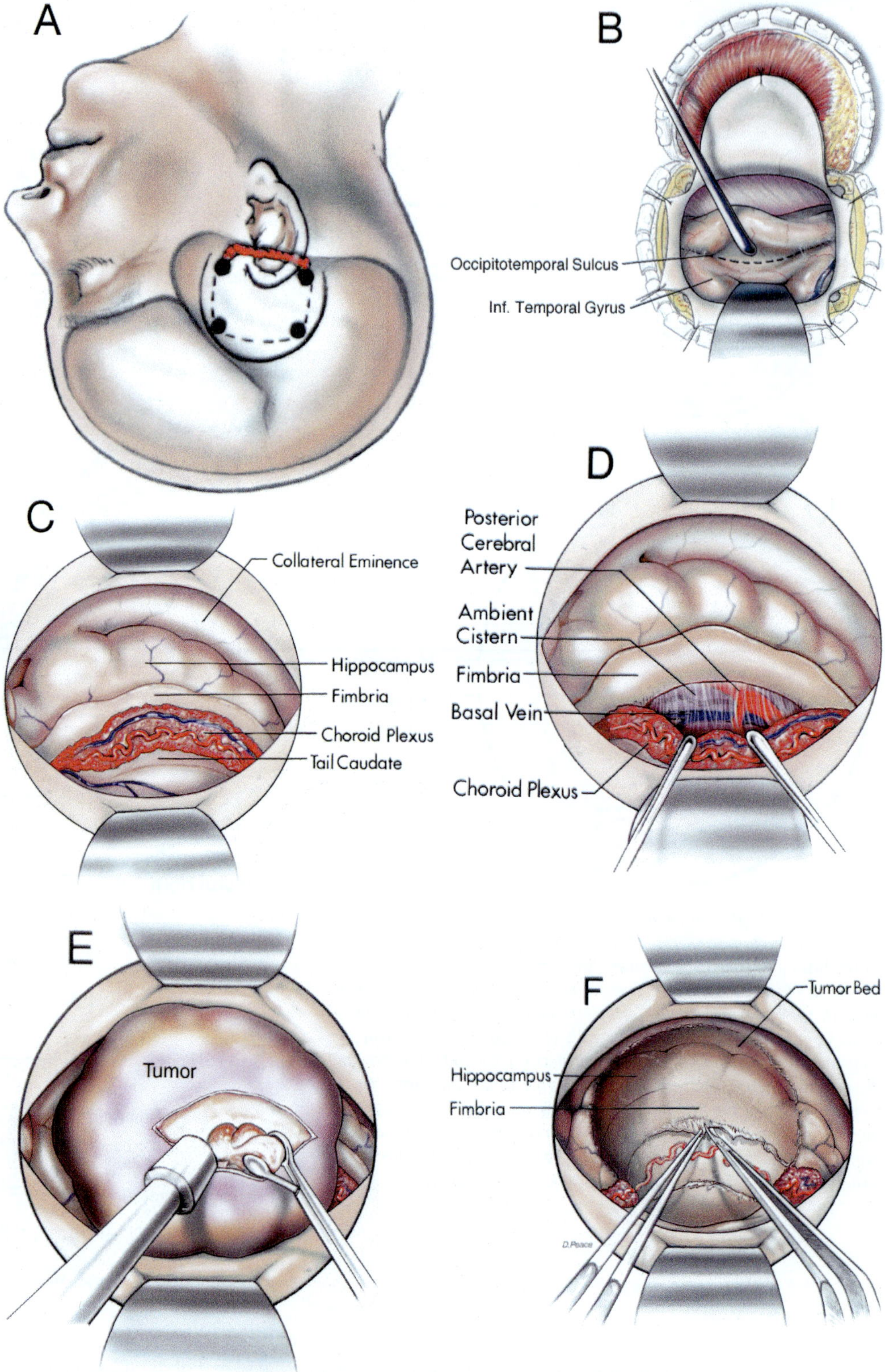

FIGURE 5.31. *Subtemporal approach to the temporal horn and basal cisterns.* A, *right temporal scalp* (solid line) *and bone flaps* (broken line) *are elevated. A small craniectomy* (cross-hatched area) *at the lower margin of the exposure gives access to the floor of the middle fossa.* B, *the dura has been opened with the pedicle inferiorly. The temporal horn is approached through a cortical incision* (broken line) *in the occipitotemporal sulcus between the inferior temporal and occipitotemporal gyri.* C *and* D, *normal anatomy of the temporal horn and ambient cistern.* C, *the temporal horn has been opened to expose the collateral eminence, hippocampus, fimbria, choroid plexus, and the tail of the caudate nucleus.* D, *the choroidal fissure has been opened by incising the attachment of the choroid plexus to the fimbria to expose the posterior cerebral artery and basal veins in the ambient cistern.* E, *an epidermoid tumor in the temporal horn has been opened and the intracapsular contents are being removed using a suction and cup forceps.* F, *a remnant of tumor capsule attached to the choroid plexus and adjacent part of the fimbria is being excised.* Inf., *inferior.*

Occipital Approach

This approach is suitable for tumors situated in the pineal region and the part of the pulvinar, medial occipital lobe, and medial atrial wall facing the quadrigeminal cistern (*Figs. 4.24 and 5.29*). See also *Figure 5.10* in the Millennium issue of *Neurosurgery* (25). It is preferred over the infratentorial supracerebellar approach for a pineal region tumor centered at the tentorial edge or above if there is no major extension to the opposite side or into the posterior fossa. It might also be considered for a lesion such as an arteriovenous malformation in which it is desirable to expose the feeding choroidal arteries in the quadrigeminal cistern before exposing the lesion in the atrium.

The patient is positioned in the three-quarter prone position with the occipital area to be operated lowermost and the face turned toward the floor. This allows the medial occipital surface along which the approach is directed to relax away from the falx, thus reducing the need for brain retraction. The procedure was first performed with the patient in a sitting position (22, 34). Some surgeons who use the park bench position place the patient's left side down and the face turned toward the floor to bring the right occipital area along which the tumor is approached uppermost (12). The occipital scalp flap and craniotomy are placed so that they will expose the margins of the transverse and sagittal sinuses and the torcular herophili. The dura mater is opened using two flaps, one based on the superior sagittal sinus and the other on the transverse sinus. The medial surface of the occipital pole is gently retracted away from the falx. The occipital pole can usually be retracted from the falx without sacrificing any bridging veins because frequently there are no bridging veins from the occipital lobe entering the part of the superior sagittal sinuses behind the lambdoid suture and parieto-occipital sulcus. The anterior calcarine (internal occipital) vein, which crosses from the anteromedial surface of the occipital lobe to the quadrigeminal cistern, is transected only when necessary because its division may produce a homonymous hemianopia.

For a tumor in the posterior third ventricle, the tentorium may be divided lateral and parallel to the straight sinus from the free edge to near the transverse sinus. The tentorium can be reflected laterally or a wedge of tentorium removed to increase the exposure. The arachnoid over the ambient and quadrigeminal cisterns is opened. A disadvantage of this approach is that the vein of Galen and internal cerebral veins are above and obstruct the approach to the pineal region, but this becomes less of a disadvantage after the tentorium is divided. The lower portion of the splenium is divided if necessary, but the splenium is usually thinned and elevated by the tumor and therefore it can routinely be spared. The ipsilateral basal vein, medial posterior choroidal and posterior cerebral arteries, and thalamus are lateral to the tumor. This exposure provides only a limited view of the contralateral half of the quadrigeminal cistern and the opposite thalamus. Meticulous attention is directed to separating the tumor from the thalamus and the quadrigeminal plate.

An atrial tumor that extends into the medial occipital cortex, near the junction of the vein of Galen and straight sinus, can be exposed from this approach by opening through the isthmus of the cingulate gyrus in front of the calcarine sulcus. The opening enters the medial wall of the atrium behind the choroidal fissure. The branches of the posterior cerebral artery and its bifurcation into the calcarine and parietooccipital branches course lateral to the pineal region tumor and medial to an atrial tumor. The lateral posterior choroidal arteries pass through the choroidal fissure in this area, and the medial posterior choroidal arteries and basal vein will be seen beside the pineal gland. The quadrigeminal plate, trochlear nerve, superior cerebellar artery, and precentral cerebellar vein may be seen in the depths of the exposure.

Infratentorial Supracerebellar Approach

This approach is suitable for tumors in the pineal region that are midline and that grow into both the posterior part of the third ventricle and the posterior fossa, displacing the quadrigeminal plate and the anterior lobe of the cerebellum. An advantage of this approach is that the deep venous system that caps the dorsal and lateral aspects of most pineal tumors does not obstruct access to the tumor (*Fig. 4.24*). *Figure 5.10* in Chapter 5 on the tentorial incisura in the Millennium issue of *Neurosurgery* also provides a review of this approach (25).

The operation is performed with the patient in the three-quarter prone position, although some may be performed in the semi-sitting or full prone position. The neck is flexed to optimize the view under the tentorium. A vertical midline incision is used. The suboccipital craniectomy extends above the lower edge of the torcular herophili and both transverse sinuses. A Y-shaped dural incision, with upper limits that extend up to the inferior margin of the transverse sinus near the midline, allows the midline dura to be reflected upward without impediment. The straight sinus and tentorium may be elevated with a retractor, and the vermis may be retracted gently downward. Bridging veins over the superior surface of the cerebellum may be transected with minimal risk. This exposure may be enlarged beyond the tentorial notch by sectioning the tentorial edge through the infratentorial approach. Incision of the arachnoid over the quadrigeminal cistern brings the deep venous system and the tumor into view. The vein of Galen and the internal cerebral veins are above the pineal gland; the superior vermian vein is posterior; the thalamus, the medial posterior choroidal and posterior cerebral arteries, and the basal veins are lateral; and the quadrigeminal plate, trochlear nerves, superior cerebellar arteries, and superior vermis are below.

The superior vermian vein may need to be transected. The superior vermis, particularly the culmen, often conceals the quadrigeminal plate when the view is directed over the apex of the tentorial cerebellar surface, but moving the retractor lateral to the apex of the tentorial surface provides a better view around the culmen to the quadrigeminal plate. Most pineal tumors are not highly vascular. Their arterial supply is from the medial and lateral posterior choroidal branches of the posterior cerebral arteries and occasionally from the superior cerebellar arteries. The tumor is removed according to the principles outlined previously. The most difficult dissection is often along the quadrigeminal plate. The tumor removal may extend into the posterior third ventricle, thus communicating the ventricle with the quadrigeminal cistern. This approach permits the placement of a Silastic tube from the posterior part of the third ventricle to the cisterna magna if the third ventricle is opened.

Lateral Approaches

The lateral approaches directed through the lower part of the lateral hemispheric surface or below the lateral hemispheric border are the frontotemporal (pterional), posterior frontotemporal, transtemporal, and subtemporal approaches (*Fig. 5.21*). The posterior frontotemporal approach exposes the anterior temporal pole and permits the anterior part of the temporal horn to be exposed through a small cortical incision or a temporal lobectomy. The transtemporal and subtemporal exposures conducted through a posterior frontotemporal craniotomy or a temporal craniotomy centered above the ear permit the full length of the temporal horn to be exposed through the lateral or inferior surfaces of the temporal lobe.

Frontotemporal (Pterional) and Posterior Frontotemporal Exposures

The frontotemporal (pterional) craniotomy may be selected for the removal of some third ventricular tumors (*Fig. 5.30*). The posterior frontotemporal approach is similar to the conventional pterional craniotomy, except that it extends further posteriorly in the temporal region. We would use these approaches only if a tumor involving the third ventricle is centered lateral to the sella or extends into the middle cranial fossa. The posterior frontotemporal exposure is selected if an anterior transtemporal or anterior subtemporal exposure is needed.

For the frontotemporal approach, the patient is placed in the supine position and the head is tilted a bit backward and turned 30 degrees away from the side of operation. Small scalp and bone flaps are elevated for the frontotemporal (pterional) approach. For the posterior frontotemporal approach, the flap extends further posteriorly above the ear. The scalp, temporalis muscle and fascia, and pericranium may be reflected as a single layer but more commonly an interfascial approach in which the scalp, galea, and lower part of the superficial temporal fascia with the superficial fat pad and nerves to the frontalis muscle are reflected as one layer and the temporalis muscle is reflected as a second layer. The lateral aspect of the sphenoid ridge is removed with a rongeur or a drill. The dura is opened, with the main flap pulled down anteroinferiorly along the region of the pterion. The frontal and temporal lobes are elevated to expose the area along the sphenoid ridge. The bridging veins from the sylvian fissure and temporal tip are coagulated and divided only if necessary. It may be possible to preserve these bridging veins if the frontotemporal approach is entirely above the sphenoid ridge or if the subtemporal approach is entirely below the sphenoid ridge. The arachnoid membrane is opened to expose the carotid artery, optic nerve, and origin of the posterior communicating and anterior choroidal arteries. The tumor is exposed through the triangle between the optic nerve and the internal carotid and anterior cerebral arteries in the frontotemporal approach or below the floor of the third ventricle through the interval between the carotid artery and the oculomotor nerve. The third ventricle may be entered through the floor if the nuclear masses are pushed laterally by the tumor and the floor consists of only a glial membrane.

The posterior frontotemporal approach is used for a lesion involving the anterior portion of the temporal horn that can be exposed through an anterior temporal lobectomy or a small cortical incision in the anterior part of the temporal lobe or a lesion involving the third ventricle extends laterally below the temporal lobe. The patient is placed in the supine position with a sandbag under the shoulder on the side to be operated. The head is tilted a bit backward and turned 45 degrees away from the side of the operation. The scalp incision begins in the frontal area and extends in a question-mark configuration back to the area above the ear and then downward to the zygoma in front of the ear. The scalp, temporalis muscle and fascia, and pericranium are reflected as a single layer. A free frontotemporal bone flap that will expose the anterior half of the lateral surface of the temporal lobe is elevated, and the lateral aspect of the sphenoid ridge is removed with a rongeur or a drill. The dura mater is opened with the main flap pulled anteroinferior along the region of the pterion. The tip of the temporal lobe may be elevated to expose the edge of the tentorium cerebelli. The temporal lobe may be elevated in the subtemporal approach to expose as far posterior as the anterior and lateral aspect of the midbrain and the upper part of the basilar artery. The tumor, once exposed, is removed according to the principles outlined previously. A decision is made as to whether to enter the temporal horn through a cortical incision or through a temporal lobectomy. The cortical incision would be selected if the lesion is strictly localized to the region of the tip of the temporal lobe. The temporal lobectomy would be considered if the lesion not only involved the temporal pole but also extended into the temporal horn. For the transcortical approach, the lower part of the middle temporal gyrus or the upper part of the inferior temporal gyrus is opened in the long axis of the gyrus and the incision is directed backward through the temporal lobe to the anterior part of the temporal horn.

To use a temporal lobectomy, the vertical incision through the temporal lobe would be situated no more than 4 cm from the temporal tip to avoid the optic radiations; the horizontal incision paralleling the sylvian fissure is directed medially through the lower part of the superior temporal gyrus or the upper part of the middle temporal gyrus. Medially, an incision through the superior temporal gyrus encounters the pia arachnoid on the medial surface of the lower lip of the sylvian fissure that covers the lower branches of the middle cerebral artery as they course over the insula. This incision paralleling the sylvian fissure is extended anteriorly and medially into the temporal pole just below the sylvian fissure and sphenoid ridge. The depths of the cortical incision will encounter the uncus and the parahippocampal gyrus, which are removed using subpial dissection to avoid injury to the branches of the middle cerebral artery that supply the internal capsule. The cortical incision extending around the temporal tip can often be completed without sacrificing the major sylvian veins, which usually enter the sphenoparietal sinus just below the edge of the sphenoid ridge. These approaches will expose the anterior part of the temporal horn as far back as the site where the anterior choroidal artery passes through the choroidal fissure near the inferior choroidal point. The prominence over the hippocampus and the collateral eminence will be seen in the floor of the temporal horn, and the inferior ventricular vein may be seen in the roof. The amygdala lies directly anterior and slightly above the tip of the temporal horn and is directly lateral to the cisternal surface of the uncus. This exposure is sufficiently anterior that it does not permit more than minimal opening of the choroidal fissure to expose the ambient cistern. It will expose the anterior choroidal artery passing through the inferior choroidal point behind the head of the hippocampus. It is satisfactory for removing a lesion in the region of the anterior wall of the temporal horn and the amygdala. Opening through the amygdala and uncus exposes the structures in the crural and ambient cisterns.

Transtemporal and Subtemporal Approaches

A temporal craniotomy and a transtemporal or subtemporal cortical incision are used for a lesion in the middle or posterior third of the temporal horn or for selected lesions of the third ventricle that extend into the ambient and crural cisterns (*Fig. 5.31*). For the temporal craniotomy centered above the ear, the patient is positioned in the supine position with the shoulder on the side of the lesion elevated and the head tilted 60 to 80 degrees away from the side of the operation. The scalp incision extends from above the zygoma anterior to the ear to the area above the ear and then posteriorly and downward to the region of the asterion posterior to the ear. The scalp, temporalis muscle and fascia, and pericranium are reflected as a single layer. The bone flap is cut low or a small craniectomy below the flap is carried down to the floor of the fossa. This may open the mastoid air cells. Care should be taken not to open the attic of the middle ear. Transient deafness from effusion of fluid into the middle ear may follow this approach. The temporal horn of the nondominant hemisphere may be exposed using a cortical incision in the middle or inferior temporal gyrus anterior to the optic radiations. An alternative and often preferable route, which minimizes the possibility of damage to the optic radiations and speech centers of the dominant hemisphere, is the subtemporal route, in which an incision is made in the inferior temporal or occipitotemporal gyrus or the collateral sulcus on the lower surface of the temporal lobe. The risk of hemorrhage, venous infarction, and edema after retraction of the temporal lobe is reduced by avoiding occlusion of the bridging veins, especially the vein of Labbé.

The opening into the temporal horn will expose the choroidal fissure and the branches of the anterior and lateral posterior choroidal arteries as they enter the choroid plexus (*Figs. 5.3, 5.6,* and *5.9*). An approach through the temporal part of the choroidal fissure is used for lesions in the medial part of the temporal lobe and ambient cistern. The choroid plexus is elevated toward the thalamus and the fissure is opened by incising along the tenia fimbriae, thus avoiding damage to vessels that pass through the tenia thalami. Opening the choroidal fissure between the tenia fimbriae and the choroid plexus permits the arteries and veins that pass through the tenia thalami, and are larger than those passing through the tenia fornix, to be preserved and retracted upward with the choroid plexus. The main advantage of this approach is that it exposes the posterior cerebral and the anterior and posterior choroidal arteries, and the basal vein without extensive retraction of the temporal lobe. The approach is especially useful for exposing arteriovenous malformations of the temporal horn, hippocampus, and medial part of the temporal lobe that are fed by the arteries entering and drained by the veins exiting the choroidal fissure (17, 22, 31). The transchoroidal approach to the basal cisterns reduces the risks of injury to the vein of Labbé and the swelling and hematoma of the temporal lobe that may result from the extensive retraction required to reach the ambient cistern by the subtemporal extracerebral approach.

SELECTION OF OPERATIVE APPROACHES

The selection of the best operative approach for a tumor of the lateral and third ventricle depends on the site of origin, path of growth, and location of the tumor, the site of compression of the third ventricle, and whether there is ventricular obstruction (*Figs. 5.21* and *5.22*). Lesions within the anterior portion of the lateral and anterosuperior part of the third ventricles are most commonly reached by the anterior transcallosal and anterior transcortical approaches. This anterior transcallosal approach is suitable for lesions in the frontal horn and body of the lateral ventricles and for reaching the anterosuperior part of the third ventricle through the lateral ventricle. The transcallosal approach is easier to perform than the transcortical approach if the ventricles are of a normal size or are minimally enlarged. The transcortical approach is suitable for reaching tumors in the anterior part of the ipsilateral lateral ventricle and the anterosuperior part of the third ventricle. It is more difficult to expose the lateral ventricle on the opposite side through the transcortical than through the transcallosal approach. The transcortical approach is facilitated if the lateral ventricles are enlarged.

Routes through the lateral ventricles to the anterior part of the third ventricle, other than by incising the ipsilateral column of the fornix, are by the transchoroidal approach in which the choroidal fissure is opened along the tenia fornix, thus allowing the fornix to be pushed to the opposite side to expose the structures in the roof of the third ventricle, and the interforniceal approach in which the body of the fornix is split longitudinally in the midline. The transchoroidal approach is preferable to those approaches involving an incision in the fornix. The transchoroidal approach has the advantage of allowing access to the central portion of the third ventricle behind the foramen of Monro by displacing, rather than transecting, the fibers in the fornix. The transchoroidal and transforniceal routes provide a satisfactory view into the third ventricle when the ventricle is exposed through the corpus callosum. The transchoroidal opening provides a better view into the third ventricle than the transforniceal approach when the ventricle is exposed through the middle frontal gyrus.

An anterior interhemispheric approach may infrequently be considered for a lesion involving the rostrum and lower half of the genu of the corpus callosum or for a lesion that extends from the rostrum into the third ventricle behind the lamina terminalis. This approach is not suitable for reaching a lesion in the region of the posterior part of the frontal horn near the foramen of Monro, in the floor of the body of the lateral ventricle, or in the superior part of the third ventricle behind the foramen of Monro.

The posterior transcortical approach directed through the superior parietal lobule is the preferred route for exposing lesions situated within the posterior part of the body and the atrium or arising in the glomus of the choroid plexus. It may also be selected for a tumor involving the posterior third ventricle if it extends into the posterior thalamic surface facing the atrium and quadrigeminal cistern. Selected lesions within the atrium may be exposed by the posterior transcallosal or the occipital interhemispheric approaches. The posterior transcortical approach, directed through the superior parietal lobule, exposes the interior of the atrium and posterior part of the body and the thalamic surface facing the posterior third ventricle, atrium, and quadrigeminal cisterns. The posterior transcallosal approach directed along the medial occipital surface may be selected for a lesion that extends upward from the atrium through the posterior part of the splenium, or that arises in the splenium and extends into the roof or the upper part of the medial wall of the atrium, or that arises in the splenium and extends into the posterior third ventricle.

Tumors in the posterior part of the third ventricle are usually approached by the occipital transtentorial or infratentorial supracerebellar approaches, but they may also be reached through the posterior part of the lateral ventricle or corpus callosum if they also involve the medial atrial wall or corpus callosum. The infratentorial supracerebellar approach is best suited to tumors in the midline below the vein of Galen that grow into both the posterior part of the third ventricle and the posterior fossa, displacing the quadrigeminal plate and the anterosuperior part of the cerebellum. An advantage of this approach to pineal tumors is that the deep venous system that caps the dorsal and lateral aspects of pineal tumors does not obstruct access to the tumor. A disadvantage of the approach, especially if it is directed over the apex of the vermis, is that it is difficult to expose the area deep in the fissure between the midbrain and cerebellum behind the colliculi; however, the exposure in this deep cleft can be increased by directing the exposure over the cerebellar hemisphere in a paramedian site lateral to the cerebellar apex (25). The infratentorial supracerebellar approach is not well suited to the tumor with a significant extension above the tentorium or growing from the thalamus or corpus callosum into the third ventricle. The occipital transtentorial approach is preferred for tumors centered at or above the tentorial edge if there is not a major extension of tumor to the opposite side or into the posterior fossa and for those located above the vein of Galen.

The temporal horn and selected lesions of the third ventricle may be approached by the frontotemporal (pterional), posterior frontotemporal, temporal, or subtemporal approach. The frontotemporal approach is selected for a lesion involving the third ventricle that extends into the interval between the optic nerve and carotid artery or between the carotid artery and oculomotor nerve. The posterior frontotemporal approach, in which the pterional flap is extending backward to the area above the ear, is used for a lesion involving the anterior portion of the temporal horn, which can be exposed through a small cortical incision in the anterior part of the temporal lobe or through a temporal lobectomy. The temporal and subtemporal routes to the temporal horn are used for a lesion in the middle or posterior third of the temporal horn or for selected lesions in the cisterns medial to the temporal horn. In the direct transtemporal approach, the temporal horn of the nondominant hemisphere is exposed by an incision in the middle or inferior temporal gyrus anterior to the optic radiations. A preferable route is the subtemporal route, which minimizes the possibility of damage to the optic radiations and speech centers of the dominant hemisphere. In the subtemporal approach, the cortical incision is in the occipitotemporal gyrus, or collateral sulcus, on the inferior surface of the temporal lobe. The opening into the temporal horn will expose the choroidal fissure. Opening through the choroidal fissure in the temporal horn by incising the tenia fornix will provide transventricular access to the area along the posterior cerebral artery and basal vein in the ambient cistern.

The most common third ventricular tumors begin in the pituitary gland and grow upward to compress the anteroinferior part of the third ventricle. The transsphenoidal approach is preferred for all tumors involving the anteroinferior part of the third ventricle that are located above a pneumatized sphenoid sinus and extend upward out of an enlarged sella turcica. The subfrontal intracranial approach is used for those tumors involving the anteroinferior part of the third ventricle that are not accessible by the transsphenoidal route because they do not extend into the sella turcica, are separated from the sella by a layer of neural tissue, are located entirely within the third ventricle, extend upward out of a normal or small sella, or are located above a nonpneumatized (conchal) type of sphenoid sinus. The subfrontal and transsphenoidal approaches, are reviewed in Chapter 8.

REFERENCES

1. Apuzzo MLJ, Giannotta SL: Transcallosal interforniceal approach, in Apuzzo MLJ (ed): *Surgery of the Third Ventricle*. Baltimore, Williams & Wilkins, 1987, pp 354–379.
2. Apuzzo MLJ, Chikovani OK, Gott PS, Teng EL, Zee CS, Giannotta SL, Weiss MH: Transcallosal, interfornicial approaches for lesions affecting the third ventricle: Surgical considerations and consequences. **Neurosurgery** 10:547–554, 1982.
3. Dandy WE: An operation for the removal of pineal tumors. **Surg Gynecol Obstet** 33:113–119, 1921.
4. Dandy WE: *Benign Tumors in the Third Ventricle of the Brain: Diagnosis and Treatment*. Springfield, Charles C Thomas, 1933.
5. Dandy WE: Operative experience in cases of pineal tumor. **Arch Surg** 33:19–46, 1936.
6. Delandsheer JM, Guyot JF, Jomin M, Scherpereel B, Laine E: Interthalamo-trigonal approach to the third ventricle [in French]. **Neurochirurgie** 24:419–422, 1978.

7. Fujii, K, Lenkey C, Rhoton AL Jr: Microsurgical anatomy of the choroidal arteries: Lateral and third ventricles. **J Neurosurg** 52:165–188, 1980.
8. Gibo H, Carver CC, Rhoton AL Jr, Lenkey C, Mitchell RJ: Microsurgical anatomy of the middle cerebral artery. **J Neurosurg** 54:151–169, 1981.
9. Gibo H, Lenkey C, Rhoton AL Jr: Microsurgical anatomy of the supraclinoid portion of the internal carotid artery. **J Neurosurg** 55:560–574, 1981.
10. Hardy DG, Peace DA, Rhoton AL Jr: Microsurgical anatomy of the superior cerebellar artery. **Neurosurgery** 6:10–28, 1980.
11. Hirsch JF, Zouaoui A, Renier D, Pierre-Kahn A: A new surgical approach to the third ventricle with interruption of the striothalamic vein. **Acta Neurochir (Wien)** 47:135–147, 1979.
12. Jamieson KG: Excision of pineal tumors. **J Neurosurg** 35:550–553, 1971.
13. Lavyne MH, Patterson RH Jr: Subchoroidal trans-velum interpositum approach to mid-third ventricular tumors. **Neurosurgery** 12:86–94, 1983.
14. Matsushima T, Rhoton AL Jr, de Oliveira EP, Peace DA: Microsurgical anatomy of the veins of the posterior fossa. **J Neurosurg** 59:63–105, 1983.
15. Nagata S, Rhoton AL Jr, Barry M: Microsurgical anatomy of the choroidal fissure. **Surg Neurol** 30:3–59, 1988.
16. Narabayashi H, Nagao T, Saito Y, Yoshida M, Nagahara M: Stereotactic amygdalotomy for behavior disorders. **Arch Neurol** 9:1–16, 1983.
17. Oka K, Rhoton AL Jr, Barry M, Rodriguez R: Microsurgical anatomy of the superficial veins of the cerebrum. **Neurosurgery** 17:711–748, 1985.
18. Ono M, Ono M, Rhoton AL Jr, Barry M: Microsurgical anatomy of the region of the tentorial incisura. **J Neurosurg** 60:365–399, 1984.
19. Ono M, Rhoton AL Jr, Peace D, Rodriguez RJ: Microsurgical anatomy of the deep venous system of the brain. **Neurosurgery** 15:621–657, 1984.
20. Perlmutter D, Rhoton AL Jr: Microsurgical anatomy of the anterior cerebral-anterior communicating-recurrent artery complex. **J Neurosurg** 45:259–272, 1976.
21. Perlmutter D, Rhoton AL Jr: Microsurgical anatomy of the distal anterior cerebral artery. **J Neurosurg** 49:204–228, 1978.
22. Poppen JL: The right occipital approach to a pinealoma. **J Neurosurg** 25: 706–710, 1966.
23. Renn WH, Rhoton AL Jr: Microsurgical anatomy of the sellar region. **J Neurosurg** 43:288–298, 1975.
24. Rhoton AL Jr: Microsurgical anatomy of the region of the third ventricle, in Apuzzo MLJ (ed): *Surgery of the Third Ventricle*. Baltimore, Williams & Wilkins, 1987, pp 92–166.
25. Rhoton AL Jr: Tentorial incisura. **Neurosurgery** 47[Suppl 1]:S131–S153, 2000.
26. Rhoton AL Jr, Fujii K, Fradd B: Microsurgical anatomy of the anterior choroidal artery. **Surg Neurol** 12:171–187, 1979.
27. Rhoton AL Jr, Hardy DG, Chambers SM: Microsurgical anatomy and dissection of the sphenoid bone, cavernous sinus and sellar region. **Surg Neurol** 12:63–104, 1979.
28. Rhoton AL Jr, Yamamoto I, Peace DA: Microsurgery of the third ventricle: Part 2—Operative approaches. **Neurosurgery** 8:357–373, 1981.
29. Rosner SS, Rhoton AL Jr, Ono M, Barry M: Microsurgical anatomy of the anterior perforating arteries. **J Neurosurg** 61:468–485, 1984.
30. Saeki N, Rhoton AL Jr: Microsurgical anatomy of the upper basilar artery and the posterior circle of Willis. **J Neurosurg** 46:563–578, 1977.
31. Shucart WA, Stein BM: Transcallosal approach to the anterior ventricular system. **Neurosurgery** 3:339–343, 1978.
32. Symon L: The intracranial approach to tumours in the area of the sella turcica, in Symon L (ed): *Operative Surgery: Neurosurgery*. London, Butterworth, 1979, pp 181–186.
33. Timurkaynak E, Rhoton AL Jr, Barry M: Microsurgical anatomy and operative approaches to the lateral ventricles. **Neurosurgery** 19:685–723, 1986.
34. VanWagenen WP: A surgical approach for the removal of certain pineal tumors. **Surg Gynecol Obstet** 53:216–220, 1931.
35. Viale GL, Turtas S, Pau A: Surgical removal of striate arteriovenous malformations. **Surg Neurol** 14:321–324, 1980.
36. Wen HT, Rhoton AL Jr, de Oliveira EP: Transchoroidal approach to the third ventricle: An anatomic study of the choroidal fissure and its clinical application. **Neurosurgery** 42:1205–1219, 1998.
37. Yamamoto I, Rhoton AL Jr, Peace DA: Microsurgery of the third ventricle: Part 1—Microsurgical anatomy. **Neurosurgery** 8:334–356, 1981.
38. Zeal AA, Rhoton AL Jr: Microsurgical anatomy of the posterior cerebral artery. **J Neurosurg** 48:534–559, 1978.

Figure from D'Agoty Gautier's Essai d'anatomie, en tableaux imprimés. *Paris, 1748.*

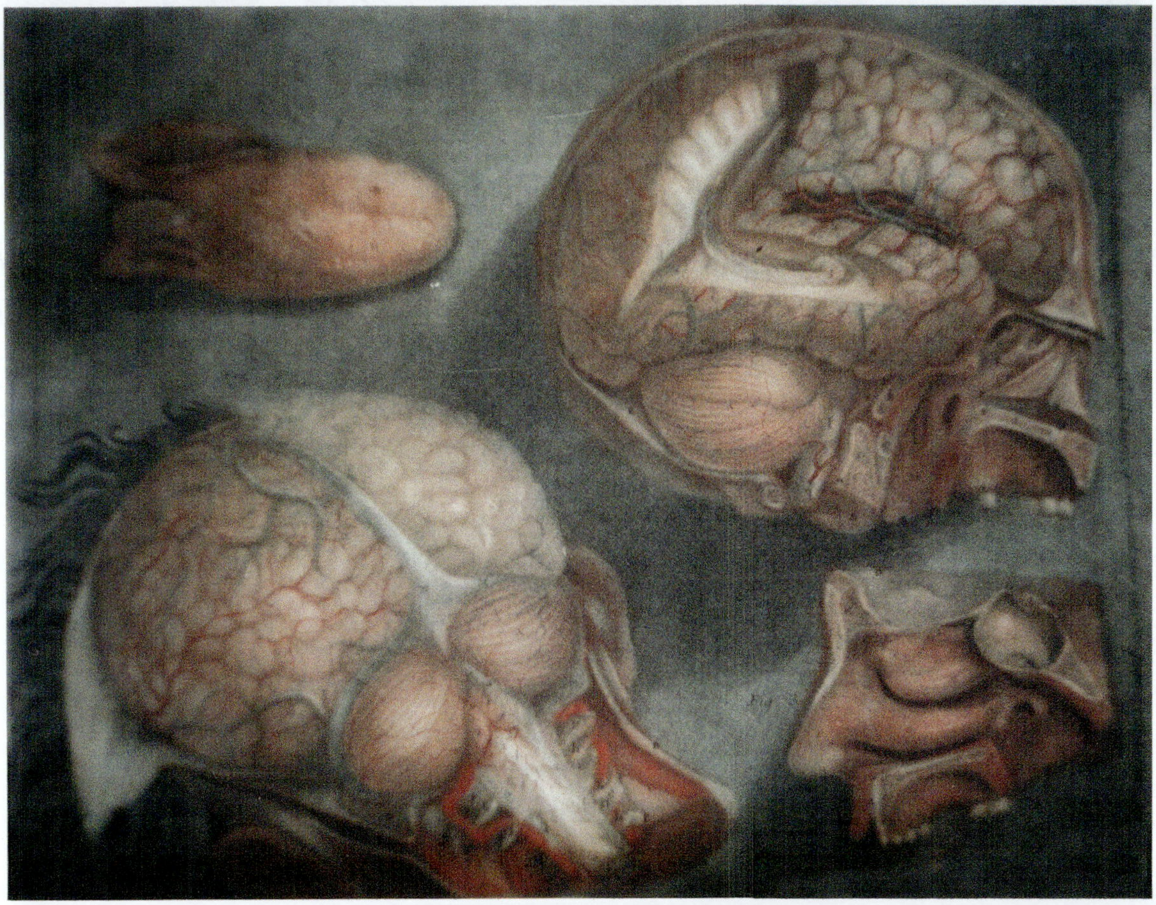

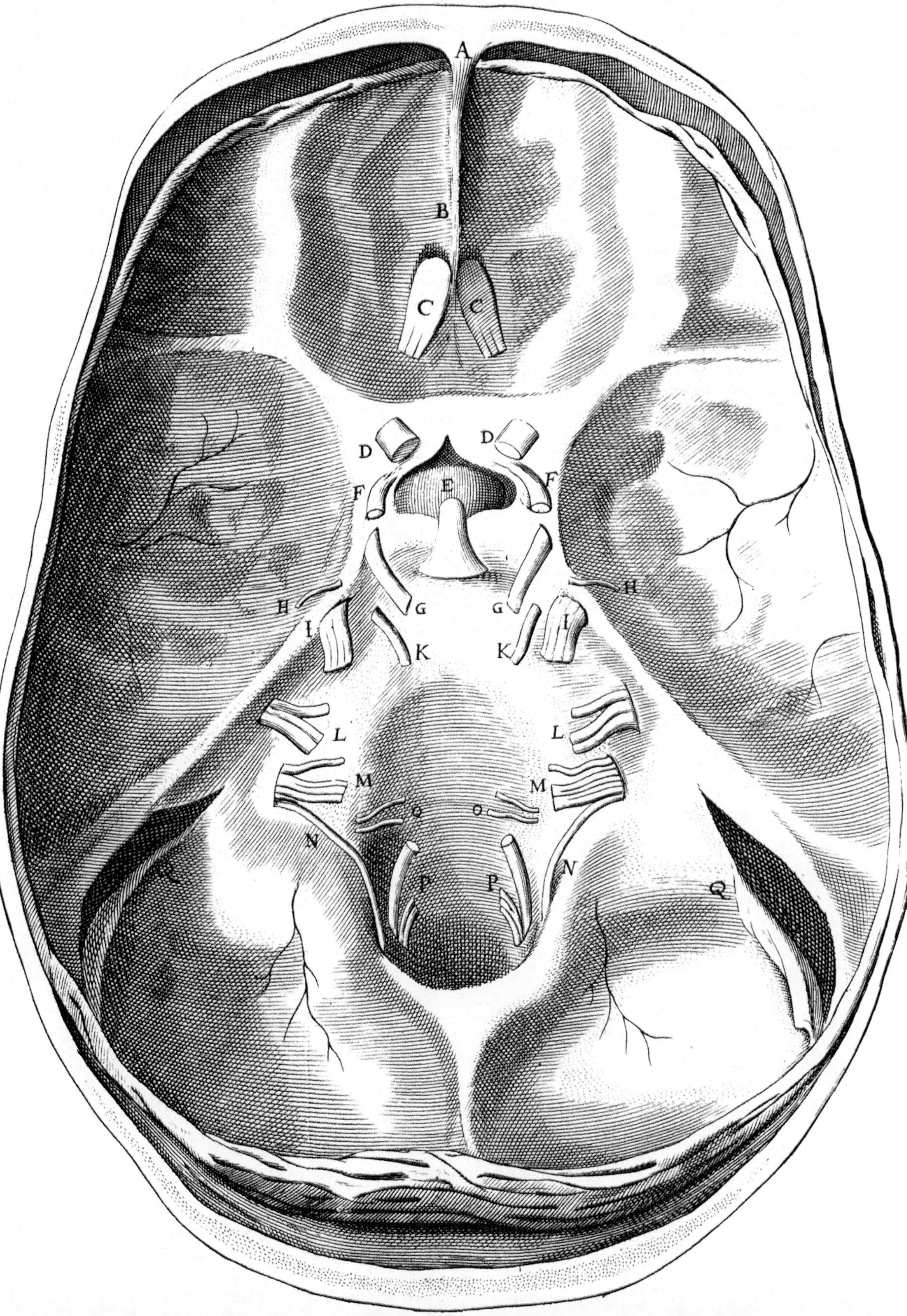

Image of the cranial base from Thomas Willis' Cerebri Anatome. *London, 1664.*

The Anterior and Middle Cranial Base

Albert L. Rhoton, Jr., M.D.
Department of Neurological Surgery, University of Florida, Gainesville, Florida

Correspondence:
Albert L. Rhoton, Jr., M.D., Department of Neurological Surgery, University of Florida McKnight Brain Institute, P.O. Box 100265, 100 South Newell Drive, Building 59, L2-100, Gainesville, FL 32610-0265.
Email:
rhoton@neurosurgery.ufl.edu

KEY WORDS: Anterior fossa, Cranial base, Cranial nerves, Infratemporal fossa, Microsurgical anatomy, Middle fossa, Nasal cavity, Orbit, Paranasal sinuses, Pterygopalatine fossa, Skull base, Surgical approaches

OVERVIEW

No part of the cranial base is immune to surgical pathology or to its use as a pathway to access lesions in the intra- or extracranial spaces. Tumors and many other lesions can involve any of the intracranial fossae, and can appear in the paranasal sinuses, nasal cavity, infratemporal and pterygopalatine fossae, orbit, and in the retropharyngeal and craniocervical regions (*Fig. 6.1*). Managing these lesions requires an extensive knowledge of the cranial base and its intra- and extracranial relationships. This chapter provides a concise review of the cranial base, focusing largely on the anterior and middle cranial base; the Millennium issue of *Neurosurgery* focused on the posterior cranial fossa (8). The chapters that follow provide a more focused review of the orbit, sella, and cavernous sinus.

The skull is divided into the cranium and the facial skeleton. The cranium is divided into the calvarium and the cranial base. The cranial base has an endocranial surface, which faces the brain, and an exocranial surface, which faces the nasal cavity and sinuses, orbits, pharynx, infratemporal and pterygopalatine fossae, and the parapharyngeal and infrapetrosal spaces (*Fig. 6.2*). Both surfaces are connected by canals, foramina, and fissures through which numerous neural and vascular structures pass. Both the endocranial and exocranial cranial base surfaces are divided into anterior, middle, and posterior parts, each of which have a central and paired lateral portions. On the intracranial side, the three parts correspond to the anterior, middle, and posterior cranial fossae (*Figs. 6.2* and *6.3*). On the endocranial side, the border between the anterior and middle cranial bases is the sphenoid ridge joined medially by the chiasmatic sulcus, and the border between the middle and posterior cranial bases is formed by the petrous ridges joined by the dorsum sellae and posterior clinoid processes. On the exocranium side, the anterior and middle cranial bases are divided at the level of a transverse line extending through the pterygomaxillary fissures and the pterygopalatine fossae at the upper level and the posterior edge of the alveolar process of the maxilla at a lower level. Medially, this corresponds to the anterior part of the attachment of the vomer to the sphenoid bone. The middle and posterior cranial bases are separated by a transverse line crossing at or near the posterior border of the vomer-sphenoid junction, the foramen lacerum, carotid canal, jugular foramen, styloid process, and the mastoid tip. The osseous structures, their foramina and fissures, canals and their muscular, and neural and vascular relationships are described in this chapter.

ANTERIOR CRANIAL BASE

Endocranial Surface

The anterior endocranial surface, formed by the ethmoid, sphenoid, and frontal bones, is divided into medial and lateral portions (*Figs. 6.3–6.5*). The medial part, covering the upper nasal cavity and the sphenoid sinus, is formed by the crista galli and the cribriform plate of the ethmoid bone anteriorly and the planum of the sphenoid body posteriorly. The lateral part, which covers the orbit and the optic canal, is formed by the frontal bone and the lesser wing of the sphenoid bone, which blends medially into the anterior clinoid process (*Figs. 6.3* and *6.4*). The foramen caecum in the midline serves as the site of passage of an emissary vein and the cribriform plate is pierced by the filaments of the olfactory nerve. The optic canal transmits the optic nerve and the ophthalmic artery. The anterior cranial base faces the frontal lobes with the gyri recti medially and the orbital gyri laterally, along with the branches of the anterior cerebral arteries medially and middle cerebral arteries laterally.

Exocranial Surface

On the exocranial side, the anterior cranial base is divided into a medial part related to the ethmoidal and sphenoid sinuses with the nasal cavity below, and a lateral part that corresponds to the orbit and maxilla (*Figs. 6.2, 6.6, 6.7,* and *6.8*) (2). The ethmoid bone forms the anterior and middle thirds and the sphenoid body forms the posterior third of the medial part. The ethmoid is formed by the cribriform plate, with the olfactory fila traveling through it, the perpendicular plate that joins the vomer in forming the nasal septum, and two lateral plates located in the medial walls of the orbits. The lateral plates separate the lateral wall of the nasal cavity and the orbit. The superior turbi-

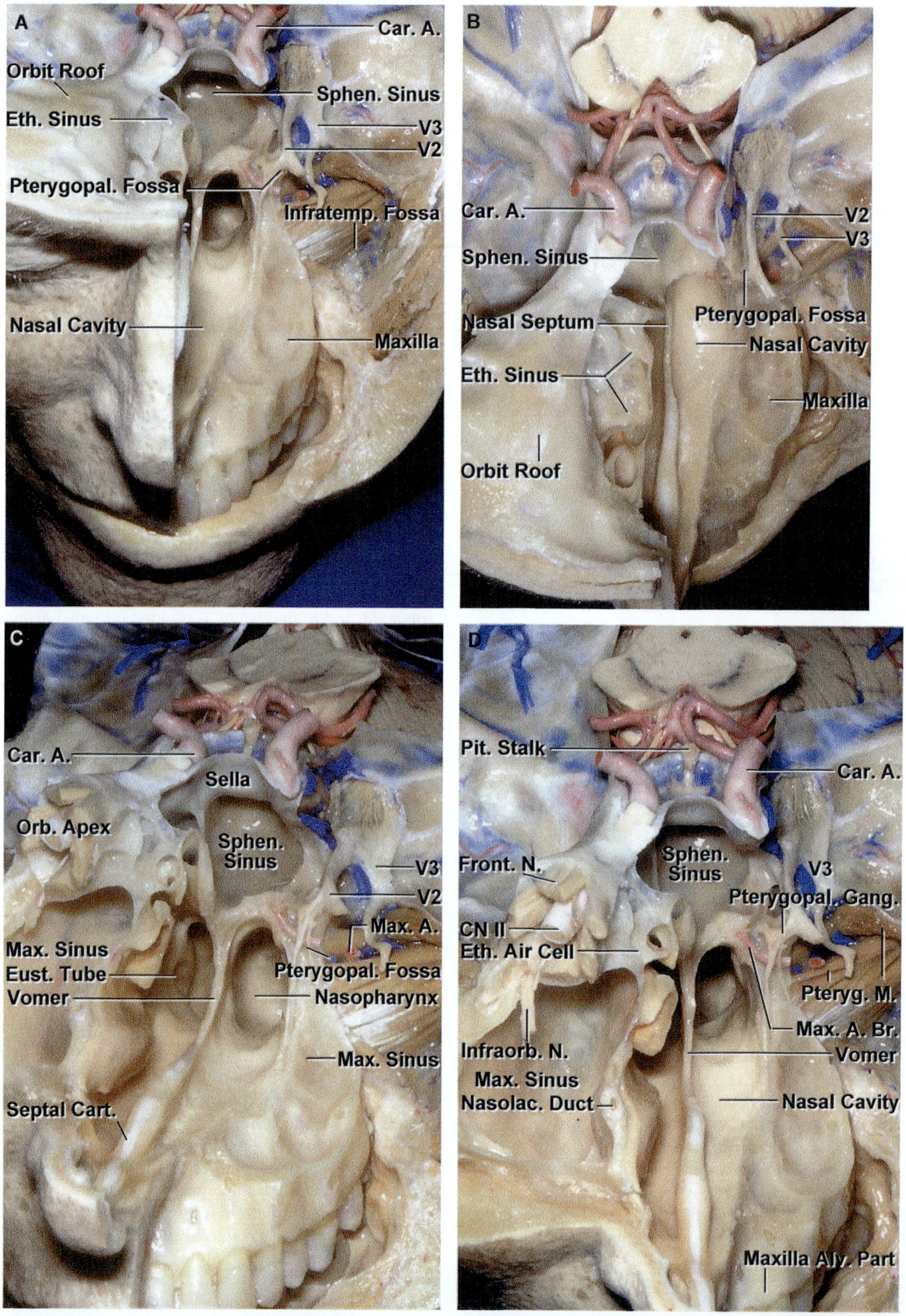
A
Car. A.
Orbit Roof
Sphen. Sinus
Eth. Sinus
V3
V2
Pterygopal. Fossa
Infratemp. Fossa
Nasal Cavity
Maxilla
B
Car. A.
V2
V3
Sphen. Sinus
Pterygopal. Fossa
Nasal Septum
Nasal Cavity
Eth. Sinus
Maxilla
Orbit Roof
C
Car. A.
Sella
Orb. Apex
Sphen. Sinus
V3
V2
Max. A.
Max. Sinus
Eust. Tube
Pterygopal. Fossa
Vomer
Nasopharynx
Max. Sinus
Septal Cart.
D
Pit. Stalk
Car. A.
Sphen. Sinus
Front. N.
V3
Pterygopal. Gang.
CN II
Eth. Air Cell
Pteryg. M.
Max. A. Br.
Infraorb. N.
Vomer
Max. Sinus
Nasolac. Duct
Nasal Cavity
Maxilla Alv. Part

FIGURE 6.1.

nate, an appendage of the ethmoid bone, projects into the superior part of the nasal cavity. The body of the sphenoid bone harbors the sphenoid sinus just below the planum sphenoidale, with the anterior orifices located above the superior turbinate. The orbital roof is formed by the lesser sphenoid wing and by the orbital plate of the frontal bone; the lateral wall is formed by the greater sphenoid wing and the zygomatic bone; the inferior wall is formed by the zygomatic, maxillary, and palatine bones; and the medial wall is formed by maxillary, lacrimal, and ethmoid bones (9). The main foramina of the region are the anterior and posterior ethmoidal foramen located in the superomedial orbital wall, transmitting the anterior and posterior ethmoidal nerves and arteries; the supraorbital and supratrochlear notches or foramina, transmitting the arteries and nerves of the same name; and the optic canal, through which the optic nerve and ophthalmic artery pass (*Figs. 6.4, 6.5,* and *6.7*). The superior orbital fissure is located between the lesser and greater wing of the sphenoid bone on the lateral side of the optic canal. The inferior orbital fissure, located between the greater sphenoid wing behind and the maxillary and palatine bones anteriorly, is closed by a fibrous tissue and orbital muscle. Covered with periorbita and filled with a great amount of fat, the orbit is divided into an anterior space where the globe lies and a posterior space that shelters the nerves, vessels, and muscles behind the globe (4). The annular tendon of Zinn, a fibrous ring that surrounds the central part of the superior orbital fissure and the optic canal, gives attachment to the superior, medial, inferior, and lateral rectus muscles (*Figs. 6.3* and *6.4*). The superior oblique attaches above the annular tendon and the inferior oblique arises from the inferomedial orbital wall just behind the rim. The oculomotor foramen, located inside the annular tendon and through which the oculomotor nerve passes, is located between the upper and lower attachment of the lateral rectus muscle. Just before passing through the superior orbital fissure and the oculomotor foramen in the annular tendon, the oculomotor nerve divides into an upper division supplying the superior rectus and levator muscles and a lower division to the medial and inferior rectus and inferior oblique muscles. The oculomotor nerve gives rise to the parasympathetic motor root to the ciliary ganglion that lies lateral to the optic nerve. The abducens nerve passes through the oculomotor foramen and enters the medial surface of the lateral rectus muscle. The ophthalmic nerve divides just behind the annular tendon into lacrimal and frontal nerves that pass outside the annular tendon, and the nasociliary nerve that passes through the annular tendon. The ophthalmic nerve gives rise to the long ciliary nerves and the sensory root to the ciliary ganglion; the former conveys the sympathetic pupillomotor fibers and the latter conveys corneal sensation. The trochlear nerve passes above and outside the superomedial edge of the annular tendon. The optic nerve passes superior and medial from the globe to reach the optic canal and divides the retro-orbital space into medial and lateral parts. The main arterial supply to the orbit is by the ophthalmic artery and its branches. This artery courses below the optic nerve in the optic canal, crosses to the lateral side of the nerve at the orbital apex, and then courses from lateral to medial above the optic nerve. The main branches are the central retinal artery and the lacrimal, ciliary, ethmoidal, supraorbital, and dorsal nasal arteries, plus numerous muscular branches. The main venous drainage of the orbit is through the superior and inferior ophthalmic veins that exit the orbit by passing outside the annular tendon and through the superior orbital fissure. The lacrimal gland, located in the superolateral part of the orbit, receives its sensory innervation from the lacrimal nerve and its parasympathetic and sympathetic innervation from the greater

FIGURE 6.1. *Anterior and middle cranial base.* A, *on the left side, the floor of the anterior fossa and the upper portion of the maxilla have been removed to expose the structures deep to the anterior and middle cranial fossa. The frontal, ethmoidal, and sphenoid sinuses and the nasal cavity lie below the medial part of the anterior cranial base. The orbit and maxilla are located below the lateral part of the anterior cranial base. The sphenoid sinus and sella are located in the medial part of the middle cranial base, and the infratemporal and pterygopalatine fossa are located below the lateral part of the middle cranial base. The carotid arteries pass upward on the medial part of the middle cranial base and are intimately related to the sphenoid and cavernous sinuses. The infratemporal fossa, which contains branches of the mandibular nerve, pterygoid muscles, pterygoid venous plexus, and maxillary artery, is located below the middle cranial base and greater sphenoid wing. The alveolar process of the maxilla, which encloses the roots of the upper teeth, has been preserved on the left side. The maxillary nerve enters the pterygopalatine fossa, which is located medial to the infratemporal fossa between the posterior wall of the maxilla and the pterygoid process of the sphenoid bone.* B, *superior view of the anterior and middle cranial base. The infratemporal fossa is located posterolateral to the maxilla. The right ethmoid air cells are exposed on the medial side of the right orbit. The nasal cavity extends upward between the ethmoidal sinuses.* C, *oblique anterior view. The facial structures on the right side have been removed to expose the orbital apex located above the maxillary sinus. The walls of the right maxillary sinus form the floor of the orbit, much of the lateral wall of the nasal cavity, and the anterior wall of the pterygopalatine and infratemporal fossa. On the left side, the mandibular nerve enters the infratemporal fossa. The maxillary nerve enters the pterygopalatine fossa, which is located in the lateral wall of the nasal cavity and contains the maxillary nerve, pterygopalatine ganglion, and terminal branches of the maxillary artery.* D, *anterior view. The orbital apex is located above the pterygopalatine fossa. The frontal branch of the ophthalmic nerve passes along the roof of the orbit, and the infraorbital branch of the maxillary nerve courses in the floor of the orbit. The posterior ethmoid air cells are located medial to the orbital apex. The vomer forms the posterior part of the nasal septum and attaches to the maxilla and palatine bones below and to the body of the sphenoid bone above. The sphenoid sinus is located in the middle cranial base below the sella turcica. The upper brainstem is seen in the posterior part of the exposure.* A., *artery;* Alv., *alveolar;* Br., *branch;* Car., *carotid;* Cart., *cartilage;* CN, *cranial nerve;* Eth., *ethmoid;* Eust., *eustachian;* Foss., *fossa;* Front., *frontal;* Gang., *ganglion;* Infraorb., *infraorbital;* Infratemp., *infratemporal;* M., *muscle;* Max., *maxillary;* N., *nerve;* Nasolac., *nasolacrimal;* Orb., *orbital;* Pit., *pituitary;* Pteryg., *pterygoid;* Pterygopal., *pterygopalatine;* Sphen., *sphenoid.*

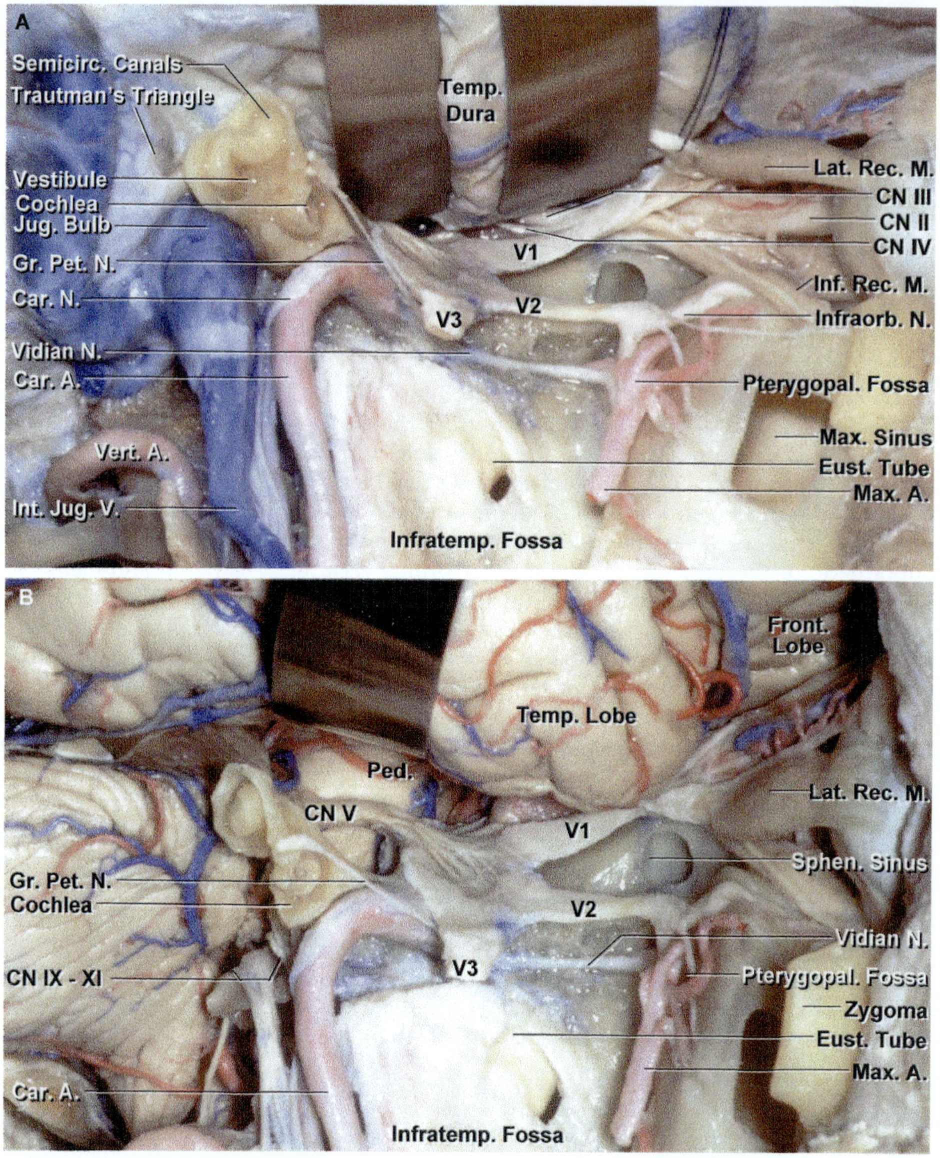

FIGURE 6.2. *Lateral view of the anterior, middle, and posterior cranial base. A, the bone and structures lateral to the orbit, infratemporal, and pterygopalatine fossa, and the parapharyngeal space and petrous part of the temporal bone have been removed to expose the structures below the anterior, middle, and posterior cranial base. The orbit and maxillary sinus are located below the anterior cranial base. The infratemporal and pterygopalatine fossae and the parapharyngeal space are located below the middle cranial base, and the suboccipital area is located below the temporal and occipital bones. The first trigeminal division is related to the upper part of the orbit. The second trigeminal branch is related to the lower part of the orbit and maxilla. The mandibular nerve exits the cranium through the foramen ovale and enters the infratemporal fossa. The pterygoid and levator and tensor veli palatini muscles have been removed to expose the eustachian tube and its opening into the nasal pharynx. The lateral part of the temporal bone has been removed to expose the cochlea, vestibule, and semicircular canals. The petrous carotid passes upward and turns medially below the cochlea. The sigmoid sinus turns downward under the semicircular canals and vestibule where the jugular bulb is located. The segment of the vertebral artery passing behind the atlanto-occipital joint is located below the posterior cranial base. B, the dura has been opened to show the relationships of the frontal and temporal lobes and the cerebellum to the cranial base. The orbit is exposed below the frontal lobe. The pterygopalatine and infratemporal fossae and the temporal bone are located below the temporal lobe. The jugular bulb and internal jugular vein have been removed to show Cranial Nerves IX through XII exiting the jugular foramen.* A., *artery;* Car., *carotid;* CN, *cranial nerve;* Eust., *eustachian;* Front., *frontal;* Gr., *greater;* Inf., *inferior;* Infraorb., *infraorbital;* Infratemp., *infratemporal;* Int., *internal;* Jug., *jugular;* Lat., *lateral;* M., *muscle;* Max., *maxillary;* N., *nerve;* Ped., *peduncle;* Pet., *petrosal;* Pterygopal., *pterygopalatine;* Rec., *rectus;* Semicirc., *semicircular;* Sphen., *sphenoid;* Temp., *temporal;* V., *vein;* Vert., *vertebral.*

FIGURE 6.3. *Osseous relationships of the anterior and middle cranial base. A, on the endocranial surface, the anterior and middle cranial base corresponds to the anterior and middle fossae. The anterior part of the cranial base is separated from the middle fossa by the sphenoid ridge and the chiasmatic sulcus. The middle cranial base is separated from the posterior cranial base by the dorsum sellae and the petrous ridges. The upper surface of the anterior cranial base is formed by the frontal bone, which roofs the orbit; the ethmoid bone, which is interposed between the frontal bones and is the site of the cribriform plate; and the lesser wing and anterior part of the body of the sphenoid, which forms the posterior part of the floor of the anterior fossa. The upper surface of the middle cranial base floor is formed by the greater sphenoid wing and posterior two-thirds of the sphenoid body anteriorly and the upper surface of the temporal bone posteriorly. The posterior part of the cranial base is formed by the temporal and occipital bones. The cribriform plate, sella, and clivus are located in the medial part of the cranial base. The lateral part of the cranial base is located above the orbits, pterygopalatine and infratemporal fossae, and the subtemporal and lateral part of the suboccipital areas. B, exocranial surface of the cranial base. This surface is more complicated than the endocranial surface. It is not demarcated into three well-defined fossae as is the endocranial surface. The exocranial surface is formed by the maxilla, the zygomatic, palatine, sphenoid, temporal, and occipital bones, and the vomer. The maxilla, orbits, and nasal cavity are located below the anterior fossa. The anterior part of the hard palate is formed by the maxilla and the posterior part is formed by the palatine bone. The anterior part of the zygomatic arch is formed by the zygoma and the posterior part by the squamosal part of the temporal bone. The mandibular fossa on the lower surface of the temporal squama is located below the posterior part of the middle fossa. The vomer attaches to the lower part of the body of the sphenoid and forms the posterior part of the nasal septum. C, anterior view. The orbital rim is formed by the frontal bone, zygoma, and maxilla. The roof of the orbit is formed by the frontal and sphenoid bones; the lateral wall by the greater sphenoid wing and the zygomatic bone; the*

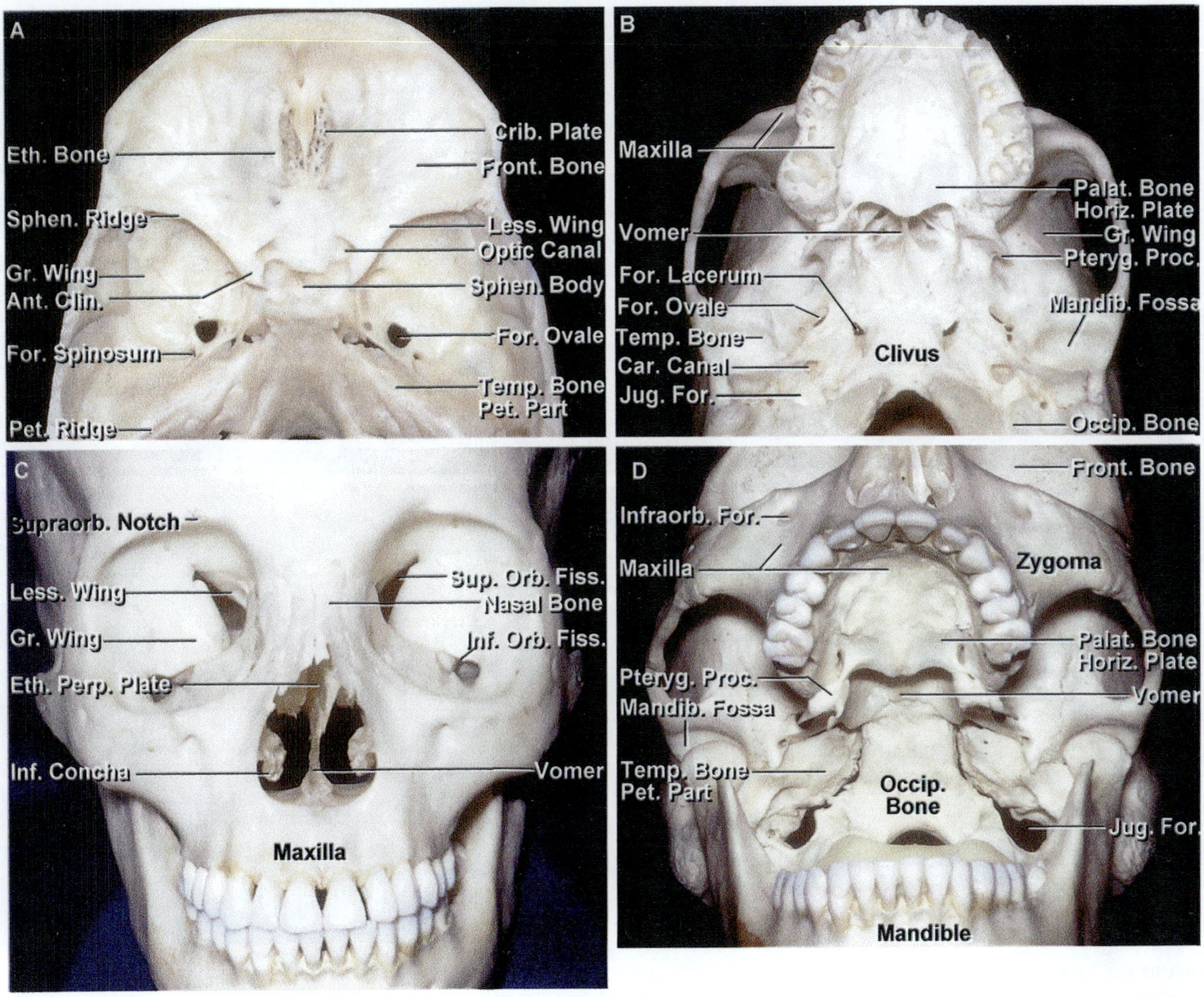

FIGURE 6.3. *Continued*
floor by the maxilla, except for a small part of the posterior floor formed by the palatine bone; and the medial wall of the orbit by the maxilla and lacrimal and ethmoid bones. The nasal bone is interposed above the anterior nasal aperture between the maxillae. The nasal cavity is located between the ethmoid bones above and the maxillae, palatine bones, and sphenoid pterygoid process below. It is roofed by the frontal and ethmoid bones and the floor is formed by the maxillae and palatal bones. The osseous nasal septum is formed by the perpendicular ethmoid plate and the vomer. The inferior concha is a separate bone, and the middle and superior conchae are appendages of the ethmoid bone. The orbit opens through the superior orbital fissure into the middle fossa and through the inferior orbital fissure into the pterygopalatine and infratemporal fossae. D, *anteroinferior view of the cranial base. The anterior part of the hard palate is formed by the maxillae and the posterior part is formed by the horizontal plate of the palatine bone. The vomer forms the posterior part of the nasal septum and divides the posterior nasal aperture in the midline. The infratemporal fossa is located below the greater sphenoid wing. The clivus is formed above by the body of the sphenoid bone and below by the basal part of the occipital bone. The petrous apex is interposed between the greater sphenoid wing and the clival part of the occipital bone. The mandibular condyles are set in the mandibular fossa, located below the posterior part of the middle fossa on the inferior surface of the squamosal part of the temporal bone.* E, *the cranial base is formed, in the lateral view, from anterior to posterior, by the maxilla and the frontal, zygomatic, sphenoid, temporal, and occipital bones. The zygomatic and frontal bones form the lateral part of the orbital rim. The pterion on the greater sphenoid wing marks the lateral end of the sphenoid ridge. The keyhole, a burr hole that exposes the dura of the anterior fossa and the periorbita in its depth, is located just above the frontozygomatic suture, behind the superior temporal line. The zygomatic arch is formed by the zygomatic bone and the squamosal part of the temporal bone. The condylar fossa, in which the mandibular condyle sits, is positioned above on the lower surface of the squamosal part of the temporal bone and posteriorly on the tympanic part of the temporal bone. The lower end of the pterygoid process unites with the posterior maxilla, but above, the process separates from the maxilla to create the pterygomaxillary fissure, which opens medially into the pterygopalatine fossa.* F, *inferior view of a cross extending through the maxillae. The maxilla, which contains a large air-filled sinus, forms the anteromedial wall of the infratemporal fossa, the anterior wall of the pterygopalatine fossa, the lateral wall of the nasal cavity, the anterior portion of the hard palate, and much of the floor of the orbit. The pterygopalatine fossa is located between the pterygoid process and the posterior maxillary wall. The nasal septum is formed anteriorly and above by the perpendicular ethmoid plate and posteriorly and below by the vomer.* G, *the right half of the maxilla and zygomatic arch has been removed. The inferior orbital fissure is located between the greater sphenoid wing and the maxilla. The right orbital roof and ethmoid air cells have been preserved. The right pterygoid process has been removed at its junction with the sphenoid body. The roof of the vidian canal, which extends through the base of the pterygoid process, has been preserved.* H, *anteroinferior view of the cranial base. The midline of the cranial base is formed, from anterior to posterior, by the frontal, ethmoid, sphenoid, and (Legend continues on next page.)*

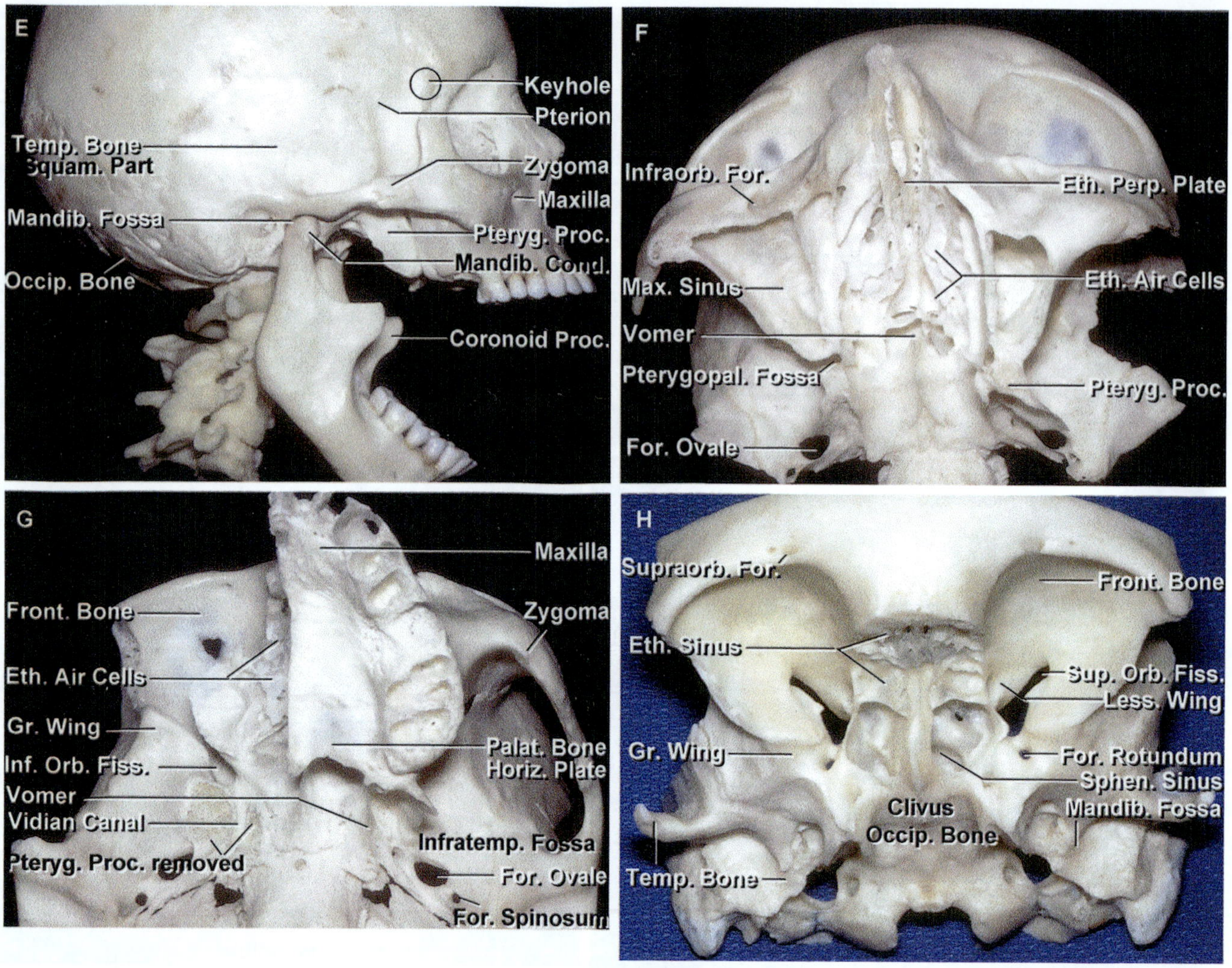

FIGURE 6.3. *Continued*

occipital bones. The roof the orbit is formed by the frontal bone and lesser sphenoid wing. The ethmoidal sinuses are located anterior to the sphenoid sinus between the orbits. I, *lateral view of the pterygomaxillary fissure. The pterygomaxillary fissure is located between the posterior maxillary wall and the pterygoid process. The pterygomaxillary fissure opens from the infratemporal fossa into the pterygopalatine fossa. The mandibular fossa is formed above by the squamosal part of the temporal bone and posteriorly by the tympanic part of the temporal bone, which also forms the anterior and lower wall of the external auditory meatus.* J, *anterior view through the maxillary sinus. The anterior and posterior walls of the maxillary sinus have been removed to expose the pterygoid process, which forms the posterior wall of the pterygopalatine fossa. The lower part of the superior orbital fissure is seen through the upper part of the maxillary sinus. The foramen rotundum opens into the pterygopalatine fossa and is separated from the superior orbital fissure by the maxillary strut. The vidian canal opens through the pterygoid process below the medial to the foramen rotundum.* K, *anterior view of a cranium sectioned through the posterior part of the ethmoid and maxillary sinuses. The ethmoidal sinuses are located anterior to the sphenoid body and sphenoid sinus. The part of the posterior wall of the maxilla forming the anterior wall of the pterygopalatine fossa has been preserved. The perpendicular plate of the palatine bone forms the medial wall of the pterygopalatine fossa. The ethmoidal sinus overlaps the lateral margin of the sphenoid ostia. The superior orbital fissure is located between the lesser and greater sphenoid wing and sphenoid body. The infratemporal fossa is located below the greater wing of the sphenoid. The temporal fossa, which contains the temporalis muscle, is located between the greater wing and the zygomatic arch.* L, *the posterior wall of the maxilla and ethmoidal sinuses have been removed to expose the sphenoid sinus and pterygopalatine fossa. The lateral wing of the sphenoid sinus extends laterally into the pterygoid process below the foramen rotundum. Septae divide the sphenoid sinus. The vidian canal opens through the base of the pterygoid process into the pterygopalatine fossa.* M, *the osseous cross section has been extended posteriorly to just in front of the superior orbital fissure. The optic strut extends from the base of the anterior clinoid to the sphenoid body and separates the optic canal from the superior orbital fissure. The foramen rotundum is located below the medial part of the superior orbital fissure. The vidian canal opens into the pterygopalatine fossa below and medial to the foramen rotundum.* N, *posterior view of the specimen in K showing the anterior part of the middle fossa from behind. The superior orbital fissure is positioned below the lesser sphenoid wing. The optic strut extends from the base of the anterior clinoid to the sphenoid body and separates the optic canal from the superior orbital fissure. The greater wing extends laterally to form part of the floor and anterior and lateral wall of the middle fossa. The medial and lateral pterygoid plates project backward from the pterygoid process. The horizontal plate of the palatine bone forms the posterior part of the hard plate. The posterior opening into the vidian canal is located above the medial pterygoid plate and extends forward through the pterygoid process at its junction with the shenoid body.* Ant., *anterior;* Car., *carotid;* Clin., *clinoid;* Cond., *condyle;* Crib., *cribriform;* Eth., *ethmoid;* Fiss., *fissure;* For., *foramen;* Front., *frontal;* Gr., *greater;* Horiz., *horizontal;* Inf., *inferior;* Infraorb., *infraorbital;* Infratemp., *infratemporal;* Jug., *jugular;* Lat., *lateral;* Less., *lesser;* Mandib., *mandibular;* Max., *maxillary;* Med., *medial;* Occip., *occipital;* Orb., *orbital;* Palat., *palatine;* Perp., *perpendicular;* Pet., *petrosal;* Post., *posterior;* Proc., *process;* Pteryg., *pterygoid;* Pterygomax., *pterygomaxillary;* Pterygopal., *pterygopalatine;* Sphen., *sphenoid;* Squam., *squamosal;* Sup., *superior;* Supraorb., *supraorbital;* Temp., *temporal.* *(Figure continues on next page.)*

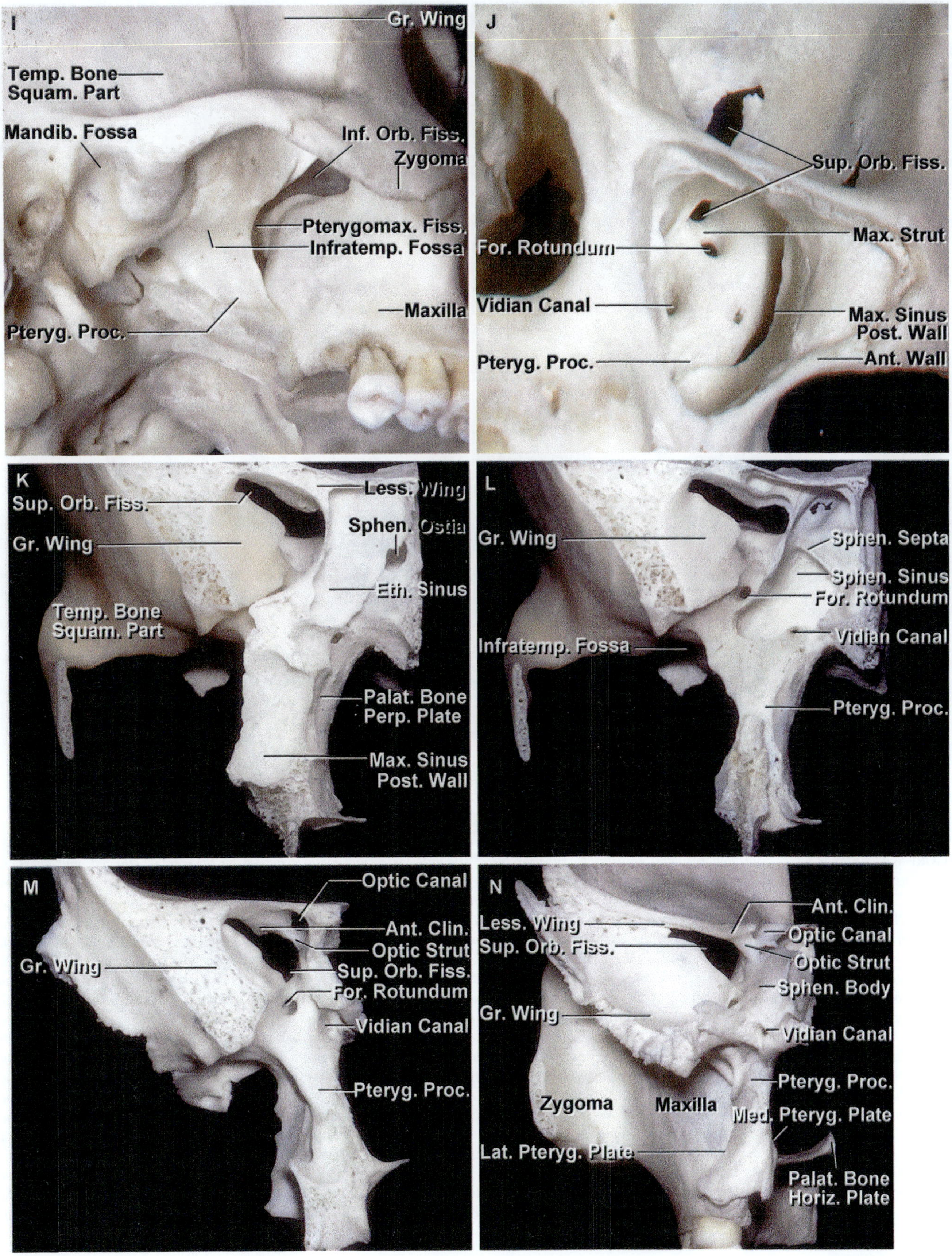

FIGURE 6.3. *Continued*

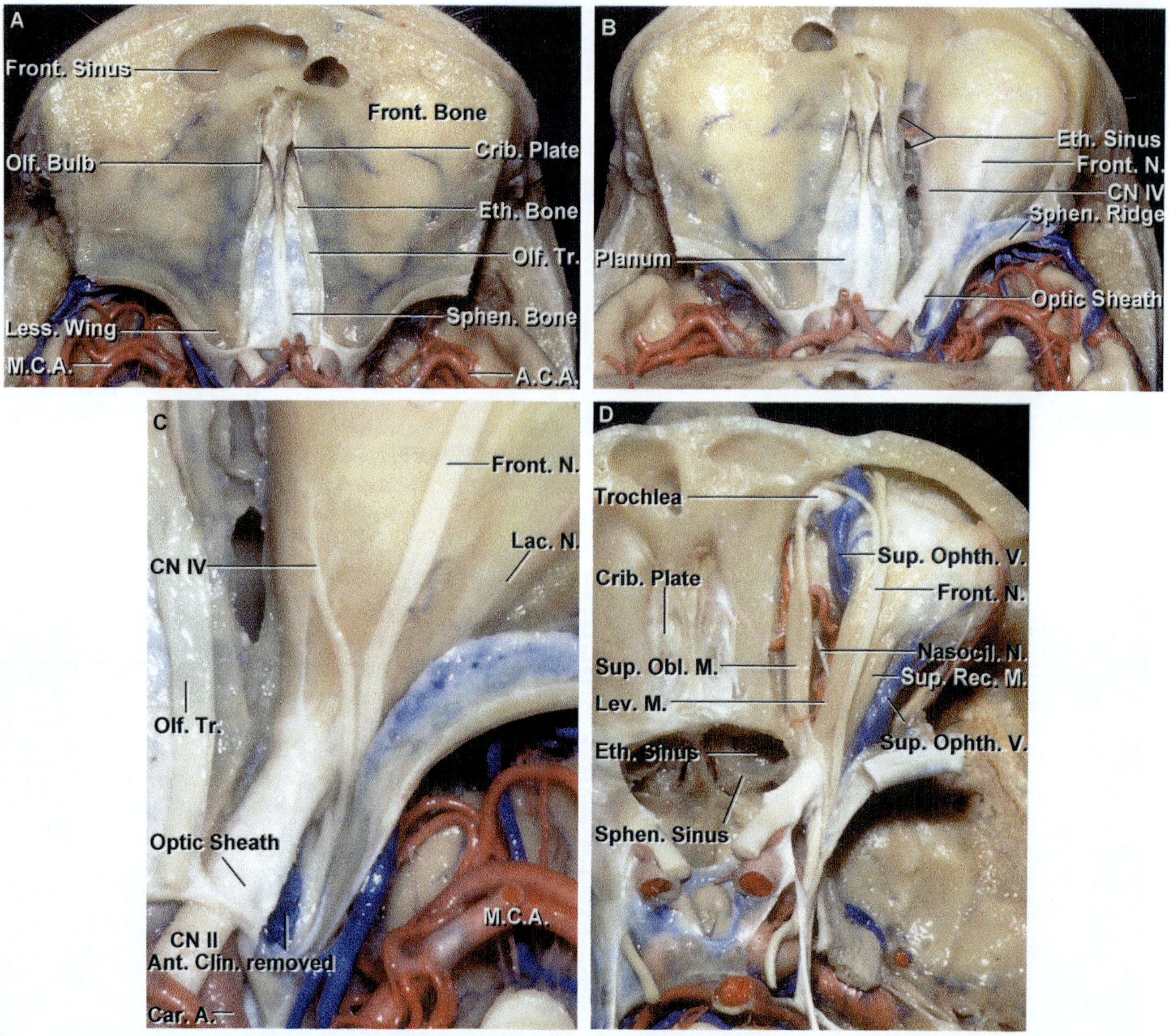

FIGURE 6.4. *Anterior fossa, orbit, and perinasal sinuses. A, superior view. The anterior cranial fossa is formed by the frontal, ethmoid, and sphenoid bones. The frontal bone splits anteriorly into two laminae, which enclose the frontal sinus. The ethmoid bones, which contain the ethmoid air cells and are the site of the crista galli and cribriform plate, are interposed between the frontal bones. Posteriorly, the frontal and ethmoid bones join the sphenoid bone, which encloses the sphenoid sinus and has the pituitary fossa on its upper surface. The olfactory bulbs and tracts have been preserved. B, the roof of the right orbit has been removed to expose the periorbita. The right anterior clinoid process and roof of the optic canal have been removed to expose the optic nerve enclosed within the optic sheath as it passes through the optic canal to reach the orbital apex. C, the frontal, trochlear, and lacrimal nerves can be seen through the periorbita. The trochlear nerve crosses above the orbital apex to reach the superior oblique muscle. D, the orbital fat has been removed and the sphenoid sinus opened. The frontal branch of the ophthalmic nerve courses above the levator muscle. The ophthalmic artery, nasociliary nerve, and superior ophthalmic vein are located medially in the anterior part of the orbit and cross between the optic nerve and superior rectus muscle to be situated on the lateral side of the optic nerve at the orbital apex. E, enlarged view. The superior oblique muscle has been retracted medially to expose the anterior and posterior ethmoidal branches of the ophthalmic artery and nasociliary nerve entering the anterior and posterior ethmoidal canal. The trochlea of the superior oblique muscle is attached to the superomedial margin of the orbit just behind the orbital rim. The frontal nerve divides into supraorbital and supratrochlear branches. F, the levator and superior rectus muscle have been retracted posteriorly to expose the nasociliary nerve, ophthalmic artery, and superior ophthalmic vein passing above the optic nerve. G, superior view of the anterior fossa in another specimen. The nasal cavity, sphenoid sinus, and orbit have been unroofed. The dura has been removed from the roof and lateral wall of the cavernous sinus. The medial strip below the anterior cranial base is formed, from anterior to posterior, by the frontal, ethmoidal, and sphenoid sinuses. The orbital fat has been removed to expose the intraorbital structures. The frontal nerve courses above the levator muscle. The trochlear nerve passes above the annular tendon to reach the superior oblique muscle. The trochlea of the superior oblique muscle is attached in the superomedial part of the anterior orbit. The lacrimal nerve courses above the lateral rectus muscle. The ophthalmic artery and superior ophthalmic vein are seen in the interval between the levator and superior oblique muscle. The anterior and posterior eth-*

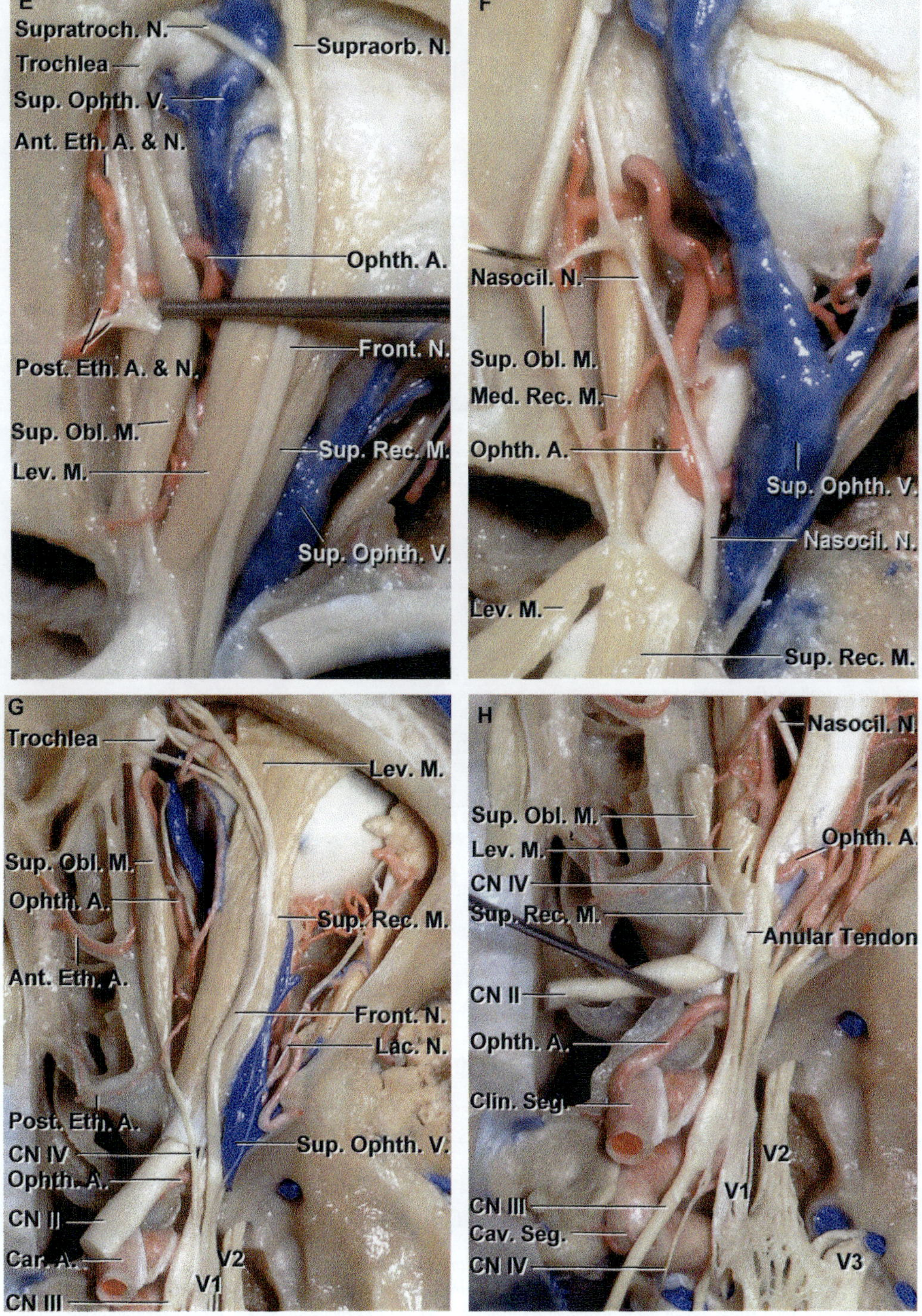

FIGURE 6.4. *Continued*
moidal branches of the ophthalmic artery course through the anterior and posterior ethmoidal canals. H, *enlarged view of cavernous sinus, superior orbital fissure, and orbital apex. The superior oblique, levator, and superior rectus muscles have been removed. The ophthalmic artery and nasociliary nerve enter the orbital apex on the lateral side of the optic nerve and cross between the optic nerve and superior rectus muscle to reach the medial part of the orbit. The optic nerve has been elevated to expose the ophthalmic artery, which courses through the optic canal on the lower side of the optic nerve and enters the orbital apex on the lateral side of the optic nerve. The ophthalmic artery then crosses medially between the optic nerve and superior rectus muscle, as does the nasociliary nerve. The maxillary nerve exits the foramen rotundum to enter the pterygopalatine fossa, and the mandibular nerve exits the foramen ovale to enter the infratemporal fossa.* A., *artery;* A.C.A., *anterior cerebral artery;* Ant., *anterior;* Car., *carotid;* Cav., *cavernous;* Clin., *clinoid;* CN, *cranial nerve;* Crib., *cribriform;* Eth., *ethmoid, ethmoidal;* Front., *frontal;* Lac., *lacrimal;* Less., *lesser;* Lev., *levator;* M., *muscle;* M.C.A., *middle cerebral artery;* Med., *medial;* N., *nerve;* Nasocil., *nasociliary;* Obl., *oblique;* Olf., *olfactory;* Ophth., *ophthalmic;* Post., *posterior;* Rec., *rectus;* Seg., *segment;* Sphen., *sphenoid;* Sup., *superior;* Supraorb., *supraorbital;* Supratroch., *supratrochlear;* Tr., *tract;* V., *vein.*

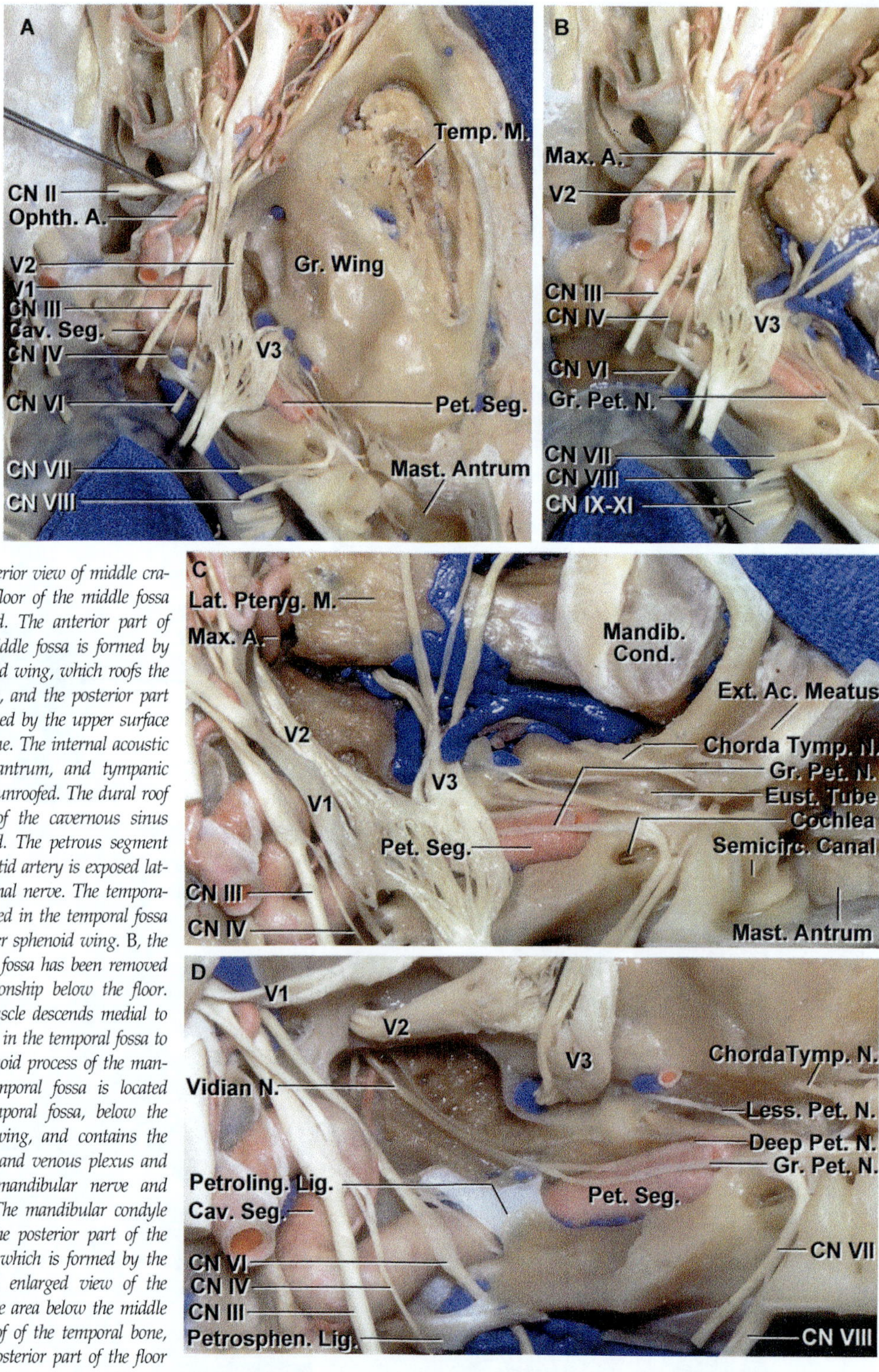

FIGURE 6.5. *Superior view of middle cranial base.* A, *the floor of the middle fossa has been preserved. The anterior part of the floor of the middle fossa is formed by the greater sphenoid wing, which roofs the infratemporal fossa, and the posterior part of the floor is formed by the upper surface of the temporal bone. The internal acoustic meatus, mastoid antrum, and tympanic cavities have been unroofed. The dural roof and lateral wall of the cavernous sinus have been removed. The petrous segment of the internal carotid artery is exposed lateral to the trigeminal nerve. The temporalis muscle is exposed in the temporal fossa lateral to the greater sphenoid wing.* B, *the floor of the middle fossa has been removed to show the relationship below the floor. The temporalis muscle descends medial to the zygomatic arch in the temporal fossa to insert on the coronoid process of the mandible. The infratemporal fossa is located medial to the temporal fossa, below the greater sphenoid wing, and contains the pterygoid muscles and venous plexus and branches of the mandibular nerve and maxillary artery. The mandibular condyle is located below the posterior part of the middle fossa floor, which is formed by the temporal bone.* C, *enlarged view of the posterior part of the area below the middle fossa floor. The roof of the temporal bone, which forms the posterior part of the floor of the middle fossa, has been opened to expose the mastoid antrum, eustachian tube, semicircular canals, cochlea, the nerves in the internal acoustic meatus, and the mandibular condyle.* D, *the trigeminal nerve has been reflected forward. The abducens nerve passes below the petrosphenoid ligament and through Dorello's canal. The petrous segment of the carotid passes below the petrolingual ligament to enter the cavernous sinus. The greater petrosal nerve is joined by the deep petrosal branch of the carotid sympathetic plexus to form the vidian nerve, which passes forward in the vidian canal, which has been unroofed. The lesser petrosal nerve arises from the tympanic branch of the glossopharyngeal nerve, which passes across the promontory in the tympanic nerve plexus and regroups to cross the floor of the middle fossa, exiting the cranium to provide parasympathetic innervation through the otic ganglion to the parotid gland. The tensor tympani muscle and eustachian are layered, with the former above the latter, along and separated from the anterior surface of the petrous carotid by a thin layer of bone.* A., *artery;* Ac., *acoustic;* Cav., *cavernous;* CN, *cranial nerve;*

and deep petrosal nerves. The petrosal nerves join to form the vidian nerve that enters the pterygopalatine ganglion, which sends branches to the zygomatic nerve that anastomoses with the lacrimal nerve to reach the gland.

MIDDLE CRANIAL BASE

Endocranial Surface

The endocranial surface of the middle portion of the middle cranial base, formed by the sphenoid and temporal bones, has medial and lateral parts (*Figs. 6.2, 6.3, 6.5,* and *6.9*). The medial part is formed by the body of the sphenoid bone, the site of the tuberculum sellae, pituitary fossa, middle and posterior clinoid processes, the carotid sulcus, and the dorsum sellae (*Fig. 6.8*). The lateral part is formed by the lesser and greater sphenoid wings, with the superior orbital fissure between them (*Figs. 6.3* and *6.5*). The lesser wing is connected to the body of the sphenoid bone by an anterior root, which forms the roof of the optic canal, and by a posterior root, also called the optic strut, which forms the floor of the optic canal and separates the optic canal from the superior orbital fissure (*Fig. 6.3*). The greater wing forms the largest part of the endocranial surface of the middle fossa, with the squamosal and the petrosal parts of the temporal bone completing this surface. The superior orbital fissure transmits the oculomotor, trochlear, ophthalmic, and abducens nerves, a recurrent meningeal artery, and the superior and inferior ophthalmic veins (5). The maxillary and mandibular nerves pass through the foramen rotundum and ovale, both located in the greater wing of the sphenoid. The not infrequently occurring sphenoidal emissary foramen, located anteromedial to the foramen spinosum, gives passage to a vein connecting the cavernous sinus and the pterygoid venous plexus. The upper surface of the petrous bone is grooved along the course of the greater and lesser petrosal nerves (*Fig. 6.5*) (6). The carotid canal extends upward and medially and provides passage to the internal carotid artery and carotid sympathetic nerves in their course to the cavernous sinus. The posterior trigeminal root reaches the middle fossa and the impression on the upper surface of the petrous bone where Meckel's cave and the semilunar ganglion sit. The roof of the carotid canal opens below the trigeminal ganglion near the distal end of the carotid canal (*Figs. 6.5, 6.6,* and *6.9*). The arcuate eminence approximates the position of the superior semicircular canal. A thin lamina of bone, the tegmen tympani, roofs the area above the middle ear and auditory ossicles on the anterolateral side of the arcuate eminence. The internal auditory canal can be identified below the floor of the middle fossa by drilling along a line approximately 60 degrees medial to the arcuate eminence, near the middle portion of the angle between the greater petrosal nerve and arcuate eminence (*Fig. 6.5*). The petrous apex, medial to the internal acoustic meatus, is free of important structure.

The middle cranial base can be divided into a lateral portion, containing the middle cranial fossa and the upper surface of the temporal bone, and a medial portion, the sellar and the parasellar region, where the pituitary gland and cavernous sinus are located (*Figs. 6.3* and *6.8*). The basal temporal lobe, formed by the parahippocampal, occipitotemporal, inferotemporal gyri, and uncus and supplied by branches of the anterior choroidal, posterior cerebral, and middle cerebral arteries, rests on the middle fossa floor. The cavernous sinus, situated between two layers of dura, is formed by an outer layer facing the brain, and an inner or periosteum layer, covering the bone of the middle fossa (3). The inner layer splits into two parts when it reaches the cavernous sinus; one invests the nerves and forms the inner layer of the lateral wall, and the medial layer faces the sphenoid body and forms the medial wall of the sinus. The same inner layer invests the oculomotor, trochlear, and ophthalmic nerves and the distal part of the abducens nerve in their course through the lateral wall of the cavernous sinus. The internal carotid artery, with its vertical posterior bend, horizontal anterior bend, and clinoidal segments, runs inside the cavernous sinus. The clinoidal segment of the internal carotid artery is between the distal and proximal dural rings and is covered by a layer of dura, which forms a collar, the carotid collar, around the artery (11). In a previous study, we found that the venous plexus, forming the cavernous sinus, extends through the lower ring, inside the collar of dura, and around the clinoid segment to the level of the upper ring. The meningohypophyseal trunk, with its tentorial, inferior hypophyseal, and dorsal meningeal branches, and the inferolateral trunk, also called the artery of the inferior cavernous sinus, arise from the intracavernous carotid artery. The proximal abducens nerve passes through Dorello's canal, located below the petrosphenoid ligament, and receives sympathetic branches from the internal carotid nerve, which pass to the ophthalmic nerve to enter the orbit.

The main venous afferents to the cavernous sinus are the superior and inferior ophthalmic veins and the sphenoparietal sinus (*Figs. 6.4* and *6.7*). Several venous compartments, named according to their relationship to the cavernous carotid artery, empty mainly into the basilar and superior and inferior petrosal sinuses, or, by way of the foramina in the middle fossa floor, into the pterygoid venous plexus (10). The sella houses the pituitary gland and is partially closed above by the diaphragma sellae. Anterolateral to the diaphragm, the carotid cave, a dural depression at the level of the distal dural ring, extends downward medial to the initial intradural segment of the internal carotid artery. The tensor tympani muscle and the eustachian tube cross medial to the foramen spinosum, below the floor of the middle fossa, and anterior to the horizontal segment of the petrous carotid (*Fig. 6.5*). The greater petrosal nerve crosses the area above and parallel to the petrous carotid artery, laterally joins the geniculate ganglion, and medi-

Cond., *condyle;* Eust., *eustachian;* Ext., *external;* Gr., *greater;* Lat., *lateral;* Less., *lesser;* Lig., *ligament;* M., *muscle;* Mandib., *mandibular;* Mast., *mastoid;* Max., *maxillary;* N., *nerve;* Ophth., *ophthalmic;* Pet., *petrosal;* Petroling., *petrolingual;* Petrosphen., *petrosphenoid;* Plex., *plexus;* Pteryg., *pterygoid;* Seg., *segment;* Semicirc., *semicircular;* Temp., *temporalis;* Tymp., *tympani.*

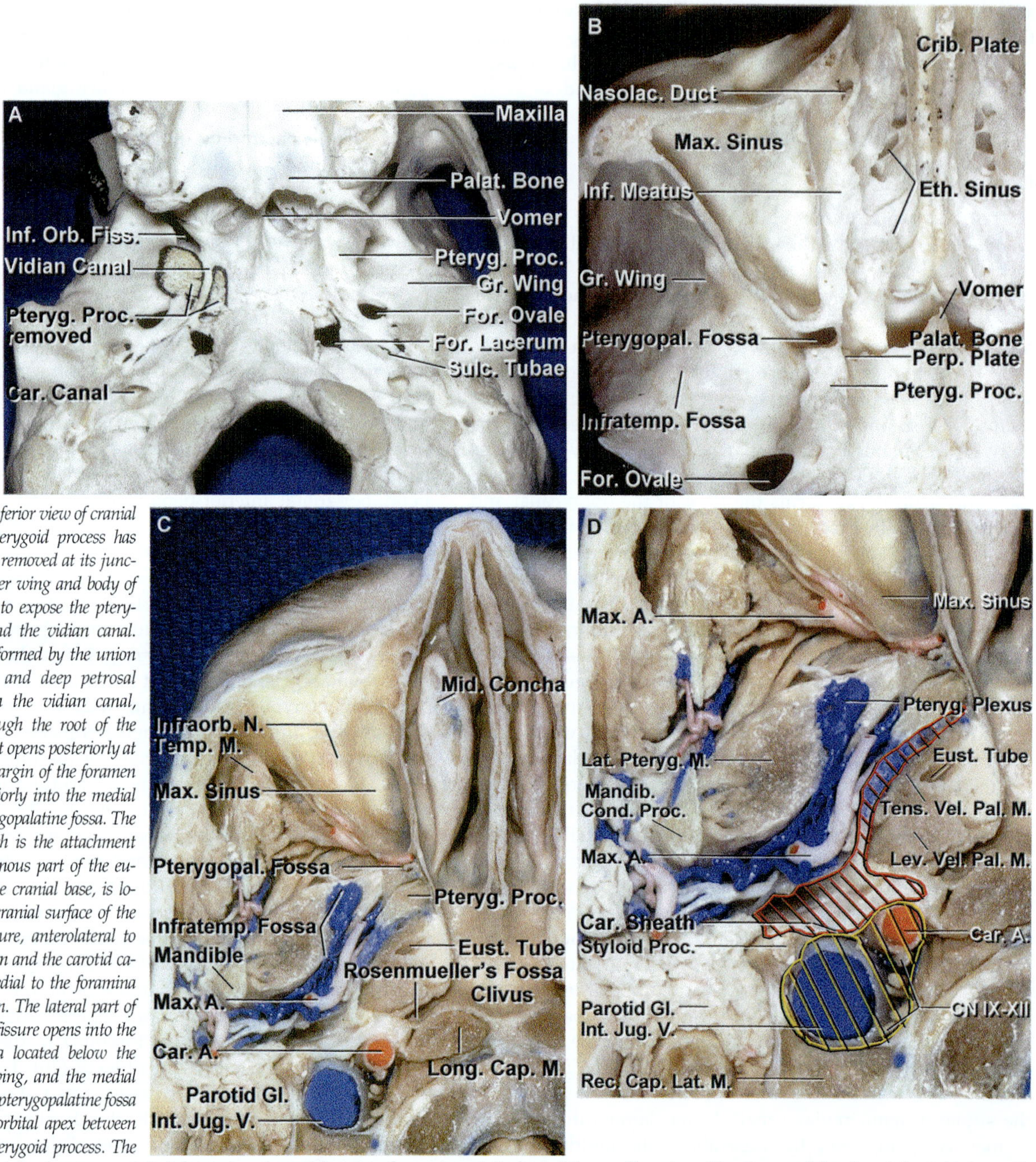

FIGURE 6.6. A, *inferior view of cranial base. The right pterygoid process has been sectioned and removed at its junction with the greater wing and body of the sphenoid bone to expose the pterygopalatine fossa and the vidian canal. The vidian nerve, formed by the union of the superficial and deep petrosal nerves, courses in the vidian canal, which passes through the root of the pterygoid process. It opens posteriorly at the anterolateral margin of the foramen lacerum and anteriorly into the medial portion of the pterygopalatine fossa. The sulcus tubae, which is the attachment site of the cartilaginous part of the eustachian tube to the cranial base, is located on the extracranial surface of the sphenopetrosal fissure, anterolateral to the foramen lacerum and the carotid canal, and posteromedial to the foramina ovale and spinosum. The lateral part of the inferior orbital fissure opens into the infratemporal fossa located below the greater sphenoid wing, and the medial part opens into the pterygopalatine fossa located below the orbital apex between the maxilla and pterygoid process. The right zygomatic arch has been removed.* B, *inferior view of an axial section of a cranium at the level of the maxillary sinus. The pterygopalatine fossa is located between the posterior wall of the maxillary sinus and the pterygoid process. The roof of the maxillary sinus forms the floor of the orbit. The infratemporal fossa is located below the greater wing of the sphenoid and opens medially into the pterygopalatine fossa. The medial wall of the pterygopalatine fossa is formed by the perpendicular plate of the palatine bone, which has an opening, the sphenopalatine foramen, through which branches of the maxillary artery and nerve reach the nasal cavity. The ethmoid air cells are located medial to the orbit.* C, *inferior views of an axial section of the cranial base. The infratemporal fossa is surrounded by the maxillary sinus anteriorly, the mandible laterally, the pterygoid process anteromedially, and the parapharyngeal space posteromedially. It contains the mandibular nerve and maxillary artery and their branches, the medial and lateral pterygoid muscles, and the pterygoid venous plexus. The posterior nasopharyngeal wall is separated from the lower clivus by the longus capitis, and the nasopharyngeal roof rests against the upper clivus and floor of the sphenoid sinus.* D, *enlarged view with highlighting of the pre-* (red) *and poststyloid* (yellow) *compartments of the parapharyngeal space. The styloid diaphragm, formed by the anterior part of the carotid sheath, separates the parapharyngeal space into pre- and poststyloid parts. The prestyloid compartment, a narrow fat-containing space between the medial pterygoid and tensor veli palatini muscle, separates the infratemporal fossa from the medially located lateral nasopharyngeal region containing the tensor and levator veli palatini and the eustachian tube. The poststyloid compartment, located behind the prestyloid part, contains the internal carotid artery, internal jugular vein, and the Cranial Nerves IX through XII.* E, *some of the lateral pterygoid muscle has been removed to expose the branches of the mandibular nerve in the*

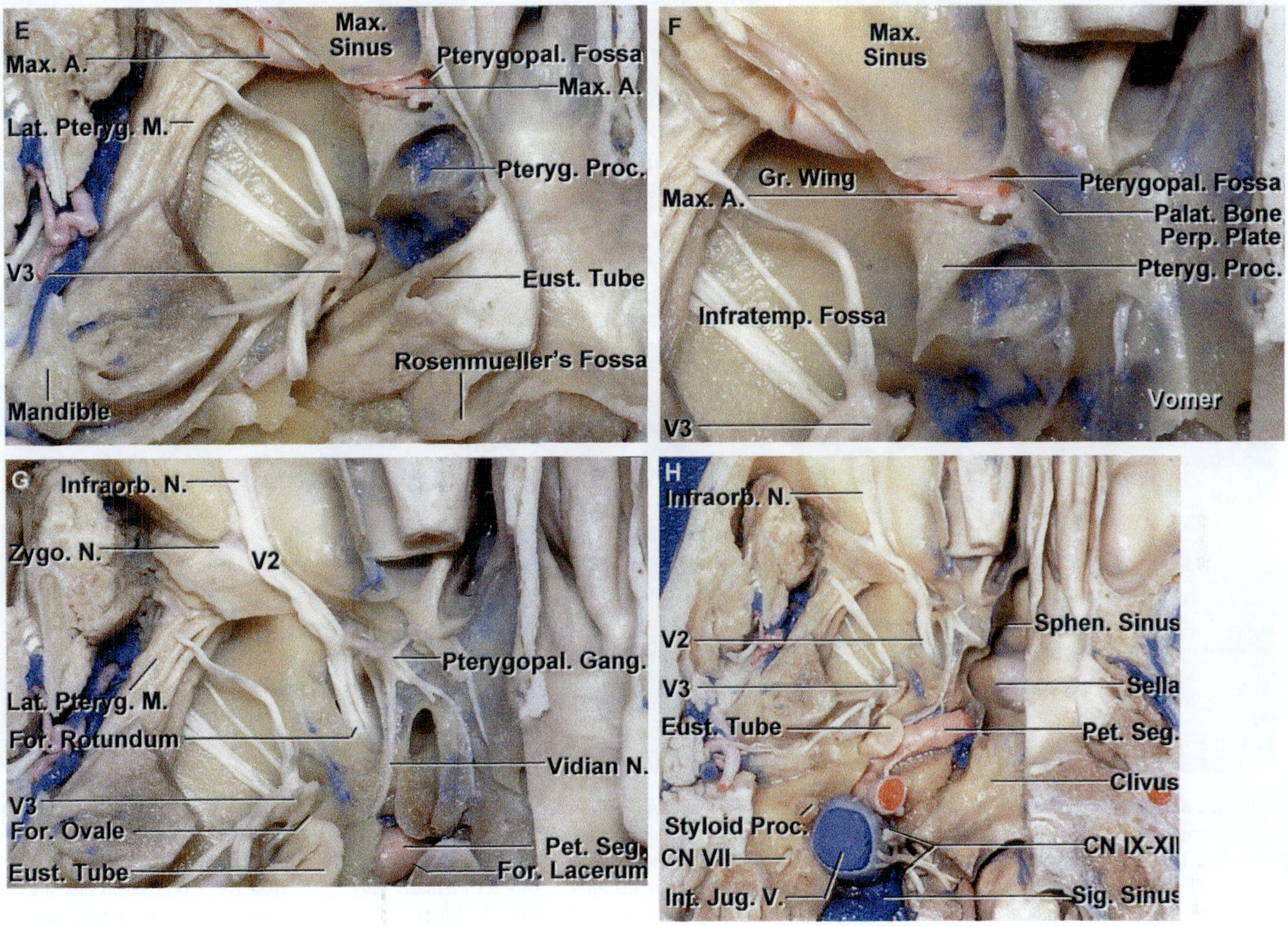

FIGURE 6.6. *Continued*
infratemporal fossa. The lower part of the pterygoid process has been removed to expose the maxillary artery in the pterygopalatine fossa. The pharyngeal recess (fossa of Rosenmüller) projects laterally from the posterolateral corner of the nasopharynx below the foramen lacerum. F, *enlarged view. The pterygopalatine fossa is located between the posterior maxillary wall anteriorly, the sphenoid pterygoid process posteriorly, the perpendicular plate of the palatine bone medially, and the infratemporal fossa laterally. The medial part of the eustachian tube has been removed.* G, *the pterygoid process has been removed to expose the maxillary nerve passing through the foramen rotundum to enter the pterygopalatine fossa, where it gives rise to the infraorbital and zygomatic nerves and communicating rami to the pterygopalatine ganglion. The vidian nerve exits the vidian canal and joins the pterygopalatine ganglion. The terminal part of the petrous carotid is exposed above the foramen lacerum.* H, *enlarged view of the region of the carotid canal and jugular foramen. The bone below the carotid canal has been removed to expose the petrous carotid. The deep portion of the parotid gland has been removed to expose the facial nerve at the styloid foramen. The sigmoid sinus hooks downward from the posterior fossa and opens into the internal jugular vein. A portion of the occipital condyle has been removed to expose the hypoglossal nerve joining the nerves exiting the jugular foramen to pass downward in the carotid sheath. The styloid process and facial nerve at the stylomastoid foramen are located on the lateral side of the internal jugular vein. The right half of the floor of the sphenoid sinus has been removed to expose the sella.* A., *artery;* Cap., *capitis;* Car., *carotid;* CN, *cranial nerve;* Cond., *condylar;* Crib., *cribriform;* Eth., *ethmoid;* Eust., *eustachian;* Fiss., *fissure;* For., *foramen;* Gang., *ganglion;* Gl., *gland;* Gr., *greater;* Inf., *inferior;* Infraorb., *infraorbital;* Infratemp., *infratemporal;* Int., *internal;* Jug., *jugular;* Lat., *lateral, lateralis;* Lev., *levator;* Long., *longus;* M., *muscle;* Max., *maxillary;* Mid., *middle;* N., *nerve;* Nasolac., *nasolacrimal;* Orb., *orbital;* Pal., *palatini;* Palat., *palatine;* Perp., *perpendicular;* Pet., *petrosal;* Plex., *plexus;* Proc., *process;* Pteryg., *pterygoid;* Pterygopal., *pterygopalatine;* Rec., *rectus;* Seg., *segment;* Sig., *sigmoid;* Sphen., *sphenoid;* Sulc., *sulcus;* Temp., *temporalis;* Tens., *tensor;* V., *vein;* Vel., *veli;* Zygo., *zygomatic.*

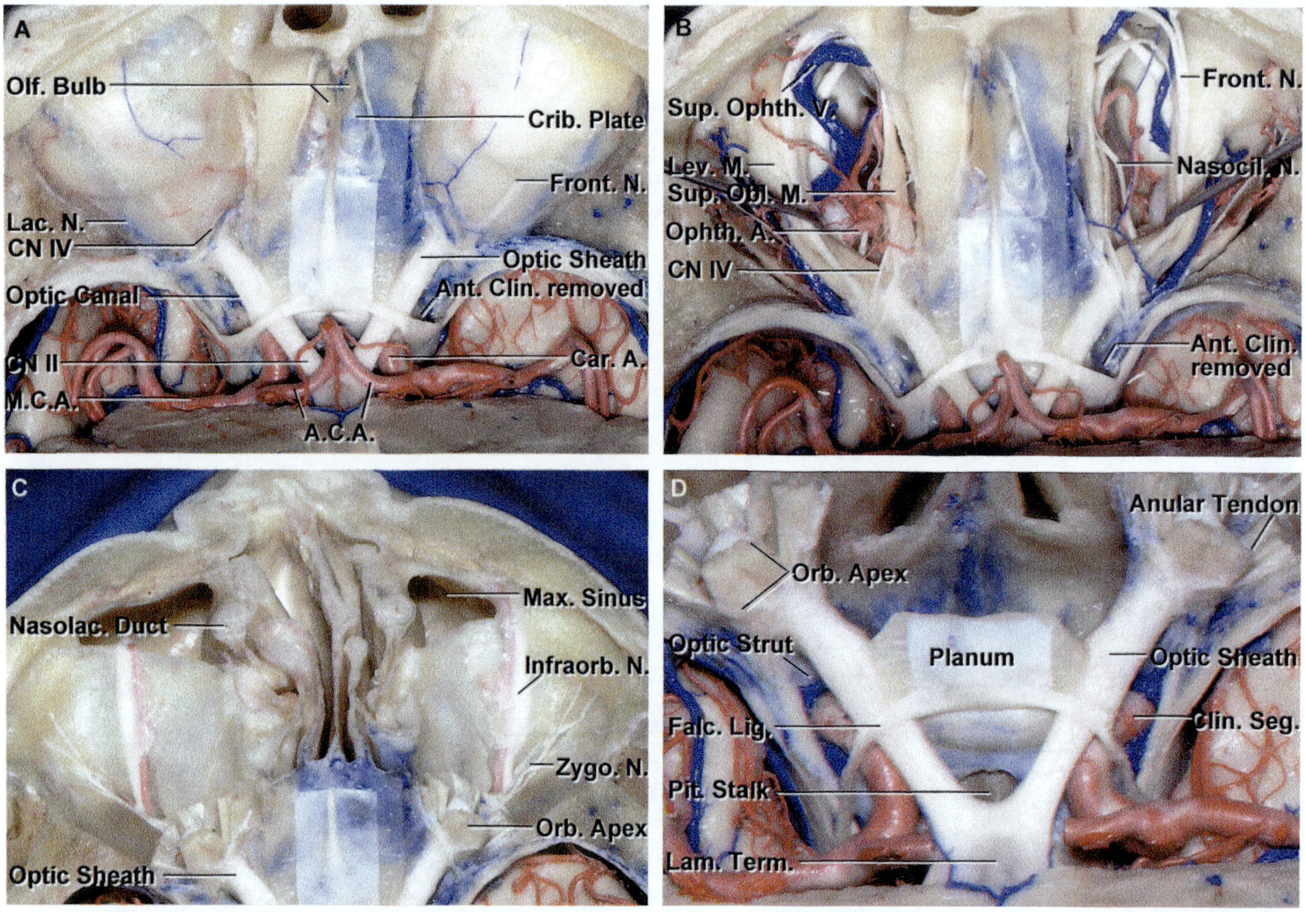

FIGURE 6.7. *Superior view of the anterior cranial base. A, both orbits have been unroofed to expose the periorbita. The optic canals have been unroofed and the anterior clinoids removed to expose the optic nerves, which are enclosed in the optic sheath within the optic canal. The frontal, trochlear, and lacrimal nerves can be seen through the periorbita. The roof of the ethmoidal sinuses and the olfactory bulbs sitting on the cribriform plate have been preserved. The anterior cerebral arteries course above the optic chiasm. B, the intraorbital fat has been removed and the levator and superior rectus muscles have been retracted laterally to expose both globes, ophthalmic arteries, superior ophthalmic veins, and nasociliary nerves. C, the orbital contents have been removed to expose the lateral wall and floor of the orbit. The maxillary sinuses are exposed below the orbital floors. The maxillary nerves give rise to the infraorbital nerve, which courses along the floor of the orbit to reach the cheek, and the zygomatic nerve, which courses along the lateral wall of the orbit to reach the malar eminence and temple. D, enlarged view. The optic nerves are enclosed within the optic sheath as they course through the optic canal. The annular tendon, from which the rectus muscles arise, surrounds the optic nerve and medial portion of the superior orbital fissure. Removal of the anterior clinoid exposes the clinoid segment of the carotid artery. The optic strut, which separates the optic canal and superior orbital fissure, has also been removed. The segment of anterior cerebral arteries passing above the chiasm has been removed to expose the lamina terminalis. The falciform dural fold extends across the optic nerve at the entrance into the optic canal.* A., *artery;* A.C.A., *anterior cerebral artery;* Ant., *anterior;* Car., *carotid;* Clin., *clinoid;* CN, *cranial nerve;* Crib., *cribriform;* Falc., *falciform;* Front., *frontal;* Infraorb., *infraorbital;* Lac., *lacrimal;* Lam., *lamina;* Lev., *levator;* Lig., *ligament;* M., *muscle;* Max., *maxillary;* M.C.A., *middle cerebral artery;* N., *nerve;* Nasocil., *nasociliary;* Nasolac., *nasolacrimal;* Obl., *oblique;* Olf., *olfactory;* Ophth., *ophthalmic;* Orb., *orbital;* Pit., *pituitary;* Seg., *segment;* Sup., *superior;* Term., *terminalis;* V., *vein;* Zygo., *zygomatic.*

FIGURE 6.8. *Structures below the medial part of the anterior and middle cranial fossae. A, midsagittal section of the anterior and middle cranial base to the right of the nasal septum. The area below the medial part of the anterior cranial fossa is formed by the frontal and ethmoidal sinuses and the nasal cavity. The nasal cavity is divided into the inferior, middle, and superior meatus and the sphenoethmoidal recess by the inferior, middle, and superior cochlea. The inferior meatus is located below the inferior turbinate, and the sphenoethmoidal recess, into which the sphenoid sinus opens, is located above the superior turbinate. The central part of the middle cranial base is formed by the body of the sphenoid bone, which contains the sphenoid sinus and sella with the pituitary gland. The cribriform plate is located in the roof of the nasal cavity. The nasopharynx and the opening of the eustachian tube are located below the sphenoid sinus. B, some of the mucosa has been removed from the concha. The inferior concha is a separate bone attached to the maxilla. The middle and superior concha are appendages of the ethmoid bone. The carotid artery courses along the lateral margin of the sphenoid sinus. The prominence within the sphenoid sinus, formed by the superior orbital fissure, is located anterior to the intracavernous carotid, and the prominence overlying the maxillary nerve is located below the intracavernous carotid. C, the middle and superior turbinates have been removed to expose the ostia of the maxillary and frontal sinuses. Both open into the middle meatus below the middle turbinate. The nasolacrimal duct opens below the inferior concha. Rosenmüller's fossa is*

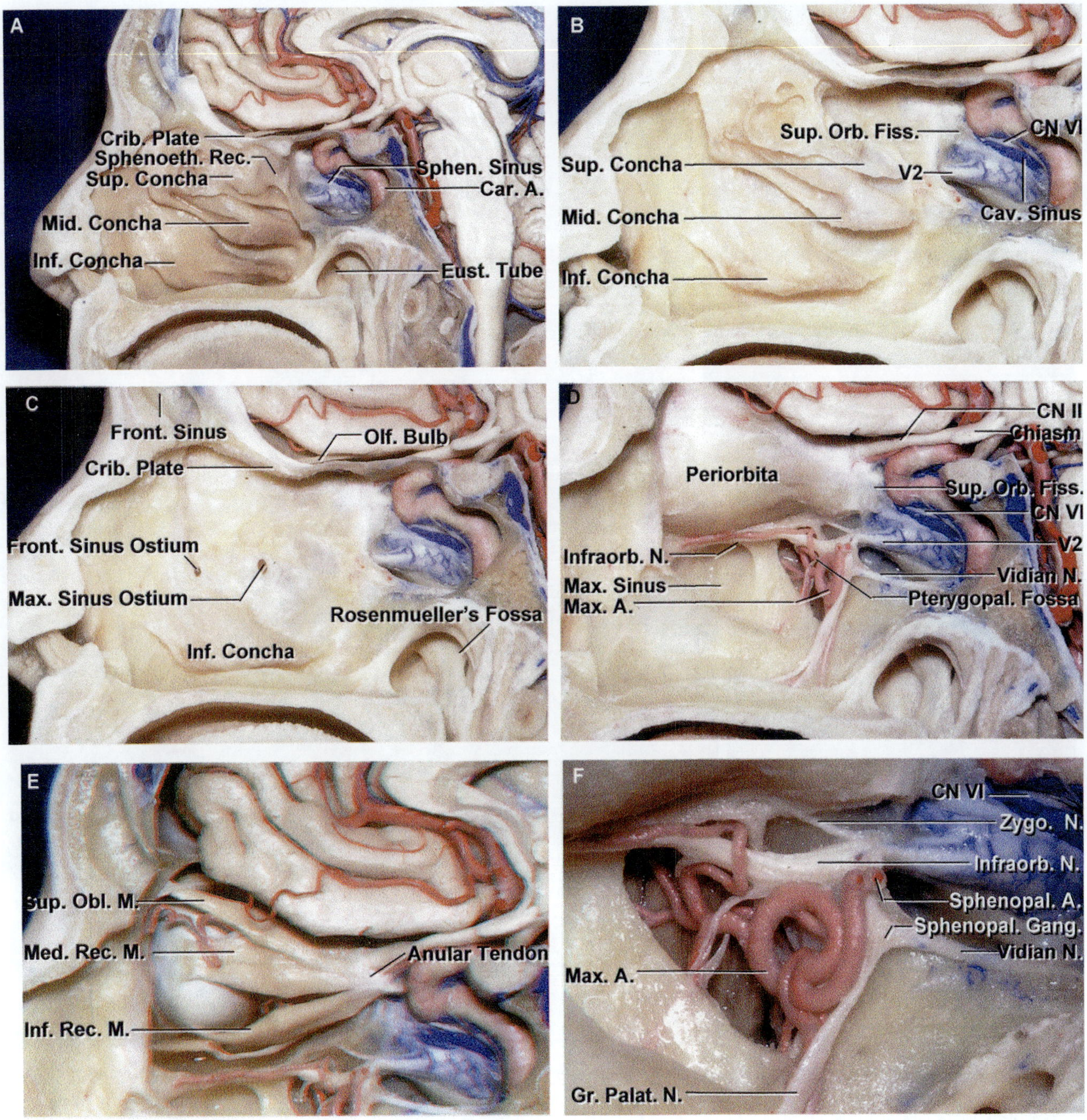

FIGURE 6.8. *Continued*

located behind the eustachian tube. D, *the medial wall of the maxillary sinus and the ethmoid air cells have been removed to expose the orbit. The optic nerve enters the orbit above the superior orbital fissure. The maxillary nerve exits the foramen rotundum to enter the pterygopalatine fossa. The vidian nerve passes through the vidian canal and enters the posterior margin of the sphenopalatine ganglion in the pterygopalatine fossa. The floor of the anterior cranial fossa forms much of the roof of the orbit, and the maxillary sinus forms most of the floor of the orbit. The abducens nerve is seen below the intracavernous segment of the internal carotid artery. The pterygopalatine fossa is located anterior to the sphenoid sinus and below the orbital apex.* E, *the intraorbital fat has been removed to expose the superior oblique and medial and inferior rectus muscles.* F, *enlarged view of the pterygopalatine fossa. The maxillary nerve exits the foramen rotundum to enter the pterygopalatine fossa, where it gives rise to the infraorbital, zygomatic, and palatine nerves and communicating rami to the pterygopalatine ganglion. The vidian nerve exits the vidian canal to enter the pterygopalatine ganglion. The pterygopalatine fossa contains branches of the maxillary nerve, the junction of the vidian nerve with the pterygopalatine ganglion, and terminal branches of the maxillary artery.* A., *artery;* Car., *carotid;* Cav., *cavernous;* CN, *cranial nerve;* Crib., *cribriform;* Eust., *eustachian;* Fiss., *fissure;* Front., *frontal;* Gang., *ganglion;* Gr., *greater;* Inf., *inferior;* Infraorb., *infraorbital;* M., *muscle;* Max., *maxillary;* Med., *medial;* Mid., *middle;* N., *nerve;* Obl., *oblique;* Olf., *olfactory;* Orb., *orbital;* Palat., *palatine;* Pterygopal., *pterygopalatine;* Rec., *recess, rectus;* Sphen., *sphenoid;* Sphenoeth., *sphenoethmoid;* Sphenopal., *sphenopalatine;* Sup., *superior;* Zygo., *zygomatic.*

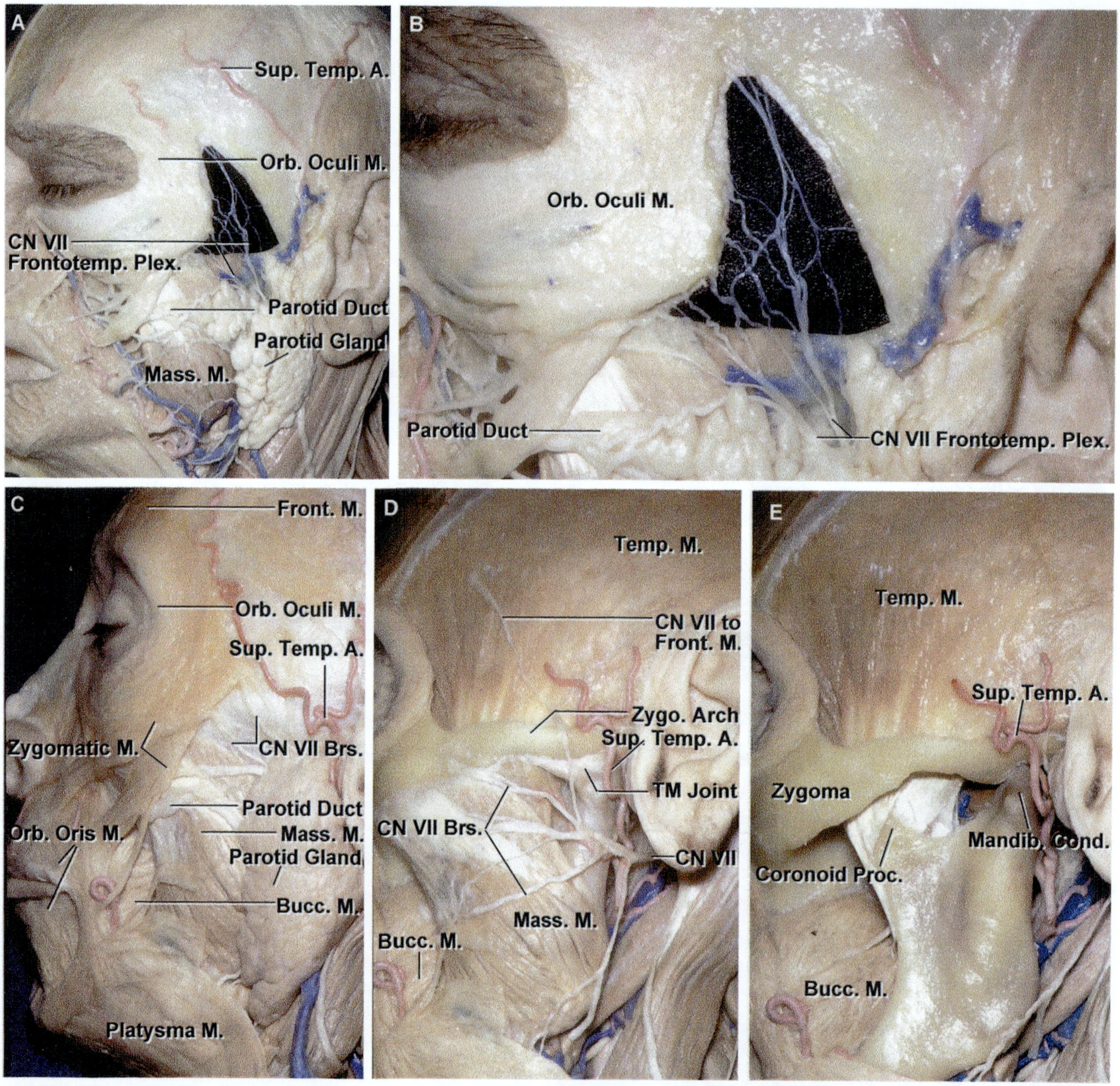

FIGURE 6.9. A, *the branches of the facial nerve, which form a fine plexus in the fat pad overlying the temporalis fascia and are directed to the orbicularis oculi and frontalis muscle, have been dissected free and a small piece of black material placed deep to their fine branches to highlight this neural network in the fat pad.* B, *enlarged view of the facial nerve plexus innervating the orbicularis oculi and frontalis muscle.* C, *lateral view of the structures superficial to the anterior and middle cranial base. The frontotemporal and zygomatic branches of the facial nerve are exposed anterior to the parotid gland. The orbicularis oculi surrounds the orbit, and the frontalis muscle extends upward from the superior orbital rim. The levators of the lip and zygomaticus muscles are located in front of the maxilla. The orbicularis oris surrounds the mouth and the buccinator muscle surrounds the oral cavity deep to the masseter muscle. The parotid duct crosses the masseter muscle. The superficial temporal artery divides into anterior and posterior branches. The parotid gland has been removed to show the branches of the facial nerve.* D, *the parotid gland has been removed to expose the facial nerve exiting the stylomastoid foramen. The facial nerve branch to the frontalis muscle has been preserved in the dissection and has been laid back against the temporalis muscle to show it crossing the zygomatic arch in its course to the forehead. The superficial temporal artery passes deep to the facial nerve in front of the ear.* E, *the masseter muscle has been removed to expose the temporalis muscle inserting on the coronoid process. The buccinator muscle, which surrounds the oral cavity, is situated on the deep side of the masseter muscle.* F, *the coronoid process and lower part of the temporalis muscle have been removed to expose the deep temporal branches of both the maxillary artery and mandibular nerve passing upward along the greater sphenoid wing and temporal squama to enter the deep side of the temporalis muscle. The lateral pterygoid muscles extend backward from the pterygoid process and greater wing of the sphenoid to insert along the mandibular condyle and temporomandibular joint.* G, *a craniotomy has been performed to expose the floor of the middle fossa, and the lateral wall of the orbital has been removed to expose the extraocular muscles. The mandibular condyle has been removed and the pterygoid muscles reflected to expose the mandibular nerve at the foramen ovale. The pterygopalatine fossa is located behind the maxilla. The floor of the orbit and the upper part of the maxilla have been removed to expose the nasal cavity.* H, *enlarged view after resection of the floor of the middle fossa*

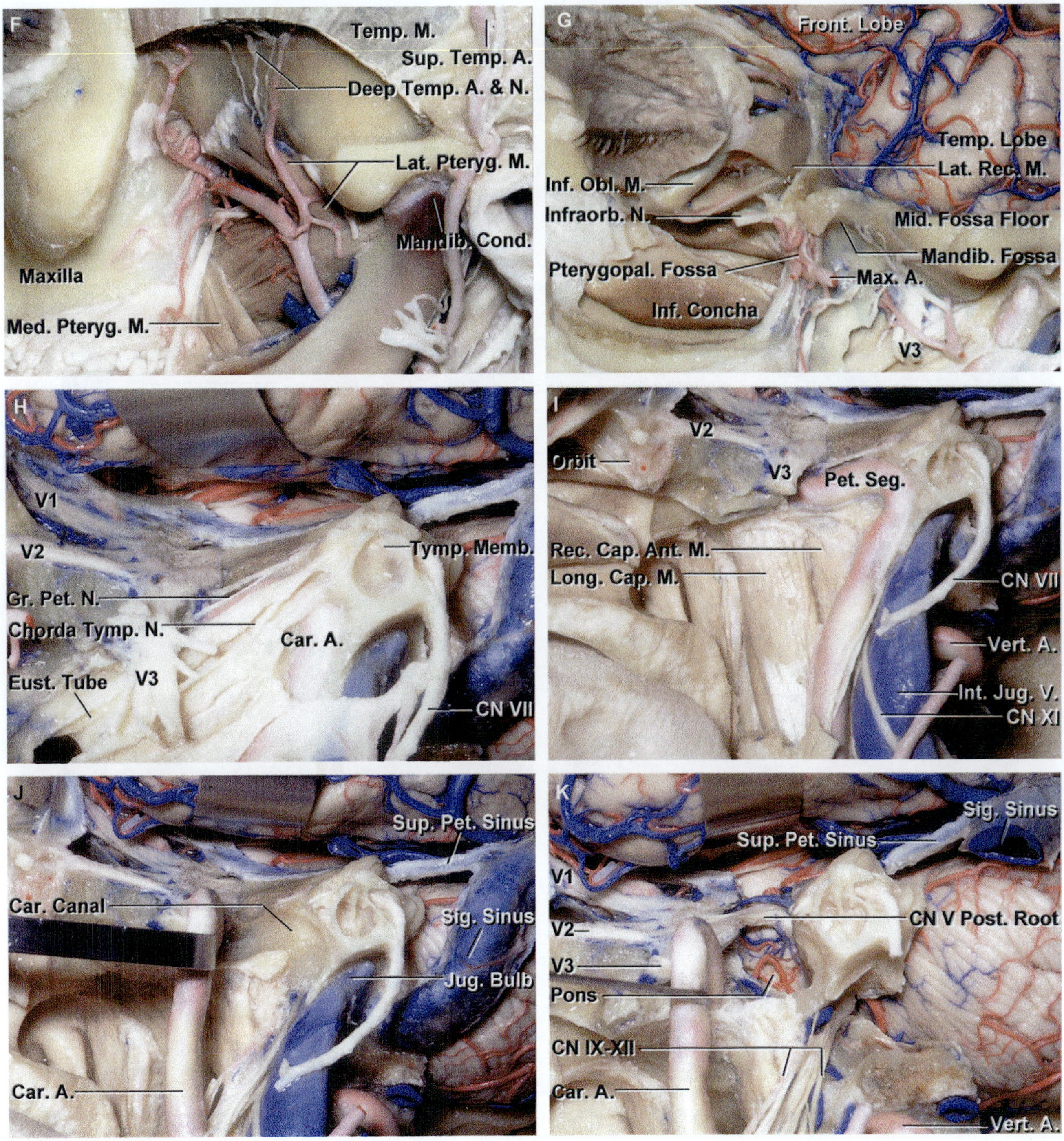

FIGURE 6.9. *Continued*
and the external auditory canal to expose the tympanic membrane and the mandibular nerve below the foramen ovale. The mastoid segment of the facial nerve has been preserved. The greater petrosal nerve crosses above the petrous carotid. The tensor tympani muscle and eustachian tube are layered along the anterior margin of the petrous carotid. I, the eustachian tube and tensor tympani have been resected to expose the upper cervical and petrous carotid. The nasopharyngeal mucosa has been opened to expose the longus capitis and rectus capitis anterior muscles. J, the carotid artery has been reflected forward out of the carotid canal. This exposes the petrous apex in front of the jugular foramen on the medial side of the internal carotid artery. K, the petrous apex has been drilled and the dura opened below the trigeminal nerve to expose the upper anterior part of the posterior cranial fossa. A segment of the internal jugular vein and jugular bulb have been resected to expose the IXth through XIIth cranial nerves below the jugular foramen and hypoglossal canal. A., *artery;* Ant., *anterior;* Brs., *branches;* Bucc., *buccinator;* Cap., *capitis;* Car., *carotid;* CN, *cranial nerve;* Cond., *condyle;* Coron., *coronoid;* Eust., *eustachian;* Front., *frontal;* Frontotemp., *frontotemporal;* Gr., *greater;* Inf., *inferior;* Infraorb., *infraorbital;* Int., *internal;* Jug., *jugular;* Lat., *lateral;* Long., *longus;* M., *muscle;* Mandib., *mandibular;* Mass., *masseter;* Max., *maxillary;* Med., *medial;* Memb., *membrane;* Mid., *middle;* N., *nerve;* Obl., *oblique;* Orb., *orbital;* Pet., *petrosal;* Plex., *plexus;* Post., *posterior;* Proc., *process;* Pteryg., *pterygoid;* Pterygopal., *pterygopalatine;* Rec., *rectus;* Seg., *segment;* Sig., *sigmoid;* Sup., *superior;* Temp., *temporal, temporalis;* TM, *temporomandibular;* Tymp., *tympani, tympanic;* V., *vein;* Vert., *vertebral;* Zygo., *zygomatic.*

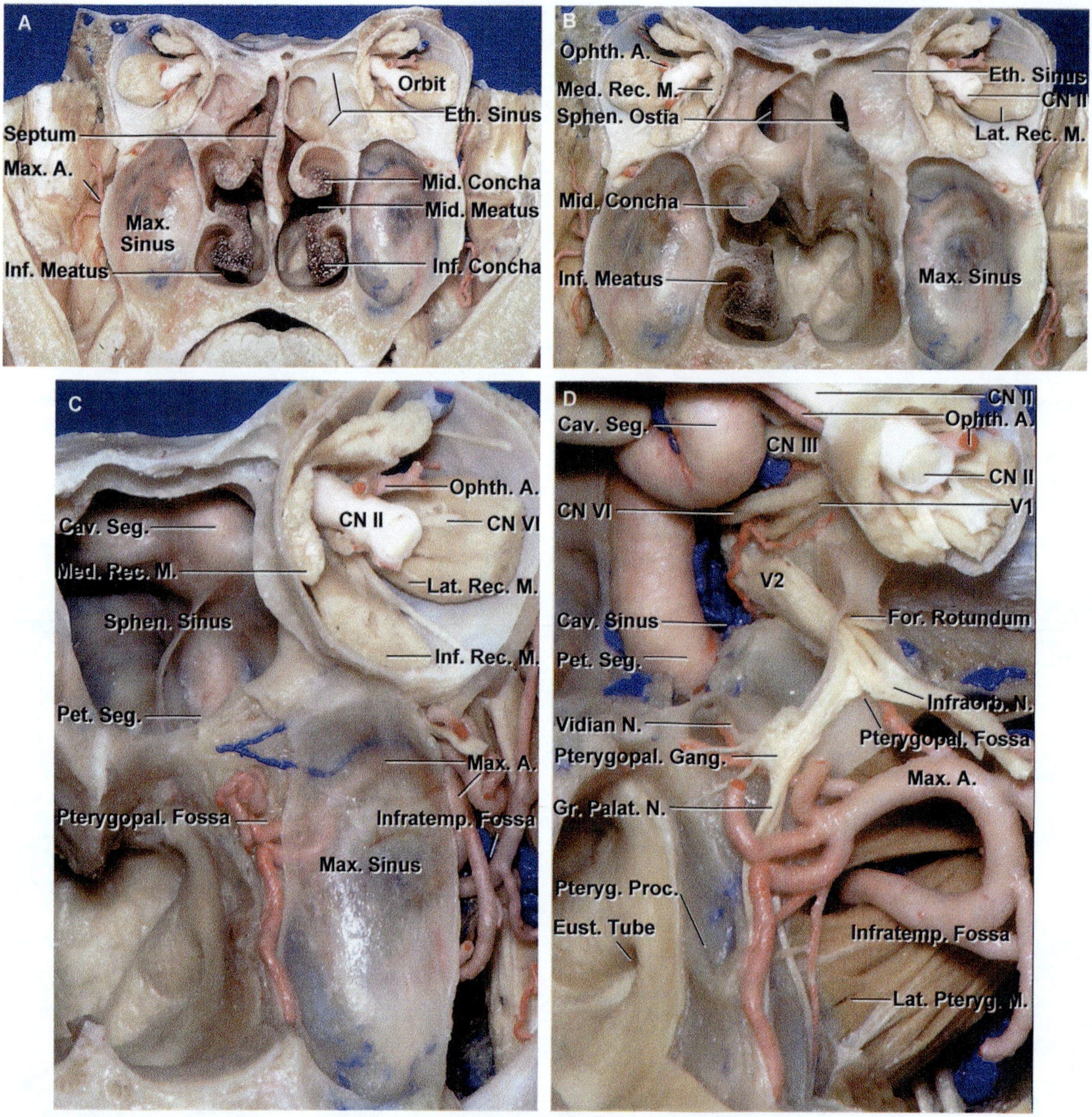

FIGURE 6.10. A, *anterior view of a coronal section, anterior to the sphenoid sinus, through the nasal cavity, orbits, and maxillary sinuses. The upper part of the nasal cavity is separated from the orbits by the ethmoidal sinuses. The lower part of the nasal cavity is bounded laterally by the maxillary sinuses. The middle concha projects medially from the lateral nasal wall at the junction of the roof of the maxillary and ethmoidal sinuses. The posterior ethmoid air cells are located in front of the lateral part of the sphenoid sinus.* B, *the middle and inferior nasal conchae on the left side and the nasal septum and the posterior ethmoidal sinuses on both sides have been removed to expose the posterior nasopharyngeal wall, the anterior aspect of the sphenoid body, and the sphenoid ostia. The posterior ethmoid air cells overlap the lateral margin of the sphenoid ostia.* C, *enlarged view showing the relationships of the nasal cavity, pterygopalatine and infratemporal fossae, orbit, and sphenoid sinus. The nasopharynx is located below the sphenoid sinus. The pterygopalatine fossa is located in the lateral wall of the nasal cavity behind the upper part of the maxillary sinus and below the orbital apex. The posterior maxillary wall is so thin that the maxillary artery coursing in the pterygopalatine fossa can be seen through the bone. The sphenopalatine branch of the maxillary artery passes through the sphenopalatine foramen to reach the walls of the nasal cavity and the sphenoid face.* D, *the posterior wall of the maxillary sinus has been removed to expose the pterygopalatine and infratemporal fossae and*

ally joins the deep petrosal branch of the carotid sympathetic nerves to form the vidian nerve, which enters the pterygopalatine ganglion (*Figs. 6.2, 6.5,* and *6.6*). The lesser petrosal nerve runs anterior to the greater petrosal nerve and exits the cranium, passing through the foramen spinosum to join the otic ganglion. The cochlea is situated below the floor of the middle cranial fossa, at the apex of the angle between the greater petrosal and labyrinthine segment of the facial nerve.

Exocranial Surface

The exocranial surface of the middle cranial base is also divided into central and lateral parts (*Figs. 6.2, 6.3, 6.6,* and *6.9*). The central part encompasses the sphenoid body and the upper part of the basal (clival) part of the occipital bone and corresponds to the sphenoid sinus and the nasopharynx. The lateral part is formed by the greater sphenoid wing, the petrous, tympanic, and squamous parts of the temporal bone, the styloid process, and the zygomatic, palatine, and maxillary bones. The medial and lateral parts are separated by a parasagittal plane passing through the medial pterygoid plate. The foramen lacerum is located at the union of the sphenoid, occipital, and petrous bones and is enclosed on its lower side by fibrocartilaginous tissue to form the inferior wall of the carotid canal. Structures transversing the lateral part include the carotid artery in the carotid canal, the glossopharyngeal, vagus, and accessory nerves in the jugular foramen, the third trigeminal division in the foramen ovale, the middle meningeal artery in the foramen spinosum, and the facial nerve in the facial canal. The pterygomaxillary fissure is the lateral opening of the pterygopalatine fossa into the infratemporal fossa. The glenoid fossa harbors the mandibular condyle. The roof of the fossa is divided into anterior and posterior parts by the squamotympanic fissure, along which the chorda tympani passes.

The area below the middle portion includes the infratemporal fossa, parapharyngeal space, infrapetrosal space, and pterygopalatine fossa (*Figs. 6.6,* and *6.9–6.11*). The boundaries of the infratemporal fossa are the middle pterygoid muscle and the pterygoid process medially, the mandible laterally, the posterior wall of the maxillary sinus anteriorly, the greater wing of the sphenoid superiorly, and the medial pterygoid muscle joining the mandible and the pterygoid fascia posteriorly. The fossa opens into the neck below. The infratemporal fossa contains the branches of mandibular nerve, the maxillary artery, and the pterygoid muscles and venous plexus. The mandibular nerve, after exiting the foramen ovale, lies anterolateral to the otic ganglion and divides immediately into its terminal branches: the pterygoid, buccal, masseteric, and temporal branches along the superior wall of the fossa; the inferior alveolar and the lingual branches, after being joined by the chorda tympani, descend between both pterygoid muscles; and the auriculotemporal branch with the maxillary artery course between the mandible and the sphenomandibular ligament. The auriculotemporal nerve carries the parasympathetic innervation of the parotid gland, which travels through the tympanic branch of the glossopharyngeal nerve that forms the lesser petrosal nerve, to reach the otic ganglion before joining the auriculotemporal nerve. The maxillary artery, which arises as a terminal branch of the external carotid artery with the superficial temporal artery, is divided into three segments. The first, or mandibular segment, passes between the sphenomandibular ligament and the mandibular neck and gives rise to the deep auricular, anterior tympanic, middle meningeal, accessory middle meningeal (enters through the foramen ovale) and the inferior alveolar artery. The second, or pterygoid segment, courses through the middle of the infratemporal fossa and gives rise to the posterosuperior alveolar, infraorbital, masseteric, pterygoid, temporal, and buccal branches. The third, or pterygopalatine segment, courses in the fossa of the same name. The pterygoid venous plexus connects through the middle fossa foramina and inferior orbital fissure with the cavernous sinus and empties into the retromandibular and facial veins.

The pterygopalatine fossa is located between the maxillary sinus in the front, the pterygoid process behind, the palatine bone medially and the body of the sphenoid bone above (*Figs. 6.3, 6.6, 6.10,* and *6.11*). The fossa opens laterally through the pterygomaxillary fissure into the infratemporal fossa and medially through the sphenopalatine foramen to the nasal cavity. Both the foramen rotundum for the maxillary nerve and the pterygoid canal for the vidian nerve open through the posterior wall of the fossa formed by the sphenoid pterygoid process. The palatovaginal canal carrying the pharyngeal nerve and artery and the greater and lesser palatine canals conveying the greater and lesser palatine arteries open into the pterygopalatine fossa. The inferior orbital fissure, across which the orbital muscle stretches, lies in front of the pterygopalatine fossa. The fossa contains branches of the maxillary nerve, vidian nerve, the pterygopalatine ganglion, and the pterygopalatine segment of the maxillary artery. The maxillary nerve passes through the foramen rotundum to enter the fossa and, after giving communicating rami to the pterygopalatine ganglion, divides into the posterosuperior alveolar, infraorbital, and zygomatic nerves. The zygomatic nerve, in addition to its sensory fibers, carries the parasympathetic fibers from the pterygopalatine ganglion to the lacrimal gland. The vidian (nerve of the pterygoid canal) ends in the pterygopalatine ganglion, which sends rami to the maxillary nerve and gives

the internal carotid artery and nerves coursing through the cavernous sinus. The maxillary artery passes through the infratemporal fossa and enters the pterygopalatine fossa, where it gives rise to branches that follow the branches of the maxillary nerve. Some of these arteries course along the sphenoid face where careful hemostasis during transsphenoidal surgery reduces the need for nasal packing after transsphenoidal operations. The maxillary nerve exits the foramen rotundum to enter the pterygopalatine fossa, where it gives rise to the infraorbital and greater palatine nerves and communicating rami to the pterygopalatine ganglion. The eustachian tube opens into the nasopharynx along the posterior edge of the medial pterygoid plate. A., *artery;* Cav., *cavernous;* CN, *cranial nerve;* Eth., *ethmoid;* Eust., *eustachian;* For., *foramen;* Gr., *greater;* Inf., *inferior;* Infraorb., *infraorbital;* Infratemp., *infratemporal;* Lat., *lateral;* M., *muscle;* Max., *maxillary;* Med., *medial;* Mid., *middle;* N., *nerve;* Ophth., *ophthalmic;* Palat., *palatine;* Pet., *petrosal;* Proc., *process;* Pteryg., *pterygoid;* Pterygopal., *pterygopalatine;* Rec., *rectus;* Seg., *segment;* Sphen., *sphenoid.*

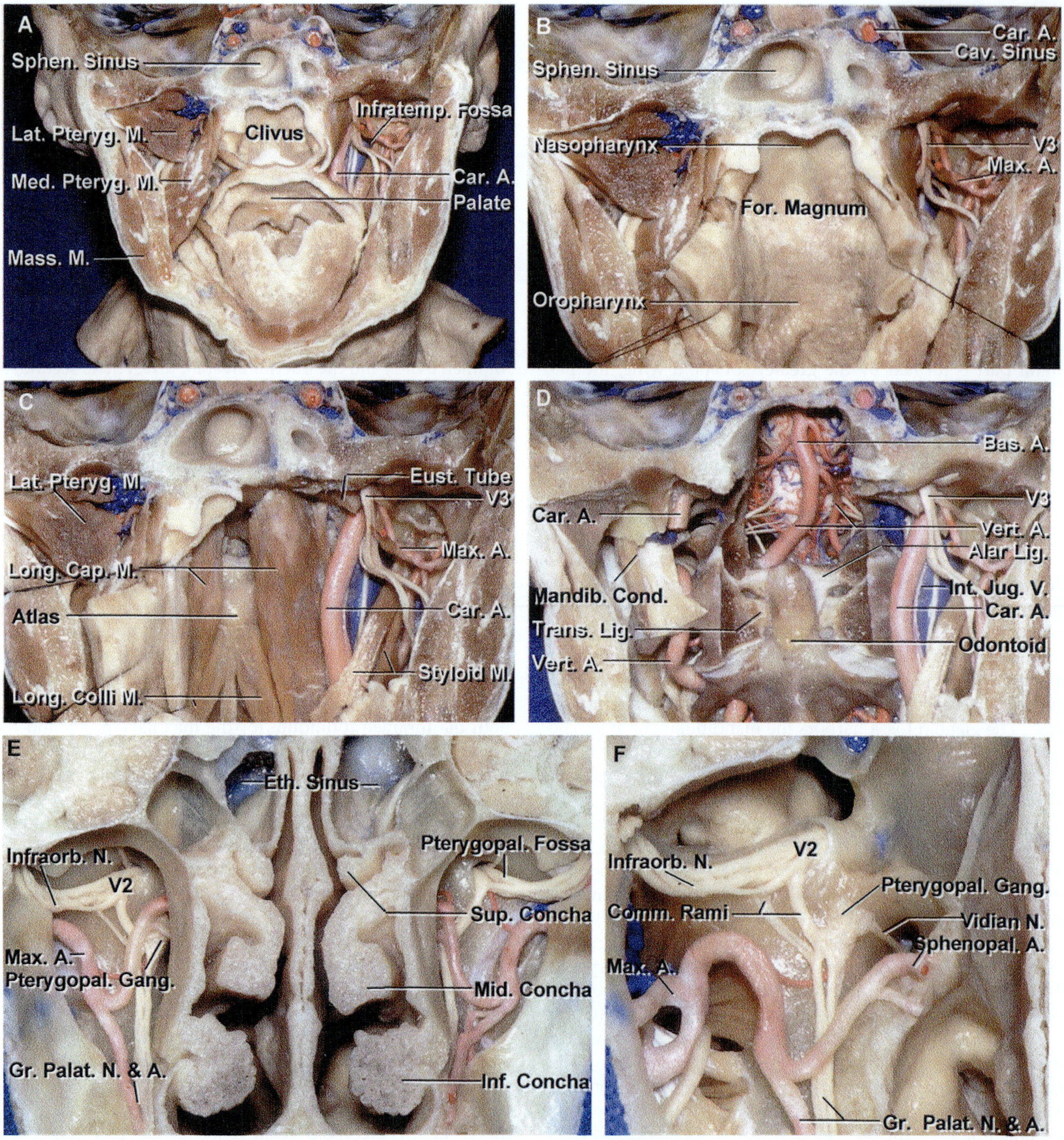

FIGURE 6.11. *Anterior view. Stepwise dissection of a cross section showing the relationships below the middle cranial base. A, the soft palate, which has been preserved, is located at the level of the foramen magnum. The infratemporal fossa, located below the greater sphenoid wing and middle cranial fossa, contains the pterygoid muscles, maxillary artery, mandibular nerve branches, and the pterygoid venous plexus, and opens posteriorly into the area around the carotid sheath, as shown on the left side. B, enlarged view. The soft palate has been divided in the midline, and the leaves reflected laterally. The atlanto-occipital joints and the foramen magnum are located at approximately the level of the hard palate. The anterior arch of C1 and the dens are located behind the oropharynx, and the clivus is located behind the nasopharynx and sphenoid sinus. The prominence over the longus capitis and the anterior arch of C1 are seen through the pharyngeal mucosa. C, the mucosa lining the posterior pharyngeal wall has been reflected to the right, exposing the longus capitis that attaches to the clivus and the part of the longus colli that attaches to the anterior arch of C1. The left eustachian tube has been divided. D, the clivus and anterior arch of C1 have been removed. The dura has been opened to expose the vertebral and basilar arteries. The dens has been preserved. The structures in the right infratemporal fossa and a segment of the right carotid artery and mandible have been removed to expose the right vertebral artery*

rise to the greater and lesser palatine and pharyngeal nerves and nasal branches. The third part of the maxillary artery enters the fossa and divides into its terminal lesser and greater palatine, sphenopalatine, vidian, and pharyngeal branches.

The parapharyngeal space lies between the structures in the pharynx wall medially, the medial pterygoid muscle and the parotid fascia laterally, and the styloid fascia investing the styloglossus, stylopharyngeal, and stylohyoid muscles posteriorly (*Fig. 6.6*). In its upper medial wall, the eustachian tube, covered below by the tensor and levator veli palatine muscles, runs from the tympanic cavity to the pharyngeal wall. This is predominantly a fat-filled space, but also contains pharyngeal branches of the ascending pharyngeal and facial arteries and branches from the glossopharyngeal nerve.

The last of the four spaces below the middle fossa is the infrapetrosal space, also referred to as the poststyloid part of the parapharyngeal space. It is located behind the styloid fascia, below the petrous bone, and medial to the mastoid process (*Figs. 6.2, 6.6,* and *6.9*). Among the foramina in the area connecting the intra- and extracranial spaces is the jugular foramen containing the jugular bulb and lower end of the inferior petrosal sinus. It also contains branches of the ascending pharyngeal artery, the glossopharyngeal, vagus, and accessory nerves, and the opening of the carotid canal through which the carotid artery and the carotid sympathetic nerves pass. Two tiny foramina located between the jugular foramen and carotid canal carry the tympanic branch of the glossopharyngeal nerve and the auricular branch of the vagus nerve. The stylomastoid foramen, conveying the facial nerve and the stylomastoid artery, opens between the mastoid tip and styloid processes. The main fissure in the area is the petroclival fissure on the upper and lower side of which courses the inferior petrosal sinus and the inferior petroclival vein, respectively. The main nerves of the area are the glossopharyngeal nerve coursing below the styloglossus muscle, the vagus nerve descending between the internal carotid artery and the jugular vein, and the accessory nerve passing lateral to the jugular vein on its way to the sternocleidomastoid muscle. The facial nerve runs to the parotid gland, where it divides into cervicofacial and temporofacial trunks. The hypoglossal nerve, after exiting the hypoglossal canal, descends between the carotid artery and the jugular vein, turning anteriorly across the lateral wall of the artery below the level of the digastric muscle. The main arteries in the area are the internal carotid artery and its cervical and petrous segments. The branches of the petrous segment are the caroticotympanic and vidian arteries. The ascending pharyngeal artery ascends medial to the carotid artery, giving meningeal branches that pass through the hypoglossal canal and jugular foramen, as well as pharyngeal branches. The occipital artery passes posteriorly on the medial side of the posterior belly of the digastric muscle. The veins in the area are the internal jugular vein, which receives drainage from the inferior petrosal sinus, and the venous plexus of the hypoglossal canal outside the jugular foramen. The main structures in the area are the styloglossus, stylopharyngeal, and stylohyoid muscles, the digastric nerve, and the stylomandibular ligament.

The medial part of the temporal bone is constituted mainly by the internal auditory canal, the carotid canal, and the petrous apex. Laterally, within the petrous part of the temporal bone on the medial side of the mastoid antrum, lies the semicircular canals and vestibule enclosed within the otic capsule (*Fig. 6.5*).

The tympanic segment of the facial nerve passes below the lateral semicircular canal, and the mastoid segment descends to the stylomastoid foramen. The vestibule (vestibular cavity), which communicates with both ends of the semicircular canals, is situated medial to the lateral semicircular canal and below the superior semicircular canal. The aditus of the mastoid antrum opens into the tympanic cavity, which contains the malleus, incus, and stapes, the chorda tympani and tympanic nerve, and the tensor tympani and stapedius muscles. The tympanic cavity is limited laterally by the tympanic membrane, medially by the bone over the cochlea, and opens anteriorly into the eustachian tube. The arteries feeding the area arise from the stylomastoid, anterior tympanic, petrosal, and caroticotympanic arteries. Posterolateral to the otic capsule, anterior to the sigmoid sinus, and inferior to the superior petrosal sinus lies the presigmoid dura, referred to as Trautmann's triangle, under which the endolymphatic sac sits.

POSTERIOR CRANIAL BASE

The endocranial surface of the posterior cranial base corresponds to the floor of the posterior fossa and area around the foramen magnum (*Figs. 6.2* and *6.3*). It is formed by the sphenoid, temporal, and occipital bones. Medially, it is formed by the dorsum sellae, basilar (clival) portion of the

ascending between the C2 and C1 transverse processes. E, *cross section through the ethmoidal and maxillary sinuses and the nasal cavity in front of the posterior maxillary wall. The posterior wall of the maxillary sinus has been removed to expose the pterygopalatine fossa and ganglia on both sides. The maxillary nerves enter the pterygopalatine fossa by passing through the foramen rotundum. The maxillary arteries enter the pterygopalatine fossa from laterally by passing through the pterygomaxillary fissure and give rise to its terminal branches in the pterygopalatine fossa. Another branch enters the greater palatine canal with the greater palatine nerves.* F, *enlarged view of the pterygopalatine fossa. The vidian nerve exits the vidian canal to enter the pterygopalatine ganglion, which receives communicating rami from the maxillary nerve. The sphenopalatine branch passes through the sphenopalatine foramen to enter the lateral nasal cavity.* A., *artery;* Bas., *basilar;* Cap., *capitis;* Car., *carotid;* Cav., *cavernous;* Comm., *communicating;* Cond., *condyle;* Eth., *ethmoid;* Eust., *eustachian;* For., *foramen;* Gang., *ganglion;* Gr., *greater;* Inf., *inferior;* Infraorb., *infraorbital;* Infratemp., *infratemporal;* Int., *internal;* Jug., *jugular;* Lat., *lateral;* Lig., *ligament;* Long., *longus;* M., *muscle;* Mandib., *mandibular;* Mass., *masseter;* Max., *maxillary;* Med., *medial;* Mid., *middle;* N., *nerve;* Palat., *palatine;* Pteryg., *pterygoid;* Pterygopal., *pterygopalatine;* Sphen., *sphenoid;* Sphenopal., *sphenopalatine;* Sup., *superior;* Trans., *transverse;* V., *vein;* Vert., *vertebral.*

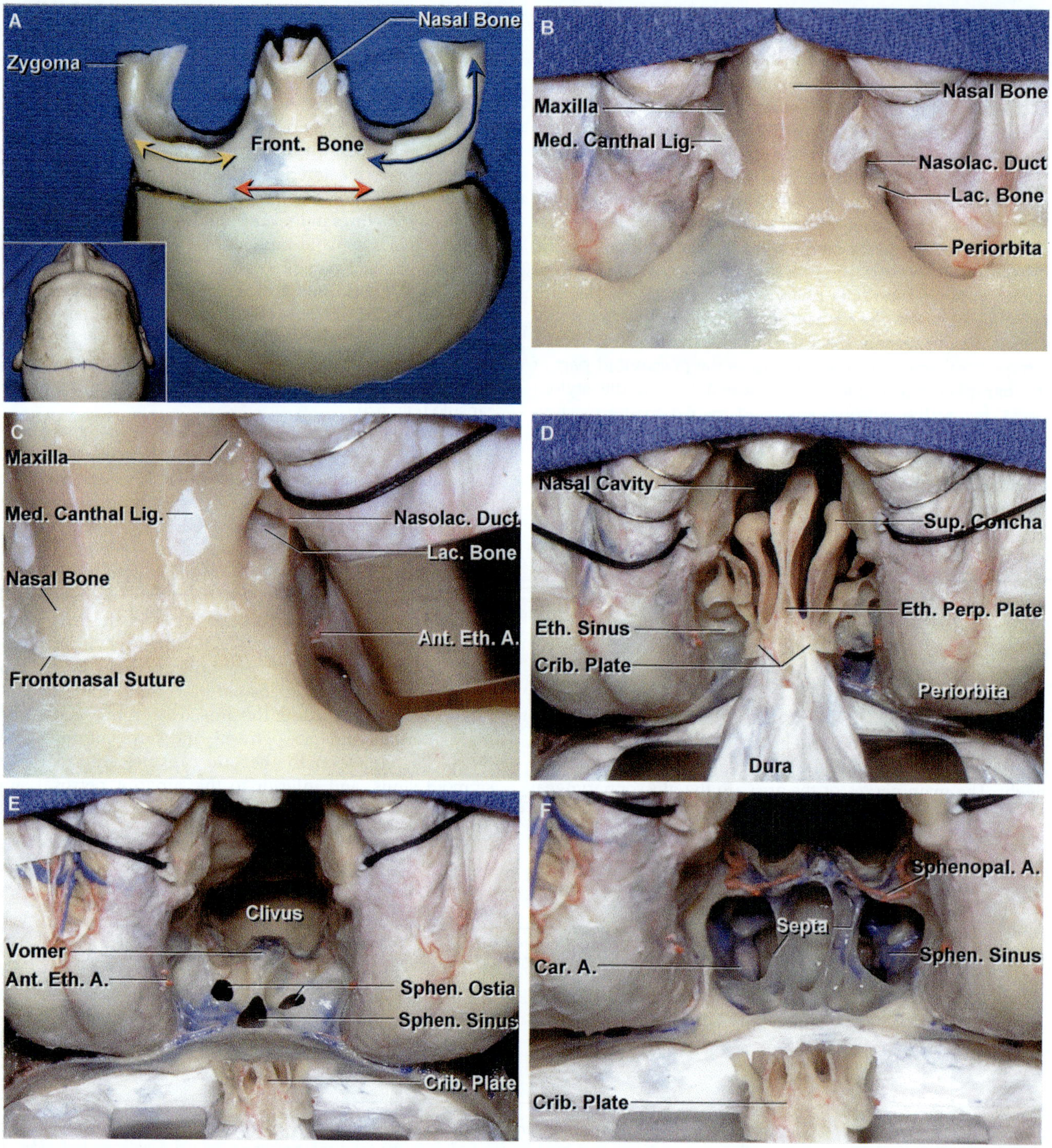

FIGURE 6.12. A–F, *relationships in the transbasal and extended frontal approaches. A, the inset shows the bicoronal scalp incision. A large bifrontal craniotomy and a fronto-orbitozygomatic osteotomy have been completed. The osteotomized segment may extend through the nasal bone and from one to the other lateral orbital rims, as shown. However, for most lesions, a more limited bone flap and osteotomy will suffice and can be tailored as needed to deal with the involvement of the cranial base, nasal cavity, paranasal sinuses, or orbit. For an orbital lesion, an orbitofrontal craniotomy, elevating only the superior orbital rim* (yellow arrows) *and orbital roof, is all that is needed. For a cavernous sinus or unilateral lesions of the anterior or middle fossa, an orbitozygomatic osteotomy will usually suffice* (blue arrow). *For a clival lesion, a more limited bifrontal approach* (red arrow) *will suffice. B, the periorbita has been separated from the walls of the orbit in preparation for the osteotomies. Division of the medial canthal ligament is not necessary for most lesions, but may be required for lesions extending into the lower nasal cavity or orbit. The ligaments should be re-approximated at the end of the operation.*

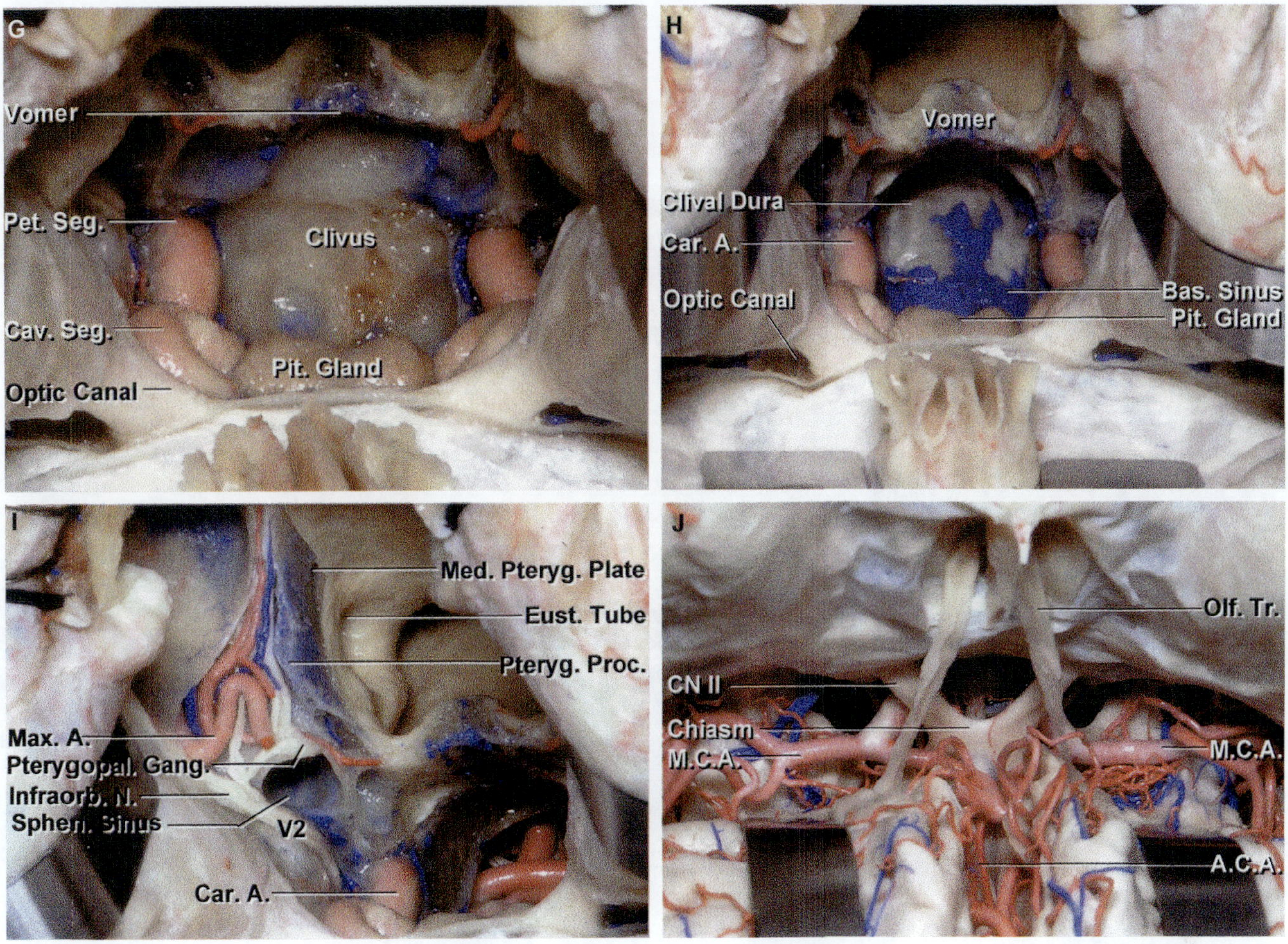

FIGURE 6.12. *Continued*
C, the right medial canthal ligament has been divided and the orbital contents retracted laterally to expose the nasolacrimal duct and the anterior ethmoidal branch of the ophthalmic artery at the anterior ethmoidal foramen. D, the osteotomies have been completed and the frontal dura elevated. The dura remains attached at the cribriform plate. The upper parts of both orbits are exposed. E, an osteotomy around the cribriform plate leaves it attached to the dura and olfactory bulbs, a maneuver that has been attempted to preserve olfaction but has not been commonly successful. The anterior face of the sphenoid sinus and both sphenoid ostia are exposed between the orbits. F, the sphenoid sinus has been opened to expose the septa within the sinus. The sphenopalatine arteries cross the anterior face of the sphenoid. G, the septa within the sphenoid sinus, the sellar floor, and the lateral sinus wall have been removed to expose the intracavernous carotid, pituitary gland, and optic canals. H, the clivus has been opened to expose the dura facing the brainstem. The basilar sinus, which interconnects the posterior parts of the cavernous sinus, is situated between the layers of dura on the upper clivus. I, the exposure has been extended laterally by opening the medial and posterior wall of the maxillary sinus to expose the branches of the maxillary nerve and artery in the pterygopalatine fossa, located behind the posterior maxillary wall. The posterior wall of the pterygopalatine fossa is formed by the pterygoid process. The maxillary nerve enters the pterygopalatine fossa where it gives rise to the infraorbital nerve, which courses along the floor of the orbit and to the palatine nerves, which descend to the palatal area. The eustachian tube opens into the nasopharynx by passing along the posterior edge of the medial pterygoid plate. The lateral wing of the sphenoid sinus extends laterally below the maxillary nerve. J, the frontal dura has been opened and the frontal lobes elevated to expose the olfactory and optic nerves and the internal carotid and anterior and middle cerebral arteries. A., *artery;* A.C.A., *anterior cerebral artery;* Ant., *anterior;* Bas., *basilar;* Car., *carotid;* Cav., *cavernous;* CN, *cranial nerve;* Crib., *cribriform;* Eth., *ethmoid, ethmoidal;* Eust., *eustachian;* Front., *frontal;* Gang., *ganglion;* Infraorb., *infraorbital;* Lac., *lacrimal;* Lig., *ligament;* Max., *maxillary;* M.C.A., *middle cerebral artery;* Med., *medial;* N., *nerve;* Nasolac., *nasolacrimal;* Olf., *olfactory;* Perp., *perpendicular;* Pet., *petrosal;* Pit., *pituitary;* Proc., *process;* Pteryg., *pterygoid;* Pterygopal., *pterygopalatine;* Seg., *segment;* Sphen., *sphenoid;* Sphenopal., *sphenopalatine;* Sup., *superior;* Tr., *tract.*

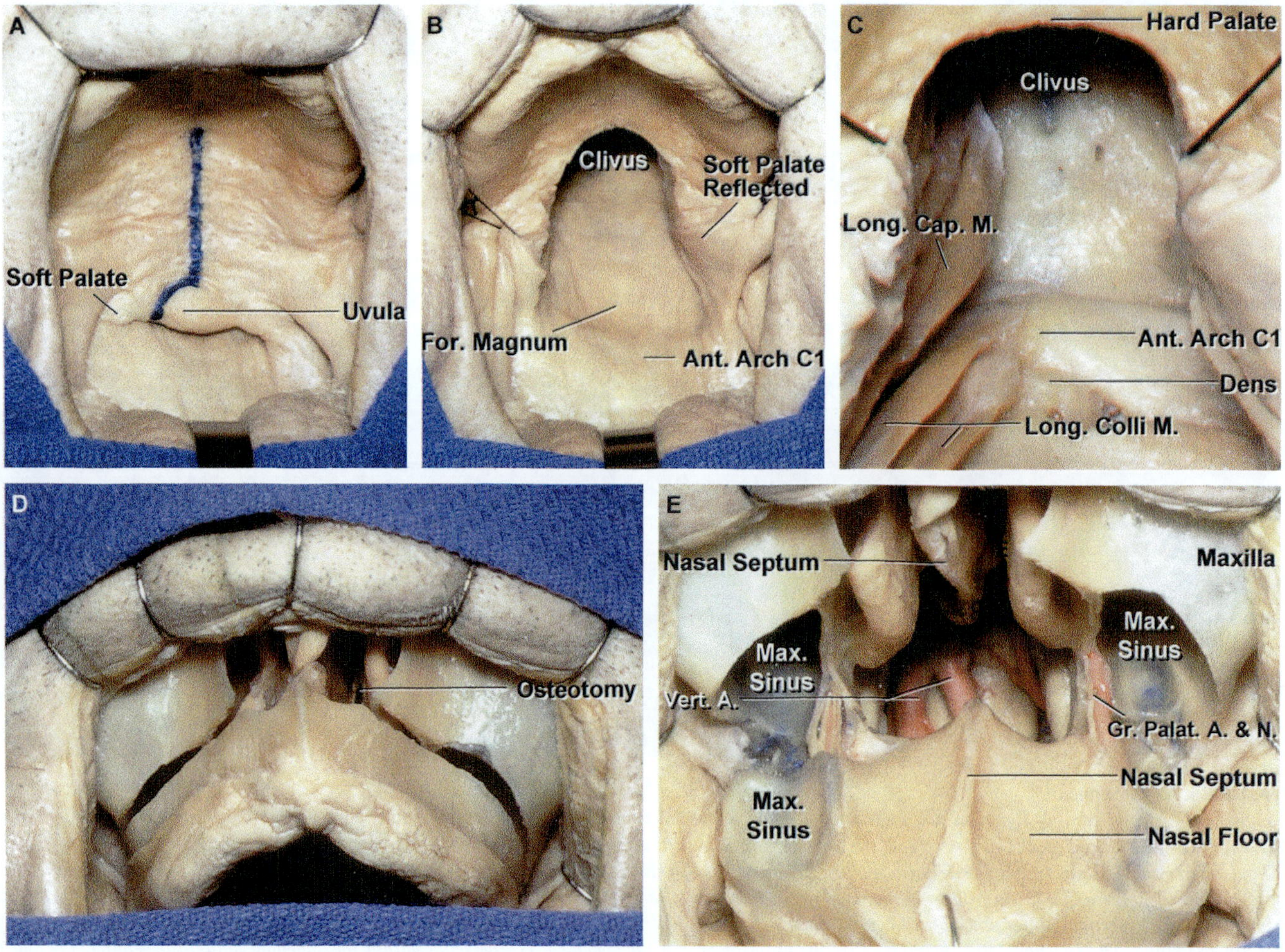

FIGURE 6.13. A, *anterior view through the open mouth. The soft palate, which extends backward from the hard palate, will block the view of the upper clivus. An incision has been outlined in the midline of the soft palate.* B, *the soft palate has been divided to expose the mucosa lining the lower clivus.* C, *the pharyngeal mucosa has been opened in the midline and the left longus capitis and longus colli have been reflected laterally.* D, *the transverse maxillary (Le Fort I) osteotomy extends through the maxillary sinus above the apex of the teeth and below the infraorbital canals.* E, *the lower maxilla has been displaced downward. A clival window and vertebral arteries are seen through the exposure.* A., *artery;* Ant., *anterior;* Cap., *capitis;* For., *foramen;* Gr., *greater;* Long., *longus;* M., *muscle;* Max., *maxillary;* N., *nerve;* Palat., *palatine;* Vert., *vertebral.*

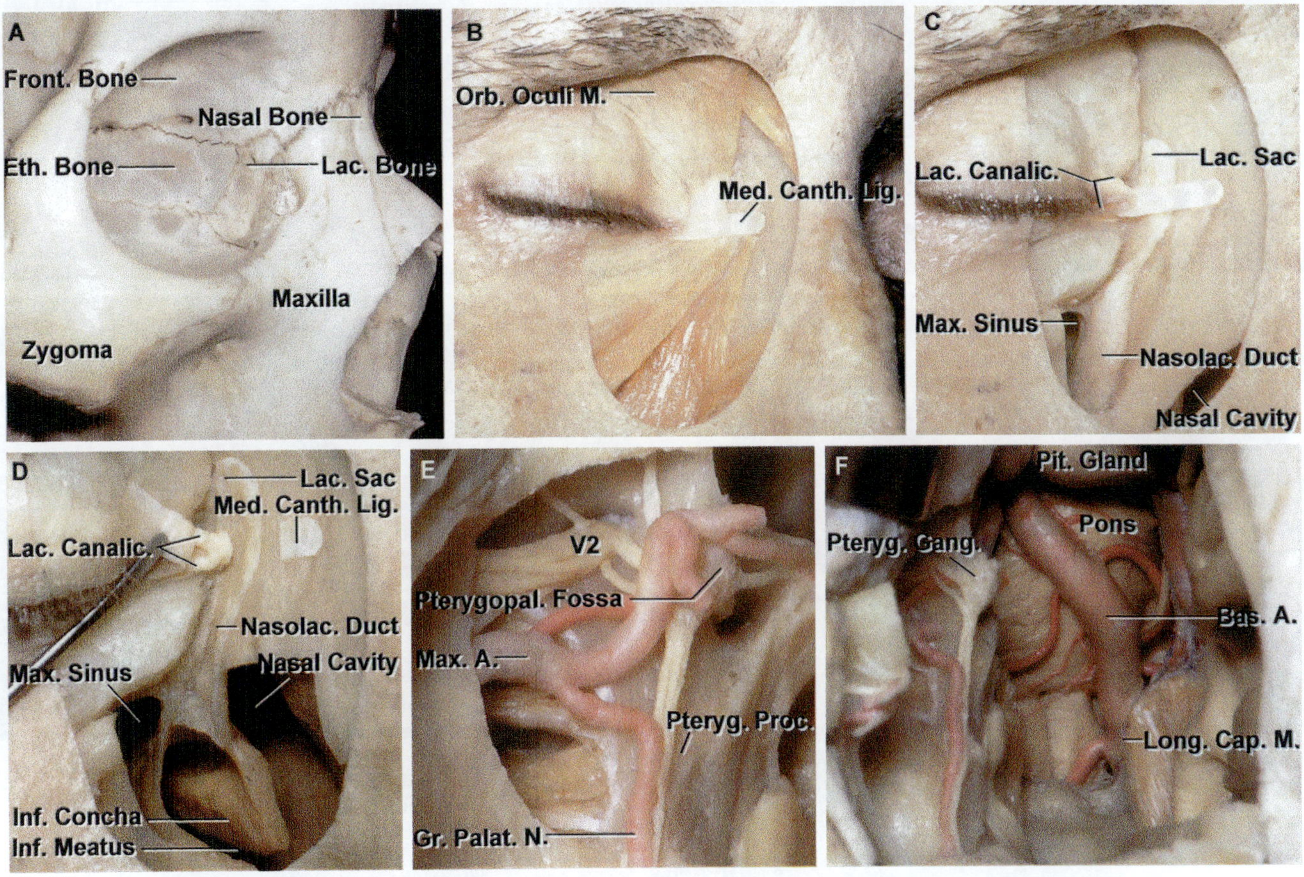

FIGURE 6.14. *Relationships of the medial orbit. A, the medial part of the orbital rim is formed by the frontal bone and maxilla. The anterior part of the nasolacrimal canal is formed by the maxilla and the posterior part by the lacrimal bone, which joins the ethmoid bone posteriorly and the frontal bone above. B, the medial part of the orbicularis oculi muscle has been exposed. The anterior band of the medial canthal ligament, which crosses in front of the lacrimal sac, is attached to the frontal process of the maxilla medially and to the superior and inferior tarsi laterally. C, the medial part of the orbicularis oculi muscle and some of the maxilla have been removed to expose the lacrimal sac, nasolacrimal duct, and a small part of the nasal cavity and maxillary sinus. D, the anterior band of the medial canthal ligament has been reflected laterally to expose the superior and inferior lacrimal canaliculi joining the lacrimal sac. Additional maxilla has been removed to expose the nasal cavity and inferior turbinate medially and the maxillary sinus laterally. The nasolacrimal duct opens into the inferior nasal meatus. E, some of the posterior and medial wall of the maxillary sinus has been removed to expose the pterygopalatine fossa, which contains the maxillary nerve and artery and their branches and the pterygopalatine ganglion. F, the approach has been directed through the nasal cavity medial to the pterygopalatine ganglion and fossa to the clivus, which has been opened to expose the basilar artery.* A., *artery;* Bas., *basilar;* Canalic., *canaliculi;* Cap., *capitis;* Eth., *ethmoid;* Front., *frontal;* Gang., *ganglion;* Gr., *greater;* Inf., *inferior;* Lac., *lacrimal;* Lig., *ligament;* Long., *longus;* M., *muscle;* Max., *maxillary;* Med., *medial;* N., *nerve;* Nasolac., *nasolacrimal;* Orb., *orbital;* Palat., *palatine;* Pit., *pituitary;* Proc., *process;* Pteryg., *pterygoid, pterygopalatine;* Pterygopal., *pterygopalatine.*

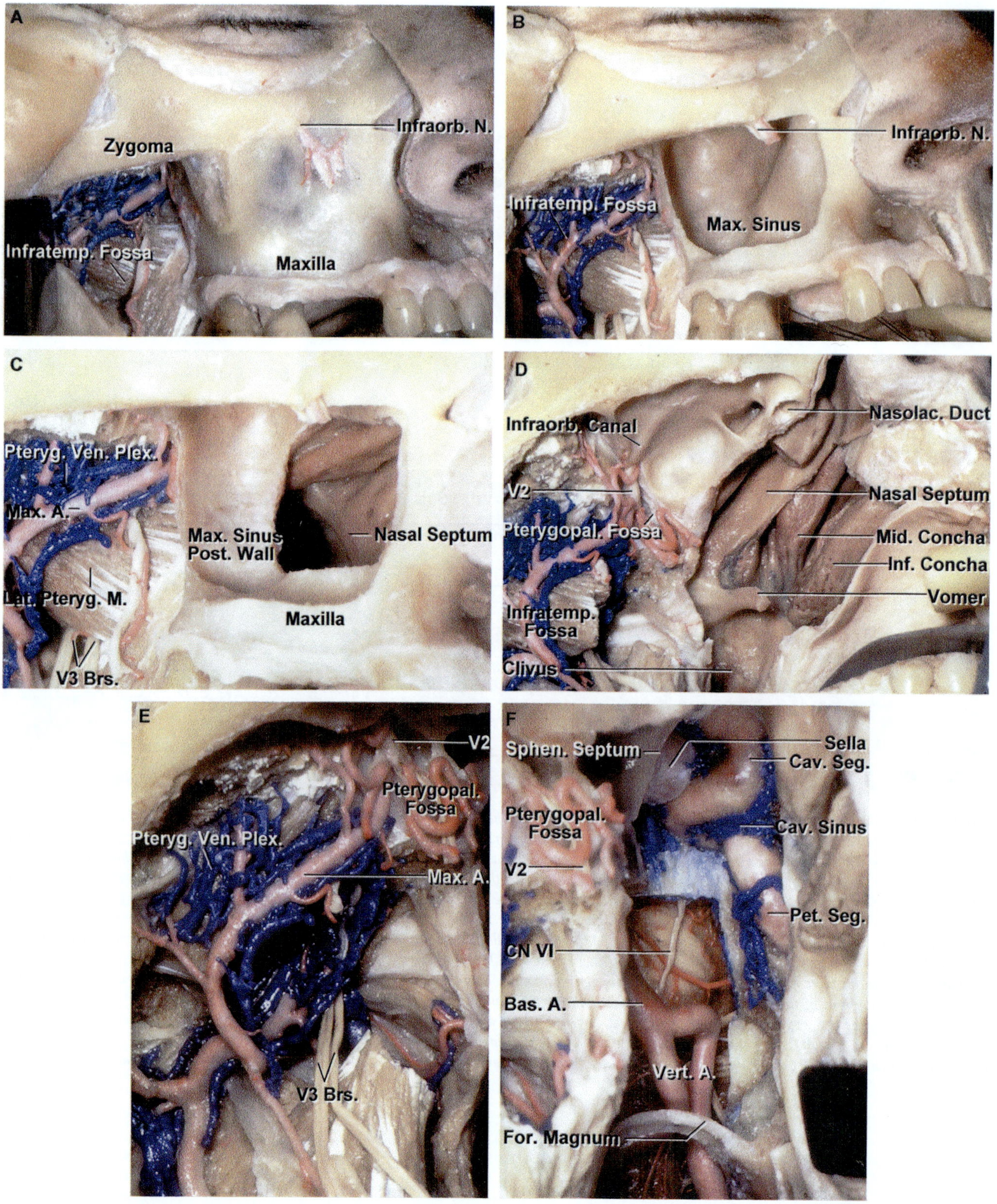
A
Infraorb. N.
Zygoma
Infratemp. Fossa
Maxilla
B
Infraorb. N.
Infratemp. Fossa
Max. Sinus
C
Pteryg. Ven. Plex.
Max. A.
Max. Sinus Post. Wall
Nasal Septum
Lat. Pteryg. M.
Maxilla
V3 Brs.
D
Nasolac. Duct
Infraorb. Canal
V2
Nasal Septum
Pterygopal. Fossa
Mid. Concha
Inf. Concha
Vomer
Infratemp. Fossa
Clivus
E
V2
Pterygopal. Fossa
Pteryg. Ven. Plex.
Max. A.
V3 Brs.
F
Sphen. Septum
Sella
Cav. Seg.
Pterygopal. Fossa
Cav. Sinus
V2
Pet. Seg.
CN VI
Bas. A.
Vert. A.
For. Magnum

FIGURE 6.15.

occipital bone, and the foramen magnum. Laterally, the endocranial surface is formed by the posterior surface of the temporal and occipital bones, with the petro-occipital fissure and the jugular foramen lying between the occipital and temporal bones.

This exocranial surface is divided into central and lateral portions. The center portion is formed by the basal (clival) part of the occipital bone, which slopes upward from the foramen magnum and the occipital condyles, lateral to its lower portion at the anterolateral margin of the foramen magnum. Lateral to the condyle lies the jugular process of the occipital bone, which forms the posterior edge of the jugular foramen and connects the squamosal and basal parts of the occipital bone. The relationships in the cranial base are not reviewed in detail in this issue; they were covered in the Millennium issue of *Neurosurgery* (8).

DISCUSSION

With the development of the combination of micro-operative techniques and cranial-base surgery, it has become possible to access all parts of the cranial base. Approaches to the posterior fossa, including the foramen magnum, clivus, and approaches directed through the temporal bone, were reviewed in the Millennium issue of *Neurosurgery* (8). The anterior and middle cranial base offers the possibility of numerous approaches from above or below, or as combined procedures.

Lesions involving the medial parts of the anterior and middle cranial base can be accessed through an intracranial or subcranial route, or a combination of the two routes. From above, the transcranial-transbasal approach, involving a bifrontal craniotomy with preservation of the supraorbital rim, can be used to access the ethmoidal and sphenoid sinuses, sella, and clivus in the medial part of the cranial base, plus the adjacent lateral part of the anterior cranial base (7). Extending the transcranial-transbasal approach by removing the supraorbital rims provides greater access to the frontal, ethmoid, and sphenoid sinuses, medial orbit, nasal cavity, and clivus (*Fig. 6.12*). The supraorbital osteotomy can be tailored to include not only the midline and adjacent part of the supraorbital rims, but can include the area extending from one lateral orbital rim to the other, so that the lateral wall and roof of the orbits plus the roof of the nasal cavity can be elevated in a single osteotomy. However, it is important that the approach be tailored to the site, size, and nature of the pathology. A limited orbitofrontal approach, in which only the superior orbital rim is elevated in conjunction with a small frontal bone flap, provides access to the orbit and intracranial area around the optic canal. A further extension of the approach involving an osteotomy of the superior orbital rim is the orbitozygomatic craniotomy in which the superior and lateral orbital rims are elevated in conjunction with a frontotemporal bone flap. The orbitozygomatic approach is selected for lesions involving the lateral orbital wall and superior orbital fissure, cavernous sinus, middle fossa, and paraclinoid area. The orbitozygomatic approach can be extended further posteriorly by elevating the zygomatic arch with the osteotomy to access the middle and infratemporal fossae. A more strictly localized approach to the middle cranial base would be through a preauricular subtemporal approach in which a temporal or frontotemporal craniotomy is combined with an extradural middle fossa exposure to access the internal auditory canal. This approach is used for removal of small acoustic neuromas or removal of the petrous apex (anterior petrosectomy) for exposure of the clivus and upper part of the posterior fossa including the upper trunk and apex of the basilar artery. The approach, directed through the middle fossa floor lateral to the internal acoustic meatus with exposure or removal of the semicircular canals, thus completing a middle fossa translabyrinthine approach, provides an extended middle fossa exposure of the posterior fossa.

The anterior and middle cranial base can also be approached from below. The most localized of the approaches

FIGURE 6.15. A–C, *transmaxillary exposure of the cranial base.* A, *in this dissection, a midfacial soft tissue flap has been reflected laterally to expose the anterior surface of the right maxilla. The operative approach to the maxillary sinus is more commonly performed using a sublabial incision in the gingivobuccal margin rather than through an incision on the face. The approach can be completed without dividing the infraorbital nerve, but in this dissection, it was divided below the infraorbital foramen. The nerve, if divided, can be resutured at the time of closing. The infratemporal fossa, which is situated below the greater sphenoid wing, has been exposed by removing the coronoid process of the mandible and a narrow wedge of zygoma.* B, *the anterior wall of the maxillary sinus has been removed. The roof of the maxillary sinus forms the majority of the floor of the orbit. The infratemporal fossa contains the pterygoid muscles, mandibular nerve, maxillary artery, and the pterygoid venous plexus.* C, *the medial and lateral walls of the maxillary sinus have been opened, but the posterior part of the sinus wall, which forms the anterior wall of the pterygopalatine fossa, has been preserved. Removing the medial wall of the sinus exposes the nasal cavity, turbinates, and nasal septum. The maxillary artery crosses the lateral pterygoid muscle to reach the pterygopalatine fossa, which is located behind the upper part of the posterior wall of the maxillary sinus and below the orbital apex.* D, *the posterior wall of the maxillary sinus has been removed to expose the pterygopalatine fossa and orbital floor. The pterygopalatine fossa is located below the orbital apex and the posteromedial part of the inferior orbital fissure. The maxillary nerve enters the pterygopalatine fossa by passing through the foramen rotundum. The maxillary nerve gives rise to the infraorbital nerve, which passes forward in the infraorbital canal in the sinus roof and orbital floor.* E, *enlarged view of infratemporal and pterygopalatine fossae. Distally, the maxillary artery enters the pterygopalatine fossa, which is located in the lateral wall of the nasal cavity below the orbital apex.* F, *the exposure has been directed medially through the nasal cavity to the clivus, which has been opened to expose the vertebral and basilar arteries and the front of the brainstem. The exposure has been extended upward by opening the sphenoid sinus and exposing the left intracavernous carotid. The margin of the foramen magnum has been preserved.* A., *artery;* Bas., *basilar;* Brs., *branches;* Cav., *cavernous;* CN, *cranial nerve;* For., *foramen;* Inf., *inferior;* Infraorb., *infraorbital;* Infratemp., *infratemporal;* Lat., *lateral;* M., *muscle;* Max., *maxillary;* Mid., *middle;* N., *nerve;* Nasolac., *nasolacrimal;* Pet., *petrosal;* Plex., *plexus;* Post., *posterior;* Pteryg., *pterygoid;* Pterygopal., *pterygopalatine;* Seg., *segment;* Sphen., *sphenoid;* Ven., *venous;* Vert., *vertebral.*

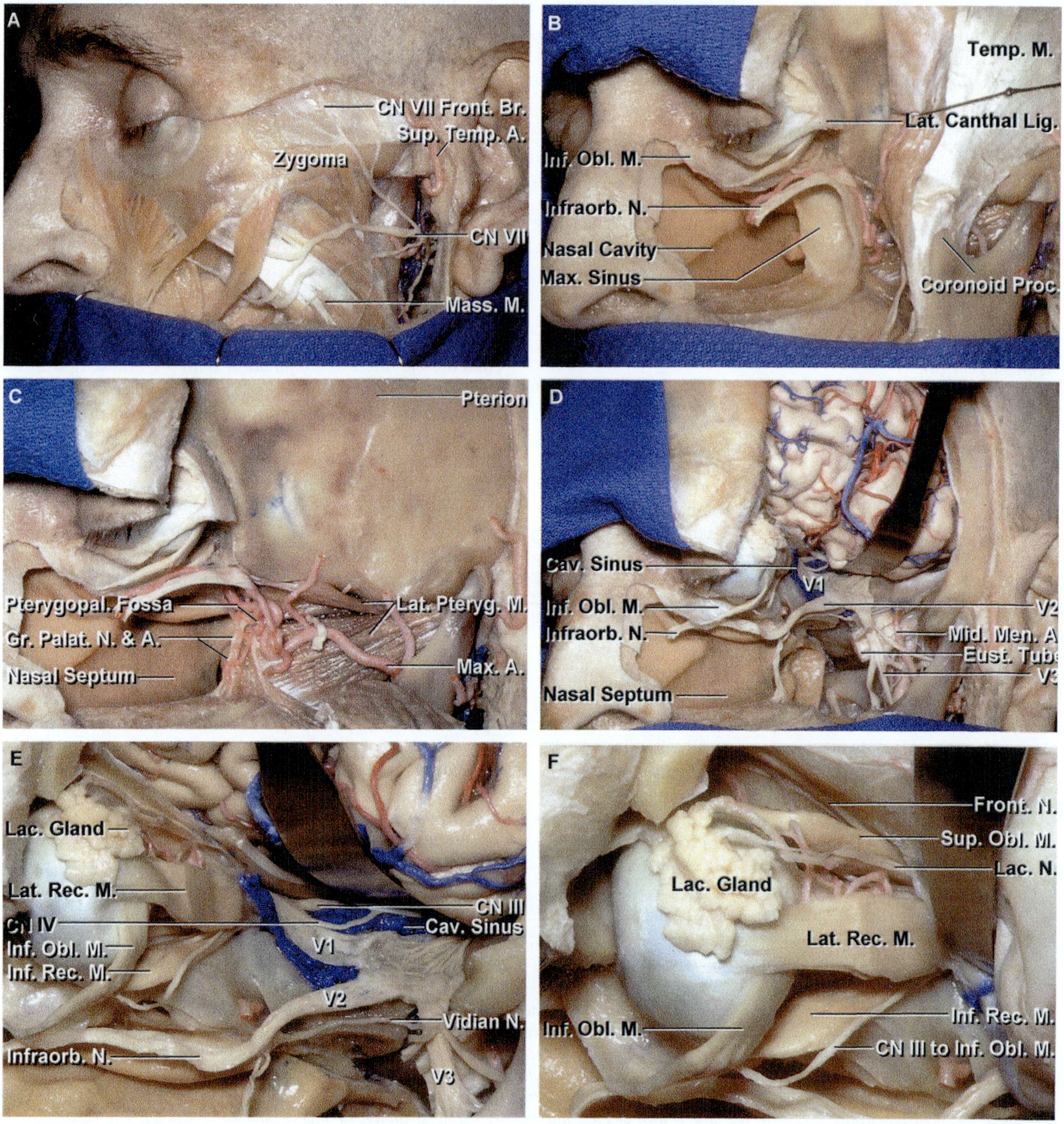

FIGURE 6.16. *Upper subtotal maxillotomy. Exposure obtained with mobilization of the upper part of the maxilla.* A, *this approach uses paranasal, lower conjunctival, transverse temporal, and preauricular incisions. In the usual approach, the cheek flap is elevated as a single layer using subperiosteal dissection. In this dissection, the layers of the cheek flap were dissected separately to illustrate the structures in the flap. The facial muscles and branches of the facial nerve are exposed. The parotid gland has been removed. The frontal branch of the facial nerve crosses the middle portion of the zygomatic arch. If facial nerve branches are transected in the approach, they are tagged in preparation for reapproximation at closure.* B, *a hemicoronal scalp incision and reflection of the temporalis muscle exposes the lateral orbital rim. The cheek flap containing the facial muscles, branches of the facial nerve, parotid gland, and masseter muscle have been reflected inferiorly to the level of the maxillary attachment of the buccinator muscle. The orbital, maxillary, and zygomatic osteotomies have been completed and the lower half of the orbital rim, the anterior, medial, and lateral walls of the maxillary sinus, and the zygomatic arch have been reflected. The lower horizontal cut, located at the Le Fort I level, extends above the apical dental roots and hard palate and along the inferior nasal meatus medially. The maxillotomy, at this stage, does not include the posterior maxillary wall or cross the greater and lesser palatine canals. The lat-*

from below is the transsphenoidal approach that can be performed either through a sublabial incision, a small incision along the side of the nasal septum, or as an endonasal or endoscopic approach directed through the nasal cavity between the nasal concha and septum (*Fig. 6.8*). Another relatively focal midline subcranial exposure is the transoral approach, which can be tailored to reach not only the clivus and upper cervical spine, but can be extended with division of the soft palate or removal of a part of the hard palate to access the sphenoid sinus superiorly or the midcervical levels below, if combined with midline transection of the tongue, mandible, or both (*Fig. 6.13*). The area below the anterior and middle cranial base can also be approached through a lateral rhinotomy incision, along the side of the nose, so that the nose can be reflected to provide access to the nasal cavity, medial orbit, the maxillary, ethmoidal, and sphenoid sinuses, and the clivus (*Fig. 6.14*). The transmaxillary approaches, either unilateral or bilateral as with the Le Fort osteotomy, can be used to provide access to the anterior and middle part of the lateral cranial base (*Figs. 6.13–6.15*). All of the central cranial base back to the foramen magnum can be accessed using the Le Fort I maxillotomy extending through the maxilla bilaterally above the dental apices and below the infraorbital canals with down-fracture of the maxillae (*Fig. 6.15*). If greater exposure is needed, the down-fractured bimaxillary segment can be divided in the midline, and the maxillae reflected laterally. There is also the possibility of using a unilateral upper or lower subtotal transmaxillary approach to access the anterior and middle cranial base (1, 2). In the lower subtotal maxillotomy approach, the portion of one maxilla located below the infraorbital canal is folded down into the floor of the mouth, thus providing access to the nasal cavity medially, the pterygopalatine fossa posteriorly, and infratemporal fossa posterolaterally (*Fig. 6.15*). The portion of the route directed through the nasal cavity can be used to reach the medial wall of the orbit and the paranasal sinuses, clivus, and upper cervical region. Another variant of the transmaxillary approach is the upper subtotal maxillotomy, in which one maxilla above the dental apex and including the orbital floor and lateral wall is mobilized to provide access to the parapharyngeal space, orbit, and upper part of the infratemporal fossa (*Fig. 6.16*) (1, 2). The upper maxillotomy approach can be combined with a frontotemporal craniotomy to yield intracranial access similar to that obtained with an orbitozygomatic craniotomy in addition to that obtained with the upper maxillotomy.

A preauricular infratemporal approach, using a preauricular skin incision, can also be used to access the middle cranial base, and infratemporal fossa and upper cervical carotid, plus the clivus and structures on the anterior side of the jugular foramen and foramen magnum (*Fig. 6.9*). The mandibular condyle can be displaced downward or resected to gain access to the upper cervical segment of the internal carotid artery and can be combined with a craniotomy to expose the middle fossa floor. The approach allows the petrous carotid to be reflected forward out of the carotid canal after resection of the eustachian tube and tensor tympani. After reflecting the carotid artery forward out of the carotid canal, the petrous apex on the medial side of the carotid canal can be removed for exposure of the upper medial part of the posterior fossa.

Because these lesions do not strictly adhere to the anatomic subdivisions of the cranial base, variations of the transcranial, subcranial, and combined approaches must often be innovatively combined for tumors of the cranial base that extend along the intracranial and subcranial structures and along the foramina and fissures in the cranial base. The approaches can be combined to provide access to virtually all of the anterior, middle, and posterior cranial base and should be tailored accurately so that they are not overly extensive and yet are sufficient to deal optimally with the pathology in a manner achieving the least disfiguring and most cosmetically and therapeutically acceptable results.

eral nasal wall was included with the maxillotomy to expose the nasal cavity. The infraorbital nerve, which crosses the orbital floor, may be preserved for reconstruction. C, *the posterior wall of the maxillary sinus has been removed to expose the pterygopalatine fossa and the palatine nerves and arteries. The base of the coronoid process was divided, and the temporalis reflected downward to expose the lateral pterygoid muscle and maxillary artery in the infratemporal fossa.* D, *a frontotemporal bone flap has been elevated, the dura covering the frontal and temporal lobes and lateral wall of the cavernous sinus have been opened, and the temporal lobe has been elevated. The pterygoid muscles, the pterygoid process and plates, and the part of the middle fossa floor formed by the greater sphenoid wing have been removed to expose the nerves passing through the foramina rotundum and ovale. The eustachian tube is exposed behind the mandibular nerve and the middle meningeal artery.* E, *magnified view of the cavernous sinus, superior orbital fissure, and orbit. The oculomotor, trochlear, and ophthalmic nerves course through the lateral wall of the cavernous sinus. The ophthalmic nerve sends its branches along the upper part of the orbit. The maxillary nerve exits the foramen rotundum and passes through the pterygopalatine fossa, where it gives rise to the infraorbital nerve that courses along the floor of the orbit. The mandibular nerve passes through the foramen ovale and sends its branches through the infratemporal fossa. The vidian nerve passes forward in the vidian canal below the maxillary nerve to join the pterygopalatine ganglion in the pterygopalatine fossa.* F, *enlarged view of the orbital exposure. The lacrimal gland sits on the superolateral margin of the globe. The lacrimal nerve courses above the lateral rectus muscle. The inferior oblique muscle passes below the attachment of the inferior rectus muscle and upward between the globe and lateral rectus muscle to insert on the globe near the tendon of insertion of the superior oblique muscle.* A., *artery;* Br., *branch;* Cav., *cavernous;* CN, *cranial nerve;* Eust., *eustachian;* Front., *frontal;* Gr., *greater;* Inf., *inferior;* Infraorb., *infraorbital;* Lac., *lacrimal;* Lat., *lateral;* Lig., *ligament;* M., *muscle;* Mass., *masseter;* Max., *maxillary;* Men., *meningeal;* Mid., *middle;* N., *nerve;* Obl., *oblique;* Palat., *palatine;* Proc., *process;* Pteryg., *pterygoid;* Pterygopal., *pterygopalatine;* Rec., *rectus;* Sup., *superior;* Temp., *temporal, temporalis.*

REFERENCES

1. Hitotsumatsu T, Rhoton AL Jr: Unilateral upper and lower subtotal maxillectomy approaches to the skull base: Microsurgical anatomy. **Neurosurgery** 46:1416–1453, 2000.
2. Hitotsumatsu T, Matsushima T, Rhoton AL Jr: Surgical anatomy of the midface and the midline skull base, in Spetzler RF (ed): *Operative Techniques in Neurosurgery*. Philadelphia, W.B. Saunders Co., vol 2, 1999, pp 160–180.
3. Inoue T, Rhoton AL Jr, Theele D, Barry ME: Surgical approaches to the cavernous sinus: A microsurgical study. **Neurosurgery** 26:903–932, 1990.
4. Natori Y, Rhoton AL Jr: Transcranial approach to the orbit: Microsurgical anatomy. **J Neurosurg** 81:78–86, 1994.
5. Natori Y, Rhoton AL Jr: Microsurgical anatomy of the superior orbital fissure. **Neurosurgery** 36:762–775, 1995.
6. Pait TG, Zeal AA, Harris FS, Paullus WS, Rhoton AL Jr: Microsurgical anatomy and dissection of the temporal bone. **Surg Neurol** 8:363–391, 1977.
7. Rhoton AL Jr: The foramen magnum. **Neurosurgery** 47[Suppl 1]:S155–S193, 2000.
8. Rhoton AL Jr: The posterior cranial fossa: Microsurgical anatomy and surgical approaches. **Neurosurgery** 47[Suppl 1]:S1–S298, 2000.
9. Rhoton AL Jr, Natori Y: *The Orbit and Sellar Region: Microsurgical Anatomy and Operative Approaches*. New York, Thieme Medical Publishers, Inc., 1996, pp 3–25.
10. Rhoton AL Jr, Harris FS, Renn WH: Microsurgical anatomy of the sellar region and cavernous sinus. **Clin Neurosurg** 24:54–85, 1977.
11. Seoane E, Rhoton AL Jr, de Oliveira EP: Microsurgical anatomy of the dural collar (carotid collar) and rings around the clinoid segment of the internal carotid artery. **Neurosurgery** 42:869–886, 1998.

Figure from D'Agoty Gautier's Essai d'anatomie, en tableaux imprimés. *Paris, 1748.*

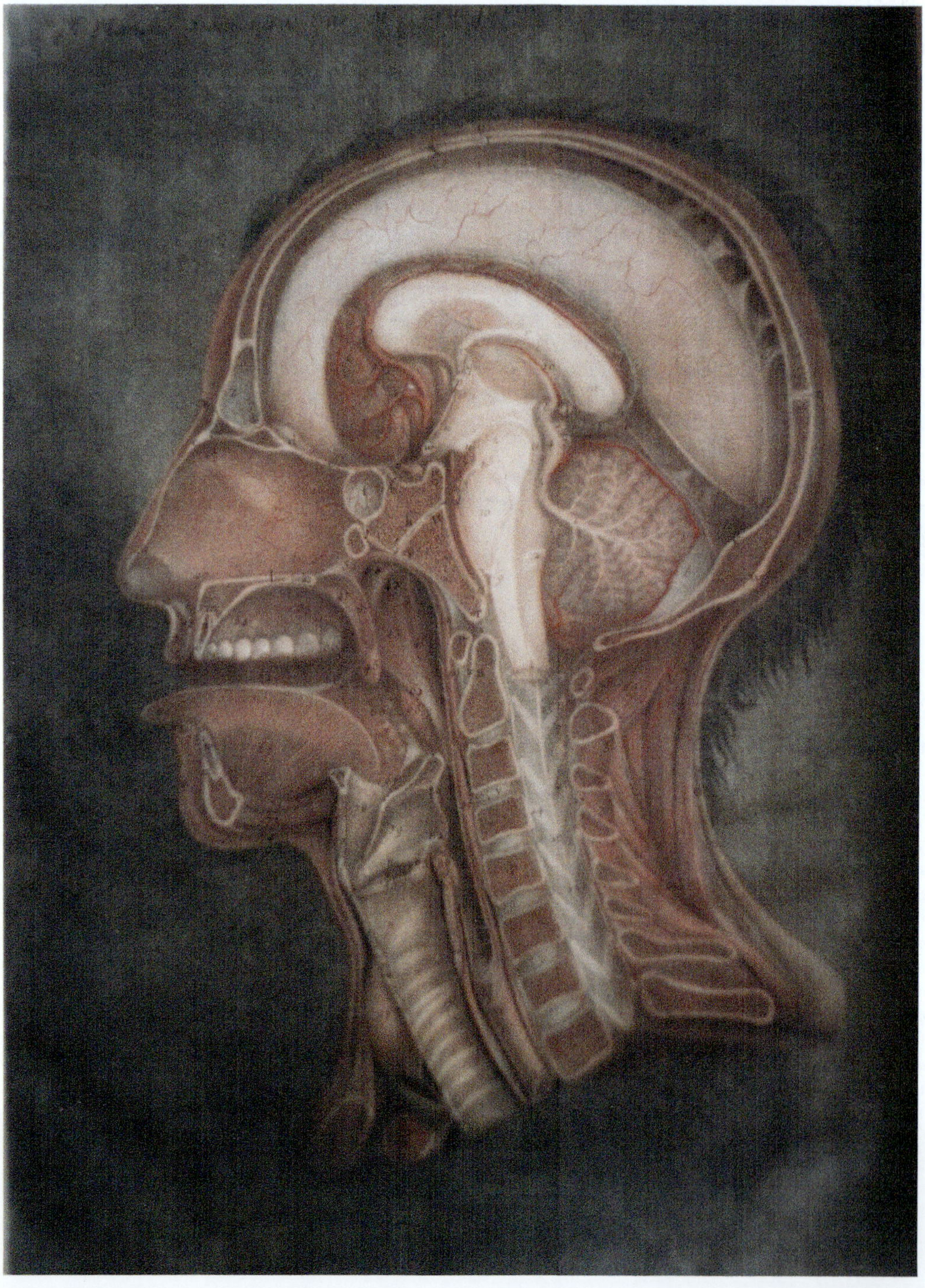

THE ORBIT

Albert L. Rhoton, Jr., M.D.

Department of Neurological Surgery, University of Florida, Gainesville, Florida

Correspondence:
Albert L. Rhoton, Jr., M.D., Department of Neurological Surgery, University of Florida McKnight Brain Institute, P.O. Box 100265, 100 South Newell Drive, Building 59, L2-100, Gainesville, FL 32610-0265.
Email: rhoton@neurosurgery.ufl.edu

KEY WORDS: Cranial base, Cranial nerves, Extraocular muscles, Microsurgical anatomy, Ophthalmic artery, Ophthalmic veins, Optic nerve, Orbit, Skull base, Surgical approach

OVERVIEW

The orbit is the complexly organized group of neural, vascular, muscular, ligamentous, and osseous structures that opens onto the face and external world to collect and provide binocular visual information to the brain. The retina, which captures visual information, is protected from external trauma, overexposure, and excessive light by the eyelids and a precisely organized mechanism for modulating light reaching the biological visual screen. The globe is surrounded by a precisely coordinated group of muscles encased in fat to allow free movement of the globe and muscles, but limited at the extremes by ligamental structures to prevent excessive mobility. Nearly all of the bones forming the anterior and middle cranial base contribute to the formation of the orbit's walls. The orbit communicates posteriorly with the anterior and middle cranial fossae and inferiorly with the pterygopalatine and infratemporal fossa. The nerves and vessels entering and exiting the orbit pass through the optic canal and superior orbital fissure, which are partially surrounded by an annular tendon, from which the rectus muscles arise. The fact that many of the neural and vascular structures entering the orbit pass through not only an osseous channel, but also through the annular tendon, creates an added complexity when considering approaches to the orbit and especially those involving the orbital apex. The orbit can be approached surgically from anteriorly through the face and conjunctivae or through any of its walls and from intracranially. The most common neurosurgical approaches are directed through the superior and lateral walls to lesions located deep in the orbit near the apex or involving the optic canal, superior orbital fissure, and adjacent areas (21, 22, 24).

OSSEOUS RELATIONSHIPS

The walls of the orbit are formed by seven bones: frontal, zygomatic, sphenoid, lacrimal, ethmoid, and palatine bones and the maxilla (*Fig. 7.1*). The upper border of the orbital opening is formed by the frontal bone, which is notched or is the site of one or several small foramina that transmit the supraorbital and supratrochlear nerves and vessels. The lateral border of the orbital opening is formed by the frontal process of the zygomatic bone, except for the upper part, which is formed by the zygomatic process of the frontal bone. The lower margin of the orbital opening is formed laterally by the zygomatic bone and medially by the maxilla. The upper part of the medial border is formed by the frontal bone and the lower part is formed by the frontal process of the maxilla. The medial part of the upper border contains the frontal sinus.

The anterior part of the orbital roof is formed by the orbital plate of the frontal bone, and the posterior part is formed by the lesser wing of the sphenoid bone, which also forms most of the sphenoid ridge (*Figs. 7.1* and *7.2*). The sphenoid and ethmoid bones are interposed between the orbital roofs. The ethmoid bone is the site of the cribriform plate and the upward-projecting crista galli to which the falx attaches. Anteriorly, the frontal bone splits into two laminae, which enclose the frontal sinuses. The lacrimal fossa, the depression in which the lacrimal gland rests, is located below the anterolateral part of the roof. Another small depression in the anteromedial part of the roof, the trochlear fossa, serves as the attachment for the trochlea of the superior oblique muscle.

The floor of the orbit is formed by the orbital plate of the maxilla, the orbital surface of zygomatic bone, and the orbital process of the palatine bone. The orbital floor, which is very thin, forms the roof of the maxillary sinus. The floor is continuous with the medial wall, except in the most anterior part, where the floor is perforated by the nasolacrimal canal. The anterior part of the floor is continuous with the lateral wall, but posteriorly, the floor and lateral wall are separated by the inferior orbital fissure. The infraorbital groove, which transmits the infraorbital branch of the maxillary nerve, leads forward out of the inferior orbital fissure to cross the floor to reach the infraorbital canal, which ends below the lower orbital rim in the infraorbital foramen.

The lateral wall consists predominantly of the greater sphenoid wing and the frontal process of the zygomatic bone. The greater sphenoid wing also forms much of the middle fossa floor and the roof of the infratemporal fossa. Superiorly, the anterior part of the lateral orbital wall is continuous with the roof, but the posterior part of the lateral wall is separated from the roof by the superior orbital fissure. The lacrimal foramen, which transmits the recurrent meningeal branch of the ophthalmic artery, is located anterior to the superior orbital fissure along the superior edge of the lateral wall. The zygomatico-

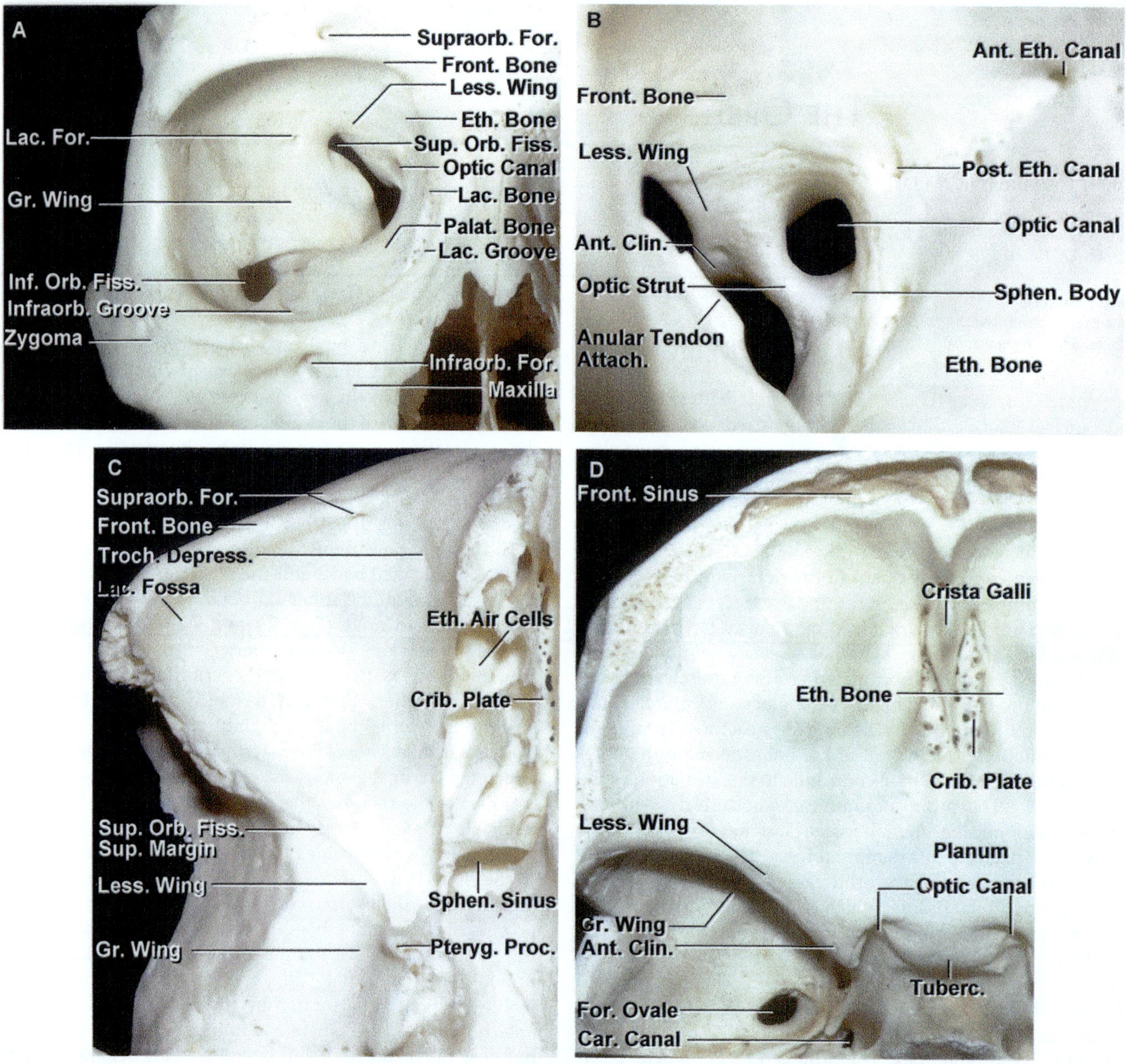

FIGURE 7.1. *Osseous relationships of the orbit.* A, *anterior view of the right orbit. The walls of the orbit are formed by seven bones. They are the frontal, zygomatic, sphenoid, lacrimal, ethmoid, and palatine bones, and the maxilla. The lateral border of the orbital opening is formed by the frontal process of the zygoma, except the upper part, which is formed by the zygomatic process of the frontal bone. The lower margin of the orbital opening is formed laterally by the zygoma and medially by the maxilla. The upper part of the medial border is formed by the frontal bone and the lower part is formed by the frontal process of the maxilla. The medial part of the upper border contains the frontal sinus. The superior orbital fissure is bounded above by the lesser wing of the sphenoid bone, below by the greater wing, and medially by the sphenoid body. The frontal bone forms the narrow lateral apex of the superior orbital fissure. The inferior orbital fissure is bounded posteriorly by the greater sphenoid wing and anteriorly by the maxilla. The supraorbital margin is notched or is the site of one or several small foramina that transmit the supraorbital nerves and vessels. The infraorbital groove, which transmits the infraorbital branch of the maxillary nerve, leads forward out of the inferior orbital fissure to cross the floor to reach the infraorbital canal, which ends in the infraorbital foramen.* B, *anterior aspect of the right optic canal. The optic canal, which transmits the optic nerve and ophthalmic artery, opens into the superomedial corner of the orbital apex. The optic canal is situated at the junction of the lesser wing with the sphenoid body. It is separated from the superior orbital fissure by the optic strut, a bridge of bone, which extends from the lower margin of the anterior clinoid to the sphenoid body. The optic strut is also referred to as the posterior root of the lesser wing. The tendinous ring, referred to as the annular tendon, from which the four rectus muscles arise, is attached to the upper, lower, and medial margin of the optic canal. The lateral edge of the annular tendon is attached to the midportion of the lateral edge*

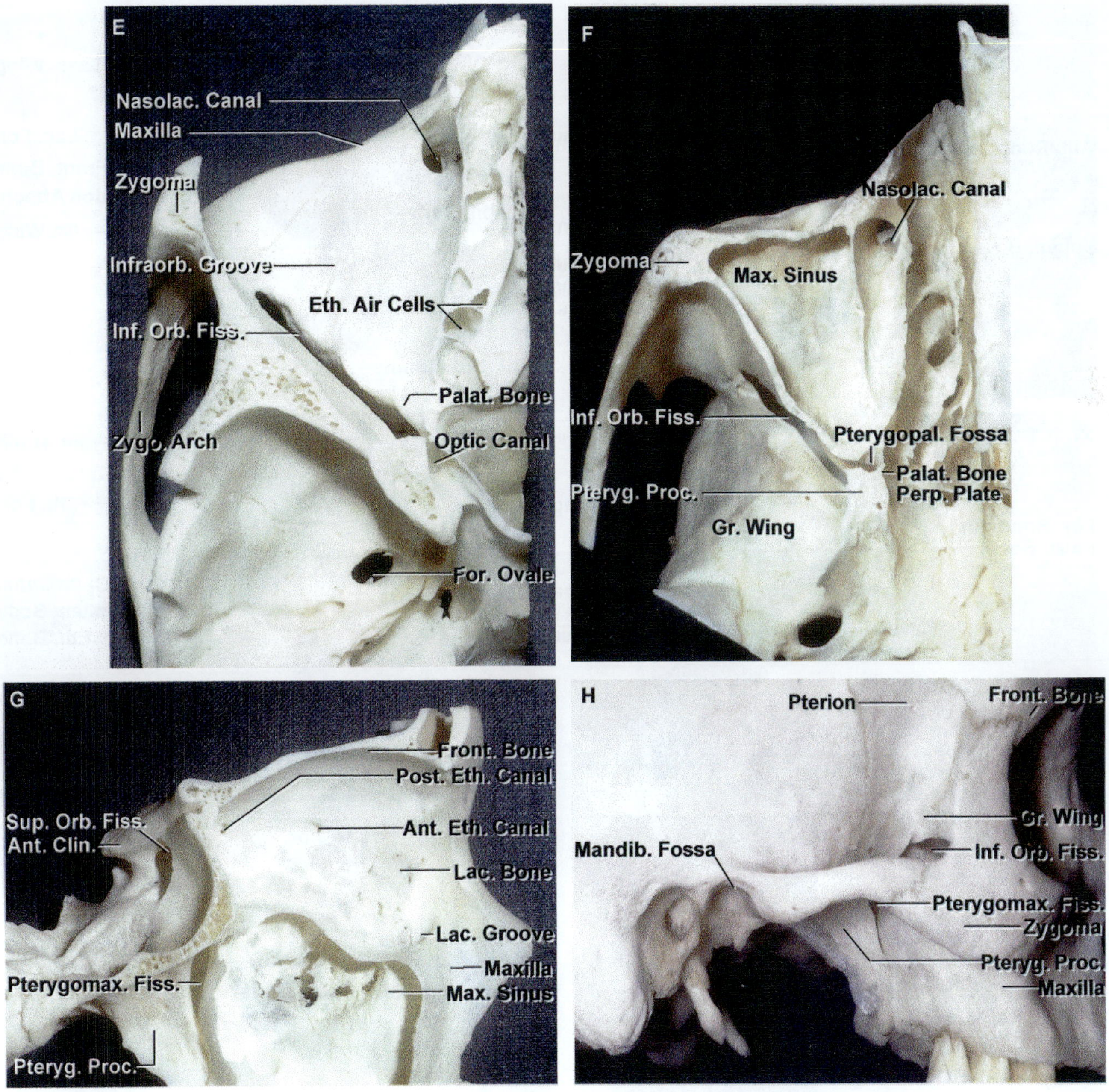

FIGURE 7.1. *Continued*
of the superior orbital fissure, where a bony prominence on the greater wing marks the junction of medial and lateral parts of the fissure. C, *roof of the right orbit viewed from below. The roof of the orbit is formed by the orbital plate of the frontal bone anteriorly and the lesser sphenoid wing posteriorly. The lacrimal fossa is the depression in the anterolateral part of the roof in which the lacrimal gland rests. There is another small depression on the anteromedial part of the roof that serves as the attachment for the trochlea of the superior oblique muscle. The optic foramen is situated posteriorly at the junction of the roof and medial wall. The ethmoid air cells and sphenoid sinus are located along the medial edge of the orbital roof.* D, *superior aspect of the floor of the anterior cranial fossae that forms the roof of both orbits. The cribriform plate of the ethmoid bone is situated in the midline between the orbital roofs. The crista galli serves as the site of attachment of the cerebral falx. Anteriorly, the frontal sinus splits into two laminae that enclose the frontal sinuses. The internal carotid artery exits the carotid canal above the foramen lacerum and passes forward in the carotid sulcus on the lateral part of the sphenoid body.* E, *floor of the right orbit viewed from above. The orbital floor is formed by the orbital plate of the maxilla, the orbital surface of the zygoma, and the orbital process of the palatine bone. The orbital floor, which is very thin, forms most of the roof of the maxillary sinus. The floor is continuous with the medial wall, except in the most anterior part where the floor is perforated by the nasolacrimal canal. The anterior part of the floor is continuous with the lateral wall, but posteriorly, the floor and lateral wall are separated by the inferior orbital fissure. The infraorbital groove, which transmits the infraorbital branch of the maxillary nerve, leads forward out of the inferior orbital fissure to cross the floor to reach the infraorbital canal, which ends in*
(Legend continues on next page.)

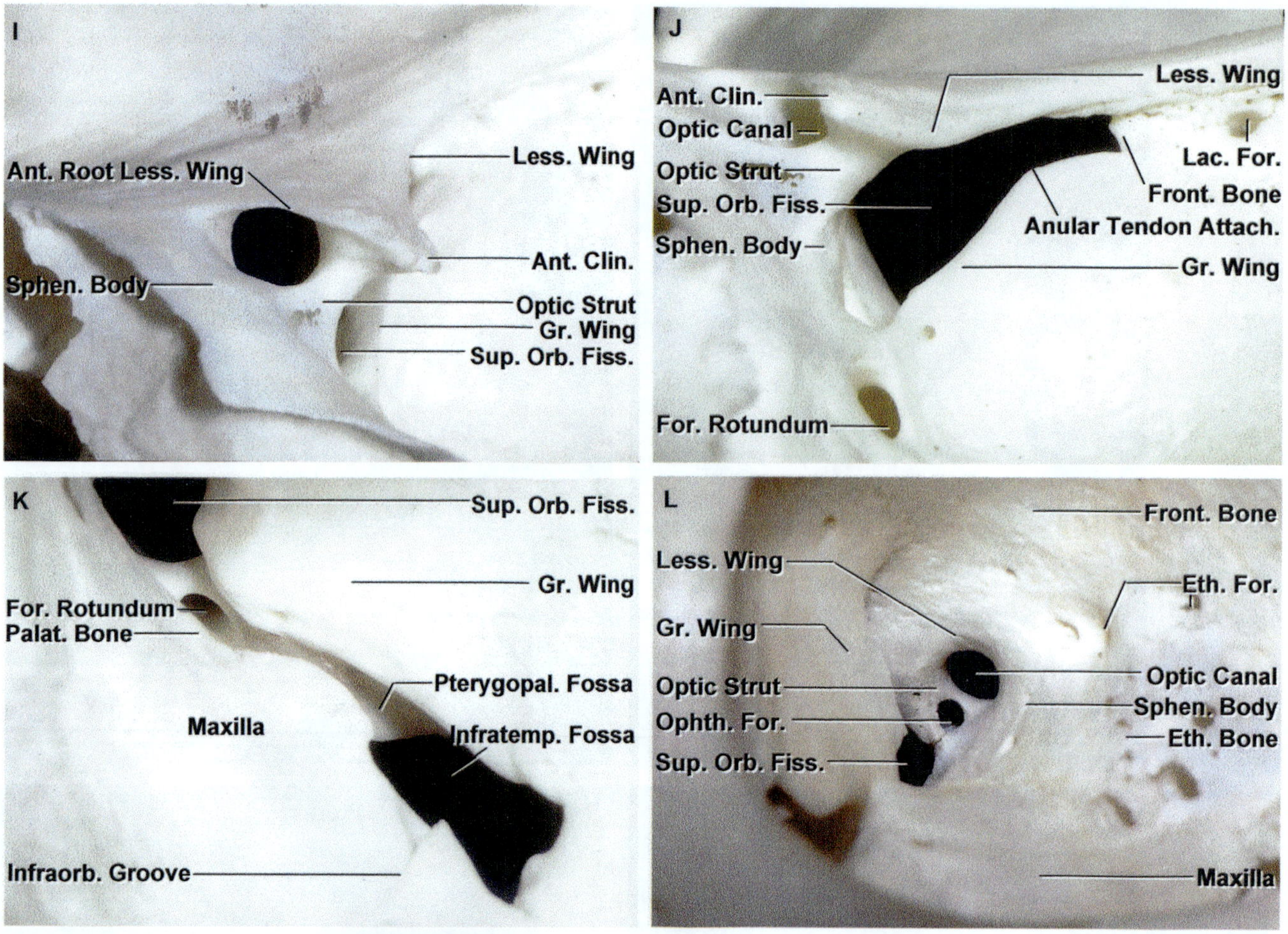

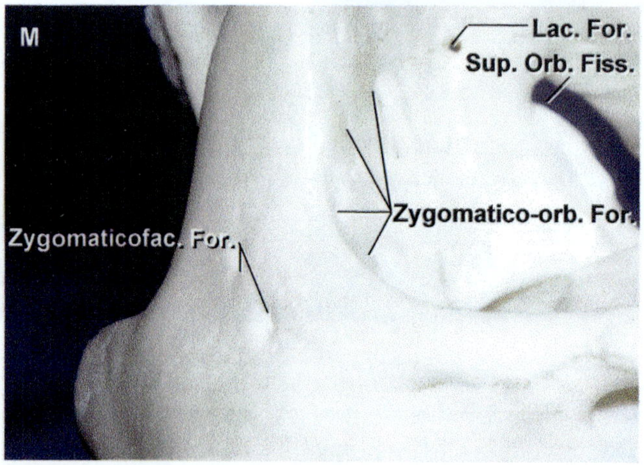

FIGURE 7.1. *Continued* *the infraorbital foramen. The posterior part of the inferior orbital fissure communicates below with the pterygopalatine fossa, and the anterior part communicates with the infratemporal fossa.* F, *inferior aspect of the roof of the maxillary sinus, which also forms the floor of the orbit. The greater sphenoid wing forms much of the middle fossa floor and the posterior part of the lateral orbital wall. The pterygopalatine fossa is located behind the maxillary sinus and contains the terminal part of the maxillary artery, the maxillary nerve, and the pterygopalatine ganglion and some branches of all three structures. The pterygopalatine fossa opens through the pterygomaxillary fissure into the infratemporal fossa, which is located below the greater sphenoid wing and contains the pterygoid muscles, a segment of the maxillary artery, branches of the mandibular nerve and the pterygoid venous plexus. The medial wall of the pterygopalatine fossa is formed by the perpendicular plate of the palatine bone and contains an opening, the sphenopalatine foramen, that communicates with the nasal cavity.* G, *lateral view of the medial wall of the right orbit. The medial wall is formed by the frontal process of the maxilla, the lacrimal bone, the orbital plate of the ethmoid bone, and the sphenoid body. The medial wall is extremely thin in the area of the orbital plate of the ethmoid bone, which separates the orbit and ethmoidal sinuses. The lacrimal sac, which sits in the lacrimal groove, drains into the nasal cavity through the nasolacrimal canal. The lacrimal groove is formed by the frontal process of the maxilla anteriorly and the lacrimal bone posteriorly. The anterior and posterior ethmoidal foramina, which transmit the anterior and posterior ethmoidal branches of the ophthalmic artery and the anterior and posterior ethmoidal branches of the nasociliary nerve, pass through the frontoethmoidal suture or the adjacent part of the frontal bone and open into the anterior cranial fossa along the lateral edge of the cribriform plate. The pterygomaxillary fissure opens into the pterygopalatine fossa.* H, *lateral aspect of the lateral wall of the right orbit. The zygoma forms the lateral*

orbital foramina on the anterolateral part of the intraorbital surface of the lateral wall transmit the zygomaticofacial and zygomaticotemporal nerves, which exit the external surface of the zygoma at the zygomaticofacial and zygomaticotemporal foramina to reach the skin of the cheek and temple.

The medial wall is formed, from anterior to posterior, by the frontal process of the maxilla, the lacrimal bone, the orbital plate of the ethmoid bone, and the body of the sphenoid bone. The medial wall is extremely thin, especially in the area of the orbital plate of the ethmoid bone, which separates the orbit and ethmoid air cells. The lacrimal sac, which sits in the lacrimal groove formed by the frontal process of the maxilla anteriorly and the lacrimal bone posteriorly, opens into the nasal cavity through the nasolacrimal canal. The anterior and posterior ethmoidal foramina, which transmit the anterior and posterior ethmoidal branches of the ophthalmic artery and the nasociliary nerve, are located at the junction of the roof and medial wall of the orbit and pass through the frontoethmoidal suture or the adjacent part of the frontal bone and open into the anterior cranial fossa along the lateral edge of the cribriform plate.

The optic canal, through which the optic nerve and ophthalmic artery pass, opens into the superomedial corner of the orbital apex at the junction of the roof and medial wall. The optic canal is situated at the junction of the lesser wing with the body of the sphenoid bone. It is separated from the superior orbital fissure by the optic strut, a bridge of bone, also referred to as the posterior root of the lesser wing, which extends from the lower margin of the base of the anterior clinoid process to the sphenoid body. The tendinous ring (annular tendon) from which the superior, inferior, medial, and lateral rectus muscles arise, is attached to the upper, lower, and medial margin of the optic canal. The anterior clinoid process projects backward from the lesser wing of the sphenoid bone into the interval between where the optic nerve enters the optic canal and where the oculomotor nerve enters the superior orbital fissure.

The intracranial end of the optic canal has an ovoid shape with a slightly greater diameter in the mediolateral than in the superior-inferior dimension. It is situated medial to the anterior clinoid process and optic strut. The medial margin is formed by the body of the sphenoid bone. The upper margin is formed by the anterior root of the lesser wing of the sphenoid bone. The lateral margin is formed by the optic strut. The lower margin of the foramen is formed by the optic strut and the adjacent part of the body of the sphenoid bone. The optic strut blends superolaterally into the base of the anterior clinoid process and inferiorly and medially into the body of the sphenoid bone. The anterior bend of the intracavernous segment of the internal carotid artery rests against the posterior surface of the optic strut and ascends on the medial side of the anterior clinoid process. The body of the sphenoid bone contains the sphenoid sinus. The chiasmatic sulcus is a shallow groove situated on the intracranial surface of the sphenoid

rim and the anterior part of the lateral wall of the orbit. Behind the zygoma, the lateral wall of the orbit is formed by the greater sphenoid wing. The temporal fossa is located between the zygomatic arch and the greater wing. The temporalis muscle arises in the temporal fossa and extends downward medial to the zygomatic arch to attach to the coronoid process of the mandible. The infratemporal fossa is located medial to the temporal fossa, below the greater sphenoid wing. The pterygomaxillary fissure, located between the posterior maxilla and the pterygoid process, opens into the pterygopalatine fossa. I, *intracranial aspect of the right optic canal. The intracranial end of the optic canal has an ovoid shape with a slightly greater diameter in the mediolateral than in the superoinferior dimension. It is situated medial to the anterior clinoid and optic strut. The medial margin is formed by the sphenoid body. The upper margin is formed by the anterior root of the lesser sphenoid wing. The lateral margin is formed by the optic strut, which is also referred to as the posterior root of the lesser wing. The lower margin of the foramen is formed by the optic strut and the adjacent part of the sphenoid body.* J, *intracranial aspect of the right superior orbital fissure. The superior orbital fissure provides a communication between the orbit and the middle fossa. It is bounded above by the lesser wing, below by the greater wing, and medially by the sphenoid body. A small portion of the lateral apex of the fissure is formed by the frontal bone. The midportion of the lateral margin of the fissure, at the junction of the fissure's narrow lateral and larger medial part, is the site of a prominence that serves as the lateral attachment of the annular tendon.* K, *orbital aspect of the right inferior orbital fissure. The inferior orbital fissure has long anterior and posterior borders and narrow medial and lateral ends. The long posterior edge is formed by the greater wing. The long anterior wall is formed by the orbital surface of the maxilla, except for a short posterior segment formed by the orbital process of the palatine bone. The narrow lateral end is formed by the zygomatic bone, and the narrow medial end is formed by the sphenoid body. The posteromedial part of the fissure communicates below with the pterygopalatine fossa, and the anterolateral part communicates with the infratemporal fossa. The orbital smooth muscle spans the upper part of the fissure.* L, *anterior aspect of the right optic canal and an anomalous ophthalmic foramen. In this specimen there is a foramen in the optic strut, referred to as an ophthalmic foramen, that transmits the ophthalmic artery.* M, *anterolateral view of the right zygomaticofacial foramina. The zygomaticofacial foramina transmit the zygomaticofacial branches of the maxillary nerve. The zygomatic nerve arises from the maxillary nerve in the pterygopalatine fossa and passes through the inferior orbital fissure to course along the lateral wall of the orbit, where it divides into zygomaticofacial and zygomaticotemporal branches. The branches enter the zygomatico-orbital foramina on the orbital surface of the zygomatic bone. The zygomaticofacial branches exit the zygomaticofacial foramina to supply the cheek. The zygomaticotemporal nerve gives a branch to the lacrimal nerve as it passes along the inferolateral margin of the orbit. It enters the zygomatico-orbital foramen on the orbital surface and exits the zygomaticotemporal foramina to reach the temporal fossa above the zygomatic arch where it is distributed to the skin of the temple. The lacrimal foramen transmits a branch of the recurrent branch of the ophthalmic or lacrimal artery, which exits the orbit through the superior orbital fissure, courses laterally below the sphenoid ridge, and turns forward through the lacrimal foramen to supply the periorbita.* Ant., *anterior;* Attach., *attachment;* Car., *carotid;* Clin., *clinoid;* Crib., *cribriform;* Depress., *depression;* Eth., *ethmoid, ethmoidal;* Fiss., *fissure;* For., *foramen;* Front., *frontal;* Gr., *greater;* Inf., *inferior;* Infraorb., *infraorbital;* Infratemp., *infratemporal;* Lac., *lacrimal;* Less., *lesser;* Mandib., *mandibular;* Max., *maxillary;* Nasolac., *nasolacrimal;* Ophth., *ophthalmic;* Orb., *orbital;* Palat., *palatine;* Perp., *perpendicular;* Post., *posterior;* Proc., *process;* Pteryg., *pterygoid;* Pterygomax., *pterygomaxillary;* Pterygopal., *pterygopalatine;* Sphen., *sphenoid;* Sup., *superior;* Supraorb., *supraorbital;* Troch., *trochlear;* Tuberc., *tuberculum;* Zygo., *zygomatic;* Zygomaticofac., *zygomaticofacial;* Zygomatico-orb., *zygomatico-orbital.*

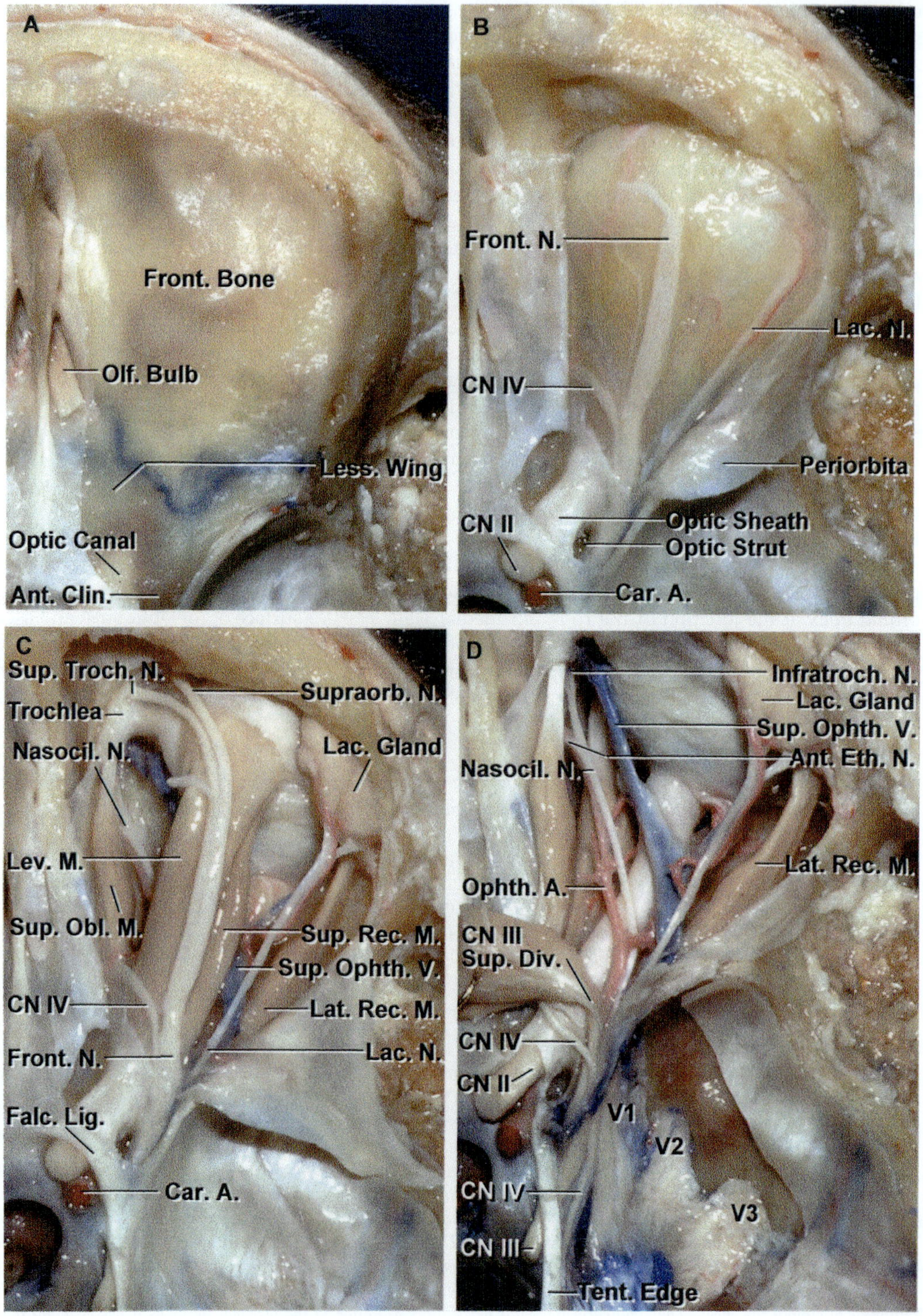

FIGURE 7.2. *Superior view of a stepwise dissection of the neural structures in the orbit and superior orbital fissure. A, the dura has been removed from the part of the frontal and sphenoid bones forming the orbital roof. The olfactory bulb rests on the cribriform plate. B, the orbit and optic canal have been unroofed, the anterior clinoid process removed, and the periorbita opened to expose the trochlear, frontal, and lacrimal nerves coursing in the orbital fat just beneath the periorbita. The optic strut, which has been partially removed, separates the optic canal and superior orbital fissure. C, the orbital fat has been removed. The ophthalmic nerve divides into the lacrimal, frontal, and nasociliary nerves. The frontal nerve passes through the superior orbital fissure and courses on the levator muscle where it divides into a supratrochlear nerve, which passes above the trochlea of the superior oblique muscle, and the supraorbital nerve, which passes through a foramen or notch in the supraorbital margin. The lacrimal nerve passes above the lateral rectus muscle to innervate the lacrimal gland and convey sensation to the area around the lateral part of the supraorbital margin. The trochlear nerve passes medially above the levator muscle to reach the superior oblique muscle. The nasociliary branch of the ophthalmic nerve passes between the superior rectus muscle and the optic nerve to reach the medial side of the orbit. The tendon of the superior oblique muscle passes through the trochlea and below the superior rectus muscle to insert on the globe between the attachment of the superior and lateral rectus muscles. D, the frontal nerve and the levator and superior rectus muscles have been divided and reflected. This exposes the superior ophthalmic vein, ophthalmic artery, and nasociliary nerve as they pass above the optic nerve. The dura lining the middle cranial fossa has been removed to expose the oculomotor, trochlear, and ophthalmic nerves as they course in the lateral wall of the cavernous sinus, and the maxillary and mandibular nerves in the middle fossa. The trochlear nerve passes forward in the wall of the cavernous sinus between the oculomotor and ophthalmic nerves and turns medially at the level of the superior orbital fissure to pass above the levator muscle. The optic nerve and ophthalmic artery pass through the optic canal and the medial part of the annular tendon. The trochlear, lacrimal, and frontal nerves and the superior ophthalmic vein pass through the narrow lateral part of the superior orbital fissure above and outside the annular tendon. The superior and inferior divisions of the oculomotor nerve, and the nasociliary and abducens nerves pass through the larger medial part of the superior orbital fissure and the annular tendon. E, the annular tendon has been divided in the interval between the origin of the superior and lateral rectus muscles. The oculomotor, abducens, and nasociliary nerves pass through the*

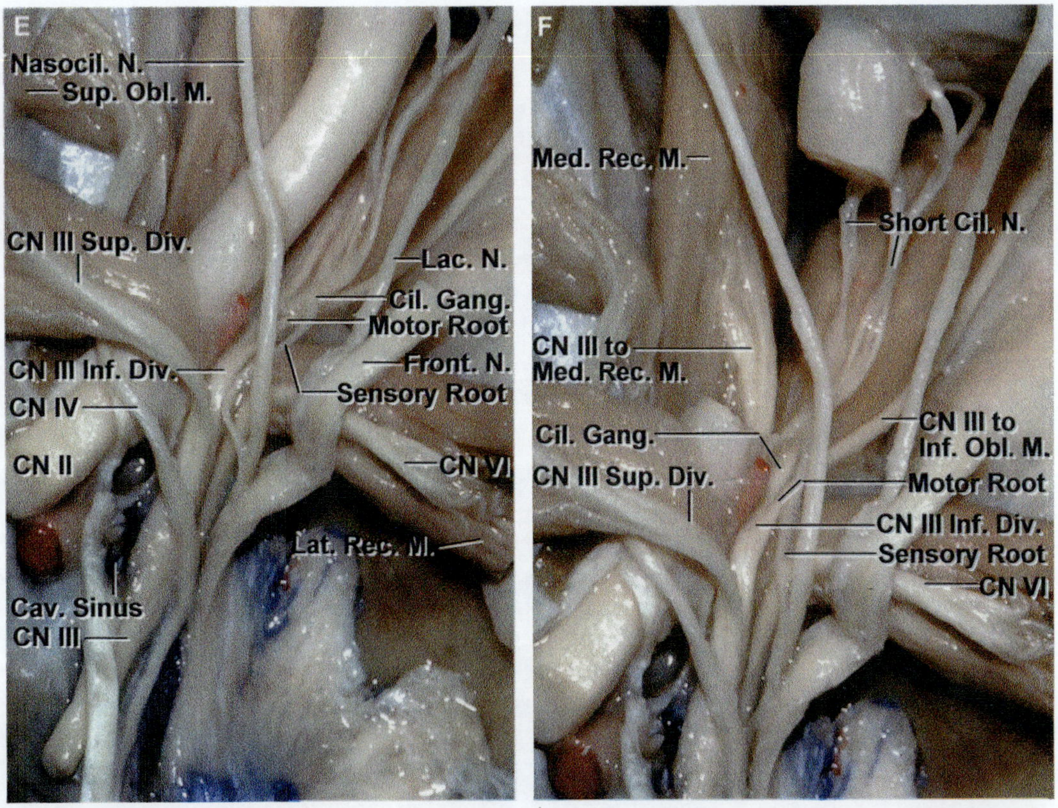

FIGURE 7.2. *Continued* *superior orbital fissure and annular tendon. The oculomotor nerve splits into superior and inferior divisions. The superior division branches on the lower surface of the superior rectus and sends branches along the medial margin of the superior rectus muscle to enter the levator muscle. The fibers of the inferior division give rise to three branches. One passes below the optic nerve to supply the medial rectus muscle, another enters the superior surface of the inferior rectus muscle, and the third branch courses along the lateral margin of the inferior rectus muscle to innervate the inferior oblique muscle. The branch to the inferior oblique muscle gives rise to the motor (parasympathetic) root to the ciliary ganglion. The nasociliary nerve arises from the medial surface of the ophthalmic nerve and gives rise to the sensory root of the ciliary ganglion. Short ciliary nerves arise from the ciliary ganglion and enter the globe around the optic nerve. The abducens nerve courses on the medial side of the ophthalmic nerve in the cavernous sinus, but it passes below the ophthalmic nerve in the superior orbital fissure to enter the medial surface of the lateral rectus muscle.* F, *a segment of the orbital portion of the optic nerve has been removed. This exposes the branch of the inferior division of the oculomotor nerve, which passes below the optic nerve and enters the medial rectus muscle. The short ciliary nerves arise from the ciliary ganglion and enter the globe around the margin of the optic nerve.* A., *artery;* Ant., *anterior;* Car., *carotid;* Cav., *cavernous;* Cil., *ciliary;* Clin., *clinoid;* CN, *cranial nerve;* Div., *division;* Eth., *ethmoidal;* Falc., *falciform;* Front., *frontal;* Gang., *ganglion;* Inf., *inferior;* Infratroch., *infratrochlear;* Lac., *lacrimal;* Lat., *lateral;* Less., *lesser;* Lev., *levator;* Lig., *ligament;* M., *muscle;* Med., *medial;* N., *nerve;* Nasocil., *nasociliary;* Obl., *oblique;* Olf., *olfactory;* Ophth., *ophthalmic;* Rec., *rectus;* Sup., *superior;* Supraorb., *supraorbital;* Sup. Troch., *supratrochlear;* Tent., *tentorial;* Troch., *trochlear;* V., *vein.*

body between the optic canals. The tuberculum sellae is located in the midline along the posterior margin of the chiasmatic sulcus.

The superior orbital fissure provides a communication between the orbit and the middle cranial fossa (*Figs. 7.1* and *7.3*) (22). The cavernous sinus is situated behind and fills the posterior margin, and the contents of the orbital apex are located in front of and fill the anterior margin of the fissure. The superior orbital fissure is situated between the greater and lesser wings and body of the sphenoid bone (22). It has a somewhat triangular shape, having a wide base medially on the sphenoid body and a narrow apex situated laterally between the lesser and greater wings. The frontal bone forms a small portion of the lateral apical margin of the fissure, because the greater and lesser wings approach, but do not meet at the narrow lateral apex. The fissure slopes gently downward from its lateral to medial border. The fissure is not oriented in a strictly coronal plane, but is directed forward so that the lateral apex is slightly forward of the medial margin.

The lateral edge of the superior orbital fissure, formed by the thin edge of the greater wing, is the sharpest and best-defined border. The lateral border slopes downward from its lateral to medial end. The upper half of this border is located in a more horizontal plane, and the lower half has a more vertical orientation. The junction of the upper and lower segments of the lateral edge is the site of a bony prominence that serves as the site of attachment of the lateral edge of the annular tendon, from which the four rectus muscles arise. This bony prominence can vary from narrow and pointed to broad and flat.

The superior wall of the fissure is formed by the lower surfaces of the lesser wing, the anterior clinoid process, and the adjacent part of the optic strut. The upper edge of the fissure is situated below the medial half of the sphenoid ridge. The anterior clinoid process projects backward above the junction of the narrow lateral and broader medial part of the fissure. The optic strut forms the upper medial border of the fissure. The strut forms the lateral edge of the optic foramen and the junction of the upper and medial walls of the superior orbital fissure.

The medial margin of the fissure is less sharply defined than the lateral margin. The upper part of the medial edge is

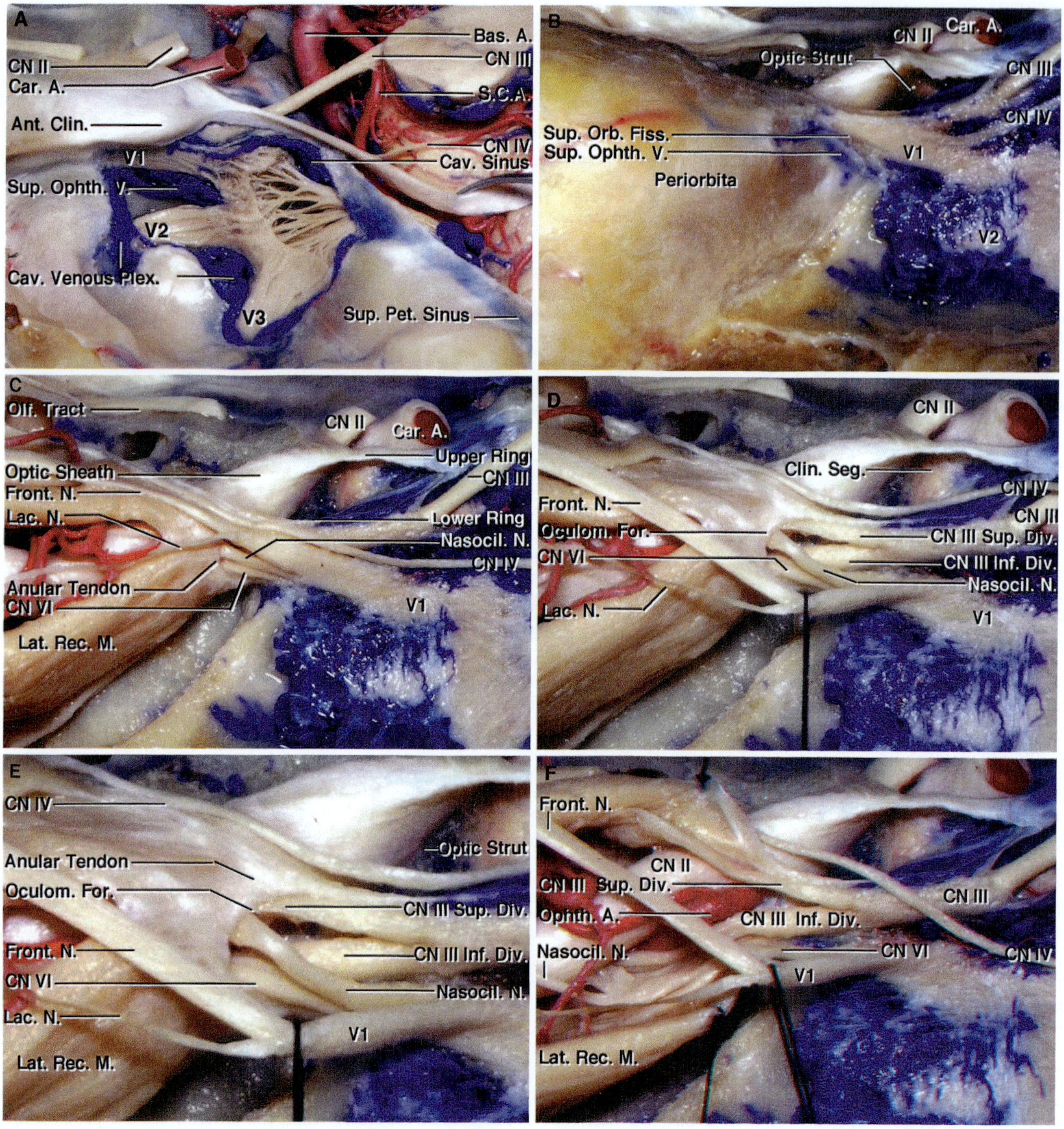

FIGURE 7.3. *Left lateral view of a stepwise dissection of the superior orbital fissure and adjacent part of the cavernous sinus and orbit.* A, *the dura covering Meckel's cave and cavernous sinus has been removed. The cavernous sinus is located medial to the upper third of the gasserian ganglion and extends down to the lower margin of the ophthalmic nerve. The superior ophthalmic vein exits the orbit and passes below the ophthalmic nerve to enter the anterior part of the cavernous sinus. The superior petrosal sinus passes above the porus of Meckel's cave to join the posterior part of the cavernous sinus. The superior orbital fissure is filled on its posterior side by the cavernous sinus and on its anterior margin by the fat in the orbital apex.* B, *the anterior clinoid, lateral orbital wall, and roof have been removed. The optic strut separates the optic nerve in the optic canal from the nerves passing through the superior orbital fissure. The superior ophthalmic vein can be seen through the periorbita as it exits the muscle cone to pass along the lateral margin of the superior orbital fissure and below the ophthalmic nerve to enter the anterior part of the cavernous sinus.* C, *the orbital fat has been removed to expose the nerve passing through the superior orbital fissure and the annular tendon from which the rectus muscles arise. The trochlear nerve passes medially above the oculomotor and ophthalmic nerves to reach the superior oblique muscles. The frontal, lacrimal, and trochlear nerves pass outside the annular tendon, and*

formed by the lateral surface of the optic strut, and the lower part is formed by the body of the sphenoid bone. The anterior part of the carotid sulcus, the shallow groove marking the course of the intracavernous segment of the carotid artery, is situated just inside and behind the medial edge of the fissure and continues upward along the posterior margin of the optic strut and the medial side of the anterior clinoid process. The lower margin of the fissure is formed by the junction of the greater wing with the sphenoid body and is located at the level of the lower edge of the cavernous sinus and the floor of the middle fossa. The lower edge of the fissure is separated from the foramen rotundum by a narrow bridge of bone, referred to as the maxillary strut. The lower end of the superior orbital fissure is located above and blends into the medial end of the inferior orbital fissure.

The inferior orbital fissure is a narrow crevasse with long anterior and posterior borders and narrow medial and lateral ends. The long posterior edge is formed by the greater wing of the sphenoid bone. The long anterior wall is formed by the orbital surface of the maxilla, except for a short segment formed by the orbital process of the palatine bone. The narrow lateral end is formed by the zygomatic bone, and the narrow medial end is formed by the sphenoid body. The posteromedial part of the fissure communicates below with the pterygopalatine fossa and the anterolateral part communicates with the infratemporal fossa, which is located below the greater sphenoid wing. The structures passing through the fissure are the zygomatic and the infraorbital and zygomatic branches of the maxillary nerve, some branches of the internal maxillary artery, and the branches of the inferior ophthalmic vein, which communicate with the pterygoid plexus. The orbital smooth muscle spans the upper part of the fissure.

The pterygomaxillary fissure is the narrow cleft between the posterior surface of the maxilla and the anterior surface of the pterygoid process of the sphenoid bone. The pterygomaxillary fissure opens into the pterygopalatine fossa, which is located below and communicates through the medial part of the inferior orbital fissure with the orbital apex. The upper part of the pterygoid process is penetrated by the foramen rotundum, through which the maxillary nerve passes to reach the pterygopalatine fossa, where it gives rise to the infraorbital and zygomatic nerves, which course in the floor and lateral orbital wall. The ostium of the vidian canal, which transmits the vidian nerve, is located below the foramen rotundum. The medial wall of the pterygopalatine fossa is formed by the perpendicular plate of the palatine bone.

PERIORBITA, DURA, AND ANNULAR TENDON

At the superior orbital fissure, the dura covering the middle fossa and cavernous sinus blends into the periorbita of the orbital apex and into the annular tendon from which the rectus muscles arise (*Figs. 7.3* and *7.4*). The annular tendon surrounds the orbital end of the optic foramen and the adjacent part of the superior orbital fissure. The fibrous components, which blend together to form the annular tendon, are the periorbita covering the orbital apex, the dura lining the superior orbital fissure and optic canal, and the optic sheath. The annular tendon is attached along the upper, medial, and lower margins of the optic canal, and to a bony prominence at the midportion of the lateral edge of the superior orbital fissure, at the junction of the fissure's narrow lateral and larger medial parts. The annular tendon does not surround the whole superior orbital fissure, but encompasses only the upper-medial portion, which is situated lateral to the optic strut and optic foramen. The lower portion of the annular tendon, the site of origin of the inferior rectus muscle, extends horizontally from the sphenoid body below the optic strut and optic foramen to an attachment on the lateral edge of the fissure. From its attachment to the greater wing, the annular tendon is directed upward to blend into the periorbita and dura, which meet on the lower margin of the lesser sphenoid wing. The segment of the annular tendon passing from the greater to the lesser wing separates the narrow lateral part of the fissure from the larger medial part and serves as the site of origin of the lateral rectus muscle.

The annular tendon and the connective tissue layer extending backward divide the superior orbital fissure into three sectors: lateral, central, and inferior. The lateral sector is quite narrow, being bounded above by the lesser wing of the sphenoid bone, below by the part of the greater wing lateral to the site of attachment of the annular tendon, and medially by the annular tendon and the origin of the lateral rectus muscle. The lateral sector transmits the trochlear, frontal, and lacrimal nerves, all of which pass through the fissure outside the annular tendon. The lacrimal nerve occupies the most lateral part of the fissure, the frontal nerve is more medial. The trochlear

the nasociliary, oculomotor, and abducens nerves pass through the tendon. D, *the frontal and lacrimal nerves have been depressed to show the nasociliary nerve arising from the medial side of the ophthalmic nerve. The oculomotor foramen is the portion of the opening in the annular tendon lateral to the optic foramen through which the superior and inferior divisions of the oculomotor nerve and the nasociliary nerve and abducens nerve pass. The oculomotor nerve divides into superior and inferior divisions just behind the superior orbital fissure. The abducens nerve courses on the medial side of the ophthalmic nerve in the cavernous sinus, but in the fissure, it turns laterally below the nerve to enter the medial side of the lateral rectus muscle.* E, *enlarged view of the oculomotor foramen.* F, *the annular tendon has been divided between the origin of the superior and lateral rectus muscles. The abducens nerve enters the medial aspect of the lateral rectus muscle. The superior division of the oculomotor nerve passes upward to innervate the levator and superior rectus muscles. The inferior division innervates the inferior oblique, inferior rectus, and medial rectus muscles and gives rise to the motor parasympathetic pupilloconstrictor fibers to the ciliary ganglion.* A., *artery;* Ant., *anterior;* Bas., *basilar;* Car., *carotid;* Cav., *cavernous;* Clin., *clinoid;* CN, *cranial nerve;* Div., *division;* Fiss., *fissure;* For., *foramen;* Front., *frontal;* Inf., *inferior;* Lac., *lacrimal;* Lat., *lateral;* M., *muscle;* N., *nerve;* Nasocil., *nasociliary;* Oculom., *oculomotor;* Olf., *olfactory;* Ophth., *ophthalmic;* Orb., *orbital;* Pet., *petrosal;* Plex., *plexus;* Rec., *rectus;* Seg., *segment;* S.C.A., *superior cerebellar artery;* Sup., *superior;* V., *vein.*

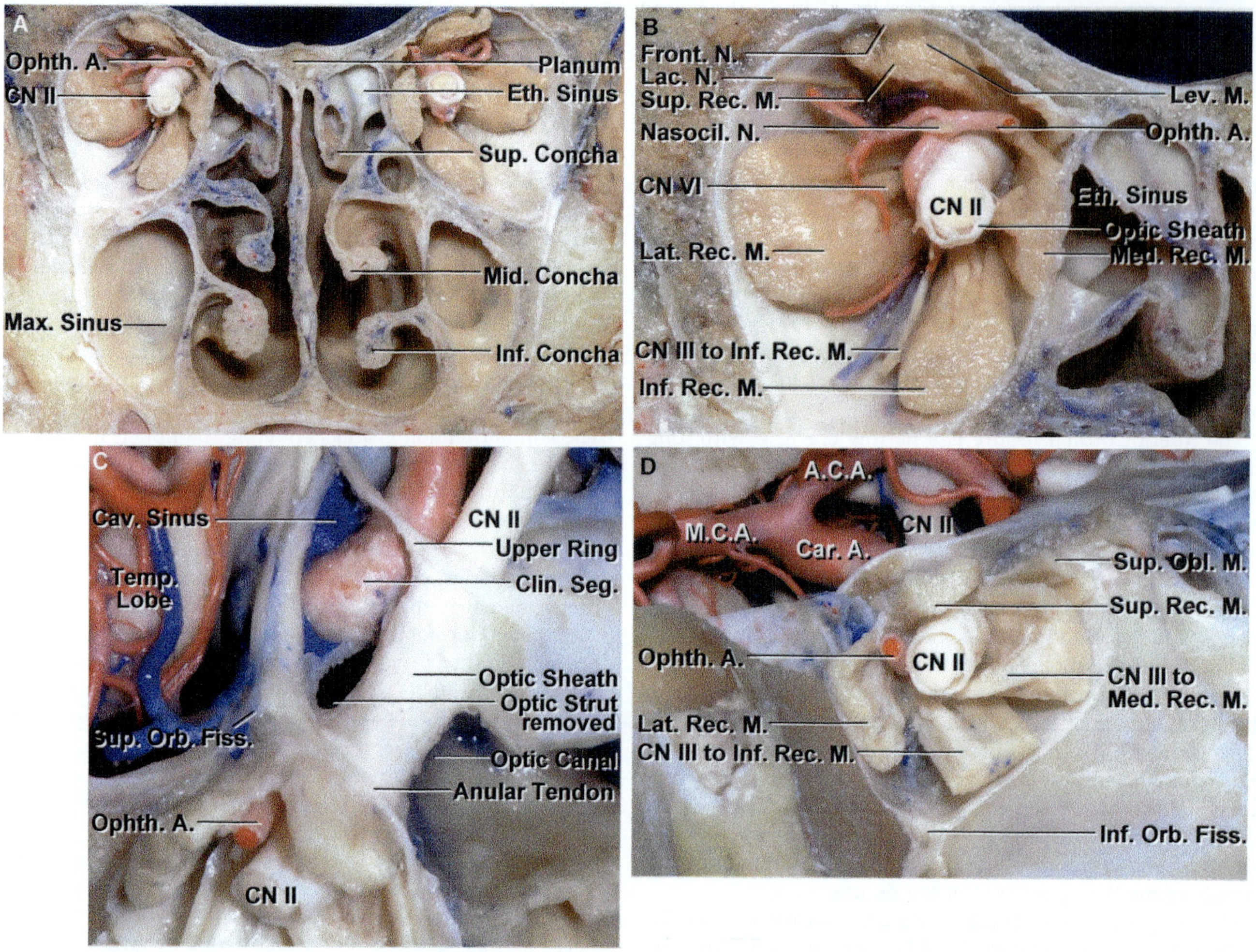

FIGURE 7.4. A, *coronal section of orbits and cranial base anterior to the orbital apex. The floor of the orbit faces the maxillary sinus and the medial wall faces the ethmoid air cells. The inferior concha is a separate bone attached to the medial maxillary wall. The middle turbinate, an appendage of the ethmoid bone, attaches to the lateral nasal wall at the level of the roof of the maxillary sinus.* B, *enlarged view of right side shown in* A. *The ophthalmic artery enters the orbit on the lateral side of the optic nerve and crosses medially above the nerve. The abducens nerve enters the medial surface of the lateral rectus muscle. The optic nerve is enclosed in the optic sheath. The nerve to the inferior oblique muscle courses along the lateral edge of the inferior rectus muscle.* C, *anterosuperior view showing the relationship of the orbital apex to the optic strut, optic canal, and superior orbital fissure. The optic strut, which has been removed, separates the optic nerve in the optic canal from the superior orbital fissure. The optic nerve enters the orbit on the medial side of the optic strut and the oculomotor, trochlear, abducens, and ophthalmic nerves enter the orbit on the lateral side of the strut. The rectus muscles arise from the annular tendon, which encircles the optic canal and the central part of the superior orbital fissure. The anterior clinoid process has been removed to expose the clinoid segment of the internal carotid artery. The upper dural ring surrounds the carotid artery at the upper edge of the clinoid segment.* D, *cross section of right orbit just in front of the apex. The ophthalmic artery enters the orbit on the lateral side of the optic nerve. The branch of the inferior division of the oculomotor nerve to the medial rectus muscle passes below the optic nerve.* E, *superior view of the floor of both orbits. The roof of the maxillary sinus forms the orbital floors. The infraorbital and zygomatic branches of the maxillary nerve enter the orbit by passing through the inferior orbital fissure. The zygomatic nerve courses along the lateral wall of the orbit to give rise to the zygomaticofacial and zygomaticotemporal nerves, which innervate the skin over the malar eminence and temporal region, respectively. The infraorbital nerve and artery course along the floor of the orbit to reach the cheek.* F, *enlarged view of the right orbit showing the course along the orbital walls taken by the zygomaticofacial, zygomaticotemporal, and infraorbital nerves. The zygomaticofacial nerves pierce the lateral orbital rim to reach the malar eminence and the zygomaticotemporal branches pass upward to reach the temple.* G, *anterior view of both orbits in another specimen. A portion of the floor of both orbits has been removed to expose the maxillary sinus while preserving the infraorbital and zygomatic nerves. The rectus muscles arise in the orbital apex from the annular tendon, which surrounds the optic canal and adjacent part of the superior orbital fissure. The ethmoidal sinuses are located on the medial side of the orbit.* H, *enlarged view. Some of the posterior wall of the maxillary sinus has been removed to expose the pterygopalatine fossa and the origin of the infraorbital and zygomatic nerves from the maxillary nerve. The structures in the pterygopalatine fossa are the maxillary nerve and its terminal branches, the pterygopalatine ganglion, and the terminal branches of the maxillary artery. The maxillary nerve gives rise to communicating rami to the pterygopalatine ganglion.* A., *artery;* A.C.A., *anterior cerebral artery;* Car., *carotid;* Cav., *cavernous;* Clin., *clinoid;* CN, *cranial nerve;* Eth., *ethmoid;* Fiss., *fissure;* Front., *frontal;* Gang., *ganglion;* Inf., *inferior;* Infraorb., *infraorbital;* Lac., *lacrimal;* Lat., *lateral;* Lev., *levator;* M., *muscle;* Max., *maxillary;* M.C.A., *middle cerebral artery;* Med., *medial;* Mid., *middle;* N., *nerve;* Nasocil., *nasociliary;* Obl., *oblique;* Ophth., *ophthalmic;* Orb., *orbital;* Pterygopal., *pterygopalatine;* Rec., *rectus;* Seg., *segment;* Sup., *superior;* Temp., *temporal;* Zygo., *zygomatic;* Zygomaticofac., *zygomaticofacial.*

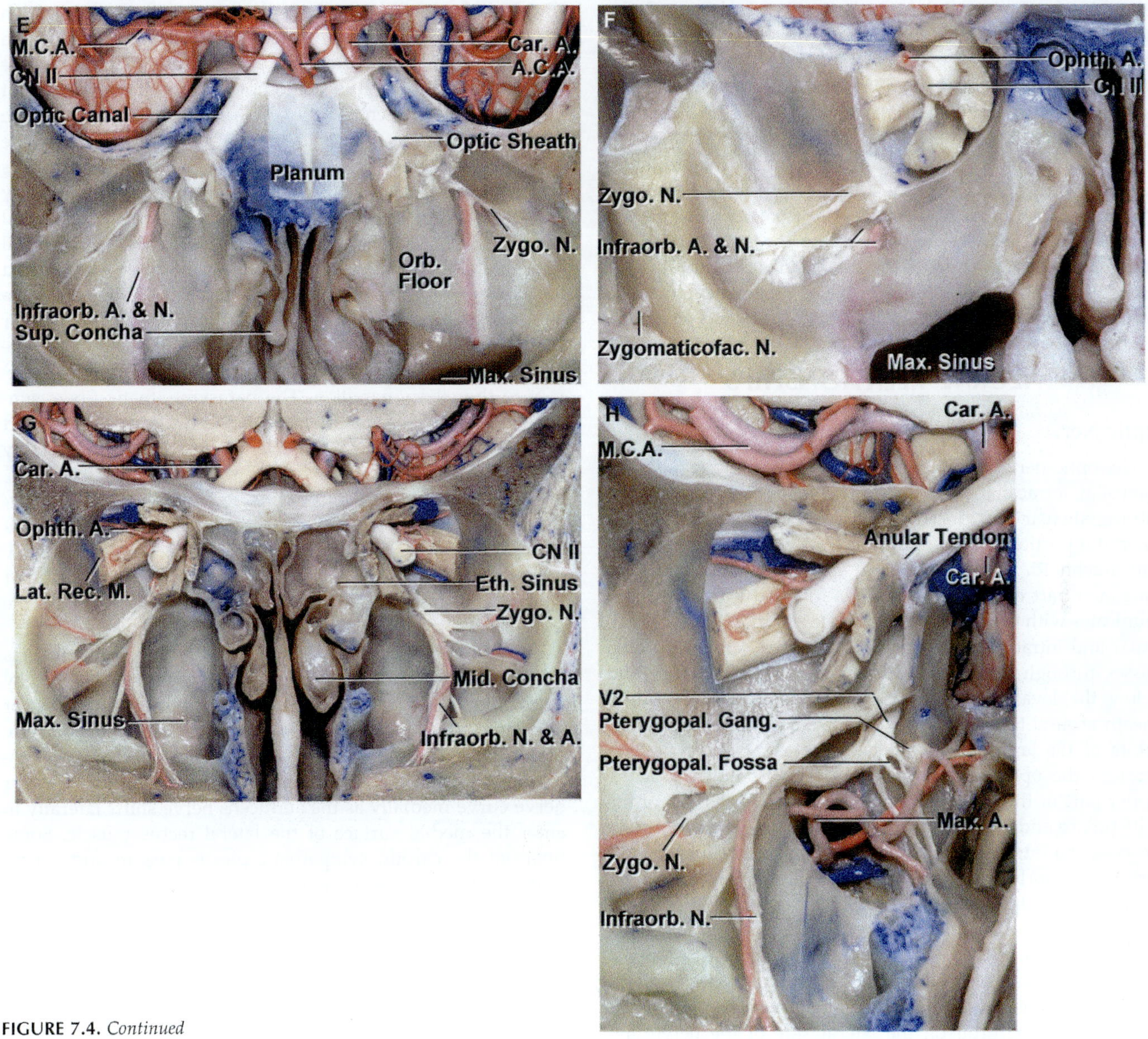

FIGURE 7.4. *Continued*

nerve passes through the fissure on the superomedial margin of the frontal nerve. The superior ophthalmic vein also passes through this sector by coursing along the lower side of the lacrimal and frontal nerves to reach the cavernous sinus.

The central sector of the superior orbital fissure, referred to as the oculomotor foramen because it is the part of the fissure through which the oculomotor nerve passes, is bounded above by the annular tendon and adjacent part of the lesser wing, medially by the optic strut and sphenoid body, laterally by the annular tendon and the prominence on the lateral margin of the fissure to which the annular tendon attaches, and below by the segment of the annular tendon spanning the interval between the sphenoid body and the bony prominence on the lateral edge of the fissure. The inferior rectus muscle arises from the annular tendon at the lower margin of this sector. The oculomotor, nasociliary, and abducens nerves and the sensory and sympathetic roots of the ciliary ganglion pass through this sector. The optic nerve and ophthalmic artery pass medially to the oculomotor foramen through the part of the annular tendon attached to the upper, lower, and medial margins of the optic foramen. The connective tissue membrane, which extends posteriorly from the annular tendon, separates the nerves passing through the lateral and central sectors of the fissure. This connective tissue extends backward from the annulus between the frontal branch of the ophthalmic nerve, which passes through the lateral sector outside the annular tendon, and the nasociliary nerve, which passes through the central sector and the annular tendon.

The inferior sector of the superior orbital fissure is situated below the annular tendon. It is bounded below by the junction of the body and greater wing of the sphenoid bone, above by the annular tendon, laterally by the part of the greater wing below the attachment of the annular tendon, and medially by the sphenoid body. The inferior rectus muscle arises from the annular tendon at the upper margin of this sector. Orbital fat extends backward below the inferior rectus muscle into this part of the fissure. The lower margin of this sector contains a posterior extension of the orbital smooth muscle, which spans the upper margin of the inferior orbital fissure. The orbital fat extends backward between the inferior rectus muscle and the orbital smooth muscle and medial to the segment of the abducens and nasociliary nerves passing through the fissure. Removal of this fat exposes the fine branches of the carotid sympathetic plexus entering the orbit, some of which form the sympathetic root of the ciliary ganglion.

NEURAL RELATIONSHIPS

Optic Nerve

The optic nerve is divided into four parts: intraocular, intraorbital, intracanalicular, and intracranial (*Figs. 7.2–7.5*). The intracanalicular part, located in the optic canal, and the intraorbital portions of the optic nerve are surrounded by dura and arachnoid. The subarachnoid space surrounding the intracranial part of the nerve extends forward from and communicates with the subarachnoid space around the intracanalicular and intraorbital portions of the nerve. The optic nerve passes through the medial part of the annular tendon and below the levator and superior rectus muscles. The dural sheath around the optic nerve blends smoothly into the periorbita at the anterior end of the optic canal. After passing through the optic canal, which forms a prominence in the upper part of the sphenoid sinus immediately in front of the sella turcica and along the medial aspect of the anterior clinoid process, the intracranial portion of the nerve is directed posterior, superiorly, and medially toward the optic chiasm.

The intraocular portion of the optic nerve, which includes the optic disc, lies within the sclera. The intraorbital portion of the optic nerve is surrounded by orbital fat and follows a slightly tortuous course. The ciliary nerves and arteries pierce the sclera in the area around the optic nerve. The ophthalmic artery enters the orbit on the lateral side of the nerve and passes above the nerve to reach the medial sides of the orbit. The superior ophthalmic vein arises in the anteromedial part of the orbit and crosses above the nerve to reach the orbital apex. Both the artery and vein course between the superior rectus muscle and the optic nerve. The branch of the inferior division of the oculomotor nerve to the medial rectus muscle passes below the optic nerve at about the same level that the ophthalmic artery and nasociliary nerve pass above the optic nerve.

Oculomotor, Trochlear, and Abducens Nerves

The oculomotor nerve enters the orbit by passing through the medial part of the fissure on the lateral surface of the optic strut (*Fig. 7.3*). At the level of the posterior margin of the fissure, in the area medial to the trochlear and nasociliary nerves, the oculomotor nerve splits into superior and inferior divisions that course one above the other as they pass through the central sector of the fissure and the oculomotor foramen on the medial side of the branches of the ophthalmic nerve. The superior division of the oculomotor nerve enters the orbit below the attachment of the superior rectus muscle to the annular tendon and sends its branches upward lateral to the optic nerve to reach the lower surface of the superior rectus and levator muscles. The inferior division courses inferiorly and medially as it proceeds through the fissure on the medial side of the nasociliary and abducens nerves. At the orbital apex, it splits into three individual branches: two are directed forward to reach the inferior rectus and inferior oblique muscles, and one passes medially below the optic nerve to enter the medial rectus muscle. In addition, the branch to the inferior oblique muscle gives rise to the motor (parasympathetic) root to the ciliary ganglion. The parasympathetic fibers synapse in the ciliary ganglion, which gives rise to the short ciliary nerves that pierce the sclera to reach the ciliary body and iris.

The trochlear nerve courses in the lateral wall of the cavernous sinus below the oculomotor nerve and above the ophthalmic nerve. It passes through the upper edge of the narrow lateral part of the superior orbital fissure outside the annular tendon and passes medially above the frontal nerve and the levator muscle to reach the superior oblique muscle.

The abducens nerve travels forward in the cavernous sinus on the medial side of the ophthalmic nerve and shifts laterally below the nasociliary nerve as it passes through the superior orbital fissure and annular tendon to enter the medial surface of the lateral rectus muscle. At the apex of the orbit, the nasociliary nerve and the inferior division of the oculomotor nerve curve medially as the abducens nerve shifts laterally to enter the medial surface of the lateral rectus muscle. Some fibers of the carotid sympathetic plexus pass to and course within the abducens nerve in the cavernous sinus.

Trigeminal Nerve

The ophthalmic branch of the trigeminal nerve is the smallest of the three trigeminal divisions (*Figs. 7.2* and *7.3*). It is inclined upward as it passes forward near the medial surface of the dura forming the lower part of the lateral wall of the cavernous sinus to reach the superior orbital fissure. It is flattened in the wall of the cavernous sinus, but at the superior orbital fissure, it takes on an oval configuration. The ophthalmic nerve splits into the lacrimal, frontal, and nasociliary nerves as it approaches the superior orbital fissure.

The lacrimal nerve arises at the level of or just behind the superior orbital fissure from the lateral edge of the ophthalmic nerve and passes through the lateral edge of the fissure on the lateral side of the frontal nerve and above the superior ophthalmic vein. On entering the orbit, the lacrimal nerve courses along the superior margin of the lateral rectus muscles, where it receives secretory fibers conveyed initially in the zygomatic nerve from the pterygopalatine ganglion and distributed through the lacrimal nerve to the lacrimal gland. The lacrimal nerve conveys sensation from the area in front of the lacrimal gland.

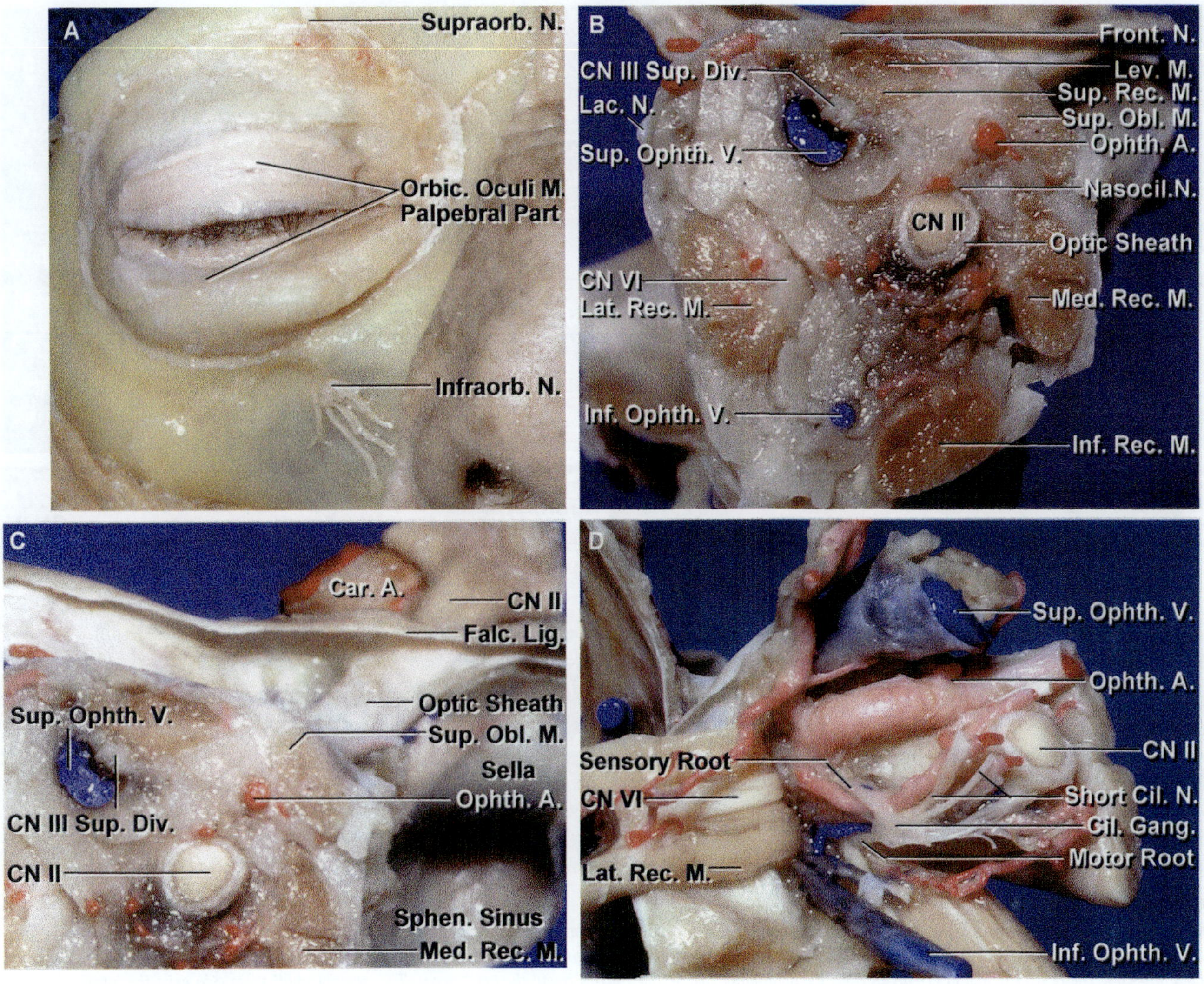

FIGURE 7.5. A, *the orbital part of the orbicularis oculi muscle has been removed and the palpebral part preserved. The supraorbital nerves carry sensation from the skin of the forehead and the infraorbital nerve carries sensation from the cheek, upper lip, and adjacent part of the nose. The supraorbital nerves reach the skin of the forehead by passing through a notch or foramen in the superior orbital rim. The infraorbital nerve arises from the maxillary nerve and passes through the inferior orbital fissure and along the infraorbital groove and canal in the orbital floor to reach the infraorbital foramen.* B–H, *anterior views of cross sections of the orbit at progressively deeper levels.* B, *anterior aspect of a coronal section through the right orbit just posterior to the globe and the inferior oblique muscle. The intraorbital part of the optic sheath, an anterior extension of the dura lining the optic canal, surrounds the optic nerve. At this level, the ophthalmic artery has crossed from lateral to medial and the superior ophthalmic has crossed from medial to lateral above the optic nerve.* C, *enlarged view of* B *to show the relationship of the cisternal and canalicular segments of the optic nerve to the intraorbital part. The cisternal segment of the optic nerve courses medial to the supraclinoid segment of the internal carotid artery. The optic sheath surrounds the intracanalicular segment in the optic canal. The optic sheath and the periorbita fuse at the orbital apex to form the annular tendon from which the rectus muscles arise. Fibers from the superior division of the oculomotor nerve enter the lower surface of the levator and superior rectus muscles. The sphenoid sinus and sella are on the medial side of the optic canal.* D, *the orbital fat has been removed and the lateral rectus muscle has been reflected to expose the ciliary ganglion, which is located inferolateral to the optic nerve. The inferior division of the oculomotor nerve sends individual branches to the inferior and medial rectus and the inferior oblique muscles. The ciliary ganglion has sensory, parasympathetic, and sympathetic roots. The motor (parasympathetic) root of the ciliary ganglion arises from the branch of the inferior oculomotor division to the inferior oblique muscle. Sensory fibers from the globe pass through the short ciliary nerves to reach the ciliary ganglion, where they form the sensory root of the ciliary ganglion, which joins the nasociliary branch of the ophthalmic nerve. Sympathetic fibers reach the ciliary ganglion from the carotid plexus. The ciliary ganglion gives rise to numerous short ciliary nerves that pierce the sclera and terminate in the pupillary sphincter and ciliary muscle.* E, *anterior aspect of a coronal section at the level of the ciliary ganglion. The inferior division of the oculomotor nerve splits into three branches that innervate the inferior and medial rectus and inferior oblique muscles. The nasociliary branch of the ophthalmic nerve passes through the annular tendon, and the frontal and lacrimal branches pass outside the annular tendon through the lateral part of the superior orbital fissure. The nasociliary nerve and ophthalmic artery course above the optic nerve at this level.* F, *section located just anterior to the lateral end of superior orbital fissure at the level of the posterior ethmoidal canal. At this level, the ophthalmic artery courses on the lateral side of the optic nerve and the nasociliary nerve courses between the optic nerve and ophthalmic artery. The recurrent meningeal artery passes above the ophthalmic artery. The* (Legend continues on next page.)

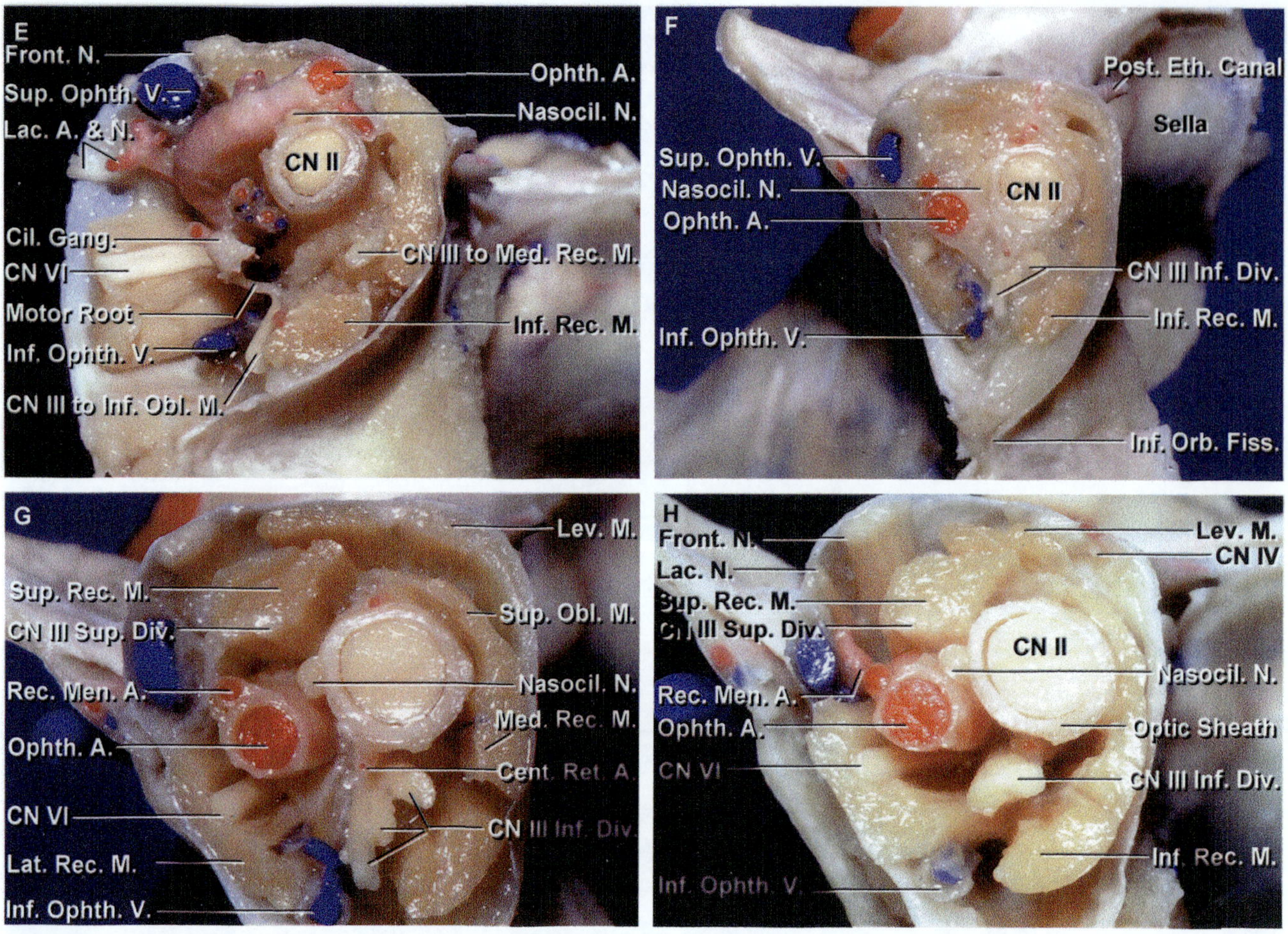

FIGURE 7.5. *Continued*
orbital smooth muscle spans the inferior orbital fissure. G, enlarged view of the section shown in F after removal of the orbital fat. At this level, the oculomotor nerve has split into a superior division that supplies the superior rectus and levator muscles and an inferior division that innervates the inferior rectus, medial rectus, and inferior oblique muscles. The central retinal artery arises from the ophthalmic artery and courses below the optic nerve. The superior ophthalmic vein exits the intraconal area by passing between the heads of the superior and lateral rectus muscles, and the inferior ophthalmic vein passes between the heads of the lateral and inferior rectus muscles. H, section through the orbital apex immediately in front of the superior orbital fissure. The annular tendon is divided into medial and lateral parts. The medial part is located in front of the optic canal and the lateral part is situated in front of the superomedial part of the superior orbital fissure. The optic nerve and ophthalmic artery pass through the medial part. The superior and inferior divisions of the oculomotor nerve and the abducens and nasociliary nerves and the sensory root of the ciliary ganglion pass through the lateral part. The superior ophthalmic vein and the recurrent meningeal artery course between the superior and lateral rectus muscles and exit the superior orbital fissure by passing outside the annulus. The inferior ophthalmic vein has exited the intraconal area at this level and is coursing below the lateral rectus muscle on its way to the cavernous sinus. This section crosses the inferior division of the oculomotor nerve proximal to its subdivision into individual branches. A., *artery;* Car., *carotid;* Cent., *central;* Cil., *ciliary;* CN, *cranial nerve;* Div., *division;* Falc., *falciform;* Front., *frontal;* Gang., *ganglion;* Inf., *inferior;* Infraorb., *infraorbital;* Lac., *lacrimal;* Lat., *lateral;* Lev., *levator;* Lig., *ligament;* M., *muscle;* Med., *medial;* Men., *meningeal;* N., *nerve;* Nasocil., *nasociliary;* Obl., *oblique;* Ophth., *ophthalmic;* Orbic., *orbicularis;* Rec., *rectus, recurrent;* Ret., *retinal;* Sphen., *sphenoid;* Sup., *superior;* Supraorb., *supraorbital;* V., *vein.*

The remainder of the ophthalmic nerve splits into the frontal nerve, which passes through the lateral sector of the fissure, and the nasociliary nerve, which passes through the central sector on the medial side of the origin of the lateral rectus muscle from the annular tendon. The frontal branch of the ophthalmic nerve arises in the lateral wall of the cavernous sinus and passes through the narrow lateral part of the superior orbital fissure on the medial side of the lacrimal nerve and superior ophthalmic vein and below the trochlear nerve. The frontal nerve courses outside and superolateral to the annular tendon and divides into the supratrochlear and supraorbital nerves within the orbit. The supratrochlear nerve runs anteriorly above the trochlea of the superior oblique muscle with the supratrochlear artery. The supraorbital nerve courses above the levator muscle with the supraorbital artery. It conveys sensation from the upper eyelid and forehead and may also carry some sympathetic fibers to the globe and pupillary dilator.

The nasociliary nerve arises from the medial side of the ophthalmic nerve and is situated above and lateral to the abducens nerve in the anterior part of the cavernous sinus. Both the abducens and the nasociliary nerves course medial to the part of the ophthalmic nerve from which the lacrimal and frontal nerves arise. At the level of the fissure, the nasociliary nerve gently ascends laterally to the inferior division of the oculomotor nerve and then crosses medially between the two divisions of the oculomotor nerve and above the optic nerve to reach the medial part of the orbit, where it gives rise to the anterior and posterior ethmoidal and infratrochlear nerves. The sensory root of the ciliary ganglion arises from the lower edge of the nasociliary nerve during passage through the lateral wall of the cavernous sinus or within the fissure. The sensory root may infrequently arise as far forward as the anterior margin of the fissure. Within the fissure, it courses between the abducens nerve laterally and the inferior oculomotor division medially and passes forward to join the posterior edge of the ciliary ganglion. The fibers from the sensory root are distributed to the globe with the short ciliary nerves and convey sensation from the cornea and globe. The nasociliary nerve also gives rise to the long ciliary nerves that enter the sclera around the optic nerve with the short ciliary nerves. The long ciliary nerve conveys sympathetic fibers to the globe and pupillary dilator and may also carry some sensation from the globe and cornea.

The maxillary nerve passes through the foramen rotundum to enter the pterygopalatine fossa, where it gives rise the infraorbital and zygomatic nerves and communicating rami to the sphenopalatine ganglion. The infraorbital and zygomatic branches pass through the inferior orbital fissure to course within the orbit. The infraorbital nerve courses along the orbital floor in the infraorbital groove and canal to reach the infraorbital foramen, where its branches are distributed to the cheek. The zygomatic branch passes through the inferior orbital fissure and courses just inside the lateral wall of the orbit, where it divides into zygomaticofacial and zygomaticotemporal branches. These branches enter the zygomatico-orbital foramina on the intraorbital surface of the zygoma and exit the zygoma at the zygomaticofacial and zygomaticotemporal foramina to reach the skin of the cheek and temple, respectively.

Ciliary Ganglion

The ciliary ganglion is situated on the inferolateral aspect of the optic nerve and on the medial side of the lateral rectus muscle (*Figs. 7.2* and *7.5*). It receives three branches: the motor (parasympathetic) root from the inferior division of the oculomotor nerve, the sensory root from the nasociliary nerve, and sympathetic fibers from the plexus around the internal carotid artery. The sympathetic fibers sometimes blend with the sensory root in the orbit. The parasympathetic fibers synapse in the ciliary ganglion. The sympathetic fibers arise in the cervical sympathetic ganglia and pass through the ciliary ganglion without synapsing. The short ciliary nerves pass from the ganglion to the globe.

Sympathetic Fibers

Sympathetic fibers ascend on the surface of the internal carotid artery, pass through the medial part of the superior orbital fissure and the oculomotor foramen, and course with the abducens and ophthalmic nerves in the cavernous sinus and also with the ophthalmic artery. Some of these fibers collect together to form the sympathetic root of the ciliary ganglion, which courses as an independent branch surrounded by orbital fat. The fibers forming the sympathetic root run forward and upward along the medial margin of the abducens nerve to reach the area lateral to the inferior division of the oculomotor nerve, where they pass through the central sector of the superior orbital fissure. Some sympathetic fibers join the ophthalmic division and are distributed to the pupil in the long ciliary and sensory root of the ciliary ganglion, both of which arise from the nasociliary nerve. Others pass directly through the fissure and orbit to the globe. Some sympathetic fibers from the carotid plexus accompany the ophthalmic artery.

Vidian Nerve and Pterygopalatine Ganglion

The vidian nerve, formed by the union of the greater petrosal branch of the facial nerve and the deep petrosal nerve from the carotid plexus, exits the vidian canal and enters the posterior aspect of the sphenopalatine ganglion in the pterygopalatine fossa. Parasympathetic fibers are conveyed in the greater petrosal nerve and sympathetic fibers are conveyed in the deep petrosal nerve. Communicating branches, typically two in number, arise from the inferior portion of the maxillary nerve and descend to join the sphenopalatine ganglion, which is located anterior to the aperture of the vidian canal. The parasympathetic fibers synapse in the ganglion and the sympathetic fibers pass through the ganglion without synapse. Fibers exiting the ganglion join the nasal, nasopalatine, and palatine nerves to convey secretory impulses to the nasal and palatine glands. The secretory fibers to the lacrimal gland pass from the ganglion via the maxillary nerve to join the zygomatic nerve, which sends a communication to the gland via the lacrimal nerve. In addition, sensory fibers, which pass through the pterygopalatine ganglion, reach the maxillary nerve and convey sensation from the ethmoidal and sphenoid sinuses, nasal cavity, nasal septum, hard palate, and roof of the pharynx.

ARTERIAL RELATIONSHIPS

Internal Carotid Artery

The anterior bend of the intracavernous segment of the internal carotid artery courses along the posterior edge of the medial margin of the superior orbital fissure and rests against the posterior surface of the optic strut (*Figs. 7.3–7.5*). After ascending along the posterior margin of the optic strut, the artery turns upward along the medial margin of the anterior clinoid process to reach the subarachnoid space. The segment of the artery coursing along the medial margin of the clinoid process is referred to as the clinoid segment.

Ophthalmic Artery

The ophthalmic artery usually arises just above the cavernous sinus from the medial half of the superior aspect of the anterior bend of the internal carotid artery (*Figs. 7.6* and *7.7*).

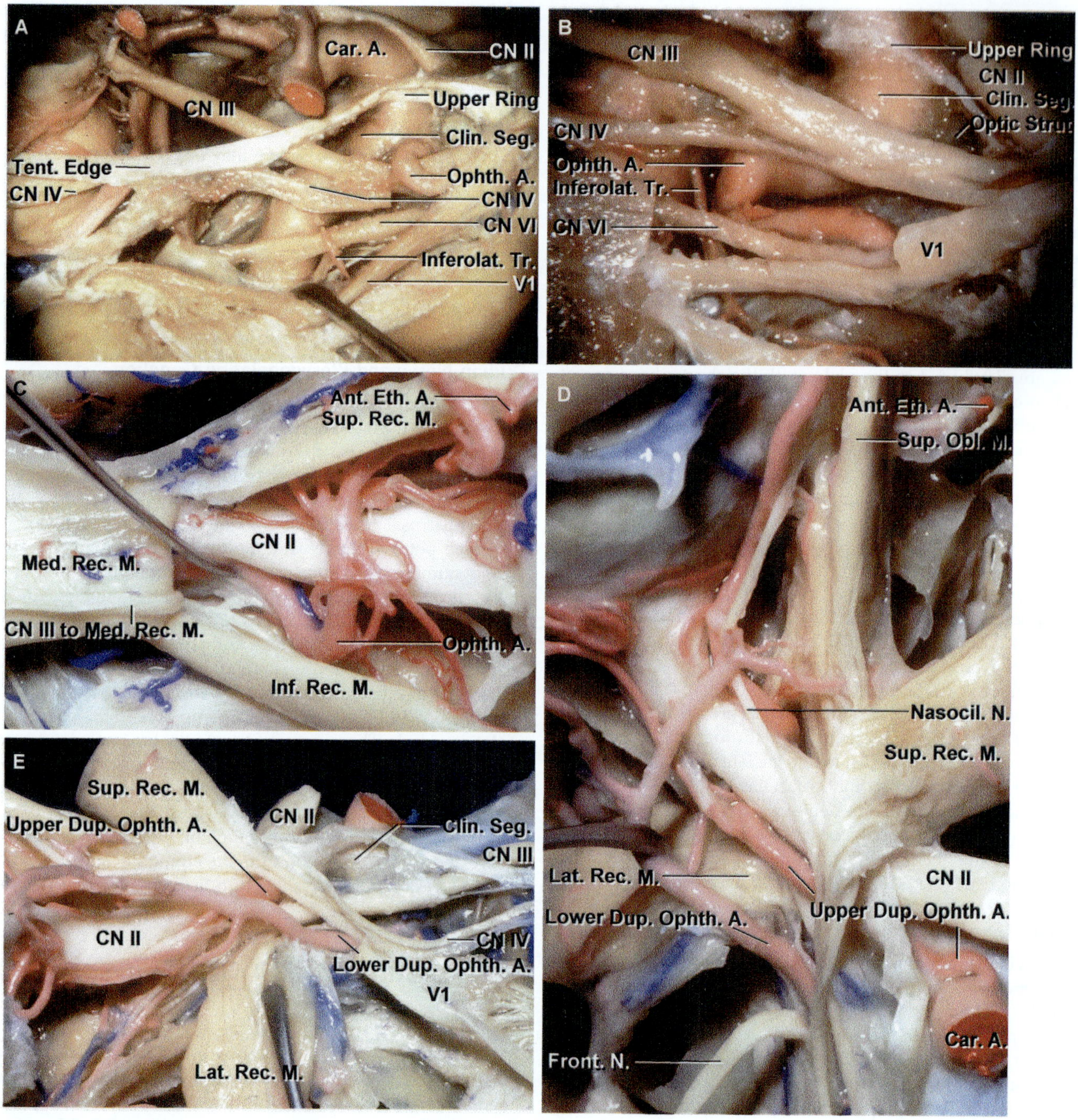

FIGURE 7.6. *Anomalies of the ophthalmic artery. A, right ophthalmic artery origin from the clinoid segment of the internal carotid artery. The ophthalmic artery usually arises just above the clinoid segment, but in this case, the artery arises from the clinoid segment below the anterior clinoid process, which has been removed. The artery passes through the superior orbital fissure between the oculomotor and ophthalmic nerves. The lateral wall of the right cavernous sinus and the anterior clinoid process have been removed to expose the intracavernous and clinoid segments of the internal carotid artery, and the ophthalmic nerve has been retracted to expose the inferolateral trunk. B, ophthalmic artery origin in the cavernous sinus. Lateral aspect of a right ophthalmic artery that arises from the intracavernous segment of the left internal carotid artery. The upper half of a segment of the ophthalmic nerve has been removed to expose an ophthalmic artery. The anterior clinoid artery has been removed to expose the clinoid segment in the interval between the optic and oculomotor nerves. C, the medial rectus muscle has been divided near the globe and reflected posteriorly to expose an ophthalmic artery that courses below the optic nerve to reach the medial part of the orbit, as occurs in approximately 15% of orbits. The branch of the inferior division of the oculomotor nerve to the medial rectus muscle enters the medial side of the muscle. The anterior ethmoidal artery courses below the superior oblique muscle to reach the anterior ethmoidal canal. D and E, duplicate left ophthalmic arteries. D, superior aspect of a duplicate ophthalmic artery. The levator and superior rectus muscles have been reflected medially and the lateral rectus muscle has been reflected laterally to expose the left optic nerve and the duplicate arteries. The upper*

Its origin is located under the medial part of the optic nerve, just behind the optic canal. In the optic canal, the ophthalmic artery courses within the optic sheath below the optic nerve and through the annular tendon. It exits the optic canal and penetrates the optic sheath to enter the orbital apex on the inferolateral aspect of the optic nerve. In the optic canal, the ophthalmic artery sometimes gives a recurrent branch to the intracranial segment of the optic nerve. Approximately 8% of ophthalmic arteries arise in the cavernous sinus rather than in the subarachnoid space (5). Those ophthalmic arteries arising in the cavernous sinus pass through the superior orbital fissure, rather than the optic canal, to reach the orbit. In some cases in which the larger ophthalmic artery passes through the superior orbital fissure, a second, smaller or hypoplastic ophthalmic artery may arise in the supraclinoid area and course in the usual manner through the optic foramen to reach the orbit. In other cases, with a normal-sized ophthalmic artery passing through the optic foramen, a smaller artery that arises from the intracavernous carotid may pass through the fissure, usually supplying the territory normally supplied by the lacrimal artery.

The ophthalmic artery may also arise as duplicate arteries of nearly equal size (24). The upper duplicate artery usually arises from the supraclinoid portion of the internal carotid artery and passes through the optic canal to enter the orbital apex on the lateral side of the optic nerve (*Fig. 7.6*). The lower duplicate artery usually arises from the internal carotid artery in the cavernous sinus and passes through the superior orbital fissure between the oculomotor nerve laterally and the abducens and ophthalmic nerves medially. Both usually cross the optic nerve, one above and one below, to reach the medial part of the orbit. The ophthalmic artery may infrequently arise from the clinoid segment, in which case it passes through the superior orbital fissure to reach the orbit (*Fig. 7.6A*). A few will pass through an accessory foramen, called the ophthalmic foramen, which pierces the optic strut (*Fig. 7.1L*). It may also infrequently arise as a branch of the middle meningeal artery (*Fig. 7.8*) (15).

The ophthalmic artery, after passing through the optic foramen and annular tendon and reaching the lateral aspect of the optic nerve may give rise to a recurrent meningeal artery that passes backward through the superior orbital fissure to reach the dura. The ophthalmic artery passes above the optic nerve in approximately 85% of orbits. In the remainder, it passes below the nerve. After passing the optic nerve, the artery courses between the superior oblique and the medial rectus muscles, where it gives rise to the anterior and posterior ethmoidal arteries that pass through the anterior and posterior ethmoidal canals with the anterior and posterior ethmoidal nerves.

The ophthalmic artery gives rise to the central retinal, lacrimal, long and short ciliary, supraorbital, medial palpebral, infratrochlear, supratrochlear, and dorsal nasal arteries, plus muscular branches to the extraocular muscles and meningeal branches that pass through the ethmoidal or lacrimal foramina or superior orbital fissure to reach the meninges. The palpebral branches of the ophthalmic artery plus the supratrochlear, infratrochlear, supraorbital, dorsal nasal, and lacrimal branches supply the skin and soft tissues of the eyelids and area around the orbital rim.

The central retinal artery, which is the first and one of the smallest branches of the ophthalmic artery, arises medial to the ciliary ganglion, pierces the lower surface of the nerve, and courses a short distance inside the dural sheath of the nerve before passing to the center of the nerve and forward to the retina in the center of the nerve. The central retinal artery is a terminal branch without anastomotic connections (*Fig. 7.7*). Its loss results in blindness.

The lacrimal artery, one of the largest and earliest branches of the ophthalmic artery, accompanies the lacrimal nerve and is distributed to the lacrimal gland and the lateral part of the eyelids and conjunctiva. A recurrent branch may also arise from the lacrimal artery or adjacent part of the ophthalmic artery and pass through the superior orbital fissure to reach the dura, only to return to the periorbita by passing through the lacrimal foramen located lateral to the superior orbital fissure on the greater sphenoid wing. The supraorbital artery arises from the ophthalmic artery as it crosses the optic nerve and runs along the medial side of the levator and superior rectus muscles to course with the supraorbital nerves. The supratrochlear artery courses with the supratrochlear nerve. The short and long posterior ciliary arteries arise from the ophthalmic artery, course with the short and long ciliary nerves, pierce the sclera around the optic nerve, and supply the choroidal coat and ciliary processes. The anterior ciliary arteries are derived from the branches to the extraocular muscles and run to the front of the globe with the tendons of the extraocular muscles, where they pierce the sclera and end in the greater arterial circle of the iris.

The anterior and posterior ethmoidal branches of the ophthalmic artery, of which the anterior is the larger, arise beneath the superior oblique muscle and pass through the anterior and posterior ethmoidal canal to reach the dura beside the cribriform plate (*Figs. 7.2* and *7.7*). The anterior ethmoidal artery crosses near the anterior edge of the cribriform plate. The posterior ethmoidal artery crosses near the posterior edge of

duplicate artery arises from the supraclinoid segment of the internal carotid artery, passes through the optic canal to enter the orbital apex on the lateral side of the optic nerve, and courses below the optic nerve to reach the medial part of the orbit. The lower duplicate artery arises from the internal carotid artery in the cavernous sinus, passes through the superior orbital fissure on the lateral side of the optic nerve, and crosses above the nerve to reach the medial part of the orbit. E, lateral view. The annular tendon has been opened between the superior and lateral rectus muscles. The duplicate artery arising above the cavernous sinus passes forward and downward to course below the optic nerve. The duplicate artery arising in the cavernous sinus passes above the optic nerve. A., *artery;* Ant., *anterior;* Car., *carotid;* Clin., *clinoid;* CN, *cranial nerve;* Dup., *duplicate;* Eth., *ethmoidal;* Front., *frontal;* Inf., *inferior;* Inferolat., *inferolateral;* Lat., *lateral;* M., *muscle;* Med., *medial;* N., *nerve;* Nasocil., *nasociliary;* Obl., *oblique;* Ophth., *ophthalmic;* Rec., *rectus;* Seg., *segment;* Sup., *superior;* Tent., *tentorial;* Tr., *trunk.*

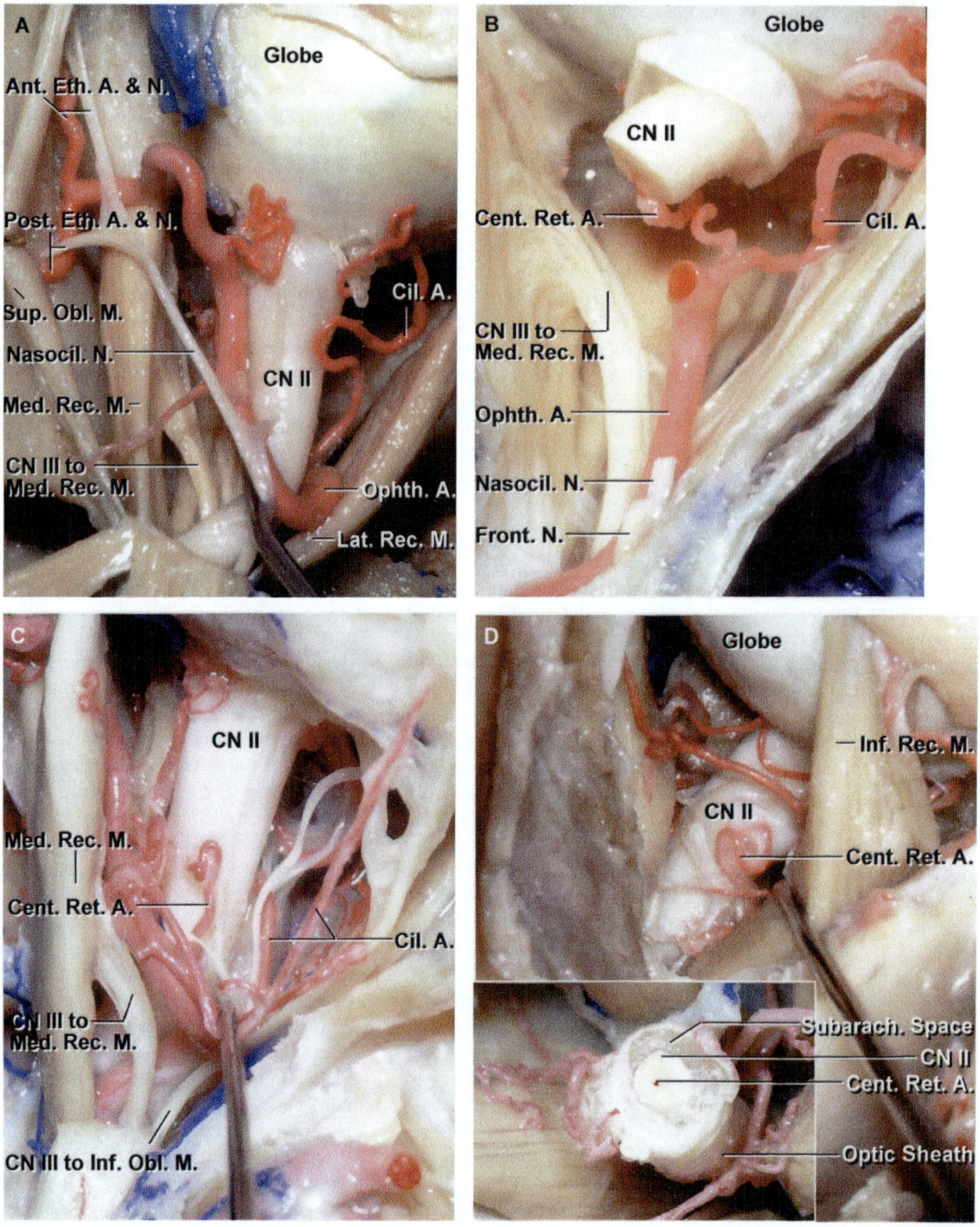

FIGURE 7.7. *Ophthalmic and central retinal arteries.* A, *superior view of the right orbit. The levator, superior rectus, and superior oblique muscles have been reflected to expose the ophthalmic artery coursing above the optic nerve. The ophthalmic artery passes above the optic nerve and between the superior oblique and the medial rectus muscles, where it gives rise to the anterior and posterior ethmoidal arteries. The anterior and posterior ethmoidal arteries pass through the anterior and posterior ethmoidal canals with the anterior and posterior ethmoidal nerves to supply the dura in the region of the cribriform plate and send branches that descend to supply the upper part of the nasal cavity.* B, *a segment of the optic nerve and ophthalmic artery have been removed to expose the central retinal artery arising as one of the first branches of the ophthalmic artery and entering the lower surface of the optic nerve.* C, *central retinal artery, inferior view. An ophthalmic artery, which courses below the optic nerve, has been retracted posteriorly to show the tortuous course of the central retinal artery before penetrating the optic nerve. The central retinal artery, which is the first or one of the earliest and smallest branches of the ophthalmic artery, pierces the lower surface of the nerve and courses a short distance inside the dural sheath of the nerve before passing to the center of the nerve, where it courses to the retina.* D, *inferior view. The inferior rectus has been retracted to expose a tortuous central retinal artery.* Inset: *Anterior view of the right orbit after removal of the globe. The central retinal artery, after penetrating the optic nerve, passes forward in the center of the nerve. The central retinal artery is a terminal branch without anastomotic connections. The ciliary arteries, coursing around the nerve, are divided into long and short and anterior ciliary arteries. The long and short ciliary arteries pierce the sclera around the optic nerve and supply the choroidal coat and ciliary processes. The anterior ciliary arteries are derived from the muscular branches of the ophthalmic artery and run to the front of the globe with the tendons of the extraocular muscles, where they pierce the sclera and end in the greater arterial circle of the iris. The subarachnoid space extends forward between the nerve and sheath.* A., *artery;* Ant., *anterior;* Cent., *central;* Cil., *ciliary;* CN, *cranial nerve;* Eth., *ethmoidal;* Front., *frontal;* Inf., *inferior;* Lat., *lateral;* M., *muscle;* Med., *medial;* N., *nerve;* Nasocil., *nasociliary;* Obl., *oblique;* Ophth., *ophthalmic;* Post., *posterior;* Rec., *rectus;* Ret., *retinal;* Subarach., *subarachnoid;* Sup., *superior.*

the cribriform plate a few millimeters anterior to the orbital end of the optic canal. As the anterior ethmoidal artery passes across the floor of the anterior cranial fossa near the cribriform plate, it gives rise to the anterior falx artery, which runs between and supplies the anterior portion of the falx and walls of the superior sagittal sinus. The anterior and posterior ethmoidal arteries then pass through the cribriform plate area to supply the ethmoidal sinuses, the infundibulum of the frontal sinus, the anterior nasal cavity, and the skin over the cartilaginous part of the nose.

Arteries that supply the margins of the superior orbital fissure and may be recruited to supply tumors in the region include the anterior branch of the middle meningeal artery, the recurrent meningeal branches of the ophthalmic and lacrimal arteries, the meningeal branches of the internal carotid artery, the tentorial branch of the meningohypophyseal trunk, the anterior branch of the inferolateral trunk, and the terminal branches of the internal maxillary artery.

VENOUS RELATIONSHIPS

The venous spaces of the cavernous sinus fill the posterior margin of the superior orbital fissure and may extend forward along the medial and lower edges of the fissure (*Figs. 7.2* and *7.3*). The veins passing through the fissure empty into the cavernous sinus. The dural sinuses into which the sylvian veins empty commonly pass below the sphenoid ridge and along the intracranial edge of the lateral margin of the superior orbital fissure to reach the cavernous sinus. These sinuses are encountered in exposures directed through the lateral margin of the fissure.

The superior ophthalmic vein arises from tributaries in the superomedial part of the orbit, and the inferior ophthalmic vein arises from tributaries in the inferolateral part of the orbit (*Figs. 7.2, 7.3,* and *7.5*). These veins are connected along the anterior margin of the orbit by large anastomotic channels formed by the facial and angular veins. This inferior ophthalmic vein may empty directly into the cavernous sinus, but more commonly, joins the superior ophthalmic vein to form a common stem that drains into the cavernous sinus.

The superior ophthalmic vein arises in the upper medial part of the orbit, passes backward on the lateral side of the superior oblique muscle, and crosses above the optic nerve to reach the lateral part of the orbit. It exits the muscle cone by passing between the heads of the superior and lateral rectus muscles and outside the annular tendon, through the narrow lateral part of the superior orbital fissure. It passes downward along the lateral margin of the annular tendon at the level of the superior orbital fissure, where it is commonly joined by the inferior ophthalmic vein to form a common trunk that enters the anteroinferior part of the cavernous sinus. Both the superior ophthalmic vein and the ophthalmic artery course along the superolateral aspect of the optic nerve in the orbital apex, but the vein passes outside the annular tendon and through the narrow lateral part of the superior orbital fissure, whereas the artery passes through the annular tendon and the optic foramen. The superior ophthalmic vein is anchored in the lateral corner of the superior orbital fissure by several fibrous bands that form a hammock around the vein, creating an obstacle to approaches to the lateral part of the orbital apex.

The inferior ophthalmic vein originates from tributaries on the anterior part of the floor and lateral wall of the orbit. It drains the inferior rectus and inferior oblique muscles, the lacrimal sac, and eyelids. It courses medially and posteriorly between the lateral and inferior rectus muscles with the branch of the oculomotor nerve to the inferior oblique muscle. It communicates with the pterygoid venous plexus through the inferior orbital fissure. It exits the muscle cone by passing between the origin of the lateral and inferior rectus muscles and the orbit, coursing below the annular tendon and through the inferior sector of the superior orbital fissure. It commonly joins the superior ophthalmic vein on the lateral aspect the annular tendon as it passes through the superior orbital fissure. The common trunk passes backward to enter the anteroinferior part of the cavernous sinus.

MUSCULAR AND TENDINOUS RELATIONSHIPS

The orbicularis oculi muscle surrounds the circumference of the orbit and spreads out on the temple and cheek (*Fig. 7.9*). It has orbital, palpebral, and lacrimal parts. The orbital part spreads in a wide band around the margin of the orbit. The palpebral part is located in the margins of the eyelids. The orbital part arises from the nasal process of the frontal bone, the frontal process of the maxilla, and the medial palpebral ligament. On the lateral side, it blends with the occipitofrontalis and the corrugator muscles. Many of the upper orbital fibers are inserted into the skin and subcutaneous tissues of the eyebrow. The palpebral part arises from the medial palpebral ligament and the bone above and below the ligament. Some of its fibers lie close to the margin of the eyelid behind the eyelashes. The lacrimal part extends behind the lacrimal sac and attaches to the lacrimal bone. The orbital part is the sphincter muscle of the eyelids. The palpebral portion closes the eyelids. The actions of the lacrimal part are important in tear transport.

The tarsi are two thin plates of dense fibrous tissue situated deep to the palpebral part of the orbicularis oculi muscle. The tarsi are placed in and give support and shape to each eyelid. Some of the fibers of the levator muscle are attached to the upper tarsus. The medial ends of the tarsi are attached by a tendinous band, the medial palpebral ligament, to the upper part of the lacrimal crest and the adjoining part of the frontal process of the maxilla in front of the lacrimal crest. The lateral ends of the tarsi are attached by a band, the lateral palpebral ligament, to a tubercle on the zygomatic bone immediately within the orbital margin. The orbital septum is a membranous sheet attached to the orbital margin where it is continuous with the periosteum along the anterior edge of the orbit. It separates the facial from the orbital structures. In the upper eyelid, the septum blends with the superficial part of the aponeurosis of the superior levator, and in the lower eyelid, it blends with the anterior surface of the tarsus. The medial and

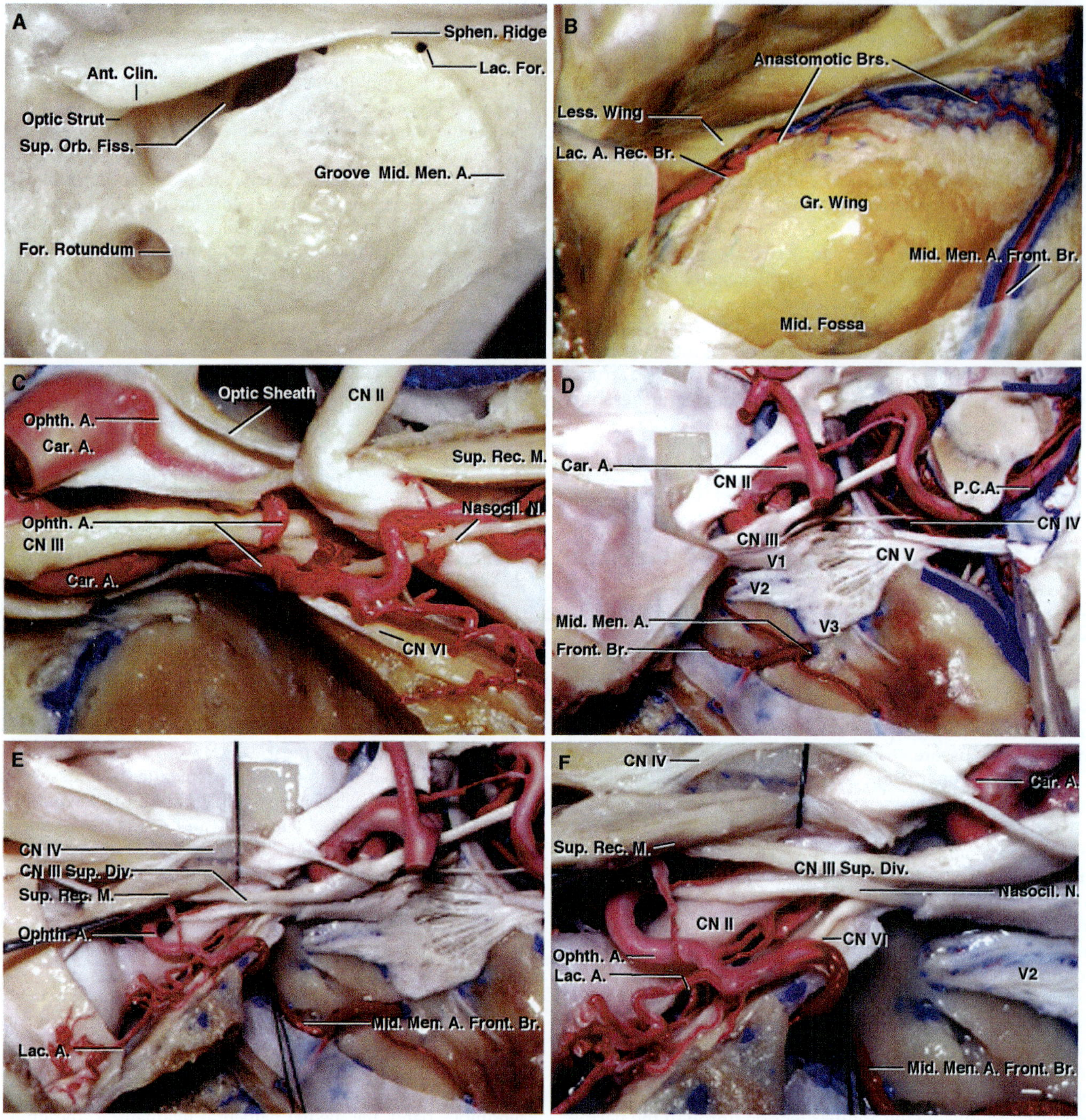

FIGURE 7.8. *Middle meningeal origin of the ophthalmic artery.* A, *posterior view of the right superior orbital fissure and the sphenoid ridge. The lacrimal foramen, through which the recurrent branch of the ophthalmic or lacrimal artery enters the orbit, is situated lateral to the superior orbital fissure. The recurrent branch frequently passes through the lateral margin of the superior orbital fissure, courses laterally below the sphenoid ridge, and turns forward through the meningolacrimal foramen to supply the periorbita in the roof of the orbit. Anastomosis from the frontal branch of the middle meningeal artery frequently contributes to the branch that passes through the lacrimal foramen.* B, *area just below the sphenoid ridge where there are often anastomoses between the recurrent branch of the lacrimal artery and the frontal branch of the middle meningeal artery.* C, *the right ophthalmic artery in the specimen with the anomalous left ophthalmic artery, shown in* D–F, *has a normal origin from the internal carotid artery. It arises below the optic nerve, which has been reflected forward, and passes forward under the optic nerve to penetrate the dura lining the optic canal, reaching the orbital apex on the lateral side of the optic nerve. The annular tendon, from which the rectus muscles arise, has been opened and the lateral rectus muscle and the nerves passing through the superior orbital fissure have been folded downward with the lateral rectus muscle to expose the artery at the orbital apex.* D, *the dura covering the left cavernous sinus has been removed. The frontal branch of the left middle meningeal artery has been exposed up to where it passes through the superior*

lateral cheek ligaments are fibrous expansions extending from sheaths of the lateral and medial rectus muscles that attach to the zygomatic and lacrimal bone, respectively. The cheek ligaments limit the actions of the lateral and medial rectus muscles.

The four rectus muscles arise from the annular tendon and form a cone around the neural and vascular structures passing through the annulus. The annular tendon is adherent to the dural sheath of the optic nerve and the periosteum above, below, and medial to the optic canal and to the lateral margin of the superior orbital fissure. The superior rectus muscle arises from the annular tendon, passes forward, and attaches to the sclera posterior to the margin of the cornea. The line of attachment is slightly oblique and curved. The superior oblique muscle arises from the periorbita covering the body of the sphenoid bone superomedial to the optic canal and runs forward, ending in a tendon that loops through the trochlea, a round tendon that attaches to the trochlear fossa of the frontal bone. After looping through the trochlea, the tendon passes laterally and posteriorly below the superior rectus muscle to insert on the sclera between the superior and lateral rectus muscles. The lateral rectus muscle arises from the annular tendon and adjacent part of the greater wing of the sphenoid bone and has a vertical line of attachment to the sclera posterior to the margin of the cornea. The inferior rectus muscle arises from the annular tendon and has an oblique line of attachment, with the medial side slightly anterior to the lateral side of the attachment. The inferior oblique muscle arises from the part of the orbital floor formed by the orbital surface of the maxilla in the area just lateral to the nasolacrimal duct, not from the orbital apex. It runs laterally and posteriorly, passing between the inferior rectus muscle and the orbital floor, and then between the lateral rectus muscle and the globe, to insert into the sclera between the superior and lateral rectus muscles near the insertion of the superior oblique muscle. The medial rectus muscle arises from the annular tendon, runs forward, and has a vertical line of attachment to the sclera. The orbital smooth muscle (Müller's muscle) spans the upper margin of the inferior orbital fissure, and blends into the periorbita, the periosteum of the maxillary bone, and the perineurium of the infraorbital nerve.

SURGICAL CONSIDERATIONS

The earliest reports of surgery for orbital lesions involved approaches directed through the lateral wall of the orbit (14, 18). The first report of a transcranial approach to the orbit was published in 1922 by Dandy (2). Since then, both extra- and intracranial routes to orbital lesions have been developed (1, 9, 12). The transcranial approach is commonly selected for tumors located in the orbital apex and/or optic canal, or involving both the orbit and adjacent intracranial areas (2, 6, 10). Tumors confined within the periorbita in the anterior two-thirds of the orbit can often be approached extracranially, but those located in the apical area, and especially those on the medial side of the optic nerve, often require a transcranial approach. An approach directed through the lateral orbital wall, involving an osteotomy of lateral rim and wall, is commonly selected for tumors confined to the superior, lateral, or inferior compartment of the orbit and those in the lateral part of the apex (14, 18). An approach directed along the medial orbital wall may be used for tumors located medial to the optic nerve that are not located deep in the apex (13, 18, 23).

The transcranial surgical approaches to the orbit may be arbitrarily divided into two types based on whether the orbital rim is or is not elevated in exposing the orbital lesion. Early approaches involved removal of a frontal or frontotemporal bone flap, with preservation of the supraorbital rim, and opening of the orbit behind the rim (3, 4, 9, 11, 16, 17, 19, 20). The transcranial approach can be tailored to the site of the lesion. For limited lesions, an approach directed through a small frontal craniotomy or frontotemporal craniotomy, with removal of the orbital roof and/or lateral wall, will provide access. However, for larger lesions, it is advantageous to elevate the orbital rim with the bone flap as is performed in the orbitofrontal or orbitozygomatic approach. In the orbitofrontal approach, only the upper rim of the orbit is elevated, and in the orbitozygomatic approach, the superior and lateral parts of the orbital rim are elevated. The orbitofrontal craniotomy would be selected for lesions involving the optic canal and orbital apex. The orbitozygomatic craniotomy would be selected for orbital lesions involving the middle fossa or superior orbital fissure, in addition to the orbit. In the one-piece orbitozygomatic approach, the orbital rim and frontotemporal bone flap are elevated together as a single bone flap. In the two-piece approach, the frontotemporal bone flap is elevated as the first piece and the osteotomy of the orbital rim and zygoma are elevated as the second piece. The orbitozygomatic approaches are reviewed in detail in Chapter 9.

Orbitofrontal Craniotomy

A bicoronal scalp flap is reflected to expose the site of the craniotomy, which includes the upper rim of the orbit (*Fig. 7.10*) (21, 22). The pericranium is reflected forward to expose the frontal bone and supraorbital margin. The supraorbital and supratrochlear nerves are exposed as they pass through a notch or foramina in the supraorbital rim. The supraorbital nerve may be released by removing bone with a drill or chisel from the lower margin of their foramen. The anterior edge of the temporalis muscle is reflected backward to expose the

orbital fissure. E, *the levator and superior rectus muscles have been elevated to show the anomalous ophthalmic artery coursing in the orbit.* F, *enlarged view of the junction of the frontal branch of the middle meningeal artery with the ophthalmic artery. The wall of the middle meningeal artery embedded in the dura is thinner than after entering the orbit where it courses in the intraorbital fat.* A., *artery;* Ant., *anterior;* Br., *branch;* Brs., *branches;* Car., *carotid;* Clin., *clinoid;* CN, *cranial nerve;* Div., *division;* Fiss., *fissure;* For., *foramen;* Front., *frontal;* Gr., *greater;* Lac., *lacrimal;* Less., *lesser;* M., *muscle;* Men., *meningeal;* Mid., *middle;* Nasocil., *nasociliary;* Ophth., *ophthalmic;* Orb., *orbital;* P.C.A., *posterior cerebral artery;* Rec., *recurrent;* Sphen., *sphenoid;* Sup., *superior.*

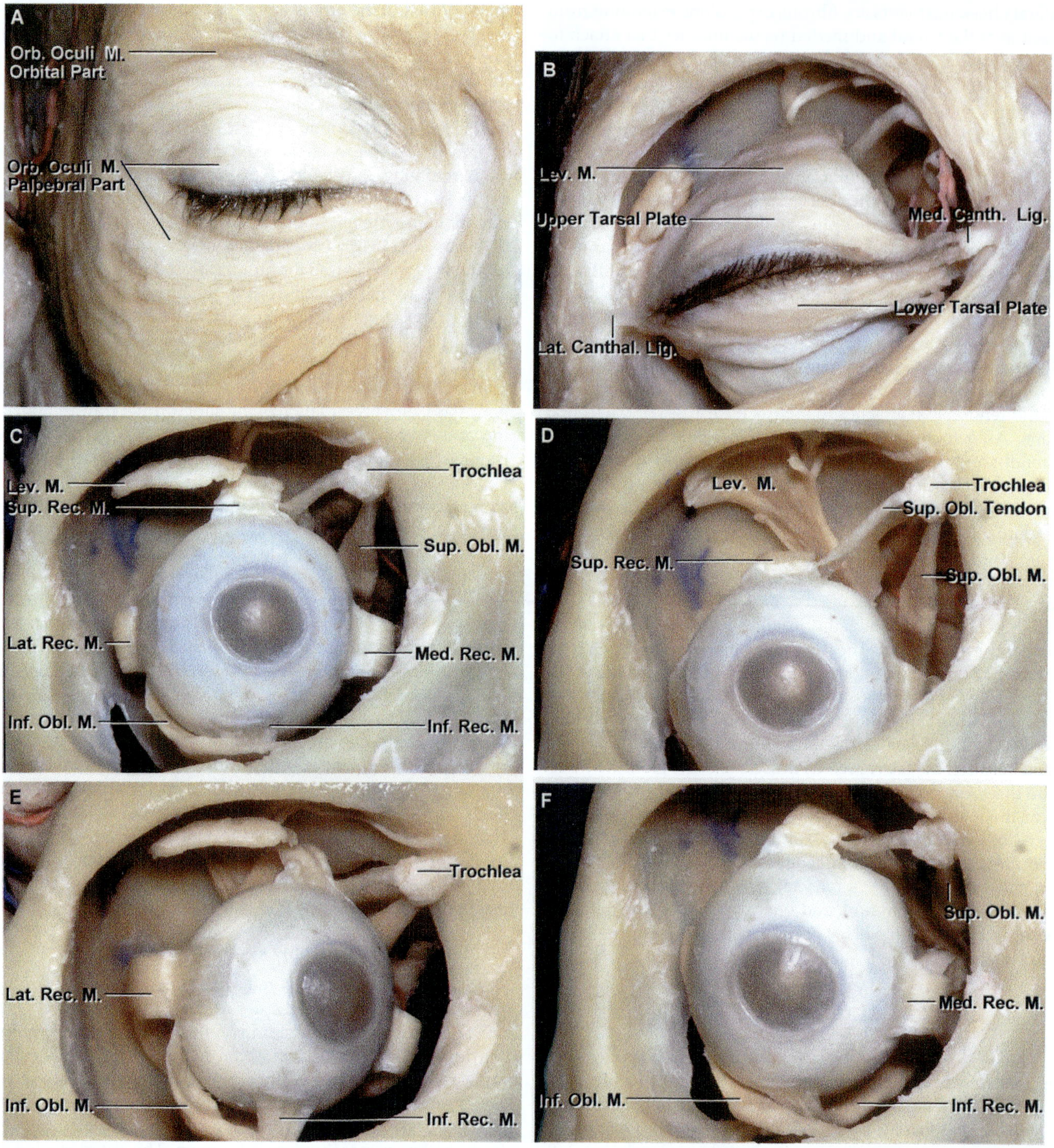

FIGURE 7.9. *Anterior view of orbit and extraocular muscles. A, the skin around the right orbit has been removed to expose the orbicularis oculi muscle. This muscle surrounds the circumference of the orbit and spreads out on the temple and cheek. It has orbital, palpebral, and lacrimal parts. The orbital part of the orbicularis oculi spreads in a wide band around the margin of the orbit. The palpebral part is located in the margins of the eyelids. The orbital part arises from the nasal process of the frontal bone, the frontal process of the maxilla, and the medial palpebral ligament. On the lateral side, it blends with the occipitofrontalis and the corrugator muscles. Many of the upper orbital fibers are inserted into the skin and subcutaneous tissues of the eyebrow. The palpebral part arises from the medial palpebral ligament and the bone above and below the ligament. Some of its fibers lie close to the margin of the eyelid behind the eyelashes. The lacrimal part extends behind the lacrimal sac and attaches to the lacrimal bone. The orbicularis oculi is the sphincter muscle of the eyelids. The palpebral portion closes the eyelids. The actions of the lacrimal part are important in tear transport. B, the orbicular muscle has been removed to expose the upper and lower tarsi, thin plates of dense fibrous tissue situated deep to the palpebral part of the orbicularis oculi muscle. The tarsi*

keyhole, the site of a burr hole that straddles the orbit and anterior cranial fossa, and which, at its depth, will expose periorbita on its lower edge and frontal dura on its upper edge. A zygomatic-temporal branch of the zygomatic nerve may be exposed on the zygomatic process of the frontal bone. The orbitofrontal bone flap includes the superior rim of the orbit and part of the orbital roof. The medial edge of the bone cut commonly extends through the frontal sinus. The thin part of the roof of the orbit behind the orbital rim is opened to prevent the fracture across the orbital roof, which occurs as the bone flap is elevated, from extending medially into the cribriform plate or ethmoid air cells.

The orbitofrontal craniotomy can be performed either as a one-piece exposure, in which the superior rim is elevated with the bone flap, or as a two-piece exposure, in which the small frontal bone flap above the supraorbital rim is elevated as the first piece and the superior rim is removed as the second piece. Approaching it in a two-piece manner allows more of the orbital roof to be preserved, because the bone cuts through the rim and roof can be performed under direct vision after the dura has been elevated from the orbital roof. In the one-piece exposure, the bone cuts through the orbital roof are made by depressing the periorbita and making the cut in the roof through the narrow space between the bone and periorbita. In addition, in the one-piece approach, it is not uncommon to have to fracture the last segment of the orbital roof between the medial and the lateral margins of the cuts in the roof, with the risk that the roof fracture can extend into the ethmoid air cells. This can be avoided if a burr hole is placed at the keyhole and the lateral part of the roof is opened through the keyhole. Another burr hole is then placed just above the medial part of the superior rim and opens through the anterior and posterior walls of the frontal sinus at the medial edge of the flap. The medial burr hole allows the medial part of the orbital rim and adjacent part of the orbital roof to be divided so that the bone flap can be elevated without having to fracture through the medial part of the roof. However, the two-piece approach obviates this, because the bone cuts in the orbital roof can be made extradurally under direct vision after elevating the dura from the roof.

Elevation of the bone flap exposes the periorbita of the orbital roof and the dura covering the anterior pole of the frontal lobe. Some lesions confined entirely to the orbit can be removed without opening the dura, but an intradural exposure is required for those lesions involving the optic canal, superior orbital fissure, or those involving the intradural surface of the orbital walls. The remaining roof of the orbit and optic canal are removed as needed. The dura can be opened and the frontal lobe elevated to expose the optic canal and optic nerve as needed. The olfactory tract is exposed above the cribriform plate. One olfactory nerve may have to be sacrificed. The falciform ligament, a dural fold that extends from the anterior clinoid process across the top of the optic nerve just proximal to the optic canal to the tuberculum sellae, may be opened (*Figs. 7.2* and *7.10*). At the site of this dural fold, the nerve is covered only by dura, rather than by dura and bone, as it is within the optic canal. The optic canal is opened to expose the intracanicular segment of the optic nerve. Opening the periorbita exposes the trochlear nerve and the supraorbital and supratrochlear branches of the frontal nerve, all of which course immediately beneath and can often be seen through the periorbita. The trochlear nerve passes medially above the levator muscle to reach the superior oblique muscle. Three routes through an orbitofrontal craniotomy can be taken to the orbital contents: medial, lateral, and central. These approaches can also be used with an orbitozygomatic craniotomy.

are placed in and give support and shape to each eyelid. Some of the fibers of the levator muscle are attached to the upper tarsus. The medial ends of the tarsi are attached by a tendinous band, the medial canthal ligament, to the upper part of the lacrimal crest and the adjoining part of the frontal process of the maxilla in front of the lacrimal crest. The lateral ends of the tarsi are attached by a band, the lateral canthal ligament, to a tubercle on the zygomatic bone immediately within the orbital margin. The orbital septum that separates the facial from the orbital structures has been removed. It attaches to the orbital margin where it is continuous with the periosteum along the anterior edge of the orbit. In the upper eyelid it blends with the superficial part of the aponeurosis of the superior levator, and in the lower eyelid, it blends with the anterior surface of the tarsus. C, *the globe and the optic nerve are surrounded by the four rectus, the levator, and two oblique muscles. The four rectus muscles arise from the annular tendon that surrounds the optic canal and adjunct part of the superior orbital fissure. The levator muscle arises from the lesser wing of the sphenoid above and anterior to the optic canal and fans out to have a broad attachment to the superior tarsus and the skin of the upper lid. The superior oblique muscle arises from the body of the sphenoid superomedial to the optic canal. The inferior oblique muscle arises from the orbital surface of the maxilla lateral to the nasolacrimal groove. The medial and lateral cheek ligaments (not shown) are fibrous expansions extending from sheaths of the lateral and medial rectus muscles that attach to the zygomatic and lacrimal bone, respectively, and limit the actions of the lateral and medial rectus muscles.* D, *globe depressed to show the insertion of the superior rectus muscle and the trochlea and distal tendon of the superior oblique muscle. The superior rectus muscle arises from the annular tendon, passes forward, and attaches to the sclera posterior to the margin of the cornea. The superior oblique muscle arises from the periorbita covering the body of the sphenoid bone superomedial to the optic canal and runs forward, ending in a tendon that loops through the trochlea, a round tendon that attaches to the trochlear fossa of the frontal bone. After looping through the trochlea, the tendon passes laterally and posteriorly below the superior rectus muscle to insert on the sclera between the superior and lateral rectus muscles.* E, *globe adducted to show the insertion of the lateral rectus muscle. The lateral rectus muscle arises from the annular tendon and adjacent part of the greater wing of the sphenoid bone and has a vertical line of attachment to the sclera.* F, *globe positioned to show the relationship of the inferior rectus and inferior oblique muscles. The inferior rectus muscle arises from the annular tendon and has an oblique line of attachment, with the medial side slightly anterior to the lateral side of the attachment. The inferior oblique muscle arises from the part of the orbital floor formed by the orbital surface of the maxilla in the area just lateral to the nasolacrimal duct, not from the orbital apex, and runs laterally and posteriorly, passing between the inferior rectus muscle and the orbital floor, and then between the lateral rectus muscle and the globe, to insert into the sclera between the superior and lateral rectus muscles near the insertion of the superior oblique muscle.* Canth., *canthal;* Inf., *inferior;* Lat., *lateral;* Lev., *levator;* Lig., *ligament;* M., *muscle;* Med., *medial;* Obl., *oblique;* Orb., *orbit;* Rec., *rectus;* Sup., *superior.*

The Medial Orbitofrontal Approach

The medial approach is directed through the space between the superior oblique muscle, which is retracted medially, and the levator and superior rectus muscles, both of which are retracted laterally (*Fig. 7.10, E* and *F*). This approach exposes the optic nerve throughout the interval from the globe to the optic canal. It is the most direct surgical approach to the apical part of the optic nerve.

Four structures are located on the lateral side of the optic nerve near the orbital apex that pass above the optic nerve to reach the medial part of the orbit. These structures, the trochlear nerve, ophthalmic artery, nasociliary nerve, and superior ophthalmic vein, cross above the nerve an average of 3.2 mm, 10.6 mm, 10.0 mm, and 23.9 mm distal to the anterior opening of the optic canal, respectively (21). In approximately 15% of orbits, the ophthalmic artery will pass below rather than above the optic nerve. The incision for opening the annular tendon, if needed, is directed between the attachment of the superior and medial rectus muscles. Before the annulus is opened, the trochlear nerve is separated from the adjacent tissues above the orbital apex to prevent its damage in opening the optic sheath. Opening the annular tendon and optic sheath exposes the medial and superior surface of the optic nerve from the globe to the optic chiasm. This incision provides excellent exposure of the optic nerve and the ophthalmic artery in the optic canal and orbital apex, but yields limited access to the structures passing through the superior orbital fissure on the lateral side of the optic nerve.

The following structures are on the medial side of the optic nerve: anteriorly near the globe, the ophthalmic artery, the nasociliary nerve, and the superior ophthalmic vein; and posteriorly near the orbital apex, the trochlear nerve and the posterior ethmoidal artery. The interval between the anteriorly and posteriorly situated structures is free of important structures, thus providing a route to the optic nerve. However, the space between the superior oblique and the levator muscles is much narrower than the space between the levator and the lateral rectus muscles used for the lateral approach. The angle through which the approach can be made is also limited in width by the medial margin of the frontal craniotomy.

The medial approach is selected for lesions located superomedial to the optic nerve or for cases in which there is a need to expose the optic nerve from the optic canal to the globe. It is the approach most commonly selected for tumors of the optic sheath or optic nerve. The medial approach is not suitable for lesions located on the lateral side of the optic nerve or for those involving the superior orbital fissure and the cavernous sinus.

The Central Orbitofrontal Approach

In the central approach, the levator muscle is retracted medially and the superior rectus muscle is retracted laterally (*Fig. 7.10, J* and *K*). The central approach, which is the least used of the three approaches directed through an orbitofrontal craniotomy, is the most direct and shortest way to the midportion of the intraorbital segment of the optic nerve. There are two variants of this approach; the choice depends on whether the frontal nerve is retracted medially with the levator muscle or laterally with the superior rectus muscle. The second variant, in which the frontal nerve is retracted laterally with the superior rectus muscle, provides a wider exposure of the orbital apex than the exposure in which the frontal nerve is retracted medially with the levator muscle.

The approach in which the frontal nerve is retracted medially with the levator muscle carries less risk of damaging the frontal nerve, because the frontal nerve and the levator muscle, on which the frontal nerve courses, do not have to be separated as they do when the frontal nerve is retracted laterally with the superior rectus muscle. On the other hand, maintaining the frontal nerve on the levator muscle blocks the approach to the deep apical region lateral to the optic nerve and yields access to only the midportion of the intraorbital segment of the optic nerve. Even when the frontal nerve is retracted laterally with the superior rectus muscle, the view into the orbital apex may be limited by the overlap of the origin of the levator and superior rectus muscles, which are located one above the other. Another disadvantage of this approach is that the orbital septum that covers the lower side of the superior rectus muscle must be opened, thus risking damage to the ophthalmic artery and the nasociliary nerve, which cross the optic nerve just beneath the septum. Structures seen in the exposure between the retracted muscles include the superior ophthalmic vein, ciliary arteries and nerves, nasociliary nerve, branch of the oculomotor nerve to the levator muscle, and the ophthalmic artery and its branches to the levator and superior rectus muscles. The many structures in the exposure create a complicated field, requiring considerable care to avoid injuring the exposed structures. However, this route is the shortest, most direct one to the middle third of the optic nerve in its intraorbital portion.

The central approach may be selected for biopsy or removal of lesions located in the midportion of the intraorbital segment of the optic nerve. The variant in which the frontal nerve is retracted laterally provides access to the posterior third of the intraorbital portion of the optic nerve.

The Lateral Orbitofrontal Approach

For the lateral approach, the optic nerve is approached between the lateral rectus muscle, which is retracted laterally, and the superior rectus and levator muscles, both of which are retracted medially (*Fig. 7.10, G–I*). The lateral approach provides a wider working space than the medial or central approach. The wider angle of access allows the approach to be directed through all parts of the orbitofrontal exposure. It is the best of the three orbitofrontal routes for exposing the deep apical area on the lateral side of the optic nerve. It is possible to expose the superior orbital fissure and adjacent part of the cavernous sinus in combination with the lateral approach if it is combined with an orbitozygomatic craniotomy, in which the superior and lateral part of the orbital rim and the roof and lateral wall of the orbit are elevated with a frontotemporal bone flap. This orbitozygomatic craniotomy in combination with the lateral approach is suitable for lesions that involve the area along the anterior clinoid process and sphenoid ridge and

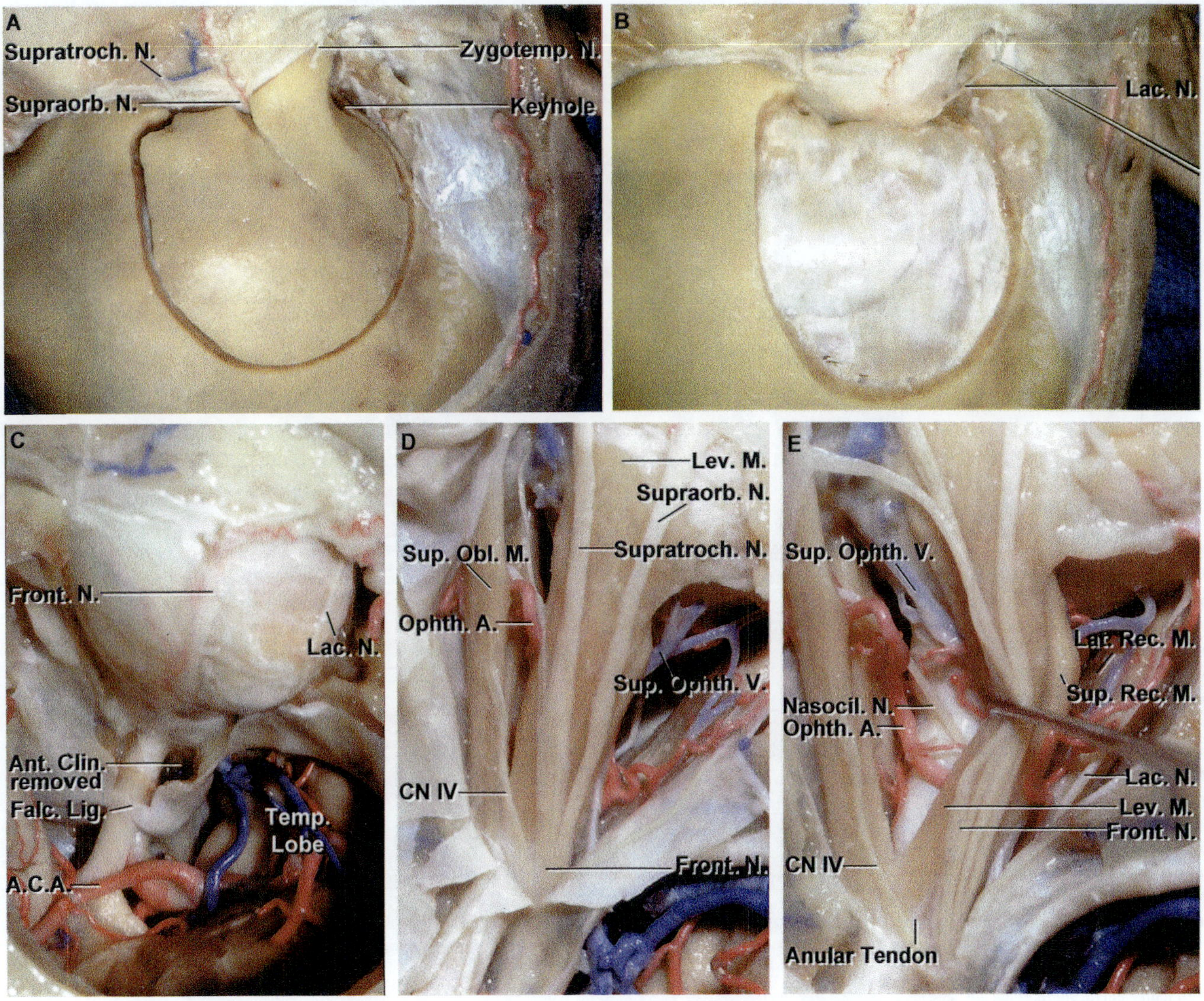

FIGURE 7.10. *Orbitofrontal craniotomy in which the supraorbital rim and the anterior part of the orbital roof are elevated with the frontal bone flap. A, a bicoronal scalp flap has been reflected forward to expose the frontal bone and supraorbital margin. The supraorbital nerve has been released by removing bone from the lower margin of the supraorbital foramen. The craniotome has cut around the margin of the orbitofrontal bone flap, which includes the supraorbital ridge and part of the orbital roof. The temporalis muscle has been reflected backward to expose the keyhole, the site of a burr hole, which at its depth will expose periorbita in its lower edge and frontal dura in its upper edge. A zygomatic-temporal branch of the zygomatic nerve is exposed on the zygomatic process of the frontal bone. B, removal of the bone flap exposes the periorbita of the orbital roof and the dura covering the frontal lobe. The medial edge of the bone cut should extend completely through the orbital rim and partially divide the thin part of the roof of the orbit behind the orbital rim to prevent the fracture across the orbital roof, which occurs as the bone flap is elevated, from extending medially into the cribriform plate or ethmoid air cells. C, the roof of the orbit has been removed, the frontal lobe elevated, and the dura and arachnoid opened to expose the optic nerve intracranially and in the optic canal. The optic canal has been unroofed to expose the intracanicular segment of the optic nerve. The falciform ligament is a dural fold, which extends from the anterior clinoid across the top of the optic nerve just proximal to the optic canal to the tuberculum sellae. At the site of this dural fold, the nerve is covered only by dura, rather than by dura and bone, as it is within the optic canal. The anterior clinoid artery, situated on the lateral side of the optic nerve, has been removed. The anterior cerebral artery courses above the optic chiasm. D, the periorbita has been opened and the orbital fat removed to expose the trochlear nerve, the supraorbital and supratrochlear branches of the frontal nerve, and the levator and superior oblique muscles. The trochlear nerve passes medially above the levator muscle to reach the superior oblique muscle. The superior ophthalmic vein passes through the lateral part of the superior orbital fissure. E and F, medial route to the optic nerve. E, the medial approach is directed through the interval between the superior oblique and the levator muscles. In the medial route there are no neural and vascular structures between the ophthalmic artery and orbital apex, except the trochlear nerve, which crosses above the levator muscle in the extraconal area. The ophthalmic artery, superior ophthalmic vein, and nasociliary nerve are situated on the lateral side of the optic nerve at the orbital apex, but further forward they cross above the nerve to reach the medial part of the orbit. F, an incision has been extended backward through the annular tendon between the superior and medial rectus muscles and through the optic sheath to expose the full length of the optic nerve. The trochlear nerve passes above the levator muscle at the orbital apex in its passage to the superior oblique muscle and should be protected in completing the incision through the annular tendon and along the optic sheath. This type of incision in the annular tendon can be combined with the medial supraorbital approach to provide access to the optic nerve from the optic chiasm to the globe. The sphenoid and ethmoidal sinuses are exposed on the medial side of the orbit. G and H, lateral route to the intraconal and apical area. The lateral route to the optic nerve is directed through the interval between the levator and superior rectus muscle medially and the lateral rectus muscle laterally. This route is often selected for lesions that involve the area lateral to the optic nerve or those extending through the superior orbital fissure. G, the levator and superior rectus muscles and the superior ophthalmic vein have been retracted medially to expose the intraorbital part*
(Legend continues on next page.)

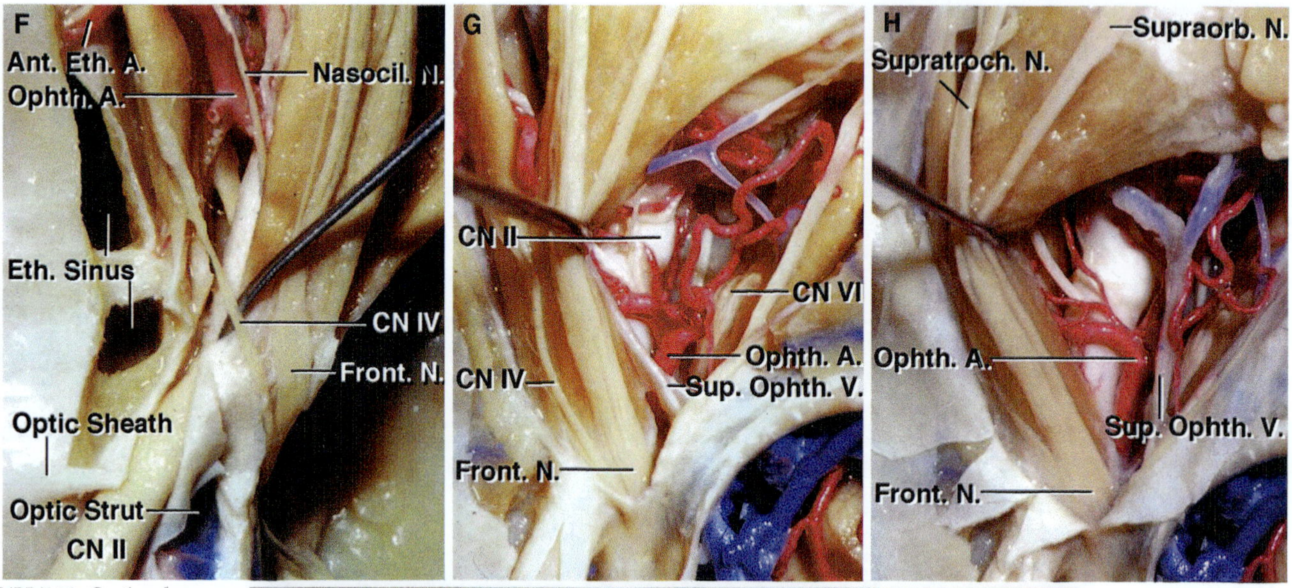

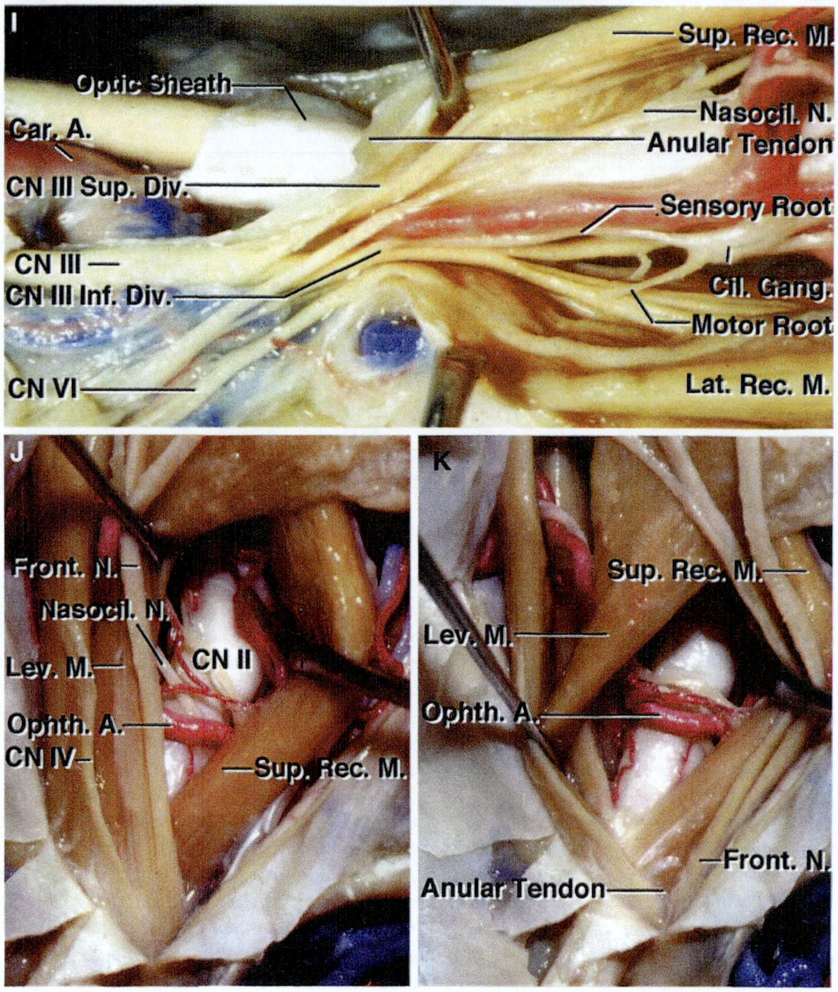

FIGURE 7.10. *Continued* *of the optic nerve. The superior ophthalmic vein blocks the view of the deep apical area.* H, *the superior ophthalmic vein has been displaced laterally to expose the deep apical area. It blocks the view of the apical area, as shown in* G, *when it is retracted medially.* I, *the annular tendon has been divided between the origin of the lateral and superior rectus muscles, as can be performed in the lateral approach. The origin of the superior rectus muscle from the annular tendon has been retracted medially and the origin of the lateral rectus muscle has been retracted laterally. This incision can be combined with a lateral supraorbital approach to increase access to the structures in the superior orbital fissure. The nasociliary nerve crosses above the optic nerve in front of the annular tendon and orbital apex. The superior division of the oculomotor nerve sends branches into the lower surface of the superior rectus and levator muscle. The abducens nerve passes through the superior orbital fissure below the nasociliary nerve and enters the medial surface of the lateral rectus muscle. The ophthalmic artery courses on the lateral side of the optic nerve at the orbital apex. The sensory root to the ciliary ganglion arises from the nasociliary nerve and the motor parasympathetic root arises from the branch of the inferior division to the inferior oblique muscle.* J *and* K, *central route to the optic nerve. This route is directed between the levator and superior rectus muscles.* J, *the levator and the frontal nerve are retracted medially, and the superior rectus muscle is retracted laterally. This exposes the middle third of the intraorbital portion of the optic nerve. It is the shortest route through the orbital roof to the optic nerve. The ophthalmic artery and the nasociliary nerve cross above the optic nerve. The branch of the*

middle fossa and extend through the superior orbital fissure into the orbit on the lateral side of the optic nerve.

There are two variants of the lateral approach; the choice is determined by whether the superior ophthalmic vein is retracted medially or laterally. If the superior ophthalmic vein is retracted medially with the superior rectus and levator muscles, it is not necessary to dissect the vein from the connective tissue, which forms a hammock around the vein adjacent to the superior fissure. It is easy to expose the optic nerve lateral to the fibrous hammock without risk of damage to the intraorbital connective tissue, which contains the ciliary nerves. However, access to the deep apical area is limited because the superior ophthalmic vein blocks the line of view. The superior ophthalmic vein enters the superior orbital fissure an average of 9.7 mm lateral to the anterior edge of the optic strut (21). It commonly passes through the superior edge of the fissure, but it may also pass through the fissure below the superior margin, in which case it is difficult to approach the deep apical area because the vein blocks access to the area on the medial side of the superior orbital fissure.

The variant in which the superior ophthalmic vein and connective tissue hammock are dissected free of adjacent structures and retracted laterally with the lateral rectus muscle provides access to lesions in the lateral part of the deep apical area that may also involve the superior orbital fissure and cavernous sinus. To retract the superior ophthalmic vein laterally, the orbital septum (which runs under the surface of the superior rectus muscle and connects to the superior ophthalmic vein) must be opened, thus risking damage to the cranial nerves that pass through the superior orbital fissure and to the ciliary ganglion, which are normally protected beneath the orbital septum. In the approach in which the vein is retracted laterally, the annular tendon is easily visualized between the origins of the superior and lateral rectus muscles. Dividing the annular tendon between the superior and lateral rectus muscles exposes the deep apical area at its junction with the superior orbital fissure.

Lateral Wall Approach (Sphenozygomatic Approach)

An approach directed through the lateral orbital wall, involving an osteotomy of the lateral orbital rim and wall, is selected for tumors confined to the superior, temporal, or inferior compartment of the orbit and those in the lateral part of the apex (14, 18) (*Fig. 7.11*). The curved skin incision begins in front of the ear, extends forward along the upper edge of the zygoma, and turns upward along the lateral rim of the orbit to expose the superficial temporal artery and the vein and zygomaticotemporal nerve. Opening the skin and subcutaneous tissues over the lateral wall of the orbit exposes the branches of the superficial temporal artery, the branches of the facial nerve to the orbicularis and frontalis muscles, the zygomaticotemporal branch of the maxillary nerve, and the auriculotemporal branch of the mandibular nerve, all of which course in the subcutaneous tissues superficial to the temporalis muscle. The branches of the facial nerve should be protected and preserved, and if divided in the exposure they should be reapproximated at the time of closure.

Elevating the lateral rim and wall exposes the periorbita anterior to the lateral edge of the superior orbital fissure. Opening the periorbita exposes the lateral rectus muscle, the lacrimal artery and nerve, and the lacrimal gland. Retracting the orbital fat exposes the structures lateral to and above and below the optic nerve, and the insertion of the lateral rectus and inferior oblique muscles on the globe. The lateral orbital rim and wall, which has been elevated in a single piece, is replaced after removing an orbital lesion.

The orbitozygomatic craniotomy, which is reviewed in Chapter 9, can be used if the lateral orbital exposure needs to be combined with the extradural exposure of the superior orbital fissure, orbital roof, anterior clinoid process, and cavernous sinus, and intradural exposure of the optic nerve, internal carotid artery and its branches, and the roof and lateral wall of the cavernous sinus. The orbitozygomatic approach can also be tailored to include only the lateral wall and not the orbital roof.

Exposing the superior orbital fissure and its sectors requires at least limited exposure of the cavernous sinus posteriorly and the orbit anteriorly. This is usually achieved with an orbitozygomatic craniotomy. Fortunately, all of the nerves of the cavernous sinus, except the abducens nerve, can be exposed by peeling away the outer layer of dura in the lateral sinus wall, while leaving the inner layer investing the nerves intact. It is possible to expose the full course of the oculomotor and trochlear nerves from their entrance into the roof of the sinus and the ophthalmic nerve from its origin through the fissure and into the orbit without opening into the major venous spaces of the sinus, because these nerves course in the inner dural layer of the lateral sinus wall. Exposure of the abducens nerve is more hazardous, because it courses within the sinus and is adherent to the lateral surface of the intracavernous carotid artery. Removing the bony margins of the superior orbital fissure without exposing the neural structures will often suffice in dealing with tumors, such as sphenoid ridge or clinoidal meningiomas, that have grown through the greater and lesser sphenoid wings to compress but not infiltrate the structures coursing through the fissure. In other cases, tumors such as schwannomas and meningiomas may grow along the nerves, requiring that the various sectors of the

superior division of the oculomotor nerve, which enters the lower surface of the superior rectus and levator muscles, crosses the field. K, *a second variant of the central approach, in which the frontal nerve is retracted laterally with the superior rectus muscle. This approach provides a wider exposure of the optic nerve in the orbital apex than the exposure in which the branches of the frontal nerve are retracted medially with the levator muscle as shown in* J. *The site at which the medial and superior rectus muscles arise from the annular tendon is also exposed.* A., *artery;* A.C.A., *anterior cerebral artery;* Ant., *anterior;* Car., *carotid;* Cil., *ciliary;* Clin., *clinoid;* CN, *cranial nerve;* Div., *division;* Eth., *ethmoid, ethmoidal;* Falc., *falciform;* Front., *frontal;* Gang., *ganglion;* Inf., *inferior;* Lac., *lacrimal;* Lat., *lateral;* Lev., *levator;* Lig., *ligament;* M., *muscle;* N., *nerve;* Nasocil., *nasociliary;* Obl., *oblique;* Ophth., *ophthalmic;* Rec., *rectus;* Sup., *superior;* Supraorb., *supraorbital;* Supratroch., *supratrochlear;* Temp., *temporal;* V., *vein;* Zygotemp., *zygotemporal.*

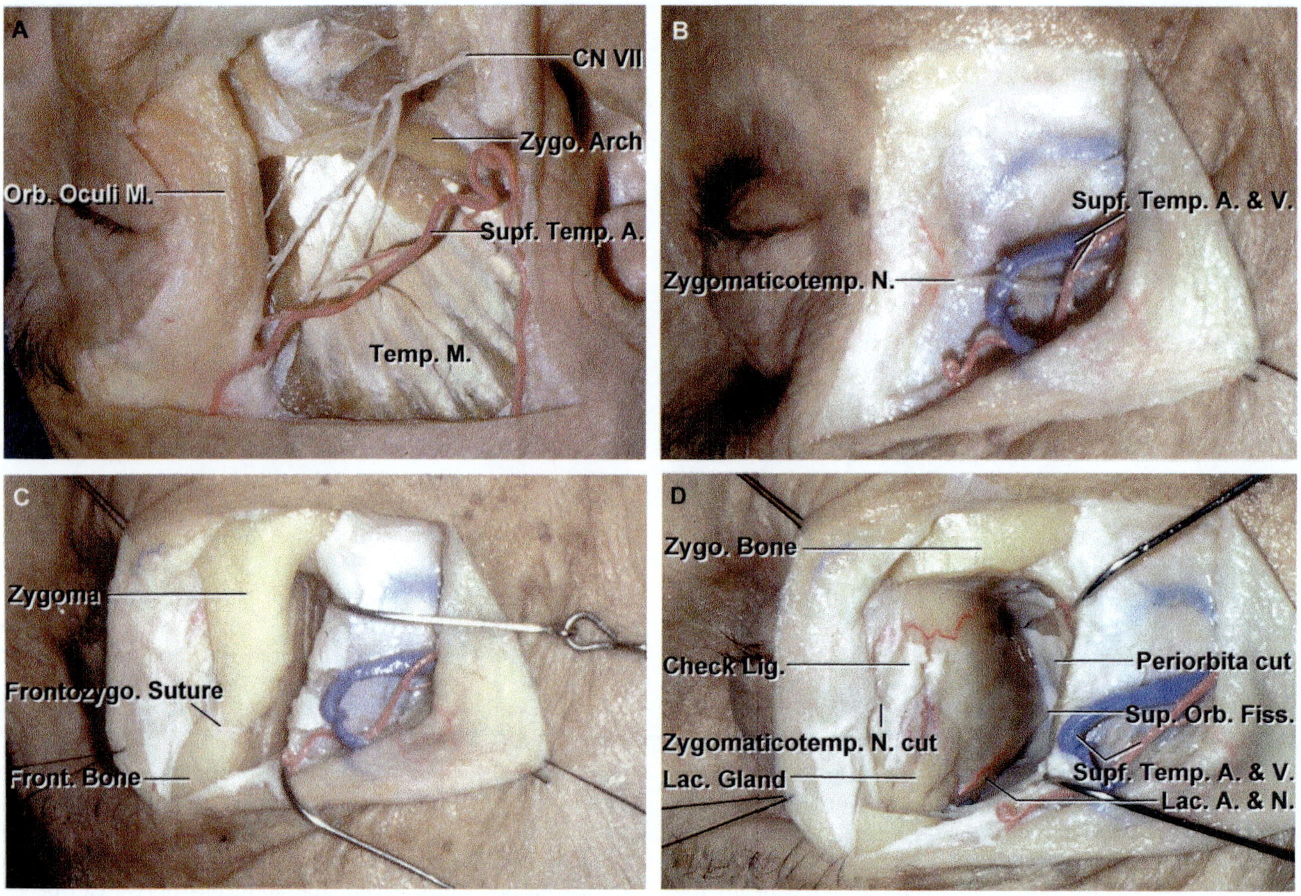

FIGURE 7.11. *Lateral orbital approach. A, structures superficial to the lateral orbital wall include the branches of the facial nerve to the orbicularis oculi and frontalis muscles, which cross the midportion of the zygomatic arch; the anterior branch of the superficial temporal artery; and the temporalis muscle, which passes medial to the zygomatic arch to insert on the coronoid process of the mandible. B–E, exposure obtained with a lateral orbitotomy. B, the curved skin incision begins in front of the ear, extends forward along the upper edge of the zygoma, and turns upward along the lateral rim of the orbit. The superficial temporal artery and vein are exposed. A zygomaticotemporal nerve branch of the maxillary nerve passes through the lateral orbital wall to convey sensation to the temple. Care is required to preserve the branches of the facial nerve to the orbicularis oculi and frontalis muscles and, if transected, reapproximation should be attempted at the end of the operation. C, the lateral orbital rim formed by the frontal process of the zygomatic bone and the zygomatic process of the frontal bone has been exposed. The temporalis muscle has been elevated from the lateral orbital wall. D, the part of the lateral wall of the orbit formed by the frontal and zygomatic bones and the adjacent part of the sphenoid wings has been elevated as a small bone flap to expose the periorbita of the anterior two-thirds of the orbital wall. The lacrimal artery and nerve course in the orbital fat above the lateral rectus muscle. The orbital part of the lacrimal gland is exposed outside the orbital fat. The lateral orbital rim, which has been removed in a single piece, is replaced after removing the orbital lesion. E, the orbital fat has been removed to expose the optic nerve and insertion of the lateral rectus and inferior oblique muscles on the globe. The superior ophthalmic vein, the nasociliary nerve, and the lacrimal and ciliary arteries and nerves are exposed above the lateral rectus muscle. F, combining the lateral orbital exposure with a frontotemporal craniotomy permits exposure of the superior orbital fissure, anterior cavernous sinus, and the frontal and temporal lobes adjoining the sylvian fissure. The lateral orbital wall has been removed to expose the periorbita. G, the combined craniotomy and lateral orbitotomy exposures include the anterior part of cavernous sinus, the superior orbital fissure, and the lateral orbit. The anterior clinoid process and a portion of the optic strut have been removed. The bone around the optic canal has been removed to expose the optic sheath. H, the periorbita has been opened to expose the lateral rectus muscle. The lacrimal and frontal nerves course through the lateral part of the superior orbital fissure. The superior ophthalmic vein courses along the lateral margin of the annular tendon. I, the lateral rectus muscle has been reflected posteriorly. The ciliary ganglion is located on the lateral side of the ophthalmic artery and optic nerves. The abducens nerve enters the medial side of the lateral rectus muscle. The motor root of the ciliary ganglion arises from the branch of the inferior oculomotor division to the inferior oblique muscle. The sensory root of the ciliary ganglion arises from the nasociliary. The ciliary ganglion gives rise to short ciliary nerves.* A., *artery;* Car., *carotid;* Cil., *ciliary;* CN, *cranial nerve;* Fiss., *fissure;* Front., *frontal;* Frontozygo., *frontozygomatic;* Gang., *ganglion;* Inf., *inferior;* Lac., *lacrimal;* Lat., *lateral;* Lig., *ligament;* M., *muscle;* N., *nerve;* Nasocil., *nasociliary;* Obl., *oblique;* Ophth., *ophthalmic;* Orb., *orbital;* Rec., *rectus;* Sup., *superior;* Supf., *superficial;* Temp., *temporal, temporalis;* V., *vein;* Zygo., *zygomatic;* Zygomaticotemp., *zygomaticotemporal.*

fissure be opened. Removal of the bone in the margin of the superior orbital fissure and anterior clinoid process are frequent steps in exposing tumors and aneurysms in the region. Care is required in removing the anterior clinoid process to avoid damaging the optic and oculomotor nerves. Both the anterior clinoid process and the optic strut may contain air

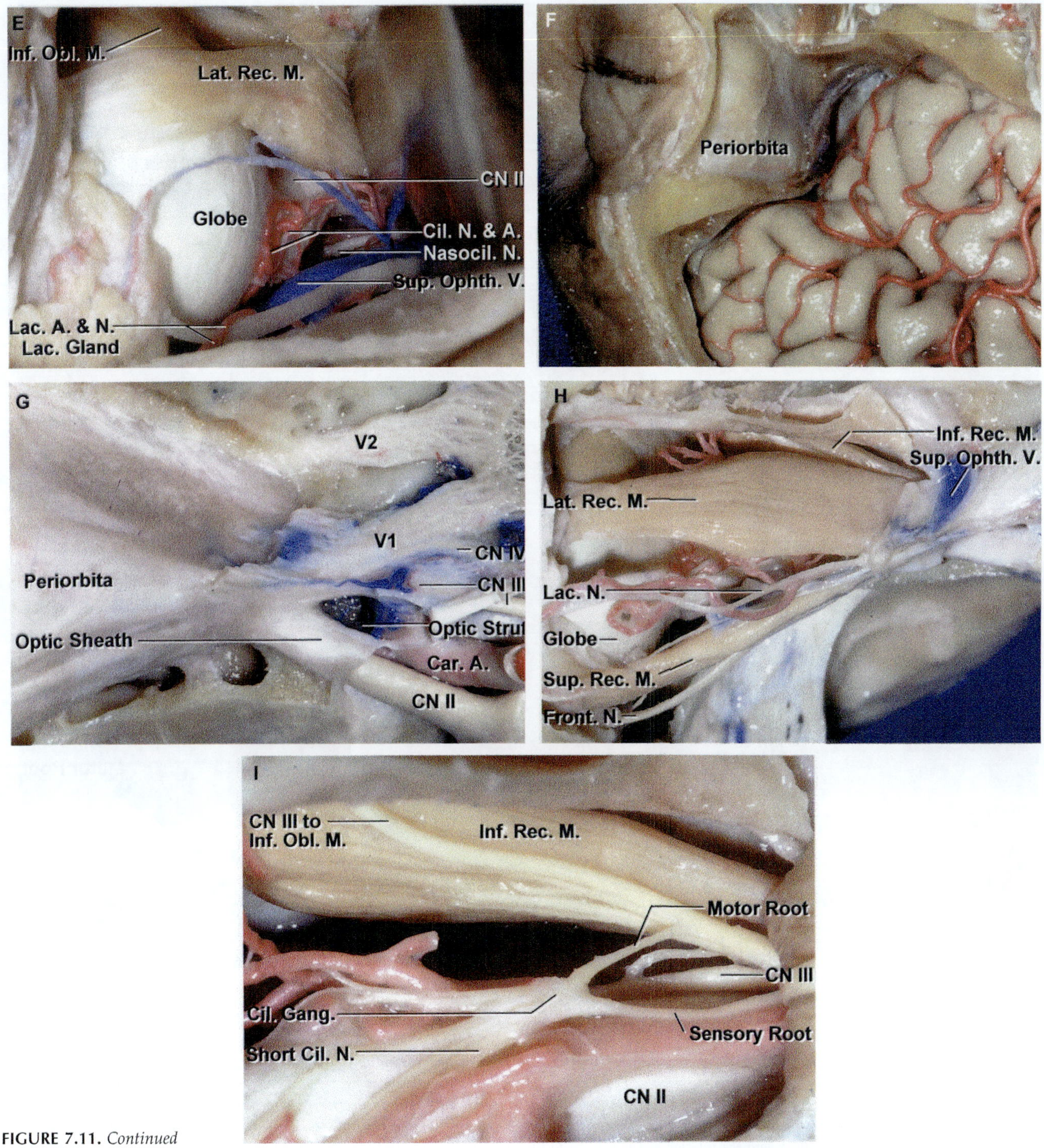

FIGURE 7.11. *Continued*

cells that communicate with the sphenoid sinus and must be closed, if opened, to prevent cerebrospinal fluid rhinorrhea.

The periosteal margins of the superior orbital fissure may be opened at several sites with or without opening the annular tendon (21, 22). The fissure's central sector and the oculomotor foramen can be opened with an incision directed through the annular tendon between the origin of the superior and lateral rectus muscles (*Fig. 7.3* and *7.10, F* and *I*). It is important to remember that the superior ophthalmic vein exits the extraocular muscle cone by passing between the origin of the superior and lateral rectus muscles (*Fig. 7.5*). The trochlear, frontal, and lacrimal nerves course lateral to this opening through the annular tendon. Openings into the lateral sector are best directed through the upper margin of the fissure, because the

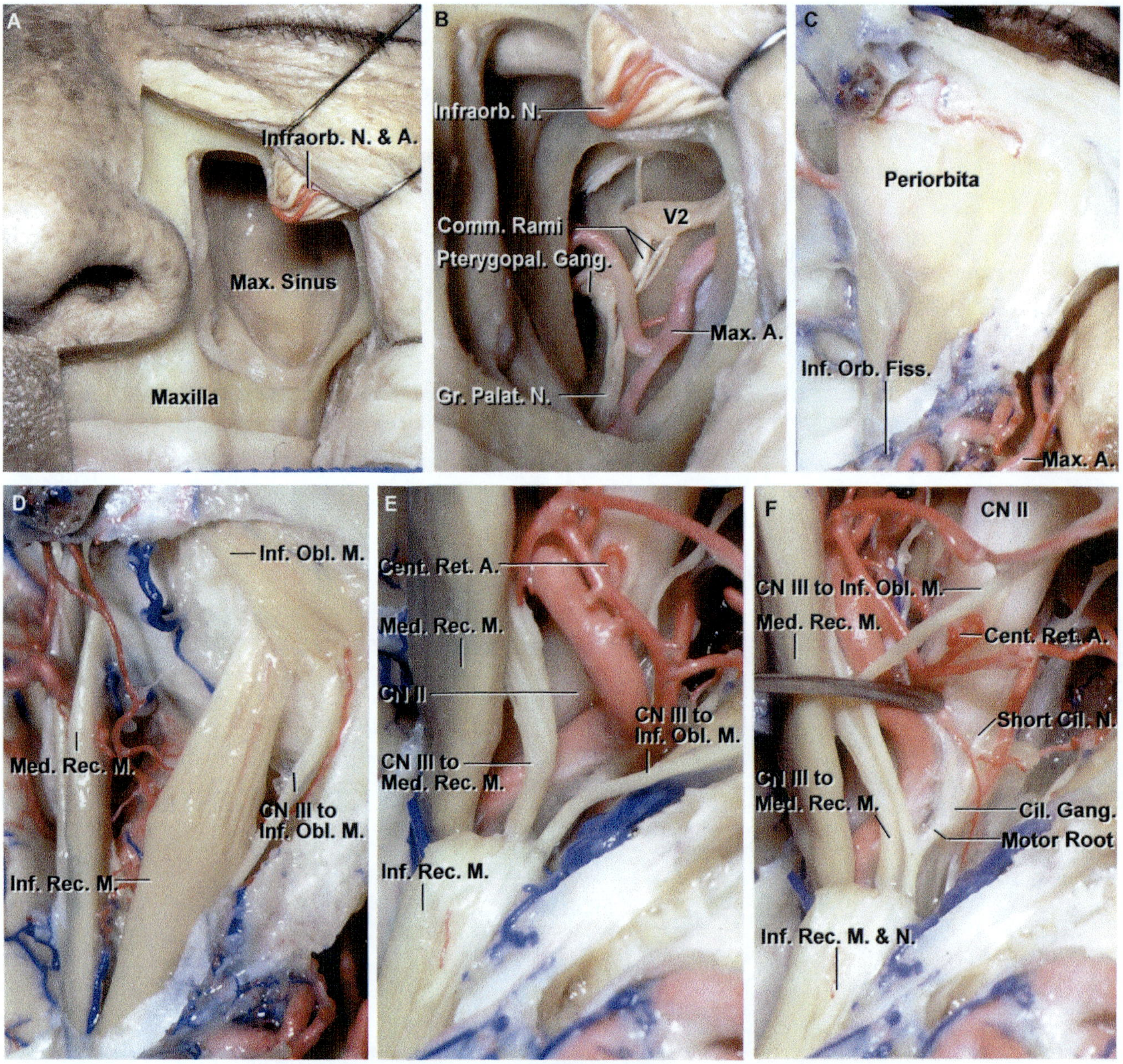

FIGURE 7.12. *Transmaxillary exposure of the orbit. A, this approach is usually performed through a degloving incision in the buccogingival junction rather than through an incision along the margin of the nose. The upper lip and cheek flap have been reflected laterally and the anterior wall of the maxilla has been opened to expose the maxillary sinus. B, enlarged view. The posterior wall of the maxillary sinus has been removed to expose the pterygopalatine fossa. The maxillary nerve enters the pterygopalatine fossa by passing through the foramen rotundum, where it gives rise to communicating rami to the pterygopalatine ganglion and infraorbital and palatine nerves. The terminal branches of the maxillary artery also course through the pterygopalatine fossa. C, inferior view of another orbit after the orbital floor has been removed and the infraorbital nerve reflected posteriorly to expose the periorbita and orbital fat. D, the orbital fat has been removed to expose the medial and inferior rectus and inferior oblique muscles. The inferior oblique muscle arises from the medial orbital wall and passes laterally below the inferior rectus muscle to insert on the sclera. The branch of the inferior division of the oculomotor nerve to the inferior oblique muscle courses along the lateral side of the inferior rectus muscle. E, the inferior rectus muscle has been divided and reflected backward. The ophthalmic artery, in this case, courses below the optic nerve, as occurs in approximately 15% of orbits. The inferior division of the oculomotor nerve gives rise to individual branches to the medial rectus, inferior oblique, and inferior rectus muscles. A tortuous central retinal artery arises below and enters the lower margin of the optic nerve. F, the ophthalmic artery has been retracted medially to expose the origin of the parasympathetic motor root to the ciliary ganglion, which courses from the branch of the inferior oculomotor division to the inferior oblique. The ganglion gives rise to short ciliary nerves, which are distributed to the globe.* A., *artery;* Cent., *central;* Cil., *ciliary;* CN, *cranial nerve;* Comm., *communicating;* Fiss., *fissure;* Gang., *ganglion;* Gr., *greater;* Inf., *inferior;* Infraorb., *infraorbital;* M., *muscle;* Max., *maxillary;* Med., *medial;* N., *nerve;* Obl., *oblique;* Orb., *orbital;* Palat., *palatine;* Pterygopal., *pterygopalatine;* Rec., *rectus;* Ret., *retinal.*

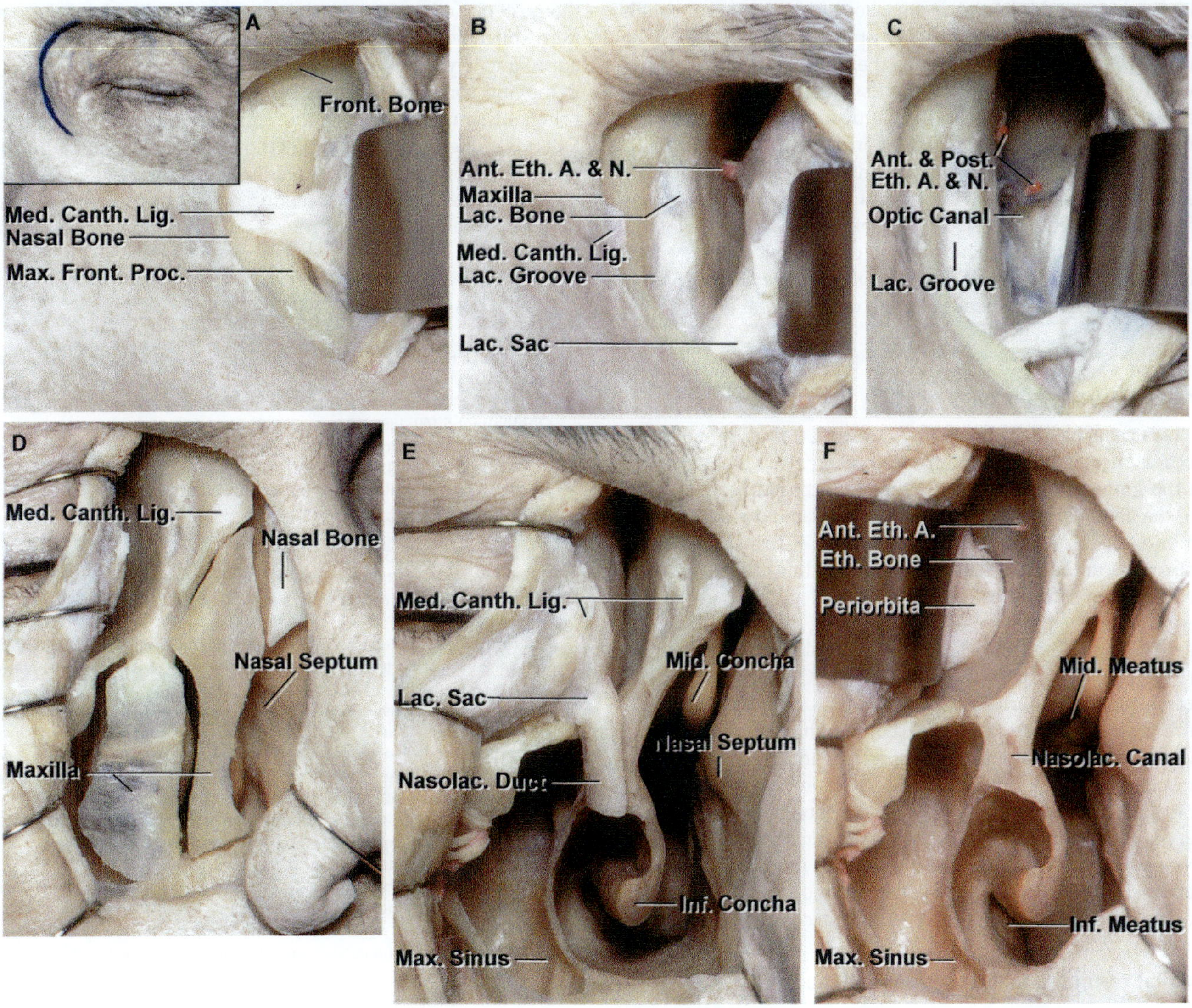

FIGURE 7.13. *Medial orbital approach. A–C, medial orbital exposure. A, the medial orbital incision on the left side is shown in the inset. The approach exposes the medial orbital wall, ethmoid air cells, and sphenoid sinus back to the level of the optic canal. The periorbita has been elevated from the frontal process of the maxillary bone and adjacent frontal bone forming the medial part of the orbital rim to expose the medial canthal ligament, which, if divided, should be reapproximated at the end of the procedure to maintain canthal balance. B, the medial palpebral ligament has been divided and the edges of the divided ligament have been preserved for re-approximation at the end of the procedure. The lacrimal sac has been retracted laterally. The exposure extends backward along the lacrimal and ethmoid bones to the level where the anterior ethmoidal artery enters the anterior ethmoidal canal. The lacrimal groove, in which the lacrimal sac sits, is formed anteriorly by the maxilla and posteriorly by the lacrimal bone. C, the exposure has been extended backward along the ethmoid, lacrimal, and frontal bones, past the level where the anterior and posterior ethmoidal arteries enter the anterior and posterior ethmoidal canal to the orbital apex and anterior end of the optic canal. The medial ethmoid air cells and adjacent part of the sphenoid sinus can be removed to expose the optic nerve in the optic canal. This approach is sometimes used to decompress the optic canal. D–F, combined medial orbital and maxillary exposures. D, the exposure includes not only the medial orbital wall, but also the adjacent part of the floor. Two small maxillary osteotomies have been completed. The medial one includes the part of the maxilla forming the anterior wall of the nasal cavity. The lateral osteotomy exposes the anterior part of the maxillary sinus. The medial palpebral ligament has been divided to expose the medial wall of the orbit. E, removing the medial osteotomy fragment exposes the nasal cavity and the nasal septum and inferior and middle conchae. Removing the lateral osteotomy fragment exposes the maxillary sinus, medial part of the orbital floor, and the nasolacrimal duct, which courses along the medial maxillary wall and opens below the inferior concha into the inferior meatus. F, the nasolacrimal duct and lacrimal sac have been retracted laterally and the exposure extended along the medial orbital wall to the area posterior to where the anterior ethmoidal artery was divided. The posterior part of the osseous nasolacrimal canal has been exposed.* A., *artery;* Ant., *anterior;* Canth., *canthal;* Eth., *ethmoid, ethmoidal;* Front., *frontal;* Inf., *inferior;* Lac., *lacrimal;* Lig., *ligament;* Max., *maxillary;* Med., *medial;* Mid., *middle;* N., *nerve;* Nasolac., *nasolacrimal;* Post., *posterior;* Proc., *process.*

superior ophthalmic vein courses along the lower margin of the lateral sector. The large sylvian veins that empty into the cavernous sinus also pass downward along the lower edge of the lateral sector. Care is required to avoid injury to the trochlear nerve when opening the upper margin of the lateral sector because this nerve hugs the upper margin of this sector.

The opening in the lateral sector should be directed through the area medial to the superior ophthalmic vein. Another incision that may be used to open the central sector is directed through the lateral margin of the fissure and annular tendon between the origins of the lateral and inferior rectus muscles. This incision is more difficult to complete than the opening between the origin of the lateral and superior rectus muscles because of the attachment of the annular tendon and a portion of the lateral rectus muscle to the prominence on the lateral margin of the fissure. The inferior ophthalmic vein is commonly encountered in this opening, because it exits the muscle cone by coursing between the origin of the lateral and inferior rectus muscles.

Transmaxillary Approach

This transmaxillary approach, directed through the orbital floor, is most commonly performed using a sublabial incision in the gingivobuccal margin rather than through an incision on the face (7, 8). Soft tissues are elevated to expose the anterior surface of the right maxilla (*Figs. 7.12* and *7.13*). The approach can be completed without dividing the infraorbital nerve at the infraorbital foramen, but if divided, it can be resutured at the time of closing. Removing the anterior wall of the maxillary sinus exposes the infraorbital canal in the roof of the sinus, which forms the orbital floor. Opening the orbital floor exposes the periorbita covering the orbital floor and the infraorbital artery and nerve. Structures that may be exposed include the inferior and medial rectus and inferior oblique muscles, the inferior division of the oculomotor nerve and its branches, the ciliary ganglion and its roots, plus short ciliary nerves that arise in the ciliary ganglion and pierce the sclera around the optic nerve and the central retinal artery. This approach may be used to reconstruct the orbital floor after trauma or to open the floor for orbital decompression.

Medial Orbital and Transethmoidal Approaches

The medial orbital incision can be used to provide access to the area lateral to the lacrimal and ethmoid bones back to the orbital apex, and with removal with some of the ethmoid air cells and sphenoid sinus facing the orbit, the optic canal can be exposed or decompressed (*Fig. 7.13*) (7, 8). The medial orbital incision extends between the medial orbit and nose along the frontal process of the maxillary bone. The exposure is extended using subperiosteal and subperiorbital dissection except at the medial canthal ligament, which is attached to the anterior and posterior margins of the lacrimal groove, and which should be divided or elevated in such a way that it can be preserved and reapproximated if divided. The lacrimal sac, which sits in the lacrimal groove, can usually be elevated. Behind this, the anterior ethmoidal branch of the ophthalmic artery is encountered as it penetrates the periorbita to enter the anterior ethmoidal canal. This artery is divided if a more posterior exposure is needed. As the exposure proceeds, posteriorly along the orbital plate of the ethmoid, the posterior ethmoidal artery is encountered entering the posterior ethmoidal canal. It passes medially along the planum sphenoidale and can be divided. The optic canal is found approximately 7 mm behind the posterior ethmoidal canal (8). Removing some of the ethmoid plate and adjacent part of the sphenoid sinus will expose the optic nerve in the optic canal. Extending the medial orbital incision downward, lateral to the nose, will allow access to the anterior part of the maxilla. Removing the medial part of the anterior wall of the maxillary sinus bordering the nasal cavity provides access to the medial orbital floor.

REFERENCES

1. Al-Mefty O, Fox JL: Superolateral orbital exposure and reconstruction. **Surg Neurol** 23:609–613, 1985.
2. Dandy WE: Prechiasmal intracranial tumors of the optic nerves. **Am J Ophthalmol** 5:169–188, 1922.
3. Frazier CH: An approach to the hypophysis through the anterior cranial fossa. **Ann Surg** 57:145–150, 1913.
4. Hamby WB: Pterional approach to the orbits for decompression or tumor removal. **J Neurosurg** 21:15–18, 1964.
5. Harris FS, Rhoton AL Jr: Anatomy of the cavernous sinus: A microsurgical study. **J Neurosurg** 45:169–180, 1976.
6. Hassler W, Eggert HR: Extradural and intradural microsurgical approaches to lesions of the optic canal and the superior orbital fissure. **Acta Neurochir (Wien)** 74:87–93, 1985.
7. Hitotsumatsu T, Rhoton AL Jr: Unilateral upper and lower subtotal maxillectomy approaches to the cranial base: Microsurgical anatomy. **Neurosurgery** 46:1416–1453, 2000.
8. Hitotsumatsu T, Matsushima T, Rhoton AL Jr: Surgical anatomy of the midface and the midline skull base, in Spetzler RF (ed): *Operative Techniques in Neurosurgery*. W.B. Saunders Co., 1999, vol 2, pp 160–180.
9. Housepian EM: Surgical treatment of unilateral optic nerve gliomas. **J Neurosurg** 31:604–607, 1969.
10. Housepian EM: Microsurgical anatomy of the orbital apex and principles of transcranial orbital exploration. **Clin Neurosurg** 25:556–573, 1978.
11. Jackson H: Orbital tumours. **Proc R Soc Med** 38:587–594, 1945.
12. Jane JA, Park TS, Pobereskin LH, Winn HR, Butler AB: The supraorbital approach: Technical note. **Neurosurgery** 11:537–542, 1982.
13. Kelman SE, Heaps R, Wolf A, Elman MJ: Optic nerve decompression surgery improves visual function in patients with pseudotumor cerebri. **Neurosurgery** 30:391–395, 1992.
14. Krönlein RU: Zur Pathologie und operativen Behandlung der Dermoidcysten der Orbita. **Beitr Klin Chir** 4:149–163, 1889.
15. Liu Q, Rhoton AL Jr: Middle meningeal origin of the ophthalmic artery. **Neurosurgery** 49:401–407, 2001.
16. Love JG, Benedict WL: Transcranial removal of intraorbital tumors. **Jour AMA** 129:777–784, 1945.
17. MacCarty CS, Brown DN: Orbital tumors in children. **Clin Neurosurg** 11:76–93, 1964.
18. Maroon JC, Kennerdell JS: Surgical approaches to the orbit: Indications and techniques. **J Neurosurg** 60:1226–1235, 1984.
19. McArthur LL: An aseptic surgical access to the pituitary body and its neighborhood. **Jour AMA** 58:2009–2011, 1912.
20. Naffziger HC: Progressive exophthalmos following thyroidectomy: Its pathology and treatment. **Ann Surg** 94:582–586, 1931.
21. Natori Y, Rhoton AL Jr: Transcranial approach to the orbit: Microsurgical anatomy. **J Neurosurg** 81:78–86, 1994.
22. Natori Y, Rhoton AL Jr: Microsurgical anatomy of the superior orbital fissure. **Neurosurgery** 36:762–775, 1995.
23. Niho S, Niho M, Niho K: Decompression of the optic canal by the transethmoidal route and decompression of the superior orbital fissure. **Can J Ophthalmol** 5:22–40, 1970.
24. Rhoton AL Jr, Natori Y: *The Orbit and Sellar Region: Microsurgical Anatomy and Operative Approaches*. New York, Thieme Medical, 1996, pp 3–25.

The Sellar Region

Albert L. Rhoton, Jr., M.D.
Department of Neurological Surgery, University of Florida, Gainesville, Florida

Correspondence:
Albert L. Rhoton, Jr., M.D., Department of Neurological Surgery, University of Florida McKnight Brain Institute, P.O. Box 100265, 100 South Newell Drive, Building 59, L2-100, Gainesville, FL 32610-0265.
Email: rhoton@neurosurgery.ufl.edu

KEY WORDS: Carotid artery, Cranial base, Microsurgical anatomy, Nasal cavity, Pituitary gland, Sella, Skull base, Sphenoid sinus, Surgical approach, Transsphenoidal surgery

The pituitary gland and sella are located below the center of the brain in the center of the cranial base (*Fig. 8.1*). Access to the sella is limited from above by the optic nerves and chiasm and the circle of Willis, from laterally by the cavernous sinuses and internal carotid arteries, and from behind by the brainstem and basilar artery. The vital structures protecting its superior, lateral, and posterior borders have led to the preferred surgical routes to tumors of the gland being from below through the nasal cavity and sphenoid sinus or from anteriorly between the frontal lobe and the floor of the anterior cranial fossa. This chapter focuses on the microsurgical anatomy important in performing the various subcranial and transcranial approaches to the sellar region. The chapter is divided into two sections: the first section deals with the relationships in the cranial base around and below the sella, and the second section deals with the relationships in the suprasellar and third ventricular regions (17). Special emphasis is placed on the transnasal route to the sella, because this route is the one most commonly selected for dealing with pituitary tumors.

SUBCRANIAL RELATIONSHIPS

Nasal Cavity

The sella can be reached by several routes through the nasal cavity (11, 17). The nasal cavity, wider below than above, is bounded above by the anterior cranial fossa, laterally by the orbit and the maxillary sinus, and below by the hard palate (*Figs. 8.2* and *8.3*). This cavity is divided sagittally by the nasal septum, which is formed anteriorly and superiorly by the perpendicular plate of the ethmoid and inferiorly and posteriorly by the vomer, with an anterior bony deficiency occupied by septal cartilage. The nasal cavity opens anteriorly onto the face through the anterior nasal aperture and posteriorly into the nasopharynx by way of the posterior nasal apertures. Each posterior nasal aperture, measuring approximately 25 mm vertically and 13 mm transversely, is bordered above by the anterior aspect of the sphenoid body, below by the posterior margin of the hard palate formed by the horizontal plate of the palatine bones, medially by the nasal septum formed by the vomer, and laterally by the medial pterygoid plate.

The lateral nasal wall usually has three medially directed projections: the superior, middle, and inferior nasal conchae, below each of which is a corresponding superior, middle, or inferior nasal meatus (*Figs. 8.2* and *8.3*). The paired sphenoethmoidal recesses, located above and behind the superior nasal conchae and in front of the upper anterior aspect of the sphenoid body, are the site of the paired sphenoid ostia, which communicate between the nasal cavity and the sphenoid sinus. The upper half of the lateral nasal wall, corresponding to the medial orbital wall, is composed, from anterior to posterior, of the frontal process of the maxilla, the lacrimal bone, and the orbital plate of the ethmoid bone. The extremely thin lacrimal and ethmoid bones, occupied by the ethmoid air cells, separate the nasal cavity from the orbit. The nasolacrimal groove and canal, the site of the lacrimal sac and nasolacrimal duct, respectively, pass downward in front of the anterior end of the middle nasal concha and open into the inferior nasal meatus. The frontoethmoidal suture, located at the junction of the roof and medial orbital wall, is situated at the level of the roof of the nasal cavity and the cribriform plate. The anterior and posterior ethmoidal foramina, which transmit the anterior and posterior ethmoidal arteries and nerves, are located in or just above the frontoethmoidal suture. These arteries and nerves exit the ethmoidal foramina and enter the anterior cranial fossa at the lateral edge of the cribriform plate. The anterior ethmoidal artery, a terminal branch of the ophthalmic artery, supplies the mucosa of the anterior and middle ethmoidal sinuses and the dura covering the cribriform plate and the planum sphenoidale. It gives rise to the anterior falcine artery intracranially. The posterior ethmoidal artery, usually smaller than the anterior ethmoidal artery and absent in up to 30% of the ophthalmic arteries, feeds the mucosa of the posterior ethmoidal sinus and the dura of the planum sphenoidale. The average distance between the anterior lacrimal crest of the maxilla's frontal process and the anterior ethmoidal foramen is 22 to 24 mm; between the anterior and posterior ethmoidal foramina, 12 to 15 mm; and between the posterior ethmoidal foramen and the optic canal, 3 to 7 mm (11). In midline transfacial procedures, these arteries may be divided between the periorbita and the medial orbital wall. Care should be taken to prevent damaging the optic nerve, which is sometimes located immediately behind the posterior ethmoidal foramen.

The lower part of the lateral nasal wall is formed, from anterior to posterior, by the maxilla, the perpendicular plate of the palatine bone, and the medial pterygoid plate. The eusta-

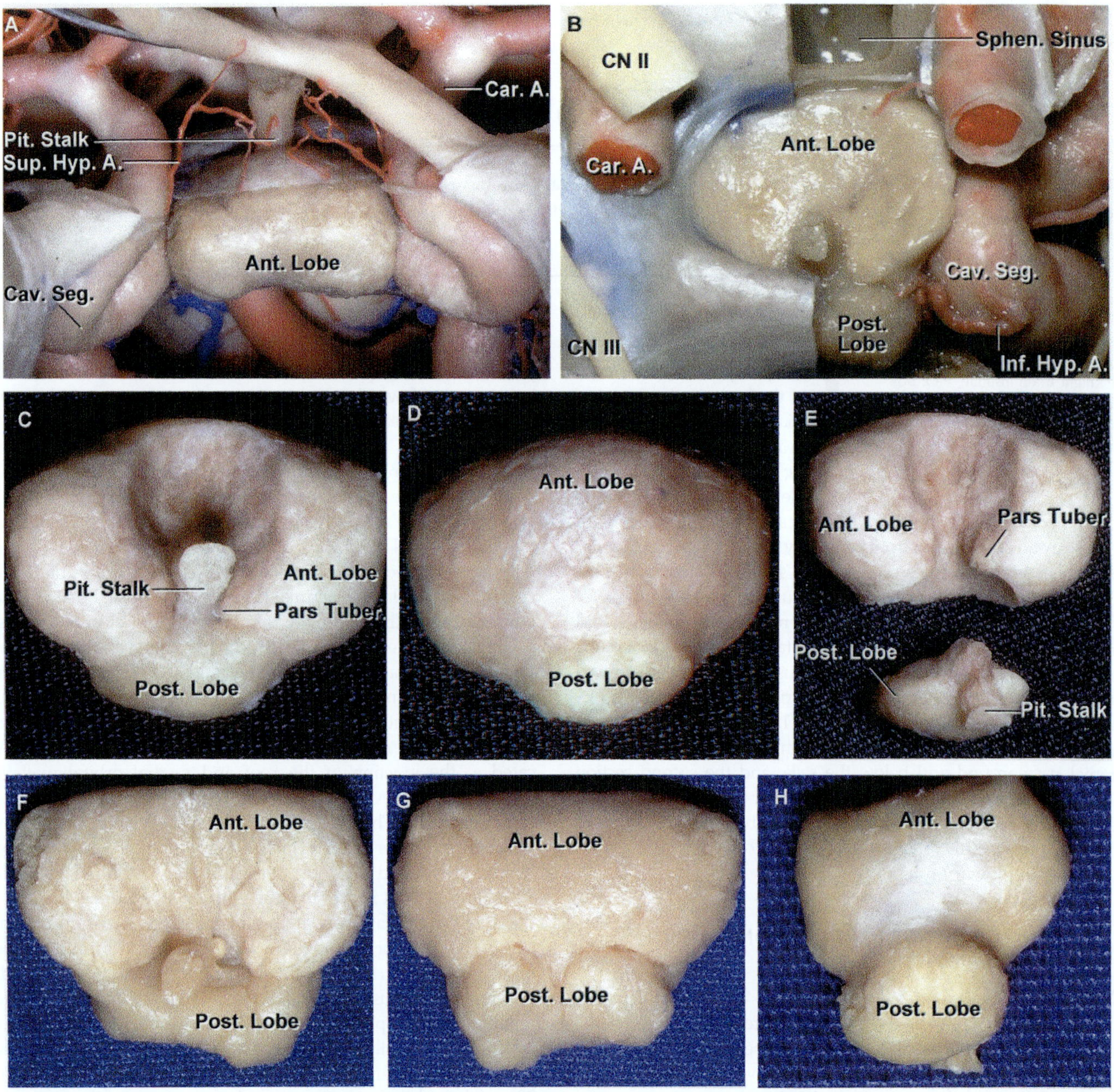

FIGURE 8.1. *The pituitary gland and its relationships. A, anterior view of the pituitary gland. The gland is located below the optic nerves and chiasm and between the cavernous segments of the internal carotid arteries. The right optic nerve has been elevated to expose the pituitary stalk. The superior hypophyseal arteries arise from the medial side of the supraclinoid portion of the internal carotid artery and pass medially to the pituitary stalk and optic chiasm. B, superior view of pituitary gland. In this case, the diaphragm was largely absent, so that the subarachnoid space extended across and was separated from the top of the anterior lobe only by arachnoid membrane. The right half of the dorsum sellae has been removed to expose the posterior lobe, which was hidden under the dorsum. The inferior hypophyseal artery travels medially from the intracavernous carotid to the posterior lobe. C and D, superior and inferior surfaces of a gland in which the anterior and posterior lobes form a relatively ovoid structure. The pars tuberalis wraps partially around the stalk. E, the anterior and posterior lobes have been separated. The stalk joins the anterosuperior surface of the posterior lobe and is partially surrounded by the pars tuberalis. F and G, superior and inferior surfaces of another gland. The posterior lobe is multinodular and the right half of the posterior lobe seems larger than the left half. H, inferior surface of another pituitary. The anterior and posterior lobes form separate distinct nodules. The posterior lobe forms a nodule attached to the posterior edge of the anterior lobe. I, midsagittal section of the sella extending through the anterior and posterior lobes and sphenoid sinus. The intercavernous carotid produces prominences in the lateral wall of the sphenoid sinus below and anterior to the gland. The sella extends forward to the anterior edge of the intracavernous carotid only if greatly expanded by tumor. Intercavernous sinuses courses along the anterior and posterior margin of the diaphragm. The basilar sinus, located on the back of the dorsum, is the largest connection across the midline between the posterior edge of the paired cavernous sinuses. The inferior hypophyseal artery arises from the posterior bend of the intercavernous carotid and is directed medially toward the posterior lobe. J, posterosuperior view of another gland deeply indented on its lateral surface by the intercavernous*

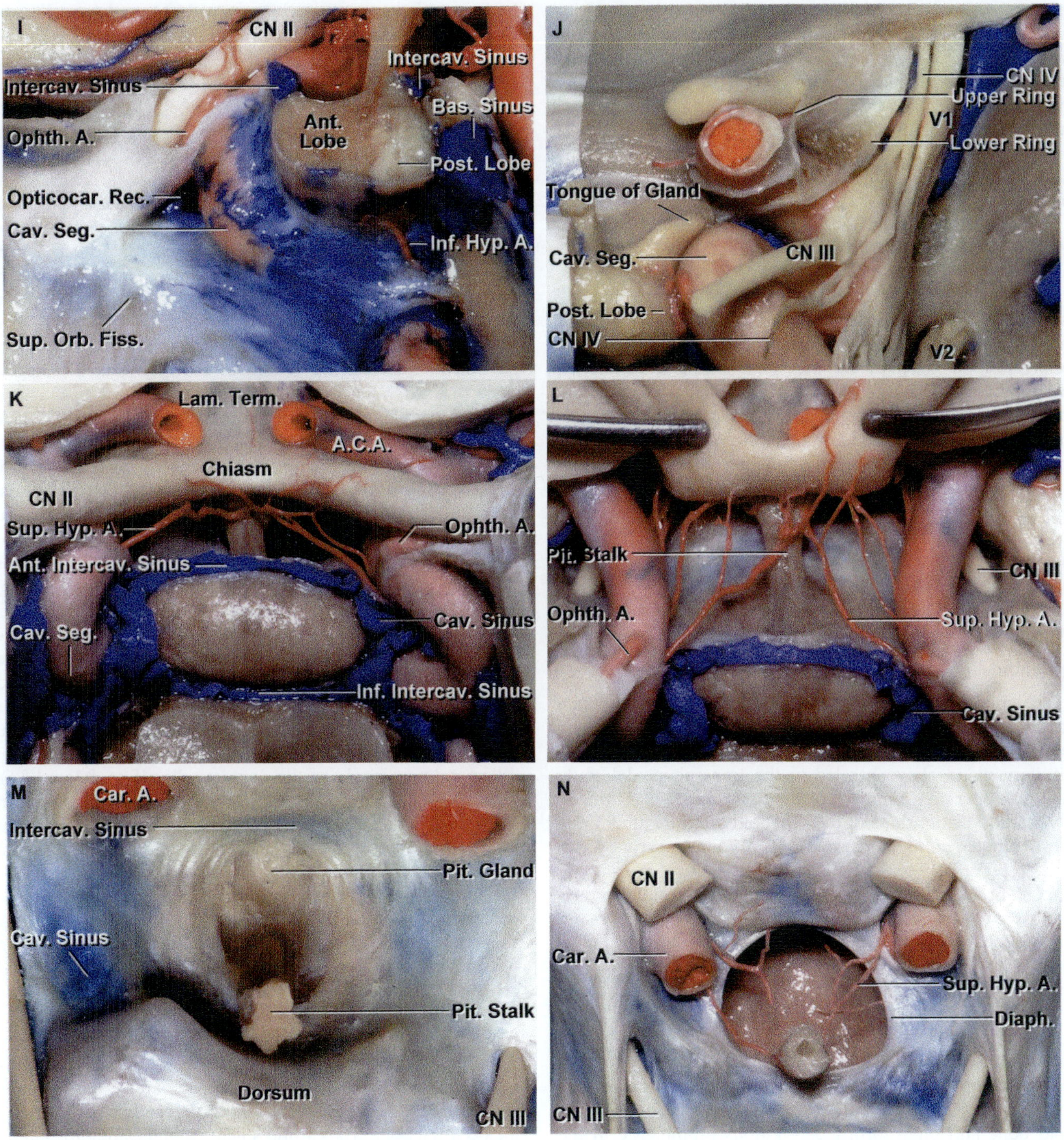

FIGURE 8.1. *Continued*
carotid. A tongue of gland extends laterally above the artery. The anterior clinoid has been removed and the nerves in the wall of the cavernous sinus exposed. K, anterior view of another gland. The cavernous sinuses are located on the lateral side of the gland and separate the gland from the intracavernous carotids. The superior hypophyseal arteries arise from the medial side of the supraclinoid carotid and pass to the chiasm and stalk. The anterior intercavernous sinus crosses the anterosuperior margin of the gland, and the inferior intracavernous sinus extends below the gland interconnecting the cavernous sinuses. L, the optic nerves and chiasm have been elevated to expose the pituitary stalk, superior hypophyseal, and ophthalmic arteries. M, another gland and sella viewed from superiorly. The diaphragm partially covers the upper surface of the gland, but the opening in the diaphragm is larger than the pituitary stalk. The posterior lobe (not shown) was entirely hidden below the dorsum sellae. An intercavernous sinus passes across the upper anterior surface of the gland. N, superior view of another gland exposed below a large natural opening in the diaphragm. A., *artery;* A.C.A., *anterior cerebral artery;* Ant., *anterior;* Bas., *basilar;* Car., *carotid;* Cav., *cavernous;* CN, *cranial nerve;* Diaph., *diaphragm;* Fiss., *fissure;* Hyp., *hypophyseal;* Inf., *inferior;* Intercav., *intercavernous;* Lam., *lamina;* Ophth., *ophthalmic;* Opticocar., *opticocarotid;* Orb., *orbital;* Pit., *pituitary;* Post., *posterior;* Rec., *recess;* Seg., *segment;* Sphen., *sphenoid;* Sup., *superior;* Term., *terminalis;* Tuber., *tuberalis.*

chian tube opens into the nasopharynx along the posterior edge of the medial pterygoid plate. The root of the middle nasal concha attaches to the lateral nasal wall near the junction of the orbit and the maxillary sinus. Thus, the medial wall of the maxillary sinus is bounded medially by the middle and inferior nasal meatus and the inferior nasal concha (*Figs. 8.2* and *8.3*). The maxillary sinus communicates with the middle nasal meatus through an opening located in the medial wall just below the roof of the sinus.

The pterygopalatine fossa is situated just outside the lateral wall of the nasal cavity between the posterior wall of the maxillary sinus anteriorly and the pterygoid process posteriorly (*Figs. 8.2–8.4*). The pterygopalatine fossa contains the pterygopalatine ganglion, which receives the vidian nerve (nerve of the pterygoid canal), the segment of the maxillary nerve and its branches located just anterior to the foramen rotundum, and the internal maxillary artery and its terminal branches. This fossa communicates laterally with the infratemporal fossa through the pterygomaxillary fissure and medially with the nasal cavity via the sphenopalatine foramen, which transmits the corresponding nerve and vessels. The internal maxillary artery exits the infratemporal fossa to enter the pterygopalatine fossa by passing through the pterygomaxillary fissure. The greater and lesser palatine arteries and nerves arise from the maxillary artery and nerve and descend in the greater and lesser palatine canals, which are separated medially from the nasal cavity by the thin perpendicular plate of the palatine bone.

Sphenoid Bone

The sphenoid bone is located in the center of the cranial base (*Figs. 8.3* and *8.5*) (21, 22). The intimate contact of the body of the sphenoid bone with the nasal cavity below and the pituitary gland above has led to the transsphenoidal route being the operative approach of choice for most sellar tumors. The neural relationships of the sphenoid bone are among the most complex of any bone. The olfactory tracts, gyrus rectus, and posterior part of the frontal lobe rest against the smooth upper surface of the lesser wing; the temporal lobe rests against the inner surface of the greater wing; the pons and mesencephalon lie posterior to the clival portion; the optic chiasm lies posterior to the chiasmatic sulcus; and the IInd through VIth cranial nerves are intimately related to the sphenoid bone and all exit the cranium through the optic canal, superior orbital fissure, foramen rotundum, or foramen ovale, all foramina located in the sphenoid bone (*Fig. 8.6*).

The sphenoid bone has many important arterial and venous relationships: the carotid arteries groove each side of the sphenoid bone and often form a serpiginous prominence in the lateral wall of the sphenoid sinus, the basilar artery rests against its posterior surface, the circle of Willis is located above its central portion, and the middle cerebral artery courses parallel to the sphenoid ridge of the lesser wing. The cavernous sinuses rest against the sphenoid bone, and intercavernous venous connections line the walls of the pituitary fossa and dorsum sellae.

In the anterior view, the sphenoid bone resembles a bat with wings outstretched (*Fig. 8.5*). It has a central portion called the body; two lesser wings, which spread outward from the superolateral part of the body; two greater wings, which spread upward from the lower part of the body; and two pterygoid processes with their medial and lateral pterygoid plates directed downward from the body. The body of the sphenoid bone is more or less cubical and contains the sphenoid sinus. The superior orbital fissure, through which the oculomotor, trochlear, abducens, and ophthalmic nerves pass, is formed on its inferior and lateral margins by the greater wing and on its superior margin by the lesser wing. The inferior surface of the lesser wing forms the posterior part of the roof of each orbit, and the exposed surface of the greater wing forms a large part of the lateral wall of the orbit, the floor of the middle fossa, and the roof of the infratemporal fossa. The optic canals are situated above and are separated from the superomedial margin of the superior orbital fissure by the optic strut, a bridge of bone that extends from the lower margin of the base of the anterior clinoid process to the body of the sphenoid. The narrowest part of the optic canal is closer to the orbital than the intracranial end. The optic canals average 5 mm in length, and are of a conical configuration, tapering to a narrow waist near the orbit end. The sphenoid ostia open from the nasal cavity into the sinus. The infratemporal crest divides the inferior from the lateral parts of the greater wing and separates the temporal fossae. The lateral pterygoid muscles arise between the infratemporal crest and the lateral pterygoid plate. The area lateral to the infratemporal line gives origin to the temporalis muscle. The pterygoid (vidian) canal courses from anterior to posterior through the junction of the pterygoid process and the sphenoid body.

In the superior view, the pituitary fossa occupies the central part of the body and is bounded anteriorly by the tuberculum sellae and posteriorly by the dorsum sellae (*Figs. 8.1* and *8.6*). The chiasmatic groove (sulcus), a shallow depression between the optic foramina, is bounded posteriorly by the tuberculum sellae and anteriorly by the planum sphenoidale. The frontal lobes and the olfactory tracts rest against the smooth upper surface of the lesser wing and the planum sphenoidale. The posterior margin of the lesser wing forms a free edge, the sphenoid ridge, which projects into the sylvian fissure to separate the frontal and temporal lobes. The anterior clinoid processes are located at the medial end of the lesser wings, the middle clinoid processes are lateral to the tuberculum sellae, and the posterior clinoid processes are situated at the superolateral margin of the dorsum sellae. The dorsum sellae is continuous with the clivus. The upper part of the clivus is formed by the sphenoid bone, and the lower part is formed by the occipital bone. The carotid sulcus extends along the lateral surface of the body of the sphenoid.

The depth of the sella turcica is the greatest distance between the floor and a perpendicular line connecting the tuberculum and dorsum. Sellar length, defined as the greatest anterior-posterior diameter of the pituitary fossa, may occur at the level of the tuberculum sellae or below. Sellar width is defined as the width of the horizontal plateau of the sellar floor between the carotid sulcus. The volume is calculated by applying the simplified mathematical formula for the volume

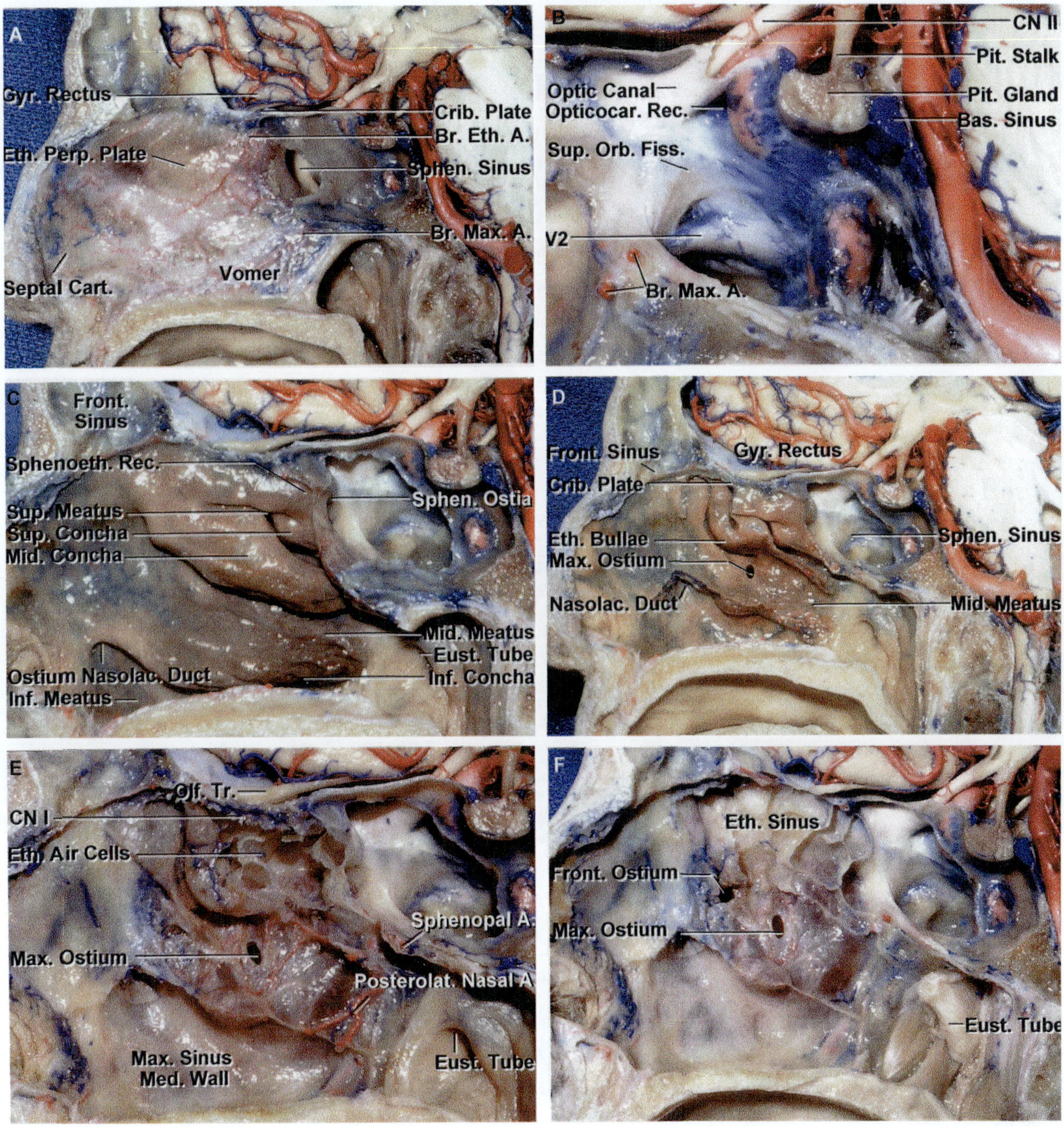

FIGURE 8.2. *Stepwise dissection of the nasal pathway along which the transsphenoidal surgery is directed.* A, *sagittal section to the left of the midline and nasal septum. The nasal septum is formed anteriorly by the septal cartilage, above by the perpendicular plate of the ethmoid, and below and posteriorly by the vomer. The posteroinferior part of the septum is supplied by the branches of the sphenopalatine artery, a terminal branch of the maxillary artery. The upper part of the septum, below the cribriform plate, is supplied by the branches of the ethmoidal arteries, which arise from the ophthalmic artery. A septum divides the sphenoid sinus near the midline. The optic chiasm, optic and oculomotor nerves, third ventricle, and pituitary stalk are located above the pituitary gland. The gyrus rectus of the frontal lobe is located above the cribriform plate and olfactory tract.* B, *midsagittal section of the sphenoid sinus and pituitary gland. Prominences overlie the optic canal, internal carotid artery, superior orbital fissure, and maxillary nerve in the wall of the sphenoid sinus. The opticocarotid recess extends laterally between the optic nerve, internal carotid artery, and the prominence passing through the superior orbital fissure, and extends into the optic strut, which separates the optic canal from the superior orbital fissure. The serpiginous prominence overlying the internal carotid artery is located anterior to and below the pituitary gland.* C, *the lateral wall of the nasal cavity is constituted below by the nasal surface of the maxilla and above by the nasal surface of the ethmoidal sinuses. The inferior concha (turbinate) is an independent bone, that articulates with the nasal surface of the maxilla and the perpendicular plate of the palatal bone. The middle and superior concha are appendages of the ethmoid bone. The lacrimal duct opens below the anterior part of the inferior concha. The inferior, middle, and* *(Legend continues on next page.)*

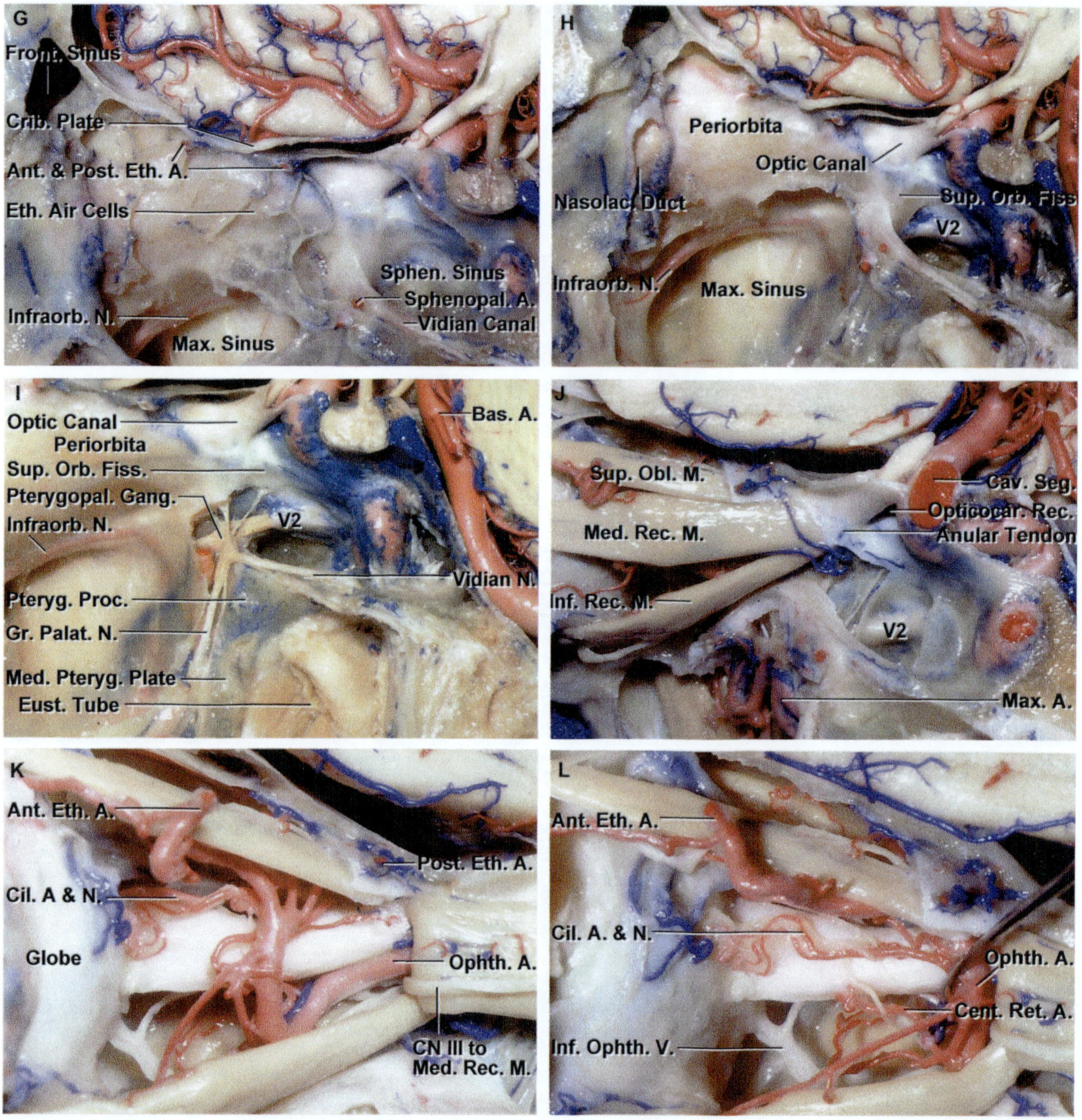

FIGURE 8.2. *Continued*

superior nasal meatus are located below their respective concha. The superior meatus is located between the middle and superior concha. The sphenoethmoidal recess, a narrow cleft located above the superior concha, separates the superior concha from the anterior surface of the sphenoid sinus and is the site of the ostium communicating the sphenoid sinus and nasal cavity. The eustachian tube opens into the nasopharynx in front of Rosenmüller's fossa. D, *the concha has been removed. The maxillary and frontal sinuses drain into the middle meatus. The lacrimal duct opens below the inferior turbinate into the inferior meatus. The ethmoid bullae are rounded prominences overlying the middle ethmoid air cells. The anterior ethmoid air cells drain into the superior meatus. The posterior ethmoid air cells and the sphenoid sinus drain into the sphenoethmoidal recess.* E, *enlarged view after removal of the nasal mucosa. The olfactory fila pass through the small openings in the cribriform plate to innervate the olfactory mucosa. The sphenopalatine artery, the terminal branch of the maxillary artery, passes through the sphenopalatine foramen in the medial wall of the pterygopalatine fossa and gives rise to the posterior lateral nasal arteries.* F, *the cribriform plate and medial wall of the ethmoid air cells have been removed. The thin lateral wall of the ethmoidal and sphenoid sinuses forms the medial wall of the orbit. The frontal sinus opens into the anterior part of the middle meatus.* G, *the medial wall of the maxillary sinus has been removed to expose the sinus roof, which forms the orbital floor. The infraorbital sulcus and canal, which are situated in the floor of the orbit, form a prominence in the roof of the maxillary sinus. The anterior and posterior ethmoidal arteries arise from the ophthalmic artery and pass through the anterior and posterior ethmoidal canals to reach the floor of the anterior fossa* of an ellipsoid, namely, volume (cm^3) = 0.5 (length × width × depth in mm)/1000. The upper limit of normal depth is 13 mm; length, 17 mm; width, 15 mm; and volume, 1100 mm (15).

The superior aspect of each greater wing is concave upward and is filled by the pole of each temporal lobe. The foramen rotundum, ovale, and spinous are located, from anterior to posterior, near the junction of the body and greater wing. When viewed from inferiorly, the vomer, a separate bone, frequently remains attached to the anterior half of the body of the sphenoid, and its most anterior portion separates the sphenoid ostia.

The pterion and the keyhole are two important anatomic landmarks in the region of the greater wing in the lateral view (*Fig. 8.5*). The pterion is located over the upper part of the greater wing and approximates the site of the lateral end of the sphenoid ridge. The keyhole is located just behind the junction of the temporal line and the zygomatic process of the frontal bone, several centimeters anterior to the pterion. A burr hole placed over the pterion will be located at the lateral end of the sphenoid ridge. A burr hole placed at the keyhole will expose the orbit in its lower part and dura over the frontal lobe in its upper part.

Sphenoid Sinus

The sphenoid sinus separates the cavernous sinuses, the cavernous segments of the carotid arteries, and the optic, extraocular, and trigeminal nerves. In addition, it separates the pituitary gland from the nasal cavity. The sphenoid sinus is subject to considerable variation in size and shape and to variation in the degree of pneumatization (*Figs. 8.5, 8.7,* and *8.8*) (4, 8). It is present as minute cavities at birth, but its main development takes place after puberty. In early life, it extends backward into the presellar area and subsequently expands into the area below and behind the sella turcica, reaching its full size during adolescence. As the sinus enlarges, it may partially encircle the optic canals. When the sinus is exceptionally large, it extends into the roots of the pterygoid processes or greater wing of the sphenoid bone and may even extend into the basilar part of the occipital bone. As age advances, the sinus frequently undergoes further enlargement associated with absorption of its bony walls. Occasionally there are gaps in its bone, with the mucous membrane lying directly against the dura mater.

There are three types of sphenoid sinus in the adult: conchal, presellar, and sellar types, depending on the extent to which the sphenoid bone is pneumatized (*Fig. 8.5*). In the conchal type, the area below the sella is a solid block of bone without an air cavity. In the presellar type of sphenoid sinus, the air cavity does not penetrate beyond a vertical plane parallel to the anterior sellar wall. The sellar type of sphenoid sinus is the most common, and here the air cavity extends into the body of sphenoid below the sella and as far posteriorly as the clivus. In our previous study in adult cadavers, this sinus was of a presellar type in 24% and of the sellar type in 76% (15). The conchal type is most common in children before the age of 12 years, at which time pneumatization begins within the sphenoid sinus. In the conchal type, which is infrequent in the adult, the thickness of bone separating the sella from the sphenoid sinus is at least 10 mm.

The depth of the sphenoid sinus is defined as the distance from the ostium of the sphenoid sinus to the closest part of the sella (*Fig. 8.8*). In the adult, the average anterior-posterior diameter of the cavity has been found to be 17 mm (range, 12–23 mm) (4). This measurement defines the length of the path within the sinus through which instruments must pass to reach the sellar wall and is important when selecting instruments for transsphenoidal surgery. The speculum most commonly used for transsphenoidal surgery is 9 cm in length and its tip should be placed anterior to the sphenoid sinus. In reaching the floor of the sella turcica, the depth of the sphenoid sinus (2 cm or more) is added to the 9 cm length of the speculum. Thus, after traversing a distance of 11 to 12 cm, the dissecting instruments must then enter the sella turcica and be able to reach above the sella if a suprasellar tumor is present. The distance may be greater in the presence of acromegaly; therefore, it is important that transsphenoidal instruments have shafts at least 12 cm in length. Some transsphenoidal

beside the cribriform plate, where they again penetrate the bone to reach the walls of the nasal cavity. The vidian canal is the site of passage of the vidian nerve to the pterygopalatine ganglion. The vidian nerve is formed by parasympathetic fibers from the greater petrosal nerve and sympathetic fibers from the deep petrosal branch of the carotid plexus. H, removing the lateral wall of the ethmoid air cells, which forms the medial wall of the orbit, exposes the periorbita. The frontal sinus is situated at the upper anterior part of the medial wall. The medial wall of the nasolacrimal duct has been removed to expose the interior of the duct. I, enlarged view. The pterygoid process extends downward and forms the posterior wall of the pterygopalatine fossa. The medial pterygoid plate is situated beneath the nasopharyngeal mucosa just in front of the orifice of the eustachian tube. The greater and lesser palatine nerves arise from the pterygopalatine ganglion in the pterygopalatine fossa and are distributed to the palate, tonsil, and lining of the nasal cavity. J, the periorbita has been opened and some of the orbital fat removed to expose the medial and inferior rectus and superior oblique muscles. The annular tendon is the condensation of periorbita from which the rectus muscles arise. It surrounds the optic foramen and medial part of the superior orbital fissure. The lateral wall of the nasal cavity has been opened to expose the terminal part of the maxillary artery in the pterygopalatine fossa. K, the medial rectus muscle has been divided near the globe and reflected posteriorly. In this case, the ophthalmic artery courses below the optic nerve to reach the medial part of the orbit. The branch of the inferior division of the oculomotor nerve to the medial rectus muscle enters the medial side of the muscle. The ophthalmic artery gives rise to the anterior and posterior ethmoidal arteries as it courses near the superior oblique muscle. L, the ophthalmic artery has been retracted posteriorly to show the central retinal artery coursing below the optic nerve. Short ciliary arteries and nerves pass to the globe. A., *artery;* Ant., *anterior;* Bas., *basilar;* Br., *branch;* Cart., *cartilage;* Cav., *cavernous;* Cent., *central;* Cil., *ciliary;* CN, *cranial nerve;* Crib., *cribriform;* Eth., *ethmoid, ethmoidal;* Eust., *eustachian;* Fiss., *fissure;* Front., *frontal;* Gang., *ganglion;* Gr., *greater;* Gyr., *gyrus;* Inf., *inferior;* Infraorb., *infraorbital;* Lat., *lateral;* M., *muscle;* Max., *maxillary;* Med., *medial;* Mid., *middle;* N., *nerve;* Nasolac., *nasolacrimal;* Obl., *oblique;* Olf., *olfactory;* Ophth., *ophthalmic;* Opticocar., *opticocarotid;* Orb., *orbital;* Pal., *palatine;* Perp., *perpendicular;* Pit., *pituitary;* Post., *posterior;* Proc., *process;* Pteryg., *pterygoid;* Pterygopal., *pterygopalatine;* Rec., *recess, rectus;* Ret., *retinal;* Seg., *segment;* Sept., *septal;* Sphen., *sphenoid;* Sphenoeth., *sphenoethmoidal;* Sphenopal., *sphenopalatine;* Sup., *superior;* Tr., *tract;* V., *vein.*

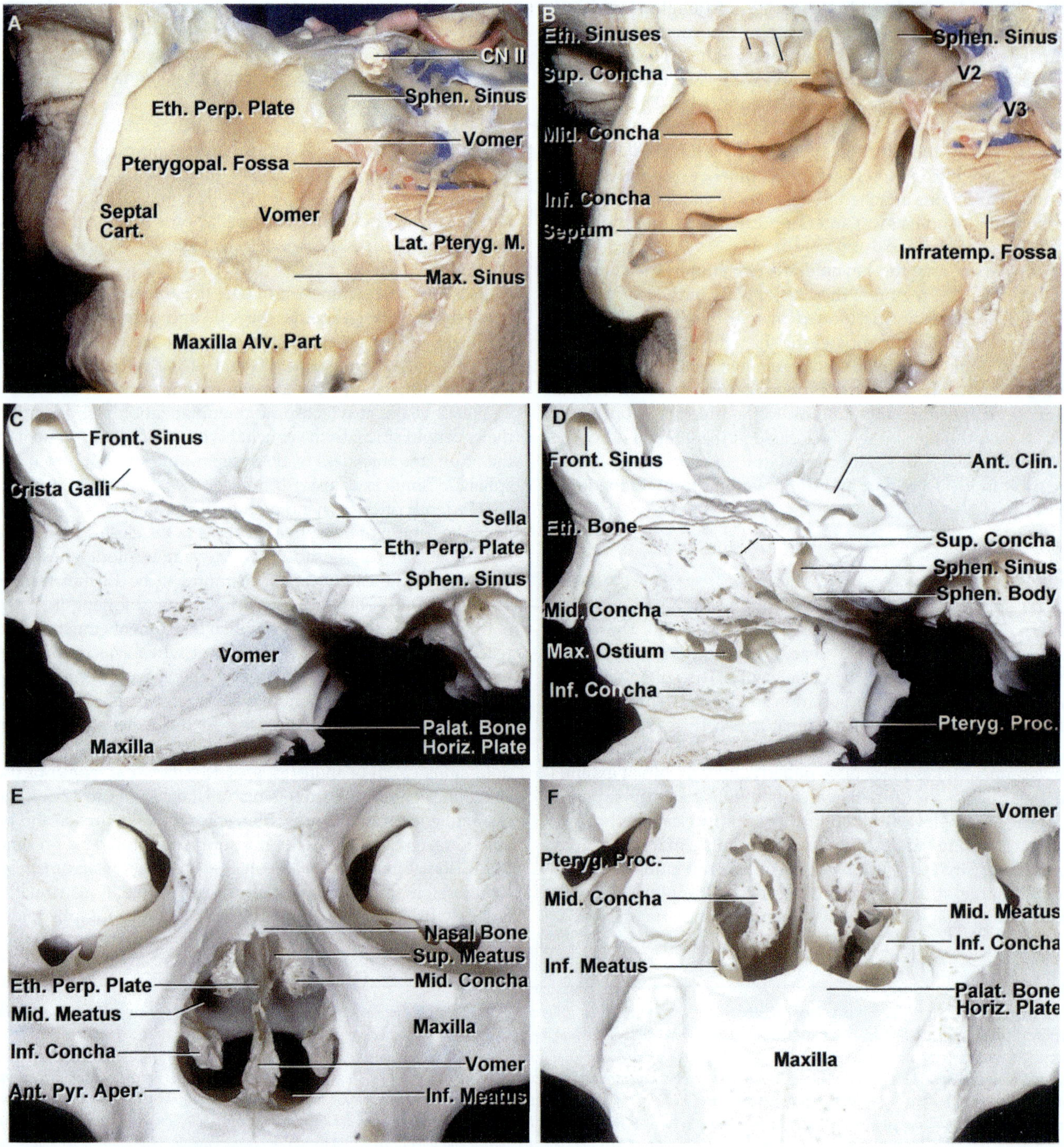

FIGURE 8.3. A–D, *comparison of osseous and mucosal structures in the nasal septum and conchae.* E–J, *osseous relationships along the transsphenoidal and endonasal approaches to the sella.* A, *the structures anterior to the left orbital apex and the portion of the maxilla above the alveolar process have been removed to expose the nasal septum, which is formed posteriorly by the vomer, above by the perpendicular plate of the ethmoid, and anteriorly by the septal cartilage.* B, *the nasal septum and anterior wall of the sphenoid sinus have been removed. This exposes the superior, middle, and inferior conchae and a midline septum within the sphenoid sinus. The ethmoid air cells are exposed in the medial wall of the right orbit. The part of the sphenoid sinus medial to and below the orbital apex has been opened.* C, *the left half of the facial skeleton, including the left half of the maxilla and orbit, has been removed to expose the left side of the nasal septum, which is formed above by the perpendicular plate of the ethmoid bone and below by the vomer. The palate is formed anteriorly by the maxilla and posteriorly by the horizontal plate of the palatine bone.* D, *the nasal septum has been removed. The inferior concha is a separate bone, which protrudes into the nasal cavity from the maxilla. The middle and superior concha are appendages of the ethmoid bone. The maxillary ostium is located between the perpendicular plate of the palatine bone behind, the ethmoid superiorly, and the medial maxillary wall below. The maxillary and frontal sinus and the anterior ethmoid air cells drain into the middle meatus, and the posterior ethmoid air cells drain into the superior meatus.* E, *the anterior nasal aperture is formed above by the nasal*

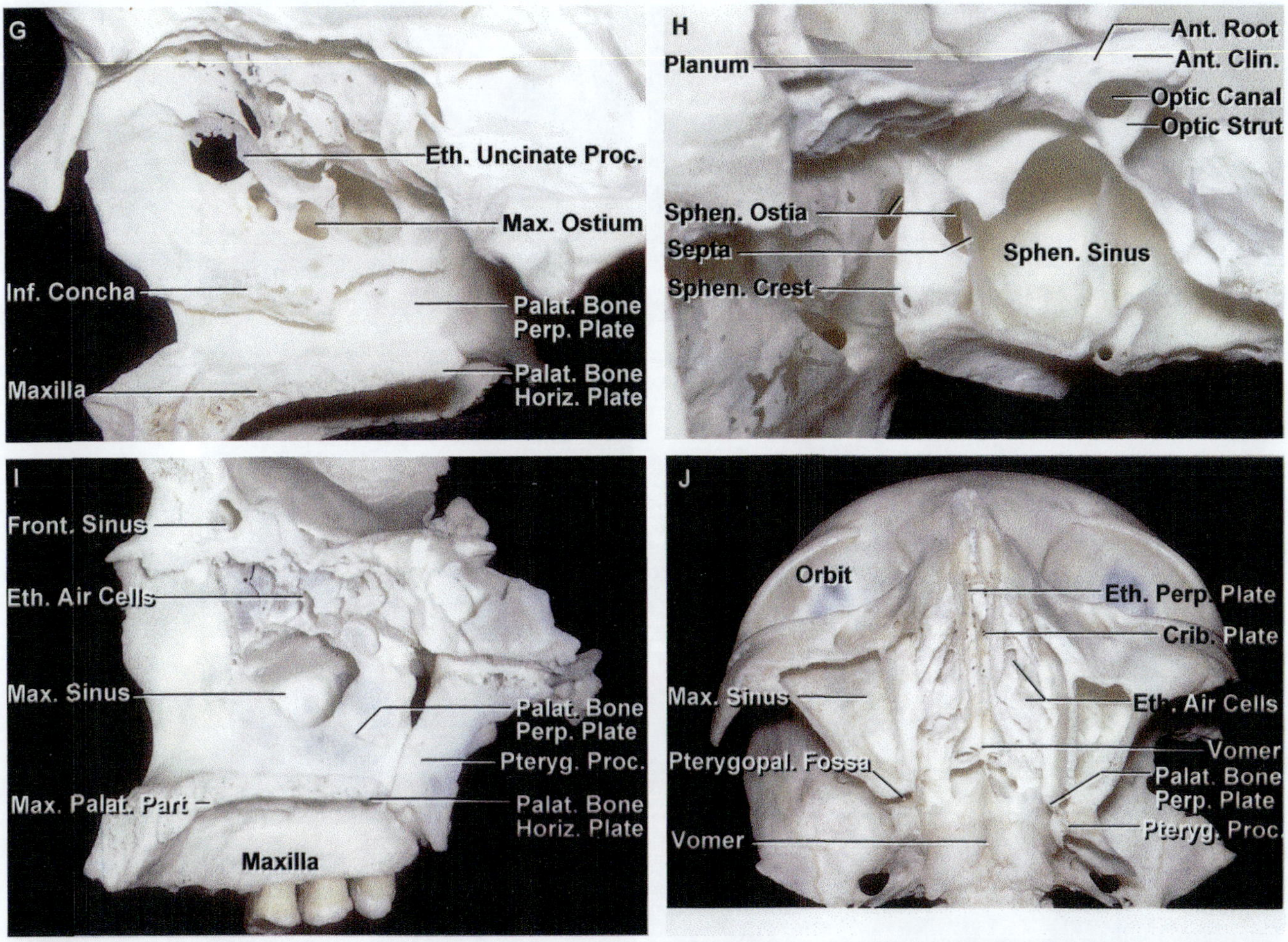

FIGURE 8.3. *Continued*
bones and laterally and below by the maxilla. The anterior part of the osseous nasal septum is formed above by the perpendicular ethmoid plate and below by the vomer. The inferior concha, a separate bone, and the middle concha, an appendage of the ethmoid bone, are visible through the aperture. F, *posterior view of the posterior nasal aperture. The floor of the posterior aperture is formed by the horizontal plate of the palatine bone. The lateral margin is formed by the medial plate of the pterygoid process and is joined anteriorly by the perpendicular plate of the palatine bone, which forms the part of the lateral nasal wall between the maxilla and the medial pterygoid plate. Posteriorly, the middle concha is much more prominent than the inferior concha and often must be displaced laterally in the transsphenoidal approach to the sphenoid sinus. The vomer extends from the upper surface of the hard palate to the body of the sphenoid bone and separates the paired nasal cavities at the posterior aperture.* G, *the middle concha has been removed. This exposes the uncinate process of the ethmoid bone. The ethmoid infundibulum, which drains the anterior ethmoid air cells and sometimes joins the frontal duct, opens downward above the uncinate process.* H, *oblique anterior view of the sphenoid sinus. The anterior wall of the left half of the sphenoid sinus has been removed. The optic canal is located between the body of the sphenoid, the optic strut, the anterior clinoid process, and the anterior root of the lesser sphenoid wing. The sphenoid ostia open, just above the superior concha, into the nasal cavity.* I, *lateral wall of the nasal cavity after removal of the concha. The upper part of the lateral wall of the nasal cavity is formed by the ethmoid air cells. The lower part of the lateral wall is formed, from anterior to posterior, by maxilla, perpendicular palatal plate, and the pterygoid process and medial pterygoid plate. The palate is formed anteriorly by the palatal plate of the maxilla and posteriorly by the horizontal plate of the palatine bone.* J, *section through the nasal cavity and both maxillae. The maxillary sinuses form part of the lateral wall of the nasal cavity and drain through the middle meatus into the nasal cavity. The cribriform plate is located above the nasal cavity in the midline. The part of the nasal septum below the cribriform plate is formed by the perpendicular ethmoid plate. The vomer forms the lower and posterior parts of the nasal septum. The wings of the vomer spread laterally along the lower surface of the sphenoid body. The ethmoid air cells are in the upper part of the lateral wall of the nasal cavity.* Alv., *alveolar;* Ant., *anterior;* Aper., *aperture;* Cart., *cartilage;* Clin., *clinoid;* CN, *cranial nerve;* Crib., *cribriform;* Eth., *ethmoid;* Front., *frontal;* Horiz., *horizontal;* Inf., *inferior;* Infratemp., *infratemporal;* Lat., *lateral;* M., *muscle;* Max., *maxilla, maxillary;* Med., *medial;* Mid., *middle;* Palat., *palatal, palatine;* Perp., *perpendicular;* Proc., *process;* Pteryg., *pterygoid;* Pterygopal., *pterygopalatine;* Pyr., *pyriform;* Sphen., *sphenoid;* Sup., *superior.*

instruments have shafts 9.5 cm in length, barely long enough to reach through the speculum into the sphenoid sinus. The fact that important neural and vascular structures are exposed either in the lateral sinus wall, directly lateral to the sella, or above the diaphragma sellae, especially if the latter is defective, has led the author to prefers blunt rather than sharp ring curettes for dissection in these areas.

Another measurement important in transsphenoidal surgery is the thickness of the anterior sellar wall and sellar floor. In our previous study, in the sellar type of sinus, the thickness

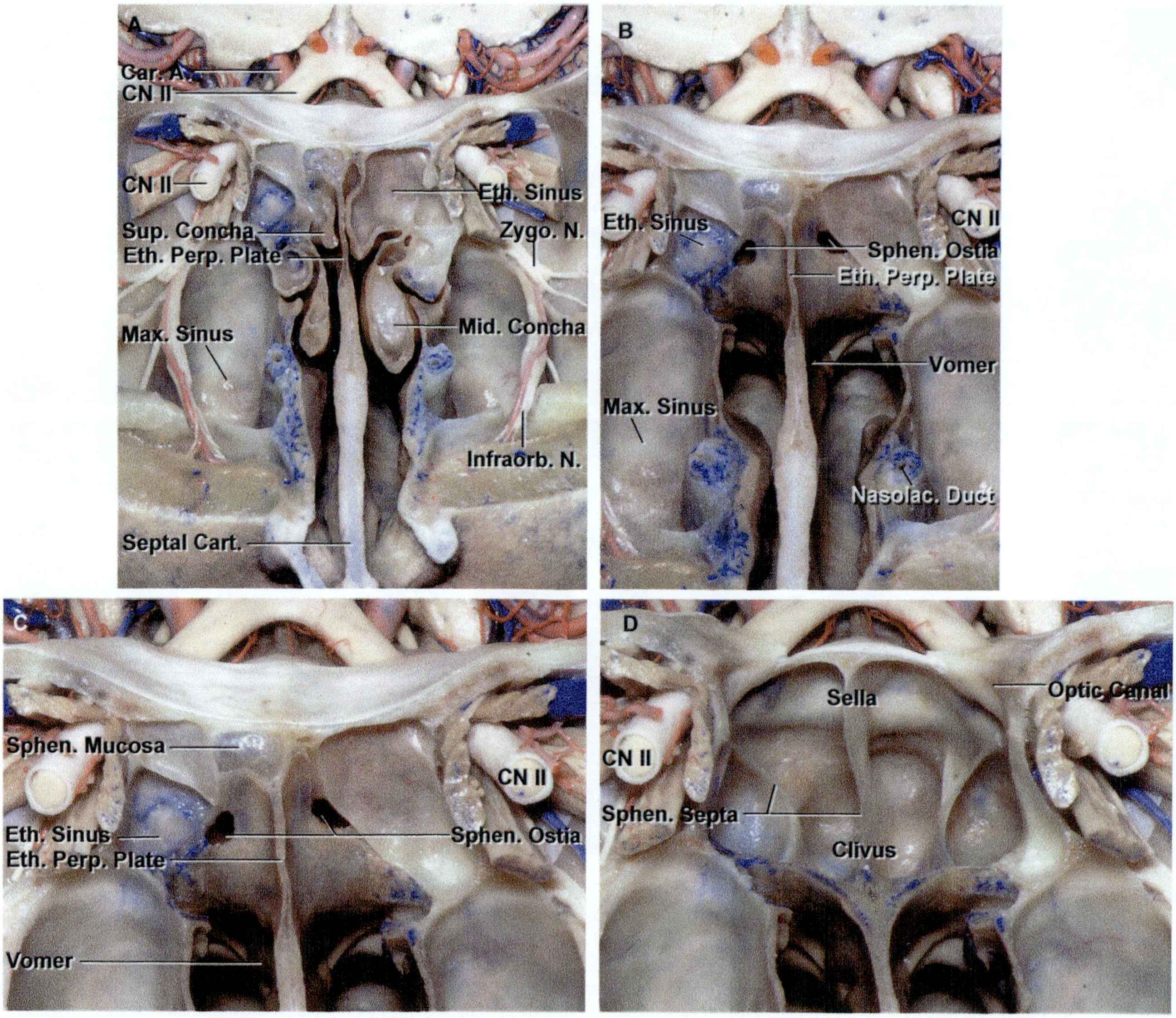

FIGURE 8.4. *Transnasal route to the sphenoid sinus and sella. A, the cross section extends across the nasal cavity, superior and middle turbinates, maxillary sinuses, the orbits near the apex and the ethmoidal sinuses in front of the sphenoid sinus. The zygomatic and infraorbital nerves arise from the maxillary nerve in the pterygopalatine fossa, which is located behind the posterior maxillary wall. The nasal septum is formed above by the perpendicular ethmoid plate, below by the vomer, and anteriorly by the cartilaginous septum. B, the concha and posterior ethmoid air cells have been removed to expose the vomer and the anterior wall of the sphenoid sinus and the sphenoid ostia. The nasolacrimal duct descends along the lateral wall of the nasal cavity. C, enlarged view. The perpendicular ethmoid plate joins the anterior sphenoid face, and the vomer extends upward to join the inferior sphenoid wall, both in the midline. The posterior ethmoid air cells are located anterior to the lateral part of the sphenoid face and overlap the superolateral margins of the sphenoid ostia. D, the anterior face of the sphenoid has been removed to expose the multiseptated sphenoid sinus and the anterior wall of the sella. The bony prominences over the optic canals are situated in the superolateral margins of the sinus. E, the anterior wall of the sella and the lateral wall of the sphenoid sinus have been removed to expose the petrous and cavernous segments of the carotid artery and the pituitary gland. The posterior wall of the maxillary sinus has been removed to expose the maxillary nerve and artery and the pterygopalatine ganglion in the pterygopalatine fossa. F, enlarged view of the right orbit and pterygopalatine fossa. The maxillary nerve gives rise to the infraorbital and zygomatic nerves and communicating rami to the pterygopalatine ganglion. Branches of the maxillary artery course through the pterygopalatine fossa. The posterior wall of the pterygopalatine fossa is formed by the pterygoid process. G, enlarged view. The branches of the maxillary artery penetrate the lateral wall of the nasal cavity to course along the sphenoid face. The maxillary nerve sends communicating rami to the sphenopalatine ganglion. The vidian nerve enters the posterior aspect of the sphenopalatine ganglion. The pituitary gland is surrounded by the cavernous sinuses laterally and an anterior intercavernous sinus above. H, the optic nerves have been elevated to show the suprasellar area and the relationships between the orbital apex, optic canals, nasal cavity, pterygopalatine fossa, and the petrous and intracavernous segments of the internal carotid artery. The superior hypophyseal arteries pass to the lower margin of the optic chiasm and the pituitary stalk. A., artery;* Car., *carotid;* Cart., *cartilage;* Cav., *cavernous;* CN, *cranial nerve;* Eth., *ethmoid;* Gang., *ganglion;* Hyp., *hypophyseal;* Infraorb., *infraorbital;* Max., *maxillary;* Mid., *middle;* N., *nerve;* Nasolac., *nasolacrimal;* Ophth., *ophthalmic;* Perp., *perpendicular;* Pet., *petrous;* Pit., *pituitary;* Proc., *process;* Pteryg., *pterygoid;* Pterygopal., *pterygopalatine;* Seg., *segment;* Sept., *septal;* Sphen., *sphenoid;* Sup., *superior.*

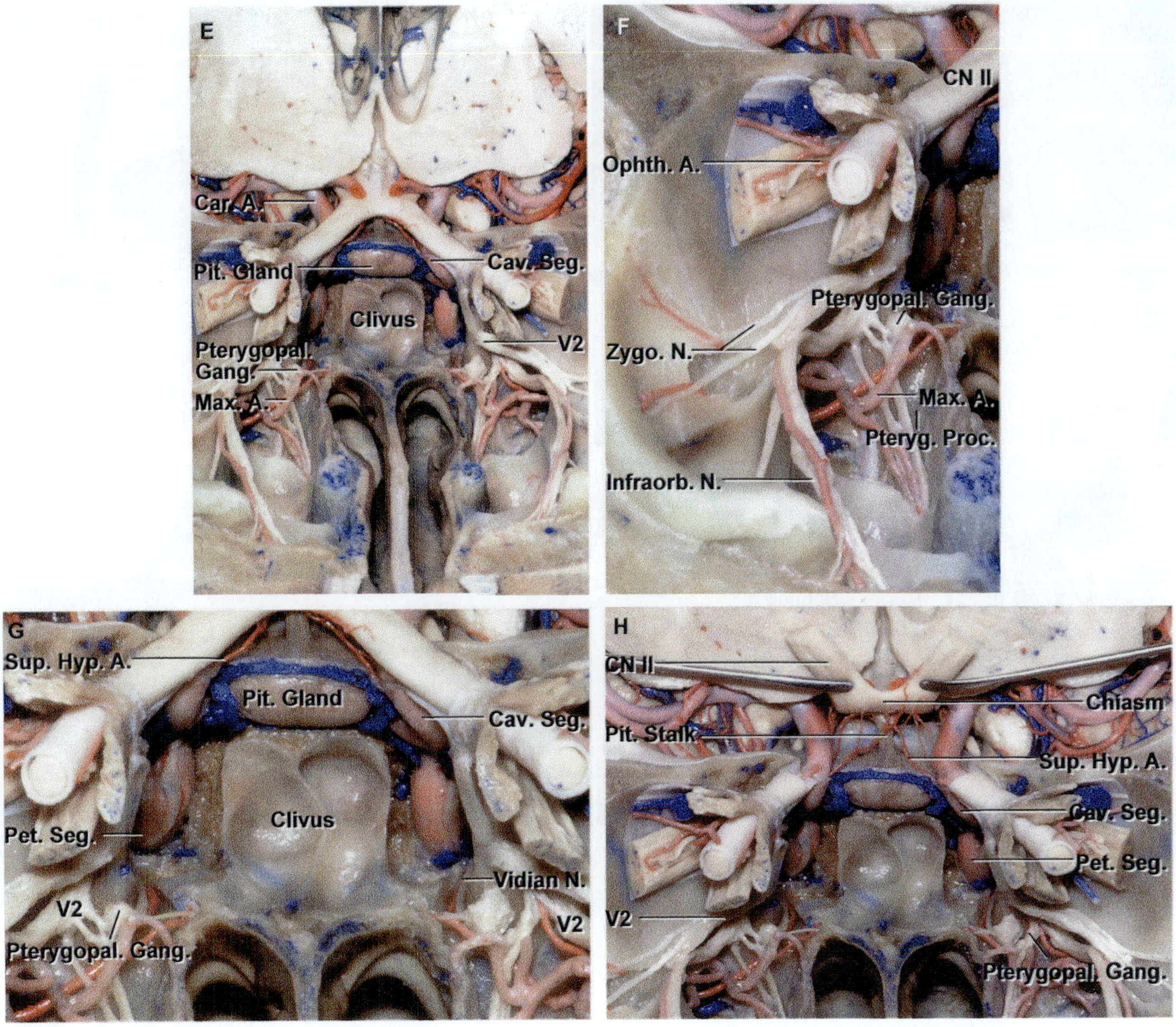

FIGURE 8.4. *Continued*

of the anterior sellar wall ranged from 0.1 to 0.7 mm (mean, 0.4 mm) as compared with 0.3 to 1.5 mm (mean, 0.7 mm) for the presellar type. The thickness of bone covering the sinus was defined at the planum sphenoidale, tuberculum sellae, anterior sellar wall, sellar floor, and the clivus. The thickest bone was found at the clivus and tuberculum sellae and the thinnest along the anterior sellar wall (15, 21).

The septae within the sphenoid sinus vary greatly in size, shape, thickness, location, completeness, and relation to the sellar floor (*Fig. 8.9*). The cavities within the sinus are seldom symmetrical from side to side and are often subdivided by irregular minor septae. The septae are often located off the midline as they cross the floor of the sella. In our previous study, a single major septum separated the sinus into two large cavities in only 68% of specimens, and even in these cases, the septae were often located off the midline or were deflected to one side (15). The most common type of sphenoid sinus has multiple small cavities in the large paired sinuses. The smaller cavities are separated by septae oriented in all directions. Computed tomography or magnetic resonance imaging of the sella provide the definition of the relationship of the septae to the floor of the sella needed for transsphenoidal surgery. Major septae may be found as far as 8 mm off the midline (15).

The internal carotid artery rests directly against the lateral surface of the body of the sphenoid bone, and its course is marked by a groove in the bone, the carotid sulcus, that defines the course of the intracavernous portion of the carotid artery. As the sphenoid sinus expands and its walls resorb, the carotid sulcus produces a prominence within the sinus wall below the floor and along the anterior margin of the sella (*Figs. 8.6, 8.8,* and *8.10*) (4, 15). This prominence is most pronounced

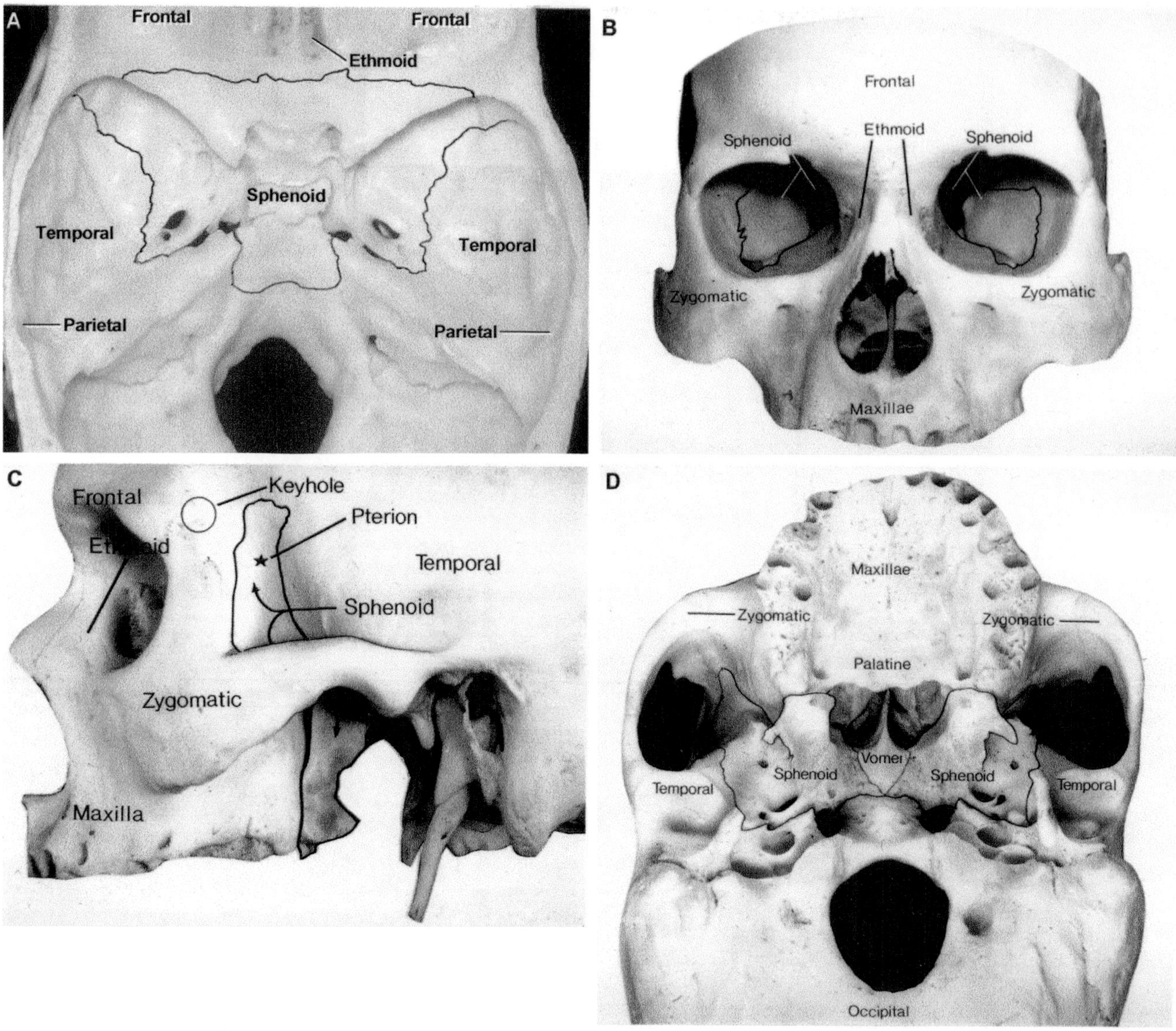

FIGURE 8.5. *Osseous relationships of the sphenoid bone. The sphenoid bone is outlined in each view.* A, *superior view.* B, *anterior view.* C, *lateral view.* D, *inferior view.* E–H, *anterior views.* E, *conchal type sphenoid bone.* F, *bone with presellar type sphenoid sinus.* G, *bone with sellar type sphenoid sinus and well-defined sphenoid ostia.* H, *bone with sellar type sphenoid sinus with poorly defined sphenoid ostia and obliquely oriented sphenoidal septae.* For., *foramen;* Lat., *lateral;* Med., *medial;* Pal., *palato-;* Sup., *superior;* Temp., *temporal.* (From, *Rhoton AL Jr, Hardy DG, Chambers SM: Microsurgical anatomy and dissection of the sphenoid bone, cavernous sinus and sellar region.* **Surg Neurol** *12:63–104, 1979 [21].)*

with maximal pneumatization of the sphenoid and varies from a small focal bulge to a serpiginous elevation marking the full course of the carotid artery along the lateral wall of the sphenoid sinus. The carotid prominence can be divided into three parts: the retrosellar, infrasellar, and presellar segments. The first part, the retrosellar segment, is located in the posterolateral part of the sinus. This segment of the prominence is present only in well-pneumatized sellar-type sinuses in which the air cavity extends laterally in the area below the dorsum. The second part, the infrasellar segment, is located below the sellar floor. The third part, the presellar segment, is located anterolateral to the anterior sellar wall. Of the 50 specimens we examined, 98% had presellar, 80% had infrasellar, and 78% had retrosellar prominences (15, 17). Any part of the prominence may be present and the others absent. If all three parts are present and connected, they form a serpiginous bulge marking the full course of the carotid artery. In the normal sinus, the presellar part extends to the anterior sellar wall. The anterior sellar wall is located anterior to the carotid prominence when the sella is greatly expanded by tumor.

Only the presellar part of the carotid prominence is present in a presellar type of sphenoid sinus, and it is this part that is also most frequently present in the sellar type of sinus. The corresponding arterial segments are slightly longer than the segments of the prominence because of tortuosity of the artery. This tortuosity, although present, is limited by the dural

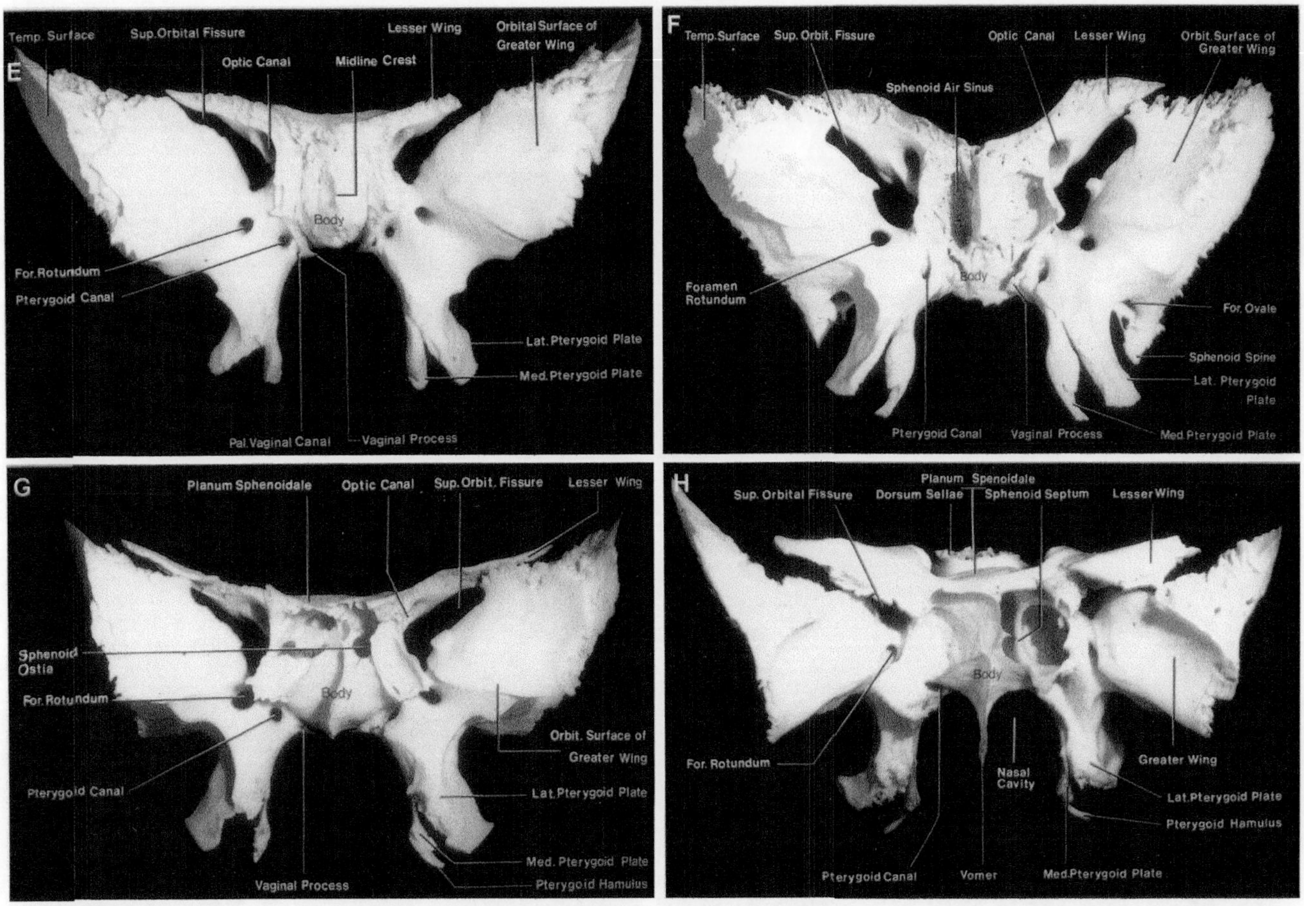

FIGURE 8.5. *Continued*

walls of the cavernous sinus, particularly if the artery is encircled by a ring of bone formed by the union of the anterior and middle clinoid processes. Serial coronal sections through the cavernous sinus show that the artery does not always nestle into the bony carotid sulcus on the intracranial surface of the sphenoid bone, but is separated from it by an extension of the cavernous sinus.

The bone separating the artery and the sphenoid sinus is thinner over the anterior than the posterior parts of the carotid prominence and is thinnest over the part of the artery just below the tuberculum sellae. In our study, a layer of bone less than 0.5 mm thick separated the artery and sinus in nearly 90% of sinuses, and areas of absence of bone between the artery and the sinus were present in nearly 10%. Such defects in the bone separating the sphenoid sinus and carotid arteries may occur bilaterally. In our study of 50 sinuses, the bone separating the artery and the sinus was as thick as 1.0 mm (4). The bone over the carotid arteries was frequently as thin or thinner than that separating the anterior surface of the pituitary gland and the sphenoid sinus. The intracranial surface of the sphenoid bone was covered by periosteum, and this and the sinus mucosa separated the air cavity and carotid arteries if no bone was present.

The proximity of the carotid prominences to the midline is important in pituitary surgery. The transverse separation between the carotid prominences of each side was measured at the level of the tuberculum sellae, anterior sellar wall, sellar floor, dorsum sellae, and clivus. The shortest distance between both carotid bulges into the sphenoid sinus is usually located at the level of the tuberculum sellae (*Figs. 8.4, 8.7,* and *8.10*). In our specimens, the shortest distance between both carotid prominences of each side was located just below the tuberculum in 72%, at the level of the floor of the sella in 20%, and at the clivus in 8% (4).

The optic canals protrude into the superolateral portion of the sinus. The superior orbital fissure produces a smooth wide prominence in the midlateral wall below the optic canal, and the maxillary nerve frequently protrudes into the inferolateral part. There are areas where no bone separates the optic sheath and sinus mucosa (*Figs. 8.2, 8.10,* and *8.11*). In nearly 80% of the optic nerves, less than 0.5 mm of bone separated the optic nerve and sheath from the sinus. Care must be taken to avoid

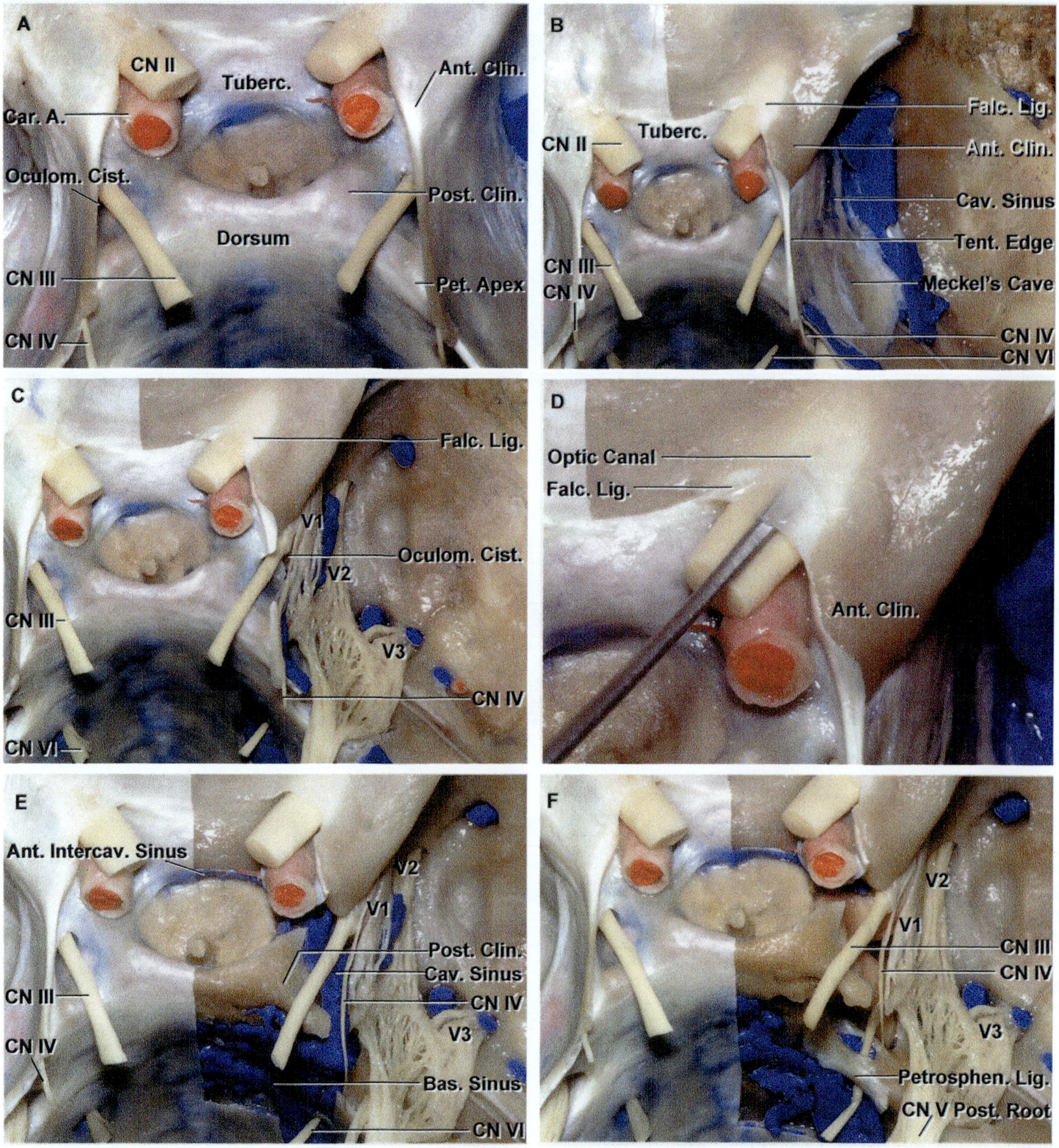

FIGURE 8.6. *Superior view of the sellar region. A, the sella is located between the cavernous sinuses. The diaphragm, which usually separates the sella from the suprasellar cisterns, is absent in this case. The oculomotor nerves enter the roof of the cavernous sinus where there is a narrow cistern around the nerve. The oculomotor triangle, the triangular patch of dura through which the oculomotor nerve enters the dura in the cavernous sinus roof, is positioned between the anterior and posterior clinoid processes and the petrous apex. The roof of the cavernous sinus extends forward under the anterior clinoid process. B, the dura covering the anterior clinoid process and optic canal has been removed. The outer layer of dura in the lateral wall of the cavernous sinus has been removed to expose the thin inner layer of the lateral sinus wall and the lateral surface of Meckel's cave. The falciform ligament, the dural fold extending above the optic nerve proximal to the nerve's entrance into the optic canal, extends from the anterior clinoid to the tuberculum. C, the inner layer of the lateral sinus wall has been removed to expose the nerves coursing in the wall of the cavernous sinus and middle fossa. The oculomotor nerve enters the narrow oculomotor cistern in the sinus roof and passes forward along the lower margin of the anterior clinoid process. D, enlarged view. A probe has been passed between the optic nerve and the falciform ligament. The dissector can be seen through the dura proximal to the osseous optic canal. The anterior clinoid is located lateral to the*

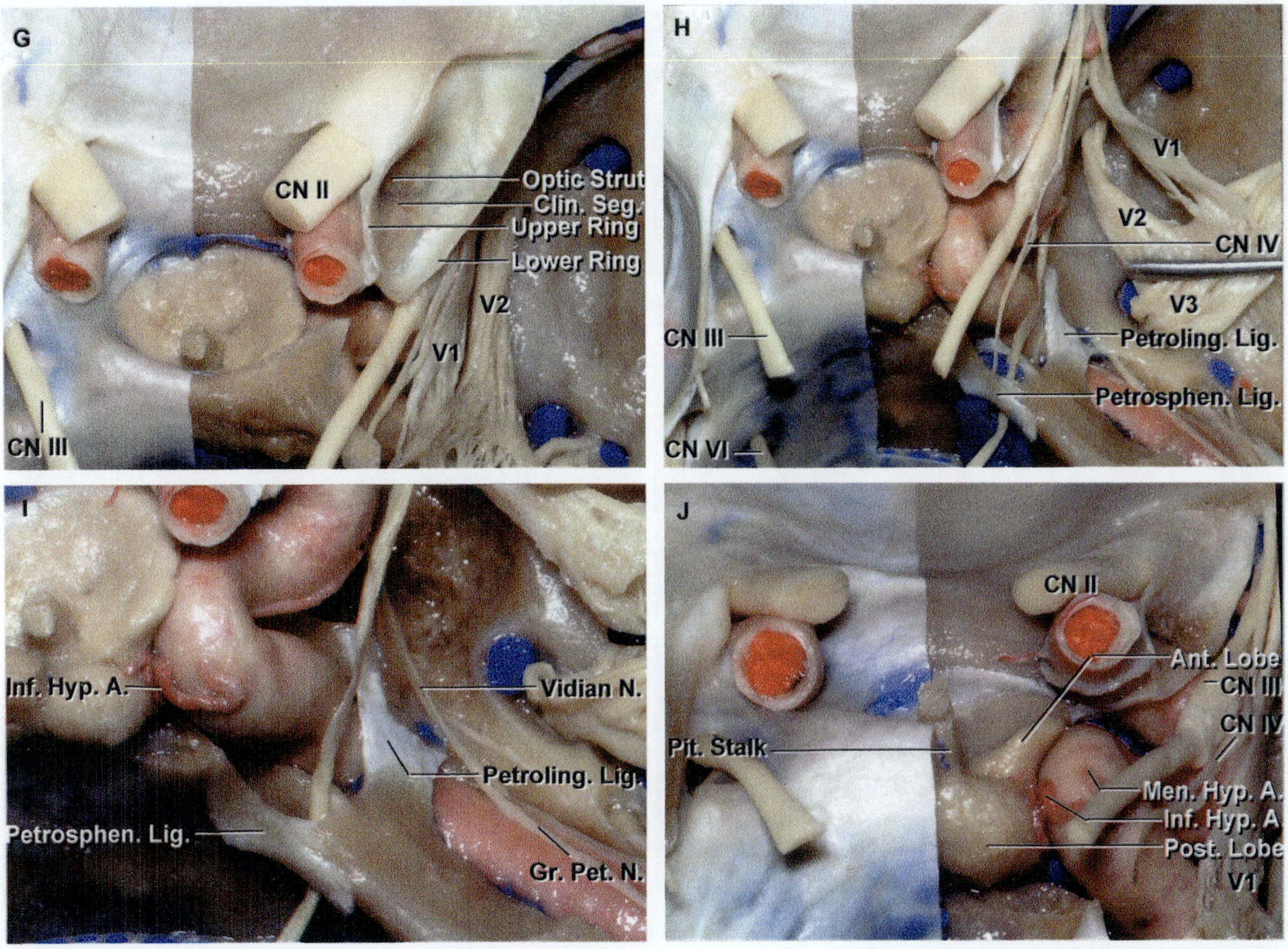

FIGURE 8.6. *Continued*
optic nerve and internal carotid artery and above the oculomotor nerve. E, *the dura covering the dorsum sellae, basilar sinus, and posterior clinoid process has been removed. The oculomotor nerve passes forward lateral to the posterior clinoid and below the anterior clinoid. An abnormal bony projection extends laterally from the right posterior clinoid below the oculomotor nerve toward the petrous apex. The basilar sinus crosses the back of the dorsum and upper clivus and communicates widely with the posterior edge of the paired cavernous sinuses. The abducens nerve passes through the lower margin of the basilar sinus. An anterior intercavernous passes along the anterior margin of the sella.* F, *the posterior part of the cavernous sinus has been cleared to expose the abducens passing through Dorello's canal, which is roofed by the petrosphenoid ligament.* G, *the anterior clinoid process has been removed to expose the clinoid segment of the internal carotid artery defined by the upper and lower dural rings. The upper ring is formed by the dura extending medially from the upper surface of the anterior clinoid. The lower dural ring is formed by the dura, which extends medially from the lower margin of the anterior clinoid and separates the lower clinoid margin from the oculomotor nerve.* H, *posterosuperior view of the sella. The dorsum and posterior clinoid have been removed to expose the posterior lobe of the pituitary, which was hidden below the dorsum. The abducens nerve is exposed below the petrosphenoid ligament. The trigeminal nerve has been reflected forward to expose the petrolingual ligament, which extends above the internal carotid artery just proximal to the artery's entry into the cavernous sinus.* I, *enlarged view of the petrolingual and petrosphenoid ligaments. The inferior hypophyseal artery passes to the capsule of the posterior lobe. The greater petrosal nerve courses medially and is joined by the deep petrosal branch of the periarterial carotid plexus to form the vidian nerve.* J, *enlarged view. The carotid artery protrudes medially to deform the lateral surface of the anterior lobe of the pituitary gland. A tongue of anterior lobe extends laterally above the intercavernous carotid.* A., *artery;* Ant., *anterior;* Bas., *basilar;* Car., *carotid;* Cav., *cavernous;* Cist., *cistern;* Clin., *clinoid;* CN, *cranial nerve;* Falc., *falciform;* Gr., *greater;* Hyp., *hypophyseal;* Inf., *inferior;* Intercav., *intercavernous;* Lig., *ligament;* Men. Hyp., *meningohypophyseal;* N., *nerve;* Oculom., *oculomotor;* Pet., *petrous;* Petroling., *petrolingual;* Petrosphen., *petrosphenoid;* Pit., *pituitary;* Post., *posterior;* Seg., *segment;* Tent., *tentorial;* Tuberc., *tuberculum.*

damage to the nerves in the transsphenoidal approach, if a dehiscence of the bone covering exposes them in the sinus. Injury to nerves exposed in the sinus wall may explain some cases of unexpected visual loss after transsphenoidal surgery (13, 20).

A pneumatized diverticulum of the sinus, called the opticocarotid recess, often extends laterally into the optic strut between the optic canal and the prominence overlying the carotid artery and superior orbital fissure (*Figs. 8.2, 8.10,* and *8.11*). This pneumatization may extend through the optic strut into the anterior clinoid process, thus creating a channel through which cerebrospinal fluid can leak into the sinus after an anterior clinoidectomy with resulting cerebrospinal fluid rhinorrhea.

The segment of the maxillary branch of the trigeminal nerve just peripheral to the foramen rotundum frequently produces

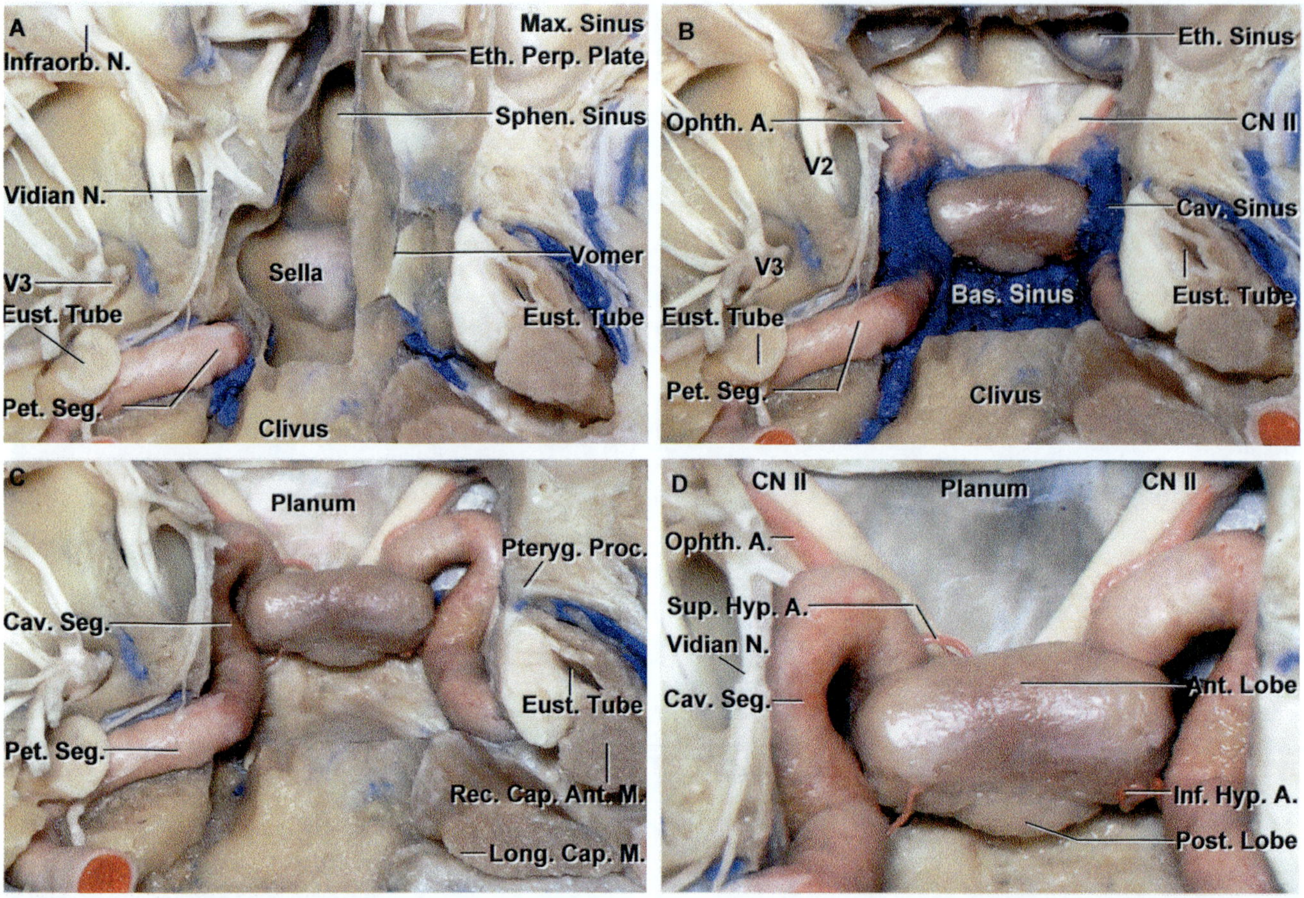

FIGURE 8.7. A–D, *inferior view of the sellar region and surrounding cranial base.* A, *the right half of the floor of the sphenoid sinus has been removed to expose the sellar floor and the part of the sphenoid sinus below the planum and tuberculum. On the specimen's left side, the eustachian tube, pterygoid process, and posterior part of the maxillary sinus have been preserved. On the right side, the medial portion of the eustachian tube and the pterygoid process have been removed. This exposes the right mandibular nerve exiting the foramen ovale and the maxillary nerve exiting the foramen rotundum and passing forward as the infraorbital nerve. The pterygopalatine ganglion is located in the pterygopalatine fossa behind the maxillary sinus in the lateral wall of the nasal cavity. The right pterygoid process has been removed to expose the vidian canal, in which the vidian nerve travels to reach the pterygopalatine ganglion. The bone below the petrous carotid has been removed up to the point where the artery turns upward to enter the posterior part of the cavernous sinus.* B, *part of the vomer, perpendicular ethmoid plate, and floor of the sphenoid sinus have been removed to expose the cavernous sinus, intracavernous carotid, and the pituitary gland. The floor of the optic canals have been removed to expose the ophthalmic arteries coursing below the optic nerves. The cavernous sinus surrounds the intracavernous carotid. An anterior intercavernous sinus crosses the anterior margin of the gland. Some of the upper clivus has been removed to expose the basilar sinus, which sits on the back of the dorsum and is the largest connection between the cavernous sinuses.* C, *the venous spaces around the pituitary gland have been cleared to expose the petrous and intracavernous carotid segments.* D, *enlarged view of the pituitary gland, intracavernous carotid, and the optic nerves and ophthalmic arteries. The inferior hypophyseal arteries pass to the posterior lobe. The superior hypophyseal arteries arise in the chiasmatic cistern and pass medially to reach the stalk and chiasm.* A., *artery;* Ant., *anterior;* Bas., *basilar;* Cap., *capitus;* Cav., *cavernous;* CN, *cranial nerve;* Eth., *ethmoid;* Eust., *eustachian;* Hyp., *hypophyseal;* Inf., *inferior;* Infraorb., *infraorbital;* Long., *longus;* M., *muscle;* Max., *maxillary;* N., *nerve;* Ophth., *ophthalmic;* Perp., *perpendicular;* Pet., *petrous;* Post., *posterior;* Proc., *process;* Pteryg., *pterygoid;* Rec., *rectus;* Seg., *segment;* Sphen., *sphenoid;* Sup., *superior.*

FIGURE 8.8. *Nasal pathway to the sphenoid sinus. Stepwise dissections showing the structures that form the lateral limit of the transnasal route to the sphenoid sinus and sella.* A, *sagittal section to right of the midline. The nasal septum, along which the transsphenoidal approach is directed, is formed above by the perpendicular plate of the ethmoid, anteriorly by the nasal septal cartilage, and below by the vomer. The vomer articulates with the anteroinferior part of the sphenoid body, and the perpendicular plate articulates with the anterior face. The sphenoid sinus is located in the body of the sphenoid bone.* B, *the sagittal section has been extended to the right of the midline. The nasal concha and meatus and the eustachian tubes are in the lateral margin of the exposure.* C, *a portion of the middle and inferior turbinates has been removed. The ostia of the maxillary and frontal sinuses opens into the middle meatus located below the middle turbinate. The nasolacrimal duct opens below the lower turbinate into the inferior meatus. Rosenmüller's fossa is located behind the eustachian tube.* D, *the mucosa in the lateral margin of the nasal cavity and the posterior part of the inferior and middle turbinates have been removed to expose the pterygoid process and the posterior maxillary wall, which form the posterior and anterior boundaries of the pterygopalatine fossa, respectively. The eustachian tube opens into the nasopharynx at the posterior edge of the pterygoid process. The terminal branches of the maxillary artery pass through the pterygopalatine fossa, located between*

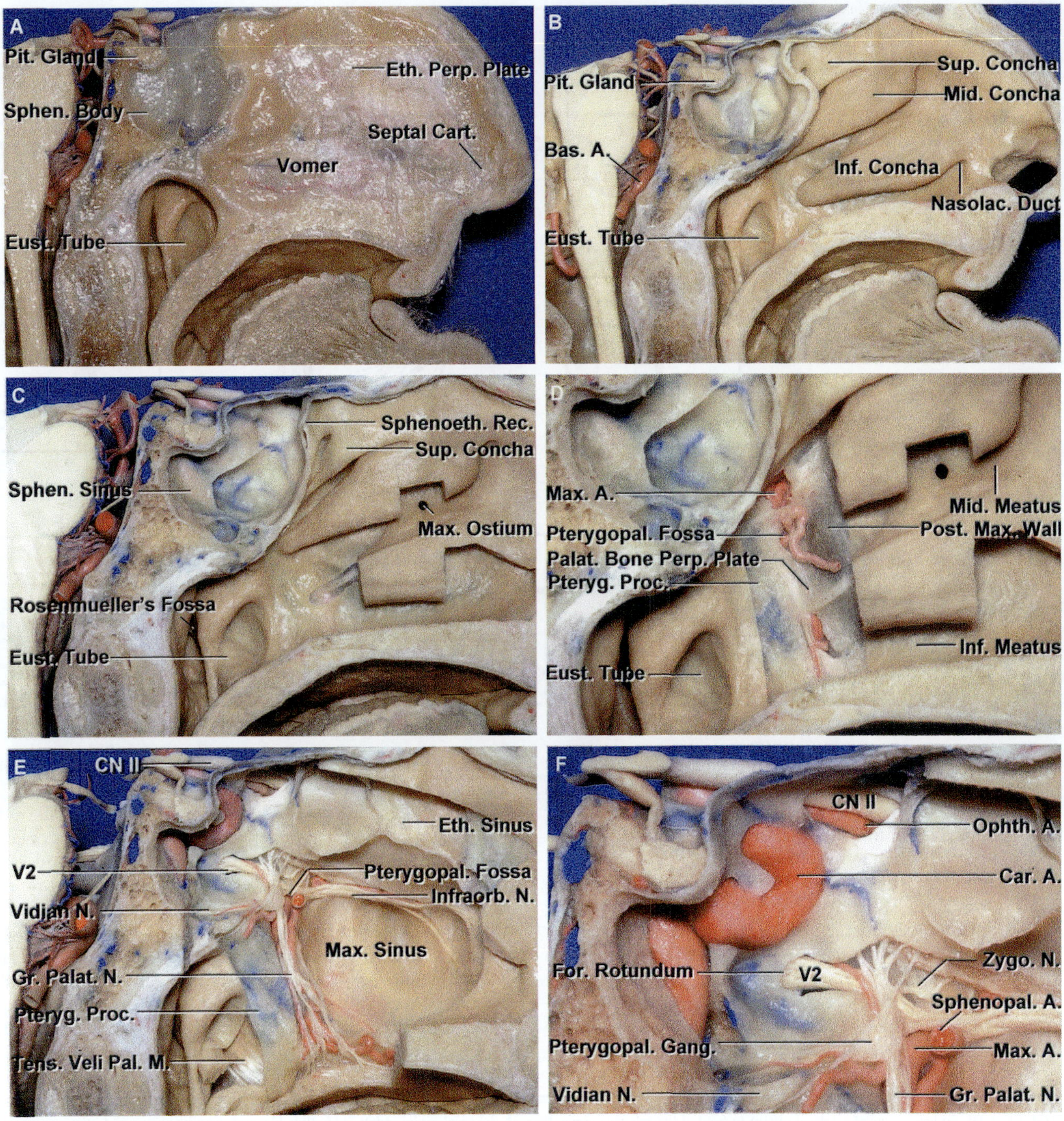

FIGURE 8.8. *Continued*
the posterior maxillary wall and the pterygoid process, to enter the posterosuperior part of the nasal cavity at the anteroinferior margin of the sphenoid sinus. The medial wall of the pterygopalatine fossa is formed by the perpendicular plate of the palatine bone. E, the medial wall of the maxillary sinus has been opened to expose the infraorbital nerve, which arises in the pterygopalatine fossa and passes forward in the sinus roof. The maxillary nerve passes through the foramen rotundum to enter the pterygopalatine, where it gives rise to the infraorbital, zygomatic, and greater palatine nerves, plus communicating rami to the pterygopalatine ganglion. F, enlarged view. The bone and dura covering the optic canal in the superolateral part of the sphenoid sinus has been opened to expose the optic nerve and ophthalmic artery in the optic canal. The junction of the petrous and cavernous carotid limits the exposure below the level of the sella. Terminal branches of the maxillary artery intermingle with the neural structures in the pterygopalatine fossa and exit the fossa to supply the tissues on the sphenoid face. A., *artery;* Bas., *basilar;* Car., *carotid;* Cart., *cartilage;* CN, *cranial nerve;* Eth., *ethmoid;* Eust., *eustachian;* For., *foramen;* Gang., *ganglion;* Gr., *greater;* Inf., *inferior;* Infraorb., *infraorbital;* M., *muscle;* Max., *maxillary;* Mid., *middle;* N., *nerve;* Nasolac., *nasolacrimal;* Ophth., *ophthalmic;* Pal., *palatini;* Palat., *palatine;* Perp., *perpendicular;* Pit., *pituitary;* Post., *posterior;* Proc., *process;* Pteryg., *pterygoid;* Pterygopal., *pterygopalatine;* Rec., *recess;* Sphen., *sphenoid;* Sphenoeth., *sphenoethmoid;* Sphenopal., *sphenopalatine;* Sup., *superior;* Tens., *tensor.*

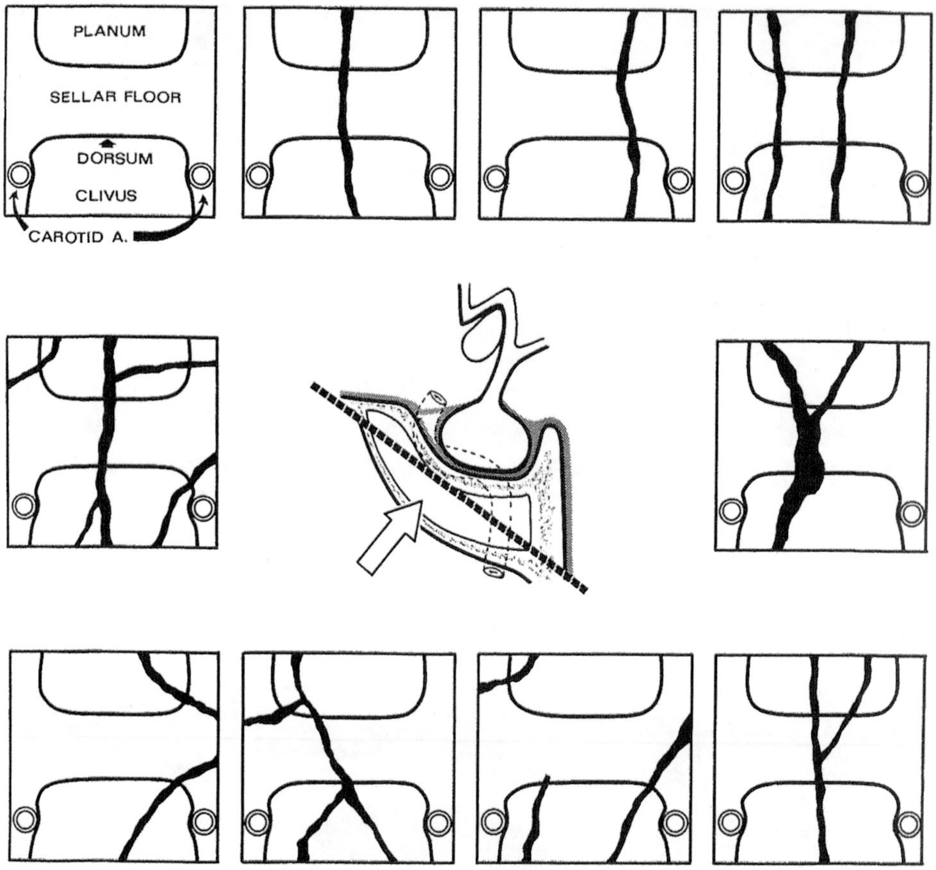

FIGURE 8.9. *Septa in the sphenoid sinus. The* heavy broken line *on the central diagram shows the plane of the section of each specimen from which the drawings were taken, and the* large arrow *shows the direction of view. The planum is above, the dorsum and clivus are below, and the sella is in an intermediate position on each diagram. The* heavy dark lines *on the drawings show the location of the septae in the sphenoid sinus. A wide variety of septae separate the sinus into cavities that vary in size and shape, seldom being symmetrical from side to side.* (From, *Renn WH, Rhoton AL Jr: Microsurgical anatomy of the sellar region.* ***J Neurosurg*** *43:288–298, 1975 [15].)*

a prominent bulge into the lateral sinus wall below the sellae, especially if the sinus is well pneumatized. This trigeminal prominence is less common with a presellar than with a sellar type of sinus. There may also be areas where no bone separates the nerve from the sinus mucosa and the presence of less than a 0.5-mm thickness of bone separating the nerve from the sinus is common. The length of maxillary division bulging into the sinus ranges from 7.0 to 15.0 mm (mean, 10.9 mm) (4). The sphenoid sinus frequently extends laterally below the maxillary nerve into the medial part of the greater sphenoid wing, which forms the floor of the middle fossa. The trigeminal ganglion and the first and third trigeminal divisions are separated from the lateral wall of the sphenoid sinus by the carotid artery.

Removing the mucosa and bone from the lateral wall of the sinus exposes the dura mater covering the medial surface of the cavernous sinus and optic canals (*Figs. 8.8, 8.10,* and *8.11*). Opening this dura exposes the carotid arteries and optic and trigeminal nerves within the sinus. The abducent nerve is located between the lateral side of the carotid artery and the medial side of the first trigeminal division. The second and third trigeminal divisions are seen in the lower margin of the opening through the lateral wall of the sphenoid sinus. In half of the cases, the optic and trigeminal nerves and the carotid

FIGURE 8.10. *Anterior view of a coronal section in front of the sphenoid sinus, through the nasal cavity, orbits, and ethmoidal and maxillary sinuses. A, the upper part of the nasal cavity is separated from the orbits by the ethmoidal sinuses. The lower part of the nasal cavity is bounded laterally by the maxillary sinuses. The middle concha projects medially from the lateral nasal wall at the junction of the roof of the maxillary and ethmoidal sinuses. The posterior ethmoid air cells are located in front of the lateral part of the face of the sphenoid sinus. B, the middle and inferior nasal conchae on the left side and the nasal septum and the posterior ethmoidal sinuses on both sides have been removed to expose the posterior nasopharyngeal wall, the anterior aspect of the sphenoid body, and the sphenoid ostia. The posterior ethmoid air cells overlap the lateral margin of the sphenoid ostia. C, the anterior wall of the sphenoid sinus has been opened and the sphenoid septa has been removed to expose the anterior sellar wall in the midline and the prominences over the optic canal and carotid arteries in the lateral walls of this well-pneumatized sphenoid sinus. The medial part of the posterior wall of the left maxillary sinus has been removed to expose branches of the maxillary artery in the pterygopalatine fossa. The opticocarotid recesses extend laterally between the prominences over the carotid arteries and optic nerves. D, the pituitary gland, intracavernous carotids, optic nerves, ophthalmic arteries, and cavernous sinuses have been exposed by removing the bone of the sinus wall. The inferolateral trunk passes above and lateral to the abducens nerve. The shortest distance between the paired carotid arteries is usually located just below the tuberculum selle. A capsular artery arises from the intercavernous carotid and passes upward and medially. E, oblique view. The bony prominences overlying the optic*

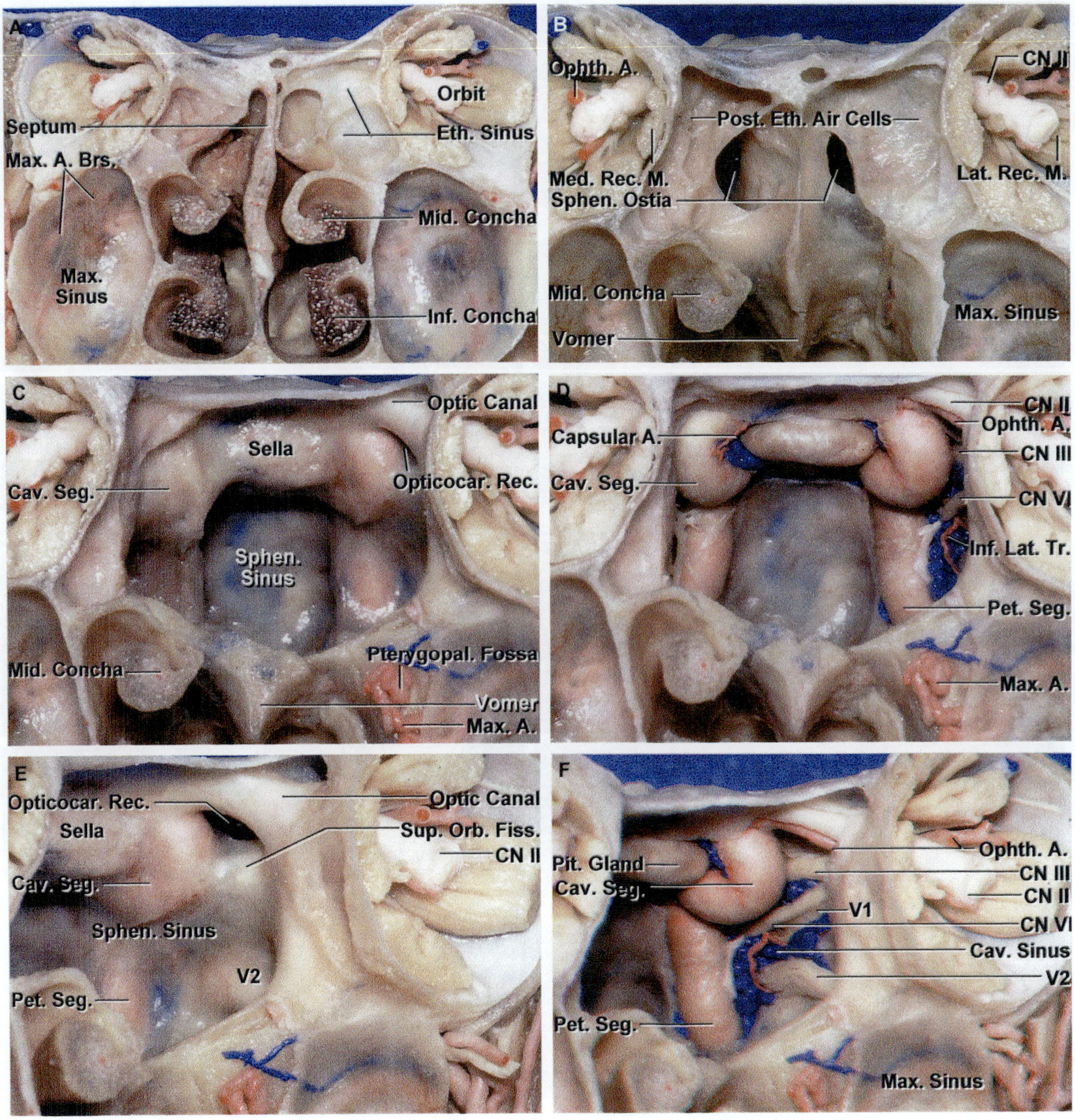

FIGURE 8.10. *Continued*
canal, superior orbital fissure, intracavernous carotid artery, and the maxillary nerve are exposed in the lateral wall of the sphenoid sinus. The bony depression between the carotid prominence and the optic canal, the opticocarotid recess, extends into the medial end of the optic strut. The broad round prominence below the opticocarotid recess is produced by the structures passing through the superior orbital fissure. F, *oblique view. The pituitary gland, intracavernous carotid artery, ophthalmic artery, and optic, ophthalmic, maxillary, oculomotor, and abducens nerves have been exposed. The abducens nerve courses medial to the ophthalmic nerve.* A., *artery;* Brs., *branches;* Cav., *cavernous;* CN., *cranial nerve;* Eth., *ethmoid;* Fiss., *fissure;* Inf., *inferior;* Lat., *lateral;* M., *muscle;* Max., *maxillary;* Med., *medial;* Mid., *middle;* Ophth., *ophthalmic;* Opticocar., *opticocarotid;* Orb., *orbital;* Pet., *petrous;* Pit., *pituitary;* Post., *posterior;* Pterygopal., *pterygopalatine;* Rec., *recess, rectus;* Seg., *segment;* Sphen., *sphenoid;* Sup., *superior;* Tr., *trunk.*

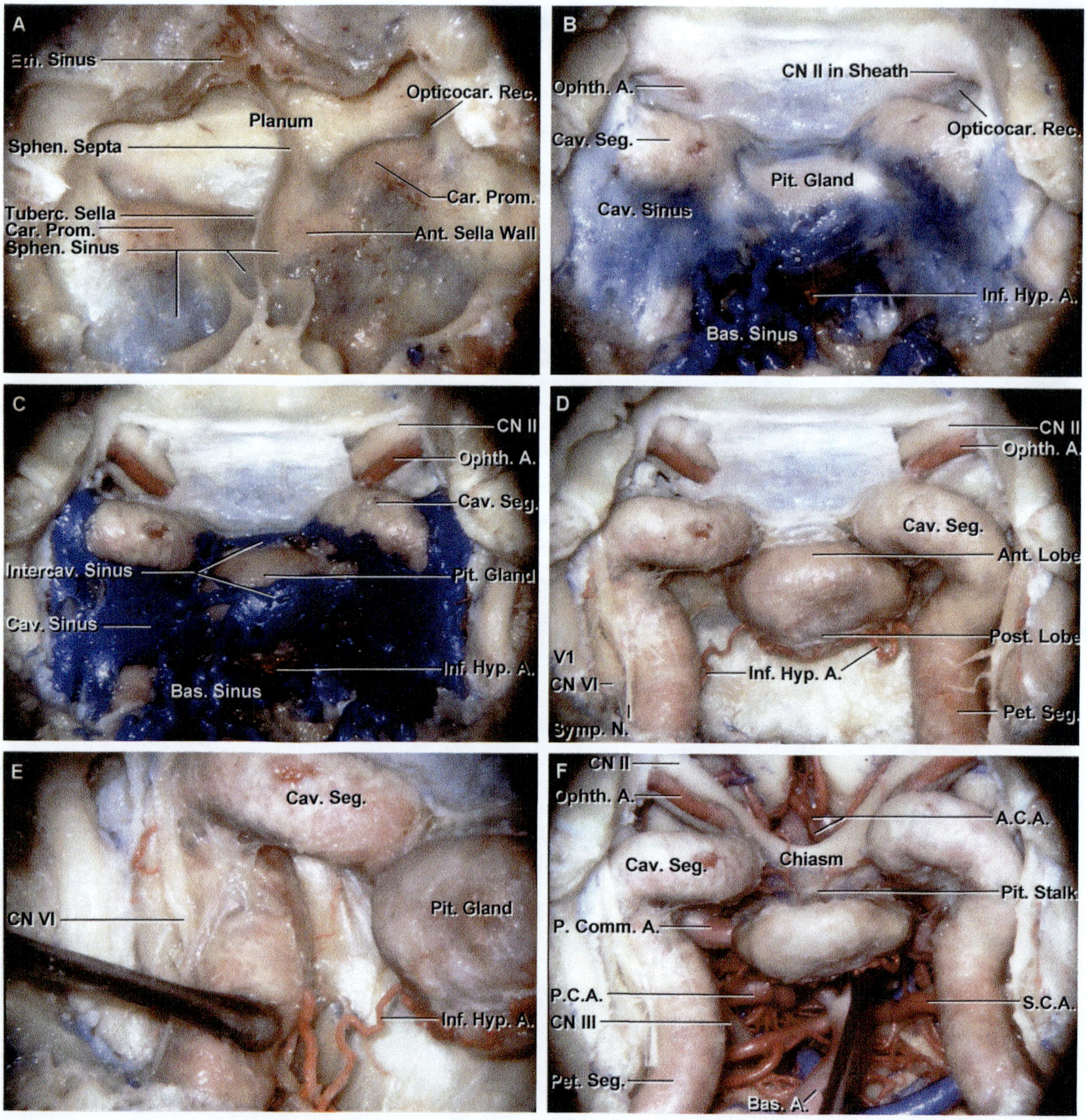

FIGURE 8.11. *Stepwise dissection examining the relationship of the sphenoid sinus to the pituitary fossa, cavernous sinus, and sellar region. A, anterior view into a sphenoid sinus with the mucosa removed to show the relationships of the structures that can be exposed by the transsphenoidal approach. The structures in the exposure include the major sphenoidal septum, anterior sellar wall, and the prominences over the carotid arteries and optic canals. The tuberculum sellae and planum sphenoidale are located above the anterior sellar wall. The opticocarotid recess extends laterally between the carotid artery and optic canal. B, the bone in the walls of the sphenoid sinus has been removed while preserving the dura. The optic nerves, intracavernous carotids, and the pituitary gland are seen through the dura. The anterior bend of the intracavernous carotid bulges forward inside the dura immediately below the optic canals. The basilar sinus, which forms the largest connection between the paired cavernous sinuses, is situated behind the clivus and dorsum sellae. The inferior hypophyseal artery passes to the capsule of the posterior lobe. The optic nerve and ophthalmic artery can be seen through the optic sheath. C, the dura forming the medial and lower walls of the cavernous sinuses has been removed. Intercavernous sinuses connect the paired cavernous sinuses across the midline. The dura in the floor of the optic canals has been opened to expose the ophthalmic arteries and the optic nerves. The basilar sinus sits on the dorsum sellae and clivus and interconnects the posterior end of the paired cavernous sinuses. D, the venous space has been cleared to expose the intracavernous carotid and the anterior and posterior pituitary lobes. The inferior hypophyseal arteries arise from the meningohypophyseal branch of the intracavernous carotid and pass to the capsule of the posterior lobe. Sympathetic nerves ascend on the carotid arteries. The abducens nerve passes through the cavernous sinus on the lateral side of the internal carotid artery and medial to the ophthalmic nerve. E, oblique*

arteries have areas where bone 0.5 mm or less in thickness separates them from the mucosa of the sphenoid sinus, and in a few cases, the bone separating these structures from the sinus is absent (5, 15).

The absence of such bony protection within the walls of the sinus may explain some of the cases of cranial nerve deficits and carotid artery injury after transsphenoidal operations (13). The bone is often thinner over the carotid arteries than over the anterior margin of the pituitary gland. Injury to the lateral wall of the sphenoid sinus offers the potential for causing blindness, extraocular muscle palsies, or facial numbness (20). Forced opening of a transsphenoidal speculum against the lateral walls of the sphenoid sinus could cause injury to the optic, trigeminal, and extraocular nerves. Extreme care should be taken to make certain that the tips of the speculum used for transsphenoidal pituitary operations are not forcefully opened within the sinus, but rather are opened anterior to the sphenoid bone. Forced opening of the speculum within the sinus could crush the thin bone over the maxillary, optic nerves and medial edge of the superior orbital fissure. Vigorous curetting of the walls of the sphenoid sinus could also cause damage to exposed arterial neural structures. The carotid arteries always project anterior to the plane of the anterior sellar wall unless the sella has been greatly expanded by tumor.

Diaphragma Sellae

The diaphragma sellae forms the roof of the sella turcica (*Fig. 8.1*). It covers the pituitary gland, except for a small central opening in its center, which transmits the pituitary stalk. The diaphragma is more rectangular than circular, tends to be convex or concave rather than flat, and is thinner around the infundibulum and somewhat thicker at the periphery. It frequently is a thin, tenuous structure that would not be an adequate barrier for protecting the suprasellar structures during transsphenoidal operation. In an earlier anatomic study, Renn and Rhoton (15) found that the diaphragma was at least as thick as one layer of dura in 38% and in most cases it furnishes an adequate barrier during transsphenoidal hypophysectomy. In the remaining 62%, the diaphragma was extremely thin over some portion of the pituitary gland. It was concave when viewed from above in 54% of the specimens, convex in 4%, and flat in 42%. Even when flat, it lies below the plane of the upper surface of the anterior clinoid process so that a medially projecting supradiaphragmatic lesion, such as an aneurysm, may seem on neuroradiological studies to be located below the anterior clinoid and within the cavernous sinus when they are above the diaphragm in the subarachnoid space.

The opening in the diaphragm's center is large when compared with the size of the pituitary stalk. The diaphragmal opening was 5 mm or more in 56% of our cases, and in these, it would not form a barrier during transsphenoidal pituitary surgery. The opening was round in 54% of the cases, and elliptical with the short diameter of the ellipse oriented in an anterior-posterior direction in 46%. A deficiency of the diaphragma sellae is assumed to be a precondition to formation of an empty sella. An outpouching of the arachnoid protruded through the central opening in the diaphragma into the sella turcica in approximately half of the patients. This outpouching, if opened, represents a potential source of postoperative cerebrospinal fluid leakage (13).

Pituitary Gland

When exposed from above by opening the diaphragma, the superior surface of the posterior lobe of the pituitary gland is lighter in color than the anterior lobe (*Fig. 8.1*). The anterior lobe wraps around the lower part of the pituitary stalk to form the pars tuberalis (16, 21). The posterior lobe is softer, almost gelatinous, and is more densely adherent to the sellar wall. The anterior lobe is firmer and is more easily separated from the sellar walls. The gland's width is the same or more than either its depth or its length in most patients. Its inferior surface usually conforms to the shape of the sellar floor, but its lateral and superior margins vary in shape because these walls are composed of soft tissue rather than bone. If there is a large opening in the diaphragma, the gland tends to be concave superiorly in the area around the stalk. The superior surface may become triangular as a result of being compressed laterally and posteriorly by the carotid arteries. As the anterior lobe is separated from the posterior lobe, there is a tendency for the pars tuberalis to be retained with the posterior lobe. Small intermediate lobe cysts are frequently encountered during separation of the anterior and posterior lobes.

Pituitary Gland and Carotid Artery

The distance separating the medial margin of the carotid artery and the lateral surface of the pituitary gland is an important consideration in transsphenoidal surgery (*Figs. 8.6, 8.7,* and *8.10*). There is often a separation between the lateral surface of the gland and the carotid artery. In our cases where the artery did not indent the gland, the distance between the gland and artery varied from 1 to 7 mm (average, 2.3 mm); however, in approximately one in four cases, the artery protruded through the medial wall of the cavernous sinus to indent the gland (*Fig. 8.1J*) (9, 15). In these cases, the gland

view of the intracavernous carotid showing the inferior hypophyseal artery passing to the capsule of the posterior lobe. F, *the dura has been removed to expose the intradural structures. The anterior cerebral arteries are situated above and the pituitary gland is situated below the optic chiasm. The basilar apex is located behind the gland. The oculomotor nerve passes forward between the posterior cerebral and superior cerebellar arteries.* A., *artery;* A.C.A., *anterior cerebral artery;* Ant., *anterior;* Bas., *basilar;* Car., *carotid;* Cav., *cavernous;* CN, *cranial nerve;* Comm., *communicating;* Eth., *ethmoid;* Hyp., *hypophyseal;* Inf., *inferior;* Intercav., *intercavernous;* N., *nerve;* Ophth., *ophthalmic;* Opticocar., *opticocarotid;* P.C.A., *posterior cerebral artery;* Pet., *petrosal;* Pit., *pituitary;* Post., *posterior;* Prom., *prominence;* Rec., *recess;* S.C.A., *superior cerebellar artery;* Seg., *segment;* Sphen., *sphenoid;* Symp., *sympathetic;* Tuberc., *tuberculum.*

loses its spherical shape and conforms to the wall of the artery, often developing protrusions above or below the artery. In these cases, it would be difficult to remove the entire gland during transsphenoidal hypophysectomy. Such residual fragments may explain the pituitary function that remains after attempted hypophysectomy. Intrasellar tumors are subjected to the same forces, which prevent them from being spherical, and the increased pressure within the tumor increases the degree to which the tumor insinuates into surrounding crevices and tissue planes. Separation of these extensions from the main mass of gland or tumor may explain cases in which the tumor and elevated pituitary hormone levels persist or recur after adenoma removed.

The proximity of the carotid arteries to the midline is extremely important in pituitary surgery. In a previous study, the shortest distance between the two carotid arteries was found in the supraclinoid area in 82% of the cases, in the cavernous sinus along the side of the sella in 14%, and in the sphenoid sinus in 4% (15). Arterial bleeding during transsphenoidal surgery has been reported as due to carotid artery injury, but may also have arisen from a tear in an arterial branch of the carotid, such as the inferior hypophyseal artery, or by avulsion of a small capsular artery from the carotid artery (13).

Intercavernous Venous Connections

Venous sinuses that interconnect the paired cavernous sinuses may be found in the margins of the diaphragma and around the gland (*Figs. 8.1, 8.6, 8.11,* and *8.12*) (15). The intercavernous connections within the sella are named on the basis of their relationship to the pituitary gland; the anterior intercavernous sinuses pass anterior to the hypophysis, and the posterior intercavernous sinuses pass behind the gland. Actually, these intercavernous connections can occur at any site along the anterior, inferior, or posterior surface of the gland, or all connections between the two sides may be absent. The anterior intercavernous sinus may cover the whole anterior wall of the sella. The anterior sinus is usually larger than the posterior sinus, but either or both may be absent. If the anterior and posterior connections coexist, the whole structure constitutes the "circular sinus." Entering an anterior intercavernous connection that extends downward in front of the gland during transsphenoidal operation may produce brisk bleeding. However, this usually stops with tem-

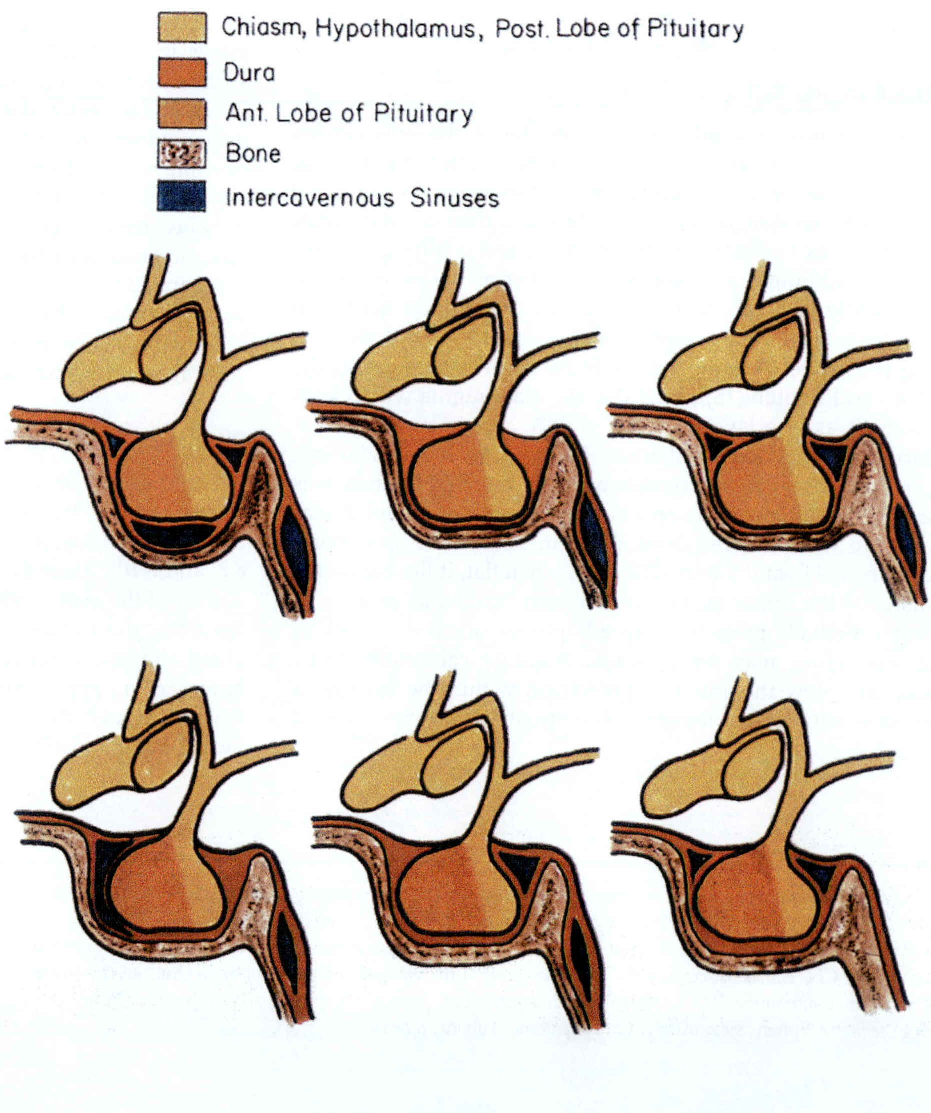

FIGURE 8.12. *Six sagittal sections of the sellar region showing variations in the intercavernous venous connections within the dura. The variations shown include combinations of anterior, posterior, and inferior intercavernous connections and the frequent presence of a basilar sinus posterior to the dorsum. Either the anterior* (lower center) *or posterior* (lower left) *intercavernous connections or both* (top center) *may be absent. The anterior intercavernous sinus may extend along the whole anterior margin of the gland* (lower left). *The basilar sinus may be absent* (lower right). (From, *Renn WH, Rhoton AL Jr: Microsurgical anatomy of the sellar region. J* **Neurosurg** *43:288–298, 1975 [15].)*

porary compression of the channel with hemostatic foam or with light coagulation, which serves to glue the walls of the channel together.

A large intercavernous venous connection called the basilar sinus passes posterior to the dorsum sellae and upper clivus connecting the posterior aspect of both cavernous sinuses (*Figs. 8.6, 8.7,* and *8.11*). The basilar sinus is the largest and most constant intercavernous connection across the midline. The superior and inferior petrosal sinuses join the basilar sinus. The abducent nerve often enters the posterior part of the cavernous sinus by passing through the basilar sinus.

Cavernous Sinus

The cavernous sinuses are located on each side of the sphenoid sinus, sella, and pituitary gland (*Figs. 8.6, 8.7,* and *8.11*). They extend from the superior orbital fissure in front to the petrous apex behind and surround the horizontal portion of the carotid artery. The medial wall of the paired cavernous sinuses form the lateral boundary of the sella. Sellar tumors frequently extend into the cavernous sinus (9). The cavernous sinuses are described in greater detail in Chapter 9.

The intracavernous portion of the carotid artery begins lateral to the posterior clinoid process where it leaves the foramen lacerum and turns abruptly forward to enter into the cavernous sinus (*Figs. 8.6–8.8, 8.10,* and *8.11*). It then passes forward in a horizontal direction for approximately 2 cm and terminates by passing upward along the medial side to the anterior clinoid process, where it penetrates the roof of the cavernous sinus. The cavernous carotid is relatively fixed by the bony ring formed by the anterior and middle clinoid processes and the carotid sulcus, but despite this, large extensions of pituitary tumor may produce lateral displacement of the artery.

The branches of the intracavernous portion of the carotid artery that supply the sellar contents are the meningohypophyseal trunk, the largest intracavernous branch, which gives rise to the inferior hypophyseal artery, and McConnell's capsular arteries, which arise directly from the internal carotid artery (*Figs. 8.6, 8.7,* and *8.11*). The meningohypophyseal trunk arises at the level of the dorsum sellae at or just before the apex of the first curve of the carotid where it turns forward after leaving the carotid canal. The inferior hypophyseal artery arises from the meningohypophyseal trunk and passes medially to the posterior pituitary capsule and lobe, and anastomoses with its mate of the opposite side after supplying the dura of the sellar floor. McConnell's capsular arteries are frequently absent and, if present, arise from the medial side of the carotid artery and pass to the capsule of the gland or the dura lining the anterior wall and floor of the sella.

The location of the nerves in the wall of the cavernous sinus are, from superior to inferior, the IIIrd cranial nerve superiorly and then the trochlear, ophthalmic, and abducens nerves (*Figs. 8.6* and *8.10*). The oculomotor, trochlear, and ophthalmic nerves lie between the two dural leaves of the lateral sinus wall. The abducens courses within the sinus on the medial side of the ophthalmic nerve and is adherent to the carotid artery medially and the ophthalmic nerve laterally. The IIIrd and IVth cranial nerves enter the dural roof of the cavernous sinus with the IIIrd nerve in front and medial to the IVth nerve. The IIIrd nerve enters the cavernous sinus slightly lateral and anterior to the dorsum sellae, almost directly above the meningohypophyseal trunk. The ophthalmic nerve enters the cavernous sinus wall inferiorly and slopes slightly upward to depart through the superior orbital fissure (*Fig. 8.6*). The VIth cranial nerve enters the lower part of the posterior wall of the sinus, bends laterally around the proximal portion of the intracavernous carotid, and runs parallel to the ophthalmic nerve between the ophthalmic nerve and intercavernous carotid. It usually enters the sinus as a single bundle, but may also be split into two bundles in the subarachnoid space before reaching the sinus. After entering the sinus, it may split into multiple, as many as five, rootlets as it courses between the internal carotid artery and ophthalmic nerve, but these collect together to form a single bundle that passes through the superior orbital fissure.

SUPRASELLAR AND THIRD VENTRICULAR REGION

This section of the chapter deals with the neural, arterial, and venous relationships in the suprasellar and third ventricular regions that are important in planning surgery for pituitary adenomas and tumors arising in the sella. The anatomy important to dealing with tumors within the third ventricle is dealt with in Chapter 5.

Ventricular and Cisternal Relationships

Tumors arising in the sella often extend upward into the suprasellar cisterns to compress the floor of the third ventricle and involve the circle of Willis and deep cerebral venous system (*Fig. 8.13*) (25). The area involved by those tumors arising in the sellae corresponds to the anterior incisural space located between the free edges of the tentorium and the front of the midbrain. The anterior incisural space corresponds roughly to the suprasellar area. From the front of the midbrain it extends obliquely forward and upward around the optic chiasm to the subcallosal area. It opens laterally into the sylvian fissure and posteriorly between the uncus and the brainstem.

The part of the anterior incisural space located below the optic chiasm has posterior and posterolateral walls (14, 19). The posterior wall is formed by the cerebral peduncles. The posterolateral wall is formed by the anterior third of the uncus, which hangs over the free edge above the oculomotor nerve. The infundibulum of the pituitary gland crosses the anterior incisural space to reach the opening in the diaphragma sellae. The part of the anterior incisural space situated above the optic chiasm is limited superiorly by the rostrum of the corpus callosum, posteriorly by the lamina terminalis, and laterally by the part of the medial surfaces of the frontal lobes located below the rostrum.

The anterior incisural space opens laterally into the part of the sylvian fissure situated below the anterior perforated substance. The anterior limb of the internal capsule, the head of the caudate nucleus, and the anterior part of the lentiform nucleus are located above the anterior perforated substance. The interpeduncular cistern, which sits in the posterior part of

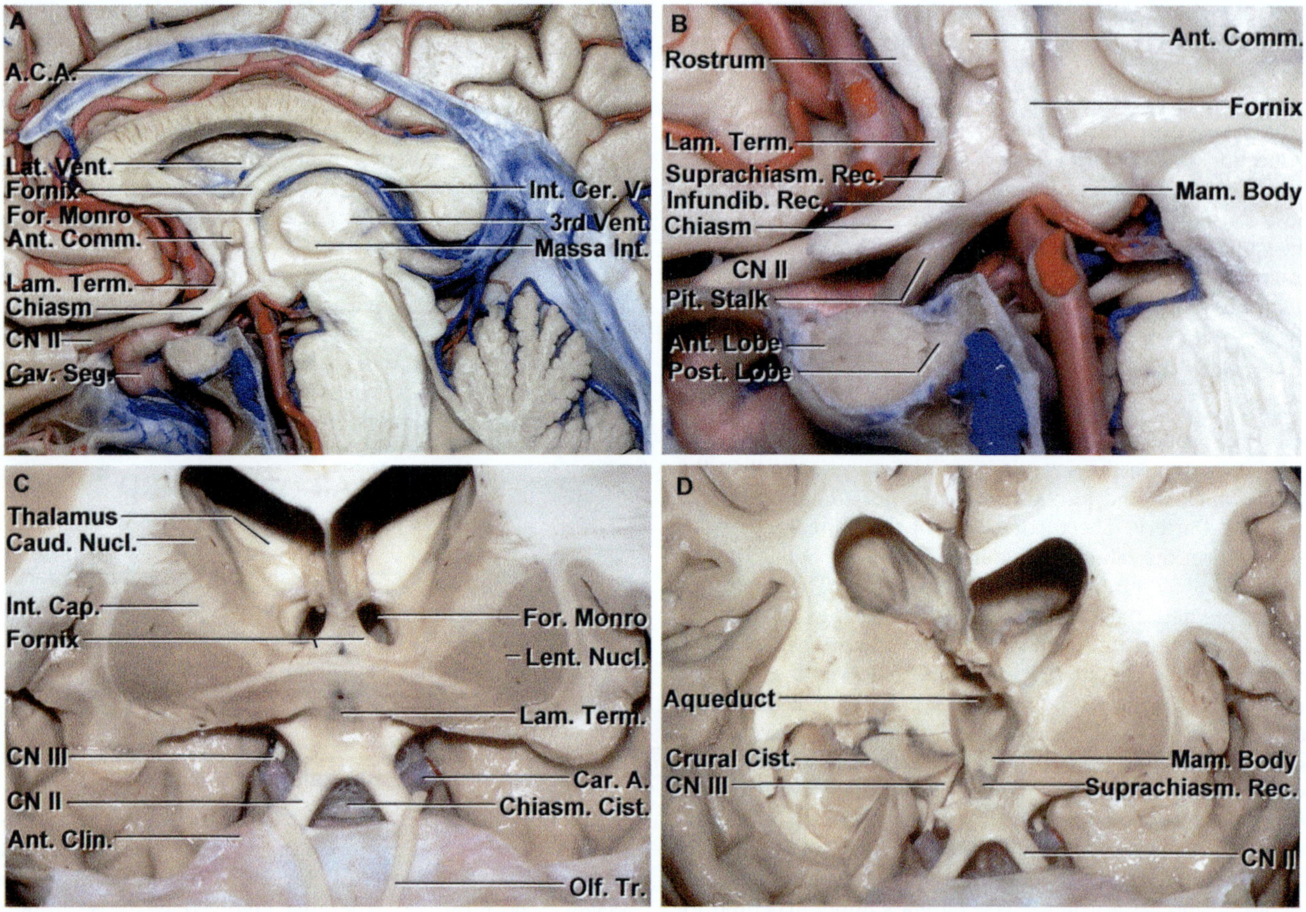

FIGURE 8.13. *Neural relationships in the suprasellar area. A, midsagittal section of the sella, pituitary gland, sphenoid sinus and third ventricle. The anterior part of the third ventricle is located above the sella. The columns of the fornix descend along the superior and anterior margins of the foramen of Monro to reach the mamillary bodies. The optic chiasm and stalk are located above the sella. The internal cerebral veins course in the roof of the third ventricle. B, enlarged view. The suprachiasmatic recess of the third ventricle is located between the lamina terminalis and the chiasm. The infundibular recess extends into the stalk in the area behind the chiasm. The lamina terminalis extends upward and is continuous with the rostrum of the corpus callosum. The thin part of the third ventricular floor between the chiasm and the mamillary bodies is suitable for a third ventriculostomy. The anterior commissure crosses the wall of the third ventricle in front of the columns of the fornix. The massa intermedium crosses the midportion of the third ventricle. C, the anterior part of the hemisphere has been removed to expose the lateral ventricles and suprasellar area. The optic nerve and chiasm are located above the sella. The chiasmatic cistern is located below the optic chiasm and opens upward between the optic nerves to the area in front of the lamina terminalis. The anterior commissure crosses the anterior wall of the third ventricle above the lamina terminalis. The anterior part of the third ventricle is located above the sella. The body of the lateral ventricle is situated above the third ventricle. The columns of the fornix form the superior and anterior margins of the foramen of Monro. The olfactory tracts pass above the optic nerves and the optic tracts pass above the oculomotor nerves. D, the cross section on the right hemisphere has been extended backward to the midportion of the temporal horn and thalamus. This exposes the oculomotor nerve arising on the medial surface of the cerebral peduncle and passing below the floor of the third ventricle and lateral to the sella. The crural cistern is located between the uncus and the cerebral peduncle. The mamillary bodies are positioned in the floor of the third ventricle. The posterior commissure sits above the aqueduct. E, the full length of the floor of the third ventricle has been exposed by removing the thalami bilaterally. The mamillary bodies are located at the junction of the anterior and middle thirds of the floor. The floor behind the mamillary bodies is formed by the upper midbrain. The floor in front of the mamillary bodies is very thin and serves as a suitable site for a third ventriculostomy. F, the floor of the third ventricle has been removed to expose the oculomotor nerves exiting the interpeduncular fossa below the posterior part of the floor of the third ventricle. The tentorial edge sweeps downward along the lateral margin of the midbrain. The upper pons is exposed behind the optic chiasm and between the oculomotor nerves. The crural cistern is located between the uncus and cerebral peduncle. G, anterior oblique view with the arteries preserved. The chiasm forms the upper margin of the chiasmatic cistern, which opens laterally into the carotid cistern surrounding the internal carotid arteries and upward around the optic chiasm to the cistern of the lamina terminalis. The anterior cerebral arteries ascend in front of the lamina terminalis. The anterior commissure crosses in the upper part of the anterior third ventricular wall. The columns of the fornix form the superior and anterior margins of the foramen of Monro. H, anterosuperior view. The upper part of the left thalamus has been removed to expose the optic tract, which extends backward above the oculomotor nerve in the lateral part of the suprasellar area to reach the lateral geniculate body. The chiasm and posterior part of the optic nerves are located directly above the sella. The anterior cerebral arteries pass above the chiasm. The left anterior cerebral artery is hypoplastic.* A., *artery;* A.C.A., *anterior cerebral artery;* Ant., *anterior;* Cap., *capsule;* Car., *carotid;* Caud., *caudate;* Cav., *cavernous;* Cer., *cerebral;* Chiasm., *chiasmatic;* Chor., *choroidal;* Cist., *cistern;* Clin., *clinoid;* CN, *cranial nerve;* Comm., *commissure;* For., *foramen;* Gen., *geniculate;* Infundib., *infundibular;* Int., *intermedia, internal;* Lam., *lamina;* Lat., *lateral;* Lent., *lenticular;* Mam., *mamillary;* M.C.A., *middle cerebral artery;* Nucl., *nucleus;* Olf., *olfactory;* P.C.A., *posterior cerebral artery;* Ped., *peduncle;* Pit., *pituitary;* Post., *posterior;* Rec., *recess;* Seg., *segment;* Suprachiasm., *suprachiasmatic;* Tent., *tentorial;* Term., *terminalis;* Tr., *tract;* V., *vein;* Vent., *ventricle.*

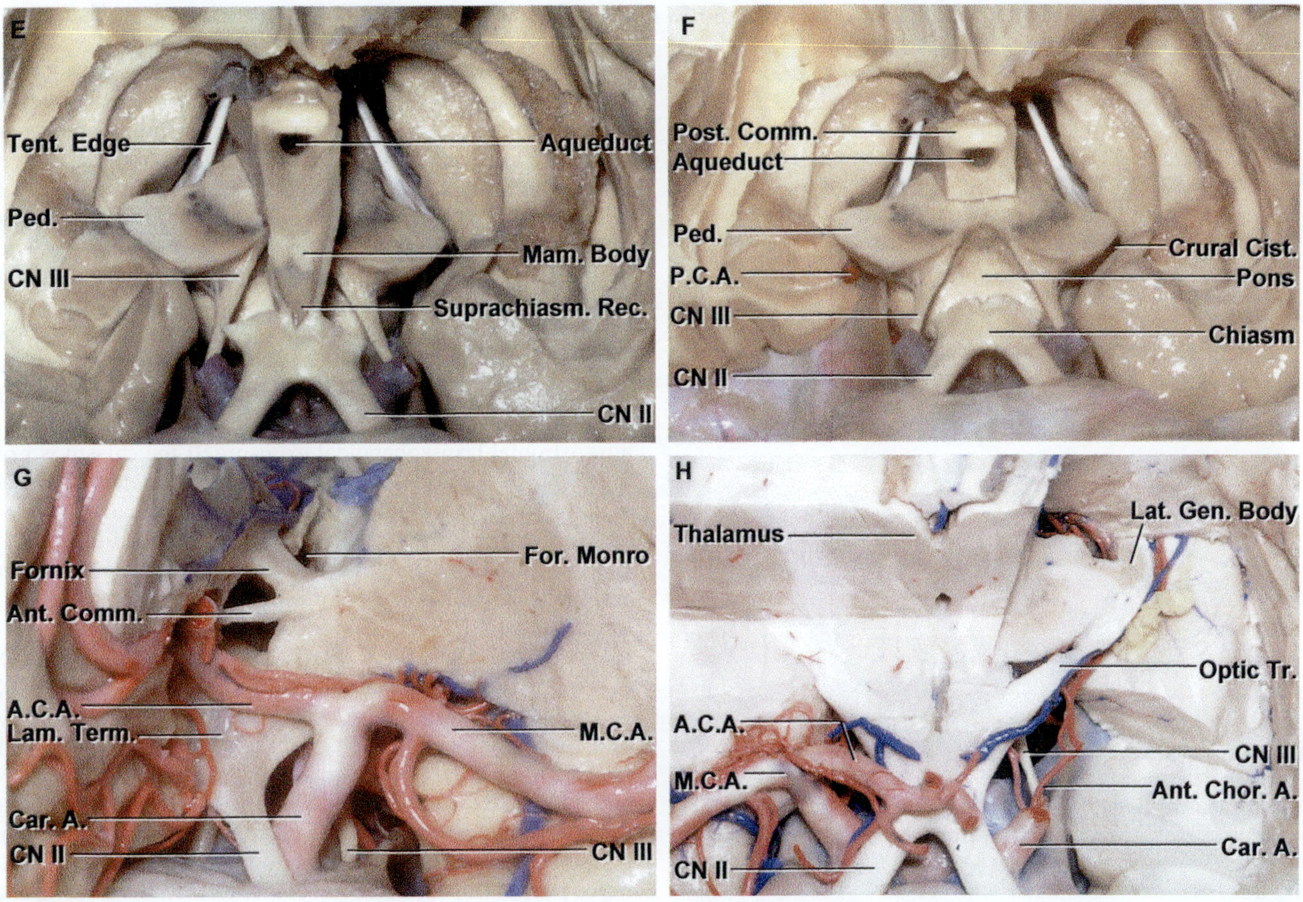

FIGURE 8.13. *Continued*

the anterior incisural space between the cerebral peduncles and the dorsum sellae, communicates anteriorly with the chiasmatic cistern, which is located below the optic chiasm. The interpeduncular and chiasmatic cisterns are separated by Liliquist's membrane, an arachnoidal sheet extending from the dorsum sellae to the anterior edge of the mamillary bodies. The chiasmatic cistern communicates around the optic chiasm with the cisterna laminae terminalis, which lies anterior to the lamina terminalis.

Cranial Nerves

The optic and oculomotor nerves and the posterior part of the olfactory tracts pass through the suprasellar region and anterior incisural space (*Figs. 8.6, 8.11,* and *8.13*). Each olfactory tract runs posteriorly and splits just above the anterior clinoid process to form the medial and lateral olfactory striae, which course along the anterior margin of the anterior perforated substance.

The optic nerves and chiasm and the anterior part of the optic tracts cross the anterior incisural space. The optic nerves emerge from the optic canals medial to the attachment of the free edges to the anterior clinoid processes and are directed posteriorly, superiorly, and medially toward the optic chiasm. From the chiasm, the optic tracts continue in a posterolateral direction around the cerebral peduncles to enter the middle incisural spaces. The optic nerve proximal to its entrance into the optic canal is covered by a reflected leaf of dura mater, the falciform process, which extends medially from the anterior clinoid process across the top of the optic nerve. The length of nerve covered only by the dura of the falciform process at the intracranial end of the optic canal may vary from less than 1 mm to as much as 1 cm (15). Coagulation of the dura above the optic nerve just proximal to the optic canal on the assumption that bone separates the dura mater from the nerve could lead to nerve injury. Compression of the optic nerve against the sharp edge of the falciform process may result in a visual field deficit, even if the compressing lesion does not damage the nerve enough to cause visual loss. Normally, the optic nerve is separated medially from the sphenoid sinus by a thin layer of bone, but if the sinus is well pneumatized, this bone is absent, and the optic nerves may protrude directly into the sphenoid sinus, separated from the sinus by only mucosa and the dural sheath of the nerve (4, 15).

Optic Chiasm

The optic chiasm is situated at the junction of the anterior wall and floor of the third ventricle (*Fig. 8.13*). The anterior cerebral and anterior communicating arteries, the lamina terminalis, and the third ventricle are located above the chiasm.

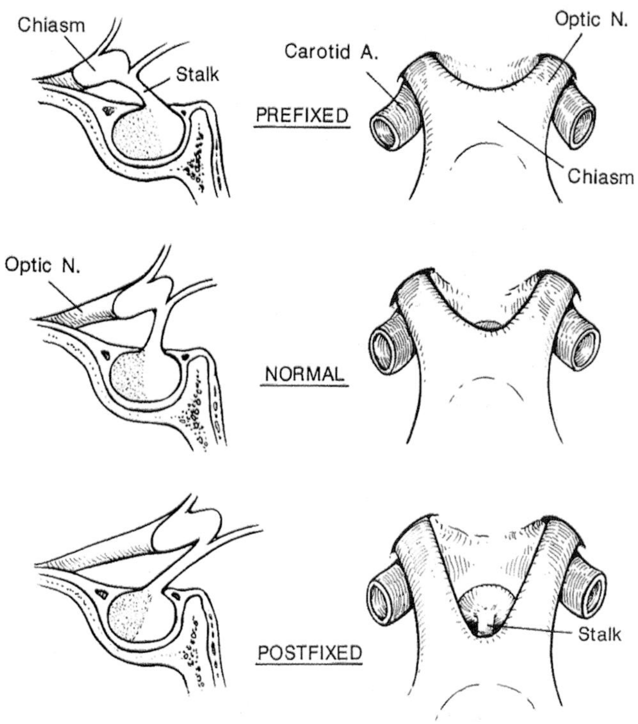

FIGURE 8.14. *Sagittal sections* (left) *and superior views* (right) *of the sellar region showing the optic nerve and chiasm, and carotid artery. The prefixed chiasm is located above the tuberculum. The normal chiasm is located above the diaphragma. The postfixed chiasm is situated above the dorsum. A., artery; N., nerve.* (From, *Rhoton AL Jr: Anatomy of the pituitary gland and sellar region, in Thapar K, Kovacs K, Scheithauer BW, Lloyd RV (eds):* Diagnosis and Management of Pituitary Tumors. *Totowa, Humana Press Inc., 2000 [17].)*

The tuber cinereum and the infundibulum are posterior to, the internal carotid arteries are lateral to, and the diaphragma sellae and pituitary gland are below the optic chiasm. The suprachiasmatic recess of the third ventricle is located between the chiasm and lamina terminalis. The infundibular recess extends into the base of the pituitary stalk behind the optic chiasm. The relationship of the chiasm to the sella is an important determinant of the ease with which the pituitary fossa can be exposed by the transfrontal surgical route (*Figs. 8.13* and *8.14*). The normal chiasm overlies the diaphragma sellae and the pituitary gland, the prefixed chiasm overlies the tuberculum, and the postfixed chiasm overlies the dorsum. In approximately 70% of our cases, the chiasm is in the normal position; of the remaining 30%, approximately half are "prefixed" and half "postfixed" (15).

A prominent tuberculum sellae may restrict access to the sellae, even in the presence of a normal chiasm. The tuberculum may vary from being almost flat to protruding upward as much as 3 mm, and it may project posteriorly to the margin of a normal chiasm (15). A prefixed chiasm, a normal chiasm with a small area between the tuberculum and the chiasm, and a superior protruding tuberculum sellae do not limit exposure by the transsphenoidal approach, but they limit the access to the suprasellar area provided by the transcranial approach. There are several methods of gaining access to the suprasellar area when these variants are present. One is to expose the sphenoid sinus from above by opening through the tuberculum and planum sphenoidale, thus converting the approach to a transfrontal-transsphenoidal exposure. If the chiasm is prefixed and the tumor is seen through a thin, stretched arterial wall of the third ventricle, the lamina terminalis may be opened to expose the tumor, but this exposure is infrequently used for pituitary adenomas, and they more commonly form craniopharyngiomas and gliomas involving the third ventricle. If the space between the carotid artery and the optic nerve has been enlarged, by a lateral or parasellar extension of tumor, the tumor may be removed through this space (16, 23).

An understanding of the relationship of the carotid artery, optic nerve, and anterior clinoid process is fundamental to all surgical approaches to the sellar and parasellar areas (*Figs. 8.6* and *8.13*). The carotid artery and the optic nerve are medial to the anterior clinoid process. The artery exits the cavernous sinus beneath and slightly lateral to the optic nerve. The optic nerve pursues a posteromedial course toward the chiasm, and the carotid artery pursues a posterolateral course toward its bifurcation below the anterior perforated substance into the anterior and middle cerebral arteries in the area.

Oculomotor Nerve

The oculomotor nerve arises in the interpeduncular cistern from the midbrain on the medial side of the cerebral peduncle and courses between the posterior cerebral and superior cerebellar arteries (*Figs. 8.6* and *8.13*). The oculomotor nerve courses in the lateral wall of the interpeduncular cistern and forms the pillars to which Liliquist's membrane attaches. Liliquist's membrane arises from the arachnoid membrane covering the dorsum sellae and separates the chiasmatic and interpeduncular cisterns. The uncus of the temporal lobe is situated lateral to the oculomotor nerve. The oculomotor

FIGURE 8.15. *Vascular relationships in the suprasellar area.* A, *the anterior cerebral arteries course above the optic chiasm and in front of the lamina terminalis. The carotid arteries exit the cavernous sinus and pass upward in the lateral margins of the suprasellar area. The superior hypophyseal arteries cross the chiasmatic cistern to reach the lower margin of the chiasm and pituitary stalk.* B, *superior view of the suprasellar region. The floor of the third ventricle has been exposed from the suprachiasmatic recess anteriorly to the level of the aqueduct posterior. The anterior cerebral arteries pass above the chiasm. The posterior communicating arteries pass backward below the floor of the third ventricle. The basilar artery bifurcates into the posterior cerebral arteries below the floor of the third ventricle.* C, *superior view of the suprasellar region. The carotid arteries course along the lateral margin of the chiasmatic cistern. The basilar bifurcation is located above and behind the sella. The posterior communicating arteries travel backward across the dorsum to join the posterior cerebral arteries. The posterior communicating arteries usually course above and medial to the oculomotor nerves.* D, *the optic chiasm is positioned above the diaphragm and sella. The optic tracts extends backward and laterally above the posterior cerebral arteries and oculomotor nerves toward the lateral geniculate bodies. The basilar bifurcation has been retracted forward to show the perforating arteries entering the midbrain, which can be dam-*

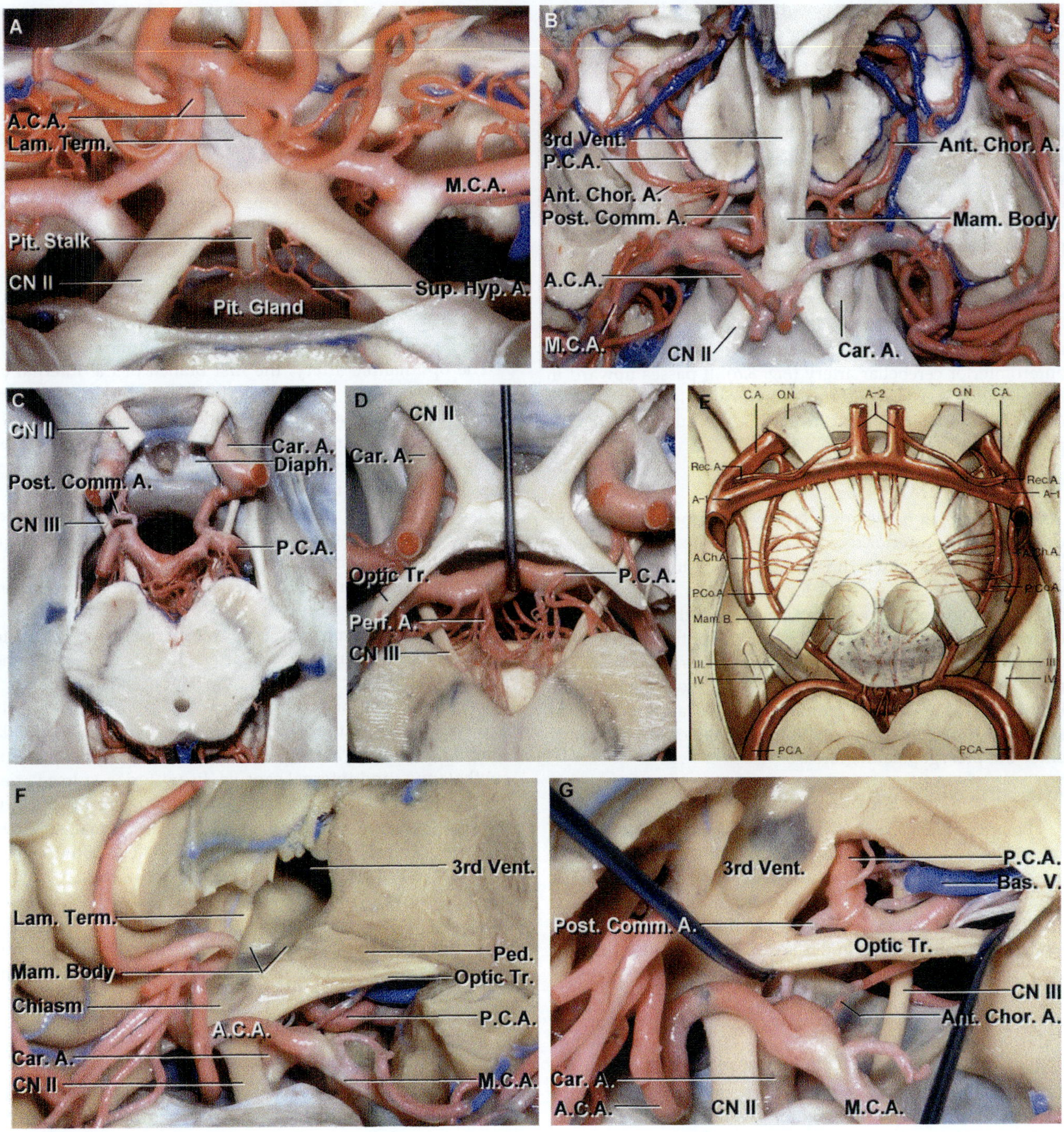

FIGURE 8.15. *Continued*
aged in the transsphenoidal approach if the posterior wall of the capsule of a pituitary adenoma is opened. E, diagrammatic view of the arteries in the suprasellar area, which can be stretched over the margin of a large tumor with suprasellar extension. All of the components of the circle of Willis and their perforating branches can be stretched over the dome of these tumors. F, superolateral view of the left optic nerve, chiasm, and tract and the floor of the third ventricle. The optic tract extends backward from the optic chiasm, around the upper edge of the cerebral peduncle, and above the posterior cerebral artery. The anterior cerebral arteries pass in front of the lamina terminalis and around the corpus callosum. G, some of the anterior part of the left cerebral peduncle has been removed while preserving the optic tract. The posterior cerebral and terminal part of the posterior communicating artery can be seen through the interval between the floor of the third ventricle and the optic tract. A., *artery;* A.C.A., *anterior cerebral artery;* A.Ch.A., *anterior choroidal artery;* Ant., *anterior;* B., *body;* Bas., *basal;* C.A., *carotid artery;* Car., *carotid;* Chor., *choroidal;* CN, *cranial nerve;* Comm., *communicating;* Diaph., *diaphragm;* Hyp., *hypophyseal;* Lam., *lamina;* Mam., *mamillary;* M.C.A., *middle cerebral artery;* O.N., *optic nerve;* P.C.A., *posterior cerebral artery;* P.Co.A., *posterior communicating artery;* Ped., *peduncle;* Perf., *perforating;* Pit., *pituitary;* Post., *posterior;* Rec., *recurrent;* Sup., *superior;* Term., *terminalis;* Tr., *tract;* V., *vein;* Vent., *ventricle.*

nerve pierces the roof of the cavernous sinus and slopes downward in the superolateral corner of the cavernous sinus.

Trochlear Nerve

The trochlear nerve is the longest and thinnest cranial nerve (*Fig. 8.6*). It arises from the midbrain below the inferior colliculi and passes around the brainstem near the junction of the midbrain and pons to reach the lower margin of the tentorial edge. The trochlear nerve pierces the medial edge of the tentorium and enters the roof of the cavernous sinus just behind the anterior tentorial attachment.

Abducens Nerve

The abducens nerve arises at the lower margin of the pons and passes above, below, or is split into two bundles by the anteroinferior cerebellar artery (*Fig. 8.6*). It passes upward in the prepontine cistern and turns forward at the upper border of the petrous apex, where it pierces the dura to enter the posterior part of the cavernous sinus.

Trigeminal Nerve

The trigeminal nerve arises on the posterior fossa from the midpons. The posterior root passes above the petrous apex to enter Meckel's cave, which is located lateral to the cavernous sinus. Meckel's cave extends forward to the level of the trigeminal ganglion. The nerve divides into the three divisions at the anterior edge of the ganglion. The ophthalmic division courses in the lower anterior part of the cavernous sinus. The maxillary nerve courses just below the cavernous sinus, where its medial side produces a prominence in the lateral wall of the sphenoid sinus, just before exiting the foramen rotundum, to enter the pterygopalatine fossa.

Arterial Relationships

The arterial relationships in the suprasellar area are among the most complex in the head, because this area contains all the components of the circle of Willis (6) (*Figs. 8.15* and *8.16*). Numerous arteries, including the internal carotid and basilar arteries and the circle of Willis and its branches, may be stretched around tumors in this area. The posterior part of the circle of Willis and the apex of the basilar artery are located in the anterior incisural space below the floor of the third ventricle; the anterior part of the circle of Willis and the anterior cerebral and anterior communicating arteries are intimately related to the anterior wall of the third ventricle; both the anterior and posterior cerebral arteries send branches into the roof of the third ventricle; the internal carotid, anterior choroidal, anterior and posterior cerebral, and anterior and posterior communicating arteries give rise to perforating branches that reach the walls of the third ventricle and anterior incisural space; and all the arterial components of the circle of Willis and the adjacent segments of the carotid and basilar arteries and their perforating branches may be stretched around suprasellar extensions of pituitary tumors (17).

The carotid artery is the most medial structure within the cavernous sinus. The internal carotid artery exits the cavernous sinus along the medial surface of the anterior clinoid process to reach the anterior incisural space (*Figs. 8.4, 8.6, 8.15,* and *8.16*). After entering this space, it courses posteriorly, superiorly, and laterally to reach the site of its bifurcation below the anterior perforated substance. It is first below and then lateral to the optic nerve and chiasm. It sends perforating branches to the optic nerve, chiasm, and tract and to the floor of the third ventricle. These branches pass across the interval between the internal carotid artery and the optic nerve and may serve as an obstacle to the operative approaches directed through the triangular space between the internal carotid artery, the optic nerve, and the anterior cerebral artery. The internal carotid artery also gives off the superior hypophyseal artery, which runs medially below the floor of the third ventricle to reach the tuber cinereum and joins its mate of the opposite side to form a ring around the infundibulum.

The ophthalmic artery, the first branch of the internal carotid artery above the cavernous sinus, usually arises and enters the optic canal below the optic nerve (*Figs. 8.7, 8.8, 8.10,* and *8.11*). Its origin and proximal segment may be visible below the optic nerve without retracting the nerve, although elevation of the optic nerve away from the carotid artery is usually required to see the segment proximal to the optic foramen. The artery arises from the supraclinoid segment of the carotid artery in most cases, but some arise within the cavernous sinus or rarely as a branch of the middle meningeal artery (9, 12, 15).

The posterior communicating artery arises from the posterior wall of the internal carotid artery and courses posteromedially below the optic tracts and the floor of the third ventricle to join the posterior cerebral artery (*Figs. 8.15* and *8.16*). Its branches penetrate the floor between the optic chiasm and the cerebral peduncle and reach the thalamus, hypothalamus, subthalamus, and internal capsule. Its posterior course varies, depending on whether the artery provides the major supply to the distal posterior cerebral artery. If it is normal, with the posterior cerebral artery arising predominately from the basilar artery, it is directed posteromedially above the oculomotor nerve toward the interpeduncular fossa. If the posterior cerebral artery has a fetal-type configuration in which it arises predominantly from the carotid artery, the posterior communicating artery is directed posterolaterally above or below and lateral to the oculomotor nerve.

The anterior choroidal artery arises from the posterior surface of the internal carotid artery above the origin of the posterior communicating artery (*Figs. 8.15* and *8.16*). It is directed posterolaterally below the optic tract between the uncus and cerebral peduncle. It passes through the choroidal fissure behind the uncus to supply the choroid plexus in the temporal horn, sending branches into the optic tract and posterior part of the third ventricular floor that reach the optic radiations, globus pallidus, internal capsule, midbrain, and thalamus.

The anterior cerebral artery arises from the internal carotid artery below the anterior perforated substance and courses anteromedially above the optic nerve and chiasm to reach the interhemispheric fissure, where it is joined to the opposite anterior cerebral artery by the anterior communicating artery

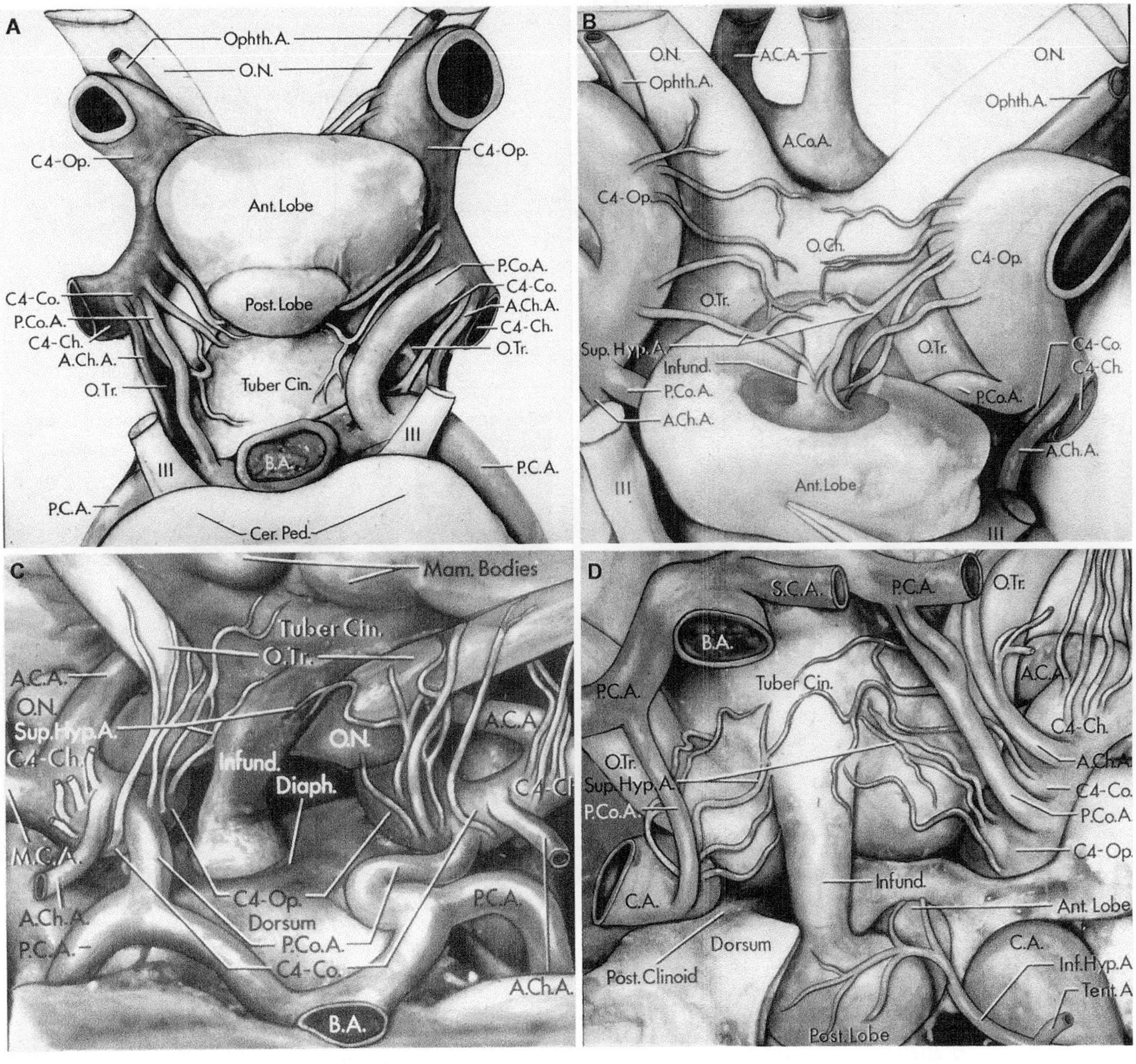

FIGURE 8.16. *Relationships in the sellar and suprasellar areas.* A, *inferior view. The supraclinoid portion of the carotid artery is divided into three segments based on the site of origin of its major branches: the ophthalmic segment extends from the origin of the ophthalmic artery to the origin of the posterior communicating artery; the communicating segment extends from the origin of the posterior communicating artery to the origin of the anterior choroidal artery; and the choroidal segment extends from the origin of the anterior choroidal artery to the bifurcation of the carotid artery. The optic nerves are above the ophthalmic arteries. The optic chiasm and optic tracts are above the anterior and posterior lobes of the pituitary gland. The tuber cinereum is anterior to the apex of the basilar artery. The posterior cerebral arteries pass around the cerebral peduncles above the oculomotor nerves. The perforating branches arising from the ophthalmic segment pass to the anterior lobe, optic nerve, and chiasm and to the anterior part of the tuber cinereum. A single perforating branch arises from the communicating segment on each side and passes upward to the optic tract and the floor of the third ventricle.* B, *the pituitary gland has been reflected backward to show the superior hypophyseal arteries passing from the ophthalmic segments to the infundibulum. The anterior cerebral and the anterior communicating arteries pass above the optic chiasm.* C, *posterior view. The basilar artery and brainstem have been divided and the floor of the third ventricle elevated to provide this posterior view of the arteries in the suprasellar area. The tuber cinereum and mamillary bodies are exposed between the optic tracts.* D, *the right half of the dorsum and the right posterior clinoid process have been removed to expose the anterior and posterior lobes of the pituitary gland. The basilar, posterior cerebral, and superior cerebellar arteries have been elevated to expose the pituitary stalk and floor of the third ventricle. The inferior hypophyseal and the tentorial arteries arise from the carotid artery.* A., *artery;* A.C.A., *anterior cerebral artery;* A.Ch.A., *anterior choroidal artery;* A.Co.A., *anterior communicating artery;* Ant., *anterior;* B.A., *basilar artery;* C.A., *carotid artery;* Cer., *cerebral;* Ch., *chiasm, choroidal;* Cin., *cinereum;* Co., *communicating;* Diaph., *diaphragm;* Hyp., *hypophyseal;* Inf., *inferior;* Infund., *infundibulum;* Mam., *mamillary;* M.C.A., *middle cerebral artery;* O.Ch., *optic chiasm;* O.N., *optic nerve;* Op., Ophth., *ophthalmic;* O.Tr., *optic tract;* P.C.A., *posterior cerebral artery;* Post., *posterior;* S.C.A., *superior cerebellar artery;* Sup., *superior;* Tent., *tentorial.* (From, *Gibo H, Lenkey C, Rhoton AL Jr: Microsurgical anatomy of the supraclinoid portion of the internal carotid artery.* ***J Neurosurg*** *55:560–574, 1981 [6].*)

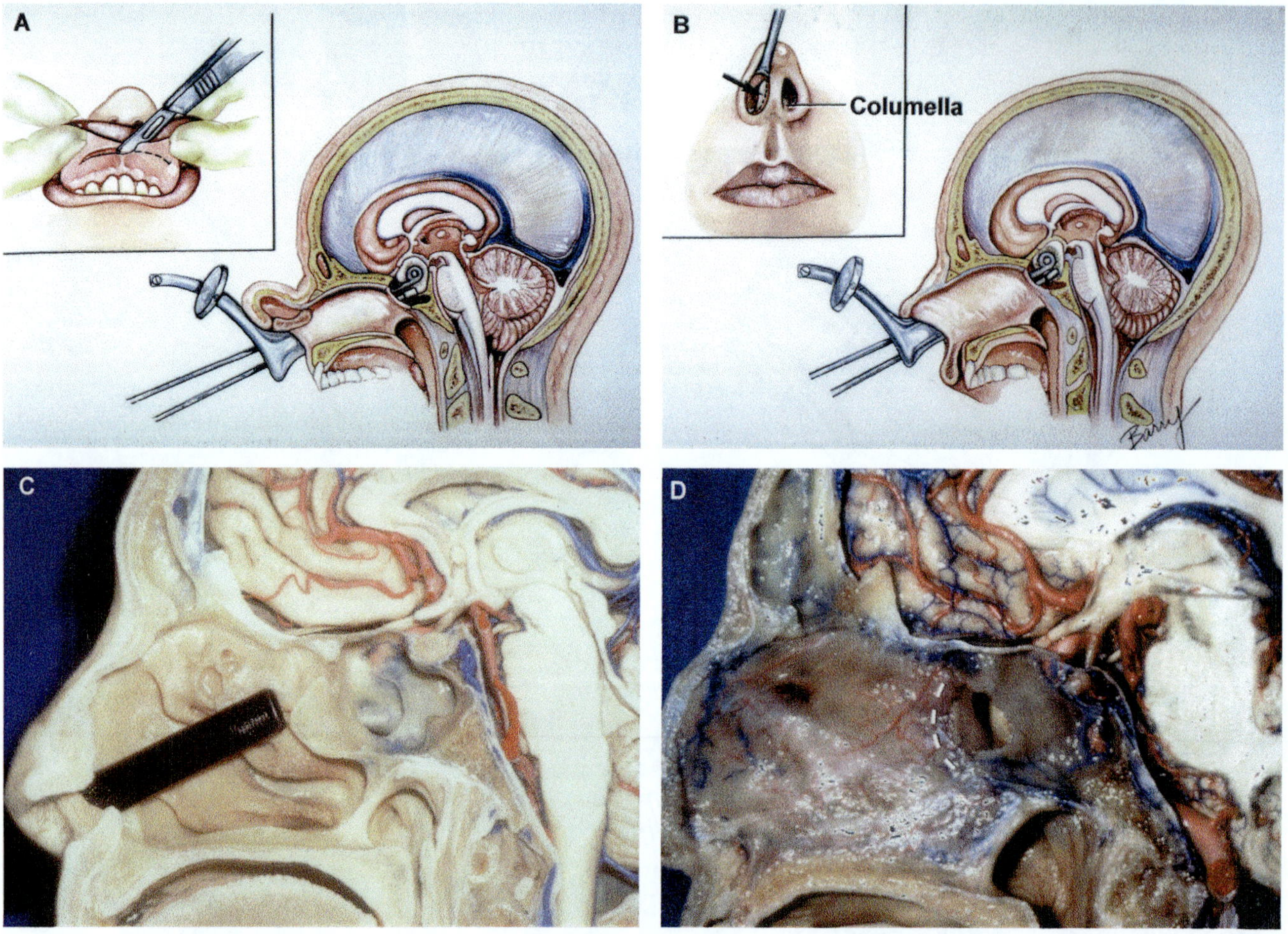

FIGURE 8.17. *Sublabial, transseptal, and endonasal approaches to the sphenoid sinus.* A, *the sublabial approach is directed under the lip and submucosally along the side of the nasal septum to the face of the sphenoid. The* inset *shows the site of the gingivobuccal incision and the direction of insertion of the speculum under the lip to reach the nasal cavity.* B, *the transseptal approach is directed through a small incision in the mucocutaneous junction along the side of the columella and submucosally along the septum to the sphenoid face.* C, *the Rhoton endonasal transsphenoidal speculum has been inserted along the route of the endonasal transsphenoidal approach directed through one nostril, between the conchae laterally and the nasal septum medially.* D, *the* broken line *shows the area where the posterior septum is separated from the face of the sphenoid sinus.* E, *superior view of the nasal cavity* (left side). *The speculum is advanced in one nostril between the septum and turbinates to the sphenoid face. The mucosa is opened on the sphenoid face to the left of the septum* (yellow arrow) *and the mucosa is elevated and the posterior septum separated from the face of the sphenoid* (red arrow) (right side). *The speculum blades have been advanced submucosally along the face of the sphenoid sinus.* F, upper left, *lateral view of the exposure of the endonasal exposure of the sphenoid sinus.* Lower right, *a small osteotome is used to open the face of the sphenoid. No bone is removed from the septum and the bone taken from the face of the sphenoid is preserved to serve as a stent for closing the anterior sellar wall.* G, *variations of transsphenoidal speculums. The speculum on the* left *has blades that are tapered so that the opening at the nostril is greater than the exposure obtained at the sphenoid face. The Rhoton speculum on the* right *was designed for endonasal transsphenoidal surgery. It has parallel blades that open so that the exposure at the sphenoid face is slightly greater than the opening of the speculum at the anterior nasal aperture.* H, *the* upper right *shows the thicker, wider blades on the traditional transsphenoidal speculum. The* lower left *shows the Rhoton modified endonasal speculum with smaller, thinner blades that open like the parallel blades shown in* G. Sphen., *sphenoid.*

(*Figs. 8.15* and *8.16*). The junction of the anterior communicating artery with the right and left A1 segments is usually above the chiasm rather than above the optic nerves. The shorter A1 segments are stretched tightly over the chiasm, and the larger ones pass anteriorly over the nerves. Displacement of the chiasm against these arteries may result in visual loss before that caused by direct compression of the visual pathways by the tumor. The arteries with a more forward course are often tortuous and elongated, and some may course forward and rest on the tuberculum sellae or planum sphenoidale. The anterior cerebral and anterior communicating arteries give rise to perforating branches that terminate in the whole anterior wall of the third ventricle and reach the adjacent parts of the hypothalamus, fornix, septum pellucidum, and striatum. The recurrent branch of the anterior cerebral artery, frequently encountered in the area, arises from the anterior cerebral artery in the region of the anterior communicating artery, courses laterally above the bifurcation of the internal carotid artery, and enters the anterior perforated substance.

The bifurcation of the basilar artery into the posterior cerebral arteries is located in the posterior part of the suprasellar area below the posterior half of the floor of the third ventricle

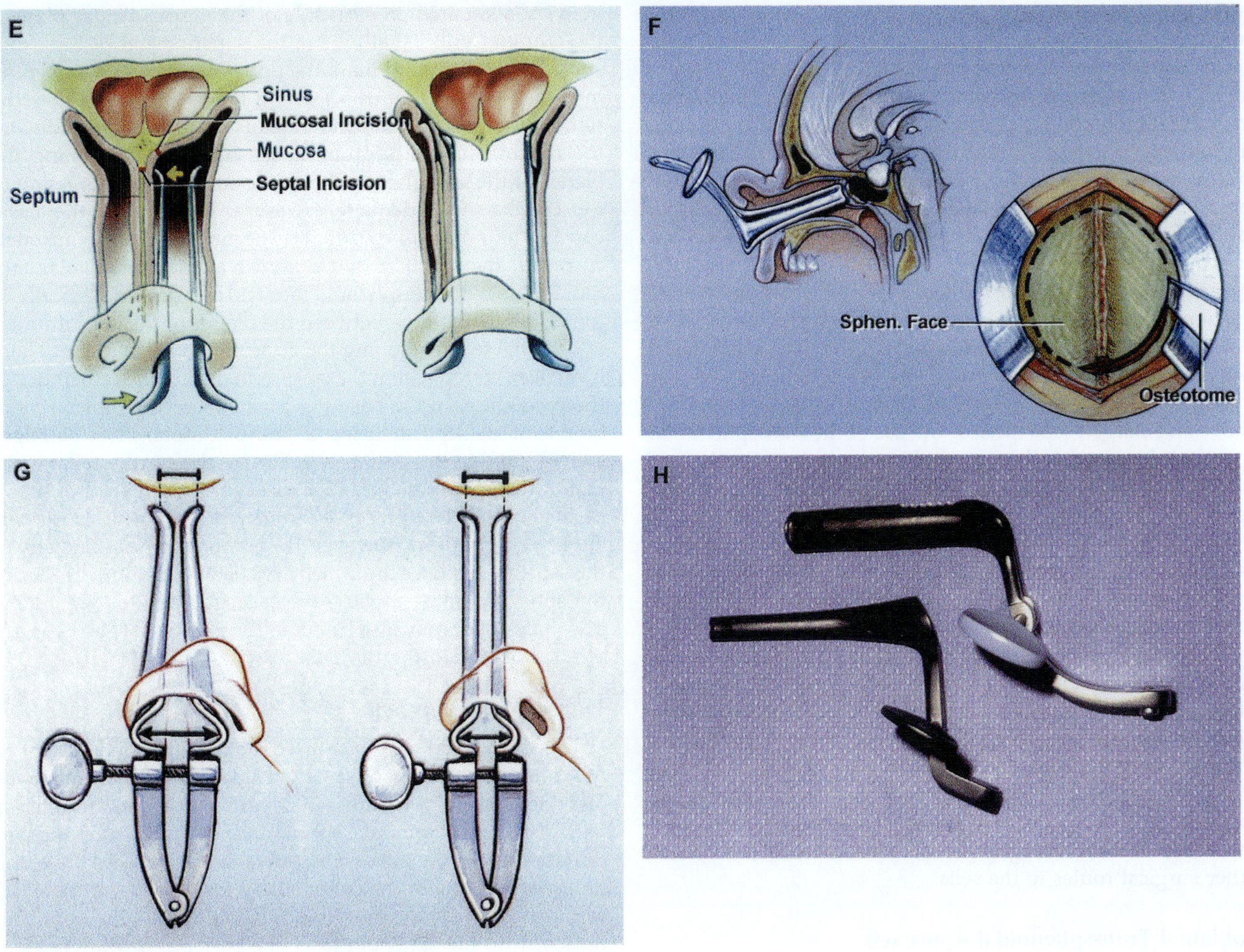

FIGURE 8.17. *Continued*

(*Figs. 8.11, 8.15,* and *8.16*). A high basilar bifurcation may indent the floor. The posterior cerebral artery courses laterally around the cerebral peduncle, above the oculomotor nerve, and passes between the uncus and the cerebral peduncle to reach the quadrigeminal cistern. Its branches reach the floor, roof, and posterior and lateral walls of the third ventricle. The thalamoperforating arteries are a pair of larger perforating branches that arise from the proximal part of the posterior cerebral artery in the sellar region and enter the brain through the posterior part of the third ventricular floor and the lateral walls. The author is aware of several cases in which damage to the thalamoperforating branches occurred during transsphenoidal surgery after opening of the posterosuperior part of the tumor capsule, with resulting coma and death.

Venous Relationships

Veins do not pose a formidable obstacle to operative approaches to the suprasellar area and lower part of the third ventricle as they do in the region of the roof and posterior third ventricle, because the veins in the suprasellar region are small. The suprasellar area is drained, almost totally, by tributaries of the basal vein. The basal veins are formed by the union of veins draining the suprasellar area, and proceed posteriorly between the midbrain and the temporal lobes to empty into the internal cerebral or great vein. The internal cerebral veins course in the roof of the third ventricle and are only infrequently involved in pituitary adenomas. They originate just behind the foramen of Monro and course posteriorly within the velum interpositum. They join above or posterior to the pineal body to form the great vein.

DISCUSSION AND OPERATIVE APPROACHES

The fact that the pituitary fossa is usually separated from the sphenoid sinus by only a thin layer of bone led to the transsphenoidal route being used for operations on sellar tumors as early as 1907 (*Figs. 8.2, 8.8, 8.10,* and *8.11*) (2, 10, 24). The approach subsequently fell into disfavor because of the high incidence of complications and the difficulty in operating through such a deep, narrow exposure. The modern redevelopment of this approach began with Dott and Bailey of Edinburgh (3) who learned the technique from Cushing and later taught it to Guiot of France (7). Guiot reintroduced this technique, using radiofluoroscopy to visualize the depth and position of the surgical instruments, and this, in combination with the illumination and magnification provided by the operating microscope, afforded the possibility of a safer approach and more accurate visualization of normal and pathological tissues (7, 8). Guiot taught the method to Hardy of Montreal (8) and both Guiot and Hardy's work reflects the improvement in the procedure brought about by the use of the operating microscope and radiofluoroscopy. Since its reintroduction, it has become the method of choice for removal of nearly all micro- and macroadenomas of the pituitary gland and selected other sellar tumors, including tumors with suprasellar extensions if they extend from and are centered above an enlarged sella turcica. The use of the transsphenoidal approach for clival and upper midline posterior fossa lesions is reviewed in Chapter 6 of the Millennium issue of *Neurosurgery* (18).

Several routes through the nasal cavity have been used to reach the sphenoid sinus (*Fig. 8.17*). The sublabial approach is directed under the lip and submucosally along the nasal septum to the sphenoid sinus. The transseptal approach avoids the oral cavity and is directed through a small incision along one side of the columella and submucosally along the septum. The endonasal approach, used in recent years by the author, is directed through one nostril, between the concha laterally and the nasal septum medially, and does not require an incision in the nose before reaching the anterior face of the sphenoid. This discussion, in addition to examining the sellar anatomy, also focuses on the microsurgical anatomy of the nasal cavity and other surgical routes to the sella.

Sublabial Transsphenoidal Approach

The head is positioned in a pinion head holder, with lateral fluoroscopy, with the head tilted or rotated so that the surgeon's direction of view is through the patient's nasal cavity sphenoid face in front of the sella. The whole procedure is performed using the operating microscope. The upper lip is elevated to expose the buccogingival margin, which is incised transversely from one canine fossa to the other. In the subperiosteal dissection, the upper lip is elevated to expose the osseous nasal floor, the nasal spine, and the lower edge of the lateral rami of the maxilla. The nasal spine and the lateral rami are preserved. With experience, the surgeon can work around rather than removing the nasal spine. We also avoid breaking off the thin edge of the lateral rami during the opening of the speculum, because healing may produce an annoying callus beside the nose. Using subperiosteal and subperichondral dissection, the mucosa is elevated from the nasal septum along the path directed to the sphenoid face.

The nasal speculum is inserted under fluoroscopic control between the septal mucosa on one side and the adjacent septum, with the handle facing superiorly (*Figs. 8.17* and *8.18*). Dissection misdirected into the area of the cribriform plate may result in a leak of cerebrospinal fluid or a loss of the sense of smell. When the speculum is correctly positioned, the sphenoid ostia situated on each side of the perpendicular plate of the ethmoid will usually lie at the superior end of the exposure. The ostia should mark the upper margins of the opening into the sphenoid sinus. Opening the speculum pushes the remaining cartilaginous and osseous septum to one side and the mucosa on the septum to the other side. Opening the blades of the speculum will provide sufficient compression of the conchae for adequate exposure. Removal of the nasal conchae is not required. If the speculum has been inserted correctly, the junction of the vomer and perpendicular ethmoid plate with the sphenoid face will be oriented vertically in the center of the area between the blades of the speculum, as is essential to maintaining the approach in the midline. There is no need to reposition the speculum during the remainder of the procedure. In the past, it was common to remove a piece of the nasal septum using a knife, scissors, or a Ballinger swivel knife to be used as a splint for closing the sella at the end of the operation, in which case, an anterior strut of septal cartilage should be preserved to maintain a normal postoperative nasal contour. However, the author avoids taking any of the septum and uses the bone harvested in opening the face of the sphenoid sinus to close the sella. A small biodegradable burr hole cover may also be cut to the appropriate size for use as a splint for closing the sella.

Transseptal Approach

The transseptal approach used a short incision adjacent to the columella, usually on the right side, at the mucocutaneous junction (*Fig. 8.17*). The incision is carried down to the anterior part of the cartilaginous septum and, by using subperichondral dissection, the exposure is advanced submucosally along the anterior edge of the columella to the left side of the nasal septum. The submucosal dissection is directed, by using fluoroscopy, to the sphenoid face. The posterior septum is separated from the sphenoid face in an area of sufficient size, usually 1.0 to 1.5 cm, to allow the tips of the speculum blades to be advanced submucosally along the sphenoid face. With an osteotome, a piece of bone large enough to serve as a splint for sellar closure can usually be harvested from the sphenoid face at the time of opening the sphenoid sinus.

Endonasal Approach

The author has used this type of transsphenoidal approach for the last four years. The view of the microscope is directed through one nostril between the nasal septum and nasal conchae to the sphenoid face below the ostia (*Figs. 8.4* and *8.17–8.19*). No incision is needed in the anterior part of the nasal cavity. In the endonasal approach, a hand-held nasal speculum, inserted under fluoroscopy into one nostril between the conchae and nasal septum, is opened to compress the conchae and septum sufficiently that the endonasal transsphenoidal speculum can be advanced through one nostril to the sphenoid face. Removal of the conchae is not required. The junction of the nasal septum with the sphenoid face is the most reliable landmark for maintaining the exposure in the midline. The sphenoid ostia are situated on each side of the perpendicular ethmoid plate and mark the upper limit of the opening

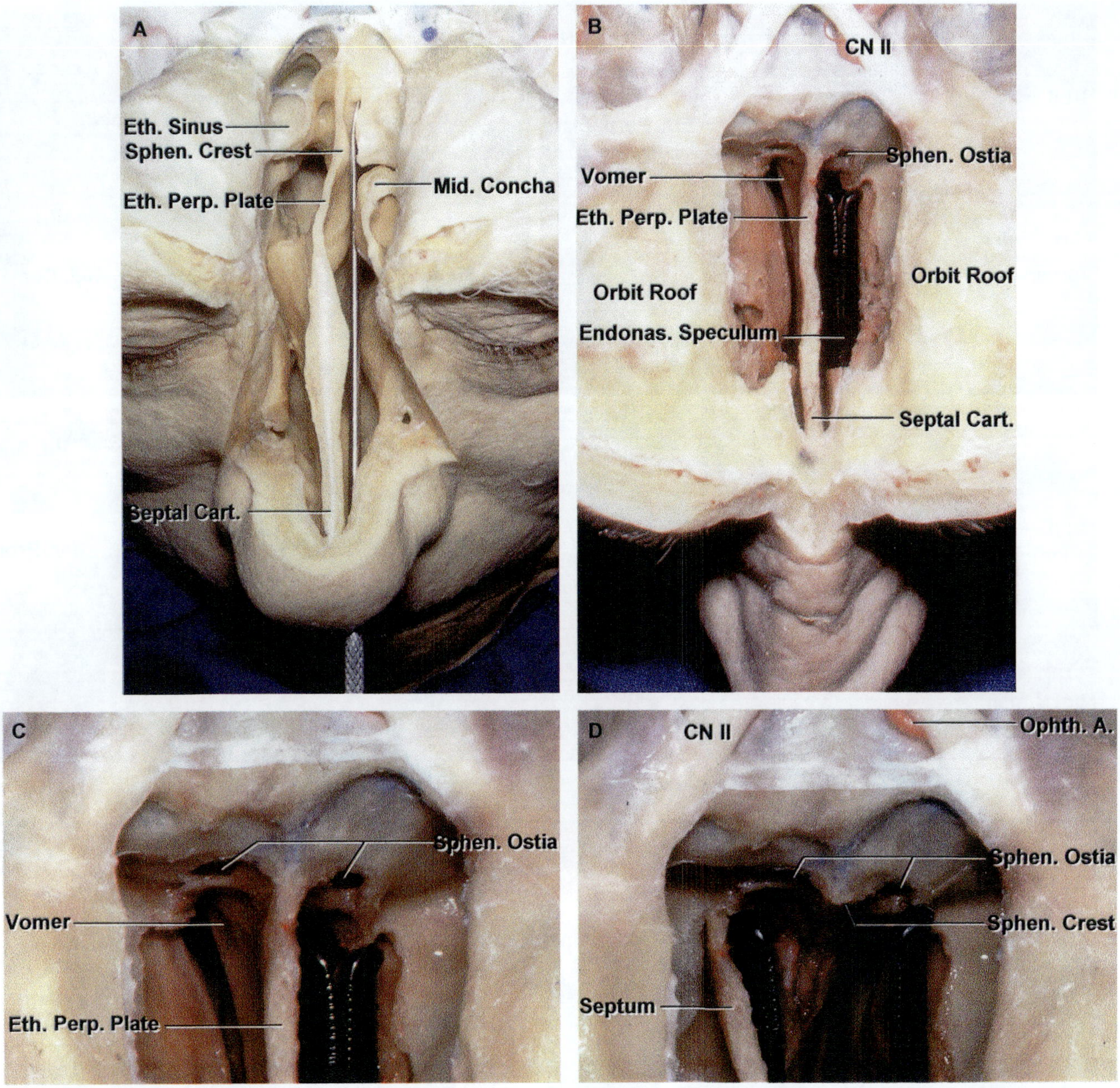

FIGURE 8.18. *Anterosuperior view of the endonasal route to the sphenoid sinus and sellar region.* A, *the roof of the nasal cavity and medial part of the floor of the anterior fossa have been removed to expose the endonasal route to the sellar region. The speculum in the endonasal approach is advanced along the course of the probe. It is advanced in one nostril and passed upward between the nasal septum and the concha to the sphenoid face. The posterior part of the middle concha provides a relative obstacle to exposing the face of the sphenoid in this case, but the concha can be displaced laterally by the blades of the speculum. A prominent concha, like this, may tend to deflect the speculum to the opposite side, unless care is taken to center the speculum blades on each side of the midline vertical crest on the sphenoid face. The posterior ethmoid air cells are positioned anterior to the lateral part of the sphenoid face. The nasal septum, in this case, is deviated to the right.* B, *the endonasal speculum has been advanced to the sphenoid face in the area below the sphenoid ostia. The septum at this level is formed by the perpendicular plate of the ethmoid. The septum below is formed by the vomer.* C, *enlarged view of the speculum blades at the face of the sphenoid. The mucosa is opened in the area below the sphenoid ostia and elevated in a small area so that the blades can be inserted submucosally.* D, *opening the speculum separates a small section of the septum from the sphenoid face and displaces the septum to the opposite side. The speculum blades can then be advanced submucosally along the sphenoid face bilaterally. The crest on the sphenoid face formed by the ethmoid perpendicular plate and vomer should be positioned in the midline between the blades of the speculum.* A., *artery;* Cart., *cartilage;* CN, *cranial nerve;* Endonas., *endonasal;* Eth., *ethmoid;* Mid., *middle;* Ophth., *ophthalmic;* Perp., *perpendicular;* Sept., *septal;* Sphen., *sphenoid.*

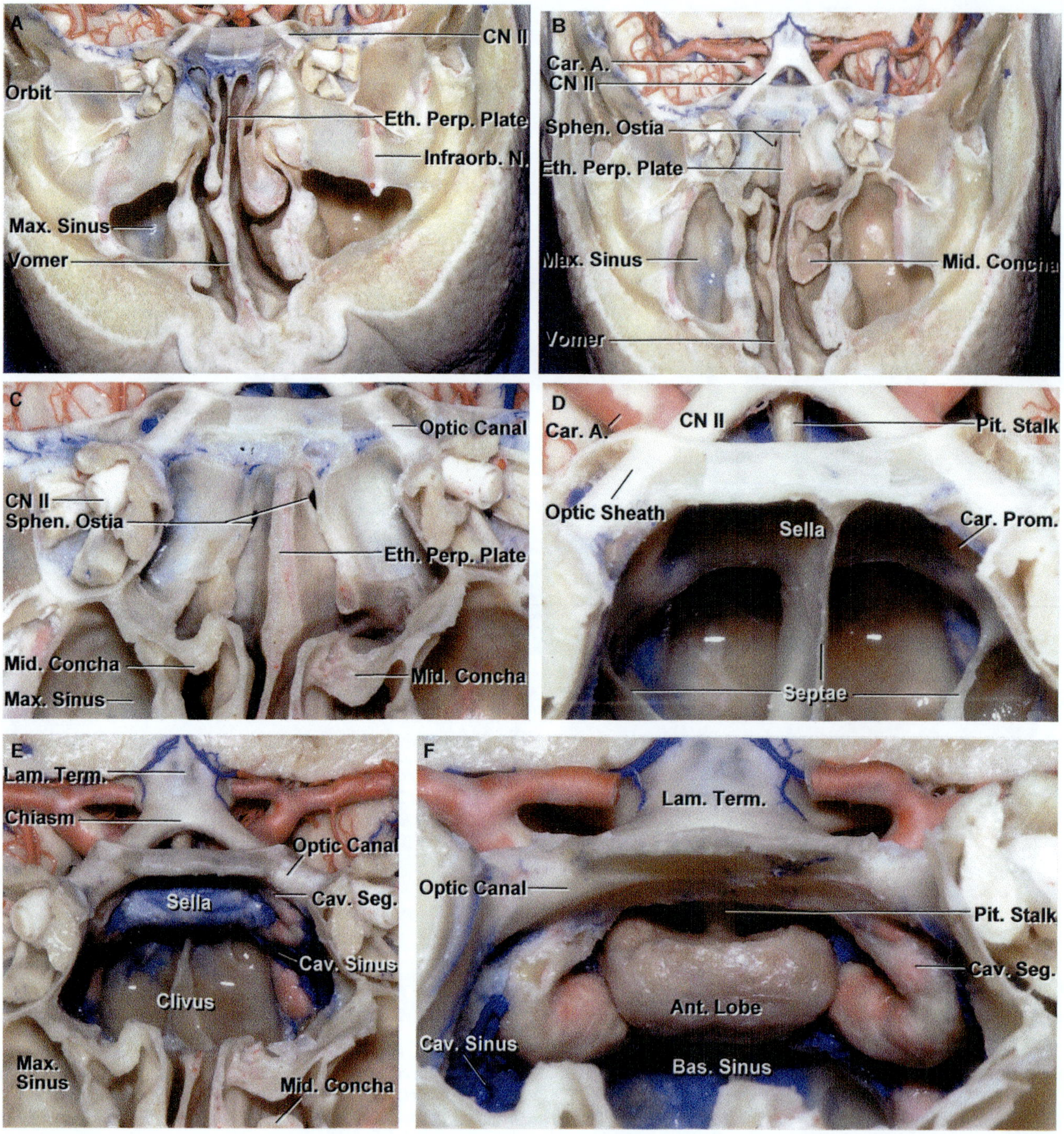

FIGURE 8.19. *Anterior view of transnasal route to the sellar region. A, this oblique cross section extends along the route used for transsphenoidal surgery. The cross section slopes upward and backward from the anterior part of the nasal cavity below to the area in front of the sphenoid sinus and orbital apex above. The roof of the orbit has been removed, leaving some of the floor and lateral wall of the orbit. The maxillary sinuses are exposed below the orbital floor. The conchae extend medially from the lateral nasal wall. The orbital apices are located lateral to the ethmoidal sinuses. The lower part of the nasal septum is formed by the vomer and the upper part is formed by the perpendicular ethmoid plate. B, the cross section has been extended backward to just in front of the sphenoid sinus. The nasal septum deviates to the right. The ethmoidal sinuses are located anterior to the lateral part of the sphenoid sinus. The maxillary sinuses are exposed below the floor of the orbits. C, enlarged view. The posterior ethmoid air cells are located in front of the upper lateral part of the sphenoid sinus and overlap the lateral margin of the sphenoid ostia. The middle concha, which block the view of the sphenoid face, must be displaced laterally in the transsphenoidal approach. D, the anterior wall of the sphenoid sinus has been removed to expose the sphenoid septi and sella. The carotid prominences are located forward and lateral to the anterior sellar wall. E, the sphenoid septi and osseous wall of the sphenoid sinus and the dural wall of the cavernous sinus have been removed to expose the cavernous sinuses and the dura lining the sella. The cavernous sinus and intracavernous carotid are exposed lateral to*

into the sphenoid sinus. Dissection misdirected into the area of the cribriform plate is to be avoided. The endonasal speculum is placed in the nasal cavity so that the crest on the sphenoid face at the septum's junction with the perpendicular ethmoid plate is positioned vertically between the tips of the speculum blades.

At the junction of the septum and sphenoid body, on the side of the nostril selected for the approach, the mucosa is incised vertically in an area long enough to accommodate the tips of the speculum blades, and the blade tips are positioned between the lips of the opened mucosa (*Figs. 8.17* and *8.18*). Opening the speculum usually separates the portion of the nasal septum at the tips of the speculum from the sphenoid face and displaces the septum to the opposite side. The mucosa on the face of the opposite side elevates away from the sphenoid face as the speculum is advanced submucosally along the sphenoid face bilaterally, with the septal crest oriented vertically in the midline.

It is important to remember that the blood supply to the tissues along the sphenoid face is from the branches of the maxillary arteries that arise in the pterygopalatine fossae and pass through the sphenopalatine foramen in the lateral walls of the nasal cavity to course along the sphenoid face (*Figs. 8.4* and *8.8*). Careful hemostasis along the anteroinferior margins of the sphenoid sinus where these arteries exit the pterygopalatine fossae is essential if postoperative packing of the nasal cavity is to be avoided. The opening in the sphenoid sinus is positioned on lateral fluoroscopy so that a small opening in the sphenoid face will provide direct access through the anterior sellar wall and the tumor.

Management of Sphenoid Sinus and Sella

The anterior wall of the sinus is opened with a small bayonetted osteotome to yield an exposure in the anterior wall approximately 1.0 to 1.5 cm in diameter. The opening may be tailored to extend predominantly to either side, depending on the size, shape, and location of the tumor. The opening is enlarged to allow passage of instruments of sufficient size and angle to remove the tumor.

The configuration of the interior of the sinus and the location of the septa are noted. The septae may vary in number and position and frequently deviate from the midline (*Figs. 8.4, 8.9,* and *8.19*). The septae are not to be used as a guide to the midline, but may be used as landmarks based on where the preoperative computed tomography or magnetic resonance imaging show them to be located in relation to the sella and the tumor. The mucosa of the sphenoid sinus is pushed laterally from the septae as needed to expose the anterior sellar wall. The mucosa is preserved because it facilitates normal sinus drainage. Usually, the mucosa on each side of the septae near the midline of the sinus can be pushed laterally to obtain a clear view of the sinus cavity and the anterior sellar wall. The floor of the sella turcica is usually seen as a smooth bulge in the superior part of the sinus if the opening into the sinus has been positioned correctly based on fluoroscopy. The sella should lie directly ahead of the tips of the speculum on fluoroscopy. The chiasmatic sulcus may produce a subsidiary bulge into the sinus and this, lying superior to the sellar floor, should not be mistaken for the sella turcica.

The prominences overlying the optic canals, superior orbital fissure, and maxillary nerve, located in the lateral part of the presellar portion of the sphenoid sinus, are not normally visible with the operating microscope and should not be searched for if the exposure is in the midline; however, they can often be identified using straight and angled endoscopes (*Figs. 8.2, 8.8, 8.10,* and *8.20*). The prominences in the sinus walls overlying the carotid arteries are frequently exposed at the lateral edge of the anterior sellar wall and are not to be confused with the prominence overlying a tumor. The carotid prominences are located just lateral and anterior to the anterior wall of the sella (*Figs. 8.2, 8.8,* and *8.10*). In a few cases, the nerves and arteries will be covered by only sinus mucosa and dura, and in others, the bone covering the optic nerves will be very thin. Therefore, the nerves passing through the optic canal, superior orbital fissure, and foramen rotundum could be injured in the transsphenoidal approach if vigorous attempts are made to strip or curette the mucosa from the walls of the sinus, or if the nasal speculum is advanced to lie within the sinus and is forcefully opened against its lateral walls. The nasal speculum should not be advanced into the sinus, because this does not increase the exposure and may cause damage to the poorly protected arteries and nerves within the sinus walls. Septae within the sinus are removed as needed to expose the anterior sellar wall. The bulge of the sellar floor is usually identifiable, unless the sinus is of a presellar or conchal type, in which case the sellar bulge may not be apparent. However, the floor of the sella turcica should be directly ahead of the long axis of the blades if the speculum has been positioned correctly on lateral fluoroscope and the vertical septal crest is positioned between the tips of the speculum blades.

A thin sellar floor facilitates the transsphenoidal approach. In nearly all adults, the floor will be less than 1 mm thick, and in two-thirds of adults, it will be less than 0.5 mm thick (1, 15). In the latter case, breaching the floor is accomplished by pressure on the bone with a small dissector, curette, or gentle tap on an osteotome. If the bone is thicker than 1 mm, it may be necessary to use the firm, but controlled, tap of a hammer against the osteotome or to remove the anterior wall with a drill.

If a drill is used to breach the sellar floor, the drilling is stopped while there is still a thin plate of bone that can be removed with a small bayonetted bone curette. The sellar

the sella. The lamina terminalis is exposed above the chiasm. F, *enlarged view. The dura lining the sella has been removed to expose the pituitary gland, the intracavernous carotid, and the cavernous sinuses. The optic canals are exposed in the superolateral part of the sphenoid sinus.* A., *artery;* Ant., *anterior;* Bas., *basilar;* Car., *carotid;* Cav., *cavernous;* CN, *cranial nerve;* Eth., *ethmoid;* Infraorb., *infraorbital;* Lam., *lamina;* Max., *maxillary;* Mid., *middle;* N., *nerve;* Perp., *perpendicular;* Pit., *pituitary;* Prom., *prominence;* Seg., *segment;* Sphen., *sphenoid;* Term., *terminalis.*

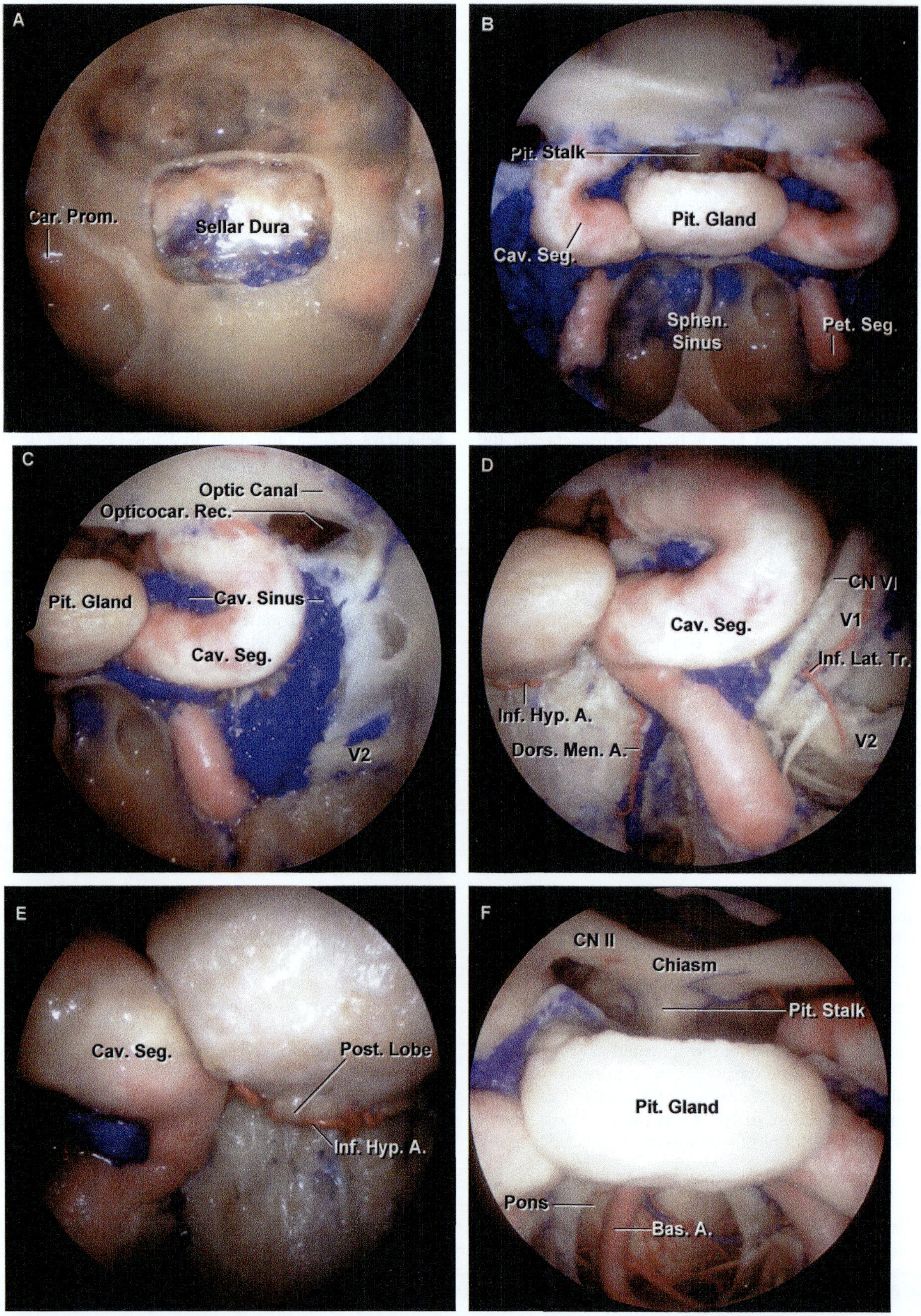
A
Car. Prom.
Sellar Dura
B
Pit. Stalk
Pit. Gland
Cav. Seg.
Sphen. Sinus
Pet. Seg.
C
Optic Canal
Opticocar. Rec.
Pit. Gland
Cav. Sinus
Cav. Seg.
V2
D
CN VI
V1
Cav. Seg.
Inf. Lat. Tr.
Inf. Hyp. A.
Dors. Men. A.
V2
E
Cav. Seg.
Post. Lobe
Inf. Hyp. A.
F
CN II
Chiasm
Pit. Stalk
Pit. Gland
Pons
Bas. A.

FIGURE 8.20.

opening should not extend along the anterior wall to the chiasmatic sulcus or tuberculum sellae, because an opening in this area is difficult to close, and may be associated with a high incidence of cerebrospinal fluid leakage. The opening in the sellar wall may be enlarged with a Kerrison rongeur if needed. The bone from the face of the sphenoid is saved for use in closing the sella.

By using a No. 11 scalpel blade on a bayonet knife handle, a short vertical incision is made in the dura in the midline. A small blunt right-angled ring curette is inserted through the small vertical dural opening, and the dura is separated from the anterior surface of the gland or tumor. After freeing the dura, a 45-degree-angle alligator scissor, rather than a knife, is selected to open the dura in an x-shaped cut from corner to corner, because a pointed knife may damage the carotid arteries in the far lateral corners of the exposure. The sellar dura is lifted away from the gland or tumor with the distal blade of the 45-degree-angled scissors, so that it can be seen that the cut does not extend into any structure deep to the dura. In some cases, the carotid artery may protrude through the medial wall of the cavernous sinus and indent the tumor and the gland and should not be mistaken for the tumor. Incising the dura on the diagonal from corner to corner provides a wider opening than a cruciate incision directed vertically and horizontally. The upper leaf of dura may be further incised in the midline if exposure over the top of the gland is needed.

After removing the tumor, the thickness of the diaphragma, the size of its opening, and the arrangement of the arachnoid around the pituitary stalk may be apparent. Excessive exploration and dissection, after the tumor is removed, is not a necessary part of most operations for pituitary adenomas and is to be avoided if possible because it may open into the cerebrospinal fluid-filled cisterns. In closing, the sella is filled with a pledget of crushed fat taken through a small skin incision from the subcutaneous tissues of the abdomen. A stent of thin bone, taken from the sphenoid face, is fashioned to fit through the sellar opening to close the defect in the sellar floor. The stent is fitted inside the sellar opening so that it fits snugly inside and overlaps the margin of the sellar opening from inside so that intrasellar and intracranial pressure will press the bone against the opening. The author avoids taking any nasal septum and uses a biodegradable burr hole corner, cut to the appropriate size and shape, if the bone from the sphenoid face is not available, as is frequent with reoperations. The sphenoid mucosa is repositioned and the ostia are inspected to make sure they are open. The sphenoid ostia may be enlarged if they seem small. No packing is placed in the sphenoid sinus unless the tumor has eroded the sellar walls and has filled the sphenoid sinus.

The transsphenoidal speculum is removed after the surgeon has ascertained that hemostasis in the sella and sphenoid sinus is satisfactory. The long hand-held speculum is reinserted, and the walls of the nasal passage on the side of the approach is inspected to make sure that hemostasis in the nasal mucosa is satisfactory and that there is an adequate opening in the anterior wall of the sphenoid sinus, preferably at the site of the ostia, for drainage of sinus secretions. The handheld speculum is then inserted into the opposite nasal passage to make certain there is no bleeding on that side. If hemostasis is excellent, as is almost always the case, no packing is left in the nose. The sphenoid ostia are also inspected to make sure the sphenoid ostia are of adequate size to promote sinus drainage, because an inadequate route of sinus drainage may lead to infection or development of a mucocele. The sinus mucosa is preserved, if possible, because it is essential to normal sinus drainage. Secretions collect in a sinus from which all the mucosa has been stripped unless the sinus has been obliterated with fat and closed.

The posterior wall of the sphenoid sinus forming the clivus may also be opened in the area below the sella with an osteotome or drill (*Figs. 8.2* and *8.20*). After the initial opening is completed, it can be enlarged with a Kerrison rongeur. If necessary, the clival opening can be extended upward by removing the floor of the sella turcica and downward by removing the floor of the sphenoid sinus.

All of these procedures are performed by using the magnified view and intense light provided by the operating microscope, which may at times be supplemented with the use of endoscopes advanced into the sphenoid, where they are helpful in identifying the structures in the wall of the sphenoid sinus. Advancing the endoscope into the sella is of less value because the tumor, bleeding, and the downwardly herniating diaphragm often obscure the endoscopic view (*Fig. 8.20*).

Subfrontal Exposure of the Suprasellar Region

A tumor situated between, above, or below the optic nerves and chiasm in the chiasmatic and lamina terminalis cisterns may be approached through a small frontal bone flap with

FIGURE 8.20. *Endoscopic views of sellar region.* A, *endoscopic view of sphenoid sinus. The carotid prominences are seen lateral to the anterior wall of the sella. The anterior sellar wall has been opened to expose the dura lining the anterior wall of the sella.* B, *the dura lining the sella and covering the intracavernous carotids and the cavernous sinuses has been removed. The pituitary stalk is exposed above the gland.* C, *view with the 30-degree-angle endoscope. The optic strut, which separates the optic canal and the superior orbital fissure, has been removed. The opticocarotid recess, which has been opened, extends into the strut. The cavernous sinus surrounds the intracavernous carotid.* D, *the venous material in the cavernous sinus has been cleared to expose the nerves coursing in the walls of the cavernous sinus. The abducens nerve courses on the medial side of the ophthalmic nerve. The maxillary nerve is in the lower margin of the exposure. The inferolateral trunk arises from the cavernous carotid artery and passes between the abducens and ophthalmic nerves.* E, *enlarged view of the inferior hypophyseal artery passing from the intracavernous carotid to the posterior lobe.* F, *the tuberculum and planum sphenoidale have been removed to expose the optic nerves and chiasm and the pituitary stalk. In addition, the clivus and the clival dura have been opened to expose the basilar artery and pons below the gland.* A., *artery;* Bas., *basilar;* Car., *carotid;* Cav., *cavernous;* CN, *cranial nerve;* Dors., *dorsal;* Hyp., *hypophyseal;* Inf. Lat., *inferolateral;* Men., *meningeal;* Opticocar., *opticocarotid;* Pet., *petrous;* Pit., *pituitary;* Post., *posterior;* Prom., *prominence;* Rec., *recess;* Seg., *segment;* Sphen., *sphenoid;* Tr., *trunk.*

frontal lobe elevation to expose the involved optic nerves and chiasm (*Figs. 8.21* and *8.22*). The bicoronal (Souttar) scalp incision from the subfrontal approach is located behind the hairline. The scalp flap is reflected forward as a single layer and a small frontal bone flap is positioned just above the supraorbital margin and extending up to the lateral edge of the superior sagittal sinus. The lateral burr hole, above the orbital rim, is positioned at the keyhole site and the medial burr hole usually extends through the front and back wall of the frontal sinus.

This approach is selected for a pituitary adenoma only if the sphenoid sinus is not pneumatized, the sella is small or not of sufficient size to reach the suprasellar extension of the tumor, or if there is an unusual suprasellar extension of the tumor that cannot be reached by the transsphenoidal approach. The subfrontal approach is most commonly used for lesions located between the upper surface of the pituitary gland and lower surface of the optic nerves and chiasm. A pterional craniotomy would be performed if there was a need to expose the area lateral to the anterior clinoid process and supraclinoid segment of the internal carotid artery, and an orbitozygomatic craniotomy might be considered if there was major involvement of the cavernous sinus.

After the area below the frontal lobe is reached, one of four routes may be followed to the tumor. The most commonly used route is the subchiasmatic approach directed between the optic nerves and below the chiasm (*Figs. 8.21* and *8.22*). Other routes that may be used are the opticocarotid approach directed between the carotid artery and the optic nerve; the transfrontal-transsphenoidal approach achieved by drilling

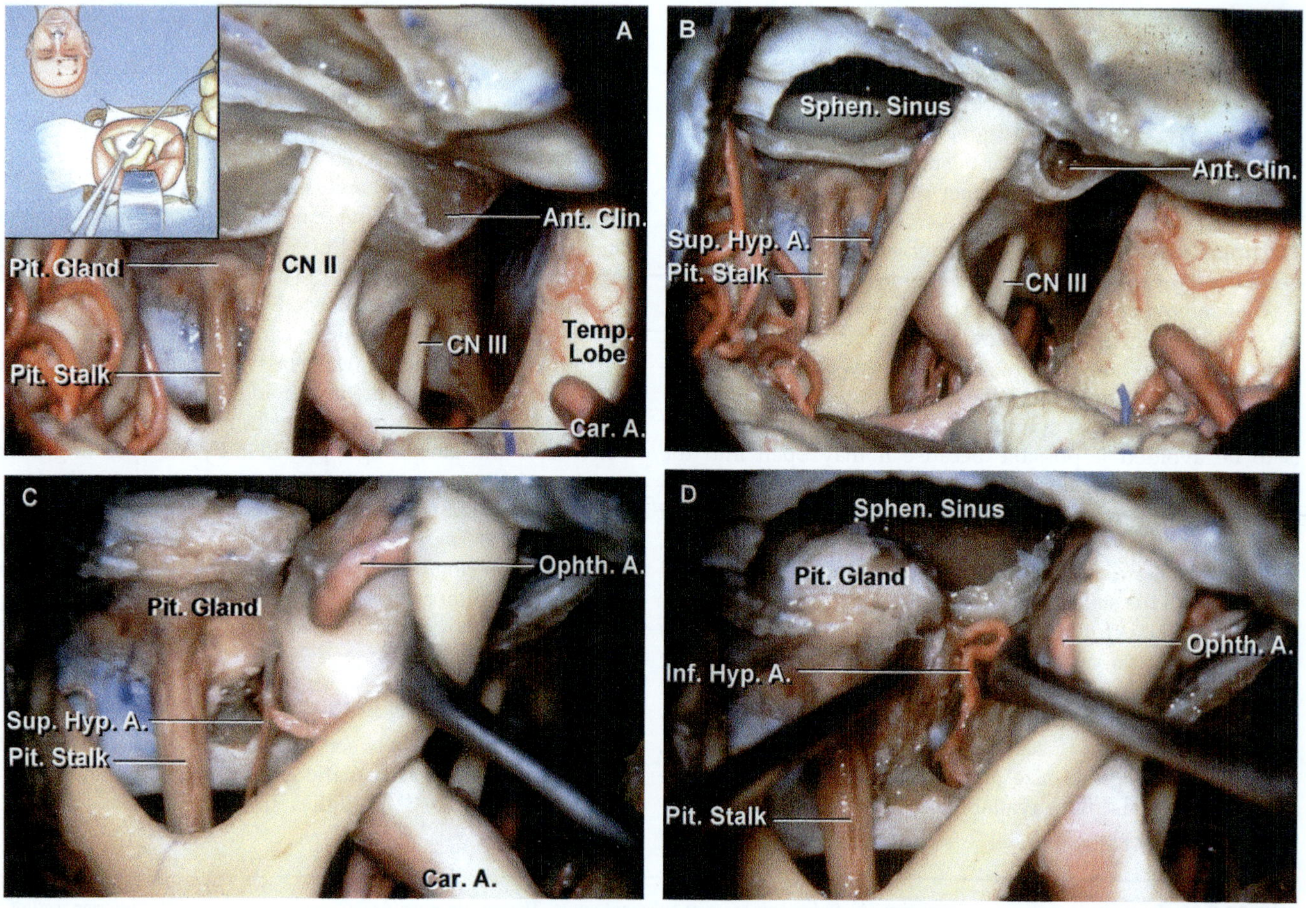

FIGURE 8.21. A–D, *subfrontal exposure of the suprasellar region.* A, *the* inset *shows the small right frontal craniotomy. The frontal lobe has been elevated to expose the right optic nerve and chiasm as shown in the* inset. *This approach is most commonly selected for lesions situated between and behind the optic nerves in the chiasmatic cistern. The dura has been removed from the upper surface of the planum sphenoidale, optic canal, and anterior clinoid process. In most cases for which this approach is selected, there is no need to expose the sphenoid sinus or remove the anterior clinoid process.* B, *the subfrontal exposure has been converted into a transfrontal-transsphenoidal approach to the sellar region by removing the roof of the sphenoid sinus. The anterior sellar wall is seen through the opening in the planum sphenoidale. The superior hypophyseal artery arises from the supraclinoid carotid and passes to the pituitary stalk.* C, *the optic nerve has been displaced laterally to show the origin of the ophthalmic artery. The anterior sellar wall has been removed to expose the anterior surface of the pituitary gland.* D, *the pituitary gland has been displaced to the left to open the space between the lateral surface of the pituitary gland and the medial surface of the intracavernous carotid. The inferior hypophyseal artery, which arises from the meningohypophyseal trunk of the intracavernous carotid, passes to the capsule of the posterior lobe.* A., *artery;* Ant., *anterior;* Car., *carotid;* Clin., *clinoid;* CN, *cranial nerve;* Hyp., *hypophyseal;* Inf., *inferior;* Ophth., *ophthalmic;* Pit., *pituitary;* Sphen., *sphenoid;* Sup., *superior;* Temp., *temporal.*

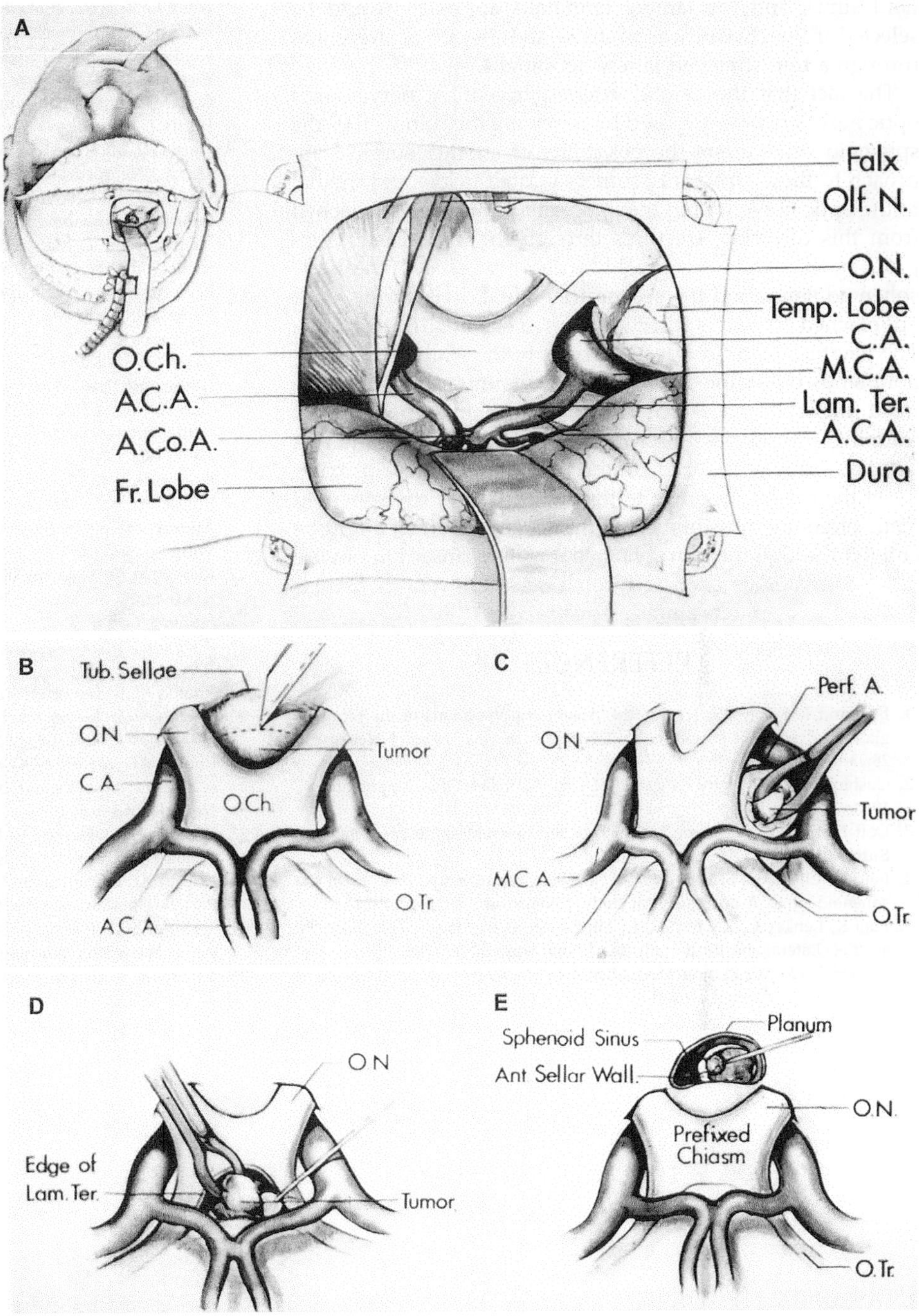

FIGURE 8.22. *Subfrontal approach to the anteroinferior part of the third ventricle. A,* Left: *Scalp incision, right frontal bone flap, dural incision, and placement of self-retaining retractor.* Right: *Intracranial exposure with the frontal lobe retracted. The optic nerves, optic chiasm, and optic tracts are stretched upward if a tumor is present. The right olfactory nerve has been divided, but the left one is intact. The anterior cerebral and anterior communicating arteries cross the optic tracts and the lamina terminalis. The temporal lobe and the carotid and middle cerebral arteries are lateral to the optic chiasm. B–E, different subfrontal approaches to the anteroinferior part of the third ventricle. B, subchiasmatic approach. The tumor is exposed between the optic nerves, the optic chiasm, and the tuberculum sellae. A knife incises the tumor capsule. C, opticocarotid approach. This approach is directed through the interval between the optic nerve and the anterior cerebral and carotid arteries. A cup forceps reaches through a hole in the tumor capsule. Perforating arteries cross the interval between the carotid artery and the optic nerve. D, lamina terminalis approach. The lamina terminalis is above the optic chiasm and between the optic tracts. The lamina terminalis has been opened, and a cup forceps reaches between its edges to remove tumor in the anteroinferior part of the third ventricle. E, transfrontal-transsphenoidal approach. A prefixed optic chiasm blocks the subchiasmatic approach to a tumor. The tumor is exposed by removing the posterior part of the planum sphenoidale and the tuberculum sellae to expose the sphenoid sinus. The sinus mucosa is depressed inferiorly and the anterior sellar wall is removed to expose the tumor. A., artery; A.C.A., anterior cerebral artery; A.Co.A., anterior communicating artery; Ant., anterior; C.A., carotid artery; Fr., frontal; Lam., lamina; M.C.A., middle cerebral artery; N., nerve; O.Ch., optic chiasm; Olf., olfactory; O.N., cranial nerve; O.Tr., optic tract; Perf., perforating; Temp., temporal; Ter., terminalis; Tub., tuberculum. (From, Rhoton AL Jr, Yamamoto I, Peace DA: Microsurgery of the third ventricle: Part 2—Operative approaches.* **Neurosurgery** *8:357–373, 1981 [23].)*

off the planum sphenoidale to approach the sella by a combined route; and the lamina terminalis approach directed above the chiasm, medial to the optic tracts, and usually above the anterior communicating artery (20). The subchiasmatic approach is most commonly used because most tumors elevate the chiasm and open the space between the optic nerves and chiasm. The optic carotid approach would be used if the tumor opened or protruded through the space between the optic nerve and carotid artery and the tumor was difficult to reach by the suprachiasmatic approach. The transfrontal-transsphenoidal approach would be used if the chiasm was prefixed and there was a large amount of tumor in the sphenoid sinus, and the lamina terminalis approach would be selected if the chiasm was prefixed and the tumor presented through a thin stretched lamina terminalis.

The fact that the carotid arteries, trigeminal nerves, and optic nerves may be exposed by removing the thin wall of the sphenoid sinus offers the possibility of another surgical approach to these structures; tumors located below and medial to the optic nerve within the optic canal could be approached from this direction; fractures through the optic canal compressing the optic nerve might be decompressed through the sphenoid sinus; and the second trigeminal division might be approached from this direction (*Figs. 8.4, 8.8, 8.10,* and *8.19*). The length of carotid artery exposed in the wall of the sphenoid sinus offers the possibility that the intracavernous segment might be exposed by the transsphenoidal approach for trapping procedures, inserting catheters for obliteration of fistulas, or for specialized contrast studies. The close proximity of the cavernous sinus to the lateral wall of the sphenoid sinus offers the possibility that the cavernous sinus might be entered through the thin sphenoidal wall for insertion of wire or other materials used to thrombose arteriovenous fistulas within the cavernous sinus.

REFERENCES

1. Bergland RM, Ray BS, Torack RM: Anatomical variations in the pituitary gland and adjacent structures in 225 human autopsy cases. **J Neurosurg** 28:93–99, 1968.
2. Cushing H: *The Pituitary Body and Its Disorders*. Philadelphia, Lippincott Co., 1912.
3. Dott NM, Bailey D: A consideration of the hypophysial adenomata. **Br J Surg** 13:314–366, 1925.
4. Fujii K, Chambers SM, Rhoton AL Jr: Neurovascular relationships of the sphenoid sinus: A microsurgical study. **J Neurosurg** 50:31–39, 1979.
5. Fujii K, Lenkey C, Rhoton AL Jr: Microsurgical anatomy of the choroidal arteries: Lateral and third ventricles. **J Neurosurg** 52:165–188, 1980.
6. Gibo H, Lenkey C, Rhoton AL Jr: Microsurgical anatomy of the supraclinoid portion of the internal carotid artery. **J Neurosurg** 55:560–574, 1981.
7. Guiot G: Transsphenoidal approach in surgical treatment of pituitary adenomas: General principles and indications in non-functioning adenomas, in Kohler PO, Ross GT (eds): *Diagnosis and Treatment of Pituitary Tumors: Proceedings of a Conference*. Amsterdam, Excerpta Medica, 1973, International Congress Series No.303, pp 159–179.
8. Hardy J: Transsphenoidal hypophysectomy. **J Neurosurg** 34:582–594, 1971.
9. Harris FS, Rhoton AL Jr: Anatomy of the cavernous sinus: A microsurgical study. **J Neurosurg** 45:169–180, 1976.
10. Hirsch O: Endonasal method of removal of hypophyseal tumors: With report of two successful cases. **Jour AMA** 55:772–774, 1910.
11. Hitotsumatsu T, Matsushima T, Rhoton AL Jr: Surgical anatomy of the midface and the midline skull base, in Spetzler RF (ed): *Operative Techniques in Neurosurgery*. Philadelphia, W.B. Saunders Co., 1999, vol 2, pp 160–180.
12. Inoue T, Rhoton AL Jr, Theele D, Barry ME: Surgical approaches to the cavernous sinus: A microsurgical study. **Neurosurgery** 26:903–932, 1990.
13. Laws ER Jr, Kern EB: Complications of trans-sphenoidal surgery. **Clin Neurosurg** 23:401–416, 1976.
14. Ono M, Ono M, Rhoton AL Jr, Barry M: Microsurgical anatomy of the region of the tentorial incisura. **J Neurosurg** 60:365–399, 1984.
15. Renn WH, Rhoton AL Jr: Microsurgical anatomy of the sellar region. **J Neurosurg** 43:288–298, 1975.
16. Rhoton AL Jr: Microsurgical anatomy of the region of the third ventricle, in Apuzzo MLJ (ed): *Surgery of the Third Ventricle*. Baltimore, Williams & Wilkins, 1987, pp 92–166.
17. Rhoton AL Jr: Anatomy of the pituitary gland and sellar region, in Thapar K, Kovacs K, Scheithauer BW, Lloyd RV (eds): *Diagnosis and Management of Pituitary Tumors*. Totowa, Humana Press Inc, 2000, pp 13–40.
18. Rhoton AL Jr: The foramen magnum. **Neurosurgery** 47[Suppl 1]:S155–S193, 2000.
19. Rhoton AL Jr: Tentorial incisura. **Neurosurgery** 47[Suppl 1]:S131–S153, 2000.
20. Rhoton AL Jr, Maniscalco JE: Microsurgery of the sellar region, in Glaser JS (ed): *Neuro-Ophthalmology*. St. Louis, C.V. Mosby, 1977, pp 106–127.
21. Rhoton AL Jr, Hardy DG, Chambers SM: Microsurgical anatomy and dissection of the sphenoid bone, cavernous sinus and sellar region. **Surg Neurol** 12:63–104, 1979.
22. Rhoton AL Jr, Harris FS, Renn WH: Microsurgical anatomy of the sellar region and cavernous sinus. **Clin Neurosurg** 24:54–85, 1977.
23. Rhoton AL Jr, Yamamoto I, Peace DA: Microsurgery of the third ventricle: Part 2—Operative approaches. **Neurosurgery** 8:357–373, 1981.
24. Schloffer H: Erfolgreiche Operation eines hypophysentumors auf nasalem Wege. **Wein Klin Wochenschr** 20:621–624, 1907.
25. Yamamoto I, Rhoton AL Jr, Peace DA: Microsurgery of the third ventricle: Part 1—Microsurgical anatomy. **Neurosurgery** 8:334–356, 1981.

The Cavernous Sinus, the Cavernous Venous Plexus, and the Carotid Collar

Albert L. Rhoton, Jr., M.D.
Department of Neurological Surgery, University of Florida, Gainesville, Florida

Correspondence:
Albert L. Rhoton, Jr., M.D., Department of Neurological Surgery, University of Florida McKnight Brain Institute, P.O. Box 100265, 100 South Newell Drive, Building 59, L2-100, Gainesville, FL 32610-0265.
Email: rhoton@neurosurgery.ufl.edu

KEY WORDS: Cavernous sinus, Cerebral veins, Cranial base surgery, Cranial nerves, Craniotomy, Internal carotid artery, Intracranial vascular system, Microsurgical anatomy, Middle cranial fossa, Skull base surgery

The paired cavernous sinuses are located near the center of the head on each side of the sella, pituitary gland, and sphenoid sinus. Each sinus has dural walls that surround a venous space through which a segment of the internal carotid artery courses. The sinus extends from the superior orbital fissure in front to the area lateral to the dorsum sellae behind (*Fig. 9.1*). Its anterior edge is attached to the margins of the superior orbital fissure and its posterior wall is located between the dorsum sellae medially and the ostium of Meckel's cave laterally. The oculomotor, trochlear, and ophthalmic nerves course in the lateral wall. The abducens nerve courses on the medial side of the ophthalmic nerve between it and the internal carotid artery. The lateral wall faces the temporal lobe, the roof faces the basal cisterns, the medial wall faces the sella, pituitary gland, and body of the sphenoid bone, and the lower edge is located below the horizontal portion of the intracavernous segment of the internal carotid artery. The cavernous sinus has venous connections with the cerebrum, cerebellum, brainstem, face, eye, orbit, nasopharynx, mastoid, and middle ear (6, 7). These connections and the relationships of the cavernous sinus to the carotid artery, extraocular nerves, and pituitary gland make the sinus of special interest to neurologists, ophthalmologists, otolaryngologists, and endocrinologists, in addition to neurosurgeons (1).

THE SINUS

The cavernous sinus is defined as the dural envelope in which the cavernous segment of the internal carotid artery courses (*Fig. 9.2*). The dural envelope contains not only the cavernous carotid artery, but is also the site of a venous confluence that receives the terminal end of multiple veins draining the orbit, sylvian fissure, and middle and anterior fossae and has free communication with the basilar, superior and inferior petrosal, and intercavernous sinuses. Overall, the sinus is shaped like a boat with its narrow keel located at the superior orbital fissure and its broader bow (posterior wall) located lateral to the dorsum sellae above the petrous apex. It has four walls: a roof and lateral, medial, and posterior walls. The deck or roof of the sinus faces upward and the lower edge, formed at the junction of the medial and lateral walls below the intracavernous segment of the internal carotid artery, gives the sinus a triangular shape in cross section (*Fig. 9.3*). The roof is formed by the dura lining the lower margin of the anterior clinoid process anteriorly and the patch of dura, called the oculomotor triangle, between the anterior and posterior clinoid processes and the petrous apex through which the oculomotor nerve penetrates the sinus roof. The medial edge of the occulomotor triangle is formed by the interclinoid dural fold, which extends from the anterior to the posterior clinoid process; the lateral margin is formed by the anterior petroclinoid fold, which extends from the anterior clinoid process to the petrous apex; and the posterior margin is formed by the posterior petroclinoid fold, which extends from the posterior clinoid process to the petrous apex.

The cavernous sinus has a wide posterior dural wall that it shares with the lateral part of the posterior wall of the basilar sinus, the venous connection extending across the back of the upper clivus and dorsum sellae. The basilar sinus is the largest venous connection between the paired cavernous sinuses. The cavernous sinus opens into and communicates widely at its posterior end with the basilar sinus. The superior and inferior petrosal sinuses also open into the lateral part of the basilar sinus, thus creating a large venous confluence along the posterior wall of the cavernous sinus at the area where the cavernous, basilar, and superior and inferior petrosal sinuses converge. This part of the posterior wall of the cavernous sinus that it shares with the basilar sinus is located lateral to the dorsum sellae, where the basilar sinus opens into the cavernous sinus and communicates with the superior and inferior petrosal sinuses. The lower margin of the posterior wall of the cavernous sinus is located at the upper margin of the petroclival fissure at the junction of the temporal and sphenoid bones. The abducens nerve passes through the lower margin of the posterior wall and under the petrosphenoid ligament to enter the sinus. The upper edge of the posterior wall is located at the level of the posterior petroclinoid dural fold, which extends from the petrous apex to the posterior clinoid process. The lateral edge of the posterior wall is located just medial to the ostium of Meckel's cave, and the medial edge is located at the lateral margin of the dorsum sellae.

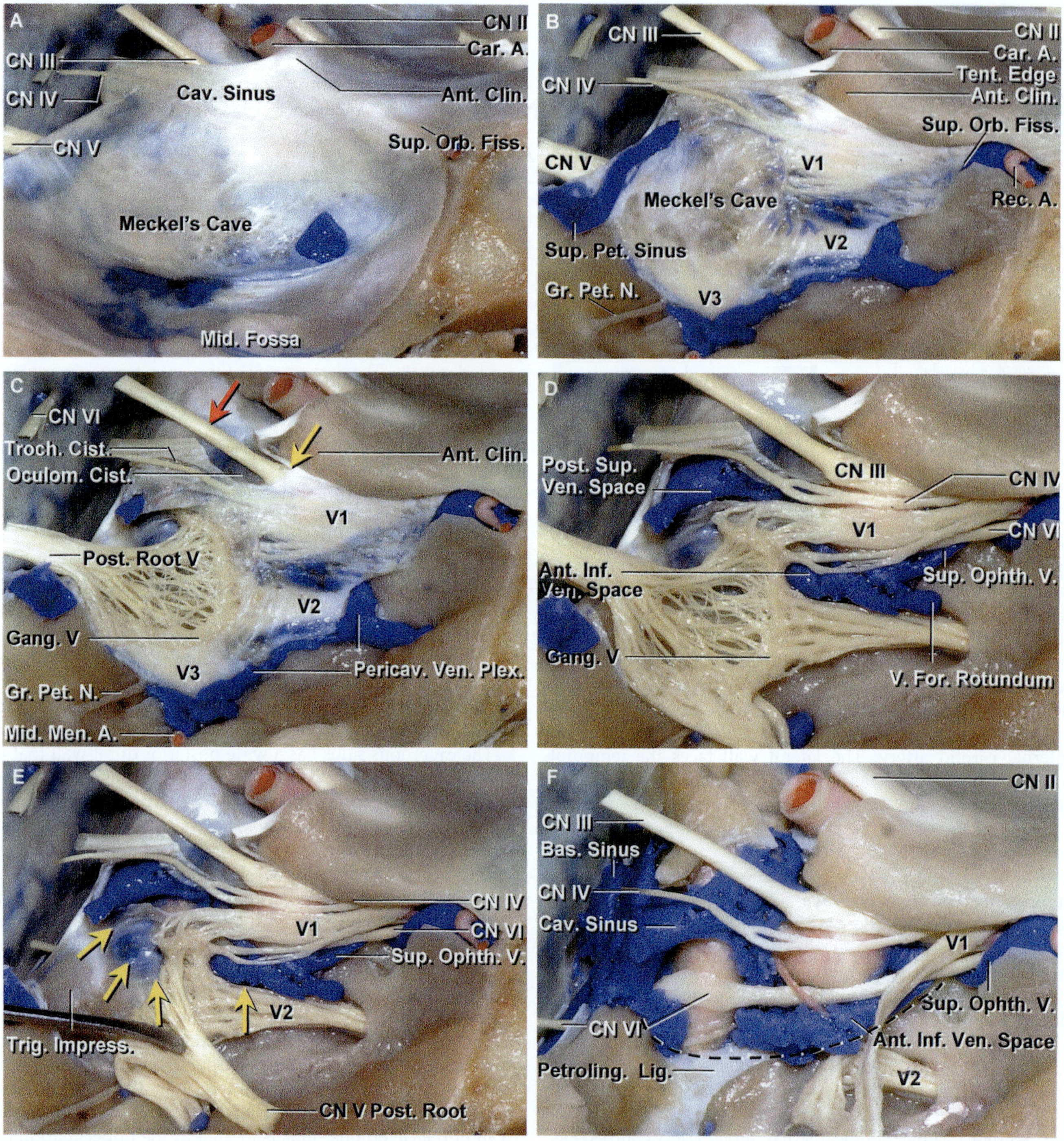

FIGURE 9.1. *Stepwise dissection of the right cavernous sinus. A, the lateral wall of the cavernous sinus extends downward from the tentorial edge and blends into the dura covering Meckel's cave and the middle fossa. The oculomotor and trochlear nerves enter the roof of the cavernous sinus. The carotid artery exits the cavernous sinus on the medial side of the anterior clinoid process. B, the outer layer of dura has been peeled away from the lateral wall of the cavernous sinus and Meckel's cave. This exposes the oculomotor and trochlear nerves entering the roof of the cavernous sinus and passing forward through the superior orbital fissure. The thin layer covering Meckel's cave consists in part of the arachnoid membrane extending forward from the posterior fossa and surrounding trigeminal nerve to the level of the trigeminal ganglion. The superior petrosal sinus passes above the ostium of Meckel's cave and joins the posterior part of the cavernous sinus. C, the oculomotor nerve enters a short cistern in the sinus roof* (red arrow) *and does not become incorporated into the lateral wall until it reaches the lower margin of the anterior clinoid process* (yellow arrow). *The arachnoid covering of Meckel's cave, which extends forward around the posterior trigeminal root to the level of the midportion of the ganglion, has been removed. The cavernous sinus extends from the superior orbital fissure to the petrous apex. It is located medial to the upper third of the gasserian ganglion. The pericavernous venous plexus surrounds the maxillary and mandibular nerves in the region of the foramen rotundum and foramen ovale. D, the remaining dura covering the lateral wall has*

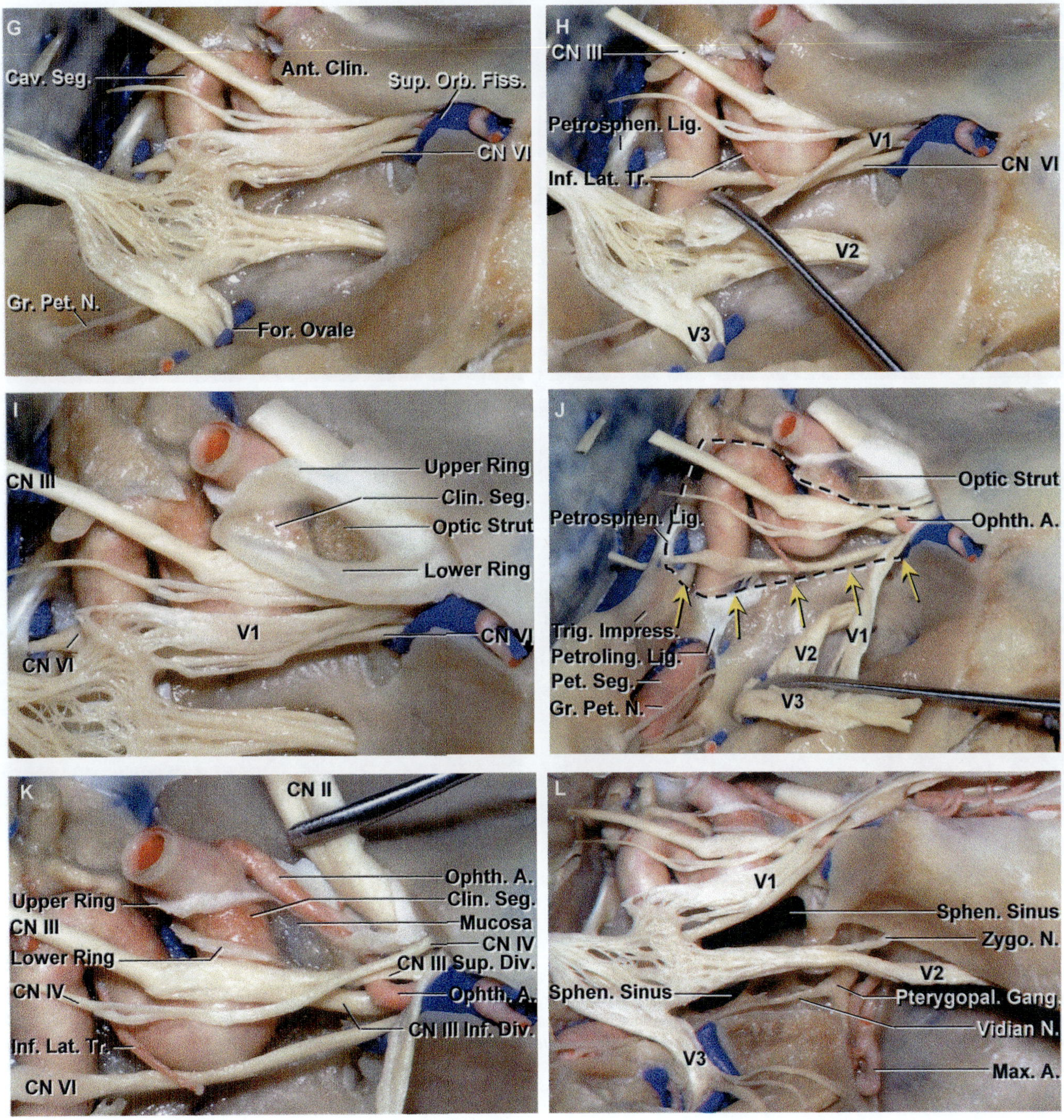

FIGURE 9.1. *Continued*

been removed. The oculomotor, trochlear, and ophthalmic nerves pass forward to converge on the superior orbital fissure. The segment of the superior petrosal sinus above the posterior trigeminal root has been removed. E, the posterior trigeminal root has been reflected forward to expose the posterior part of the lower margin of the cavernous sinus (yellow arrow) in the area medial to the trigeminal impression on the petrous apex, in which Meckel's cave sits. The superior ophthalmic vein exits the orbit through the superior orbital fissure and passes posteriorly below the ophthalmic nerve to enter the cavernous sinus. F, the trigeminal nerve and its three divisions have been reflected forward to expose the venous spaces of the cavernous sinus. The lower margin of the cavernous sinus (broken line) is located at the site where the internal carotid artery exits the carotid canal by passing below the petrolingual ligament. The venous spaces in the cavernous sinus communicate posteriorly with the inferior and superior petrosal and basilar sinuses. In addition, the cavernous sinus communicates with the superior ophthalmic veins and the venous plexus around the maxillary and mandibular nerves and pituitary gland. G, the venous plexus surrounding the nerves has been removed to expose the trigeminal divisions and the nerves coursing in the wall of the cavernous sinus. H, the ophthalmic nerve has been depressed to expose the abducens nerve, which passes under the petrosphenoid ligament roofing Dorello's canal, and courses medial to the ophthalmic nerve. The abducens nerve crosses laterally below the ophthalmic nerve as it passes through the superior orbital fissure. I, the

(Legend continues on next page.)

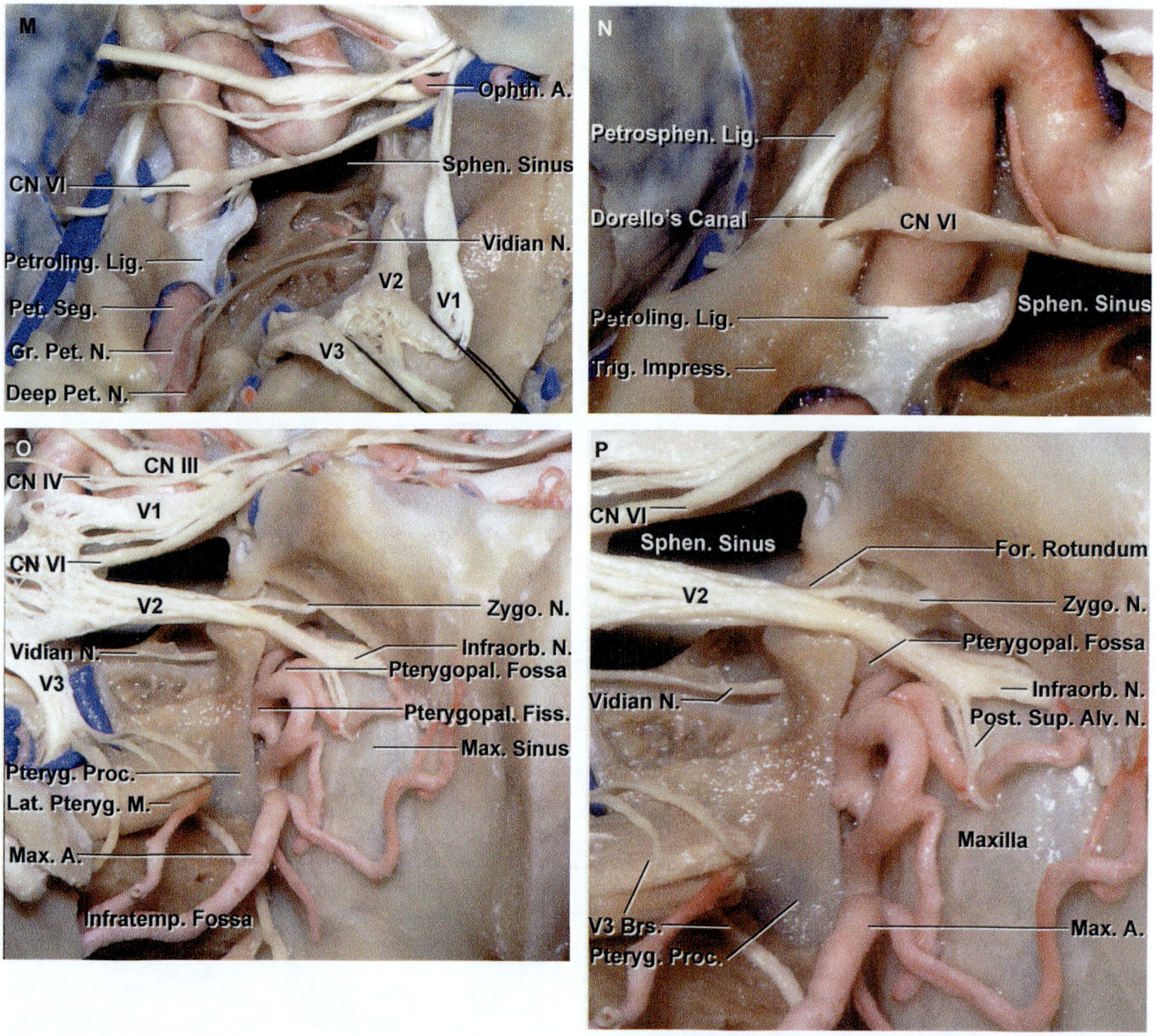

FIGURE 9.1. *Continued*

anterior clinoid process has been removed. The optic strut separates the optic canal and superior orbital fissure. The dura extending medially off the upper surface of the anterior clinoid forms the upper dural ring around the internal carotid artery, and the dura lining the lower margin of the clinoid extends medially to form the lower dural ring. The clinoid segment of the carotid artery, located between the upper and lower ring, is enclosed in the dura sheath, referred to as the carotid collar. J, the trigeminal nerve has been folded downward to expose the petrolingual ligament, which extends above the internal carotid artery, just proximal to where the artery enters the cavernous sinus. The abducens nerve passes around the internal carotid artery and courses medial to the ophthalmic nerve in the lower part of the cavernous sinus. The margins of the cavernous sinus are shown with an broken line. *The cavernous sinus does not extend laterally into the area of the trigeminal impression where Meckel's cave sets. K, enlarged view. The optic nerve has been elevated to expose the ophthalmic artery coursing within the optic sheath. At the orbital apex, the artery penetrates the optic sheath and enters the orbital apex on the lateral side of the optic nerve. Removal of additional optic strut exposes the mucosa lining the sphenoid sinus on the medial side of the optic strut. L, the bone between the first and second and the second and third trigeminal divisions has been drilled to expose the lateral wing of the sphenoid sinus. The vidian nerve, which passes forward to enter the sphenopalatine ganglion in the pterygopalatine fossa, is exposed between the second and third trigeminal divisions. M, the trigeminal nerve has been reflected forward to expose the opening into the lateral wing of the sphenoid sinus. The vidian nerve, formed by the union of the greater and deep petrosal nerves, courses forward in the vidian canal to reach the pterygopalatine fossa. N, enlarged view of the petrolingual and petrosphenoid ligaments. The petrosphenoid ligament extends from the lower part of the lateral margin of the dorsum sellae above the abducens nerve to the petrous apex. The lower margin of the posterior wall of the cavernous sinus is located at the lower margin of Dorello's canal. Anteriorly, the lower margin of the cavernous sinus is located at the level that the internal carotid artery exits the area below the petrolingual ligament and enters the posterior part of the cavernous sinus. O, the exposure has been extended down to the infratemporal and pterygopalatine fossae. The infratemporal fossa*

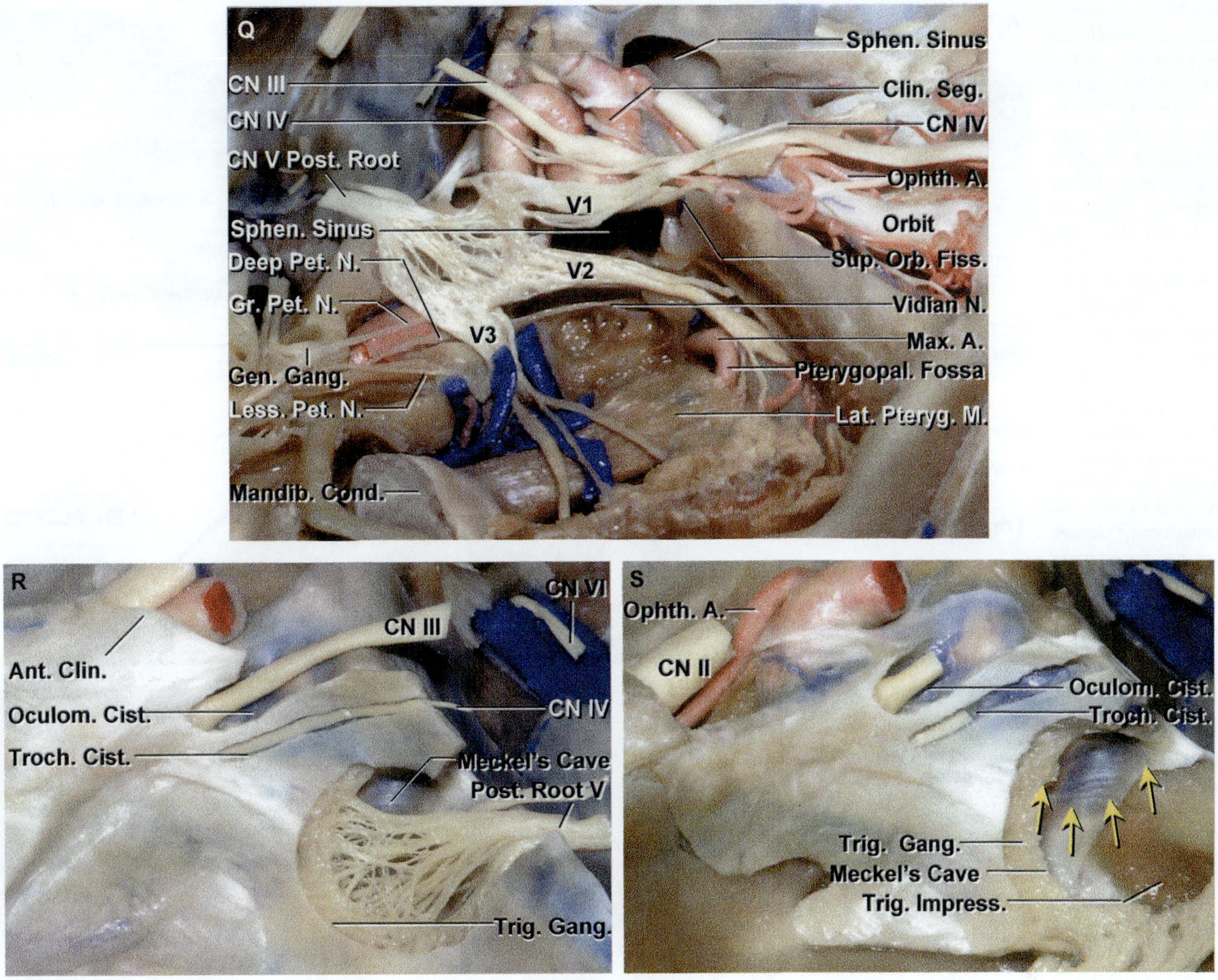

FIGURE 9.1. *Continued*
contains branches of the mandibular nerve and maxillary artery, the pterygoid muscles, and the pterygoid venous plexus. The maxillary nerve passes through the foramen rotundum to enter the pterygopalatine fossa. P, *enlarged view. The pterygopalatine fossa is located between the posterior maxillary wall and the pterygoid process. The vidian nerve penetrates the upper part of the pterygoid process and the area below the foramen rotundum to enter pterygopalatine fossa. The maxillary nerve gives rise to zygomatic, infraorbital, and posterosuperior alveolar nerves, and branches and rami to the pterygopalatine ganglion.* Q, *overview. The posterior wall of the cavernous sinus extends laterally from the dorsum sellae to the medial edge of the ostium of Meckel's cave. The floor of the middle fossa has been removed to expose the infratemporal fossa, which contains the branches of the maxillary artery and the mandibular nerve, the pterygoid venous plexus, and the pterygoid muscles. The infratemporal fossa opens medially into the pterygopalatine fossa. The maxillary nerve passes through the foramen rotundum to enter the pterygopalatine fossa and send branches along the orbital floor. The ophthalmic nerve passes through the superior orbital fissure and sends branches along the orbital roof.* R, *lateral view of the left cavernous sinus. The oculomotor, trochlear, and trigeminal nerves are all enclosed in an arachnoid sac that surrounds the nerve for a short distance after they enter into the dura. The lateral wall of all three cisterns has been removed. Meckel's cave, the cistern around the posterior trigeminal root, extends forward to the middle portion of the gasserian ganglion. The oculomotor cistern extends forward in the roof of the cavernous sinus to where the nerve passes under the anterior clinoid process. The thin cistern around the trochlear nerve extends forward below the oculomotor cistern.* S, *the posterior trigeminal root has been removed to expose the trigeminal impression and the lower margin of the cavernous sinus, which is located at the level of the upper and middle thirds of the trigeminal ganglion* (arrows). A., *artery;* Alv., *alveolar;* Ant., *anterior;* Bas., *basilar;* Brs., *branches;* Car., *carotid;* Cav., *cavernous;* Cist., *cistern;* Clin., *clinoid;* CN, *cranial nerve;* Cond., *condyle;* Div., *division;* Fiss., *fissure;* For., *foramen;* Gang., *ganglion;* Gen., *geniculate;* Gr., *greater;* Impress., *impression;* Inf., *inferior;* Inf. Lat., *inferolateral;* Infraorb., *infraorbital;* Infratemp., *infratemporal;* Lat., *lateral;* Less., *lesser;* Lig., *ligament;* M., *muscle;* Mandib., *mandibular;* Max., *maxillary;* Men., *meningeal;* Mid., *middle;* N., *nerve;* Oculom., *oculomotor;* Ophth., *ophthalmic;* Orb., *orbital;* Pericav., *pericavernous;* Pet., *petrosal, petrous;* Petroling., *petrolingual;* Petrosphen., *petrosphenoid;* Plex., *plexus;* Post., *posterior;* Proc., *process;* Pteryg., *pterygoid;* Pterygopal., *pterygopalatine;* Rec., *recurrent;* Seg., *segment;* Sphen., *sphenoid;* Sup., *superior;* Tent., *tentorial;* Tr., *trunk;* Trig., *trigeminal;* Troch., *trochlear;* V., *vein;* Ven., *venous;* Zygo., *zygomatic.*

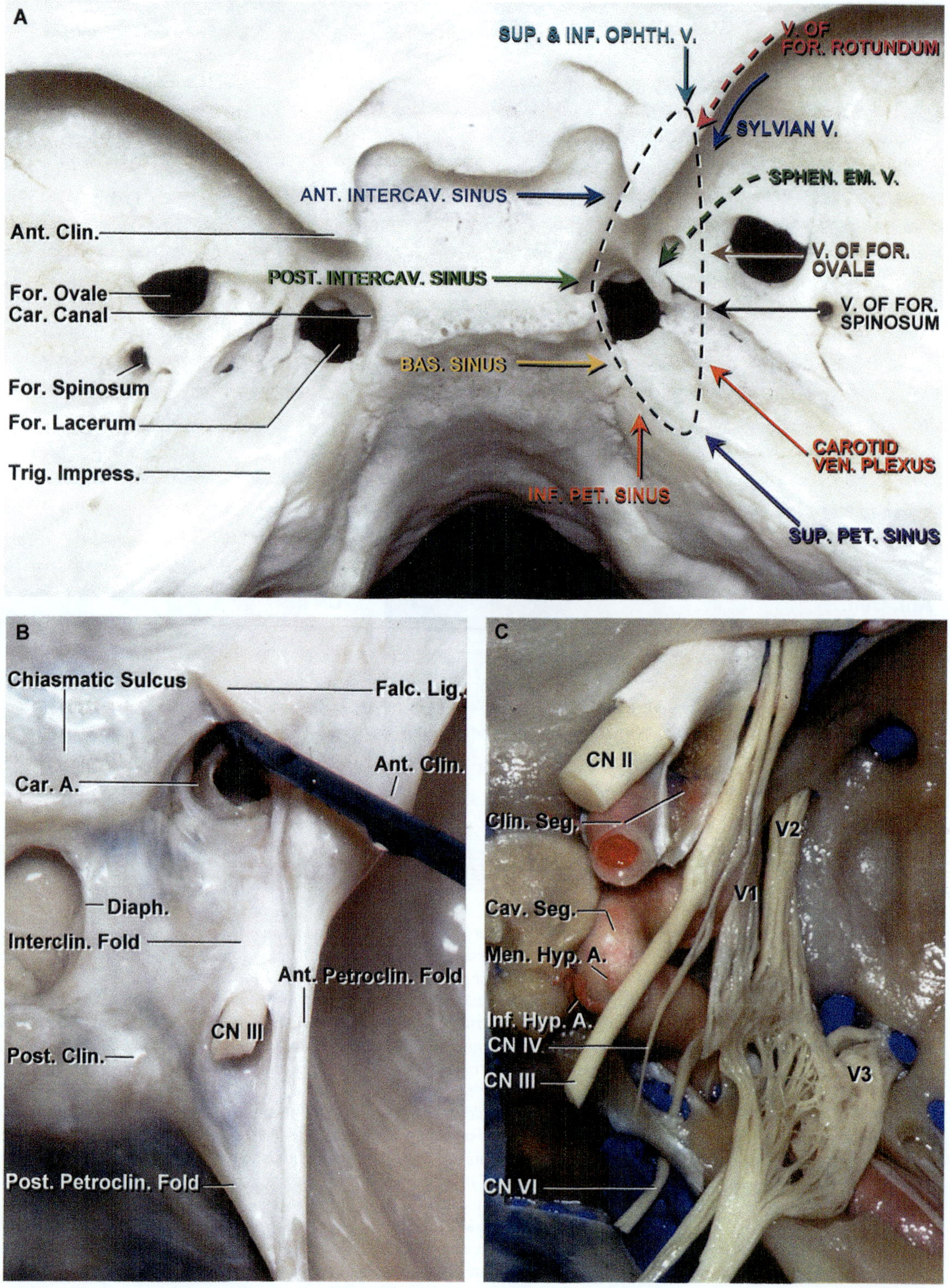

FIGURE 9.2. A, *superior view of the cranial base in the region of the cavernous sinus. The cavernous sinus extends from the superior orbital fissure anteriorly, to the petrous apex posteriorly, and it is bordered by the sella medially and the middle fossa laterally. It fills the posterior margin of the superior orbital fissure, which is located below the anterior clinoid process and its posterior wall, extends from the lateral edge of the dorsum sellae to the medial margin of the trigeminal impression and Meckel's cave. Numerous venous channels open into the cavernous sinus. These include the basilar, anterior and posterior intercavernous, and the superior and inferior petrosal sinuses; the sylvian and ophthalmic veins, and the veins exiting the foramen ovale, rotundum, and spinosum; and the carotid canal and the sphenoidal emissary foramen. Each structure is shown by* colored ar*rows. The basilar sinus is the largest communicating channel between the cavernous sinuses.* B, *superior view of the roof of the cavernous sinus. The oculomotor triangle, through which the oculomotor enters the roof of the cavernous sinus, is located between the anterior and posterior petroclinoid and the interclinoid dural folds. The interclinoid fold extends from the anterior to the posterior clinoid process. The anterior petroclinoid fold extends from the petrous apex to the anterior clinoid process and the posterior petroclinoid fold extends from the petrous apex to the posterior clinoid process. The internal carotid artery has been divided at the point it exits the roof of the cavernous sinus. A probe has been inserted under the falciform dura fold, which extends medially from the anterior clinoid process and above the optic canal to the chiasmatic sulcus.* C, *the dura has been removed from the roof and lateral wall of another cavernous sinus. The anterior clinoid process has been preserved. The abducens nerve passes around the lateral surface of the internal carotid artery. The oculomotor and ophthalmic nerves have been divided to expose the floor of the cavernous sinus, which is located at the level of the lower edge of the carotid sulcus on the sphenoid body below the intracavernous carotid.* D, *superior view of the cavernous sinus with the anterior clinoid process and roof removed. The roof of*

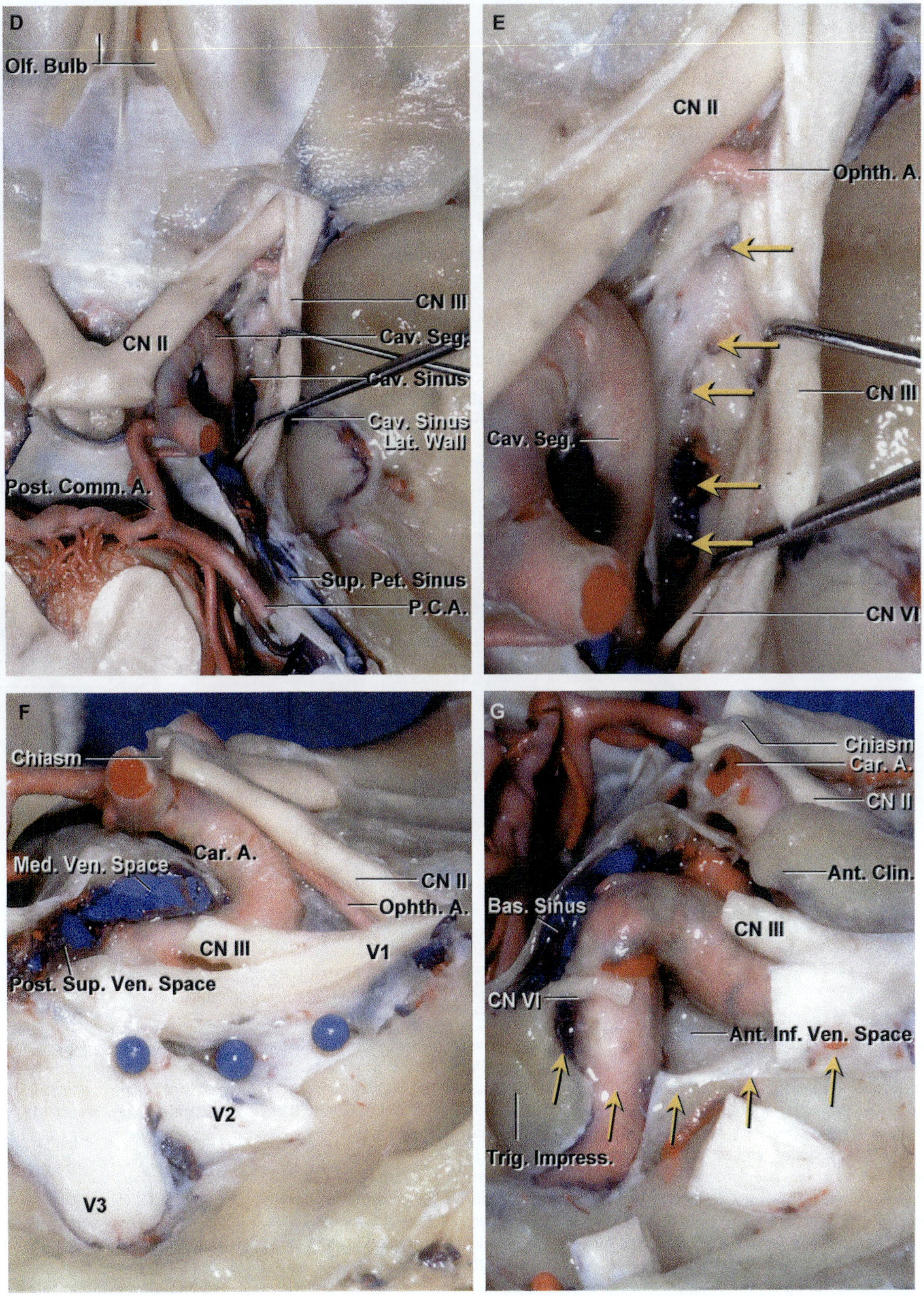

FIGURE 9.2. *Continued the sinus extends backward from the area below the anterior clinoid process, which has been removed, into the area between the middle fossa and sella and posteriorly, to the area lateral to the dorsum sellae. The lateral wall of the cavernous sinus, in which the oculomotor, ophthalmic, and trochlear nerves course, has been retracted laterally to show the lower margin of the sinus from inside.* E, *enlarged view of the sinus opened from above. Numerous ostia of veins drain the surrounding areas, which open into the cavernous sinus* (arrows). *The ophthalmic artery enters the optic canal.* F, *the cavernous sinus shown in* C *and* D *is viewed from laterally.* The pins *have been inserted along the lower edge of the interior of the sinus shown in* E. *The lower edge of the sinus is located medial to the upper third of Meckel's cave and trigeminal ganglion and extends forward below the ophthalmic nerve, but does not include the area of the maxillary nerve.* G, *lateral view of the specimen shown in* C. *A segment of the oculomotor, trigeminal, trochlear, and abducens nerves has been removed.* The arrows *have been placed along the lower margin of the dural envelope forming the lower margin of the cavernous sinus. The cavernous sinus does not extend laterally to the mandibular and maxillary nerves, but extends down to just below the carotid sulcus on the body of the sphenoid bone.* A., *artery;* Ant., *anterior;* Bas., *basal;* Car., *carotid;* Cav., *cavernous;* Clin., *clinoid;* CN, *cranial nerve;* Comm., *communicating;* Diaph., *diaphragm;* Em., *emissary;* Falc., *falciform;* For., *foramen;* Hyp., *hypophyseal;* Impress., *impression;* Inf., *inferior;* Intercav., *intercavernous;* Interclin., *interclinoid;* Lat., *lateral;* Lig., *ligament;* Med., *medial;* Men., *meningeal;* Men. Hyp., *meningohypophyseal;* Olf., *olfactory;* Ophth., *ophthalmic;* P.C.A., *posterior cerebral artery;* Pet., *petrosal;* Petroclin., *petroclinoid;* Post., *posterior;* Seg., *segment;* Sphen., *sphenoid;* Sup., *superior;* Trig., *trigeminal;* V., *vein;* Ven., *venous.*

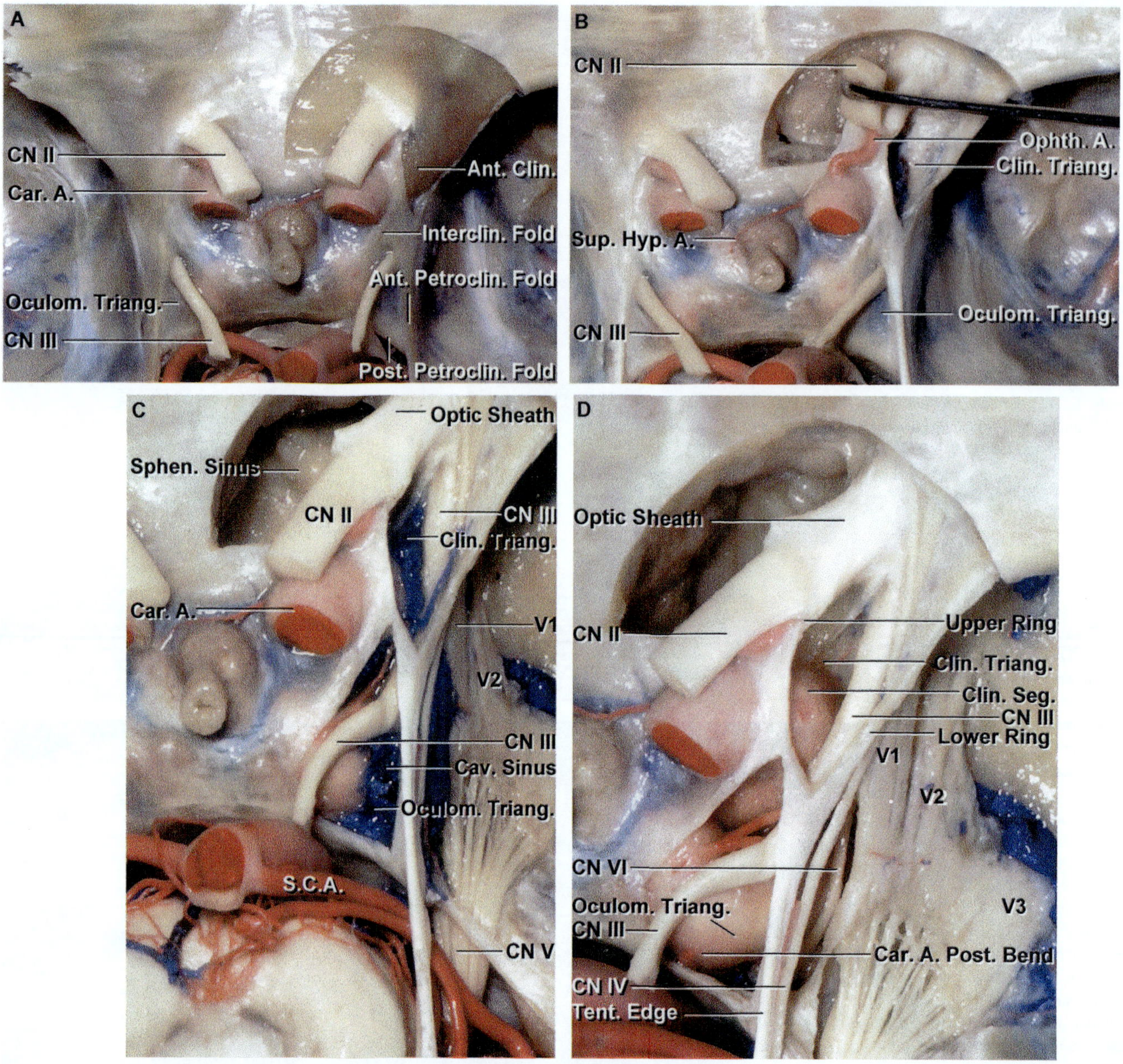

FIGURE 9.3. *Stepwise dissection of the roof of the cavernous sinus. A, superior view. The dura covering the upper surface of the right anterior clinoid process, optic canal, and adjacent part of the planum has been removed. The roof of the cavernous sinus is formed anteriorly by the dura lining the lower margin of the anterior clinoid and posteriorly by the dura covering the oculomotor triangle located between the anterior and posterior petroclinoidal and intraclinoidal dural folds. The oculomotor nerve enters the roof of the cavernous sinus through the oculomotor triangle. B, the anterior clinoid and roof of the optic canal has been removed. The optic nerve has been elevated to expose the ophthalmic artery entering the optic foramen. Removing the anterior clinoid exposes the floor of the clinoidal triangle located between the optic and oculomotor nerves. The dura separating the lower surface of the clinoid from the oculomotor nerve and extending medially around the carotid artery, referred to as the carotidoculomotor membrane, forms the floor of the clinoidal triangle and the anterior part of the roof of the cavernous sinus. The dura extending medially off the upper surface of the clinoid forms the upper dural ring, and the carotidoculomotor membrane extending medially from the lower surface of the clinoid forms the lower dural ring. C, the dura in the floor of the clinoidal triangle and roof of the oculomotor triangle, which together form the roof of the cavernous sinus, have been removed to expose the upper part of the cavernous sinus. The dura has been elevated from the lateral wall of the cavernous sinus and middle fossa floor to expose the nerves coursing in the lateral wall of the cavernous sinus. D, the sinus has been cleared to expose the clinoid segment of the internal carotid artery in the clinoidal triangle and the posterior bend of the intercavernous carotid below the oculomotor triangle. The anterior part of the roof is formed by the dura that separates the anterior clinoid and oculomotor nerve and that extends medially to form the lower dural ring. The posterior part of the roof is formed by the dura forming the oculomotor triangle. A., artery;* Ant., *anterior;* Car., *carotid;* Cav., *cavernous;* Clin., *clinoid;* CN, *cranial nerve;* Hyp., *hypophyseal;* Interclin., *interclinoid;* Oculom., *oculomotor;* Ophth., *ophthalmic;* Petroclin., *petroclinoid;* Post., *posterior;* S.C.A., *superior cerebellar artery;* Seg., *segment;* Sphen., *sphenoid;* Sup., *superior;* Tent., *tentorial;* Triang., *triangle.*

The lateral wall extends from the medial edge of Meckel's cave posteriorly to the lateral margin of the superior orbital fissure anteriorly, and from the anterior petroclinoid dural fold above to the lower margin of the carotid sulcus below. The carotid sulcus is the groove on the lateral aspect of the body of the sphenoid along which the internal carotid artery courses (*Fig. 9.4*). The sheet of dura forming the posterior part of the lateral wall of the sinus also forms the upper third of the medial wall of Meckel's cave, which is located lateral to and is separated from the posterior part of the cavernous sinus by their shared dural wall. The medial wall is formed by the dura that constitutes the lateral wall of the sella turcica and covers the lateral surface of the body of the sphenoid bone. The medial wall extends from the lateral edge of the dorsum sellae posteriorly to the medial edge of the superior orbital fissure anteriorly, and from the interclinoid dural fold above to the lower margin of the carotid sulcus below. Anteriorly, the lower edge of the sinus, where the medial and lateral walls meet, is located just below where the ophthalmic nerve courses in the lateral sinus wall; proceeding posteriorly, it is located medial to the junction of the upper and middle third of the gasserian ganglion. Finally, at the posterior part, it slopes upward medial to the upper part of Meckel's cave (*Fig. 9.1E*). Behind the site where the ophthalmic nerve arises from the trigeminal ganglion, the lower edge of the medial and lateral walls of the sinus come together at the lateral edge of the carotid sulcus on the medial side of the upper part of Meckel's cave. Only the upper part of the medial wall of Meckel's cave and the upper part of the gasserian ganglion are located directly lateral to the cavernous sinus; thus almost all of Meckel's cave is located below and lateral to the posterior part of the cavernous sinus (*Figs. 9.1* and *9.2*). Meckel's cave extends forward from the posterior fossa, where its ostium is located between the medial part of the petrous ridge below, the superior petrosal sinus above, and the lateral edge of the cavernous sinus medially. The subarachnoid space extends forward within Meckel's cave to approximately the level of the midportion of the gasserian ganglion. The terminal part of the petrous carotid exits the carotid canal and passes under the trigeminal nerve and the petrolingual ligament, where it turns upward to enter the posterior part of the cavernous sinus. The artery becomes enclosed in the dural envelope of the cavernous sinus only when it exits the region of the foramen lacerum and turns upward, after traveling below the petrolingual ligament to reach the carotid sulcus on the lateral surface of the sphenoid body (*Fig. 9.1*).

The maxillary nerve does not course in the lateral wall of the dural envelop of the sinus as does the ophthalmic nerve. It courses beneath the dura of the middle fossa, below the level where the medial and lateral walls of the cavernous sinus join at the lower edge of the ophthalmic nerve. The superior ophthalmic vein usually courses posteriorly along the sphenoid body in the interval between the ophthalmic and maxillary nerves to reach the anteroinferior part of the sinus. As the dura is elevated from the floor of the middle fossa, it can be stripped upward off the lateral aspects of both the maxillary and ophthalmic nerves, but only the ophthalmic nerve has the venous space of the cavernous sinus on its medial side. The medial side of the maxillary nerve sits against the bone and is located below the lower edge of the anterior part of the sinus.

Numerous venous channels course along the lateral margin of the sella, the medial part of the middle fossa, the superior and inferior orbital fissures, the foramina ovale, rotundum, and spinosum and surrounding the pituitary gland. These channels converge on the cavernous sinus and may be, mistakenly, considered to be part of the cavernous sinus (*Fig. 9.2*). However, they course outside the dural envelope containing the internal carotid artery and open into the sinus through discrete ostia. They are part of the pericavernous venous plexus, but are not within the sinus. There is a tendency in classifying tumors in the region to include those tumors along the anterior clinoid process and in the region of Meckel's cave and petrous apex as cavernous sinus tumors; however, the author would not define those as cavernous sinus tumors. Those tumors that involve this region, but do not involve or extend into the dural envelope around the carotid artery, are much more amenable to resection than those involving and extending inside the dural envelope.

The important osseous relationships in the area are reviewed before the dural relationships in the area are considered.

OSSEOUS RELATIONSHIPS

The cavernous sinus sits on the lateral aspect of the body of the sphenoid bone (*Figs. 9.2* and *9.4*) (19). The posterior part of the lower edge of the sinus is located above the junction of the petrous apex and body of the sphenoid bone at the upper end of the petroclival fissure, and the posterior edge of the medial wall rests against the lateral edge of the dorsum sellae. The cavernous sinus extends downward and laterally from the lateral margin of the sella, across the sphenoid body to the junction of the body and greater sphenoid wing of the sphenoid, but does not extend laterally to include the margins of the foramina ovale, rotundum, or spinosum, although venous channels coursing through and around these foramina empty into the sinus and are part of the pericavernous venus plexus. The inconsistently occurring sphenoid emissary foramen, situated medial to the foramen ovale, transmits an emissary vein from the cavernous sinus.

The carotid sulcus is the shallow groove on the lateral aspect of the body of the sphenoid bone along which the internal carotid courses in the cavernous sinus. The intracavernous carotid sits against and is separated from the carotid sulcus by the dura of the medial sinus wall (*Fig. 9.4*). The carotid sulcus begins below and lateral to the dorsum sellae at the intracranial end of the carotid canal, turns forward to groove the body of the sphenoid immediately below the lateral edge of the floor of the sella, and turns upward to end medial to the anterior clinoid process. The segment of the internal carotid artery that courses along the medial side of the clinoid is referred to as the clinoid segment. The carotid sulcus, in well-pneumatized sphenoid bones, forms a serpiginous prominence that can be seen in the lateral wall of the sphenoid sinus

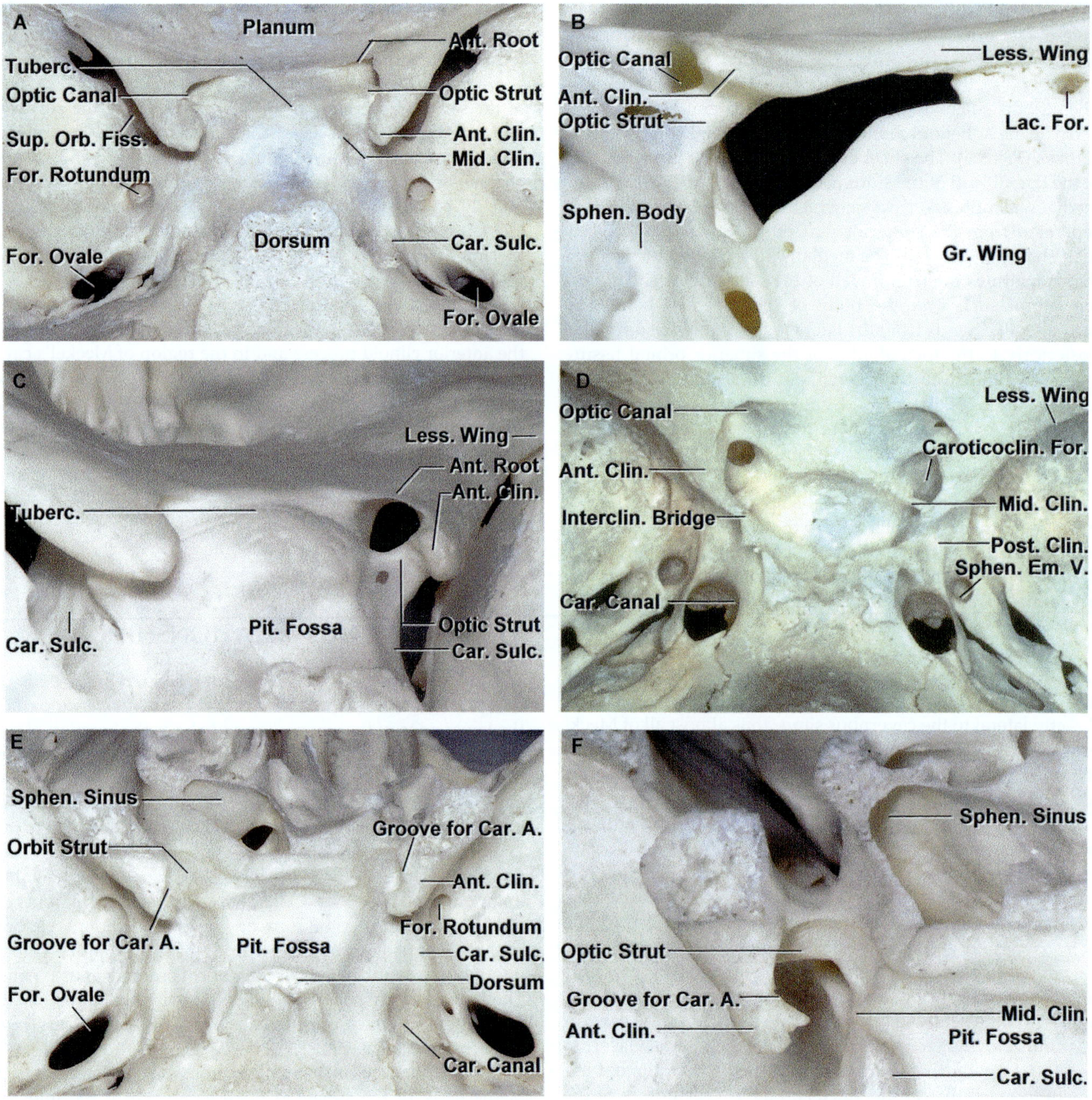

FIGURE 9.4. *Osseous relationships of the cavernous sinus and carotid collar. A, superior view. The osseous structures, which nearly encircle the clinoid segment of the internal carotid artery, include the anterior clinoid laterally, the optic strut anteriorly, and the carotid sulcus medially. The carotid sulcus begins lateral to the dorsum sellae at the intracranial end of the carotid canal, extends forward just below the sellar floor, and turns upward along the posterior surface of the optic strut. The anterior clinoid process projects backward from the lesser wing of the sphenoid bone, often overlapping the lateral edge of the carotid sulcus. The anterior root of the lesser sphenoid wing extends medially to form the roof of the optic canal. The posterior root of the lesser wing, referred to as the optic strut, extends from the inferomedial aspect of the anterior clinoid to the sphenoid body. The bony collar around the carotid artery formed by the anterior clinoid, optic strut, and carotid sulcus is inclined downward as it slopes medially from the upper surface of the anterior clinoid to the carotid sulcus. Another small prominence, the middle clinoid process, situated on the medial side of the carotid sulcus at the level of the tip of the anterior clinoid process, projects upward and laterally. In some cases, there is an osseous bridge extending from the tip of the middle clinoid to the tip of the anterior clinoid. In well-pneumatized sphenoid bones, the carotid sulcus is seen as a prominence in the lateral wall of the sphenoid sinus just below the floor of the sella. B, posterior view of the optic strut, optic canal, and the superior orbital fissure. The optic strut separates the optic canal and superior orbital fissure and forms the floor of the optic canal and the superomedial part of the roof of the superior orbital fissure. The posterior surface of the strut is shaped to accommodate the anterior wall of the clinoid segment. The artery courses along and may groove the medial half of the lower aspect of the ante-*

below the pituitary fossa. The bone in the lateral wall of the sphenoid sinus may be thin or even absent in some areas, thus allowing the artery to be observed through the sinus wall.

Anterior and Middle Clinoid Processes

The anterior clinoid process projects posteriorly from the lesser wing of the sphenoid bone above the anterior part of the roof of the sinus (*Fig. 9.4*). The base of the clinoid has three sites of continuity with the adjacent part of the sphenoid bone. The base is attached anteriorly at the medial edge of the sphenoid ridge, formed by the lesser sphenoid wing, and is attached medially to the anterior and posterior roots of the lesser wing. The anterior root of the lesser wing extends medially from the base of the anterior clinoid to the body of the sphenoid bone and forms the roof of the optic canal. The posterior root of the lesser wing, called the optic strut, extends medially below the optic nerve to the sphenoid body and forms the floor of the optic canal. The base of the anterior clinoid forms the lateral margin of the optic canal. The segment of the internal carotid artery that courses along the medial aspect of and is exposed by removing the anterior clinoid is referred to as the clinoid segment. The clinoid segment courses below the medial half of the lower margin of the clinoid, where it grooves the bone before coursing upward along the medial edge of the clinoid (*Fig. 9.4F*). The medial edge of the clinoid, just behind the base, is frequently the site of a shallow rounded indention that accommodates the lateral surface of the clinoid segment. The posterior tip of the clinoid often projects medially behind the lateral part of the clinoid segment. The anterior clinoid is the site of attachment of the anteromedial part of the tentorium and the anterior petroclinoid and interclinoid dural folds. Another dural fold, the falciform ligament, extends from the base of the clinoid across the roof of the optic canal to the planum sphenoidale. The chiasmatic sulcus is a shallow trough on the upper surface of the sphenoid bone between the intracranial end of the optic canals. The tuberculum sellae is located in the midline along the ridge forming the posterior margin of the chiasmatic sulcus. The anterior clinoid has a dense surface of cortical bone and a weak diploe of cancellous bone that is sometimes crossed by small venous channels that communicate with the cavernous sinus and the diploic veins of the orbital roof. The air cells in the sphenoid sinus may also extend through the optic strut into the anterior clinoid.

There is another small prominence, the middle clinoid process, that projects upward on the medial side of the terminal part of the carotid sulcus and medial to the tip of the anterior clinoid process (*Fig. 9.3*). An osseous bridge may extend from the tip of the middle clinoid to the tip of the anterior clinoid, thus converting the roof of the anterior part of the cavernous sinus into a bony ring or foramen, referred to as a caroticoclinoidal foramen, through which the internal carotid artery passes (*Fig. 9.4D*). This type of variant may infrequently occur bilaterally (15). There may also be interclinoidal osseous bridges that extend from the anterior to the posterior clinoid unilaterally or bilaterally (*Fig. 9.4D*). Such bridges make it difficult to remove the anterior clinoid process.

Optic Strut

The optic strut (posterior root of the lesser wing) is a small bridge of bone that extends from the inferomedial aspect of the base of the anterior clinoid process to the body of the sphenoid just in front of the carotid sulcus (*Figs. 9.1* and *9.4*) (18). The strut, from its junction with the clinoid, slopes gently downward as it approaches the body of the sphenoid. The strut separates the optic canal and superior orbital fissure. The superior surface of the strut, which slopes downward and forward from its intracranial edge, forms the floor of the optic canal. The inferior surface of the optic strut forms the medial part of the roof of the superior orbital fissure and the anterior part of the roof of the cavernous sinus. The strut sits at the junction of the orbital apex anteriorly, with the superior orbital fissure and optic canal posteriorly. The anterior edge of the strut is a narrow ridge located at the junction of its superior and inferior surfaces. The posterior face of the optic strut, which faces slightly downward, is shaped to accommodate the

rior clinoid before turning upward along the medial edge of the clinoid. The air cells in the sphenoid sinus may extend into the optic strut and anterior clinoid. In this case, the sphenoid sinus has pneumatized to a degree that bone is absent over the anterior part of the carotid sulcus, just medial to where the optic strut attaches to the body of the sphenoid bone. The maxillary strut is the bridge of bone separating the superior orbital fissure from the foramen rotundum. C, *oblique posterior view of the right optic strut. The lateral part of the bony collar around the clinoid segment is formed by the anterior clinoid, the anterior part is formed by the posterior surface of the optic strut and the part of the carotid sulcus located medial to the anterior clinoid process. The posterior surface of the optic strut is wider medially adjacent to the carotid sulcus than it is laterally at the site of attachment to the anterior clinoid process. The optic strut slopes downward from its lateral end so that the medial part of the bony collar is located below the level of the part of the collar joining the anterior clinoid. The inferomedial aspect of the right anterior clinoid is grooved by the artery.* D, *superior view of specimen with bilateral caroticoclinoidal foramen and interclinoidal osseous bridges. An osseous bridge connects the tips of the anterior and middle clinoid processes bilaterally, thus creating a bony ring around the artery, called a caroticoclinoidal foramen, on each side. There is also an interclinoidal osseous bridge connecting the anterior and posterior clinoid processes on both sides.* E, *superior view of another specimen, in which the lesser sphenoid wings and the base of the anterior clinoids and roof of the optic canals have been removed. The remaining part of the anterior clinoid is held in place by its attachment to the optic strut. The medial side of the anterior clinoid is grooved to accommodate the clinoid segment.* F, *enlarged view of the left half of* E. *The posterior face of the optic strut is shaped to accommodate the anterior surface, and the medial aspect of the anterior clinoid is grooved to accommodate the lateral surface of the clinoid segment. The tip of the anterior clinoid process is the site of a small bony projection directed toward the middle clinoid process, with the anterior and middle clinoids nearly completing a ring around the clinoid segment at the level of the cavernous sinus roof.* A., *artery;* Ant., *anterior;* Car., *carotid;* Caroticoclin., *caroticoclinoid;* Clin., *clinoid;* Em., *emissary;* Fiss., *fissure;* For., *foramen;* Gr., *greater;* Interclin., *interclinoid;* Lac., *lacrimal;* Less., *lesser;* Mid., *middle;* Orb., *orbital;* Pit., *pituitary;* Post., *posterior;* Sphen., *sphenoid;* Sulc., *sulcus;* Sup., *superior;* Tuberc., *tuberculum;* V., *vein.*

anterior surface of the anterior bend of the intracavernous carotid, which rests against the posterior surface of the optic strut as it ascends on the medial side of the anterior clinoid process. The posterior face of the strut also widens as it slopes medially. The site at which the strut blends into the sphenoid body is marked on the surface of the sphenoid bone facing the sphenoid sinus by a recess, the opticocarotid recess, which extends laterally from the superolateral part of the sphenoid sinus between the prominences in the sinus wall overlying the carotid sulcus and optic canal. This recess may extend deeply into the strut, so that the strut is partially or completely aerated by a lateral extension of the sphenoid sinus. The aeration may extend through the strut into the anterior clinoid process. Venous channels connecting the cavernous sinus with diploic veins of the orbital roof and anterior clinoid process may extend into or through the optic strut.

DURAL RELATIONSHIPS

The dural relationships of the anterior clinoid process are especially important in planning surgical approaches to the area (*Figs. 9.1–9.5*). The dura lining and extending medially from the upper surface of the anterior clinoid forms the lateral part of a dural ring, referred to as the upper or distal ring, which defines the upper margin of the carotid's clinoid segment (22). The dura forming the lateral part of the upper ring extends forward and medially below the optic nerve to line the upper surface of the optic strut and form the anterior part of the upper ring. The dura lining the upper surface of the optic strut extends medially and posteriorly at the level of the upper part of the carotid sulcus to form the medial part of the upper ring. Further medially, the dura forming the upper ring blends into the diaphragma sellae. The dura, extending medially above the optic nerve from the clinoid process to line the anterior root of the lesser wing and attaching to the posterior edge of the planum sphenoidale, is located at the horizontal level of the upper surface of the clinoid. However, the dura that extends medially off the upper surface of the clinoid to line the upper surface of the optic strut and form the upper dural ring slopes downward as it proceeds medially, so that the medial part of the upper dural ring actually lies at the level of the lower rather than the upper surface of the anterior clinoid and optic canal.

The layer of dura that lines the lower margin of the anterior clinoid and extends medially to form the lower or proximal dural ring is called the carotidoculomotor membrane because it separates the lower margin of the clinoid from the oculomotor nerve and extends medially around the carotid artery (*Figs. 9.5* and *9.6*). This membrane extends medially and forward to line the lower surface of the optic strut and forms the anterior part of the lower ring. The dura lining the lower margin of the optic strut blends medially and backward into the dura lining the carotid sulcus, but does not form as distinct a lower ring on the medial side of the artery as it does along the anterior and lateral margins. The medial part of the lower ring is located at the level of a line extending from the lower margin of the optic strut to the floor of the sella (*Fig. 9.6H*). This line approximates the lower margin of the segment of the artery, which tightly hugs the carotid sulcus. Below the level of the sellar floor, the artery, not being enclosed in the bony ring formed by the clinoid and strut, becomes more widely separated from the carotid sulcus and its dural lining to admit the large venous channels forming the medial venous space of the cavernous sinus.

The segment of the internal carotid artery located between the upper and lower dural rings, which is exposed by removing the anterior clinoid process, is referred to as the clinoid segment. It may be necessary to divide the dural rings to mobilize the carotid artery for dealing with aneurysms arising at the level of the roof of the cavernous sinus from the internal carotid artery at the origin of the ophthalmic artery.

Carotid Collar

The dura forming the lateral and anterior edges of the lower ring, as it approaches the clinoid segment, turns upward inside the bony ring to form a collar (carotid collar) around the artery, which does not adhere or fuse to the wall of the artery until it reaches the level of the upper ring (*Figs. 9.4* and *9.6*) (22). The site at which the dura forming the lower ring turns upward to form the collar around the clinoid segment is not attached to the arterial wall, but is separated from the artery by a narrow space through which course venous channels communicating with the anterior part of the cavernous sinus. These venous channels extend to just below the level of the upper dural ring. The dura forming the collar is so thin that the artery and the thin venous channels, referred to as the clinoid venous plexus, can be seen through the collar (*Fig. 9.6*). The transition between the medial side of the carotid collar and the lower ring, which is located at the level of the floor of the pituitary fossa, is not as sharply defined as it is on the anterior and lateral sides, where the dura forming the lower ring turns sharply upward around the artery at the edge of the optic strut and anterior clinoid.

The dural collar and the upper and lower rings slope downward as they extend medially from the clinoid (*Fig. 9.6*). The upper and lower rings also diverge as they slope medially, making the collar wider in the area facing the carotid sulcus and the medial end of the optic strut than in the areas facing the anterior clinoid. The carotid collar disappears posterior to the tip of the anterior clinoid process, where the dura lining the upper and lower surfaces of the clinoid process fuse into a single dural layer that forms the oculomotor triangle and posterior part of the roof of the cavernous sinus. The anterior part of the roof is formed by the dura lining the lower margin of the anterior clinoid.

The upper dural ring, at its junction with the collar, is adherent to the surface of the artery and serves as a barrier between the intra- and extradural spaces. In contrast, the lower dural ring and lower part of the collar are separated from the wall of the artery, creating a narrow space in which courses a thin layer of venous channels that are continuous through the lower part of the collar and lower dural ring with the venous channels within the cavernous sinus.

NEURAL RELATIONSHIPS

The nerves in the sinus wall or sinus are, from superior to inferior, the IIIrd cranial nerve followed by the trochlear, ophthalmic, and abducens nerves (*Figs. 9.1, 9.5,* and *9.7–9.9*) (6, 7, 17). The oculomotor, trochlear, and ophthalmic nerves

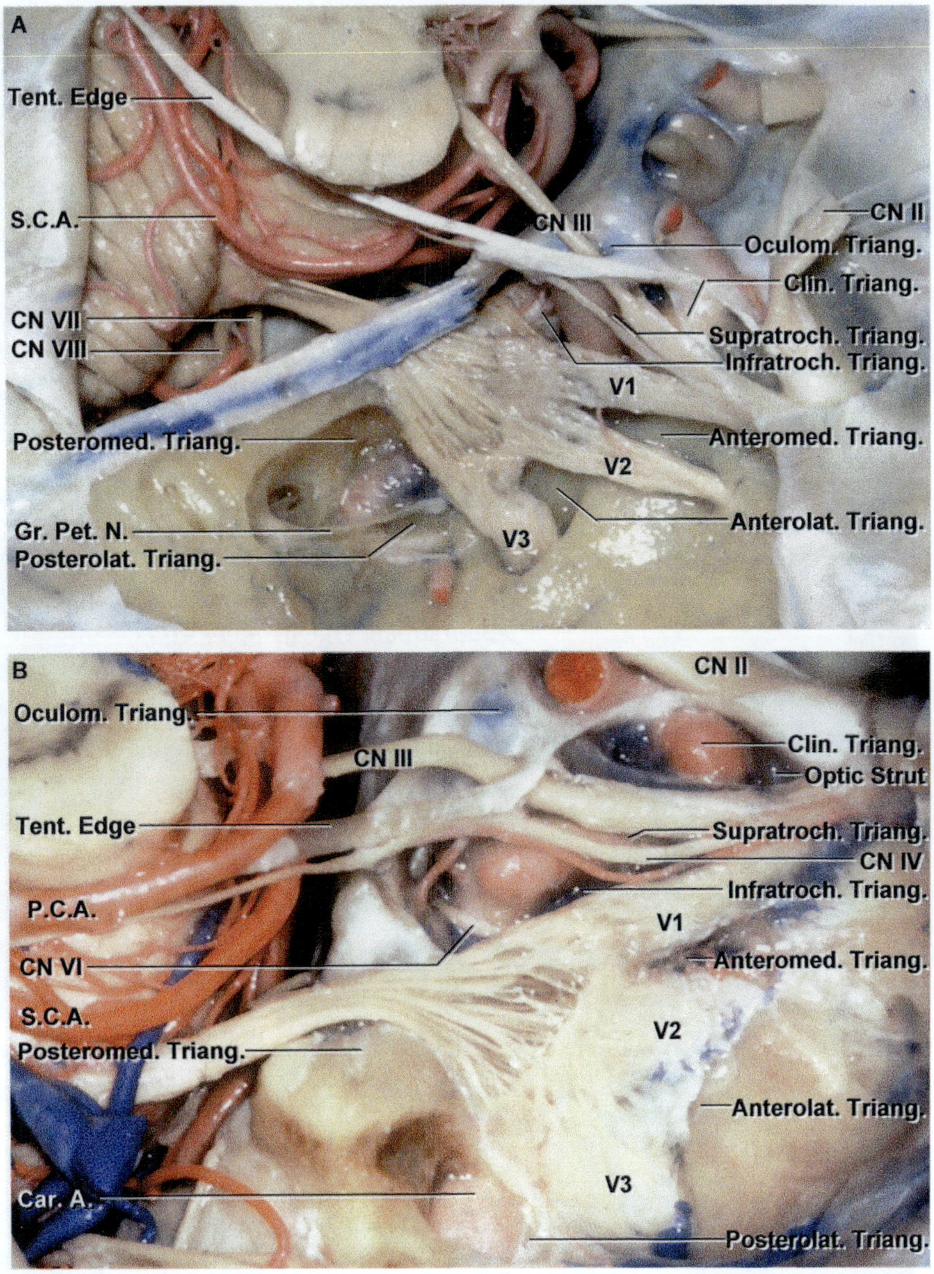

FIGURE 9.5. *Triangles in the region of the cavernous sinus and middle fossa formed by the convergence and divergence of the cranial nerves. A–B, lateral aspect of brainstem and posterior fossa showing the brainstem origin of the cranial nerves, which form the margins of the cavernous sinus and middle fossa triangles. The tentorial edge was preserved in A and removed in B. There are four cavernous sinus triangles, four middle fossa triangles, and two paraclival triangles. The cavernous sinus triangles are the clinoidal, oculomotor, supratrochlear, and infratrochlear triangle. The clinoidal triangle, exposed by removing the anterior clinoid process, is situated in the interval between the optic and oculomotor nerves. The optic strut is in the anterior part, the clinoid segment is in the midportion and the thin roof of the cavernous sinus is in the posterior part of this triangle. The oculomotor triangle is the triangular patch of dura through which the oculomotor nerve enters the roof of the cavernous sinus. The posterior margin of this triangle is formed by the posterior petroclinoid dural fold, which extends from the petrous apex to the posterior clinoid process. The lateral margin is formed by the anterior petroclinoid dural fold, which extends from the petrous apex to the anterior clinoid process. The medial margin is formed by the intraclinoid dural fold, which extends from the anterior to the posterior clinoid. The supratrochlear triangle is situated between the lower surface of the oculomotor nerve and the upper surface of the trochlear nerve, and has a line joining the points of entrance of these nerves into the dura as its third margin. This triangle is very narrow. The infratrochlear triangle (Parkinson's triangle) is located between the lower margin of the trochlear nerve and the upper margin of the ophthalmic nerve, and has a third margin formed by a line connecting the point of entry of the trochlear nerve into the dura to the site where the trigeminal nerve enters Meckel's cave. The posterior bend of the carotid artery and the origin of the meningohypophyseal trunk are located in this triangle. The middle fossa triangles are the anteromedial, anterolateral, posterolateral, and the posteromedial triangles. The anteromedial triangle is situated between the lower margin of the ophthalmic and the upper margin of the maxillary nerves, and has a third edge formed by a line connecting the point where the ophthalmic nerve passes through the superior orbital fissure and the maxillary nerve passes through the foramen rotundum. Removing bone in the medial wall of this triangle will create an opening into the sphenoid sinus. The anterolateral triangle is located between the lower surface of the maxillary nerve, the upper surface of the mandibular nerve, and a line connecting the foramen ovale and rotundum. Opening the bone in the medial wall of this triangle exposes the sphenoid sinus. The posterolateral triangle (Glasscock's triangle) is formed on the anterolateral side by the lateral surface of the mandibular nerve distal to the point at which the greater petrosal nerve crosses below the lateral surface of the trigeminal nerve, and on the posterolateral side is formed by the anterior margin of the greater petrosal nerve. This triangle encompasses the floor of the middle cranial fossa between these two structures. The middle meningeal artery passes through the foramen spinosum in this triangle. Opening the floor of the middle fossa in this triangle exposes the infratemporal fossa. The posteromedial triangle (Kawase's triangle) is located between the greater petrosal nerve and the lateral edge of the trigeminal nerve behind the point where the greater petrosal nerve passes below the lateral edge of the trigeminal nerve, and a line along the connecting hiatus falopi to the dural ostium of Meckel's cave. The petrous carotid crosses the anterior margin of this triangle. The cochlea is located below the floor of the middle fossa in the lateral apex of the triangle. Drilling the bony floor of the triangle in the area behind the internal carotid artery and medial to the cochlea exposes the lateral edge of the clivus. The paraclival triangles are the inferomedial and inferolateral triangles. The inferolateral paraclival triangle is located on the posterior surface of the clivus and temporal bone. The medial margin is formed by a line connecting the dural entry sites of the trochlear and abducens nerves; the upper margin extends from the dural entrance of the trochlear nerve to the point at which the first petrosal vein lateral to Meckel's cave joins the superior petrosal sinus (removed); and the lower margin is formed by a line connecting the point at which the abducens nerve enters the dura to the site at which the first petrosal vein, lateral to the trigeminal nerve, joins the superior petrosal sinus. The porus, through which the posterior trigeminal root enters Meckel's cave, is situated in the center of the inferolateral paraclival triangle. The inferomedial paraclival triangle is formed above by a line extending from the posterior clinoid process to the dural entrance of the trochlear nerve, laterally by a line connecting the dural* *(Legend continues on next page.)*

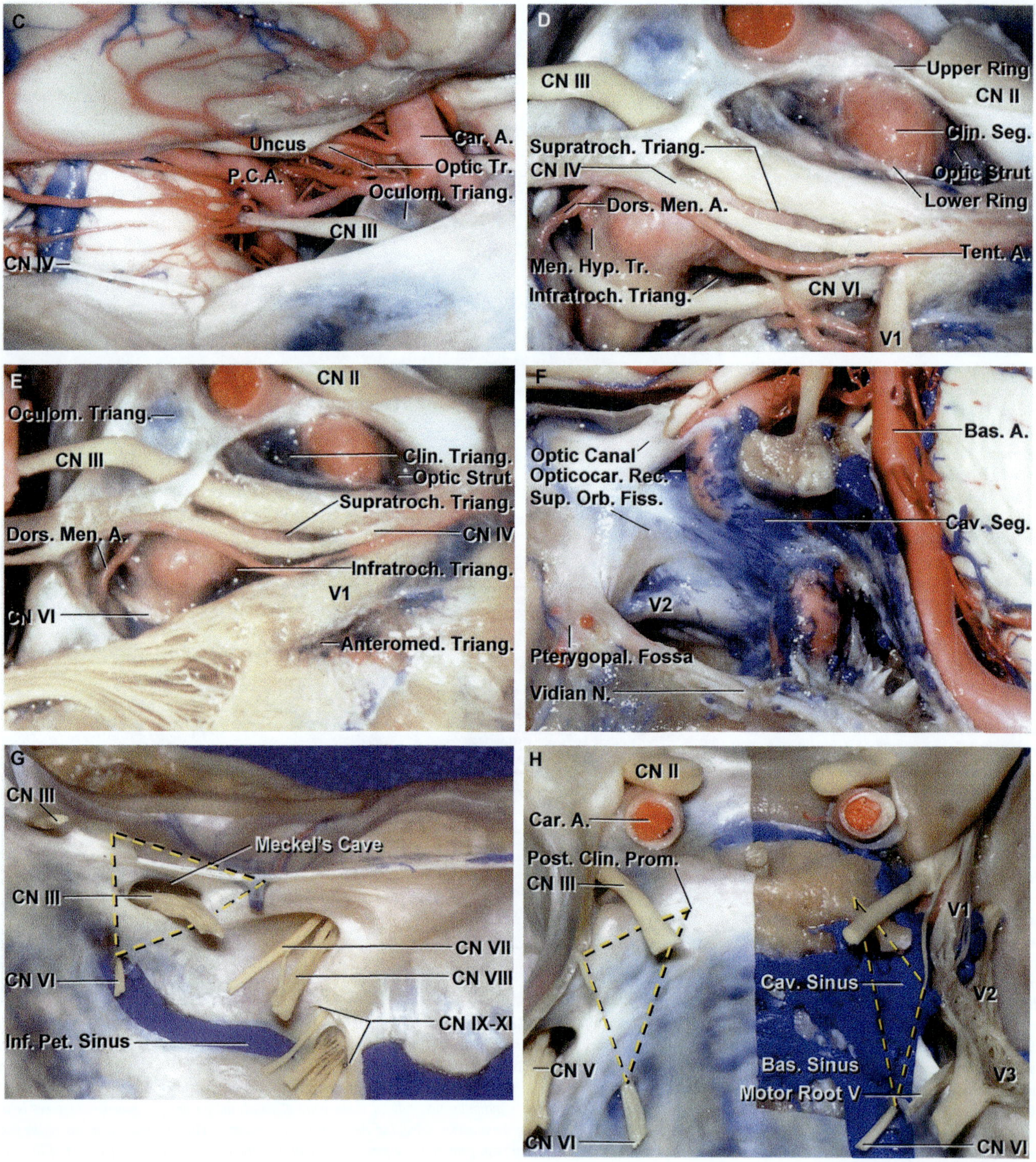

FIGURE 9.5. *Continued*

entrances of the trochlear and abducens nerves, and medially by a line extending from the dural entrance of the abducens nerve to the posterior clinoid process. The dura in this triangle forms the posterior wall of cavernous sinus. C, lateral view of the parasellar area and the oculomotor triangle. The temporal lobe has been elevated to expose the oculomotor and trochlear nerves as they enter the roof of the cavernous sinus. The oculomotor triangle is the triangular patch of dura through which the oculomotor nerve enters the roof of the cavernous sinus. The optic tract passes backward on the medial side of the uncus. D, enlarged view of the clinoidal, oculomotor, supratrochlear, and infratrochlear cavernous sinus triangles. The optic strut is exposed in the anterior part of the clinoidal triangle, the clinoid segment is exposed in the midportion and the roof of the cavernous sinus is exposed in the posterior part. The upper margin of the clinoid segment is surrounded by the upper dural ring, which is formed by the dura extending medially from the upper surface of the anterior clinoid. The lower margin of the clinoid segment is defined by the lower dural ring, which is formed by the dura extending medially from the course in the inner part of the lateral sinus wall. The abducens courses medial to the ophthalmic nerve and is adherent to the lateral surface of the intracavernous carotid medially, but it also is adherent laterally to the medial surface of the ophthalmic nerve and the inner part of the lateral sinus wall.

The oculomotor nerve pierces the roof of the cavernous sinus near the center of the oculomotor triangle, and the IVth nerve enters the dura at the posterolateral edge of the triangle. A short length of both trochlear and oculomotor nerves are surrounded by a dural and arachnoid cuff to create the oculomotor and trochlear cisterns as they pass through the roof of the cavernous sinus and below the anterior clinoid process. Both nerves are situated medial to and slightly beneath the level of the free edge of the tentorium at their point of entry.

The oculomotor nerve enters the cavernous sinus slightly lateral and anterior to the dorsum sellae, almost directly above the origin of the meningohypophyseal trunk from the intracavernous carotid, and courses along the lower margin of the anterior clinoid and the carotidoculomotor membrane. The oculomotor nerve pierces the sinus roof between 2 and 7 mm posterior to the initial supraclinoid segment of the carotid artery; the average separation is 5 mm (6).

The trochlear nerve enters the roof of the sinus posterolateral to the IIIrd nerve and courses below the oculomotor nerve in the posterior part of the lateral wall. Anteriorly, below the base of the anterior clinoid process, it passes upward along the lateral surface of the oculomotor nerve. From there, the trochlear nerve passes medially between the oculomotor nerve and dura lining the lower margin of the anterior clinoid and optic strut to reach the medial part of the orbit and the superior oblique muscle.

The ophthalmic nerve is the smallest of the three trigeminal divisions. It is inclined upward as it passes forward near the medial surface of the dura, forming the lower part of the lateral wall of the cavernous sinus, to reach the superior orbital fissure. It is flattened in the wall of the cavernous sinus, but at the superior orbital fissure, it takes on an oval configuration. The ophthalmic nerve splits into the lacrimal, frontal, and nasociliary nerves as it approaches the superior orbital fissure.

The superior petrosal sinus passes above the posterior root of the trigeminal root to form the upper margin of the ostium of Meckel's cave, the dural and subarachnoid cavern, which communicates with the subarachnoid space in the posterior fossa (*Figs. 9.1* and *9.8*). The cave extends forward around the posterior trigeminal root to the midportion of the ganglion. The motor root of the trigeminal nerve courses on the medial side of the sensory fibers at the level of Meckel's cave (*Fig. 9.7*).

The abducens nerve pierces the dura forming the lower part of the posterior wall of the sinus at the upper border of the petrous apex and enters a dural cave, referred to as Dorello's canal, where it passes below the petrosphenoid ligament (Gruber's ligament) that extends from the lower part of the lateral edge of the dorsum sellae to the petrous apex, to enter the cavernous sinus (*Figs. 9.1, 9.7,* and *9.8*). The nerve bends laterally around the proximal portion of the intercavernous carotid and gently ascends as it passes forward inside the cavernous sinus medial to the ophthalmic nerve, on the lateral side of the internal carotid artery, and below and medial to the nasociliary nerve. It has the most medial site of entry of the nerves coursing in the sinus wall and maintains that position in its course through the sinus. The nerve usually enters the sinus as a single bundle, but may persist as two bundles in the subarachnoid space. After entering the sinus, it may split into as many as five rootlets as it courses between the internal carotid artery and ophthalmic nerve. In a study of 50 sinuses, the intracavernous segment of the nerve consisted of a single rootlet in 34 specimens, two rootlets in 13, three rootlets in 2, and five rootlets in 1 specimen (6).

Sympathetic fiber bundles large enough to be recognized without a surgical microscope travel on the surface of the carotid as it emerges from the foramen lacerum. Some of the bundles join the VIth nerve within the sinus before ultimately being distributed to the first trigeminal division, which sends sympathetic fibers that reach the pupillodilator through the

lower margin of the anterior clinoid. The dura on the lower margin of the anterior clinoid, referred to as the carotidoculomotor membrane, separates the lower surface of the anterior clinoid from the upper surface of the oculomotor nerve and extends medially to form the lower dural ring. The posterior bend of the internal carotid artery and the origin of the meningohypophyseal trunk, which gives rise to the tentorial and dorsal meningeal arteries, are exposed in the infratrochlear triangle. The abducens nerve passes through Dorello's canal and between the lateral surface of the intracavernous carotid and the medial side of the ophthalmic nerve. The inferolateral trunk arises from the horizontal segment of the intracavernous carotid and passes above the abducens nerve. E *and* F, *side by side comparison of medial and lateral aspects of the cavernous sinus.* E, *lateral view of cavernous sinus.* F, *view, through the sphenoid sinus, of the medial side of the cavernous sinus. The optic nerve is exposed at the upper margin of the clinoidal triangle and above the optic strut. On the sphenoid sinus side of the specimen, the optic canal is seen above the opticocarotid recess, which leads into the optic strut. The clinoid segment rests against the posterior aspect of the optic strut in both views. In the lateral view, the superior orbital fissure through which the ophthalmic, trochlear, abducens nerves pass is seen below the optic strut. In the view through the sphenoid sinus, the medial edge of the superior orbital fissure produces a wide rounded prominence below the optic strut, and the maxillary nerve produces a prominence in the lower part of the sphenoid sinus just distal to the foramen rotundum. The lateral wing of the sphenoid sinus extends laterally under the maxillary nerve into the medial part of the floor of the middle fossa. Opening the middle fossa floor in the anteromedial and anterolateral triangles exposes the sphenoid sinus.* G, *posterior view of the inferolateral triangle. The medial edge of the inferolateral triangle extends between the dural entrances of the IVth and VIth nerves. The inferior limb extends from the VIth nerve to where the first vein lateral to Meckel's cave joins the superior petrosal sinus and the superior limb extends from that vein to the dural entrance of the IVth nerve. The ostium of Meckel's cave is located within the inferolateral triangle.* H, *posterior view of the inferomedial triangles. The medial limb of the inferomedial triangle extends from the posterior clinoid to the dural entrance to the abducens nerve. The lateral limb extends between the dural entrances of the IVth and VIth nerves and the superior limb extends from the IVth nerve to the posterior clinoid. On the right side, there is an abnormal projection of the posterior clinoid process, which extends below the oculomotor nerve toward the petrous apex.* A., *artery;* Anterolat., *anterolateral;* Anteromed., *anteromedial;* Bas., *basilar;* Car., *carotid;* Cav., *cavernous;* Clin., *clinoid;* CN, *cranial nerve;* Dors., *dorsal;* Fiss., *fissure;* Gr., *greater;* Inf., *inferior;* Infratroch., *infratrochlear;* Men., *meningeal;* Men. Hyp., *meningohypophyseal;* N., *nerve;* Oculom., *oculomotor;* Opticocar., *opticocarotid;* Orb., *orbital;* P.C.A., *posterior cerebral artery;* Pet., *petrosal;* Post., *posterior;* Posterolat., *posterolateral;* Posteromed., *posteromedial;* Prom., *prominence;* Pterygopal., *pterygopalatine;* Rec., *recess;* S.C.A., *superior cerebellar artery;* Seg., *segment;* Sup., *superior;* Supratroch., *supratrochlear;* Tent., *tentorial;* Tr., *tract, trunk;* Triang., *triangle.*

long ciliary nerves and by passing through the ciliary ganglion (8, 12). Some sympathetic fibers pass directly from the carotid plexus to the ciliary ganglion and others may travel along the ophthalmic artery to the globe (23).

CAVERNOUS SINUS AND MIDDLE FOSSA TRIANGLES

Parkinson (13) described a triangle within the lateral wall of the cavernous sinus through which the intracavernous portion of the carotid artery and its branches might be exposed for the surgical treatment of carotid-cavernous fistulae (*Fig. 9.5*). Since his pioneering work, a number of significant triangular relationships formed by the convergence and divergence of the cranial nerves in the region of the cavernous sinus and middle fossa have been defined. There are four triangles in the cavernous sinus, four middle fossae lateral to the cavernous sinus, and two fossae in the paraclival area that are helpful in understanding and planning approaches to the cavernous sinus. The cavernous sinus triangles are formed by the optic, oculomotor, trochlear, and ophthalmic nerves converging on the optic canal and superior orbital fissure. The middle fossa triangles are formed by the trigeminal divisions diverging as they pass from the gasserian ganglion to reach their foramina (17).

Cavernous Sinus Triangles

Clinoidal Triangle

This triangle is situated in the interval between the optic and oculomotor nerves. This triangle is exposed by removing the anterior clinoid process. The optic strut is in the anterior part, the clinoid segment of the internal carotid artery is in the midportion, and the thin roof of the cavernous sinus is in the posterior part of this triangle.

Oculomotor Triangle

This triangle is formed by the triangular patch of dura through which the oculomotor nerve enters the roof of the cavernous sinus. Two margins of this triangle are formed by the anterior and posterior petroclinoidal dural folds that extend, respectively, from the anterior and posterior clinoid processes to the petrous apex. The third side is formed by the interclinoidal dural fold that extends from the anterior to the posterior clinoid process.

Supratrochlear Triangle

This triangle is situated between the lower surface of the oculomotor nerve and the upper surface of the trochlear nerve. A line joining the points of entrance of these nerves into the dura forms the third margin. This triangle is very narrow.

Infratrochlear Triangle (Parkinson's Triangle)

This triangle is located between the lower margin of the trochlear nerve and the upper margin of the ophthalmic nerve. The third margin is formed by a line connecting the point of entry of the trochlear nerve into the dura to the site where the trigeminal nerve enters Meckel's cave. The posterior bend of the internal carotid artery and the origin of the meningohypophyseal trunk from the posterior bend are located in this triangle, except when the carotid artery is elongated and tortuous. In that case, the origin may be pushed upward into the oculomotor triangle. Parkinson (12–14) first described the surgical exposure of the intercavernous portion of the carotid artery through this triangle for the treatment of carotid-cavernous fistulas. In an earlier study, we found that the superior margin of the triangle formed by the lower margin of the IVth nerve averaged 13 mm (range, 8–20 mm); the inferior margin formed by the upper margin of the Vth cranial nerve

FIGURE 9.6. *Stepwise dissection of the carotid collar.* A, *lateral view of the paraclinoidal area. The anterior clinoid process projects backward from its base on the lesser wing. The carotid artery passes upward, and the optic nerve enters the optic canal on the medial side of the anterior clinoid. The origin of the ophthalmic artery bulges upward, below the optic nerve. The oculomotor nerve enters the roof of the cavernous sinus and passes along the lower margin of the anterior clinoid process.* B, *the anterior clinoid and the bone forming the roof and lateral wall of the optic canal have been removed. The clinoid segment of the internal carotid artery is located in the medial wall of the space created by removal of the anterior clinoid. The dura that covers the medial and lower surfaces of the anterior clinoid has been preserved. The layer of dura that covers the medial side of the anterior clinoid forms the lateral part of the carotid collar. The upper surface of the optic strut forms the floor of the optic canal. The anterior wall of the clinoid segment rests against the posterior surface of the optic strut. The dura lining the upper and lower surfaces of the optic strut extends backward to form the anterior part of the upper and lower dural rings and the dura lining the posterior surface of the strut forms the anterior part of the carotid collar. The falciform ligament is a dural fold, which extends above the optic nerve at the posterior edge of the optic canal.* C, *enlarged view of the lateral aspect of the carotid collar and optic strut. The anterior surface of the clinoid segment rests against the posterior surface of the optic strut. This strut is triangular in cross section. The upper surface of the optic strut, which forms of the lower margin of the optic canal, slopes forward and downward from its intracranial edge. The lower surface of the optic strut forms part of the upper margin of the superior orbital fissure. The posterior surface of the optic strut is contoured to accommodate the anterior wall of the clinoid segment. The dura that lines the lower margin of the anterior clinoid process and extends medially above the oculomotor nerve to surround the internal carotid artery and form the lower dural ring is referred to as the carotidoculomotor membrane. The lower ring does not tightly adhere to the surface of the artery, as does the upper ring. The lower ring admits venous tributaries of the cavernous sinus, referred to as the clinoid venous plexus, which course between the clinoid segment and the carotid collar and can be seen through the collar. Thus, the clinoid segment of the internal carotid artery, which was once considered to lie outside the cavernous sinus, is partially surrounded by the venous tributaries of the cavernous sinus.* D, *the optic strut has been removed. The layer of dura that lines the posterior surface of the optic strut forms the anterior part of the carotid collar. The medial end of the strut attaches to the body of the sphenoid bone immediately in front of the carotid sulcus. In some cases, the interior of the optic strut is aerated by a lateral extension of the sphenoid sinus, which may also extend through the strut into the anterior clinoid. The dura lining the lower margin of the anterior clinoid, which forms the carotidoculomotor membrane, also forms the most anterior portion of the roof of the cavernous sinus. The venous channels of the cavernous sinus extend upward between the carotid collar and the clinoid segment. The layers of dura lining the upper and lower surfaces of the clinoid process come together at the posterior tip of the anterior clinoid.* E, *the outer layer of dura in the lateral wall of the cavernous*

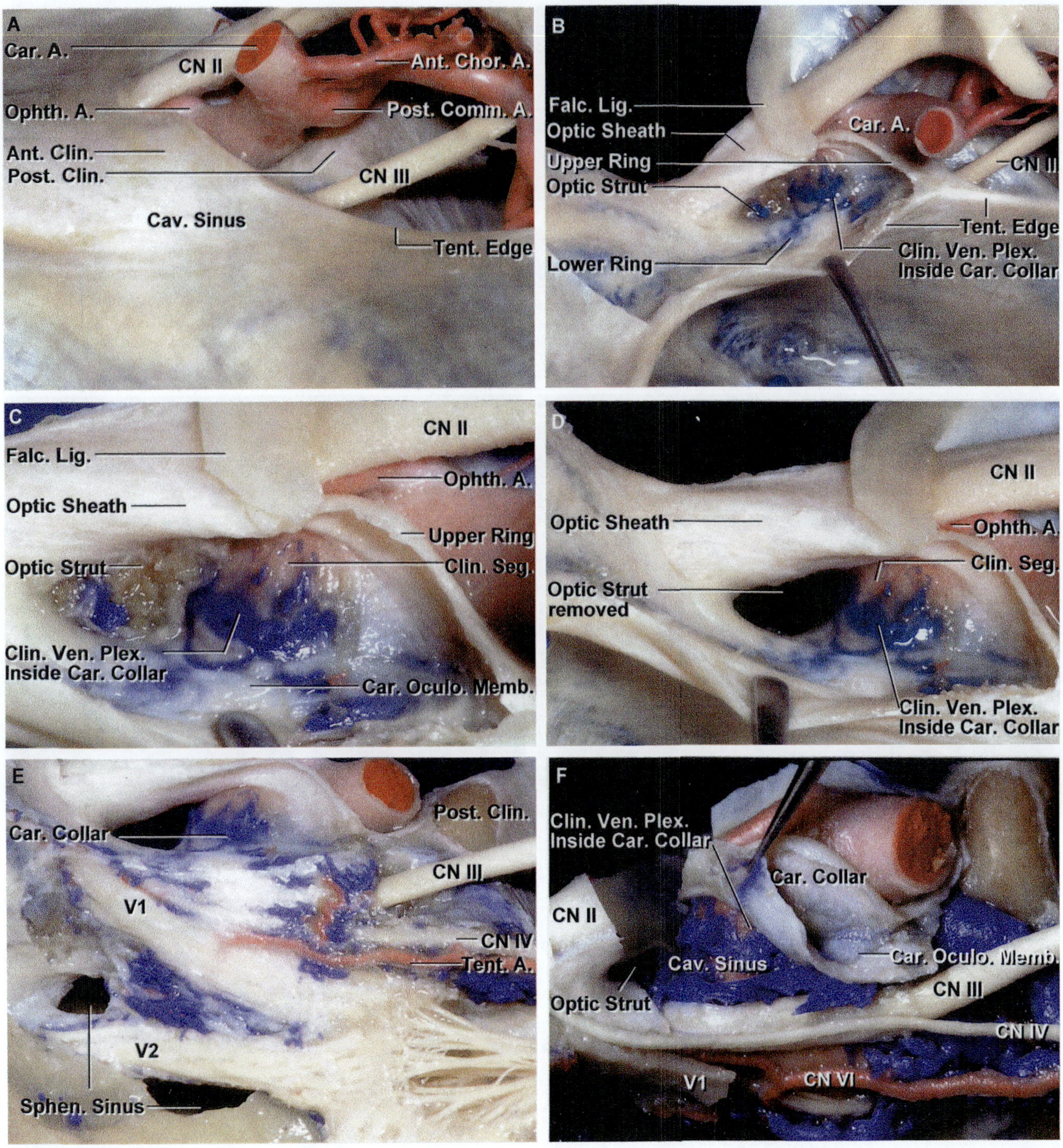

FIGURE 9.6. *Continued*
sinus has been removed to expose the trigeminal, oculomotor, and trochlear nerves, which are enmeshed in the inner layer of dura. The maxillary strut, the bridge of bone located between the superior orbital fissure and the foramen rotundum, has been removed. The oculomotor and trochlear nerves course on the lower surface of the carotid-oculomotor membrane. A tentorial artery passes above the ophthalmic nerve. The openings created by removal of the optic and maxillary struts and the bone below the maxillary nerve open into the sphenoid sinus. F, *the segment of the optic nerve that courses above the optic strut has been removed. The carotidoculomotor membrane has been separated from the oculomotor nerve and folded upward to expose the tributaries of the cavernous sinus, which course between the carotid collar and the clinoid segment, and extend upward to near the upper ring.* G, *the trigeminal, oculomotor, and trochlear nerves have been removed and the abducens nerve preserved. The dura forming the carotid collar has been folded upward after dividing the collar beginning below at the level of the lower dural ring and extending upward to just below the upper ring. The inferolateral trunk, a branch of the intracavernous carotid, passes above the abducens nerve. (Legend continues on next page.)*

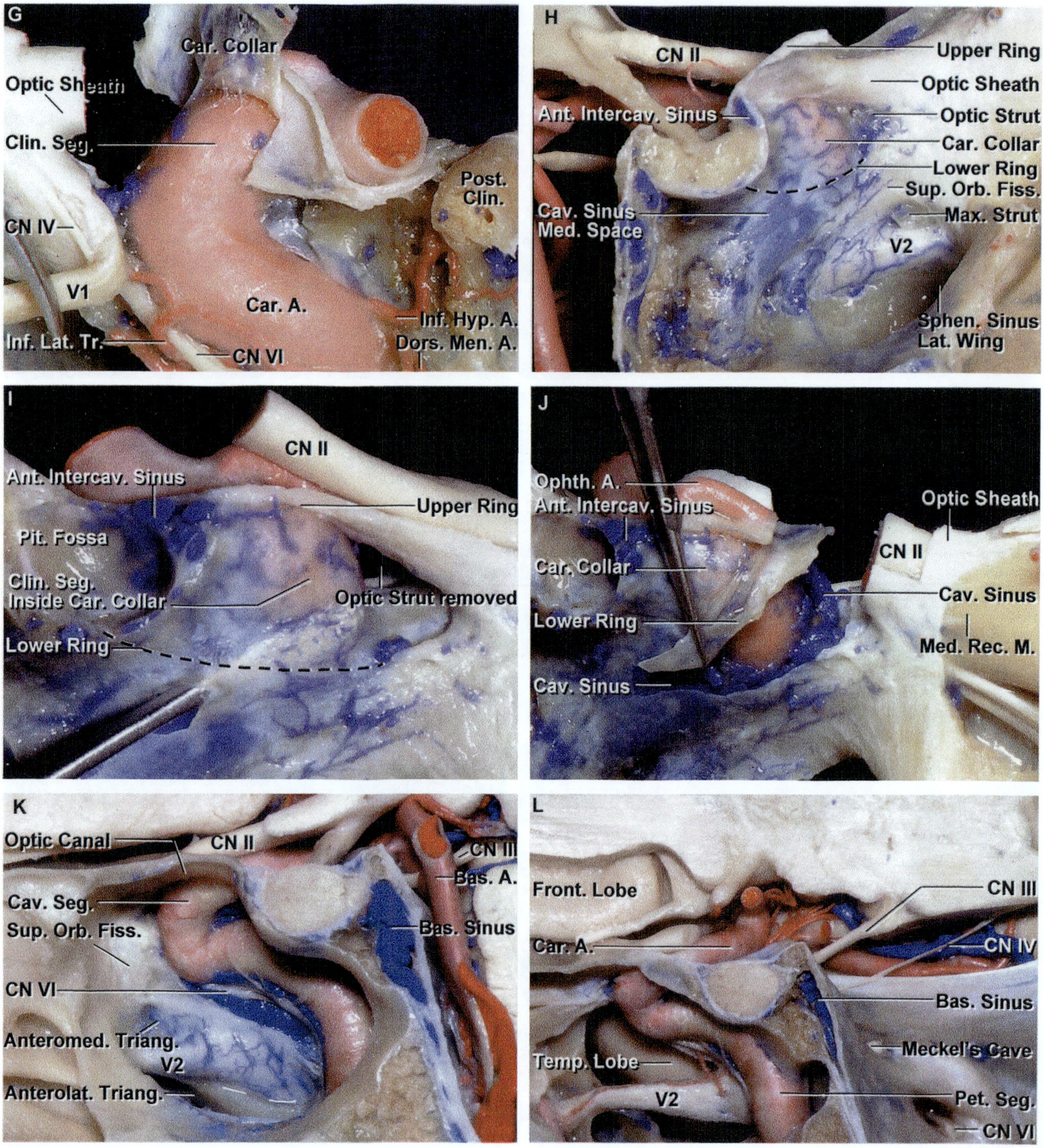

FIGURE 9.6. *Continued*

The tentorial artery arises from the inferolateral trunk, and the inferior hypophyseal artery arises directly from the internal carotid artery rather than from the meningohypophyseal artery, which is absent in this case. H, *the bone and mucosa in the lateral wall of the sphenoid sinus have been removed to expose the dura that forms the medial wall of the cavernous sinus. The optic canal and optic sheath are located in the superolateral margin of the sphenoid sinus. The optic strut forms the floor of the optic canal and separates the lower margin of the optic canal from the upper margin of the superior orbital fissure. The maxillary nerve crosses along the midportion of the lateral wall of the sphenoid sinus and is separated from the superior orbital fissure by the maxillary strut, a narrow bridge of bone between the fissure and the foramen rotundum. The medial aspect of the superior orbital fissure produces a bulge in the lateral wall of the sphenoid sinus between the optic and maxillary struts. The intracavernous carotid can be seen through the dura in the area behind the optic strut. The medial side of the carotid collar, which extends around the medial side of the artery in the area behind the optic strut, is not as well defined and is wider than on the lateral side of the artery. The lower* averaged 14 mm (range, 5–24 mm); and the posterior margin represented by the slope of the dorsum and clivus averaged 6 mm (range, 3–14 mm). The average triangle measured 13 × 14 × 6 mm; however, it could be very small, measuring only 8 × 5 × 3 mm, and it may not be large enough to provide a good surgical exposure of all of the arterial branches within the sinus (6). Parkinson (12), through an incision starting 4 mm beneath the dural entrance of the IIIrd nerve and extending anteriorly approximately 2 cm parallel to the slope of the IIIrd and IVth nerves, exposed the meningohypophyseal trunk and the artery of the inferior cavernous sinus. The VIth nerve at the bottom edge of the exposure was seen on retracting the superior aspect of the trigeminal nerve. The most anterior aspect of the cavernous carotid was not seen through this exposure unless the carotid artery was grasped and pulled backward. Parkinson thought that the triangle would provide access to most spontaneous fistulas, assuming that they are due to ruptured aneurysms developing at the point of departure of the meningohypophyseal trunk or artery of the inferior cavernous sinus.

Middle Fossa Triangles

Anteromedial Middle Fossa Triangle

This triangle is situated between the lower margin of the ophthalmic and the upper margin of the maxillary nerves. The third edge is formed by a line connecting the point where the ophthalmic nerve passes through the superior orbital fissure and the maxillary nerve passes through the foramen rotundum (*Fig. 9.5*). Removing bone in the triangular space between the ophthalmic or maxillary nerve opens into the sphenoid sinus.

Anterolateral Middle Fossa Triangle

This triangle is located between the lower surface of the maxillary nerve, the upper surface of the mandibular nerve, and a line connecting the foramen ovale and rotundum. Opening the bone in the medial wall of this triangle exposes the lateral wing of the sphenoid sinus.

Posterolateral Middle Fossa Triangle (Glasscock's Triangle)

This triangle is formed on the anteromedial side by the lateral surface of the mandibular nerve distal to the point at which the greater petrosal nerve crosses below the lateral surface of the trigeminal nerve. On the posterolateral side, it is formed by the anterior margin of the greater petrosal nerve. This triangle opens laterally to encompasses the floor of the middle cranial fossa between these two structures. The middle meningeal artery passes through the foramen spinosum in this triangle. Opening the floor of the middle fossa in this triangle exposes the infratemporal fossa.

Posteromedial Middle Fossa Triangle (Kawase's Triangle)

This triangle is located between the greater petrosal nerve, and the lateral edge of the trigeminal nerve behind the point where the greater petrosal nerve passes below its lateral surface, and a line along the connecting hiatus fallopii to the dural ostium of Meckel's cave. The petrous segment of the internal carotid artery crosses the anterior margin of this triangle. The cochlea is located below the floor of the middle fossa in the lateral apex of the triangle. Removing the bone in the lateral

margin of the collar on the medial side of the clinoid segment is located at approximately the level of the broken line *extending from the lower margin of the optic strut to the floor of the sella. The small venous channels within the collar can be seen through the dura. The anterior intracavernous sinus courses at the posterior margin of the upper dural ring. The lateral wing of the sphenoid sinus extends below the maxillary nerve and below the middle fossa floor.* I, *the optic strut has been removed. A small opening in the dura admits a probe that has been passed forward between the dura and the internal carotid artery along the lower margin of the carotid collar. The dura that lines the upper surface of the optic strut and the lower part of the optic sheath is continuous posteriorly with the upper ring. The lower margin of the collar is located at approximately the level of the* broken line *extending from the lower margin of the optic strut to the floor of the sella.* J, *the segment of the optic nerve coursing above the optic strut has been removed, but the segment passing through the annular tendon, from which the rectus muscles arise, has been preserved. The dura has been opened along the margin of the lower ring to expose the venous spaces within the cavernous sinus which extend upward inside the carotid collar. The venous spaces inside the envelope of the cavernous sinus increase in size in the area below the collar.* K *and* L, *medial aspect of another cavernous sinus on the right side.* K, *the bone in the lateral wall of the sphenoid sinus has been removed to expose the medial aspect of the optic canal, superior orbital fissure, the prominence over the maxillary nerve, and the middle fossa dura. The dura in the medial wall of the cavernous sinus has been removed to expose the intercavernous carotid and the abducens nerve. The lower margin of the cavernous sinus is marked with* yellow arrows *and is located below the intracavernous segment of the carotid and the abducens nerve. The optic canal and opticocarotid recess are located above the superior orbital fissure and anterior bend of the cavernous carotid. The prominence of the superior orbital fissure is located below the opticocarotid recess. Another recess extends laterally into the maxillary strut, the bridge of bone that separates the superior orbital fissure and the foramen rotundum. The maxillary nerve produces a prominence in the lateral wall of the sphenoid sinus below which is located the lateral wing of the sphenoid, which extends below the floor of the middle fossa in the region of the anterolateral triangle. The basilar sinus is the largest connection across the midline between the cavernous sinuses.* L, *the middle fossa dura, lateral to the sphenoid sinus and between the superior orbital fissure and maxillary nerve, has been opened to expose the medial aspect of the temporal lobe. Bone has been removed below the maxillary nerve to expose the floor of the middle fossa below the temporal lobe. The optic, oculomotor, and trochlear nerves and the internal carotid artery are exposed above the sella.* A., *artery;* Ant., *anterior;* Anterolat., *anterolateral;* Anteromed., *anteromedial;* Bas., *basilar;* Car., *carotid;* Car. Oculo., *carotidoculomotor;* Cav., *cavernous;* Chor., *choroid;* Clin., *clinoid;* CN, *cranial nerve;* Comm., *communicating;* Dors., *dorsal;* Falc., *falciform;* Fiss., *fissure;* Front., *frontal;* Hyp., *hypophyseal;* Inf., *inferior;* Inf. Lat., *inferolateral;* Intercav., *intercavernous;* Lat., *lateral;* Lig., *ligament;* M., *muscle;* Max., *maxillary;* Med., *medial;* Memb., *membrane;* Men., *meningeal;* Ophth., *ophthalmic;* Orb., *orbital;* Pet., *petrous;* Pit., *pituitary;* Plex., *plexus;* Post., *posterior;* Rec., *rectus;* Seg., *segment;* Sphen., *sphenoid;* Sup., *superior;* Temp., *temporal;* Tent., *tentorial;* Tr., *trunk;* Ven., *venous.*

part of the posteromedial triangle exposes the cochlea and the anterior wall of the internal auditory canal, and removing the bone in the medial part of the posteromedial triangle exposes the side of the clivus and the inferior petrosal sinus. The approach directed through the temporal bone in this triangle is referred to as an anterior petrosectomy.

Paraclinoid Triangles

Inferolateral Paraclival Triangle

This triangle is located on the posterior surface of the clivus and temporal bone (*Fig. 9.5*). The medial margin is formed by a line connecting the dural entry sites of the trochlear and abducens nerves; the upper margin extends from the dural entrance of the trochlear nerve to the point at which the first petrosal vein lateral to Meckel's cave joins the superior petrosal sinus; and the lower margin is formed by a line connecting the point at which the abducens nerve enters the dura to the site at which the first petrosal vein, lateral to the trigeminal nerve, joins the superior petrosal sinus. The porus through which the posterior trigeminal root enters Meckel's cave is situated in the center of the inferolateral paraclival triangle.

Inferomedial Paraclival Triangle

This triangle is formed above by a line extending from the posterior clinoid process to the dural entrance of the trochlear nerve; laterally by a line connecting the dural entrances of the trochlear and abducens nerves; and medially by a line extending from the dural entrance of the abducens nerve to the posterior clinoid process. The abducens nerve enters the cavernous sinus at the lower edge of this triangle. This triangle extends along the posterior sinus wall. Removing the medial part of the inferomedial triangle behind the internal carotid artery exposes the lateral edge of the dorsum sellae, the upper end of the petroclival suture, and the VIth nerve passing below Gruber's ligament.

ARTERIAL RELATIONSHIPS

The internal carotid artery exits the foramen lacerum lateral to the posterior clinoid process where it passes under the petrolingual ligament and turns abruptly forward to course along the carotid sulcus and lateral part of the body of the sphenoid. It passes forward in a horizontal direction for approximately 2 cm and terminates by passing upward along the medial side to the anterior clinoid process and the posterior surface of the optic strut where it penetrates the roof of the cavernous sinus. The clinoid segment of the carotid artery is tightly surrounded by the anterior clinoid process laterally, the optic strut anteriorly, and the carotid sulcus medially, leaving only a narrow space between the bone and artery (*Figs. 9.1, 9.5,* and *9.6*). The dura lining the surface of these osseous structures facing the clinoid segment forms the carotid collar around the clinoid segment. The intracavernous carotid is relatively fixed by the bony ring, but despite this, large extensions of pituitary tumor may produce lateral displacement of the artery.

Just proximal to the cavernous sinus in the foramen lacerum the artery lies beneath the trigeminal nerve (6). In surgical approaches to the trigeminal nerve directed through the middle cranial fossa, there is a tendency to assume that the carotid artery is distant from the trigeminal nerve. However, nearly 85% of carotid arteries are exposed under some portion of Meckel's cave and the trigeminal nerve with only dura, and no bone, separating the nerve from the artery (*Figs. 9.1* and *9.5*) (6). In the remainder, the bone separating the nerve and artery is often paper-thin. The absence of bone over the carotid often extends to the lateral edge of the trigeminal nerve and, in more than a third, the bone covering the carotid is defective lateral to the edge of the third division. The maximum length of artery exposed lateral to the nerve was 7 mm in our study.

The branches of the intracavernous carotid are the meningohypophyseal trunk, the largest branch, present in 100% of our specimens; the artery of the inferior cavernous sinus, present in 84%; and McConnell's capsular arteries, present in 28% (*Fig. 9.1*). Less frequent branches of the intracavernous carotid were the ophthalmic artery (8%) and the dorsal meningeal artery (6%) (6).

Ophthalmic Artery

The ophthalmic artery commonly arises just above the upper ring from the medial half of the anterior wall of the internal carotid artery (*Figs. 9.1* and *9.6–9.8*). From its origin, it runs anteriorly and laterally on the upper surface of the optic strut and below the optic nerve. It runs freely above the optic strut inside the posterior part of the optic canal, but anteriorly it pierces the dura on the upper surface of the optic strut and exits the optic canal outside the optic sheath to course on the inferolateral aspect of the optic nerve and sheath at the orbital apex. The ophthalmic artery may also arise in the cavernous sinus or from the clinoid segment, in which case it usually passes through the superior orbital fissure. It may rarely arise from the middle meningeal artery (10).

Intracavernous Branches

The meningohypophyseal trunk, the most proximal intracavernous branch, arises lateral to the dorsum sellae at or just before the apex of the first curve of the intracavernous carotid where it turns forward after leaving the foramen lacerum (*Figs. 9.1* and *9.8*). It is approximately the same size as the ophthalmic artery. The IIIrd and IVth nerves enter the dural roof of the cavernous sinus just above or slightly behind the trifurcation of the meningohypophyseal trunk. The meningohypophyseal trunk divides near the roof of the cavernous sinus and typically gives rise to three branches: 1) the tentorial artery, also called the artery of Bernasconi-Cassinari, which courses lateral to the tentorium; 2) the inferior hypophyseal, which travels medially to supply the posterior pituitary capsule; and 3) the dorsal meningeal artery, which enters the dura of the posterior sinus wall and supplies the clival dura and VIth nerve. The artery of the inferior cavernous sinus, also called the inferolateral trunk, may infrequently arise from the meningohypophyseal trunk (6).

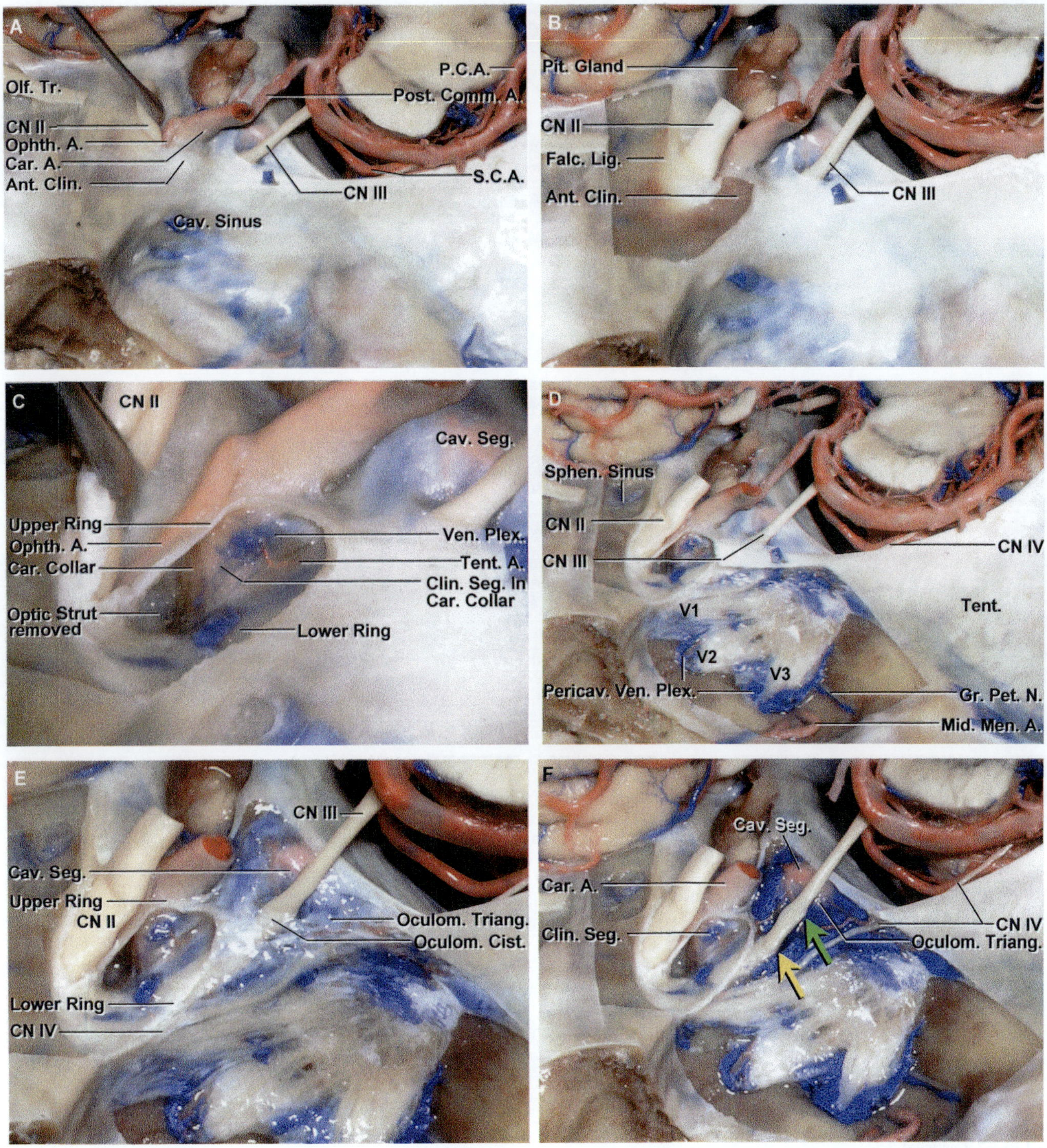

FIGURE 9.7. *Intradural approach to the cavernous sinus. A, this is the dissection that the participants complete in our microsurgery courses to demonstrate the intradural approach to the cavernous sinus. At this stage of the course, the cerebral hemisphere has been removed and the suprasellar area and the lateral wall of the cavernous sinus have been exposed. The optic nerve has been elevated to expose the ophthalmic artery entering the optic canal. B, the dura over the upper surface of the anterior clinoid, optic canal, and planum has been removed in preparation for anterior clinoidectomy and removal of the roof of the optic canal. The falciform ligament extends across the optic nerve just proximal to the nerve's entrance to the optic canal. C, the anterior clinoid and optic strut have been removed to expose the clinoid segment of the carotid artery enclosed in the dural carotid collar. The carotid artery, within this cavernous sinus, is quite tortuous and bulges upward medial to the oculomotor nerve to distort the roof of the sinus. Removal of the optic strut exposed the sphenoid sinus mucosa extending into the base of the strut. The carotid collar is the cuff of dura that encloses the clinoid segment between the upper and lower dural rings. The lower dural ring is loosely adherent to the artery, but the upper dural ring adheres tightly to the artery. D, a dural incision extending around the margin of the lateral wall of the cavernous sinus and the trigeminal nerve has been completed, and the outer layer of dura in the lateral sinus wall has been removed to expose the thin inner layer in which the nerves course. The pericavernous venous plexus extends around all three trigeminal* *(Legend continues on next page.)*

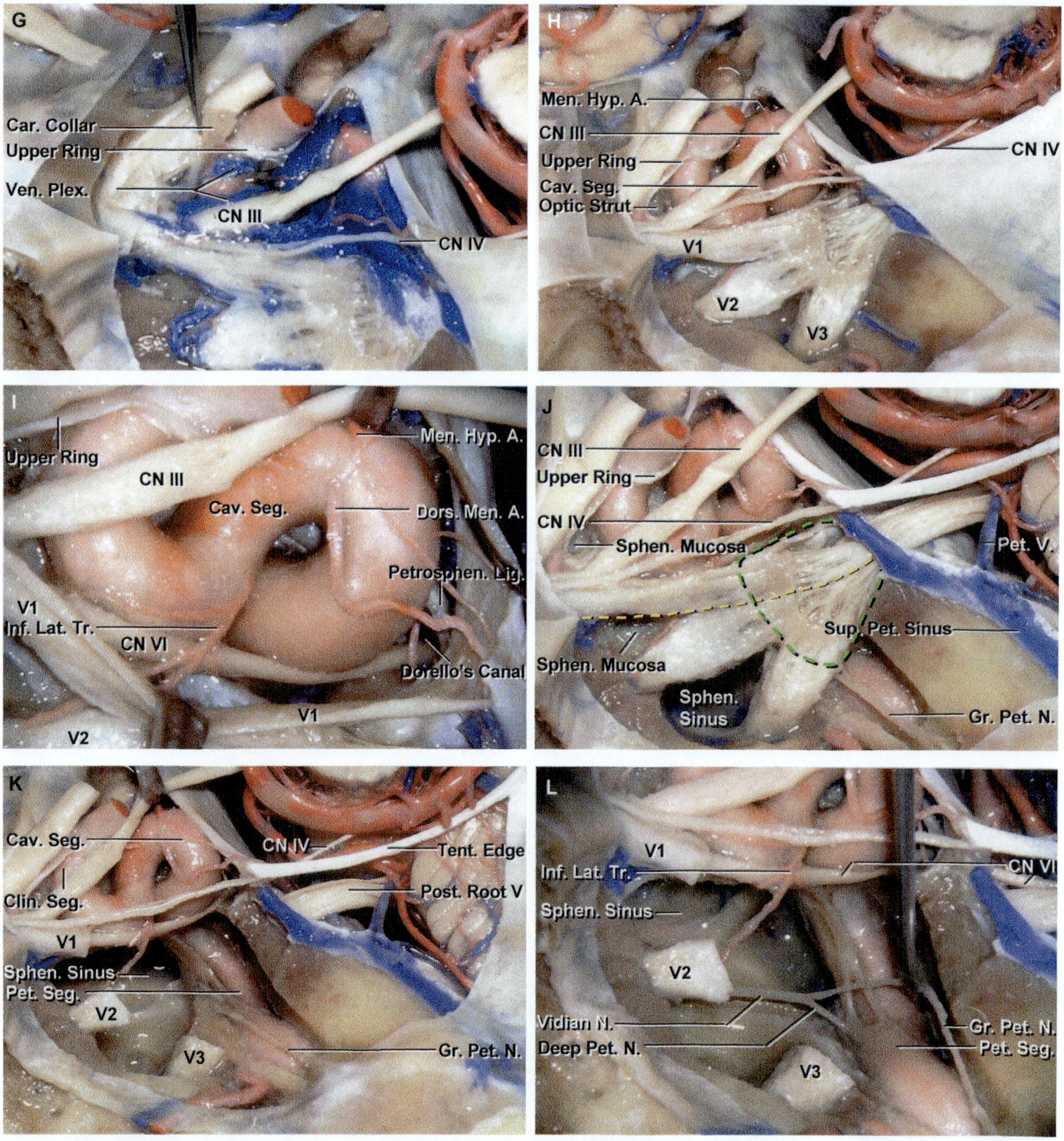

FIGURE 9.7. *Continued*
divisions. The greater petrosal nerve is exposed lateral to the trigeminal ganglion. E, the outer layer of the dural roof of sinus has been removed, while the thin layer investing the nerves has been preserved. The oculomotor nerve enters the dura through the oculomotor triangle located between the anterior and posterior clinoid processes and the petrous apex, and sits in a narrow cistern in the sinus roof that extends a variable length along the course of the nerve. The dura, which lines the lower surface of the anterior clinoid and separates the clinoid and the oculomotor nerve, referred to as the carotidoculomotor membrane, extends medially around the lower edge of the clinoid segment to form the lower dural ring. F, the thin inner layer of dura remaining over the lateral wall of the oculomotor triangle has been removed. The dura covering the lower margin of the anterior clinoid process and in the oculomotor triangle forms the roof of the cavernous sinus. The level at which the oculomotor nerve enters the oculomotor cistern is marked with a green arrow *and the level at which the cistern ends and the nerve become tightly invested by dura is shown with a* yellow arrow. *G, the dura between the upper and lower dural ring that forms the carotid collar has been separated from the internal carotid artery and folded upward to expose the thin venous plexus extending inside the carotid collar. H, the venous space surrounding the carotid artery and the trigeminal nerve has been cleared. This exposes the full course of the intracavernous carotid, which is quite tortuous and bulges upward to elevate the roof of the cavernous sinus. The upper dural ring, which is tightly adherent to the artery,*

The tentorial artery, the most constant branch of the meningohypophyseal trunk, present in 100% of instances, passes forward to the roof of the cavernous sinus and then posterolaterally along the free edge of the tentorium (*Figs. 9.5* and *9.6*). It sends branches to the IIIrd and IVth cranial nerves, and anastomoses with the meningeal branches of the ophthalmic artery and its mate of the opposite side. Bernasconi and Cassinari (2) first reported the angiographic visualization of a tentorial artery supplying tentorial meningiomas. It has a wavy appearance and ranges in length from 5 to 35 mm in normal angiograms. If longer than 40 mm, a pathological lesion, usually a tumor, is considered probable, although it may be seen angiographically in arteriovenous malformations (26).

The dorsal meningeal artery arises from the meningohypophyseal trunk in 90% of cavernous sinuses (*Figs. 9.5* and *9.8*). It passes posteriorly through the cavernous sinus with the abducent nerve to reach the dura over the dorsum and clivus. It sends a branch to the VIth cranial nerve and anastomoses with its mate of the opposite side. Six percent of dorsal meningeal arteries arise directly from the intracavernous carotid, below the meningohypophyseal trunk.

The inferior hypophyseal artery, the least frequent of the three common branches of the meningohypophyseal trunk, arises from the meningohypophyseal trunk in 80% of cavernous sinuses (6, 7). It passes medially to the posterior pituitary capsule and lobe and anastomoses with its mate of the opposite side after supplying the dura of the sellar floor. It may supply pituitary adenomas and tumors of the sphenoid sinus. It may also arise directly from the intracavernous carotid.

The inferolateral trunk (artery of the inferior cavernous sinus) arises from the lateral side of the midportion of the horizontal segment of the intracavernous carotid approximately 5 to 8 mm distal to the origin of the meningohypophyseal trunk (*Figs. 9.1* and *9.8*). It arises directly from the carotid artery in 84% of cavernous sinuses and from the meningohypophyseal artery in another 6% (6, 7). It passes above or below the VIth nerve and downward medial to the first trigeminal division to supply the dura of the inferior lateral wall of the cavernous sinus and the area of the foramina rotundum and ovale. It may anastomose with the middle meningeal artery at the foramen spinosum. Some branches pass to the trigeminal ganglion.

McConnell's capsular arteries arise from the medial side of the carotid artery and pass to the capsule of the gland or the dura lining the anterior wall and floor of the sella. They are frequently absent, being found in approximately a quarter of cavernous sinus (6). They arise approximately distal to the origin of the artery of the inferior cavernous sinus. Some run medially in the dura covering the sellar floor and the anterior lobe of the pituitary and anastomose with the branches of the inferior hypophyseal artery. Others originate just before the carotid artery pierces the dural roof of the cavernous sinus and run medially in the dura of the anterior sellar wall, anastomosing with its opposite mate (11).

The branches of the intracavernous carotid anastomose with carotid branches from the opposite side and provide an important collateral pathway in occlusion of the internal carotid artery below the cavernous sinus. These branches also enlarge and are of significance in the diagnosis and management of carotid-cavernous fistulas. The demonstration of these arteries does not necessarily indicate the presence of a lesion, but their presence should precipitate careful review of the base of the cranium and tentorium.

Parkinson (14) noted that spontaneous carotid-cavernous fistulas, which are presumed to be due to aneurysm rupture, tend to occur at the junction of one of the branches with the intracavernous carotid. Traumatic fistulas due to tears of the carotid and / or one or more of its intracavernous branches may have several sources, and are commonly located anteriorly in the sinus. Another artery, larger than the meningohypophyseal trunk, that may pass through the cavernous sinus, is a persistent trigeminal artery. This artery arises from the carotid artery in the cavernous sinus proximal to the origin of the meningohypophyseal trunk and joins the basilar artery between the superior cerebellar and anteroinferior cerebellar arteries.

Arteriovenous fistulae between the branches of the meningohypophyseal trunk, especially the dorsal meningeal branch and the basilar sinus, may produce all the signs and symptoms associated with a fistula between the internal carotid artery

extends below the optic nerve and across the upper surface of the optic strut. I, enlarged view of the intravenous carotid artery. The ophthalmic nerve has been depressed to expose the abducens nerve as it passes around the lateral margin of the carotid artery. The inferolateral trunk arises from the intracavernous carotid, passes above the VIth nerve, and gives rise to a branch that passes forward toward the foramen rotundum. The meningohypophyseal artery has been distorted by the tortuous course of the internal carotid artery. The dorsal meningeal branch of the meningohypophyseal trunk passes backward toward Dorello's canal and the clivus. The petrosphenoid ligament (Gruber's ligament) roofs Dorello's canal through which the abducens nerve enters the lower margin of the sinus. J, the lower margin of the cavernous sinus is marked with a yellow line, *and Meckel's cave, the arachnoid cistern around the trigeminal nerve, is outlined with a* green line. *The lower edge of the cavernous sinus is located medial to the junction of the upper and middle third of Meckel's cave. The bone in the anteromedial and anterolateral triangles has been opened to expose the lateral wing of the sphenoid sinus extending laterally below the trigeminal nerve. K, the trigeminal ganglion and the adjacent part of the posterior root and division have been removed to expose the petrous segment of the internal carotid artery and the lateral wing of the sphenoid sinus. L, bone has been removed in the floor of the sphenoid sinus to "unroof" the vidian canal in which the vidian nerve courses. The vidian nerve is formed by the union of the greater petrosal nerve and the deep petrosal nerve, the latter arising from the periarterial carotid plexus. The two roots join in the region of the foramen lacerum and enter the vidian canal to reach the pterygopalatine ganglion in the pterygopalatine fossa. A., artery;* Ant., *anterior;* Car., *carotid;* Cav., *cavernous;* Cist., *cistern;* Clin., *clinoid;* CN, *cranial nerve;* Comm., *communicating;* Dors., *dorsal;* Falc., *falciform;* Gr., *greater;* Inf. Lat., *inferolateral;* Lig., *ligament;* Men., *meningeal;* Men. Hyp., *meningohypophyseal;* Mid., *middle;* N., *nerve;* Oculom., *oculomotor;* Olf., *olfactory;* Ophth., *ophthalmic;* P.C.A., *posterior cerebral artery;* Pericav., *pericavernous;* Pet., *petrosal, petrous;* Petrosphen., *petrosphenoid;* Pit., *pituitary;* Plex., *plexus;* Post., *posterior;* S.C.A., *superior cerebellar artery;* Seg., *segment;* Sphen., *sphenoid;* Sup., *superior;* Tent., *tentorial, tentorium;* Tr., *tract, trunk;* V., *vein;* Ven., *venous.*

and the cavernous sinus (6). A fistula between the dorsal meningeal branch of the meningohypophyseal trunk and the basilar sinus may be of the low-flow type. The fistulas, because of a communication between a branch of the intracavernous carotid or a branch of the external carotid artery in the floor of the middle fossa on one of the venous channels, will be more amenable to direct occlusion of the fistula than one in which there has been a traumatic rupture of the carotid artery into a large venous cavern. In dealing with a carotid-cavernous fistula, it is important to remember that the proptosis may occur on the side opposite the cavernous sinus harboring the fistula. Proptosis may also occur with arteriovenous fistulas in intracranial locations other than the cavernous sinus. Proptosis may result from fistulas between the branches of the external carotid artery and the lateral sinus, caused by high-pressure flow from the fistula through the vein of Labbé to the sylvian veins and then into the cavernous sinus and ophthalmic veins or through the petrosal sinuses into the cavernous sinus and then to the orbit.

VENOUS RELATIONSHIPS

The cavernous sinus is narrowest anteriorly adjacent to the superior orbital fissure and widest posteriorly lateral to the dorsum sellae where it opens into the venous confluence formed by the junction of the basilar, cavernous, and superior and inferior petrosal sinuses (*Fig. 9.2* and *9.3*). The sinus is connected to the orbit by the superior and inferior ophthalmic veins, to the cerebral hemispheres through the middle and inferior cerebral veins, to the retina by the central retinal vein, to the dura by tributaries of the middle meningeal veins, to the transverse sinus via the superior petrosal sinus, to the jugular bulb by way of the inferior petrosal sinus, to the pterygoid venous plexus by the emissary veins passing through the cranial foramina, and to the facial veins through the ophthalmic veins. The basilar sinus, the largest and most constant intercavernous connection across the midline, passes posterior to the dorsum sellae and upper clivus and connects the posterior aspect of both cavernous sinuses.

The three main venous spaces within the sinus, identified by their relation to the carotid artery, are the medial, the anteroinferior, and the posterosuperior compartments (*Figs. 9.1–9.3*). The widest spaces are located posteriorly near the junction with the basilar sinus and anteriorly near the superior orbital fissure. The medial compartment is situated between the pituitary gland and the carotid artery. The medial space may be as wide as 7 mm, but may be obliterated by a tortuous carotid that indents the pituitary gland (6). The anteroinferior space is located in the concavity below the first curve of the intracavernous carotid where the superior and inferior ophthalmic veins commonly open into the sinus (*Fig. 9.1*). The VIth nerve enters the anteroinferior space after passing laterally around the intracavernous portion of the carotid (6). The superior or common trunk of the superior and inferior ophthalmic veins commonly empties into this space. The posterosuperior space is located between the carotid and the posterior half of the roof of the sinus (*Fig. 9.1*). The basilar sinus opens into the posterosuperior space. The meningohypophyseal artery arises in this space. A tortuous elongated intracavernous carotid may obliterate the posterosuperior space (*Fig. 9.8*). These three venous spaces are larger than the lateral space located between the carotid artery and the lateral sinus wall. The lateral space is usually so narrow that the VIth nerve that passes through it is adherent to the carotid on its medial side and to the sinus wall on its lateral side. Venous spaces that extend lateral to the carotid artery and VIth nerve are found in less than 10% of sinuses (1). The fact that the medial or posterior spaces are the largest make them the most suitable areas for entering the sinus. The medial space can be entered through the roof on the medial side of the oculomotor nerve. Attempting to enter the sinus through the roof on the lateral side of the oculomotor nerve carries a greater risk of damaging the abducens nerve than entry on the medial side, because the lateral space in which the abducens nerve courses is very narrow.

Intercavernous Sinus

The venous sinuses commonly found in the margins of the diaphragma and sella and connecting both cavernous sinuses are termed the intercavernous sinuses (*Figs. 9.1, 9.2, 9.7,* and *9.8*) (16). These intercavernous connections within the sella are named on the basis of their relationship to the pituitary gland; the anterior intercavernous sinuses pass anterior to the hypophysis, and the posterior intercavernous sinuses pass behind the gland. These transsellar connections between the cavernous sinuses may exist at any point from the anterior to posterior wall of the sella, including the diaphragma, or all connections between the two sides may be absent. They can occur at any site along the anterior, inferior, or posterior surface of the gland. The anterior intercavernous sinuses are usually larger than the posterior ones and may cover the whole anterior wall of the sella, but either the anterior or posterior connections, or both, may be absent. If the anterior and posterior connections coexist and join with the cavernous sinus to form a venous ring around the gland, the whole structure constitutes the "circular sinus." Entering an anterior intercavernous connection that extends downward in front of the gland during transsphenoidal operation may produce brisk bleeding. However, this usually stops with temporary compression of the channel or with gentle coagulation, which serves to glue the walls of the channel together. The anterior intercavernous sinus, which crosses the upper anterior margin of the sella, joins the cavernous sinus immediately behind the site at which the upper and lower rings fuse at the posterior tip of the clinoid process (*Fig. 9.6*) (22).

Clinoid Venous Space

The clinoid venous space, the upward extension of the cavernous sinus through the lower dural ring and inside the carotid collar, is widest at the level of the lower ring through which it communicates with the larger venous channels in the anterior part of the cavernous sinus and narrows superiorly to

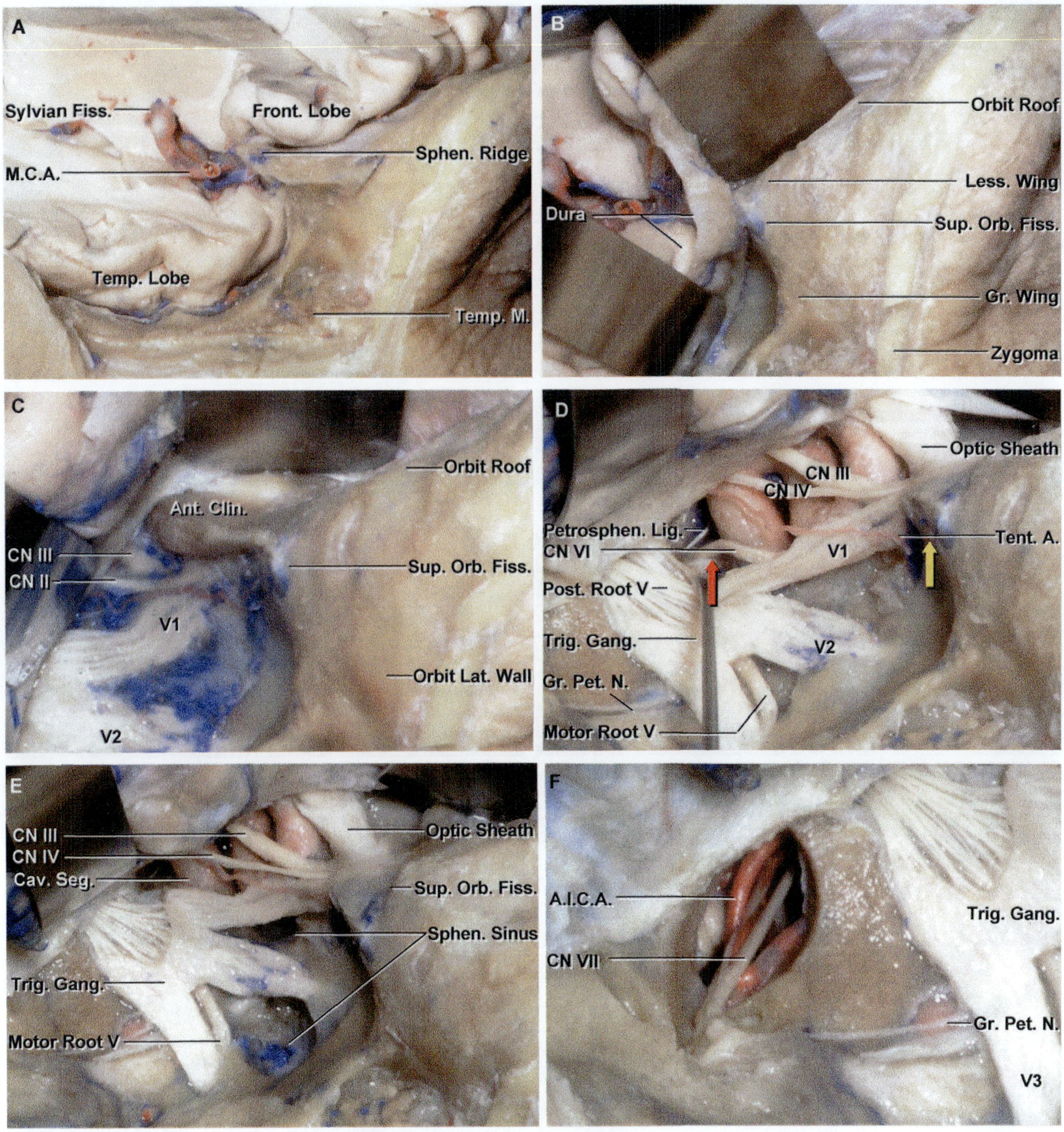

FIGURE 9.8. *Extradural approach to the cavernous sinus. This is the dissection participants complete in our microsurgery courses to demonstrate the intradural approach to the cavernous sinus.* A, *at this stage of the course, part of the frontal and temporal lobes has been removed and the sylvian fissure has been exposed.* B, *the sphenoid ridge has been removed and dura has been elevated from the superior and lateral wall of the orbit to expose the superior orbital fissure. At the lateral margin of the superior orbital fissure, the dura becomes thick and tough at the point it blends into the periorbita, making it necessary to make a sharp shallow cut in this dura at the lateral margin of the fissure to continue peeling the outer layer of dura away from the wall of the cavernous sinus.* C, *the outer layer of dura has been pealed back to expose the anterior clinoid process and the oculomotor and trochlear nerves and trigeminal divisions. The nerves course in the thin inner layer of the lateral wall of the cavernous sinus.* D, *the anterior clinoid has been removed to expose the clinoid segment of the internal carotid artery. The thin inner layer of dura within the wall of the sinus has been removed and the ophthalmic nerve has been depressed to expose the abducens nerve coming through Dorello's canal, located below the petrosphenoid (Gruber's) ligament. The lower margin of the posterior wall of the sinus is located at the petrous apex just below where the abducens nerve enters Dorello's canal* (red arrow). *The anterior edge of the*
(Legend continues on next page.)

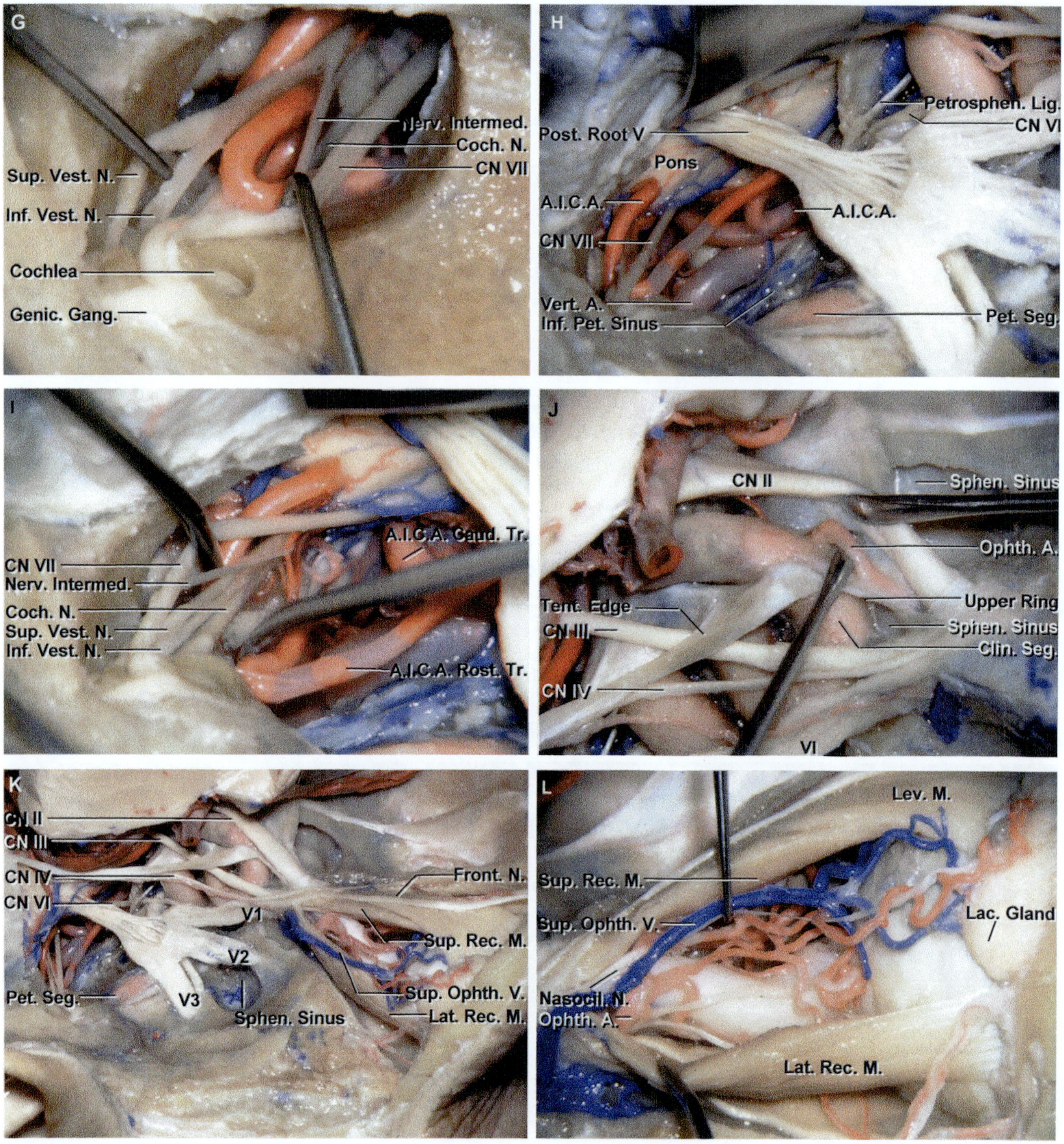

FIGURE 9.8. *Continued*

lower margin is located at the lower margin of the superior orbital fissure (yellow arrow). *E, the bone in the anteromedial and anterolateral middle fossa triangles has been drilled to open into the lateral wing of the sphenoid sinus. The motor root of the trigeminal nerve courses along the medial side of the trigeminal ganglion and enters the medial part of the foramen ovale with the mandibular nerve. F, the bone behind the greater petrosal nerve and lateral to the trigeminal nerve in Kawase's triangle has been drilled to expose the nerves and anteroinferior cerebellar artery in the internal acoustic meatus. G, the superior vestibular and facial nerves have been retracted to expose the superior and inferior vestibular nerves posteriorly and the facial and cochlear nerves anteriorly within the meatus. The anteroinferior cerebellar artery loops into the meatus. The nervus intermedius courses with the VIIIth nerve near the brainstem and jumps to the facial nerve, either in the cerebellopontine angle or internal acoustic meatus. H, the petrous apex has been drilled downward to the level of the inferior petrosal sinus and medially to the lateral edge of Dorello's canal. This exposure includes the anteroinferior cerebellar artery bifurca-*

a thin serpiginous venous plexus, which disappears as the upper ring is approached, thus demonstrating that the clinoid segment is intracavernous (*Fig. 9.6*). The clinoid venous space has connections with the diploic veins of the orbital roof by way of small emissary veins that pass through small foramina in the surface of the anterior clinoid process and the optic strut facing the dural collar.

DISCUSSION

A controversy has arisen as to whether the sinus is an unbroken, trabeculated, venous cavern or a plexus of various-sized veins that divide and coalesce and incompletely surround the carotid artery (1, 14, 24). Both concepts are, in part, correct. Numerous veins, such as those from the orbit, middle fossa dura, and sylvian fissure, maintain their integrity as they wind their way around the carotid arteries and nerves in the sinus wall before opening into the sinus. In other areas, numerous dural sinuses converge and form large venous spaces in the sinus, such as in the area where the basilar and the superior and inferior petrosal sinuses open into the posterior part of the cavernous sinus, or on the medial side of the carotid artery where the intercavernous sinus joins the cavernous sinus. The degree to which a cavern or a venous plexus will predominate varies from sinus to sinus and from one area to another in the same sinus. A dural venous plexus, which is referred to here as the pericavernous venus plexus and not the cavernous sinus, predominates in the middle fossa dura lateral to the cavernous sinus and anteriorly near the orbital apex and superior orbital fissure, but becomes a cavern where these numerous venous channels join with the dural envelope defining the sinus (*Figs. 9.2, 9.3,* and *9.5*). The cavern is largest at the junction of the basilar and superior and inferior petrosal sinuses with the cavernous sinus and on the medial side of the carotid where the intercavernous sinus joins the paired cavernous sinuses. Parkinson's observations are valuable in that they form the basis for carefully examining the anatomy of the carotid-cavernous fistulae and identifying those involving the veins in the area that can be repaired with a single clip while preserving the carotid artery.

Operative Considerations

The walls of the cavernous sinus are exposed in the operative approaches that reach the intra-, supra-, and parasellar areas (3, 4, 20, 21). A pterional (frontotemporal) or orbitozygomatic craniotomy is commonly selected to expose the roof and lateral wall of the sinus and also to provide access to the adjoining orbit and suprasellar area (*Fig. 9.9*). The lateral sinus wall can also be exposed by the subtemporal route, but reaching the sinus roof by this route often requires significant temporal lobe retraction, and the angle of view is not suitable for examining the roof. The orbitozygomatic approach is a variant of the frontotemporal craniotomy in which a variable amount of the upper and lateral orbital rim and zygomatic arch are elevated as a single piece in continuity with the bone flap or as a second step after elevation of a frontotemporal (pterional) bone flap (*Figs. 9.10* and *9.11*). The orbitozygomatic craniotomy provides an excellent exposure of the cavernous sinus and orbital contents and the structures passing through the optic canal and superior orbital fissure (*Figs. 9.7* and *9.9*). The exposure of the orbital contents by this approach is reviewed in Chapter 7. The frontotemporal approach without the orbitozygomatic osteotomy is suitable for lesions that are more strictly intracranial in the supra- and parasellar areas.

The nerves in the lateral sinus wall can be exposed using a pterional or orbitozygomatic extradural approach, in which the outer layer of dura in the lateral wall is peeled from the thin, fragile inner layer, investing the nerves that separate easily from the thicker outer layer (25). The peeling is begun laterally and anteriorly near the sphenoid ridge where the dura is elevated from the osseous surface of the greater and lesser wings of the sphenoid. At the lateral edge of the superior orbital fissure, where the middle fossa dura blends into the periorbital, the dura becomes resistant to being separated. A shallow, sharp cut in the fibrous band at the lateral edge of the fissure allows the dural elevation to proceed posteriorly along the lateral wall of the sinus, where the thicker outer layer of dura separates from the thin inner part of the lateral wall that encases the oculomotor, trochlear, and ophthalmic nerves. The upper limit of the dural separation is the anterior petroclinoid dural fold at the lateral edge of the sinus roof, and

tion and extends down to the level of the vertebral artery. I, the facial nerve has been retracted backward to expose the nervous intermedius and the superior and inferior vestibular and cochlear nerves. The rostral trunk of the anteroinferior cerebellar artery loops into the internalacoustic meatus, and the caudal trunk passes downward to the inferolateral part of the cerebellum. J, the roof of the cavernous sinus is located medial to the tentorial edge and includes the oculomotor triangle, through which the oculomotor nerve passes, and the dura lining the lower margin of the anterior clinoid. The optic nerve has been elevated to expose the origin of the ophthalmic artery, which enters the optic canal and penetrates the optic sheath to enter the orbit on the lateral side of the optic nerve. K, the roof and lateral wall of the orbit have been removed to expose the orbital contents. L, enlarged view of the structures in the upper part of the orbit. The levator and superior rectus muscles have been elevated and the lateral rectus muscle has been depressed. The superior ophthalmic vein passes backward and empties into the cavernous sinus after passing downward along the lower margin of the ophthalmic nerve. The nasociliary nerve, ophthalmic artery, and superior ophthalmic vein course above the optic nerve and are located on the lateral side of the optic nerve at the orbital apex. A.I.C.A., *anteroinferior cerebellar artery;* Ant., *anterior;* Caud., *caudal;* Cav., *cavernous;* Clin., *clinoid;* CN, *cranial nerve;* Coch., *cochlear;* Fiss., *fissure;* Front., *frontal;* Gang., *ganglion;* Genic., *geniculate;* Gr., *greater;* Inf., *inferior;* Intermed., *intermedius;* Lac., *lacrimal;* Lat., *lateral;* Less., *lesser;* Lev., *levator;* Lig., *ligament;* M., *muscle;* M.C.A., *middle cerebral artery;* N., *nerve;* Nasocil., *nasociliary;* Nerv., *nervus;* Ophth., *ophthalmic;* Orb., *orbital;* Pet., *petrosal, petrous;* Petrosphen., *petrosphenoid;* Post., *posterior;* Rec., *rectus;* Rost., *rostral;* Seg., *segment;* Sphen., *sphenoid;* Sup., *superior;* Temp., *temporal, temporalis;* Tent., *tentorial;* Tr., *trunk;* Trig., *trigeminal;* V., *vein;* Vert., *vertebral;* Vest., *vestibular.*

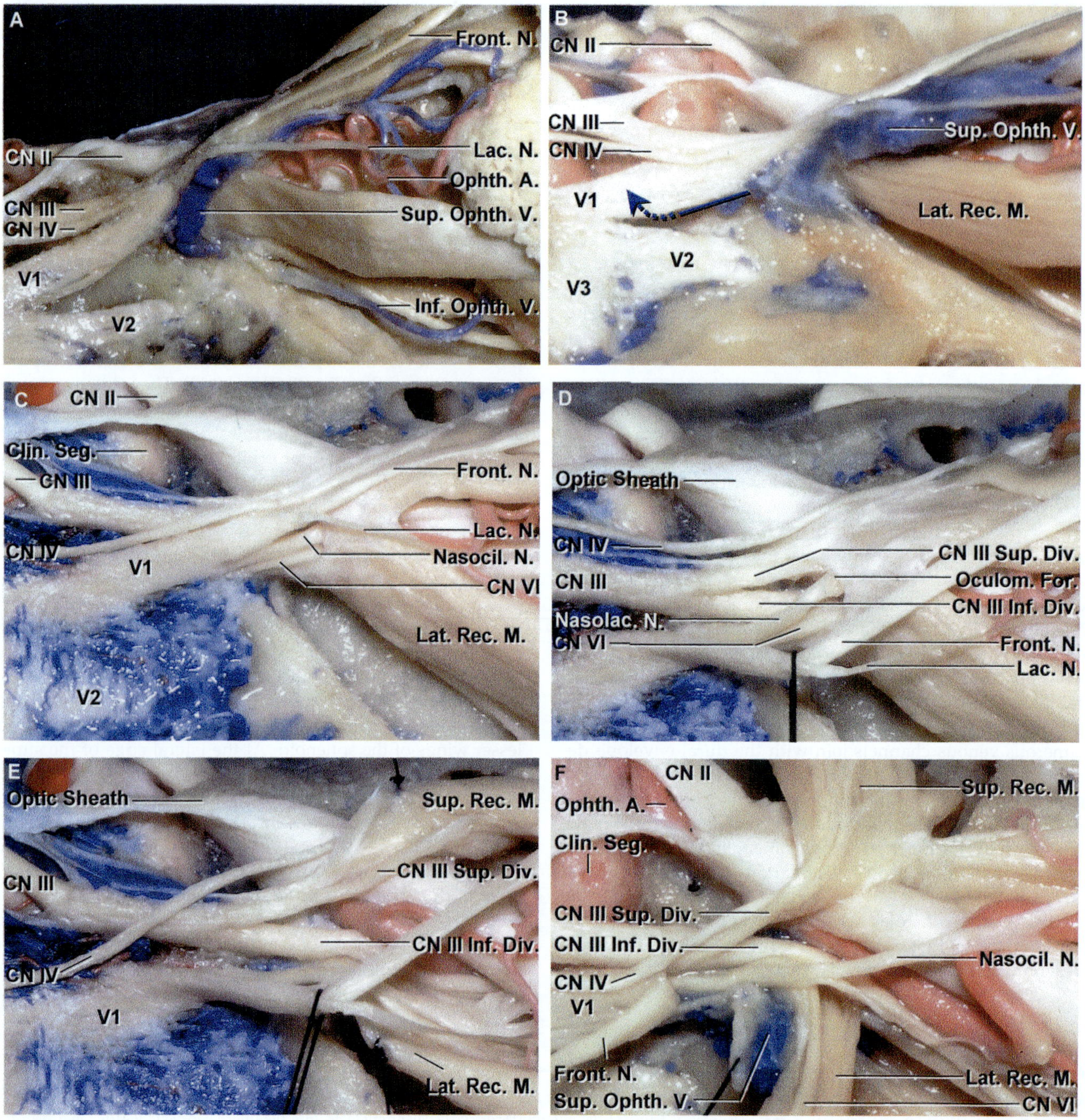

FIGURE 9.9. *Lateral aspect of the left cavernous sinus, superior orbital fissure, and orbit.* A, *the lateral wall and roof of the right orbit and the intraorbital fat have been removed. The anterior clinoid process and dura in the lateral wall of the cavernous sinus have been preserved. The oculomotor, trochlear, and ophthalmic nerves have been exposed by removing the dura in the lateral wall of the cavernous sinus. The superior and inferior ophthalmic veins arise inside the muscle cone, but exit the intraconal area as they converge on the orbital apex. The superior ophthalmic vein passes downward along the origin of the lateral rectus muscle from the annular tendon, where it is joined by the inferior ophthalmic vein to form a common trunk that passes backward below and medial to the ophthalmic nerve to enter the cavernous sinus.* B, *another specimen with the anterior clinoid, lateral wall of the orbit, and cavernous sinus removed. The superior ophthalmic vein exits the muscle cone to pass along the lateral margin of the superior orbital fissure and below the ophthalmic nerve* (blue arrow) *to enter the anteroinferior part of the cavernous sinus on the medial side of the ophthalmic nerve.* C, *the superior ophthalmic vein has been removed. The trochlear nerve passes medially above the oculomotor and ophthalmic nerves to reach the superior oblique muscles. The frontal, lacrimal, and trochlear nerves pass outside the annular tendon, and the nasociliary, oculomotor, and abducens nerves pass through the tendon.* D, *the frontal and lacrimal nerves have been depressed to show the nasociliary nerve arising from the medial side of the ophthalmic nerve. The oculomotor*

the posterior limit is the petrous ridge. At the posteromedial aspect of the exposure, the dura is elevated from the middle fossa floor to expose the mandibular and greater petrosal nerves and the lateral wall of Meckel's cave. The upper part of Meckel's cave is located lateral to the posterior part of the cavernous sinus. The petrous segment of the internal carotid artery and the greater petrosal nerve may be exposed in the floor of the middle fossa lateral to Meckel's cave and the trigeminal ganglion.

In the orbitozygomatic approach, a frontotemporal scalp flap is reflected to expose the superior and lateral orbital margins, the zygomatic arch, temporal fascia, and frontozygomatic suture. The upper edge of the temporal fat pad above the zygoma, which overlies the temporal fascia and contains the frontal branches of the facial nerve, comes into the exposure as the scalp flap is being elevated (*Fig. 9.11*). The superficial layer of temporalis fascia is incised at the upper edge of the fat pad so that the fat pad and the underlying temporal fascia can be reflected downward in a single layer with the scalp flap to protect the branches of the facial nerve. The temporalis muscle deep to the superficial fascial incision is not incised in completing the fascial incision above the fat pad. The pericranium in the frontal region may be elevated with the scalp flap or as a separate layer that can be used in closing the anterior fossa.

In some cases, the orbitozygomatic osteotomy needs to include only the superior and lateral orbital rims and not the zygomatic arch. If an osteotomy of the zygomatic arch is needed, an alternative to elevating it with the superior and lateral orbital rims is to divide its anterior or posterior margin so that it can be reflected inferiorly with the temporalis muscle. In the orbitozygomatic exposure, the periorbita is separated from the anterior part of the roof and lateral orbital wall before completing the orbitozygomatic osteotomy. The one-piece orbitozygomatic bone flap includes part of the upper and lateral orbital rim, and possibly the zygomatic arch with the pterional flap. In the two-piece orbitozygomatic approach the frontotemporal bone flap is elevated as the initial step and the orbitozygomatic osteotomy is performed as the second step. The site of the osteotomy in the roof and lateral orbital wall are more easily completed in the two-piece approach because the site of the orbital bone cuts can be easily visualized from intracranially after the dura has been elevated from the orbital roof and lateral wall (*Fig. 9.12*). In the one-piece approach, the site of the cut in the orbital roof is visualized in the narrow space between the periorbita and bone, and there is the added risk that the dura is not elevated from the orbital roof before making the bone cuts as it can be with the two-piece approach. An important step is accurate placement of the keyhole burr hole, which has the frontal dura and periorbita exposed in the depths of its upper and lower margin, respectively. The keyhole is located just behind the junction of the anterior end of the superior temporal line with the upper part of the lateral orbital rim just above and behind the frontozygomatic suture. Having the keyhole properly placed facilitates the cuts along the lateral wall and roof of the orbit. A cuff of temporalis fascia is left along the temporal line during the opening to serve as a site for anchoring the temporalis muscle and fascia at the time of closing. Elevating the bone flap exposes the frontal and temporal dura and the periorbita. The orbitozygomatic exposure commonly includes nearly 180 degrees of the orbital rim, and provides excellent access to the superior and lateral aspects of the orbit. The recurrent meningeal branch of the ophthalmic artery courses along the temporal dura near the junction of the roof and the lateral wall of the orbit. In a rare case, the ophthalmic artery will arise from the anterior branch of the middle meningeal artery in the region of the sphenoid ridge; occlusion of this anomalous artery results in blindness (10).

Opening the dura and the sylvian fissure, if needed, exposes both optic nerves, the optic chiasm, ipsilateral optic tract, oculomotor nerve, and the carotid bifurcation, in addition to the lateral wall and roof of the sinus. This exposure allows access to the optic nerve from the chiasm to the globe, and permits the orbital contents to be exposed from above or laterally. Elevating the orbital surface of the frontal lobe and displacing the anterior pole of the temporal lobe posteriorly provides a pretemporal exposure of the basal cisterns. The large sylvian veins coursing along the sylvian fissure and emptying into the cavernous sinus should be preserved if possible. Elevating the internal carotid artery so as to open the interval between the artery and the oculomotor nerve exposes the basilar, posterior cerebral, superior cerebellar, and posterior communicating arteries.

Exposing the superior orbital fissure and its sectors requires at least limited exposure of the cavernous sinus posteriorly and the orbit anteriorly (*Fig. 9.9*). Fortunately, all of the nerves of the cavernous sinus, except the abducens nerve, can be exposed by opening or elevating the outer layer of dura in the lateral sinus wall while leaving the inner layer intact. It is possible to expose the oculomotor, trochlear, and ophthalmic nerves from their entrance into the sinus roof and through the fissure into the orbit without opening into the major venous spaces of the sinus, because these nerves course in the inner part of the dura forming the lateral sinus wall. Exposure of the abducens nerve is more hazardous because it courses medial to the ophthalmic nerve and is adherent to the lateral surface of the horizontal segment of the intracavernous carotid.

foramen is the portion of the opening in the annular tendon lateral to the optic foramen through which the superior and inferior divisions of the oculomotor nerve and the nasociliary and abducens nerves pass. The oculomotor nerve divides into superior and inferior divisions just behind the superior orbital fissure and annular tendon. The abducens nerve courses on the medial side of the ophthalmic nerve in the cavernous sinus, but in the fissure, it turns laterally below the nerve to enter the medial side of the lateral rectus muscle. E, *the annular tendon has been divided between the origin of the superior and lateral rectus muscles. The superior division of the oculomotor nerve passes upward to innervate the levator and superior rectus muscles. The inferior division innervates the inferior oblique, inferior rectus, and medial rectus muscles and gives rise to the parasympathetic pupilloconstrictor fibers to the ciliary ganglion.* F, *another specimen to show the oculomotor nerve splitting into the superior and inferior divisions at the anterior edge of the cavernous sinus just behind the superior orbital fissure.* A., *artery;* Clin., *clinoid;* CN, *cranial nerve;* Div., *division;* For., *foramen;* Front., *frontal;* Inf., *inferior;* Lac., *lacrimal;* Lat., *lateral;* M., *muscle;* N., *nerve;* Nasocil., *nasociliary;* Oculom., *oculomotor;* Ophth., *ophthalmic;* Rec., *rectus;* Seg., *segment;* Sup., *superior;* V., *vein.*

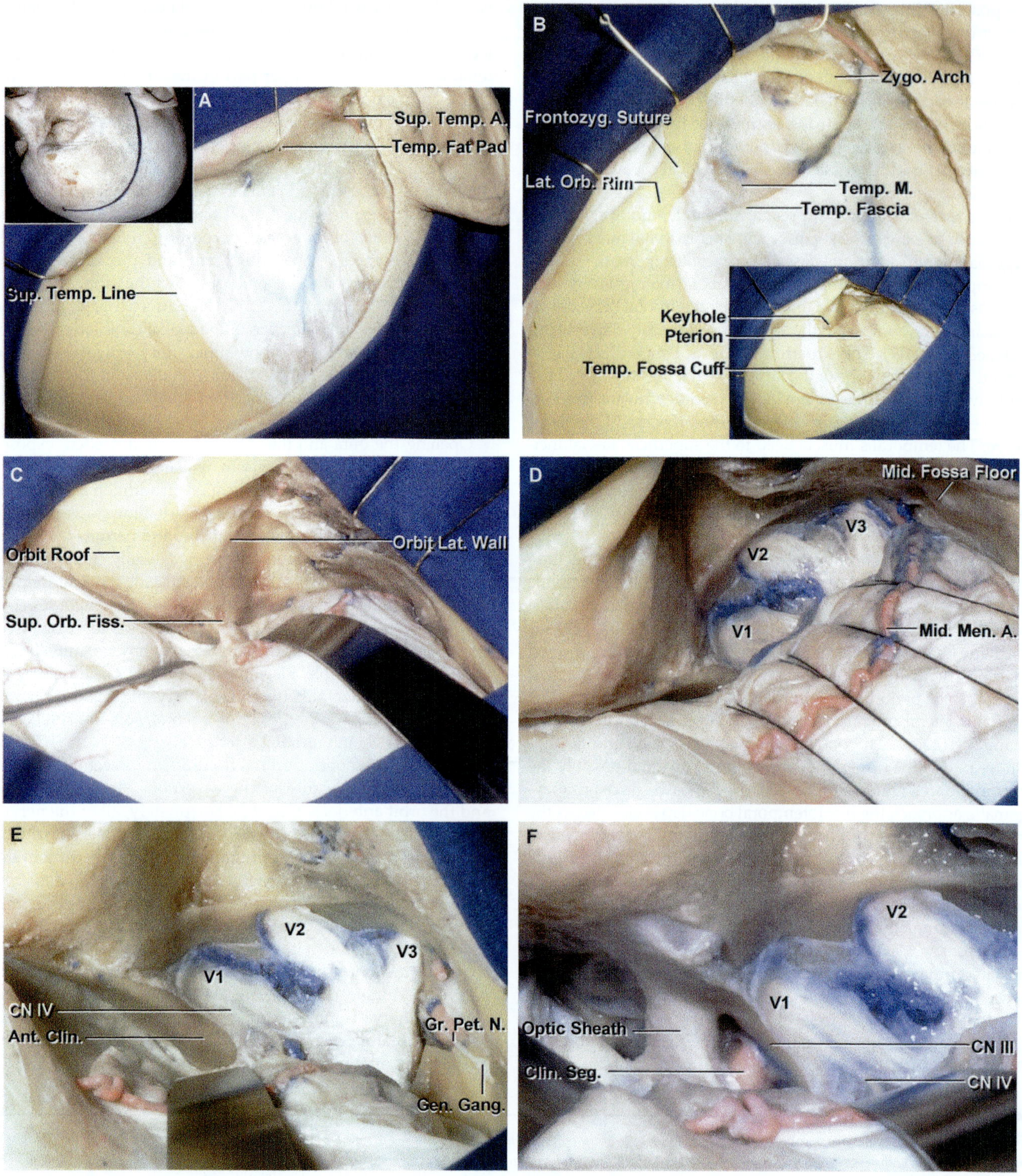

FIGURE 9.10. *Pterional craniotomy and extradural approach to the cavernous sinus. A, the* inset (upper left) *shows the site of the scalp incision. The scalp has been reflected using subgaleal dissection to expose the frontal bone and the temporalis muscle and fascia. The facial nerve branches to the frontalis muscle course in the fat pad above the zygomatic arch. B, the superficial layer of temporalis fascia has been divided just above the fat pad so that the superficial layer of temporalis fascia and the fat pad can be folded downward with the scalp flap to protect the branches of the facial nerve. The* inset *shows the burr holes and craniotome cuts for the bone flap. A cuff of temporalis fascia is preserved along the superior temporal line to aid in anchoring the temporal muscle to the line at the time of closure. The keyhole burr hole is located above and behind the frontozygomatic suture. C, the sphenoid ridge has*

Removal of the bone in the margin of the superior orbital fissure is a frequent step in exposing tumors and aneurysms in the region. The anterior clinoid process and the adjacent part of the lesser wing are frequently removed in dealing with ophthalmic and superior hypophyseal aneurysms and in removing tumors involving the cavernous sinus, anterior clinoid process, and medial sphenoid ridge. The greater wing may also be removed in dealing with tumors involving the middle fossa and cavernous sinus. Removing the bony margins of the fissure without exposing the neural structures will often suffice in dealing with tumors, such as meningiomas, that have grown through the bone to compress but not infiltrate the structures in the fissure. In other cases, tumors such as schwannomas and meningiomas may grow along the nerves, requiring that the various sectors of the fissure be opened, as described in Chapter 7.

In removing the anterior clinoid to expose the clinoid segment, it is important to remember that the carotid artery passes not only along the medial edge of the clinoid, but also courses upward against, often grooving, the medial half of the lower surface of the clinoid. The posterior tip of the clinoid may also project medially behind the clinoid segment toward the middle clinoid, to which it may be united by an osseous bridge, thus forming a complete bony ring around the clinoid segment. There may also be an interclinoidal osseous bridge joining the anterior and posterior clinoid process.

Care is required in removing the anterior clinoid process to avoid damaging the optic nerve on its medial side and the oculomotor nerve on its lower side, because these nerves are separated from the clinoid by only the thin layer of dura on the surface of the clinoid (*Figs. 9.5–9.8*). The segment of the trochlear nerve crossing medially between the upper surface of the oculomotor nerve and the lower surface of the clinoid can also be damaged in removing the anterior clinoid or the upper margin of the superior orbital fissure lateral to the clinoid. Similar care must be exercised when removing the optic strut to avoid injury to the optic nerve, which passes along the upper margin, and the oculomotor nerve, which passes along the lower margin of the strut (*Figs. 9.5–9.8*). Exposure or removal of the optic strut can be helpful when exposing the internal carotid artery for proximal control when dealing with lesions located at the roof of the cavernous sinus. Both the anterior clinoid and the strut may contain air cells that communicate with the sphenoid sinus and must be repaired, if opened, to prevent cerebrospinal fluid rhinorrhea.

The finding that the clinoid segment is intracavernous, being located within a collar of dura in which venous tributaries of the cavernous sinus course, has important implications for surgery in the region. The lateral margins of the carotid collar and the dural rings are the easiest to expose because these margins are accessed by removing the anterior clinoid process. The anterior and medial part of the carotid collar and rings, on the other hand, are more difficult to access because of their deeper location. It is important to note that the anterior part of the upper dural ring, which forms the roof of the cavernous sinus, does not extend across the top of the optic canal, but is located below the optic nerve on the upper surface of the optic strut, which forms the floor of the optic canal. The dura covering the anterior part of the upper surface of the anterior clinoid process also extends medially to cover the roof of the optic canal. However, it is the dura extending below the optic nerve that forms the anterior part of the upper ring.

Removing the anterior clinoid aids in visualization of the origin of the ophthalmic artery, which arises medial to and below the level of the upper edge of the anterior clinoid. However, removing the clinoid provides only limited access to the part of the upper dural ring formed by the dura extending posteriorly from the upper surface of the optic strut. Gaining access to the upper surface of the optic strut and the anterior part of the upper ring usually requires that the roof of the optic canal and the adjacent posterior part of the roof of the orbit be removed. This allows the falciform dural fold, which extends medially above the optic nerve from the upper surface of the anterior clinoid process to the chiasmatic sulcus at the posterior edge of the planum sphenoidale, and also the posterior part of the optic sheath, to be opened, so that the optic nerve can be elevated for a more adequate exposure of the upper ring at the level of the floor of the optic canal. The falciform ligament usually covers several millimeters of the optic nerve just proximal to where it passes below the intracranial edge of the roof of the optic canal. Elevating the optic nerve aids in visualization of the origin of the ophthalmic artery, which most commonly arises just above the upper dural ring and passes forward below the optic nerve on the superior surface of the dura lining the optic strut.

Opening some part of the upper ring aids in exposing the segment of the internal carotid artery located immediately proximal to lesions involving the origin of the ophthalmic artery. It is best to open the dura just outside the junction of the upper ring with the carotid collar, leaving a small cuff of dura attached to the artery rather than separating the upper ring from the arterial wall, which may create an opening into the venous spaces inside the carotid collar. The incision in the upper ring is usually confined to the area lateral, anterior, and anteromedial to the internal carotid artery, which may yield an exposure adequate to place a clip across the neck of an ophthalmic aneurysm or a temporary clip on the carotid artery below the origin of the ophthalmic artery. Opening the pos-

been flattened and a thin shell of bone has been left along the roof and lateral wall of the orbit. The dura has been elevated from the orbital root and lateral wall to the lateral edge of the superior orbital fissure, where the dura blends into the periorbita. It is often necessary to make a shallow cut in the dura at this lateral apex of the fissure to continue to peel the thick outer layer of dura in the lateral sinus wall from the inner layer investing the nerves. D, the outer layer of dura in the lateral sinus wall and covering Meckel's cave has been elevated to expose the three trigeminal divisions, which course in the thin inner layer of the lateral wall. E, the dura has been elevated from the anterior clinoid process and backward along the sinus wall to expose the greater petrosal nerve and petrous ridge. F, the anterior clinoid process has been removed to expose the clinoid segment and the anterior part of the sinus roof formed by the dura lining the lower surface of the clinoid. A., *artery;* Ant., *anterior;* Clin., *clinoid;* CN, *cranial nerve;* Fiss., *fissure;* Frontozyg., *frontozygomatic;* Gang., *ganglion;* Gen., *geniculate;* Gr., *greater;* Lat., *lateral;* M., *muscle;* Men., *meningeal;* Mid., *middle;* N., *nerve;* Orb., *orbital;* Pet., *petrosal;* Seg., *segment;* Sup., *superior;* Temp., *temporal, temporalis;* Zygo., *zygomatic.*

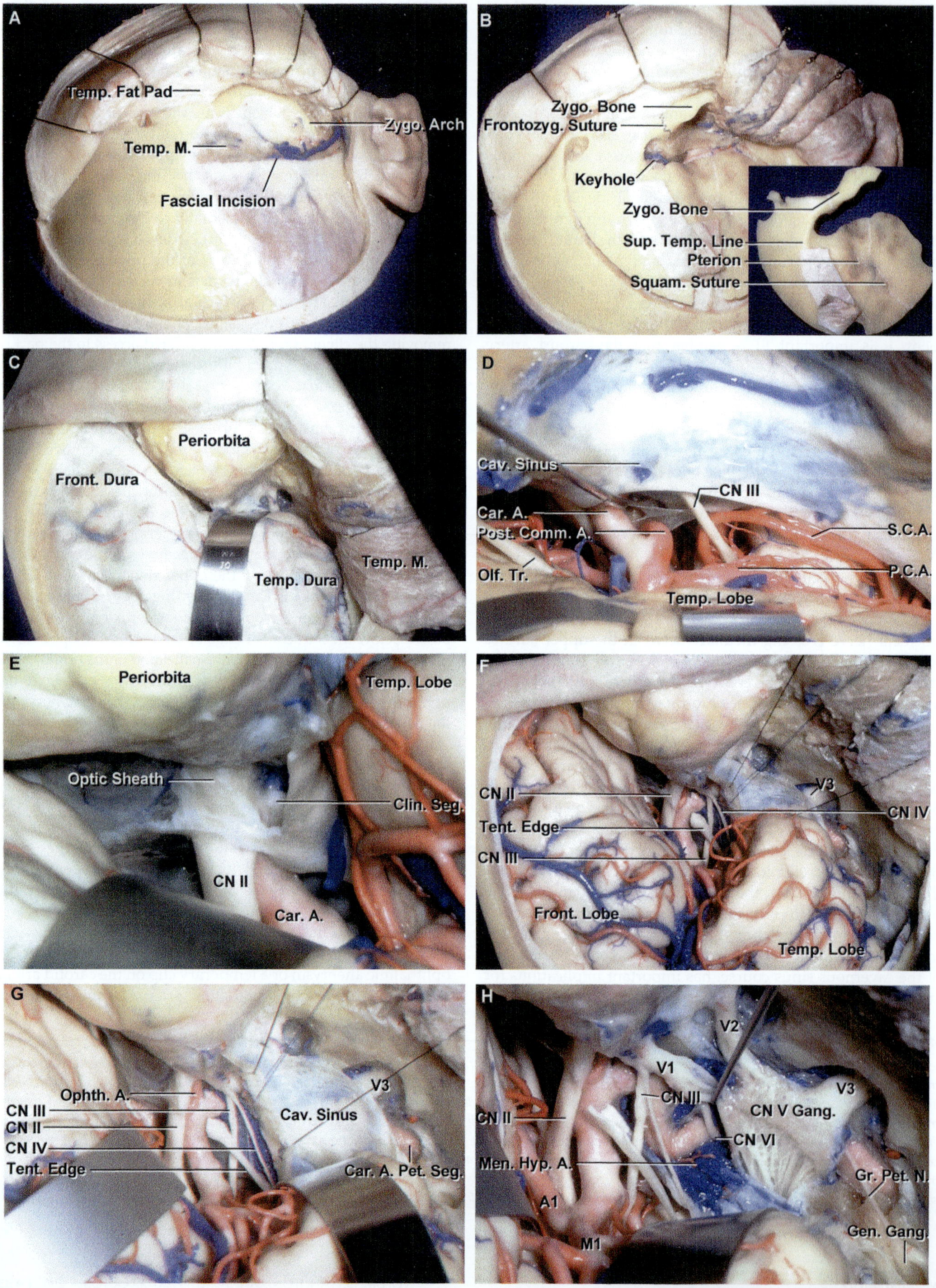
A
Temp. Fat Pad
Zygo. Arch
Temp. M.
Fascial Incision
B
Zygo. Bone
Frontozyg. Suture
Keyhole
Zygo. Bone
Sup. Temp. Line
Pterion
Squam. Suture
C
Periorbita
Front. Dura
Temp. M.
Temp. Dura
D
Cav. Sinus
CN III
Car. A.
Post. Comm. A.
S.C.A.
Olf. Tr.
P.C.A.
Temp. Lobe
E
Periorbita
Temp. Lobe
Optic Sheath
Clin. Seg.
CN II
Car. A.
F
V3
CN II
CN IV
Tent. Edge
CN III
Front. Lobe
Temp. Lobe
G
V3
Ophth. A.
CN III
Cav. Sinus
CN II
CN IV
Tent. Edge
Car. A. Pet. Seg.
H
V2
V1
V3
CN III
CN V Gang.
CN II
CN VI
Men. Hyp. A.
Gr. Pet. N.
A1
Gen. Gang.
M1

teromedial part of the upper ring will commonly open into the junction of the anterior intercavernous sinus with the cavernous sinus, with resultant brisk bleeding that can usually be controlled with gentle packing with a hemostatic agent.

The dura forming the upper part of the carotid collar can usually be opened with minimal bleeding because the venous channels within the clinoid venous space are small. However, opening the dura at the lower margin of the carotid collar or the lower dural ring formed by the carotidoculomotor membrane may be associated with more brisk venous bleeding, but it is usually easily controlled with gentle packing unless there is an arteriovenous fistula in the sinus. Removing the anterior clinoid and lateral part of the optic strut may also lead to easily controllable venous bleeding, caused by opening the small veins that drain the diploe of the anterior clinoid, optic strut, and posterior orbital roof and penetrate the carotid collar to enter directly into the venous channels within the collar.

There is the possibility of placing a temporary clip across the clinoid segment of the carotid artery for proximal control without opening the collar, if the extradural plane between the dural collar and the bony surface of the optic strut and carotid sulcus is developed after removing the anterior clinoid process (*Fig. 9.6*). Developing the plane between the collar and the optic strut on the anterior side and between the collar and the carotid sulcus on the medial side of the clinoid segment will allow a curved clip to be applied, placing one blade of the clip through the opening created by elevating the dura from the optic strut and carotid sulcus and placing the blades of the clip to close on the medial and lateral side of the artery across and outside the collar. Removing the optic strut facilitates this clip placement by creating a space through which one blade of the clip can be advanced to reach the medial side of the artery.

That the collar and the upper ring slope downward as they proceed medially from the upper surface of the anterior clinoid allows lesions located on the medial side of the clinoid segment in the area below the optic chiasm to project below the level of the anterior clinoid on radiological studies, even though they are located intradurally. Aneurysms, such as those arising at the origin of the superior hypophyseal artery, that project medially between the diaphragm and the chiasm and which might be considered to be intracavernous on the lateral angiogram because they project below the upper edge of the clinoid, are actually intradural within the subarachnoid space.

The medial wall of the cavernous sinus wall may also be exposed in the lateral margin of the transsphenoidal approach by extending the bone removal laterally from the anterior sellar wall to the area of the prominences overlying the carotid arteries, superior orbital fissure, and the maxillary nerve (*Figs. 9.5* and *9.6*) (5, 9). Some of the posterior ethmoid air cells often have to be removed to gain the lateral exposure in the sphenoid sinus needed to see the wall of the cavernous sinus because the posterior ethmoid air cells are located in front of the upper part of the lateral wing of the sphenoid sinus. Removing the posterior part of the middle turbinate may also assist in the exposure. Care is required to avoid injury to the optic nerve in the superolateral part of the sphenoid sinus, the nerves passing through the superior orbital fissure in the midportion, and the maxillary nerve in the lower portion, where they may occasionally be exposed directly under the sphenoid mucosa. The length of carotid artery exposed in the

FIGURE 9.11. *One-piece orbitozygomatic craniotomy and intradural approach to the cavernous sinus.* A, *a frontotemporal scalp flap has been reflected forward to expose the superior and lateral orbital rim and the zygomatic arch. An incision has been made in the superficial temporalis fascia along the upper margin of the temporal fat pad, which overlies the lower part of the temporalis fascia and contains the frontal branches of the facial nerve, so that the fat pad can be reflected downward with the scalp to protect the branches of the facial nerve as the flap is elevated. The temporalis muscle, under the fascial incision, has not been incised. The pericranium in the frontal region has been elevated with the scalp flap.* B, *the bone flap, which includes part of the upper and lateral orbital rim and the zygomatic arch, has been outlined with the craniotome. The periorbita has been separated from the orbital roof and lateral wall, and the zygomatic arch at the lower margin of the bone flap has been divided. The keyhole, located just behind the junction of the temporal line with the lateral orbital rim and just above and behind the frontozygomatic suture, is the site of a burr hole that will have the frontal dura and periorbita exposed in the depths of its upper and lower margin, respectively. The bone flap is shown in the* inset. *In closing the incision, the temporalis muscle and fascia are anchored to the cuff of temporal fascia remaining along the temporal line. The pterion marks the lateral margin of the sphenoid ridge and sylvian fissure.* C, *the bone flap has been elevated to expose the frontal and temporal dura and the periorbita. The flap includes almost 180 degrees of the orbital rim and provides excellent access to the superior and lateral aspects of the orbit.* D, *the temporal lobe has been elevated to expose the lateral wall of the cavernous sinus. The oculomotor nerve passes forward between the posterior cerebral and superior cerebellar arteries to enter the roof of the cavernous sinus.* E, *the sylvian fissure has been opened and the remaining part of the orbital roof, the anterior clinoid, and the roof of the optic canal have been removed. The clinoid segment of the internal carotid artery is exposed in the clinoidal triangle. The optic sheath surrounds the optic nerve in the optic canal.* F, *some of the dura forming the roof of the cavernous sinus and lining the floor of the middle cranial fossa has been removed, while preserving some of the dura forming the lateral sinus wall.* G, *enlarged view. The site at which the oculomotor nerve passes through the sinus roof medial to the tentorial edge has been preserved. Removing the dura from the lateral part of the floor of the middle cranial fossa exposes the petrous segment of the carotid artery and the mandibular nerve entering the foramen ovale.* H, *the dura has been elevated from the lateral wall of the cavernous sinus to expose the trigeminal ganglion and the ophthalmic, maxillary, and mandibular nerves. Bone has been drilled from the floor of the middle fossa to expose the facial nerve and geniculate ganglion. The ophthalmic nerve has been depressed to expose the abducens nerve coursing around the lateral surface of the intracavernous carotid. The meningohypophyseal trunk arises from the posterior bend of the internal carotid artery within the cavernous sinus.* A., *artery;* Car., *carotid;* Cav., *cavernous;* Clin., *clinoid;* CN, *cranial nerve;* Comm., *communicating;* Front., *frontal;* Frontozygo., *frontozygomatic;* Gang., *ganglion;* Gen., *geniculate;* Gr., *greater;* M., *muscle;* Men. Hyp., *meningohypophyseal;* N., *nerve;* Olf., *olfactory;* Ophth., *ophthalmic;* P.C.A., *posterior cerebral artery;* Pet., *petrosal, petrous;* Post., *posterior;* S.C.A., *superior cerebellar artery;* Seg., *segment;* Squam., *squamous;* Sup., *superior;* Temp., *temporal, temporalis;* Tent., *tentorial;* Tr., *tract;* Zygo., *zygomatic.*

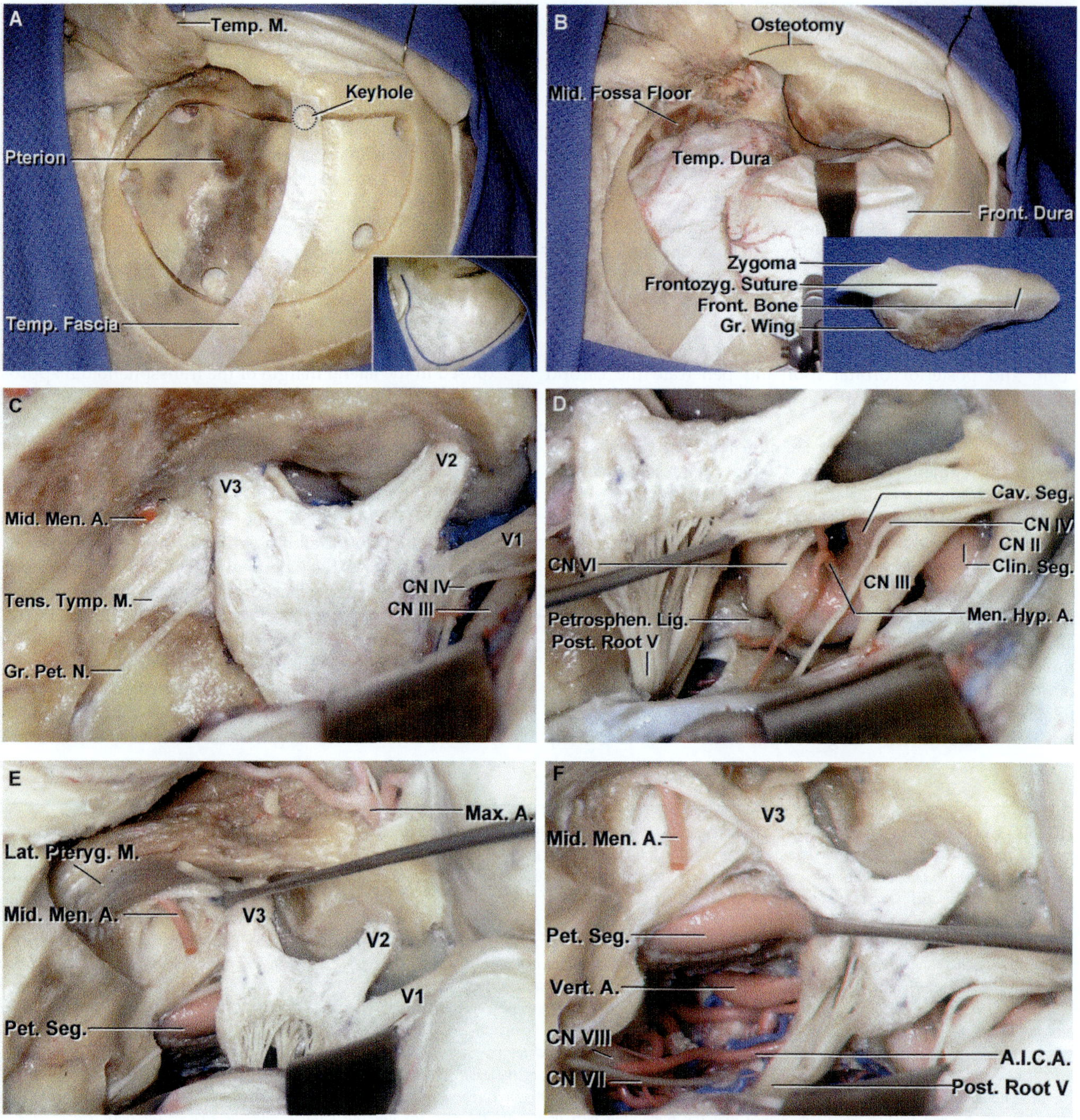

FIGURE 9.12. *Three-piece orbitozygomatic craniotomy. A, the inset shows the site of the skin incision. The first set of osteotomies divides the anterior and posterior end of the zygomatic arch so that the arch can be folded downward with the temporalis muscle. The second bone cut is the pterional bone flap, which is outlined, and the third piece is the orbitozygomatic osteotomy. B, the dura has been elevated from the roof and lateral wall of the orbital roof and the sphenoid ridge has been removed. The third piece, the orbitozygomatic osteotomy, includes the roof and the portion of the lateral wall of the orbit as outlined. The inset shows the orbitozygomatic osteotomy. Completing the bone cuts from intracranially allows more of the roof and lateral wall of the orbit to be preserved than with the one-piece orbitozygomatic craniotomy. C, the dura has been elevated from the lateral sinus wall to expose the oculomotor, trochlear, and ophthalmic nerves entering the superior orbital fissure and the maxillary and mandibular nerves exiting the foramen rotundum and ovale. The extradural exposure extends backward across the greater petrosal nerve to the petrous ridge. D, the ophthalmic nerve has been depressed to expose the abducens nerve and the intracavernous carotid. The anterior clinoid has been removed to expose the clinoid segment. E, the floor of the middle fossa has been removed to expose the mandibular nerve, lateral pterygoid muscle, and terminal part of the maxillary artery in the infratemporal fossa. F, the petrous apex behind the petrous segment of the carotid has been removed to expose the anteroinferior cerebellar artery and the cranial nerves in the cerebellopontine angle. G, the cervical carotid artery and the branches of the mandibular nerve have been extended in the infratemporal fossa. The eustachian*

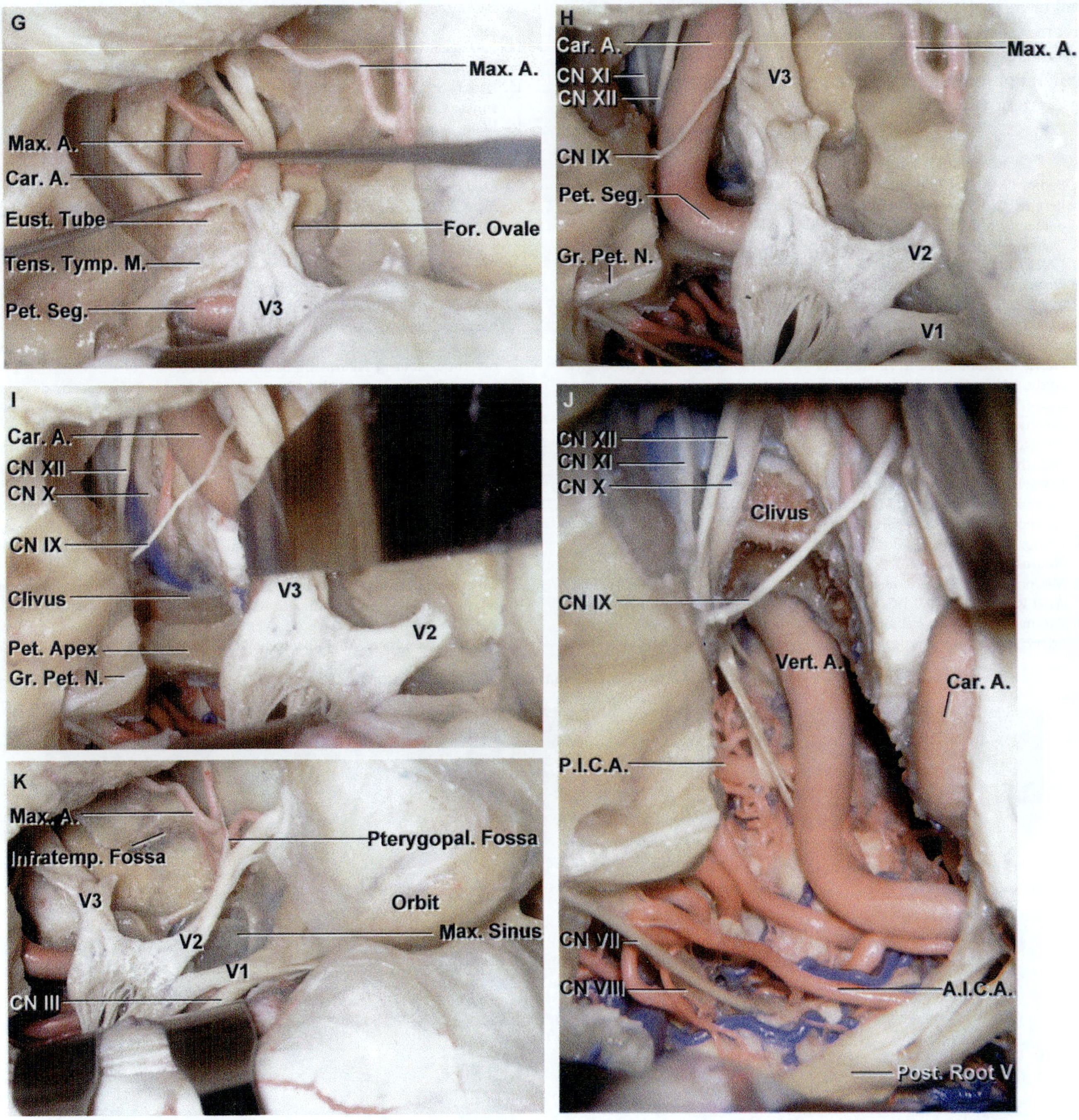

FIGURE 9.12. *Continued*
tube and tensor tympani muscle are layered along the anterior margin of the petrous carotid. H, the tensor tympani and eustachian tube have been resected to expose the upper cervical and petrous carotid. I, the carotid artery has been reflected forward to expose the petrous apex and clivus on the medial side of the carotid canal. J, the petrous apex and lateral part of the clivus have been removed and the dura opened, exposing the anterior and posteroinferior cerebellar and vertebral arteries and the facial and hypoglossal nerves. The opening through the petrous apex and clivus is located medial to where the lower cranial nerves exit the jugular foramen. K, the exposure has been carried forward to where the maxillary artery and nerve cross the pterygopalatine fossa. A., artery; A.I.C.A., *anteroinferior cerebellar artery;* Car., *carotid;* Cav., *cavernous;* Clin., *clinoid;* CN, *cranial nerve;* Eust., *eustachian;* For., *foramen;* Front., *frontal;* Frontozyg., *frontozygomatic;* Gr., *greater;* Infratemp., *infratemporal;* Lat., *lateral;* Lig., *ligament;* M., *muscle;* Max., *maxillary;* Men., *meningeal;* Men. Hyp., *meningohypophyseal;* Mid., *middle;* N., *nerve;* Pet., *petrosal, petrous;* Petrosphen., *petrosphenoid;* P.I.C.A., *posteroinferior cerebellar artery;* Post., *posterior;* Pteryg., *pterygoid;* Pterygopal., *pterygopalatine;* Seg., *segment;* Temp., *temporal, temporalis;* Tens., *tensor;* Tymp., *tympani;* Vert., *vertebral.*

wall of the sphenoid sinus offers the possibility that the intracavernous segment might be exposed by the transsphenoidal approach for trapping procedures, inserting catheters for obliteration of fistulas, or for insertion of material to thrombose arteriovenous fistulas in the sinus.

REFERENCES

1. Bedford MA: The "cavernous" sinus. **Br J Ophthalmol** 50:41–46, 1966.
2. Bernasconi V, Cassinari V: Caratteristische angiografiche dei meningiomi del tentorio. **Radiol Med (Torino)** 43:1015–1026, 1957.
3. Dolenc VV: Direct microsurgical repair of intracavernous vascular lesions. **J Neurosurg** 58:824–831, 1983.
4. Dolenc VV: A combined epi- and subdural direct approach to carotid-ophthalmic artery aneurysms. **J Neurosurg** 62:667–672, 1985.
5. Fujii K, Chambers SM, Rhoton AL Jr: Neurovascular relationships of the sphenoid sinus: A microsurgical study. **J Neurosurg** 50:31–39, 1979.
6. Harris FS, Rhoton AL Jr: Anatomy of the cavernous sinus: A microsurgical study. **J Neurosurg** 45:169–180, 1976.
7. Inoue T, Rhoton AL Jr, Theele D, Barry ME: Surgical approaches to the cavernous sinus: A microsurgical study. **Neurosurgery** 26:903–932, 1990.
8. Johnston JA, Parkinson D: Intracranial sympathetic pathways associated with the sixth cranial nerve. **J Neurosurg** 40:236–243, 1974.
9. Laws ER Jr, Onofrio BM, Pearson BW, McDonald TJ, Dirrenberger RA: Successful management of bilateral carotid-cavernous fistulae with a transsphenoidal approach. **Neurosurgery** 4:162–167, 1979.
10. Liu Q, Rhoton AL Jr: Middle meningeal origin of the ophthalmic artery. **Neurosurgery** 49:401–407, 2001.
11. McConnell EM: The arterial blood supply of the human hypophysis cerebri. **Anat Rec** 115:175–203, 1953.
12. Parkinson D: A surgical approach to the cavernous portion of the carotid artery: Anatomical studies and case report. **J Neurosurg** 23:474–483, 1965.
13. Parkinson D: Transcavernous repair of carotid cavernous fistula: Case report. **J Neurosurg** 26:420–424, 1967.
14. Parkinson D: Carotid cavernous fistula: Direct repair with preservation of the carotid artery—Technical note. **J Neurosurg** 38:99–106, 1973.
15. Parkinson D: Surgical anatomy of the lateral sellar compartment (cavernous sinus). **Clin Neurosurg** 36:219–239, 1990.
16. Renn WH, Rhoton AL Jr: Microsurgical anatomy of the sellar region. **J Neurosurg** 43:288–298, 1975.
17. Rhoton AL Jr, Natori Y: Neural structures, in Rhoton Al Jr, Natori Y (eds): *The Orbit and Sellar Region: Microsurgical Anatomy and Operative Approaches.* New York, Thieme Medical Publishers, Inc., 1996, pp 28–77.
18. Rhoton AL Jr, Natori Y: The skull, in Rhoton Al Jr, Natori Y (eds): *The Orbit and Sellar Region: Microsurgical Anatomy and Operative Approaches.* New York, Thieme Medical Publishers, Inc., 1996, pp 4–25.
19. Rhoton AL Jr, Hardy DG, Chambers SM: Microsurgical anatomy and dissection of the sphenoid bone, cavernous sinus and sellar region. **Surg Neurol** 12:63–104, 1979.
20. Sekhar LN, Møller AR: Operative management of tumors involving the cavernous sinus. **J Neurosurg** 64:879–889, 1986.
21. Sekhar LN, Burgess J, Akin O: Anatomical study of the cavernous sinus emphasizing operative approaches and related vascular and neural reconstruction. **Neurosurgery** 21:806–816, 1987.
22. Seoane ER, Rhoton AL Jr, de Oliveira EP: Microsurgical anatomy of the dural collar (carotid collar) and rings around the clinoid segment of the internal carotid artery. **Neurosurgery** 42:869–886, 1998.
23. Sunderland S, Hughes ESR: The pupilloconstrictor pathway and the nerves to the ocular muscles in man. **Brain** 69:301–309, 1946.
24. Taptas JN: The so-called cavernous sinus: A review of the controversy and its implications for neurosurgeons. **Neurosurgery** 11:712–717, 1982.
25. Umansky F, Nathan H: The lateral wall of the cavernous sinus: With special reference to the nerves related to it. **J Neurosurg** 56:228–234, 1982.
26. Wallace S, Goldberg HI, Leeds NE, Mishkin MM: The cavernous branches of the internal carotid artery. **Am J Roentgenol Radium Ther Nucl Med** 101:34–46, 1967.

Figure from D'Agoty Gautier's Essai d'anatomie, en tableaux imprimés. *Paris, 1748.*

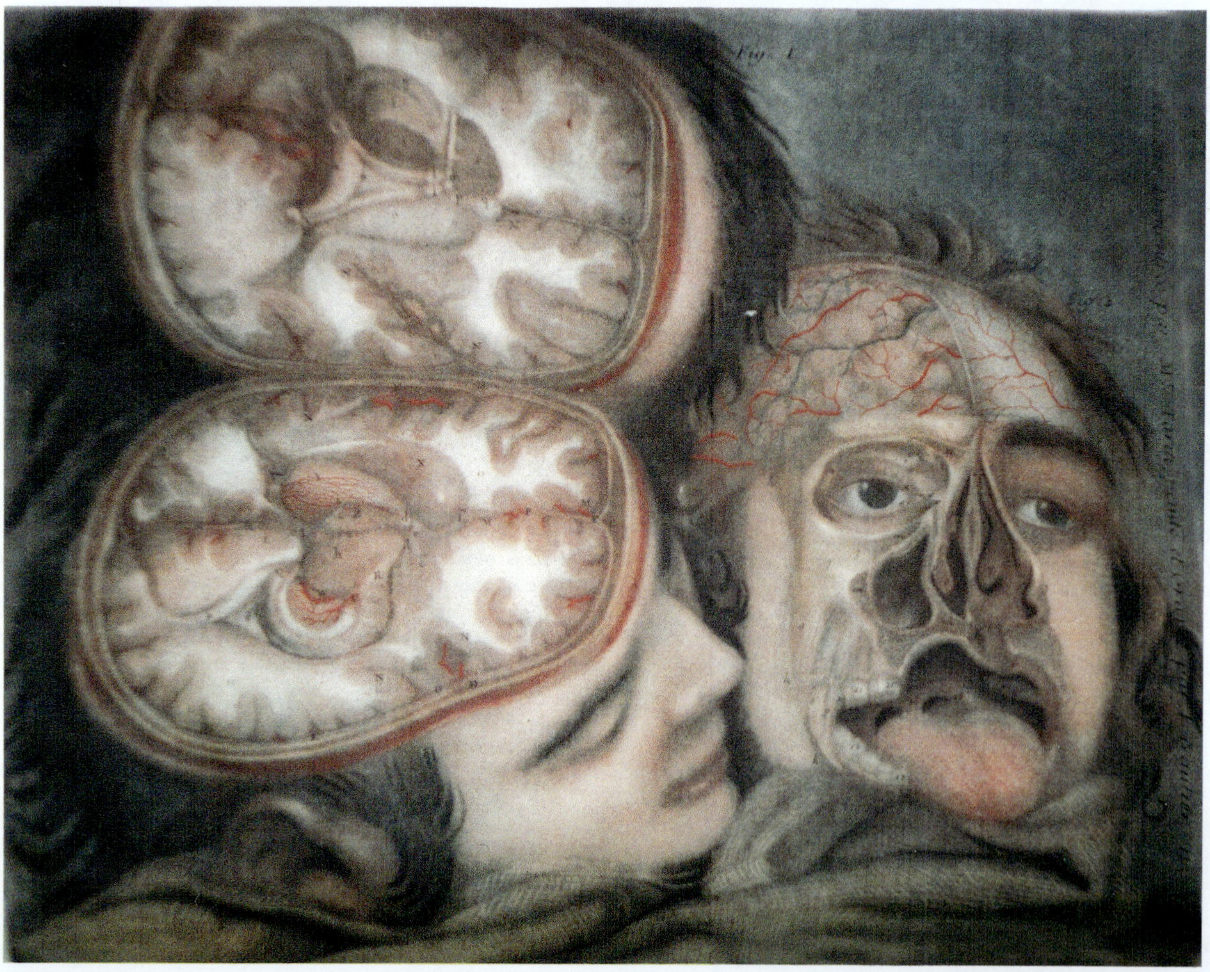

PART 3

The Posterior Cranial Fossa: Microsurgical Anatomy & Surgical Approaches

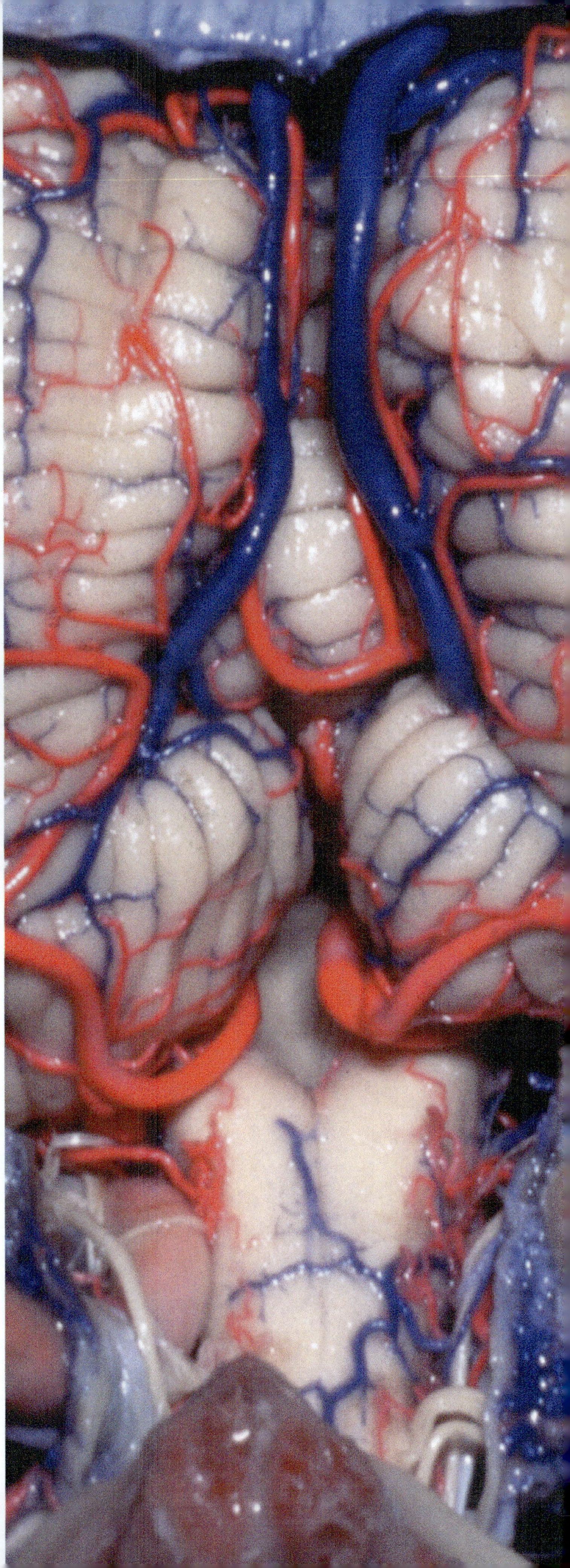

CHAPTER 1

Cerebellum and Fourth Ventricle

Albert L. Rhoton, Jr., M.D.

Department of Neurological Surgery, University of Florida, Gainesville, Florida

Key words: Cerebellar artery, Cranial nerve, Fourth ventricle, Intracranial vein, Microsurgical anatomy

The posterior cranial fossa, the largest and deepest of the three cranial fossae, contains the most complex intracranial anatomy. Here, in approximately one-eighth the intracranial space, are found the pathways regulating consciousness, vital autonomic functions, and motor activities and sensory reception for the head, body, and extremities, in addition to the centers for controlling balance and gait. Only 2 of the 12 pairs of cranial nerves are located entirely outside the posterior fossa; the 10 other pairs have a segment within the posterior fossa (22, 25) (*Fig. 1.1*). The posterior fossa is strategically situated at the outlet of the cerebrospinal fluid flow from the ventricular system. The arterial relationships are especially complex, with the vertebral and basilar arteries having relatively inaccessible segments deep in front of the brainstem and the major cerebellar arteries coursing in relation to multiple sets of cranial nerves before reaching the cerebellum (9, 10, 18, 19).

The posterior fossa extends from the tentorial incisura, through which it communicates with the supratentorial space, to the foramen magnum, through which it communicates with the spinal canal. It is surrounded by the occipital, temporal, parietal, and sphenoid bones (*Fig. 1.1*). It is bounded in front by the dorsum sellae, the posterior part of the sphenoid body, and the clival part of the occipital bone; behind by the lower portion of the squamosal part of the occipital bone; and on each side by the petrous and mastoid parts of the temporal bone, the lateral part of the occipital bone, and above and behind by a small part of the mastoid angle of the parietal bone. Its intracranial surface is penetrated by the jugular foramen, internal acoustic meatus, hypoglossal canal, the vestibular and cochlear aqueducts, and several venous emissary foramina, all of which will be explored in greater detail. The upper surface of the cerebellum is separated from the supratentorial space by the tentorium cerebelli. Optimizing an operative approach to the posterior fossa requires an understanding of the relationships of the cerebellum, cranial nerves, brainstem, the cerebellar arteries, veins, and peduncles, and the complex fissures between the cerebellum and brainstem. The relationships of the fourth ventricle to the cerebellar surfaces and the fissures through which the ventricle is approached surgically are among the most complex in the brain. This section on the cerebellum and fourth ventricle will begin at the cerebellar surfaces and progress to the deeper neural structures.

CEREBELLAR SURFACES

The cortical surfaces are divided on the basis of the structures they face, or along which they may be exposed, to make this description more readily applicable to the operative setting (*Fig. 1.2*). The first surface, the tentorial surface, faces the tentorium and is retracted in a supracerebellar approach; the second surface, the suboccipital surface, is located below and between the lateral and sigmoid sinuses and is exposed in a suboccipital craniectomy; and the third surface, the petrosal surface, faces forward toward the posterior surface of the petrous bone and is retracted to expose the cerebellopontine angle. Each of the surfaces has the vermis in the midline and the hemispheres laterally and is divided by a major fissure named on the basis of the surface that it divides. The hemispheric lobules forming each of the three surfaces commonly overlap onto and form a part of the adjacent surfaces (22). The fissures dividing the three cortical surfaces are to be distinguished from the fissures between the cerebellum and the brainstem.

Tentorial surface

The tentorial surface faces and conforms to the lower surface of the tentorium (*Figs. 1.2–1.4*). The anteromedial part of this surface, the apex, formed by the anterior vermis, is the highest point on the cerebellum. This surface slopes downward from its anteromedial to its posterolateral edge. On the tentorial surface, the transition from the vermis to the hemispheres is smooth and not marked by the deep fissures on the suboccipital surface between the vermis and hemispheres. Deep notches, the anterior and posterior cerebellar incisurae, groove the anterior and posterior edges of the tentorial surface in the midline. The brainstem fits into the anterior cerebellar incisura and the falx cerebelli fits into the posterior incisura (*Fig. 1.2*).

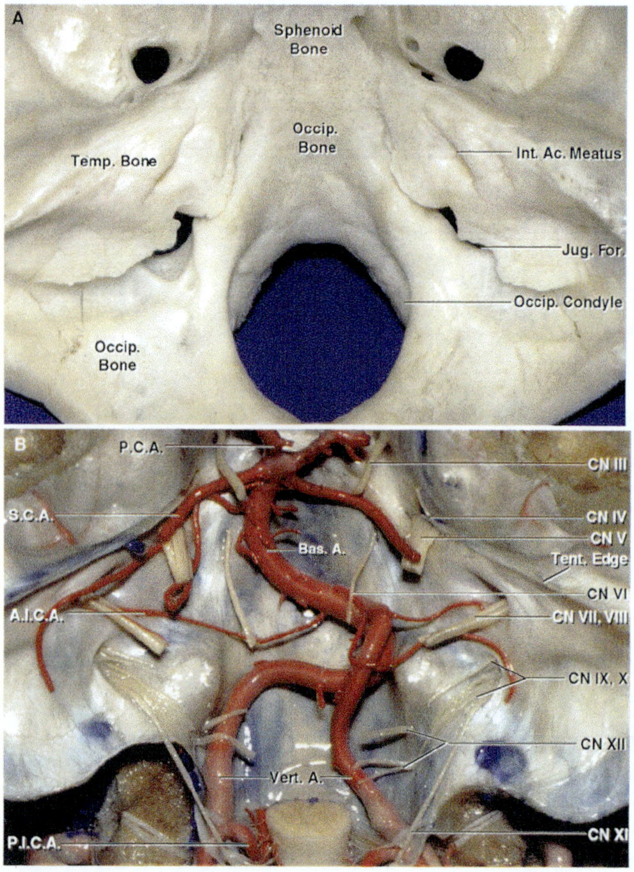

FIGURE 1.1. ***A*, superior view of the posterior cranial fossa. The osseus walls of the posterior fossa are formed by the occipital, temporal, and sphenoid bones. The fossa is bounded in front by the dorsum sellae and posterior part of the sphenoid bone and the clival part of the occipital bone; behind by the lower portion of the squamosal part of the occipital bone; and on each side by the petrous and mastoid parts of the temporal bone, and the lateral part of the occipital bone. One small part above the temporal bone is formed by the inferior angle of the parietal bone. *B*, nerves and arteries of the posterior fossa. Only 2 of the 12 pairs of cranial nerves course entirely outside the posterior fossa. The tentorium, which is attached along the petrous ridges, roofs the posterior fossa. *A.*, artery; *Ac.*, acoustic; *A.I.C.A.*, anteroinferior cerebellar artery; *Bas.*, basilar; *CN*, cranial nerve; *For.*, foramen; *Int.*, internal; *Jug.*, jugular; *Occip.*, occipital; *P.C.A.*, posterior cerebral artery; *P.I.C.A.*, posteroinferior cerebellar artery; *S.C.A.*, superior cerebellar artery; *Temp.*, temporal; *Tent.*, tentorial; *Vert.*, vertebral.**

The anterior border, separating the tentorial and petrosal surfaces, has a lateral part (the anterolateral margin) that is parallel to the superior petrosal sinus and separates the hemispheric part of the tentorial and petrosal surfaces, and a medial part (the anteromedial margin) that faces the midbrain and forms the posterior border of the fissure between the midbrain and cerebellum. The anterior angle formed by the junction of the anterolateral and anteromedial margins is directed anteriorly above the origin of the posterior root of the trigeminal nerve. The posterior border between the tentorial and the suboccipital surfaces also has a lateral and a medial part. The lateral part (the posterolateral margin) is parallel and adjacent to the lateral sinus and separates the hemispheric part of the suboccipital and tentorial surfaces, and the short medial part (the posteromedial margin) faces the posterior cerebellar incisura and separates the vermic part of the two surfaces. The lateral angle, formed by the junction of the anterolateral and posterolateral margins, is located at the junction of sigmoid, lateral, and superior petrosal sinuses. Veins often converge on the anterior and lateral angles.

The hemispheric part of the tentorial surface includes the quadrangular, simple, and superior semilunar lobules, and the vermian part includes the culmen, declive, and folium. The vermian and the related hemispheric parts from above to below in sequence are the culmen and the quadrangular lobule, the declive and the simple lobule, and the folium and the superior semilunar lobule. The tentorial surface is divided at the site of its major fissure, the tentorial fissure, into anterior and posterior parts. This fissure, located between the quadrangular and the simple lobules on the hemisphere and the culmen and the declive on the vermis, has also been called the primary fissure. The postclival fissure separates the simple and the superior semilunar lobules. The interfolial fissures on this surface pass anterolaterally from the midline and are continuous with the fissures on the superior half of the petrosal surface.

Suboccipital surface

The suboccipital surface, located below and between the lateral and sigmoid sinuses, is the most complex of the three surfaces (*Figs. 1.2* and *1.5*). Operative approaches to the fourth ventricle and most cerebellar tumors are commonly directed around or through this surface. It has a deep vertical depression, the posterior cerebellar incisura, which contains a fold of dura, the falx cerebelli. The vermis is folded into and forms the cortical surface within this incisura. The lateral walls of the incisura are formed by the medial aspects of the cerebellar hemispheres. Deep clefts, the vermohemispheric fissures, separate the vermis from the hemispheres. The vermian surface within the incisura has a diamond shape. The upper half of the diamond-shaped formation has a pyramidal shape and is called the pyramid. The folium and the tuber, superior to the pyramid, form the apex of the suboccipital part of the vermis. The lower half of the diamond-shaped formation, the uvula, projects downward between the tonsils, thus mimicking the situation in the oropharynx. The rostromedial margin of the tonsils borders the tapering edges of the uvula. The nodule, the lowermost subdivision of the vermis, is hidden deep to the uvula. The strip of vermis within the incisura is broadest at the junction of the pyramid and uvula. Inferiorly, the posterior cerebellar incisura is continuous with the vallecula cerebelli, a cleft between the tonsils that leads through the foramen of Magendie into the fourth ventricle.

The hemispheric portion of the suboccipital surface is formed by the superior and inferior semilunar and biventral

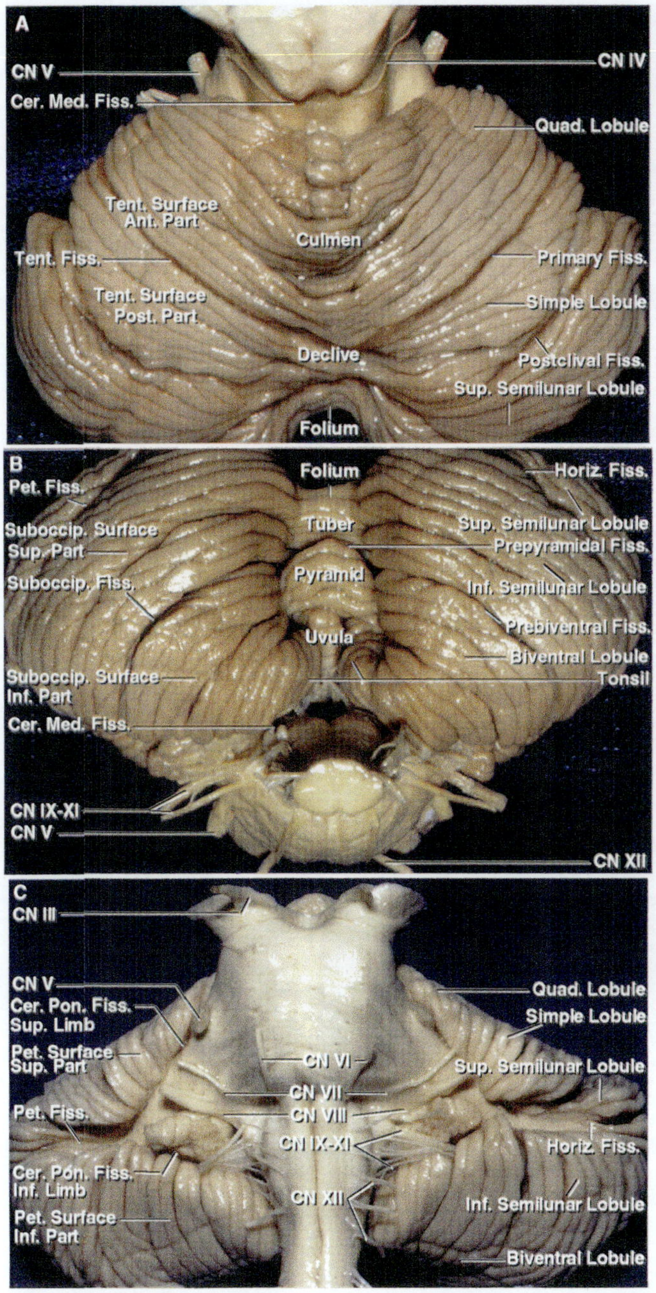

FIGURE 1.2. Tentorial, suboccipital, and petrosal cerebellar surfaces. *A*, the tentorial surface faces the lower surface of the tentorium. The anterior vermis is the most superior part of the tentorial surface. This surface slopes downward to its posterior and lateral margins. The vermian subdivisions of this surface are superior to their corresponding hemispheric parts. The classical nomenclature applied to the vermian and hemispheric subdivisions of the tentorial surface is listed on the *right*, and our simplified nomenclature is listed on the *left*. The culmen and quadrangular lobules correspond to the anterior part of the tentorial surface, and the declive, simple lobules, and part of the superior semilunar lobules correspond to the posterior part of the tentorial surface. The fissure separating the tentorial surface into anterior and posterior parts is referred to as the tentorial fissure in our nomenclature, but is the primary fissure in older nomenclature. This fissure separates the hemispheric surface between the quadrangular and simple lobules and the vermis between the declive and culmen. The anterior part of the superior surface of the cerebellum surrounds the posterior half of the midbrain to form the cerebellomesencephalic fissure. *B*, suboccipital surface. The suboccipital surface is located below and between the sigmoid and lateral sinuses and is the surface that is exposed in a wide bilateral suboccipital craniectomy. The classical nomenclature applied to this surface is shown on the *right*, and our simplified nomenclature is on the *left*. The vermis sits in a large median depression, the posterior cerebellar incisura, between the cerebellar hemispheres. According to classical nomenclature, the portions of the vermis within the incisura from above to below are the folium, tuber, pyramid, and uvula. The parts of the hemispheric surface from above to below are the superior and inferior semilunar and biventral lobules and the tonsils. These lobules extend beyond the suboccipital surface to the other surfaces of the cerebellum. The prebiventral fissures between the inferior semilunar and the biventral lobules separate the hemispheres into superior and inferior parts, and the prepyramidal fissure between the pyramid and tuber separates the vermis into superior and inferior parts. We refer to the union of the prebiventral and the prepyramidal fissures that divide the suboccipital surface into superior and inferior parts as the suboccipital fissure. From below to above the corresponding vermian and hemispheric parts are the uvula and the tonsils, the pyramid and the biventral lobules, the tuber and inferior semilunar lobules, and the folium and the superior semilunar lobules. The petrosal (horizontal) fissure, the most prominent fissure on the petrosal surface, extends onto the suboccipital surface and divides the superior half of the suboccipital surface between the superior and inferior semilunar lobules. The cerebellomedullary fissure extends superiorly between the cerebellum and medulla. *C*, petrosal surface. The petrosal surface faces forward toward the petrous temporal bone and is the surface that is retracted to surgically expose the cerebellopontine angle. The classical nomenclature applied to this surface is shown on the *right*, and our simplified nomenclature is on the *left*. The petrosal fissure divides the petrosal surface into superior and inferior parts. The superior part is formed by the quadrangular, simple, and a small part of the superior semilunar lobules. The inferior part is formed by the inferior semilunar and biventral lobules and the tonsil. The cerebellopontine fissures are V-shaped fissures formed where the cerebellum wraps around the pons and the middle cerebellar peduncles. These fissures have a superior and an inferior limb, which meet at a lateral apex. The petrosal fissure extends laterally from the apex of the cerebellopontine fissures. *Ant.*, anterior; *Cer.Med.*, cerebellomedullary; *Cer.Pon.*, cerebellopontine; *CN*, cranial nerve; *Fiss.*, fissure; *Horiz.*, horizontal; *Inf.*, inferior; *Pet.*, petrosal; *Post.*, posterior; *Quad.*, quadrangular; *Suboccip.*, suboccipital; *Sup.*, superior; *Tent.*, tentorial.

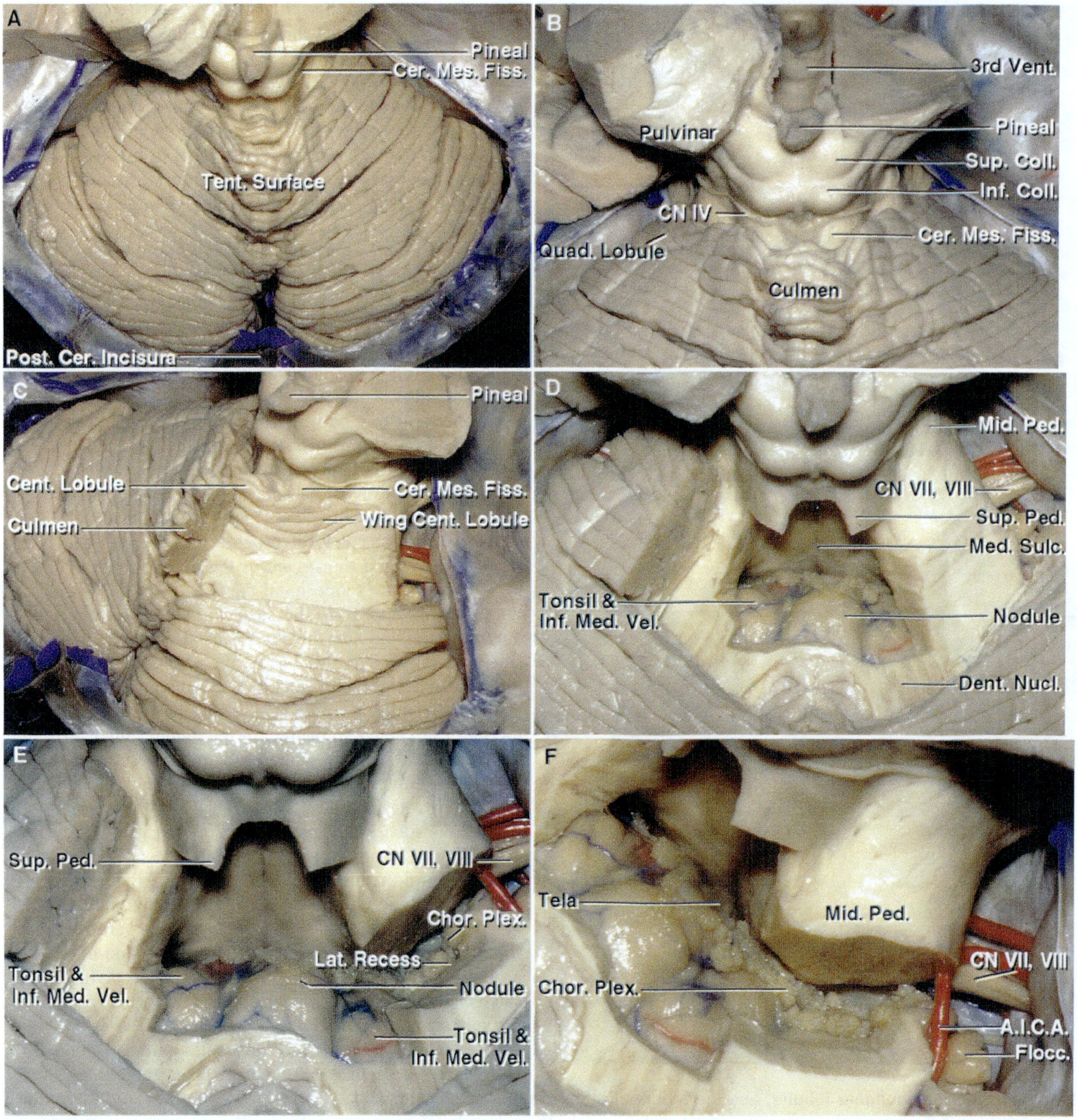

FIGURE 1.3. Tentorial surface and cerebellomesencephalic fissure. *A*, the tentorial surface faces the tentorium, which has been removed. The surface slopes downward from the apex to the posterior and lateral margins. The upper part of the tentorial surface surrounds the posterior half of the midbrain and forms the posterior lip of the cerebellomesencephalic fissure. The anterior cerebellar incisura, the notch where the brainstem fits into the anterior part of the tentorial surface, is located anteriorly and the posterior cerebellar incisura, the notch where the falx cerebelli fits into the cerebellum, is located posteriorly. *B*, enlarged view of the cerebellomesencephalic fissure, which extends downward between the midbrain and the cerebellum. The superficial part of the posterior lip is formed by the culmen in the midline and the quadrangular lobule laterally. The quadrigeminal cistern extends caudally from the pineal into the cerebellomesencephalic fissure. *C*, the culmen has been removed to expose the central lobule and its wings, which form part of the posterior lip of the cerebellomesencephalic fissure. *D*, the central lobule and its wings, the lingula, the superior medullary velum, and medial part of the superior cerebellar peduncles have been removed to expose the fourth ventricle. The lower half of the roof is formed in the midline by the

lobules and the tonsils, and the vermic portion is formed by the folium, tuber, pyramid, and uvula. The vermian and the related hemispheric parts from above to below are the folium and the superior semilunar lobules, the tuber and the inferior semilunar lobules, the pyramid and the biventral lobules, and the uvula and the tonsils.

The suboccipital surface is divided at its major fissure, the suboccipital fissure, into superior and inferior parts. The suboccipital fissure has a vermian and a hemispheric part. The vermian part of this fissure, the prepyramidal fissure, separates the tuber and the pyramid, and the hemispheric part, the prebiventral fissure, separates the biventral and the inferior semilunar lobules. The prebiventral and prepyramidal fissures are continuous at the vermohemispheric junction, and together they form the suboccipital fissure. The petrosal fissure, the major fissure on the petrosal surface, extends from the petrosal surface onto the suboccipital surface, and separates the superior and inferior semilunar lobules laterally and the folium and the tuber medially. The tonsillobiventral fissure separates the tonsil and the biventral lobule.

The tonsils, the most prominent structure blocking access to the caudal part of the fourth ventricle, are a hemispheric component (*Figs. 1.5* and *1.6*). Each tonsil is an ovoid structure in the inferomedial part of the suboccipital surface that is attached to the remainder of the cerebellum along its superolateral border by a white matter bundle called the tonsillar peduncle. The remaining tonsillar surfaces are free surfaces. The inferior pole and posterior surface face the cisterna magna and are visible inferomedial to the remainder of the suboccipital surface. The lateral surface of each tonsil is covered by, but is separated from, the biventral lobule by a narrow cleft, except superiorly at the level of the tonsillar peduncle. The medial, anterior, and superior surfaces all face other neural structures, but are separated from them by narrow fissures. The anterior surface of each tonsil faces and is separated from the posterior surface of the medulla by the cerebellomedullary fissure. The medial surfaces of the tonsils face each other across a narrow cleft, the vallecula, which leads into the fourth ventricle. The ventral aspect of the superior pole of each tonsil faces the three structures (tela choroidea, inferior medullary velum, and nodule) forming the lower half of the roof of the fourth ventricle. The superior pole is separated from the surrounding structures by a posterior extension of the cerebellomedullary fissure, called either the telovelotonsillar or supratonsillar cleft. The posterior aspect of the superior pole faces the uvula medially and the biventral lobule laterally.

Petrosal surface

The petrosal or anterior surface faces the posterior surface of the petrous bones, the brainstem, and the fourth ventricle (*Figs. 1.2* and *1.7*). The lateral or hemispheric part of the petrosal surface rests against the petrous bone and is retracted to expose the cerebellopontine angle. The median or vermian part of the petrosal surface has a deep longitudinal furrow, the anterior cerebellar incisura, that wraps around the posterior surface of the brainstem and fourth ventricle. The right and left halves of the petrosal surfaces are not connected from side to side by a continuous strip of vermis, as are the suboccipital and tentorial surfaces, because of the interposition of the fourth ventricle between the superior and inferior part of the vermis. The vermal components rostral to the fourth ventricle are the lingula, the central lobule, and the culmen, and those caudal to the fourth ventricle are the nodule and the uvula. The hemispheric surfaces are formed by the wings of the central lobule and the anterior surfaces of the quadrangular, simple, biventral, and superior and inferior semilunar lobules, the tonsils, and the flocculi. The vermian and related hemispheric parts are the central lobule and the wings of the central lobule, the culmen and the quadrangular lobules, the nodule and the flocculi, and the uvula and the tonsils. The major fissure on this surface, the petrosal fissure, also called the horizontal fissure, splits the petrosal surface into superior and inferior parts and extends onto the suboccipital surface between the superior and inferior semilunar lobules.

THE FOURTH VENTRICLE AND THE CEREBELLAR-BRAINSTEM FISSURES

Fourth ventricle

The fourth ventricle is a broad, tent-shaped midline cavity located between the cerebellum and the brainstem. It is connected rostrally through the aqueduct with the third ventricle, caudally through the foramen of Magendie with the cisterna magna, and laterally through the foramina of Luschka with the cerebellopontine angles. Most of the cranial nerves arise near its floor. It has a roof, a floor, and two lateral recesses. It is ventral to the cerebellum, dorsal to the pons and medulla, and medial to the cerebellar peduncles.

nodule and laterally by the inferior medullary velum, which passes laterally above, but is separated from the rostral pole of the tonsils by the cerebellomedullary fissure. *E*, some of the middle peduncle has been removed to expose the choroid plexus extending through the lateral recess into the cerebellopontine angle below the facial and vestibulocochlear nerves. *F*, oblique view of the lower half of the roof formed by the inferior medullary velum and the tela choroidea in which the choroid plexus arises. The inferior medullary velum arises on the surface of the nodule and extends laterally to blend into the flocculus and, with the flocculus and nodule, forms the flocculonodular lobe of the cerebellum. *A.I.C.A.*, anteroinferior cerebellar artery; *Cent.*, central; *Cer.*, cerebellar; *Cer.Mes.*, cerebellomesencephalic; *Chor.*, choroid; *CN*, cranial nerve; *Coll.*, colliculus; *Dent.*, dentate; *Fiss.*, fissure; *Flocc.*, flocculus; *Inf.*, inferior; *Lat.*, lateral; *Mid.*, middle; *Med.*, median, medullary; *Nucl.*, nucleus; *Ped.*, peduncle; *Plex.*, plexus; *Post.*, posterior; *Quad.*, quadrangular; *Sulc.*, sulcus; *Sup.*, superior; *Tent.*, tentorial; *Vel.*, velum; *Vent.*, ventricle.

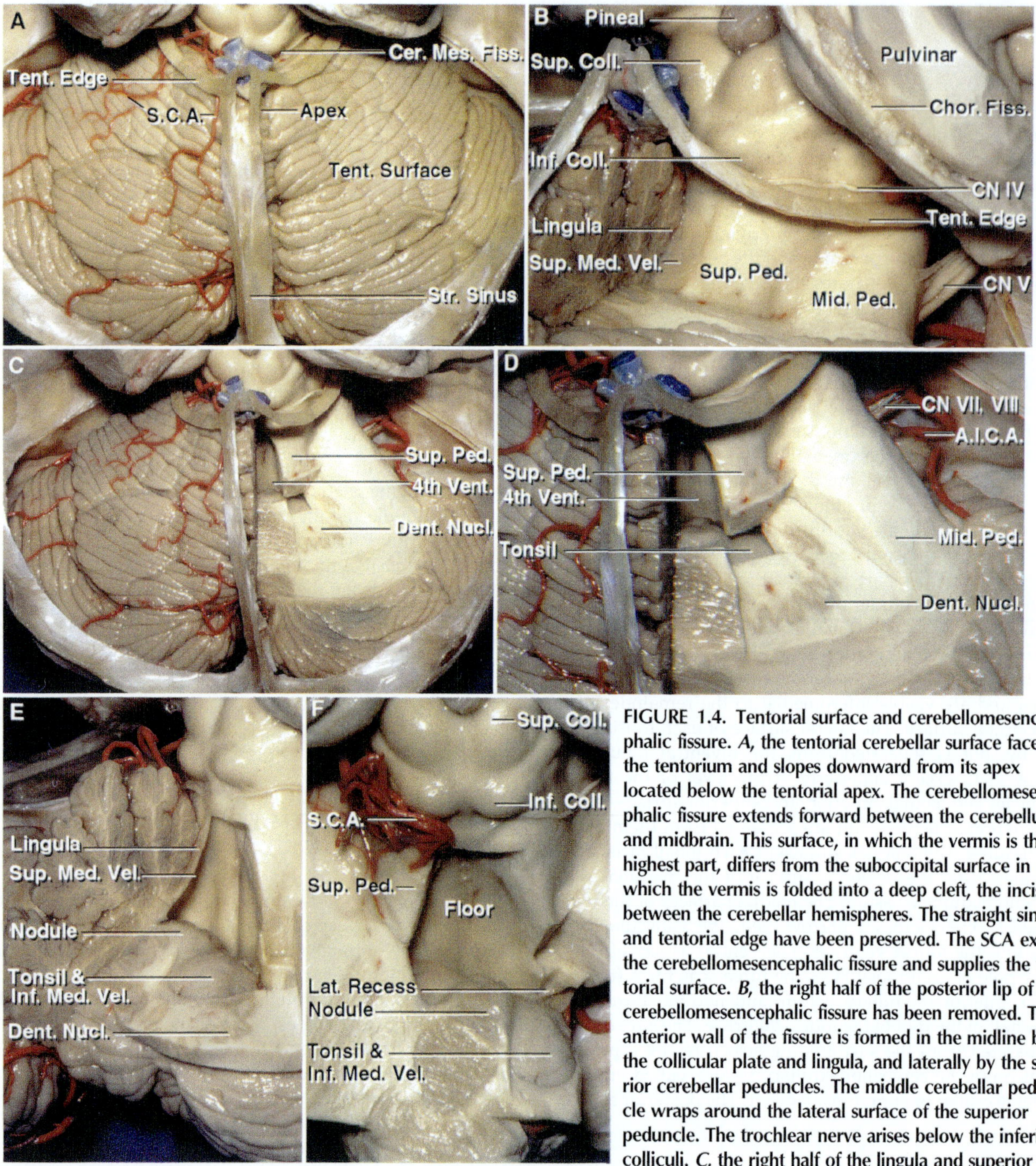

FIGURE 1.4. Tentorial surface and cerebellomesencephalic fissure. *A*, the tentorial cerebellar surface faces the tentorium and slopes downward from its apex located below the tentorial apex. The cerebellomesencephalic fissure extends forward between the cerebellum and midbrain. This surface, in which the vermis is the highest part, differs from the suboccipital surface in which the vermis is folded into a deep cleft, the incisura, between the cerebellar hemispheres. The straight sinus and tentorial edge have been preserved. The SCA exits the cerebellomesencephalic fissure and supplies the tentorial surface. *B*, the right half of the posterior lip of the cerebellomesencephalic fissure has been removed. The anterior wall of the fissure is formed in the midline by the collicular plate and lingula, and laterally by the superior cerebellar peduncles. The middle cerebellar peduncle wraps around the lateral surface of the superior peduncle. The trochlear nerve arises below the inferior colliculi. *C*, the right half of the lingula and superior medullary velum have been removed to expose the fourth ventricle. Additional white matter has been removed below the right superior peduncle to expose the dentate nucleus in which the superior peduncular fibers arise. *D*, enlarged view. The dentate nucleus appears to wrap around the rostral pole of the tonsil. *E*, oblique view into the fourth ventricle. Additional cerebellum has been removed to expose the nodule and rostral pole of the tonsil. The dentate nucleus wraps around the rostral pole of the tonsil. The upper half of the roof is formed by the superior medullary velum, which has the lingula layered on its outer surface. The upper part of the lower half of the roof is formed by the nodule in the midline and by the inferior medullary velum laterally. The inferior medullary velum, an almost transparent membrane, stretches laterally across the upper pole of the tonsil. *F*, the left half of the upper part of the roof has been removed. The velum arises on the nodule and sweeps laterally above both tonsils. The SCA courses within the cerebellomesencephalic fissure. *A.I.C.A.*, anteroinferior cerebellar artery; *Cer.Mes.*, cerebellomesencephalic; *Chor.*, choroidal; *CN*, cranial nerve; *Coll.*, colliculus; *Dent.*, dentate; *Fiss.*, fissure; *Inf.*, inferior; *Lat.*, lateral; *Med.*, medullary; *Mid.*, middle; *Nucl.*, nucleus; *Ped.*, peduncle; *S.C.A.*, superior cerebellar artery; *Str.*, straight; *Sup.*, superior; *Tent.*, tentorial; *Vel.*, velum; *Vent.*, ventricle.

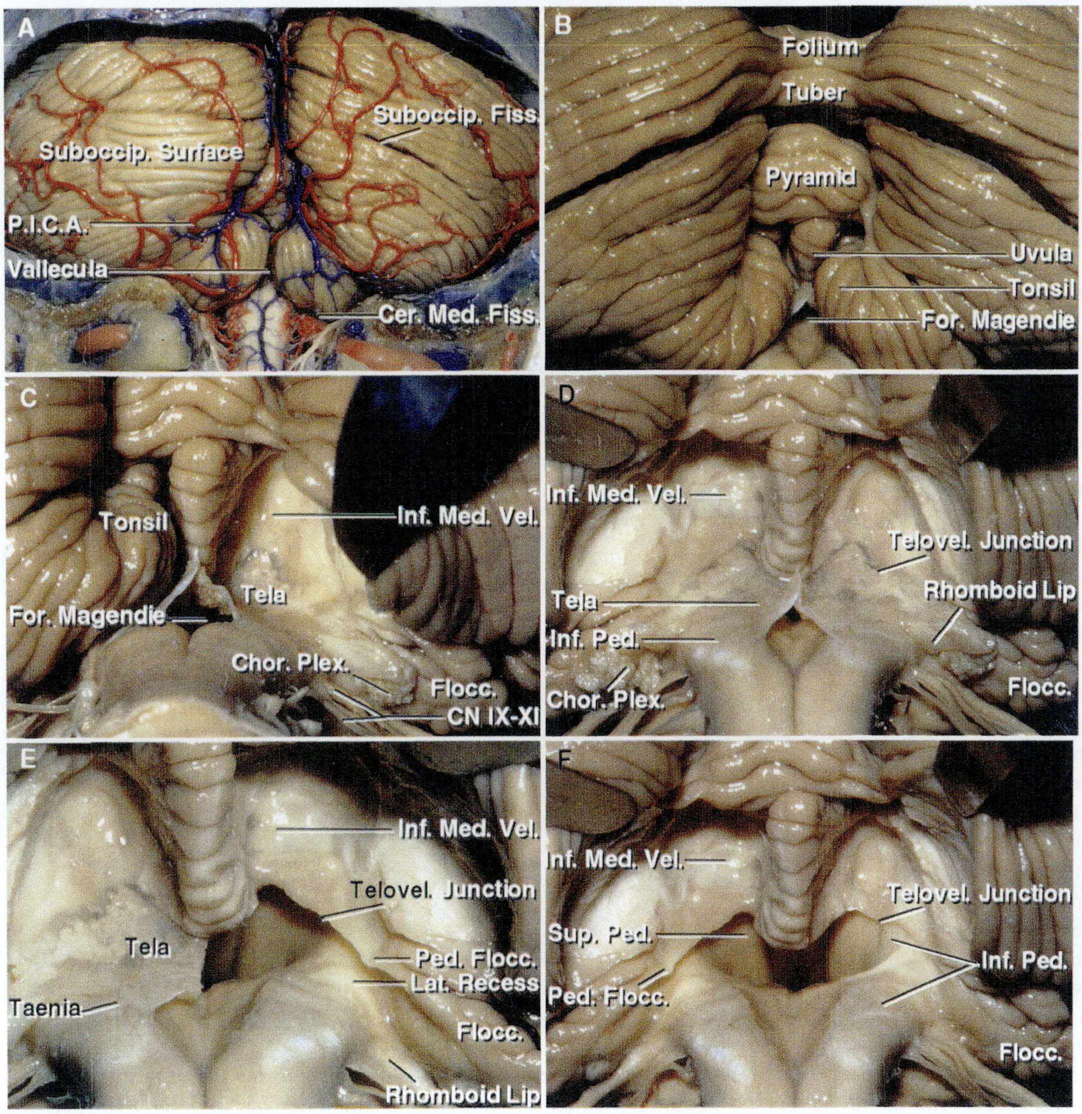

FIGURE 1.5. Suboccipital surface of the cerebellum and the cerebellomedullary fissure. *A*, the suboccipital surface is located below and between the sigmoid and lateral sinuses and is the surface that is exposed in a wide suboccipital craniectomy. The vermis sits in a depression, the posterior cerebellar incisura, between the hemispheres. The cerebellomedullary fissure extends superiorly between the cerebellum and medulla along the inferior half of the ventricular roof. The vallecula extends upward between the tonsils and communicates through the foramen of Magendie with the fourth ventricle. The PICA supplies the suboccipital surface. *B*, enlarged view. The lower parts of the vermis behind the ventricle are the pyramid and uvula. *C*, the right tonsil has been removed to expose the lower part of the roof formed by the inferior medullary velum and tela choroidea. The nodule on which the velum arises is hidden in front of the uvula. The uvula hangs downward between the tonsils, thus mimicking the situation in the oropharynx. The choroid plexus arises on the inner surface of the tela and extends through the foramen of Luschka behind the glossopharyngeal and vagus nerve. The inferior medullary velum arises on the surface of the nodule, drapes across the superior pole of the tonsil, and blends into the flocculus laterally. *D*, both tonsils have been removed to expose the inferior medullary velum and tela choroidea bilaterally. The telovelar junction is the junction between the velum and tela. The cerebellomedullary fissure extends upward between the rostral pole of the tonsil on one side and the tela choroidea and inferior medullary velum on the opposite side. The segment of the PICA passing through this cleft is called the telovelotonsillar segment. The rhomboid lip is a sheet-like layer of neural tissue attached to the lateral margin of the ventricular floor, which extends posterior to the glossopharyngeal and vagus nerves and joins the tela choroidea to form a pouch at the outer extremity of the lateral recess. *E*, the right half of the tela has been removed to expose the ventricle and the lateral recess. The inferior medullary velum extends laterally to form a peduncle, the peduncle of the flocculus, which blends into the flocculus at the outer margin of the lateral recess. *F*, the tela has been removed on both sides. The lateral wall of the upper half of the ventricle is formed by the superior cerebellar peduncles. The inferior cerebellar peduncles ascend along the dorsolateral medulla and form the anterior and rostral margins of the lateral recess. *Cer.Med.*, cerebellomedullary; *Chor.*, choroid; *CN*, cranial nerve; *Fiss.*, fissure; *Flocc.*, flocculus; *For.*, foramen; *Inf.*, inferior; *Lat.*, lateral; *Med.*, medullary; *Ped.*, peduncle; *P.I.C.A.*, posteroinferior cerebellar artery; *Plex.*, plexus; *Suboccip.*, suboccipital; *Sup.*, superior; *Telovel.*, telovelar; *Vel.*, velum.

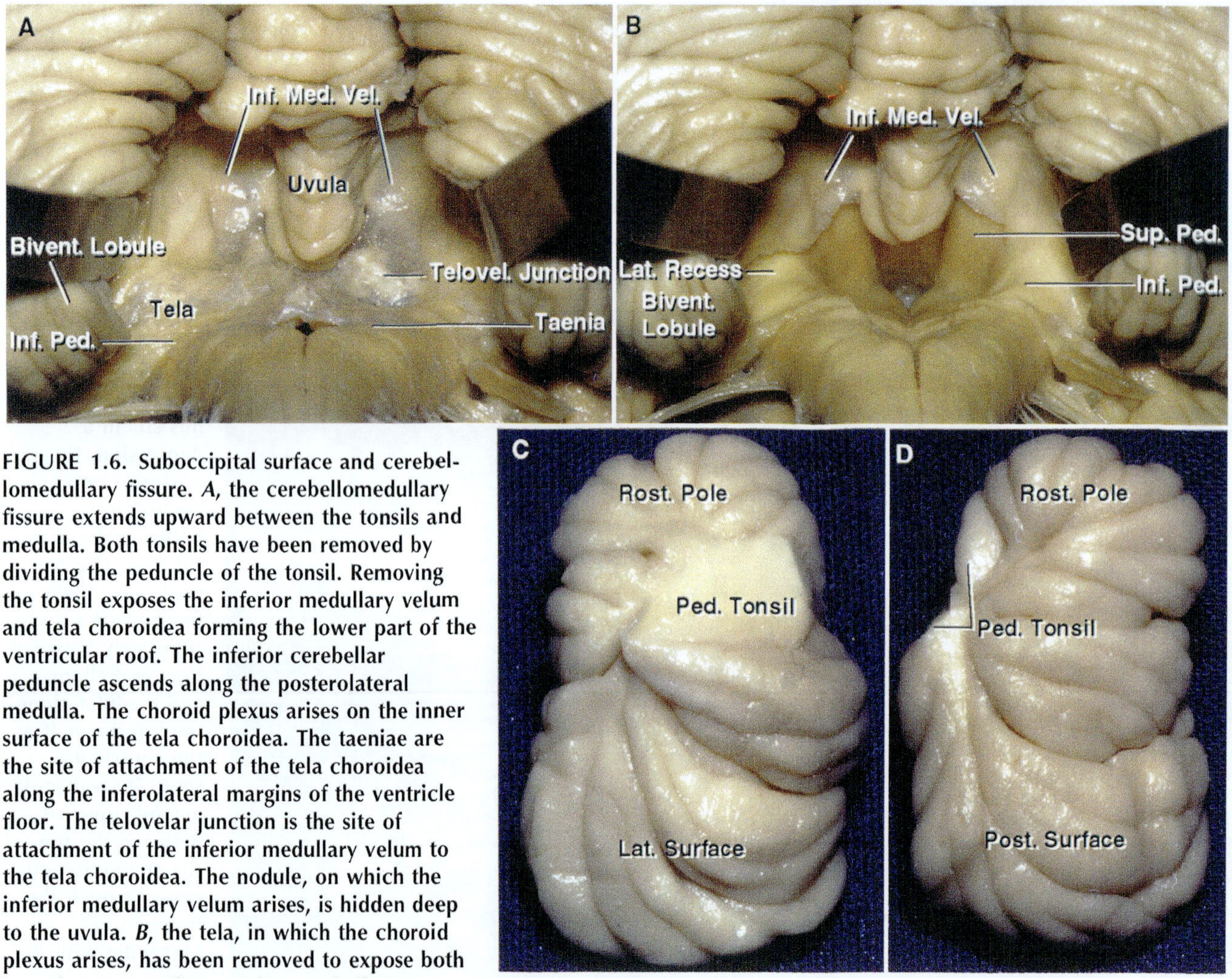

FIGURE 1.6. Suboccipital surface and cerebellomedullary fissure. *A*, the cerebellomedullary fissure extends upward between the tonsils and medulla. Both tonsils have been removed by dividing the peduncle of the tonsil. Removing the tonsil exposes the inferior medullary velum and tela choroidea forming the lower part of the ventricular roof. The inferior cerebellar peduncle ascends along the posterolateral medulla. The choroid plexus arises on the inner surface of the tela choroidea. The taeniae are the site of attachment of the tela choroidea along the inferolateral margins of the ventricle floor. The telovelar junction is the site of attachment of the inferior medullary velum to the tela choroidea. The nodule, on which the inferior medullary velum arises, is hidden deep to the uvula. *B*, the tela, in which the choroid plexus arises, has been removed to expose both lateral recesses. The superior cerebellar peduncle forms the lateral wall of the upper half of the ventricle. The inferior cerebellar peduncle forms the anterior and upper margin of the lateral recess. The middle cerebellar peduncle, which forms a large prominence on the lateral surface of the pons, is separated from the ventricular surface by the superior and inferior cerebellar peduncles. *C*, lateral surface of the left tonsil. All of the tonsillar surfaces, except at the superolateral margin, are free surfaces. The peduncle of the tonsil, located along the superolateral margin of the tonsil, attaches the tonsil to the remainder of the cerebellum. The posterior surface of the tonsil faces the cisterna magna. The medial surface faces the other tonsil. The anterior surface faces the posterior medulla. The rostral pole faces the inferior medullary velum and tela choroidea. The lateral surface below the peduncle of the tonsil faces the biventral lobule. *D*, posterior view of the left tonsil. The peduncle of the tonsil is located along the superolateral margin. Dividing the narrow peduncle allows the tonsil to be separated from the remaining cerebellum. *Bivent.*, biventral; *Inf.*, inferior; *Lat.*, lateral; *Med.*, medullary; *Ped.*, peduncle; *Post.*, posterior; *Rost.*, rostral; *Sup.*, superior; *Telovel.*, telovelar; *Vel.*, velum.

The ventricular roof is tent-shaped (*Figs. 1.8* and *1.9*). The roof expands laterally and posteriorly from its narrow rostral end just below the aqueduct to the level of the fastigium and lateral recess, the site of its greatest height and width, and from there it tapers to a narrow caudal apex at the level of the foramen of Magendie. The apex of the roof, the fastigium, divides it into superior and inferior parts. The superior part is distinctly different from the inferior part, in that the inferior part is formed largely by thin membranous layers and the superior part is formed by thicker neural structures.

The external or cisternal surfaces of the structures forming the roof are intimately related to the fissures between the cerebellum and brainstem. The three fissures formed by the embryological folding of the cerebellum around the brainstem are the cerebellomesencephalic fissure, which extends inferiorly between the cerebellum and mesencephalon and is inti-

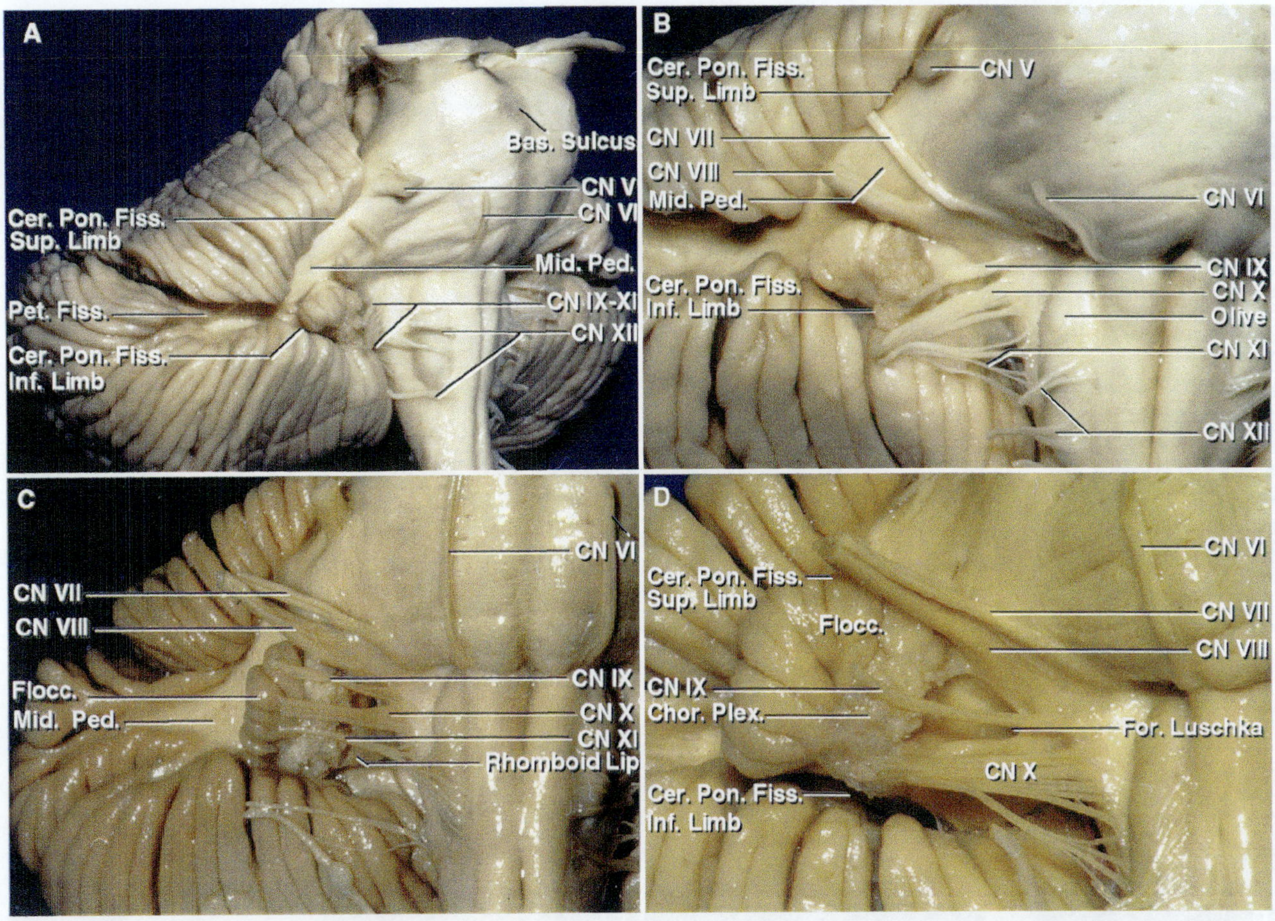

FIGURE 1.7. Brainstem, petrosal surface, and cerebellopontine fissure. *A*, oblique view. The petrosal surfaces of the cerebellum face forward toward the petrous bone and is the surface that is retracted to expose the cerebellopontine angle. The cerebellopontine fissure, which might also be referred to as the cerebellopontine angle, is a V-shaped fissure formed where the cerebellum wraps around the pons and middle cerebellar peduncle. The superior and inferior limbs meet laterally at the apex located at the anterior end of the petrosal fissure that divides the petrosal surface into superior and inferior parts. Cranial nerves V through XI arise within the margins of the cerebellopontine fissure. The flocculus and choroid plexus extend laterally from the foramen of Magendie above the lower limb of the fissure. The basilar sulcus is a shallow longitudinal groove on the anterior surface of the pons, which accommodates the basilar artery. *B*, enlarged view. The petrosal fissure extends laterally from the apex of the cerebellopontine fissure. The abducens nerve arises in the medial part of the pontomedullary sulcus rostral to the medullary pyramids. The facial and vestibulocochlear nerves arise just rostral to the foramen of Luschka near the flocculus at the lateral end of the pontomedullary sulcus. The hypoglossal nerves arise anterior to and the glossopharyngeal, vagus, and accessory nerves arise posterior to the olives. Choroid plexus protrudes from the foramen of Luschka behind the glossopharyngeal and vagus nerves. *C*, enlarged view of another brainstem. The facial and vestibulocochlear nerves join the brainstem 2 or 3 mm rostral to the glossopharyngeal nerve on a line drawn dorsal to the olive along the origin of the rootlets of the glossopharyngeal, vagus, and accessory rootlets. The rhomboid lip, a thin neural membrane in the ventral margin of the lateral recess, extends laterally behind the glossopharyngeal, vagus, and accessory nerves with the choroid plexus. *D*, enlarged view of another cerebellopontine fissure. The cerebellopontine angle is the area situated between the superior and inferior limbs of the cerebellopontine fissure. The glossopharyngeal, vagus, and accessory nerves arise near the inferior limb, dorsal to the olive, and anterior to the choroid plexus protruding from the foramen of Luschka. The facial and vestibulocochlear nerves arise in the midportion of the fissure and the trigeminal nerve near the superior limb of the fissure. The hypoglossal rootlets arise in front of the olive and the cranial rootlets of the accessory nerve. *Bas.*, basilar; *Cer.Pon.*, cerebellopontine; *Chor.*, choroid; *CN*, cranial nerve; *Fiss.*, fissure; *Flocc.*, flocculus; *For.*, foramen; *Inf.*, inferior; *Mid.*, middle; *Ped.*, peduncle; *Pet.*, petrosal; *Plex.*, plexus; *Sup.*, superior.

mately related to the superior half of the roof (*Figs. 1.3* and *1.4*); the cerebellopontine fissures, which are formed by the folding of the cerebellum around the lateral sides of the pons and are intimately related to the lateral recesses (*Figs. 1.7* and *1.8*); and the cerebellomedullary fissure, which extends superiorly between the cerebellum and the medulla and is intimately related to the inferior half of the roof (*Figs. 1.5* and *1.6*).

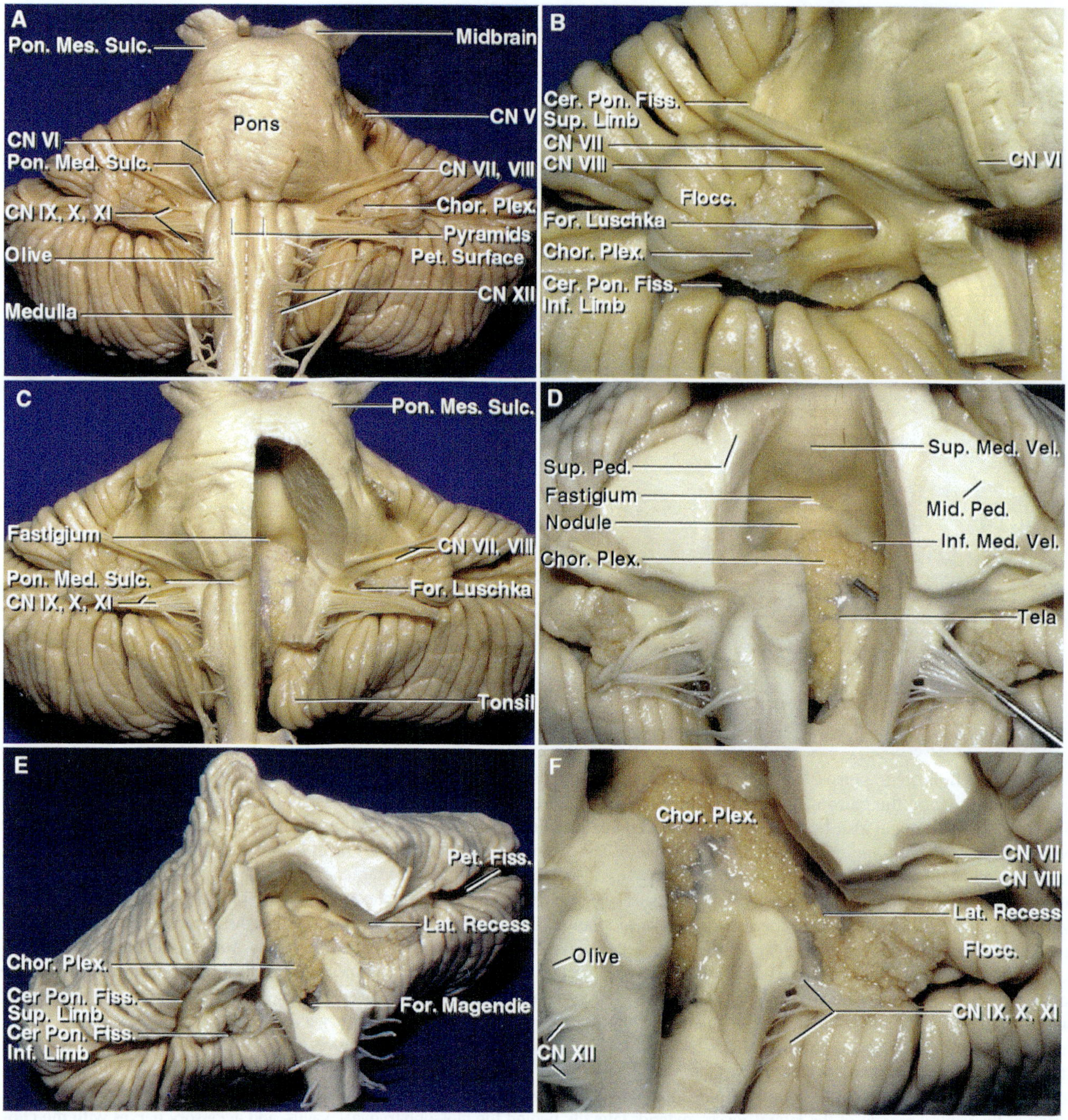

FIGURE 1.8. *A–F.* Brainstem, fourth ventricle, and petrosal cerebellar surface. Stepwise anterior exposure. *A*, the petrosal surface faces forward toward the posterior surface of the temporal bone. The fourth ventricle is located behind the pons and medulla. The midbrain and pons are separated by the pontomesencephalic sulcus and the pons and medulla by the pontomedullary sulcus. The trigeminal nerves arise from the midpons. The abducens nerve arises in the medial part of the pontomedullary sulcus, rostral to the medullary pyramids. The facial and vestibulocochlear nerves arise at the lateral end of the pontomedullary sulcus immediately rostral to the foramen of Luschka. The hypoglossal nerves arise anterior to the olives and the glossopharyngeal, vagus, and accessory nerves arise posterior to the olives. Choroid plexus protrudes from the foramen of Luschka behind to the glossopharyngeal and vagus nerves. *B*, right cerebellopontine angle following removal of some of the medulla. The foramen of Luschka opens into the cerebellopontine angle below the junction of the facial and vestibulocochlear nerves with the lateral end of the pontomedullary sulcus. Choroid plexus protrudes from the lateral recess and foramen of Luschka behind the glossopharyngeal, vagus, and accessory nerves. The cerebellopontine fissure, a V-shaped fissure formed by the cerebellum wrapping around the pons and middle cerebellar peduncle, has a superior and inferior limb that

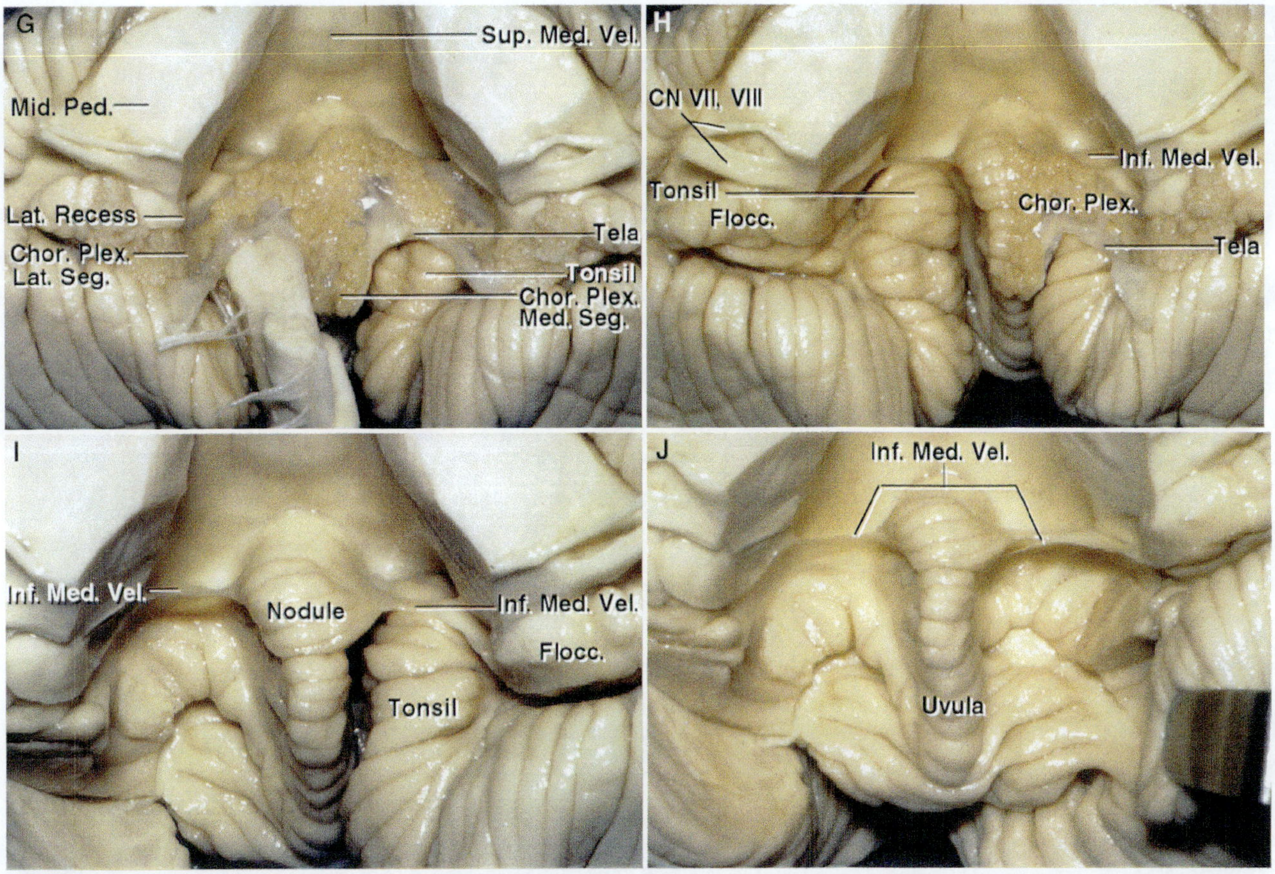

FIGURE 1.8. *G–J.* Brainstem, fourth ventricle, and petrosal cerebellar surface. *G*, the left half of the medulla has been removed. The superior half of the roof is formed by the superior medullary velum, which has the lingula of the vermis layered on its outer surface. The lower half of the roof is formed by the inferior medullary velum, which arises on the surface of the nodule, and the tela choroidea in which the choroid plexus arises. The choroid plexus is composed of paired L-shaped fringes, which have medial and lateral segments. The lateral segments extend laterally through the foramen of Luschka and the medial segments extend longitudinally through the foramen of Magendie. *H*, the right half of the tela choroidea and choroid plexus have been removed to expose the upper pole of right tonsil. *I*, the right cerebellar tonsil has been removed. All of the surfaces of the tonsils are free surfaces except the superolateral margin, the site of the tonsillar peduncle, a bundle of white matter, which attaches the tonsil to the remainder of the cerebellum. The inferior medullary velum is a thin membranous layer of neural tissue that arises on the nodule and extends laterally above the rostral pole of the tonsil to blend into the flocculus and form the flocculonodular lobe of the cerebellum. The cranial loop of the PICA courses between the rostral pole of the tonsil and the inferior medullary velum. *J*, both tonsils have been removed. The inferior medullary velum sweeps laterally from the surface of the nodule.

define the margins of the cerebellopontine angle. The superior limb extends above the trigeminal nerve and the inferior limb passes below the flocculus and the nerves that pass to the jugular foramen. *C*, the part of the pons and medulla forming the left half of the floor of the ventricle has been removed to expose the fastigium, which divides the ventricular roof into superior and inferior parts. *D*, the right half of the pons has been removed to expose the upper half of the roof. The superior part of the roof is formed by the superior medullary velum. The rostral part of the lower half of the roof is formed by the nodule and inferior medullary velum and the caudal part is formed by the tela choroidea, a thin arachnoid-like membrane, in which the choroid plexus arises. *E*, the cerebellopontine fissure has upper and lower limbs, which meet at a later apex located at the medial end of the petrosal fissure, also called the horizontal fissure, which divides the petrosal surface into upper and lower halves. The junction of the pons and medulla, which forms the anterior wall of the left lateral recess, has been removed to expose the choroid plexus protruding through the lateral recess into the cerebellopontine angles. *F*, enlarged view. The choroid plexus protrudes laterally through the foramen of Luschka into the cerebellopontine angle below the flocculus. *Cer.Pon.*, cerebellopontine; *Chor.*, choroid; *CN*, cranial nerve; *Fiss.*, fissure; *Flocc.*, flocculus; *For.*, foramen; *Inf.*, inferior; *Lat.*, lateral; *Med.*, medial, medullary; *Mid.*, middle; *Ped.*, peduncle; *Pet.*, petrosal; *Plex.*, plexus; *Pon.Med.*, pontomedullary; *Pon.Mes.*, pontomesencephalic; *Seg.*, segment; *Sulc.*, sulcus; *Sup.*, superior; *Vel.*, velum.

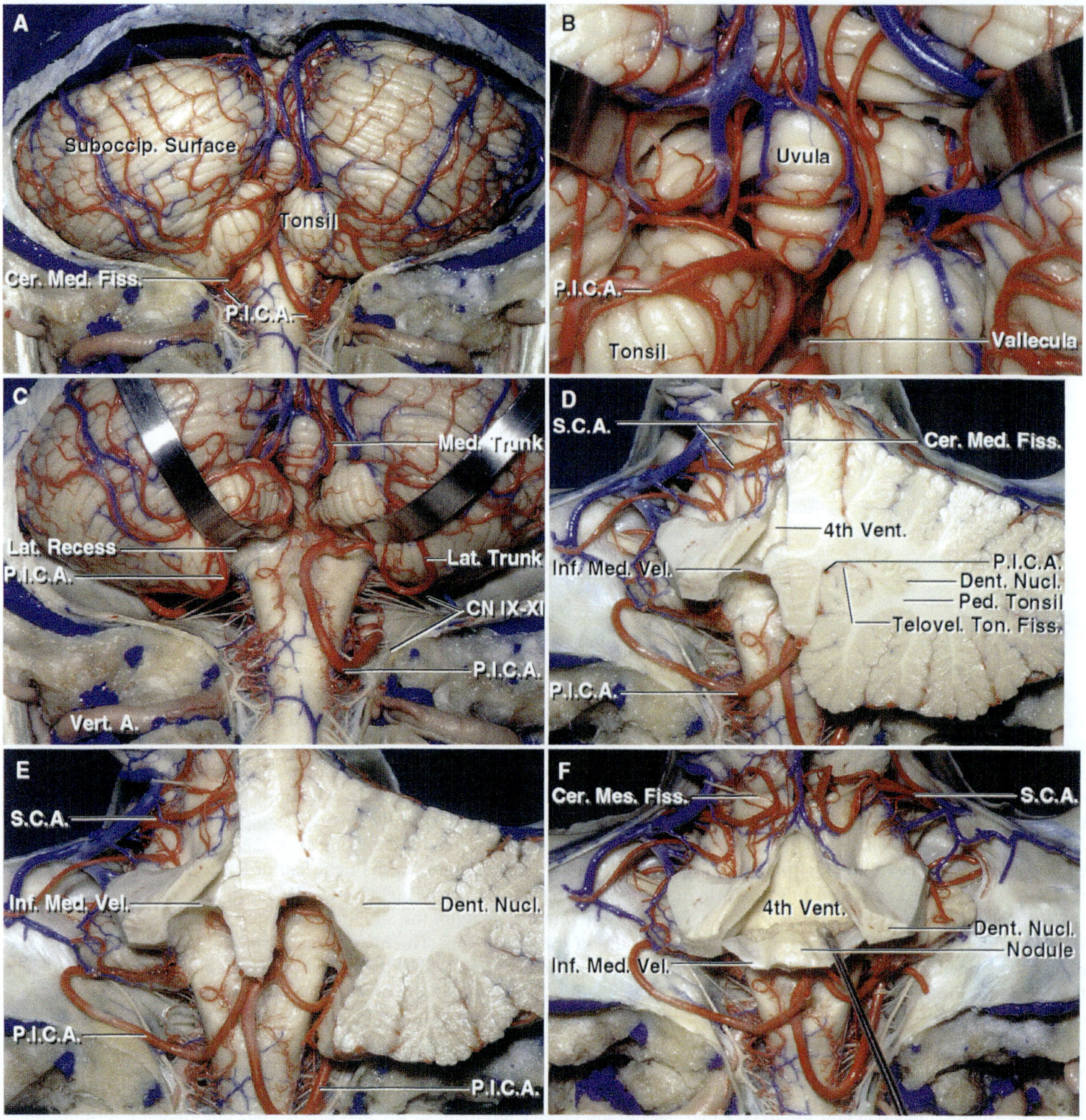

FIGURE 1.9. *A–F.* Posterior views. Stepwise dissection examining the relationships of the inferior medullary velum, dentate nucleus, tonsil, and the cerebellomedullary and cerebellomesencephalic fissures. *A*, the PICAs pass around the posterior medulla to reach the lower margin of the cerebellomedullary fissure. The left PICA courses around the lower pole of the tonsil. The right PICA descends well below the tonsil to the level of the foramen magnum before ascending along the medial tonsillar surface. *B*, the PICAs ascend between the tonsils and medulla to reach the interval between the tonsil and uvula and to supply the suboccipital surface. *C*, the posterior medullary segment of the right PICA divides into a medial trunk supplying the vermis and paravermian area and a lateral trunk supplying the hemisphere. *D*, the cerebellum has been sectioned in an oblique coronal plane to show the relationship of the rostral pole of the tonsil to the inferior medullary velum and dentate nucleus. The dentate nucleus is located above the posterolateral part of the ventricular roof, near the fastigium, where it wraps around, and is separated from, the rostral pole of the tonsil by the inferior medullary velum. The left tonsil has been removed while preserving the left half of the inferior medullary velum. The SCAs course in the cerebellomesencephalic fissure. The PICA passes between the walls of the cerebellomedullary fissure formed above by the inferior medullary velum and

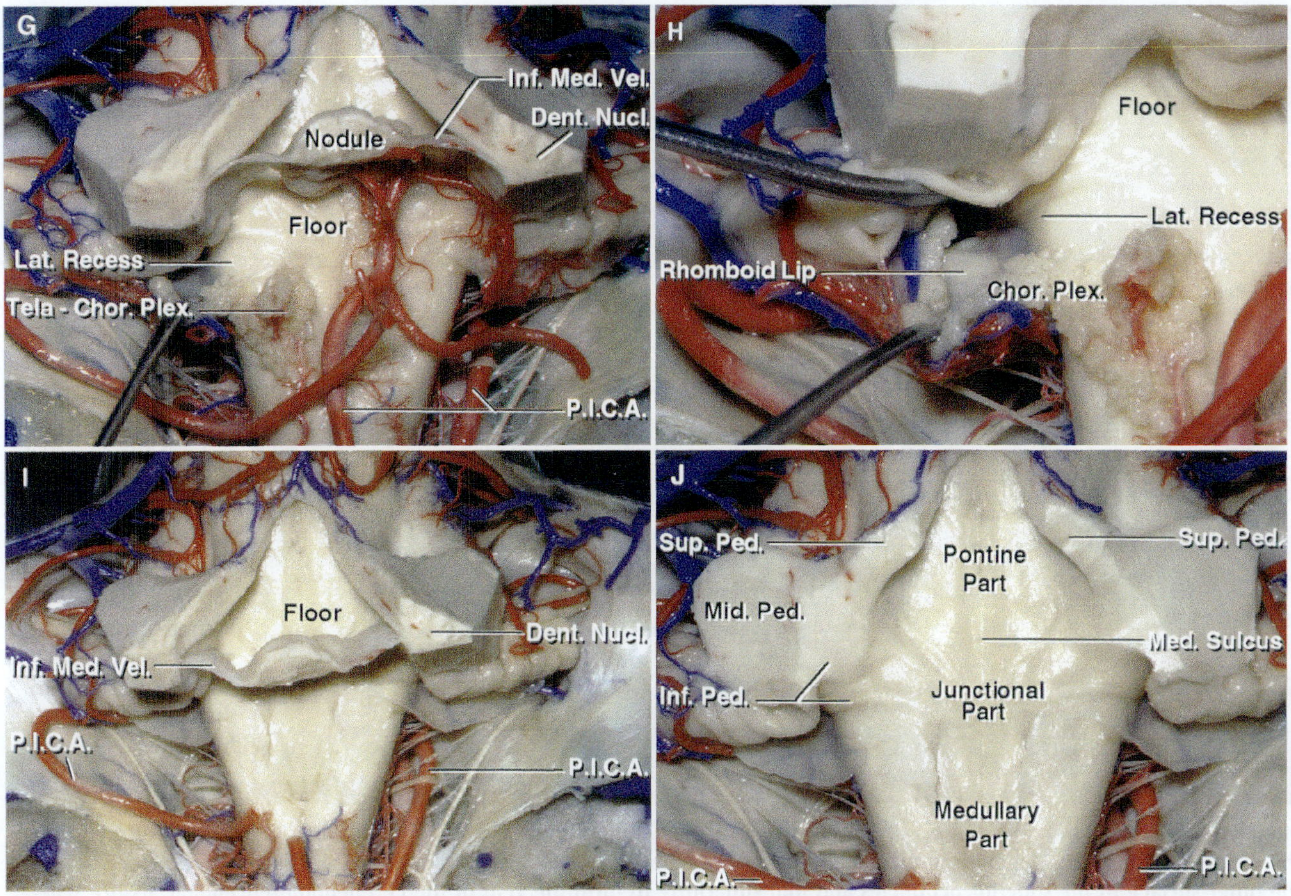

FIGURE 1.9. ***G–J.*** **Posterior views. *G,* the tela choroidea, in which the choroid plexus arises, has been folded downward to expose the lower part of the floor. *H,* enlarged view of the left lateral recess and the foramen of Luschka. The rhomboid lip is a thin layer of neural tissue, which extends laterally from the anterior margin of the lateral recess and, with the tela choroidea, forms a pouch at the outer edge of the lateral recess. Choroid plexus extends through the lateral recess and foramen of Luschka into the cerebellopontine angle. *I,* the tela has been removed to expose the parts of the floor located above and below the nodule and inferior medullary velum. *J,* the nodule and the inferior medullary velum have been removed to expose the full length of the floor, which is divided in the midline by the median sulcus and craniocaudally into pontine, junctional, and medullary parts. The superior and inferior peduncles face the ventricular surface. The middle cerebellar peduncle is separated from the ventricular surface by the superior and inferior peduncles. *Chor.,* choroid; *Dent.,* dentate; *Inf.,* inferior; *Lat.,* lateral; *Med.,* median, medullary; *Mid.,* middle; *Nucl.,* nucleus; *P.I.C.A.,* posteroinferior cerebellar artery; *Ped.,* peduncle; *Plex.,* plexus; *Sup.,* superior; *Vel.,* velum.**

A major cerebellar artery and vein course in each fissure. The superior cerebellar artery (SCA) and the vein of the cerebellomesencephalic fissure course within the cerebellomesencephalic fissure, the anteroinferior cerebellar artery (AICA) and the vein of the cerebellopontine fissure are related to the cerebellopontine fissure, and the posteroinferior cerebellar artery (PICA) and the vein of the cerebellomedullary fissure are intimately related to the cerebellomedullary fissure. These arteries and veins will be reviewed in the next two chapters on the cerebellar arteries and posterior fossa veins (10, 18, 19).

Each fissure communicates with the adjacent fissure. The cerebellopontine fissures are continuous around the rostral surface of the middle cerebellar peduncles with the caudal

below by the upper pole of the tonsil. *E,* both tonsils have been removed. The PICAs ascend through the cleft between the inferior medullary velum and rostral pole of the tonsil. *F,* the superior part of the ventricular roof has been removed and the nodule and the inferior medullary velum has been folded downward to expose the floor. *A.,* artery; *Cer. Med.,* cerebellomedullary; *Cer.Mes.,* cerebellomesencephalic; *CN,* cranial nerve; *Dent.,* dentate; *Fiss.,* fissure; *Inf.,* inferior; *Lat.,* lateral; *Med.,* medial, medullary; *Nucl.,* nucleus; *Ped.,* peduncle; *P.I.C.A.,* posteroinferior cerebellar artery; *S.C.A.,* superior cerebellar artery; *Suboccip.,* suboccipital; *Telovel. Ton.,* telovelotonsillar; *Vel.,* velum; *Vent.,* ventricle; *Vert.,* vertebral.

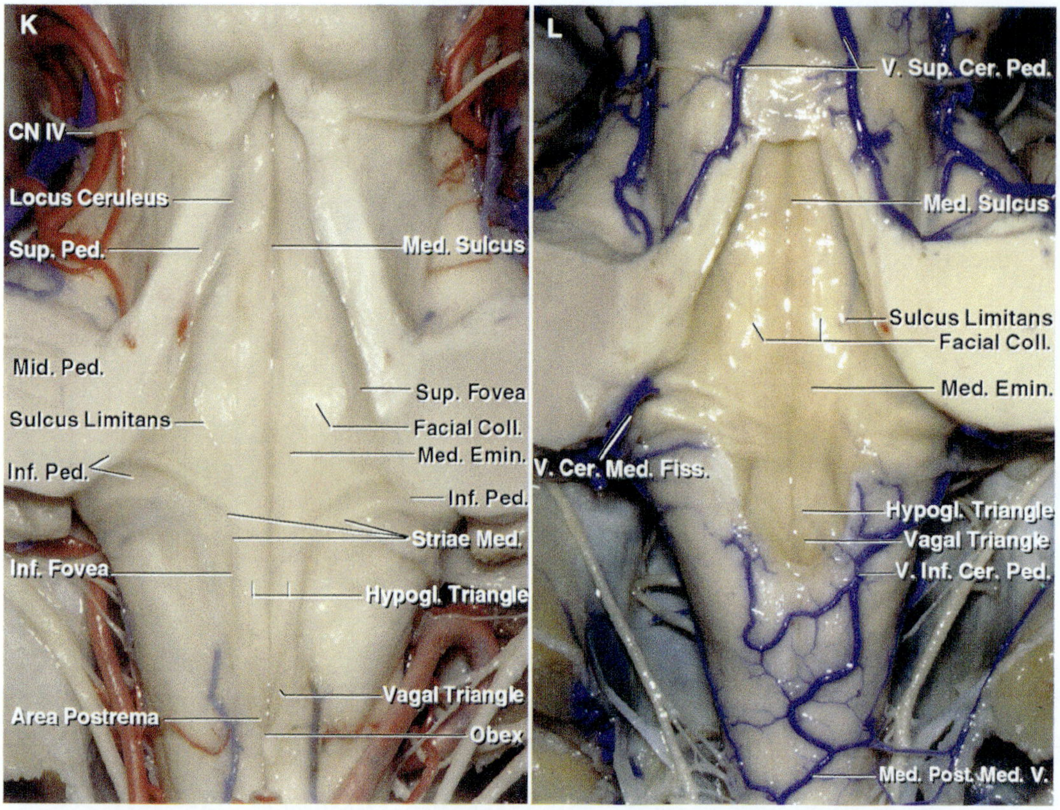

FIGURE 1.9. ***K*** **and** ***L.*** **Posterior views.** ***K,*** **enlarged view of the floor of the fourth ventricle. The median sulcus divides the floor longitudinally in the midline. Each half of the floor is divided longitudinally by an irregular sulcus, the sulcus limitans, which deepens lateral to the facial colliculus and hypoglossal triangles to form the superior and inferior foveae. A darkened area of cells, the locus ceruleus, is located at the rostral end of the sulcus limitans. The stria medullaris crosses the floor at the level of the lateral recess. The hypoglossal and vagal nuclei and the area postrema are stacked one above the other in the lower part of the floor to give the configuration of a pen nib and, thus, the area is referred to as the calamus scriptorius.** ***L,*** **another fourth ventricular floor. The paired veins of the superior cerebellar peduncle course on the outer surface of the superior peduncles and join superiorly to form the vein of the cerebellomesencephalic fissure. The median posterior medullary vein ascends on the medulla and splits into the paired veins of the inferior cerebellar peduncle at the caudal margin of the floor. That left vein is hypoplastic. The left vein of the cerebellomedullary fissure passes along the lateral recess and ascends to join the petrosal group of veins in the cerebellopontine angle.** ***Cer.Med.,*** **cerebellomedullary;** ***Cer.,*** **cerebellar;** ***CN,*** **cranial nerve;** ***Coll.,*** **colliculus;** ***Emin.,*** **eminence;** ***Fiss.,*** **fissure;** ***Hypogl.,*** **hypoglossal;** ***Inf.,*** **inferior;** ***Med.,*** **median, medullary;** ***Mid.,*** **middle;** ***Ped.,*** **peduncle;** ***Post.,*** **posterior;** ***Striae Med.,*** **Stria medullaris;** ***Sup.,*** **superior;** ***V.,*** **vein.**

edges of the cerebellomesencephalic fissure and around the caudal margin of the middle cerebellar peduncles with the rostral limits of the cerebellomedullary fissure. These fissures will be reviewed in greater detail in the discussion of the roof and lateral recesses of the fourth ventricle.

Upper ventricular roof and the cerebellomesencephalic fissure

The ventricular surface of the superior part of the roof of the fourth ventricle is divided into a single median and two lateral parts (*Figs. 1.3* and *1.4*). The median part is formed by the superior medullary velum, and the lateral parts (also referred to as the lateral walls) are formed by the inner surface of the cerebellar peduncles. The superior medullary velum is a thin lamina of white matter that spans the interval between the superior cerebellar peduncles and has the lingula, the uppermost division of the vermis, on its outer surface. It is continuous at the fastigium with the inferior medullary velum. The rostral portion of the ventricular surface of each lateral wall is formed by the medial surface of the superior cerebellar peduncle, and the caudal part is formed by the inferior cerebellar peduncle.

The middle cerebellar peduncle, although it is the largest component of the fiber bundle formed by the union of the three cerebellar peduncles, is separated from the ventricular surface by the fibers of the inferior and superior peduncles on its medial surface (*Fig. 1.9*). The fibers of the inferior cerebellar peduncle ascend in the posterolateral medulla and turn posteriorly in the inferomedial part of the fiber bundle formed by the union of the three peduncles to line the ventricular surface of the superior margin of the lateral recess and the inferior part of the lateral wall. The fibers of the superior cerebellar peduncle arise in the dentate nucleus and ascend on the medial side of the middle cerebellar peduncle to form the ventricular surface of the superior part of the lateral wall.

The cisternal (external) surface of the structures forming the superior part of the roof also form the anterior wall of the cerebellomesencephalic fissure. This fissure, which extends inferiorly between the cerebellum and midbrain, is V-shaped when viewed from superiorly (*Figs. 1.3* and *1.4*). This fissure has also been referred to as the precentral cerebellar fissure. The dorsal half of the midbrain sits within the limbs of the V-shaped notch, and the cerebellum forms the outer margin, with the apex being posterior. The inner wall of the fissure, which forms the outer surface of the superior part of the roof, is composed of the lingula, the dorsal surface of the superior cerebellar peduncles, and the rostral surface of the middle cerebellar peduncles. The lingula, a thin, narrow tongue of vermis, sits on the outer surface of the superior medullary velum. The superior cerebellar peduncles form smooth longitudinal prominences on each side of the lingula before disappearing into the midbrain beneath the colliculi. The rostral surface of the middle cerebellar peduncles appear to wrap around the caudal margin of the superior cerebellar peduncles. A shallow groove, the interpeduncular sulcus, marks the junction of the superior and the middle cerebellar peduncles. The interpeduncular sulcus is continuous anteriorly with the pontomesencephalic sulcus, a transverse groove between the pons and midbrain, and superiorly with the lateral mesencephalic sulcus, a longitudinal fissure dorsal to the cerebral peduncle. The trochlear nerves arise in the cerebellomesencephalic fissure below the inferior colliculi and pass anterolateral to exit the anterior part of the fissure. The outer wall of the cerebellomesencephalic fissure is formed by the culmen and the central lobule and its wings.

The neural structures separating the ventricular and cisternal surfaces of the superior part of the roof are thinnest in the area of the superior medullary velum and lingula and thickest in the area of the cerebellar peduncles. The rostral portion of each lateral wall, formed by only the superior cerebellar peduncle, is thinner than the caudal portion, which is formed by the three cerebellar peduncles after they have united.

Lower roof and cerebellomedullary fissure

The inferior portion of the roof slopes sharply ventral and slightly caudal from the fastigium to its attachment to the inferolateral borders of the floor (*Figs. 1.3–1.6*). The ventricular and cisternal surfaces are formed by the same structures, the tela choroidea and the inferior medullary velum, except in the rostral midline, where the ventricular surface is formed by the nodule and the cisternal surface is formed by the uvula. The choroid plexus is attached to the ventricular surface of the tela choroidea.

The ventricular surface is divided into a cranial part formed by the nodule and the inferior medullary velum and a caudal part formed by the tela choroidea. The inferior medullary velum is a membranous layer and is all that remains of the connection between the nodule and the flocculi that form the flocculonodular lobe of the primitive cerebellum (14) (*Figs. 1.8* and *1.9*). It is a thin bilateral semitranslucent butterfly-shaped sheet of neural tissue that blends into the ventricular surface of the nodule medially and stretches laterally across, but is separated from, the superior pole of the tonsil by a narrow, rostral extension of the cerebellomedullary fissure. It blends into the dorsal margin of each lateral recess and forms the peduncle of each flocculus. The inferior medullary velum is continuous at the level of the fastigium with the superior medullary velum. Caudally it is attached to the tela choroidea.

The tela choroidea forms the caudal part of the inferior portion of the roof and the inferior wall of each lateral recess (*Figs. 1.5, 1.6,* and *1.9*). It consists of two thin, semitransparent membranes, each having a thickness comparable to arachnoid, between which is sandwiched a vascular layer composed of the choroidal arteries and veins. The choroid plexus projects from the ventricular surface of the tela choroidea into the fourth ventricle. The line of attachment of the inferior medullary velum to the tela choroidea, the telovelar junction, extends from the nodule into each lateral recess. The tela choroidea sweeps inferiorly from the telovelar junction around the superior pole of each tonsil to its attachment to the inferolateral edges of the floor along narrow white ridges, the taeniae, which meet at the obex. Cranially, the taeniae turn laterally over the inferior cerebellar peduncles and pass horizontally along the inferior borders of the lateral recesses. The tela choroidea does not completely enclose the inferior half of the fourth ventricle, but has three openings into the subarachnoid space: the paired foramina of Luschka located at the outer margin of the lateral recesses and the foramen of Magendie located at the caudal tip of the fourth ventricle.

The cisternal (external) surface of the caudal half of the roof faces and is intimately related to the cerebellomedullary fissure (*Figs. 1.6, 1.8,* and *1.9*). This fissure is one of the most complex fissures in the brain. The ventral wall of the fissure is formed by the posterior surface of the medulla, the inferior medullary velum, and the tela choroidea. The dorsal wall of the fissure is formed by the uvula in the midline and the tonsils and biventral lobules laterally. It extends superiorly to the level of the lateral recesses and communicates around the superior poles of the tonsils with the cisterna magna, through the foramen of Magendie with the fourth ventricle, and around the foramina of Luschka with the cerebellopontine fissures. The rostral pole of the tonsils faces the inferior medullary velum, the tela choroidea, and the peritonsillar part of the uvula and the biventral lobule in the superior part of the fissure (*Figs. 1.3–1.6*). The portion of the fissure between the tonsil, the tela choroidea, and the inferior medullary velum is called the telovelotonsillar cleft, and the superior extension of this cleft over the superior pole of the tonsil has been called the supratonsillar cleft.

LATERAL RECESS AND CEREBELLOPONTINE FISSURE

The lateral recesses are narrow, curved pouches formed by the union of the roof and the floor. They extend laterally below the cerebellar peduncles and open through the foramina of Luschka into the cerebellopontine angles (*Figs. 1.3, 1.5, 1.6,* and *1.8*). The ventral wall of each lateral recess is formed by the junctional part of the floor and the rhomboid lip, a sheetlike layer of neural tissue that extends laterally from the floor and unites with the tela choroidea to form a pouch at the outer extremity of the lateral recess. The rostral wall of each lateral recess is formed by the caudal margin of the cerebellar peduncles. The inferior cerebellar peduncle courses upward in the floor ventral to the lateral recess and turns posteriorly at the lower part of the pons to form the ventricular surface of the rostral wall. The peduncle of the flocculus interconnecting the inferior medullary velum and the flocculus crosses in the dorsal margin of the lateral recess. The caudal wall is formed by the tela choroidea that stretches from the lateral part of the taenia to the peduncle of the flocculus. The biventral lobule is dorsal to the lateral recess. The flocculus is superior to the outer extremity of the lateral recess. The rootlets of the glossopharyngeal and vagus nerves arise ventral to and the facial nerve arises rostral to the lateral recess. The fibers of the vestibulocochlear nerve cross the floor of the recess.

Each lateral recess opens into the cerebellopontine angle along the cerebellopontine fissure (*Fig. 1.7*). This V-shaped fissure is formed by the folding of the cerebellar hemisphere around the lateral side of the pons and the middle cerebellar peduncle. It has a superior limb between the rostral half of the middle cerebellar peduncle and the superior part of the petrosal surface and an inferior limb between the caudal half of the middle cerebellar peduncle and the inferior part of the petrosal surface. The middle cerebellar peduncle fills the interval between the two limbs. The apex of the fissure is located laterally where the superior and inferior limbs meet. The petrosal fissure extends laterally from the apex. The lateral recess and the foramen of Luschka open into the medial part of the inferior limb. Other structures located along the inferior limb are the flocculus, the rhomboid lip, the choroid plexus protruding from the foramen of Luschka, and the facial, vestibulocochlear, glossopharyngeal, and vagus nerves. The trigeminal nerve arises from the pons along the superior limb of the fissure.

The superior limb of the cerebellopontine fissure communicates above the trigeminal nerve with the lateral part of the cerebellomesencephalic fissure, and the inferior limb communicates with the lateral part of the cerebellomedullary fissure at the level of the lateral recess. The flocculus projects into the cerebellopontine angle at the confluence of the cerebellopontine and cerebellomedullary fissures. The vestibulocochlear and facial nerves enter the brainstem anterosuperior to the flocculus, and the fila of the glossopharyngeal and the vagal nerves cross anteroinferiorly to it.

CHOROID PLEXUS

The choroid plexus of the posterior fossa is composed of two inverted L-shaped fringes that arise on the ventricular surface of the tela choroidea and are located on each side of the midline (7) (*Figs. 1.3* and *1.8*). The paired longitudinal limbs bordering the median plane are the medial segments. The transverse limbs that originate from the rostral ends of the medial segments are the lateral segments. The entire structure presents the form of a letter T, the vertical limb of which, however, is double.

The medial segments are located in the roof near the midline, and the lateral segments extend through the lateral recesses and the foramina of Luschka into the cerebellopontine angles. The medial segments stretch from the level of the nodule anterior to the tonsils to the level of the foramen of Magendie. Each medial segment is subdivided into a rostral or nodular part and a caudal or tonsillar part. The nodular parts are widest at their junction with the lateral segments. The tonsillar parts are anterior to the tonsils and extend inferiorly through the foramen of Magendie. The rostral and caudal ends of the medial segments are often fused.

The lateral segments form a transversely oriented fringe that attach to the rostral part of the medial segments and extend parallel to the telovelar junction through the lateral recesses into the cerebellopontine angles. Each lateral segment is subdivided into a medial or peduncular part and a lateral or floccular part. The peduncular part forms a narrow fringe that is continuous with the rostral part of the medial segment and is attached to the tela choroidea covering the lateral recess inferior to the cerebellar peduncles. The floccular part is continuous with the peduncular part at the lateral margin of the cerebellar peduncles and protrudes through the foramen of Luschka into the cerebellopontine angle below the flocculus.

BRAINSTEM AND FLOOR

Brainstem

The brainstem and ventricle floor are considered together because the brainstem forms the fourth ventricular floor. The brainstem in the posterior fossa is composed of the mesencephalon, pons, and medulla (*Figs. 1.7–1.9*). The mesencephalon consists of the cerebral peduncles, the tegmentum, and the tectum. It is demarcated superiorly from the diencephalon by the sulcus between the optic tracts and the cerebral peduncles, and inferiorly from the pons by the pontomesencephalic sulcus. The interpeduncular fossa, a wedge-shaped depression between the cerebral peduncles, has the posterior perforated substance in its floor. The rootlets of the oculomotor nerves arise in the depths of the interpeduncular fossa and form the fossa's walls lateral to the posterior perforated substance. A small depression, the superior foramen cecum, is located in the caudal part of the interpeduncular fossa. The pontomesencephalic sulcus runs from the superior foramen cecum around the cerebral peduncles to join the lateral mesencephalic sulcus, a vertical sulcus between the tegmentum and the cerebral peduncle.

The belly of the pons is convex from side to side, as well as from top to bottom, and is continuous on each side with the middle cerebellar peduncles. It has a shallow midline groove, the basilar sulcus, which extends from its superior to its inferior border. The posterior root of the trigeminal nerve emerges from the upper portion of the middle cerebellar peduncle just below the anterior angle of the cerebellum. The pons is demarcated inferiorly from the medulla by the pontomedullary sulcus, which extends laterally from the inferior foramen cecum (a midline dimple) to the supraolivary fossette (a depression located rostral to the olive). The rootlets of the facial and the vestibulocochlear nerves arise superior to this fossette and the rootlets of the glossopharyngeal and the vagal nerves originate dorsal to it.

The anterior surface of the medulla is formed by the medullary pyramids, which face the clivus, the anterior edge of the foramen magnum, and the rostral part of the odontoid process (*Figs. 1.7* and *1.8*). The anteromedian sulcus divides the upper medulla in the anterior midline between the pyramids and disappears on the lower medulla at the level of the decussation of the pyramids, but it reappears below the decussation and is continuous caudally with the anteromedian fissure of the spinal cord. The lateral surface of the medulla is formed predominantly by the inferior olives, which are situated lateral to and separated from the pyramids by the anterolateral (preolivary) sulcus. The rootlets of the hypoglossal nerves arise in the anterolateral sulcus. The lateral surface is demarcated posteriorly by the exits of the rootlets of the glossopharyngeal, vagus, and accessory nerves just dorsal to the posterolateral (postolivary) sulcus, which courses along the dorsal margin of the olive and is continuous below with the posterolateral sulcus of the spinal cord. The abducens nerves emerge from the pontomedullary sulcus rostral to the pyramids. The posterior surface of the medulla is divided into superior and inferior parts. The superior part is composed in the midline of the inferior half of the floor of the fourth ventricle and laterally by the inferior cerebellar peduncles. The inferior part of the posterior surface is divided into two halves in the midline by the posteromedian sulcus, and each half is composed of the gracile fasciculus and tubercle medially, and the cuneate fasciculus and tubercle laterally. The posteromedian sulcus of the medulla, which separates the paired gracile fasciculi in the midline, ends superiorly at the obex of the fourth ventricle and is continuous inferiorly with the posteromedian sulcus of the spinal cord. The posterior intermediate sulcus, which separates the gracile and cuneate fasciculi, is continuous inferiorly with the posterior intermediate sulcus of the spinal cord. The lower medulla blends indistinguishably into the upper spinal cord at the level of the C1 nerve roots (*Figs. 1.5–1.7*).

Floor

The floor has a rhomboid shape (*Fig. 1.9*). The rostral two-thirds of the floor is posterior to the pons and the caudal one-third is posterior to the medulla. Its cranial apex is at the level of the cerebral aqueduct; its caudal tip, the obex, is located at the rostral end of the remnant of the spinal canal, anterior to the foramen of Magendie; and its lateral angles open through the lateral recesses and foramina of Luschka into the cerebellopontine angles. A line connecting the orifices of the lateral recesses is located at the level of the junction of the caudal and the middle third of the length of the floor and also at the level of the junction of the pons and the medulla.

The floor is divided into three parts: a superior or pontine part, an intermediate or junctional part, and an inferior or medullary part. The superior part has a triangular shape: its apex is at the cerebral aqueduct, its base is represented by an imaginary line connecting the lower margin of the cerebellar peduncles, and its lateral limbs are formed by the medial surfaces of the cerebral peduncles. The intermediate part is the strip between the lower margin of the cerebellar peduncles and the site of attachment of the tela choroidea to the taeniae just below the lateral recesses. The intermediate part extends into the lateral recesses. The inferior part has a triangular shape and is limited laterally by the taeniae marking the inferolateral margins of the floor. Its caudal tip, the obex, is anterior to the foramen of Magendie.

The floor is divided longitudinally from the rostral apex to the caudal tip into symmetrical halves by the median sulcus. The sulcus limitans, another longitudinal sulcus, divides each half of the floor into a raised median strip, called the median eminence, that borders the midline and a lateral region called the vestibular area.

Each median eminence, the strip between the sulcus limitans and the median sulcus, from above to below contains the facial colliculus, a rounded prominence related to the facial nerve, and three triangular areas overlying the hypoglossal and vagus nuclei and the area postrema. The three triangular areas are paired and are stacked along the median sulcus to give the caudal part of the floor a feather or pen nib configuration; thus, the area is called the calamus scriptorius. At the pontine level the median eminence has a width equal to that of the full half of the floor and thus the sulcus limitans corresponds with the lateral limit of this part of the floor.

The sulcus limitans is discontinuous and is most prominent in the pontine and medullary portions of the floor, where it deepens at two points to form dimples called foveae, and is least distinct in the junctional part of the floor. One of the two dimples, the superior fovea, is located in the pontine portion of the floor and the other, the inferior fovea, is located in the medullary part of the floor. At the level of the superior fovea, the median eminence forms an elongated swelling, the facial colliculus, which overlies the nucleus of the abducens nerve and the ascending section of the root of the facial nerve. At the rostral tip of each sulcus limitans in the lateral margin of the floor is a bluish gray area, the locus ceruleus, which owes its color to a group of pigmented nerve cells. The hypoglossal triangle is medial to the inferior fovea and overlies the nucleus of the hypoglossal nerve. Caudal to the inferior fovea and between the hypoglossal triangle and the lower part of the vestibular area is a triangular dark field, the vagal triangle, that overlies the dorsal nucleus of the vagus nerve. A translucent ridge, the funiculus separans, crosses the lower part of the vagal triangle. The area postrema forms a small tongue-shaped area between the funiculus separans and the gracile tubercle in the lower limit of the median eminence immediately rostral to the obex.

The vestibular area, the portion of the floor lateral to the median eminence and sulcus limitans, is widest in the intermediate part of the floor, where it forms a rounded elevation that extends into the lateral recess. White strands, the striae medullaris, course transversely from the region of the lateral recess across the inferior cerebellar peduncles above the hypoglossal triangles toward the midline and disappear in the median sulcus. The vestibular nuclei lie beneath the vestibular area. The auditory tubercle produced by the underlying dorsal cochlear nucleus and the cochlear part of the vestibulocochlear nerve forms a prominence in the lateral part of the vestibular area.

VASCULAR RELATIONSHIPS

Each wall of the fourth ventricle has surgically important arterial relationships: the SCA is intimately related to the superior half of the roof; the PICA is intimately related to the inferior half of the roof; the AICA is intimately related to the lateral recess and the foramen of Luschka; and the basilar and vertebral arteries give rise to many perforating branches that reach the floor of the fourth ventricle (5, 7, 9, 10, 18, 19) (*Figs. 1.9* and *1.10*). The choroidal branches of the AICA supply the portion of the choroid plexus in the cerebellopontine angle and the adjacent part of the lateral recess, and the PICA supplies the choroid plexus in the roof and the medial part of the lateral recess (7).

There are no major veins within the cavity of the fourth ventricle. The veins most intimately related to the fourth ventricle are those in the fissures between the cerebellum and the brainstem and on the cerebellar peduncle (21). The veins of the cerebellomesencephalic fissure and the superior cerebellar peduncle course on the superior part of the roof, the veins of the cerebellomedullary fissure and the inferior cerebellar peduncle drain the inferior half of the roof, and the veins of the cerebellopontine fissure and the middle cerebellar peduncle drain the lateral wall and the cerebellopontine angle around the lateral recess. These vascular relationships will be explored in greater detail in the next two chapters on the cerebellar arteries and posterior fossa veins.

DISCUSSION

Effects of neural injury

The operative approaches to the cerebellum and fourth ventricle may require splitting of the vermis, resection of part

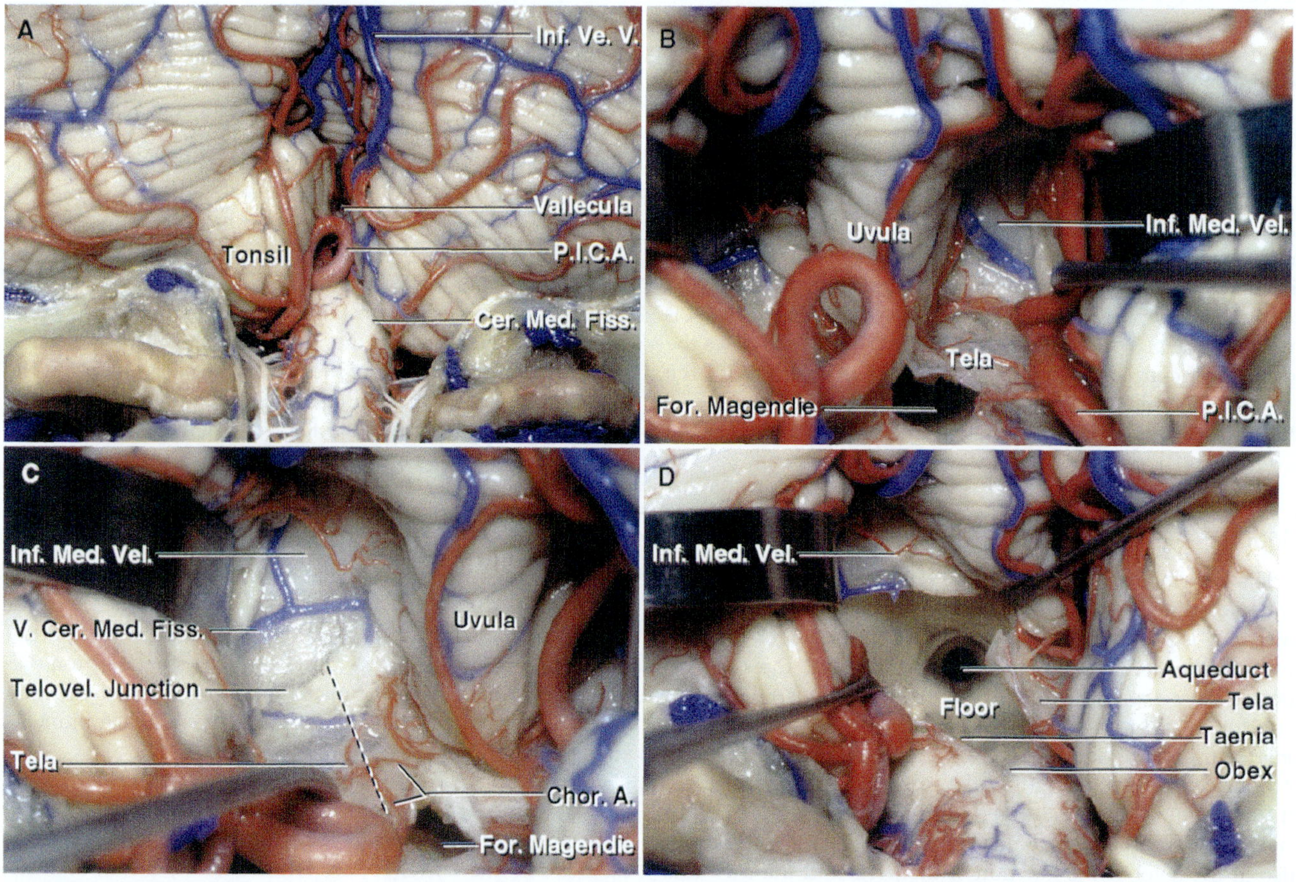

FIGURE 1.10. ***A–D.*** **Telovelar approach to the fourth ventricle.** ***A*****, the cerebellomedullary fissure extends upward between the tonsils posteriorly and the medulla anteriorly. The vallecula opens between the tonsils into the fourth ventricle.** ***B*****, both tonsils have been retracted laterally to expose the inferior medullary velum and tela choroidea that form the lower part of the ventricular roof. The nodule of the vermis, on which the inferior medullary arises, is hidden deep to the uvula.** ***C*****, enlarged view of the left half of the cerebellomedullary fissure. The choroidal arteries course along the tela choroidea from which the choroid plexus projects into the roof of the fourth ventricle. The vein of the cerebellomedullary fissure, which crosses the inferior medullary velum, is the largest vein in the cerebellomedullary fissure. The interrupted line shows the site of the incision in the tela to provide the exposure seen in the next step. The telovelar junction is the line of attachment of the tela to the velum.** ***D*****, the tela choroidea has been opened extending from the foramen of Magendie to the junction with the inferior medullary velum. The uvula has been displaced to the right side to provide this view extending from the aqueduct to the obex.** ***A.*****, artery;** ***Cer.Med.*****, cerebellomedullary;** ***Chor.*****, choroidal;** ***Fiss.*****, fissure;** ***For.*****, foramen;** ***Inf.*****, inferior;** ***Med.*****, medullary;** ***P.I.C.A.*****, posteroinferior cerebellar artery;** ***Telovel.*****, telovelar;** ***V.*****, vein;** ***Ve.*****, vermian;** ***Vel.*****, velum.**

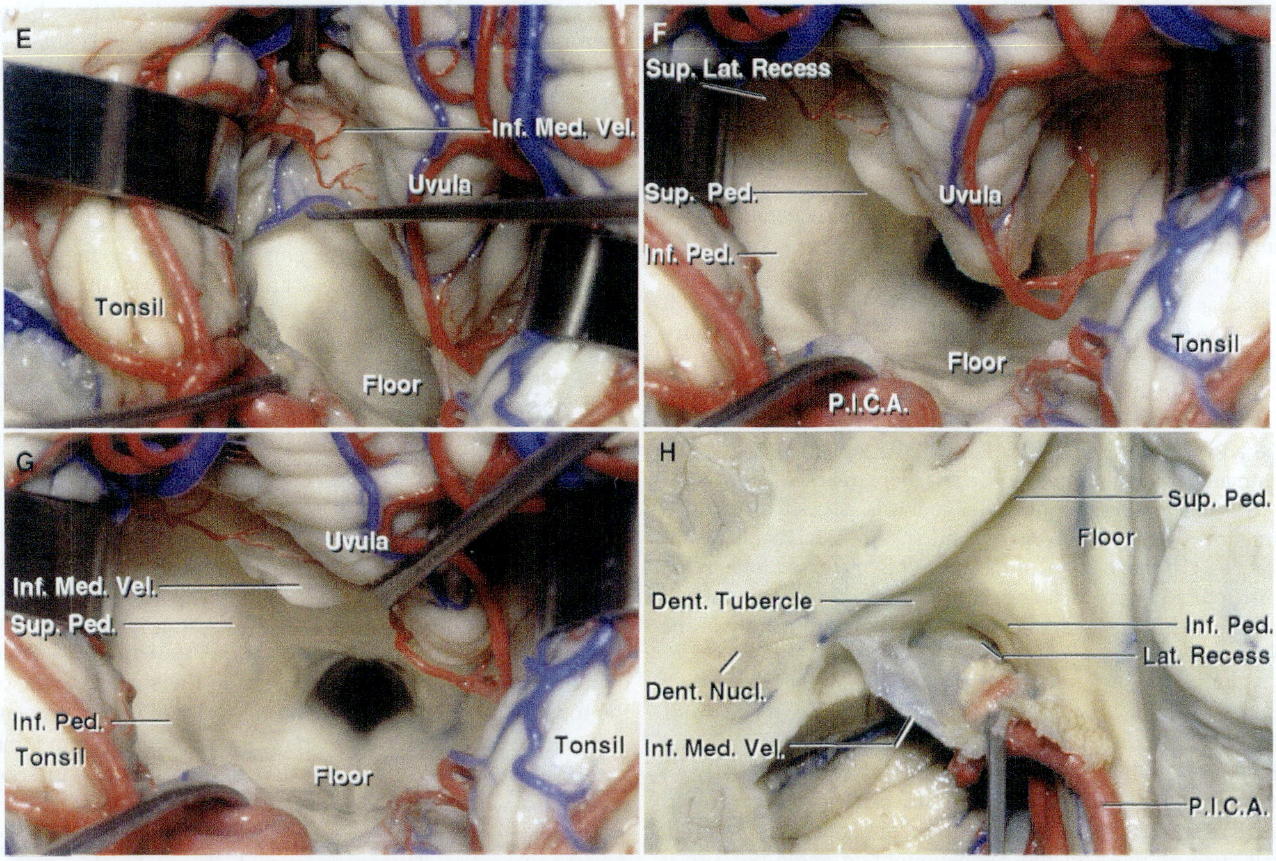

FIGURE 1.10. ***E–H.*** **Telovelar approach to the fourth ventricle.** ***E,*** **the tip of a nerve hook placed inside the fourth ventricle is seen through the paper-thin inferior medullary velum.** ***F,*** **the left half of the inferior medullary velum has been divided to expose the superolateral recess and the ventricular surface formed by the superior and inferior peduncles.** ***G,*** **the uvula has been retracted to the right to expose all of the floor and much of the roof of the ventricle.** ***H,*** **the right half of the cerebellum was removed by dividing the vermis sagittally and the cerebellar peduncles transversely. The tonsil has been removed and the inferior medullary velum and the cranial loop of the PICA have been displaced downward to expose the opening into the lateral recess. The dentate nucleus forms a prominence, the dentate tubercle, in the superolateral recess of the roof of the fourth ventricle near the site of attachment of the inferior medullary velum.** ***Dent.,*** **dentate;** ***Inf.,*** **inferior;** ***Lat.,*** **lateral;** ***Med.,*** **medullary;** ***Nucl.,*** **nucleus;** ***P.I.C.A.,*** **posteroinferior cerebellar artery;** ***Ped.,*** **peduncle;** ***Sup.,*** **superior;** ***Vel.,*** **velum.**

of the hemisphere, removal of the tonsil, opening of the inferior medullary velum, separation of tumor from the floor and roof, dissection in the region of the cerebellar peduncles and deep cerebellar nuclei, and retraction or removal of the flocculus. Horsley pointed out that large amounts of cerebellar tissue could be sacrificed with little or no demonstrable loss of function (13). A common approach to the fourth ventricle is by splitting the vermis on the suboccipital surface, as recommended by Dandy (3) and Kempe (15). Dandy stated that the vermis could be opened at its center to gain access to fourth ventricular tumors without causing a disturbance of function, provided that the operator carefully avoided the dentate nuclei (3). Small lesions in the vermis caused no symptoms or deficit, but larger lesions of the uvula, nodule, and flocculus, involving cerebellar fibers related to the vestibular system, cause equilibratory disturbances, with truncal ataxia, staggering gait, and oscillation of the head and trunk on assumption of the erect position without ataxia on voluntary movement of the extremities (8, 11, 12, 16). Injury to the vestibular projections from the brainstem to the flocculonodular lobe also causes nystagmus that is present in all directions of gaze. Cerebellar mutism is a transient complication that may appear after removal of cerebellar tumors, usually in children, characterized by lack of speech output in the awake patient, with intact speech comprehension, sometimes associated with oropharyngeal apraxia (2, 4, 24). Although the exact anatomic substrate for the mutism remains unknown, the majority occurred after removal of midline tumors involving the vermis (2, 4, 24, 26). The inferior part of the vermis, including the pyramid, uvula, and nodule has been implicated.

Hemispheric resection may be required to reach lesions of the lateral part of the roof or the lateral recess of the fourth ventricle. Frazier resected the lateral part of the hemisphere without permanent sequelae (6). Unilateral resection of the part of the hemisphere lateral to the dentate nuclei results in ataxia of voluntary movement, hypotonia, and adiadochokinesia in the ipsilateral limbs with errors in rate, range, direction, and force of movement, which are often transient (8, 11, 12, 16). If the ablation involves the dentate nucleus, these disturbances are more severe and enduring and there is, in addition, intention tremor with voluntary movement of the extremities. During an operation on the caudal part of the roof, one should remember that the denate nuclei are located just rostral to the superior pole of the tonsils and are wrapped around the superolateral recess of the ventricle near the inferior medullary velum. Dysarthria results when resection extends into the paravermian part of the cerebellar hemisphere and occurs more frequently from left hemisphere injury than from vermal or right hemisphere injury (17). Nystagmus with hemispheric lesions is associated with an ocular rest point 10 to 30 degrees toward the unaffected side, with greater oscillation upon looking to the side of the lesion. The addition of a vermian lesion or a lesion extending to the contralateral hemisphere produces more marked symptoms than a unilateral hemispheric lesion and is associated with disturbances of standing, walking, and speech. Lesions of the anterior part of the tentorial surface result in increased tone in the muscles used for maintaining the erect posture. If the lateral half of this area is damaged, the hypertonia is predominantly in the ipsilateral extremities.

All of the cerebellar peduncles converge on the lateral wall and roof and may be damaged here. The inferior and superior cerebellar peduncles are more likely to be injured during procedures within the ventricle because they abut directly on the ventricular surface; the middle cerebellar peduncle would be more susceptible to injury in procedures near the external wall such as those in the cerebellopontine angle because it forms a major part of the cisternal surface of the ventricular wall. Lesions of the middle cerebellar peduncle cause ataxia and dysmetria during voluntary movement of the ipsilateral extremities with hypotonia similar to that produced by damage to the lateral part of the hemisphere. Lesions of the superior cerebellar peduncle cause severe ipsilateral intention tremor, dysmetria, and decomposition of movement. The syndrome is mild and subsides rapidly if there is only a partial section of the peduncle. Section of the inferior cerebellar peduncle causes disturbances of equilibrium similar to those produced by ablation of the flocculonodular lobe, with truncal ataxia and staggering gait.

The consequences of removal or gentle manipulation of tumors attached to the floor of the fourth ventricle include intraoperative blood pressure decrease, apnea, and/or respiratory rate increase and postoperative diplopia, disturbances of speech and swallowing, and poor cough reflex associated with incidental disturbances of gastrointestinal bleeding, aspiration pneumonia, and electrolyte disturbances (1).

Telovelar approach to fourth ventricle

Lesions of the fourth ventricle have posed a special challenge to neurosurgeons because of the severe deficits that may follow injury to the structures in the ventricular walls and floor. In the past, operative access to the fourth ventricle was obtained by splitting the cerebellar vermis or removing part of a cerebellar hemisphere (1, 3, 15). In examining the clefts and walls of the cerebellomedullary fissure, we have found that opening the tela alone will provide adequate ventricular exposure in most cases without splitting the vermis (20, 22, 23) (*Fig. 1.10*). The inferior medullary velum, another paper-thin layer, can also be opened if opening the tela does not provide adequate exposure. Opening the tela alone provides access to the full length of the floor and all of the ventricular cavity except, possibly, the fastigium, superolateral recess, and the superior half of the roof. Opening the inferior medullary velum accesses the latter areas and the superior half of the roof. Extending the telar opening laterally toward the foramen of Luschka opens the lateral recess and exposes the peduncular surfaces bordering the recess. Tumors in the fourth ventricle may stretch and thin these two semi-translucent membranes to a degree that one may not be aware that they are being opened in exposing a fourth ventricular tumor. There are no reports of deficits following isolate opening of the tela and velum. However, other structures exposed in the ventricle walls and at risk for producing the deficits described above include the dentate nuclei, cerebellar peduncles, floor of the fourth ventricle, and the PICA. During an operation on the caudal part of the roof, one should remember that the dentate nuclei are located just rostral to the superior pole of the tonsils underlying the dentate tubercles in the posterolateral part of the roof where they are wrapped around the superolateral recesses near the lateral edges of the inferior medullary velum (*Figs. 1.9* and *1.10*). All of the cerebellar peduncles converge on the lateral wall and roof where they may be damaged. The superior cerebellar peduncle is more likely to be injured during operations on lesions involving the superior part of the roof above the level of the dentate tubercles; the inferior peduncles are most susceptible to damage in exposing lesions within the lateral recess; and the middle cerebellar peduncle is susceptible to injury in procedures near the external wall of the superior half of the roof, such as those in the cerebellopontine angle, because the middle peduncle forms a major part of the cisternal surface of the ventricular wall. The consequences of removal or gentle manipulation of tumors attached to the floor of the fourth ventricle have been reviewed.

The PICA is frequently exposed in approaches directed through the tela choroidea or inferior medullar velum, but only infrequently occluded during operative approaches to the fourth ventricle. Occlusion of the branches of the PICA distal to the medullary branches at the level of roof of the fourth ventricle avoids the syndrome of medullary infarction but produces a syndrome resembling labyrinthitis, which includes rotatory dizziness, nausea, vomiting, inability to stand or walk unaided, and nystagmus without appendicular dysmetria (11). The main trunk of the AICA is infrequently exposed in opening the cerebellomedullary fissure, but it may also send choroidal branches to the tela and choroid plexus in the lateral recess.

Reprint requests: Albert L. Rhoton, Jr., M.D., Department of Neurological Surgery, University of Florida, Brain Institute, P.O. Box 100265, 100 South Newell Drive, Building 59, L2-100, Gainesville, FL 32610-0265.

REFERENCES

1. Baker GS: Physiologic abnormalities encountered after removal of brain tumors from the floor of the fourth ventricle. **J Neurosurg** 23:338–343, 1965.
2. Dailey AT, McKahann GM, Berger MS: The pathophysiology of oral pharyngeal apraxia and mutism following posterior fossa tumor resection in children. **J Neurosurg** 83:467–475, 1995.
3. Dandy WE: *The Brain*. Hagerstown, WF Prior Co., 1966, pp 452–458.
4. Dietze DD, Mickle JP: Cerebellar mutism after posterior fossa surgery. **Pediatr Neurosurg** 16:25–31, 1990–1991.
5. Duvernoy HM: *Human Brainstem Vessels*. Berlin, Springer-Verlag, 1978.
6. Frazier CH: Remarks upon the surgical aspects of tumors of the cerebellum. **N Y State J Med** 18:272–280, 332–337, 1918.
7. Fujii K, Lenkey C, Rhoton AL Jr: Microsurgical anatomy of the choroidal arteries: Fourth ventricle and cerebellopontine angles. **J Neurosurg** 52:504–524, 1980.
8. Fulton JF, Dow RS: The cerebellum: A summary of functional localization. **Yale J Biol Med** 10:89–119, 1937.
9. Hardy DG, Rhoton AL Jr: Microsurgical relationship of the superior cerebellar artery and the trigeminal nerve. **J Neurosurg** 49: 669–678, 1978.
10. Hardy DG, Peace DA, Rhoton AL Jr: Microsurgical anatomy of the superior cerebellar artery. **Neurosurgery** 6:10–28, 1980.
11. Holmes G: The Croonian lectures on the clinical symptoms of cerebellar disease and their interpretation. **Lancet** 1:1177–1182, 1231–1237, 1922.
12. Holmes G: The Croonian lectures on the clinical symptoms of cerebellar disease and their interpretation. **Lancet** 2:59–65, 111–115, 1922.
13. Horsley V: On the technique of operations on the central nervous system. **Br Med J** 2:411–423, 1906.
14. Johnston TB: A note on the peduncle of the flocculus and the posterior medullary velum. **J Anat** 68:471–479, 1934.
15. Kempe LG: *Operative Neurosurgery*. New York, Springer-Verlag, 1970, vol 2, pp 14–17.
16. Larsell O: The cerebellum: A review and interpretation. **Arch Neurol Psychiatry** 38:580–607, 1937.
17. Lechtenberg R, Gilman S: Speech disorders in cerebellar disease. **Ann Neurol** 3:285–290, 1978.
18. Lister JR, Rhoton AL Jr, Matsushima T, Peace DA: Microsurgical anatomy of the posterior inferior cerebellar artery. **Neurosurgery** 10:170–199, 1982.
19. Martin RG, Grant JL, Peace D, Theiss C, Rhoton AL Jr: Microsurgical relationships of the anterior inferior cerebellar artery and the facial-vestibulocochlear nerve complex. **Neurosurgery** 6:483–507, 1980.
20. Matsushima T, Fukui M, Inoue T, Natori Y, Baba T, Fujii K: Microsurgical and magnetic resonance imaging anatomy of the cerebellomedullary fissure and its application during fourth ventricle surgery. **Neurosurgery** 30:325–330, 1992.
21. Matsushima T, Rhoton AL Jr, de Oliveira E, Peace D: Microsurgical anatomy of the veins of the posterior fossa. **J Neurosurg** 59:63–105, 1983.
22. Matsushima T, Rhoton AL Jr, Lenkey C: Microsurgery of the fourth ventricle: Part I—Microsurgical anatomy. **Neurosurgery** 11:631–667, 1982.
23. Mussi A, Rhoton AL Jr: Telovelar approach to the fourth ventricle: Microsurgical anatomy. **J Neurosurg** 92:812–823, 2000.
24. Pollack IF, Polinko P, Albright L, Towbin R, Fitz C: Mutism and pseudobulbar symptoms after resection of posterior fossa tumors in children: Incidence and pathophysiology. **Neurosurgery** 37: 885–893, 1995.
25. Rhoton AL Jr: Microsurgical anatomy of posterior fossa cranial nerves, in Barrow DL (ed): *Surgery of the Cranial Nerves of the Posterior Fossa: Neurosurgical Topics*. Chicago, AANS, 1993, pp 1–103.
26. Van Calenbergh F, Van de Laar A, Plets C, Goffin J, Casaer P: Transient cerebellar mutism after posterior fossa surgery in children. **Neurosurgery** 37:894–898, 1995.

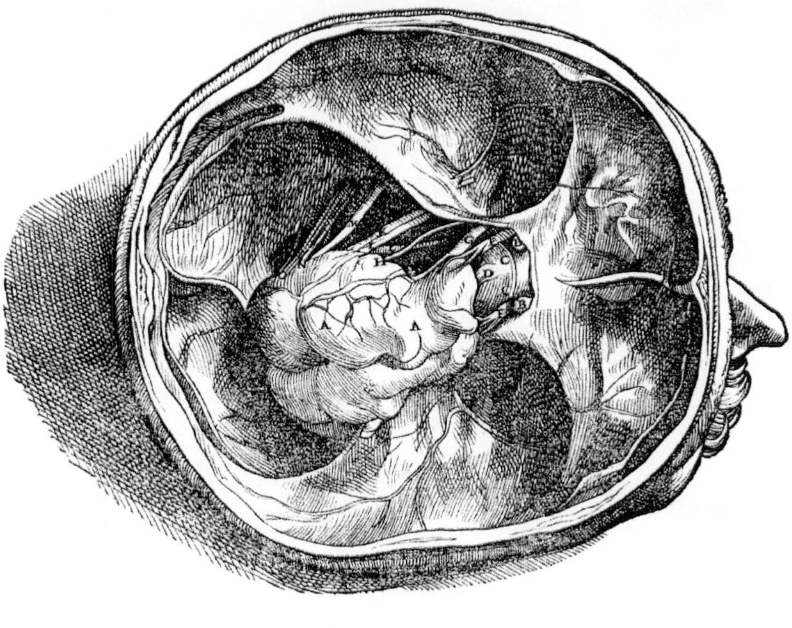

Cranial floor and contents of the posterior fossa. Vesalius (1514–1564) was only 28 years old when his publication was printed. The woodcuts, with their innovative landscape background, were by Jan Stephan Kalkar. From, Andreas Vesalius, *De Humani Corporis Fabrica*. Basel, Ex officina Ioannis Oporini, 1543. Courtesy, Rare Book Room, Norris Medical Library, Keck School of Medicine, Los Angeles, California.

DECIMAE QVARTAE FIGVRAE, EIVSDEMQVE characterum Index.

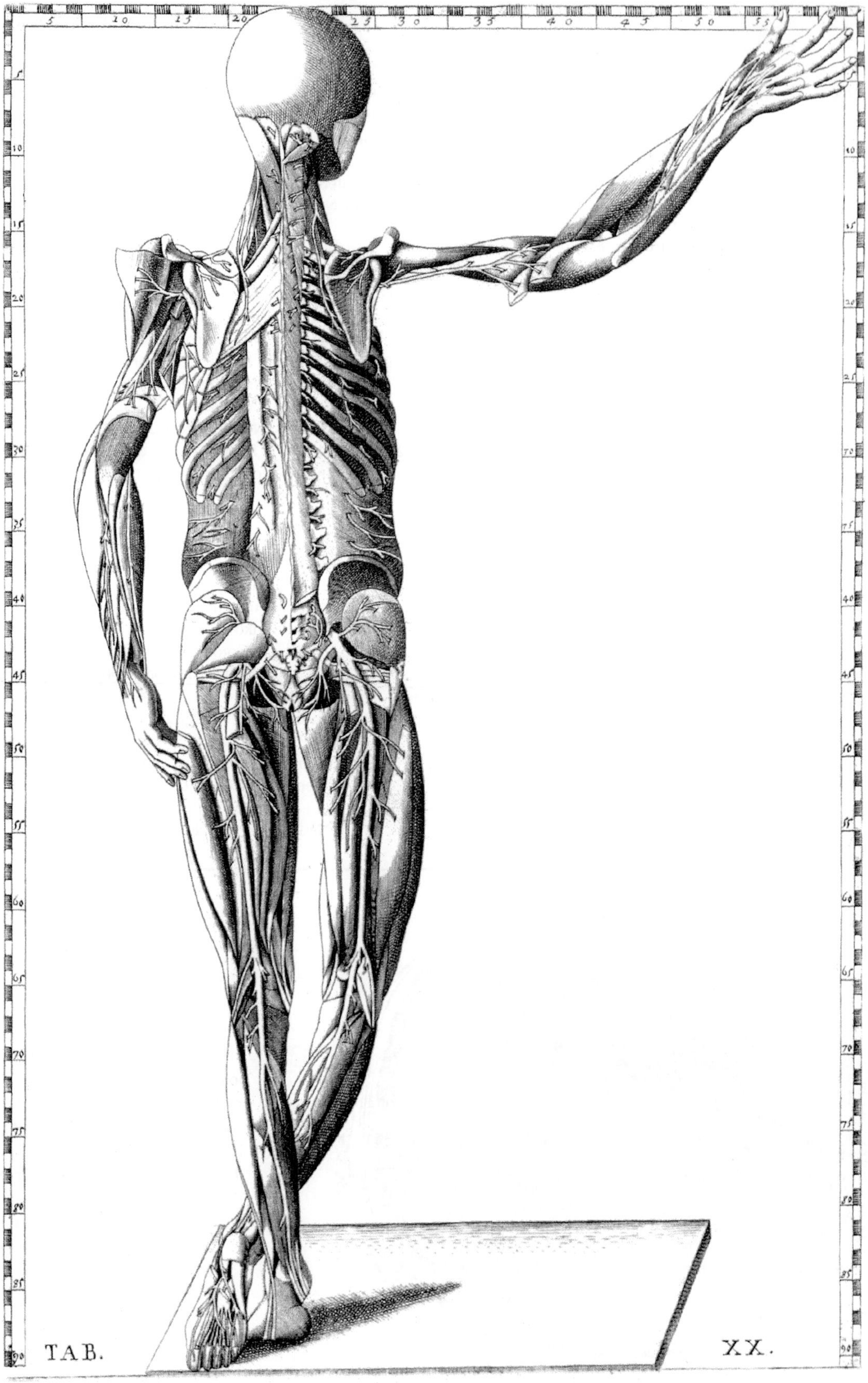

Deep dissection exposing posterior skeletal and neural structures. Although Eustachio's anatomical plates were originally engraved in 1552, they were not printed until 160 years later. From, Bartolommeo Eustachio, *Tabulae anatomicae*. Rome, Sumptibus Laurentii & Thomae Pagliarini, 1728. Courtesy, Rare Book Room, Norris Medical Library, Keck School of Medicine, Los Angeles, California.

CHAPTER 2

The Cerebellar Arteries

Albert L. Rhoton, Jr., M.D.

Department of Neurological Surgery, University of Florida, Gainesville, Florida

Key words: Anteroinferior cerebellar artery, Cerebellum, Cerebrovascular disease, Cranial nerves, Microneurosurgery, Posterior cranial fossa, Posteroinferior cerebellar artery, Superior cerebellar artery

Optimizing operative approaches to the posterior fossa requires an understanding of the relationship of the cerebellar arteries to the cranial nerves, brainstem, cerebellar peduncles, fissures between the cerebellum and brainstem, and the cerebellar surfaces (45). When examining these relationships, three neurovascular complexes are defined: an upper complex related to the superior cerebellar artery (SCA); a middle complex related to the anteroinferior cerebellar artery (AICA); and a lower complex related to the posteroinferior cerebellar artery (PICA) (*Figs. 2.1* and 2.2) (35).

Other structures, in addition to the three cerebellar arteries, occurring in sets of three in the posterior fossa that bear a consistent relationship to the SCA, AICA, and PICA are the parts of the brainstem (midbrain, pons, and medulla); the cerebellar peduncles (superior, middle, and inferior); the fissures between the brainstem and the cerebellum (cerebellomesencephalic, cerebellopontine, and cerebellomedullary); and the surfaces of the cerebellum (tentorial, petrosal, and suboccipital). Each neurovascular complex includes one of the three parts of the brainstem, one of the three surfaces of the cerebellum, one of the three cerebellar peduncles, and one of the three major fissures between the cerebellum and the brainstem. In addition, each neurovascular complex contains a group of cranial nerves. The upper complex includes the oculomotor, trochlear, and trigeminal nerves that are related to the SCA. The middle complex includes the abducens, facial, and vestibulocochlear nerves that are related to the AICA. The lower complex includes the glossopharyngeal, vagus, accessory, and hypoglossal nerves that are related to the PICA.

In summary, the upper complex includes the SCA, midbrain, cerebellomesencephalic fissure, superior cerebellar peduncle, tentorial surface of the cerebellum, and the oculomotor, trochlear, and trigeminal nerves. The SCA arises in front of the midbrain, passes below the oculomotor and trochlear nerves and above the trigeminal nerve to reach the cerebellomesencephalic fissure, where it runs on the superior cerebellar peduncle and terminates by supplying the tentorial surface of the cerebellum.

The middle complex includes the AICA, pons, middle cerebellar peduncle, cerebellopontine fissure, petrosal surface of the cerebellum, and the abducens, facial, and vestibulocochlear nerves. The AICA arises at the pontine level, courses in relationship to the abducens, facial, and vestibulocochlear nerves to reach the surface of the middle cerebellar peduncle, where it courses along the cerebellopontine fissure and terminates by supplying the petrosal surface of the cerebellum.

The lower complex includes the PICA, medulla, inferior cerebellar peduncle, cerebellomedullary fissure, suboccipital surface of the cerebellum, and the glossopharyngeal, vagus, spinal accessory, and hypoglossal nerves. The PICA arises at the medullary level, encircles the medulla, passing in relationship to the glossopharyngeal, vagus, accessory, and hypoglossal nerves to reach the surface of the inferior cerebellar peduncle, where it dips into the cerebellomedullary fissure and terminates by supplying the suboccipital surface of the cerebellum.

THE SUPERIOR CEREBELLAR ARTERY

Overview

The SCA or its branches are exposed in surgical approaches to the basilar apex, tentorial incisura, trigeminal nerve, cerebellopontine angle, pineal region, clivus, and the upper part of the cerebellum (18, 19).

The SCA is intimately related to the cerebellomesencephalic fissure, the superior half of the fourth ventricular roof, the superior cerebellar peduncle, and the tentorial surface (*Figs. 2.3-2.5*). The SCA arises in front of the midbrain, usually from the basilar artery near the apex, and passes below the oculomotor nerve, but may infrequently arise from the proximal PCA and pass above the oculomotor nerve. It dips caudally and encircles the brainstem near the pontomesencephalic junction, passing below the trochlear nerve and above the trigeminal nerve. Its proximal portion courses medial to the free edge of the tentorium cerebelli, and its distal part passes below the tentorium, making it the most rostral of the infratentorial arteries. After passing above the trigeminal nerve, it enters the cerebellomesencephalic fissure, where its branches make several sharp turns and give rise to the precerebellar arteries, which pass to the deep cerebellar white matter and the dentate nucleus. On leaving the cerebellomesencephalic fissure where its branches are again medial to the tentorial edge, its branches pass posteriorly under the tentorial edge

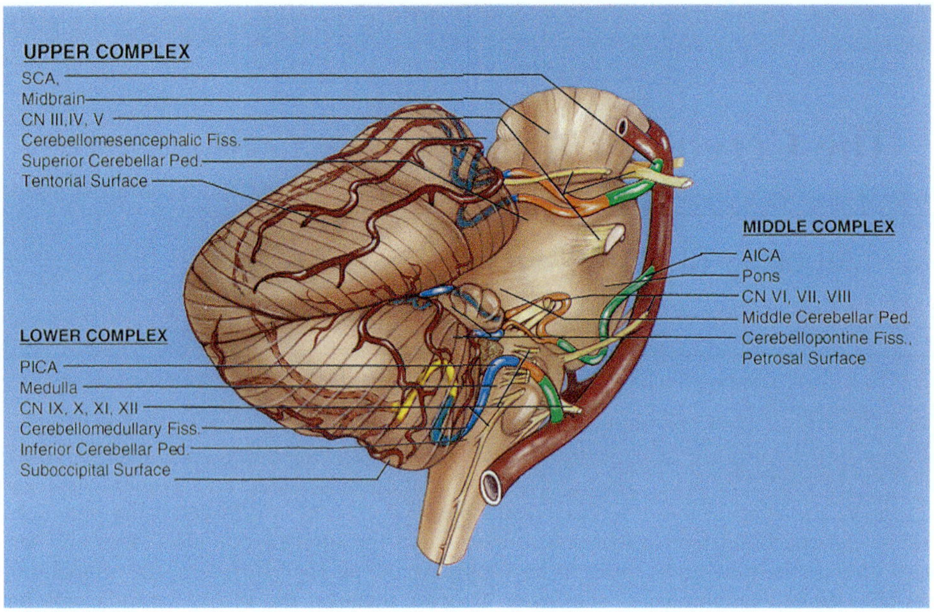

FIGURE 2.1. Each of the three neurovascular complexes in the posterior fossa includes one of the three cerebellar arteries, one of the three parts of the brainstem, one of the three cerebellar peduncles, one of the three cerebellar surfaces, one of the three fissures between the brainstem and the cerebellum, and one of the three groups of cranial nerves. The upper complex is related to the SCA, the middle complex is related to the AICA, and the lower complex is related to the PICA. The upper complex includes the SCA, midbrain, superior cerebellar peduncle, cerebellomesencephalic fissure, tentorial cerebellar surface, and the oculomotor, trochlear, and trigeminal nerves. The middle complex includes the PICA, pons, middle cerebellar peduncle, cerebellopontine fissure, petrosal surface, and the abducens, facial, and vestibulocochlear nerves. The lower complex includes the PICA, medulla, inferior cerebellar peduncle, cerebellomedullary fissure, suboccipital surface, and the glossopharyngeal, vagus, accessory, and hypoglossal nerves. The SCA is divided into four segments: anterior pontomesencephalic (*green*), lateral pontomesencephalic (*orange*), cerebellomesencephalic (*blue*), and cortical (*red*). Each segment may be composed of one or more trunks, depending on the level of bifurcation of the main trunk. The AICA is divided into four segments: anterior pontine (*green*), lateral pontomedullary (*orange*), flocculonodular (*blue*), and cortical (*red*). The PICA is divided into five segments: anterior medullary (*green*), lateral medullary (*orange*), tonsillomedullary (*blue*), telovelotonsillar (*yellow*), and cortical (*red*). *A.I.C.A.*, anteroinferior cerebellar artery; *CN*, cranial nerve; *Fiss.*, fissure; *Ped.*, peduncle; *P.I.C.A.*, posteroinferior cerebellar artery; *S.C.A.*, superior cerebellar artery.

and are distributed to the tentorial surface. It usually arises as a single trunk, but may also arise as a double (or duplicate) trunk. The SCAs arising as a single trunk bifurcate into a rostral and a caudal trunk. The SCA gives off perforating branches to the brainstem and cerebellar peduncles. Precerebellar branches arise within the cerebellomesencephalic fissure. The rostral trunk supplies the vermian and paravermian area and the caudal trunk supplies the hemisphere on the suboccipital surface. The SCA frequently has points of contact with the oculomotor, trochlear, and trigeminal nerves.

Segments

The SCA is divided into four segments: anterior pontomesencephalic, lateral pontomesencephalic, cerebellomesencephalic, and cortical (*Fig. 2.1*). Each segment may be composed of one or more trunks, depending on the level of bifurcation of the main trunk (*Fig. 2.6*).

Anterior pontomesencephalic segment

This segment is located between the dorsum sellae and the upper brainstem. It begins at the origin of the SCA and extends below the oculomotor nerve to the anterolateral margin of the brainstem. Its lateral part is medial to the anterior half of the free tentorial edge.

Lateral pontomesencephalic segment

This segment begins at the anterolateral margin of the brainstem and frequently dips caudally onto the lateral side of the upper pons (*Figs. 2.1, 2.7,* and *2.8*). Its caudal loop projects toward and often reaches the root entry zone of the trigeminal nerve at the midpontine level. The trochlear nerve passes above the midportion of this segment. The anterior part of this segment is often visible above the tentorial edge, but the caudal loop usually carries it below the tentorium. This segment terminates at the anterior margin of the cerebellomesencephalic fissure. The basal vein and the PCA course above and parallel to this SCA.

Cerebellomesencephalic segment

This segment courses within the cerebellomesencephalic fissure (*Figs. 2.7-2.9*). The SCA branches enter the shallowest part of the fissure located above the trigeminal root entry zone and again course medial to the tentorial edge with its branches intertwined with the trochlear nerve. The fissure in which the SCA proceeds progressively deepens medially and is deepest in the midline behind the superior medullary velum. Through a series of hairpin-like curves, the SCA loops deeply into the fissure and passes upward to reach the anterior edge of the tentorial surface. The trunks and branches of the SCA are held in the fissure by branches that penetrate the

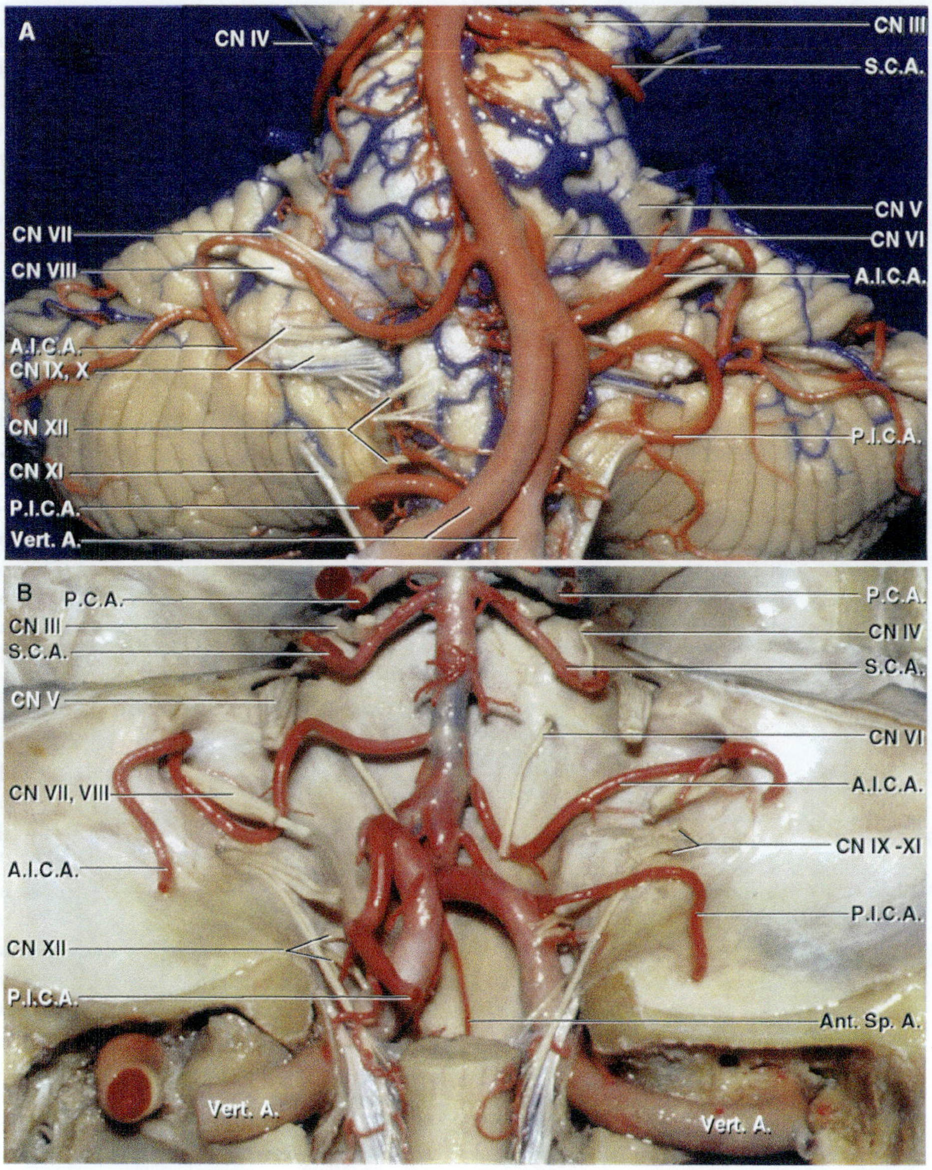

FIGURE 2.2. *A*, anterior view of the brainstem and cerebellar arteries. *B*, posterior view of the cranial base with the cranial nerves and arteries preserved. *A* and *B*, the SCA arises at the midbrain level and encircles the brainstem near the pontomesencephalic junction. The SCA courses below the oculomotor and trochlear nerves and above the trigeminal nerve. The SCA loops down closer to the trigeminal nerve in *B* than in *A*. The AICA arises at the pontine level and courses by the abducens, facial, and vestibulocochlear nerves. In *A*, both AICAs pass below the abducens nerves. In *B*, the left abducens nerve passes in front of the AICA and the right abducens nerve passes behind the AICA. The PICAs arise from the vertebral artery at the medullary level and course in relation to the glossopharyngeal, vagus, accessory, and hypoglossal nerves. The origin of the SCAs are quite symmetrical from side to side. There is slight asymmetry in the level of origin of the AICAs and marked asymmetry in the level of the origin of the PICAs, especially in *A*. *A.*, artery; *A.I.C.A.*, anteroinferior cerebellar artery; *Ant.*, anterior; *CN*, cranial nerve; *P.C.A.*, posterior cerebral artery; *P.I.C.A.*, posteroinferior cerebellar artery; *S.C.A.*, superior cerebellar artery; *Sp.*, spinal; *Vert.*, vertebral.

fissure's opposing walls. Identification of individual branches of the SCA within this fissure is made difficult by the sharp curves of the branches and by the large number of intermingled arterial loops.

Cortical segment

This segment includes the branches distal to the cerebellomesencephalic fissure that pass under the tentorial edge and are distributed to the tentorial surface and, if a marginal branch is present, to the upper part of the petrosal surface (*Figs. 2.6-2.9*).

Origin

The SCA is the most consistent of the infratentorial cerebellar arteries in its presence and area of supply (49). Absence of the SCA, although rare, has been reported (50). In our previous study of 50 SCAs, 43 arose as a single trunk and 7 arose as two (duplicate) trunks (19). Duplicate trunks were present bilaterally in only one of the brains we examined. Triplication of the origin is rare. All but 2 of the 50 SCAs examined arose from the basilar artery. The two exceptions arose solely or in part from the posterior cerebral artery and passed above the oculomotor nerve, after which they followed the typical distal course. The solitary trunk of nonduplicated SCAs and the rostral trunk of duplicate SCAs usually arise from the basilar artery below, but directly adjacent to, the origin of the PCA. The arteries not arising adjacent to the origin of the PCA arise within 2.5 mm of the PCA origin.

The origin of the right and left SCAs and PCAs frequently takes a cruciate configuration in which the limbs cross at the apex of the basilar artery (*Fig. 2.2*). The height of the bifurca-

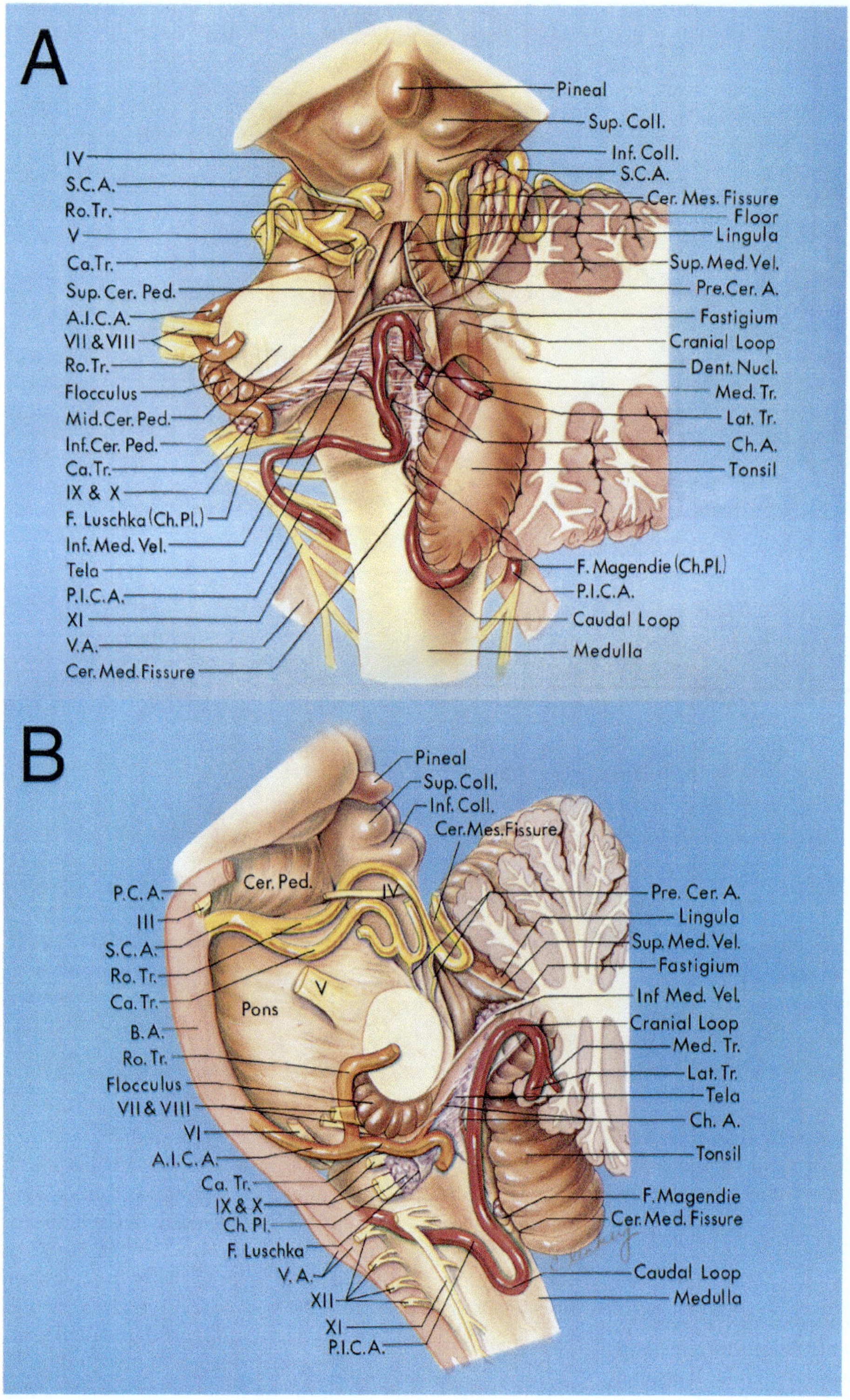

FIGURE 2.3. Relationships of the cerebellar arteries. *A*, posterior view with the left and part of the right half of the cerebellum removed. *B*, lateral view with the left half of the cerebellum removed to expose the fourth ventricle. The SCAs (*yellow*) are intimately related to the superior half of the fourth ventricular roof and the cerebellomesencephalic fissure; the AICAs (*orange*) are intimately related to the cerebellopontine fissures and the lateral recesses; and the PICAs (*red*) are intimately related to the caudal half of the roof and the cerebellomedullary fissure. The SCAs pass around the midbrain above the trigeminal nerve and divide into rostral and caudal trunks. The branches of these trunks loop deeply into the cerebellomesencephalic fissure and give off the precerebellar arteries, which pass along the superior cerebellar peduncles to the dentate nuclei. The PICAS arise from the vertebral arteries and pass between the glossopharyngeal, vagus, and accessory nerves to reach the cerebellomedullary fissure. After passing near the caudal pole of the tonsils, where they form a caudal loop, they ascend through the cerebellomedullary fissure, where they are intimately related to the caudal part of the ventricular roof. They pass around the rostral pole of the tonsil and through the telovelotonsillar cleft, where they form a cranial loop. In their course around the tonsils, they divide into medial and lateral trunks. They give off branches to the dentate nuclei near the superior pole of the tonsils. The AICAs arise from the basilar artery and pass near or between the facial and vestibulocochlear nerves and are intimately related to the cerebellopontine fissures, the flocculi, and the lateral recesses. The AICAs divide into rostral and caudal trunks before reaching the facial and vestibulocochlear nerves. The rostral trunk passes between the nerves and along the middle cerebellar peduncle near the cerebellopontine fissure. The caudal trunk passes below the nerves and near the lateral recess to supply the lower part of the petrosal surface. The AICA and the PICA give rise to the choroidal arteries, which supply the tela choroidea and attached choroid plexus. (From, Matsushima T, Rhoton AL Jr, Lenkey C: Microsurgery of the fourth ventricle: Part I—Microsurgical anatomy. Neurosurgery 11:631–667, 1982 [35].) *A.*, artery; *A.I.C.A.*, anteroinferior cerebellar artery; *B.*, basilar; *Ca.*, caudal; *Cer.*, cerebellar; *Cer. Med.*, cerebellomedullary; *Cer. Mes.*, cerebellomesencephalic; *Ch.*, choroid, choroidal; *Coll.*, colliculus; *Dent.*, dentate; *F.*, foramen; *Inf.*, inferior; *Lat.*, lateral; *Med.*, medial, medullary; *Mid.*, middle; *Nucl.*, nucleus; *P.C.A.*, posterior cerebral artery; *Ped.*, peduncle; *P.I.C.A.*, posteroinferior cerebellar artery; *Pl.*, plexus; *Ro.*, rostral; *S.C.A.*, superior cerebellar artery; *Sup.*, superior; *Tr.*, trunk; *V.*, vein; *V.A.*, vertebral artery; *Vel.*, velum.

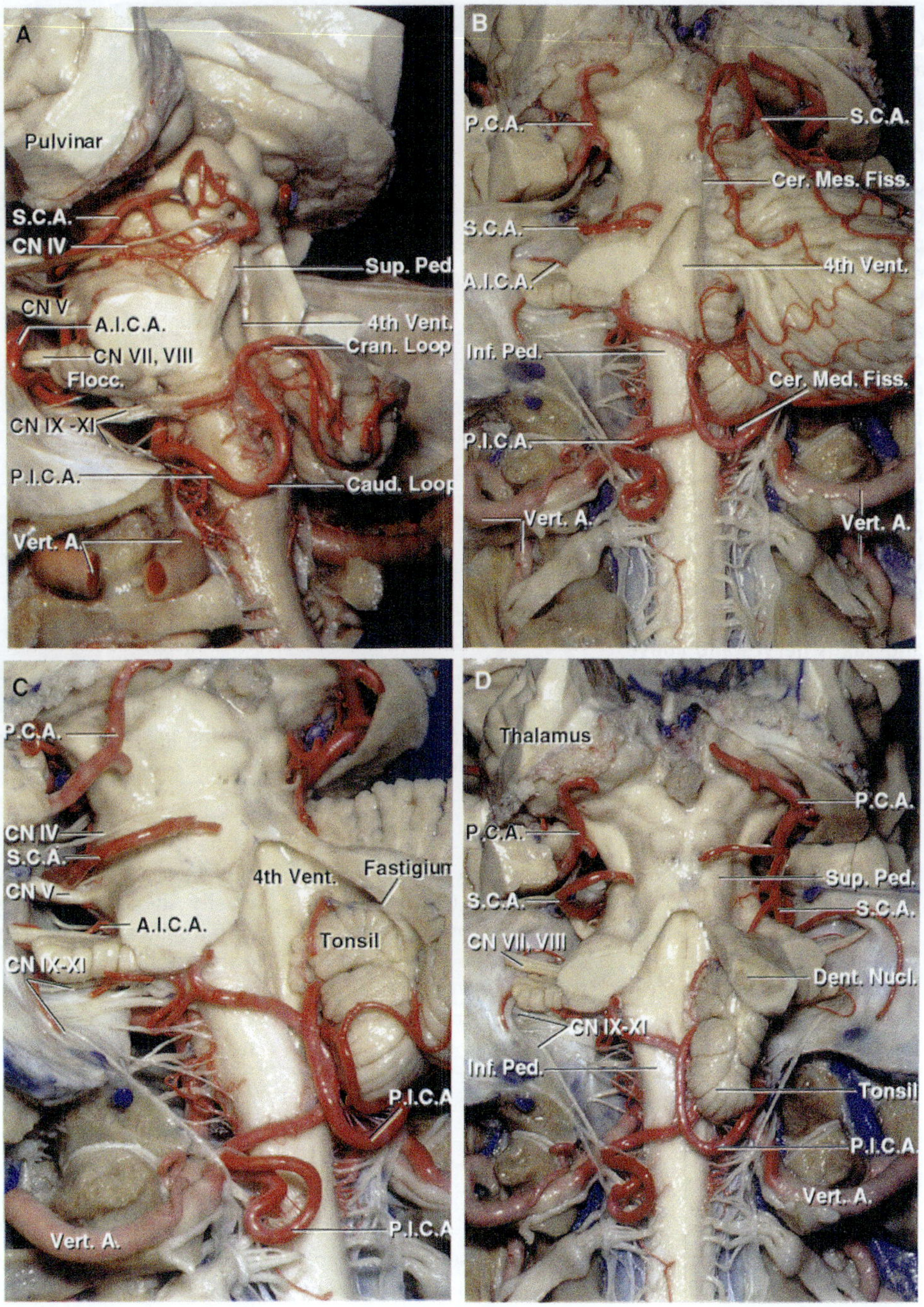

FIGURE 2.4. *A–D.* **Cerebellar arteries, brainstem, and cerebellar-brainstem fissures.** *A,* **posterolateral view. The SCA passes around the midbrain to enter the cerebellomesencephalic fissure, where it sends perforating branches into the posterior midbrain below a line between the superior and inferior colliculi, and down the superior peduncle to the dentate nucleus. The AICA loops around the flocculus and the facial and vestibulocochlear nerves. The left PICA passes between the rootlets of the nerves entering the jugular foramen and turns caudally around the lower pole of the left tonsil, which has been removed, and then ascends to form a cranial loop at the upper pole of the tonsil bordering the inferior half of the ventricular roof.** *B,* **another specimen. The left half of the cerebellum has been removed. The SCA passes around the midbrain below the PCA in the lower part of the ambient and quadrigeminal cisterns, enters the cerebellomesencephalic fissure, and loops over the posterior lip of the fissure to supply the tentorial surface. The PICA arises from the vertebral artery, passes around the medulla, crosses the inferior cerebellar peduncle, and enters the cerebellomedullary fissure, where it passes along the inferior half of the ventricular roof, and exits the fissure to supply the suboccipital surface. The AICA passes laterally around the pons and above the flocculus.** *C,* **enlarged oblique view. The right PICA loops around the caudal and rostral poles of the tonsil. The left PICA dips below the level of the foramen magnum.** *D,* **posterior view after removing all of the cerebellum except for the right tonsil and dentate nucleus.** *A.,* artery; *A.I.C.A.,* anteroinferior cerebellar artery; *Caud.,* caudal; *Cer. Med.,* cerebellomedullary; *Cer. Mes.,* cerebellomesencephalic; *Chor.,* choroid; *CN,* cranial nerve; *Cran.,* cranial; *Dent.,* dentate; *Fiss.,* fissure; *Flocc.,* flocculus; *Inf.,* inferior; *Mid.,* middle; *Nucl.,* nucleus; *P.C.A.,* posterior cerebral artery; *Ped.,* peduncle; *P.I.C.A.,* posteroinferior cerebellar artery; *Plex.,* plexus; *S.C.A.,* superior cerebellar artery; *Sup.,* superior; *Vent.,* ventricle; *Vert.,* vertebral.

tion of the basilar artery is an important determinant of the initial course (47, 59). The level of the bifurcation of the basilar artery is normal if the bifurcation occurs at the pontomesencephalic junction, high if it occurs anterior to the mesencephalon, and low if it is anterior to the pons. The origin of the SCA is above the edge of the tentorium if the bifurcation is high, medial to the free edge if it is normal, and below the tentorium if it is low. In our study, the bifurcation was in a

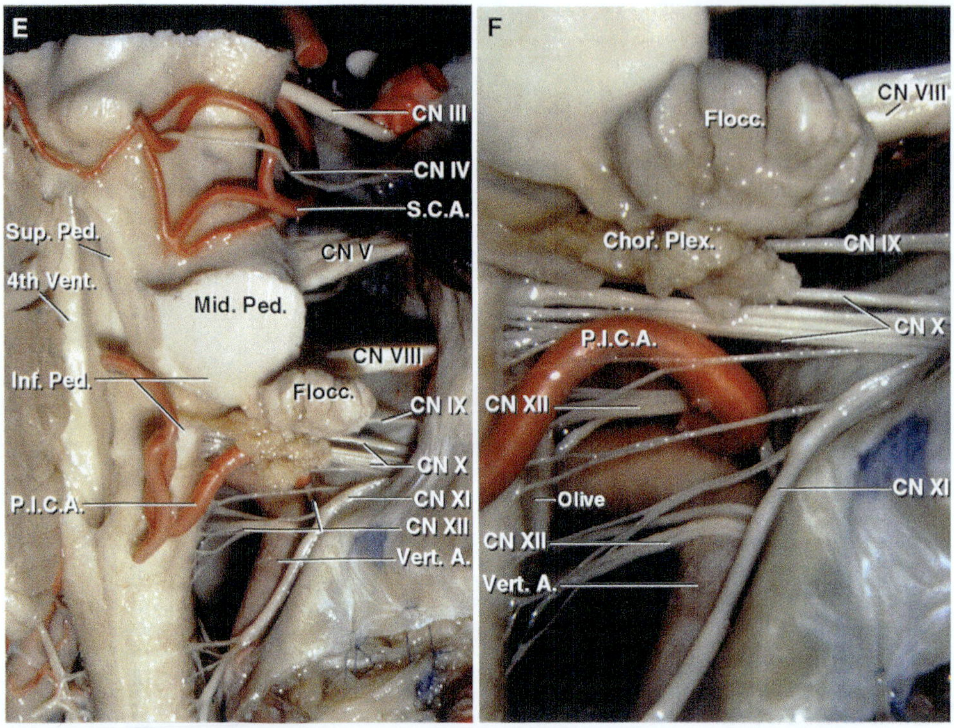

FIGURE 2.4. *E* **and** *F.* **Cerebellar arteries, brainstem, and cerebellar-brainstem fissures.** *E,* **the SCA passes above the trigeminal nerve and enters the cerebellomesencephalic fissure, where it sends branches down the superior peduncle to the dentate nucleus. The PICA passes between the vagus and accessory nerves and courses on the inferior peduncle to reach the cerebellomedullary fissure.** *F,* **enlarged view of the lateral recess. The flocculus and choroid plexus project laterally from the margin of the foramen of Luschka into the cerebellopontine angle, behind the glossopharyngeal and vagus nerves and above the PICA. The hypoglossal rootlets arises from the medulla in front of the glossopharyngeal and vagus nerves and cross the posterior surface of the vertebral artery. Some hypoglossal rootlets pass above and others below the PICA origin.**

normal position in 18 of the 25 brains that we examined, high in 6, and low in 1. Three of the six arteries with a high bifurcation were associated with a fetal origin of the PCA (47).

The length of the basilar artery ranges from 20 to 40 mm (average, 30) and its diameter is greater at its origin from the vertebral arteries, range from 3 to 8 mm (average, 5–6 mm) than at its apex (range, 3–7 mm; mean, 4–5 mm). The basilar artery is usually straight or deviates a short distance off the midline, but a few will deviate laterally as far as the origin of the abducens nerve or the facial and vestibulocochlear nerves (18, 19).

Bifurcation

All of the SCAs that arise as a single vessel bifurcate into two major trunks, one rostral and one caudal (*Fig. 2.10*). This bifurcation occurs between 0.6 and 34.0 mm (average, 19 mm) from the origin, most commonly near the point of maximal caudal descent of the artery on the lateral side of the brainstem. Rostral and caudal trunks are present in nearly every hemisphere as a result of either a duplicate origin or the bifurcation of a main artery. The rostral and caudal trunks formed by a duplicate origin, referred to as rostral and caudal duplicate SCAs, have a distribution equivalent to that of the rostral and caudal trunks formed by the bifurcation of a solitary SCA.

The rostral trunk terminates by supplying the vermis and a variable portion of the adjacent hemisphere. The caudal trunk supplies the hemispheric surface lateral to the area supplied by the rostral trunk. The diameters of the rostral and caudal trunks are approximately equal, but if one is smaller, it is usually the caudal trunk. If one trunk is small, the other supplies a larger area. The caudal trunk rarely sends branches to the vermis.

Branches

Perforating arteries

These perforating branches are divided into a direct and circumflex type (*Fig. 2.7*). The direct type pursues a straight course to enter the brainstem. The circumflex type winds around the brainstem before terminating in it. The circumflex perforating arteries are subdivided into short and long types. The short circumflex type travels 90 degrees or less around the circumference of the brainstem. The long circumflex type travels a greater distance to reach the opposite surface. Both types of circumflex arteries send branches into the brainstem along their course.

Perforating branches arise from the great majority of main, rostral, and caudal trunks. Most trunks give rise to two to five perforating branches, although some may give rise to no perforators and others to as many as 10. The most common type of perforating artery arising from the main trunk is the long circumflex type, but it also gives rise to direct and short circumflex branches. In descending order, the main trunk branches terminate in the tegmentum in the region of the junction between the superior and middle cerebellar pe-

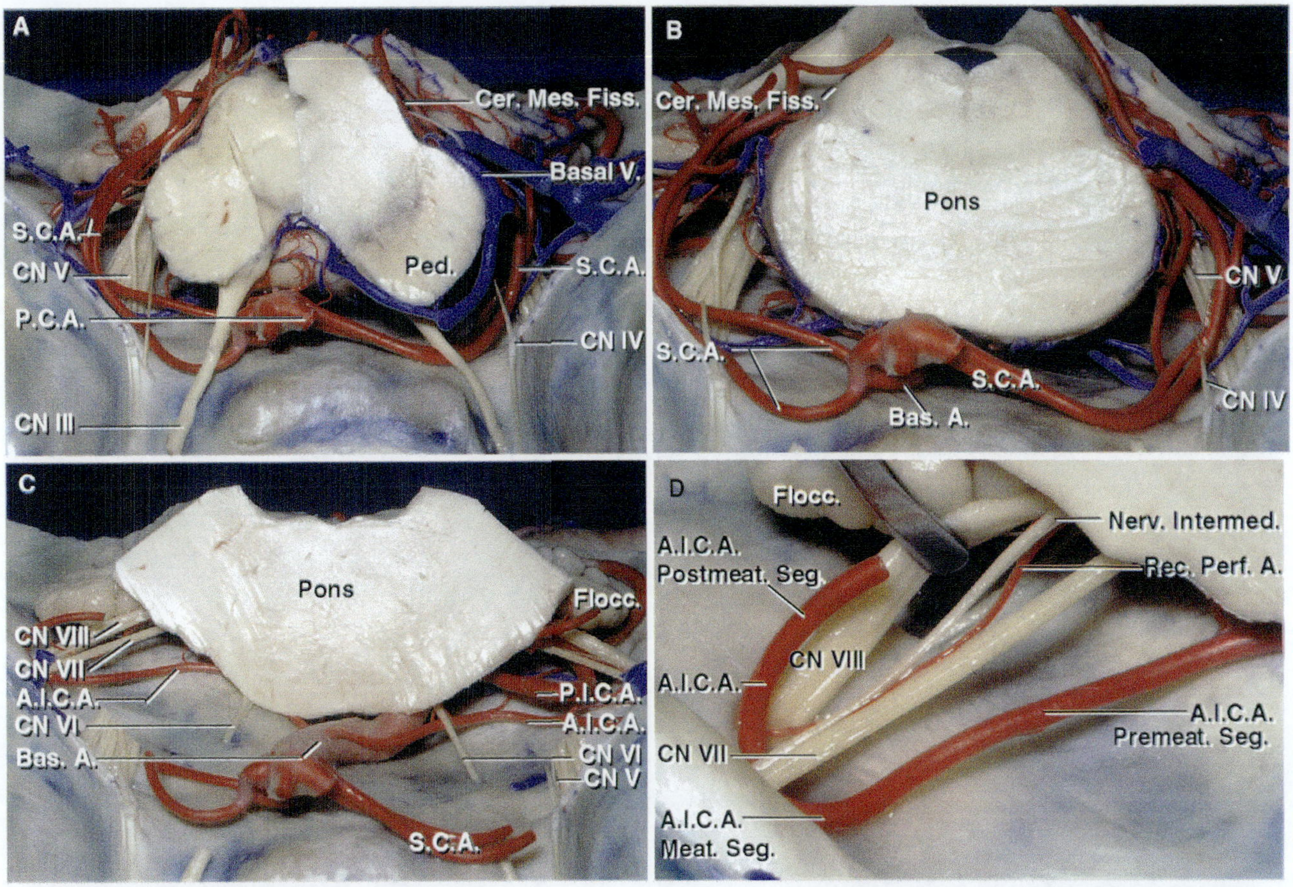

FIGURE 2.5. ***A–D.*** **Cerebellar arteries. Superior views.** ***A,*** **both SCAs arise as duplicate arteries at the midbrain level and accompany the basal vein around the brainstem to enter the cerebellomesencephalic fissure. They pass below the oculomotor and trochlear nerves and above the trigeminal nerves. The SCA trunks are intertwined with the trochlear nerve on the posterolateral brainstem.** ***B,*** **the level of the brainstem section has been extended downward to the pons. The rostral and caudal trunks of the duplicate SCAs arise directly from the side of the basilar artery and pass laterally above the trigeminal nerve.** ***C,*** **the brainstem section has been extended downward to the midpons. The trigeminal, oculomotor, and trochlear nerves have been divided so that the brainstem could be reflected backward to expose the AICA and the facial and vestibulocochlear nerves. Both AICAs pass below the abducens nerves and loop laterally toward the internal acoustic meatus. The left PICA loops upward in front of the pons between the facial and vestibulocochlear nerves and the AICA before turning downward to encircle the medulla.** ***D,*** **enlarged view. The right AICA loops laterally into the porus of the internal acoustic meatus, as occurs in approximately half of cases. The AICA has a premeatal segment that passes toward the meatus, a meatal segment that loops into the porus in about half of cerebellopontine angles, and a postmeatal segment that loops back to the brainstem. The vestibulocochlear nerve has been retracted to expose the nervus intermedius, which arises at the brainstem along the anterior surface of the vestibulocochlear nerve, has a free segment in the cerebellopontine angle, and joins the facial nerve as it proceeds laterally toward the meatus. The AICA gives rise to a recurrent perforating branch to the brainstem.** ***A.,*** **artery;** ***A.I.C.A.,*** **anteroinferior cerebellar artery;** ***Bas.,*** **basilar;** ***Bridg.,*** **bridging;** ***Cer. Mes.,*** **cerebellomesencephalic;** ***CN,*** **cranial nerve;** ***Fiss.,*** **fissure;** ***Flocc.,*** **flocculus;** ***Intermed.,*** **intermedius;** ***Meat.,*** **meatal;** ***Mes.,*** **mesencephalic;** ***Nerv.,*** **nervus;** ***P.C.A.,*** **posterior cerebral artery;** ***Ped.,*** **peduncle;** ***Perf.,*** **perforating;** ***P.I.C.A.,*** **posteroinferior cerebellar artery;** ***Premeat.,*** **premeatal;** ***Rec.,*** **recurrent;** ***S.C.A.,*** **superior cerebellar artery;** ***Seg.,*** **segment;** ***V.,*** **vein;** ***Vent.,*** **ventrical;** ***Vert.,*** **vertebral.**

duncles, the interpeduncular fossa (usually the direct type), the cerebral peduncle, and the collicular region.

The branches from the rostral and caudal trunk are most frequently circumflex. They course around the brainstem to reach two main areas: the region of the junction of the superior and middle cerebellar peduncles and the quadrigeminal cistern below the sulcus between the superior and inferior colliculi. In descending order, they terminate in the junction between the superior and middle cerebellar peduncles, the inferior colliculus, the cerebral peduncle, and the interpeduncular fossa.

The basilar artery also gives rise to multiple perforating branches to the brainstem. Those arising near the origin of the SCA intermingle with the direct perforating branches arising

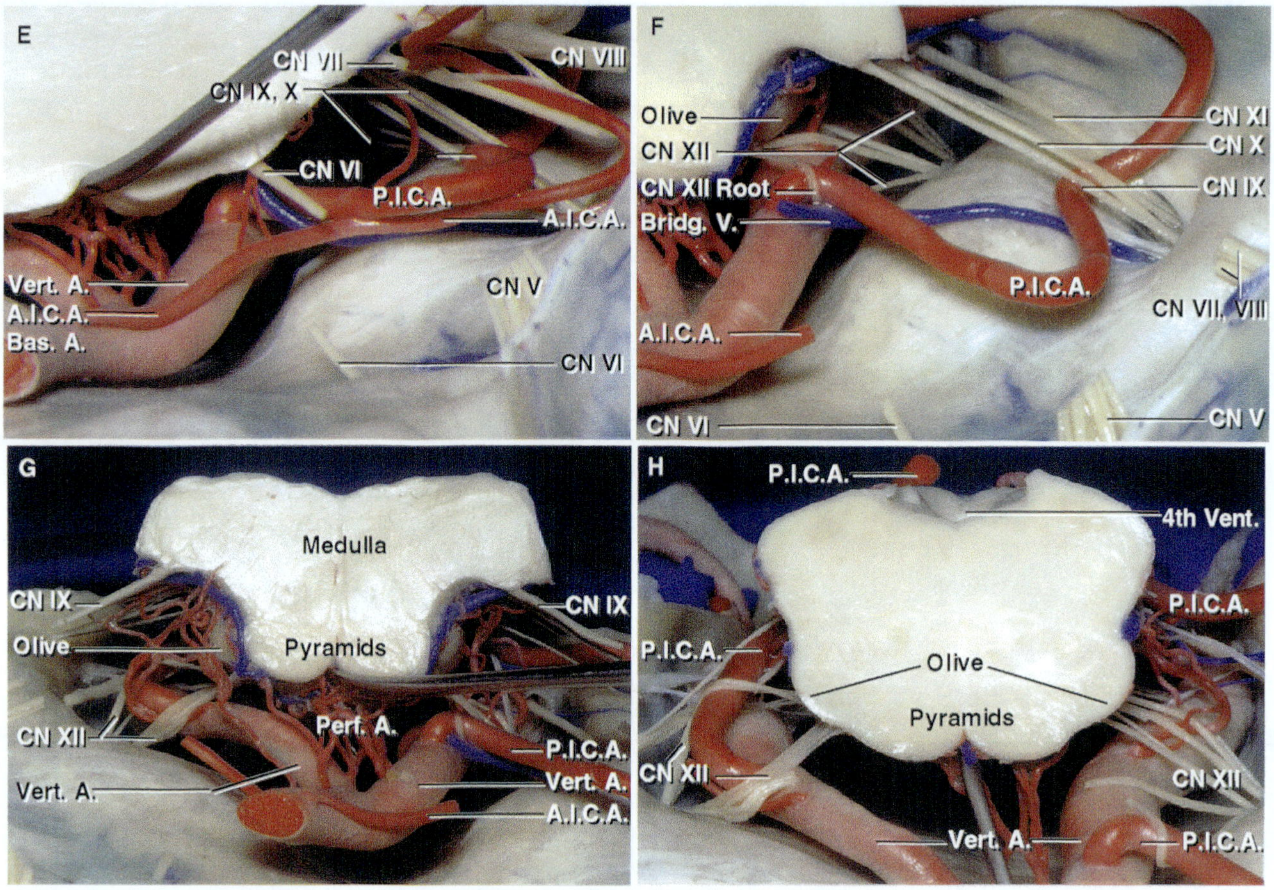

FIGURE 2.5. ***E–H.*** **Cerebellar arteries.** ***E,*** **enlarged view. The left AICA arises from the basilar artery and passes laterally toward the porus of the internal acoustic meatus before turning medially between the facial and vestibulocochlear nerves. The tortuous PICA loops upward between the AICA and the facial nerve before turning downward.** ***F,*** **the AICA and the nerves entering the internal acoustic meatus have been divided. The PICA loops upward before turning caudally and passing between the rootlets of the vagus and accessory nerves. The hypoglossal nerve arises from the brainstem in front of the olive. One of the rootlets of the hypoglossal nerve loops upward around the origin of the PICA before descending to join the other rootlets at the hypoglossal canal. A bridging vein passes from the medulla to the jugular bulb.** ***G,*** **the section has been extended downward to the level of the medulla to show the perforating branches of the vertebral and basilar arteries entering the medullary pyramids and the lateral medulla. The glossopharyngeal, vagus, and accessory nerves arise dorsal to the olives. The hypoglossal nerve arises ventral to the olives and passes behind the vertebral arteries.** ***H,*** **the medullary section has been extended caudally. The level of the PICA origins from the vertebral arteries are asymmetric. The right PICA intermingles with multiple rootlets of the hypoglossal nerve, while the left PICA, which arises at a higher level, has only the upper hypoglossal rootlet stretched around it. The PICAs encircle the medulla and appear on the dorsal surface behind the fourth ventricle. The left is larger than the right vertebral artery.**

from the proximal SCA. Those arising above the origin of the SCA enter the interpeduncular fossa.

Precerebellar branches

The precerebellar arteries arise from the trunks and cortical branches within the cerebellomesencephalic fissure (*Figs. 2.7-2.9*). As many as eight precerebellar arteries may arise within the fissure and these, along with the trunks and cortical branches and their sharp turns in the fissure, create a complexity that makes arterial dissection and identification difficult. These precerebellar branches tether the distal parts of the trunks and the proximal parts of the cortical arteries in the fissure. The precerebellar arteries consist of a medial group of small branches that pass between the superior medullary velum and the central lobule and a lateral group of larger branches that course between the superior and middle cerebellar peduncles and the wings of the central lobule. The cortical arteries supplying the hemispheric surface lateral to the vermis send precerebellar branches that reach the dentate and deep cerebellar nuclei, and those terminating in the vermis send branches to the inferior colliculi and the superior medullary velum.

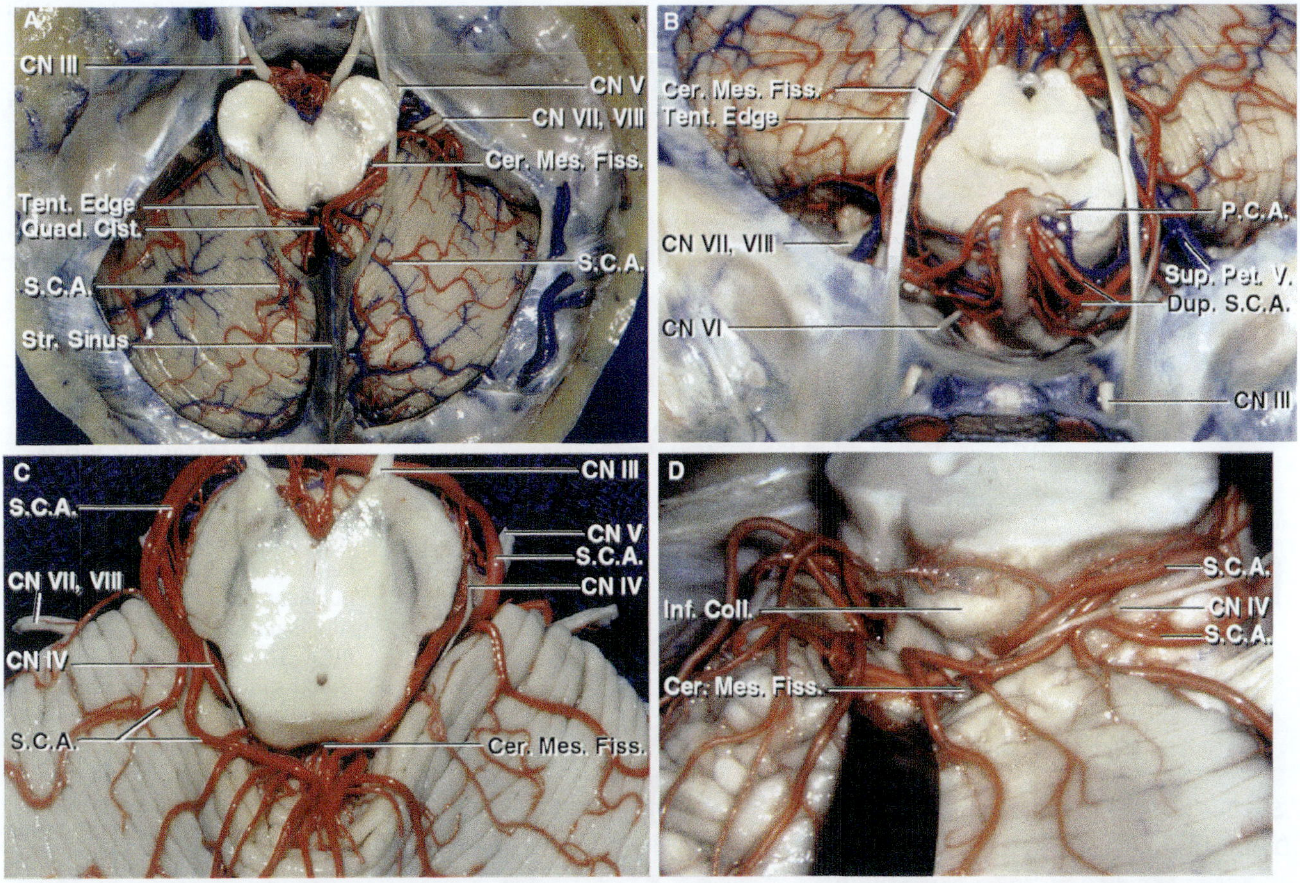

FIGURE 2.6. The SCA, cerebellomesencephalic fissure, and tentorial surface. Superior views. *A*, the SCAs pass around the midbrain to enter the cerebellomesencephalic fissure and, after a series of hairpin turns in the fissure, loop over the posterior lip of the fissure to reach the tentorial surface. The lower part of the quadrigeminal cistern extends in the cerebellomesencephalic fissure. The tentorial surface slopes downward from the apex just behind the fissure. *B*, anterosuperior view. The left SCA arises on a duplicate artery. In their initial course, the SCAs loop laterally below the tentorial edge, but further posteriorly, they pass medially under the tentorial edge to enter the cerebellomesencephalic fissure. *C*, another cerebellum. The SCAs loop into the cerebellomesencephalic fissure, where they undergo a series of hairpin turns before exiting the fissure to supply the tentorial surface. *D*, the posterior lip of the fissure has been retracted to expose the branches of the SCA within the fissure. *Cer. Mes.*, cerebellomesencephalic; *Cist.*, cistern; *CN*, cranial nerve; *Coll.*, colliculus; *Dup.*, duplicate; *Fiss.*, fissure; *Inf.*, inferior; *P.C.A.*, posterior cerebral artery; *Pet.*, petrosal; *Quad.*, quadrigeminal; *S.C.A.*, superior cerebellar artery; *Str.*, straight; *Sup.*, superior; *Tent.*, tentorial; *V.*, vein.

Cortical arteries

The most constant cortical supply of the SCA is to the tentorial surface (*Figs. 2.6-2.9*). The cortical territory of the SCA is more constant than that of the AICA and PICA, but is reciprocal with them. The SCA usually supplies the majority of the tentorial surface and frequently the adjacent upper part of the petrosal surface. The maximal field of supply includes a full half of the tentorial surface with overlap onto the opposite half of the vermis, the superior part of the suboccipital surface, and the upper two-thirds of the petrosal surface, including both lips of the petrosal fissure. The smallest field of supply includes only the part of the tentorial surface that lies anterior to the tentorial fissure.

The cortical branches are divided into hemispheric and vermian groups (*Fig. 2.7*). The cortical surface of each half of the vermis is divided into medial and paramedian segments and each hemisphere lateral to the vermis is divided into medial, intermediate, and lateral segments, because the most frequent pattern includes two vermian arteries and three hemispheric arteries corresponding to these segments.

Hemispheric arteries

The hemispheric branches arise from the rostral and caudal trunks in the depths of the cerebellomesencephalic fissure. They give rise to the precerebellar arteries, which bind their proximal parts within the cerebellomesencephalic fissure. After leaving the fissure, the hemispheric branches proceed to supply the tentorial surface lateral to the vermis. The rostral and caudal trunks together most commonly give rise to three, but sometimes as many as five, hemispheric

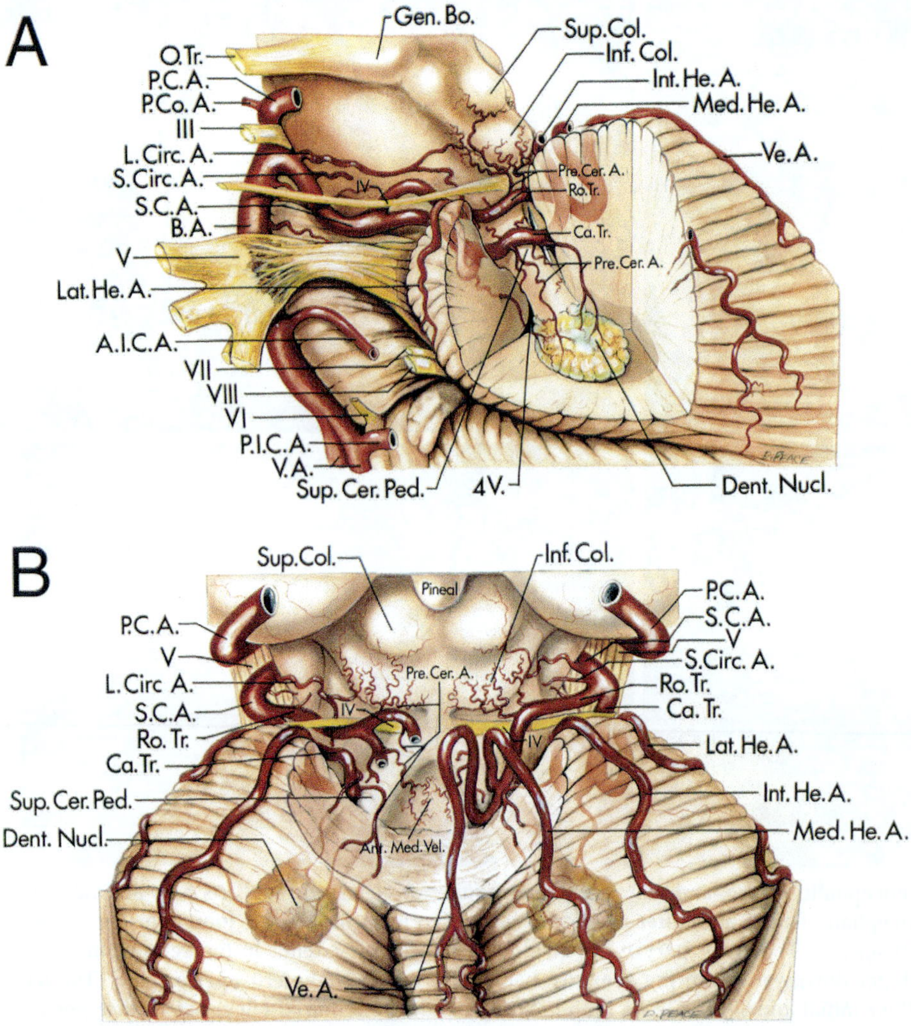

FIGURE 2.7. Relationships of the SCA. *A*, left lateral view of the SCA with part of the cerebellum removed to show the termination of the superior cerebellar peduncle in the dentate nucleus. The main trunk of the SCA passes below the oculomotor and trochlear nerves and above the trigeminal nerve and splits into rostral and caudal trunks. The optic tract and short circumflex arteries pass around the brainstem. The precerebellar arteries arise in the cerebellomesencephalic fissure, supply the adjoining cerebellum and the inferior colliculus, and send branches along the superior cerebellar peduncle to the dentate nucleus. The superior colliculus is supplied predominantly by the PICA. The rostral and caudal trunks split into vermian and lateral, medial, and intermediate hemispheric arteries. *B*, superior view with the superior lip of cerebellomesencephalic fissure removed to show branches within the fissure. The circumflex perforating arteries terminate in the inferior colliculus and the region of the junction of the superior and middle cerebellar peduncles. The precerebellar branches pass along the superior cerebellar peduncles to the dentate nucleus. The right half of the vermis is supplied by a large vermian artery and the hemispheric surface is supplied by medial, intermediate, and lateral hemispheric arteries. (From, Hardy DG, Peace DA, Rhoton AL Jr: Microsurgical anatomy of the superior cerebellar artery. Neurosurgery 6:10–28, 1980 [19].) *A.*, artery; *A.I.C.A.*, anteroinferior cerebellar artery; *Ant.*, anterior; *B.*, basilar; *Bo.*, body; *Ca.*, caudal; *Cer.*, cerebellar; *Circ.*, circumflex; *Co.*, communicating; *Coll.*, colliculus; *Dent.*, dentate; *Gen.*, geniculate; *He.*, hemispheric; *Inf.*, inferior; *Int.*, intermediate; *L.*, long; *Lat.*, lateral; *Med.*, medial; *Nucl.*, nucleus; *O.*, optic; *P.*, posterior; *P.C.A.*, posterior cerebral artery; *Ped.*, peduncle; *Ro.*, rostral; *S.*, short; *Sup.*, superior; *Tr.*, trunk; *V.*, ventricle or vertebral; *Ve.*, vermian.

branches. There is a reciprocal relationship between the hemispheric arteries. If one is small, the adjacent ones are large and supply the territory normally supplied by the more rudimentary vessel.

The most common pattern is three hemispheric branches: lateral, intermediate, and medial corresponding to the third of the hemispheric surface that they supply. Each branch supplies approximately one-third of the tentorial surface of the hemisphere. However, there are frequent exceptions in which the hemispheric areas are supplied by two branches or by branches from the adjacent hemispheric segments. The medial segment is most frequently supplied from the rostral trunk and the lateral segment is most often supplied from the caudal trunk. The vermian arteries occasionally overlap onto the medial hemispheric segment, and the marginal artery (to be described later) overlaps the lateral hemispheric segment. The whole tentorial hemispheric surface was supplied by a branch of the caudal trunk in one hemisphere and by branches arising from the rostral trunk in one other hemisphere. On reaching the tentorial surface, the hemispheric arteries split into one to seven (average, three) sub-branches, which arborize over the tentorial surface and terminate by disappearing between the cerebellar folia.

Vermian arteries

The vermian arteries arise from the rostral trunk within the cerebellomesencephalic fissure. The rostral trunk most commonly gives rise to two vermian arteries (maximum four). If the vermian branches on one side are hypoplastic, their area is supplied by branches from the contralateral SCA. The most common pattern is two vermian arteries: one distributed to a medial strip bordering the midline and one distributed to a paramedian strip bordering the hemispheric surface. Anastomoses between vermian branches from the two sides are frequent near the apex of the tentorial surface.

Marginal branch

About half of the proximal SCA trunks give rise to a marginal branch to the adjacent petrosal surface (*Figs. 2.9* and *2.10*). When present, the marginal branch is the first cortical branch. It usually arises from the lateral pontomesencephalic segment and does not enter the cerebellomesencephalic fissure, as do the other cortical branches, but passes from its origin to the cortical surface. It may also arise from the caudal or main trunk or from the basilar artery as a variant of a duplicate origin of the SCA. Its most constant supply is to the part of the petrosal surface adjoining the tentorial surface. Its largest area of supply includes the full extent of the superior part of the petrosal surface and both lips of the petrous fissure. Its area of supply is inversely related to the size of the petrosal surface area supplied by the AICA. The AICA or its branches supply the majority of the petrosal fissure if the marginal artery is small or absent. Anastomoses between the marginal artery and the AICA are frequent and are most prominent if the marginal branch is large. Perforating branches arising from the marginal branch terminate in the region of the middle cerebellar peduncle.

Relationship to the cranial nerves

The SCA passes near and frequently has points of contact with the oculomotor, trochlear, or trigeminal nerves (*Figs. 2.2, 2.5,* and *2.8*).

Oculomotor nerve

The proximal part of the SCA passes below and is separated from the PCA by the oculomotor nerve (*Fig. 2.5*). Nearly two-thirds of SCAs have a point of contact with the oculomotor nerve, usually on the inferior surface. The point of contact usually involves the main trunk or, less commonly, the rostral trunk if there is an early bifurcation. This is a contact on the superior surface of the nerve only if the SCA arises from the PCA, as occurs infrequently. Sunderland suggests that the oculomotor nerve may occasionally be constricted between the PCA and SCA (52).

The length of vessel between its origin and its point of contact with the oculomotor nerve averages 4.5 mm (range, 1–9 mm) and the length of the nerve between its origin from the midbrain and the point of contact with the SCA averages 5 mm (range, 1–10 mm) (19). The diameter of the artery at the point of contact averages 2 mm (range, 1–3 mm). There is less likely to be a point of contact with the oculomotor nerve if there is a duplicate origin, a low origin from the basilar artery, or a fetal configuration of the PCA.

Trochlear nerve

The trochlear nerve arises below the inferior colliculus and passes forward in the cerebellomesencephalic fissure (*Figs. 2.4, 2.5,* and *2.10*). It passes from the medial to the lateral side of the branches of the rostral and caudal trunks as it passes forward within the fissure. On reaching the lateral side of the brainstem, it courses between the lower surface of the tentorium and the SCA. The nerve has points of contact with the SCA trunks in almost all cases. This contact may involve the main, rostral, or caudal trunk, or both the rostral and caudal trunks. The point of contact with the nerve averages 17 mm (range, 4–30 mm) from the origin of the nerve and 24 mm (range, 13–38 mm) from the origin of the SCA (18).

Trigeminal nerve

The trigeminal nerve arises from the lateral part of the pons and runs obliquely upward (*Figs. 2.8* and *2.10*). It exits the posterior cranial fossa by passing forward beneath the tentorial attachment to enter Meckel's cave. The SCA encircles the brainstem above the trigeminal nerve, making a shallow caudal loop on the lateral side of the pons (18). Contact occurs between the SCA and the trigeminal nerve in those cases with the most prominent caudally projecting loops. About half of the SCAs have a point of contact with the SCA, which, depending on the site of bifurcation, may involve the main, rostral, caudal or both the rostral and caudal trunks, or a marginal hemispheric branch. The diameter of the vessel at the point of contact averages 1 to 2 mm, but may range from less than 2 to nearly 3 mm. The distance between the origin of the vessel and the point of contact with the trigeminal nerve varies from 15 to 33 mm (average, 21 mm). The separation between the SCA and the 24 trigeminal nerves, without a neurovascular contact ranges from less than 1 to 8 mm (average, 3 mm).

The point of contact with the SCA is usually on the superior or superomedial aspect of the nerve. Often a few fascicles of the nerve are indented or distorted by the vessel 3 to 4 mm, but as much as 12 mm peripheral to the point of entry into the pons. In 6 of the 50 specimens we examined, the contact was located at the pontine root entry zone, usually by a loop tucked into the axilla formed between the brainstem and the medial side of the trigeminal nerve. There is no correlation between the configuration of the SCA at its origin and the presence or absence of loops impinging upon the trigeminal nerve; however, the point of bifurcation of the SCA did affect the caliber of the vessel that made contact with the nerve. The contacting vessel is of a smaller caliber if there is an early SCA bifurcation. The significance of these contacts in trigeminal neuralgia is reviewed in the chapter on the cerebellopontine angle (7, 16, 22, 45).

Relationship to the tentorium cerebelli

The tentorium incisura (notch), the opening through the tentorium cerebelli, is triangular with the base on the clivus (*Figs. 2.6, 2.8,* and *2.9*) (41). The other two limbs are formed by the right and left free edges that join at an apex located between the colliculi below the occipital lobes above.

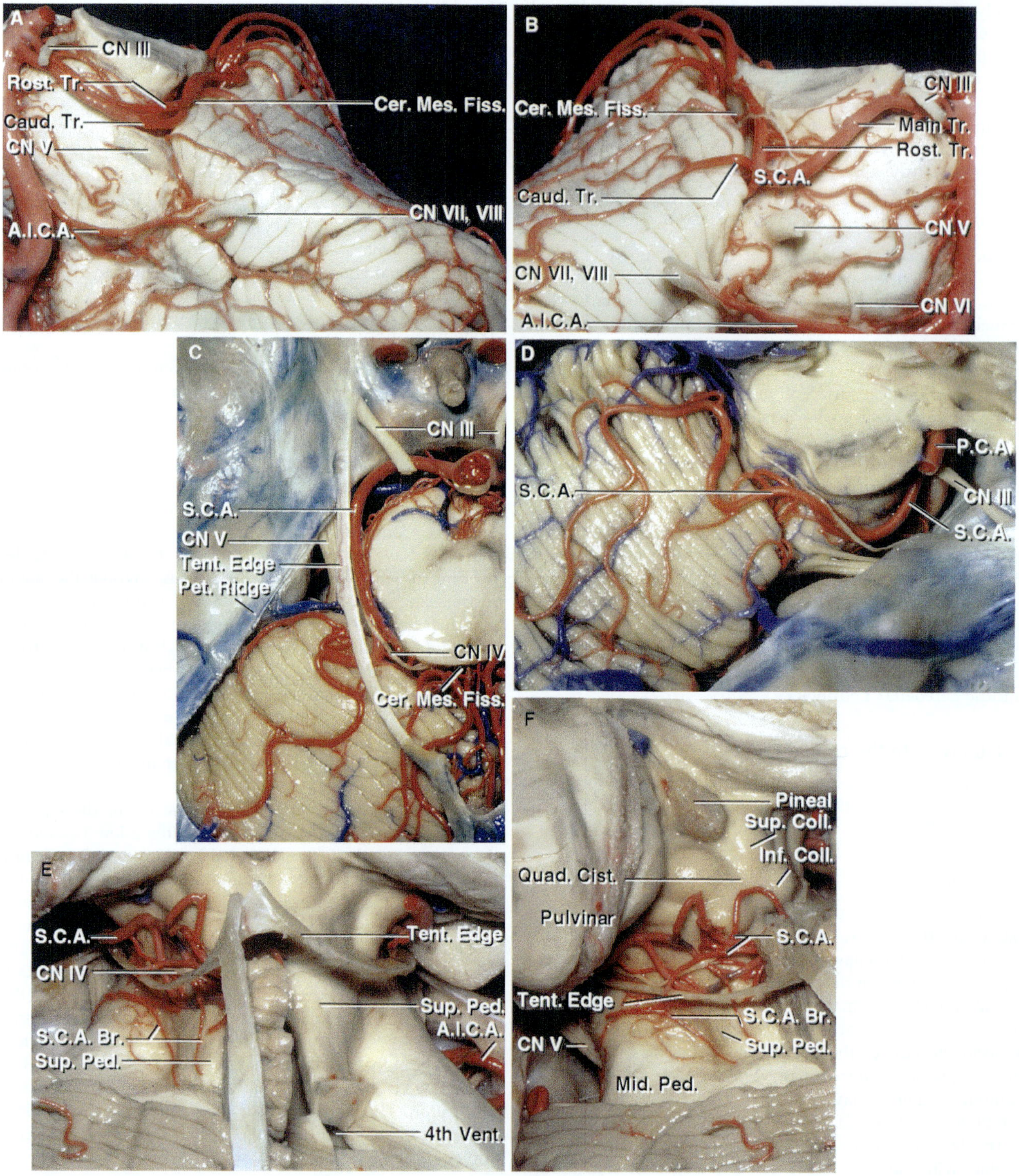

FIGURE 2.8. SCA relationships. *A*, the left SCA arises as a duplicate artery. The caudal duplicate trunk crosses the rostral surface of the trigeminal nerve before entering the cerebellomesencephalic fissure. *B*, the right SCA does not divide into rostral and caudal trunks until it reaches the anterior edge of the cerebellomesencephalic fissure. *C*, near its origin, the SCA courses below the oculomotor nerve and distally, near its entrance into the cerebellomesencephalic fissure, passes under the trochlear nerve. *D*, another SCA. A large trunk passes directly from the side of the brainstem to the hemispheric surface without entering the fissure, although it does give off some smaller branches to the fissure. *E*, the posterior lip of the cerebellomesencephalic fissure has been removed and the upper half of the roof of the fourth ventricle opened. The SCA gives rise

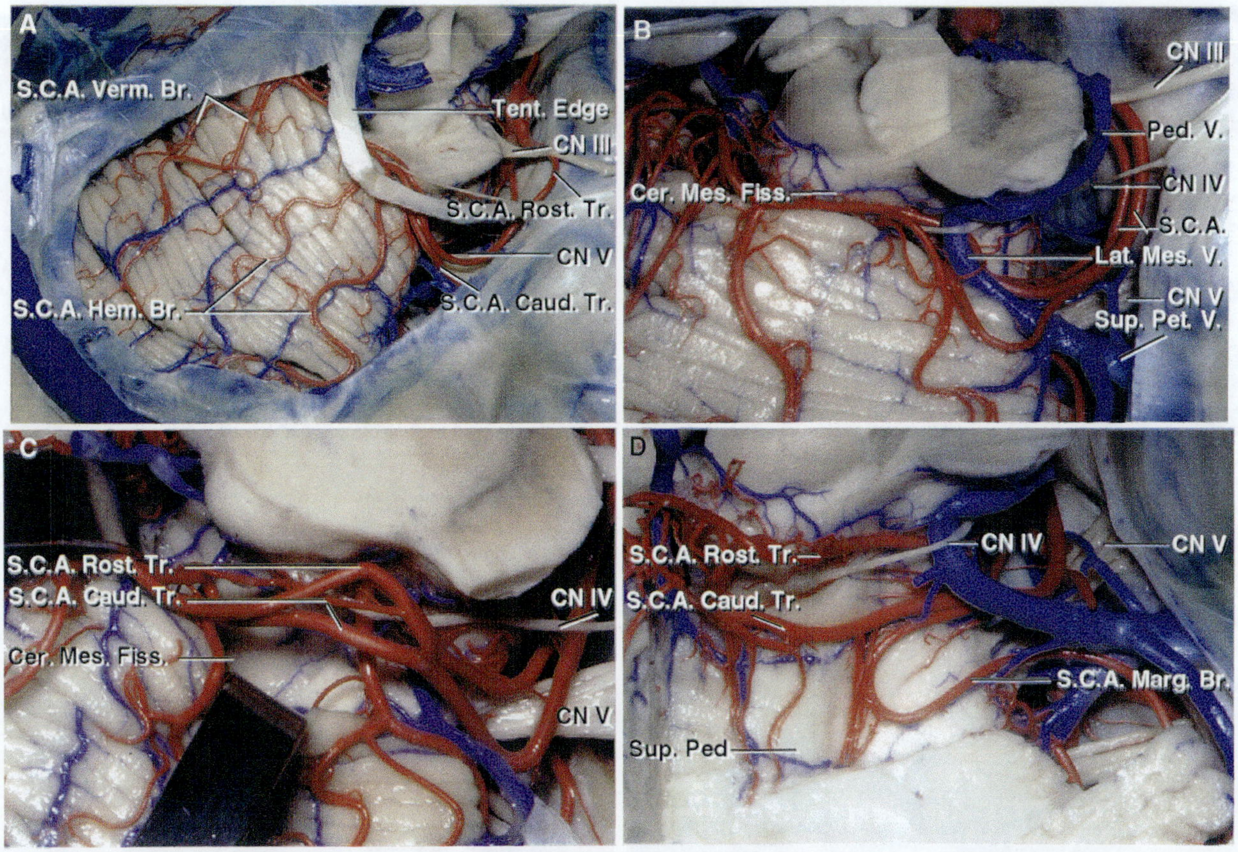

FIGURE 2.9. *A*, the right SCA arises from the basilar artery as a duplicate artery. The rostral duplicate trunk gives rise to vermian branches that supply the vermis and the adjacent part of the hemisphere. The caudal duplicate trunk gives rise to hemispheric branches. *B*, enlarged view. Care is required in occluding and dividing the superior petrosal veins around the trigeminal nerve, because the branches of the SCA may be intertwined with the tributaries of the veins, as in this example. The peduncular vein, which usually empties into the basal vein, joins the lateral mesencephalic vein, and empties into the superior petrosal sinus. *C*, the lip of the fissure has been retracted to expose the SCA trunks and branches. *D*, the posterior lip of the cerebellomesencephalic fissure has been removed. Within the fissure, the SCA branches pass down the superior cerebellar peduncle. Some SCA branches pass above and some below the trochlear nerve. The SCA gives rise to a marginal branch that supplies some of the petrosal surface bordering the tentorial surface. *Br.*, branch; *Caud.*, caudal; *Cer. Mes.*, cerebellomesencephalic; *CN*, cranial nerve; *Fiss.*, fissure; *Hem.*, hemispheric; *Lat.*, lateral; *Marg.*, marginal; *Mes.*, mesencephalic; *Ped.*, peduncle; *Pet.*, petrosal; *Rost.*, rostral; *S.C.A.*, superior cerebellar artery; *Sup.*, superior; *Tent.*, tentorial; *Tr.*, trunk; *V.*, vein; *Verm.*, vermian.

The proximal portion of the SCA, usually the main trunk unless there is a duplicate origin or an early bifurcation, courses medial to the anterior third of the free edge. The SCAs with a high origin arise superior to the level of the tentorial edge, but the initial course of all of these slopes caudally. Nearly 20% of SCAs have a point of contact with the free edge of the anterior half of the tentorium. Distally, the SCA loops caudally and passes beneath, sometimes contacting the middle third of the free edge of the tentorium. The interval between the free edge and the SCA as the SCA passes below the free edge averages 3 mm (range, 0–5 mm). The part nearest the lower surface of the free edge is the main trunk in most cases, but may be the rostral or caudal trunk if there is an early bifurcation. Further distally, branches pass

to perforating branches that pass down the superior cerebellar peduncle to supply the dentate nucleus. *F*, oblique posterior view of the SCA branches within the cerebellomesencephalic fissure and the quadrigeminal cistern. The SCA supplies the cisternal walls below the sulcus between the superior and inferior colliculi, and the PCA supplies the wall above this level. *A.I.C.A.*, anteroinferior cerebellar artery; *Br.*, branch; *Caud.*, caudal; *Cer. Mes.*, cerebellomesencephalic; *Cist.*, cistern; *CN*, cranial nerve; *Coll.*, colliculus; *Fiss.*, fissure; *Inf.*, inferior; *Mid.*, middle; *P.C.A.*, posterior cerebral artery; *Ped.*, peduncle; *Pet.*, petrosal; *Quad.*, quadrigeminal; *Rost.*, rostral; *S.C.A.*, superior cerebellar artery; *Sup.*, superior; *Tent.*, tentorial; *Tr.*, trunk; *Vent.*, ventricle.

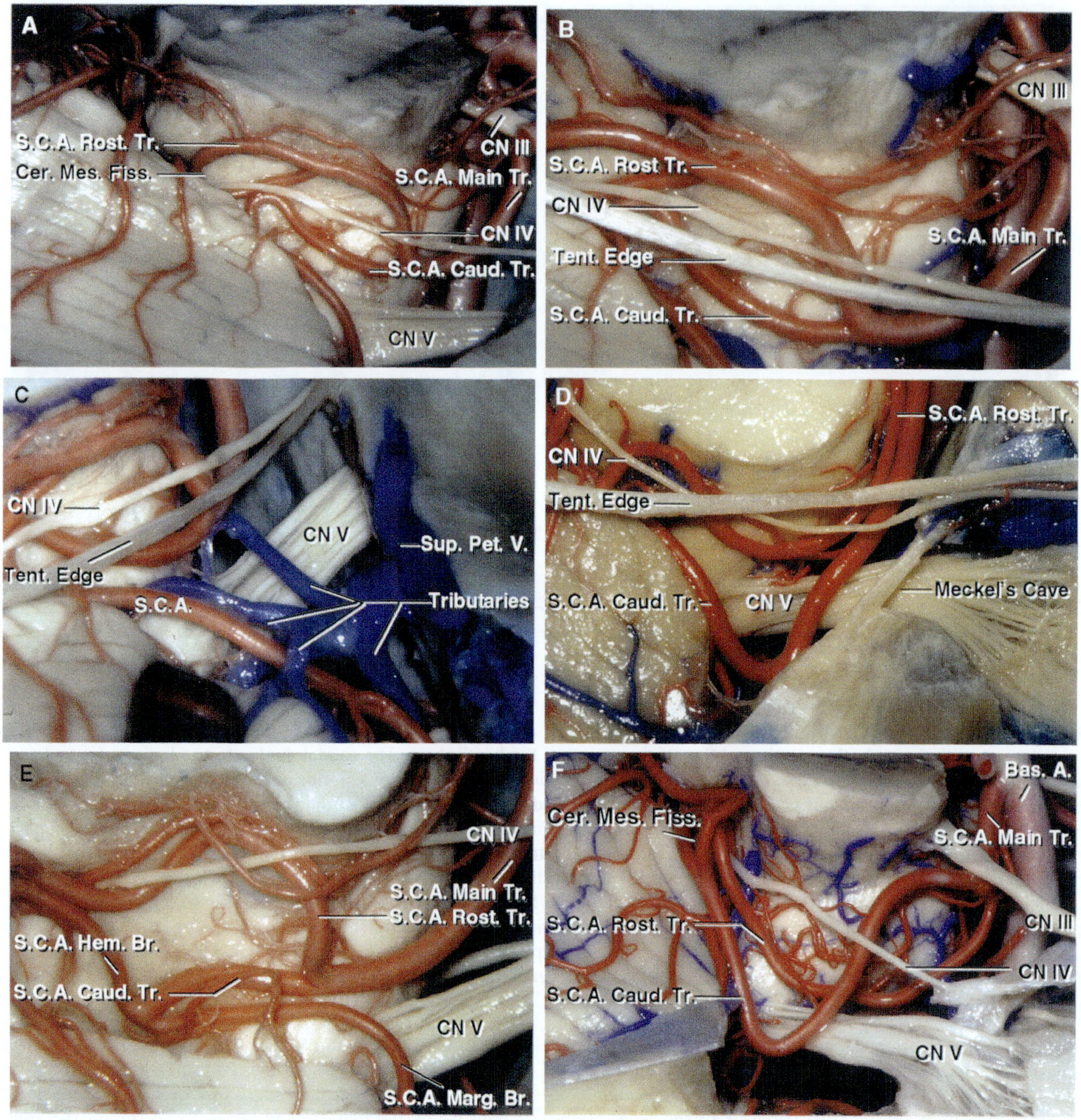

FIGURE 2.10. SCA trunks. *A*, the main trunk of the SCA bifurcates above the trigeminal nerve into a rostral and caudal trunk. The main trunk passes below the trochlear nerve and tentorial edge at the anterolateral brainstem, but distally the rostral trunk passes above and the caudal trunk below the trochlear nerve and tentorial edge. *B*, view after removing the tentorial edge. The most common compression of the trigeminal nerve in trigeminal neuralgia is by the SCA at the junction of the main with the rostral and caudal trunks, which in this case is located above the trigeminal nerve. Both trunks dip into the cerebellomesencephalic fissure before reaching the tentorial surface. *C*, this superior petrosal vein has multiple tributaries that have become entwined with the branches of the SCA. These veins often need to be coagulated and divided in reaching the trigeminal nerve. The SCA could be obliterated in coagulating the tributaries of the superior petrosal vein unless care is taken to carefully separate the arterial trunks from the venous tributaries. *D*, this SCA has a duplicate origin in which both the rostral and caudal trunks arise directly from the basilar artery. Both trunks, at the anterolateral brainstem, pass below the tentorial edge and trochlear nerve and above the trigeminal nerve. At the posterolateral margin of the brainstem, the rostral trunk loops above the level of the trochlear nerve and tentorial edge. The caudal trunk rests against the posterior trigeminal

medial to the posterior third of the free edge as they enter and exit the cerebellomesencephalic fissure. These branches remain caudal to the level of the free edge in the interval between the colliculi and the occipital lobe, but distally, pass below the tentorium to reach the superior surface of the cerebellum.

DISCUSSION

The effects of occlusion of a cerebellar artery range from clinical silence to infarction of portions of the brainstem or cerebellum with swelling, hemorrhage, and death (3, 18, 19, 30). Occlusion of the SCA, although uncommon, produces a distinctive clinical picture that results from infarction of the cerebellum, dentate nucleus, brachium conjunctivum, and long sensory pathways in the tegmentum of the rostral pons (32). The onset is marked by vomiting, sudden dizziness, and the inability to stand or walk. Occlusion may result in cerebellar dysfunction caused by involvement of the cerebellum and its deep nuclei and peduncles; ipsilateral intention tremor caused by involvement of the dentate nucleus and the superior cerebellar peduncle; ipsilateral Horner's syndrome caused by involvement of the descending oculosympathetic fibers; contralateral loss of pain and temperature sensation caused by involvement of the lateral spinothalamic and quintothalamic tracts; nystagmus caused by involvement of the medial longitudinal fasciculus and cerebellar pathways; contralateral disturbance of hearing caused by involvement of the crossed fibers of the lateral lemniscus; and loss of emotional expression on the analgesic side caused by damage to the involuntary mimetic pathways in the upper brainstem. Although a specific clinical syndrome may result from an SCA occlusion, it is worth emphasizing that in the posterior fossa, a given area of parenchyma cannot be as predictably allotted to a specific vessel as in the cerebral circulation, because of the extensive anastomoses over the cerebellum and the variation in arterial distribution.

The recovery and survival of many patients after the intentional occlusion of a major cerebellar artery is attributed to adequacy of the collateral circulation. If the adjacent arteries are unusually small and the artery occluded is large, the collateral circulation is likely to be poor, creating an unfavorable and dangerous situation. Arterial spasm caused by mechanical irritation induced by brain retraction may render the collateral supply less effective. Acute occlusion of any one of the cerebellar arteries is frequently associated with vomiting, dizziness, and the inability to stand or walk.

The SCA is important in both hemorrhagic and ischemic cerebrovascular disease of the posterior fossa. The dentate nucleus, the most common site of spontaneous cerebellar hemorrhage, is supplied by the precerebellar and the penetrating cortical branches of the SCA (8, 49). The area supplied by the SCA is postulated to be the most vulnerable to damage by decreased blood flow in the posterior fossa, because it represents the distal borderline of the vertebral and basilar arteries (49). Infarcts may occur in the area supplied by the SCA in the absence of its occlusion, after occlusion of the vertebral or basilar arteries.

The SCA and its branches may be stretched against the tentorial edge by expanding lesions in the posterior fossa that cause a rostral protrusion of the upper surface of the cerebellum through the tentorial opening. The surface of the vermis and adjacent parts of the lateral lobes are grooved by the free edge of the tentorium, and branches of the SCA may thus be compressed. Symmetrical softening of the cerebellar cortex in the area of supply will result, and similar changes may be found in the dentate nuclei that are supplied by the deep branches (46).

Operative exposure

The SCA is exposed in dealing with neoplasms involving the cerebellum, posterior cavernous sinus, tentorial incisura, and cerebellopontine angle; with aneurysms arising at the basilar apex, origin of the SCA and PCA, and, although rare, on the distal SCA; less commonly in dealing with arteriovenous malformations; during vascular decompression of the trigeminal nerve in trigeminal neuralgia; and during a revascularization bypass procedure for posterior fossa ischemia.

Selecting an operative approach to a lesion involving the SCA requires that the arterial segments involved be accurately defined. Lesions located at the front of the brainstem near the origin require a different approach from those located on the back of the brainstem in the quadrigeminal cistern or cerebellomesencephalic fissure. The only supratentorial approach that provides exposures to the SCA origin, anterior and lateral pontomesencephalic and cerebellomesencephalic segments, and the proximal cortical branches is a temporal craniotomy with elevation of the temporal and occipital lobes combined with division and retraction of the tentorium. Extending this approach backward to the quadrigeminal cistern often necessitates obliteration of some of the veins draining the lower surface of the temporal and occipital lobes, with the risk of venous infarction and edema. A similar

root as the nerve passes below the anterior edge of the tentorium to enter Meckel's cave. *E*, another SCA. The main trunk passes above the trigeminal nerve before bifurcating into rostral and caudal trunks. The main trunk courses below the trochlear nerve, but the rostral trunk loops upward medial to the nerve. The caudal trunk divides into a large hemispheric branch that supplies the tentorial surface and a marginal branch, which supplies some of the upper part of the petrosal surface. *F*, another SCA. The artery bifurcates below the oculomotor nerve. Both trunks pass below the trochlear nerve at the anterolateral margin of the brainstem and above the trochlear nerve distally at the entrance into the cerebellomesencephalic fissure. *A.*, artery; *Bas.*, basilar; *Br.*, branch; *Caud.*, caudal; *Cer. Mes.*, cerebellomesencephalic; *CN*, cranial nerve; *Fiss.*, fissure; *Hem.*, hemispheric; *Marg.*, marginal; *Pet.*, petrosal; *Rost.*, rostral; *S.C.A.*, superior cerebellar artery; *Sup.*, superior; *Tent.*, tentorial; *Tr.*, trunk; *V.*, vein.

or even greater exposure of the SCA is achieved with the supra-infratentorial presigmoid approach with tentorial splitting, but this is a much more extensive operation. When the tentorium is divided in either of the above approaches, care must be taken to prevent injury to the trochlear nerve that passes between the lateral pontomesencephalic segment and the tentorial edge. The SCA origin, along with the basilar apex, if located above the dorsum sellae, can be reached through a pterional craniotomy with opening of Liliequist's membrane. Exposing a low SCA origin by the pterional route may require that the dura roof of the cavernous sinus be opened, a so-called transcavernous approach, and that the posterior clinoid and upper part of the dorsum sellae be removed. Resecting the petrous apex in the subtemporal anterior petrousectomy approach will also aid in exposing a low SCA origin, if it cannot be exposed by dividing the tentorium. A lateral suboccipital craniectomy or, as this writer prefers, a craniotomy, done through a vertical lateral suboccipital incision and extending to the edge of the transverse and sigmoid sinuses, provides excellent exposure of the SCA in the region of the trigeminal nerve and the anterior part of the cerebellomesencephalic fissure. This approach provides satisfactory exposure of the lateral pontomesencephalic segment, but not of the origin or of other segments. An infratentorial-supracerebellar approach directed through a suboccipital craniectomy provides satisfactory exposure of the cortical branches, but not those within the depths of the cerebellomesencephalic fissure or lateral to the brainstem. The occipital transtentorial approach provides a more favorable angle for exposing the branches ipsilateral to the craniotomy near the midline, below the pineal within the cerebellomesencephalic fissure, and in the posterior part of the ambient cistern.

ANTEROINFERIOR CEREBELLAR ARTERY

Overview

The AICA courses through the central part of the cerebellopontine angle near the facial and vestibulocochlear nerve (*Figs. 2.5* and *2.11*). It or its branches may be exposed in surgical approaches to cerebellopontine angle, basilar or vertebral arteries, clivus, the fourth ventricle and cerebellum, and during approaches directed through the temporal and occipital bones.

The AICA is intimately related to the pons, lateral recess, foramen of Luschka, cerebellopontine fissure, middle cerebellar peduncle, and petrosal cerebellar surface (*Figs. 2.1-2.3* and *2.11*). The AICA originates from the basilar artery, usually as a single trunk, and encircles the pons near the abducent, facial, and vestibulocochlear nerves. After coursing near and sending branches to the nerves entering the acoustic meatus and to the choroid plexus protruding from the foramen of Luschka, it passes around the flocculus on the middle cerebellar peduncle to supply the lips of the cerebellopontine fissure and the petrosal surface. It commonly bifurcates near the facial-vestibulocochlear nerve complex to form a rostral and a caudal trunk. The rostral trunk sends its branches laterally along the middle cerebellar peduncle to the superior lip of the cerebellopontine fissure and the adjoining part of the petrosal surface, and the caudal trunk supplies the inferior part of the petrosal surface, including a part of the flocculus and the choroid plexus. The AICA gives rise to perforating arteries to the brainstem, choroidal branches to the tela and choroid plexus, and the nerve-related arteries, including the labyrinthine, recurrent perforating, and subarcuate arteries (34).

Segments

The AICA is divided into four segments: anterior pontine, lateral pontine, flocculonodular, and cortical. Each segment may include more than one trunk, depending on the level of bifurcation of the artery (*Fig. 2.1*).

Anterior pontine segment

This segment, located between the clivus and the belly of the pons, begins at the origin and ends at the level of a line drawn through the long axis of the inferior olive and extending upward on the pons. This segment usually lies in contact with the rootlets of the abducent nerve.

Lateral pontine segment

This segment begins at the anterolateral margin of the pons and passes through the cerebellopontine angle above, below, or between the facial and vestibulocochlear nerves and is intimately related to the internal auditory meatus, the lateral recess, and the choroid plexus protruding from the foramen of Luschka (*Figs. 2.11* and *2.12*). This segment gives rise to the nerve-related branches that course near or within the internal acoustic meatus in close relationship to the facial and vestibulocochlear nerves. This segment is divided into premeatal, meatal, and postmeatal parts, depending on their relationship to the porus of the internal acoustic meatus (*Fig. 2.5*). These nerve-related branches are the labyrinth artery, which supplies the facial and vestibulocochlear nerves and vestibulocochlear labyrinth; the recurrent perforating arteries, which pass toward the meatus, but turn medially to supply the brainstem; and the subarcuate artery, which enters the subarcuate fossa. This segment not uncommonly dips below the pontomedullary junction, especially if it is tortuous.

Flocculopeduncular segment

This segment begins where the artery passes rostral or caudal to the flocculus to reach the middle cerebellar peduncle and the cerebellopontine fissure (*Fig. 2.11*). The trunks that course along the peduncle may be hidden beneath the flocculus or the lips of the cerebellopontine fissure.

Cortical segment

This segment supplies predominantly the petrosal surface.

Origin

The AICA usually originates from the basilar artery as a single vessel, but may also arise as two (duplicate) or three (triplicate) arteries (*Figs. 2.2, 2.3,* and *2.11*). It can arise at any point along the basilar artery, but most commonly arises from

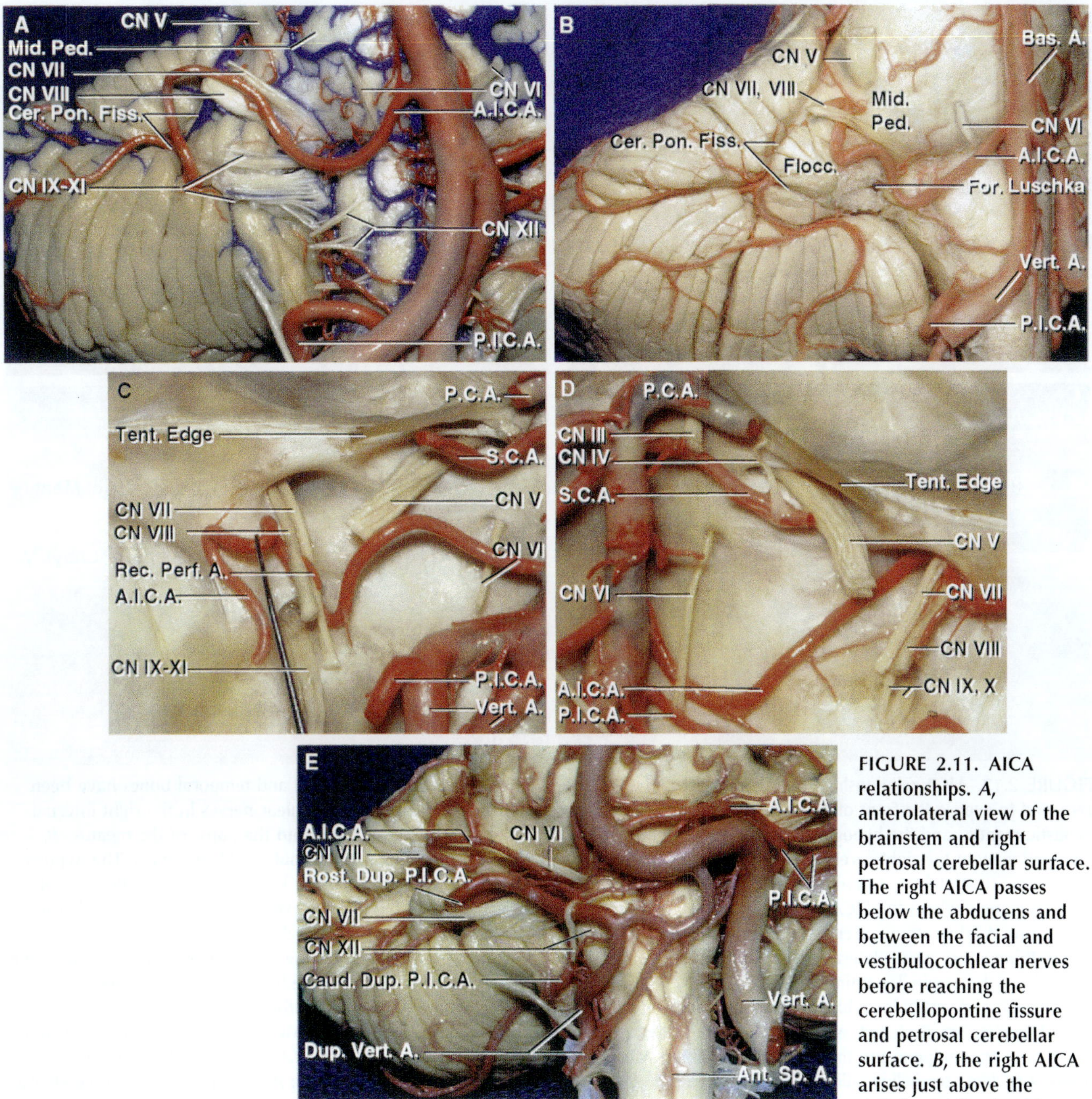

FIGURE 2.11. AICA relationships. *A*, anterolateral view of the brainstem and right petrosal cerebellar surface. The right AICA passes below the abducens and between the facial and vestibulocochlear nerves before reaching the cerebellopontine fissure and petrosal cerebellar surface. *B*, the right AICA arises just above the vertebrobasilar junction and passes below the pontomedullary junction before turning upward to reach the surface of the middle cerebellar peduncle. It passes above the floccular and along the cerebellopontine fissure to reach the petrosal surface. *C* and *D*, the cerebellum and brainstem have been removed to show the relationship of the AICAs to the cranial nerves and internal acoustic meatus. *C*, the left AICA passes above the abducens nerve and below the facial and vestibulocochlear nerves, where it gives rise to a recurrent perforating branch to the brainstem. The SCA passes above the posterior trigeminal root. *D*, the right AICA loops into the porus of the meatus and between the facial and vestibulocochlear nerves. *E*, another brainstem and cerebellum. The right vertebral artery is a duplicate artery and gives rise to duplicate PICAs. The AICAs arise from the lower part of the basilar artery. The left AICA is larger than the right. The rostral duplicate PICA loops upward into the cerebellopontine angle. The left vertebral artery loops upward into the left cerebellopontine angle. *A.*, artery; *A.I.C.A.*, anteroinferior cerebellar artery; *Ant.*, anterior; *Bas.*, basilar; *Caud.*, caudal; *Cer. Pon.*, cerebellopontine; *CN*, cranial nerve; *Dup.*, duplicate; *Fiss.*, fissure; *Flocc.*, flocculus; *For.*, foramen; *Mid.*, middle; *P.C.A.*, posterior cerebral artery; *Ped.*, peduncle; *Perf.*, perforating; *P.I.C.A.*, posteroinferior cerebellar artery; *Pon.*, pontine; *Rec.*, recurrent; *Rost.*, rostral; *S.C.A.*, superior cerebellar artery; *Sp.*, spinal; *Tent.*, tentorial; *Vert.*, vertebral.

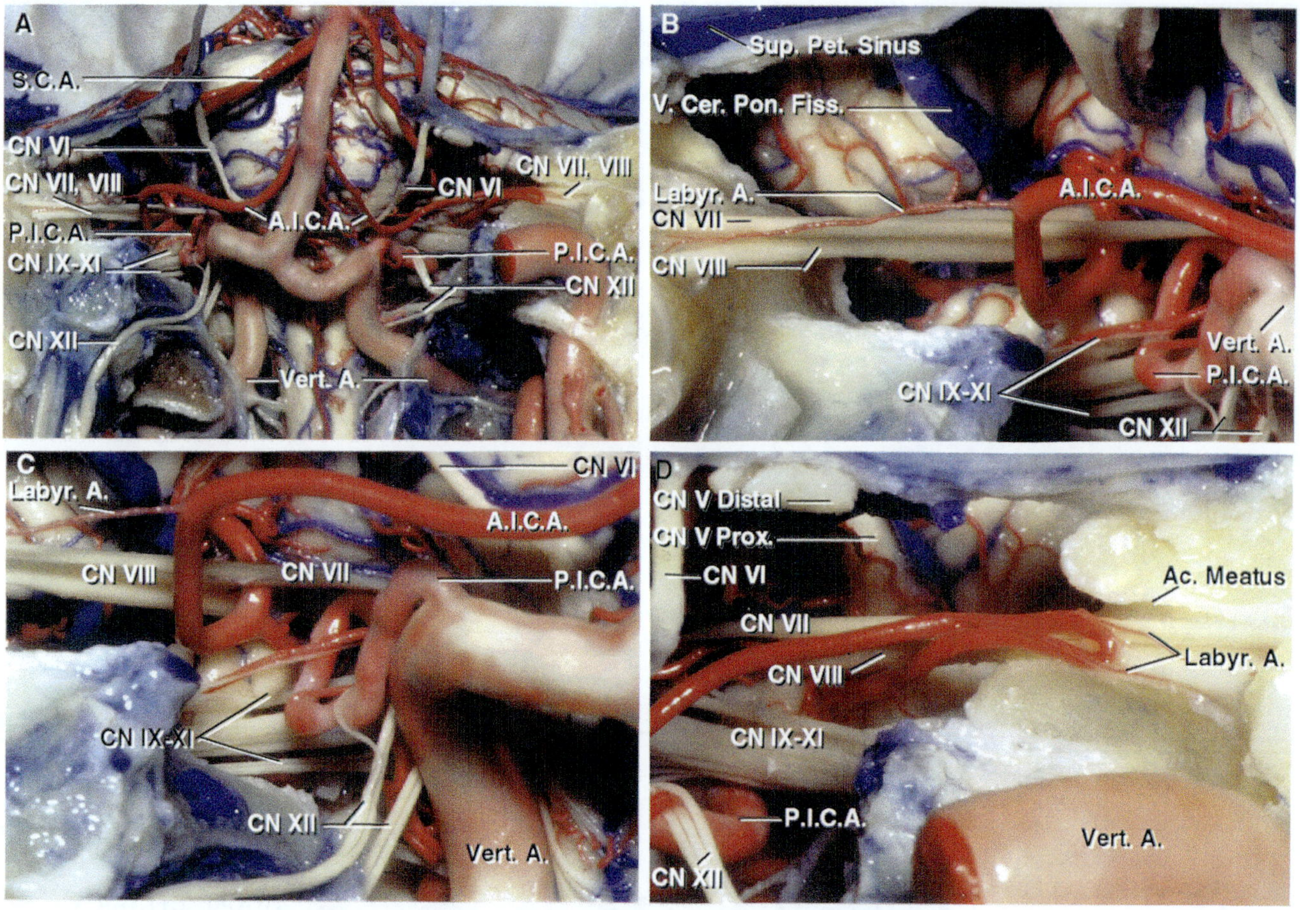

FIGURE 2.12. AICA relationships. *A*, anterior view. The clivus and adjacent part of the occipital and temporal bones have been removed to expose the front of brainstem, vertebral and basilar arteries, facial and vestibulocochlear nerves in the right internal acoustic meatus, and the hypoglossal nerve in the right hypoglossal canal. The left AICA loops into the porus of the meatus. *B*, enlarged view of the right cerebellopontine angle. The AICA passes between the facial and vestibulocochlear nerves. The hypoglossal nerves are stretched around the posterior surface of the vertebral artery. The vertebral artery kinks upward into the cerebellopontine angle where the PICA arises in close relationship to the root exit zone of the facial nerve, a common finding in hemifacial spasm. A labyrinthine artery arises from the AICA. *C*, another enlarged view of the right cerebellopontine angle. The labyrinthine artery passes laterally with the facial nerve. The PICA loops upward and contacts the lower margin of the facial nerve. The vein of the cerebellopontine fissure ascends to empty into the superior petrosal sinus. *D*, the left AICA passes below the abducens, facial, and vestibulocochlear nerves and loops into the porus where it gives off two labyrinthine branches. Some of the hypoglossal rootlets are stretched over the PICA. The posterior trigeminal nerve was divided behind Meckel's cave. The proximal stump arises from the midpons and the distal portion enters Meckel's cave. *A.*, artery; *Ac.*, acoustic; *A.I.C.A.*, anteroinferior cerebellar artery; *Cer. Pon.*, cerebellopontine; *CN*, cranial nerve; *Fiss.*, fissure; *Labyr.*, labyrinthine; *Pet.*, petrosal; *P.I.C.A.*, posteroinferior cerebellar artery; *Prox.*, proximal; *S.C.A.*, superior cerebellar artery; *Sup.*, superior; *V.*, vein; *Vert.*, vertebral.

the lower half. There is frequent asymmetry in the level of origin from side to side, with one arising significantly above the level of the other. In our previous study, we found that of 50 AICAs 72% arose as a single trunk, 26% as two (duplicate) arteries, and 2% as three (triplicate) arteries (34). From its origin, the AICA courses backward around the pons toward the CPA. Its proximal part lays in contact with either the dorsal or the ventral aspect of the abducens nerve. After passing the abducens nerve, it proceeds to the CPA where one or more of its trunks course in close relationship to the facial and vestibulocochlear nerves and thus are said to be nerve-related.

Bifurcation

The AICAs arising as a single trunk usually bifurcate into a rostral and a caudal trunk. The duplicate AICAs referred to as rostral and caudal duplicate AICAs have a distribution similar to the distribution of the rostral and caudal trunks formed by the bifurcation of a single AICA. Approximately two-thirds bifurcated before and one-third bifurcated after crossing the facial and vestibulocochlear nerves. The segment proximal to the bifurcation is the main trunk, and the two trunks formed by the bifurcation are the rostral and the caudal trunks. If the bifurcation is proximal to the facial and vestibulocochlear nerves, either the rostral trunk alone or both of the postbifurcation trunks may be nerve-related. The rostral duplicate AICAs give rise to nerve-related branches more often than the caudal duplicate AICAs. The main trunk of the duplicate AICAs also commonly bifurcate to form rostral and caudal trunks that sent branches to the cerebellum.

After crossing the nerves, the rostral trunk usually courses laterally above the flocculus to reach the surface of the middle cerebellar peduncle and the petrosal fissure to be distributed to the superior lip of the cerebellopontine fissure and the adjoining part of the petrosal surface. The caudal trunks are frequently related to the lateral portion of the fourth ventricle. If the bifurcation is proximal to the facial and vestibulocochlear nerve, the caudal trunk courses caudal to the flocculus to supply the inferior part of the petrosal surface, including a part of the flocculus and the choroid plexus. If the bifurcation is distal to the nerves, the caudal trunk courses posteriorly in the inferior limb of the cerebellopontine fissure near the foramen of Luschka. The caudal trunks often enter the lateral portion of the cerebellomedullary fissure just below the lateral recess before turning laterally to supply the inferior part of the petrosal surface. The distal branches of the caudal trunk often anastomose with the PICA, and those from the rostral trunk anastomose with the SCA. The AICA gives rise to perforating arteries to the brainstem, choroidal branches to the lateral segment of the choroid plexus, and the nerve-related arteries described above.

Nerve-related branches

The nerve-related branches are those that course in or near the porus of the meatus and by the facial and vestibulocochlear nerves (*Figs. 2.5* and *2.11-2.14*) (34). Each nerve-related segment is composed of one or two arterial trunks. One was most common. The single nerve-related segments were formed from either the main or a rostral trunk, which arise, in decreasing order of frequency, from a solitary AICA, a rostral duplicate AICA, or a caudal duplicate AICA. The double segments result from the presence of one of two anatomic configurations: a) both the rostral and caudal trunks of a solitary AICA or of one duplicate AICA are nerve-related, or b) one trunk from each of duplicate AICAs or one trunk from two of three triplicate AICAs is nerve related.

Premeatal segment

This segment begins at the basilar artery and courses around the brainstem to reach the facial and vestibulocochlear nerves and the anterior edge of the meatus. The premeatal segment is composed of one or two arterial trunks. In the 50 CPAs we examined, there were 56 nerve-related premeatal segments, 44 CPAs (88%) had solitary, and 6 (12%) had double premeatal segments (34). Most of the premeatal segments, 46 of the 56, were anteroinferior to the nerves. The remainder were anterior, inferior, or anterosuperior to the nerves (*Fig. 2.14*).

Meatal segment

This segment, located in the vicinity of the internal auditory meatus, often forms a laterally convex loop, the medial loop, directed toward or through the meatus. The medial segment was located medial to the porus in about half of CPAs and formed a loop that reached the porus or protruded into the canal in the other half. Sunderland and Mazzoni found the meatal segment at the porus or within the canal in 64 and 67% of CPAs, respectively (36, 51). Mazzoni found that the meatal segment was medial to the porus in 33%, reached the porus in 27%, and entered the canal in 40%, rarely going beyond the medial half of the canal (36).

In the 50 CPAs examined, we found there were 59 nerve-related meatal segments; 41 CPAs (82%) had one, and 9 (18%) had two meatal segments. The majority of the meatal segments coursed below or between the facial and vestibulocochlear nerves (*Fig. 2.14*). There were three more meatal segments than premeatal segments, because in three CPAs, a premeatal segment bifurcated near the nerves to yield two nerve-related meatal segments. The majority of meatal loops coursed in a horizontal plane above or below the nerves, but some, mostly those passing between the facial and vestibulocochlear nerves, coursed in a vertical or oblique plane.

Subarcuate loop

In some CPAs, the nerve-related loop formed a second laterally convex curve that gave the loop an "M" configuration. This second loop was called the subarcuate loop, because it was directed toward the subarcuate fossa, a small depression in the bone superolateral to the meatus. This loop was located either posterior, posteroinferior, or posterosuperior to the vestibulocochlear nerve. The apex of the loop was occasionally adherent to the dura over the subarcuate fossa at the point where the subarcuate artery arose.

Postmeatal segment

This segment begins distal to the nerves and courses medially to supply the brainstem and the cerebellum. The 59 meatal segments found in our previous study of 50 CPAs gave rise to 60 postmeatal segments; 80% of the CPAs had one, and 10 (20%) had two postmeatal segments. There was one more postmeatal segment than meatal segment, because one meatal segment bifurcated to form two postmeatal segments. The postmeatal segments were most commonly posteroinferior, superior, or posterior to or between the nerves (*Fig. 2.14*); none were anterior to the nerves. Each of the vessels forming a double segment might pursue similar or separate courses in relation to the nerves.

Branches of nerve-related AICAs

In their course through the CPA, the nerve-related trunks gives off four branches (*Figs. 2.12-2.14*): 1) labyrinthine (internal auditory) arteries, which enter the internal auditory canal and reached the inner ear; 2) recurrent perforating arteries, which course medially from their origin to supply the brainstem; 3) subarcuate arteries, which passed through the subarcuate fossa to reach the subarcuate canal; and 4) cerebellosubarcuate arteries, which terminated by sending one branch to the subarcuate canal and one to the cerebellum.

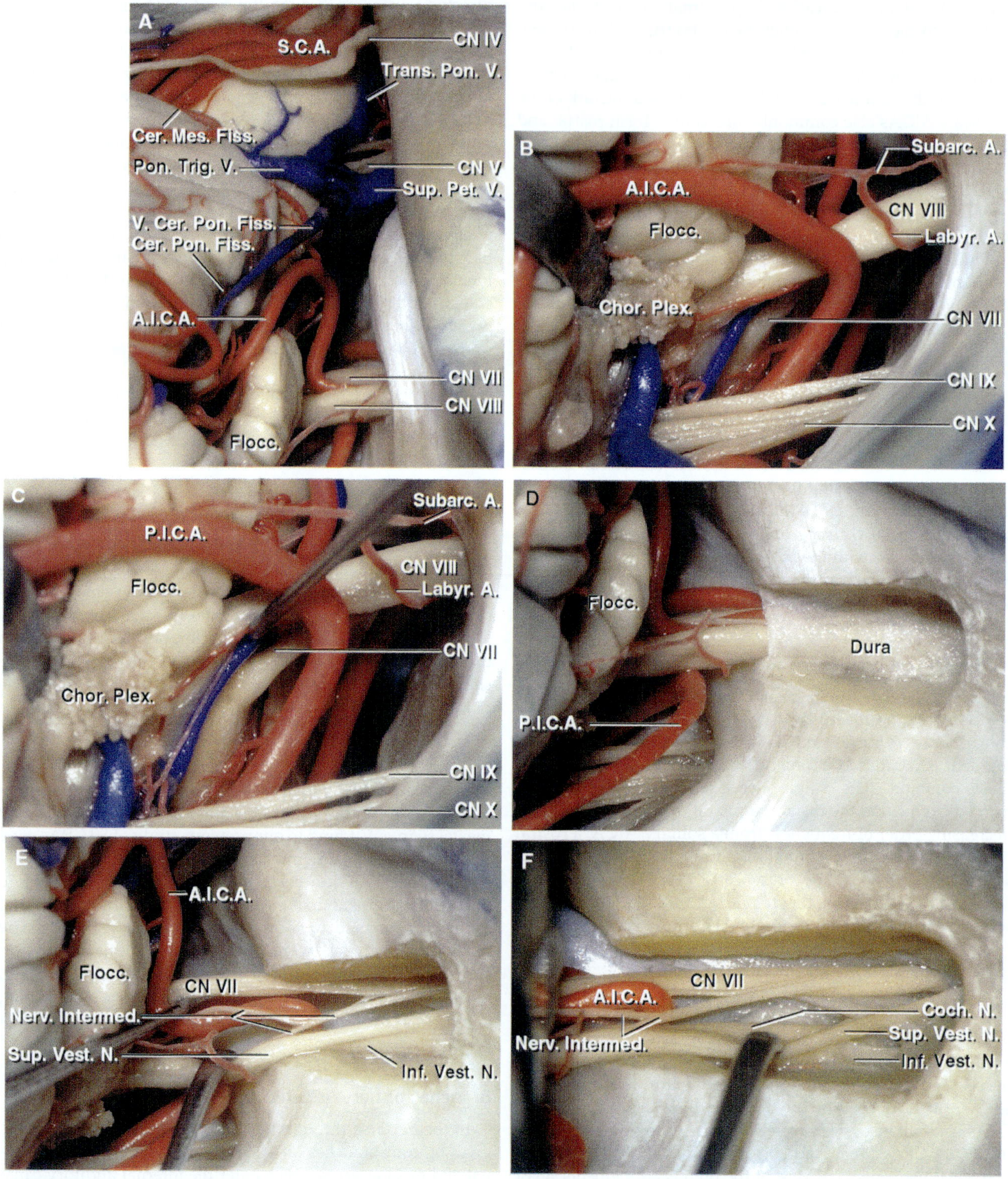

FIGURE 2.13. *A*, AICA relationships in the right CPA by retrosigmoid approach. The AICA passes laterally between the facial and vestibulocochlear nerves and turns medially to course along the middle cerebellar peduncle and cerebellopontine fissure. A large superior petrosal vein with multiple tributaries, including the pontotrigeminal and transverse pontine veins and the vein of the cerebellopontine fissure, passes behind the trigeminal nerve. The flocculus hides the junction of the facial and vestibulocochlear nerves with the brainstem. *B*, the flocculus and choroid plexus, which protrudes from the foramen of Luschka, have been elevated to expose the junction of the facial and vestibulocochlear nerves with the brainstem, where the facial

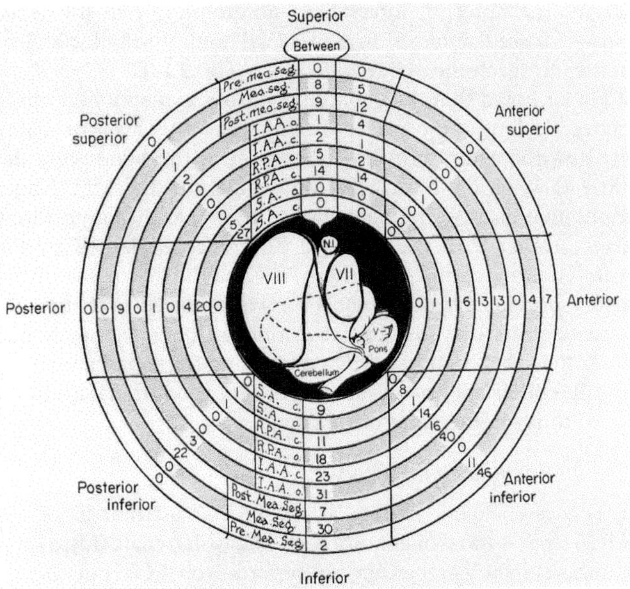

FIGURE 2.14. Diagram showing the relationship of nerve-related arteries to the nerves in the cerebellopontine angle. The nerves are oriented as shown in the central diagram of the right side of the brainstem. The trigeminal nerve arises from the pons. The facial and vestibulocochlear nerves and the nervus intermedius are oriented as shown. The terms superior, anterosuperior, and so on, refer to the relationship of the arteries to the nerves. The number of arteries and arterial segments found in 50 CPAs are listed according to their location in relationship to the nerves. The most common locations were premeatal segment, anteroinferior; meatal segment, inferior; postmeatal segment, posteroinferior; internal auditory artery origin and course, inferior and anteroinferior; recurrent perforating artery origin, inferior and anteroinferior, and course, superior and between; and subarcuate artery origin, posterior, and course, posterosuperior. (From, Martin RG, Grant JL, Peace DA, Theiss C, Rhoton AL Jr: Microsurgical relationships of the anterior inferior cerebellar artery and the facial-vestibulocochlear nerve complex. Neurosurgery 6:483–507, 1980 [34].) *c.*, course; *I.A.A.*, internal auditory artery; *Mea.*, meatal; *o.*, origin; *R.P.A.*, recurrent perforating artery; *S.A.*, subarcuate artery; *Seg.*, segment.

Labyrinthine (internal auditory) arteries

These arteries are the one or more branches of the AICA that enter the internal auditory canal and send branches to the bone and dura lining the internal auditory canal, to the nerves within the canal, and terminate by giving rise to the vestibular, cochlear, and vestibulocochlear arteries that supply the organs of the inner ear (*Figs. 2.12-2.14*) (34).

The labyrinthine arteries almost always arise from the AICA or one of its branches, although a few have been reported to arise from the basilar artery. In one study, as many as 17% were found to arise from the basilar artery (40, 51, 56). We believe that this discrepancy is explained by differences in the definition of the internal auditory artery and the AICA used in the various studies. In this study and those of Adachi and Fisch, the trunk of origin on the basilar artery of an artery sending a branch to the internal auditory canal was called an AICA if it sent branches, although small, to the cerebellum. The site of origin of the internal auditory artery was defined as the point where the branch to the internal auditory canal arose from the trunk of the AICA sending branches to the cerebellum (1, 13). On the other hand, Nager and Sunderland called a trunk arising from the basilar artery a labyrinthine artery rather than an AICA if the branch entering the meatus was larger than the branch reaching the cerebellum (40, 51). Adachi and Fisch, who did not find a single internal auditory artery that arose from the basilar artery, were always able to find a cerebellar branch, although small, on the vessel entering the meatus (1, 13). Mazzoni reported that the internal auditory artery arose from the PICA in a few cases (36), a finding not confirmed in our study or in the other studies mentioned above. In our study, there was one internal auditory artery in 30% of the CPAs, two in 54%, three in 14%, and four in 2%.

Of the 94 internal auditory arteries found in our study, in 50 CPAs, 72 (77%) originated from the premeatal segment, 20 (21%) from the meatal segment, and 2 (2%) from the postmeatal segment (34). They arose proximal to the subarcuate loop in each CPA in which the latter loop was present. Fifty-four percent originated from a solitary AICA, 23% from a duplicate or triplicate AICA, and 23% from a recurrent perforating artery. Mazzoni and Hansen also noted that the internal auditory artery may arise from the recurrent perforating, subarcuate, or cerebellosubarcuate arteries (37).

nerve is seen below the vestibulocochlear nerve. An AICA branch gives rise to both the subarcuate and labyrinthine arteries. *C*, a dissector elevates the vestibulocochlear nerve to more clearly define the junction of the facial nerve with the brainstem. The junction of the facial nerve with the brainstem is easier to expose below rather than above the vestibulocochlear nerve. *D*, the posterior meatal wall has been removed to expose the dura lining the meatus. *E*, the meatal dura has been opened and the vestibulocochlear nerve displaced downward to expose the facial nerve coursing anterior and superior within the meatus. The nervus intermedius, which arises on the anterior surface of the vestibulocochlear nerve and passes laterally to join the facial nerve, is composed of several rootlets, as is common. *F*, the cleavage plane between the superior and inferior vestibular nerves has been developed. The cochlear nerve is located anterior to the inferior vestibular nerve. *A.*, artery; *A.I.C.A.*, anteroinferior cerebellar artery; *Cer. Mes.*, cerebellomesencephalic; *Cer. Pon.*, cerebellopontine; *Chor.*, choroid; *CN*, cranial nerve; *Coch.*, cochlear; *Fiss.*, fissure; *Flocc.*, flocculus; *Inf.*, inferior; *Intermed.*, intermedius; *Labyr.*, labyrinthine; *N.*, nerve; *Nerv.*, nervus; *Pet.*, petrosal; *P.I.C.A.*, posteroinferior cerebellar artery; *Plex.*, plexus; *Pon.*, pontine; *S.C.A.*, superior cerebellar artery; *Subarc.*, subarcuate; *Sup.*, superior; *Trans.*, transverse; *Trig.*, trigeminal; *V.*, vein; *Vest.*, vestibular.

The internal auditory arteries are divided into two approximately equal-sized groups based on their relationship to the meatus. One group originates medial to the porus and the other arises at the porus or within the auditory canal. Those arising medial to the porus most commonly originate and course anterior, anteroinferior, or inferior to the nerves. Fisch noted that the internal auditory arteries often entered the canal by crossing the anteroinferior rim of the porus (13). Those arising at the porus or within the canal most commonly originate inferior or anteroinferior to the nerves.

Recurrent perforating arteries

These perforating arteries arise from the nerve-related vessels and often travel from their origin toward the meatus, occasionally looping into the meatus before taking a recurrent course along the facial and vestibulocochlear nerves to reach the brainstem (*Figs. 2.5* and *2.14*). They send branches to these nerves and to the brainstem surrounding the entry zone of those nerves. They also send branches, in decreasing order of frequency, to the middle cerebellar peduncle and the adjacent part of the pons, the pons around the entry zone of the trigeminal nerve, the choroid plexus of the CPA, the superolateral medulla, and the glossopharyngeal and vagus nerves. The recurrent perforating arteries give rise to about one-fourth of the internal auditory arteries and 10% of subarcuate arteries.

In our study, recurrent perforating arteries were present in 41 (82%) of the CPAs; one was present in 37 CPAs (74%), two in 3 (6%), and three in 1 (2%) (34). Most arose from the premeatal segment, but they also arose from the meatal loop and the postmeatal segment. There was marked variability in their relationship to the facial and vestibulocochlear nerves. Most originated inferior, anteroinferior or anterior to or between the nerves and coursed medially between or above or below the nerves (*Fig. 2.14*).

Subarcuate artery

The subarcuate artery usually originates medial to the porus, penetrates the dura covering the subarcuate fossa, and enters the subarcuate canal (*Figs. 2.13* and *2.14*). In a few cases, it originates in the internal auditory canal. The subarcuate arteries originating in the auditory canal take one of two courses to reach the subarcuate canal; some take a recurrent course through the porus to reach the subarcuate fossa, and others penetrated the meatal wall to reach the subarcuate canal. The artery supplies the petrous bone in the region of the semicircular canals (43). The subarcuate canal is recognized as a potential route of extension of infections from the mastoid region to the meninges and the superior petrosal sinus (40). The AICA is adherent to the dura lining the subarcuate fossa at the site of origin of the subarcuate artery in a few CPAs.

In our study, a subarcuate artery was present in 36 (72%) of the 50 CPAs; 13 (26%) originated from the premeatal segment, 2 (4%) from the meatal segment, and 21 (42%) from the postmeatal segment (34). When present, there was only one subarcuate artery. Most originated posterior and coursed posterosuperior to the nerves to reach the subarcuate fossa. Those originating anterior, inferior, or anteroinferior to the facial nerve crossed inferior to the facial and vestibulocochlear nerves to reach the subarcuate fossa (*Fig. 2.14*).

Nager noted that the subarcuate artery is mentioned rarely in descriptions of the arteries in this area (40). This is probably because the artery and its connection to the bone were destroyed when the brain was removed from the skull. Nager found that its most frequent site of origin was the labyrinthine artery rather than the AICA, a difference explained by the difference in definitions of the AICA and the internal auditory artery previously mentioned (40). He reported that the subarcuate artery may also have a double origin; one branch may enter the subarcuate canal by penetrating the subarcuate fossa and the other may penetrate the wall of the internal auditory canal to reach the subarcuate canal.

Cerebellosubarcuate artery

The cerebellosubarcuate artery is a small branch of the AICA that sends one branch to the subarcuate fossa and another to the cerebellum, as reported by Mazzoni (37). It usually originates proximal to the meatal loop, passing inferior to the facial and vestibulocochlear nerves before coursing superolateral to reach the subarcuate fossa. At the fossa, it gives rise to a subarcuate artery and turns medially to supply the cerebellum. A cerebellosubarcuate artery was present in four of the CPAs we investigated (34). The artery originates anteroinferior or inferior to the nerves entering the meatus. The cerebellar branch terminates on the flocculus and on the adjacent cerebellar cortex below the flocculus.

Cortical branches

The most common pattern is for the AICA to supply the majority of the petrosal surface, but the cortical area of the supply is quite variable (*Fig. 2.11*). It can vary from a small area on the flocculus and adjacent part of the petrosal surface to include the whole petrosal surface and adjacent part of the tentorial and suboccipital surfaces. After crossing the nerves, the rostral trunk usually courses above the flocculus to be distributed to the superior lip of the cerebellopontine fissure, and the caudal trunks course caudal to the flocculus to supply the inferior part of the petrosal surface. If the PICA is absent, the caudal trunk may supply almost all of the ipsilateral suboccipital hemisphere and vermis. Overlap of the SCA onto the upper part of the petrosal surface and the PICA onto the lateral part of the suboccipital surface in not uncommon.

DISCUSSION

Occlusion of the AICA results in syndromes related predominantly to softening of the lateral portions of the brainstem and cerebellar peduncles, rather than to involvement of the cerebellar hemisphere, including palsies of the facial and vestibulocochlear nerves caused by involvement of the nerves and their nuclei; vertigo, nausea, vomiting, and nystagmus caused by lesions of the vestibular nuclei and their connections with the nuclei of the vagus nerves; ipsilateral loss of pain and temperature sensation on the face and corneal hypesthesia caused by interruption of the spinal tract and nucleus of the trigeminal nerve; Horner's syndrome caused by interruption of the descending pupillodilator fibers in the lateral portion of the pons and medulla; cerebellar ataxia and asynergia ascribed to a lesion in the cerebellar peduncles; and an incomplete loss of pain and temperature sensation on the contralateral half of the body (the absence of a complete contralateral hypalgesia is caused by the extreme lateral and posterior position of the lesion, which spares a portion of the lateral spinothalamic tract) (2, 3). All of the syndromes caused by its occlusion are not identical, because of the variability of the AICA. The symptoms usually are sudden in onset and unaccompanied by a loss of consciousness (2). The most prominent symptom is vertigo, often associated with nausea and vomiting, followed by a facial paralysis, deafness, sensory loss, and cerebellar disorders. Notable by their absence are signs of involvement of the corticospinal tract and medial lemniscus, which are nourished from midline tributaries of the vertebral and basilar arteries.

The recovery and survival of many patients after the intentional occlusion of the AICA at operation is attributed to adequacy of the collateral circulation from the other cerebellar arteries (34). The size of the area of infarction after AICA occlusion is inversely related to the size of the PICA and SCA and to the size of the anastomoses with those arteries. If the PICA is unusually small and the AICA is large, the collateral circulation is likely to be poor, creating an unfavorable and dangerous situation in the event of AICA occlusion. Arterial spasm caused by mechanical irritation induced by the brain retractor used during tumor removal may render the collateral supply less effective.

Operative exposure

The AICA is most commonly exposed in operations for tumors of the cerebellopontine angle. Aneurysms involving the AICA are rare and if not located at the origin, are most likely located at or near the internal acoustic meatus (25, 31). The displacement and management of the nerve-related arteries with acoustic neuromas are reviewed in greater detail in the chapter on the cerebellopontine angle. Arteriovenous malformations located infratentorially are uncommon compared with those in supratentorial locations, and not infrequently involve the other cerebellar arteries, in addition to the AICA and the brainstem, thus increasing the management risk (9, 39, 44). Compression of the facial and vestibulocochlear nerves by tortuous arteries is postulated to cause dysfunction of these nerves, a concept that is reviewed in Chapter Four on the cerebellopontine angle (18, 19, 34).

The AICA may be approached by a lateral suboccipital (retrosigmoid), middle fossa, translabyrinthine or combined supra-infratentorial presigmoid approach. The suboccipital exposure is excellent for lesions involving the meatal and postmeatal segments of the AICA, the lateral part of the mid- and lower brainstem below the trigeminal nerve, and the area near the internal acoustic meatus. A subtemporal middle fossa approach, with division of the tentorium and possibly combined with a medial petrosectomy, may be selected for lesions in which the AICA has a high origin, or also involves the SCA and basilar arteries and is medial to the trigeminal nerve. In the middle fossa approach to the internal meatus, only a short segment of the artery located near the meatus is exposed and sometimes only if the artery loops into the meatal perus. The translabyrinthine approach exposes the AICA, at and for a short distance proximal and distal to the internal acoustic meatus and along the anterior part of the petrosal surface. The supra-infratentorial presigmoid approaches with various degrees of resection of the semicircular canals, vestibule, and cochlea may be selected for lesions located deep in front of the brainstem, especially those located near the AICA origin. The AICA origin may be exposed in the anterior approaches directly through the clivus only if the origin is near the midline, but not if the origin is from a tortuous basilar artery that loops laterally into the cerebellopontine angle lateral to the medial aspect of the cavernous sinus and petrous carotid, which limit the lateral extent of the anterior exposures of the prepontine cistern.

POSTEROINFERIOR CEREBELLAR ARTERY

Overview

The PICA has the most complex, tortuous, and variable course and area of supply of the cerebellar arteries. It may be exposed in surgical approaches to the foramen magnum, fourth ventricle, cerebellar hemisphere, brainstem, jugular foramen, cerebellopontine angle, petrous apex, and clivus (30).

The PICA is intimately related to the cerebellomedullary fissure, the inferior half of the ventricular roof, the inferior cerebellar peduncle, and the suboccipital surface (*Figs. 2.1-2.5*). The PICA, by definition, arises from the vertebral artery near the inferior olive and passes posteriorly around the medulla. At the anterolateral margin of the medulla, it passes rostral or caudal to or between the rootlets of the hypoglossal nerve, and at the posterolateral margin of the medulla it courses rostral to or between the fila of the glossopharyngeal, vagus, and accessory nerves. After passing the latter nerves, it courses around the cerebellar tonsil and enters the cerebellomedullary fissure and passes posterior to the lower half of the roof of the fourth ventricle. On exiting the cerebellomedullary fissure, its branches are distributed to the vermis and hemisphere of the suboccipital surface. Its area of supply is the most variable of the cerebellar arteries (26). Most PICAs bifurcate into a medial and a lateral trunk. The medial trunk supplies the vermis and adjacent part of the hemisphere, and the lateral trunk supplies the cortical surface of the tonsil and the hemisphere. The PICA gives off perforating, choroidal, and cortical arteries. The cortical arteries are divided into vermian, tonsillar, and hemispheric groups.

Segments

The PICA is divided into five segments: 1) anterior medullary, 2) lateral medullary, 3) tonsillomedullary 4) telovelotonsillar, and 5) cortical (*Figs. 2.1* and *2.15*). These segments are

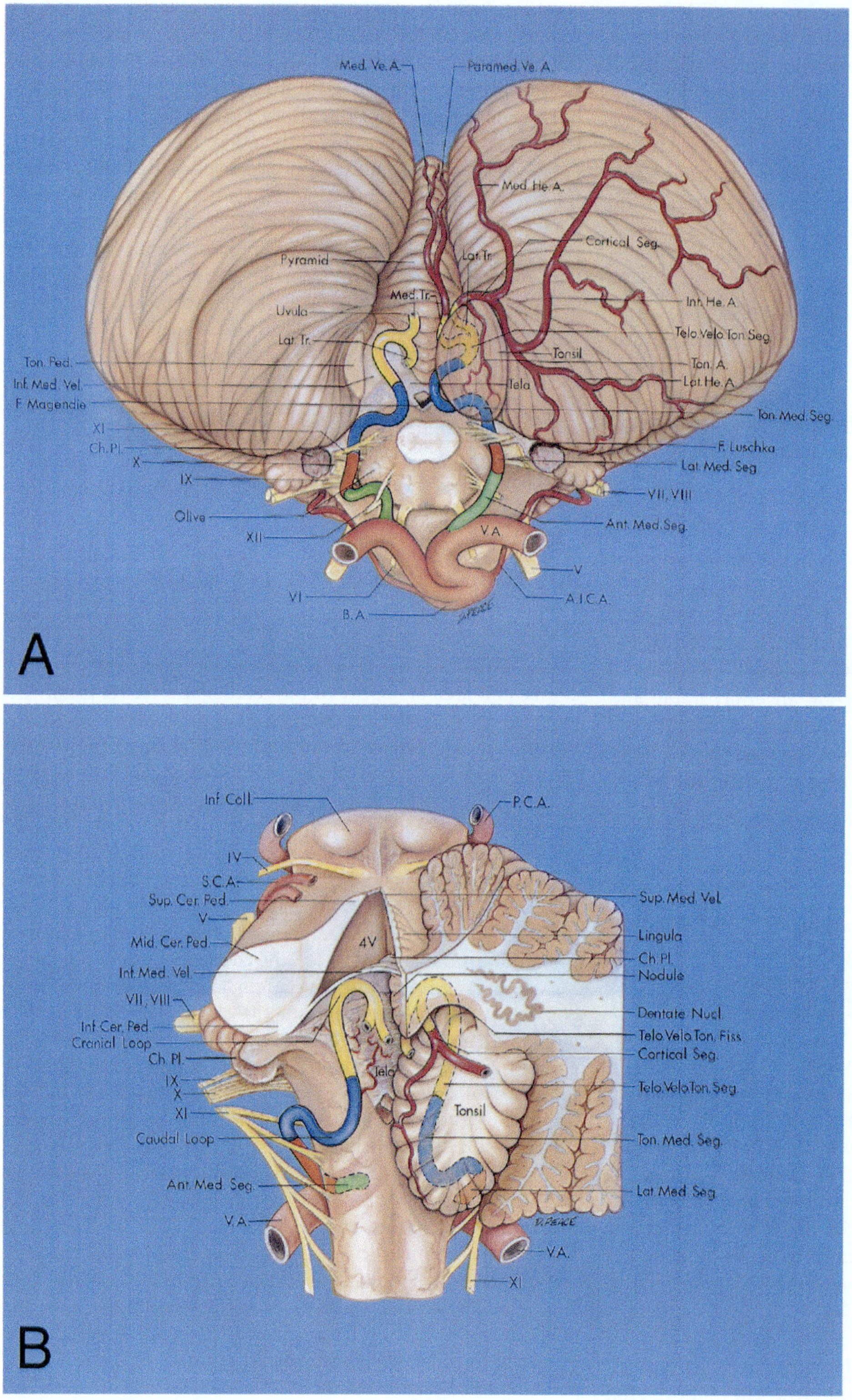

FIGURE 2.15. *A* and *B*. Segments of the PICA. *A*, inferior view. The left tonsil has been removed at the level of the tonsillar peduncle, its site of attachment to the remainder of the hemisphere. The anterior medullary segment (*green*) extends from the origin at the vertebral artery to the level of the inferior olive. This segment courses rostral or caudal to or between the rootlets of the hypoglossal nerve. The lateral medullary segment (*orange*) extends from the level of the most prominent part of the olive to the level of the rootlets of the glossopharyngeal, vagus, and accessory nerves. The tonsillomedullary segment (*blue*) extends from the level of the latter nerves around the caudal half of the tonsil and often forms a caudally convex loop. The telovelotonsillar segment (*yellow*) extends from the midlevel of the tonsil to the exit from the cleft located between the tela choroidea and the inferior medullary velum superiorly and the superior pole of the tonsil inferiorly. The cortical segment (*red*) extends from where the artery and its branches exit the fissures between the tonsil, vermis, and hemisphere to reach the cortical surface. The bifurcation of the main trunk into medial and lateral trunks is often located at the level of the tonsillomedullary or the telovelotonsillar segments. The medial trunk gives rise to median and paramedian vermian arteries. The lateral trunk gives rise to lateral, intermediate, and medial hemispheric and tonsillar arteries. *B*, enlarged posterior view. The left and part of the right halves of the cerebellum was removed to show the relationship of the PICA to the roof of the fourth ventricle. The dentate nucleus wraps around the superior pole of the tonsil. The telovelotonsillar fissure is below the inferior half of the roof of the fourth ventricle between the tonsil, tela choroidea, and inferior medullary velum. The caudal loop of the PICA is near the caudal pole of the tonsil, and the cranial loop is above the rostral pole of the tonsil. *A.*, artery; *A.I.C.A.*, anteroinferior cerebellar artery; *Ant.*, anterior; *B.A.*, basilar artery; *Cer.*, cerebellar; *Ch.*, choroid; *Coll.*, colliculus; *F.*, foramen; *Fiss.*, fissure; *He.*, hemispheric; *Inf.*, inferior; *Int.*, intermediate; *Lat.*, lateral; *Med.*, medial, medullary; *Mid.*, middle; *Nucl.*, nucleus; *Paramed.*, paramedian; *P.C.A.*, posterior cerebral artery; *Ped.*, peduncle; *Pl.*, plexus; *S.C.A.*, superior cerebellar artery; *Seg.*, segment; *Sup.*, superior; *Ton.*, tonsillar; *Tr.*, trunk; *V.A.*, vertebral artery; *Ve.*, vermian; *Vel.*, velum.

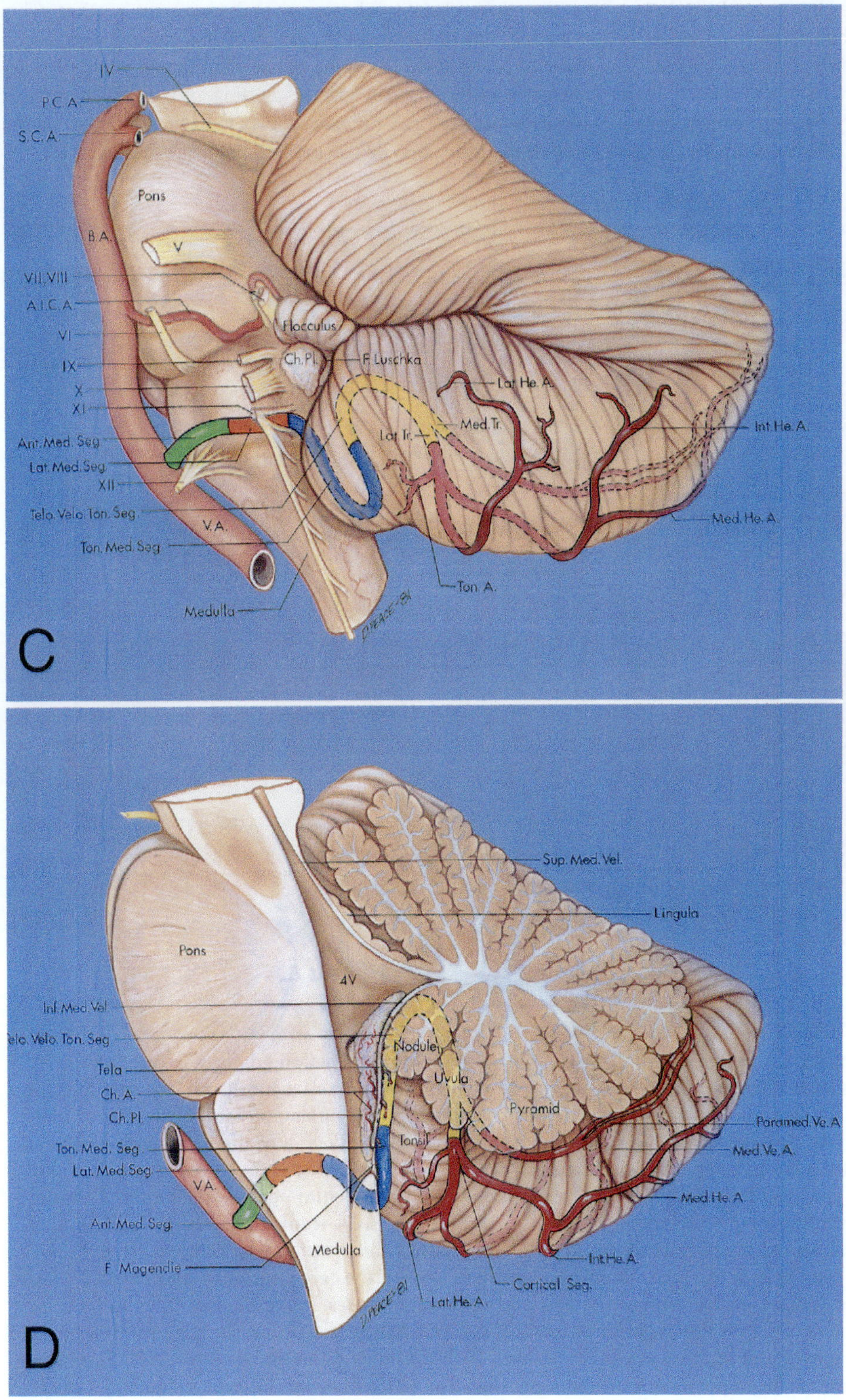

FIGURE 2.15. ***C*** **and** ***D*****. Segments of the PICA.** ***C*****, lateral view. The anterior medullary segment passes rostral to the hypoglossal nerve. The lateral medullary segment passes between the accessory rootlets. The tonsillomedullary segment forms a cranially convex loop near the inferior pole of the tonsil. The telovelotonsillar segment forms a cranially convex loop and bifurcates into medial and lateral trunks near its termination. The cortical segment spreads across the suboccipital surface.** ***D*****, midsagittal section. The tonsillomedullary and telovelotonsillar segments send choroidal branches into the choroid plexus. The telovelotonsillar segment ascends between the nodule and uvula medially and the tonsil laterally. (From, Lister JR, Rhoton AL Jr, Matsushima T, Peace DA: Microsurgical anatomy of the posterior inferior cerebellar artery. Neurosurgery 10:170–199, 1982 [30].)**

often longer than the distance around the medulla or the tonsil because the PICA frequently has a tortuous course and forms complex loops on the side of the brainstem among the lower cranial nerves, near the tonsil, and caudal to the roof of the fourth ventricle. Each segment may include more than one trunk, depending on the level of bifurcation of the artery.

Anterior medullary segment

This segment lies anterior to the medulla. It begins at the origin of the PICA anterior to the medulla and extends backward past the hypoglossal rootlets to the level of a rostrocaudal line through the most prominent part of the inferior olive that marks the boundary between the anterior and lateral surfaces of the medulla. Those PICAs arising lateral rather than anterior to the medulla do not have an anterior medullary segment. An anterior medullary segment is more likely to be present if the PICA arises from the superior part of the vertebral artery, because the vertebral artery courses from the lateral side of the medulla below to the anterior surface of the medulla above. An anterior medullary segment is present if the vertebral artery at the level of origin of the PICA has passed to the anterior surface of the brainstem. From its origin, the PICA usually passed posteriorly around or between the hypoglossal rootlets, but occasionally loops upward, downward, laterally, or medially before passing posteriorly around or between the hypoglossal rootlets.

Lateral medullary segment

This segment begins where the artery passes the most prominent point of the olive and ends at the level of the origin of the glossopharyngeal, vagus, and accessory rootlets. This segment is present in most PICAs. Its course varies from passing directly posterior to reach the glossopharyngeal, vagal, and accessory rootlets to ascending, descending, or passing laterally or medially to form one or more complex loops in the cistern on the side of the brainstem before passing between these nerves.

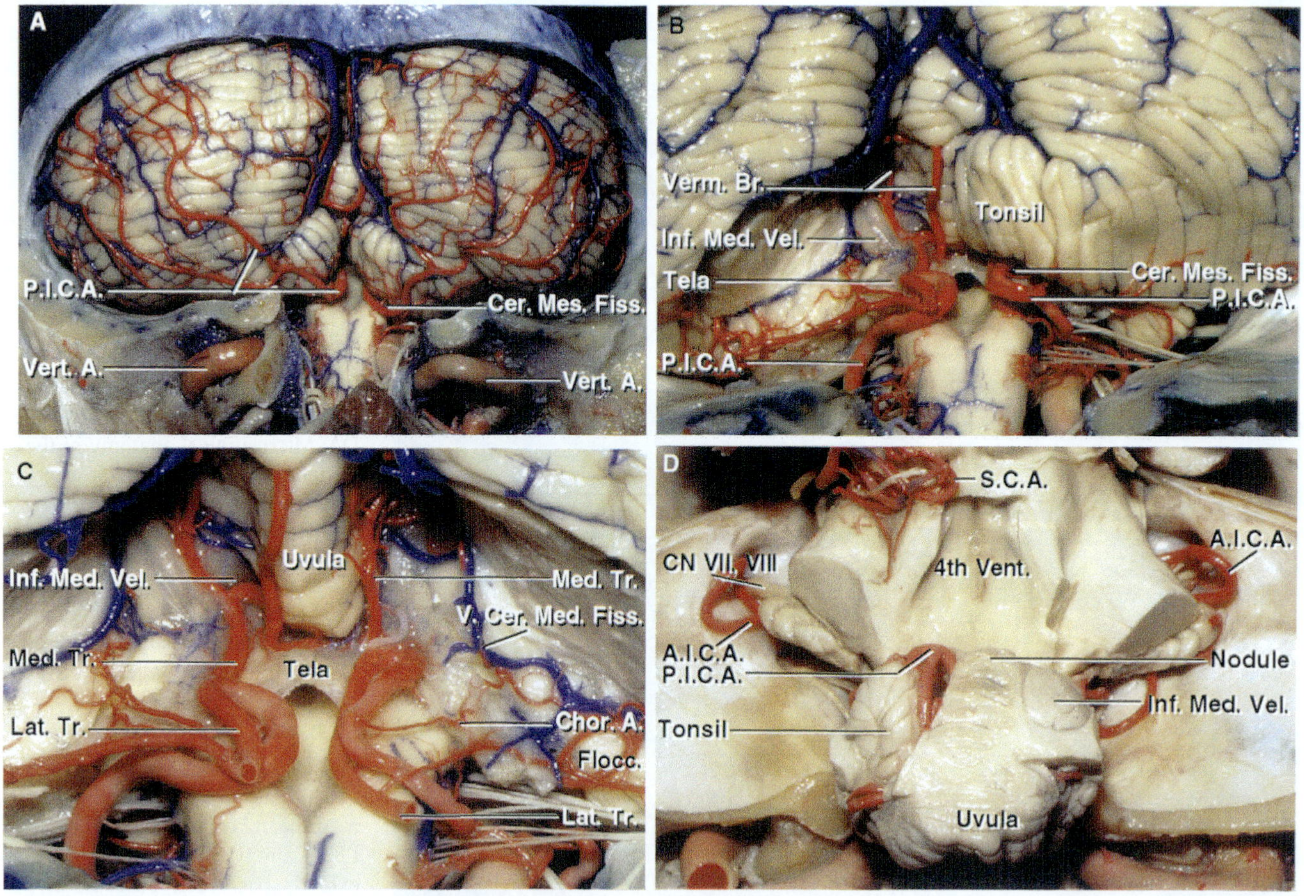

FIGURE 2.16. PICA relationships. *A*, the PICA courses around the medulla, enters the cerebellomedullary fissure, and exits the fissure to supply the suboccipital surface. The fissure extends upward between the cerebellar tonsils on one side and the medulla and inferior half of the ventricle roof on the other side. The PICAs frequently form a caudal loop at the lower pole of the cerebellar tonsils. *B*, enlarged view. The left tonsil has been removed to expose the course of the PICA within the cerebellomedullary fissure. The PICAs often loop upward around the rostral pole of the tonsil, where they course between the rostral pole of the tonsil on the lower side and the tela choroidea and inferior medullary velum on the upper side. *C*, both tonsils and the adjacent part of the biventral lobule have been removed to expose the PICA trunks. The PICAs divide into a medial trunk, which supplies the vermis and adjacent part of the hemisphere, and a caudal trunk, which loops around the tonsil to supply the largest part of the hemispheric surface. Choroidal branches pass to the tela choroidea and choroid plexus in the roof. The vein of the cerebellomedullary fissure crosses the tela and velum and passes above the flocculus to join the veins in the cerebellopontine angle that empty into the superior petrosal sinus. *D*, another dissection showing the relationship of the cranial loop of the PICA to the tonsils and inferior medullary velum. Both tonsils and the nodule and uvula have been preserved. The inferior medullary velum has been preserved on the right side. The left half of the inferior medullary velum has been removed to expose the supratonsillar loop of the PICA, which courses between the velum and the tonsil. The velum stretches laterally from the nodule across the rostral pole of the tonsil to blend into the flocculus. *A.*, artery; *A.I.C.A.*, anteroinferior cerebellar artery; *Br.*, branch; *Cer. Med.*, cerebellomedullary; *Cer. Mes.*, cerebellomesencephalic; *Chor.*, choroidal; *CN*, cranial nerve; *Fiss.*, fissure; *Flocc.*, flocculus; *Inf.*, inferior; *Lat.*, lateral; *Med.*, medial, medullary; *Mes.*, mesencephalic; *P.I.C.A.*, posteroinferior cerebellar artery; *S.C.A.*, superior cerebellar artery; *Tr.*, trunk; *V.*, vein; *Vel.*, velum; *Vent.*, ventricle; *Verm.*, vermian; *Vert.*, vertebral.

Tonsillomedullary segment

This segment begins where the PICA passes posterior to the glossopharyngeal, vagus, and accessory nerves and extends medially across the posterior aspect of the medulla near the caudal half of the tonsil (*Figs. 2.3, 2.4, 2.15,* and *2.16*). It ends where the artery ascends to the midlevel of the medial surface of the tonsil. The proximal portion of this segment usually courses near the lateral recess and then posteriorly to reach the inferior pole of the tonsil. This segment commonly passes medially between the lower margin of the tonsil and the medulla before turning rostrally along the medial surface of the tonsil. The loop passing near the lower part of the tonsil, referred to as the caudal or infratonsillar loop, has been reported to form a caudally convex loop that coincides with the caudal pole of the tonsil, but it may also course superior or inferior to the caudal pole of the tonsil without forming a loop. In some cases it dips below the caudal margin of the tonsil and even below the level of the foramen magnum. A caudally convex loop is not present if the PICA passes directly medial between the tonsil and medulla, if the PICA ascends along the lateral surface of the tonsil to reach the hemispheric surface, or if the artery has a low origin from the vertebral artery and ascends posterior to the medulla to reach the tonsil (*Fig. 2.17*).

The relationships between the tonsillomedullary segment and the cerebellar tonsil and foramen magnum varies (*Fig. 2.17*). In our previous study of 42 PICAs, the caudal limit of this segment was located superior to the caudal pole of the tonsil in 23, inferior in 8, and at the same level in 11 (30). This segment passed medially in a location 10.0 mm inferior to 13.0 mm superior (average, 1.6 mm superior) to the caudal tip of the tonsil. The caudal limit of this segment was superior to the foramen magnum in 37 PICAs, inferior in 4, and at the same level in 1. It was located 7.0 mm inferior to 18.0 mm superior (average, 6.9 mm superior) to the foramen magnum.

Telovelotonsillar segment

This is the most complex of the segments. It begins at the midportion of the PICA's ascent along the medial surface of the tonsil toward the roof of the fourth ventricle and ends where it exits the fissures between the vermis, tonsil, and hemisphere to reach the suboccipital surface (*Figs. 2.15-2.18*). In most, but not all, hemispheres, this segment often forms a loop with a convex rostral curve, called the cranial loop (20, 38, 57). This loop is located caudal to the fastigium between the cerebellar tonsil below and the tela choroidea and posterior medullary velum above. The apex of the cranial loop usually overlies the central part of the inferior medullary velum, but its location varies from the superior to the inferior margin and from the medial to the lateral extent of the inferior medullary velum. The apex of the cranial loop is inferior to the level of the fastigium of the fourth ventricle in most cases, but may also extend to the level of the fastigium. This segment gives rise to branches that supply the tela choroidea and choroid plexus of the fourth ventricle.

Cortical segment

This segment begins where the trunks and branches leave the groove between the vermis medially and the tonsil and the hemisphere laterally, and includes the terminal cortical branches. The bifurcation of the PICA often occurs near the origin of this segment. The cortical branches radiate outward from the superior and lateral borders of the tonsil to the remainder of the vermis and hemisphere.

The PICA origin and the vertebral artery

The PICA is defined here, in agreement with others, as the cerebellar artery that arises from the vertebral artery (*Figs. 2.19* and *2.20*) (49, 55). The PICA is less commonly defined as the cerebellar artery that supplies the posteroinferior part of the cerebellum and generally arises from the vertebral artery, but may also arise from the basilar artery (4, 56).

Of 50 cerebellar hemispheres examined in our previous study, all but 1 had vertebral arteries, and 42 of the 49 vertebral arteries gave rise to PICAs (30). Both a vertebral artery and the associated PICA were absent in a few hemispheres. If a PICA is present, it is the largest branch of the vertebral artery. It is rarely absent bilaterally, but may arise as a double or duplicate PICA. Forty-one of the 42 PICAs arose as a single trunk and 1 arose as a duplicate trunk. The vertebral artery sometimes terminates in a PICA.

The vertebral artery enters the dura lateral to the cervicomedullary junction, courses superior, anterior, and medial to reach the front of the medulla and joins its mate from the opposite side at approximately the level of the pontomedullary junction to form the basilar artery. The site of the origin of the PICA from the vertebral artery varies from below the foramen magnum to the vertebrobasilar junction. A few of the PICAs arising below the foramen magnum may arise from the vertebral artery in an extradural location (*Fig. 2.21*) (12). Thirty-five of the 42 PICAs examined in our previous study arose above the level of the foramen magnum, and 7 vessels originated below. The origin was located 14.0 mm below to 26.0 mm above the level of the foramen magnum (average, 8.6 mm above) (30). The origin was located 0 to 35.0 mm (average, 16.9 mm) below the junction of the vertebral and basilar arteries.

The PICA arises from the posterior or lateral surfaces of the vertebral artery more often than from the medial or anterior surfaces (*Fig. 2.19*). On leaving the parent vessel, the initial course of the PICA is posterior, lateral, or superior more often than anterior, medial, or inferior (*Fig. 2.20*). The vertebral artery's diameter is greater at its entrance through the dura (range, 1.8–6.2 mm; average, 4.4 mm) than at the PICA origin (range, 1.6–5.7 mm; average, 3.9 mm) or at its termination (range, 1.7–5.5 mm; average, 3.7 mm). The diameter of the PICA at its origin ranges from 0.5 to 3.4 mm (average, 2.0 mm). The origin was 1.0 mm or less in diameter in 4 cerebellae. The PICA has been reported to be hypoplastic in 5 to 16% of cerebellar hemispheres (33, 48).

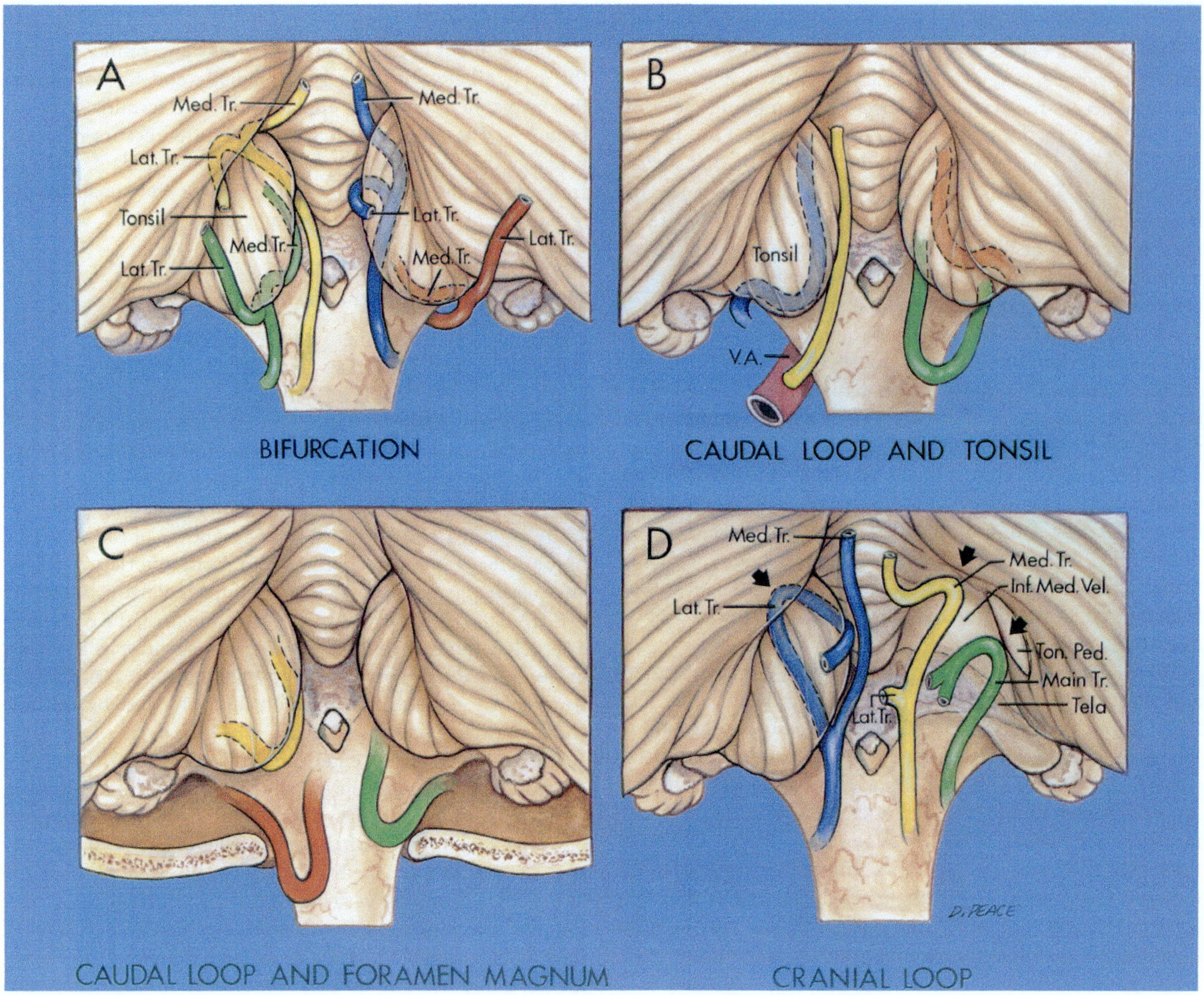

FIGURE 2.17. Locations of the PICA bifurcation, the caudal loops in relation to the tonsil and the foramen magnum, and the cranial loops. *A*, site of the bifurcation in relation to the tonsil. The main trunk of the PICA may bifurcate at any site along the margin of the tonsil. Inferolateral bifurcation (*red*): the lateral trunk passes upward lateral to the tonsil to reach the hemisphere, and the medial trunk passes along the anteromedial margin of the tonsil. Inferomedial bifurcation (*green*): the lateral trunk passes superolateral over the posterior margin of the tonsil to reach the hemispheric surface, and the medial trunk passes upward along the anteromedial margin of the tonsil. Superomedial bifurcation (*blue*): the lateral trunk passes posteriorly over the medial surface of the tonsil, and the medial trunk ascends to supply the vermis. Superolateral bifurcation (*yellow*): the lateral trunk passes out of the fissure between the tonsil and the hemisphere and proceeds to the hemispheric surface, and the medial trunk ascends to supply the vermis. *B*, location of the caudal loop in relation to the tonsil. The tonsillomedullary segment often formed a caudally convex loop (*blue, orange, green*) as it passed medially across the posterior surface of the medulla. This caudal part of the tonsillomedullary segment was located between 10.0 mm inferior and 13.0 mm superior (average, 1.6 mm superior) to the caudal tip of the tonsil. This loop could be found superior to (*orange*), inferior to (*green*), or at the level of (*blue*) the caudal tip of the tonsil. In some cases (*yellow*), the PICA ascended from the vertebral artery (V.A.) or took another course to reach the medial surface of the tonsil without forming a caudal loop. *C*, relation of the caudal loop to the foramen magnum. Most caudal loops were superior to the foramen magnum (*yellow*), but they could be inferior to (*red*) or at the level of (*green*) the foramen magnum. The caudal loop was located between 7.0 mm inferior and 18.0 mm superior (average, 6.9 mm superior) to the foramen magnum. *D*, relationship of the cranial loop (*arrow*) to the superior pole of the tonsil and the trunks of the PICA. The right tonsil was removed at the level of the tonsillar peduncle to expose the inferior medullary velum and the tela choroidea. The telovelotonsillar segment often formed a cranially convex loop. below the fastigium. The cranially convex loop could be formed by either the main (*green*), medial (*yellow*), or lateral (*blue*) trunk. On the left (*blue*), the lateral trunk (*arrow*) forms a cranially convex loop over the superior pole of the tonsil

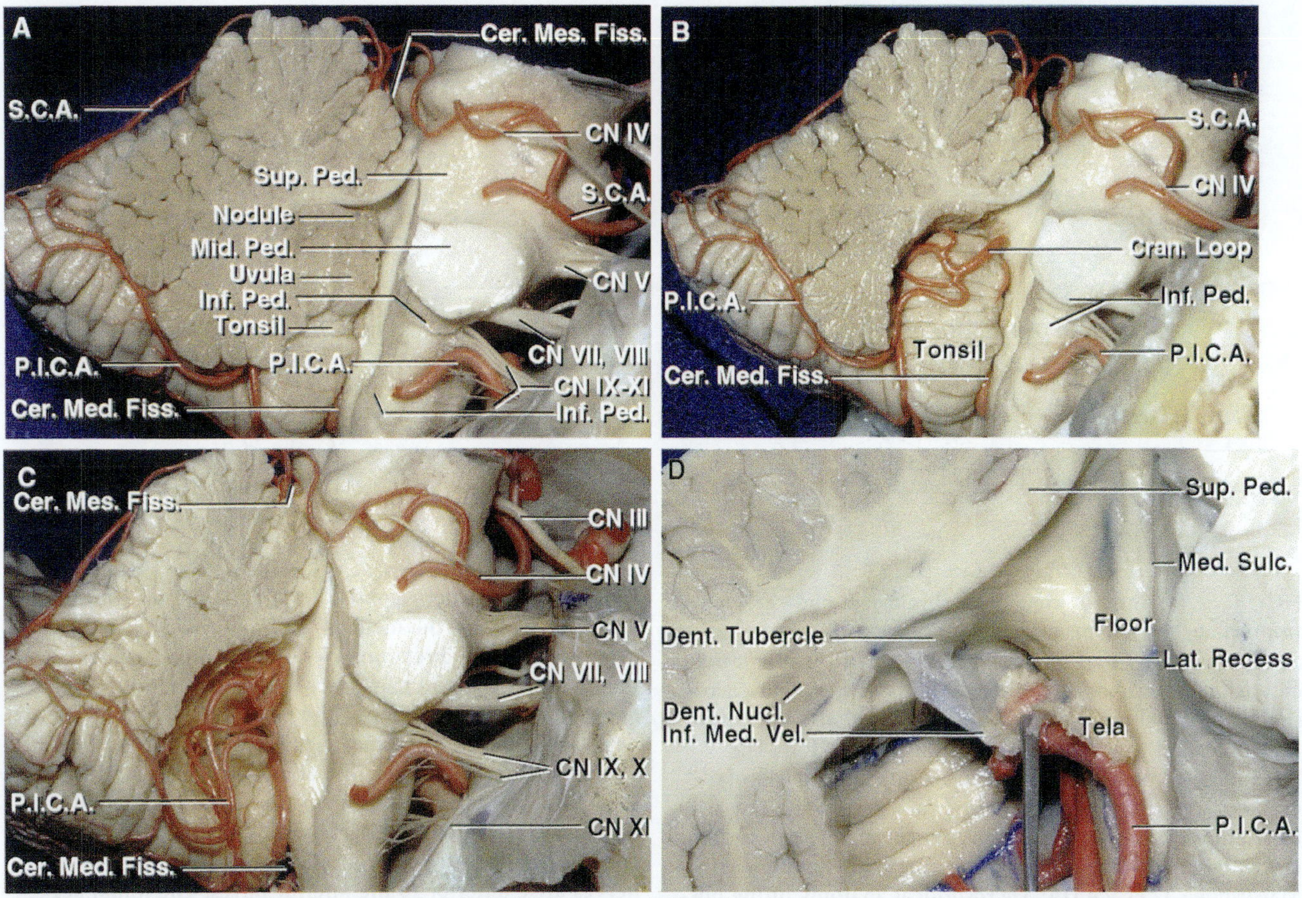

FIGURE 2.18. PICA relationships. ***A*****, the right half of the cerebellum has been removed. The right PICA passes between the rootlets of the vagus and accessory nerves to reach the surface of the inferior cerebellar peduncle. The left PICA, as it courses around the rostral pole of the tonsil, is hidden by the remaining left half of the uvula. The SCA passes around the brainstem below the oculomotor nerve and above the trigeminal nerve.** ***B*****, the part of the uvula and nodule medial to the tonsil has been removed to expose the PICAs passage through the cerebellomedullary fissure and around the tonsil. The artery frequently forms a caudal loop at the lower margin of the tonsil and a cranial or supratonsillar loop that wraps around the rostral pole of the tonsil.** ***C*****, the tonsil has been removed to expose the PICA's looping course through the cerebellomedullary fissure.** ***D*****, the inferior medullary velum, which stretches across the rostral pole of the tonsil, has been folded downward to expose the dentate tubercle, a prominence near the fastigium that underlies the dentate nucleus. The lateral recess is also exposed. The telovelotonsillar segment of the PICA courses in the cerebellomedullary fissure between the tela and velum on one side and the tonsil on the other side.** ***Cer. Med.*****, cerebellomedullary;** ***Cer. Mes.*****, cerebellomesencephalic;** ***CN*****, cranial nerve;** ***Cran.*****, cranial;** ***Dent.*****, dentate;** ***Fiss.*****, fissure;** ***Inf.*****, inferior;** ***Lat.*****, lateral;** ***Med.*****, median, medullary;** ***Mid.*****, middle;** ***Nucl.*****, nucleus;** ***Ped.*****, peduncle;** ***P.I.C.A.*****, posteroinferior cerebellar artery;** ***S.C.A.*****, superior cerebellar artery;** ***Sulc.*****, sulcus;** ***Sup.*****, superior;** ***Vel.*****, velum.**

Bifurcation

Most PICAs bifurcate into a smaller medial and a larger lateral trunk; the trunk before the bifurcation is referred to as the main trunk. The medial trunk supplies the vermis and adjacent part of the hemisphere and the lateral trunk supplies most of the hemispheric and tonsillar parts of the suboccipital surface. The PICAs that do not bifurcate are usually small and supply only a small area on the tonsil and adjacent part of the vermis and hemisphere.

and the medial trunk ascends straight to the vermis. In the center (*yellow*), the medial trunk (*arrow*) forms a cranially convex loop at the superior pole of the tonsil and the lateral trunk courses around the medial surface of the tonsil. On the right (*green*), the cranial loop is formed by the main trunk (*arrow*) and lies in the telovelotonsillar fissure anterior to the superior pole of the tonsil. (From, Lister JR, Rhoton AL Jr, Matsushima T, Peace DA: Microsurgical anatomy of the posterior inferior cerebellar artery. Neurosurgery 10:170–199, 1982 [30].) ***Inf.*****, inferior;** ***Lat.*****, lateral;** ***Med.*****, medial, medullary;** ***Ped.*****, peduncle;** ***Ton.*****, tonsillar;** ***Tr.*****, trunk;** ***V.A.*****, vertebral artery;** ***Vel.*****, velum.**

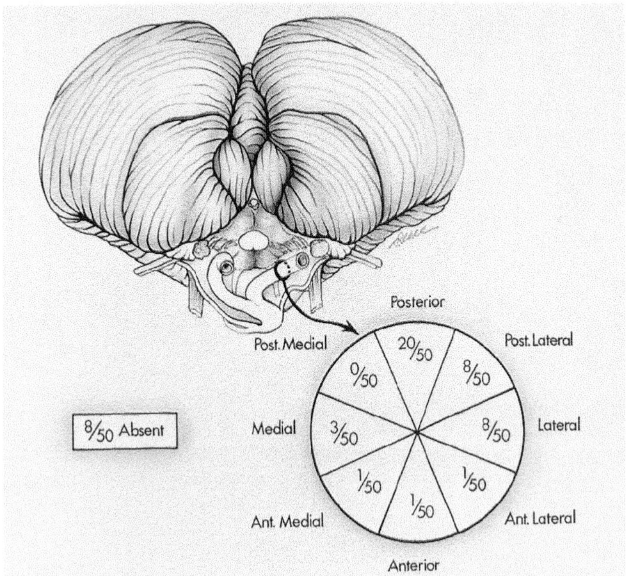

FIGURE 2.19. Inferior view of the brainstem and cerebellum (*top*) shows the site on the circumference of the vertebral artery (*lower right*) of the origin of the 42 PICAs found in 50 cerebellar hemispheres. The *circle* on the lower right corresponds to the circumference of the vertebral artery. Eight of the 50 cerebellar hemispheres did not have a PICA. The PICA most commonly arose from the posterior, posterolateral, or lateral surface of the vertebral artery, but a few sites of origin were located on the anterior or medial half of the circumference of the artery. (From, Lister JR, Rhoton AL Jr, Matsushima T, Peace DA: Microsurgical anatomy of the posterior inferior cerebellar artery. Neurosurgery 10:170–199, 1982 [30].)

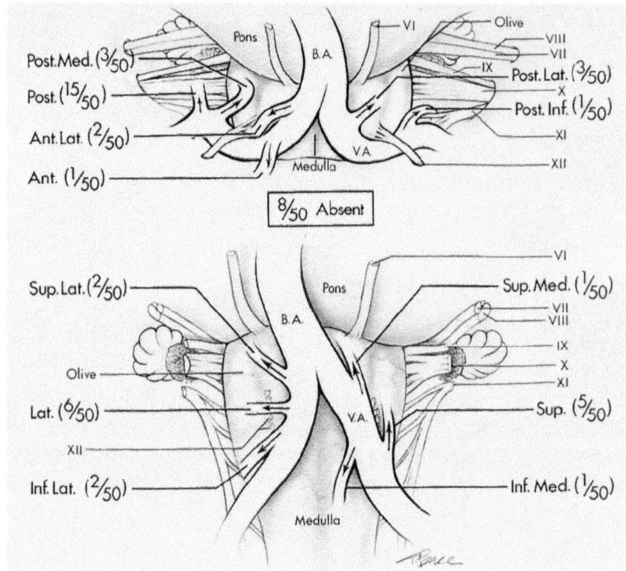

FIGURE 2.20. Anterosuperior (*top*) and anterior (*bottom*) views of the pons, the medulla, and the vertebral and basilar arteries show the direction taken by the initial segment of the PICA. Forty-two PICAs were found in the 50 cerebellar hemispheres we examined. The *arrows* are on and define the direction taken by the initial segment of the PICAs immediately distal to their origin. The abducens, facial, and vestibulocochlear nerves arise at the level of the pontomedullary junction. The glossopharyngeal, vagus, and accessory nerves arise posterior to the inferior olives, and the hypoglossal nerves arise anterior to the inferior olives. The initial segment was most commonly directed posterior, lateral superior, posterolateral, or posteromedial. A few PICAS were directed superolateral, inferolateral, anterolateral, posteroinferior, superomedial, inferomedial, or anterior. (From, Lister JR, Rhoton AL Jr, Matsushima T, Peace DA: Microsurgical anatomy of the posterior inferior cerebellar artery. Neurosurgery 10:170–199, 1982 [30].) *Ant.*, anterior; *B.A.*, basilar artery; *Inf.*, inferior; *Lat.*, lateral; *Med.*, medial; *Post.*, posterior; *Sup.*, superior; *V.A.*, vertebral artery.

The bifurcation usually occurs posterior to the brainstem as the PICA courses around the tonsil (*Figs. 2.16, 2.17,* and *2.22*). The most common site of the bifurcation is in the telovelotonsillar fissure as the artery courses around the rostral pole of the tonsil. The medial trunk usually ascends in the vermohemispheric fissure to reach the vermis, and the lateral trunk passes laterally out of the telovelotonsillar fissure to reach the hemispheric surface. If the bifurcation occurs at a more proximal site in relation to the tonsil, the medial trunk usually ascends along the medial tonsillar surface and through the vermohemispheric fissure, and the lateral trunk passes posteriorly over the tonsillar surface near the point of bifurcation to reach the hemispheric surface. If the bifurcation occurs proximal to the lateral margin of the tonsil, the medial trunk commonly pursues a course around the medial surface of the tonsil to reach the vermohemispheric fissure, and the lateral trunk passes directly to the hemispheric surface.

The medial trunk terminates by sending branches over the inferior part of the vermis and adjacent part of the tonsil and hemisphere. The lateral trunk divides into a larger hemispheric trunk that gives off multiple branches to the hemisphere and smaller tonsillar branches that supply the posterior and inferior surfaces of the tonsil. This division of the lateral trunk into tonsillar and hemispheric branches may occur at various sites in relation to the tonsil, but is most commonly located near the posterior margin of the medial surface of the tonsil. The trunks passing through the tonsillomedullary fissure send branches to the medulla, and the trunks passing through the telovelotonsillar fissure send ascending branches to the dentate nucleus (55).

Branches

The PICA gives rise to perforating branches to the medulla, choroidal arteries that supply the tela choroidea and choroid plexus, and cortical arteries. The cortical arteries are divided into median and paramedian vermian; tonsillar; and medial, intermediate, and lateral hemispheric arteries. The cortical

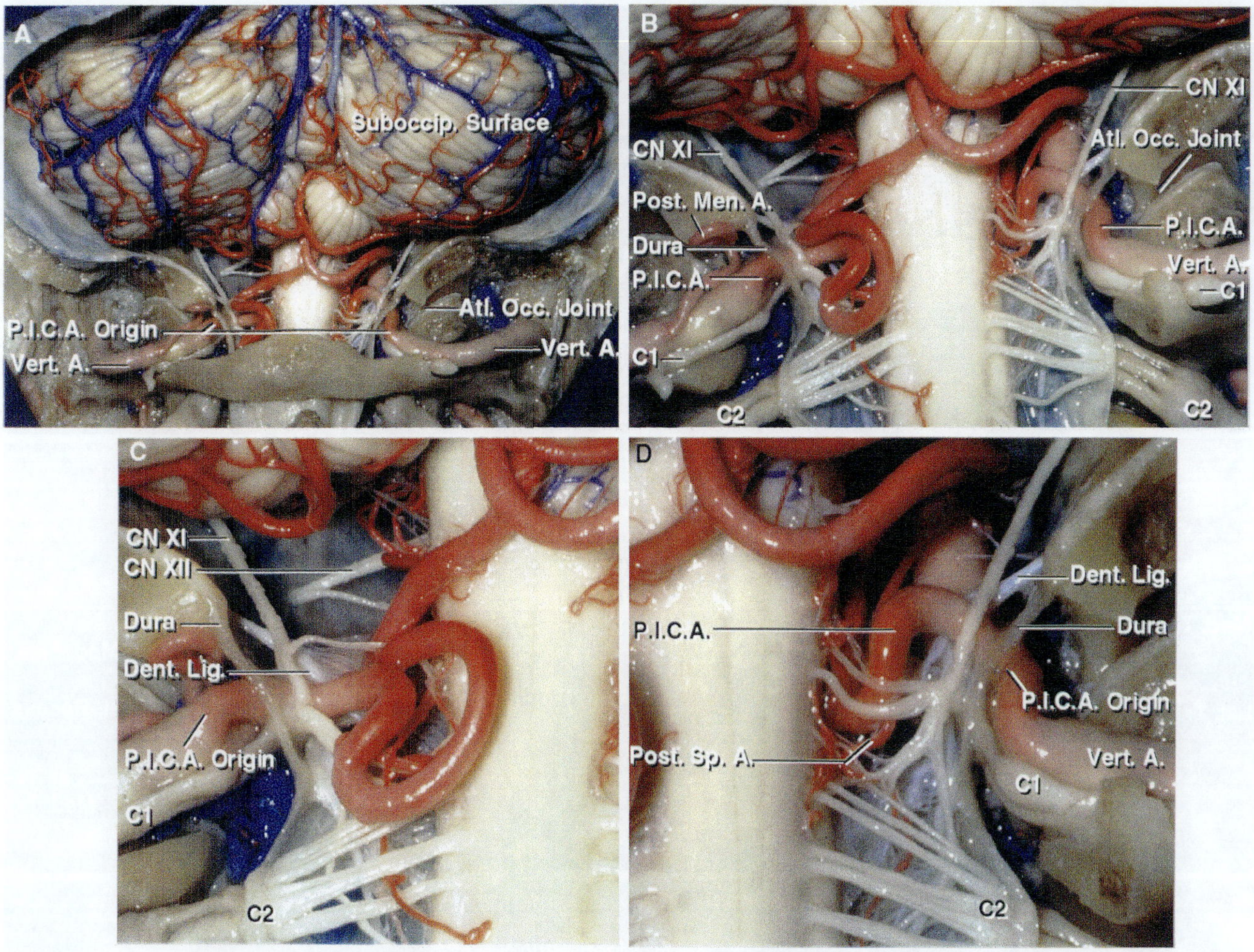

FIGURE 2.21. Bilateral PICAs with an extradural origin. *A*, both PICAs arise outside the dura as the vertebral arteries course behind the atlanto-occipital joints. The PICAs enter the dura at the level of the dorsolateral medulla and do not have an anterior medullary or a full lateral medullary segment. The left PICA loops downward in front of the posterior arch of the atlas. *B*, enlarged view. The left PICA gives off a posterior meningeal artery, penetrates the dura by passing through the dural cuff around the vertebral artery, and loops downward behind the accessory nerve and the C1 and C2 roots before ascending to enter the cerebellomedullary fissure. The right PICA passes through the dura and courses along the side of the medulla in front of the rootlets of the accessory nerve. *C*, the left PICA penetrates the dural cuff with the vertebral artery and the C1 nerve root. The accessory nerve passes posterior to both the vertebral artery and the PICA. The rostral attachment of the dentate ligament ascends between the PICA and the vertebral artery to attach to the dura at the level of the foramen magnum. *D*, the C1 nerve root passes through the dural cuff with the vertebral artery and the PICA. The accessory nerve ascends posterior to both the vertebral artery and PICA. A small posterior spinal artery arises from the PICA and courses along the dorsolateral aspect of the spinal cord. *A.*, artery; *Atl.*, atlanto; *CN*, cranial nerve; *Dent.*, dentate; *Lig.*, ligament; *Men.*, meningeal; *Occ.*, occipital; *P.I.C.A.*, posteroinferior cerebellar artery; *Post.*, posterior; *Sp.*, spinal; *Suboccip.*, suboccipital; *Vert.*, vertebral.

branches arising near the superior pole of the tonsil send branches upward to supply the dentate nucleus.

Perforating arteries

The perforating arteries are small arteries that arise from the three medullary segments and terminate in the brainstem. They are divided into direct and circumflex types. The direct type pursues a straight course to enter the brainstem. The circumflex type passes around the brainstem before terminating in it. The circumflex perforating arteries are divided into short and long types. The short circumflex type does not travel more than 90 degrees around the circumference of the brainstem. The long circumflex type travels a greater distance to reach the opposite surface. Both types of circumflex arteries send branches into the brainstem along their course. The perforating arteries have numerous branches and anastomoses that create a plexiform pattern on the medullary surface. In our previous study, the anterior medullary segments gave

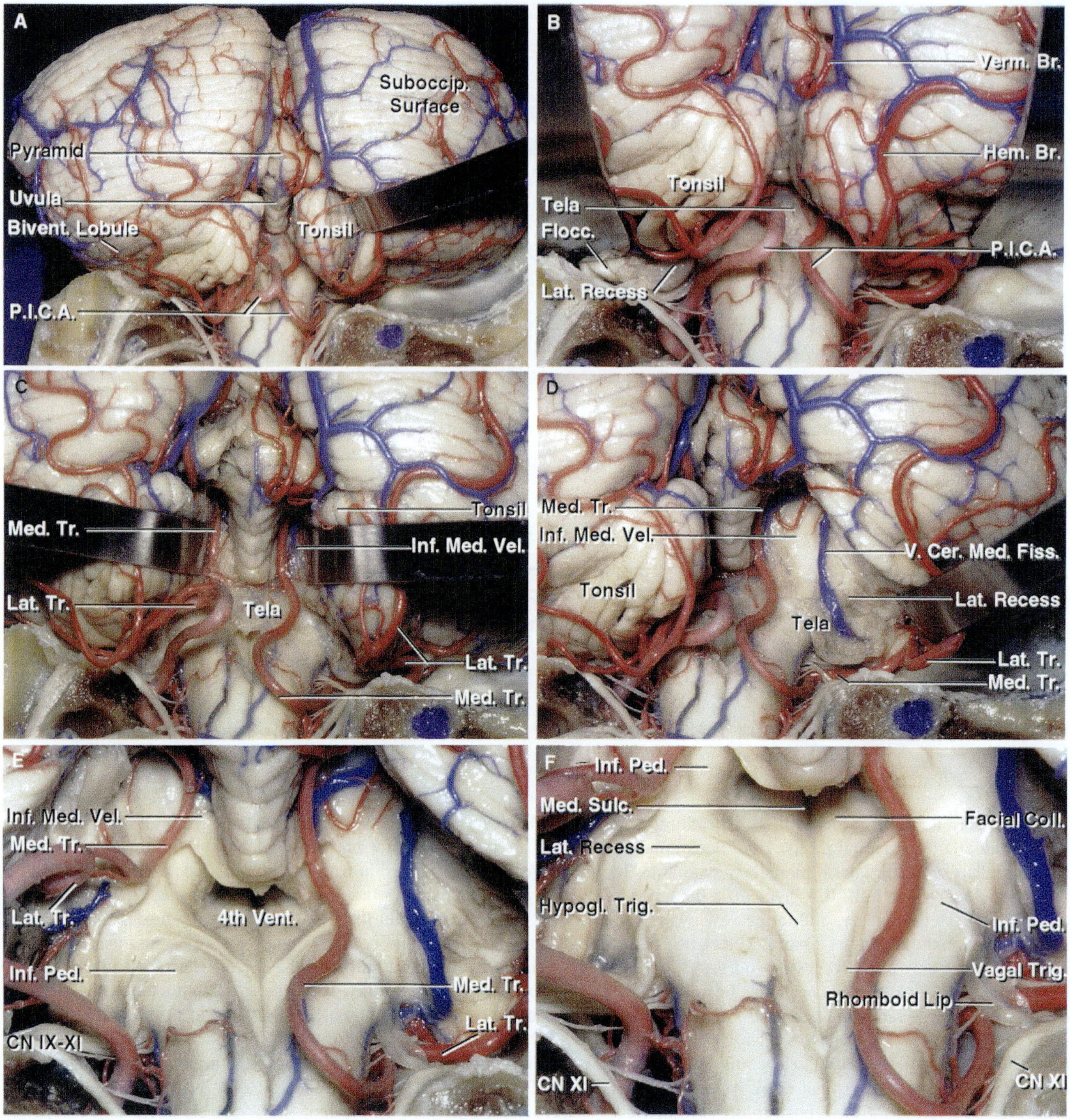

FIGURE 2.22. PICA relationships. *A*, the left PICA is larger than the right. Both PICAs enter the cerebellomedullary fissure, pass around the tonsils, and exit the fissure to supply the suboccipital surface. The natural cleft between the right tonsil and the biventral lobule has been opened. The tonsil is attached to the remainder of the cerebellum by the tonsillar peduncle, a white matter bundle along its superolateral margin. All of the other margins of the tonsils are free margins. *B*, enlarged view. The left biventral lobule has been elevated to expose the flocculus protruding from the margin of the lateral recess. *C*, the tonsils have been retracted laterally to expose the PICAs coursing in the cerebellomedullary fissure. The right PICA bifurcates into medial and lateral trunks before reaching the cerebellomedullary fissure. The left PICA bifurcates within the fissure. The medial trunks supply the vermis and adjacent part of the hemisphere and the lateral trunks supply the remainder of the hemisphere. *D*, the right tonsil has been removed to expose the lateral recess and bifurcation of the right PICA into medial and lateral trunks. *E*, both tonsils and the tela have been removed to expose the ventricular floor and walls. The left PICA divides into its trunks within the cerebellomedullary fissure. The inferior medullary velum has been preserved, but is a thin layer that

rise to 0 to 2 (average, 1.0) perforating branches per hemisphere, which were most commonly of the short circumflex posterior type and supplied the anterior, lateral, or posterior surfaces of the medulla (30). The lateral medullary segments gave rise to 0 to 5 (average, 1.8) branches per hemisphere that supplied the lateral or posterior medulla predominately as short circumflex arteries. The tonsillomedullary segment gave rise to more perforating branches than the other segments (range, 0–11 per hemisphere; average, 3.3). They were either of the direct or short circumflex type, but the former predominated. They terminated in the lateral and posterior surfaces of the medulla.

The perforating branches of the PICA intermingle and overlap with those arising from the vertebral artery (*Fig. 2.5*). The segment of the vertebral artery distal to the origin of the PICA more frequently gives rise to perforating arteries than the segment proximal to the PICA origin. The perforating branches arising between the entrance of the vertebral artery into the dura mater and origin of the PICA are most commonly of the short circumflex or direct type and terminate predominately on the lateral side of the medulla. Those arising between the PICA origin and the vertebrobasilar junction are predominately of the short circumflex type and terminate on the anterior and lateral surfaces of the medulla. The segment of the vertebral artery distal to the PICA origin also gives rise to a few branches that enter the choroid plexus protruding from the foramen of Luschka.

Choroidal arteries

The PICA gives rise to branches that supply the tela choroidea and choroid plexus of the fourth ventricle, usually supplying the choroid plexus near the midline of the roof of the fourth ventricle and in the medial part of the lateral recess (*Figs. 2.16* and *2.23*) (15). This includes all of the medial segment and the adjacent part of the lateral segment of the choroid plexus. More choroidal branches arise from the tonsillomedullary and telovelotonsillar segments than from the lateral or anterior medullary segment. The AICA usually supplies the portion of the choroid plexus not supplied by the PICA, commonly that part in the cerebellopontine angle and the adjacent part of the lateral recess.

Cortical arteries

The most constant area supplied by the PICA includes the majority of the ipsilateral half of the suboccipital surface of the cerebellum (*Figs. 2.15, 2.16,* and *2.22*). This includes the majority of the suboccipital surface of the ipsilateral hemisphere and tonsil, the ipsilateral half of the vermis, and the anterior aspect of the tonsil. The largest area supplied by a PICA includes all of the ipsilateral half of the suboccipital surface with overlap onto the contralateral half of the suboccipital surface and the adjacent parts of the tentorial and petrosal surfaces. The smallest area supplied by a PICA is confined to the inferior part of the ipsilateral cerebellar tonsil. The cortical area supplied by the PICA is more variable than that supplied by the AICA and the SCA. If the PICA is absent on one side, the contralateral PICA or the ipsilateral AICA supplies most of the area normally supplied by the absent PICA.

The cortical branches are divided into hemispheric, vermian, and tonsillar groups. The vermian branches usually arise from the medial trunk, and the hemispheric and tonsillar branches from the lateral trunk. Each half of the vermis is divided into median and paramedian segments, and the hemisphere lateral to the vermis is divided into medial, intermediate, and lateral segments. There is a reciprocal relationship with frequent overlap in the areas supplied by the tonsillar, hemispheric, and vermian branches.

Hemispheric branches

The hemispheric branches most commonly arise from the lateral trunk within or distal to the vermohemispheric fissure. They appear to radiate outward to the hemispheric surface from the superior and lateral margin of the tonsil. In our previous study, the number of hemispheric branches given off from a PICA ranged from 0 to 9 (average, 2.8). Four PICAs had no hemispheric branches (30). A common pattern was for there to be three branches with an individual branch being directed to the medial, intermediate, and lateral segments of the suboccipital surface. The medial hemispheric segment is occasionally supplied by the medial trunk. The ipsilateral AICA often gives rise to branches that overlap onto the lateral hemispheric segment, and the SCA often overlaps onto the superior part of the three hemispheric segments.

Vermian arteries

The vermian arteries usually arise from the medial trunk in the vermohemispheric fissure. A common pattern is for there to be one or two vermian branches. If two are present, they are often directed to the median and paramedian segments. If no vermian branches are present, the vermian area is usually supplied by the contralateral PICA.

Tonsillar branches

The tonsillar branches usually arise from the lateral trunk and most commonly supply the medial, posterior, inferior,

can be opened, if needed, to increase the exposure of the fourth ventricle. *F*, enlarged view showing the relationship of the PICAs to the fourth ventricle. The PICAs, after passing between the rootlets of the accessory rootlets course along the caudolateral margin of the fourth ventricle on the inferior cerebellar peduncle before entering the cerebellomedullary fissure. The left PICA has been reflected laterally. The facial colliculus is in the upper and hypoglossal and vagal nuclei are in the lower part of the floor. *Bivent.*, biventral; *Br.*, branch; *Cer. Med.*, cerebellomedullary; *CN*, cranial nerve; *Coll.*, colliculus; *Fiss.*, fissure; *Flocc.*, flocculus; *Hem.*, hemispheric; *Hypogl.*, hypoglossal; *Inf.*, inferior; *Lat.*, lateral; *Med.*, medial, medullary; *Ped.*, peduncle; *P.I.C.A.*, posteroinferior cerebellar artery; *Suboccip.*, suboccipital; *Tr.*, trunk; *Trig.*, trigeminal; *V.*, vein; *Vel.*, velum; *Vent.*, ventricle; *Verm.*, vermian.

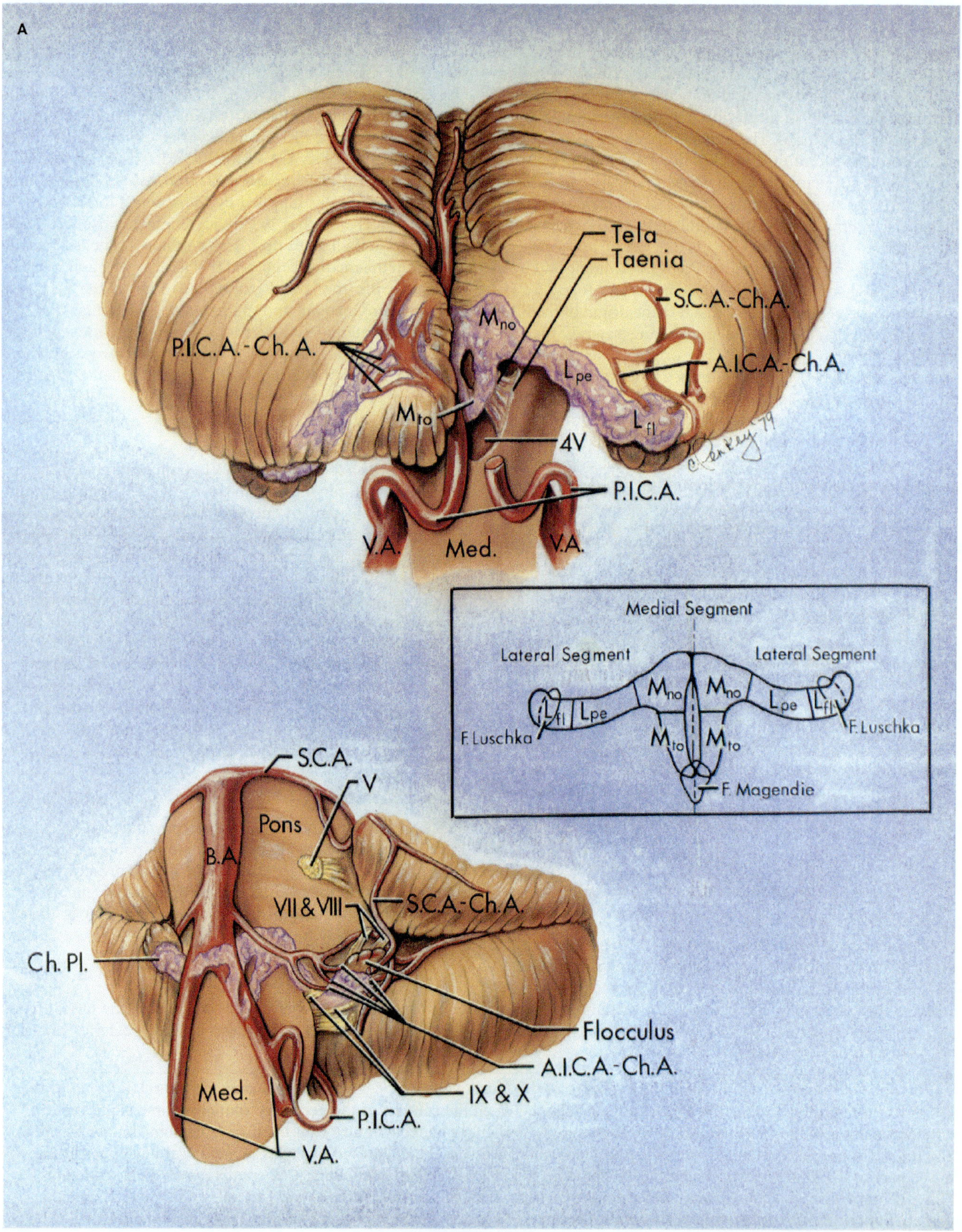
A
Tela
Taenia
S.C.A.-Ch.A.
M_{no}
P.I.C.A.-Ch. A.
L_{pe}
A.I.C.A.-Ch.A.
M_{to}
L_{fl}
4V
P.I.C.A.
V.A.
Med.
V.A.
Medial Segment
Lateral Segment
Lateral Segment
M_{no}
M_{no}
L_{fl}
L_{pe}
L_{pe}
L_{fl}
F. Luschka
F. Luschka
M_{to}
M_{to}
F. Magendie
S.C.A.
V
Pons
B.A.
VII & VIII
S.C.A.-Ch.A.
Ch. Pl.
Flocculus
A.I.C.A.-Ch.A.
IX & X
Med.
P.I.C.A.
V.A.

FIGURE 2.23A

and part of the anterior surfaces of the tonsil. If there are no branches directed predominately to the tonsil, the tonsil is supplied by the adjacent hemispheric and vermian branches.

Relationship to the cranial nerves

The PICA has the most complex relationship to the cranial nerves of any artery (27, 30, 52). The vertebral artery courses anterior to glossopharyngeal, vagus, accessory, and hypoglossal nerves, and the proximal part of the PICA passes around or between and often stretches or distorts the rootlets of these and adjacent nerves.

The inferior olive protrudes from the anterolateral surface of the medulla near the vertebral artery and the origin of the PICA (*Fig. 2.24*). The hypoglossal nerve joins the brainstem on its anterior border and the glossopharyngeal, vagus, and accessory nerves on its posterior border. Most PICAs arise at the level of the olive, but some will arise rostral or caudal to that level. The PICA origins at the level of the olive are either lateral or anterior to the olive. The PICA origin is anterior to the olive if the vertebral artery pursues its usual course anterior to the olive, but if the vertebral artery is tortuous and kinked posteriorly, the PICA origin is lateral to the olive.

Hypoglossal rootlets

The hypoglossal nerve arises as a line of rootlets that exits the brainstem along the anterior margin of the caudal two-thirds of the olive in the preolivary sulcus, a groove between the olive and the medullary pyramid (*Fig. 2.24*). The hypoglossal rootlets, in their course from the preolivary sulcus to the hypoglossal canal, pass posterior to the vertebral artery, except in the rare instance in which they pass anterior to the artery. If the vertebral artery is elongated or tortuous and courses lateral to the olive, it stretches the hypoglossal rootlets dorsally over its posterior surface. Some tortuous vertebral arteries stretch the hypoglossal rootlets so far posteriorly that they intermingle with the glossopharyngeal, vagus, and accessory nerves.

The relation of the origin and proximal part of the PICA to the hypoglossal rootlets varies markedly. The PICA arises either rostral or caudal or at the level of the hypoglossal rootlets. The majority of the PICAs arise at the level of the hypoglossal rootlets near the junction of the hypoglossal rootlets with the medulla (*Fig. 2.24*). The PICAs that arise superior or inferior to the hypoglossal rootlets usually course superior or inferior to, rather than between, the hypoglossal rootlets. The hypoglossal rootlets are frequently stretched around the origin and initial segment of the PICAs that arise at the level of the caudal two-thirds of the olive, in addition to being stretched posteriorly by the vertebral artery. About half of the PICA origins are located anterior to and half posterior to or at the level of the rostrocaudal line drawn through the exits of the hypoglossal rootlets from the medulla. The vertebral artery courses from the lateral side of the inferior part of the medulla to the anterior surface of the superior part of the medulla. Those PICAs arising inferior to the olive, arise posterior to the level of the hypoglossal rootlets if the vertebral artery at the site of origin of the PICA has not coursed far enough anterior to reach the level of the hypoglossal rootlets. The PICA origin is anterior to the hypoglossal rootlets if the vertebral artery, on reaching the hypoglossal rootlets, was anterior to the olive. The PICA origin is located at the level of or posterior to the hypoglossal rootlets if the vertebral artery at the site of origin of the PICA courses lateral to the olive and stretches the hypoglossal rootlets posteriorly.

The initial segment of the PICA has a variable course in relation to the hypoglossal rootlets. The most common course is for the PICA to arise from the vertebral artery and pass directly posteriorly around or between the hypoglossal rootlets. However, some PICAs will loop upward, downward, or laterally in front of the hypoglossal rootlets before passing posteriorly between or around them.

Glossopharyngeal, vagus, and accessory nerves

After coursing posterior to the hypoglossal rootlets, the PICA encounters the rootlets of the glossopharyngeal, vagus, and accessory nerves (*Fig. 2.25*). The glossopharyngeal, vagus, and accessory nerves arise as a line of rootlets, then exit the brainstem along the posterior edge of the olive in the retro-olivary sulcus, a shallow groove between the olive and the posterolateral surface of the medulla. The glossopharyngeal nerve arises as one or rarely two rootlets posterior to the superior third of the olive, just inferior to the pontomedullary junction and anterior to the foramen of Luschka and the rhomboid lip of the lateral recess of the fourth ventricle. The

FIGURE 2.23. *A.* Schematic illustration of choroidal arteries in the posterior fossa. *Upper*: Posterior or suboccipital view. The choroid plexus is composed of two medial and two lateral segments. Each medial segment is divided into a rostral, or nodular, and a caudal, or tonsillar, part. Each lateral segment is divided into a medial, or peduncular, and a lateral, or floccular, part. The medulla, fourth ventricle, vertebral arteries, and origin of the PICAs are below. The choroidal arteries arise from the PICA, SCA, and AICA. The choroid plexus is attached to the tela choroidea, which is attached to the taenia along the border of the floor of the fourth ventricle. *Lower*: Anterolateral view. The choroid plexus is seen through the brainstem. The AICA arises from the basilar artery and sends branches that enter the choroid plexus near the flocculus. The SCA may also send choroidal branches to the floccular part of the choroid plexus. *Right Center*: Diagram showing subdivision of the choroid plexus into medial and lateral segments. The medial segments have nodular and tonsillar parts and the lateral segments have peduncular and floccular parts. The floccular parts protrude through the foramina of Luschka, and the tonsillar parts extend through the foramen of Magendie. *A.*, artery; *A.I.C.A.*, anteroinferior cerebellar artery; *B.A.*, basilar artery; *Ch.*, choroidal; *F.*, foramen; *fl.*, floccular; *He.*, hemispheric; L., lateral; *M.*, medial; *Med.*, medulla; *no.*, nodular; *pe.*, peduncular; *P.I.C.A.*, posteroinferior cerebellar artery; *Pl.*, plexus; *S.C.A.*, superior cerebellar artery; *to.*, tonsillar; *To.*, tonsillo; *V.A.*, vertebral artery; *Ve.*, vermian.

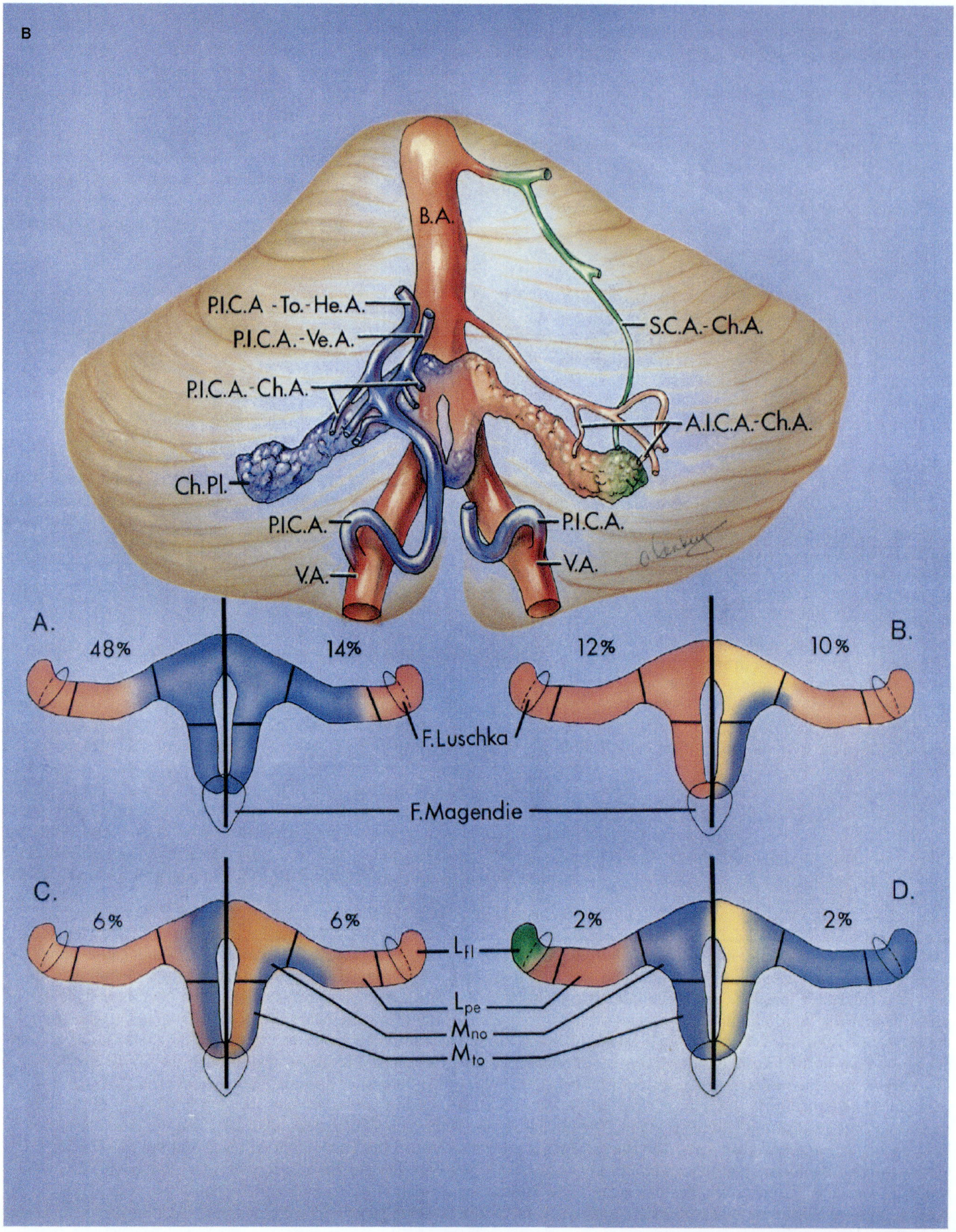
B
B.A.
P.I.C.A -To.-He.A.
P.I.C.A.-Ve.A.
P.I.C.A.-Ch.A.
S.C.A.-Ch.A.
A.I.C.A.-Ch.A.
Ch.Pl.
P.I.C.A.
P.I.C.A.
V.A.
V.A.
A.
48%
14%
12%
10%
B.
F.Luschka
F.Magendie
C.
6%
6%
2%
2%
D.
L_{Fl}
L_{pe}
M_{no}
M_{to}

FIGURE 2.23*B*.

vagus nerve arises inferior to the glossopharyngeal nerve as a line of tightly packed rootlets posterior to the superior third of the olive. The accessory nerve arises as a widely separated series of rootlets that originates from the medulla and upper cervical cord, inferior to the vagus nerve below the level of the junction of the upper and middle third of the olive. The glossopharyngeal and vagus nerves arise rostral to the level of origin of the hypoglossal rootlets. The accessory rootlets arise at both the level of and inferior to the origin of the hypoglossal rootlets.

The PICA commonly passes from the lateral to the posterior aspect of the medulla by passing between the rootlets of the glossopharyngeal, vagus, and accessory nerves. The PICA may be ascending, descending, or passing laterally, or medially or be involved in a complex loop that stretches and distorts these nerves as it passes between them. Of the 42 PICAs found in 50 cerebellae in a previous study, 16 passed between the rootlets of the accessory nerve, 10 passed between the rootlets of the vagus nerve, 13 passed between the vagus and accessory nerves, 2 passed above the glossopharyngeal nerve between the latter nerve and the vestibulocochlear nerve, and 1 passed between the glossopharyngeal and vagus nerves (30).

Facial and vestibulocochlear nerves

The facial and vestibulocochlear nerves arise superior to the glossopharyngeal nerve at the level of the pontomedullary junction. The proximal part of the PICA usually passes around the brainstem inferior to the facial and vestibulocochlear nerves. However, in some cerebellopontine angles, the proximal part of the PICA, after coursing posterior to the level of the hypoglossal rootlets, loops superiorly toward, even compressing, the facial and vestibulocochlear nerves before descending to pass between the glossopharyngeal, vagus, and accessory rootlets (*Figs. 2.11* and *2.12*).

DISCUSSION

Occlusion

The consequences of a PICA occlusion vary and may be overshadowed by the effects of occlusion of the parent vertebral artery. The effects range from a clinically silent occlusion to infarction of portions of the brainstem or cerebellum with swelling, hemorrhage, and death (53). Nearly all occlusions of the PICA, but only slightly more than half of occlusions of the vertebral artery, result in medullary or cerebellar infarction (5, 11). The incidence of medullary and cerebellar infarction in vertebral artery occlusion increases greatly if the origin of the PICA is included in the occlusion. Occlusion of the PICA is usually the result of thrombosis of a preexisting atherosclerotic stenosis and is less commonly caused by embolization (5).

Occlusion of the PICA causes an infarct in the lateral medulla, dorsal to the inferior olivary nucleus. The syndrome of occlusion of the PICA, referred to as the lateral medullary syndrome, includes ipsilateral numbness of the face caused by injury to the spinal tract of the trigeminal nerve; loss of pain and temperature on the contralateral half of the body caused by damage to the spinothalamic tract; dysphagia, dysarthria, and hoarseness as a result of homolateral weakness of the palate, pharynx, vocal cord, and occasionally the sternoclinoid muscle caused by a lesion in the nucleus ambiguis; ataxia, dizziness, vertigo, nystagmus, and homolateral cerebellar signs caused by damage to the vestibular nuclei, cerebellar tracts in the brainstem, and the cerebellum; an ipsilateral Horner's syndrome caused by disruption of the oculosympathetic fibers in the lateral medullary reticular substance; and vomiting caused by involvement of the nucleus and tractus solitarius. Other less common accompaniments include nystagmus and diplopia caused by a lesion in the dorsal medulla and the medial longitudinal fasciculus; and facial weakness caused by damage to the facial motor nucleus (10, 14, 17).

The syndrome associated with lateral medullary infarction may be caused by occlusion of either the PICA or the vertebral artery, but it is most commonly attributable to vertebral artery occlusion (14, 17). Fisher et al. noted that 75% of cases of lateral medullary syndrome were associated with a vertebral artery occlusion and that only 12% had a PICA occlusion (14). The site of the infarct with a PICA occlusion does not differ significantly from that with a vertebral artery occlusion. Symptoms, if present with the other manifestation of the lateral medullary syndrome, suggest vertebral artery rather than PICA occlusion include paresis of the trunk, limb, and tongue muscles, crossed sensory loss with dysphagia, visual loss suggesting calcarine cortex involvement, diplopia with an abducens nerve palsy, loss of hearing, or a facial palsy.

Occlusion of the branches of the PICA distal to the medullary branches produces a syndrome resembling labyrinthitis and includes rotatory dizziness, nausea, vomiting, inability to stand or walk unaided, and nystagmus without appendicular dysmetria. The dizziness, unsteadiness, and nystagmus are postulated to caused by involvement of the flocculonodular complex. The lack of brainstem signs in this syndrome indicates that the occlusion is distal to the medullary branches of the PICA. Branch occlusions are usually caused by emboli and

FIGURE 2.23. ***B.*** **Schematic illustrations of the choroid plexus of the posterior fossa showing the different patterns of blood supply.** ***Upper*****: Orienting diagram. The PICA and its plexal area of supply are shown in** ***blue*****, the AICA in** ***red*****, and the SCA in** ***green*****. The PICA divides into vermian and tonsillohemispheric branches.** ***Lower diagrams*** **(*A–D*): The size of the area supplied by the arteries arising from the AICA, PICA, and SCA is shown. Each half of the schematic diagrams shows a different pattern. Colors used to show plexal areas of supply of the different cerebellar arteries are as follows:** ***red*****: ipsilateral AICA;** ***orange*****: contralateral AICA;** ***blue*****: ipsilateral PICA;** ***yellow*****: contralateral PICA; and** ***green*****: ipsilateral SCA. (From, Fujii K, Lenkey C, Rhoton AL Jr: Microsurgical anatomy of the choroidal arteries: Fourth ventricle and cerebellopontine angles. J Neurosurg 52:504–524, 1980 [15].)**

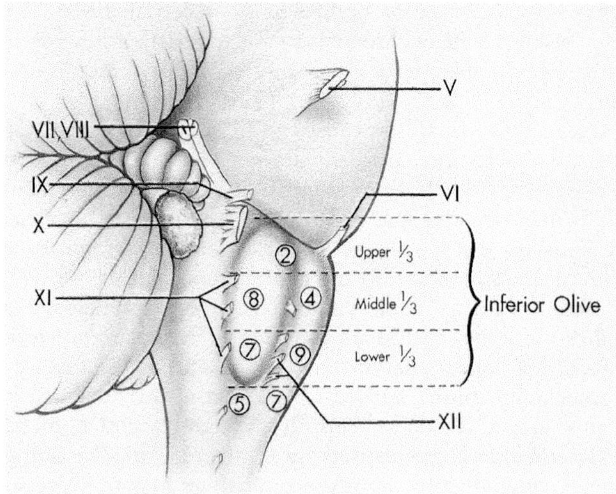

FIGURE 2.24. Lateral view of the right side of the brainstem shows the site of origin of the PICA in relation to the inferior olive and the rootlets of the hypoglossal nerve. Forty-two PICAs were found in the 50 cerebellar hemispheres we examined. The rootlets of the glossopharyngeal, vagus, and accessory nerves arose posterior to the olive. The glossopharyngeal and vagus nerves arose at the level of the upper third of the olive. The accessory rootlets arose at the level of the lower two-thirds of the olive and below. The rootlets of the hypoglossal nerve arose anterior to and slightly below the lower two-thirds of the olive. Two PICAS arose at the level of the rostral third of the olive, 12 arose at the level of the middle third, 16 arose at the level of the caudal third, and 12 arose below the olive. Twenty arose anterior to the olive, and 22 arose beside the olive. The vertebral arteries and PICA origins located beside the olive stretched the hypoglossal rootlets posteriorly because the hypoglossal rootlets always pass posterior to the vertebral artery. (From, Lister JR, Rhoton AL Jr, Matsushima T, Peace DA: Microsurgical anatomy of the posterior inferior cerebellar artery. Neurosurgery 10:170–199, 1982 [30].)

result in infarction of the suboccipital portion of the cerebellar hemisphere and vermis. Massive acute cerebellar infarction is most frequently caused by PICA or vertebral artery occlusion, with the most common site of cerebellar infarction being in the PICA territory (53).

Operative exposure

The PICA is exposed in dealing with neoplasms involving the cerebellopontine angle, foramen magnum, cervicocranial junction, clivus, jugular foramen, fourth ventricle, and cerebellum; aneurysms arising at the PICA origin, the most common site in the posterior fossa below the basilar apex, and less frequently from the distal segments (30); arterial dissections at the PICA-vertebral junction (54, 58); arteriovenous malformations, which also commonly involve the other cerebellar arteries and the brainstem as well as the cerebellum (6); posterior fossa ischemia requiring bypass because of the PICAs easy accessibility through a suboccipital craniotomy and the proximity to the occipital artery (28); anomalies at the cranio-

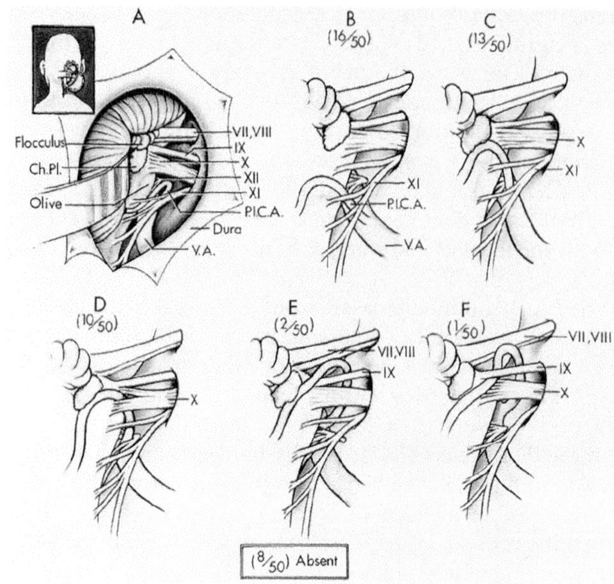

FIGURE 2.25. Relationship of the PICA to the rootlets of the glossopharyngeal, vagus, and accessory nerves. *A*, orientation of illustrations *B* through *F*. The inset shows the site of the scalp flap and the craniectomy. The large illustration shows the cerebellum retracted and the facial, vestibulocochlear, glossopharyngeal, vagus, accessory, and hypoglossal nerves. The glossopharyngeal, vagal, and accessory rootlets arise posterior to the olive, and the hypoglossal rootlets arise anterior to the olive. The choroid plexus and the flocculus project into the cerebellopontine angle posterior to the glossopharyngeal and vagus nerves. The PICA arises from the vertebral artery and passes inferior (*B* and *C*), superior (*E* and *F*), or between (*D*) the rootlets of the hypoglossal nerve. Of the 42 PICAs found in 50 cerebellar hemispheres, 16 passed between the rootlets of the accessory nerve (*B*), 13 passed between the vagus and accessory nerves (*C*), 10 passed between the rootlets of the vagus nerve (*D*), 2 passed between the glossopharyngeal and vestibulocochlear nerves (*E*), and 1 passed between the glossopharyngeal and vagus nerves (*F*). A tortuous PICA may ascend anterior to the glossopharyngeal and vagus nerves and compress and distort the facial and vestibulocochlear nerves before passing posteriorly between the glossopharyngeal, vagus, and accessory nerves (*E* and *F*). (From, Lister JR, Rhoton AL Jr, Matsushima T, Peace DA: Microsurgical anatomy of the posterior inferior cerebellar artery. Neurosurgery 10:170–199, 1982 [30].)

cervical junction, like the Chiari malformation and osseous deformities; and dysfunction of the lower cranial nerves like glossopharyngeal neuralgia (21, 23, 24, 29, 42).

The PICA can arise outside the dura, and at any point from along the intradural course of the vertebral artery. The origin can be located along the lateral side of the medulla, if the artery arises near the passage of the vertebral artery through the dura, or in front of the brainstem, if the origin is high near the vertebrobasilar junction. Exposing a low-lying PICA origin, either extra- or immediately intradurally, at the level of the foramen magnum can be achieved by a midline suboccipital or a far-lateral approach. If an artery with a low-lying origin has to be followed upward into the cerebellopontine angle or there is a need to mobilize the site of the vertebral artery's passage through the dura, a far-lateral or transcondylar modification approach are to be considered. A retrosigmoid craniotomy may be sufficient to expose a PICA arising from the midportion of the vertebral artery on the lateral side of the brainstem in the lower part of the cerebellopontine angle. If there is a need to expose the origin deep in the midline near the vertebrobasilar junction, a supra-infratentorial presigmoid approach with some added degree of labyrinth resection may be required, depending on the depth of the PICA origin and the pathology. A midline suboccipital craniectomy, possibly combined with removal of the posterior atlantal arch, is usually sufficient to expose pathology involving the tonsillomedullary and telovelotonsillar segments of the artery. Lesions involving the PICA in the walls in the fourth ventricle, vermis, and paravermian areas are usually exposed by a midline suboccipital approach. Lesions involving the hemispheric branch can be exposed through a vertical suboccipital incision and craniotomy centered over the pathology. The anatomy of PICA compression of the lower cranial nerves and medulla is reviewed in the section on the cerebellopontine angle.

Reprint requests: Albert L. Rhoton, Jr., M.D., Department of Neurological Surgery, University of Florida Brain Institute, P.O. Box 100265, 100 South Newell Drive, Building 59, L2-100, Gainesville, FL 32610-0265.

REFERENCES

1. Adachi B: *Das Artieriensystem der Japaner*. Kyoto, Kaiserlich-Japanische Universität, 1928, vol I, p 123.
2. Adams RD: Occlusion of the anterior inferior cerebellar artery. **Arch Neurol Psychiatry** 49:765–770, 1943.
3. Atkinson WJ: The anterior inferior cerebellar artery. **J Neurol Neurosurg Psychiatry** 12:137–151, 1949.
4. Burns JB, Hoffman JC, Brylski JR: Posterior inferior cerebellar artery in fourth ventricular dilatation. **Acta Radiol Diagn (Stockh)** 13:58–65, 1972.
5. Castaigne P, Lhermitte F, Gautier JC, Escourolle R, Derouesné C, Der Agopian P, Popa C: Arterial occlusions in the vertebro-basilar system: A study of 44 patients with post-mortem data. **Brain** 96:133–154, 1973.
6. Chou SN, Erickson DL, Ortiz-Suarez HJ: Surgical treatment of vascular lesions in the brain stem. **J Neurosurg** 42:23–31, 1975.
7. Dandy WE: Concerning the cause of trigeminal neuralgia. **Am J Surg** 24:447–455, 1934.
8. Dinsdale H, Logue V: Ruptured posterior fossa aneurysms and their surgical treatment. **J Neurol Neurosurg Psychiatry** 22:202–217, 1959.
9. Drake CG: Surgical removal of arteriovenous malformations from the brain stem and cerebellopontine angle. **J Neurosurg** 43:661–670, 1975.
10. Duncan GW, Parker SW, Fisher CM: Acute cerebellar infarction in the PICA territory. **Arch Neurol** 32:364–368, 1975.
11. Feely MP: Cerebellar infarction. **Neurosurgery** 4:7–11, 1979.
12. Fine AD, Cardoso A, Rhoton AL Jr: Microsurgical anatomy of the extracranial-extradural origin of the posterior inferior cerebellar artery. **J Neurosurg** 91:645–652, 1999.
13. Fisch U: The surgical anatomy of the so-called internal auditory artery, in *Proceedings of the Tenth Nobel Symposium on Disorders of the Skull Base Region*. Stockholm, Almqvist and Wiksell, pp 121–130, 1968.
14. Fisher CM, Karnes WE, Kubik CS: Lateral medullary infarction: The pattern of vascular occlusion. **J Neuropathol Exp Neurol** 20:323–379, 1961.
15. Fujii K, Lenkey C, Rhoton AL Jr: Microsurgical anatomy of the choroidal arteries: Fourth ventricle and cerebellopontine angles. **J Neurosurg** 52:504–524, 1980.
16. Gardner WJ: Concerning the mechanism of trigeminal neuralgia and hemifacial spasm. **J Neurosurg** 19:947–958, 1962.
17. Goodhart SP, Davison C: Syndrome of the posterior inferior and anterior inferior cerebellar arteries and their branches. **Arch Neurol Psychiatry** 35:501–524, 1936.
18. Hardy DG, Rhoton AL Jr: Microsurgical relationships of the superior cerebellar artery and the trigeminal nerve. **J Neurosurg** 49:669–678, 1978.
19. Hardy DG, Peace DA, Rhoton AL Jr: Microsurgical anatomy of the superior cerebellar artery. **Neurosurgery** 6:10–28, 1980.
20. Huang YP, Wolf BS: Angiographic features of fourth ventricle tumors with special reference to the posterior inferior cerebellar artery. **AJR Am J Roentgenol** 107:543–564, 1969.
21. Jannetta PJ: Neurovascular cross-compression in patients with hyperactive dysfunction symptoms of the eighth cranial nerve. **Surg Forum** 26:467–469, 1975.
22. Jannetta PJ: Microsurgical approach to the trigeminal nerve for tic douloureux. **Prog Neurol Surg** 7:180–200, 1976.
23. Jannetta PJ, Gendell HM: Clinical observations on etiology of essential hypertension. **Surg Forum** 30:431–432, 1979.
24. Jannetta PJ, Abbassy M, Maroon JC, Ramos FM, Albin MS: Etiology and definitive microsurgical treatment of hemifacial spasm: Operative techniques and results in 47 patients. **J Neurosurg** 47:321–328, 1977.
25. Johnson JH, Kline DG: Anterior inferior cerebellar artery aneurysms: Case report. **J Neurosurg** 48:455–460, 1978.
26. Kaplan HA, Ford DH: Arteria cerebelli inferior posterior, in *The Brain Vascular System*. Amsterdam, Elsevier, 1966, pp 93–95.
27. Katsuta T, Rhoton AL Jr, Matsushima T: The jugular foramen: Microsurgical anatomy and operative approaches. **Neurosurgery** 41:149–202, 1997.
28. Khodadad G, Singh RS, Olinger CP: Possible prevention of brain stem stroke by microvascular anastomosis in the vertebrobasilar system. **Stroke** 8:316–321, 1977.
29. Laha RK, Jannetta PJ: Glossopharyngeal neuralgia. **J Neurosurg** 47:316–320, 1977.
30. Lister JR, Rhoton AL Jr, Matsushima T, Peace DA: Microsurgical anatomy of the posterior inferior cerebellar artery. **Neurosurgery** 10:170–199, 1982.
31. Locksley HB: Report on the cooperative study of intracranial aneurysms and subarachnoid hemorrhage: Section V, Part II—Natural history of subarachnoid hemorrhage, intracranial aneurysms and arteriovenous malformations. **J Neurosurg** 25:321–368, 1966.
32. Luhan JA, Pollack SL: Occlusion of the superior cerebellar artery. **Neurology** 3:77–89, 1953.
33. Margolis MT, Newton TH: The posterior inferior cerebellar artery, in Newton TH, Potts DG (eds): *Radiology of the Skull and Brain, Angiography*. St. Louis, C.V. Mosby, 1974, vol 2, book 2, pp 1710–1774.
34. Martin RG, Grant JL, Peace DA, Theiss C, Rhoton AL Jr: Microsurgical relationships of the anterior inferior cerebellar artery and the facial-vestibulocochlear nerve complex. **Neurosurgery** 6:483–507, 1980.

35. Matsushima T, Rhoton AL Jr, Lenkey C: Microsurgery of the fourth ventricle: Part I—Microsurgical anatomy. **Neurosurgery** 11:631–667, 1982.
36. Mazzoni A: Internal auditory canal: Arterial relations at the porus acusticus. **Ann Otol Rhinol Laryngol** 78:797–814, 1969.
37. Mazzoni A, Hansen CC: Surgical anatomy of the arteries of the internal auditory canal. **Arch Otolaryngol** 91:128–135, 1970.
38. Megret M: A landmark for the choroidal arteries of the fourth ventricle: Branches of the posterior inferior cerebellar artery. **Neuroradiology** 5:85–90, 1973.
39. Mount LA: Arteriovenous angioma derived from the anterior inferior cerebellar artery: Its diagnosis and treatment. **J Neurosurg** 22:612–615, 1965.
40. Nager GT: Origins and relations of the internal auditory artery and the subarcuate artery. **Ann Otol Rhinol Laryngol** 63:51–61, 1954.
41. Ono M, Ono M, Rhoton AL Jr, Barry M: Microsurgical anatomy of the region of the tentorial incisura. **J Neurosurg** 60:365–399, 1984.
42. Ouaknine GE, Robert F, Molina-Negro P, Hardy J: Geniculate neuralgia and audio-vestibular disturbances due to compression of the intermediate and eighth nerves by the postero-inferior cerebellar artery. **Surg Neurol** 13:147–150, 1980.
43. Pait TG, Zeal A, Harris FS, Paullus WS, Rhoton AL Jr: Microsurgical anatomy and dissection of the temporal bone. **Surg Neurol** 8:363–391, 1977.
44. Perret G, Nishioka H: Report on the cooperative study of intracranial aneurysms and subarachnoid hemorrhage: Section VI—Arteriovenous malformations. **J Neurosurg** 25:467–490, 1966.
45. Rhoton AL Jr: Microsurgical anatomy of posterior fossa cranial nerves, in Barrow DL (ed): *Surgery of the Cranial Nerves of the Posterior Fossa: Neurosurgical Topics*. Chicago, AANS, 1993, pp 1–103.
46. Russel DS, Rubinstein LJ: *Pathology of Tumors of the Nervous System*. Baltimore, Williams & Wilkins, 1977, p 368.
47. Saeki N, Rhoton AL Jr: Microsurgical anatomy of the upper basilar artery and the posterior circle of Willis. **J Neurosurg** 46:563–578, 1977.
48. Salamon G, Huang YP: *Radiologic Anatomy of the Brain*. Berlin, Springer-Verlag, 1976, pp 305–306.
49. Stephens RB, Stilwell DL: *Arteries and Veins of the Human Brain*. Springfield, Charles C Thomas, 1969, pp 72–73, 95–96.
50. Stopford JSB: The arteries of the pons and medulla oblongata. **J Anat** 50:131–164, 1916.
51. Sunderland S: The arterial relations of the internal auditory meatus. **Brain** 68:23–27, 1945.
52. Sunderland S: Neurovascular relations and anomalies at the base of the brain. **J Neurol Neurosurg Psychiatry** 2:243–257, 1948.
53. Sypert GW, Alvord EC Jr: Cerebellar infarction: A clinicopathological study. **Arch Neurol** 32:357–363, 1975.
54. Waga S, Fujimoto K, Morooka Y: Dissecting aneurysm of the vertebral artery. **Surg Neurol** 10:237–239, 1978.
55. Warwick R, Williams PL: *Gray's Anatomy*. Philadelphia, W.B. Saunders Co., 1973, ed 35, pp 643–644.
56. Watt JC, McKillop AN: Relation of arteries to roots of nerves in posterior cranial fossa in man. **Arch Surg** 30:336–345, 1935.
57. Wolf BS, Newman CM, Khilnani MT: The posterior inferior cerebellar artery on vertebral angiography. **AJR Am J Roentgenol** 87:322–337, 1962.
58. Yonas H, Agamanolis D, Takaoka Y, White RJ: Dissecting intracranial aneurysms. **Surg Neurol** 8:407–415, 1977.
59. Zeal AA, Rhoton AL Jr: Microsurgical anatomy of the posterior cerebral artery. **J Neurosurg** 48:534–559, 1978.

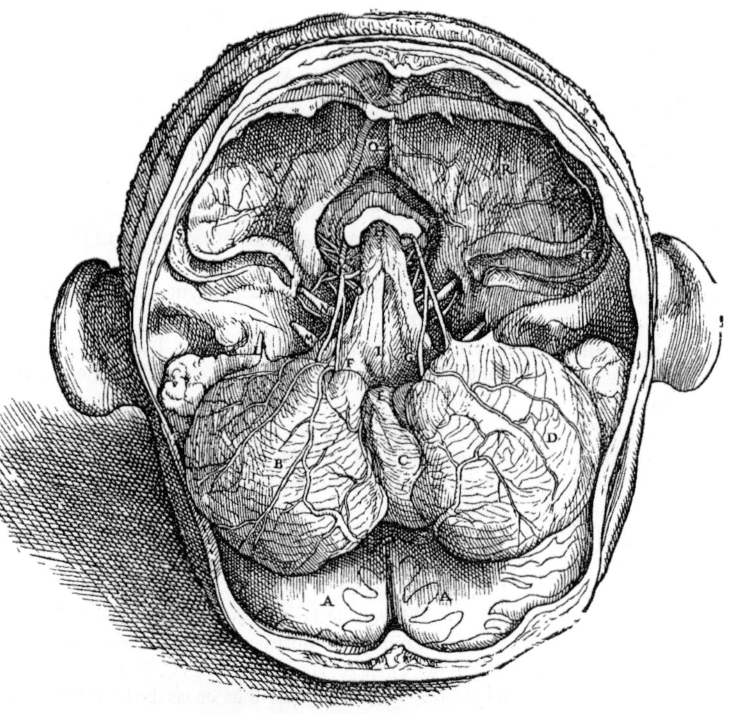

Cranial floor, cerebellum, and brain stem, from, Andreas Vesalius, *De Humani Corporis Fabrica*. Basel, Ex officina Ioannis Oporini, 1543. Courtesy, Rare Book Room, Norris Medical Library, Keck School of Medicine, Los Angeles, California.

CHAPTER 3

The Posterior Fossa Veins

Albert L. Rhoton, Jr., M.D.

Department of Neurological Surgery, University of Florida, Gainesville, Florida

Key words: Anatomic study, Brainstem, Cerebellum, Posterior fossa, Veins

The veins of the posterior fossa are divided into four groups: superficial, deep, brainstem, and bridging veins. The superficial veins are divided on the basis of which of the three cortical surfaces they drain; the tentorial surface is drained by the superior hemispheric and superior vermian veins, the suboccipital surface is drained by the inferior hemispheric and inferior vermian veins; and the petrosal surface is drained by the anterior hemispheric veins (15, 16). The deep veins course in the three fissures between the cerebellum and the brainstem and on the three cerebellar peduncles. The major deep veins in the fissures between the cerebellum and brainstem are the veins of the cerebellomesencephalic, cerebellomedullary, and cerebellopontine fissures, and those on the cerebellar peduncles are the veins of the superior, middle, and inferior cerebellar peduncles. The veins of the brainstem are named on the basis of whether they drain the midbrain, pons, or medulla and course transversely or horizontally. The veins of the posterior fossa terminate as bridging veins, which collect into three groups: a galenic group that drains into the vein of Galen; a petrosal group that drains into the petrosal sinuses; and a tentorial group that drains into the tentorial sinuses, which empty into the transverse, straight, or superior petrosal sinus (*Figs. 3.1* and *3.2*).

THE POSTERIOR FOSSA VEINS

Superficial veins

The superficial veins drain the cortical surfaces of the cerebellum. They are divided on the basis of whether they drain the tentorial, petrosal, or suboccipital surface and whether they drain the hemisphere or vermis. The tentorial surface is drained by the superior hemispheric and the superior vermian veins; the suboccipital surface is drained by the inferior hemispheric and the inferior vermian veins; and the petrosal surface is drained by the anterior hemispheric veins. In addition, selected cortical veins may be named on the basis of the vermian or hemispheric lobule that they drain, or on the basis of the fissure in which they course. The superficial tonsillar veins are also included in this group.

Deep veins

The deep veins course in the three deep fissures between the cerebellum and brainstem near the roof and walls of the fourth ventricle and on the three cerebellar peduncles that course within these fissures. The vein of the cerebellomesencephalic fissure arises in the cerebellomesencephalic fissure and is intimately related to the superior half of the roof; the vein of the cerebellomedullary fissure courses in the cerebellomedullary fissure, and is intimately related to the inferior half of the roof; and the vein of the cerebellopontine fissure courses in the cerebellopontine fissure is intimately related to the lateral recess and lateral walls of the fourth ventricle.

The major veins on the surface of the three cerebellar peduncles also course within these fissures. The vein of the superior cerebellar peduncle courses on the posterior surface of the superior cerebellar peduncle in the cerebellomesencephalic fissure; the vein of the inferior cerebellar peduncle ascends on the posterior surface of the inferior cerebellar peduncle in the cerebellomedullary fissure; and the vein of the middle cerebellar peduncle ascends on the lateral surface of the middle cerebellar peduncle in the anterior part of the cerebellopontine fissure. The deep tonsillar veins are also included in this group.

Veins of the brainstem

The veins of the brainstem are named on the basis of three characteristics: the subdivision of the brainstem drained (mesencephalon, pons, or medulla); the surface of the brainstem drained (median anterior, lateral anterior, etc.); and the direction in which they course (transverse or longitudinal).

The longitudinally oriented veins are the median anterior pontomesencephalic and the median anterior medullary veins, which course in the midline; the lateral anterior pontomesencephalic and the lateral anterior medullary veins, which course on the anterolateral surface of the brainstem; and the lateral medullary and the lateral mesencephalic veins, which course on the lateral surface of the brainstem. The transversely oriented veins running in the sulci at the junctions of the pons and mesencephalon and the pons and medulla are the veins of the pontomesencephalic and the pontomedullary sulci. The transverse pontine and transverse medullary veins course across the anterior and

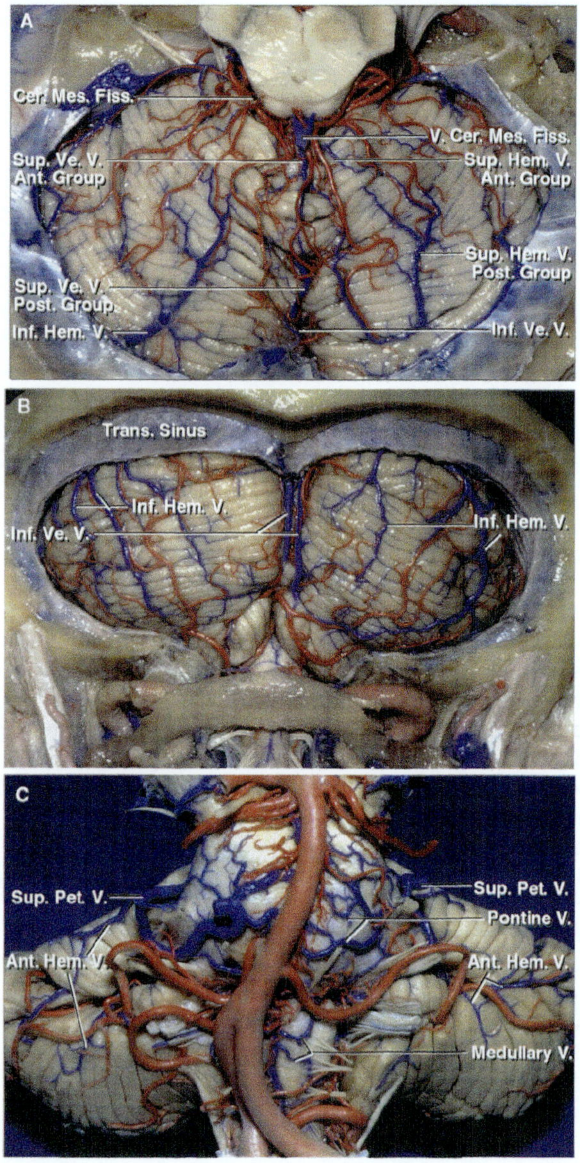

FIGURE 3.1. Drainage patterns of the cerebellar surfaces. *A*, tentorial surface. The tentorial surface is drained by the superior hemispheric and superior vermian veins, which are divided into an anterior and a posterior group. The anterior group and the veins from the cerebellomesencephalic fissure empty predominantly into the vein of Galen and its tributaries. The posterior group drains the posterior part of the tentorial surface and empties into the tentorial sinuses, which are tributaries of the straight, transverse, or superior petrosal sinus, or the torcula. Some of the inferior hemispheric veins from the suboccipital surface pass forward under the transverse sinus and cross the posterior part of the tentorial surface to empty into the tentorial sinuses. *B*, suboccipital surface. The suboccipital surface is drained by the inferior hemispheric and inferior vermian veins, which ascend toward the transverse sinus, but then turn forward below the sinus and commonly empty into the tentorial sinuses. Some of the inferior hemispheric veins from the suboccipital surface empty into the inferior vermian veins, which in turn empty into the tentorial sinuses. *C*, petrosal surface and anterior surface of the brainstem. The anterior hemispheric veins, which drain the petrosal surface, and the veins from the brainstem commonly unite to form the superior petrosal veins that empty into the superior petrosal sinus. *Ant.*, anterior; *Cer. Mes.*, cerebellomesencephalic; *Fiss.*, fissure; *Hem.*, hemispheric; *Inf.*, inferior; *Pet.*, petrosal; *Post.*, posterior; *Sup.*, superior; *Trans.*, transverse; *V.*, vein; *Ve.*, vermian.

lateral surfaces of the pons and medulla, and the peduncular veins pass around the cerebral peduncles.

Bridging veins and major draining groups

The terminal ends of veins draining the brainstem and cerebellum form bridging veins that cross the subarachnoid and subdural spaces to reach the venous sinuses in the dura (3, 6, 20, 21, 25). These bridging veins collect into three groups: a superior or galenic group that drains into the vein of Galen; an anterior or petrosal group that drains into the petrosal sinuses; and a posterior or tentorial group that drains into the sinuses converging on the torcula.

An outline of the veins is as follows (*Fig. 3.3*):

I. Superficial Veins
  A. Tentorial surface
    1. Superior vermian veins
    2. Superior hemispheric veins
  B. Suboccipital surface
    1. Inferior vermian veins
    2. Inferior hemispheric veins
    3. Retrotonsillar veins
    4. Medial and lateral tonsillar veins
  C. Petrosal surface
    1. Anterior hemispheric veins
II. Deep Veins
  A. Cerebellomesencephalic fissure
    1. Vein of superior cerebellar peduncle
    2. Vein of cerebellomesencephalic fissure
    3. Pontotrigeminal vein
    4. Tectal veins
  B. Cerebellomedullary fissure
    1. Vein of cerebellomedullary fissure
    2. Vein of inferior cerebellar peduncle
    3. Supratonsillar veins
    4. Choroidal veins
  C. Cerebellopontine fissure
    1. Vein of cerebellopontine fissure
    2. Vein of middle cerebellar peduncle
III. Veins of the Brainstem
  A. Longitudinal veins
    1. Midline
      a. Median anterior pontomesencephalic vein
      b. Median anterior medullary vein
    2. Anterolateral
      a. Lateral anterior pontomesencephalic vein
      b. Lateral anterior medullary vein

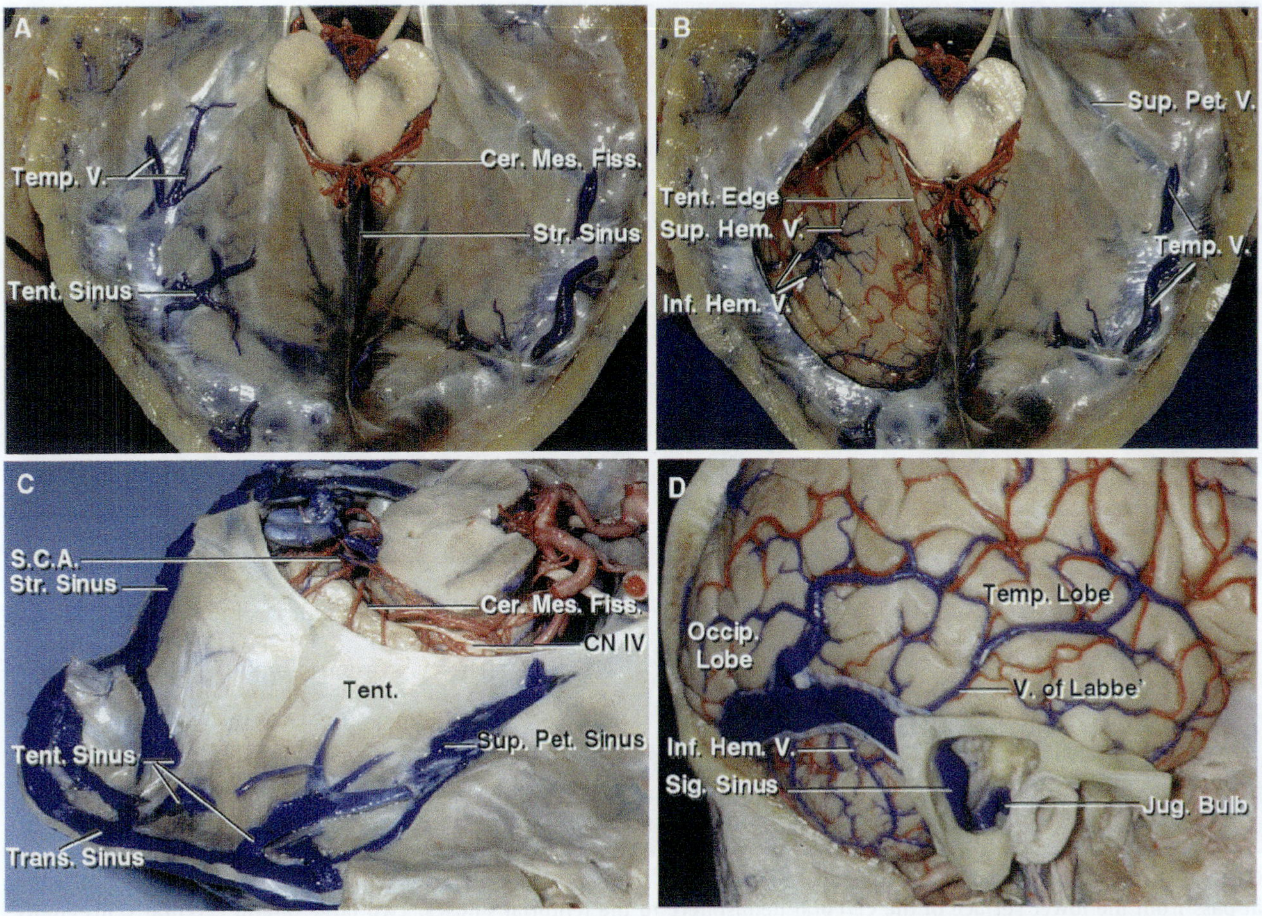

FIGURE 3.2. *A–D.* Venous drainage of the posterior fossa. *A,* superior surface of the tentorium. Some of the tentorial sinuses can be seen through the tentorial surface. Veins from both the cerebrum and cerebellum empty into the tentorial sinuses. The veins in the quadrigeminal cistern and the cerebellomesencephalic fissure empty into the vein of Galen and its tributaries. *B,* the left half of the tentorium has been removed while preserving the tentorial edge. The inferior hemispheric veins from the suboccipital surface cross the posterior part of the tentorial surface to empty into one of the tentorial sinuses with some of the superior hemispheric veins. Two veins from the right posterior temporal lobe empty into the transverse sinus. *C,* superolateral view of the tentorium. A complex and variable group of venous sinuses course within the tentorium and empty into the straight, transverse, and superior petrosal sinuses. The veins draining the suboccipital surface and posterior part of the tentorial surface empty into the tentorial sinuses. The majority of veins from the upper part of the tentorial surface drain toward the cerebellomesencephalic fissure and empty into tributaries of the vein of Galen. Some veins from the lateral part of the tentorial surface may empty into the superior petrosal sinus. *D,* lateral cerebral and cerebellar surfaces. The sinuses in the tentorium receive drainage from both the cerebrum and cerebellum. Veins from the lateral and inferior surfaces of the cerebral hemisphere pass toward, but often turn medially above the transverse sinus to join the tentorium sinuses that empty into the transverse sinus. The inferior hemispheric veins from the suboccipital surface ascend toward, but often pass below the transverse sinus to empty into the tentorial sinuses. A mastoidectomy has been completed to expose the sigmoid sinus and jugular bulb. *Cer.,* cerebellar; *Cer. Mes.,* cerebellomesencephalic; *Cist.,* cistern; *CN,* cranial nerve; *Fiss.,* fissure; *Hem.,* hemispheric; *Inf.,* inferior; *Int.,* internal; *Jug.,* jugular; *Occip.,* occipital; *Ped.,* peduncle; *Pet.,* petrosal; *Quad.,* quadrigeminal; *S.C.A.,* superior cerebellar artery; *Sig.,* sigmoid; *Str.,* straight; *Sup.,* superior; *Temp.,* temporal; *Tent.,* tentorial; *Trans.,* transverse; *V.,* vein.

3. Lateral
   a. Lateral mesencephalic vein
   b. Lateral medullary and retro-olivary veins

B. Transverse Veins
   1. Peduncular vein
   2. Posterior communicating vein
   3. Vein of pontomesencephalic sulcus
   4. Transverse pontine veins
   5. Vein of pontomedullary sulcus
   6. Transverse medullary vein

IV. Bridging Veins (Major Draining Groups)
   A. Galenic group (to vein of Galen)
   B. Tentorial group (to torcula and tentorial sinuses)
   C. Petrosal group (to petrosal sinuses)
   D. Other bridging veins

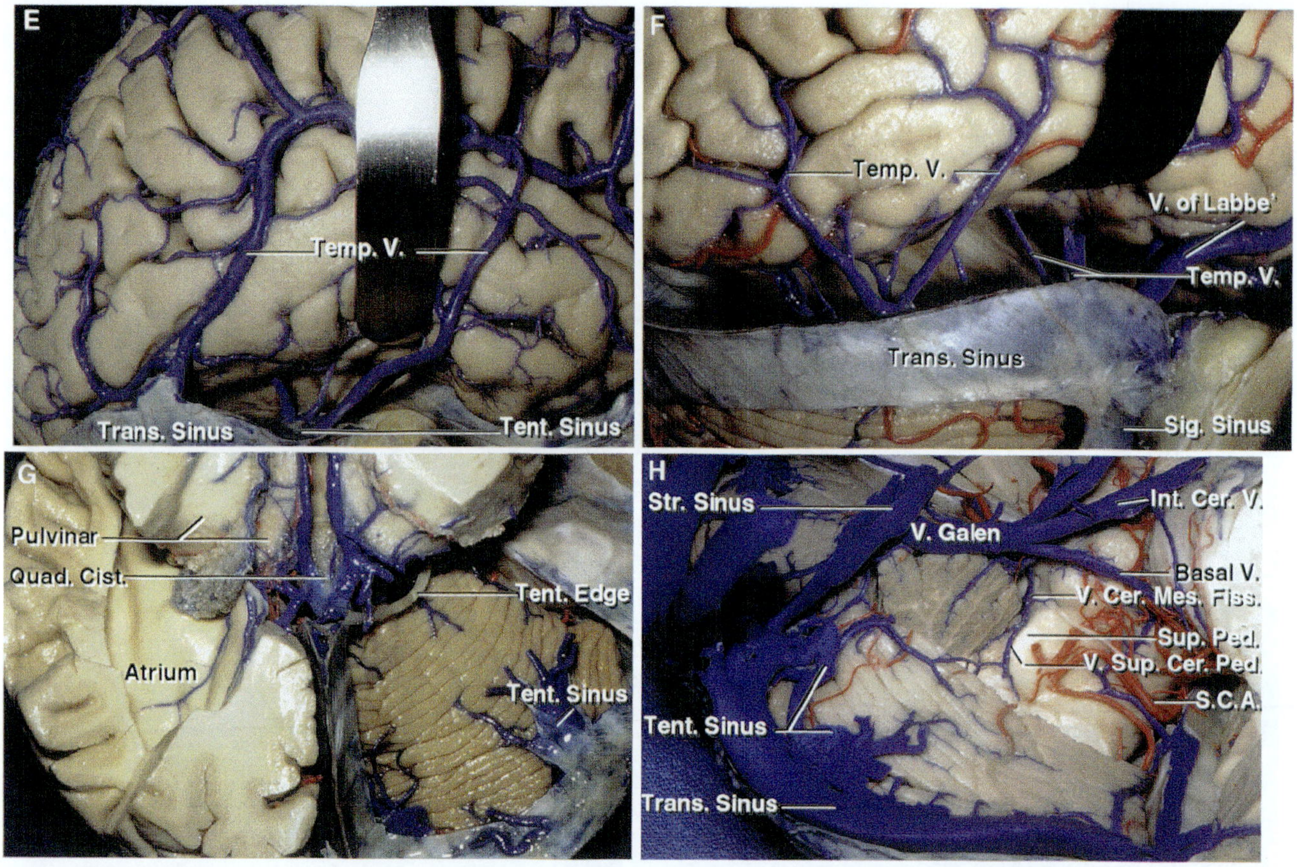

FIGURE 3.2. ***E–H.*** **Venous drainage of the posterior fossa.** ***E,*** **the temporal lobe has been elevated to show a group of veins that pass from the lower surface of the cerebral hemisphere to the tentorial sinuses. Two large lateral cerebral veins empty into the right transverse sinus, but the more medial veins exposed by eliminating the temporal lobe empty into tentorial sinuses.** ***F,*** **the posterior part of the right temporal lobe has been elevated to show the complex of veins on the inferior surface of the hemisphere that empty into the tentorial sinuses.** ***G,*** **the right half of the tentorium has been opened while preserving a large tentorial sinus, which receives drainage from the cerebrum and cerebellum. The temporal and occipital lobes have been preserved on the left side.** ***H,*** **the posterior lip of the cerebellomesencephalic fissure has been removed. The paired veins of the superior cerebellar peduncle ascend to join and form the vein of the cerebellomesencephalic fissure, which empties into the vein of Galen.**

SUPERFICIAL VEINS

The superficial veins drain the tentorial, suboccipital, and petrosal surfaces. Each surface has the vermis in the midline and the hemispheres laterally, and is divided by a major fissure named on the basis of the surface that it divides (*Figs. 3.1* and *3.3*).

The three surfaces are separated by borders that are parallel to the major venous sinuses surrounding the cerebellum. The tentorial and petrosal surfaces are separated by a border that parallels the superior petrosal sinus; the tentorial and suboccipital surfaces are separated by a border that parallels the transverse sinus; and the suboccipital and petrosal surfaces are separated by a border that parallels the sigmoid sinus. The veins from adjoining surfaces frequently join near these borders to form common trunks that terminate in a dural sinus. The veins from adjoining surfaces often anastomose across these borders. These anastomoses often take place in the fissures between the folia, which are continuous from one surface to the other. The hemispheric lobules and interfolial fissures on the tentorial surface overlap onto the superior part of the petrosal surface, and those on the suboccipital surface overlap onto the inferior part of the petrosal surface.

The cortical surfaces are drained by a mixture of longitudinal and transverse veins. On some surfaces the predominant drainage is transversely oriented along the interfolial fissures, and on others the major drainage is longitudinally oriented at right angles to these fissures. The veins within the interfolial fissures may not be visible on the cortical surface.

Tentorial surface

The tentorial surface drained by the superior hemispheric and superior vermian veins, conforms to the lower surface of the tentorium (*Figs. 3.1-3.5*).

Superior vermian veins

The veins that drain the vermian part of the tentorial surface are divided into an anterior group, which ascends toward

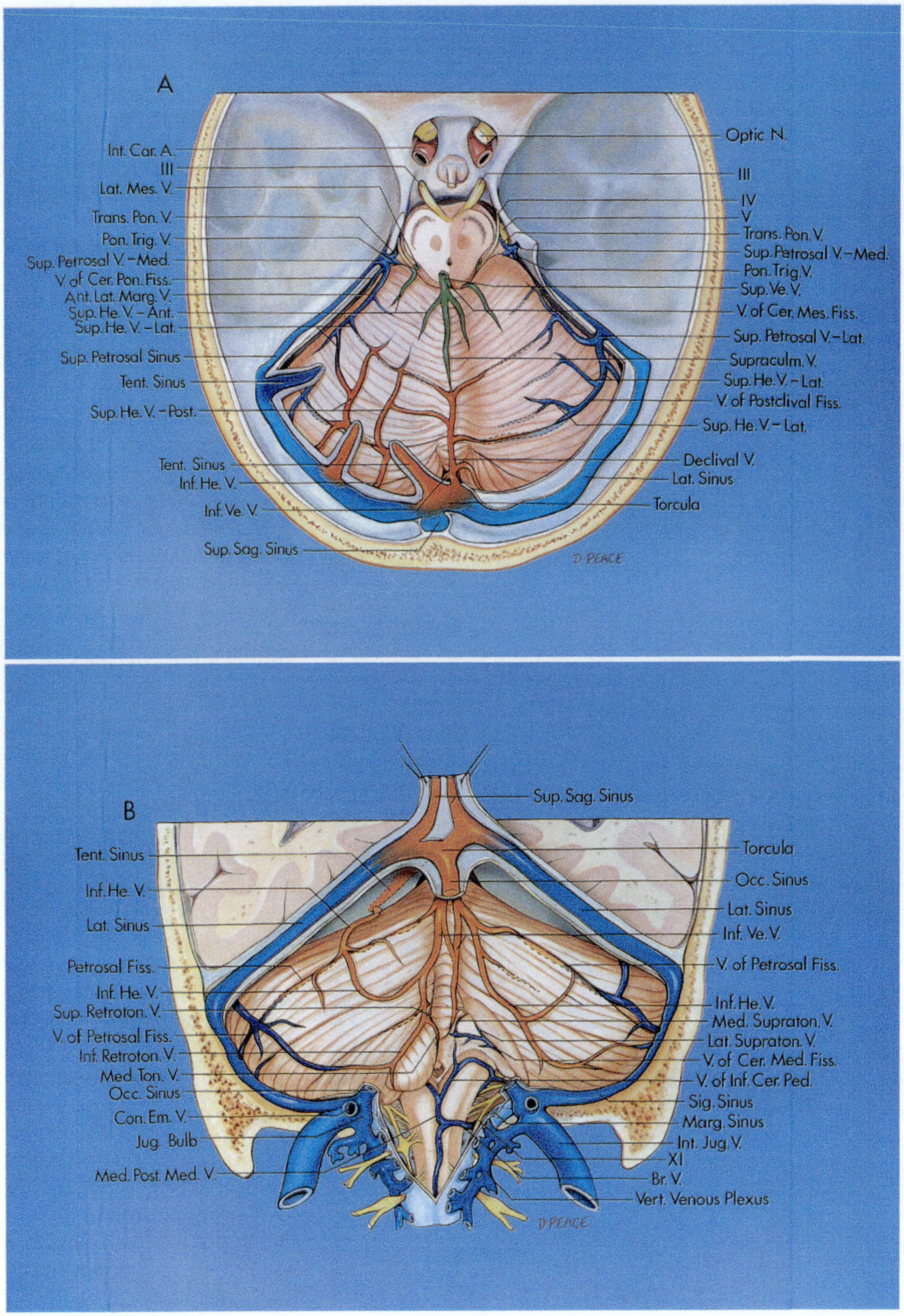

FIGURE 3.3. ***A*** **and** ***B.*** **Veins of the posterior fossa. The veins in the posterior are divided into three groups: a galenic group** ***(green)*** **that drains into the vein of Galen; a petrosal group** ***(blue)*** **that drains into the petrosal sinuses; and a tentorial group** ***(brown)*** **that drains into the sinuses near the torcula.** ***A,*** **tentorial surface, superior view. The tentorium has been removed except in the area of the tentorial sinuses.** ***B,*** **suboccipital surface, posterior view. The right tonsil and the medial part of the biventral lobule have been removed to expose the structures on the ventral wall of the cerebellomedullary fissure.** ***A.,*** **artery;** ***Ant.,*** **anterior;** ***Bas.,*** **basilar;** ***Br.,*** **bridging;** ***Car.,*** **carotid;** ***Cav.,*** **cavernous;** ***Cer.,*** **cerebellar, cerebello, cerebral;** ***Cer. Mes.,*** **cerebellomesencephalic;** ***Ch.,*** **choroidal;** ***Com.,*** **communicating;** ***Con.,*** **condylar;** ***Em.,*** **emissary;** ***Fiss.,*** **fissure;** ***He.,*** **hemispheric;** ***Inf.,*** **inferior;** ***Int.,*** **internal;** ***Jug.,*** **jugular;** ***Lat.,*** **lateral;** ***Lig.,*** **ligament;** ***Marg.,*** **marginal;** ***Med.,*** **medial, medullary;** ***Mes.,*** **mesencephalic;** ***Mid.,*** **mid, middle;** ***N.,*** **nerve;** ***Occ.,*** **occipital;** ***Olf.,*** **olfactory;** ***Ped.,*** **peduncle;** ***Pon.,*** **pontine;** ***Post.,*** **posterior;** ***Retroton.,*** **retrotonsillar;** ***Sag.,*** **sagittal;** ***Sig.,*** **sigmoid;** ***Str.,*** **straight;** ***Sulc.,*** **sulcus;** ***Sup.,*** **superior;** ***Supraculm.,*** **supraculminate;** ***Supraton.,*** **supratonsillar;** ***Tent.,*** **tentorial;** ***Ton.,*** **tonsillar;** ***Trans.,*** **transverse;** ***Trig.,*** **trigeminal;** ***V.,*** **vein;** ***Ve.,*** **vermian;** ***Vel.,*** **velum;** ***Vert.,*** **vertebral.**

the vein of Galen, and a posterior group, which descends toward the torcula (*Figs. 3.3-3.5*). The anterior, or ascending, veins originate near the tentorial fissure and join near the apex of the cerebellum to form the superior vermian vein that crosses the quadrigeminal cistern to reach the vein of Galen. The major tributaries of the superior vermian veins are the vein of the cerebellomesencephalic fissure, to be described later; the tectal veins from the quadrigeminal plate; and the hemispheric branches from the medial part of the hemisphere. The posterior, or descending, superior vermian veins originate in or near the tentorial fissure, course posteriorly, and drain alone or after joining the inferior vermian veins into the torcula or a tentorial sinus.

Superior hemispheric veins

These veins are divided into larger anterior and posterior groups and a smaller lateral group (*Figs. 3.3-3.5*). The veins in

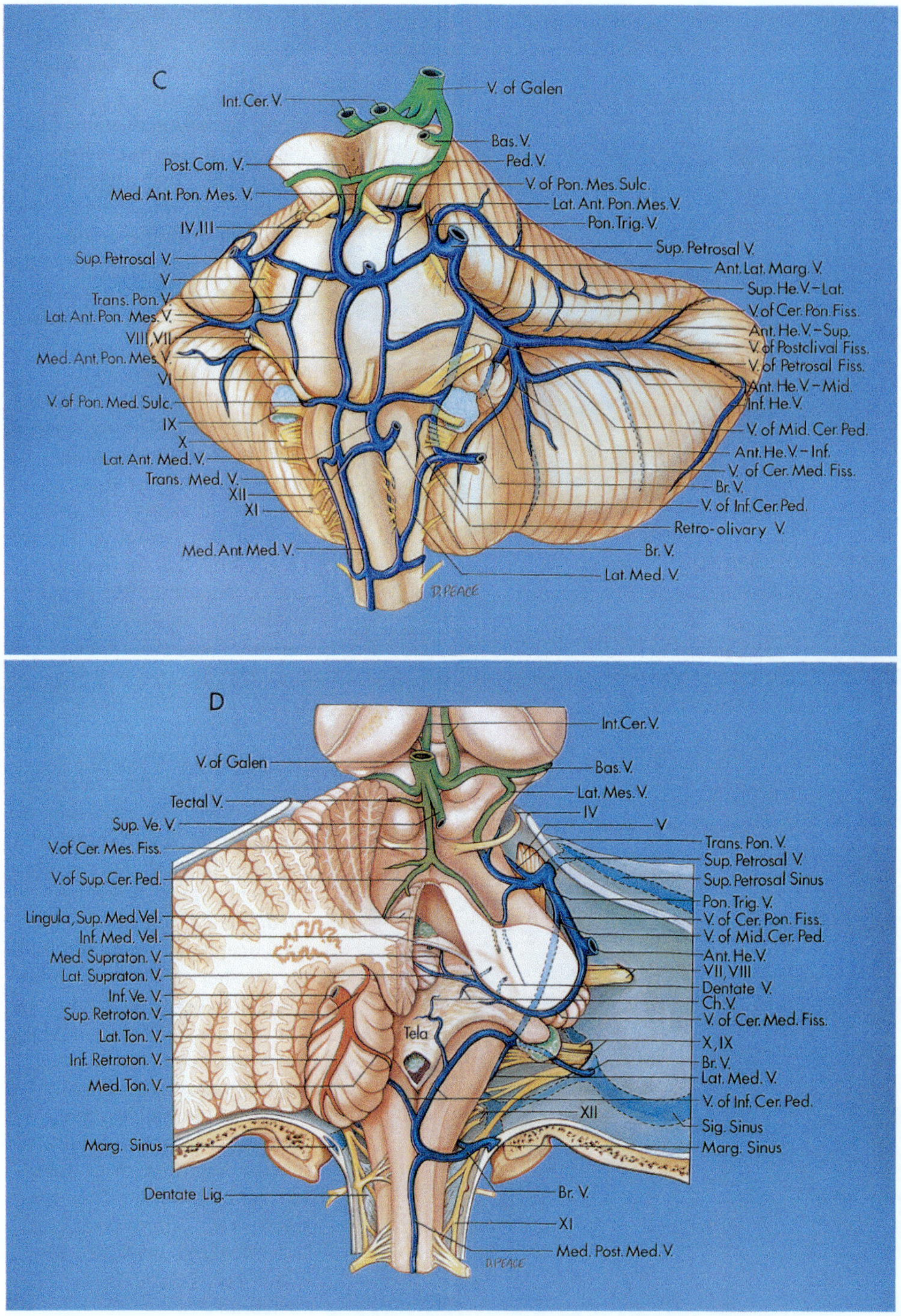

FIGURE 3.3. ***C* and *D*. Veins of the posterior fossa. *C*, petrosal surface and left side of the brainstem, anterolateral view. *D*, deep cerebellum and fourth ventricle, posterior view. The right cerebellar hemisphere and the part of the left cerebellar hemisphere posterior to the dentate nucleus and tonsil have been removed to show the roof of the fourth ventricle and the cerebellomesencephalic and cerebellomedullary fissures.**

the torcula or the superior petrosal, transverse, or tentorial sinuses. The veins in the smaller lateral group originate on the lateral part of the tentorial surface and drain directly into the superior petrosal sinus or one of its tributaries.

Suboccipital surface

The suboccipital surface, drained by the inferior hemispheric and inferior vermian veins and the superficial group of tonsillar veins, conforms to the part of the inner surface of the occipital bone located between the sigmoid sinuses (*Figs. 3.3* and *3.6-3.8*). The superficial group of tonsillar veins is composed of the retrotonsillar and the lateral and medial tonsillar veins that converge on the posterior surface of the tonsil and join to form the inferior vermian vein. There is also a deep group of tonsillar veins, the supratonsillar veins, which course in the cerebellomedullary fissure along the inferior part of the roof of the fourth ventricle and join the vein of the cerebellomedullary fissure.

the anterior group drain the anterior part of the hemispheric surface and join the superior vermian vein or the veins in the cerebellomesencephalic fissure. The other veins in the anterior group cross the anteromedial margin of the cerebellum and dip into and join the veins coursing in the cerebellomesencephalic fissure. The veins in the posterior group drain the posterior part of the tentorial surface. They usually join and form a common trunk with the inferior hemispheric veins from the suboccipital surface to form bridging veins that enter

Inferior vermian veins

The inferior vermian veins drain the vermis and the adjacent portion of the hemisphere, including part of the tonsil (*Figs. 3.3* and *3.6-3.8*). These paired veins are usually formed by the union of the retrotonsillar veins. They ascend along the vermohemispheric fissures and terminate in the straight or transverse sinuses or the torcula, either directly or through a short tentorial sinus. They may course on the vermis or the adjacent part of the hemisphere before reaching the vermohemispheric fissure. In a few cases, one inferior vermian vein will cross the vermis to terminate in the inferior vermian vein on the opposite side. There is often an anastomotic vein that crosses obliquely or transversely from one inferior vermian vein to the other. Some interconnect the veins after they leave the surface of the cerebellum to form bridging veins (24). The tributaries of the inferior vermian vein, beginning caudally, include veins from the tonsil (the superior and inferior retrotonsillar and the medial and the lateral tonsillar veins), the adjacent part of the vermis and hemisphere, and the posteromedial part of the tentorial surface.

Inferior hemispheric veins

The inferior hemispheric veins are oriented longitudinally or transversely on the suboccipital surface (*Figs. 3.3, 3.6,* and *3.7*). The majority of the longitudinal veins ascend and cross the margin between the suboccipital and tentorial surfaces to join the posterior group of superior hemispheric veins before emptying into a sinus in the tentorium. Some join the lower part of the inferior vermian vein. The transversely oriented veins course along the fissures between the folia and predominantly empty into the inferior vermian vein medially, but a few join the anterior hemisphere veins laterally.

The inferior hemispheric veins are divided into four groups: the superomedial, inferomedial, superolateral, and inferolateral veins, based on the part of the suboccipital surface that they drain. The veins in the superomedial group are the largest. The major veins in this group usually run longitudinally and drain into the torcular, a tentorial sinus, or the inferior vermian vein. Transversely oriented veins in this group, if well developed, drain into the torcula or the inferior vermian vein. The inferomedial group consists of small veins that originate and course inferiorly on the biventral lobule to join the inferior retrotonsillar or the inferior vermian veins. The veins in the superolateral group usually pass superolaterally across the posterior margin of the hemisphere and drain either directly or through a tentorial sinus into the superior petrosal or transverse sinuses, but some smaller members of this group may course around the lateral margin of the hemisphere to join the anterior hemispheric veins on the petrosal surface. The veins in the inferolateral group drain the lateral part of the biventral lobule and pass around the inferior margin of the hemisphere to join the anterior hemispheric veins.

Retrotonsillar veins

The superior and inferior retrotonsillar veins drain the superior and inferior poles and the posterior surface of the tonsils (*Figs. 3.3* and *3.8*). They receive tributaries from the medial and lateral tonsillar surfaces and the adjacent part of the vermis and hemisphere. The superior retrotonsillar vein arises near the superior pole and courses posteriorly to join the inferior retrotonsillar vein to form the inferior vermian vein. The inferior retrotonsillar vein arises near the caudal pole of the tonsil and courses superiorly to join the superior retrotonsillar vein and other tributaries from lateral and medial tonsillar surfaces.

Medial and lateral tonsillar veins

The medial tonsillar veins originate on the tonsillar surface facing the other tonsil, and the lateral tonsillar veins arise on the lateral side of the tonsil fissure between the tonsil and biventral lobule (*Fig. 3.3*). These veins usually course posteriorly and drain into the superior or inferior retrotonsillar or the inferior vermian veins.

Petrosal surface

This surface, drained by the anterior hemispheric veins, faces the posterior surface of the petrous bone (*Figs. 3.3* and *3.9*).

Anterior hemispheric veins

These veins arise near the border that separates the petrosal surface from the suboccipital and tentorial surfaces, and pass anteriorly to converge on the cerebellopontine fissure and the middle cerebellar peduncle. They are divided into superior, middle, and inferior groups. The veins in the inferior group arise on the inferior part of the petrosal surface and converge on the caudal part of the cerebellopontine fissure to form a common trunk. The vein of the cerebellomedullary fissure, if it passes dorsal to the flocculus, joins the common trunk of the inferior group. The veins in the middle group drain the middle portion of the petrosal surface and converge on the apex of the cerebellopontine fissure. The common trunk of the inferior group joins the common trunk of the middle group near the flocculus to form the vein of the cerebellopontine fissure, which passes to the superior petrosal sinus. In a few cases, the common trunk of the middle group does not join the common trunk of the inferior group, but ascends to drain directly into the superior petrosal sinus. The superior group, the smallest of the three groups, drains the rostral edge of the petrosal surface. These veins course anteriorly or posteriorly to join either the vein of the cerebellopontine fissure, the anterolateral marginal vein that courses along the junction of the tentorial and petrosal surfaces, or one of the superior hemispheric veins.

DEEP VEINS

The deep veins course in the fissures between the brainstem and the cerebellum near the roof and lateral walls of the fourth ventricle (*Fig. 3.3*). The veins most intimately related to the superior part of the roof are those that course in the cerebellomesencephalic fissure; the veins most intimately related to the inferior part of the roof are those that course in the cerebellomedullary fissure; and those most intimately related to the lateral wall and cerebellopontine angle are those that course in the cerebellopontine fissure. The structures ventral to the floor of the fourth ventricle are drained by the veins of the brainstem, which are considered in the section on the veins of the brainstem in this chapter.

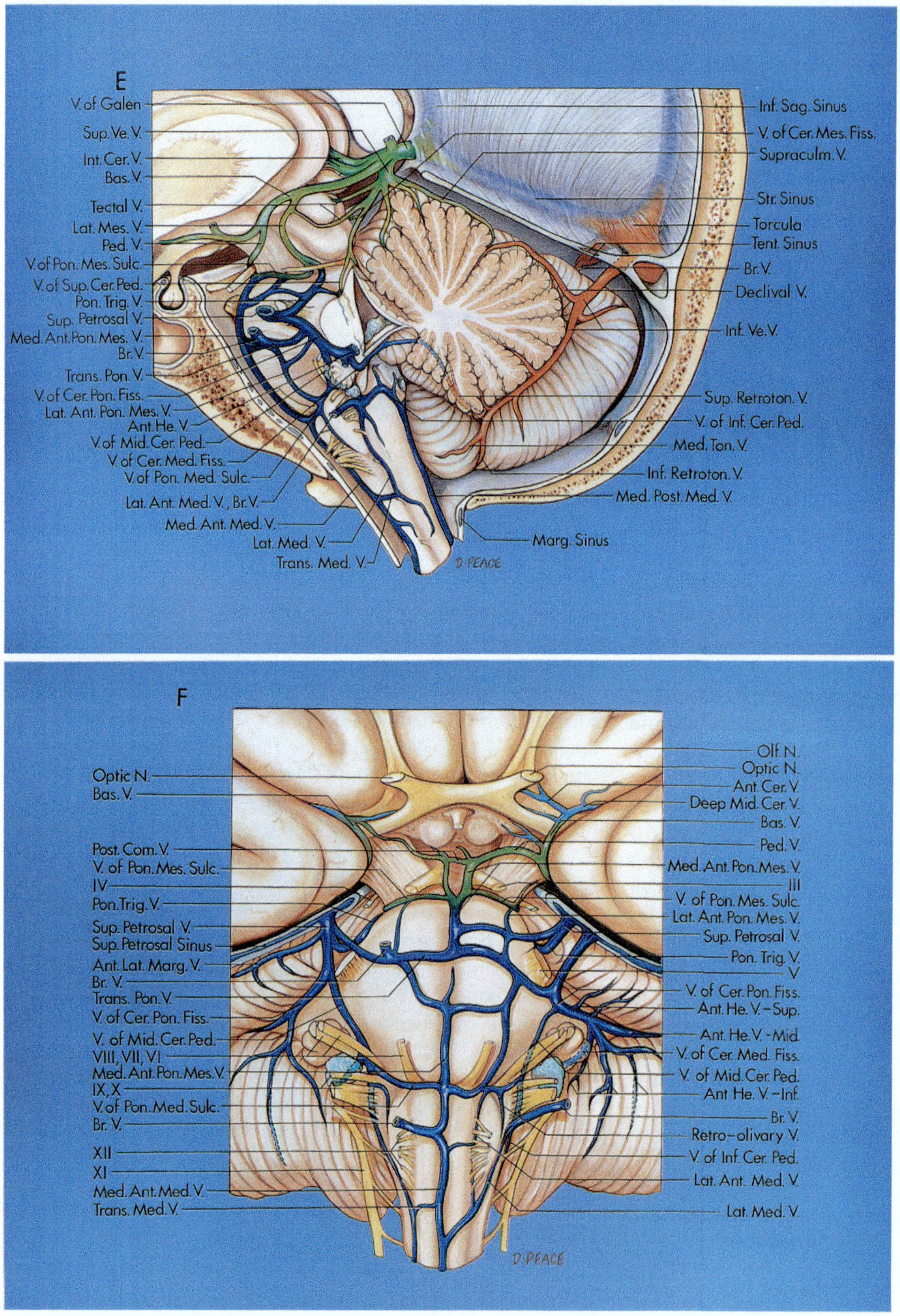

FIGURE 3.3. *E* and *F*. Veins of the posterior fossa. *E*, midsagittal section of cerebellum and fourth ventricle. Left lateral view. The left half of the cerebellum has been removed to expose the fourth ventricle. *F*, brainstem. Anterior view. The part of the tentorium between the temporal lobe and the cerebellum has been preserved. *A–F*, the inferior sagittal sinus joins the straight sinus at the apex of the tentorium. The superior sagittal sinus joins the straight sinus at the torcula. The superior petrosal sinus passes along the petrous ridge and joins the junction of the lateral (referred to here as the transverse sinus) and sigmoid sinuses posteriorly and the cavernous sinus anteriorly. The veins converging on the tentorium join to form tentorial sinuses that drain into the straight, lateral, and superior petrosal sinuses and the torcula. The marginal sinus courses in the dura at the level of the foramen magnum above the rostral attachment of the dentate ligament. The emissary vein passing through the condylar foramen joins the sigmoid sinus. The vertebral venous plexus anastomoses with the internal jugular vein. Bridging veins pass from the surface of the cerebellum and brainstem to the dural sinuses. The superior hemispheric veins are divided into three groups: an anterior group that drains toward the vein of Galen; a posterior group that drains into the veins converging on the straight sinus, torcula, and medial part of the lateral sinus; and a lateral group that drains into the superior petrosal sinus, the anterolateral marginal vein, and the lateral part of the lateral sinus. The superior vermian veins drain the tentorial part of the vermis. The veins on the superior part of the tentorial surface of the vermis ascend toward the superior vermian vein and those on the inferior part of the tentorial surface of the vermis descend toward the torcula. The tributary of the superior vermian vein draining the tentorial surface of the culmen has been called the supraculminate vein. The declival vein drains the declive and joins the inferior vermian vein or the torcula. The vein of the postclival fissure courses in the postclival fissure. The superior petrosal veins are divided into medial, intermediate, and lateral groups, depending on whether they enter the middle, intermediate, or lateral third of the superior petrosal sinus. The inferior hemispheric veins drain the hemispheric part of the suboccipital surface, and the inferior vermian veins drain the vermian part of the suboccipital

Cerebellomesencephalic fissure

The major veins in the cerebellomesencephalic fissure are the veins of the cerebellomesencephalic fissure and the superior cerebellar peduncle, and the pontotrigeminal and lateral mesencephalic veins (*Figs. 3.2-3.5* and *3.10*).

Vein of the superior cerebellar peduncle

The paired veins of the superior cerebellar peduncle originate deep in the cerebellomesencephalic fissure near the caudolateral margin of the superior cerebellar peduncles from tributaries draining the dentate nuclei, superior cerebellar peduncles, and the walls of the cerebellomesencephalic fissure (*Figs. 3.3* and *3.4*). They first course medially across the peduncles and then upward on the peduncles, just lateral to the lingula. They join near the rostral tip of the lingula to form a single trunk, the vein of the cerebellomesencephalic fissure. In a few cases, the paired veins do not join but form two separate veins of the cerebellomesencephalic fissure. Each nerve of the superior cerebellar peduncle anastomoses with the pontotrigeminal and lateral mesencephalic vein.

Vein of the cerebellomesencephalic fissure

This vein, also referred to as the precentral cerebellar vein, arises deep in the cerebellomesencephalic fissure from the union of the veins of the superior cerebellar peduncle. It crosses the quadrigeminal cistern anterior to the central lobule

surface. The inferior vermian veins drain toward the tentorium and enter the torcula or a tentorial sinus. The inferior hemispheric veins cross the posterior margin of the cerebellum to reach the tentorial surface, where they often join the superior hemispheric veins before terminating in the tentorial, lateral, or superior petrosal sinuses or the torcula. The inferior vermian vein is formed on the posterior surface of the tonsil by the union of the superior and inferior retrotonsillar veins. The medial and lateral tonsillar veins pass to the retrotonsillar or the inferior vermian veins. The vein of the petrosal fissure passes along the petrosal fissure. The anterior hemispheric veins that drain the petrosal surface of the cerebellum and are divided into superior, middle, and inferior groups, depending on whether they drain the superior, inferior, or middle third of the petrosal surface. The anterior hemispheric veins converge on the lateral cerebellar incisura and join to form the vein of the cerebellopontine fissure that ascends to enter the superior petrosal sinus. The major veins related to the superior half of the roof of the fourth ventricle are the veins of the cerebellomesencephalic fissure and the superior cerebellar peduncle; the major veins related to the inferior part of the roof are the veins of the cerebellomedullary fissure and the inferior cerebellar peduncle; and the major veins in the region of the lateral recesses and lateral walls are the veins of the cerebellopontine fissure and the middle cerebellar peduncle. In the cerebellomesencephalic fissure, the paired veins of the superior cerebellar peduncle ascend lateral to the lingula and the superior medullary velum and join to form the vein of the cerebellomedullary fissure, which ascends to join the superior vermian vein. The internal cerebral, basal, and superior vermian veins enter the vein of Galen. The lateral mesencephalic and the pontotrigeminal veins course in the cerebellomesencephalic fissure. The lateral mesencephalic vein courses in the lateral mesencephalic sulcus. The pontotrigeminal vein arises on the superior and middle cerebellar peduncles and passes rostral to the trigeminal nerve. The tectal veins arise in the region of the colliculi. The vein of the cerebellomedullary fissure arises on the lateral side of the uvula and nodule and passes laterally through the cerebellomedullary fissure, either dorsal or ventral to the flocculus, to join one of the veins in the cerebellopontine angle. The vein of the cerebellomedullary fissure receives the medial and lateral supratonsillar veins, which pass along the medial and lateral edge of the inferior medullary velum above the superior pole of the tonsil. The dentate nucleus is drained by the supratonsillar veins and the vein of the cerebellomedullary fissure. The median posterior medullary vein ascends on the posterior medulla and divides just below the obex into the paired veins of the inferior cerebellar peduncle. The veins of the inferior cerebellar peduncle ascend on the inferior cerebellar peduncles and join the lateral medullary veins. The choroidal veins draining the tela choroidea and choroid plexus are tributaries of the veins of the inferior cerebellar peduncle and the cerebellomedullary fissure. The peduncular veins arise in the interpeduncular fossa and pass laterally to join the basal veins. The posterior communicating vein interconnects the medial ends of the peduncular veins. The longitudinally oriented veins in the midline on the anterior surface of the brainstem are the median anterior medullary vein, which ascends on the medulla, and the median anterior pontomesencephalic vein that ascends in the midline on the pons and midbrain. The median anterior pontomesencephalic vein does not usually extend the full length of the pons. The ends adjoining the absent segment often join the transverse pontine veins. The transversely oriented veins coursing in the sulci between the subdivisions of the brainstem are the veins of the pontomesencephalic and the pontomedullary sulci. Each vein of the middle cerebellar peduncle arises in the region of the foramen of Luschka near the flocculus and ascends on the middle cerebellar peduncle to join the vein of the cerebellopontine fissure or one of the superior petrosal veins. The lateral anterior medullary vein courses along the preolivary sulcus near the hypoglossal nerve. The lateral anterior pontomesencephalic vein passes along the anterolateral margin of the pons and medulla. The transverse medullary veins pass transversely across the medulla. The retro-olivary vein courses along the posterior margin of the olive, and the lateral medullary vein courses slightly dorsal to the olive, along the origin of the rootlets arising from the dorsolateral surface of the medulla. There are diffuse anastomoses between the veins ventral to the diencephalon and third ventricle and those draining the midbrain. The deep middle cerebral and the anterior cerebral veins join the basal vein in the region of the anterior perforated substance. (From, Matsushima T, Rhoton AL Jr, de Oliveira E, Peace D: Microsurgical anatomy of the veins of the posterior fossa. J Neurosurg 59:63–105, 1983 [15].)

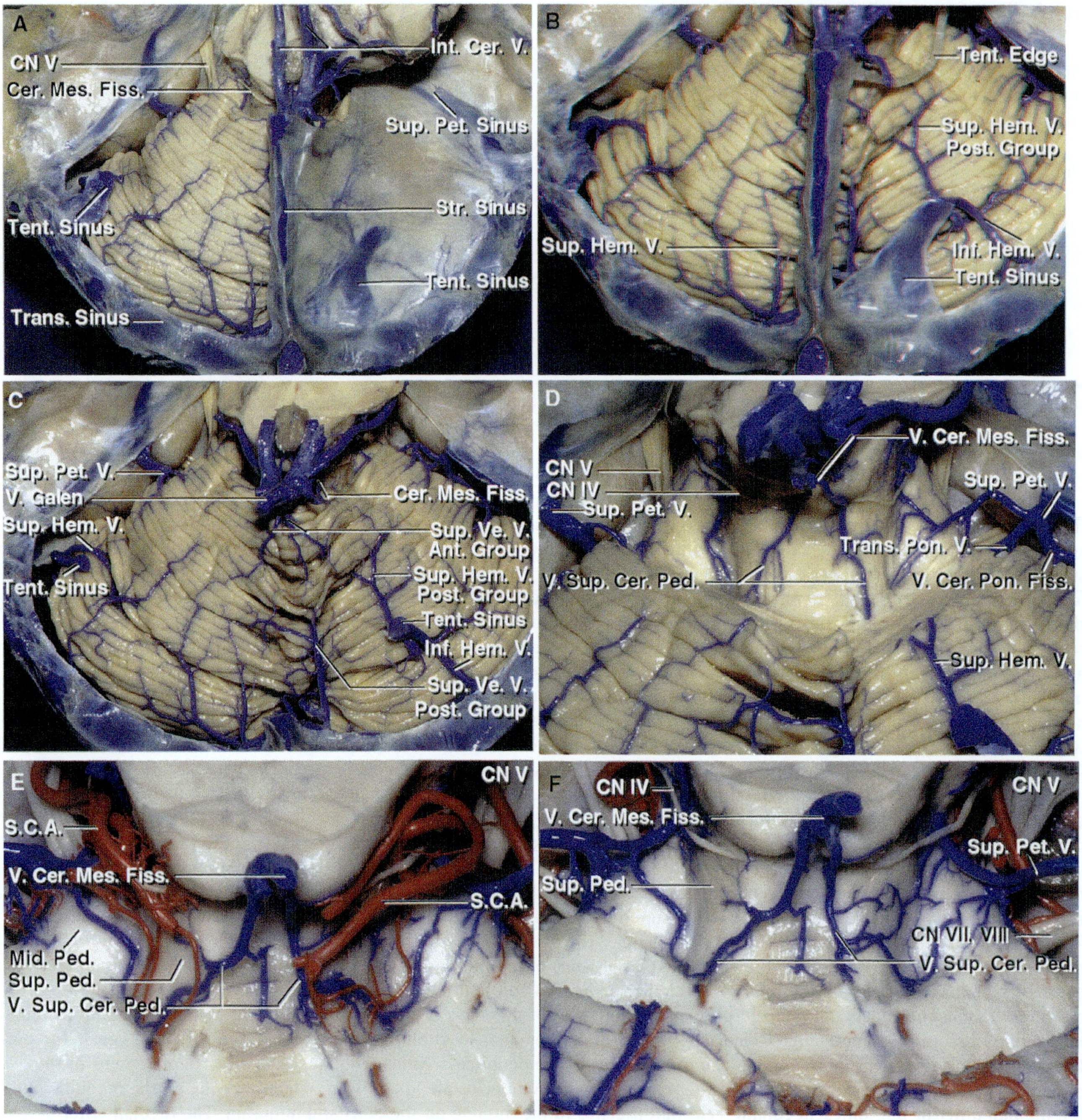

FIGURE 3.4. Tentorial surface and cerebellomesencephalic fissure. *A*, the left half of the tentorium has been removed while preserving a laterally placed tentorial sinus. A large sinus is seen through the right tentorial surface. *B*, the right half of the tentorium has been removed to expose a large inferior hemispheric vein from the suboccipital surface and a smaller superior hemispheric vein from the tentorial surface emptying into the large tentorial sinus. The superior hemispheric veins, which drain the tentorial surface, are divided into an anterior group, which empties into the Galenic system, and a posterior group, like the vein shown, which empties into the tentorial sinuses. Smaller veins from both the left tentorial and suboccipital surfaces join the laterally placed tentorial sinus near the junction of the left transverse and superior petrosal sinuses. *C*, the straight and tentorial sinuses have been removed. The anterior group drains toward the cerebellomesencephalic fissure and the vein of Galen, and the posterior group passes backward to empty into the tentorial sinuses. *D*, the posterior lip of the cerebellomesencephalic fissure has been removed to expose the veins of the superior cerebellar peduncle, which ascend to unite and form the vein of the cerebellomesencephalic fissure that empties into the vein of Galen. A transverse pontine vein and the vein of the cerebellopontine fissure join to form a superior petrosal vein that empties into the superior petrosal sinus.

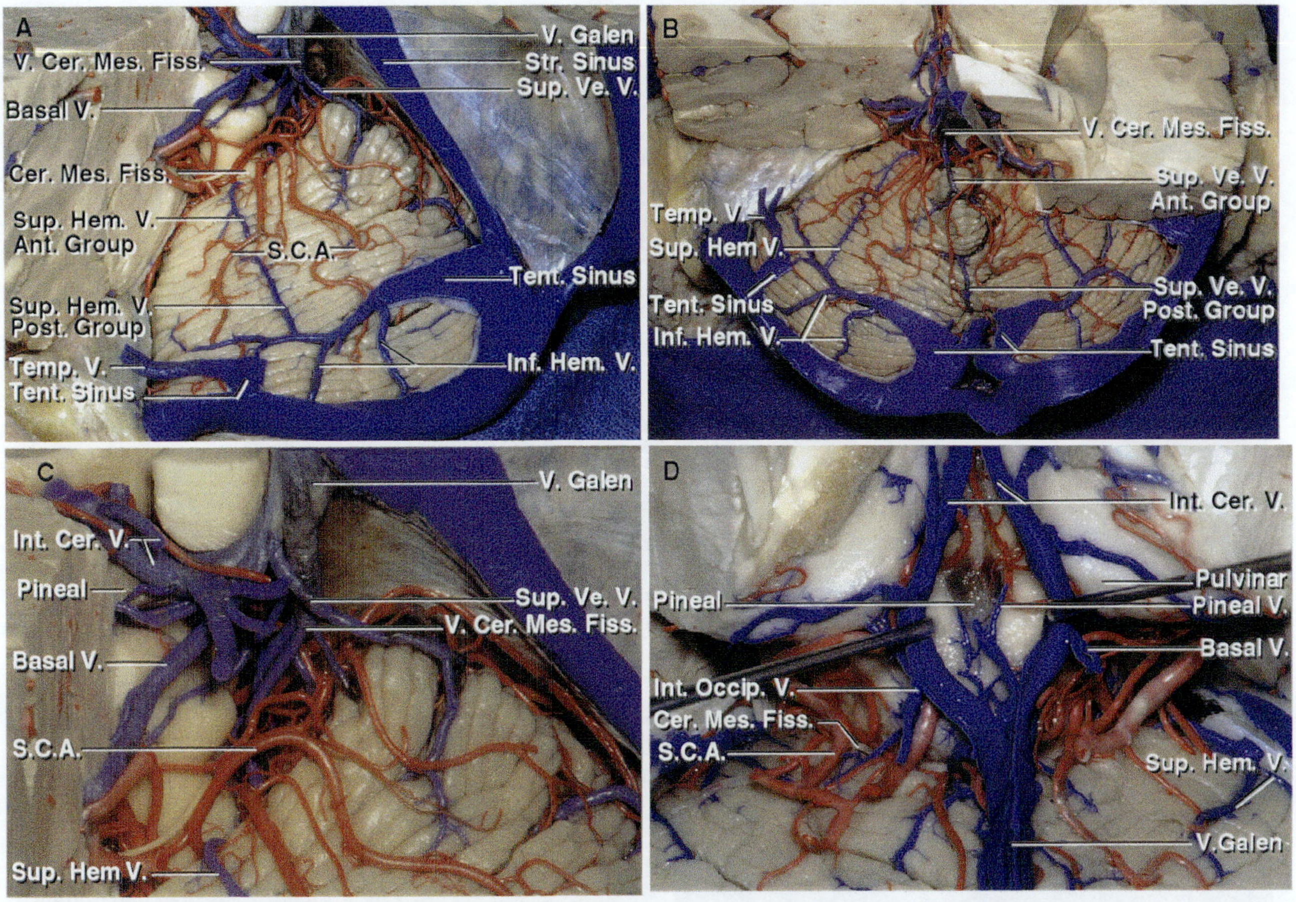

FIGURE 3.5. Tentorial surface and cerebellomesencephalic fissure. *A*, the left half of the tentorium has been removed while preserving the tentorial sinuses. The anterior group of superior vermian and superior hemispheric veins arise on the upper part of the tentorial surface and ascend to reach the veins exiting the cerebellomesencephalic fissure, which empty into the vein of Galen. The posterior group of superior vermian and superior hemispheric veins arise on the posterior part of the tentorial surface and descend to empty into tentorial sinuses. The inferior hemispheric veins, which arise on the suboccipital surface, also empty into the tentorial sinuses. *B*, both halves of the tentorium have been removed while preserving the large tentorial sinuses. The superior hemispheric veins from the posterior part of the tentorial surface and the inferior hemispheric veins from the suboccipital surface drain into the paired large tentorial sinus that join the torcula. The veins draining the anterior part of the tentorial surface empty into the tributaries of the vein of Galen. *C*, lateral view of the cerebellomesencephalic fissure. The largest vein in the fissure is the vein of the cerebellomesencephalic fissure. The internal cerebral veins pass above the pineal to join the vein of Galen. *D*, the veins draining the walls of the cerebellomesencephalic fissure join the vein of Galen, as do the internal cerebral and basal veins. A pineal vein also joins the Galenic group. *Ant.*, anterior; *Cer.*, cerebral; *Cer. Mes.*, cerebellomesencephalic; *Fiss.*, fissure; *Hem.*, hemispheric; *Inf.*, inferior; *Int.*, internal; *Occip.*, occipital; *Post.*, posterior; *S.C.A.*, superior cerebellar artery; *Str.*, straight; *Sup.*, superior; *Temp.*, temporal; *Tent.*, tentorial; *V.*, vein; *Ve.*, vermian.

◄

E–F, cerebellomesencephalic fissure from another hemisphere. *E*, the posterior lip of the cerebellomesencephalic fissure has been removed to expose the tributaries of the vein of the cerebellomesencephalic fissure and the branches of the SCA. The paired veins of the superior cerebellar peduncle unite to form the vein of the cerebellomesencephalic fissure that empties into the vein of Galen. *F*, the branches of the SCA within the cerebellomesencephalic fissure have been removed. The paired veins of the superior cerebellar peduncle ascend on the superior cerebellar peduncles and join to form the vein of the cerebellomesencephalic fissure. The veins on the surface of the middle cerebellar peduncle course laterally to join the veins emptying into the superior petrosal sinus. *A.*, artery; *Ant.*, anterior; *Cer.*, cerebral; *Cer. Mes.*, cerebellomesencephalic; *CN.*, cranial nerve; *Fiss.*, fissure; *Hem.*, hemispheric; *Inf.*, inferior; *Int.*, internal; *Mid.*, middle; *N.*, nerve; *Ped.*, peduncle; *Post.*, posterior; *Str.*, straight; *Sup.*, superior; *Tent.*, tentorial; *Trans.*, transverse; *V.*, vein; *Ve.*, vermian.

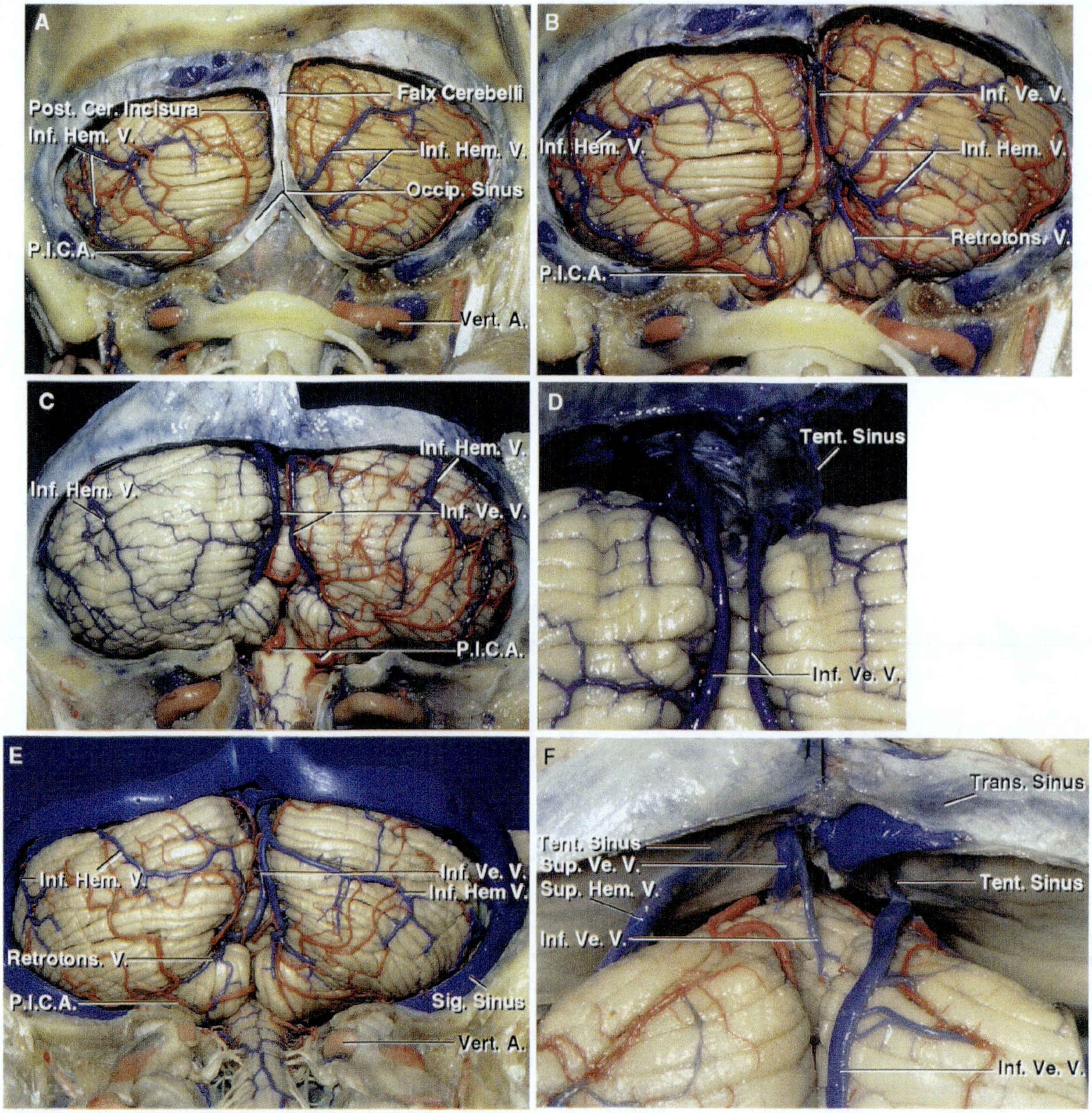

FIGURE 3.6. Suboccipital surface. *A*, the falx cerebelli, which fits into the posterior cerebellar incisura in which the vermis is partially buried, has been preserved. The inferior hemispheric veins drain the hemispheric portion of the suboccipital surface. A large left inferior hemispheric vein ascends toward a tentorial sinus. A large right inferior hemispheric vein descends medially to join an inferior vermian vein, which ascends to empty into the sinuses in the tentorium. The occipital sinus courses within the falx cerebelli and joins the torcula above and the sigmoid sinus below. *B*, the falx cerebelli has been removed to expose the inferior vermian veins, which ascend and pass below the transverse sinus to empty into the tentorial sinuses. The retrotonsillar veins and other veins around the superior pole of the tonsils ascend to join the inferior vermian veins. *C* and *D*, another cerebellum. *C*, the branches of the PICA supplying the left hemisphere have been removed, but those on the right have been preserved. The inferior vermian and hemispheric veins on both halves of the suboccipital surface ascend and pass below the transverse sinus to empty into the sinuses in the tentorium. *D*, enlarged view of the inferior vermian veins that ascend to empty into sinuses in the tentorium. *E*, another cerebellum. A large right inferior hemispheric vein joins an inferior vermian vein that crosses the upper edge of the suboccipital surface and courses for a short distance on the tentorial surface before emptying into a tentorial sinus. *F*, enlarged view of another cerebellum. The large right inferior vermian vein passes forward to join the sinuses in the tentorium. A superior hemispheric vein from the tentorial surface descends to join a tentorial sinus. In the midline, a superior and inferior vermian join to empty into a tentorial sinus. *A.*, artery; *Cer.*, cerebellar; *Hem.*, hemispheric; *Inf.*, inferior; *Occip.*, occipital; *P.I.C.A.*, posteroinferior cerebellar artery; *Post.*, posterior; *Retroton.*, retrotonsillar; *Sig.*, sigmoid; *Sup.*, superior; *Tent.*, tentorial; *Trans.*, transverse; *V.*, vein; *Ve.*, vermian; *Vert.*, vertebral.

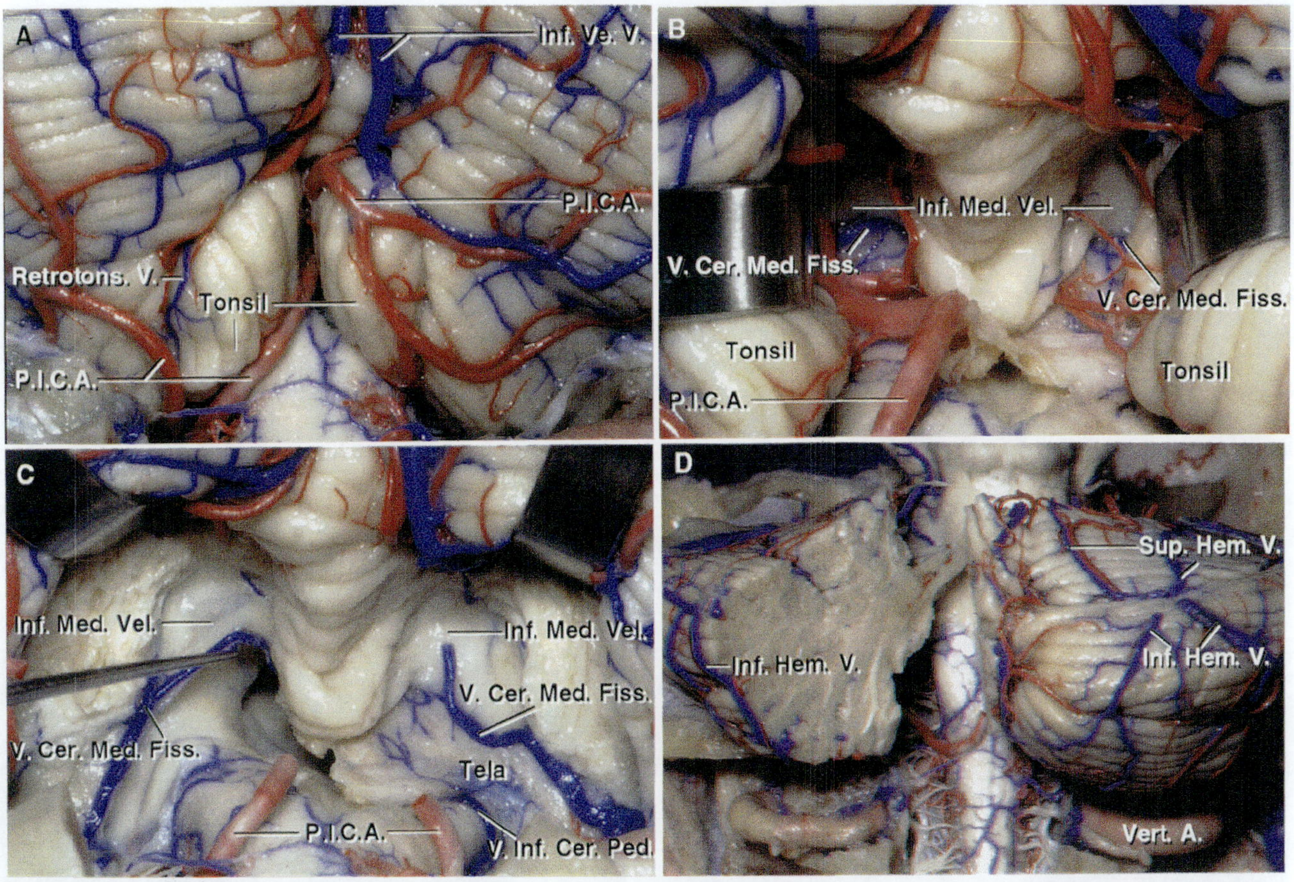

FIGURE 3.7. Suboccipital surface and cerebellomedullary fissure. *A*, the veins from the region of the tonsil empty into the inferior vermian veins that ascend toward the sinuses in the tentorium. *B*, gentle retraction of the cerebellar tonsils exposes the veins of the cerebellomedullary fissure crossing the inferior medullary velum. *C*, the cerebellar tonsils have been removed. The tela on the left side has been removed. The veins of the cerebellomesencephalic fissure cross the inferior medullary velum to join the veins in the cerebellopontine angles, which empty into the superior petrosal veins. The medial end of the veins of the cerebellomedullary fissure anastomose with the veins around the tonsil. *D*, a portion of the left half of the cerebellum has been removed. The inferior hemispheric veins from the suboccipital surface ascend and cross the junction of the suboccipital and tentorial surfaces to course on the posterior part of the tentorial surface, where they often form common stems with the superior hemispheric veins from the posterior part of the tentorial surface before emptying into the tentorial sinuses. *A.*, artery; *Cer.*, cerebellar; *Cer. Med.*, cerebellomedullary; *Fiss.*, fissure; *Hem.*, hemispheric; *Inf.*, inferior; *Med.*, medullary; *Ped.*, peduncle; *P.I.C.A.*, posteroinferior cerebellar artery; *Retrotons.*, retrotonsillar; *Sup.*, superior; *V.*, vein; *Ve.*, vermian; *Vel.*, velum; *Vert.*, vertebral.

to drain either directly or through the superior vermian vein into the vein of Galen (*Figs. 3.2-3.5* and *3.10*). Its tributaries are from the posterior aspect of the midbrain and the walls of the cerebellomesencephalic fissure, and occasionally include the tectal and preculminate veins.

Pontotrigeminal vein

This vein arises on the surface of the middle cerebellar peduncle near the interpeduncular sulcus located between the superior and middle peduncles, passes above the trigeminal nerve, and drains directly into the superior petrosal sinus or its tributaries (*Figs. 3.10* and *3.11*). Its proximal end frequently anastomoses with the vein of the superior cerebellar peduncle and the lateral mesencephalic vein. Some of the superior hemispheric and transverse pontine veins may drain into the pontotrigeminal vein.

Tectal veins

The small tectal veins originate on or near the superior and inferior colliculi and course upward in the quadrigeminal cistern to drain into the vein of the cerebellomesencephalic fissure, the superior vermian or internal cerebral vein, or the vein of Galen. These veins often anastomose with the vein of the superior cerebellar peduncle and the pineal, lateral mesencephalic, and basal veins.

Cerebellomedullary fissure

The major veins in the cerebellomedullary fissure are the veins of the cerebellomedullary fissure and the inferior cerebellar

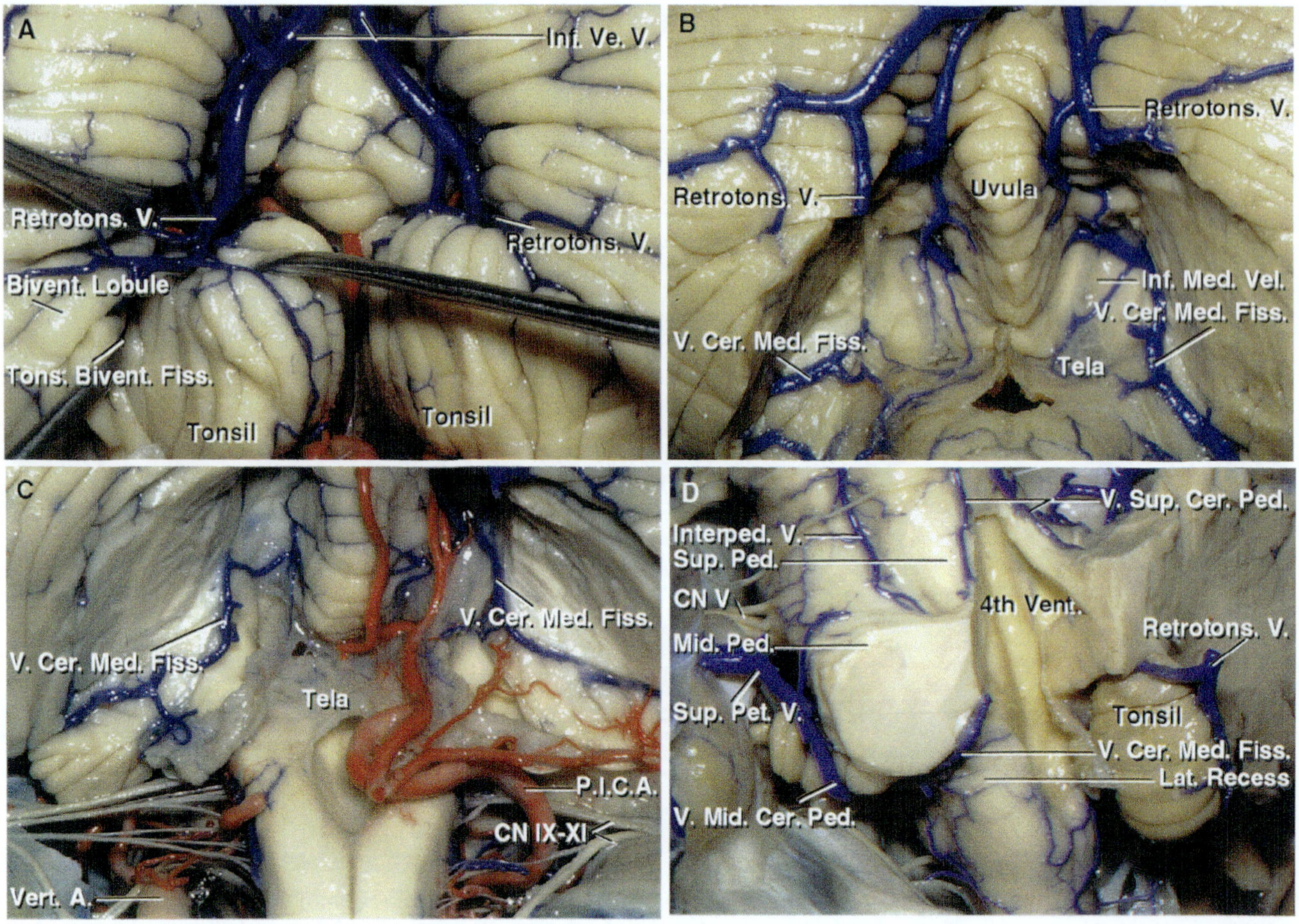

FIGURE 3.8. Suboccipital surface and the cerebellomedullary fissure. *A*, the retrotonsillar veins pass upward in the fissure between the tonsil and biventral lobule and empty into the inferior vermian veins. *B*, the tonsils have been removed to expose the veins of the cerebellomedullary fissure, which pass laterally on the inferior medullary velum and across the lateral recesses to join the veins in the cerebellopontine angles. The medial end of the veins of the cerebellomedullary fissure anastomose with the veins around the tonsil. *C*, another specimen. The tonsils and part of the biventral lobules have been removed to expose the paired veins of the cerebellomedullary fissure, which cross the inferior medullary velum to empty into the veins in the cerebellopontine angles. *D*, the cerebellar hemispheres, except for the right tonsil, have been removed. The right retrotonsillar vein courses along the posterior surface of the tonsil and empties into an inferior vermian vein. The left vein of the cerebellomedullary fissure passes through the lateral recess to join the vein of the middle cerebellar peduncle, which ascends to empty into a superior petrosal vein. The paired veins of the superior cerebellar peduncle ascend on the peduncle and join to form the vein of the cerebellomesencephalic fissure. An interpeduncular vein courses between the superior and middle cerebellar peduncles. *A.*, artery; *Bivent.*, biventral; *Cer.*, cerebellar; *Cer. Med.*, cerebellomedullary; *CN*, cranial nerve; *Fiss.*, fissure; *Inf.*, inferior; *Interped.*, interpeduncular; *Lat.*, lateral; *Med.*, medullary; *Mid.*, middle; *Ped.*, peduncle; *Pet.*, petrosal; *P.I.C.A.*, posteroinferior cerebellar artery; *Retrotons.*, retrotonsillar; *Sup.*, superior; *Tons.*, tonsillar; *V.*, vein; *Ve.*, vermian; *Vent.*, ventricle; *Vert.*, vertebral.

peduncle (*Figs. 3.3, 3.7-3.9*) (2). Both of these veins drain into the cerebellopontine angle through the communication between the cerebellomedullary and cerebellopontine fissures.

Vein of the cerebellomedullary fissure

This vein originates on the lateral edge of the nodule and uvula, courses laterally near the junction of the inferior medullary velum and tela choroidea, and passes dorsal or ventral to the flocculus to reach the cerebellopontine angle (*Figs. 3.7-3.9*). If it courses dorsal to the flocculus, it terminates in the anterior hemispheric veins or in the vein of the cerebellopontine fissure. If it courses ventral to the flocculus, it passes between the flocculus and the foramen of Luschka and joins the lateral medullary vein or the vein of the inferior cerebellar peduncle or the pontomedullary sulcus to form the vein of the middle cerebellar peduncle. The vein of the cerebellomedullary fissure frequently connects with its mate on the opposite side through a transverse vein crossing the nodule or uvula and/or with the inferior vermian vein. The medial part of the vein of the cerebellomedullary fissure is sometimes hypoplastic or absent. Its tributaries drain the inferior medullary velum, tela choroidea and attached choroid plexus, periventricular white matter, dentate nuclei, anteroinferior surface of the biventral lobule, and the inferior vermis.

Vein of the inferior cerebellar peduncle

This vein courses on the peduncle parallel and several millimeters caudal to the curved inferolateral margin of the fourth ventricle (*Figs. 3.3, 3.7*, and *3.9*). Its caudal part is visible on the posterior surface of the medulla lateral to Magendie's foramen, but its superior portion is hidden in the cerebellomedullary fissure. Inferiorly, the veins from each side join below the obex to form a single channel, the median posterior medullary vein. Superiorly, it passes below the lateral recesses and joins the vein of the pontomedullary sulcus, either directly or by first connecting with the lateral medullary vein. It often receives the vein of the cerebellomedullary fissure near the lateral end of the pontomedullary sulcus. These veins, converging on the lateral end of the pontomedullary sulcus, join to form the vein of the middle cerebellar peduncle. The vein of the inferior cerebellar peduncle drains the posterior and lateral aspects of the medulla, the tela choroidea, choroid plexus, the inferior part of the floor of the fourth ventricle, the lateral recess, and the glossopharyngeal and vagus nerves. This rostral part of the vein of the inferior cerebellar peduncle often anastomoses with the sinuses converging on the jugular foramen through a bridging vein that passes along the nerves that pass through the jugular foramen.

Supratonsillar veins

The supratonsillar veins course in the cerebellomedullary fissure near the superior pole of the tonsil (*Fig. 3.3*) (9). The name "supratonsillar" suggests that these veins drain the tonsil; however, they course on and drain the opposite side of the cerebellomedullary fissure from the tonsil. They originate in the deep nuclei and white matter of the cerebellum and drain the inferior half of the roof of the fourth ventricle rather than the tonsil. They course along the inferior medullary velum and drain into the vein of the cerebellomedullary fissure or the inferior vermian vein.

Choroidal veins

The choroidal veins drain the tela choroidea and the attached choroid plexus, and are tributaries of the veins of the cerebellomedullary fissure and the inferior cerebellar peduncle. The medial half of the vein of the cerebellomedullary fissure drains the rostral part of the medial segment and the medial part of the lateral segment of the choroid plexus. The lateral half of the vein of the cerebellomedullary fissure, and the rostral part of the vein of the inferior cerebellar peduncle drain the lateral part of the lateral segment. The caudal part of the vein of the inferior cerebellar peduncle receives the drainage of the caudal part of the medial segment (*Fig. 3.3*).

Cerebellopontine fissure

The major veins arising in this region are the veins of the cerebellopontine fissure and the middle cerebellar peduncle.

Vein of the cerebellopontine fissure

This is the largest vein draining the petrosal surface. It is formed just rostral or caudal to the flocculus by the union of the stems of the anterior hemispheric veins (*Figs. 3.9-3.11*). It courses in or near the superior limb of the cerebellopontine fissure, or on the superior part of the petrosal surface near the anterolateral margin. It crosses the subarachnoid space rostral to the facial, vestibulocochlear, and trigeminal nerves, and drains into the superior petrosal sinus either directly or after forming a common stem with other veins draining into the superior petrosal sinus. The vein of the middle cerebellar peduncle and the pontotrigeminal vein often join the vein of the cerebellopontine fissure to form one of the trunks that drain into the superior petrosal sinus near the trigeminal nerve. The vein of the cerebellomedullary fissure, if it passes dorsal to the flocculus, may drain into the vein of the cerebellopontine fissure.

Vein of the middle cerebellar peduncle

This vein originates in the fossette above the inferior olive by the union of the vein of the pontomedullary sulcus with the lateral medullary vein or the vein of the inferior cerebellar peduncle (*Figs. 3.8-3.11*). It ascends on the lateral surface of the middle cerebellar peduncle near the base of the cerebellopontine fissure to reach the area posterior to the origin of the trigeminal nerve. It drains directly into the superior petrosal sinus or joins other veins to form one of the common trunks that drain into the superior petrosal sinus. Its initial part passes either between the flocculus and the origin of the vestibulocochlear nerve or between the origins of the vestibulocochlear and the facial nerves.

The vein of the middle cerebellar peduncle receives the drainage of the rostral half of the medulla, the inferior half of the fourth ventricle, and the lateral surface of the pons. It often receives the drainage of the veins of the cerebellomedullary fissure and inferior cerebellar peduncle, some of the transverse pontine veins, and the veins draining the origins of the facial and the vestibulocochlear nerves. It is large if the vein of the cerebellomedullary fissure courses ventral to the flocculus to join it rather than passing dorsal to the flocculus to join the anterior hemispheric veins or the vein of the cerebellopontine fissure.

VEINS OF THE BRAINSTEM

The veins of the brainstem are divided into two groups based on whether they course longitudinally or transversely (*Figs. 3.3* and *3.9-3.11*). The longitudinal veins are the median anterior pontomesencephalic, median anterior medullary, lateral anterior pontomesencephalic, lateral anterior medullary (preolivary), lateral mesencephalic, lateral medullary, and retro-olivary veins. The transverse veins are the veins of the pontomesencephalic and the pontomedullary sulci, and the transverse pontine, transverse medullary, peduncular, and posterior communicating veins.

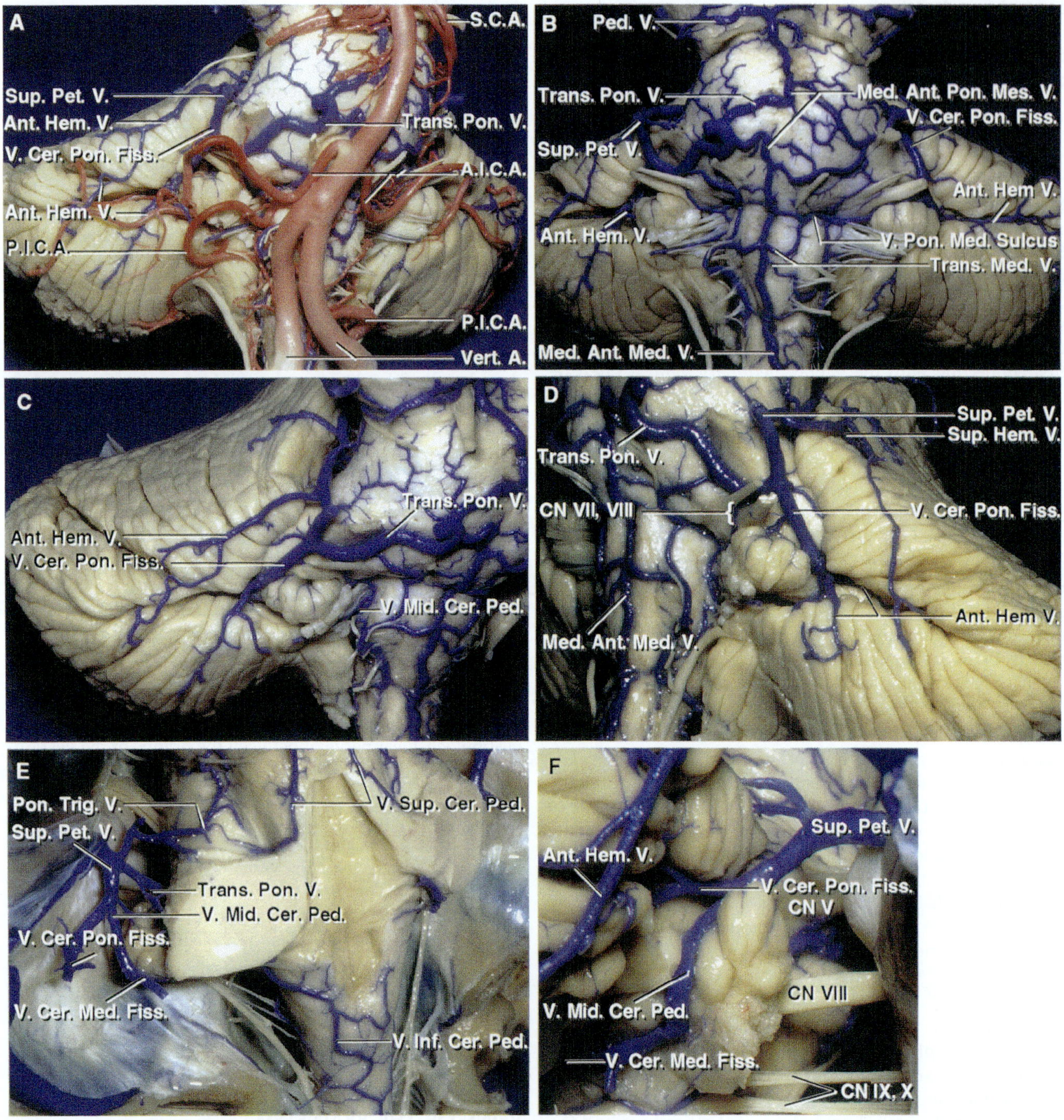

FIGURE 3.9. Brainstem and petrosal surface. *A*, the vertebral and basilar arteries and their branches course superficial to the veins. The veins on the anterior surface of the pons and medulla and the petrosal surface drain predominantly into the superior petrosal veins, which empty into the superior petrosal sinuses. *B*, the arteries have been removed. The median anterior pontomesencephalic and median anterior medullary veins ascend on the front of the brainstem. The transverse pontine and transverse medullary veins run transversely across the pons and medulla surfaces. The anterior hemispheric veins drain the petrosal surface and commonly empty into the vein of the cerebellopontine fissure, which ascends to join the superior petrosal veins. The vein of the pontomedullary sulcus passes across the pontomedullary junction. *C*, enlarged view of the right petrosal surface. The anterior hemispheric veins drain the petrosal surface and pass forward to empty into the vein of the cerebellopontine fissure or a superior petrosal vein. The vein of the cerebellopontine fissure arises at the lateral apex of the cerebellopontine fissure and crosses the middle cerebellar peduncle, where it is joined by a large transverse pontine vein. *D*, enlarged view of the left petrosal surface. The vein of the cerebellopontine fissure arises from the union of the anterior hemispheric veins at the apex of the cerebellopontine fissure

Longitudinal veins

Median anterior pontomesencephalic vein

This vein runs in or near the midline on the anterior surface of the mesencephalon and the pons (*Figs. 3.9-3.11*). It has a mesencephalic segment that courses in the interpeduncular fossa, and a pontine segment that runs in or adjacent to the basilar sulcus. The mesencephalic segment of this vein is usually composed of the two veins, which are frequently asymmetrical in size and course near the oculomotor nerves on the lateral walls of the interpeduncular fossa. They usually anastomose rostrally with the medial end of the peduncular veins and the lateral ends of the posterior communicating vein. The small veins exiting the posterior perforated substance often join this confluence. A bridging vein may arise in the interpeduncular fossa and pass to the tentorial edge. The paired mesencephalic segments join several millimeters below the pontomesencephalic sulcus on the upper surface of the pons to form the pontine segment. If the superior part of the pontine segment is absent, the mesencephalic segment divides to connect inferiorly with the lateral anterior pontomesencephalic vein or the vein of the pontomesencephalic sulcus.

The pontine segment, which connects caudally with the median anterior medullary vein and the vein of the pontomedullary sulcus, is subdivided into superior, middle, and inferior parts. One of the three parts is usually absent. If the superior portion is absent, the middle portion anastomoses superiorly with a transverse pontine vein, and the caudal part is continuous inferiorly with the median anterior medullary vein. If the middle part is absent, the caudal end of the superior part and the cranial end of the inferior part anastomose with the transverse pontine or the lateral anterior pontomesencephalic veins. The pontine segment may deviate to one side away from the basilar sulcus, especially if the transverse pontine vein gives rise to a large bridging vein to a petrosal sinus.

Median anterior medullary vein

This vein courses in the median anterior medullary fissure between the medullary pyramids (*Figs. 3.9-3.11*). It connects superiorly with the median anterior pontomesencephalic vein and the vein of the pontomedullary sulcus at the pontomedullary junction and inferiorly with the anterior spinal vein. It may join the lateral anterior pontomesencephalic vein rostrally if the inferior part of the median anterior pontomesencephalic vein is absent. A bridging vein may connect the median anterior medullary vein with the sinuses around the jugular foramen.

Lateral anterior pontomesencephalic vein

This vein on the anterolateral aspect of the brainstem is rarely continuous from the midbrain to the lower pons (*Fig. 3.3*). At the mesencephalic level it may anastomose with the basal and peduncular veins and the vein of the pontomesencephalic sulcus, and at the pontine level it anastomoses with the transverse pontine veins. Caudally, it joins the vein of the pontomedullary sulcus near the abducens nerve. It deviates medially to connect with the median anterior pontomesencephalic or the median anterior medullary veins, if the lower part of the median anterior pontomesencephalic vein is absent. It may give rise to a bridging vein to the inferior petrosal sinus.

Lateral anterior medullary vein (preolivary vein)

This vein courses in the anterolateral sulcus between the pyramid and the olive, and is partly hidden by the roots of the hypoglossal nerve (*Fig. 3.3*). A segment along the lateral border of the pyramid may be absent. It connects superiorly with the vein of the pontomedullary sulcus and inferiorly with the lateral medullary or transverse medullary vein. The median and lateral anterior medullary veins are linked together by the transverse medullary veins that cross the pyramids at various levels.

Lateral mesencephalic vein

This vein runs in or adjacent to the lateral mesencephalic sulcus and usually drains into the basal vein near the medial geniculate body (*Fig. 3.3*). It drains the posterolateral aspect of the midbrain and sometimes receives a branch from the quadrigeminal plate. Its inferior end anastomoses with the pontotrigeminal vein and the vein of the pontomesencephalic sulcus. It sometimes receives a superior hemispheric or tectal vein (1, 9, 26).

and ascends to be joined by a superior hemispheric vein from the lateral part of the tentorial surface before emptying into the superior petrosal sinus. *E*, the cerebellum has been removed to expose the veins of the superior, inferior, and middle cerebellar peduncles. The vein of the superior cerebellar peduncle ascends to join the vein of the cerebellomesencephalic fissure. The vein of the inferior cerebellar peduncle crosses the peduncle at the inferolateral margin of the fourth ventricle and passes around the lateral recess to join the veins in the cerebellopontine angle. The veins of the cerebellopontine fissure and middle cerebellar peduncle and a transverse pontine vein join to form a superior petrosal vein. The vein of the cerebellomedullary fissure empties into the vein of the middle cerebellar peduncle. *F*, posterior view of the right cerebellopontine angle. The vein of the cerebellomedullary fissure passes laterally across the lateral recess and empties into the vein of the middle cerebellar peduncle. The latter vein and the vein of the cerebellopontine fissure join to form a large superior petrosal vein. A large anterior hemispheric vein ascends along the petrosal surface. *A.*, artery; *A.I.C.A.*, anteroinferior cerebellar artery; *Ant.*, anterior; *Cer.*, cerebellar, cerebral; *Cer. Med.*, cerebellomedullary; *Cer. Pon.*, cerebellopontine; *CN*, cranial nerve; *Fiss.*, fissure; *Hem.*, hemispheric; *Inf.*, inferior; *Med.*, median, medullary; *Mid.*, middle; *Ped.*, peduncle; *Pet.*, petrosal; *P.I.C.A.*, posteroinferior cerebellar artery; *Pon.*, pontine; *Pon. Med.*, pontomedullary; *Pon. Mes.*, pontomesencephalic; *Pon. Trig.*, pontotrigeminal; *S.C.A.*, superior cerebellar artery; *Sup.*, superior; *Trans.*, transverse; *Trig.*, trigeminal; *V.*, vein; *Vert.*, vertebral.

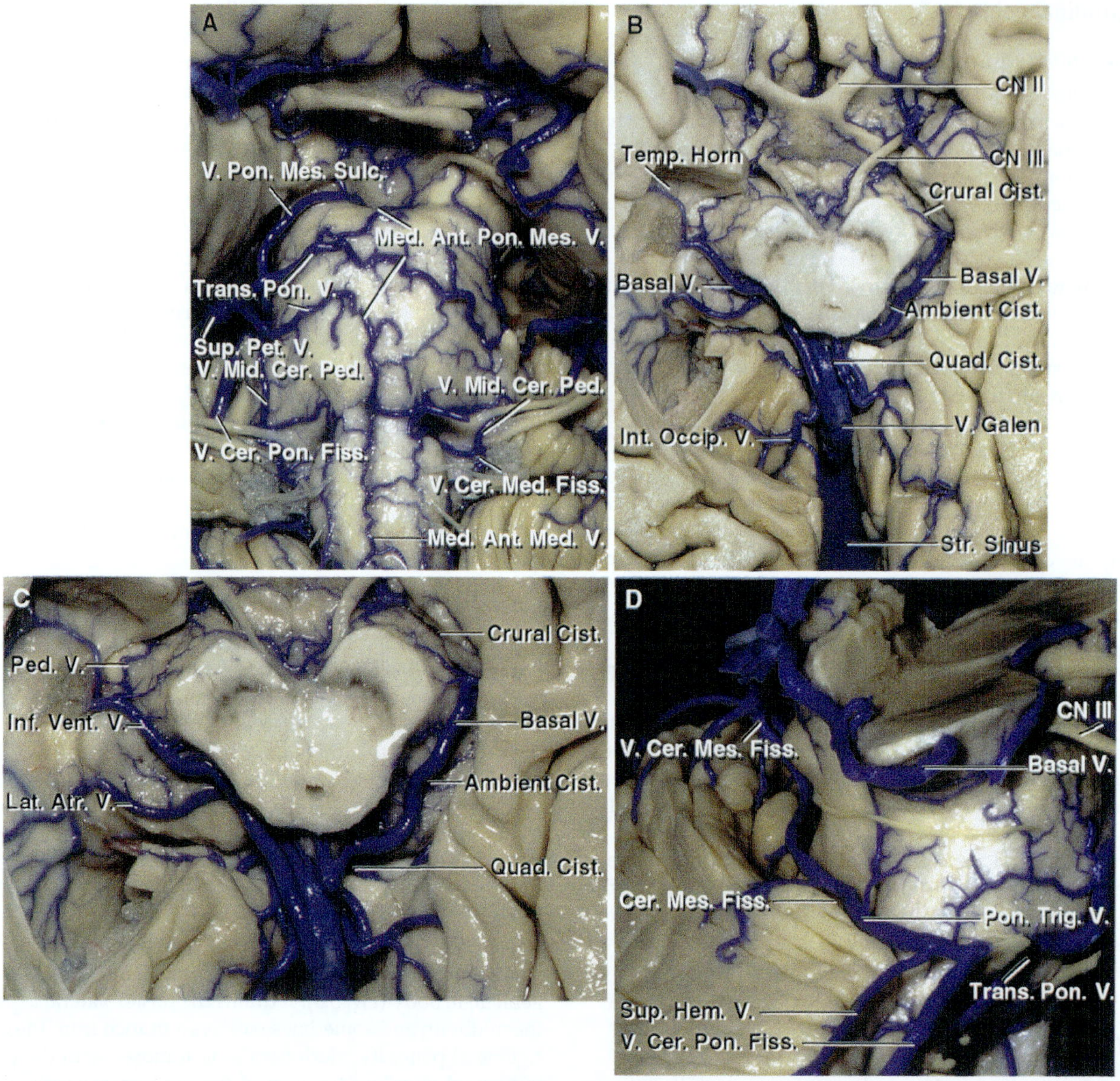

FIGURE 3.10. Upper brainstem. *A*, the veins on the anterior surface of the pons and medulla and the veins of the cerebellopontine fissure and their tributaries empty into the superior petrosal veins. The median anterior medullary vein and median anterior pontomesencephalic veins course in the midline, but often do not extend along the full length of the pons and medulla. The vein of the pontomesencephalic sulcus and the transverse pontine veins are transversely oriented. The veins of the cerebellomedullary fissure join the veins of the middle cerebellar peduncle, which ascends to join the veins of the cerebellopontine fissure. *B*, the veins in the crural and ambient cistern join the basal vein, which empties into the vein of Galen in the quadrigeminal cistern. The basal vein also drains the walls of the temporal horn, which has been opened on the right. An internal occipital vein passes from the calcarine sulcus and occipital lobe to the vein of Galen. *C*, enlarged view of the basal cisterns. The inferior ventricular vein from the temporal horn and the lateral atrial vein join the basal vein, which also drains the walls of the crural and ambient cisterns. The cerebellomesencephalic fissure, an inferior extension of the quadrigeminal cistern, is drained by tributaries of the vein of Galen. *D*, lateral view of the cerebellomesencephalic fissure. The veins in the medial portion of the cerebellomesencephalic fissure empty into the vein of Galen and those from the lateral part may join the superior petrosal veins. In this case, the vein of the cerebellomesencephalic fissure is small, resulting in most of the fissure's drainage being directed laterally through a pontotrigeminal vein, which passes above the trigeminal nerve to empty into a superior petrosal vein formed by a superior hemispheric and transverse pontine vein and the vein of the cerebellopontine fissure. *Ant.*, anterior; *Atr.*, atrial; *Cer.*, cerebellar; *Cer. Med.*, cerebellomedullary; *Cer. Mes.*, cerebellomesencephalic; *Cist.*, cistern; *CN*, cranial nerve; *Fiss.*, fissure; *Hem.*, hemispheric; *Int.*, internal; *Lat.*, lateral; *Med.*, median, medullary; *Mes.*, mesencephalic; *Mid.*, middle; *Occip.*, occipital; *Ped.*, peduncle; *Pet.*, petrosal; *Pon.*, pontine, ponto; *Quad.*, quadrigeminal; *Str.*, straight; *Sulc.*, sulcus; *Sup.*, superior; *Temp.*, temporal; *Trans.*, transverse; *Trig.*, trigeminal; *V.*, vein; *Vent.*, ventricle.

Lateral medullary and retro-olivary veins

There are usually two longitudinal veins between the lateral border of the olive and the foramen of Luschka (*Fig. 3.3*): a smaller ventral vein (the retro-olivary vein), and a larger dorsal vein (the lateral medullary vein). The lateral medullary vein courses slightly dorsal to the retro-olivary sulcus along the rootlets of the accessory, vagus, and glossopharyngeal nerves. It receives the retro-olivary vein from its ventral side and the vein of the inferior cerebellar peduncle from its dorsal side, and joins the vein of the pontomedullary sulcus to form the vein of the middle cerebellar peduncle. This vein and the vein of the inferior cerebellar peduncle often give rise to an inferior petrosal bridging vein near the foramen of Luschka, which courses along the rootlets of the nerves entering the jugular foramen to join the venous sinuses near the jugular bulb.

The retro-olivary vein usually courses along the rostral two-thirds of the retro-olivary sulcus slightly ventral to the lateral medullary vein. Although small, it may rarely replace the lateral medullary vein. It often anastomoses near the lower edge of the olive with the caudal part of the lateral medullary vein and above the olive with either the vein of the pontomedullary sulcus or the rostral end of the lateral medullary vein.

Transversely oriented veins

Peduncular vein

This vein arises in the interpeduncular fossa and courses laterally around the cerebral peduncle below the optic tract toward the basal vein (*Figs. 3.3, 3.9,* and *3.10*). It anastomoses medially with the posterior communicating vein, which links the medial ends of the peduncular veins, and with the upper end of the median anterior pontomesencephalic vein. Its medial end is located on the superomedial surface of the origin of the oculomotor nerve. The lateral end of the vein drains into the basal vein or one of its tributaries. In a few cases it drains through a bridging vein into a sinus in the edge of the tentorium.

Posterior communicating vein

This vein courses transversely across the interpeduncular fossa on the superomedial surface of the oculomotor nerves, interconnecting the medial ends of the peduncular veins and the rostral ends of the median anterior pontomesencephalic veins (*Fig. 3.3*). It usually courses in the interpeduncular cistern, bridging over rather than coursing on the floor of the interpeduncular fossa. Small veins exiting the interpeduncular fossa frequently join the posterior communicating vein.

Vein of the pontomesencephalic sulcus

This vein is usually small, and does not extend the entire length of the pontomesencephalic sulcus from the midline to the lateral mesencephalic sulcus (*Fig. 3.3* and *3.10*). It passes below the oculomotor nerves and anastomoses with the median and lateral anterior pontomesencephalic veins in most cases. The lateral mesencephalic and pontotrigeminal veins may anastomose with the lateral end of this vein near the confluence of the pontomesencephalic, lateral mesencephalic, and interpeduncular sulci.

Transverse pontine veins

This is a group of veins that cross the anterior surface of the pons at various levels (*Figs. 3.9-3.11*). They interconnect the median anterior pontomesencephalic vein and the veins on the lateral surface of the pons. The most prominent transverse pontine veins are located at the midpons. Those on the upper and lower thirds of the pons are usually small and only infrequently transverse the full width of the pons. Those on the midpons are usually present bilaterally and anastomose medially with the median anterior pontomesencephalic vein. They course laterally above or below the trigeminal nerve to drain into the superior petrosal sinus, the pontotrigeminal vein, or the vein of the cerebellopontine fissure or the middle cerebellar peduncle. They sometimes give rise to a bridging vein to the inferior petrosal sinus. If the middle third of the median anterior pontomesencephalic vein is absent, the ends adjoining the absent segments drain into the transverse pontine veins.

Vein of the pontomedullary sulcus

This vein courses in or near the pontomedullary sulcus and connects with the longitudinally oriented veins on the anterior aspect of the pons and medulla (*Figs. 3.3* and *3.9*). It joins the lateral medullary or retro-olivary veins or the vein of the inferior cerebellar peduncle above the olive to form the vein of the middle cerebellar peduncle. It may give rise to a bridging vein to the sinuses around the jugular foramen.

Transverse medullary veins

These veins cross the anterior and lateral surfaces of the medulla at the level of the medullary pyramid or below (*Fig. 3.9*). They interconnect the median anterior medullary vein with the veins on the lateral surface of the medulla. They rarely cross the full distance from the median anterior medullary vein to the lateral medullary vein, but usually consist of one or two shorter veins passing transversely across the medullary pyramid or the olive. The largest transverse medullary veins are usually situated at the level of the middle third of the pyramid. They sometimes give rise to a bridging vein to the sigmoid or marginal sinuses.

MAJOR DRAINING GROUPS

The terminal end of the veins draining the brainstem and cerebellum form bridging veins that collect into three groups: 1) a galenic group that drains into the vein of Galen; 2) a petrosal group that drains into the petrosal sinuses; and 3) a tentorial group that drains into the sinuses converging on the torcula (*Fig. 3.3*). The galenic group drains the tentorial surface, the cerebellomesencephalic fissure, and the superior half of the roof of the fourth ventricle; the petrosal group drains the petrosal surface, the cerebellomedullary and cerebellopontine fissures, the inferior half of the roof of the fourth ventricle and the lateral recesses, and the anterior and

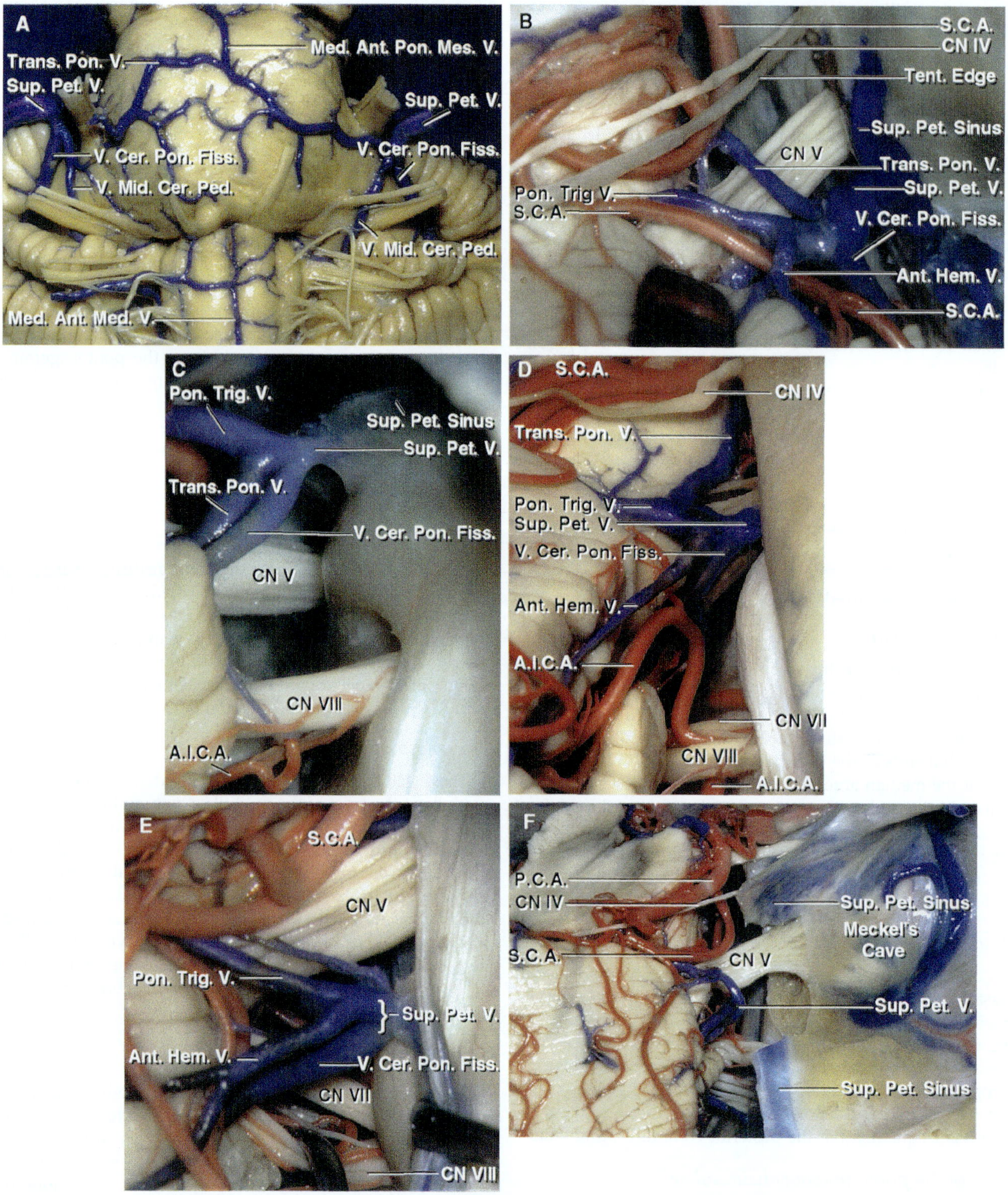

FIGURE 3.11. Superior petrosal veins. *A*, the superior petrosal veins drain the anterior and lateral surfaces of the brainstem, the petrosal surface, and some of the lateral part of the tentorial and suboccipital surfaces. The veins of the middle cerebellar peduncle ascend on the middle cerebellar peduncles and join the veins of the cerebellopontine fissure and the transverse pontine veins to form superior petrosal veins that empty into the superior petrosal sinuses. *B*, lateral view of a large superior petrosal vein formed by the union of the transverse pontine, pontotrigeminal, and anterior hemispheric veins and the vein of the cerebellopontine fissure. A large branch of the superior cerebellar artery and the trigeminal nerve are enmeshed in the tributaries of this superior

lateral sides of the pons and medulla; and the tentorial group drains the suboccipital surface. Other less frequent bridging veins pass to the cavernous, marginal, basilar, and sigmoid sinuses and the jugular bulb.

Galenic draining group

This group, formed by the veins converging on the vein of Galen, includes the superficial veins that drain the tentorial surface, the deep veins that drain the superior part of the roof of the fourth ventricle and the cerebellomesencephalic fissure, and the brainstem veins that drain the midbrain. Most of these veins drain through the superior vermian and basal veins to reach the vein of Galen (*Figs. 3.2-3.5*). The superficial group includes the superior vermian vein and the anterior group of the superior hemispheric veins; the deep group includes the vein of the cerebellomesencephalic fissure and the paired veins of the superior cerebellar peduncle; and the brainstem group includes the peduncular, posterior communicating, and tectal veins and the rostral portions of the medial and lateral anterior pontomesencephalic and the lateral mesencephalic veins. All of these brainstem veins, except for the tectal vein, join the basal vein that drains into the vein of Galen. The tectal veins join the superior vermian vein or the vein of the cerebellomesencephalic fissure.

Tentorial draining group

The tentorial draining group includes the veins that drain into the straight and lateral sinuses and the torcula, either directly or through a tentorial sinus (*Figs. 3.2-3.6*). It is composed of the superficial veins draining the suboccipital surface and the posterior part of the tentorial surface. The veins from the suboccipital surface include the inferior vermian veins and inferior hemispheric veins. The veins from the tentorial surface include the posterior groups of superior hemispheric and superior vermian veins. The inferior hemispheric veins and the posterior group of the superior hemispheric veins often join before entering the tentorial sinuses, which drain into the torcula or into the straight or lateral sinuses near the torcula.

The tentorial sinuses also receive the inferior cerebral veins, the vein of Labbé, and the bridging veins to the tentorial edge. The tentorial sinuses can course directly medially to drain into the midportion of the straight sinus, posteromedially to drain into the torcula or the straight or lateral sinus near the torcula, immediately posteriorly to drain into the middle third of the lateral sinus, or posterolaterally to drain into the lateral and superior petrosal sinuses at or near the confluence of the two sinuses. Some sinuses are formed by the union of veins draining the tentorium itself.

Petrosal draining group

The petrosal draining group includes the veins draining into the petrosal sinuses (*Figs. 3.1, 3.11,* and *3.12*) (9, 26). This draining group includes the superficial veins that drain the lateral part of the cerebellar hemisphere; a deep group that drains the cerebellopontine and cerebellomedullary and the lateral part of the cerebellomesencephalic fissures, and the inferior part of the roof and the lateral wall of the fourth ventricle; and a brainstem group that drains much of the brainstem.

The petrosal veins are divided into superior and inferior petrosal veins based on whether they enter the superior or inferior petrosal sinus. The superior petrosal veins are among the largest and most frequent veins in the posterior fossa. The inferior petrosal veins are represented by a few small bridging veins. The superior petrosal veins may be formed by the terminal segment of a single vein or by the common stem formed by the union of several veins. The most common tributaries of the superior petrosal veins are the transverse pontine and pontotrigeminal veins, the common stem of the lateral group of the superior hemispheric veins, and the veins of the cerebellopontine fissure and the middle cerebellar peduncle. The superior petrosal veins are subdivided into a lateral, intermediate, and medial group based on the relationship of their site of entry into the superior petrosal sinus to the internal acoustic meatus. The intermediate group drains into the sinus above the internal acoustic meatus, the medial group drains into the sinus medial to the meatus, and the lateral group drains into the sinus lateral to the meatus. Of 20 superior petrosal sinuses examined in our previous study, 8 received one superior petrosal vein, 10 received two, and 2 received three (15). Of the 34 superior petrosal veins, 22 (64.7%) were of the medial type, 3 (8.8%) were of the inter-

petrosal vein. Care is required to avoid occluding the superior cerebellar artery when occluding a multipronged petrosal vein. *C*, retrosigmoid view. The right cerebellopontine angle is drained by a superior petrosal vein formed by the pontotrigeminal and transverse pontine veins and the vein of the cerebellopontine fissure. *D*, the tributaries of this superior petrosal vein include the transverse pontine, pontotrigeminal, and anterior hemispheric veins and the vein of the cerebellopontine fissure. *E*, superior petrosal vein with multiple tributaries. The vestibulocochlear nerve has been depressed to expose the facial nerve. *F*, the segment of the superior petrosal sinus, which crosses above the trigeminal nerve and receives the superior petrosal veins, has been removed. The posterior trigeminal nerve passes forward below the tentorial edge and the superior petrosal sinus to enter Meckel's cave. The superior petrosal sinus extends medially through the upper edge of the porus of Meckel's cave and above the trigeminal nerve to join the cavernous sinus. Some superior petrosal veins may join the sinus on the medial side of the trigeminal nerve. *A.I.C.A.*, anteroinferior cerebellar artery; *Ant.*, anterior; *Cer.*, cerebellar; *Cer. Pon.*, cerebellopontine; *CN*, cranial nerve; *Fiss.*, fissure; *Hem.*, hemispheric; *Med.*, median, medullary; *Mid.*, middle; *P.C.A.*, posterior cerebral artery; *Ped.*, peduncle; *Pet.*, petrosal; *Pon.*, pontine; *Pon. Mes.*, pontomesencephalic; *Pon. Trig.*, pontotrigeminal; *S.C.A.*, superior cerebellar artery; *Sup.*, superior; *Tent.*, tentorial; *Trans.*, transverse; *V.*, vein.

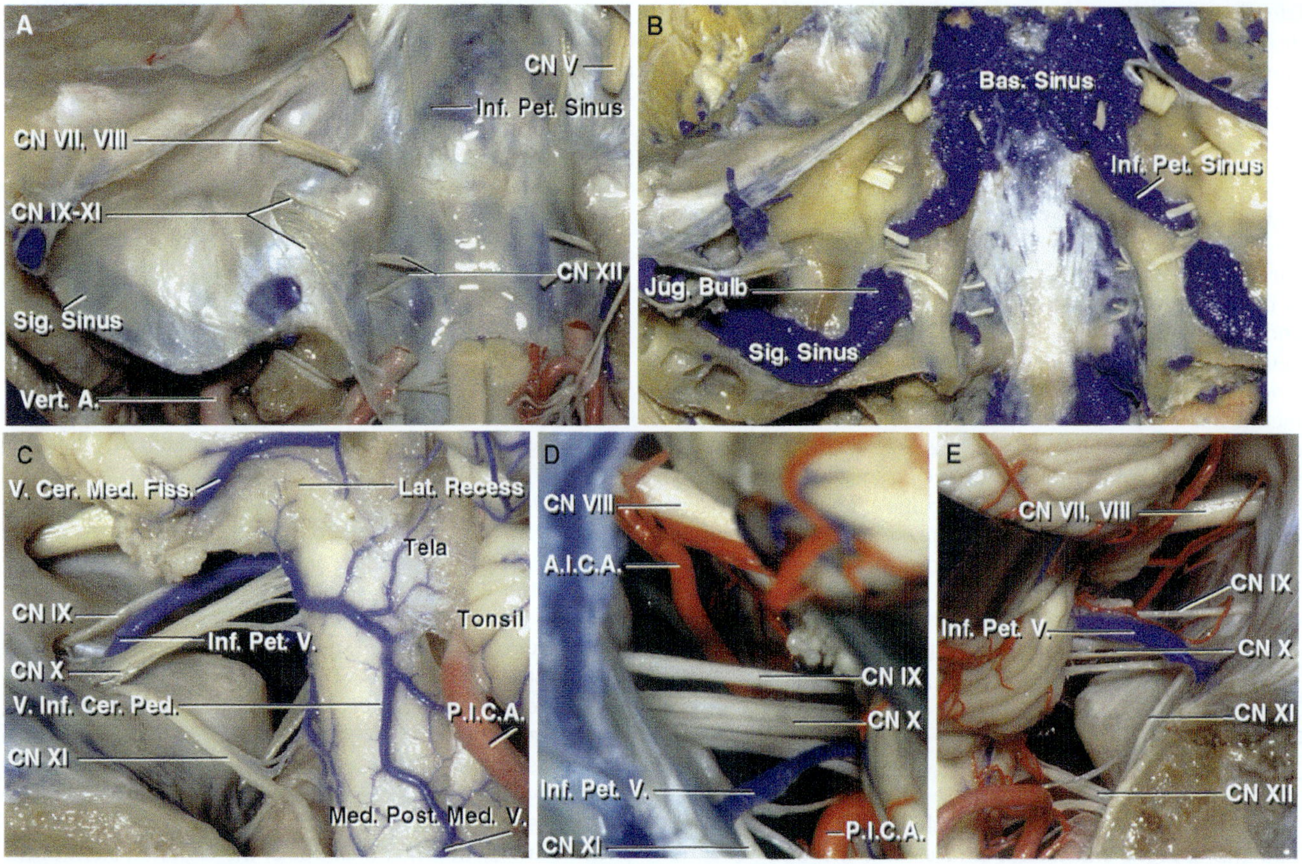

FIGURE 3.12. Inferior petrosal sinus and veins. ***A*, posterior view of the anterior portion of the posterior fossa with the brainstem and cerebellum removed. The inferior petrosal and sigmoid sinuses can be seen through the dura. *B*, the dural roof of the basilar, inferior petrosal, and sigmoid sinuses have been removed. The inferior petrosal sinuses extend from the basilar sinus above to the jugular bulbs below. The inferior petrosal veins arise on the brainstem and empty into the lower part of the inferior petrosal sinus, jugular bulb, or distal sigmoid sinus. *C–E*, posterior views into cerebellopontine angle. *C*, an inferior petrosal vein passes from the medulla between the glossopharyngeal and vagus nerves to the jugular bulb. It receives the drainage of the vein of the inferior cerebellar peduncle, which crosses the peduncle just below the lateral recess. *D*, an inferior petrosal nerve passes behind the glossopharyngeal and vagus nerves to empty into the terminal part of the sigmoid sinus. *E*, an inferior petrosal vein crosses behind the nerves entering the jugular foramen to reach the sigmoid sinus. *A.*, artery; *A.I.C.A.*, anteroinferior cerebellar artery; *Bas.*, basilar; *Cer.*, cerebellar; *Cer. Med.*, cerebellomedullary; *CN*, cranial nerve; *Fiss.*, fissure; *Inf.*, inferior; *Jug.*, jugular; *Lat.*, lateral; *Med.*, median, medullary; *Ped.*, peduncle; *Pet.*, petrosal; *P.I.C.A.*, posteroinferior cerebellar artery; *Post.*, posterior; *Sig.*, sigmoid; *V.*, vein; *Vert.*, vertebral.**

mediate type, and 9 (26.5%) were of the lateral type. Nineteen of 20 (95%) sinuses examined had veins of the medial type, 3 (15%) had veins of the intermediate type, and 9 (45%) had veins of the lateral type. The medial group of superior petrosal veins is usually a common trunk formed by the union of two or three of the following veins: transverse pontine veins, pontotrigeminal veins, and the veins of the cerebellopontine fissure and the middle cerebellar peduncle. The latter veins may also enter the sinus without joining another vein. Two of the three intermediate superior petrosal veins were formed by a single vein, the vein of the cerebellopontine fissure. The most common veins in the lateral group are the common stem formed by the union of superior and inferior hemispheric veins and the vein of the cerebellopontine fissure.

Other bridging veins

The major bridging veins have been discussed above. Other less frequent bridging veins run from the basal vein to a sinus coursing in the tentorial edge; from the peduncular vein to a sinus in the tentorial edge or the cavernous sinus; from the lateral or medial anterior pontomesencephalic or a transverse pontine vein to the posterior portion of the cavernous or the adjoining part of the inferior petrosal sinuses just below Meckel's cave; from the veins of the pontomedullary sulcus and the inferior cerebellar peduncle or the lateral medullary vein to the sigmoid and inferior petrosal sinuses near the jugular foramen or jugular bulb; from the vein of the pontomedullary sulcus, and the lateral anterior, lateral, and transverse medullary veins to a marginal sinus at the level of the foramen magnum or to the veins in the hypoglossal canal, which communicates with the marginal sinuses (*Fig. 3.12*) (13, 15).

DISCUSSION

The infrequent reports of adverse sequelae after the intraoperative occlusion of veins in the posterior fossa is caused by the diffuse anastomosis between the veins. It is not surprising that more severe sequelae have occurred after occlusion of bridging veins than after occlusion of veins on the surface of the cerebellum, since the bridging veins are formed by the terminal end of numerous surface veins. The veins crossing the cerebellopontine angle to reach the petrosal sinuses are the ones most frequently occluded in the course of operations in the posterior fossa. Bridging veins are more frequently exposed and sacrificed in the rostral part of the cerebellopontine angle during operations near the trigeminal nerve than during operations in the central or caudal part near the nerves entering the internal acoustic meatus and the jugular foramen. Exposure of the trigeminal nerve through a suboccipital craniectomy commonly requires the sacrifice of one or more bridging veins, while exposure of the nerves entering the internal acoustic meatus infrequently requires sacrifice of even a single bridging vein.

In 1929, Dandy pointed out that the petrosal vein should receive special attention during posterior fossa operations on the trigeminal nerve (4). His illustration showed a vein that coursed in the cerebellopontine angle near the rostral aspect of the trigeminal nerve to drain into the superior petrosal sinus. Later, this common stem came to be known either as the superior petrosal vein or simply as the petrosal vein (4, 5, 23). No consideration has been given in the surgical literature to the identification of the trunks that unite to form the petrosal veins, and to the size of the area drained by their tributaries. The veins converging on the trigeminal nerve to form the superior petrosal veins are the transverse pontine and the pontotrigeminal veins, and the veins of the cerebellopontine fissure and the middle cerebellar peduncle. The largest vein contributing to the formation of the petrosal vein near the trigeminal nerve is the vein of the cerebellopontine fissure, which drains most of the petrosal surface of the cerebellum and much of the lower brainstem and the cerebellopontine and cerebellomedullary fissures. Although superior petrosal veins can be located at any point along the superior petrosal sinus, most are located just lateral to the trigeminal nerve. Adverse sequelae only infrequently follow occlusion of this medial group of superior petrosal veins; however, we have seen two patients with a transient cerebellar disturbance caused by a venous infarction with hemorrhagic edema after the intraoperative occlusion of these veins lateral to the trigeminal nerve.

The exposure of lesions such as acoustic neuromas in the central part of the cerebellopontine angle near the lateral recess, by retracting the petrosal surface of the hemisphere away from the sigmoid sinus, can usually be completed without sacrificing a single bridging vein. If a vein is obliterated during acoustic tumor removal, it is usually one of the superior petrosal veins that is sacrificed near the superior pole of the tumor during the later stages of the removal of a large tumor. Smaller tumors can often be removed without sacrificing a petrosal vein. The large vein encountered around the superior pole of an acoustic neuroma is the vein of the cerebellopontine fissure, which passes from the petrosal surface and cerebellopontine fissure above the facial and vestibulocochlear nerves to the area above the trigeminal nerve. This vein has been occluded during acoustic neuroma removal without causing a deficit (14).

Compression of the trigeminal nerve by the surrounding veins is postulated to be a cause of trigeminal neuralgia (8, 11). In 411 operations for trigeminal neuralgia, Jannetta found veins compressing the nerve in 153; however, none of these veins involved in this compression was listed by name (11). Compression of the facial and glossopharyngeal nerves by veins has also been postulated to be a cause of hemifacial spasm and glossopharyngeal neuralgia (12). The venous relationships of the trigeminal nerve where numerous bridging veins converge on and cross the subarachnoid space near the posterior root is distinctly different from those in the region of the facial and vestibulocochlear nerves, where the predominant veins are on the side of the brainstem and in contact with the nerves at their junction with the brainstem. The veins coursing on or near the junction of the facial and vestibulocochlear nerves with the brainstem are the veins of the middle cerebellar peduncle, the cerebellomedullary fissure, and the pontomedullary sulcus. There are no large veins intermingling with the nerves at or within the acoustic meatus, as occurs with the arteries. The major veins near the glossopharyngeal and vagus nerves also course near the origin of the nerves on the surface of the brainstem, although there are small bridging veins that course along these nerves to the venous sinuses near the jugular bulb. The lateral medullary, retroolivary, and transverse medullary veins and the vein of the inferior cerebellar peduncle course near the origin of the rootlets of the glossopharyngeal and vagus nerves.

Bridging veins are more frequently encountered in exposing the tentorial surface of the cerebellum than in exposing the suboccipital or petrosal surfaces of the cerebellum. The bridging veins from the suboccipital surface are often encountered on the posterior part of the tentorial surface because the hemispheric veins from the suboccipital surface uniformly ascend to the tentorial surface before forming bridging veins that pass to the venous sinuses in the tentorium. Most of the veins from the petrosal surface pass to the vein of the cerebellopontine fissure and not directly to a venous sinus. The veins from the tentorial and suboccipital surface that enter the sinuses in the tentorium are obstacles in the supracerebellar approaches. In the infratentorial supracerebellar approach to the pineal region, it may be necessary to divide numerous bridging veins entering the torcula and the tentorial sinuses, including some of the superior and inferior hemispheric and vermian veins, and the vein of the cerebellomesencephalic fissure. These veins have commonly been sacrificed without adverse effect to open the quadrigeminal region and the incisura (18, 22, 27). However cerebellar swelling followed transection of one of the bridging veins by Page (17).

Bridging veins infrequently cross from the suboccipital surface, tonsils, and medulla to the venous sinuses in the dura overlying the suboccipital surface. In a few cases, an inferior vermian or hemispheric vein will give rise to a bridging vein that drains into the occipital sinuses below the torcula, and the veins on the posterior and lateral surfaces of the medulla will give rise to bridging veins to the marginal or the occipital sinuses (7, 19). In approaching the fourth ventricle, the veins around the tonsils, on the lower vermis, and near the inferior part of the roof may be sacrificed. These veins, including the vein of the cerebellomedullary fissure, have been occluded repeatedly without sequelae.

It may be necessary to divide part of the tentorium in either the occipital transtentorial or the infratentorial supracerebellar approaches (10). In the occipital transtentorial approach, the occipital lobe can often be retracted away from the falx and tentorium adjoining the straight sinus without sacrificing any veins, because only infrequently are there bridging veins from the occipital lobe near the straight sinus to the torcula, lateral, straight, and superior sagittal sinuses. The posterior 5 cm of the superior sagittal sinus is frequently devoid of bridging veins. The vein of Labbé, which drains into the lateral portion of the lateral sinus, is usually lateral to this exposure, and the internal occipital vein, which must be divided to reach the pineal region, drains not into a dural sinus, but into the internal cerebral or great vein in the quadrigeminal cistern. In the transtentorial approach the tentorium is divided adjacent to and parallel to the straight sinus beginning at the free edge and extending posteriorly (20). The tentorial sinuses in the anterior part of the tentorium are smaller and less frequent than those in the posterior part of the tentorium. Most of the tentorial sinuses found in the posterior third of the tentorium are formed by the cerebellar veins. The veins draining the lower portion of the temporal and occipital lobes empty into the more anteriorly situated tentorial sinuses that drain into the superior petrosal or adjacent part of the transverse sinus. The tentorial sinuses formed by the veins draining the cerebrum commonly course posteromedially, posterolaterally, or straight posteriorly from their origin. The sinus in the anterior part of the tentorium usually receives only small bridging veins from the midbrain, but in rare cases, the basal vein may terminate as a large bridging vein that enters the anterior part of the tentorium. The anteromedial edge of the tentorium posterior to the superior petrosal sinus may be sectioned through a subtemporal craniectomy to expose the trigeminal nerve and the surrounding superior petrosal venous complex from their superolateral side. This provides excellent exposure of the pontotrigeminal and transverse pontine veins passing above the trigeminal nerve, but some of the transverse pontine and bridging veins may be hidden below or medial to the nerve in this exposure.

Reprint requests: Albert L. Rhoton, Jr., M.D., Department of Neurological Surgery, University of Florida Brain Institute, P.O. Box 100265, 100 South Newell Drive, Building 59, L2-100, Gainesville, FL 32610-0265.

REFERENCES

1. Billewicz O: The normal and pathological radioanatomy of the lateral mesencephalic vein. **Neuroradiology** 8:295–299, 1975.
2. Braun JP, Tournade A: The veins of the lateral recess of the 4th ventricle. **Neuroradiology** 7:9–13, 1974.
3. Browder J, Kaplan HA, Krieger AJ: Anatomical features of the straight sinus and its tributaries: Clinical correlations. **J Neurosurg** 44:55–61, 1976.
4. Dandy WE: An operation for the cure of tic douloureux: Partial section of the sensory root at the pons. **Arch Surg** 18:687–734, 1929.
5. Dandy WE: Concerning the cause of trigeminal neuralgia. **Am J Surg** 24:447–455, 1934.
6. Das AC, Hasan M: The occipital sinus. **J Neurosurg** 33:307–311, 1970.
7. Duvernoy HM: *Human Brainstem Vessels*. New York, Springer-Verlag, 1977, pp 6–24.
8. Haines SJ, Jannetta PJ, Zorub DS: Microvascular relations of the trigeminal nerve: An anatomical study with clinical correlation. **J Neurosurg** 52:381–386, 1980.
9. Huang YP, Wolf BS: Veins of the posterior fossa, in Newton TH, Potts DG (eds): *Radiology of the Skull and Brain*. St Louis, C.V. Mosby, 1974, vol II, Book 3, pp 2155–2216.
10. Jamieson KG: Excision of pineal tumors. **J Neurosurg** 35:550–553, 1971.
11. Jannetta PJ: Vascular decompression in trigeminal neuralgia, in Samii M, Jannetta PJ (eds): *The Cranial Nerves: Anatomy-Pathology-Diagnosis-Treatment*. New York, Springer-Verlag, 1981, pp 331–340.
12. Jannetta PJ, Abbasy M, Maroon JC, Ramos FM, Albin MS: Etiology and definitive microsurgical treatment of hemifacial spasm: Operative techniques and results in 47 patients. **J Neurosurg** 47:321–328, 1977.
13. Katsuta T, Rhoton AL Jr, Matsushima T: The jugular foramen: Microsurgical anatomy and operative approaches. **Neurosurgery** 41:149–202, 1997.
14. Kempe LG: *Posterior Fossa, Spinal Cord and Peripheral Nerve Disease: Operative Neurosurgery*. New York, Springer-Verlag, 1970, vol 2, pp 34–45.
15. Matsushima T, Rhoton AL Jr, de Oliveira E, Peace D: Microsurgical anatomy of the veins of the posterior fossa. **J Neurosurg** 59:63–105, 1983.
16. Matsushima T, Rhoton AL Jr, Lenkey C: Microsurgery of the fourth ventricle: Part 1—Microsurgical anatomy. **Neurosurgery** 11:631–667, 1982.
17. Page LK: The infratentorial-supracerebellar exposure of tumors in the pineal area. **Neurosurgery** 1:36–40, 1977.
18. Pendl G: Infratentorial approach to mesencephalic tumors, in Koos WT, Böck FW, Spetzler RF (eds): *Clinical Microneurosurgery*. Stuttgart, Georg Thieme, 1976, pp 143–150.
19. Perese DM: Superficial veins of the brain from a surgical point of view. **J Neurosurg** 17:402–412, 1960.
20. Rhoton AL Jr, Yamamoto I, Peace DA: Microsurgery of the third ventricle: Part 2—Operative approaches. **Neurosurgery** 8:357–373, 1981.
21. Saxena RC, Beg MAQ, Das AC: The straight sinus. **J Neurosurg** 41:724–727, 1974.
22. Stein BM: The infratentorial supracerebellar approach to pineal lesions. **J Neurosurg** 35:197–202, 1971.
23. Takahashi M, Wilson G, Hanafee W: The significance of the petrosal vein in the diagnosis of cerebellopontine angle tumors. **Radiology** 89:834–840, 1967.
24. Wackenheim A, Braun JP: *The Veins of the Posterior Fossa: Normal and Pathologic Findings*. New York, Springer-Verlag, 1978, pp 1–23.
25. Waltner JG: Anatomic variations of the lateral and sigmoid sinuses. **Arch Otolaryngol** 39:307–312, 1944.
26. Wolf BS, Huang YP, Newman CM: The lateral anastomotic mesencephalic vein and other variations in drainage of the basal cerebral brain. **AJR Am J Roentgenol** 89:411–422, 1963.
27. Yamamoto I, Kageyama N: Microsurgical anatomy of the pineal region. **J Neurosurg** 53:205–221, 1980.

CHAPTER 4

The Cerebellopontine Angle and Posterior Fossa Cranial Nerves by the Retrosigmoid Approach

Albert L. Rhoton, Jr., M.D.

Department of Neurological Surgery, University of Florida, Gainesville, Florida

Key words: Acoustic neuroma, Cerebellopontine angle, Cranial nerves, Hemifacial spasm, Microsurgery, Microsurgical anatomy, Surgical approach, Trigeminal neuralgia

The cerebellopontine angle is located between the superior and inferior limbs of the angular cerebellopontine fissure formed by the petrosal cerebellar surface folding around the pons and middle cerebellar peduncle (*Fig. 4.1*). The cerebellopontine fissure opens medially and has superior and inferior limbs that meet at a lateral apex. The fourth through the eleventh cranial nerves are located near or within the angular space between the two limbs commonly referred to as the cerebellopontine angle (*Fig. 4.1*). The trochlear and trigeminal nerves are located near the fissure's superior limb and the glossopharyngeal, vagus, and accessory nerves are located near the inferior limb. The abducens nerve is located near the base of the fissure, along a line connecting the anterior ends of the superior and inferior limbs.

This description of the cranial nerves and operative approaches to the cerebellopontine angle is organized around the three neurovascular complexes, defined in the chapter on the cerebellar arteries, and focuses on the retrosigmoid approach, which is the most frequently selected approach for lesions in the angle. The microsurgical anatomy of acoustic neuromas, vascular compression syndromes, and other disorders involving the nerves in the cerebellopontine angle are the subjects of this section.

UPPER NEUROVASCULAR COMPLEX

The most common operation directed to the upper neurovascular complex is the exposure of the posterior root of the trigeminal nerve. The posterior trigeminal root joins the brainstem about halfway between the lower and upper borders of the pons (*Fig. 4.2*). Frequently, a lip of cerebellum projects forward and obscures the junction of the posterior root with the pons. In its intradural course, the trigeminal nerve uniformly runs obliquely upward from the lateral part of the pons toward the petrous apex. It exits the posterior fossa to enter the middle cranial fossa by passing forward beneath the tentorial attachment to enter Meckel's cave, which sits in the trigeminal impression on the upper surface of the petrous part of the temporal bone.

Trigeminal root anatomy

The fibers from the third division remain in a caudolateral position in the posterior root throughout the interval from the ganglion to the pons, the first division rostromedial, with second-division fibers in an intermediate position (*Figs. 4.2* and *4.3*). Conclusions that the third-division fibers remain caudolateral and that the first-division fibers remain rostromedial from the pons to the ganglion agree with data from clinical and laboratory studies (5, 8, 31). There are anastomoses between the fibers from each division in the area posterior to the ganglion (*Fig. 4.2*). Results of selective rhizotomy of the posterior root indicate that somatotopic localization with the third division inferolaterally and the ophthalmic division dorsomedially is well maintained posterior to, and despite, the prominent retrogasserian anastomoses (5).

A cross section of the sensory root between the pons and the petrous apex is elliptical. In most nerves, the angle between the longest diameter of this cross section and the long axis of the body is 40 to 50 degrees; the angle, however, can vary from 10 to 80 degrees (*Fig. 4.4*) (12). An angle of 80 degrees places the third-division fibers almost directly lateral to those of the first division; but an angle of 10 degrees places the third-division fibers almost directly caudal to those of the first division. The variability in the degree of rotation of the sensory root entering the pons may explain some differences in the quantity of sensation retained after partial section of the nerve in the posterior cranial fossa. The most frequent pattern is for the third-division fibers to be caudolateral to the first-division fibers; some nerves, however, are rotated so that third-division fibers will be almost directly lateral to the first division; others are rotated nearly 70 degrees away from this so that the third-division fibers will be directly caudal to those of the first division. Cutting into the nerve partially from a caudolateral direction would give a significantly different pattern of sensory loss if the nerve is rotated with the third division lateral to the first, than if the third division is almost directly caudal to the first division.

At the junction of the nerve with the pons, as many as 15 separate nerve rootlets may be spread around the rostral

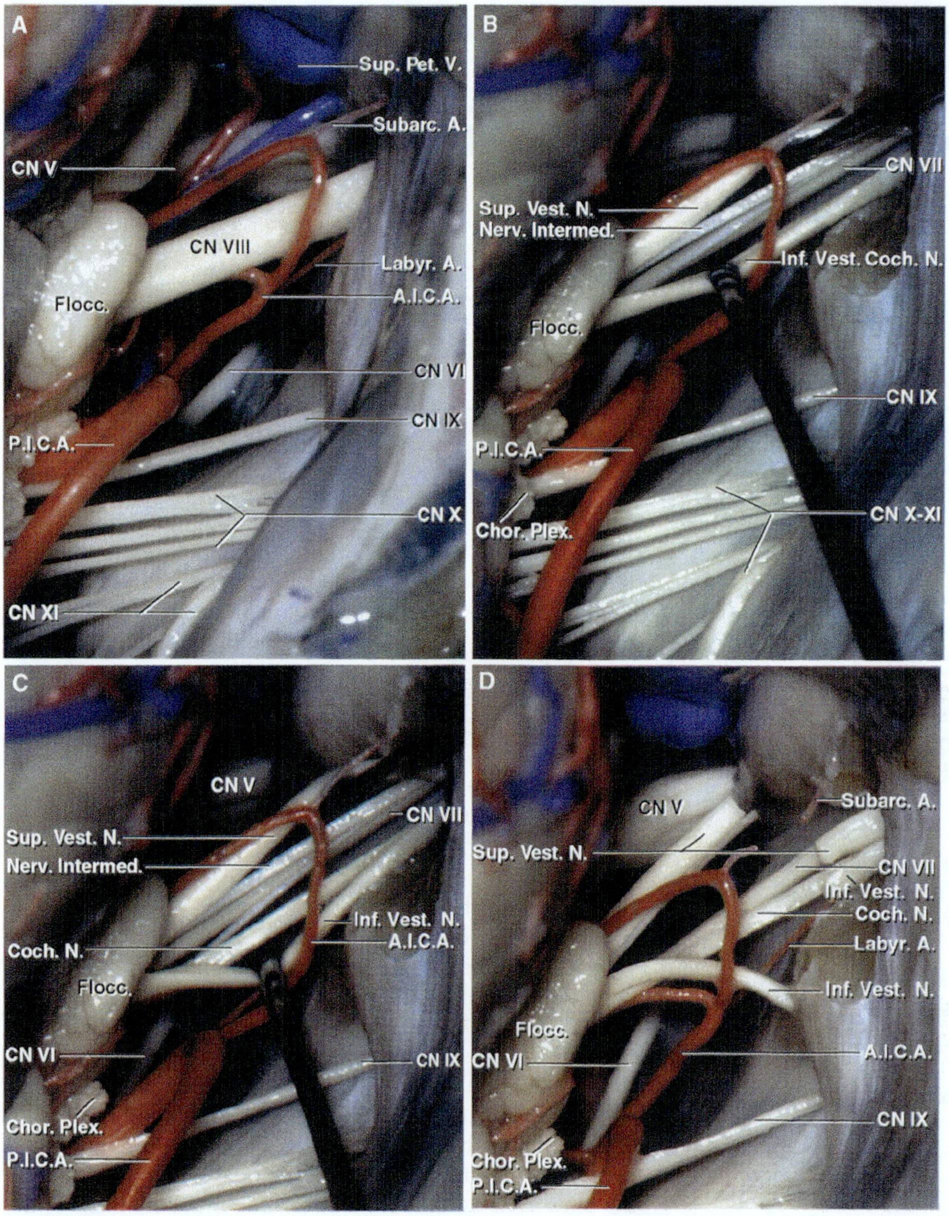

FIGURE 4.1. **Retrosigmoid exposure of the nerves in the right cerebellopontine angle. *A*, the vestibulocochlear nerve enters the internal acoustic meatus with a labyrinthine branch of the AICA. The PICA courses around the glossopharyngeal, vagus, and accessory nerves. The abducens nerve ascends in front of the pons. A subarcuate artery enters the subarcuate fossa superolateral to the porus of the meatus. Choroid plexus protrudes into the cerebellopontine angle behind the glossopharyngeal and vagus nerves. *B*, the posterior wall of the internal acoustic meatus has been removed. The cleavage plane between the upper bundle, formed by the superior vestibular nerve, and the lower bundle, formed by the inferior vestibular and cochlear nerves, was begun laterally where the nerves have separated near the meatal fundus and extended medially. The nervus intermedius arises on the anterior surface of the vestibulocochlear nerve, has a free segment in the cistern and/or meatus, and joins the facial nerve distally. The facial nerve is located anterior to the superior vestibular nerve and the cochlear nerve is anterior to the inferior vestibular nerve. *C*, the cleavage plane between the cochlear and inferior vestibular nerves, which is well developed in the lateral end of the internal acoustic meatus, has been extended medially. Within the cerebellopontine angle, the superior vestibular nerve is posterior and superior, the facial nerve anterior and superior, the inferior vestibular nerve posterior and inferior, and the cochlear nerve anterior and inferior. *D*, the superior and inferior vestibular nerves have been divided to expose the facial and cochlear nerves. A labyrinthine branch of the PICA enters the internal meatus. *A.*, artery; *A.I.C.A.*, anteroinferior cerebellar artery; *Chor. Plex.*, choroid plexus; *CN*, cranial nerve; *Coch.*, cochlear; *Flocc.*, flocculus; *Inf.*, inferior; *Intermed.*, intermedius; *Labyr.*, labyrinth; *N.*, nerve; *Nerv.*, nervus; *Pet.*, petrosal; *P.I.C.A.*, posteroinferior cerebellar artery; *Subarc.*, subarcuate; *Sup.*, superior; *V.*, vein; *Vest.*, vestibular.**

half of the site where the main sensory cone enters the pons (12). These rootlets are either motor or aberrant sensory rootlets. The aberrant sensory fibers are small rootlets that penetrate the pons outside the main sensory root (*Figs. 4.2, 4.5,* and *4.6*). The aberrant rootlets arise around the rostral two-thirds of the nerve and usually join the root a short distance from the brainstem. There may be as many as eight aberrant roots. Those arising rostral to the sensory root most frequently enter the first division, and those arising more caudally enter the second or third division. No aberrant rootlets originate around the caudal third of the sensory root. Of 66 aberrant rootlets found in our study of 50 trigeminal nerves, 49 went into the first division, 10 into the second division, and 7 into the third division (12). The findings that aberrant rootlets are

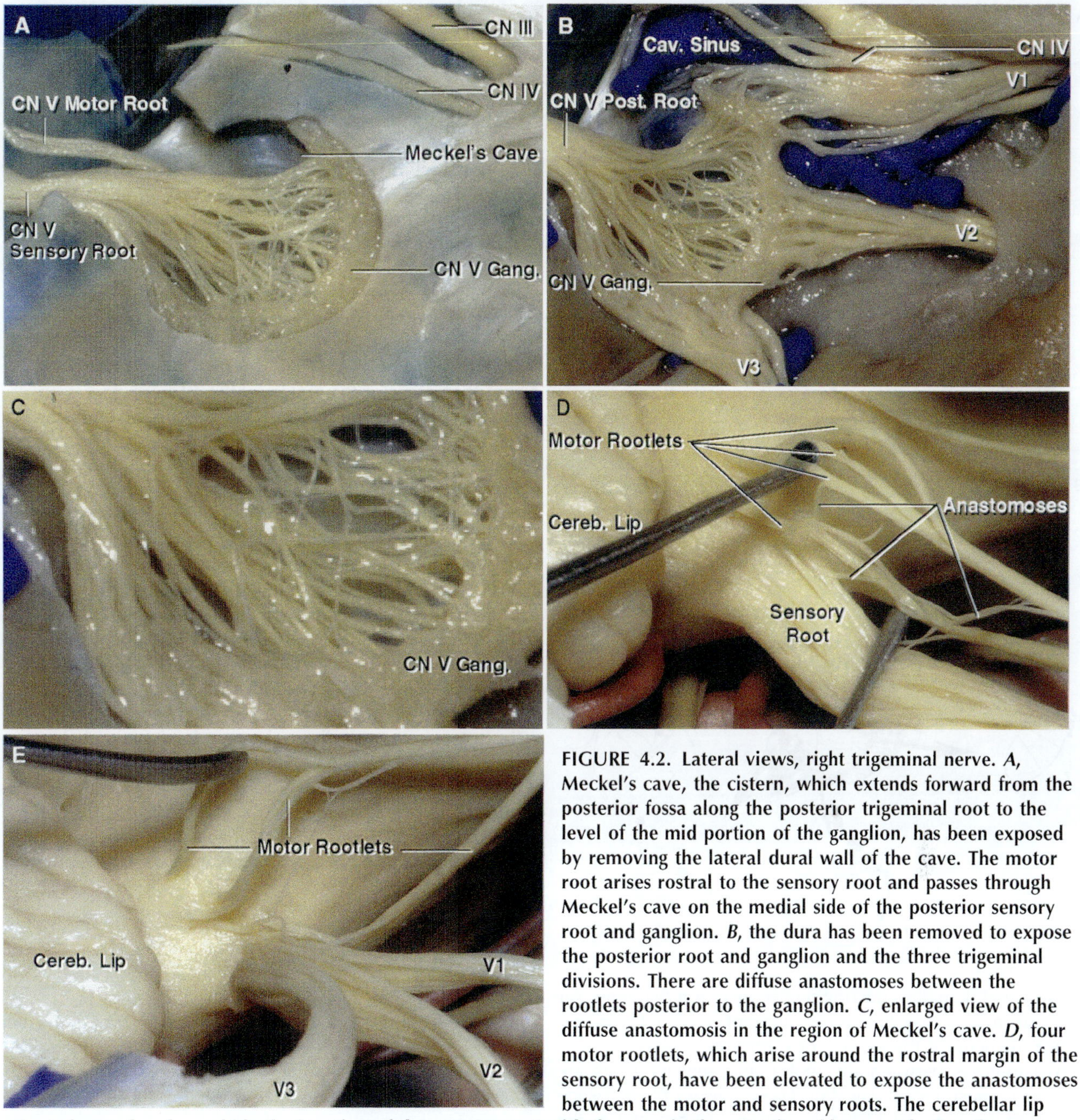

FIGURE 4.2. Lateral views, right trigeminal nerve. *A*, Meckel's cave, the cistern, which extends forward from the posterior fossa along the posterior trigeminal root to the level of the mid portion of the ganglion, has been exposed by removing the lateral dural wall of the cave. The motor root arises rostral to the sensory root and passes through Meckel's cave on the medial side of the posterior sensory root and ganglion. *B*, the dura has been removed to expose the posterior root and ganglion and the three trigeminal divisions. There are diffuse anastomoses between the rootlets posterior to the ganglion. *C*, enlarged view of the diffuse anastomosis in the region of Meckel's cave. *D*, four motor rootlets, which arise around the rostral margin of the sensory root, have been elevated to expose the anastomoses between the motor and sensory roots. The cerebellar lip projects forward and may hide the junction of the sensory root with the pons in the retrosigmoid approach. *E*, a cleavage plane has been started anteriorly and extended backward to the level of the posterior root. The first-division fibers are rostromedial within the posterior root and the third-division fibers caudolateral with the second division being in an intermediate location. *Cav.*, cavernous; *Cereb.*, cerebellar; *CN*, cranial nerve; *Gang.*, ganglion; *Post.*, posterior; *V.*, vein.

most commonly related to the first division agree with Dandy's conclusion that when the accessory fibers are spared, sensation in the first division tends to be spared (5). The aberrant rootlets appear to be nonspecific sensory fibers separated from the root by transverse pontine fibers (12, 43). Aberrant roots contribute mainly to the first division and probably do not convey a specific sensory modality from all three divisions.

Motor rootlets also arise around the rostral part of the nerve; however, they tend to arise further from the main sensory cone than do the accessory sensory rootlets. The motor root may be composed of 4 to 14 separate rootlets, each having a separate exit from the pons (*Figs. 4.2, 4.3,* and *4.7*) (12). The aberrant sensory fibers usually arise closer to the main sensory root than to the motor fibers. Some aberrant sensory fibers, however, will arise further from the main

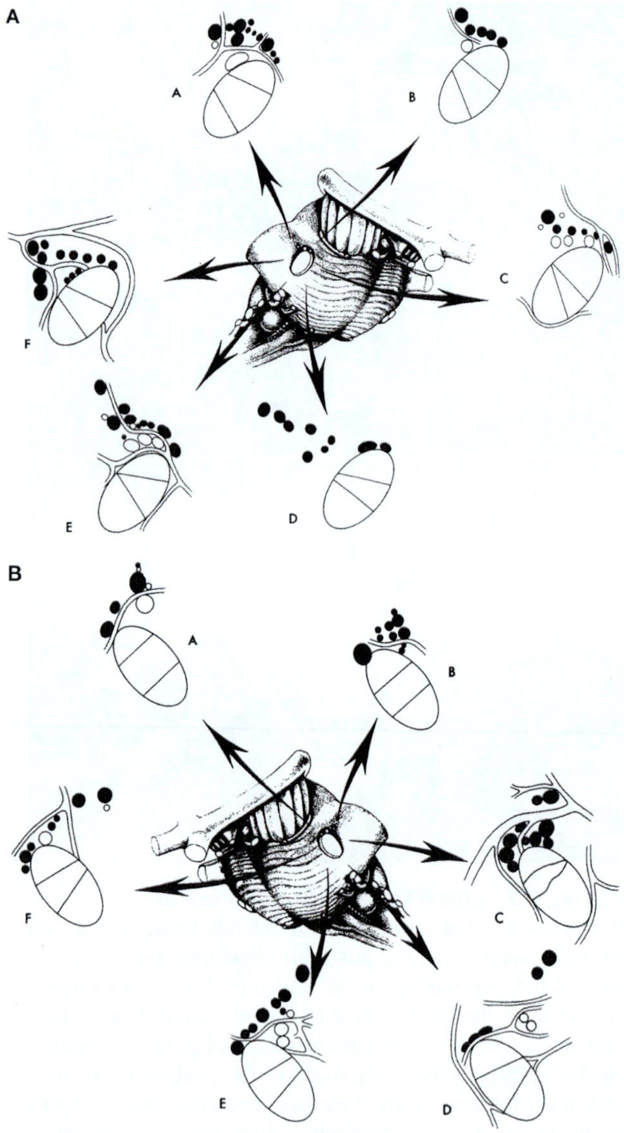

FIGURE 4.3. Diagrams of 12 trigeminal nerves showing the relationship of the trigeminal sensory root, motor rootlets, and aberrant sensory rootlets at the site of entry into the pons. The central diagrams are for orientation and show the elliptical cross section of the sensory root. The large ovals (*A–F*) represent the sensory root and are oriented in the same manner as the sensory root in the central diagram. The sites of origin of the motor rootlets are *black*. *Upper*: Nerves on the right. Only 5 motor rootlets are present in *B*, but 13 are seen in *F*. The aberrant sensory rootlets are shown by the *dark outline with clear center*. None are present in *D* and *F*. In *C* and *E*, some aberrant rootlets arise farther from the sensory root than some of the motor rootlets. *Lower*, nerves on the left. Only 4 motor rootlets are present in *A*, but there are 10 in *B* and *C*. Aberrant sensory rootlets are shown by the *dark outline with clear center*. None are present in *B* and *C*. In *A*, *D*, *E*, and *F*, some aberrant rootlets arise farther from the sensory root than some of the motor rootlets. Lines through the *oval* representing the main sensory root show portions of the nerve from each of the three divisions. In all diagrams, the rostromedial portion is from the first division, the caudolateral portion is from the third division, and the second division is in an intermediate position. In all these nerves, except *A* and *B* in the left nerve, the second division fibers make up a greater portion of the medial than the lateral portion of the sensory root. Small arteries or veins coursing between the rootlets at the level of entry into the pons are shown in all diagrams of both nerves, except *D* in the right nerve (*upper*). (From, Gudmundsson K, Rhoton AL Jr, Rushton JG: Detailed anatomy of Surgical approach, the intracranial portion of the trigeminal nerve. J Neurosurg 35:592–600, 1971 [12].)

sensory root than does the origin of some motor filaments; for this reason, it is easy to confuse aberrant sensory fibers and motor filaments at the nerve/pons junction.

Anastomoses between the motor and sensory roots are present in most nerves (*Fig. 4.2*). Those sensory fibers associated with the motor root from the pons to just proximal to the ganglion, where they anastomose with the sensory root, would be spared with a rhizotomy in the posterior fossa. Horsley et al. (15) suspected that there were sensory fibers in the trigeminal motor root, suggesting that the motor root be sectioned if trigeminal neuralgia recurred after the complete section of the sensory root. Our studies offer two explanations for the accidental preservation of sensation after posterior rhizotomy: 1) sparing of the aberrant sensory rootlets, and 2) sparing of the anastomotic sensory fibers that run with the motor root at the level of the rhizotomy (12). Anastomosis is a more likely explanation for the accidental sensory preservation and recurrence of trigeminal neuralgia after the section of the posterior root, because anastomotic rootlets are present throughout the interval from the pons to the ganglion. Aberrant sensory roots are present in only half of the nerves. They provide another explanation for the preservation of sensation after section of the main sensory root.

Anatomy of vascular compression in the upper neurovascular complex

In 1934, Dandy postulated that arterial compression and distortion of the trigeminal nerve might be the cause of trigeminal neuralgia (6). He described the superior cerebellar artery (SCA) as affecting the nerve in 30.7% of his 215 cases of trigeminal neuralgia. The vascular compression theory failed to gain acceptance at the time, but it awaited the better demonstration of these pathological changes at surgery by Jannetta (17, 21) using magnification provided by the operating microscope.

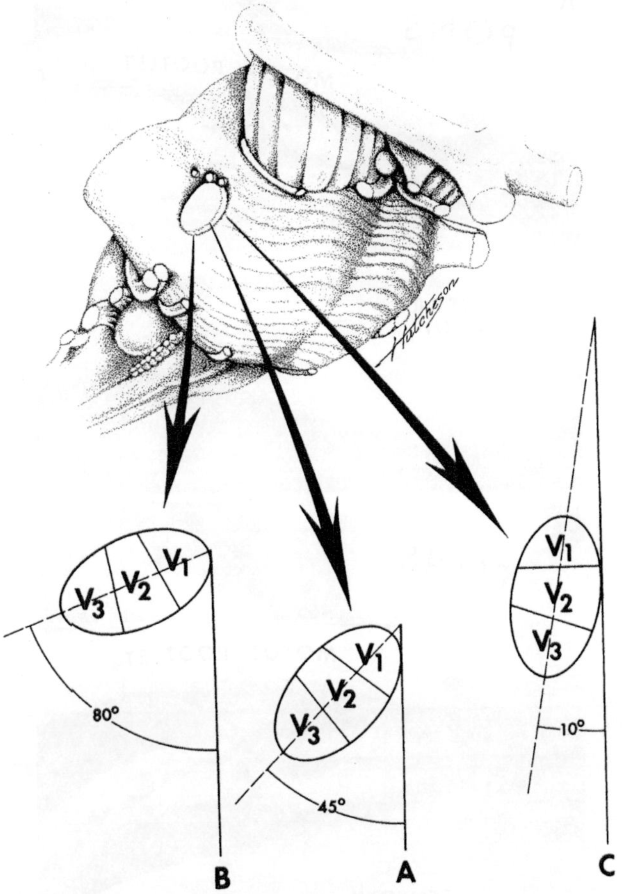

FIGURE 4.4. Variability of the longest axis of the elliptical cross section of the trigeminal nerve at the pons (*broken line*) to the longitudinal axis of the body (*solid line*). The long axis of most nerves makes a 40- to 50-degree angle with the longitudinal axis of the body (*A*); however, this can vary from 10 degrees (*C*) to 80 degrees (*B*). In *B*, the third division is almost directly lateral to the first division, and in *C*, it is almost directly caudal. (From, Gudmundsson K, Rhoton AL Jr, Rushton JG: Detailed anatomy of the intracranial portion of the trigeminal nerve. J Neurosurg 35:592–600, 1971 [12].)

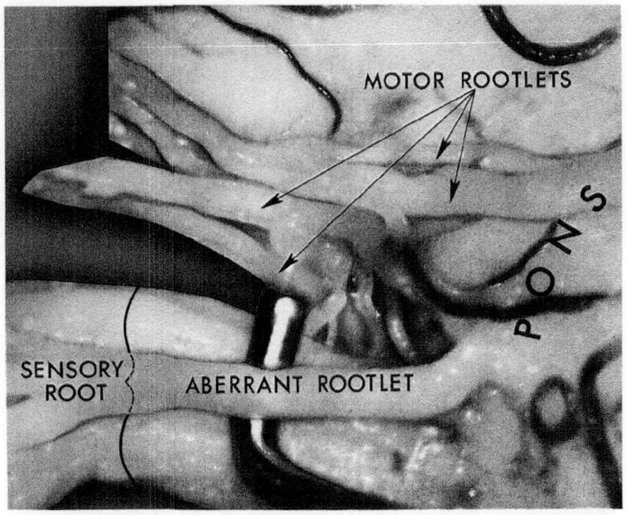

FIGURE 4.5. Lateral view of the left trigeminal nerve. A nerve hook is between the large aberrant sensory rootlet and the main sensory root. An aberrant rootlet arises from the pons directly lateral to the sensory root and joins the sensory root about 1 cm from the brainstem. Four motor rootlets are seen above the sensory root. (From, Gudmundsson K, Rhoton AL Jr, Rushton JG: Detailed anatomy of the intracranial portion of the trigeminal nerve. J Neurosurg 35:592–600, 1971 [12].)

This upper neurovascular complex, for a vascular decompression operation, is approached using a vertical scalp incision crossing the asterion, which usually overlies the junction of the lower half of the transverse and sigmoid sinuses (*Fig. 4.8*). The bone opening, a small craniotomy, located behind the upper half of the sigmoid sinus, exposes the edge of the junction of the transverse and sigmoid sinuses in its superolateral margin. The cerebellum is relaxed by opening the arachnoid and removing cerebrospinal fluid, a maneuver made safer by the use of the operating microscope. A narrow brain spatula, commonly 3 mm at the tip, is introduced parallel and just below the superior petrosal sinus to elevate the superolateral margin of the cerebellum (*Fig. 4.9*) (36). The use of a wider spatula or a lower entry point along the lateral cerebellum risks damaging the vestibulocochlear nerve. A bridging petrosal vein, which commonly blocks access to the trigeminal nerve, is coagulated with gentle bipolar coagulation and divided nearer its junction with the brain than to the superior petrosal sinus. Unexpected bleeding encountered as the superolateral margin of the cerebellum is elevated, if venous in appearance, is usually related to stretching and tearing of the petrosal veins that pass from the superior surface of the cerebellum to the venous sinus in the tentorium or, if arterial in appearance, to tearing of the subarcuate branch of the anteroinferior cerebellar artery (AICA) behind the internal auditory canal at its site of penetration of the dura covering the subarcuate fossa. The trochlear nerve is identified before opening the arachnoid behind the trigeminal nerve, because it may be difficult to see the nerve after the arachnoid has been opened and shrinks into thick white clumps that may hide the nerve. Usually, the trochlear nerve is several millimeters above the trigeminal nerve; it may be carried downward, however, if it is adherent to a segment of the SCA that has looped into the axilla of the trigeminal nerve. The overhanging lip of the cerebellomesencephalic fissure must be retracted gently to expose the junction of the nerve with the pons.

The most common finding at a vascular decompression operation for trigeminal neuralgia is a segment of the SCA compressing the trigeminal nerve (13, 18). Normally, the SCA encircles the brainstem well above the trigeminal nerve. In adults, the SCA commonly makes a shallow, caudal loop and courses inferiorly for a variable distance on the lateral side of the pons (*Figs. 4.8* and *4.10-4.12*). In those cases with the most prominent caudally projecting loop, contact be-

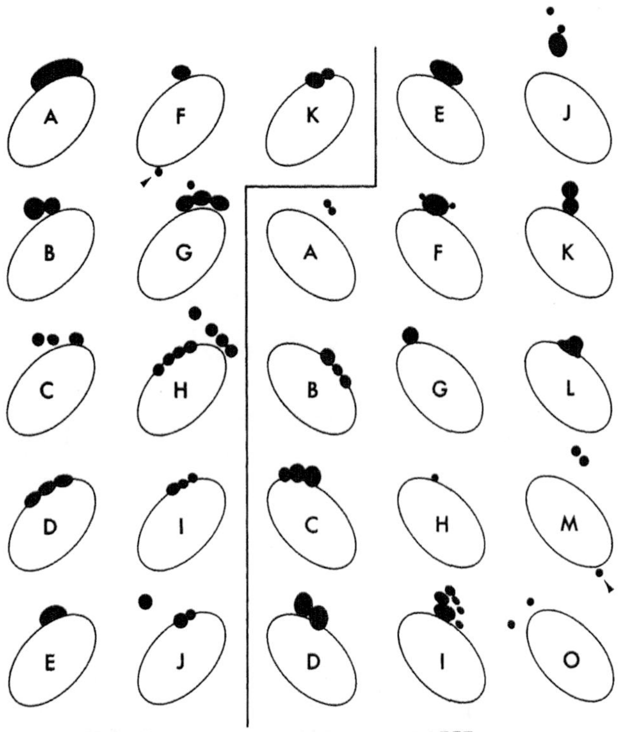

FIGURE 4.6. Origin of the aberrant sensory rootlets in relation to the main sensory root. The *large, clear oval* represents a cross section of the sensory root at the level of entry into the pons. Origin of aberrant rootlets is in *solid black.* All nerves to the left of the solid line are from the right side and are oriented the same as the nerves shown in *Figure 4.3* (upper*). Those to the right of the line are from the left side and are oriented as shown in* Figure 4.3 (*lower*). The rootlet origin shown with the *arrow* below F (*right*) goes with sensory root G, and the rootlet origin shown with the *arrow* below M (*left*) goes with sensory root O. The rostral margin of the root is superior and the caudal margin is inferior on the diagrams. No aberrant sensory root originates caudal to the main sensory root. (From, Gudmundsson K, Rhoton AL Jr, Rushton JG: Detailed anatomy of the intracranial portion of the trigeminal nerve. J Neurosurg 35:592–600, 1971 [12].)

tween the artery and the trigeminal nerve occurs. The point of contact with the SCA is usually on the superior or superomedial aspect of the nerve; and often a few fascicles of the nerve are distorted by an SCA that has looped down into the axilla between the medial side of the nerve and the pons (*Figs. 4.8* and *4.12*). An arterial loop in the axilla may not be visible from the retrosigmoid view behind the trigeminal nerve if the SCA courses around the brainstem directly in front of the nerve. The loop of the SCA also may be difficult to see if the artery passes over the rostral aspect of the nerve very close to the brainstem, where it may be hidden by the overhanging lip of the cerebellomesencephalic fissure. The loop of the SCA may be seen dangling below the lower margin of the nerve, even though it is not visible above the nerve. These loops of the SCA, however, always pass rostrally along the medial and

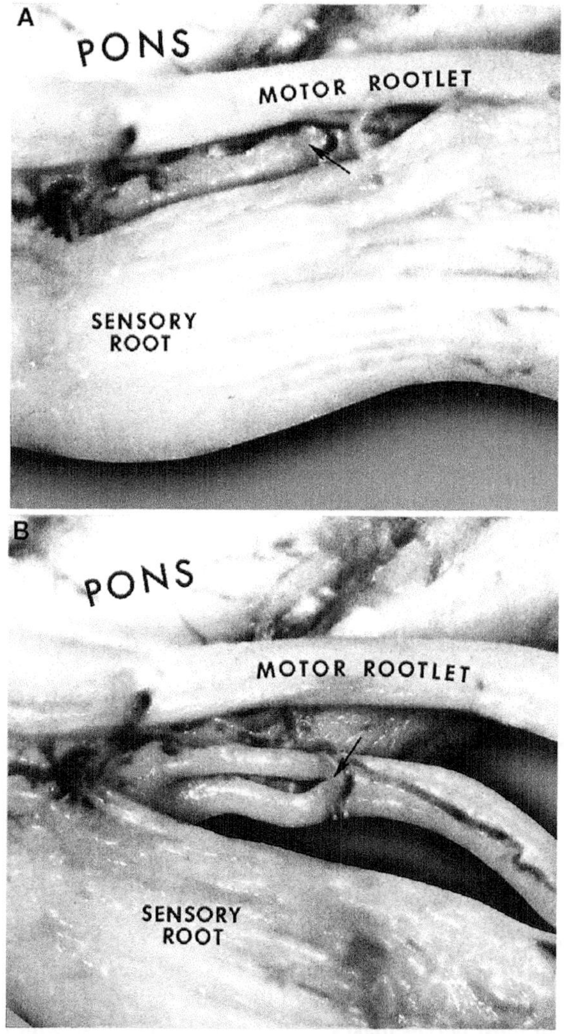

FIGURE 4.7. *A,* lateral view of the right trigeminal nerve near its junction with the pons. The *arrow* points to the intermediate group of fibers between the motor rootlet and the sensory root. *B,* the same trigeminal nerve. The *arrow* points to the intermediate group of fibers that proved to be a motor rootlet when traced distally. This illustrates the difficulty in telling whether an intermediate group of fibers is motor or sensory unless the nerve bundles can be separated and examined individually. (From, Gudmundsson K, Rhoton AL Jr, Rushton JG: Detailed anatomy of the intracranial portion of the trigeminal nerve. J Neurosurg 35:592–600, 1971 [12].)

superior surfaces of the nerve to reach the cerebellomesencephalic fissure. The medial axilla of the nerve must be carefully explored before concluding that there is no arterial loop in the axilla of the nerve. It is important to remember that the trunks do not pass directly from the side of the brainstem to the superior surface of the cerebellum; they dip into the deep fissure between the cerebellum and midbrain at the posterior margin of the trigeminal nerve. The SCA gives off perforating arteries that may limit the degree of repositioning of the artery achievable in a microvascular decompression operation.

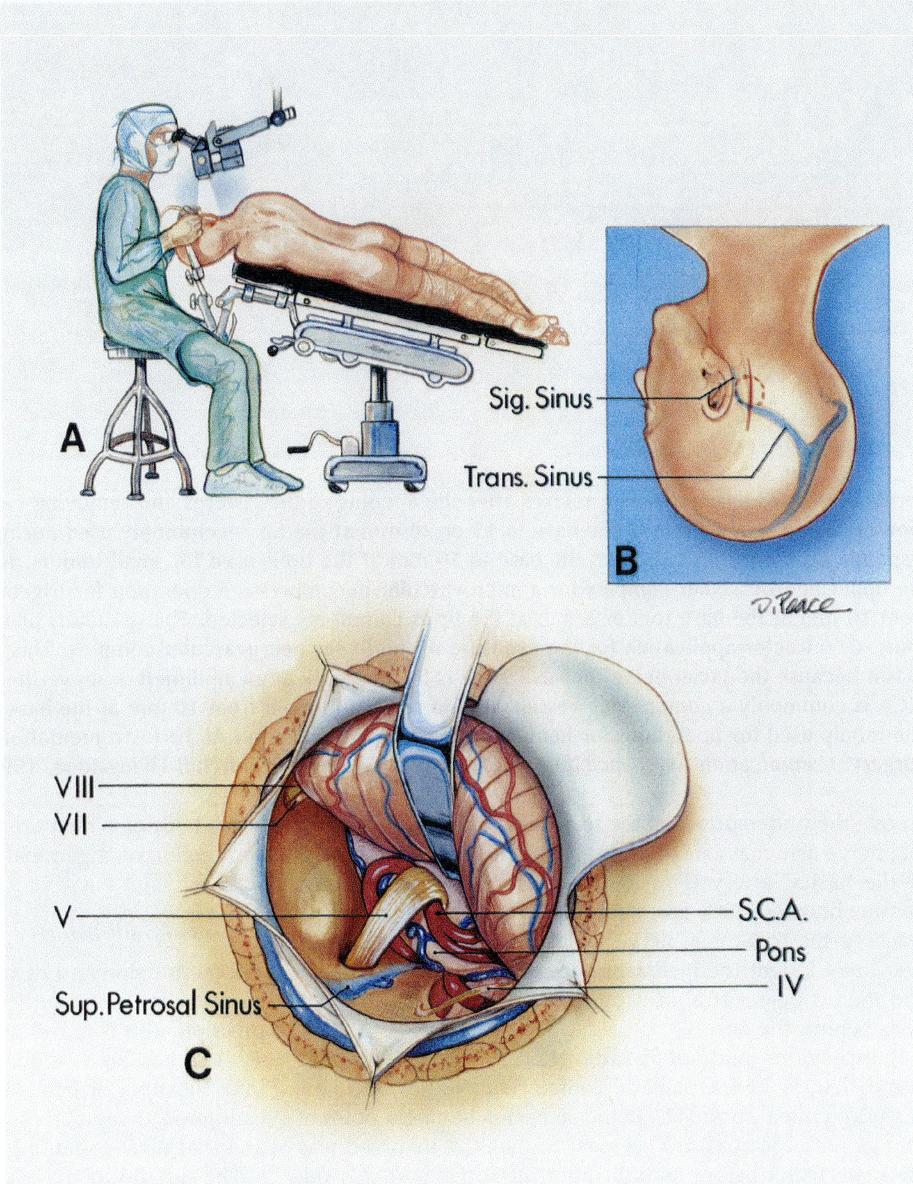

FIGURE 4.8. Retrosigmoid approach to the trigeminal nerve for a microvascular decompression operation. *A*, (*upper left*), the patient is positioned in the three-quarter prone position. The surgeon is seated at the head of the table. The table is tilted so that the feet are lower than the heart. *B*, the vertical paramedian incision crosses the asterion. The superolateral margin of the craniotomy is positioned at the junction of the transverse and sigmoid sinuses. *C*, the superolateral margin of the cerebellum is gently elevated using a brain spatula tapered from 10 mm at the base to 3 or 5 mm at the tip to expose the site at which the trigeminal nerve enters the pons. The brain spatula is advanced and aligned parallel to the superior petrosal sinus. The trochlear nerve is at the superior margin of the exposure and the facial and vestibulocochlear nerves are at the lower margin. The dura is tacked up to the adjacent muscles to maximize the exposure along the superolateral margin of the cerebellum. The main trunk of the SCA loops down into the axilla of the trigeminal nerve. (From, Rhoton AL Jr: Microsurgical anatomy of decompression operations on the trigeminal nerve, in Rovit RL, Murali R, Jannetta PJ (eds): *Trigeminal Neuralgia*. Baltimore, Williams & Wilkins, 1990, pp 165–200 [34].) *S.C.A.*, superior cerebellar artery; *Sig.*, sigmoid; *Sup.*, superior; *Trans.*, transverse.

The most common site of compression of the trigeminal nerve on the SCA is at the junction of the main trunk with the origin of the rostral and caudal trunks (*Figs. 4.11* and *4.12*) (34). However, other sites of compression are seen, depending on how far distal the artery bifurcates in relation to the trigeminal nerve. If the SCA bifurcates near the basilar artery or if there is a duplicate configuration in which the rostral and caudal trunks arise directly from the basilar artery, both trunks may loop down into the axilla and compress the nerve. Alternatively, if the artery bifurcates before reaching the nerve, the caudal trunk may compress the nerve and the rostral trunk may course well above the nerve. If the artery bifurcates distal to the nerve, only the main trunk will be involved in the compression. The point of bifurcation of the SCA does affect the caliber of the vessel that makes contact with the nerve. The contacting vessel will be of a smaller caliber if the SCA bifurcates before reaching the trigeminal nerve.

A less frequent source of compression of the trigeminal nerve is by the AICA (*Figs. 4.11* and *4.12*). Normally, the AICA passes around the pons below the trigeminal nerve with the facial and vestibulocochlear nerves. The AICA, however, may have a high origin and loop upward to indent the medial or lower surface of the trigeminal nerve before passing downward to course with the facial and vestibulocochlear nerves. A serpentine basilar artery also may wander laterally and compress the medial side of the trigeminal nerve (43). This type of basilar artery often is elongated and has a fusiform configuration. More than one artery may compress the nerve. In a few cases, the SCA will compress the rostral surface of the nerve and the AICA will compress the caudal surface. Infrequently, the posteroinferior cerebellar artery (PICA) may reach and

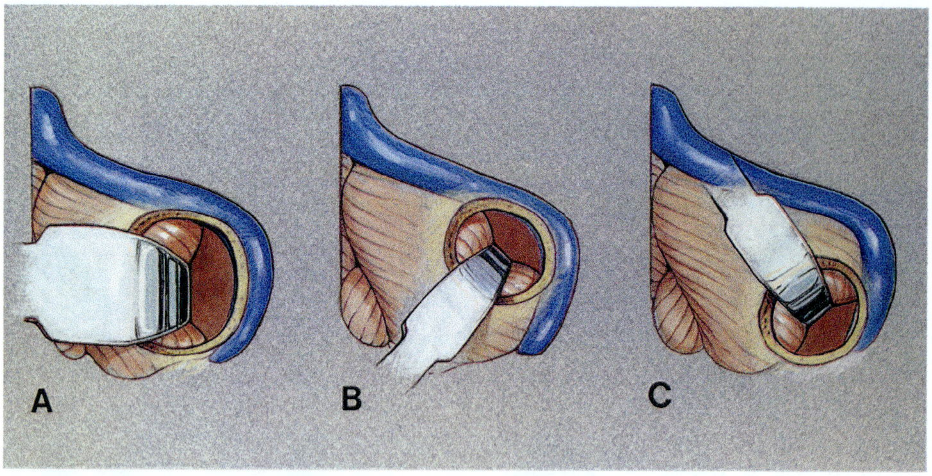

FIGURE 4.9. Direction of the application of brain spatulas for surgery in the various compartments of the cerebellopontine angle. *A*, lateral exposure for a lesion in the midportion of the cerebellopontine angle, such as an acoustic neuroma. The site of the craniotomy below the transverse sinus and medial to the sigmoid sinus is shown for removing an acoustic neuroma or other lesion involving multiple neurovascular complexes. The spatula protects the lateral surface of the cerebellum after the cerebellum relaxes after the opening of the cisterns and removing cerebrospinal fluid. A brain spatula tapered from 20 or 25 mm at the base to 15 or 20 mm at the tip is commonly used during the removal of large tumors, and a spatula tapered from 15 mm at the base to 10 mm at the tip is used for small tumors. *B*, spatula application for exposing the upper neurovascular complex for a microvascular decompression operation for trigeminal neuralgia. A spatula tapered from 10 mm at the base to 3 or 5 mm at the tip is commonly selected. The spatula is placed parallel to the superior petrosal sinus. *C*, retractor application for the exposure of the lower neurovascular complex. This approach also is used in hemifacial spasm because the facial nerve root exit zone is located only a few millimeters above the glossopharyngeal nerve and the PICA is commonly a compressing vessel. A brain spatula tapered from 10 mm at the base to 3 or 5 mm at the tip is commonly used for operations for hemifacial spasm. (From, Rhoton AL Jr: Instrumentation, in Apuzzo MLJ (ed): *Brain Surgery: Complication Avoidance and Management.* New York, Churchill-Livingstone, 1993, vol 2, pp 1647–1670 [36].)

groove the undersurface of the trigeminal nerve. The trigeminal nerve also may be compressed by a large pontine branch of the basilar artery (*Figs. 4.11* and *4.12*). Normally, these pontine branches pass around and penetrate the pons before reaching the trigeminal nerve. A large pontine artery, however, may indent the medial surface of the trigeminal nerve and then course rostral or caudal to the nerve to supply the pons behind the nerve.

In a previous study of 50 cadaveric trigeminal nerves, we found that 26 had a point of contact with the SCA in the posterior cranial fossa (14). In the 26 nerves having a point of contact with the SCA, the segment of the SCA involved was the main trunk before its bifurcation in 8, the caudal trunk distal to the bifurcation in 11, the rostral trunk in 2, both the rostral and caudal trunk in 4, and a hemispheric branch of the caudal trunk in 1. In that study, the site of vascular contact was commonly a few millimeters peripheral to the point of entry of the nerve into the pons (average, 3.7 mm) rather than at the root entry zone, as is seen in most of our cases with trigeminal neuralgia. In one cadaveric specimen, the vascular contact was more than 1 cm from the pons. In 6 of the 50 cadaveric nerves, the contact occurred at the pontine sensory root entry zone of the trigeminal nerve. The main trunk of the AICA also impinged on 4 of the 50 cadaveric trigeminal nerves that were examined, and in 3 of these, there was also a point of contact between the nerve and the SCA. One nerve also was contacted on its superior surface by the SCA and on its inferior surface by both trunks of a duplicated AICA. Not all of these contacts seen in our anatomic studies produced distortion of the nerve or occurred at the sensory root entry zone, both of which are postulated as a prerequisite for the production of trigeminal neuralgia (18).

Venous relationships

Compression and distortion of the trigeminal nerve by the surrounding veins, although less frequent than arterial compression, also is found in trigeminal neuralgia (*Figs. 4.13* and *4.14*) (2, 18, 26). It is the superior petrosal veins that empty into the superior petrosal sinus that are most frequently encountered in operative approaches to the trigeminal nerve and that most commonly compress the trigeminal nerve.

The superior petrosal veins are among the largest and most frequently encountered veins in the posterior fossa. The superior petrosal veins may be formed by the terminal segment of a single vein or by the common stem formed by the union of several veins. The most common tributaries of the superior petrosal veins are the transverse pontine and pontotrigeminal veins, the veins of the cerebellopontine fissure and the middle cerebellar peduncle, and the common stem of the veins draining the lateral part of the cerebellar hemisphere. The transverse pontine veins, which pass near the trigeminal nerve to reach the bridging veins entering the superior petrosal sinus, are the most frequent veins to compress the trigeminal nerve. They may course medially in the axilla of the nerve or they also may pass above, below, or lateral to the nerve and may indent any of its surfaces. The vein of the middle cerebellar peduncle may compress the lateral or medial surface of the trigeminal nerve before joining the petrosal veins as it ascends in the pons. The vein of the cerebellopontine fissure may

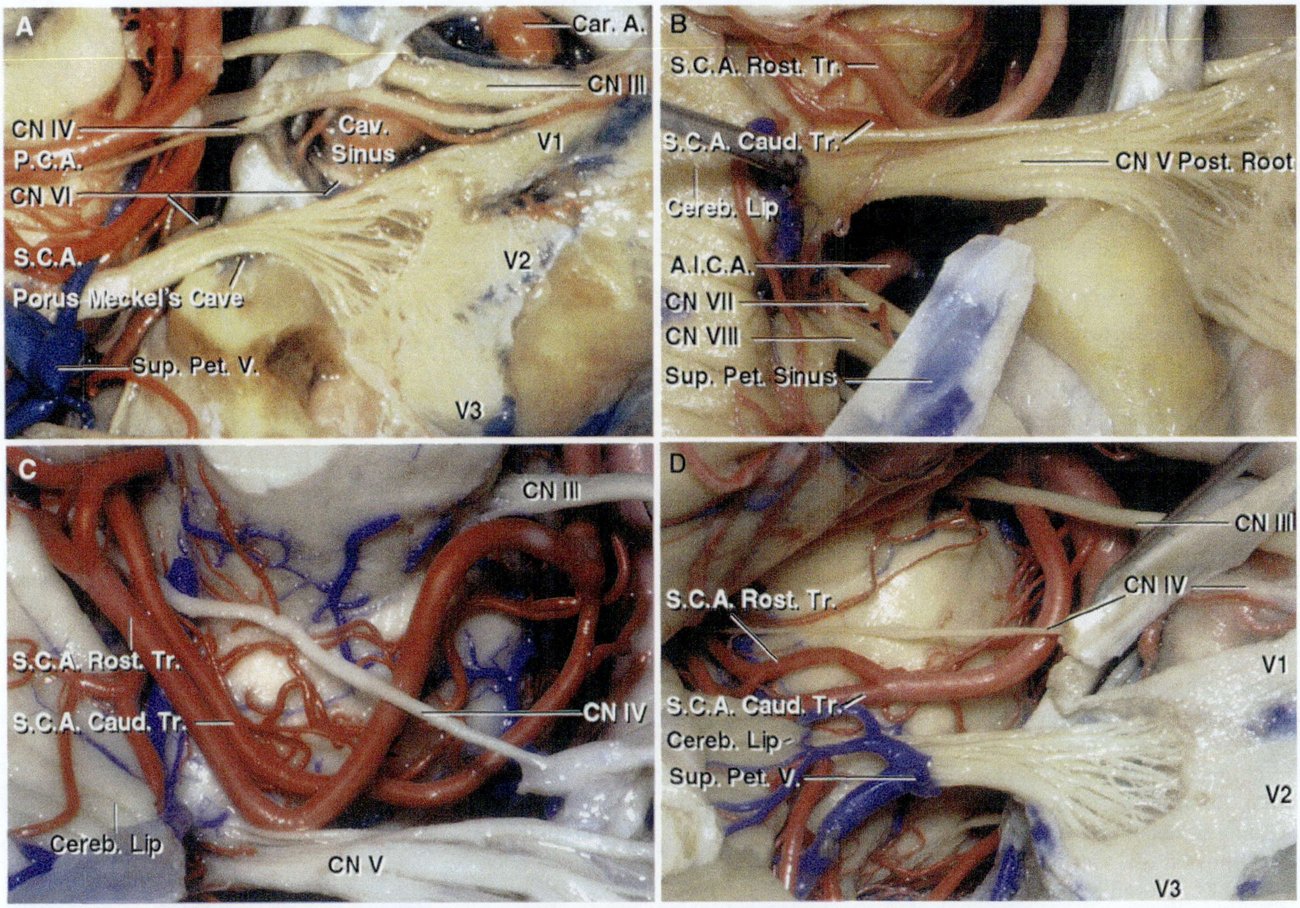

FIGURE 4.10. Trigeminal nerve and SCA relationships. ***A*, the trigeminal posterior root, ganglion, and three divisions have been exposed by removing the dura from the lateral wall of Meckel's cave and the cavernous sinus. The posterior root enters the midpons below the SCA and is intertwined with the branches of the superior petrosal vein. *B*, the SCA loops downward and, at the junction of the rostral and caudal trunks, contacts the posterior trigeminal root at the pontine junction. The cerebellar lip projects forward and may block access to the junction of the trigeminal nerve and pons in the retrosigmoid approach. *C*, SCA with an early bifurcation. The rostral trunk loops downward and indents the upper surface of the trigeminal nerve. *D*, another SCA passes around the pons and bifurcates into its rostral and caudal trunks above the trigeminal root entry zone. *A.*, artery; *A.I.C.A.*, anteroinferior cerebellar artery; *Car.*, carotid; *Caud.*, caudal; *Cav.*, cavernous; *Cereb.*, cerebellar; *CN*, cranial nerve; *Pet.*, petrosal; *Post.*, posterior; *Rost.*, rostral; *S.C.A.*, superior cerebellar artery; *Sup.*, superior; *Tr.*, trunk; *V.*, vein.**

indent the lateral margin of the trigeminal nerve as it ascends toward the superior petrosal sinus, and the pontotrigeminal vein may indent the upper margin of the nerve.

The junction of these veins, which converge and form a single trunk before entering the superior petrosal sinus, usually is lateral to the trigeminal nerve. This junction, however, may be located medial to the trigeminal nerve, in which case the common trunk must pass around the trigeminal nerve before reaching the superior petrosal sinus. These common trunks also may compress the trigeminal nerve.

Suprameatal extension of the retrosigmoid approach

The part of the posterior surface of the temporal bone that forms the superior lip of the porus of the internal acoustic meatus is the site of a prominence, the suprameatal tubercle, that blocks access to the lateral margin of the trigeminal nerve and the prepontine cistern medial to the trigeminal nerve (*Figs. 4.15* and *4.16*). Removal of the suprameatal tubercle increases access to the region of the upper neurovascular complex around the trigeminal nerve, and may possibly avoid the need for a supratentorial craniotomy in exposing tumors that are located predominantly in the cerebellopontine angle but also extend into the posterior part of the middle fossa in the region of Meckel's cave (42). The tubercle, the most prominent bony elevation around the circumference of the internal acoustic meatus, is defined below by the internal acoustic meatus, above by the petrous ridge, laterally by a vertical line crossing the posterior edge of the porus of the internal acoustic meatus, and medially by a vertical line crossing the medial edge of the trigeminal notch, a depression in the petrous ridge located below the porus of Meckel's cave. Above and medial to the suprameatal tubercle, the posteromedial part of the floor of the middle cranial fossa is

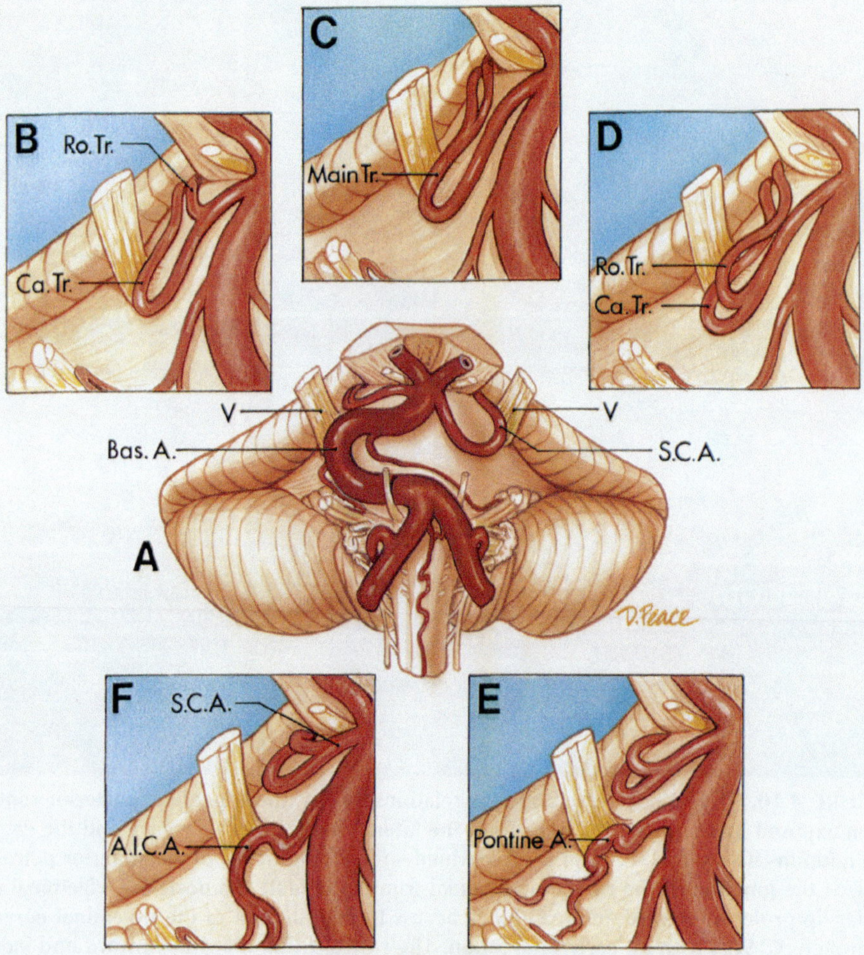

FIGURE 4.11. Sites of arterial compression of the trigeminal nerve. Orientation as shown in the central diagram. *A*, central diagram. The right trigeminal nerve is compressed by a tortuous basilar artery and the left trigeminal nerve is compressed by the main trunk of the SCA. *B*, the SCA bifurcates into rostral and caudal trunks before reaching the trigeminal nerve. The nerve is compressed by the caudal trunk. *C*, the SCA bifurcates distally to the nerve. The nerve is compressed by the main trunk. *D*, the SCA bifurcates before reaching the nerve. The nerve is compressed by both the rostral and caudal trunks. *E*, the nerve is compressed by a large pontine artery. *F*, the nerve is compressed by an AICA that has a high origin and loops upward into the medial surface of the nerve. The SCA passes around the brainstem above the nerve. (From, Rhoton AL Jr: Microsurgical anatomy of decompression operations on the trigeminal nerve, in Rovit RL, Murali R, Jannetta PJ (eds): *Trigeminal Neuralgia.* Baltimore, Williams & Wilkins, 1990, pp 165–200 [34].) *A.*, artery; *A.I.C.A.*, anteroinferior cerebellar artery; *Bas.*, basilar; *Ca.*, caudal; *Ro.*, rostral; *S.C.A.*, superior cerebellar artery; *Tr.*, tract; *V.*, vein.

the site of the depression underlying Meckel's cave in which the posterior trigeminal root sits. The most prominent posterior projection of the tubercle is located above the lateral half of the porus of the internal acoustic meatus.

The neural structures that surround and limit access to the suprameatal tubercle are the cerebellum posteriorly, the facial and vestibulocochlear nerves below, the trigeminal nerve above and medial, and the abducens nerve medially. The cerebellopontine cistern opens through the porus into Meckel's cave. Meckel's segment of the trigeminal nerve, which begins at the porus and extends to the trigeminal ganglion, is differentiated from the cavernous segment in the wall of the cavernous sinus. Meckel's segment is narrower adjacent to the porus and fans out as it approaches the posterior edge of the gasserian ganglion, which is embedded in the dura just anterior to the anterior edge of Meckel's cave.

The intraosseous structures, which limit the extent of the drilling if they are to be preserved, are the posterior part of the superior semicircular canal, the upper part of the posterior semicircular canal, and the common crus of the two canals. After removal of the suprameatal tubercle, the drilling can be extended below Meckel's cave to the edge of the petroclival fissure just in front of the inferior petrosal sinus and immediately lateral to the abducens nerve. Removing the bone in this area provides access, on average, to the posterior 10.3 mm (range, 8.0–13.0 mm) of Meckel's cave and the enclosed portion of the trigeminal nerve, and opens a 180-degree window around the lateral and lower surface of the posterior trigeminal root, which may be used for accessing the posterior part of the middle fossa (*Figs. 4.15* and *4.16*).

The size of the area created by removing the suprameatal tubercle and adjacent part of the petrous apex by the retrosig-

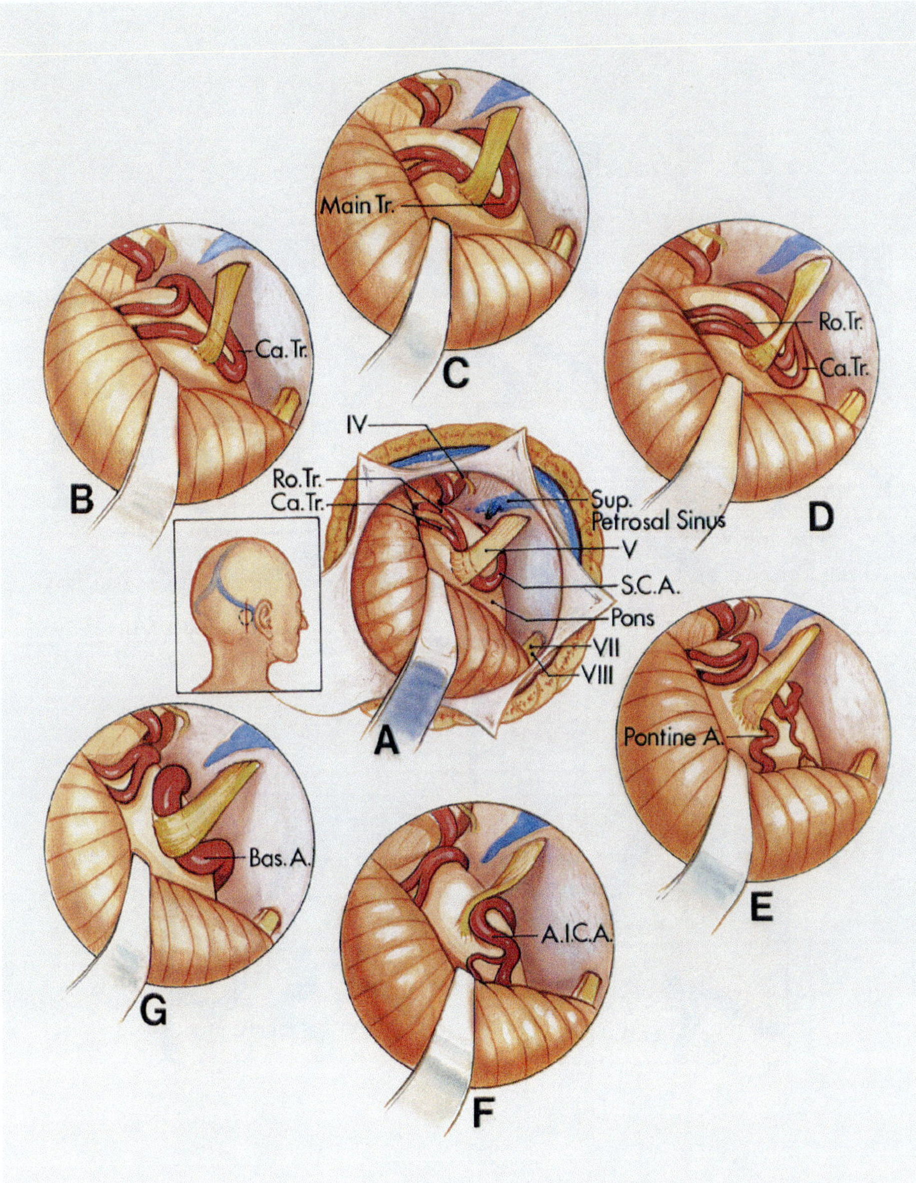

FIGURE 4.12. Sites of arterial compression of the trigeminal nerve as seen through a suboccipital craniotomy. *A*, central diagram. The site of the skin incision (*solid line*) and the craniotomy (*interrupted line*) are shown in the *insert*. The superolateral margin of the cerebellum is gently retracted to expose the trigeminal nerve and the SCA. The brain spatula is advanced parallel to the superior petrosal sinus. The trochlear nerve is at the superior margin of the exposure and the facial and vestibulocochlear nerves are at the lower margin. The trigeminal nerve is compressed by a loop of the SCA that dangles down into the axilla of the nerve. The site of compression on the artery is at the junction of the main trunk with the rostral and caudal trunks. *B*, the nerve is compressed by the caudal trunk. *C*, the nerve is compressed by the main trunk. *D*, compression by both the rostral and caudal trunks. *E*, compression by a pontine branch of the basilar artery. *F*, compression by the AICA. *G*, compression by a tortuous basilar artery. *A.*, artery; *A.I.C.A.*, anteroinferior cerebellar artery; *Bas.*, basilar; *Ca.*, caudal; *Ro.*, rostral; *S.C.A.*, superior cerebellar artery; *Sup.*, superior; *Tr.*, trunk; *V.*, vein. (From, Rhoton AL Jr: Microsurgical anatomy of decompression operations on the trigeminal nerve, in Rovit RL, Murali R, Jannetta PJ (eds): *Trigeminal Neuralgia*. Baltimore, Williams & Wilkins, 1990, pp 165–200 [34].)

moid route is limited superiorly by the superior petrosal sinus and the dura covering the upper surface of the petrous bone. The superior petrosal sinus can be divided, and Meckel's cave and the tentorium lateral to the porus of Meckel's cave can be opened to provide intradural access to the posteromedial part of the middle fossa, but cannot be extended forward to the horizontal portion of the petrous carotid.

The suprameatal extension of the retrosigmoid approach may permit removal of some tumors that are located mainly in the posterior fossa but that extend into the middle fossa in the region of Meckel's cave. The space created after drilling the suprameatal tubercle and the bone medial to the internal auditory canal and below the trigeminal nerve was enough to extend the retrosigmoid approach as far as 13.0 mm (average, 10.3 mm) anterior to what could be achieved using the retrosigmoid approach alone (42). The extent to which the bone in the region of the suprameatal tubercle could be removed using the retrosigmoid approach is defined and limited by the neural and bony structures in the region. The cerebellum, with gentle retraction, limits the angle at which the suprameatal tubercle can be drilled, although when combined with evacuation of cerebrospinal fluid, it provides a space to adequately visualize and remove lesions medial to the suprameatal tubercle. A portion of this bone is commonly removed in approaching tumors extending into the internal acoustic meatus. It is possible to remove approximately 270 degrees of the circumference of the wall of the internal acoustic meatus when using the retrosigmoid approach; however,

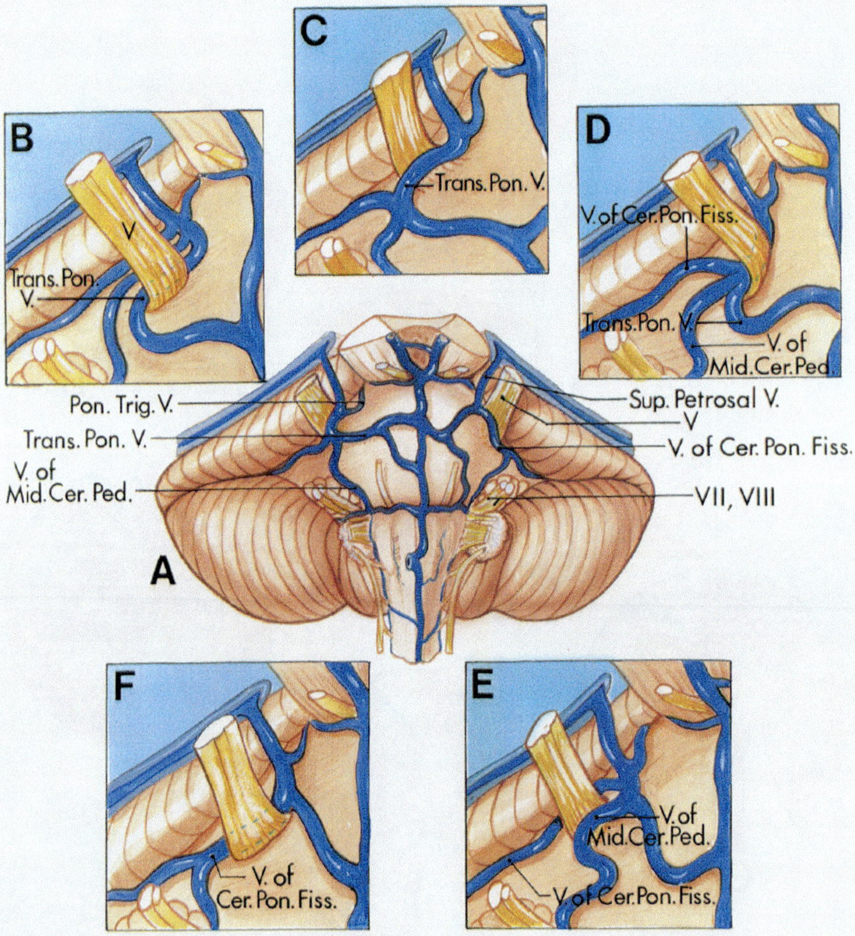

FIGURE 4.13. **Sites of venous compression of the trigeminal nerve. *A*, central diagram. Anterior view. The veins that commonly compress the trigeminal nerve are tributaries of the superior petrosal vein. The tributaries that converge on and may compress the nerve are the transverse pontine and pontotrigeminal veins and the veins of the cerebellopontine fissure and middle cerebellar peduncle. The transverse pontine veins course transversely across the pons. The vein of the middle cerebellar peduncle arises in the region of the facial and vestibulocochlear nerves and ascends on the pons. The vein of the cerebellopontine fissure arises along the cleft between the pons and the cerebellum and ascends behind the trigeminal nerve. The pontotrigeminal vein arises on the upper pons and passes above the trigeminal nerve. *B*, a transverse pontine vein compresses the lateral side of the nerve and joins the veins of the middle cerebellar peduncle and cerebellopontine fissure to empty into a superior petrosal vein. *C*, the medial side of the nerve is compressed by a tortuous transverse pontine vein. *D*, the lateral side of the nerve is compressed by the junction of the transverse pontine vein with the veins of the middle cerebellar peduncle and the cerebellopontine fissure. *E*, the nerve is compressed on the medial side by the vein of the middle cerebellar peduncle and on the lateral side by the vein of the cerebellopontine fissure. *F*, the lateral side of the nerve is compressed by the vein of the cerebellopontine fissure. (From, Rhoton AL Jr: Microsurgical anatomy of decompression operations on the trigeminal nerve, in Rovit RL, Murali R, Jannetta PJ (eds): *Trigeminal Neuralgia.* Baltimore, Williams & Wilkins, 1990, pp 165–200 [34].) *Cer.*, cerebellar; *Cer. Pon.*, cerebellopontine; *Fiss.*, fissure; *Mid.*, middle; *Ped.*, peduncle; *Pon.*, pontine; *Sup.*, superior; *Trans.*, transverse; *Trig.*, trigeminal; *V.*, vein.**

with the approach described herein, only the bone in the region of the suprameatal tubercle is removed. The drilling on the lateral side of the tubercle should avoid the posterior semicircular canal and common crus of the posterior and superior canals if hearing is to be preserved, but on the medial side, it can extend through the petrous apex into the side of the clivus.

Often, the subarcuate branch of the AICA must be obliterated to access the suprameatal tubercle. Accessing the suprameatal tubercle often requires that the superior petrosal veins be obliterated and divided. This allows the drilling to be directed medially along the lateral and lower margin of the porus of Meckel's cave. The dura along the lower and lateral margin of the porus of Meckel's cave and the tentorium lateral to the porus trigeminus can then be opened to expose the trigeminal nerve in the posterior part of Meckel's cave and the middle cranial fossa. Care is taken to protect the trochlear nerve if the tentorial incision is to be extended through the free edge.

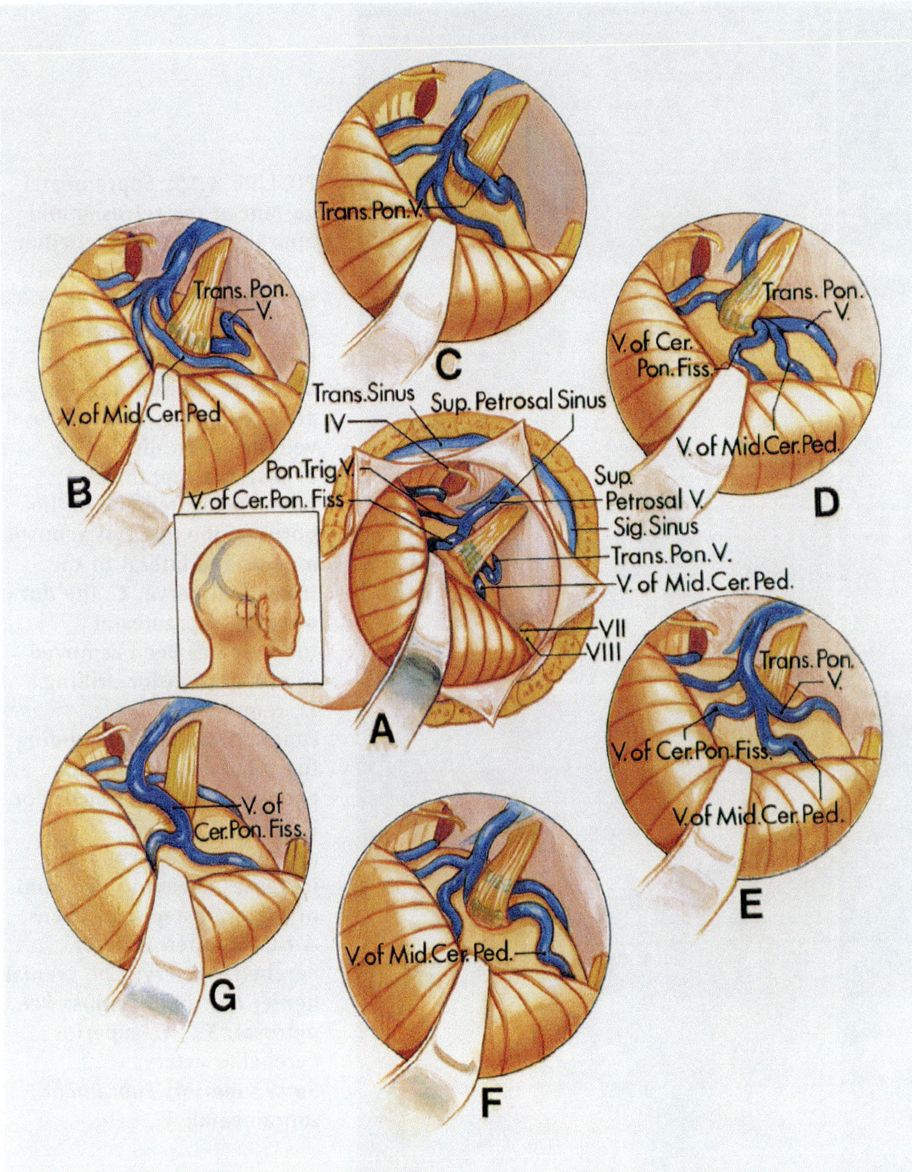

FIGURE 4.14. Sites of venous compression of the trigeminal nerve as seen through a retrosigmoid craniotomy. *A*, the insert shows the site of the scalp incision (*solid line*) and the craniotomy (*interrupted line*). The cerebellum has been elevated to expose the junction of the trigeminal nerve with the pons. The superior petrosal veins empty into the superior petrosal sinus. The trochlear nerve is at the superior margin and the facial and vestibulocochlear nerves are at the lower margin of the exposure. The craniotomy exposes the junction of the sigmoid and transverse sinuses. The trigeminal nerve is compressed by the junction of a transverse pontine vein and the vein of the middle cerebellar peduncle with the superior petrosal vein. The vein of the cerebellopontine fissure ascends behind the nerve and the pontotrigeminal vein passes above the nerve. *B*, the trigeminal nerve is compressed on its medial side by a transverse pontine vein and on its lateral side by the vein of the middle cerebellar peduncle. *C*, the lateral side of the nerve is compressed by a transverse pontine vein. *D*, the medial side of the nerve is compressed by the junction of a transverse pontine vein with the veins of the middle cerebellar peduncle and cerebellopontine fissure. *E*, the lateral side of the nerve is compressed by the junction of the transverse pontine vein with the veins of the middle cerebellar peduncle and cerebellopontine fissure. *F*, the medial side of the nerve is compressed by the vein of the middle cerebellar peduncle. *G*, the lateral side of the nerve is compressed by the vein of the cerebellopontine fissure. (From, Rhoton AL Jr: Microsurgical anatomy of decompression operations on the trigeminal nerve, in Rovit RL, Murali R, Jannetta PJ (eds): *Trigeminal Neuralgia*. Baltimore, Williams & Wilkins, 1990, pp 165–200 [34].) *Cer.*, cerebellar; *Cer. Pon.*, cerebellopontine; *Fiss.*, fissure; *Mid.*, middle; *Ped.*, peduncle; *Pon.*, pontine; *Sig.*, sigmoid; *Sup.*, superior; *Trans.*, transverse; *Trig.*, trigeminal; *V.*, vein.

MIDDLE NEUROVASCULAR COMPLEX

The middle complex includes the AICA, pons, middle cerebellar peduncle, cerebellopontine fissure, petrosal surface of the cerebellum, and the abducens, facial, and vestibulocochlear nerves (*Figs. 4.1* and *4.17*). The AICA arises at the pontine level and courses in relationship to the abducens, facial, and vestibulocochlear nerves to reach the surface of the middle cerebellar peduncle, where it courses along the cerebellopontine fissure and terminates by supplying the petrosal surface of the cerebellum. Operations directed to the middle complex are for the removal of acoustic neuromas and other tumors and for the relief of hemifacial spasm. The considerations related to acoustic neuromas will be dealt with first.

Anatomy of acoustic neuromas

Acoustic neuromas, as they expand, may involve a majority of the cranial nerves, cerebellar arteries, and parts of the brainstem. On the lateral side, in the meatus, they com-

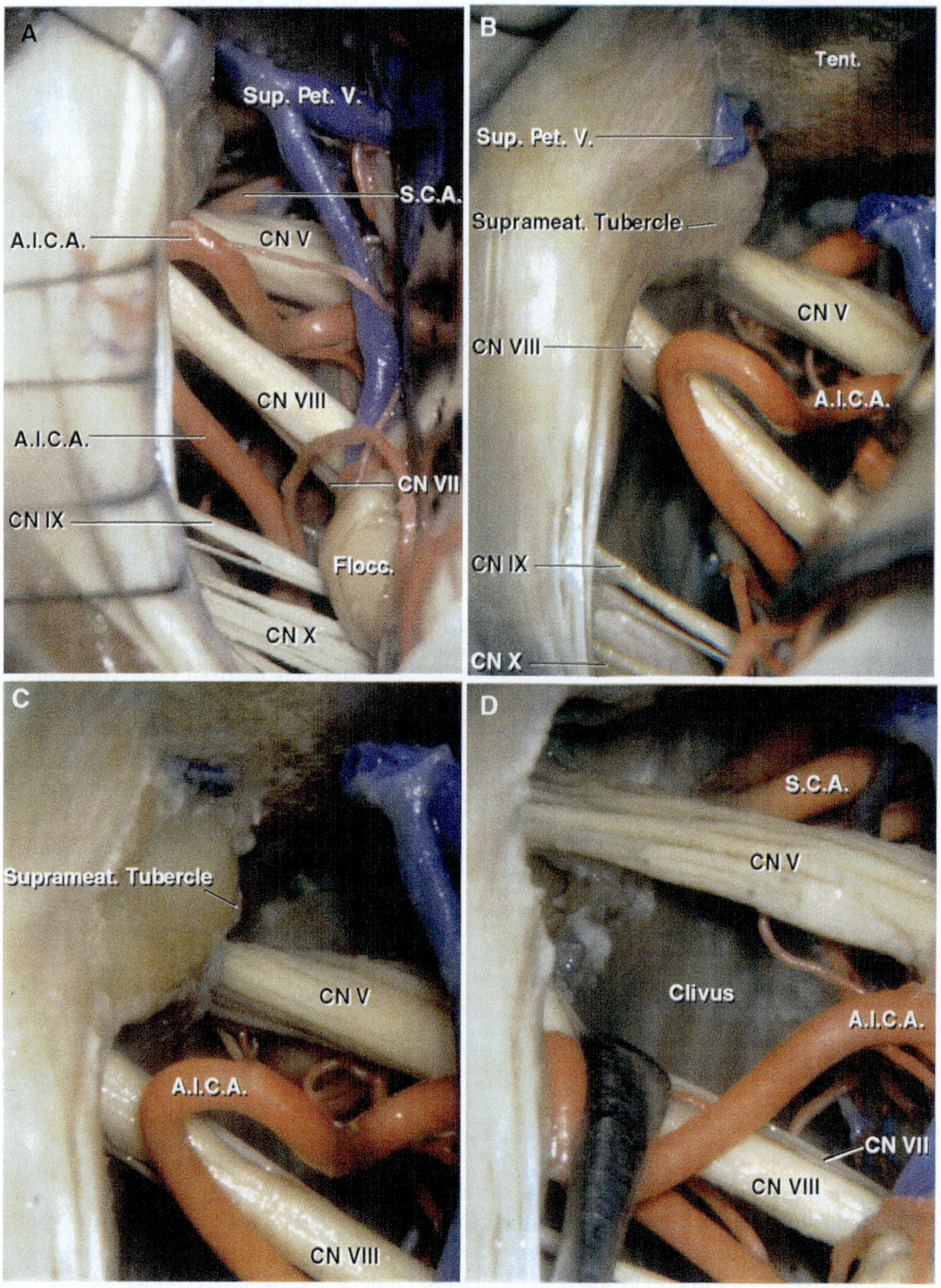

FIGURE 4.15. **Suprameatal variant of the retrosigmoid approach.** ***A,*** **the cerebellum has been elevated to expose the nerves in the cerebellopontine angle. A large petrosal vein blocks access to the suprameatal area.** ***B,*** **the superior petrosal vein has been divided to expose the suprameatal tubercle located above the porus of the internal acoustic meatus and lateral to the trigeminal nerve.** ***C,*** **the dura over the suprameatal tubercle has been removed in preparation for drilling.** ***D,*** **removing the suprameatal bone, including the tubercle, extends the exposure along the posterior trigeminal root by approximately 1 cm and increases access to the front of the brainstem and clivus.** ***A.I.C.A.,*** **anteroinferior cerebellar artery;** ***CN,*** **cranial nerve;** ***Flocc.,*** **flocculus;** ***Pet.,*** **petrosal;** ***S.C.A.,*** **superior cerebellar artery;** ***Sup.,*** **superior;** ***Suprameat.,*** **suprameatal;** ***V.,*** **vein.**

monly expand by enlarging the meatus, but infrequently erode into the vestibule and cochlea. On the medial side, they compress the pons, medulla, and cerebellum. An understanding of microsurgical anatomy is especially important in preserving the facial and adjacent cranial nerves, which are the neural structures at greatest risk during acoustic neuroma removal. A widely accepted operative precept is that a nerve involved by a tumor should be identified proximal or distal to the tumor, where its displacement and distortion is the least, before the tumor is removed from the involved segment of the nerve. Considerable attention has been directed to the early identification of the facial nerve distal to the tumor at the lateral part of the internal acoustic canal. Less attention has been directed to identification at the brainstem on the medial side of the tumor. These anatomic considerations are divided into sections dealing with the relationships at the lateral end of the tumor in the meatus and those on the medial end of the tumor at the brainstem, which follow in this chapter (33, 35, 37).

Meatal relationships

The nerves in the lateral part of the internal acoustic meatus are the facial, cochlear, and inferior and superior vestibular

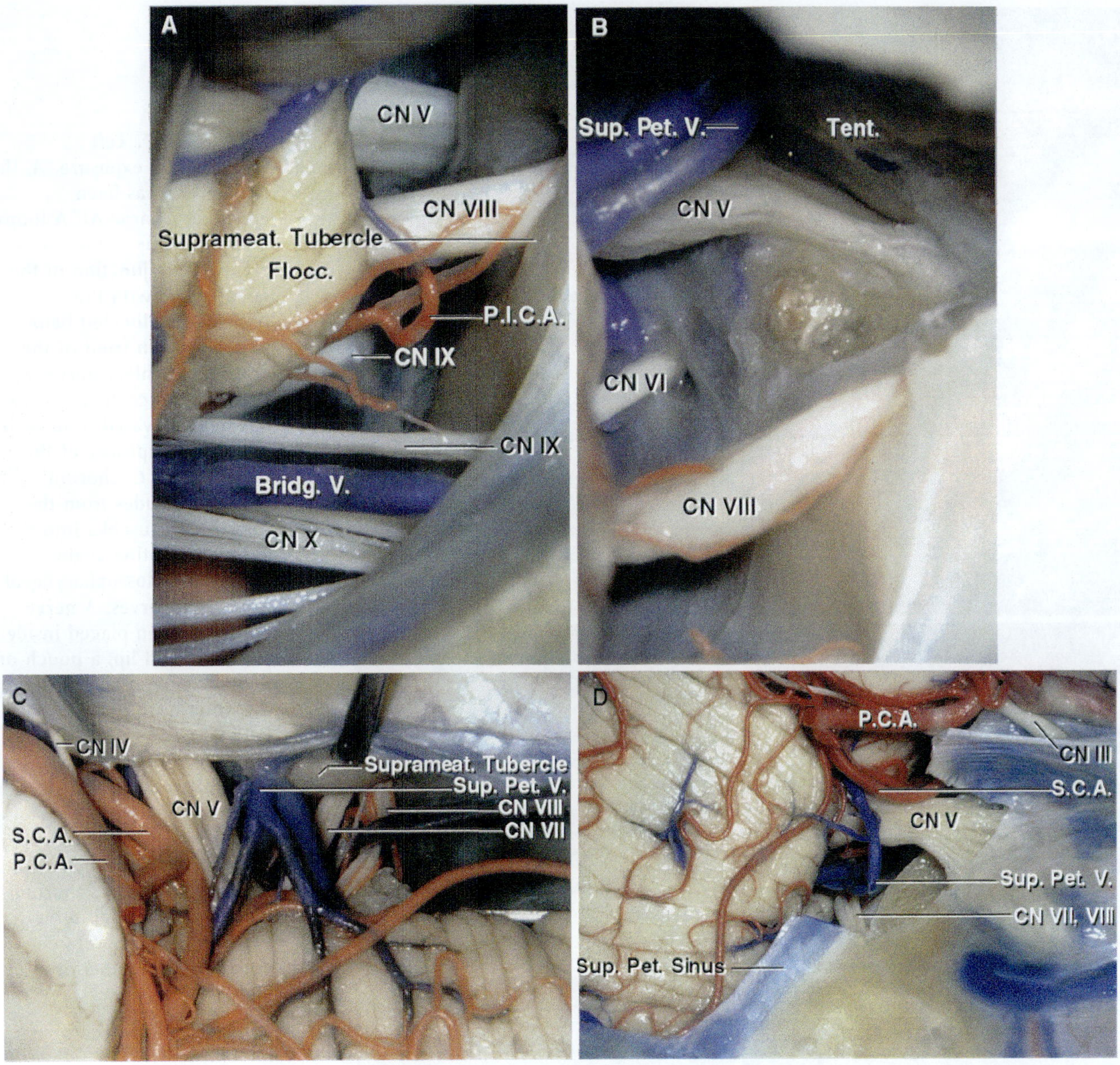

FIGURE 4.16. Suprameatal approach to the posterior part of Meckel's cave. *A*, right cerebellopontine angle. The suprameatal tubercle is located above the porus of the internal meatus. A large inferior petrosal vein passes behind the vagus nerve. *B*, the suprameatal tubercle has been removed and the dura extending anteriorly toward Meckel's cave has been opened to provide 1 cm of additional exposure along the posterior trigeminal root. In addition, access to the side of the clivus is improved. *C*, superior view of the suprameatal tubercle. The tubercle is located lateral to the trigeminal nerve, below the superior petrosal vein, and above the internal acoustic meatus and the facial and vestibulocochlear nerves. *D*, lateral view after removal of the suprameatal tubercle and the segment of the superior petrosal sinus passing above the porus of Meckel's cave. This improves the length of the posterior trigeminal root exposed by 8 to 10 mm, compared with the exposure before drilling the tubercle. *Bridg.*, bridging; *CN*, cranial nerve; *Flocc.*, flocculus; *P.C.A.*, posterior cerebral artery; *Pet.*, petrosal; *P.I.C.A.*, posteroinferior cerebellar artery; *S.C.A.*, superior cerebellar artery; *Sup.*, superior; *Suprameat.*, suprameatal; *Tent.*, tentorium; *V.*, vein.

nerves (*Figs. 4.1* and *4.18*) (30, 38). The position of the nerves is most constant in the lateral portion of the meatus, which is divided into a superior and an inferior portion by a horizontal ridge, called either the transverse or falciform crest. The facial and the superior vestibular nerves are superior to the crest. The facial nerve is anterior to the superior vestibular nerve and is separated from it at the lateral end of the meatus by a vertical ridge of bone, called the vertical crest. The vertical crest is also called "Bill's bar" in recognition of William House's role in focusing on the importance of this crest in

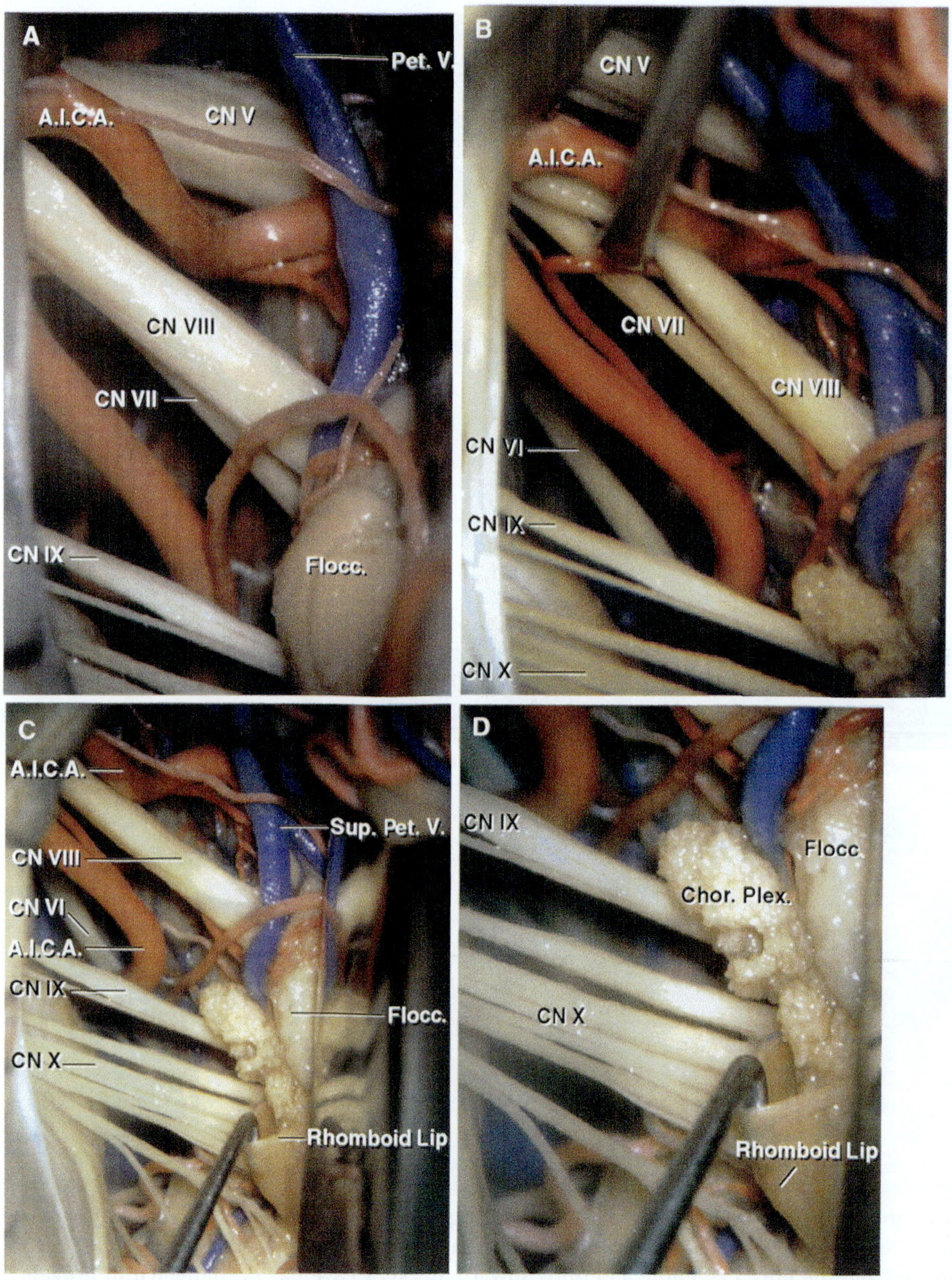

FIGURE 4.17. Left retrosigmoid exposure. *A*, the cerebellum has been elevated. A large AICA loops into the porus of the internal meatus. The junction of the facial nerve with the brainstem is located below and slightly in front of the vestibulocochlear nerve. *B*, the vestibulocochlear nerve has been elevated to provide additional exposure of the facial nerve. *C*, choroid plexus protrudes from the foramen of Luschka into the cerebellopontine angle behind the glossopharyngeal and vagus nerves. A nerve hook has been placed inside the rhomboid lip, a pouch of neural tissue attached along the anterior margin of the lateral recess and extending laterally behind the glossopharyngeal and vagus nerves. *D*, enlarged view of the rhomboid lip. *A.I.C.A.*, anteroinferior cerebellar artery; *Chor. Plex.*, choroid plexus; *CN*, cranial nerve; *Flocc.*, flocculus; *Pet.*, petrosal; *Sup.*, superior; *V.*, vein.

identifying the facial nerve in the lateral end of the canal (16). The cochlear and inferior vestibular nerves run below the transverse crest with the cochlear nerve located anteriorly. Thus, the lateral meatus can be considered to be divided into four portions, with the facial nerve being anterosuperior, the cochlear nerve anteroinferior, the superior vestibular nerve posteroinferior. The anatomy of the region offers the opportunity for three basic approaches to the tumor in the meatus and cerebellopontine angle. One is directed through the middle cranial fossa and the roof of the meatus. Another is directed through the labyrinth and posterior surface of the temporal bone. The third is directed through the posterior cranial fossa and posterior meatal lip. The translabyrinthine and middle fossa approaches are reviewed in the chapter on the temporal bone.

Retrosigmoid approach. The retrosigmoid approach to the meatus is directed through a vertical scalp incision that crosses the asterion. A burr hole is placed below the asterion and a craniotomy is performed exposing the lower margin of the transverse sinus superiorly, the posterior margin of the sigmoid sinus laterally, and the inferior portion of the squamous part of the occipital bone inferiorly. The intradural exposure is directed down the plane between the posterior face of the temporal bone and the petrosal cerebellar surface (*Figs. 4.1, 4.17,* and *4.18*) (35–37). The petrosal cerebellar surface usually relaxes away from the temporal bone after the

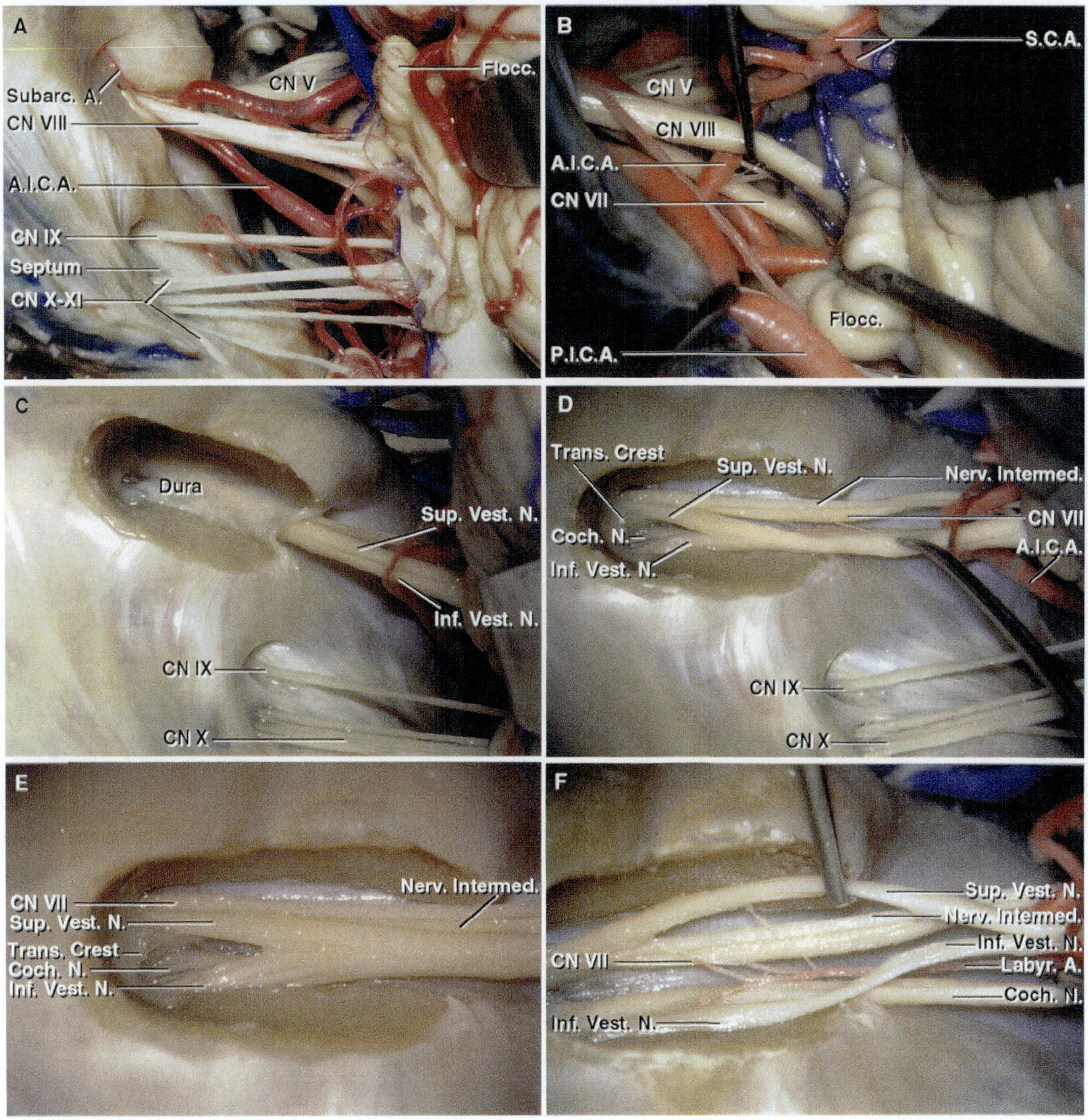

FIGURE 4.18. *A–F.* Left cerebellopontine angle. *A,* the AICA passes between the facial and vestibulocochlear nerves. A dural septum separates the glossopharyngeal and vagus nerves at the jugular foramen. *B,* the vestibulocochlear nerve and the flocculus have been elevated to expose the junction of the facial nerve with the brainstem. In the retrosigmoid approach, the facial nerve junction with the brainstem can be exposed below the vestibulocochlear nerve. *C,* the posterior wall of the internal acoustic meatus has been removed. The cleavage plane between the superior and inferior vestibular nerves is especially prominent. *D,* the dura lining the internal acoustic meatus has been opened. The transverse crest separates the superior vestibular and facial nerves above from the inferior vestibular and cochlear nerves below. *E,* enlarged view of the nerves within the meatus. The cochlear nerve is partially hidden anterior to the inferior vestibular nerve. *F,* the cleavage plane between the superior and inferior vestibular and cochlear nerves has been started laterally and extended medially to expose the individual nerve bundles. *A.,* artery; *A.I.C.A.,* anteroinferior cerebellar artery; *Arc.,* arcuate; *CN,* cranial nerve; *Coch.,* cochlear; *Emin.,* eminence; *Endolymph.,* endolymphatic; *Flocc.,* flocculus; *Inf.,* inferior; *Intermed.,* intermedius; *Jug.,* jugular; *Labyr.,* labyrinth; *N.,* nerve; *Nerv.,* nervus; *P.I.C.A.,* posteroinferior cerebellar artery; *Post.,* posterior; *S.C.A.,* superior cerebellar artery; *Subarc.,* subarcuate; *Sup.,* superior; *Trans.,* transverse; *Vert.,* vertebral; *Vest.,* vestibular.

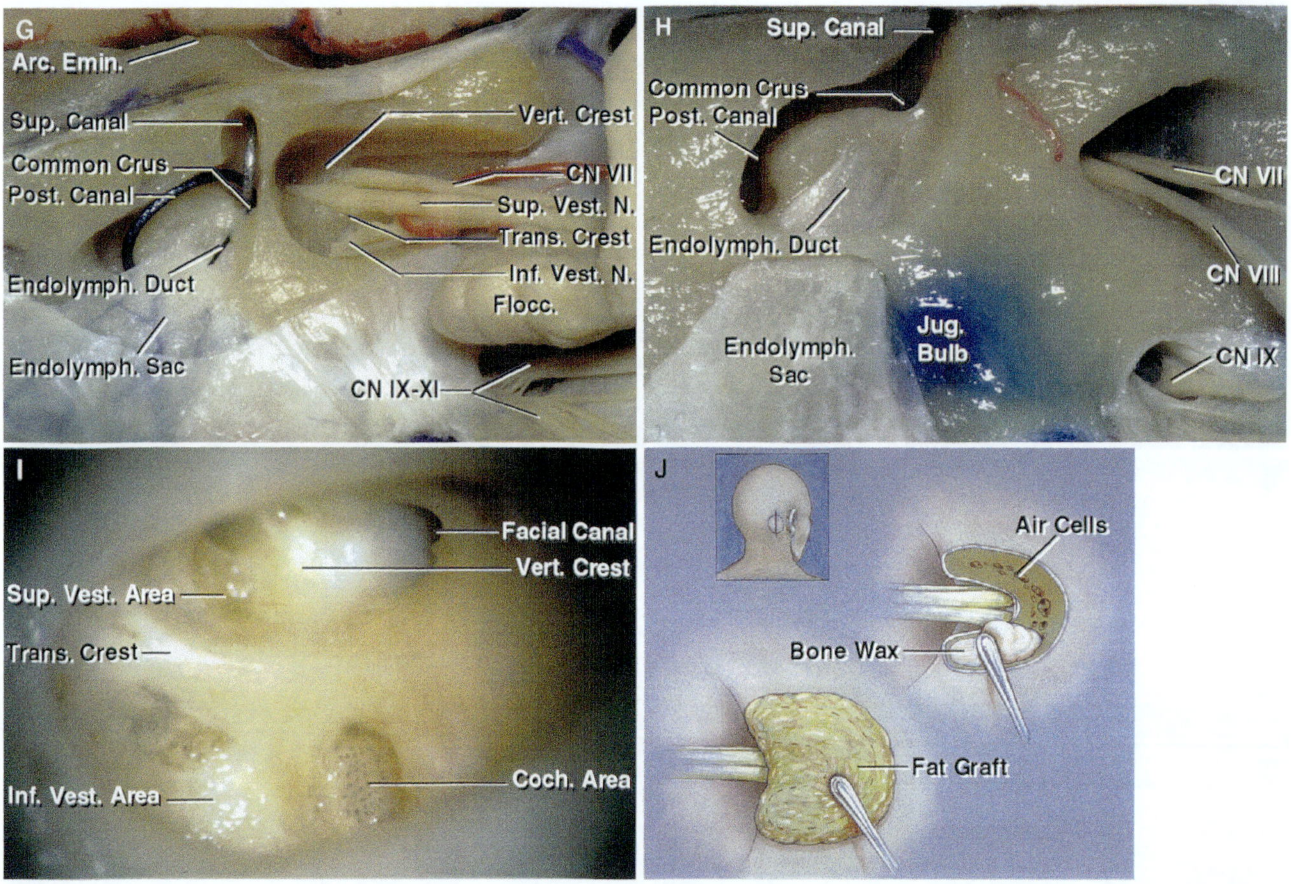

FIGURE 4.18. ***G–J.*** **Left cerebellopontine angle.** ***G,*** **the vertical and transverse crest are exposed at the meatal fundus. The common crus and adjacent part of the superior and posterior canals have been exposed. The endolymphatic duct and sac are situated inferolateral to the internal acoustic meatus.** ***H,*** **another dissection showing the relationships of the junction of the posterior and superior canals and common crus to the meatus. The endolymphatic duct extends downward and backward from the vestibule and opens into the endolymphatic sac, which sits under the dura in the area below and lateral to the meatus. The jugular bulb can be seen through the bone medial to the endolymphatic sac.** ***I,*** **fundus of the left internal acoustic meatus. The transverse crest separates the superior vestibular area and facial canal above from the inferior vestibular and cochlear areas below. The vertical crest separates the superior vestibular area from the entrance into the facial canal. The multiple cochlear nerve filaments penetrating the tiny openings in the lamina cribrosa at the meatal fundus can easily be torn with traction on the nerve from lateral to medial, therefore, we try to direct the strokes of dissection from medial to lateral when there is an opportunity to preserve hearing.** ***J,*** **closure after removing the posterior wall of the internal acoustic meatus. Bone wax on a microdissector is carefully placed into open air cells in the posterior meatal lip and then a pledget of crushed subcutaneous abdominal fat is laid over the drilled meatal area. This has prevented cerebrospinal fluid leaks after removal of the posterior wall of the internal acoustic meatus in more than 200 consecutive operations for acoustic neuroma by the author.**

arachnoid membrane over the cisterna magna has been opened and the cerebrospinal fluid allowed to escape. When removing the posterior meatal wall, it often is necessary to sacrifice the subarcuate artery because it passes through the dura on the posterior meatal wall to reach the subarcuate fossa (*Figs. 4.1* and *4.18*) (25). This artery usually has a sufficiently long stem that its obliteration does not risk damage to the AICA from which it arises. In a few cases, however, the subarcuate artery and the segment of the AICA from which it arises will be incorporated into the dura covering the subarcuate fossa. In this case, the dura and the artery will have to be separated together from the posterior meatal lip wall in preparation for opening the meatus.

The posterior semicircular canal and its common crus with the superior canal, both of which are situated just lateral to the posterior meatal lip, should be preserved when removing the posterior meatal wall if there is the possibility of preserving hearing, since hearing may be lost if damage occurs (*Fig. 4.18*). Care also is required to avoid injury to the vestibular aqueduct, which is situated inferolateral to the meatal lip, and the endolymphatic sac, which expands under the dura on the posterior surface of the temporal bone inferolateral to the meatal porus (*Fig. 4.18*). The endolymphatic sac may be entered in removing the dura from the posterior meatal lip. There is little danger of encountering the cochlear canaliculus, which has a more medial course below the internal auditory

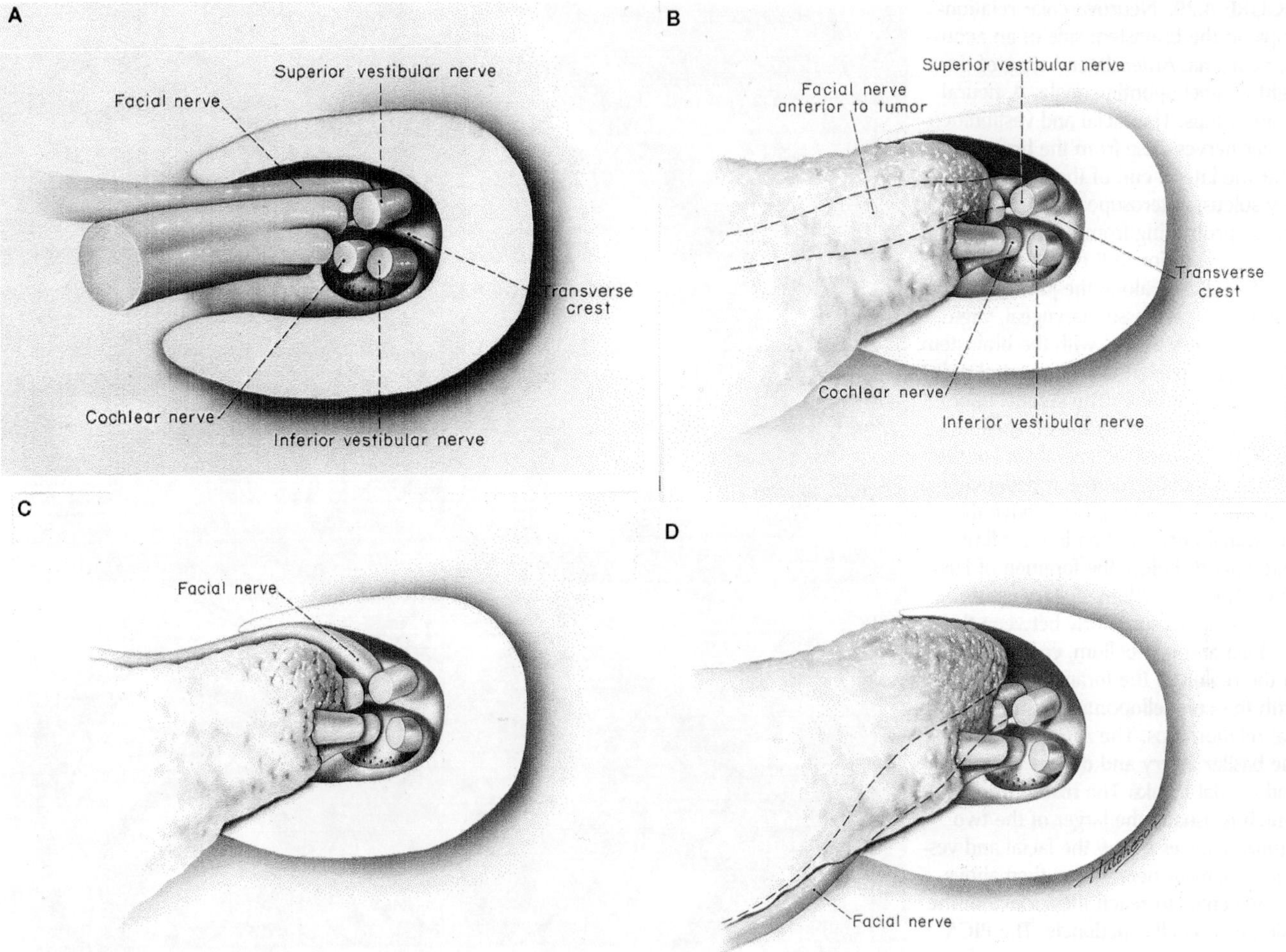

FIGURE 4.19. View of right internal acoustic meatus with the posterior lip removed to show variable direction of facial nerve displacement by acoustic neuroma. *A*, normal neural relationships with the eighth nerve dividing into its three parts in the lateral meatus. The facial and superior vestibular nerves are above the transverse crest and the cochlear and inferior vestibular nerves are below. The facial nerve occupies the anterosuperior quadrant of the lateral meatus. *B*, the facial nerve is displaced directly anteriorly. This is a frequent direction of displacement with acoustic neuroma. *C*, another frequent direction of displacement of the facial nerve is anterior and superior. *D*, the facial nerve is displaced anteriorly and inferiorly by tumor, which erodes the superior wall of the meatus above the nerves and grows into the area above the nerves, displacing them inferiorly. (From, Rhoton AL Jr: Microsurgery of the Internal Acoustic Meatus. Surg Neurol 2:311–318, 1974 [32].)

canal. An unusually high projection of the jugular bulb into the posterior wall of the meatus presents an anomaly that may block access to the posterior meatal lip. Mastoid air cells commonly are encountered in the posterior meatal lip.

After removing the posterior wall of the meatus, the dura lining the meatus is opened to expose its contents (*Figs. 4.18* and *4.19*). The facial nerve is identified near the origin of the facial canal at the anterosuperior quadrant of the meatus rather than in a more medial location where the direction of displacement is variable. If the tumor extends into the vestibule, the latter can easily be exposed by drilling and removing the posterior wall of the vestibule lateral to the meatal fundus. The strokes of the fine dissecting instruments along the vestibulocochlear nerve should be directed from medial to lateral rather than from lateral to medial, because traction medially may tear the tiny filaments of the cochlear nerve at the site where these filaments penetrate the lateral end of the meatus to enter the modiolus of the cochlea (*Fig. 4.18*).

Brainstem relationships

A consistent set of neural, arterial, and venous relationships at the brainstem facilitates the identification of the nerves on the medial side of an acoustic neuroma (*Figs. 4.20-4.22*) (33, 37, 38).

Neural relationships. The landmarks on the medial or brainstem side of structures that are helpful in guiding the surgeon to the junction of the facial nerve with the brainstem

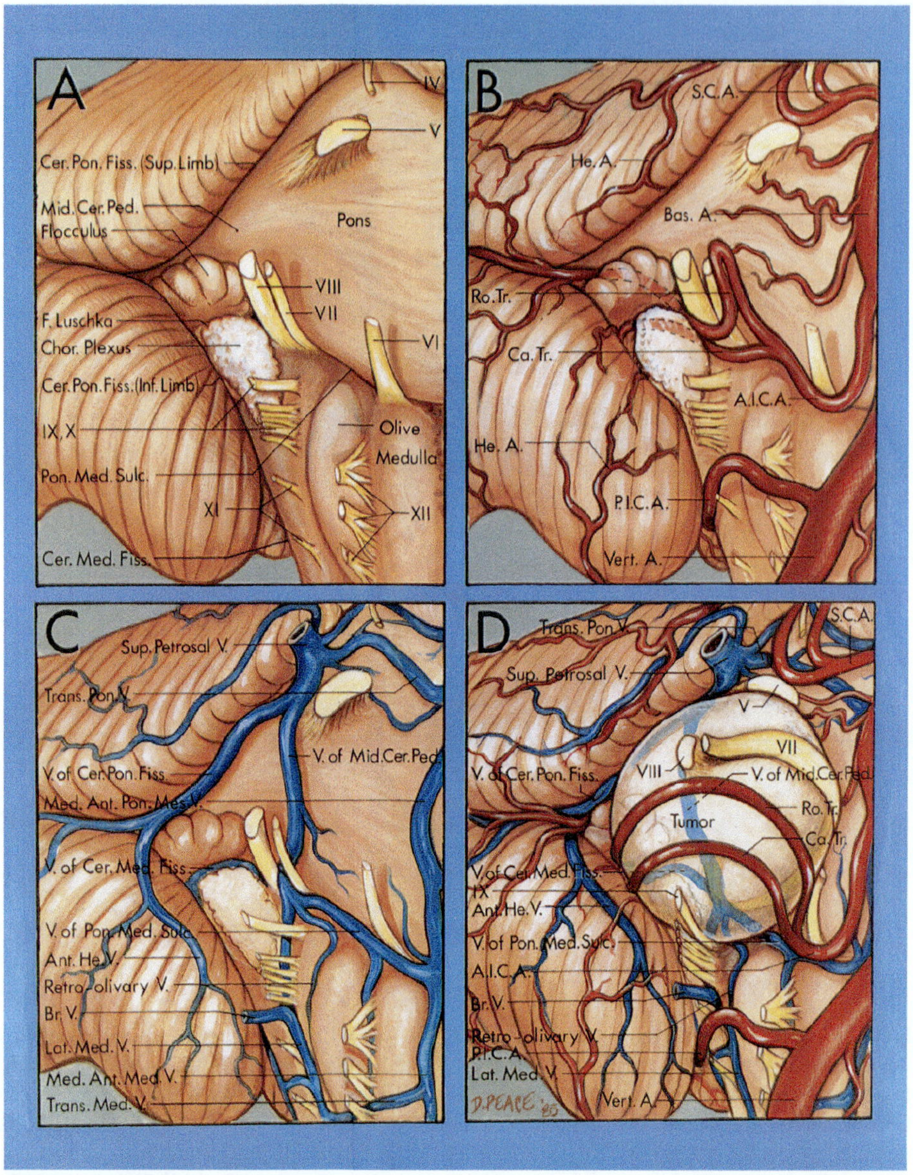

FIGURE 4.20. Neurovascular relationships on the brainstem side of an acoustic neuroma. Anterolateral view of the right cerebellopontine angle. *A*, neural relationships. The facial and vestibulocochlear nerves arise from the brainstem near the lateral end of the pontomedullary sulcus, anterosuperior to the choroid plexus protruding from the foramen of Luschka, anterior to the flocculus, rostral to a line drawn along the junction of the rootlets of the glossopharyngeal, vagus, and accessory nerves with the brainstem, and slightly posterior to the rostral pole of the inferior olive. The cerebellopontine fissure formed by the cerebellum wrapping around the lateral side of the pons and middle cerebellar peduncle has a superior limb that passes above the trigeminal nerve and an inferior limb that extends below the foramen of Luschka. The cerebellomedullary fissure, which extends superiorly between the medulla and cerebellum, communicates in the region of the foramen of Luschka with the cerebellopontine fissure. *B*, arterial relationships. The AICA arises from the basilar artery and divides into rostral and caudal trunks. The rostral trunk, which is usually the larger of the two trunks, courses below the facial and vestibulocochlear nerves, and then above the flocculus to reach the surface of the middle cerebellar peduncle. The PICA arises from the vertebral artery and passes first between the hypoglossal rootlets, and then between the vagus and accessory nerves on its way to the cerebellar hemisphere. The SCA passes above the trigeminal nerve. The cerebellar arteries give rise to hemispheric branches. *C*, venous relationships. The veins that converge on the junction of the facial and vestibulocochlear nerves with the brainstem are the veins of the pontomedullary sulcus, cerebellomedullary fissure, middle cerebellar peduncle, and the retro-olivary and lateral medullary veins. The vein of the cerebellopontine fissure, which passes above the flocculus on the middle cerebellar peduncle, is formed by the anterior hemispheric veins that arise on the cerebellum. Transverse pontine and transverse medullary veins cross the pons and medulla. The median anterior medullary and median anterior pontomesencephalic veins ascend on the anterior surface of the medulla and pons. The veins of the middle cerebellar peduncle and the cerebellopontine fissure and a transverse pontine vein join to form a superior petrosal vein, which empties into the superior petrosal sinus. A bridging vein passes below the vagal rootlets toward the jugular foramen. *D*, neurovascular relationships of an acoustic neuroma. The tumor arises from the vestibulocochlear nerve and displaces the facial nerve anteriorly, the trigeminal nerve superiorly, and the vagus and glossopharyngeal nerves inferiorly. The facial nerve, even though displaced by the tumor, enters the brainstem along the lateral margin of the pontomedullary sulcus, rostral to the glossopharyngeal and vagus nerves, anterior to the flocculus, and rostral to the choroid plexus protruding from the foramen of Luschka. The rostral trunk of the AICA, after passing below the tumor, returns to the surface of the middle cerebellar peduncle above the flocculus. The veins displaced around the medial side of the tumor are the veins of the middle cerebellar peduncle, cerebellomedullary fissure, cerebellopontine fissure, and pontomedullary sulcus, and the retro-olivary and lateral medullary veins. (From, Rhoton AL Jr: Microsurgical anatomy of the brainstem surface facing an acoustic neuroma. Surg Neurol 25:326–339, 1986 [33].) *A.*, artery; *A.I.C.A.*, anteroinferior cerebellar artery; *Ant.*, anterior; *Bas.*, basilar; *Br.*, bridging; *Ca.*, caudal; *Cer.*, cerebellar; *Cer. Pon.*, cerebellopontine; *Chor.*, choroid; *F.*, foramen; *Fiss.*, fissure; *Hem.*, hemispheric; *Lat.*, lateral; *Med.*, medial, medullary; *Mid.*, middle; *Ped.*, peduncle; *P.I.C.A.*, posteroinferior cerebellar artery; *Pon.*, pontine; *Pon. Med.*, pontomedullary; *Pon. Mes.*, pontomesencephalic; *Ro.*, rostral; *S.C.A.*, superior cerebellar artery; *Sulc.*, sulcus; *Sup.*, superior; *Tr.*, trunk; *Trans.*, transverse; *V.*, vein; *Vert.*, vertebral.

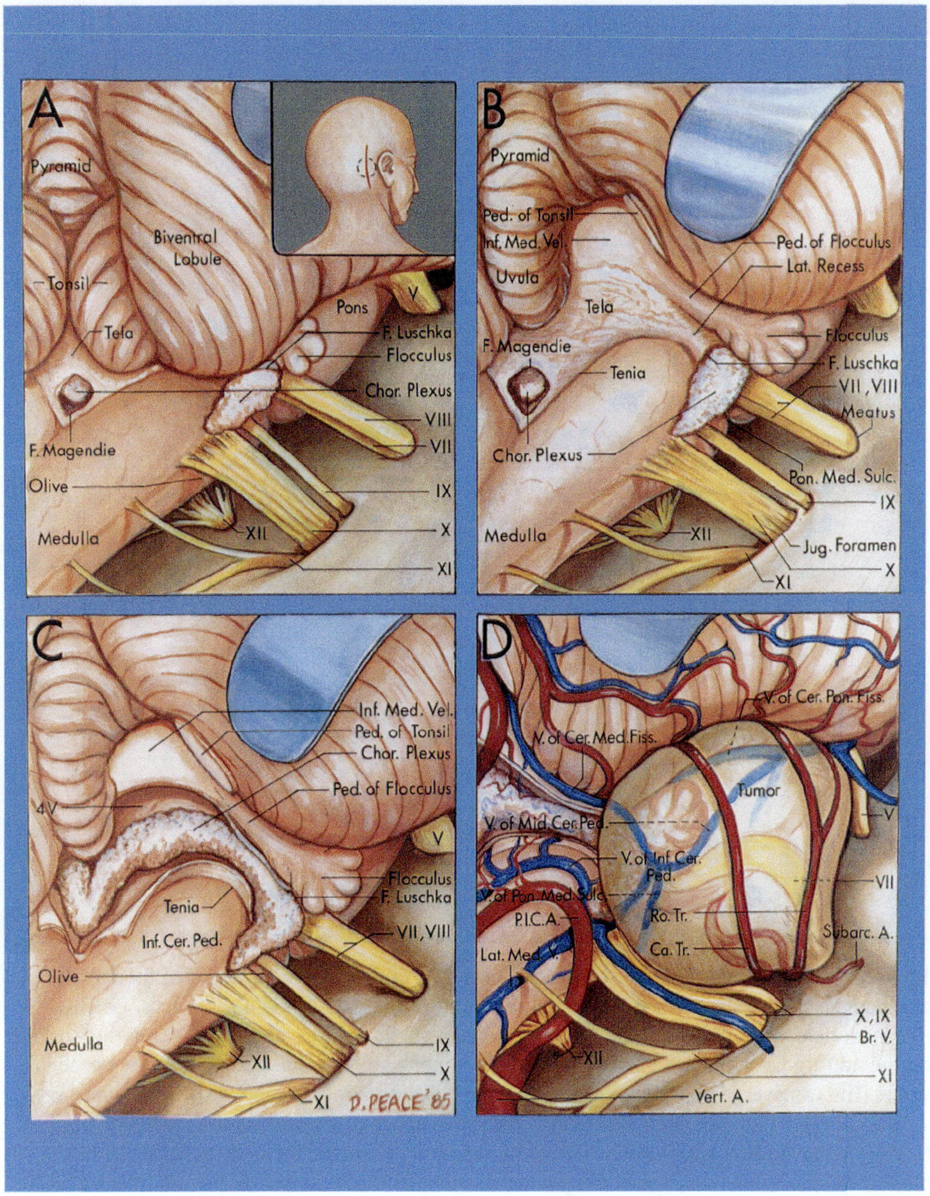

FIGURE 4.21. Relationship of the foramen of Luschka and the lateral recess of the fourth ventricle to the junction of the facial and vestibulocochlear nerves with the brainstem, as seen through a suboccipital craniotomy. *A*, the orientation, skin incision (*solid line*), and craniotomy (*interrupted line*) are shown in the *insert*. The foramen of Luschka opens into the cerebellopontine angle behind the glossopharyngeal and vagus nerves. The choroid plexus protrudes from the foramen of Luschka, slightly below and behind the facial and vestibulocochlear nerves, and behind to the glossopharyngeal and vagus nerves. The flocculus protrudes into the cerebellopontine angle above the foramen of Luschka. The accessory nerve arises below the vagus nerve. The hypoglossal rootlets arise ventral to the olive. The trigeminal nerve crosses in the upper part of the exposure. *B*, the right cerebellar tonsil has been removed by dividing the tonsillar peduncle to show the relationship of the lateral recess to the facial and vestibulocochlear nerves. The flocculus and choroid plexus protrude in the cerebellopontine angle behind the junction of the facial and vestibulocochlear nerves with the brainstem. The inferior medullary velum stretches from the lateral side of the vermis to the flocculus and is all that remains of the connection between the flocculus and the nodulus, which form the flocculonodular lobe of the cerebellum. The inferior medullary velum stretches laterally to form the peduncle of the flocculus. The tela choroidea forms the caudal part of the roof of the fourth ventricle and has the choroid plexus attached to its inner surface. The facial and vestibulocochlear nerves enter the brainstem at the lateral end of the pontomedullary sulcus. *C*, the tela choroidea has been opened, but the choroid plexus, which arises on the inner surface of the tela in the fourth ventricle, has been preserved. The fringelike choroid plexus extends through the foramen of Luschka slightly below and behind the junction of the facial and vestibulocochlear nerves with the brainstem. The inferior cerebellar peduncle ascends on the dorsolateral margin of the medulla. *D*, relationships of an acoustic neuroma. The facial nerve is displaced anteriorly and superiorly in the cerebellopontine angle and enters the brainstem at the lateral end of the pontomedullary sulcus, anterosuperior to the choroid plexus protruding from the foramen of Luschka, and near where the flocculus is attached along the margin of the lateral recess. The tumor displaces the trigeminal nerve upward and the glossopharyngeal and vagus nerves downward. The AICA gives rise to a subarcuate artery, which enters the subarcuate fossa in the posterior wall of the internal acoustic meatus and bifurcates into a rostral and a caudal trunk. The rostral trunk courses above the flocculus to reach the surface of the middle cerebellar peduncle. (From, Rhoton AL Jr: Microsurgical anatomy of the brainstem surface facing an acoustic neuroma. Surg Neurol 25:326–339, 1986 [33].) *Br.*, bridging; *Ca.*, caudal; *Cer. Med.*, cerebellomedullary; *Cer. Pon.*, cerebellopontine; *Chor.* choroid; *F.*, foramen; *Fiss.*, fissure; *Inf.*, inferior; *Jug.*, jugular; *Lat.*, lateral; *Med.*, medial, medullary; *Mid.*, middle; *Ped.*, peduncle; *P.I.C.A.*, posteroinferior cerebellar artery; *Pon. Med.*, pontomedullary; *Ro.*, rostral; *Subarc.*, subarcuate; *Sulc.*, sulcus; *Tr.*, trunk; *V.*, vein; *Vel.*, velum.

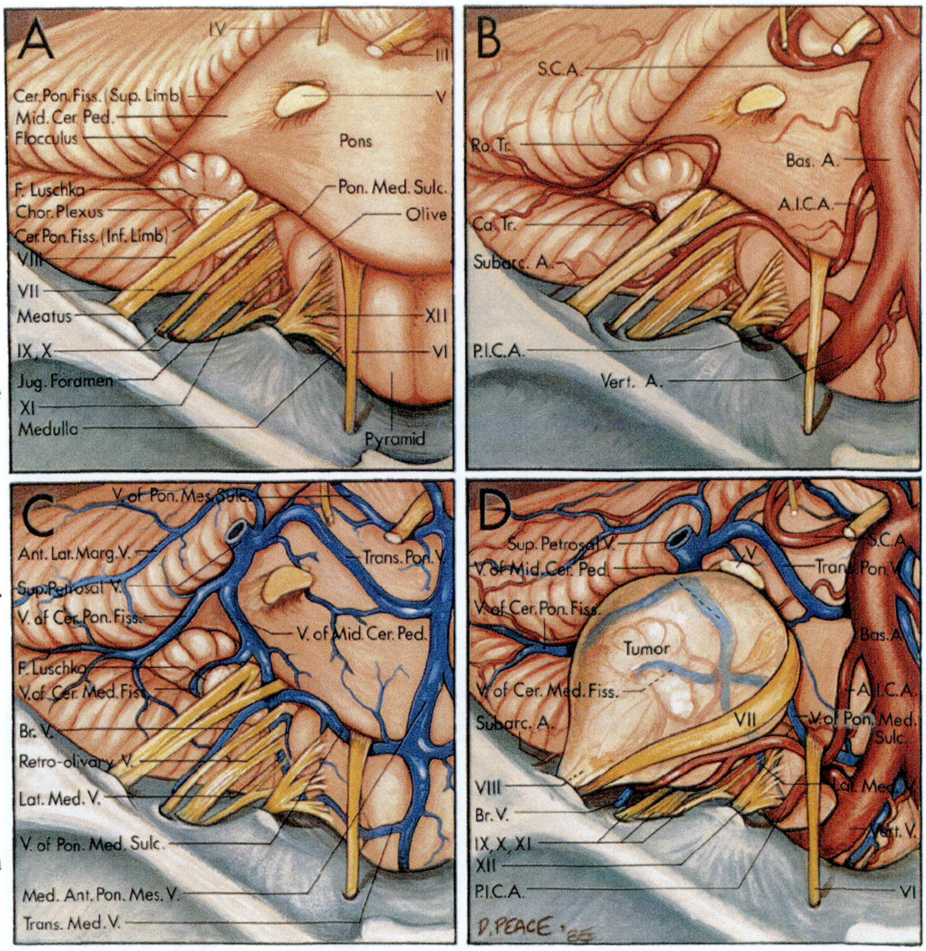

FIGURE 4.22. Neurovascular relationships on the brainstem side of an acoustic neuroma. Anterosuperior views. *A*, neural relationships. The cerebrum and tentorium cerebelli have been removed, and the trigeminal, trochlear, and oculomotor nerves have been divided to allow the brainstem to be displaced posteriorly to expose the cerebellopontine angle from above. The facial and vestibulocochlear nerves arise at the lateral end of the pontomedullary sulcus anterior to the flocculus, rostral to the glossopharyngeal, vagus, and accessory nerves, and anterosuperior to the choroid plexus protruding from the foramen of Luschka. The cerebellopontine fissure, formed where the cerebellum wraps around the lateral side of the pons and middle cerebellar peduncle, has superior and inferior limbs. The foramen of Luschka opens into the inferior limb near the facial and vestibulocochlear nerves. *B*, arterial relationships. The AICA arises from the basilar artery, passes below the facial and vestibulocochlear nerves, gives rise to the subarcuate artery, and divides into a rostral and a caudal trunk. The rostral trunk passes above the flocculus to course on the middle cerebellar peduncle, and the caudal trunk supplies the area below the flocculus. *C*, venous relationships. The veins converging on the junction of the facial nerve with the brainstem are the lateral medullary and retro-olivary veins, and the veins of the pontomedullary sulcus, cerebellomedullary fissure, and middle cerebellar peduncle. The median anterior pontomesencephalic vein ascends on the anterior surface of the brainstem, and the transverse pontine and transverse medullary veins cross the pons and medulla. The vein of the cerebellopontine fissure passes above the flocculus. The transverse pontine vein and the veins of the middle cerebellar peduncle and cerebellopontine fissure join to form one of the superior petrosal veins that empty into the superior petrosal sinus. A bridging vein passes from the side of the brainstem to the jugular foramen. The anterolateral marginal vein crosses the anterolateral margin of the cerebellum. The vein of the pontomesencephalic sulcus courses in the pontomesencephalic sulcus below the oculomotor nerve. *D*, neurovascular relationships of an acoustic neuroma. The tumor arises from the vestibulocochlear nerve and displaces the facial nerve anteriorly, the trigeminal nerve superiorly, and the glossopharyngeal and vagus nerves inferiorly. The vestibulocochlear nerve disappears into the tumor. The facial nerve enters the brainstem along the lateral margin of the pontomedullary sulcus, rostral to the glossopharyngeal nerve, anterior to the flocculus, and rostral to the choroid plexus protruding from the foramen of Luschka. The AICA is usually displaced around the lower margin of the tumor. The veins displaced around the medial side of the tumor are the veins of the pontomedullary sulcus, middle cerebellar peduncle, and cerebellomedullary fissure, and the lateral medullary and retro-olivary veins. (From, Rhoton AL Jr: Microsurgical anatomy of the brainstem surface facing an acoustic neuroma. Surg Neurol 25:326–339, 1986 [33].) *A.*, artery; *A.I.C.A.*, anteroinferior cerebellar artery; *Ant.*, anterior; *Bas.*, basilar; *Br.*, bridging; *Ca.*, caudal; *Cer.*, cerebellar; *Cer. Pon.*, cerebellopontine; *Chor.*, choroid; *F.*, foramen; *Fiss.*, fissure; *Inf.*, inferior; *Jug.*, jugular; *Lat.*, lateral; *Marg.*, marginal; *Med.*, medial, medullary; *Mid.*, middle; *Ped.*, peduncle; *P.I.C.A.*, posteroinferior cerebellar artery; *Pon.*, pontine; *Pon. Med.*, pontomedullary; *Pon. Mes.*, pontomesencephalic; *Ro.*, rostral; *S.C.A.*, superior cerebellar artery; *Subarc.*, subarcuate; *Sulc.*, sulcus; *Sup.*, superior; *Tr.*, trunk; *Trans.*, transverse; *V.*, vein; *Vert.*, vertebral.

are the pontomedullary sulcus; the junction of the glossopharyngeal, vagus, and spinal accessory nerves with the medulla; the foramen of Luschka and its choroid plexus; and the flocculus. The facial nerve arises from the brainstem near the lateral end of the pontomedullary sulcus 1 to 2 mm anterior to the point at which the vestibulocochlear nerve joins the brainstem at the lateral end of the sulcus. The interval between the vestibulocochlear and facial nerves is greatest at the level of the pontomedullary sulcus and decreases as these nerves approach the meatus.

The facial nerve enjoys a consistent relationship to the junction of the glossopharyngeal, vagus, and spinal accessory nerves with the medulla (*Figs. 4.20-4.22*). The facial nerve arises 2 to 3 mm above the most rostral rootlet contributing to these nerves. A helpful way of visualizing the point where the facial nerve will exit from the brain stern, even when displaced by a tumor, is to project an imaginary line along the medullary junction of the rootlets forming the glossopharyngeal, vagus, and spinal accessory nerves upward through the pontomedullary junction. This line, at a point 2 to 3 mm above the junction of the glossopharyngeal nerve with the medulla, will pass through the pontomedullary junction at the site where the facial nerve exits from the brainstem. The filaments of the nervus intermedius also are stretched around an acoustic neuroma.

The structures related to the lateral recess of the fourth ventricle that have a consistent relationship to the facial and vestibulocochlear nerves are the foramen of Luschka and its choroid plexus, and the flocculus (*Figs. 4.20-4.22*) (10, 27). The foramen of Luschka is situated at the lateral margin of the pontomedullary sulcus, just behind the junction of the glossopharyngeal nerve with the brainstem, and immediately posteroinferior to the junction of the facial and vestibulocochlear nerves with the brainstem. The foramen of Luschka is infrequently well visualized. A consistently identifiable tuft of choroid plexus, however, hangs out of the foramen of Luschka and sits on the posterior surface of the glossopharyngeal and vagus nerves just inferior to the junction of the facial and vestibulocochlear nerves with the brainstem. Another structure related to the lateral recess, the flocculus, projects from the margin of the lateral recess and foramen of Luschka into the cerebellopontine angle, just posterior to where the facial and vestibulocochlear nerves join the pontomedullary sulcus.

Arterial relationships. The arteries crossing the cerebellopontine angle, especially the AICA, enjoy a consistent relationship to the facial and vestibulocochlear nerves, the foramen of Luschka, and the flocculus as described elsewhere in this volume (13, 14, 24, 25). In a previous study, the author's group found that the AICA formed a loop that reached the porus or protruded into the canal in 54% of the cases (25). When opening the meatus by the middle fossa, translabyrinthine, or posterior approaches, care is required to avoid injury to the AICA if it is located at or protrudes through the porus.

In most cases, the AICA passes below the facial and vestibulocochlear nerves as it encircles the brainstem, but it also may pass above or between these nerves in its course around the brainstem (*Fig. 4.23*). In the most common case, in which the artery passes below the nerves, the tumor would displace the artery inferiorly. If the artery courses between the facial and vestibulocochlear nerves, a tumor arising in the latter nerve will displace the artery forward. Tumor growth would displace the artery superiorly if it passes above the nerves. Atkinson pointed out that those cases of acoustic neuroma appearing at necropsy after operation frequently had occlusion of the AICA (3). In three cases presented by Atkinson, an arterial branch coursing over the tumor capsule was ligated with resulting lateral pontine, tegmental, and medullary infarction in the area supplied by the AICA and death. He noted that the blood pressure rose at or near the time of occlusion of the artery, although the hypertension often subsided by the end of the operation. These tumors may also displace the PICA and insinuate themselves between the basilar artery and the pons, stretching the perforating branches of the basilar artery. The labyrinthine, recurrent perforating, and subarcuate branches arise from the AICA near the facial and vestibulocochlear nerves and are frequently stretched around a cerebellopontine angle tumor.

Venous relationships. The veins on the side of the brainstem that have a predictable relationship to the facial and vestibulocochlear nerves are the vein of the pontomedullary sulcus, the veins of the cerebellomedullary fissure, middle cerebellar peduncle, and cerebellopontine fissure (*Figs. 4.20-4.22*) (26). The identification of any of these veins during the removal of the tumor makes it easier to identify the site of the junction of the facial and vestibulocochlear nerves with the brainstem. The exposure of an acoustic neuroma in the central part of the cerebellopontine angle near the lateral recess usually can be completed without sacrificing a bridging vein. If a vein is obliterated during acoustic tumor removal, it is usually one of the superior petrosal veins, which is sacrificed near the superior pole of the tumor during the later stages of the removal of a large tumor. Small acoustic neuromas usually are removed without sacrificing a petrosal vein. The largest vein encountered around the superior pole of an acoustic neuroma is the vein of the cerebellopontine fissure.

Summary: Anatomy of acoustic neuromas

Because acoustic neuromas most frequently arise in the posteriorly placed vestibular nerves, they usually displace the facial and cochlear nerves anteriorly (*Figs. 4.19* and *4.24*). The facial nerve is stretched around the anterior half of the tumor capsule. Variability in the direction of the growth of the tumor arising from the vestibular nerves may result in the facial nerve being displaced, not only directly anteriorly, but also anterosuperiorly or anteroinferiorly. The nerve infrequently is found on the posterior surface of the tumor. Because the facial nerve always enters the facial canal at the anterosuperior quadrant of the meatal fundus, it usually is easiest to locate it here, rather than at a more medial location where the degree of displacement of the nerve is more variable. The cochlear nerve also lies anterior to the vestibular nerve and is stretched most frequently around the anterior half of the tumor. The strokes of the fine dissecting instruments used in removing the tumor should be directed along the vestibulocochlear nerve from medial to lateral rather than from lateral to medial, because traction medially may tear the tiny filaments of the cochlear nerve at the site where these filaments penetrate the lateral end of the meatus to enter the cochlea (*Figs. 4.18* and *4.25*).

The operation for a cerebellopontine angle tumor should be planned so that the tumor surface is allowed to settle away from the neural tissue rather than the neural structures being

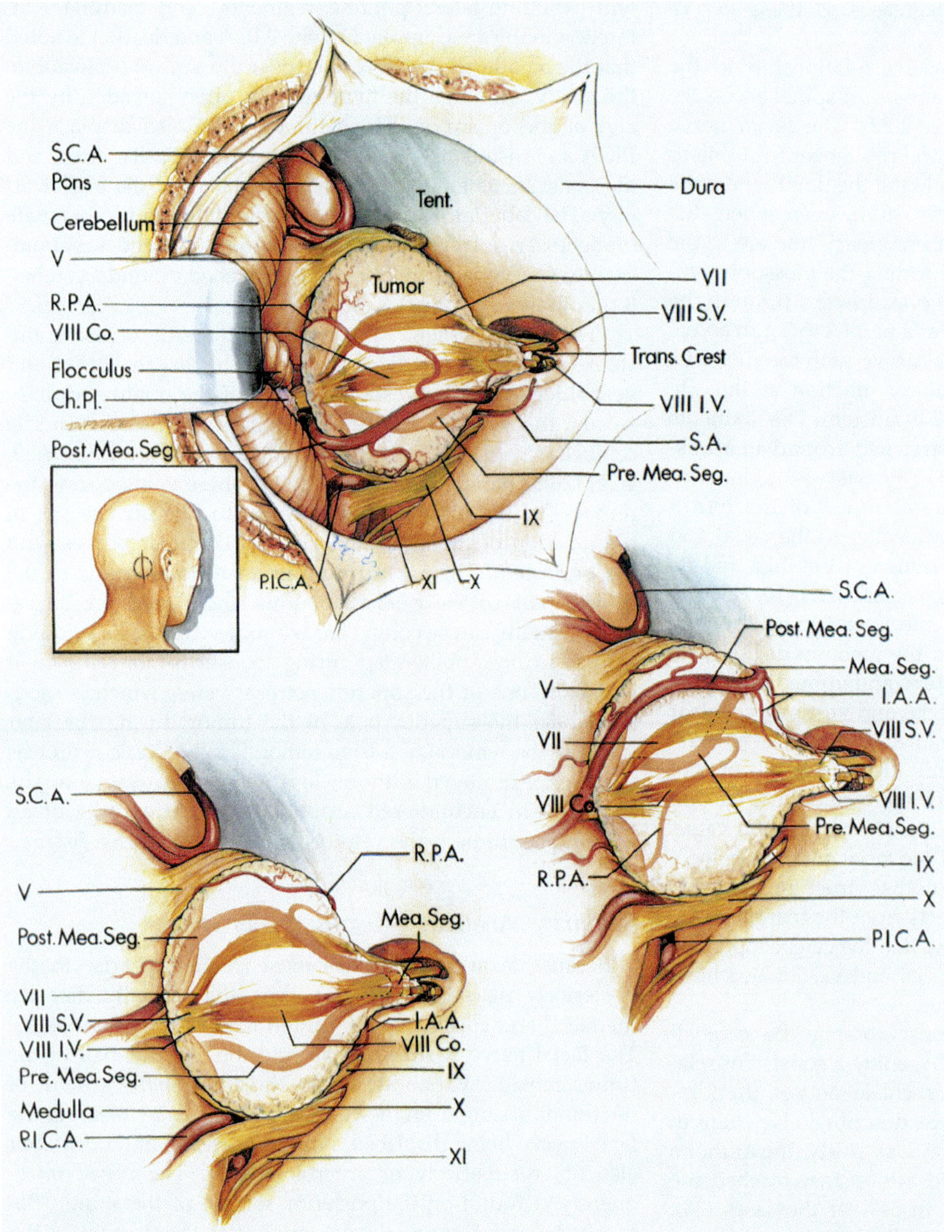

FIGURE 4.23. Posterior views of the direction of displacement of the AICA around an acoustic neuroma. *Top left,* the *insert* shows the direction of view. Both the premeatal and the postmeatal segments are in their most common locations around the lower margin of the tumor. The premeatal segment approaches the meatus from anteroinferior, and the postmeatal segment passes posteroinferior to the tumor. The SCA and the trigeminal nerve are above the tumor, and the PICA and the glossopharyngeal, vagus, and spinal accessory nerves are below the tumor. The choroid plexus protrudes into the cerebellopontine angle medial to the tumor. The posterior wall of the internal acoustic canal has been removed to expose the transverse crest and the superior vestibular and inferior vestibular nerves. The vestibular nerves disappear into the tumor; however, the cochlear and facial nerves are displaced around the anterior margin of the tumor. A subarcuate artery arises from the premeatal segment, and a recurrent perforating artery arises from the postmeatal segment. *Center right,* in a less common pattern of displacement of the AICA, the premeatal and postmeatal segments are above the tumor. The internal auditory arteries arise from the meatal segment. *Bottom left,* both the premeatal and the postmeatal segments are displaced anteriorly to the tumor. This occurs if the AICA courses between the vestibulocochlear and facial nerves. The tumor arises in the vestibular nerves, and tumor growth displaces both the premeatal and the postmeatal segments anteriorly. (From, Martin RG, Grant JL, Peace DA, Theiss C, Rhoton AL Jr: Microsurgical relationships of the anterior inferior cerebellar artery and the facial-vestibulocochlear nerve complex. Neurosurgery 6:483–507, 1980 [25].) *Ch. Pl.,* choroid plexus; *Co.,* cochlear; *I.A.A.,* internal auditory (labyrinthine) artery; *I.V.,* inferior vestibular; *Mea.,* meatal; *P.I.C.A.,* posteroinferior cerebellar artery; *Post.,* posterior; *R.P.A.,* recurrent perforating artery; *S.A.,* subarcuate artery; *S.V.,* superior vestibular; *S.C.A.,* superior cerebellar artery; *Seg.,* segment; *Tent.,* tentorium.

retracted away from the tumor (*Fig. 4.25*). No attempt is made to see the whole tumor upon initial exposure. The surface of the tumor then is opened and the intracapsular contents are removed. As the intracapsular contents are evacuated, the tumor shifts laterally, allowing more of the tumor to be removed through the small exposure. The most common reason for the tumor appearing to be tightly adherent to the neural structures is not adhesions between the capsule and surrounding tissue, but, rather, the residual tumor within the capsule wedging the tumor into position. As the intracapsular contents are removed, the tumor capsule folds laterally, revealing the structures on the brainstem side of the tumor.

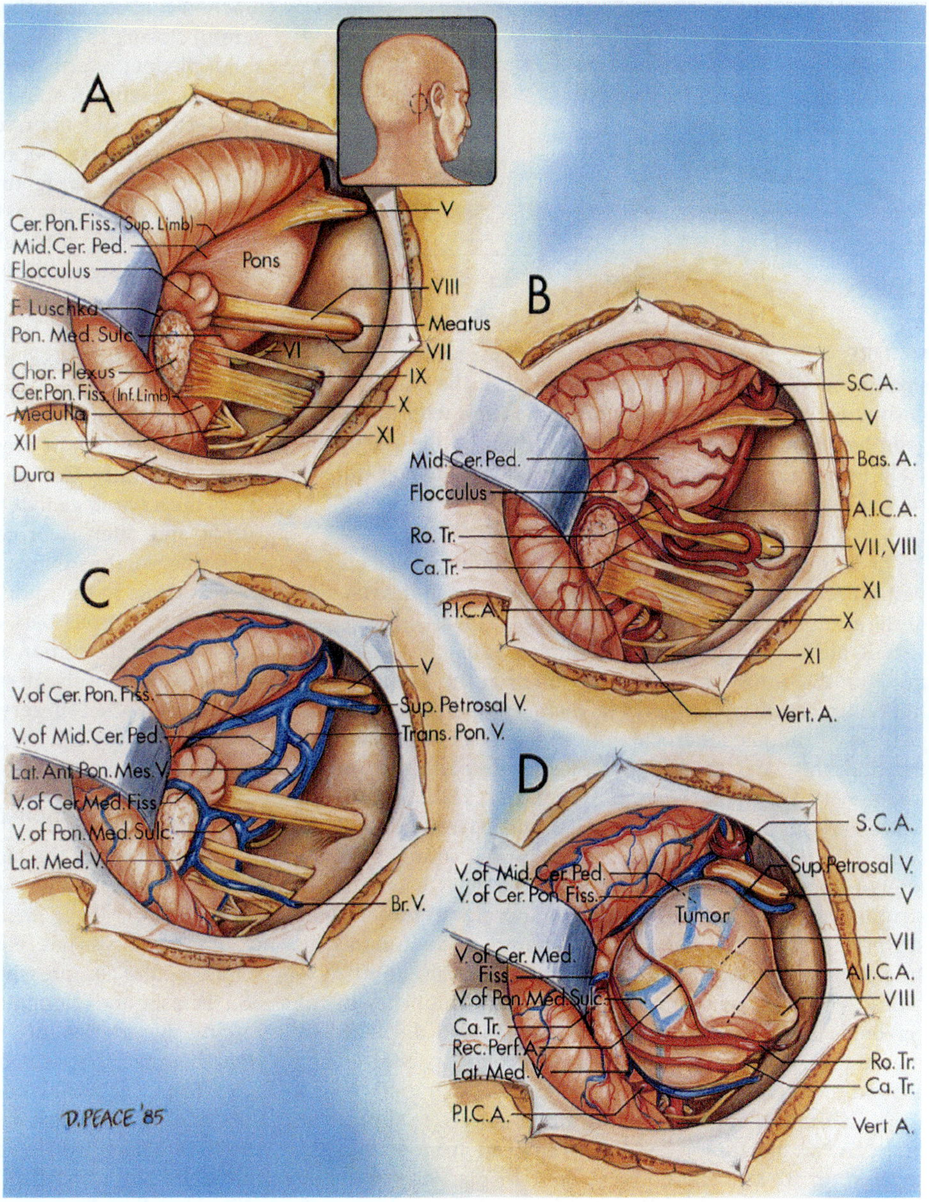

FIGURE 4.24. Neurovascular relationships on the brainstem side of an acoustic neuroma. Posterior view through a retrosigmoid craniotomy. *A*, neural relationships. The orientation, skin incision (*solid line*), and craniotomy site (*interrupted line*) are shown in the *insert*. The retractor is on the petrosal surface of the cerebellum. The facial and vestibulocochlear nerves arise at the lateral end of the pontomedullary sulcus, anterior to the flocculus, rostral to the glossopharyngeal, vagus, and accessory nerves, and anterosuperior to the choroid plexus protruding from the foramen of Luschka. The cerebellopontine fissure, formed where the cerebellum wraps around the lateral side of the pons and middle cerebellar peduncle, has superior and inferior limbs. *B*, arterial relationships. The AICA arises from the basilar artery and divides into a rostral trunk, which passes above the flocculus to reach the surface of the middle cerebellar peduncle, and a caudal trunk, which supplies the area below the flocculus. The PICA arises from the vertebral artery and passes dorsally between the vagus and accessory nerves. The SCA courses above the trigeminal nerve. *C*, venous relationships. The veins that join near the junction of the facial and vestibulocochlear nerves with the brainstem are the lateral medullary veins and the veins of the cerebellomedullary fissure, pontomedullary sulcus, and middle cerebellar peduncle. The vein of the cerebellopontine fissure passes above the flocculus along the superior limb of the cerebellopontine fissure and joins the vein of the middle cerebellar peduncle and a transverse pontine vein to form a superior petrosal vein, which empties into the superior petrosal sinus. A bridging vein passes behind the vagus nerve. The lateral anterior pontomesencephalic vein ascends on the pons. *D*, neurovascular relationships of an acoustic neuroma. The tumor arises from the vestibulocochlear nerve and displaces the facial nerve anteriorly, the trigeminal nerve superiorly, and the glossopharyngeal and vagus nerves inferiorly. The vestibulocochlear nerve disappears into the tumor. The facial nerve enters the brainstem at the lateral margin of the pontomedullary sulcus anterior to the flocculus and rostral to the choroid plexus protruding from the foramen of Luschka. The rostral trunk of the AICA courses below the tumor and above the flocculus to reach the surface of the middle cerebellar peduncle. The veins displaced around the medial side of the tumor are the lateral medullary veins and the veins of the middle cerebellar peduncle, cerebellomedullary fissure, and pontomedullary sulcus. The vein of the cerebellopontine fissure passes above the tumor. A recurrent perforating branch of the AICA passes across the tumor and supplies the brainstem. (From, Rhoton AL Jr: Microsurgical anatomy of the brainstem surface facing an acoustic neuroma. Surg Neurol 25:326–339, 1986 [33].) *A.*, artery; *A.I.C.A.*, anteroinferior cerebellar artery; *Ant.*, anterior; *Bas.*, basilar; *Br.*, bridging; *Ca.*, caudal; *Cer.*, cerebellar; *Cer. Pon.*, cerebellopontine; *Chor.*, choroid; *F.*, foramen; *Fiss.*, fissure; *Lat.*, lateral; *Med.*, medial, medulla; *Mid.*, middle; *Ped.*, peduncle; *Perf.*, perforating; *P.I.C.A.*, posteroinferior cerebellar artery; *Pon.*, pontine; *Pon. Med.*, pontomedullary; *Rec.*, recurrent; *Ro.*, rostral; *S.C.A.*, superior cerebellar artery; *Sulc.*, sulcus; *Sup.*, superior; *Tr.*, trunk; *V.*, vein; *Vert.*, vertebral.

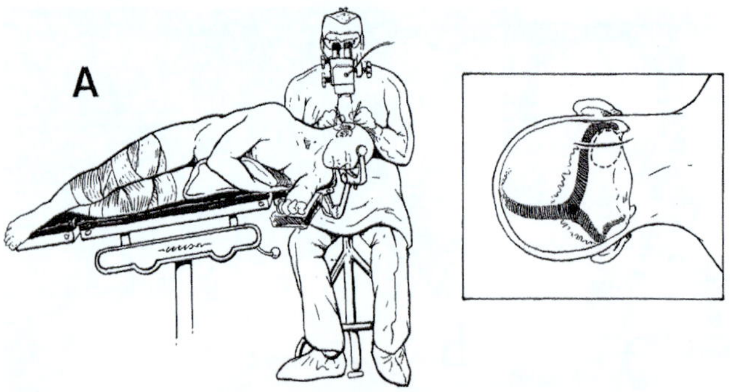

FIGURE 4.25. *A*. Retrosigmoid approach for removal of small or medium-size acoustic neuromas. *A*, the patient is positioned in the three-quarter prone position with the surgeon behind the head. The insert (*right*) shows the site of the scalp incision (*continuous line*) and the bony opening (*interrupted line*).

The landmarks that are helpful in identifying the facial and vestibulocochlear nerves at the brainstem on the medial side of the tumor have been reviewed (*Figs. 4.20-4.24*) (33). These nerves, although distorted by the tumor, usually can be identified on the brainstem side of the tumor at the lateral end of the pontomedullary sulcus, just rostral to the glossopharyngeal nerve and just anterosuperior to the foramen of Luschka, the flocculus, and the choroid plexus protruding from the foramen of Luschka. After the facial and vestibulocochlear nerves are identified on the medial and lateral sides of the tumor, the final remnants of the tumor are separated from the intervening segment of the nerves using fine dissecting instruments (*Fig. 4.25*). It is especially important to preserve the segment of the cerebellar arteries adherent to the tumor capsule because a major cause of operative mortality and morbidity is the loss of perforating arteries and branches of the cerebellar arteries that may be adherent to and displaced by the tumor. Any vessel that stands above or is stretched around the tumor capsule should be dealt with initially as if it were an artery that runs over the tumor surface to supply the brain. After the tumor has been removed from within the capsule, an attempt should be made to displace the vessel off the tumor capsule. When dissected free of the capsule, vessels that initially appeared to be adherent to the capsule often prove to be neural vessels. The number of veins sacrificed should be kept to a minimum because of the undesirable consequences of their loss. Obliteration of the petrosal veins, which pass from the surface of the cerebellum and the brainstem to the superior petrosal sinus, is inescapable when reaching and removing some cerebellopontine angle tumors. Occlusion of these veins, which drain much of the cerebellum and the brainstem, infrequently may cause hemorrhagic edema of the cerebellum and the brainstem. Some of these veins may need to be sacrificed if the tumor extends into the area above the internal acoustic meatus. Small acoustic neuromas and other tumors in the lower part of the cerebellopontine angle, however, frequently may be removed without sacrificing a petrosal vein. In removing the posterior meatal lip, a communication may be established between the subarachnoid space and the mastoid air cells that will require careful closure to prevent a cerebrospinal fluid leak. Laying a small pledget of crushed fat over the drilled meatal area has been successful in minimizing this complication (*Fig. 4.25*). The retrosigmoid approach is used by this author for most acoustic neuromas, because it is suitable for the removal of both small and large tumors. Unlike the translabyrinthine approach, described in the section on the temporal bone, which is directed through the vestibule and semicircular canals, the retrosigmoid approach is not necessarily associated with hearing loss. The retrosigmoid approach provides a broader exposure of the small tumor than does the middle fossa approach. Also, once the nerves are identified lateral to the tumor, there are advantages to being able to separate the tumor capsule off the nerves beginning medially, because this more often results in preservation of hearing than dissection starting laterally. Compared with the middle fossa approach, it has the advantage that the facial nerve is usually deep to the tumor and often is protected by a thin veil of vestibulocochlear nerve, thus increasing the opportunity for facial nerve preservation. In the middle fossa approach, the facial nerve is often in the upper part of the exposure, stretched over the upper half of the tumor, and much of the dissection is directly on the surface of the nerve, which increases the risk of facial dysfunction after surgery.

Anatomy of vascular compression in the middle neurovascular complex

Compression of the facial and vestibulocochlear nerves by tortuous arteries is postulated to cause dysfunction of these nerves, and cases in which surgical liberation of the vessels from these nerves has relieved the symptoms provide support for a vascular compressive etiology (*Figs. 4.1* and *4.20*) (11, 20, 38). Ectasia and elongation of the arteries are important in forcing the arteries into the nerves. Gardner was the first to treat hemifacial spasm by removing a compressive arterial loop from the facial nerve (11). Jannetta et al., using the suboccipital approach to the cerebellopontine angle, found mechanical compression and distortion of the root exit zone of the facial nerve in all of 47 patients with hemifacial spasm (20). The distorting vessel not only was the AICA and its branches, but in some cases was found to be the PICA, the vertebral or basilar artery, veins, or an arteriovenous malformation (*Fig. 4.26*) (20). It is expected that the AICA would be the compressing vessel in most cases because the facial nerve is located in the middle neurovascular complex. However, a tortuous PICA is an equally frequent offending vessel in hemifacial spasm, followed in order by the vertebral artery, basilar artery, veins, and a combination of these vessels (*Figs. 4.26* and *4.27*). The proximal part of the PICA usually passes around the brainstem below the facial and vestibulocochlear nerves. In some cerebellopontine angles, however, the proximal part of the PICA, after coursing posteriorly to the level of the hypoglossal rootlets, will loop superiorly toward the facial and vestibulocochlear nerves before descending to pass between the glossopharyngeal, vagus, and spinal accessory nerves.

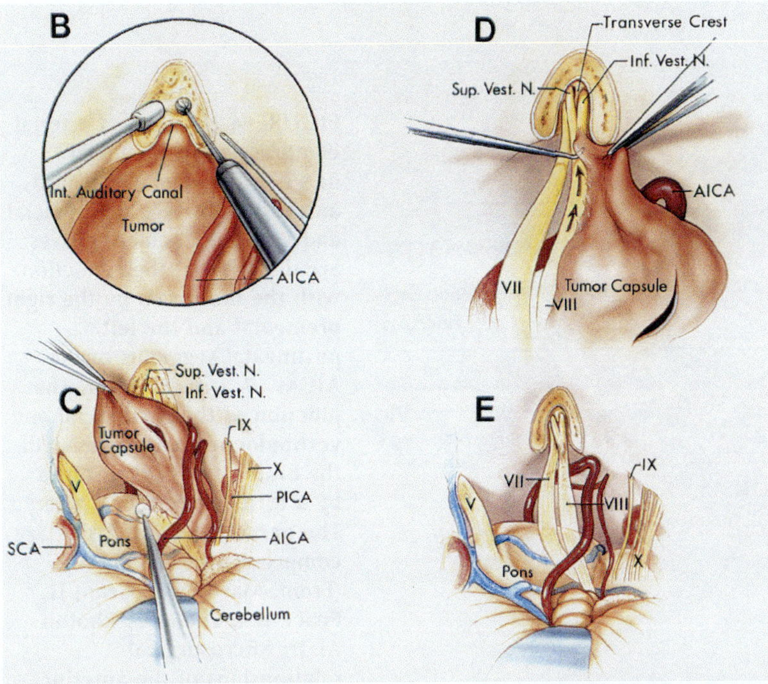

FIGURE 4.25. ***B–E.* Retrosigmoid approach for the removal of small or medium-size acoustic neuromas. *B*, the posterior wall of the internal auditory canal is removed using an irrigating drill. The AICA courses around the lower margin of the tumor. *C*, the intracapsular contents of the tumor have been removed. The capsule of the tumor is being separated from the pons and the posterior surface of the part of the facial and vestibulocochlear nerves adjacent to the brainstem. The superior and inferior vestibular nerves are seen at the lateral end of the internal auditory canal. The trigeminal nerve and SCA are above the tumor and the glossopharyngeal and vagus nerves and the PICA are below the tumor. *D*, the dissection along the eighth nerve is done in a medial to lateral direction (*arrows*) to avoid tearing the tiny filaments of the cochlear nerve in the lateral end of the canal where they pass through the lamina cribrosa. The transverse crest separates the superior and inferior vestibular nerves in the lateral end of the canal. *E*, cerebellopontine angle and internal auditory canal after tumor removal. The facial and vestibulocochlear nerves have been preserved. *A.I.C.A.*, anteroinferior cerebellar artery; *Inf.*, inferior; *Int.*, internal; *N.*, nerve; *P.I.C.A.*, posteroinferior cerebellar artery; *S.C.A.*, superior cerebellar artery; *Sup.*, superior; *Vest.*, vestibular. (From, Rhoton AL Jr: Microsurgical anatomy of acoustic neuromas, in Sekhar LN, Janecka IP (eds): *Surgery of Cranial Base Tumors*. New York, Raven Press, 1993, pp 687–713 [37].)**

The offending arterial loop may be located on either the superior or the inferior aspect of the facial nerve at its exit from the brainstem. In the most common type of hemifacial spasm, that beginning in the orbicularis oculi muscle and gradually spreading downward to involve the lower face, the anteroinferior aspect of the nerve root exit zone will commonly be compressed. Atypical hemifacial spasm, a much less common entity, beginning in the lower or midface and spreading upward to involve the frontalis muscle, will be caused by the compression of the posterosuperior aspect of the facial nerve at the brainstem. Jannetta and others thought that the arteries frequently seen coursing around or between the facial and vestibulocochlear nerves in the interval between the brainstem and porus acusticus, as found by Gardner (11), were not the cause of hemifacial spasm, but that cross-compression of the facial nerve by the same arteries coursing at right angles to the nerve at the root exit zone was the essential element (20). The craniotomy for hemifacial spasm is positioned behind the lower half of the sigmoid sinus.

The operation for hemifacial spasm is directed along the inferolateral margin of the cerebellum (*Figs. 4.28* and *4.29*). The craniotomy is located medial to the lower half of the sigmoid sinus (*Figs. 4.9, 4.28,* and *4.29*). It is not necessary to extend the bone opening downward to the foramen magnum or upward to the transverse sinus. The inferolateral margin of the cerebellum is elevated with a small brain spatula and the arachnoid behind the glossopharyngeal and vagus nerves is opened. This will expose the tuft of choroid plexus protruding from the foramen of Luschka, which sits on the posterior surface of the glossopharyngeal and vagus nerves. Commonly, the flocculus is seen protruding behind the nerves and blocks their visualization at the junction with the brainstem. It also may be difficult to see the facial nerve that is hidden in front of the vestibulocochlear nerve. At this time, it is important to recall that the facial nerve root exits the brainstem 2 to 3 mm rostral to the point at which the glossopharyngeal nerve enters the brainstem. To expose the nerve's exit zone, it may be necessary to gently separate the choroid plexus from the posterior margin of the glossopharyngeal nerve so that its junction with the brainstem can be seen. The brain spatula is advanced upwards to elevate the choroid plexus away from the posterior margin of the glossopharyngeal nerve. The exposure is then directed several millimeters above the glossopharyngeal nerve to where the facial nerve will be seen joining the brainstem below and in front of the vestibulocochlear nerve. The spatula often needs to be positioned so that it elevates the lower margin of the flocculus. Care must be taken to avoid damage to the vestibulocochlear nerve, which may be adherent to the flocculus. In the experience of this author, the most common offending artery is a PICA that loops upward before passing between the glossopharyngeal, vagus, and spinal accessory nerves. After looping into the facial nerve exit zone, the PICA then passes distally between the rootlets of the lower cranial nerves. The compressing artery may also be the premeatal or postmeatal segments of the AICA or a tortuous vertebral or basilar artery. Care is taken to explore the interval between the facial and vestibulocochlear

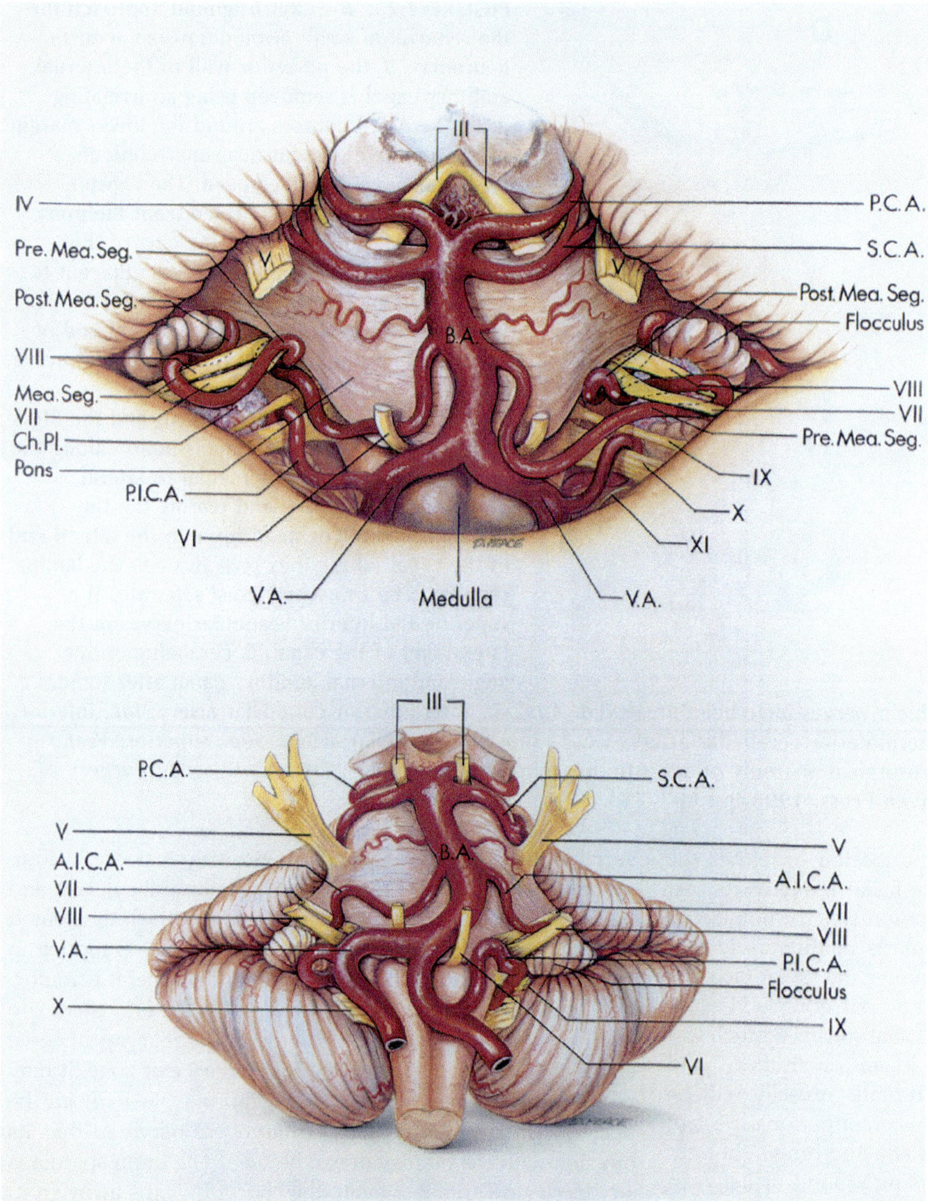

FIGURE 4.26. Sites of arterial compression of the facial nerve in hemifacial spasm. *A*, anterosuperior view. The facial and vestibulocochlear nerves are distorted at their junction with the brainstem by the right premeatal and the left postmeatal segments of the AICAs. *B*, anterior view. The junction of the right facial and vestibulocochlear nerves with the brainstem is compressed by a tortuous vertebral artery. The nerves on the left side are compressed by the PICA. (From, Martin RG, Grant JL, Peace DA, Theiss C, Rhoton AL Jr: Microsurgical relationships of the anterior inferior cerebellar artery and the facial-vestibulocochlear nerve complex. Neurosurgery 6:483–507, 1980 [25].) *A.I.C.A.*, anteroinferior cerebellar artery; *Ch. Pl.*, choroid plexus; *Mea.*, meatal; *P.C.A.*, posterior cerebral artery; *P.I.C.A.*, posteroinferior cerebellar artery; *Post.*, posterior; *S.C.A.*, superior cerebellar artery; *Seg.*, segment; *V.A.*, vertebral artery.

nerves because it would be easy to miss a vessel compressing the facial nerve in this location.

Venous compression is less commonly encountered. The most common venous compression is by the vein of the pontomedullary sulcus, the retro-olivary vein, or the vein of the middle cerebral peduncle (26). The vein of the pontomedullary sulcus and the retro-olivary vein commonly join in the region of the facial nerve to form the vein of the middle cerebellar peduncle, which ascends on the middle cerebral peduncle toward the superior petrosal sinus. The vein of the middle cerebral peduncle commonly passes between the facial and vestibulocochlear nerves. It is not uncommon to encounter a bridging vein that passes from the lateral side of the medulla to the jugular bulb. At the time of elevating the cerebellum, it is best to obliterate this vein with gentle bipolar coagulation.

Cochlear and vestibular nerve compression syndromes

Vascular compression has been reported as a cause of cochlear and vestibular nerve dysfunction manifested by tinnitus, hearing loss, dysequilibrium, and disabling positional vertigo (21, 28, 29). The site of the compressive lesion with vestibulocochlear nerve dysfunction has been reported to be more peripheral along the nerve rather than at the junction with the brainstem, as commonly seen in trigeminal neuralgia and hemifacial spasm. Jannetta and others have restricted the use of the operation for vestibulocochlear nerve symptoms to those patients who are disabled and have documented unilateral disease on neuro-otologic testing. Jannetta et al. (21) and Gardner (11) have postulated that vascular compression of a cranial nerve is more likely to be symptomatic when it is located on the nerve proximal to the Obersteiner-Redlich zone

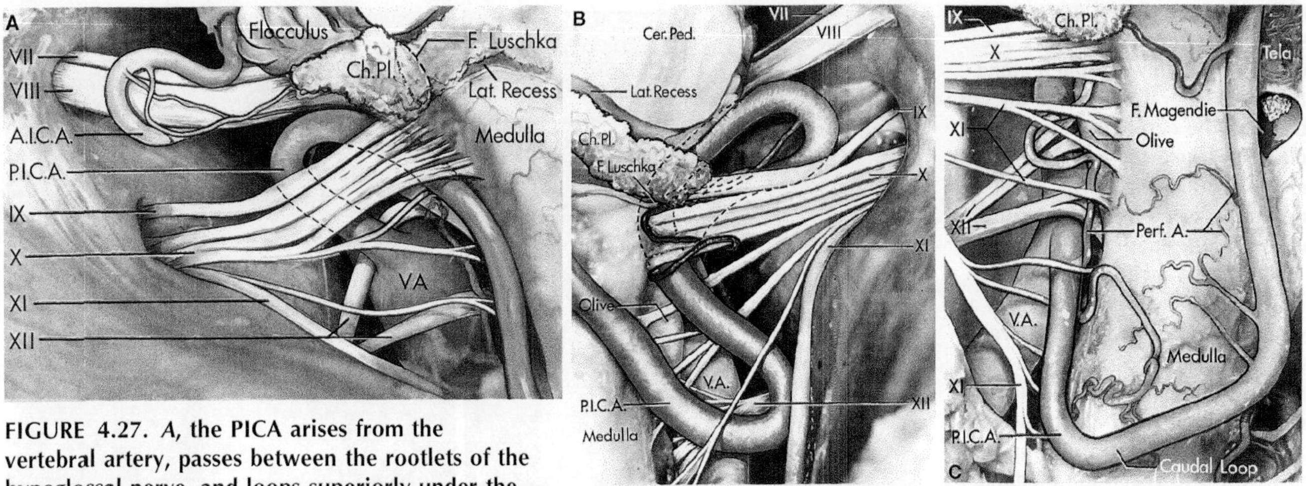

FIGURE 4.27. ***A,*** **the PICA arises from the vertebral artery, passes between the rootlets of the hypoglossal nerve, and loops superiorly under the glossopharyngeal and vagus nerves before passing posteroinferiorly between the rootlets of the vagus and spinal accessory nerves. The vertebral artery stretches the rootlets of the hypoglossal nerve posteriorly. The AICA loops posterior to the facial and vestibulocochlear nerves.** ***B,*** **a tortuous PICA arises from the vertebral artery and passes rostrally toward the vestibulocochlear and facial nerves. At the level of the vestibulocochlear nerve, it loops inferiorly and descends anterior to the glossopharyngeal and vagus nerves, and passes between the vagus and spinal accessory nerves. The PICA compresses the medulla anterior to the origin of the glossopharyngeal and vagus nerves. The choroid plexus protrudes from the foramen of Luschka posterior to the glossopharyngeal nerve. The cerebellar peduncles are above the lateral recess of the fourth ventricle.** ***C,*** **the vertebral artery displaces and stretches the hypoglossal rootlets so far posteriorly that they intermingle with the rootlets of the spinal accessory nerve. The PICA descends between the rootlets of the spinal accessory nerve. (From, Lister JR, Rhoton AL Jr, Matsushima T, Peace DA: Microsurgical anatomy of the posterior inferior cerebellar artery. Neurosurgery 10: 170–199, 1982 [24].)** ***A.,*** **artery;** ***A.I.C.A.,*** **anteroinferior cerebellar artery;** ***Cer.,*** **cerebellar;** ***Ch. Pl.,*** **choroid plexus;** ***F.,*** **foramen;** ***Lat.,*** **lateral;** ***Ped.,*** **peduncle;** ***Perf.,*** **perforating;** ***P.I.C.A.,*** **posteroinferior cerebellar artery;** ***V.A.,*** **vertebral artery.**

where the axons are insulated by central myelin produced by oligodendroglia. It is proximal to this glial-neurilemmal junction that the compression causes transaxonal excitement between the afferent and efferent fibers. This glial-neurilemmal junction on the facial and trigeminal nerves is situated at the nerve root junction with the brainstem, but the entire intracranial portion of the vestibulocochlear nerve is sensitive to compression because the glial-neurilemmal junction is located at or in the internal acoustic meatus (21).

Compression by veins is less common around the facial and vestibulocochlear nerves than in the region of the trigeminal nerve because the veins around the facial and vestibulocochlear nerves tend to be smaller. Because no large bridging veins cross the subarachnoid space around the facial and vestibulocochlear nerves, as are seen frequently around the trigeminal nerve, any vascular cross-compression of facial and vestibulocochlear nerves peripheral to the brainstem is likely to be caused by arteries that loop through the cerebellopontine angle and even into the meatus. The veins at the level of the junction of the facial and vestibulocochlear nerves with the brainstem tightly hug the pontomedullary junction where they are adhere to the pial membrane, as described earlier in the section on the middle neurovascular complex.

Geniculate neuralgia

Sectioning the nervus intermedius for geniculate neuralgia requires an understanding of the complex anatomy of this small nerve that is hidden between the vestibulocochlear and facial nerves (*Figs. 4.1* and *4.30*) (40). The nervus intermedius usually is described as a component of the facial nerve. Relatively little note has been taken of the fact that it may be closely bound to the vestibulocochlear nerve for a variable distance before it enters the brainstem, and that in the cerebellopontine angle, it may consist of as many as four rootlets. The nervus intermedius is found divisible into three parts: a medial segment that adheres closely to the vestibulocochlear nerve, an intermediate segment that lies freely between the acoustic nerve and the motor root of the facial nerve, and a distal segment that joins the motor root to form the facial nerve (40). Twenty-two percent of the nerves were adherent to the acoustic nerve for 14 mm or more (the entire course of the nerve in the posterior cranial fossa) and could be found as a separate structure only after opening the internal acoustic meatus. In most instances, the nerve was a single trunk, but in some cases, it was composed of as many as four rootlets. A single large root most frequently arises at the brainstem anterior to the superior vestibular nerve and, in the meatus, lies anterior to the superior vestibular nerve. When multiple rootlets are present, they may arise along the whole anterior surface of the vestibulocochlear nerve; however, they usually converge immediately proximal to the junction with the facial motor root to form a single bundle that lies anterior to the superior vestibular nerve.

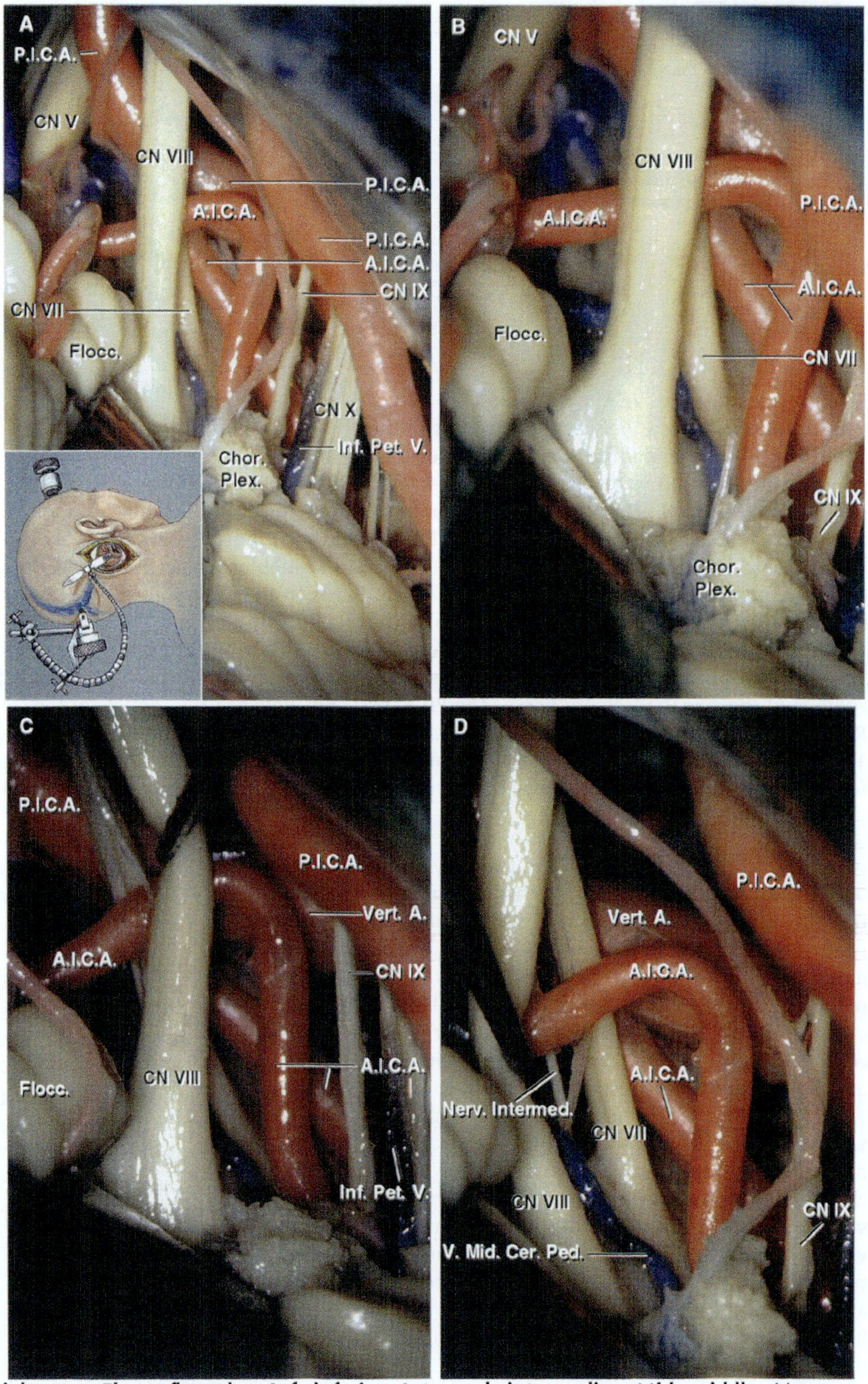

FIGURE 4.28. Facial nerve exposure in hemifacial spasm. *A*, the insert shows the approach along the inferolateral margin of the cerebellum. The cerebellum has been elevated to expose the right cerebellopontine angle. The facial nerve exit zone from the brainstem is seen along the lower margin of the vestibulocochlear nerve. The AICA passes between the facial and vestibulocochlear nerve. A large tortuous PICA loops upward anterior to the facial and vestibulocochlear nerves and behind the trigeminal nerve, before turning downward to reach the medulla. The flocculus and the choroid plexus protruding from the foramen Luschka often hide the junction of the facial and vestibulocochlear nerves with brainstem. In this case, the flocculus has been gently elevated to expose the junction of these nerves with the brainstem. *B*, enlarged view. Exposing the facial nerve exit zone from the brainstem is facilitated by directing the exposure along the inferolateral margin of the cerebellum in the area above the glossopharyngeal nerve and below the lower edge of the flocculus. *C*, the vestibulocochlear nerve has been depressed. This exposes the distal segment of the facial nerve, but does not provide access to the junction of the facial nerve with the brainstem, which should be visualized in dealing with hemifacial spasm. *D*, the vestibulocochlear nerve has been gently elevated. This exposes both the rostral and caudal margins of the facial nerve at the brainstem. A rootlet of the nervus intermedius is also exposed. The vein of the middle cerebellar peduncle passes between the facial and vestibulocochlear nerve. *A.*, artery; *A.I.C.A.*, anteroinferior cerebellar artery; *Cer.*, cerebellar; *Chor. Plex.*, choroid plexus; *CN*, cranial nerve; *Flocc.*, flocculus; *Inf.*, inferior; *Intermed.*, intermedius; *Mid.*, middle; *Nerv.*, nervus; *Ped.*, peduncle; *Pet.*, petrosal; *P.I.C.A.*, posteroinferior cerebellar artery; *V.*, vein; *Vert.*, vertebral.

It is the free segment between the facial and vestibulocochlear nerve that is divided in geniculate neuralgia. This segment, where the nervus intermedius is free of both the facial and vestibulocochlear nerves, may be located in the cerebellopontine angle or in the meatus if the nervus intermedius is composed of a single rootlet. If the nervus intermedius is composed of more than one rootlet, however, there may be free segments both in the cerebellopontine angle and in the meatus. Geniculate neuralgia with or without vestibulocochlear dysfunction also has been postulated to be caused by

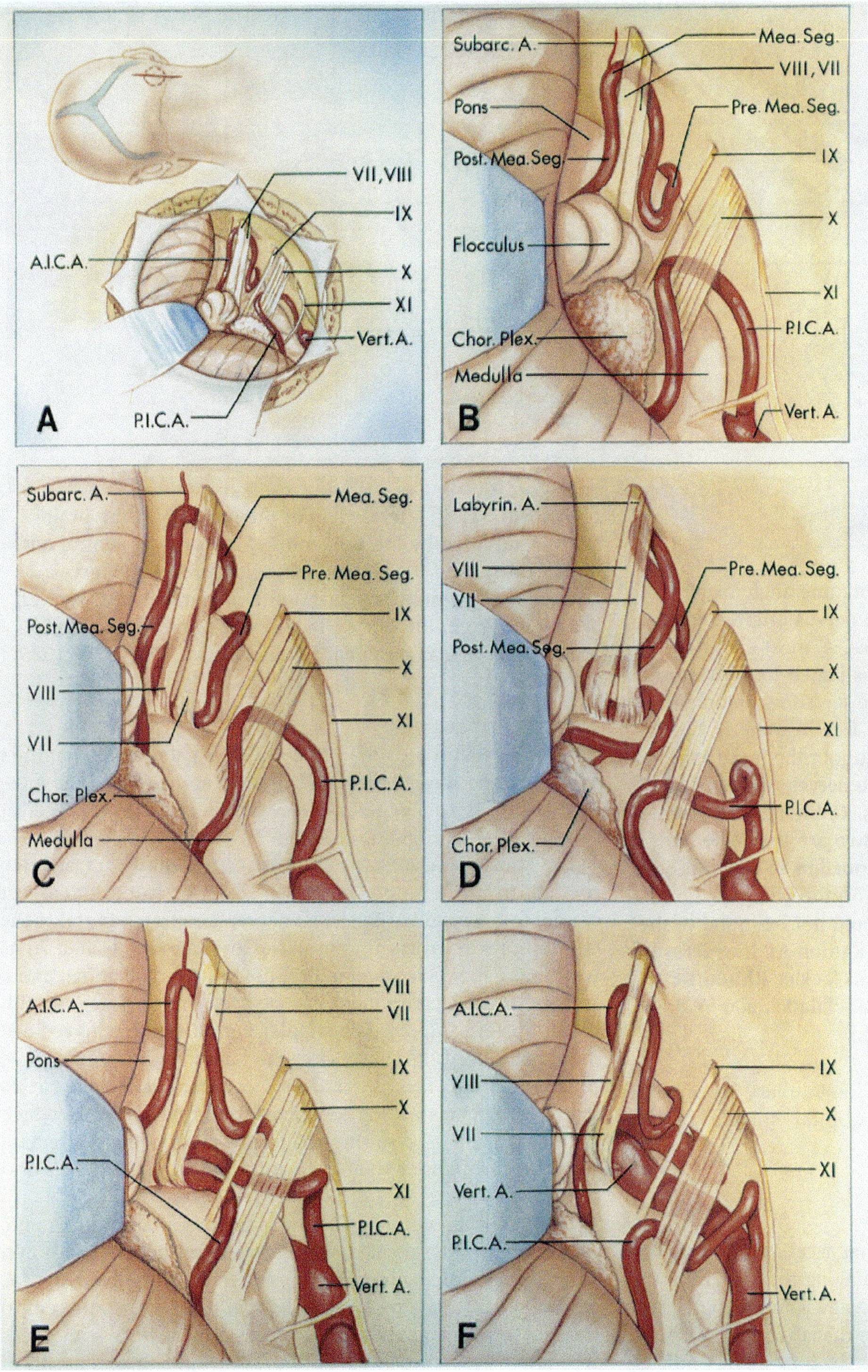

FIGURE 4.29. *A–F*, arterial compression of the facial nerve in hemifacial spasm as viewed through a retrosigmoid craniotomy performed with the patient in the three-quarter prone position. *A*, the *upper* drawing shows the site of the incision (*straight line*) and the location of the craniotomy (*broken line*). The *lower* drawing shows the surgical exposure obtained with this approach. The AICA and the facial and vestibulocochlear nerves are in the midportion of the exposure. The vertebral artery, PICA, and the glossopharyngeal, vagus, and spinal accessory nerves are below. *B*, the cerebellum is elevated to expose the facial and vestibulocochlear nerves and the premeatal, meatal, and postmeatal segments of the AICA. The flocculus and the choroid plexus block the view of the junction of the facial and vestibulocochlear nerves with the brainstem. *C*, the flocculus and the choroid plexus have been elevated to expose the root entry/exit zone of the facial and vestibulocochlear nerves. The premeatal segment compresses the nerves at the junction with the pons and the medulla. *D*, the nerve root entry/exit zone is compressed by the postmeatal segment. *E*, a tortuous PICA loops upward to compress the nerves at their junction with the brainstem before turning inferiorly to pass between the glossopharyngeal and vagus nerves. *F*, a tortuous vertebral artery compresses the nerve root entry/exit zone. *A.*, artery; *A.I.C.A.*, anteroinferior cerebellar artery; *Chor. Plex.*, choroid plexus; *Labyrin.*, labyrinthine; *Mea.*, meatal; *P.I.C.A.*, posteroinferior cerebellar artery; *Post.*, posterior; *Seg.*, segment; *Subarc.*, subarcuate; *Vert.*, vertebral.

vascular compression of the nervus intermedius or vestibulocochlear nerve (21, 29).

LOWER NEUROVASCULAR COMPLEX

The lower complex, which is related to the PICA, includes the medulla, inferior cerebellar peduncle, cerebellomedullary fissure, suboccipital surface of the cerebellum, and the glossopharyngeal, vagus, spinal accessory, and hypoglossal nerves (*Figs. 4.1, 4.17,* and *4.27*). The PICA arises at the medullary level, encircles the medulla, passing in relationship to the glossopharyngeal, vagus, spinal accessory, and hypoglossal nerves to reach the surface of the inferior cerebellar pe-

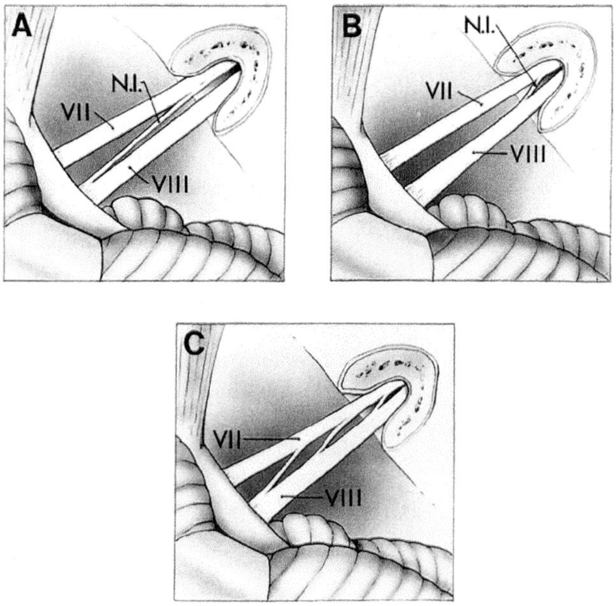

FIGURE 4.30. View of the cerebellopontine angle from above to show the relationship of the nervus intermedius to the facial and vestibulocochlear nerves. *A*, most common relationship. The nervus intermedius is joined to the ventral surface of the vestibulocochlear nerve for a few millimeters adjacent to the brainstem, then has a free segment in the cerebellopontine angle as it courses to join the facial motor root. *B*, pattern present in 20% of the nerves studied. The free segment is entirely in the meatus. *C*, the nervus intermedius consists of three free segments: two are the angle and one is in the meatus. The nervus intermedius in *A* could be exposed in the angle without drilling off the posterior lip of the meatus. In *B*, the free segment could not be found in the angle but only in the meatus. (From, Rhoton AL Jr: Microsurgical anatomy of acoustic neuromas, in Jackler RK (ed): *Otolaryngologic Clinics of North America.* Philadelphia, W.B. Saunders Co., 1992, pp 257–294 [35].)

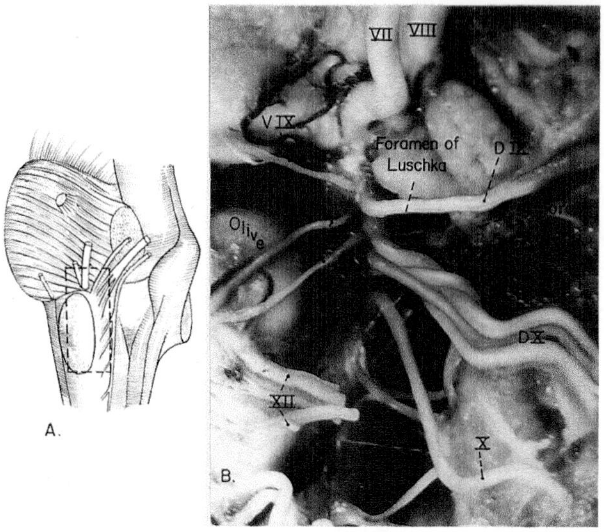

FIGURE 4.31. *A*, lateral view of the left side of the brainstem as outlined by the broken line. *B*, note the ventral and dorsal rootlets of the glossopharyngeal and vagus nerves. One ventral glossopharyngeal and two ventral vagal rootlets are seen. (From, Rhoton AL Jr, Buza R: Microsurgical anatomy of the jugular foramen. J Neurosurg 42:541–550, 1975 [39].)

duncle, where it dips into the cerebellomedullary fissure and terminates by supplying the suboccipital surface of the cerebellum.

Neural relationships

The glossopharyngeal, vagus, spinal accessory, and hypoglossal nerves arise from the medulla along the margin of the inferior olive. The glossopharyngeal, vagus, and spinal accessory nerves arise as a line of rootlets that exit the brainstem along the posterior edge of the olive in the post-olivary sulcus, a shallow groove between the olive and posterolateral surface of the medulla (*Figs. 4.1, 4.17, 4.31,* and *4.32*). The hypoglossal nerve arises as a line of rootlets that exit the brainstem along the anterior margin of the lower two-thirds of the olive in the preolivary sulcus, a groove between the olive and the medullary pyramid. The glossopharyngeal and vagus nerves arise at the level of the superior third of the olive. The spinal accessory rootlets arise along the posterior margin of the inferior two-thirds of the olive and from the lower medulla and the upper segments of the cervical spinal cord. The glossopharyngeal and vagus nerves arise rostral to the level of origin of the hypoglossal rootlets.

The glossopharyngeal nerve arises as one or rarely two rootlets from the upper medulla, posterior to the olive, just caudal to the origin of the facial nerve. It courses ventral to the choroid plexus protruding from the foramen of Luschka on its way to the jugular foramen. Frequently, a larger dorsal and a smaller ventral component can be seen at the junction with the brainstem (22, 39). The smaller ventral rootlets have been demonstrated to be motor and the larger main bundle to be sensory (7, 44). The larger dorsal component usually arises from the medulla as one root, except in a few cases in which it will originate as two rootlets. The two rootlets may remain separate throughout their course to the dura (*Figs. 4.31* and *4.32*).

The vagus nerve arises below the glossopharyngeal nerve as a line of tightly packed rootlets along a line 2 to 5.5 mm in length posterior to the superior third of the olive (*Figs. 4.1, 4.27,* and *4.32*). The most rostral vagal fibers arise adjacent to the glossopharyngeal origin, from which they are sometimes separated by as much as 2 mm. The vagus is composed of multiple combinations of large and small rootlets that pass ventral to the choroid plexus protruding from the foramen of Luschka on its way to the jugular foramen. Occasionally, several small rootlets are found originating ventral to the majority of the vagal rootlets (*Figs. 4.31* and *4.32*). These small ventral rootlets are considered to be motor (7).

The accessory nerve arises as a widely separated series of rootlets that originated from the medulla at the level of the

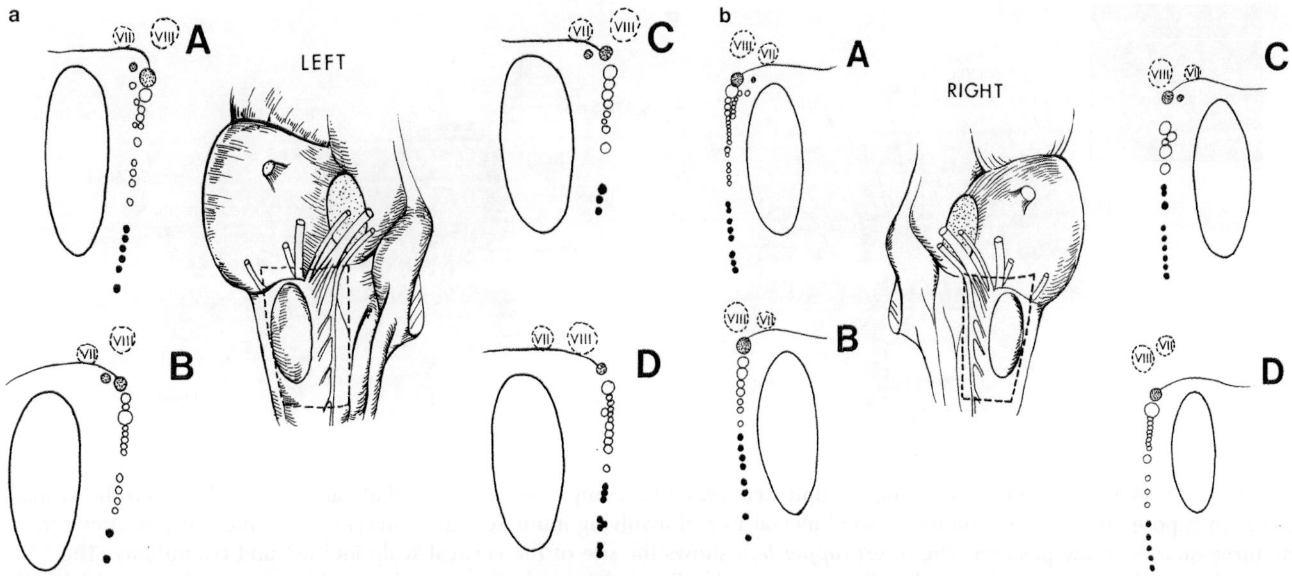

FIGURE 4.32. The *broken line* on the drawing of the lateral surface of the brainstem outlines the area shown in each diagram, demonstrating the brainstem origin and variations of the rootlet size of the glossopharyngeal, vagus, and spinal accessory nerves. The *large ovoid structure* is the inferior olive. The *broken-line circles* outline the origin of the facial and vestibulocochlear nerves. The *most cephalad, shaded circles* indicate glossopharyngeal rootlet origins, *intermediate, open circles* indicate vagal rootlet origins, and *caudal, black circles* outline spinal accessory rootlet origins. The glossopharyngeal nerve usually originates as one large rootlet, the vagus as a series of large and small rootlets, and the spinal accessory as a series of small rootlets. *Top,* note the small ventral rootlets of the glossopharyngeal nerve in *A, B,* and *C* and the small ventral rootlet between the glossopharyngeal and vagus nerves in *A.* The glossopharyngeal rootlet is larger than the rostral rootlet of the vagus nerve in all except *D,* in which the rostral vagal rootlet is larger than the glossopharyngeal nerve. *Bottom,* note the wide separation of the origin of the glossopharyngeal and vagus nerves in *C,* the small ventral rootlet of the glossopharyngeal nerve in *C,* and the small ventral rootlets of the glossopharyngeal and vagus nerves in *A.* The glossopharyngeal nerve is smaller than the upper vagal rootlet in *A* and *D.* (From, Rhoton AL Jr, Buza R: Microsurgical anatomy of the jugular foramen. J Neurosurg 42:541–550, 1975 [39].)

lower two-thirds of the olive and from the upper cervical cord. The cranial rootlets of the accessory nerve arise as a line of rootlets ranging in diameter from 0.1 to 1 mm just caudal to the vagal fibers (*Figs. 4.1, 4.17, 4.27,* and *4.32*). The cranial rootlets of the accessory nerve are more properly regarded as inferior vagal rootlets, since they arise from vagal nuclei (22, 39). It may be difficult to separate the lower vagal fibers from the upper accessory rootlets because the vagal and cranial accessory fibers usually enter the vagal meatus as a single bundle.

The upper rootlets of the spinal portion of the accessory nerve originate several millimeters caudal to the lowest cranial accessory fibers and either course to join the cranial accessory bundle or enter the lower border of the vagal meatus separate from the cranial accessory rootlets. The spinal accessory fibers pass superolateral from their origin to reach the jugular foramen. Although the cranial and spinal portion of the accessory nerve most frequently enter the vagal meatus together, they may infrequently be separated by a dural septum.

The rootlets forming the hypoglossal nerve arise from the medulla along a line that is continuous inferiorly with the line along which the ventral spinal roots arise (*Figs. 4.1, 4.17,* and *4.27*). These rootlets arise in a nucleus whose rostral part sits deep to the hypoglossal triangle in the floor of the fourth ventricle, and exit the medulla along the anterior margin of the caudal two-thirds of the olive. The hypoglossal rootlets course anterolateral through the subarachnoid space and pass behind the vertebral artery to reach the hypoglossal canal. If the vertebral artery is short and straight, it may not contact or distort the hypoglossal rootlets, but if the artery is tortuous it may stretch the hypoglossal rootlets posteriorly over its dorsal surface (38). Infrequently, the vertebral artery passes between the rootlets of the hypoglossal nerve (24). Before entering the hypoglossal canal, the rootlets collect into two bundles, and in some cases, the canal is divided by a bony septum that separates the two bundles. After passing through the canal, the bundles unite and the nerve lies medial to the internal jugular vein, and the glossopharyngeal, vagus, and accessory nerves.

Anatomy of glossopharyngeal neuralgia

Dandy (4) described endocranial sectioning of the glossopharyngeal nerve for neuralgia, but because this alone did not adequately control the neuralgia, he later advocated the additional sectioning of "perhaps 1/8 to 1/6 of the vagus" (*Figs. 4.1, 4.17, 4.27,* and *4.32*). Tarlov (44, 45) sectioned the cephalic

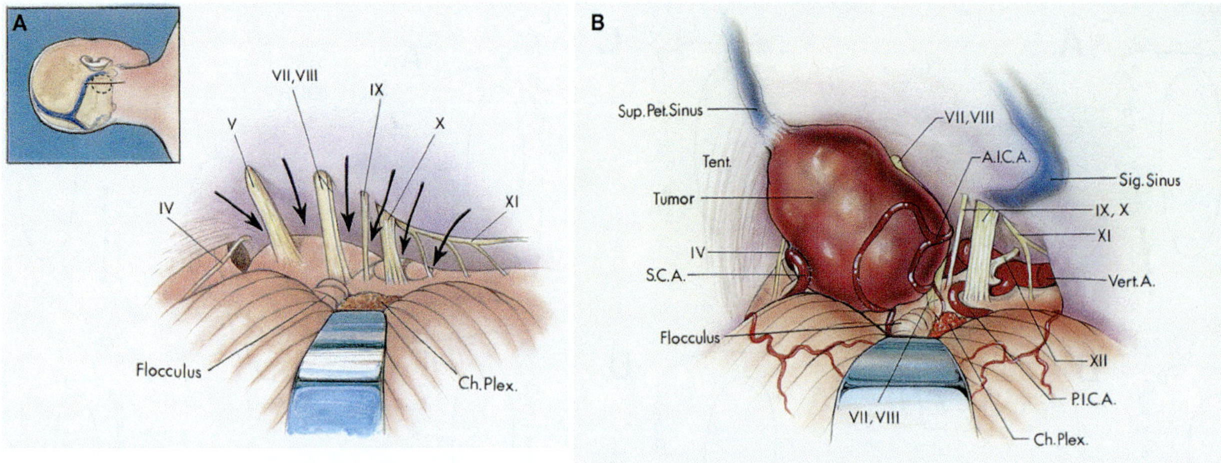

FIGURE 4.33. ***A* and *B*. Tumors involving multiple neurovascular complexes. *A*, routes that can be taken between the cranial nerves to expose and remove a tumor situated medial to and involving multiple cranial nerves. The patient is positioned in the three-quarter prone position. The *insert* (*upper left*) shows the site of the vertical scalp incision and craniotomy. The approach to pathology located medial to the nerves can be directed (*arrows*) between the trochlear nerve above and trigeminal nerve below; between the trigeminal nerve above and the facial and vestibulocochlear nerves below; between the facial and vestibulocochlear nerves above and the glossopharyngeal nerve below; between the glossopharyngeal and vagus nerves; between the vagus nerve and accessory rootlets; and between the widely separated rootlets of the accessory nerve. A tumor located medial to the nerves will often widen the intervals between the nerves, depending on the site of origin of the tumor. Choroid plexus protrudes from the foramen of Luschka. *B*, meningioma attached lateral to the trigeminal nerve in the region of the superior petrosal sinus. The trochlear nerve is elevated, the trigeminal nerve is pushed medially, and the facial and vestibulocochlear nerves are stretched below the tumor. *A.*, artery; *A.I.C.A.*, anteroinferior cerebellar artery; *Bas.*, basilar; *Ch. Plex.*, choroid plexus; *Pet.*, petrosal; *P.I.C.A.*, posteroinferior cerebellar artery; *S.C.A.*, superior cerebellar artery; *Sig.*, sigmoid; *Sup.*, superior; *Tent.*, tentorium; *Vert.*, vertebral.**

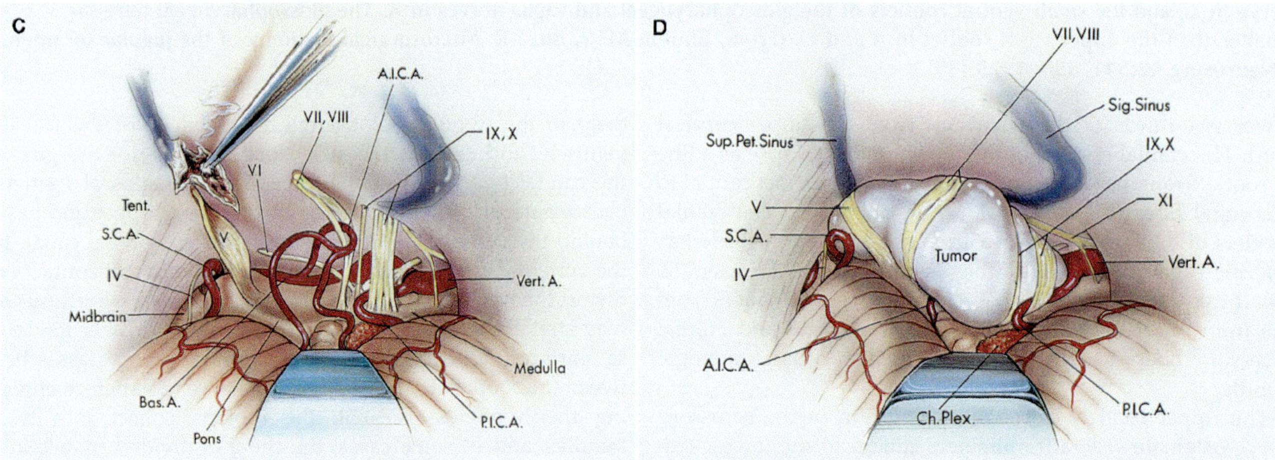

FIGURE 4.33. ***C* and *D*. Tumors involving multiple neurovascular complexes. *C*, the tumor has been removed. The thin distorted nerves have been preserved, and the remaining dural attachment is removed or cauterized with bipolar coagulation. The basilar artery and abducens nerve are exposed. *D*, a large meningioma arising from the clivus in the region of the inferior petrosal sinus with involvement of the fourth through the eleventh nerves. The nerves are displaced laterally around the tumor. The tumor is removed by working through the intervals between the nerves.**

third of the vagal-spinal accessory group and produced analgesia of the epiglottis but only hypalgesia over the mucosa of the lower pharynx and larynx. In his second case, he sectioned the cephalic half of the vagal-spinal accessory complex; this caused both analgesia and transient paralysis of the ipsilateral soft palate, pharynx, and larynx. In our study, the structure of the vagus nerve was variable, being composed of all large or all small rootlets or any combination of the two. It is suggested that fewer of the rostral rootlets be cut if the diameters of the upper rootlets are large rather than small; the

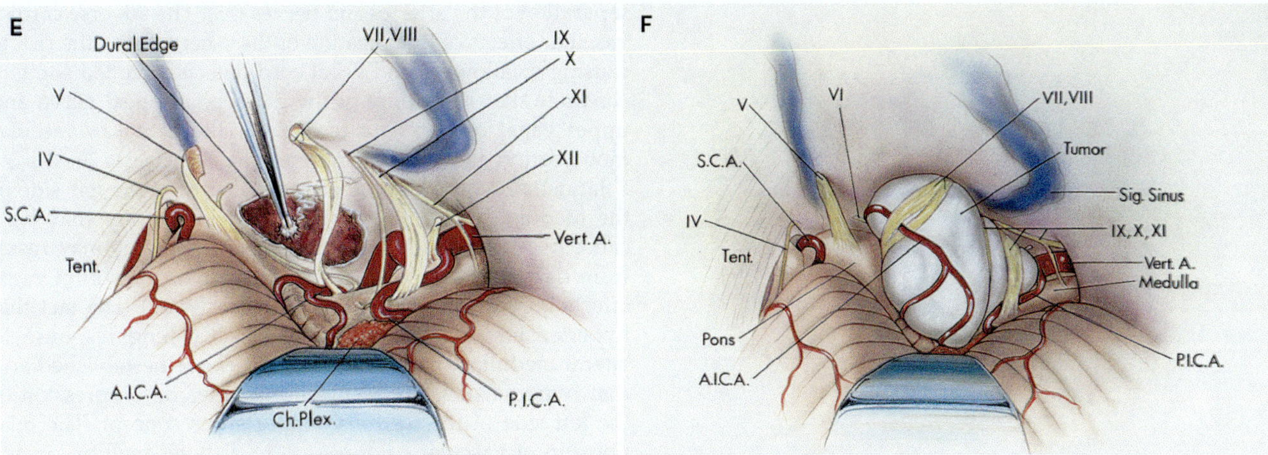

FIGURE 4.33. ***E* and *F*. Tumors involving multiple neurovascular complexes. *E*, the meningioma has been removed. The dural attachment has been partially removed and the base is being cauterized. *F*, meningioma arising medial to the jugular bulb in the region of the jugular tubercle and involving the lower cranial nerves.**

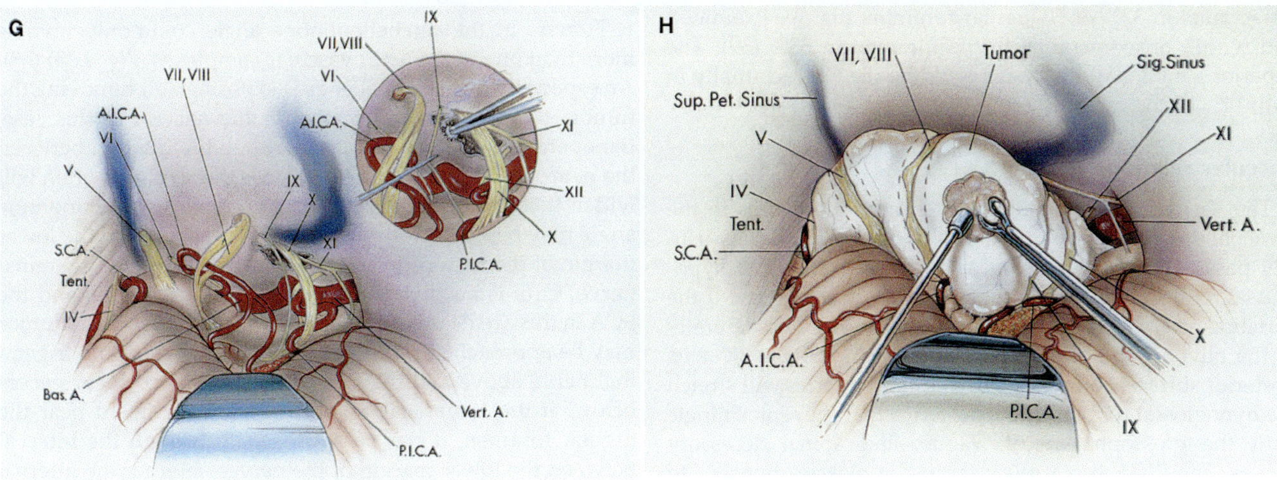

FIGURE 4.33. ***G* and *H*. Tumors involving multiple neurovascular complexes. *G*, the tumor was removed by operating through the intervals between the facial and vestibulocochlear nerves above and the glossopharyngeal nerve below and between the glossopharyngeal and vagus nerves (*round insert*). *H*, a large epidermoid tumor being removed by working through the intervals between the nerves.**

diameter of the largest rootlet is 1.5 mm and the smallest is 0.1 mm (39).

A large glossopharyngeal nerve diameter might be associated with a small diameter of the upper rootlets of the vagus nerve, or a large vagus nerve might be associated with a small glossopharyngeal nerve, because the two nerves arise from the same nuclei and have a similar function (7). This idea that more fibers might be distributed to one nerve, leaving the other smaller, was not confirmed in our studies (39). When the diameter of the dorsal root of the glossopharyngeal nerve is compared with the mean of the upper rootlets of the vagus nerve, no significant correlation is found (39). A smaller diameter of the glossopharyngeal nerve is not commonly associated with a large mean diameter of the upper rootlets of the vagus, nor is a large glossopharyngeal nerve diameter associated with a small diameter of the vagal rootlets.

The only location where the glossopharyngeal nerve can consistently be distinguished from the vagus is just proximal to the dural meati where a dural septum separates the glossopharyngeal and vagus nerves (39). This septum varies in width from 0.5 to 4.9 mm and serves to differentiate the glossopharyngeal nerve from the vagus nerve. The close medullary origin of the glossopharyngeal and vagus nerves and the frequent arachnoid adhesions between the two makes separation difficult in their course through the subarachnoid space or adjacent to the brainstem, except in the few cases in which there will be a 1- to 2-mm separation between their origin at the medulla.

The superior glossopharyngeal and vagal ganglia may be visible intracranially (22). In glossopharyngeal neuralgia, Adson (1) noted the need to section the glossopharyngeal nerve proximal to the superior ganglion. The superior ganglion was

I

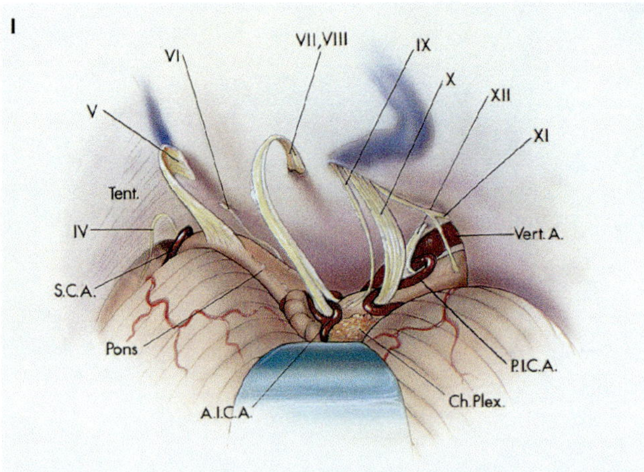

FIGURE 4.33. *I*. Tumors involving multiple neurovascular complexes. *I*, distorted nerves after the removal of the epidermoid tumor.

intracranial in 32% of 50 jugular foramina that we examined and within or extracranial to the foramen in 68% (39). The superior ganglion of the vagus could be seen intracranially in only 14% of the cases.

Vascular relationships

The vertebral artery courses anterior to the nerves in the lower neurovascular complex. The hypoglossal rootlets usually pass behind the vertebral artery, however, some hypoglossal rootlets infrequently pass anterior to the artery. If the vertebral artery is elongated or tortuous and courses laterally to the olive, it will stretch the hypoglossal rootless over its posterior surface. Some tortuous vertebral arteries will stretch the hypoglossal rootlets so far posterior that they intermingle with the glossopharyngeal, vagus, and spinal accessory nerves. The PICA has a much more complex relationship to these nerves (*Fig. 4.27*). The proximal part of the PICA passes around or between and often stretches or distorts the rootlets of the nerves in the lower complex. At the anterolateral medulla, the PICA passes around or between the rootlets of the hypoglossal nerve. At the posterolateral margin of the medulla, it passes between the fila of the glossopharyngeal, vagus, and spinal accessory nerves. The PICA may be ascending, descending, or passing laterally or medially, or may be involved in a complex loop that stretches and distorts these nerves as it passes between them (*Fig. 4.27*). The relationships of the PICA and vertebral artery to these nerves are reviewed in greater detail in the chapter on the cerebellar arteries.

Vascular compression in the lower neurovascular complex

The close relationship of the PICA and the vertebral artery to the glossopharyngeal and vagus nerves makes it logical to explore these relationships in glossopharyngeal neuralgia (23, 46). Both the glossopharyngeal and vagus nerves have been found to be compressed at their junction with the brainstem by the PICA or the vertebral artery, or both, with relief after separation of the arteries and nerves (23). The adverse cardiovascular effects of mobilization of these nerves and the risk to causing swallowing and vocal cord defects have led some to conclude that rhizotomy of the glossopharyngeal nerve and upper vagal rootlets is a reasonable alternative to vascular mobilization along the lateral medulla (19, 20, 21, 29, 41).

Jannetta has proposed that compression of the left side of the medulla by the PICA or the vertebral artery may be a cause of hypertension and that diabetes mellitus may result from right lateral medullary compression as a result of vagal effects on pancreatic islet cell secretion (9, 19). The fact that hypertension is a component of the Cushing response to lateral medullary compression has been well established and that hypertension has been relieved after decompression of the left side of the medulla supports this concept. The relationship of vascular compression to diabetes mellitus awaits further elucidation.

Tumors involving multiple neurovascular complexes

Tumors in the cerebellopontine angle commonly involve more than one of the neurovascular complexes (*Fig. 4.33*) (38). An especially difficult challenge is exposing and removing the tumors that are situated medial to the nerves. In this case, the operation must be directed through the interval between the neurovascular complexes, because these tumors often will widen these intervals. Lesions in the upper cerebellopontine angle may be exposed through the interval between the lower margin of the tentorium and the upper edge of the trigeminal nerve. Care is needed to protect the trochlear nerve and the SCA in this area. Further inferiorly, the medially placed tumor may be approached through the interval between the trigeminal nerve above and the facial and vestibulocochlear nerves below. If the tumor has an even lower attachment near the jugular foramen, it can be approached through the interval between the lower margin of the nerves entering the internal meatus and the upper margin of the glossopharyngeal nerve, or through the interval between the lower rootlets of the vagus nerve and the upper rootlets of the spinal accessory nerve. The intervals between the glossopharyngeal and vagus nerves and between the individual vagal rootless usually are too narrow to work through unless they have been opened by the tumor; however, the interval between the lower of the cranial accessory rootlets may provide access to lesions in the area. The role of procedures involving resection of parts of the temporal bone in accessing lesions in this area is reviewed in the chapter on the temporal bone.

Reprint requests: Albert L. Rhoton, Jr., M.D., Department of Neurological Surgery, University of Florida Brain Institute, P.O. Box 100265, 100 South Newell Drive, Building 59, L2-100, Gainesville, FL 32610-0265.

REFERENCES

1. Adson AW: The surgical treatment of glossopharyngeal neuralgia. **Arch Neurol Psychiatry** 12:487–506, 1924.

2. Apfelbaum RI: Microvascular decompression for tic douloureux results, in Brackmann DE (ed): *Neurological Surgery of the Ear and Skull Base*. New York, Raven Press, 1982, pp 175–180.
3. Atkinson WJ: The anterior inferior cerebellar artery: Its variations, pontine distribution, and significance in the surgery of cerebello-pontine angle tumours. **J Neurol Neurosurg Psychiatry** 12:137–151, 1949.
4. Dandy WE: Glossopharyngeal neuralgia (tic douloureux): Its diagnosis and treatment. **Arch Surg** 15:198–214, 1927.
5. Dandy WE: An operation for the cure of tic douloureux: Partial section of the sensory root at the pons. **Arch Surg** 18:687–734, 1929.
6. Dandy WE: Concerning the cause of trigeminal neuralgia. **Am J Surg** 24:447–455, 1934.
7. DuBois FS, Foley JO: Experimental studies on the vagus and spinal accessory nerves in the cat. **Anat Rec** 64:285–307, 1936.
8. Emmons WF, Rhoton AL Jr: Subdivision of the trigeminal sensory root: Experimental study in the monkey. **J Neurosurg** 35:585–591, 1971.
9. Fein JM, Frishman W: Neurogenic hypertension related to vascular compression of the lateral medulla. **Neurosurgery** 6:615–622, 1980.
10. Fujii K, Lenkey C, Rhoton AL Jr: Microsurgical anatomy of the choroidal arteries: Fourth ventricle and cerebellopontine angles. **J Neurosurg** 52:504–524, 1980.
11. Gardner WJ: Concerning the mechanism of trigeminal neuralgia and hemifacial spasm. **J Neurosurg** 19:947–958, 1962.
12. Gudmundsson K, Rhoton AL Jr, Rushton JG: Detailed anatomy of the intracranial portion of the trigeminal nerve. **J Neurosurg** 35:592–600, 1971.
13. Hardy DG, Rhoton AL Jr: Microsurgical relationships of the superior cerebellar artery and the trigeminal nerve. **J Neurosurg** 49:669–678, 1978.
14. Hardy DG, Peace DA, Rhoton AL Jr: Microsurgical anatomy of the superior cerebellar artery. **Neurosurgery** 6:10–28, 1980.
15. Horsley V, Taylor J, Coleman WS: Remarks on the various surgical procedures devised for the relief or cure of trigeminal neuralgia (tic douloureux). **Br Med J** 2:1139–1143, 1191–1193, 1249–1252, 1891.
16. House WF: Translabyrinthine approach, in House WF, Luetje CM (eds): *Acoustic Tumors: II—Management*. Baltimore, University Park Press, 1979, pp 43–87.
17. Jannetta PJ: Arterial compression of the trigeminal nerve at the pons in patients with trigeminal neuralgia. **J Neurosurg** 26:159–162, 1967.
18. Jannetta PJ: Vascular decompression in trigeminal neuralgia, in Samii M, Jannetta PJ (eds): *The Cranial Nerves: Anatomy, Pathology, Pathophysiology, Diagnosis, Treatment*. New York, Springer-Verlag, 1981, pp 331–340.
19. Jannetta PJ, Gendell HM: Clinical observations on etiology essential hypertension. **Surg Forum** 30:431–432, 1979.
20. Jannetta PJ, Abbasy M, Maroon JC, Ramos FM, Albin MS: Etiology and definitive microsurgical treatment of hemifacial spasm: Operative techniques and results in 47 patients. **J Neurosurg** 47:321–328, 1977.
21. Jannetta PJ, Møller MB, Møller AR, Sekhar LN: Neurosurgical treatment of vertigo by microvascular decompression of the eighth cranial nerve. **Clin Neurosurg** 33:645–665, 1986.
22. Katsuta T, Rhoton AL Jr, Matsushima T: The jugular foramen: Microsurgical anatomy and operative approaches. **Neurosurgery** 41:149–202, 1997.
23. Laha RK, Jannetta PJ: Glossopharyngeal neuralgia. **J Neurosurg** 47:316–320, 1977.
24. Lister JR, Rhoton AL Jr, Matsushima T, Peace DA: Microsurgical anatomy of the posterior inferior cerebellar artery. **Neurosurgery** 10:170–199, 1982.
25. Martin RG, Grant JL, Peace DA, Theiss C, Rhoton AL Jr: Microsurgical relationships of the anterior inferior cerebellar artery and the facial-vestibulocochlear nerve complex. **Neurosurgery** 6:483–507, 1980.
26. Matsushima T, Rhoton AL Jr, de Oliveira E, Peace DA: Microsurgical anatomy of the veins of the posterior fossa. **J Neurosurg** 59:63–105, 1983.
27. Matsushima T, Rhoton AL Jr, Lenkey C: Microsurgery of the fourth ventricle: Part I—Microsurgical anatomy. **Neurosurgery** 11:631–667, 1982.
28. Møller MB, Møller AR, Jannetta PJ, Sekhar L: Diagnosis and surgical treatment of disabling positional vertigo. **J Neurosurg** 64:21–28, 1986.
29. Ouaknine GE, Robert F, Molina-Negro P, Hardy J: Geniculate neuralgia and audio-vestibular disturbances due to compression of the intermediate and eighth nerves by the postero-inferior cerebellar artery. **Surg Neurol** 13:147–150, 1980.
30. Pait TG, Zeal A, Harris FS, Paullus WS, Rhoton AL Jr: Microsurgical anatomy and dissection of the temporal bone. **Surg Neurol** 8:363–391, 1977.
31. Pelletier V, Poulos DA, Lende RA: Localization in the trigeminal root. Presented at the American Association of Neurological Surgeons, Washington, DC, 1970.
32. Rhoton AL Jr: Microsurgery of the internal acoustic meatus. **Surg Neurol** 2:311–318, 1974.
33. Rhoton AL Jr: Microsurgical anatomy of the brainstem surface facing an acoustic neuroma. **Surg Neurol** 25:326–339, 1986.
34. Rhoton AL Jr: Microsurgical anatomy of decompression operations on the trigeminal nerve, in Rovit RL, Murali R, Jannetta PJ (eds): *Trigeminal Neuralgia*. Baltimore, Williams & Wilkins, 1990, pp 165–200.
35. Rhoton AL Jr: Microsurgical anatomy of acoustic neuromas, in Jackler RK (ed): *Otolaryngologic Clinics of North America*. Philadelphia, W.B. Saunders Co., 1992, pp 257–294.
36. Rhoton AL Jr: Instrumentation, in Apuzzo MLJ (ed): *Brain Surgery: Complication, Avoidance and Management*. New York, Churchill Livingstone, 1993, pp 1647–1670.
37. Rhoton AL Jr: Microsurgical anatomy of acoustic neuromas, in Sekhar LN, Janecka IP (eds): *Surgery of Cranial Base Tumors*. New York, Raven Press, 1993, pp 687–713.
38. Rhoton AL Jr: Microsurgical anatomy of posterior fossa cranial nerves, in Barrow DL (ed): *Surgery of the Cranial Nerves of the Posterior Fossa: Neurosurgical Topics*. Park Ridge, AANS, 1993, pp 1–103.
39. Rhoton AL Jr, Buza R: Microsurgical anatomy of the jugular foramen. **J Neurosurg** 42:541–550, 1975.
40. Rhoton AL Jr, Kobayashi S, Hollingshead WH: Nervus intermedius. **J Neurosurg** 29:609–618, 1968.
41. Segal R, Gendell HM, Canfield D, Dujovny M, Jannetta PJ: Cardiovascular response to pulsatile pressure applied to ventrolateral medulla. **Surg Forum** 30:433–435, 1979.
42. Seoane ER, Rhoton AL Jr: Suprameatal extension of the retrosigmoid approach: Microsurgical anatomy. **Neurosurgery** 44:553–560, 1999.
43. Sunderland S: Neurovascular relationships and anomalies at the base of the brain. **J Neurol Neurosurg Psychiatry** 11:243–257, 1948.
44. Tarlov IM: Structure of the nerve root: Part II—Differentiation of sensory from motor roots: Observations on identification of function in roots of mixed cranial nerves. **Arch Neurol Psychiatry** 37:1338–1355, 1937.
45. Tarlov IM: Section of the cephalic third of the vagus-spinal accessory complex: Clinical and histologic results. **Arch Neurol Psychiatry** 47:141–148, 1942.
46. Watt JC, McKillop AN: Relation of arteries to roots of nerves in posterior cranial fossa in man. **Arch Surg** 30:336–345, 1935.

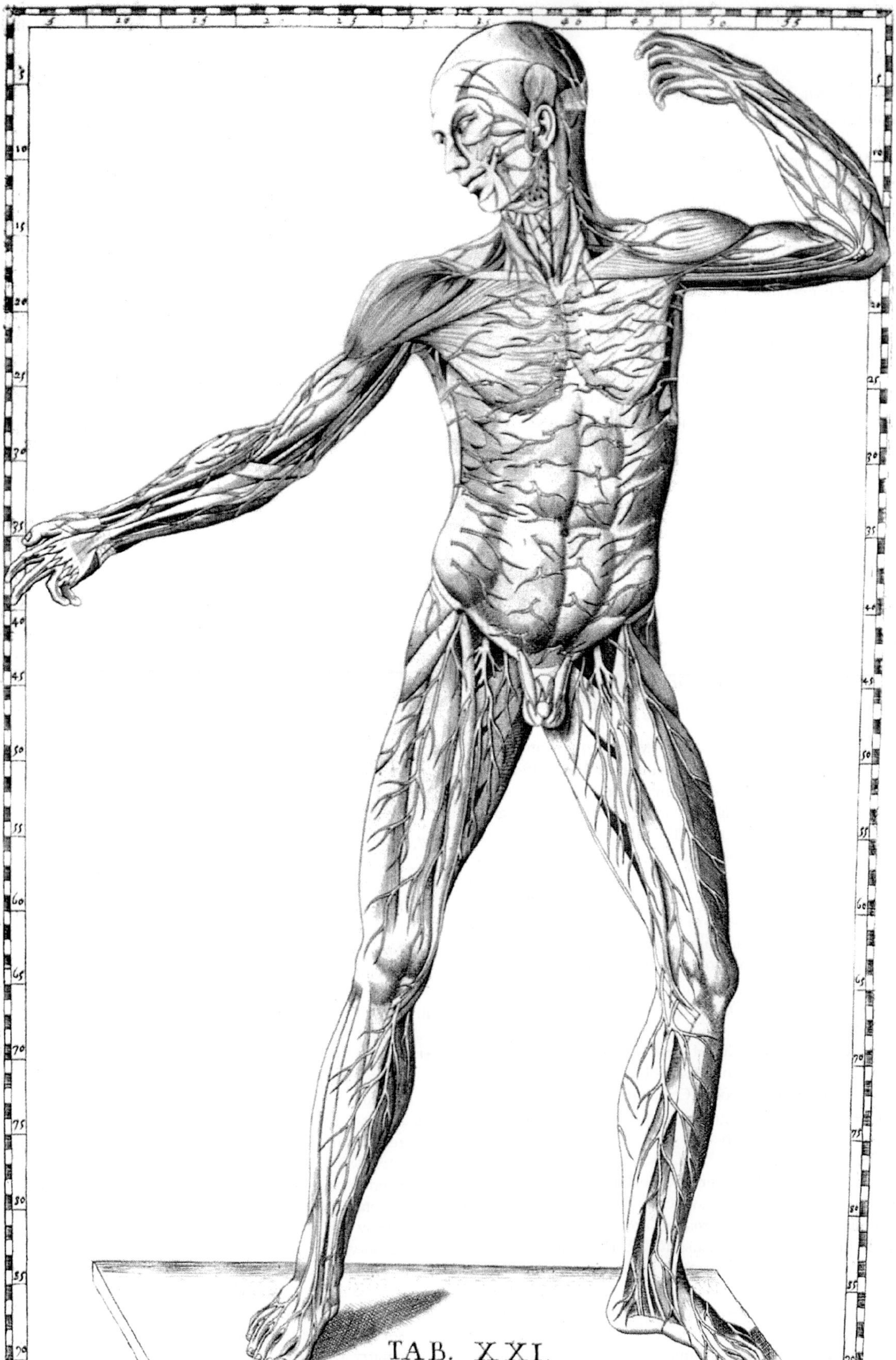

Anterior superficial neural complexes, from, Bartolommeo Eustachio, *Tabulae anatomicae*. Rome, Sumptibus Laurentii & Thomae Pagliarini, 1728. Courtesy, Rare Book Room, Norris Medical Library, Keck School of Medicine, Los Angeles, California.

CHAPTER 5

Tentorial Incisura

Albert L. Rhoton, Jr., M.D.

Department of Neurological Surgery, University of Florida, Gainesville, Florida

Key words: Anatomic study, Anatomy, Circle of Willis, Incisura, Midbrain, Neurovascular, Tentorium

The tentorial incisura provides the only communication between the supratentorial and infratentorial spaces (17) (*Fig. 5.1*). The area between the upper brainstem and the incisural edges is divided into the anterior, middle, and posterior incisural spaces (*Fig. 5.2*). The anterior incisural space is located anterior to the brainstem and extends upward around the optic chiasm to the subcallosal area; the middle incisural space is located lateral to the brainstem and is intimately related to the hippocampal formation in the medial part of the temporal lobe; and the posterior incisural space is located posterior to the midbrain and corresponds to the region of the pineal gland and vein of Galen. The arterial relationships in the anterior incisural space and the venous relationships in the posterior incisural space are extremely complex, since the anterior incisural space contains all of the components of the circle of Willis and the bifurcation of the internal carotid and basilar arteries, and the posterior incisural space contains the convergence of the internal cerebral and basal veins and many of their tributaries on the vein of Galen. The incisura is intimately related to the depths of the cerebrum and cerebellum, the first six cranial nerves, and the upper brainstem. Some part of the incisura is commonly exposed during the operations for aneurysms, deep tumors and arteriovenous malformations, trigeminal neuralgia, and epilepsy. Much attention has been focused on the distortions of this anatomy by herniation of the brain through the incisural space.

ANATOMY OF THE TENTORIUM

The tentorium covers the cerebellum, supports the cerebrum, and forms a collar around the brainstem (*Figs. 5.2* and *5.3*). The tentorium slopes downward from its apex, located at the posterior edge of the incisura, to its attachment to the temporal, occipital, and sphenoid bones. All of the tentorial margins, except the free edges bordering the incisura, are rigidly attached to the cranium. The anterior border is attached to the petrous ridge and divides to enclose the superior petrosal sinus. The lateral and posterior borders, which divide to enclose the transverse sinus and the torcula, are attached to the inner surface of the occipital and temporal bones along the internal occipital protuberance and to the edges of the shallow osseous groove for the transverse sinus.

The anterior end of each free edge is attached to the petrous apex and the anterior and posterior clinoid processes (*Figs. 5.1–5.3*). The attachment to the petrous apex and the clinoid processes forms three dural folds: the anterior and posterior petroclinoid folds and the interclinoid fold. Between these folds is located the oculomotor trigone, a shallow depressed area over the posterior part of the roof of the cavernous sinus, through which the oculomotor and trochlear nerves enter the sinus. The posterior petroclinoid fold extends from the petrous apex to the posterior clinoid process; the anterior petroclinoid fold extends from the petrous apex to the anterior clinoid process; and the interclinoid fold covers the ligament extending from the anterior to the posterior clinoid process. The oculomotor nerve penetrates the dura in the central part of this triangle, the oculomotor triangle, and the trochlear nerve enters the dura at the posterolateral edge of this triangle. The petrosphenoid ligament passes between the leaves of the posterior petroclinoid fold from the petrous apex to the lateral border of the dorsum sellae, just below the posterior clinoid process. The abducens nerve passes below the petrosphenoid ligament to enter the cavernous sinus. The dura forming the roof of the oculomotor trigones extends medially across the sella to form the diaphragma sellae, which covers the pituitary gland and contains an opening for the infundibulum.

Anterolateral to the diaphragma are two orifices: a bone orifice, the optic canal (through which the optic nerve enters the orbit), and a dural orifice through which the internal carotid artery exits the cavernous sinus (*Fig. 5.3*). From the anterior part of the free edge, the dura mater slopes steeply downward to form the lateral wall of the cavernous sinus and to cover the middle cranial fossa. Plaut reported that the attachment of the anterior end of the free edge to the petrous apex may be situated as much as 10 mm lateral and 8 mm below the level of the clinoid processes and that the low position of the free edge may facilitate descending tentorial herniations (20).

The falx cerebri fuses into the dorsal surface of the tentorium in the midline behind the apex (*Fig. 5.1*). The straight sinus, which is enclosed in the falcotentorial junction, begins at the tentorial apex, where it receives the vein of Galen and the inferior sagittal sinus, and terminates in the torcular.

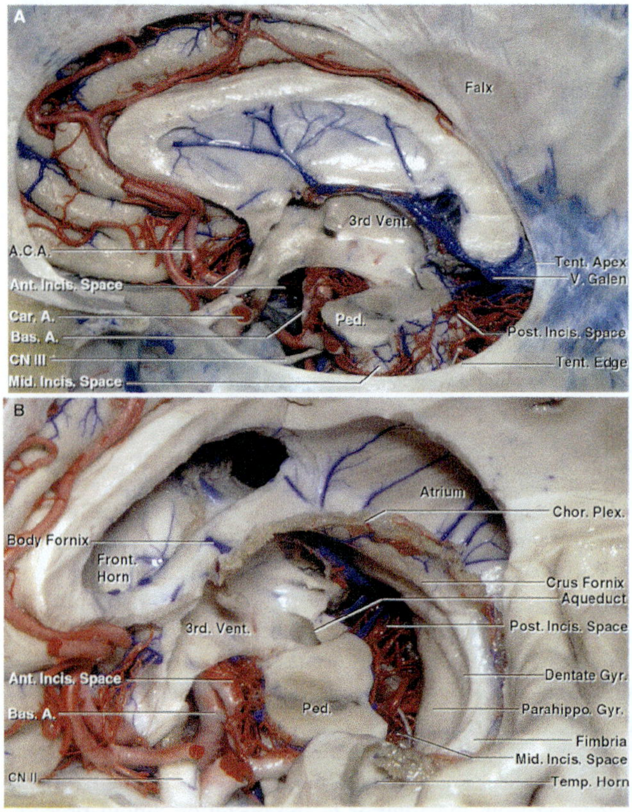

FIGURE 5.1. Tentorial incisura. ***A,*** **the left cerebral hemisphere has been removed. The tentorial incisura is located between the tentorial edges and is the only site of communication behind the supra and infratentorial spaces. The tentorial apex is located at the junction of the vein of Galen and the straight sinus. The tentorial edges slope downward from the apex. The free edge passes along the side of the brainstem and anteriorly blends into the dura covering the petrous apex and the anterior and posterior clinoid processes. The incisura, in relation to the midbrain, is divided into anterior, middle, and posterior spaces. The anterior incisural space extends above the optic chiasm to the lamina terminalis and below the chiasm and third ventricular floor to the interpeduncular fossa. The middle incisural space is located between the midbrain and tentorial edge, opens upward into the ambient and crural cisterns, and extends inferiorly into the anterior part of the cerebellomesencephalic fissure. The posterior incisural space, located between the posterior midbrain and the tentorial apex, encompasses the quadrigeminal cistern, which extends into the cerebellomesencephalic fissure and along the outer surface of the upper part of the fourth ventricular roof. The anterior incisural space, located below the frontal horn, contains the basilar bifurcation. The PCA and SCA arise in the anterior and pass around the brainstem to reach the middle and posterior incisural spaces. The branches of the PCA and SCA pass through the lateral part of the posterior incisural space, and the large venous structures converging on the vein of Galen course in the medial part of the posterior incisural space.** ***B,*** **part of the left central hemisphere and all of the left thalamus have been removed, while preserving the fornix and choroid plexus. The frontal horn and anterior part of the third ventricle is located above the anterior incisural space. The middle incisural space is located medial to the temporal horn, between the temporal lobe and midbrain. The posterior incisural space is located between the tentorial apex and posterior midbrain surface.** ***A.,*** **artery;** ***A.C.A.,*** **anterior cerebral artery;** ***Ant.,*** **anterior;** ***Bas.,*** **basilar;** ***Car.,*** **carotid;** ***Chor.,*** **choroid;** ***CN,*** **cranial nerve;** ***Front.,*** **frontal;** ***Gyr.,*** **gyrus;** ***Incis.,*** **incisural;** ***Mid.,*** **middle;** ***Parahippo.,*** **parahippocampal;** ***Ped.,*** **peduncle;** ***Plex.,*** **plexus;** ***Post.,*** **posterior;** ***Temp.,*** **temporal;** ***Tent.,*** **tentorial;** ***V.,*** **vein;** ***Vent.,*** **ventricle.**

TENTORIAL INCISURA

The incisura is roughly triangular and has its anterior edge or base on the dorsum sellae and its apex dorsal to the midbrain, just posterior to the pineal gland (*Fig. 5.2*). The incisura, when viewed from above after removal of the cerebral hemispheres, is filled by the midbrain, pons, and cerebellum, and the free edges skirt the cerebral peduncles, either touching or being separated from them by a variable distance (*Fig. 5.2*). The amount of cerebellar cortex visible between the midbrain and the free edge varies from none when the free edge hugs the tectum to a large amount when the incisura extends far posteriorly. When viewed from below after removal of the cerebellum, the incisura is filled by the midbrain and the uncus and parahippocampal gyrus (*Fig. 5.4*). The amount of parahippocampal gyrus visible from below varies from none when the free edge hugs the tectum to a large amount when the incisura is very wide. The width of the incisura varies from 26 to 35 mm (average, 29.6 mm) and the anteroposterior diameter varies from 46 to 75 mm (average, 52.0 mm) (17).

The area between the brainstem and the free edges is divided into: an anterior incisural space located in front of the brainstem; paired middle incisural spaces situated lateral to the brainstem; and a posterior incisural space located behind the brainstem (*Figs. 5.1–5.4*). The description of each incisural space is divided into sections on neural, cisternal, ventricular, cranial nerve, arterial, and venous relationships.

ANTERIOR INCISURAL SPACE

Neural relationships

The anterior incisural space is located anterior to the midbrain and pons. It extends inferiorly between the brainstem and clivus and obliquely forward and upward around the optic chiasm to the subcallosal area. It opens laterally into the medial part of the Sylvian fissure, and posteriorly between the uncus and the brainstem into the middle incisural space (*Figs. 5.3* and *5.4*).

The part of the anterior incisural space located below the optic chiasm has posterolateral and posterior walls. The posterolateral wall is formed by the bulbous prominence of the anterior third of the uncus, which hangs over the anterior part

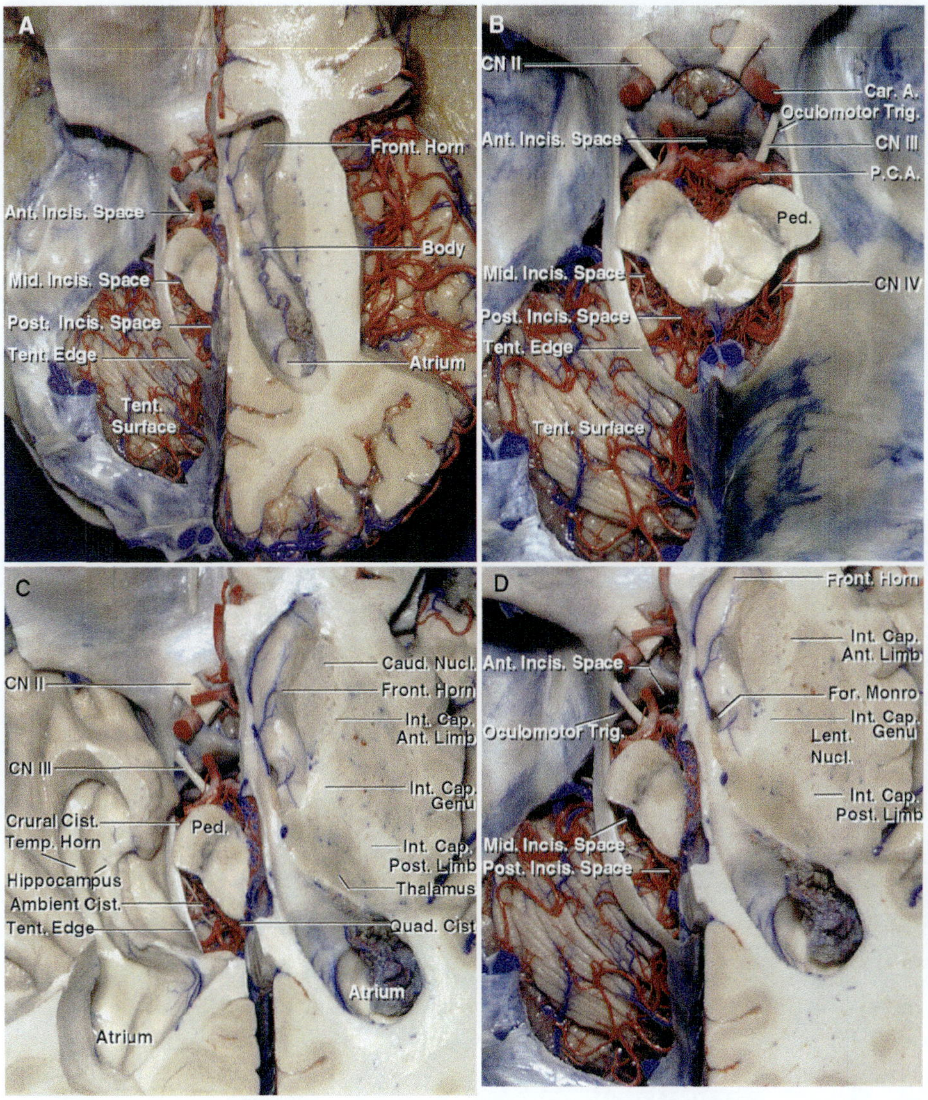

FIGURE 5.2. Tentorial incisura, superior views. *A*, the left cerebrum, above the level of the cerebral peduncle, has been removed to expose the anterior, middle, and posterior incisural spaces. The thalamus, which forms the floor of the body of the lateral ventricle, sits directly above the central part of the tentorial incisura. The right lateral ventricle and the lower wall of the sylvian fissure have been preserved. The left half of the tentorium, except the edge, has been removed to expose the tentorial cerebellar surface. The frontal horn is located above the anterior incisural space. Structures located in the anterior incisural space below the frontal horn include the optic nerves and chiasm, internal carotid arteries, and the upper part of the basilar artery and its branches. The middle incisural space, located between the midbrain and tentorial edge, opens upward into the crural and ambient cisterns and downward into the anterior part of the cerebellomesencephalic fissure. The posterior incisural space, located between the midbrain and the tentorial apex, includes the area of the quadrigeminal cistern and opens into the central part of the cerebellomesencephalic fissure. The atrium of the lateral ventricle is situated lateral to the posterior incisural space. *B*, view of the tentorial incisura after removing the cerebrum. The tentorial edges sweep along the lateral margin of the cerebral peduncle. The oculomotor nerve passes medial to the anterior edge of the tentorium and enters the cavernous sinus by passing through a triangular patch of dura called the oculomotor trigone. *C*, superior view of the tentorial incisura before removing the left temporal lobe. The crural cistern is located between the cerebral peduncle and uncus. The ambient cistern opens upward between the midbrain and the medial surface of the temporal lobe formed by the parahippocampal and dentate gyri. The thalamus and the genu of the internal capsule are located above the central part of the tentorial incisura. *D*, enlarged view after removing the temporal lobe. The internal capsule and the lentiform nucleus are located above the middle incisural space. The genu of the internal capsule abuts on the lateral ventricular wall at the level of the foramen of Monro. *A.*, artery; *Ant.*, anterior; *Cap.*, capsule; *Car.*, carotid; *Caud.*, caudate; *Cist.*, cistern; *CN*, cranial nerve; *For.*, foramen; *Front.*, frontal; *Incis.*, incisural; *Int.*, internal; *Lent.*, lentiform; *Mid.*, middle; *Nucl.*, nucleus; *P.C.A.*, posterior cerebral artery; *Ped.*, peduncle; *Post.*, posterior; *Quad.*, quadrigeminal; *Tent.*, tentorial; *Trig.*, trigone.

of the free edge above the oculomotor trigone (*Fig. 5.2*). The posterior wall is formed by the pons and cerebral peduncles. The infundibulum of the pituitary gland crosses the anterior incisural space to reach the opening in the diaphragma sellae. The part of the anterior incisural space situated above the optic chiasm is limited superiorly by the rostrum of the corpus callosum, posteriorly by the lamina terminalis, and laterally by the part of the medial surfaces of the frontal lobes located below the rostrum.

The anterior incisural space opens laterally into the part of the Sylvian fissure situated below the anterior perforated substance (*Fig. 5.4*). The anterior limb of the internal capsule, the head of the caudate nucleus, and the anterior part of the

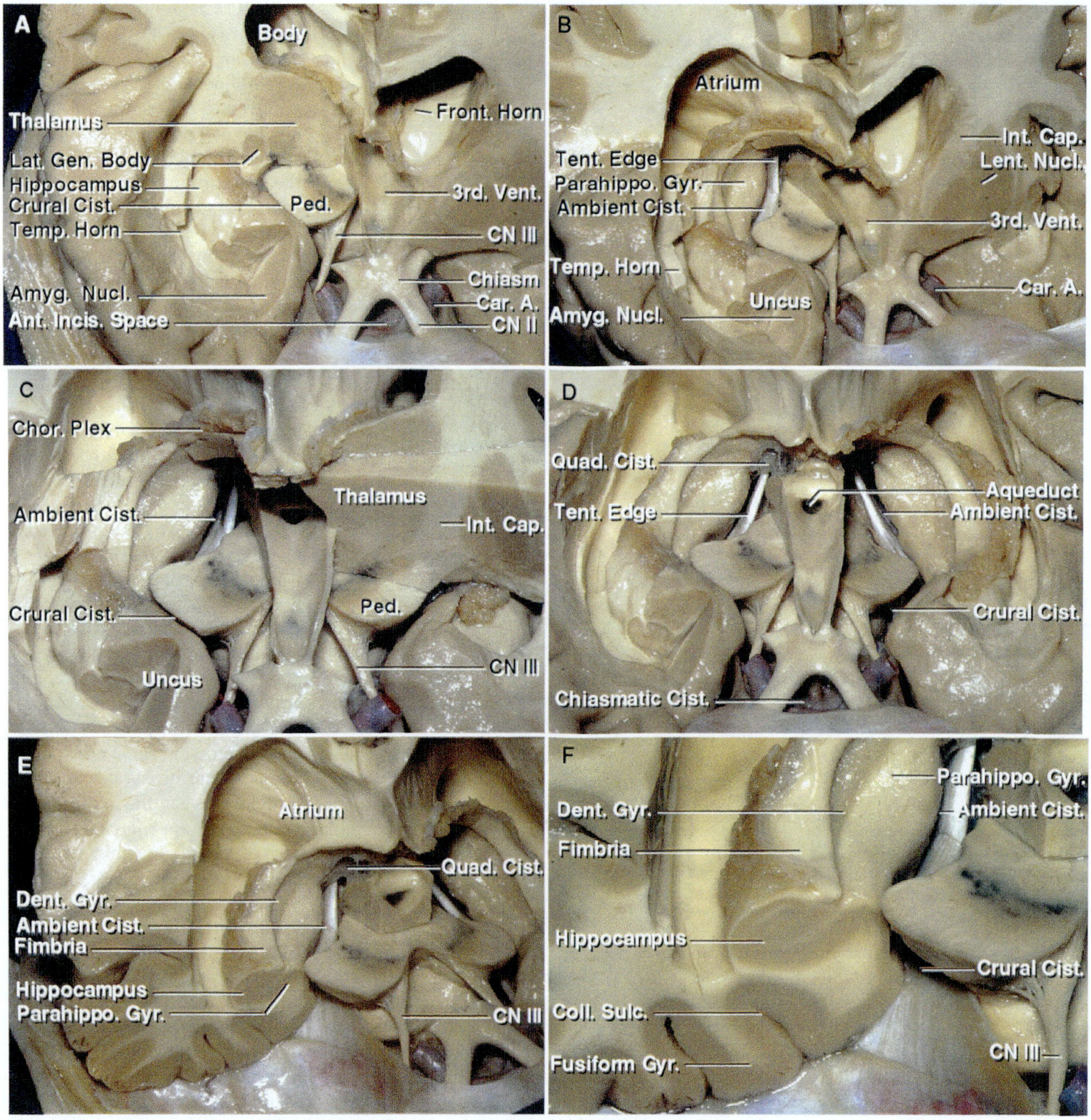

FIGURE 5.3. Stepwise dissection of the neural structures above the tentorial incisura. *A*, the coronal section of the right hemisphere crosses vertically through the thalamus and lateral geniculate body and the transverse section crosses the cerebral peduncle. The right temporal horn has been opened to expose the hippocampus and amygdaloid nucleus. The floor of the third ventricle is exposed in the midline. The coronal section of the left hemisphere crosses anterior to the thalamus near the foramen of Monro and genu of the internal capsule. The anterior incisural space extends from the interpeduncular fossa, around the chiasm, and into the suprachiasmatic area. *B*, the right thalamus has been removed while preserving the fornix, which wraps around the thalamus to form the outer edge of the choroidal fissure situated between the thalamus and fornix. The middle incisural space extends upward into the ambient and crural cisterns. The crural cistern is located between the uncus and the cerebral peduncle. The ambient cistern in located between the parahippocampal and dentate gyri and the fimbria of the fornix laterally and the midbrain medially. The posterior part of the tentorial edge is exposed. The quadrigeminal cistern is located in the posterior incisural space between the tentorial apex and the pineal. The atrium is located lateral to the quadrigeminal cistern and posterior incisural space. *C*, enlarged view. The coronal section through the left hemisphere has been extended backward to the level of the thalamus and posterior limb of the internal capsule. The left temporal horn is

lentiform nucleus are located above the anterior perforated substance (*Fig. 5.2*).

Cisternal relationships

The interpeduncular cistern, which sits in the posterior part of the anterior incisural space between the cerebral peduncles and the dorsum sellae, communicates laterally with the Sylvian cistern below the anterior perforated substance and anteriorly with the chiasmatic cistern located below the optic chiasm. The interpeduncular and chiasmatic cisterns are separated by Liliequist's membrane, an arachnoidal sheet extending from the dorsum sellae to the anterior edge of the mammillary bodies (14, 35, 36). The chiasmatic cistern communicates around the optic chiasm with the cisterna laminae terminalis, which lies anterior to the lamina terminalis.

Ventricular relationships

The anterior part of the third ventricle projects into the anterior incisural space in the medial plane, dividing it into supra and infra chiasmatic portions. The frontal horns of the lateral ventricles are located above the anterior incisural space (*Figs. 5.1–5.3*). The tip of the temporal horn is separated from the uncal surface, forming the posterolateral wall of the anterior incisural space, by the amygdaloid nucleus.

Cranial nerves

The optic and oculomotor nerves and the posterior part of the olfactory tracts pass through the anterior incisural space. Each olfactory tract runs posteriorly, and splits just above the anterior clinoid process to form the medial and the lateral olfactory striae, which course along the anterior margin of the anterior perforated substance (*Fig. 5.4*).

The optic nerves and chiasm and the anterior part of the optic tracts cross the anterior incisural space (*Fig. 5.3*). The optic nerves emerge from the optic canal medial to the attachment of the free edge to the anterior clinoid processes, and are directed posteriorly, superiorly, and medially toward the optic chiasm. The optic chiasm is usually located above the diaphragma sellae, but it may be prefixed and lie over the tuberculum sellae or postfixed and lie over the dorsum sellae. From the chiasm, the optic tract continues in a posterolateral direction around the cerebral peduncle to enter the middle incisural space (*Fig. 5.4*). The oculomotor nerve emerges from the midbrain on the medial surface of the cerebral peduncle. It crosses the anterior incisural space between the posterior cerebral artery (PCA) and the superior cerebellar artery (SCA) and passes inferomedial to the uncus to enter the roof of the cavernous sinus through the oculomotor trigone. The abducens nerve ascends from deep within the infratentorial part of the anterior incisural space. It emerges from the pontomedullary sulcus, ascends in the prepontine cistern to pierce the dura covering the clivus, and passes below the petrosphenoid ligament to enter the cavernous sinus.

Arterial relationships

The arterial relationships of the anterior incisural space are complex because it contains all of the components of the circle of Willis (4, 5, 7, 18, 19, 27, 37). The internal carotid artery enters the anterior incisural space by passing along the medial surface of the anterior clinoid process and bifurcates below the anterior perforated substance (*Figs. 5.5* and *5.6*). The posterior communicating artery arises from the posteromedial aspect of the carotid artery and courses superomedial to the oculomotor nerve to join the PCA in the anterior incisural space. The anterior choroidal artery originates from the posterior surface of the carotid artery 0.1 to 3.0 mm distal to the origin of the posterior communicating artery and courses below the optic tract before passing between the uncus and the cerebral peduncle to enter the middle incisural space (3, 24).

The proximal part of the anterior cerebral artery also courses in the anterior incisural space (*Fig. 5.6*). It arises below the anterior perforated substance and courses anteromedially above the optic chiasm, where it is joined to its mate from the opposite side by the anterior communicating artery. It then courses upward in front of the lamina terminalis. The middle cerebral artery courses laterally from its origin below the anterior perforated substance. The major bifurcation of the middle cerebral artery is usually located in the lateral part of the anterior incisural space.

The basilar artery ascends and gives rise to the PCA and SCA in the posterior part of the anterior incisural space be-

exposed below the basal ganglia. The optic nerves, chiasm, and tracts, and the oculomotor nerves cross the anterior incisural space. The middle incisural space extends into the ambient and crural cisterns, and the posterior incisural space, located in front of the tentorial apex, contains the quadrigeminal cistern. *D,* the upper parts of the anterior and middle incisural spaces have been exposed by removing the thalami on both sides. The tentorial edges extend forward from the apex, located at the posterior margin of the pineal region, along the side of the midbrain to attach to the petrous ridge and clinoid processes. *E,* the temporal lobe has been sectioned in a coronal plane and the third ventricular floor has been removed. The lateral wall of the ambient cistern is formed by the parahippocampal and dentate gyri and the fimbria of the fornix. *F,* enlarged view. The rounded medial edge of the parahippocampal gyrus, the site of the subiculum, which blends into the hippocampus, joins the dentate gyri and fimbria to form the lateral wall of the ambient cistern. The fimbria arises on the hippocampal surface. *A.,* artery; *Amyg.,* amygdaloid; *Ant.,* anterior; *Cap.,* capsule; *Car.,* carotid; *Chor.,* choroid; *Cist.,* cistern; *CN,* cranial nerve; *Coll.,* colliculus; *Dent.,* dentate; *Front.,* frontal; *Gen.,* geniculate; *Gyr.,* gyrus; *Incis.,* incisural; *Int.,* internal; *Lat.,* lateral; *Lent.,* lentiform; *Nucl.,* nucleus; *Parahippo.,* parahippocampal; *Ped.,* peduncle; *Plex.,* plexus; *Quad.,* quadrigeminal; *Sulc.,* sulcus; *Temp.,* temporal; *Tent.,* tentorial; *Vent.,* ventricle.

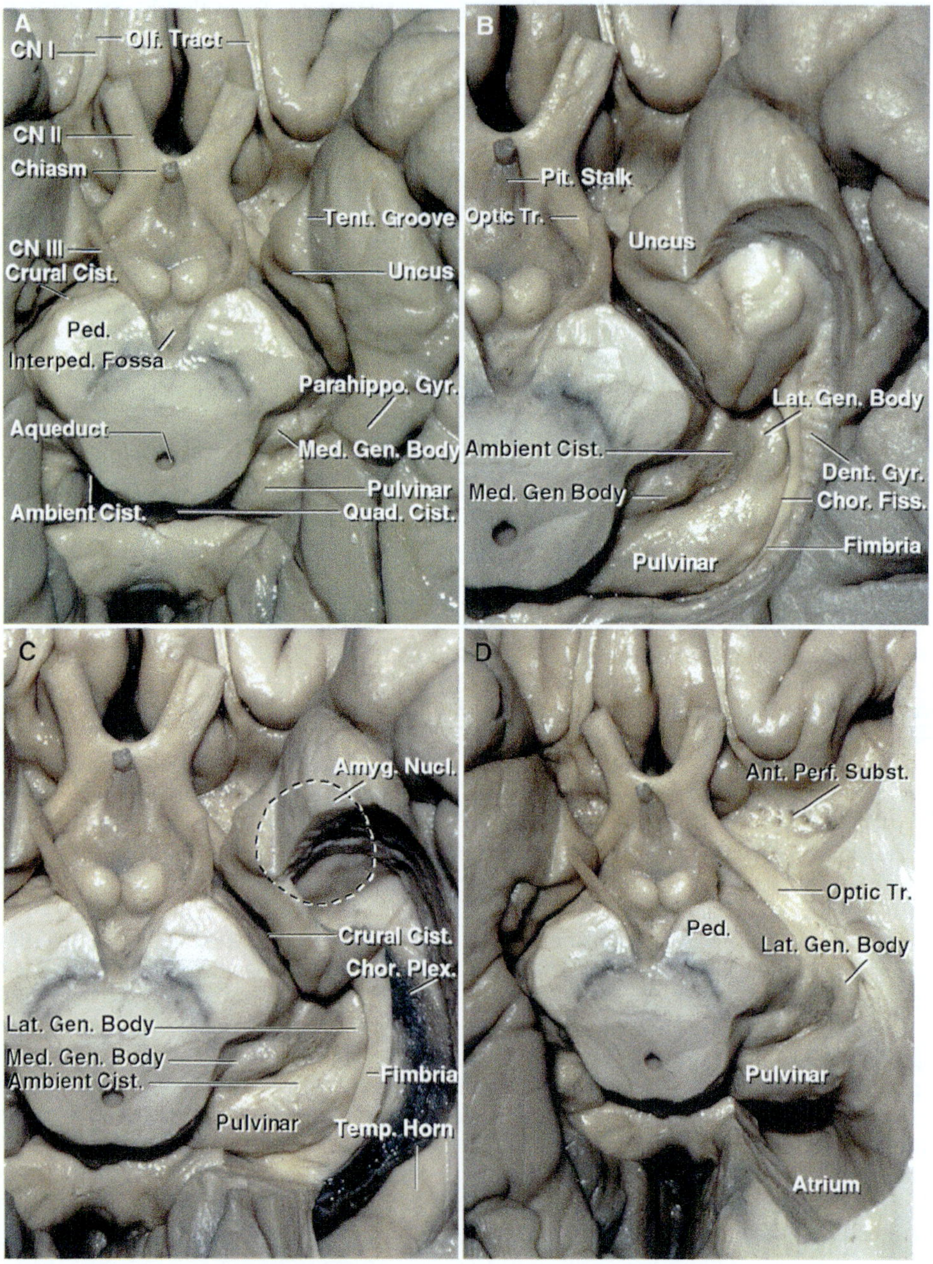

FIGURE 5.4. Neural relationships above the tentorial incisura. Stepwise dissection viewed from below. *A,* the anterior incisural space extends forward from the interpeduncular fossa below the floor of the third ventricle and around the optic chiasm to the lamina terminalis. The middle incisural space extends upward into the crural cistern located between the uncus and cerebral peduncle and the ambient cisterns located between the lateral midbrain and the temporal lobe. The posterior incisural space is located behind the midbrain and includes the quadrigeminal cistern and pineal region. The anterior part of the tentorial edge has grooved the uncus. *B,* the medial edge of the parahippocampal gyrus has been removed to expose the roof of the ambient cistern formed by the lower surface of the thalamus and the geniculate bodies. The optic tract extends posteriorly in the roof of the crural cistern and terminates in the lateral geniculate body located in the anterior part of the roof of the ambient cisterns. The dentate gyrus and the fimbria of the fornix are located in the lateral margin of the ambient cistern above the parahippocampal gyrus. *C,* the part of the parahippocampal gyrus below the temporal horn has been removed while preserving the fimbria of the fornix. The choroid plexus in the temporal horn is attached along the choroidal fissure located between the fimbria and the thalamus. *D,* all but the upper part of the left temporal lobe and fimbria has been removed. The optic tract extends posteriorly through the crural cistern to the anterior part of the ambient cistern where it terminates in the lateral geniculate body. The posterior incisural space between the midbrain and the tentorial apex borders the atrium laterally. *Amyg.,* amygdaloid; *Ant.,* anterior; *Chor.,* choroid, choroidal; *Cist.,* cistern; *CN,* cranial nerve; *Dent.,* dentate; *Fiss.,* fissure; *Gen.,* geniculate; *Gyr.,* gyrus; *Interped.,* interpeduncular; *Lat.,* lateral; *Med.,* medial; *Nucl.,* nucleus; *Olf.,* olfactory; *Parahippo.,* parahippocampal; *Ped.,* peduncle; *Perf.,* perforated; *Pit.,* pituitary; *Plex.,* plexus; *Quad.,* quadrigeminal; *Subst.,* substance; *Temp.,* temporal; *Tent.,* tentorial; *Tr.,* trunk.

tween the posterior perforated substance and the clivus (*Fig. 5.7*). The position of the basilar tip and bifurcation varies from as far caudal as 1.3 mm below the pontomesencephalic sulcus to as far rostral as the mammillary bodies (17). The PCA courses laterally around the cerebral peduncle, above the oculomotor nerve. It exits the anterior and enters the middle incisural space by coursing between the uncus and the cerebral peduncle. The SCA originates in the anterior incisural space below the PCA and courses laterally below the oculomotor nerve (*Fig. 5.7*). The origin is usually just rostral to the level of the free edge. It dips below the tentorium to reach the superior surface of the cerebellum at the junction of the ante-

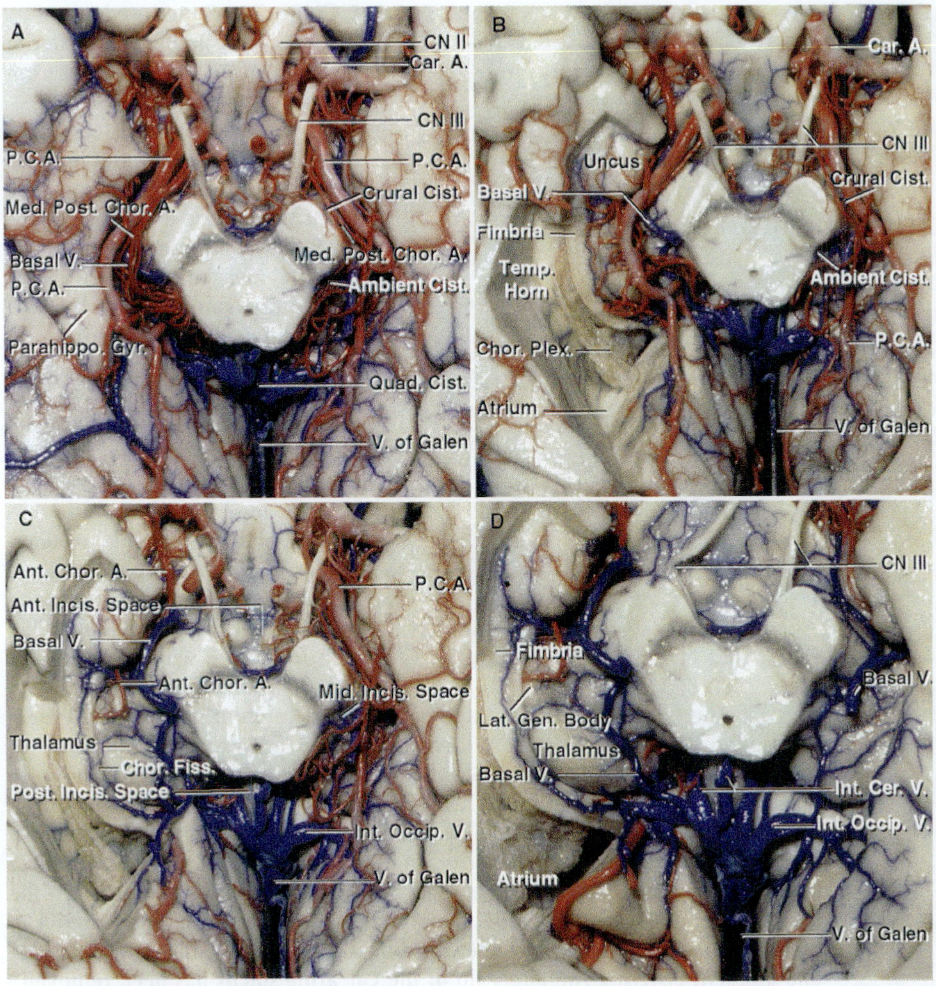

FIGURE 5.5. Tentorial incisura. ***A,*** **view from below of the cisterns bordering the tentorial incisura. The middle incisural space opens upward into the crural cistern located between the uncus and peduncle and the ambient cistern located between the parahippocampal gyrus and the lateral surface of the brainstem. The PCAs course through the crural and ambient cisterns to reach the posterior incisural space, the site of the quadrigeminal cistern. The basal vein accompanies the PCA in the upper part of the crural and ambient cisterns and empties into the vein of Galen in the quadrigeminal cistern. The medial posterior choroidal arteries course around the brainstem on the medial side of the PCAs with the long circumflex perforating branches.** ***B,*** **the medial part of the right temporal lobe has been removed to expose the temporal horn. The fimbria of the fornix, which arises on the upper surface of the hippocampus and forms the lower margin of the choroidal fissure, has been preserved. The thalamus, geniculate bodies, and optic tract are in the roof of the crural and ambient cisterns.** ***C,*** **the right PCA has been removed. The basal vein passes backward above the PCA and empties into the vein of Galen with the internal cerebral and internal occipital veins. The lower surface of the thalamus, the geniculate bodies, and the optic tract form the roof of the crural and ambient cisterns. The anterior choroidal artery passes posteriorly above the uncus and through the choroidal fissure to supply the choroid plexus in the temporal horn.** ***D,*** **both PCAs have been removed to expose the roof of the middle incisural space on both sides and the basal veins, which drain the neural structures in the region.** ***A.,*** **artery;** ***Ant.,*** **anterior;** ***Car.,*** **carotid;** ***Cer.,*** **cerebral;** ***Chor.,*** **choroid, choroidal;** ***Cist.,*** **cistern;** ***CN,*** **cranial nerve;** ***Fiss.,*** **fissure;** ***Gen.,*** **geniculate;** ***Gyr.,*** **gyrus;** ***Incis.,*** **incisural;** ***Int.,*** **internal;** ***Lat.,*** **lateral;** ***Med.,*** **medial;** ***Mid.,*** **middle;** ***Occip.,*** **occipital;** ***Parahippo.,*** **parahippocampal;** ***P.C.A.,*** **posterior cerebral artery;** ***Plex.,*** **plexus;** ***Post.,*** **posterior;** ***Quad.,*** **quadrigeminal;** ***Temp.,*** **temporal;** ***V.,*** **vein.**

rior and middle incisural spaces. The structures in the walls of the anterior incisural space receive perforating branches from all of the above arteries.

Venous relationships

The main venous trunk related to the anterior incisural space is the basal vein (*Figs. 5.5* and *5.6*) (16). It courses through the anterior, middle, and posterior incisural spaces to empty into the vein of Galen. It originates below the anterior perforated substance, courses posterolaterally around the cerebral peduncle, below the optic tract and medial to the uncus, to enter the middle incisural space.

MIDDLE INCISURAL SPACE

Neural relationships

The middle incisural space is located lateral to the brainstem (*Figs. 5.3* and *5.4*). This narrow space extends upward between the temporal lobe and the midbrain and downward between the cerebellum and the upper brainstem. It has medial and lateral walls and a roof. The medial wall, formed by the lateral surface of the midbrain and upper pons, is divided by the pontomesencephalic sulcus, which lies at the level of the free edge. The surface of the midbrain facing the middle incisural space is divided into a larger anterior part formed by the

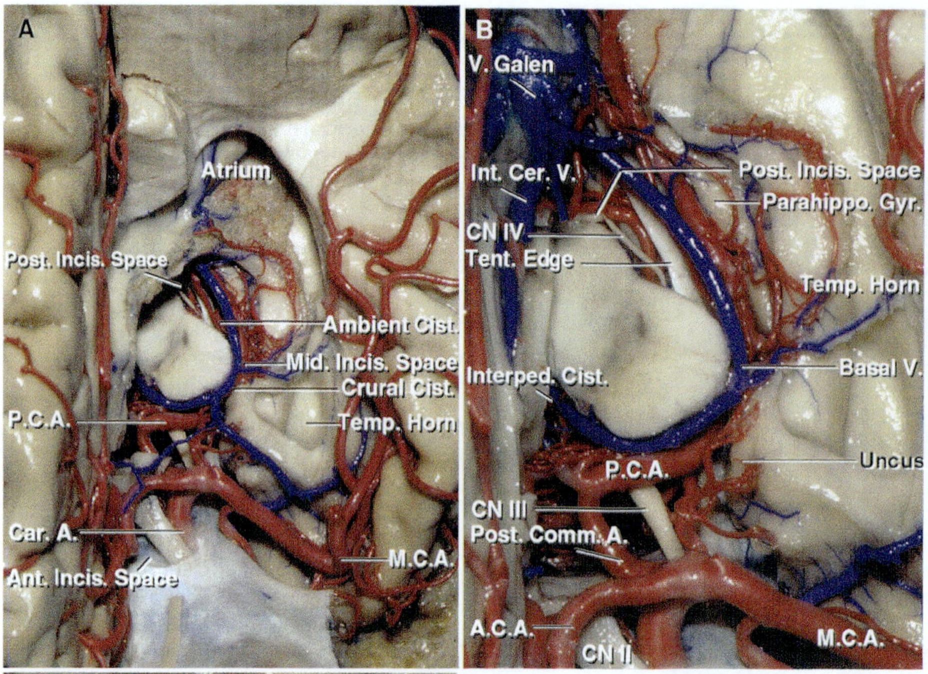

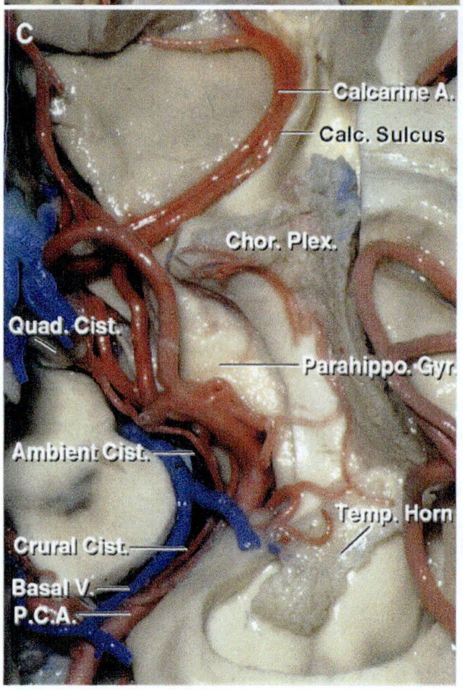

FIGURE 5.6. Superior views of the anterior, middle, and posterior incisural spaces. *A* and *B* are from one specimen and *C* is from another. *A,* the basal cisterns in the region of the tentorial incisura have been exposed by removing the thalamus and all of the left cerebral hemisphere except the occipital and temporal lobes. The roof of the temporal horn has been removed. The structures related to the anterior incisural space, located between the tuberculum sellae anteriorly, the midbrain posteriorly, and the anterior tentorial edge laterally, includes the optic nerve and chiasm, and the internal carotid, basilar, superior cerebellar, and PCAs. The anterior incisural space opens posteriorly into the middle incisural space, which extends into the crural and ambient cisterns. The crural cistern is located between the cerebral peduncle and the uncus, and the ambient cistern is located between the lateral midbrain and the medial surface of the temporal lobe. The ambient cistern opens posteriorly into the posterior incisural space, which contains the quadrigeminal cistern. The basal vein and the PCA and SCA pass around the midbrain in the middle incisural space to reach the posterior incisural space and quadrigeminal cistern. *B,* enlarged view. The preserved tentorial edge is exposed between the basal vein and trochlear nerve. *C,* superior view of the middle and posterior incisural space in another specimen. The basal vein courses through the crural and ambient cisterns. The upper lip of the calcarine sulcus has been removed but the lower lip of the sulcus has been preserved. The calcarine branch of the PCA loops laterally into the calcarine sulcus, which extends so deeply into the medial part of the hemisphere that it forms a prominence, the calcar avis, in the lower part of the medial wall of the atrium. *A.,* artery; *A.C.A.,* anterior cerebral artery; *Ant.,* anterior; *Car.,* carotid; *Calc.,* calcarine; *Cer.,* cerebral; *Chor.,* choroid, choroidal; *Cist.,* cistern; *CN,* cranial nerve; *Comm.,* communicating; *Gyr.,* gyrus; *Incis.,* incisural; *Int.,* internal; *Interped.,* interpeduncular; *M.C.A.,* middle cerebral artery; *Mid.,* middle; *Parahippo.,* parahippocampal; *P.C.A.,* posterior cerebral artery; *Plex.,* plexus; *Post.,* posterior; *Quad.,* quadrigeminal; *Sulc.,* sulcus; *Temp.,* temporal; *Tent.,* tentorial; *V.,* vein.

cerebral peduncle and a smaller posterior part formed by the tegmental surface. The optic tract forms a smooth white band at the upper edge of the cerebral peduncle that stands in sharp contrast to the vertically striated surface of the peduncle. The peduncular and tegmental surfaces are separated by the lateral mesencephalic sulcus, a vertical groove that extends from the pulvinar above to the pontomesencephalic sulcus below.

The roof of the middle incisural space has a narrow anterior part formed by the posterior part of the optic tract that is flattened between the cerebral peduncle and the uncus, and a wider posterior part formed by the inferior surface of the thalamus (*Fig. 5.4*). The lateral geniculate body protrudes from the lower surface of the thalamus just behind the uncus. The medial geniculate body bulges into the roof posteromedial to the lateral geniculate body just behind the lateral mesencephalic sulcus.

The lateral wall of the supratentorial part of the middle incisural space is composed of the hippocampal formation on the medial surface of the temporal lobe (*Figs. 5.3* and *5.4*). The uncus and parahippocampal gyri, the most inferior structures

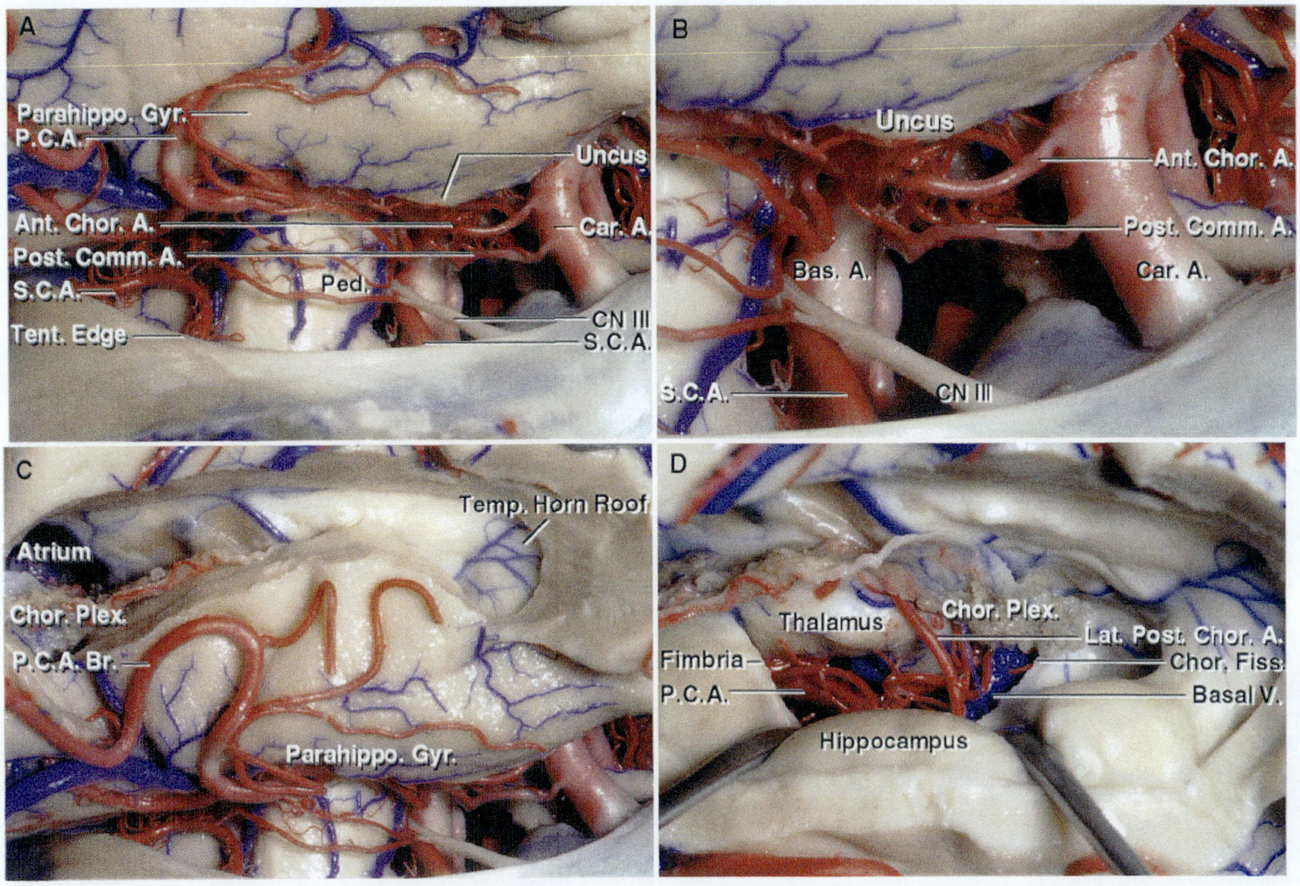

FIGURE 5.7. ***A–D.*** **Anterior and middle incisural space.** ***A,*** **the right temporal lobe has been elevated. The middle incisural space, located between the lateral surface of the midbrain and the tentorial edge, opens upward into the ambient cistern where the PCA and basal vein course. The internal carotid artery is exposed in front of the midbrain in the anterior incisural space.** ***B,*** **enlarged view of the junction of the anterior and middle incisural space. The internal carotid artery, optic nerves, and basilar bifurcation are located in the anterior incisural space. The oculomotor nerve passes forward between the PCA and SCA.** ***C,*** **the inferior temporal and fusiform gyri have been removed to expose the lateral edge of the parahippocampal gyrus above the middle incisural space. The opening into the temporal horn exposes the choroid plexus attached along the choroidal fissure. The veins draining the roof of the temporal horn empty into the basal vein.** ***D,*** **the choroidal fissure has been opened by detaching the choroid plexus from the fimbria of the fornix. Opening the fissure exposes the upper part of the ambient cistern and the branches of the PCA and basal vein.** ***A.,*** **artery;** ***Ant.,*** **anterior;** ***Bas.,*** **basilar;** ***Br.,*** **branch;** ***Car.,*** **carotid;** ***Chor.,*** **choroid, choroidal;** ***Cist.,*** **cistern;** ***CN,*** **cranial nerve;** ***Comm.,*** **communicating;** ***Coll.,*** **colliculus;** ***Fiss.,*** **fissure;** ***Gen.,*** **geniculate;** ***Gyr.,*** **gyrus;** ***Inf.,*** **inferior;** ***Lat.,*** **lateral;** ***Med.,*** **medial;** ***Mes.,*** **mesencephalic;** ***Parahippo.,*** **parahippocampal;** ***P.C.A.,*** **posterior cerebral artery;** ***Ped.,*** **peduncle;** ***Plex.,*** **plexus;** ***Post.,*** **posterior;** ***S.C.A.,*** **superior cerebellar artery;** ***Sup.,*** **superior;** ***Temp.,*** **temporal;** ***Tent.,*** **tentorial;** ***V.,*** **vein;** ***Vent.,*** **ventricular.**

in this part of the lateral wall, form a curved border around the middle incisural space. The uncus bulges medially at the anterior end of the parahippocampal gyrus. The amygdaloid nucleus is situated just lateral to the medial surface of the uncus and just anterior to the tip of the temporal horn.

The uncus commonly prolapses into the incisura anteriorly and has a groove along its undersurface marking the free edge (*Fig. 5.4*). This groove usually disappears at the lateral margin of the peduncle, because the free edge often hugs the peduncle at this site, but it may reappear posterior to the peduncle on the lower surface of the parahippocampal gyrus as the space between the brainstem and the free edge increases. In our specimens, these grooves were commonly present on the uncus and adjacent part of the parahippocampal gyrus without being observed on the posterior part of the parahippocampal gyrus, but they were only rarely present posteriorly, and not anteriorly (17). The distance from the most medial point of the uncus to this groove varied from 2 to 8.6 mm (average, 4.4 mm). Howell reported that these grooves may measure up to 15 mm in length and lie as far as 10 mm from the medial tip of the uncus (10). Klintworth (12, 13) noted unilateral uncal grooving in 88.4% of brains and bilateral grooving in 80%.

Posterior to the uncus, the surface of the temporal lobe facing the middle incisural space is formed by three longitu-

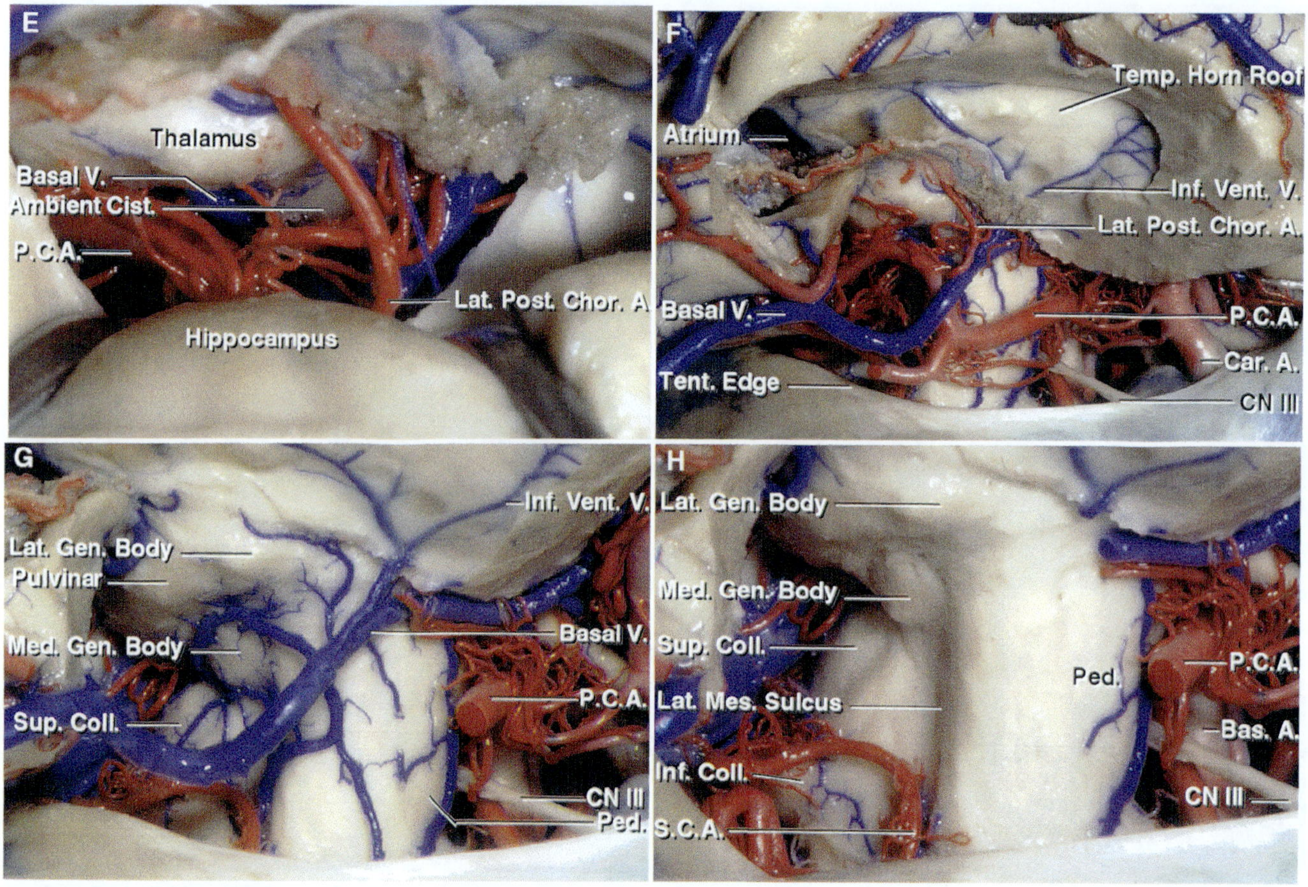

FIGURE 5.7. ***E–H. E,*** **anterior and middle incisural space, enlarged view. The opening through the choroidal fissure exposes the basal vein and branches of the PCA in the upper part of the ambient cistern. The PCA gives off numerous branches to the choroid plexus, including a large lateral posterior choroidal artery.** ***F,*** **the hippocampus and the medial part of the temporal lobe, including the parahippocampal gyrus, have been removed to expose the upper part of the middle incisural space. The PCA and basal vein course through the middle incisural space on the medial side of the parahippocampal gyrus, which has been removed. The choroid plexus remains attached along the choroidal fissure located between the fimbria and the lower surface of the thalamus. The inferior ventricular veins drain the roof of the temporal horn and empty into the basal vein.** ***G,*** **the branches of the PCA have been removed to expose the basal vein, which originates below the anterior perforated substance and courses posteriorly through the middle incisural space to gain access to the posterior incisural space and the quadrigeminal cistern. The pulvinar and lower surface of the thalamus, including the geniculate bodies, are in the upper margin of the exposure.** ***H,*** **the basal vein has been removed. This exposes the lateral aspect of the cerebral peduncle and the tegmental part of the midbrain, which are separated by the lateral mesencephalic sulcus. The medial and lateral geniculate bodies protrude downward from the lower surface of the thalamus.**

dinal strips of neural tissue, one located above the other, which are interlocked with the hippocampal formation to make an important part of the limbic system (*Figs. 5.3* and *5.4*). The most inferior strip is formed by the rounded medial edge of the parahippocampal gyrus; the middle strip is formed by the dentate gyrus, a serrated or beaded strip of gray matter located on the medial surface of the hippocampal formation; and the superior strip is formed by the fimbria of the fornix, a white band formed by the fibers emanating from the hippocampal formation that are directed posteriorly into the crus of the fornix.

The middle incisural space extends below the tentorium to communicate with the anterior part of the cerebellomesencephalic fissure, located between the anterosuperior part of the cerebellum and the lateral surface of the tegmentum.

Cisternal relationships

The supratentorial part of the middle incisural space contains the crural and ambient cisterns (*Figs. 5.2–5.6*). The crural cistern, located between the cerebral peduncle and the uncus, is a posterolateral extension of the interpeduncular cistern. The crural cistern opens posteriorly into the ambient cistern, demarcated medially by the midbrain, above by the pulvinar, and laterally by the parahippocampal and dentate gyri and fimbria of the fornix. The ambient cistern is continuous posteriorly with the quadrigeminal cistern, the major cistern in the posterior incisural space. The ambient cistern extends below the free edge into the part of the cerebellomesencephalic fissure located above the origin of the trigeminal nerve.

Ventricular relationships

The temporal horn extends into the medial part of the temporal lobe lateral to the middle incisural space and ends approximately 3 cm from the temporal pole (*Figs. 5.2–5.7*). The choroidal fissure, located between the fimbria of the fornix and the lower surface of the thalamus, is the site of attachment of the choroid plexus in the temporal horn. The paired bodies of the lateral ventricles are located directly above the central part of the incisura. They sit on and are separated from the central part of the incisura by the thalamus.

Cranial nerves

The trochlear and trigeminal nerves are related to the middle incisural space (*Fig. 5.8*). The trochlear nerve has the longest course within the incisura of any nerve and is the cranial nerve most intimately related to the free edge. The trochlear nerve arises below the inferior colliculus in the posterior incisural space and passes forward through the middle incisural space between the PCA and SCA. Its initial course around the midbrain is medial to the free edge in the space between the tectum and cerebellum. It reaches the lower margin of the free

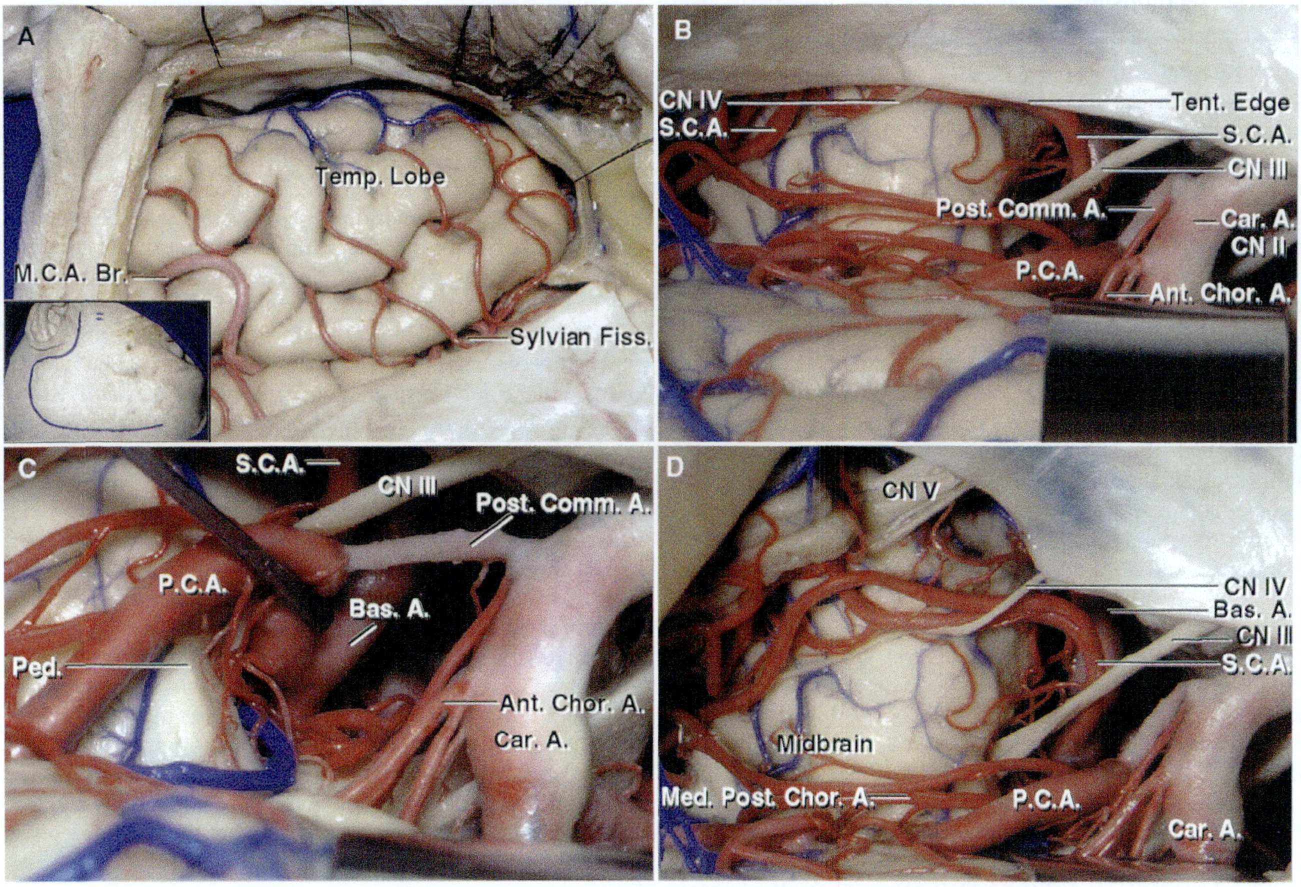

FIGURE 5.8. Anterior and middle subtemporal exposure of the anterior and adjacent part of the middle incisural space. *A*, the craniotomy flap and dural opening exposes the temporal lobe and the floor of the middle cranial fossa. The insert shows the site of the scalp incision. *B*, the temporal lobe has been elevated to expose the PCA and SCA in the anterior and middle incisural space. The PCA passes above and the SCA below the oculomotor nerve. The SCA branches course with the trochlear nerve around the side of the brainstem. *C*, the PCA has been depressed to expose the basilar artery. The anterior choroidal artery arises in the anterior incisural space and passes between the cerebral peduncle and uncus to enter the crural cistern in the middle incisural space. *D*, the tentorium has been divided behind the petrous ridge to expose the SCA and the trigeminal and trochlear nerves in the region of the middle incisural space. The SCA sends branches above the trigeminal nerve and into the anterior part of the cerebellomesencephalic fissure. The medial posterior choroidal artery also passes around the lateral side of the brainstem. *A.*, artery; *Ant.*, anterior; *Bas.*, basilar; *Br.*, branch; *Car.*, carotid; *Chor.*, choroidal, *CN*, cranial nerve; *Comm.*, communicating; *Fiss.*, fissure; *M.C.A.*, middle cerebral artery; *Med.*, medial; *P.C.A.*, posterior cerebral artery; *Ped.*, peduncle; *Post.*, posterior; *S.C.A.*, superior cerebellar artery; *Temp.*, temporal; *Tent.*, tentorial.

edge at the posterior edge of the cerebral peduncle. It pierces the free edge in the posterior part of the oculomotor trigone and runs for a short distance in the anterior petroclinoid fold before entering the lateral wall of the cavernous sinus.

The trigeminal nerve courses in the infratentorial part of the middle incisural compartment. It arises on the anterolateral aspect of the mid pons and passes above the petrous apex to enter Meckel's cave (the arachnoidal and dural cavern) where it separates into the three sensory divisions (6). The medial edge of the posterior trigeminal root is observed just medial to the tentorial edge if one looks from straight superior through the incisura with the cerebrum removed, but it is hidden below the free edge in the lateral view provided by the subtemporal operative exposure.

Arterial relationships

The major arteries in the middle incisural space, the anterior choroidal, PCA, and SCA, arise in the anterior incisural space and reach the middle incisural space by coursing around the brainstem parallel to the free edge (*Figs. 5.5–5.8*). The anterior choroidal artery enters the superior part of the middle incisural space below the optic tract and passes through the choroidal fissure near the inferior choroidal point to supply the choroid plexus in the temporal horn.

The PCA enters the middle incisural space between the cerebral peduncle and uncus and passes straight posteriorly between the tegmentum and subiculum (*Figs. 5.6* and *5.8*). It gives off several cortical branches, which cross the free edge to reach the inferior surface of the temporal and occipital lobes, and the lateral posterior choroidal and thalamogeniculate arteries, which course medial to the free edge. The lateral posterior choroidal arteries, arising in the middle incisural space, course superolaterally through the choroidal fissure and around the pulvinar to reach the choroid plexus in the temporal horn and atrium (*Fig. 5.7*). The medial posterior choroidal artery arises from the proximal part of the PCA in the anterior incisural space and courses parallel and medial to the PCA through the middle incisural space to reach the posterior incisural space (*Fig. 5.5*). The thalamogeniculate branches arise below the pulvinar and pass upward through the geniculate bodies to reach the thalamus and internal capsule.

The SCA usually passes below the level of the free edge and bifurcates into rostral and caudal trunks as it passes around the lateral margin of the cerebral peduncle to enter the middle incisural spaces (*Figs. 5.7* and *5.8*). It passes above the trigeminal nerve and enters the cerebellomesencephalic fissure in the anterior part of the middle incisural space. The walls of the supratentorial part of the middle incisural space are supplied by the perforating branches of the anterior choroidal and PCA, and the walls in the infratentorial part are supplied by the SCA.

Venous relationships

The venous relationships in the middle incisural space are relatively simple (*Figs. 5.5–5.7*). The basal vein courses along the upper part of the cerebral peduncle and below the pulvinar to reach the posterior incisural space. It may infrequently terminate in a tentorial sinus in the free edge at this level.

POSTERIOR INCISURAL SPACE

Neural relationships

The posterior incisural space lies posterior to the midbrain and corresponds to the pineal region (*Figs. 5.1–5.4*) (33). It has a roof, floor, and anterior and lateral walls, and extends backward to the level of the tentorial apex. The quadrigeminal plate is located at the center of the anterior wall. The anterior wall rostral to the colliculi is formed by the pineal body. The habenular commissure forms the upper half and the posterior commissure forms the lower half of the attachment of the pineal body to the posterior part of the third ventricle. The part of the anterior wall below the colliculi is formed in the midline by the lingula of the vermis and laterally by the superior cerebellar peduncles as they ascend beside the lingula.

The roof of the posterior incisural space is formed by the lower surface of the splenium, the terminal part of the crura of the fornices, and the hippocampal commissure (*Figs. 5.1* and *5.4*). Each crus arises as a continuation of the fimbria, passes around the posterior margin of the pulvinar, and blends into the lower margin of the splenium. The hippocampal commissure is an oblique band of fibers that courses below the splenium between the medial margins of the crura. The floor of the posterior incisural space is formed by the anterosuperior part of the cerebellum and consists of the culmen of the vermis in the midline and the quadrangular lobules of the hemispheres laterally. The posterior incisural space extends inferiorly into the cerebellomesencephalic fissure.

Each lateral wall is formed by the pulvinar, crus of the fornix, and the medial surface of the cerebral hemisphere. The anterior part of the lateral wall is formed by the part of the pulvinar located just lateral to the pineal body. The lateral wall, posterior to the pulvinar, is formed by the segment of the crus of the fornix that wraps around the posterior margin of the pulvinar (*Fig. 5.1*). The posterior part of the lateral walls is formed by the cortical areas located below the splenium on the medial surface of the hemisphere. These areas include the posterior part of the parahippocampal and dentate gyri. The posterior part of the parahippocampal gyrus usually extends medially above the posterior part of the free edge and may have shallow grooves from the free edge on its lower surface.

Cisternal relationships

The quadrigeminal cistern, situated posterior to the quadrigeminal plate, is the major cistern in the posterior incisural space (*Figs. 5.1–5.4*). The quadrigeminal cistern communicates above with the posterior pericallosal cistern; inferiorly into the cerebellomesencephalic fissure; inferolaterally into the posterior part of the ambient cistern located between the midbrain and the parahippocampal gyrus; and laterally into the retrothalamic areas medial to where the crus of the fornix wraps the posterior part of the pulvinar. The quadrigeminal cistern may communicate with the velum interpositum, a space that extends forward into the roof of the third ventricle between the splenium above and the pineal body below.

Ventricular relationships

The posterior portion of the third ventricle and the cerebral aqueduct are anterior and the atria and occipital horns of the lateral ventricles are lateral to the posterior incisural space (*Figs. 5.2–5.4*). The aqueduct passes ventral to the anterior wall of the posterior incisural space. The atrium is separated from the posterior incisural space by the crus of the fornix as it passes posterior to the pulvinar and by the cortical gyri located in the lateral wall of the posterior incisural space.

Arterial relationships

The trunks and branches of the PCA and SCA enter the posterior incisural space from anteriorly (*Figs. 5.5* and *5.6*). The PCA courses through the lateral part of the posterior incisural space and bifurcates into the calcarine and parieto-occipital arteries near where it crosses above the free edge. The medial posterior choroidal arteries enter the posterior incisural space from anteriorly, turn forward beside the pineal body, and enter the velum interpositum to supply the choroid plexus in the roof of the third ventricle and the body of the lateral ventricle. The lateral posterior choroidal arteries that arise in the posterior incisural space pass around the posteromedial surface of the pulvinar and through the choroidal fissure to supply the choroid plexus in the atrium, giving branches to the thalamus along the way.

The SCA is coursing within the cerebellomesencephalic fissure when it reaches the posterior incisural space. These branches, upon exiting the cerebellomesencephalic fissure, are anterior to the free edge, but they pass below the free edge to supply the tentorial surface of the cerebellum (*Fig. 5.2*).

The perforating branches of the PCA and SCA, and the medial posterior choroidal arteries supply the walls of the posterior incisural space. The PCAs supply the structures above the level of the lower margin of the superior colliculi and the SCAs supply the structures below the upper margin of the inferior colliculus.

Venous relationships

The posterior incisural space has the most complex venous relationships in the cranium, because the internal cerebral and basal veins and many of their tributaries converge on the vein of Galen within this area (*Figs. 5.1, 5.5,* and *5.6*). The internal cerebral veins exit the velum interpositum and the basal veins exit the ambient cistern to reach the posterior incisural space, where they join to form the vein of Galen. The vein of Galen passes below the splenium to enter the straight sinus at the tentorial apex. The junction of the vein of Galen with the straight sinus varies from being nearly flat if the tentorial apex is located below the splenium to forming a sharp angle if the apex is located above the splenium, so that the vein of Galen must turn sharply upward to reach the straight sinus at the apex. The largest vein from the infratentorial part of the posterior incisural space, the vein of the cerebellomesencephalic fissure, originates from the union of the paired veins of the superior cerebellar peduncle.

Tentorial arteries

The tentorial arteries arise from three sources (8). The first source, the cavernous segment of the carotid artery, provides two arteries: the basal tentorial artery (the artery of Bernasconi-Cassinari) from the meningohypophyseal trunk, and the marginal tentorial artery from the artery from the inferolateral trunk (also called the artery of the inferior cavernous sinus). The basal tentorial artery arises from the meningohypophyseal trunk and courses posterolaterally along the medial part of the tentorial attachment to the petrous ridge. The marginal tentorial artery arises from the inferolateral trunk, passes laterally over the abducens nerve, then superoposteriorly near the trochlear nerve to enter the tentorial edge. If this artery is absent, a branch from the meningohypophyseal artery may replace it (8, 28, 32).

The second source of tentorial arteries is from the SCA. The meningeal branch originates from the main or rostral trunk near where the artery passes under the tentorium, and it enters the free edge in the middle incisural space. In our specimens, 28% of the SCAs gave rise to a tentorial branch, and such a vessel may be encountered when the tentorium is divided through a subtemporal approach (17).

The third source is the proximal part of the PCA. The tentorial branch of the PCA arises as a long circumflex artery that courses around the brainstem and below the free edge to enter the tentorium near the apex (17, 37). This artery may also give branches to the superior vermis and inferior colliculi.

DISCUSSION

Tentorial herniation

Tentorial herniation is the most common and most important form of brain herniation (10, 12, 15). In descending herniation caused by supratentorial mass lesions, the uncus and parahippocampal gyri herniate downward through the incisura, and in ascending herniation resulting from infratentorial masses, the superior part of the cerebellum may herniate upward through the incisura. These brain herniations may cause combinations of direct effects caused by neural compression and indirect effects caused by vascular compromise. Symptoms may result from displacement, compression, and stretching of the brainstem and cranial nerves, hemorrhage and infarction caused by compression and tearing of arteries and veins, increasing edema and intracranial pressure caused by venous obstruction, hydrocephalus caused by obstruction of the aqueduct and subarachnoid space at the incisura, and strangulation of the prolapsed tissue.

The type of the tentorial herniation in each case depends on the position and rate of expansion of the lesion and the size and shape of the incisura. The signs appear early when structures are deformed rapidly, whereas advanced distortion may occur before the appearance of signs if the herniation develops slowly. A wide space between the free edge and brainstem facilitates cerebral herniation since more tissue can herniate into the space (20). A low position of the anterior portion of the free edge also facilitates descending herniation (20).

Descending herniations are divided into anterior, posterior, and complete types. In the anterior type, the uncus herniates into the interpeduncular and crural cisterns. This shift carries the brainstem to the opposite side, thus increasing the space between the free edge and the brainstem, and facilitating a further shift of tissue through the aperture. Eventually, the parahippocampal gyrus, from the splenium to the uncus, may be forced through the opening and the incisura becomes plugged with herniated temporal lobe, deformed hypothalamus, and compressed midbrain. The amygdaloid nucleus is involved with the uncus in the herniated mass. Distortion and compression of the midbrain reticular activating pathways causes a decreased level of consciousness. Compression of the ipsilateral cerebral peduncle causes contralateral pyramidal signs and, if the lateral displacement of brainstem is severe, the contralateral cerebral peduncle may be forced against the free edge, thus producing a groove on the peduncle called a Kernohan's notch, with ipsilateral pyramidal signs (30). In the terminal stage, deformation of the midbrain causes decerebrate rigidity. Distortion and compression of the posterior hypothalamus may cause cardiovascular, respiratory, and thermoregulatory disturbances. The pituitary stalk may be stretched and compressed against the dorsum sellae, causing diabetes insipidus. The oculomotor nerve courses between the medial border of the uncus and the posterior petroclinoidal fold, and may be kinked or compressed here or between the PCA and SCA, or it may be stretched as the hernia displaces the midbrain posteriorly. Initially, the pupilloconstrictor fibers, which are concentrated on the superior surface of the nerve, are compressed. Later, somatic fibers to the extraocular muscles are disturbed. In the early stages, irritation of the pupilloconstrictor fibers may cause pupillary constriction, but this usually gives way to a paralytic effect with pupillary dilation as the hernia enlarges. The optic tract is displaced medially and downward, but the resulting visual loss is often masked by deepening coma. Compression of the uncus, amygdaloid nucleus, parahippocampal gyrus, and hippocampal formation against the free edge may cause memory, behavior, and personality changes. Residual scarring of the hippocampal formation may cause seizures. The trochlear nerve usually escapes involvement in such herniations, but caudal displacement of the brainstem may result in a palsy of the abducens nerve by stretching it in the subarachnoid space or by strangling it in its course around the AICA.

Stretching or compression of the anterior choroidal and PCA between the temporal lobe and the peduncle or obstruction of the PCA as it crosses the free edge may cause visual field loss caused by ischemia of the optic tract, optic radiation, or the lateral geniculate body; contralateral hemiplegia caused by involvement of the cerebral peduncle and midbrain; or changes in personality and behavior caused by damage to the amygdaloid nucleus or hippocampal formation; unconsciousness and decerebrate rigidity caused by midbrain ischemia; and contralateral sensory loss caused by ischemia of the ventral thalamic nuclei. Brainstem hemorrhage frequently accompanies tentorial herniation.

In the posterior type of tentorial herniation, the posterior portion of the parahippocampal and lingual gyri and the isthmus of the cingular gyrus may shift through the incisura into the quadrigeminal cistern and compress and displace the dorsal half of the midbrain. Tectal compression may cause vertical gaze disturbances. Compression and obstruction of the aqueduct causes hydrocephalus and raises the intracranial pressure. In the posterior type of herniation, the PCA or its calcarine branch is pressed against the free edge and may be obstructed, causing infarction of the occipital cortex and hemianopsia. The basal vein may be compressed between the midbrain and herniated temporal lobe, and the vein of Galen may be obstructed as it curves around the splenium, thus aggravating the venous congestion, edema, and intracranial tension. The complete type of herniation yields a combination of signs and symptoms observed with anterior and posterior herniations.

Hemorrhage into the brainstem as a result of tearing of arteries and veins without cerebral herniation may occur if the incisura hugs the brainstem so tightly that it prevents cerebral herniation while allowing axial displacement of the brainstem.

In ascending herniation attributable to a posterior fossa mass lesion, the superior part of the cerebellar vermis and hemispheres herniate upward through the incisura into the quadrigeminal cistern. Cerebellar infarction may result from compression of the branches of the SCA where they pass under the free edge. The hernia may compress the great cerebral vein against the splenium, which is fixed above by the falx, thus increasing the venous congestion, edema, and intracranial pressure.

Pathology and operative approaches

Most aneurysms, many pineal, sellar, parasellar, and third ventricular tumors, and some anteriovenous malformations are approached through the incisural spaces. The arteries in the incisura have been subject to bypass procedures, and many operations for trigeminal neuralgia are directed through this area. In addition, structures bordering the area have been ablated either at craniotomy or stereotactically for the control of epilepsy. The selection of the best operative approach for a given lesion of the incisura depends on the space involved.

Anterior incisural space

Nearly 95% of saccular arterial aneurysms arise within the anterior incisural space. The basic anatomy of the common aneurysms has been reviewed elsewhere by Rhoton (23). The aneurysms arising from the part of the circle of Willis located anterior to Liliequist's membrane, and from the internal carotid and middle cerebral artery are most commonly approached through a frontotemporal (pterional) craniotomy (35) (*Fig. 5.9*). Aneurysms located behind Liliequist's membrane at the basilar apex in the interpeduncular fossa may be exposed through either a frontotemporal or subtemporal craniotomy if they are located above the dorsum sellae (35, 36)

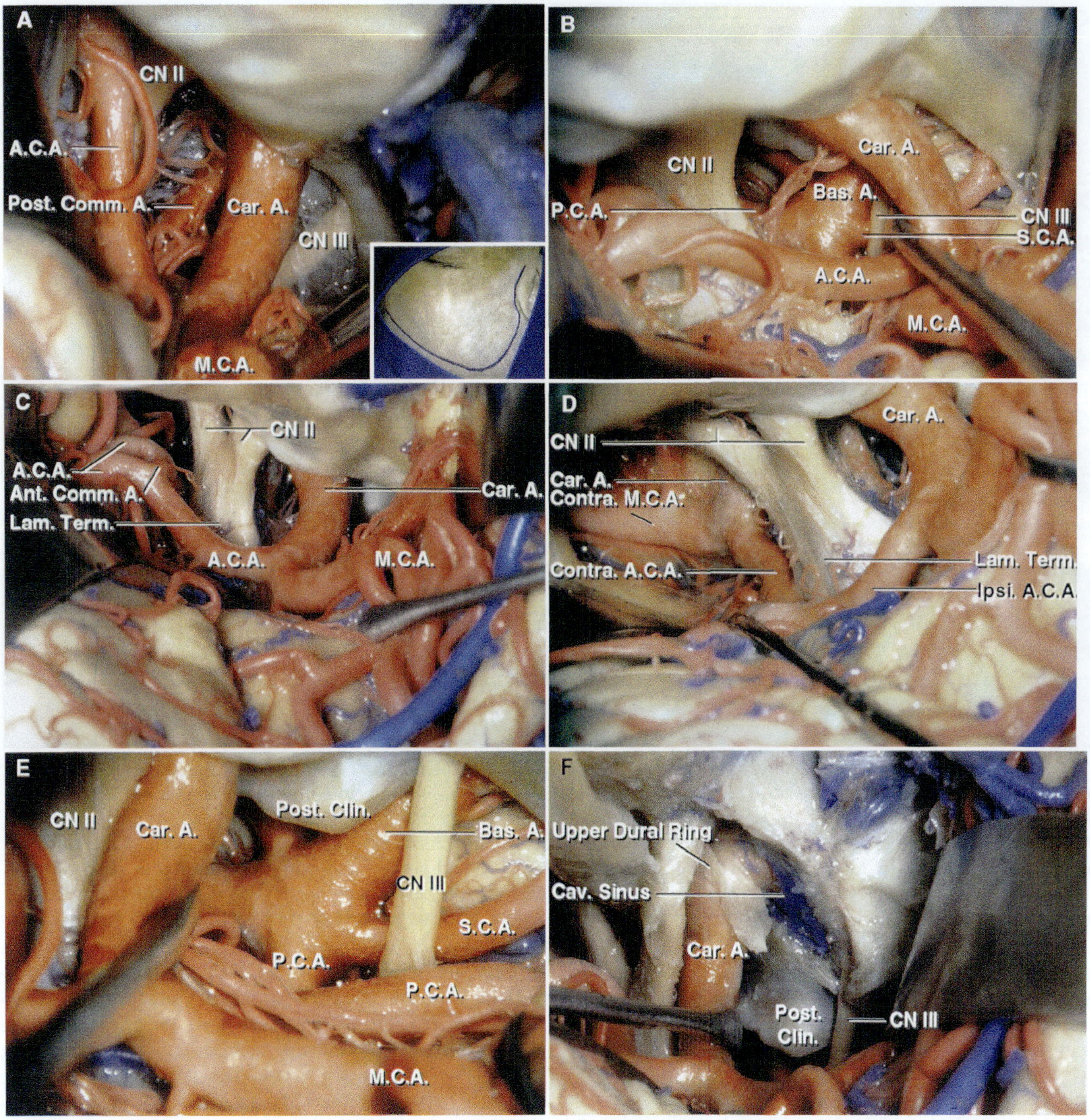

FIGURE 5.9. *A–F.* Exposure of the anterior incisural space through a frontotemporal craniotomy. *A,* the insert shows the site of the craniotomy. The frontal and temporal lobes have been retracted to expose the optic and oculomotor nerves and the anterior and middle cerebral and posterior communicating arteries. *B,* the opticocarotid triangle, located between the optic nerve and the carotid and anterior cerebral arteries, has been opened with gentle retraction to expose the basilar apex and the ipsilateral oculomotor nerve passing forward between the PCA and SCA. *C,* the exposure has been directed medially above the optic chiasm to expose the region of the anterior communicating artery. *D,* the frontal lobe has been elevated to expose the contralateral carotid and anterior and middle cerebral arteries. *E,* the carotid artery has been elevated to expose the basilar artery apex through the interval between the carotid artery and oculomotor nerve. The posterior clinoid process blocks access to the basilar artery. *F,* the anterior clinoid process and the roof of the cavernous sinus have been removed to provide access to the posterior clinoid process. The upper dural ring is located at the level of the upper margin of the anterior clinoid process. *A.,* artery; *A.C.A.,* anterior cerebral artery; *Ant.,* anterior; *Bas.,* basilar; *Car.,* carotid; *Cav.,* cavernous; *Clin.,* clinoid; *CN,* cranial nerve; *Comm.,* communicating; *Contra.,* contralateral; *Ipsi.,* ipsilateral; *Lam.,* lamina; *M.C.A.,* middle cerebral artery; *P.C.A.,* posterior cerebral artery; *Post.,* posterior; *S.C.A.,* superior cerebellar artery; *Term.,* terminalis; *V1.,* first ophthalmic branch, trigeminal nerve.

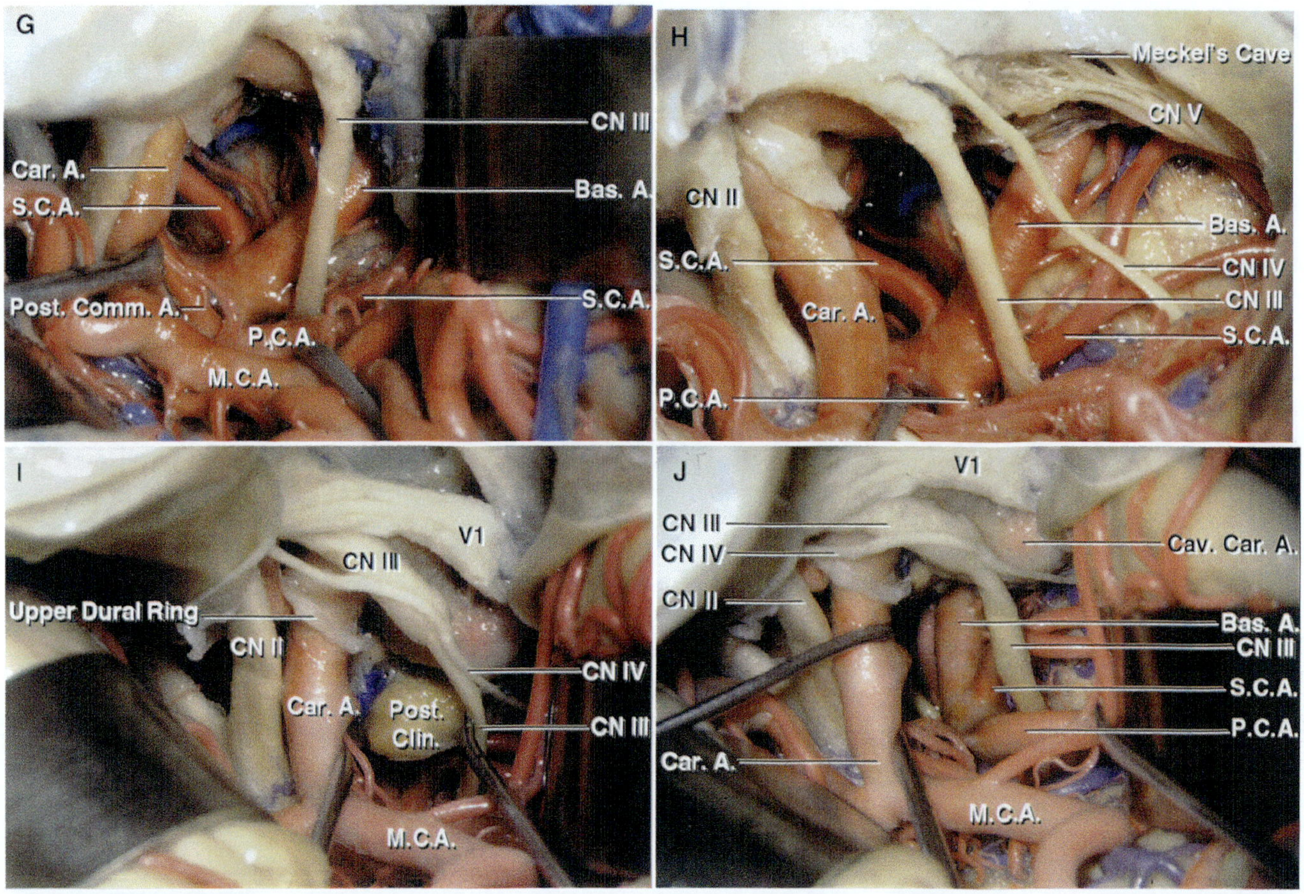

FIGURE 5.9. ***G–J.*** **Exposure of the anterior incisural space through a frontotemporal craniotomy.** ***G,*** **the posterior clinoid process has been removed to increase access to the upper portion of the basilar artery.** ***H,*** **the anterior part of the tentorial edge has been removed to expose the upper margin of the posterior trigeminal root in Meckel's cave and to provide increased access to the upper anterior part of the posterior fossa. The trochlear nerve was preserved in opening the anterior part of the tentorial edge.** ***I,*** **another dissection in which the anterior clinoid process and roof of the cavernous sinus were removed to expose the posterior clinoid process in the interval between the carotid anteriorly and the oculomotor posteriorly.** ***J,*** **the posterior clinoid was removed to provide increased access to the upper part of the basilar artery.**

(*Figs. 5.8* and *5.9*). Those located below the dorsum or in the prepontine cistern may require a pretemporal, anterior, or mid subtemporal craniotomy with incision or retraction of the tentorium (*Fig. 5.7*).

Incision and retraction of the tentorium are commonly required to gain access to lesions around the incisura. The incision in the tentorium to expose the interpeduncular and prepontine cisterns is usually located just posterior to the point where the trochlear nerve enters the free edge. The free edge may be retracted by means of sutures placed near to it, but special care is required to avoid stretching and damaging the trochlear nerve in its course inferomedial to and entering the free edge near the posterior margin of the oculomotor trigone. The tentorial arteries and venous sinuses may be encountered in sectioning the tentorium (16). Sectioning of the tentorium has been used to alleviate pressure on the brainstem caused by large incisural lesions that cannot be removed (2).

Perforating arteries to the brainstem are at greatest risk in approaches to the anterior incisural space, because they are commonly stretched around lesions in this area. Hypoplastic arterial segments in the circle of Willis should not be sacrificed during the exposure because hypoplastic segments have been found to have the same number and size of perforating branches as arteries of a normal diameter (23).

Tumors arising in or extending into the anterior incisural space include pituitary adenomas, craniopharyngiomas, clival chordomas, meningiomas arising from the tuberculum sellae, clivus, and medial part of the sphenoid ridge, gliomas of the optic nerve and hypothalamus, some dermoid cysts and teratomas, and neuromas of the oculomotor nerve. Tumors in the anterior incisural space may be approached by the bifrontal, subfrontal, frontal-interhemispheric, frontotemporal, subtemporal, and transsphenoidal routes. Tumors located anterior to Liliequist's membrane between the optic chiasm and the sellar floor are commonly operated on by the transsphenoidal or subfrontal route. The transsphenoidal approach is preferred if the tumor extends upward out of an enlarged sella turcica and is located above a pneumatized sphenoid sinus. The subfrontal intracranial approach is reserved for those tumors in the chiasmatic cistern that are not accessible by the transsphenoidal route because they are located entirely above the diaphragma sellae, or extend upward out of a normal or small sella, or are located above a nonpneumatized (conchal) type of sphenoid sinus. The subfrontal approach permits exposure of the tumor within the anterior incisural space by four routes: 1) the subchiasmatic approach between the optic nerves and below the optic chiasm; 2) the opticocarotid route directed between the optic nerve and carotid artery; 3) the lamina terminalis approach directed above the optic chiasm through a thinned lamina terminalis; and 4) the transfrontal-transsphenoidal approach obtained by entering the sphenoid sinus and sella through the transfrontal craniotomy (22, 25, 26). The subchiasmatic approach is used if the subchiasmatic opening is enlarged by the tumor. The opticocarotid route is selected if parasellar extension of the tumor widens the space between the carotid artery and the optic nerve and the tumor cannot be reached by the subchiasmatic approach. The lamina terminalis approach is selected if the tumor has pushed the chiasm into a prefixed position and extends into the third ventricle to stretch the lamina terminalis so that the tumor is visible through it. The transfrontal-transsphenoidal approach is selected if the tumor grows upward out of the sella, the sphenoid sinus is pneumatized and the tumor does not stretch the lamina terminalis or widen the opticocarotid space, and a prefixed chiasm blocks the subchiasmatic exposure. A bifrontal craniotomy may be used if the tumor extends forward in both anterior cranial fossae and cannot be reached by a unilateral subfrontal exposure. A frontal interhemispheric approach directed along the anterior part of the falx is used for lesions restricted to the part of the anterior interhemispheric space located just below the rostrum, especially if the tumor arises in the genu or rostrum of and grows into the anterior incisural space.

The frontotemporal approach is used for a tumor arising from the sphenoid ridge or anterior clinoid process, or if it arises above the diaphragma and extends along the sphenoid ridge or into the middle cranial fossa, or if the lesion is accessible through the spaces between the optic nerve and carotid artery or between the carotid artery and the oculomotor nerve (*Fig. 5.9*). Some lesions may require that the above approach be combined with resection of the cranial base if the lesion involves the paranasal sinuses, nasal cavity, pharynx, orbit, or cavernous sinus, and for those extending from the anterior incisural space into the area behind the dorsum sella or petrous apex, and those in which the lower opening provided by cranial base resection will yield a better angle of exposure or reduce the need for brain retraction. These approaches include the transcranial-transbasal, extended frontal, fronto-orbital, orbitozygomatic, transcavernous, preauricular-infratemporal, and subtemporal anterior petrousectomy, some of which are discussed more fully in the chapters on the foramen magnum and temporal bone.

Middle incisural space

Lesions in the middle incisural space include meningiomas arising from Meckel's cave, the anterior part of the free edge and the petrous apex, gliomas of the temporal lobe and thalamus, anteriovenous malformations of the medial temporal lobe, and neuromas of the trochlear and trigeminal nerves. The infrequent aneurysms arising in the middle incisural space are usually located on the PCA at the origin of its first major cortical branch or on the SCA at its bifurcation into rostral and caudal trunks. Bypass operations using vein and arterial grafts have been applied to the trunks and branches of the posterior cerebral and superior cerebellar branches in the middle incisural space bordering the incisura. The middle incisural space is exposed in performing amygdalohippocampectomy and temporal lobectomy for epilepsy since both the amygdalae and hippocampus extend medial to the free edge. The trigeminal nerve is also frequently exposed in the middle incisural space in the course of operations for trigeminal neuralgia.

Approaches to the middle incisural space include the posterior frontotemporal, subtemporal, temporal-transventricular, and the lateral suboccipital routes (*Figs. 5.7* and *5.8*). The subtemporal approach with elevation of the temporal lobe is commonly used to expose lesions in the cisterns around the incisura. Hemorrhage, venous infarction, and edema following retraction of the temporal lobe during this approach are minimized by placing the lower margin of the craniotomy and dural exposure at the cranial base so as to reduce the need for retraction, and by avoiding occlusion of the bridging veins, especially the vein of Labbé. The tentorium is frequently divided to increase the exposure or to decompress the brainstem when mass lesions are impacted in the incisura (2). Resection of part of the parahippocampal gyrus may facilitate exposure of the upper part of the middle incisural space (1). A transventricular approach using a cortical incision in the nondominant inferior or middle temporal gyrus may be used if the lesion involves the temporal horn, choroidal fissure, hippocampal formation, or the upper part of the middle incisural space (9). A cortical incision in the medial occipitotemporal gyrus on the inferior surface of the temporal lobe has been used to minimize visual and speech deficits in exposing the temporal horn of the dominant hemisphere. After entering the temporal horn, the choroidal fissure is opened to expose the middle incisural space. The subtemporal craniectomy may be combined with a suboccipital craniectomy with section of the tentorium and transverse sinus to remove lesions in the prepontine or cerebellopontine cisterns. The trochlear nerve is the cranial nerve most frequently injured in the middle incisural space. It can be injured in dividing the free edge and is so thin and friable that it may rupture from gentle retraction on the leaves formed by dividing the tentorium. The above approaches may be combined with cranial base approaches involving resection or mobilization of the orbital rim, zygomatic arch, floor of the middle fossa, or a portion of the temporal bone as are accomplished in the orbitozygomatic craniotomy, and the preauricular infratemporal or anterior petrousectomy approaches.

The posterior trigeminal root is frequently exposed through a lateral suboccipital craniectomy in the infratentorial part of the middle incisural space for rhizotomy or microvascular decompression operations. The exposure is directed along the

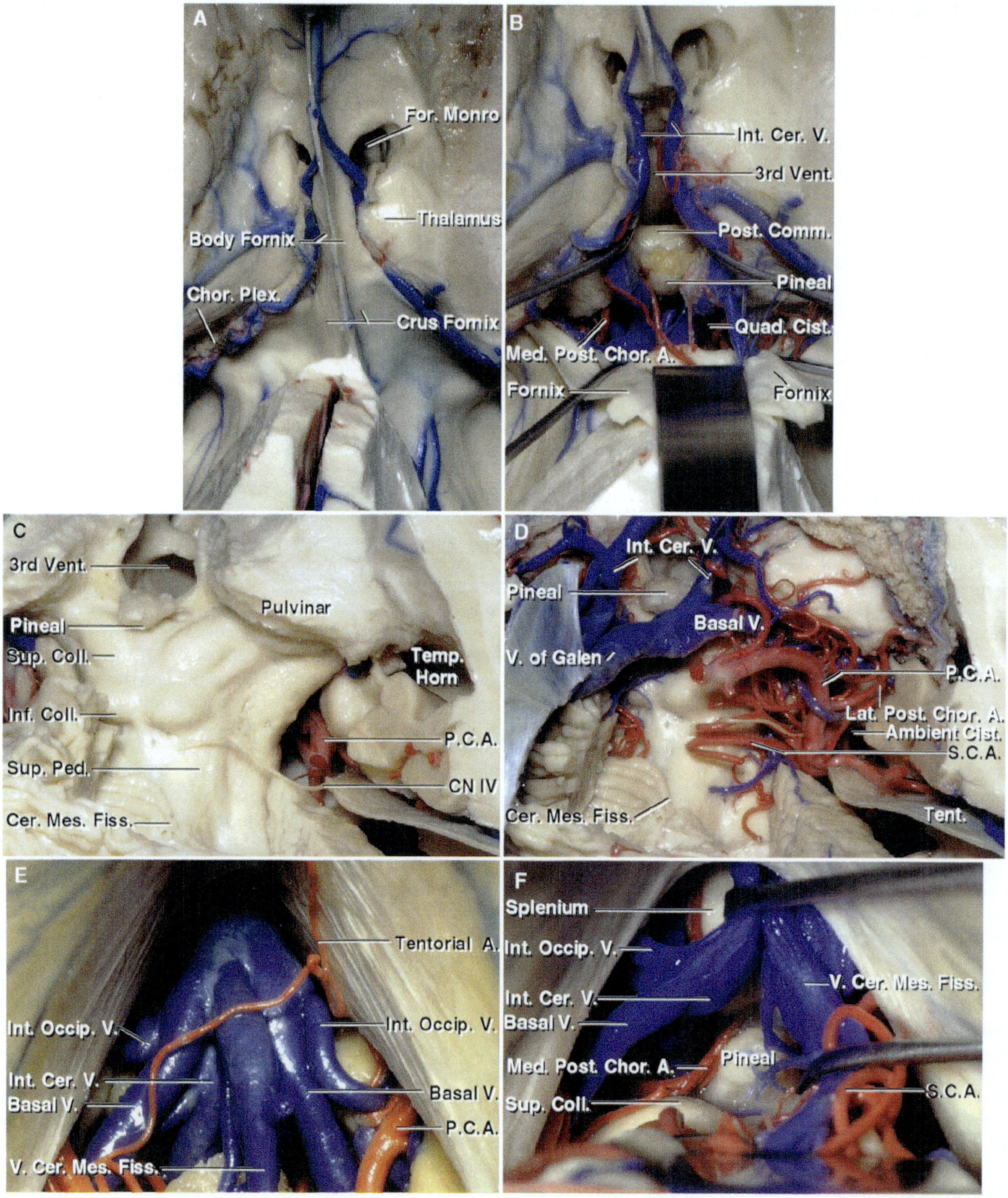

FIGURE 5.10. *A–F.* Comparison of the midline and paramedian infratentorial supracerebellar and the occipital transtentorial approaches to the quadrigeminal cistern and the posterior third ventricle. *A–D,* views of the third ventricle and quadrigeminal cistern. *A,* third ventricle from above. The body of the fornix separates the body of the lateral ventricle from the roof of the third ventricle. The body of the fornix blends posteriorly into the crus of the fornix, which is situated above the posterior part of the third ventricle. The choroidal fissure, the site of attachment of the choroid plexus, is situated between the fornix and thalamus. *B,* the fornix was divided at the level of the columns, just behind the foramen of Monro, and reflected

angle formed by the insertion of the tentorium to the petrous ridge. The posterior root proximal to Meckel's cave has also been exposed through a subtemporal craniectomy combined with incision of the tentorium (11). The posterior root may also be exposed for rhizotomy within Meckel's cave through a subtemporal extradural approach.

Posterior incisural space

Lesions in the posterior incisural space include pineal tumors; meningiomas arising at the falcotentorial junction and from the tela choroidea of the velum interpositum and atrium; gliomas of the splenium, pulvinar, quadrigeminal plate, and cerebellum; aneurysms of the vein of Galen; and anteriovenous malformations involving the medial occipital lobe and upper cerebellum.

Lesions in the posterior incisural space may be approached from above the tentorium along the medial surface of the occipital lobe using an occipital transtentorial approach, through the posterior part of the lateral ventricle using a posterior transventricular approach, and through the corpus callosum using a posterior interhemispheric transcallosal approach, or from below the tentorium through the supracerebellar space using an infratentorial supracerebellar approach (*Figs. 5.10* and *5.11*). The infratentorial supracerebellar and occipital transtentorial approaches, which are most commonly selected for pineal region tumors, may be combined with incision of the tentorium lateral to the straight sinus and less commonly with division of the tentorium and transverse sinus. A tentorial branch of the PCA or SCA may enter the dura lateral to the straight sinus. Venous sinuses are more commonly encountered in the posterior than in the anterior parts of the tentorium. Part of the tentorium may be removed in resecting tumors that arise from or invade it.

The infratentorial supracerebellar approach may be selected for lesions in the pineal region located below the vein of Galen and its major tributaries (29). The approach is best suited to tumors in the midline that grow into the lower half of the posterior incisural space, displacing the quadrigeminal plate and apex of the tentorial cerebellar surface. The occipital transtentorial approach is preferred for lesions centered at or above the tentorial edge, especially if they are located above the vein of Galen. The latter approach may also provide a better angle of access for some lesions involving the ipsilateral half of the cerebellomesencephalic fissure and posterior part of the ambient cistern, although they may be located below the level of the vein of Galen (21, 34) The posterior transcallosal approach, in which the splenium is divided, would be used only if the lesion appears to arise in the splenium above the vein of Galen and extends into the posterior incisural space. The posterior transventricular approach provides adequate exposure of the atrium and posterior portion of the body of the lateral ventricle and would be the preferred approach to a tumor involving the posterior incisural space if the tumor extends into the pulvinar or involves the atrium or the glomus of the choroid plexus. The preferable approach to the ventricle is through the superior parietal lobule, although on approach to the pineal region using a cortical incision in the superior temporal gyrus and directed through the atrium has been advocated (31).

Comparison of occipital transtentorial and infratentorial supracerebellar approaches

In examining the posterior incisural space, we compared the midline and paramedian variants of the infratentorial supracerebellar approach and the occipital transtentorial approach (*Figs. 5.10* and *5.11*). The midline infratentorial supracerebellar approach is directed steeply upward over the apex of the vermis where the large complex of veins emptying into the vein of Galen, and especially the vein of the cerebellomesencephalic fissure, blocks access to the pineal region. The venous complex could be gently displaced to expose the lower part of the splenium, the pineal, and the superior colliculus, but the prominent vermian apex forming the posterior lip of the cerebellomesencephalic fissure limits exposure below the level of the superior colliculus. In the paramedian variant of the infratentorial supracerebellar approach, the retraction was advanced above the hemisphere lateral to the vermis. This approach was not as upwardly steep as the approach above the vermian apex and provided access to the pineal region, the lower part of the splenium, and gave greater access to the ipsilateral half of the cerebellomesencephalic fissure. In addition, the approach could be advanced along the lateral part of the cerebellar surface to expose the posterior part of the ambient cistern. In the occipital

posteriorly to expose the posterior commissure, pineal, and adjacent part of the quadrigeminal cistern. *C,* the quadrigeminal cistern is located behind the pineal and the colliculi and between the pulvinars. It extends into the cerebellomesencephalic fissure. The trochlear nerves arise below the inferior colliculi. *D,* view similar to *C,* except that the vessels have been preserved. The internal cerebral and basal veins join the vein of Galen behind the pineal. The PCA and SCA exit the ambient cistern to enter the lateral part of the quadrigeminal cistern. Both the infratentorial supracerebellar and occipital transtentorial approaches are directed to this area. *E* and *F,* midline infratentorial supracerebellar approach. *E,* the venous complex emptying into the vein of Galen blocks access to the pineal region. This complex includes the internal occipital, basal and internal cerebral veins, and the vein of the cerebellomesencephalic fissure. A tentorial branch of the SCA crosses the exposure. *F,* the vein of Galen has been retracted to expose the splenium. The vein of the cerebellomesencephalic fissure has been retracted to expose the pineal. *A.,* artery; *Bridg.,* bridging; Cer., *cerebral; Cer. Mes.,* cerebellomesencephalic; *Chor.,* choroidal; *Cist.,* cistern; *CN,* cranial nerve; *Coll.,* colliculus; *Comm.,* communicating; *Fiss.,* fissure; *For.,* foramen; *Inf.,* inferior; *Int.,* internal; *Lat.,* lateral; *Med.,* medial; *Occip.,* occipital; *P.C.A.,* posterior cerebral artery; *Ped.,* peduncle; *Plex.,* plexus; *Post.,* posterior; *Quad.,* quadrigeminal; *Sag.,* sagittal; *S.C.A.,* superior cerebellar artery; *Str.,* straight; *Sup.,* superior; *Temp.,* temporal; *Tent.,* tentorial; *Trans.,* transverse; *V.,* vein; *Ve.,* vermian; *Vent.,* ventricle.

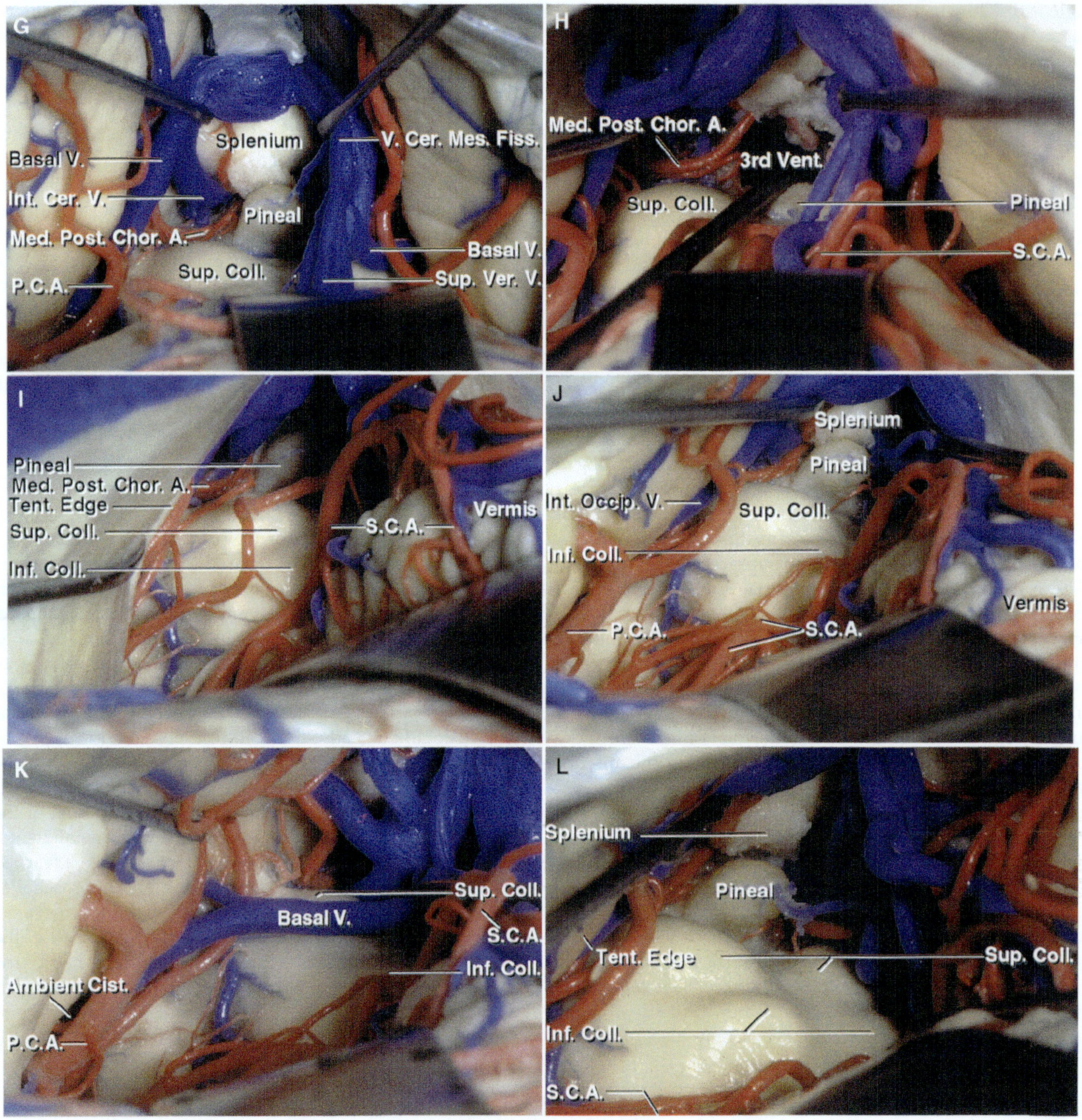

FIGURE 5.10. *G–L. G* and *H,* midline infratentorial supracerebellar approach. *G,* the left basal and internal cerebral veins have been elevated and the vein of the cerebellomesencephalic fissure, which is joined by a superior vermian vein, has been retracted to the right to expose the superior colliculus, pineal, and splenium. *H,* the tela choroidea attached to the upper surface of the pineal has been opened to expose the posterior part of the third ventricle. *I–L,* paramedian variant of the infratentorial supracerebellar approach. In this variant, the retraction of the tentorial surface is shifted off the vermis and tentorial apex to the paramedian part of the hemisphere. This paramedian variant of the approach accesses the lateral part of the quadrigeminal cistern and the posterior part of the ambient cistern and, in addition, provides a better view into the central and ipsilateral half of the cerebellomesencephalic fissure than the approach directed in the midline above the vermian apex. *I,* the retraction for the paramedian approach has been shifted to the left of the vermis. *J,* the left internal cerebral and internal occipital veins have been retracted to expose the posterior part of the splenium, the pineal and the superior and inferior colliculi, and the branches of the PCA and SCA exiting the ambient cistern. *K,* enlarged view. The exposure has been shifted to where the PCA exits the ambient cistern. *L,* the paramedian approach provides easier access to the superior and inferior colliculi and requires less retraction than is needed to expose these structures in the approach directed in the midline above the apex of the tentorial cerebellar surface.

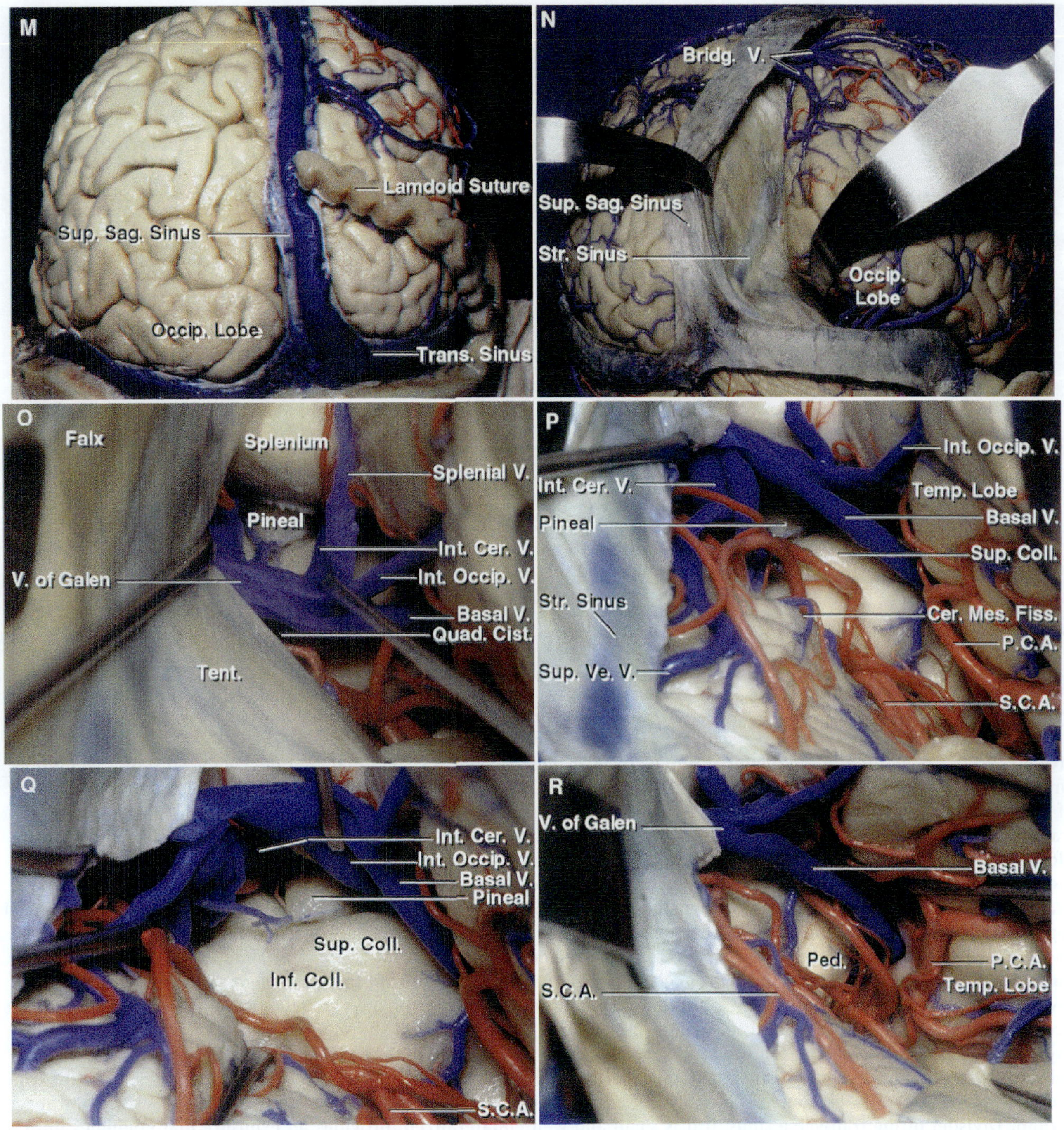

FIGURE 5.10. *M–R.* Occipital transtentorial approach. *M,* the occipital transtentorial is directed along the medial surface of the occipital lobe below the lambdoid suture. This occipital lobe below the lambdoid suture is commonly free of bridging veins to the superior sagittal sinus, making it a reasonable route for the occipital transtentorial approach. *N,* there are no large bridging veins between the posterior 6 cm of the occipital lobe and superior sagittal sinus. The first vein encountered is the internal occipital vein that passes from the anterior part of the medial occipital lobe to the vein of Galen. *O,* the vein of Galen has been retracted to expose the splenium and pineal from above. *P,* the tentorium has been opened lateral to the straight sinus, and the vein of Galen has been displaced to the left side to expose the pineal and the superior and inferior colliculi. *Q,* elevating the branches of the vein of Galen provides a satisfactory view into the quadrigeminal cistern, with a better view into the cerebellomesencephalic fissure than can be achieved with the infratentorial supracerebellar approach directed over the apex of the tentorial cerebellar surface. *R,* the exposure has been directed laterally along the side of the brainstem to the ambient cistern where the lateral margin of the cerebral peduncle is exposed.

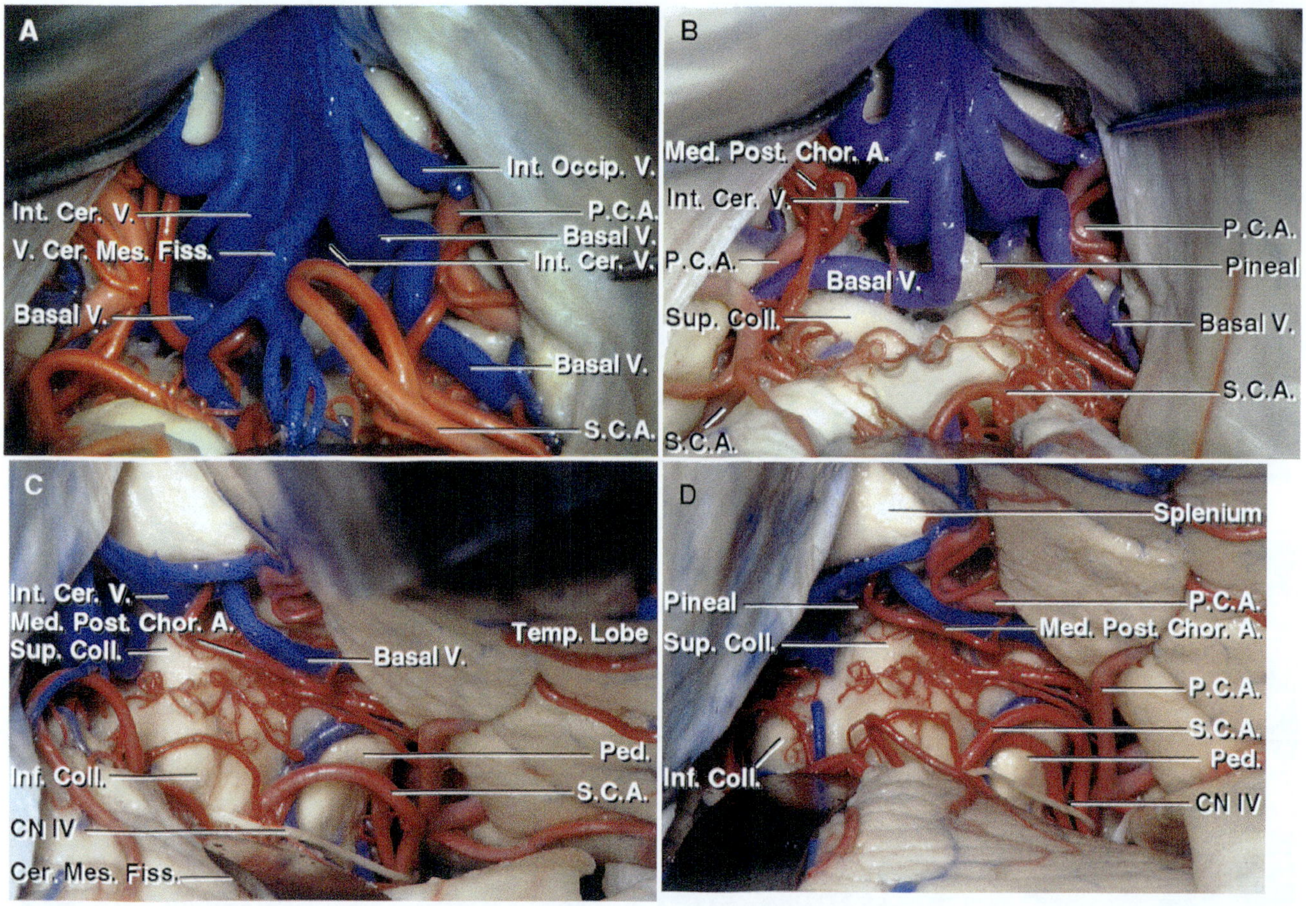

FIGURE 5.11. **Comparison of infratentorial supracerebellar, the occipital transtentorial, and the combined supra- and infratentorial approaches.** ***A,*** **infratentorial supracerebellar approach. The approach has been directed between the lower surface of the tentorium and the tentorial cerebellar surface. The large venous complex draining into the vein of Galen is in the central part of the exposure and the PCA and SCA are exposed laterally. A large vein of the cerebellomesencephalic fissure blocks access to the pineal and limits access to the cerebellomesencephalic fissure. This approach is selected for lesions located in the midline below the vein of Galen and not extending deeply into the cerebellopontine fissure. The SCA branches looping around the lip of the cerebellomesencephalic fissure may extend upward and limit access to the pineal region.** ***B,*** **the vein of the cerebellomesencephalic fissure has to be divided to expose the pineal. The medial posterior choroidal arteries are intertwined with the veins in the region.** ***C,*** **the occipital transtentorial approach has been directed along the medial side of the right occipital lobe. The tentorium behind the quadrigeminal cistern has been divided. The approach provides access to the splenium and the upper part of the cerebellomesencephalic fissure and has been extended forward to the lateral surface of the cerebral peduncles. Both the superior and inferior colliculi can be exposed and the arteries can be followed forward into the ipsilateral ambient cistern. In addition, the veins joining the vein of Galen can be elevated to expose the pineal. The trochlear nerve is exposed just distal to its brainstem exit below the inferior colliculus.** ***D,*** **combined supra and infratentorial exposure with the division of the transverse sinus and tentorium. Division of the transverse sinus, if it is small and well collateralized, provides an exposure that combines both the supra- and infratentorial approaches.** ***A.*****, artery;** **Cer.**, ***cerebral; Cer. Mes.*****, cerebellomesencephalic;** ***Chor.*****, choroidal;** ***CN,*** **cranial nerve;** ***Coll.*****, colliculus;** ***Fiss.*****, fissure;** ***Inf.*****, inferior;** ***Int.*****, internal;** ***Med.*****, medial;** ***Occip.*****, occipital;** ***P.C.A.*****, posterior cerebral artery;** ***Ped.*****, peduncle;** ***Post.*****, posterior;** ***S.C.A.*****, superior cerebellar artery;** ***Sup.*****, superior;** ***Temp.*****, temporal;** ***V.*****, vein.**

transtentorial approach, the occipital lobe was retracted and the tentorium divided along the edge of the straight sinus. This provided access to the splenium above the vein of Galen and, with gentle retraction of the venous complex in the posterior incisural space, the pineal and the upper part of the cerebellomesencephalic fissure could be visualized. The approach provided wider access to the midline and ipsilateral half of the cerebellomesencephalic fissure than did the midline infratentorial supracerebellar approach. In addition, it provided an excellent route for reaching the posterior part of the ambient cistern and even the lateral surface of the cerebral peduncle in the crural cistern. The exposure of the lateral part of the contralateral half of the quadrigeminal cistern was more limited than could be achieved with the midline infratentorial supracerebellar approach. The supra and infratentorial approaches can be converted into a combined approach by dividing the transverse sinus in addition to the tentorium, if the sinus is small and is well collateralized through the opposite side (*Fig. 5.11*).

Reprint requests: Albert L. Rhoton, Jr., M.D., Department of Neurological Surgery, University of Florida Brain Institute, P.O. Box 100265, 100 S. Newell Drive, Building 59, L2-100, Gainesville, FL 32610-0265.

REFERENCES

1. Drake CG: The treatment of aneurysms of the posterior circulation. **Clin Neurosurg** 26:96–144, 1979.
2. Fox JL: Tentorial section for decompression of the brainstem and a large basilar aneurysm: Case report. **J Neurosurg** 28:74–77, 1968.
3. Fujii Y, Lenkey C, Rhoton AL Jr: Microsurgical anatomy of the choroidal arteries: Lateral and third ventricles. **J Neurosurg** 52: 165–188, 1980.
4. Gibo H, Carver CC, Rhoton AL Jr, Lenkey C, Mitchell RJ: Microsurgical anatomy of the middle cerebral artery. **J Neurosurg** 54:151–169, 1981.
5. Gibo H, Lenkey C, Rhoton AL Jr: Microsurgical anatomy of the supraclinoid portion of the internal carotid artery. **J Neurosurg** 55:560–574, 1981.
6. Gudmundsson K, Rhoton AL Jr, Rushton JG: Detailed anatomy of the intracranial portion of the trigeminal nerve. **J Neurosurg** 35:592–600, 1971.
7. Hardy DG, Peace DA, Rhoton AL Jr: Microsurgical anatomy of the superior cerebellar artery. **Neurosurgery** 6:10–28, 1980.
8. Harris FS, Rhoton AL Jr: Anatomy of the cavernous sinus: A microsurgical study. **J Neurosurg** 45:169–180, 1976.
9. Heros RC: Arteriovenous malformations of the medial temporal lobe: Surgical approach and neuroradiological characterization. **J Neurosurg** 56:44–52, 1982.
10. Howell DA: Upper brain-stem compression and foraminal impaction with intracranial space-occupying lesions and brain swelling. **Brain** 82:525–550, 1959.
11. Jannetta PJ, Rand RW: Transtentorial retrogasserian rhizotomy in trigeminal neuralgia by microneurosurgical technique. **Bull Los Angeles Neurol Soc** 31:93–99, 1966.
12. Klintworth GK: Paratentorial grooving of human brains with particular reference to transtentorial herniation and the pathogenesis of secondary brain-stem hemorrhages. **Am J Pathol** 53:391–408, 1968.
13. Klintworth GK: The comparative anatomy and phylogeny of the tentorium cerebelli. **Anat Rec** 160:635–641, 1968.
14. Liliequist B: The subarachnoid cisterns: An anatomic and roentgenologic study. **Acta Radiol Suppl** 185:1–108, 1959.
15. Mastri AR: Brain herniations: Section I—Pathology, in Newton TH, Potts DG (eds): *Radiology of the Skull and Brain*. St Louis, CV Mosby, 1974, vol 2, book 4, pp 2659–2670.
16. Matsushima T, Rhoton AL Jr, de Oliveira E, Peace D: Microsurgical anatomy of the veins of the posterior fossa. **J Neurosurg** 59:63–105, 1983.
17. Ono M, Ono M, Rhoton AL Jr, Barry M: Microsurgical anatomy of the region of the tentorial incisura. **J Neurosurg** 60:365–399, 1984.
18. Perlmutter D, Rhoton AL Jr: Microsurgical anatomy of the anterior cerebral-anterior communicating-recurrent artery complex. **J Neurosurg** 45:259–272, 1976.
19. Perlmutter D, Rhoton AL Jr: Microsurgical anatomy of the distal anterior cerebral artery. **J Neurosurg** 49:204–228, 1978.
20. Plaut HA: Size of the tentorial incisura related to cerebral herniation. **Acta Radiol (Diagn)** 1:916–928, 1963.
21. Poppen JL: The right occipital approach to a pinealoma. **J Neurosurg** 25:706–710, 1966.
22. Renn WH, Rhoton AL Jr: Microsurgical anatomy of the sellar region. **J Neurosurg** 43:288–298, 1975.
23. Rhoton AL Jr: Anatomy of saccular aneurysms. **Surg Neurol** 14:59–66, 1980.
24. Rhoton AL Jr, Fujii K, Fradd B: Microsurgical anatomy of the anterior choroidal artery. **Surg Neurol** 12:171–187, 1979.
25. Rhoton AL Jr, Hardy DG, Chambers SM: Microsurgical anatomy and dissection of the sphenoid bone, cavernous sinus and cellar region. **Surg Neurol** 12:63–104, 1979.
26. Rhoton AL Jr, Yamamoto I, Peace DA: Microsurgery of the third ventricle: Part 2—Operative approaches. **Neurosurgery** 8:357–373, 1981.
27. Saeki N, Rhoton AL Jr: Microsurgical anatomy of the upper basilar artery and the posterior circle of Willis. **J Neurosurg** 46:563–578, 1977.
28. Schechter MM, Zingesser LH, Rosenbaum A: Tentorial meningiomas. **AJR Am J Roentgenol** 104:123–131, 1968.
29. Stein BM: Supracerebellar-infratentorial approach to pineal tumors. **Surg Neurol** 11:331–337, 1979.
30. Sunderland S: The tentorial notch and complications produced by herniations of the brain through that aperture. **Br J Surg** 45:422–438, 1958.
31. Van Wagenen WP: A surgical approach for the removal of certain pineal tumors: Report of a case. **Surg Gynecol Obstet** 53:216–220, 1931.
32. Weinstein M, Stein R, Pollock J, Stucker TB, Newton TH: Meningeal branch of the posterior cerebral artery. **Neuroradiology** 7:129–131, 1974.
33. Yamamoto I, Rhoton AL Jr, Peace DA: Microsurgery of the third ventricle: Part 1—Microsurgical anatomy. **Neurosurgery** 8:334–356, 1981.
34. Yasargil MG, Antic J, Laciga R, Jain KK, Boone SC: Arteriovenous malformations of vein of Galen: Microsurgical treatment. **Surg Neurol** 3:195–200, 1976.
35. Yasargil MG, Antic J, Laciga R, Jain KK, Hodosh RM, Smith RD: Microsurgical pterional approach to aneurysms of the basilar bifurcation. **Surg Neurol** 6:83–91, 1976.
36. Yasargil MG, Kasdaglis K, Jain KK, Weber HP: Anatomical observations of the subarachnoid cisterns of the brain during surgery. **J Neurosurg** 44:298–302, 1976.
37. Zeal AA, Rhoton AL Jr: Microsurgical anatomy of the posterior cerebral artery. **J Neurosurg** 48:534–559, 1978.

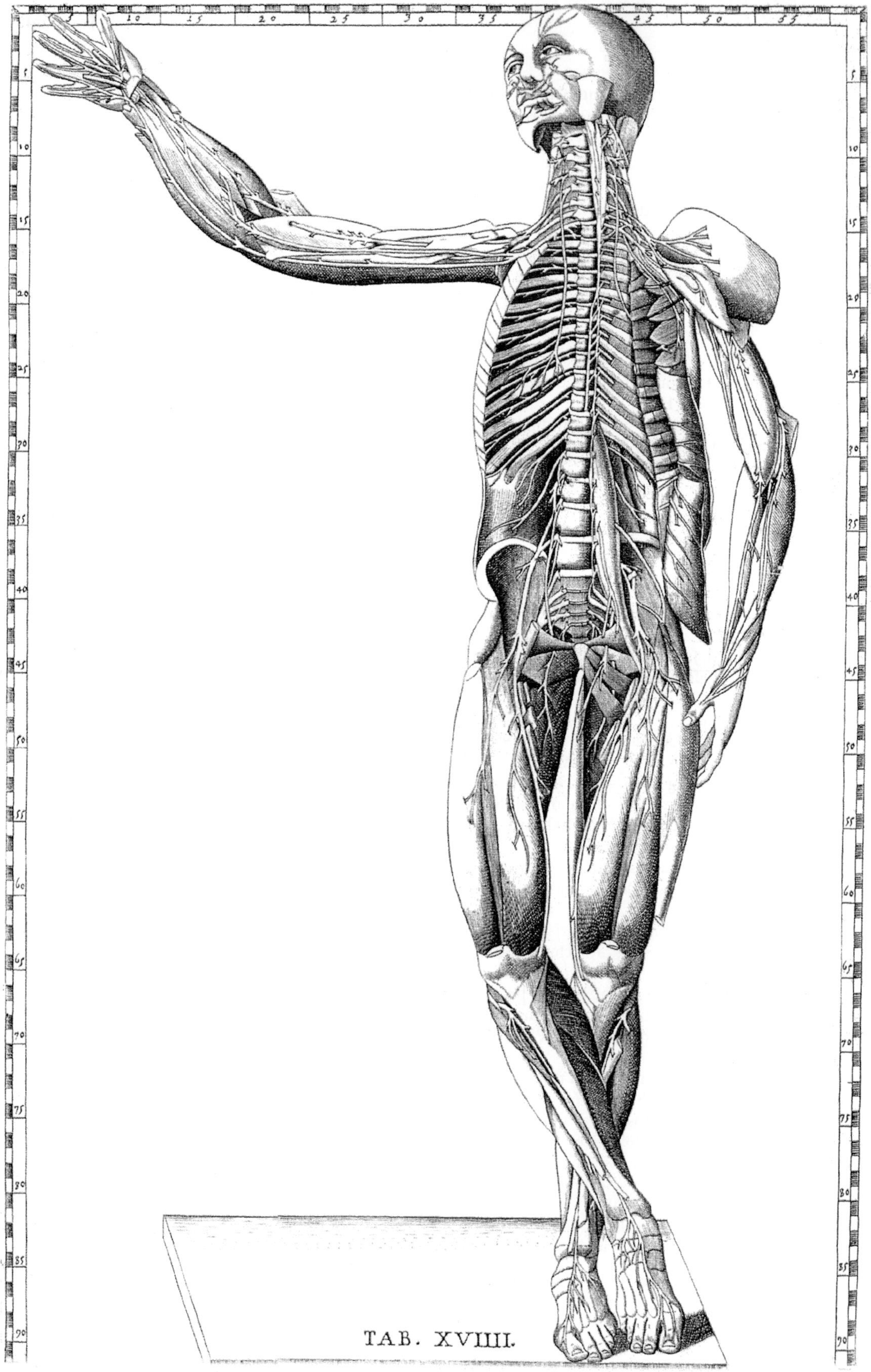

Deep thoracic and abdominal dissection revealing skeletal and neural structures, from, Bartolommeo Eustachio, *Tabulae anatomicae*. Rome, Sumptibus Laurentii & Thomae Pagliarini, 1728. Courtesy, Rare Book Room, Norris Medical Library, Keck School of Medicine, Los Angeles, California.

CHAPTER 6

The Foramen Magnum

Albert L. Rhoton, Jr., M.D.

Department of Neurological Surgery, University of Florida, Gainesville, Florida

Key words: Cranial nerves, Craniovertebral junction, Foramen magnum, Microsurgery, Vertebral artery

The foramen magnum is located in the occipital bone, which has three parts: a squamosal part located behind the foramen magnum; a basal (clival) portion located anterior to the foramen magnum; and a condylar part that connects the squamosal and clival parts (*Fig. 6.1*). The suboccipital approaches are directed through the squamosal part and the anterior approaches through the clival part. The condylar part, which includes the occipital condyle, posterior margin of the jugular foramen, and hypoglossal canal, is exposed in the far-lateral approach and its transcondylar, retrocondylar, and supracondylar modifications described in the chapter on the far lateral approach. Structures involved in foramen magnum lesions include the lower cranial and upper spinal nerves, the caudal brainstem and rostral spinal cord, the vertebral artery and its branches, the veins and dural sinuses at the craniovertebral junction, and the ligaments and muscles uniting the atlas, axis, and occipital bone (5, 26). The foramen magnum is most commonly approached from posteriorly through the suboccipital and upper cervical region or from anteriorly through the nasal and oral cavities, the pharynx, or maxilla.

THE FORAMEN MAGNUM

Osseous relationships

The osseous structures that must be considered in planning an approach to the region of the foramen magnum are the occipital bone, the atlas, and the axis.

Occipital bone

The occipital bone surrounds the foramen magnum (*Fig. 6.1*). The foraminal opening is oval shaped and is wider posteriorly than anteriorly. The wider posterior part transmits the medulla, and the narrower anterior part sits above the odontoid process. The occipital bone is divided into a squamosal part located above and behind the foramen magnum, a basal part situated in front of the foramen magnum, and paired condylar parts located lateral to the foramen magnum.

The squamous part is an internally concave plate located above and behind the foramen magnum. Its upper margins articulate with the parietal bones at the lambdoid sutures and its lower margins articulate with the mastoid portion of the temporal bones at the occipitomastoid sutures. The convex external surface has several prominences on which the muscles of the neck attach. The largest prominence, the external occipital protuberance or inion, is situated at the central part of the external surface. The inion is located an average of 1 cm below the apex of the internal occipital protuberance and the inferior margin of the confluence of the sagittal and transverse sinuses. Two parallel ridges radiate laterally from the protuberance: the highest nuchal line is the upper and thinner ridge, and the superior nuchal line is the lower and more prominent one. The area below the nuchal lines is rough and irregular and serves as the site of attachment of numerous muscles. A vertical ridge, the external occipital crest, descends from the external occipital protuberance to the midpoint of the posterior margin of the foramen magnum. The inferior nuchal lines run laterally from the midpoint of the crest.

The internal surface of the squamous part is concave and has a prominence, the internal occipital protuberance, near its center. The internal surface is divided into four unequal fossae by the sulcus of the superior sagittal sinus that extends upward from the protuberance, the internal occipital crest, a prominent ridge that descends from the protuberance, and the paired sulci for the transverse sinuses that extend laterally from the protuberance. The sulcus for the right transverse sinus is usually larger than the one on the left. The upper two fossae are adapted to the poles of the occipital lobes. The inferior two fossae conform to the contours of the cerebellar hemispheres. The internal occipital crest bifurcates above the foramen magnum to form paired lower limbs, which extend along each side of the posterior margin of the foramen. A depression between the lower limbs, the vermian fossa, is occupied by the inferior part of the vermis. The falx cerebelli is attached along the internal occipital crest.

The basilar part of the occipital bone, which is also referred to as the clivus, is a thick quadrangular plate of bone that extends forward and upward, at an angle of about 45° from the foramen magnum. It joins the sphenoid bone at the sphenoccipital synchondrosis just below the dorsum sellae (7). The superior surface of the clivus is concave from side to side and is separated on each side from the petrous part of the temporal bone by the petroclival fissure. This fissure has the inferior petrosal sinus on its upper surface and ends posteriorly at the jugular foramen. On the inferior surface of the basilar part, in

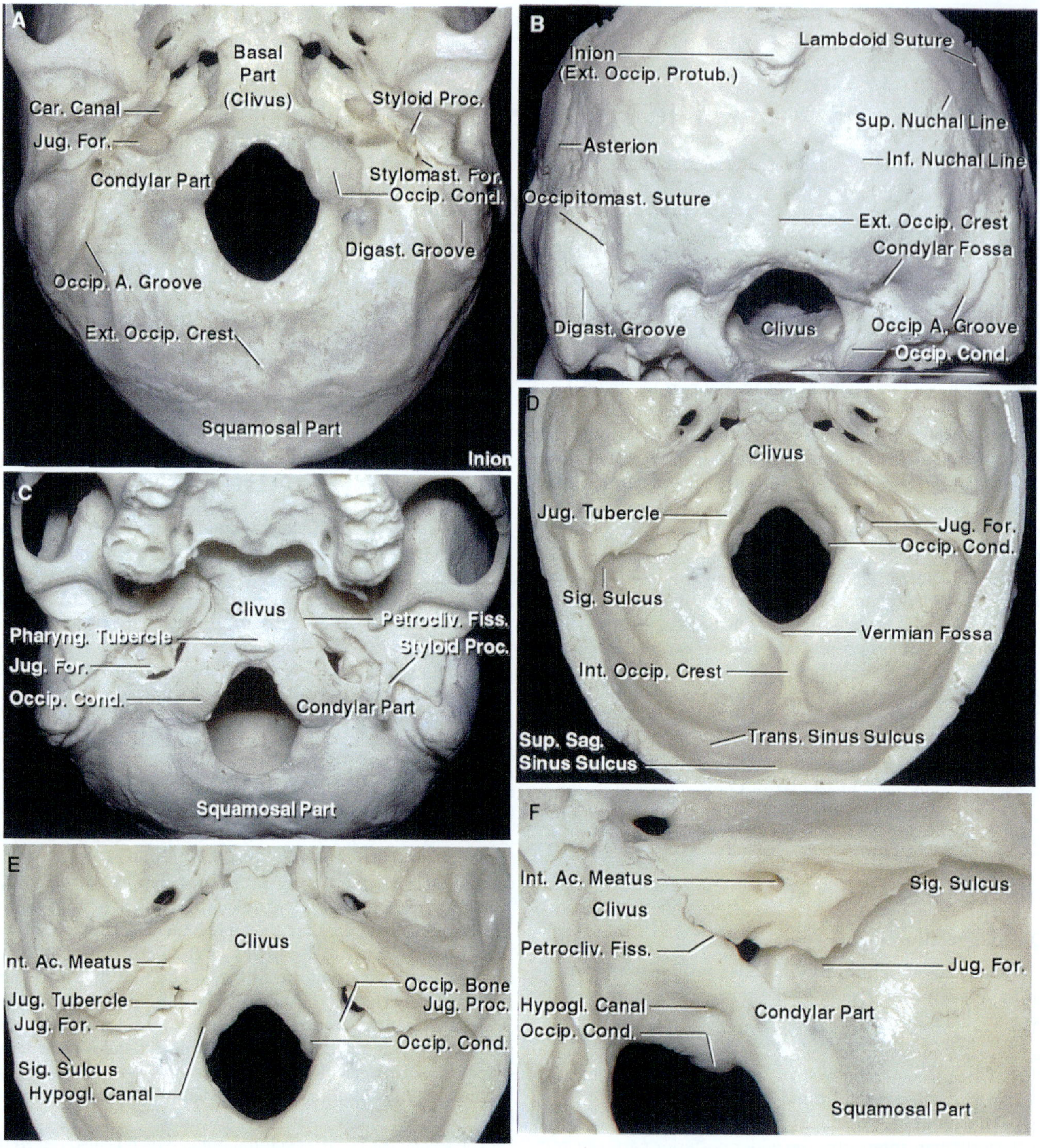

FIGURE 6.1. Occipital bone and foramen magnum. *A*, inferior view. *B*, posteroinferior view. *C*, anterior-inferior view. *D*, superior view. *E*, posterosuperior view. *F*, oblique posterosuperior view. The occipital bone surrounds the oval-shaped foramen magnum, which is wider posteriorly than anteriorly. The narrower anterior part sits above the odontoid process and it encroached on from laterally by the occipital condyles. The wider posterior part transmits the medulla. The occipital bone is divided into a squamosal part located above and behind the foramen magnum; a basal (clival) part situated in front of the foramen magnum; and paired condylar parts located lateral to the foramen magnum. The squamous part is internally concave. Its upper margin articulates with the parietal bone at the lambdoid suture, and its lower margin articulates with the mastoid portion of the temporal bone at the occipitomastoid suture. The convex external surface of the squamosal part has several prominences. The largest prominence, the external occipital protuberance (inion), is situated at the central part of the

front of the foramen magnum, a small elevation, the pharyngeal tubercle, gives attachment to the fibrous raphe of the pharynx.

The paired lateral or condylar parts are situated at the sides of the foramen magnum. The occipital condyles, which articulate with the atlas, protrude from the external surface of this part. These condyles are located lateral to the anterior half of the foramen magnum. They are oval in shape, convex downward, face downward and laterally, and have their long axes directed forward and medially. A tubercle that gives attachment to the alar ligament of the odontoid process is situated on the medial side of each condyle. The hypoglossal canal, which transmits the hypoglossal nerve, is situated above the condyle, and is directed forward and laterally from the posterior cranial fossa. The canal may be partially or completely divided by a bony septum. Septated hypoglossal canals were found on one or both sides in 6% of the dry skulls (15).

The condylar fossa, a depression located on the external surface behind the condyle, is often perforated to form the posterior condylar canal through which an emissary vein connects the vertebral venous plexus with the sigmoid sinus. One or both condylar foramina may be absent or incompletely perforated (9). The jugular process, a quadrilateral plate of bone, extends laterally from the posterior half of the condyle to form the posterior border of the jugular foramen. It serves as a bridge between the condylar and squamosal portions of the occipital bone. The jugular process articulates laterally with the jugular surface of the temporal bone. On the intracranial surface of the condylar part an oval prominence, the jugular tubercle, sits just superior to the hypoglossal canal and just medial to the lower extent of the petroclival fissure. The caudal part of the tubercle often presents a shallow furrow above which the glossopharyngeal, vagus, and accessory nerves course. The groove of the sigmoid sinus curves medially and forward around an upwardly directed, hook-shaped process, on the superior surface of the jugular process, and ends at the jugular foramen. The posterior condylar canal opens into the posterior cranial fossa close to the medial end of the groove for the sigmoid sinus.

The jugular foramen is situated lateral and slightly superior to the anterior half of the condyles. It is bordered posteriorly by the jugular process of the occipital bone, and anteriorly and superiorly by the jugular fossa of the petrous portion of the temporal bone (14). The foramen sits at the posterior end of the petroclival suture. The jugular foramen is divided into two parts by the intrajugular processes on the opposing edges of the petrous and occipital bones, which either join directly or are connected by a fibrous band. The smaller anteromedial part, the petrous part, transmits the inferior petrosal sinus, and the larger posterolateral part, the sigmoid part, transmits the sigmoid sinus. The intrajugular part, situated along the intrajugular processes, transmits the glossopharyngeal, vagus, and accessory nerves. The enlarged part of the internal jugular vein located within the foramen is referred to as the jugular bulb. The jugular process also serves as the site of attachment of the rectus capitis lateralis muscle behind the jugular foramen.

The atlas

The atlas, the first cervical vertebra, differs from the other cervical vertebrae by being ring shaped and by lacking a vertebral body and a spinous process (*Fig. 6.2*). It consists of two thick lateral masses situated at the anterolateral parts of the ring. The lateral masses are connected in front by a short anterior arch and behind by a longer curved posterior arch. The position of the usual vertebral body is occupied by the odontoid process of the axis. The anterior arch is convexed forward and has a median anterior tubercle. The posterior

external surface. The superior nuchal line radiates laterally from the protuberance. A vertical ridge, the external occipital crest, descends from the external occipital protuberance to the midpoint of the posterior margin of the foramen magnum. The inferior nuchal lines run laterally on both sides from the midpoint of the crest. The internal surface of the squamous part is concave and has a prominence, the internal occipital protuberance, near its center. The internal surface is divided into four unequal fossae by the sulcus of the superior sagittal sinus, the internal occipital crest, and the sulci for the transverse sinuses. The internal occipital crest bifurcates above the foramen magnum to form a V-shaped ridge between the limbs of which is the vermian fossa. The basilar part of the occipital bone, which is also referred to as the clivus, is a thick quadrangular plate of bone that extends forward and upward to join the sphenoid bone just below the dorsum sellae. The superior surface of the clivus slopes upward from the foramen magnum and is concave from side to side. The clivus is separated on each side from the petrous part of the temporal bone by the petroclival fissure that ends posteriorly at the jugular foramen. The occipitomastoid suture extends posterolateral from the jugular foramen. On the inferior surface of the basilar part, a small elevation, the pharyngeal tubercle, gives attachment to the fibrous raphe of the pharynx. The condylar parts of the occipital bone, on which the occipital condyles an located, are situated lateral to the foramen magnum on the external surface. The alar tubercle, which gives attachment to the alar ligament, is situated on the medial side of each condyle. The hypoglossal canal is situated above the condyle. The condylar fossa, which may be converted into a foramen for the passage of an emissary vein, is located behind the condyle. The jugular process of the occipital bone extends laterally from the posterior half of the condyle and articulates with the jugular surface of the temporal bone. The sulcus of the sigmoid sinus crosses the superior surface of the jugular process. The jugular foramen is bordered posteriorly by the jugular process of the occipital bone and anteriorly by the jugular fossa of the petrous temporal bone. The jugular tubercle lies on the internal surface above the hypoglossal canal. *A.*, artery; *Ac.*, acoustic; *Car.*, carotid; *Cond.*, condyle; *Digast.*, digastric; *Ext.*, external; *Fiss.*, fissure; *For.*, foramen; *Hypogl.*, hypoglossal; *Inf.*, inferior; *Jug.*, jugular; *Occipitomast.*, occipitomastoid; *Occip.*, occipital; *Petrocliv.*, petroclival; *Pharyng.*, pharyngeal; *Proc.*, process; *Protrub.*, protuberance; *Sag.*, sagittal; *Sig.*, sigmoid; *Sup.*, superior; *Trans.*, transverse.

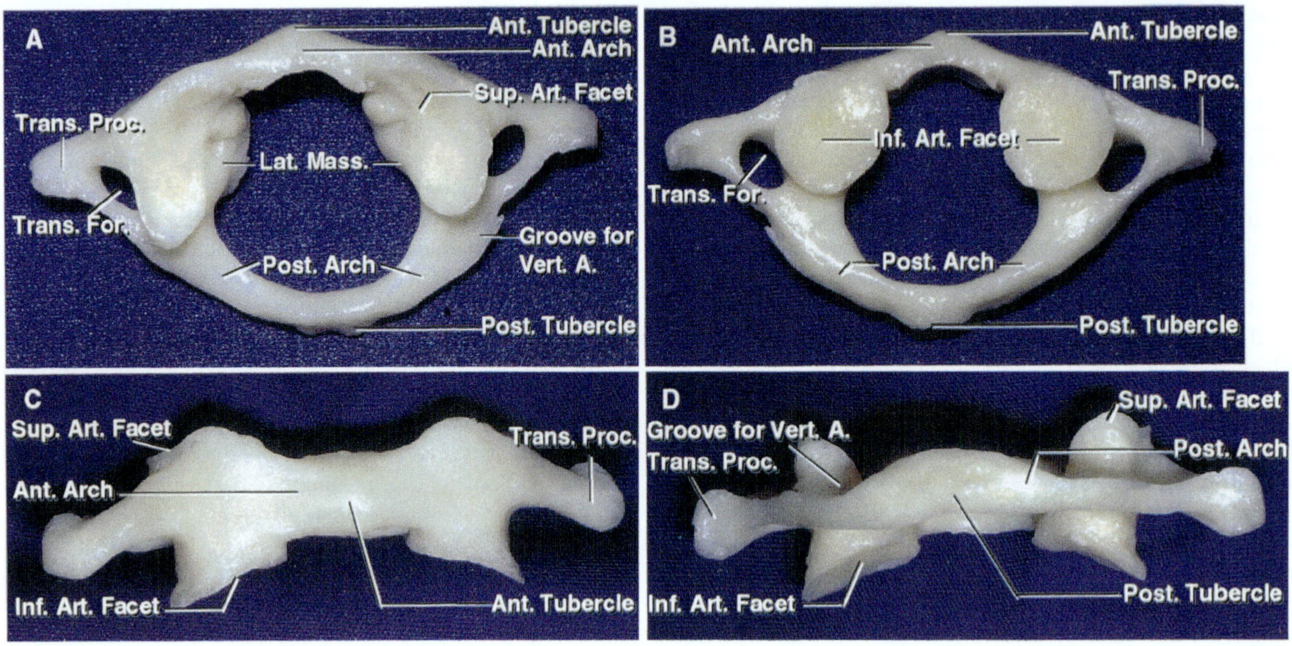

FIGURE 6.2. ***A–D.*** **The atlas.** ***A,*** **superior view;** ***B,*** **inferior view;** ***C,*** **anterior view;** ***D,*** **posterior view. The atlas consists of two thick lateral masses situated at the anteromedial part of the ring, which are connected in front by a short anterior arch and posteriorly by a longer curved posterior arch. The anterior and posterior tubercles are at the anterior and posterior midline. The superior articular facet is an oval, concave facet that faces upward and medially to articulate with the occipital condyle. The inferior articular facet is a circular, flat, or slightly concave facet that faces downward, medially, and slightly backward and articulates with the superior articular facet of the axis. The medial aspect of each lateral mass has a small tubercle for the attachment of the transverse ligament of the atlas. The transverse process projects from the lateral masses. The transverse foramina transmit the vertebral arteries. The upper surface of the posterior arch adjacent to the lateral masses has paired grooves in which the vertebral arteries course.** ***A.,*** **artery;** ***Ant.,*** **anterior;** ***Art.,*** **articular;** ***For.,*** **foramen;** ***Lat.,*** **lateral;** ***Mass.,*** **masses;** ***Post.,*** **posterior;** ***Proc.,*** **process;** ***Trans.,*** **transverse;** ***Vert.,*** **vertebral.**

arch is convex backward and has a median posterior tubercle and a groove on the lateral part of its upper-outer surface in which the vertebral artery courses. The groove may be partly or fully converted into a foramen by a bridge of bone that arches backward from the posterior edge of the superior articular facet of the atlas to its posterior arch. The first cervical spinal nerve also lies in the groove, which is located between the artery and the bone. The upper surface of each lateral mass has an oval concave facet that faces upward and medially and articulates with the occipital condyle that faces downward and laterally. The inferior surface of each lateral mass has a circular, flat, or slightly concave facet that faces downward, medially, and slightly backward, and it articulates with the superior articular facet of the axis. The medial aspect of each lateral mass has a small tubercle for the attachment of the transverse ligament of the atlas, which passes behind the dens. Each transverse foramen, which transmits a vertebral artery, and upon which the nerve root sits, is situated between the lateral mass and the transverse process.

The axis

The axis, the second cervical vertebra, more closely resembles the typical vertebrae than the atlas, but is distinguished by the odontoid process (dens), which projects upward from the body (*Fig. 6.2*). The dens is 1.0- to 1.5-cm long, and approximately 1-cm wide. On the front of the dens is an articular facet that forms a joint with the facet on the back of the anterior arch of the atlas. The dens has a pointed apex that is joined by the apical ligament, has a flattened side where the alar ligaments are attached, and is grooved at the base of its posterior surface where the transverse ligament of the atlas passes. The dens and body are flanked by a pair of large oval facets that extend laterally from the body onto the adjoining parts of the pedicles and articulate with the inferior facets of the atlas. The superior facets do not form an articular pillar with the inferior facets, but are anterior to the latter. The anterior aspect of the body is hollowed out on each side of the midline in the area where the longus colli muscles attach. The lamina are thicker than on any other cervical vertebrae, the pedicles are stout, and the spinous process is large.

The transverse processes of the axis are small. Their blunt tips present a single tubercle, the anterior tubercle, situated at or near the junction of the anterior root of the transverse process and the body. Each transverse foramen faces superolaterally, thus permitting the lateral deviation of the vertebral artery as it passes up to the more widely separated transverse foramina in the atlas. The inferior articular facets are situated at the junction of the pedicles and laminae, and face downward and forward. The spade-shaped vertebral foramen is relatively large.

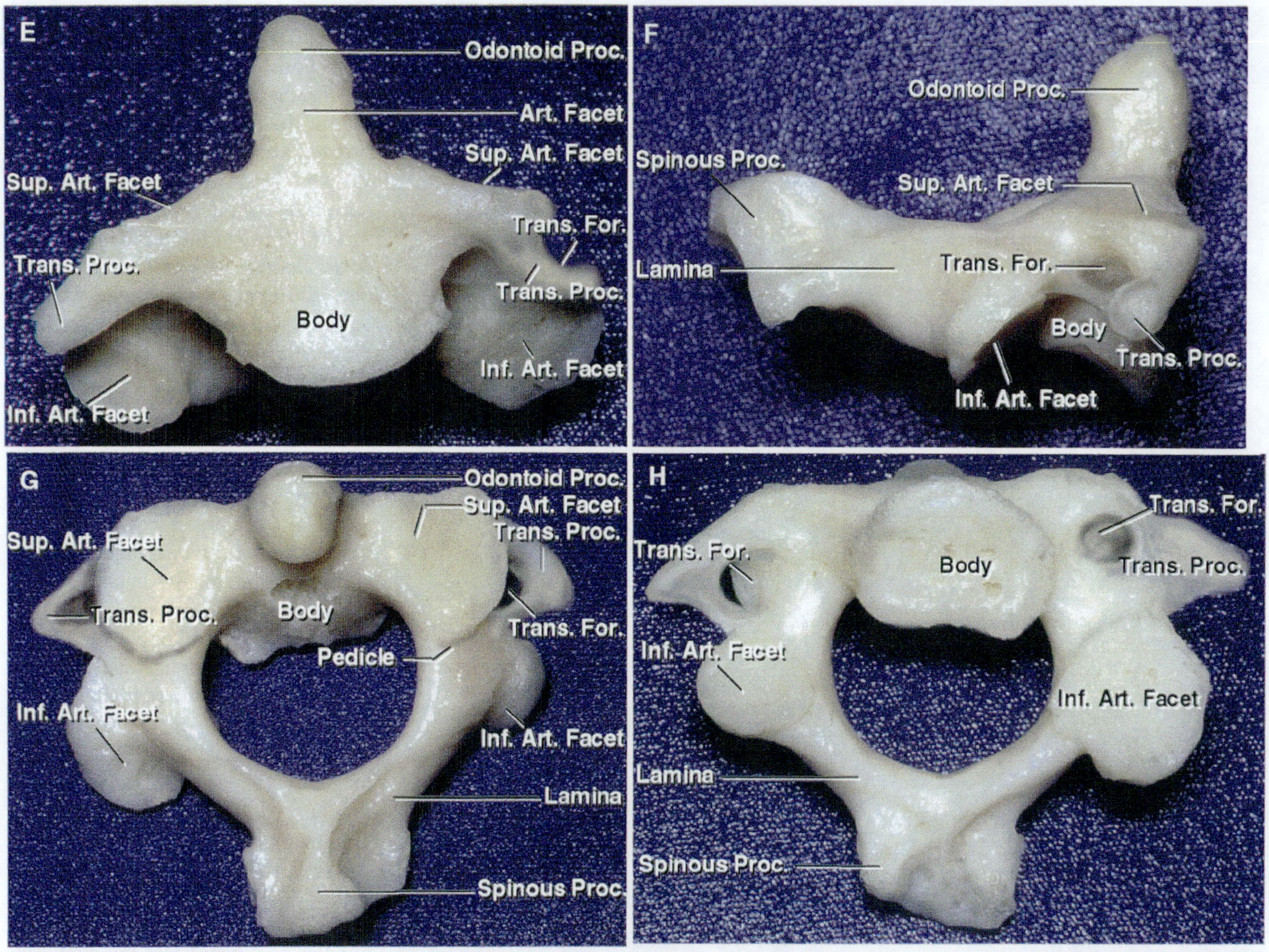

FIGURE 6.2. ***E–H.*** **The axis.** ***E,*** **anterior view;** ***F,*** **lateral view;** ***G,*** **superior view;** ***H,*** **inferior view. The axis is distinguished by the odontoid process (dens). On the front of the dens is an articular facet that forms a joint with the facet on the back of the anterior arch of the atlas. The dens is grooved at the base of its posterior surface where the transverse ligament of the atlas passes. The oval superior articular facets articulate with the inferior facets of the atlas. The superior facets are anterior to the inferior facets. The pedicles and laminae are thicker than on the other cervical vertebra and the lamina fuse behind to form a large spinous process. The transverse foramina are directed superolaterally, thus permitting the lateral deviation of the vertebral arteries as they pass up to the more widely separated transverse foramina in the atlas. The inferior articular facets face downward and forward.**

The atlantoaxial joints

The articulation of the atlas and axis comprises four synovial joints: two median ones on the front and back of the dens, and paired lateral ones between the opposing articular facets on the lateral masses of the atlas and axis (*Figs. 6.2-6.4*). Each of the median joints, situated on the front and back of the dens, has its own fibrous capsule and synovial cavity. The anterior one is situated between the anterior surface of the dens and the posterior aspect of the anterior arch of the atlas. The posterior one has an even larger synovial cavity and lies between the cartilage-covered anterior surface of the transverse ligament of the atlas and the posterior surface of the dens.

The atlas and axis are united by the cruciform ligament, the anterior and posterior longitudinal ligaments, and the articular capsules surrounding the joints between the opposing articular facets on the lateral masses. The cruciform ligament has transverse and vertical parts that form a cross behind the dens. The transverse part, called the transverse ligament, is a thick strong band that arches across the ring of the atlas behind the dens and divides the vertebral canal into a larger posterior compartment containing the dura and the spinal cord and a smaller anterior compartment containing the odontoid process. The transverse ligament is broader in the middle behind the dens than at the ends where it is attached to a tubercle on the medial side of the lateral masses of the atlas. As it crosses the dens, small longitudinal bands are directed upward and downward from its posterior surface. The cranial extension is attached to the upper surface of the clivus between the apical ligament of the dens and the tectorial membrane. The lower band is attached to the posterior surface of the body of the axis. The neck of the dens is constricted where it is embraced posteriorly by the transverse ligament.

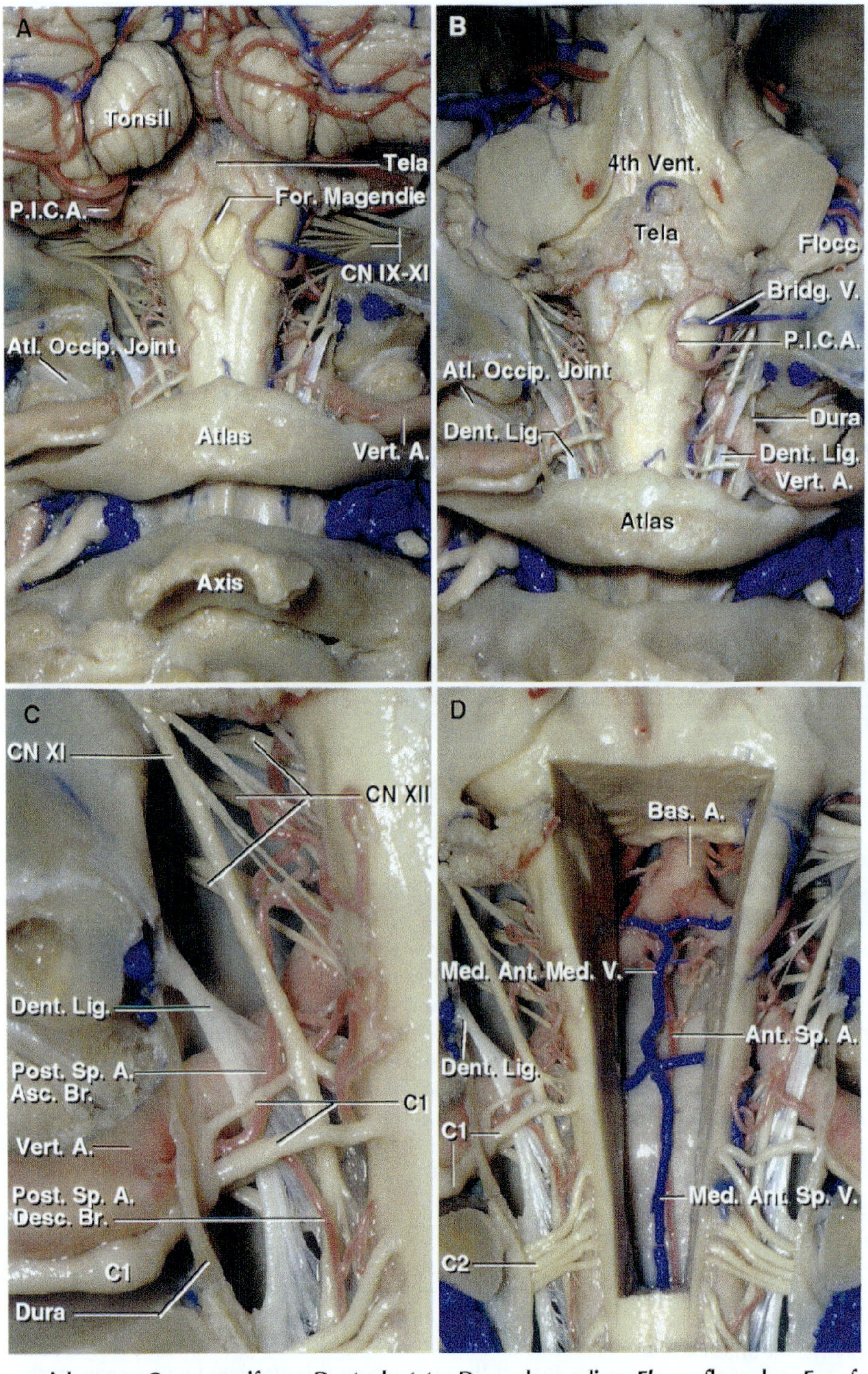

FIGURE 6.3. *A–D.* Foramen magnum. Posterior view. Stepwise dissection. *A,* the cerebellar tonsils, the foramen of Magendie, and lower part of the fourth ventricle are situated above the foramen magnum. The vertebral artery penetrates the dura below the foramen magnum and ascends through the foramen in front of the dentate ligament and accessory nerves. The glossopharyngeal, vagus, and accessory nerves pass through the jugular foramen, which is located lateral to the anterior half of the foramen magnum. *B,* the cerebellum has been removed. The vertebral arteries pass through the foramen magnum to reach the front of the medulla. *C,* enlarged view of the left half of the foramen magnum. The vertebral artery passes behind and below the atlanto-occipital joint, penetrates the dura, and passes in front of the dentate ligament and accessory nerve. The rostral end of the dentate ligament attaches to the dura at the level of the foramen magnum. The C1 nerve penetrates the dura with the vertebral artery. The hypoglossal nerve passes behind the vertebral artery and enters the hypoglossal canal. The hypoglossal nerve is separated into several bundles as it penetrates the dura. The posterior spinal artery arises as the vertebral artery enters the dura and gives rise to ascending and descending branches. *D,* a longitudinal strip of the medulla and floor of the fourth ventricle has been removed to expose the vertebrobasilar junction, the origin of the anterior spinal artery, and the median anterior medullary and median anterior spinal veins. *A.,* artery; *A.I.C.A.,* anteroinferior cerebellar artery; *Ant.,* anterior; *Asc.,* ascending; *Atl.,* atlanto-; *Bas.,* basilar; *Br.,* branch; *Bridg.,* bridging; *CN,* cranial nerve; *Cruc.,* cruciform; *Dent.,* dentate; *Desc.,* descending; *Flocc.,* flocculus; *For.,* foramen; *Horiz.,* horizontal; *Lig.,* ligament; *Med.,* median, medullary; *Memb.,* membrane; *Men.,* meningeal; *Occip.,* occipital; *P.I.C.A.,* posteroinferior cerebellar artery; *Post.,* posterior; *Sp.,* spinal; *Trans.,* transverse; *V.,* vein; *Vent.,* ventricle; *Vert.,* vertebral.

In front, the atlas and axis are connected by the anterior longitudinal ligament, which is a wide band fixed above to the lower border of the anterior arch of the atlas and below to the front of the body of the axis. The posterior longitudinal ligament is attached below to the posterior surface of the body of the axis, and above to the transverse part of the cruciform ligament and the clivus. Posterior to the spinal canal, the atlas and axis are joined by a broad, thin membrane in series with the ligamentum flavum that is attached above to the lower border of the posterior arch of the atlas, and below to the

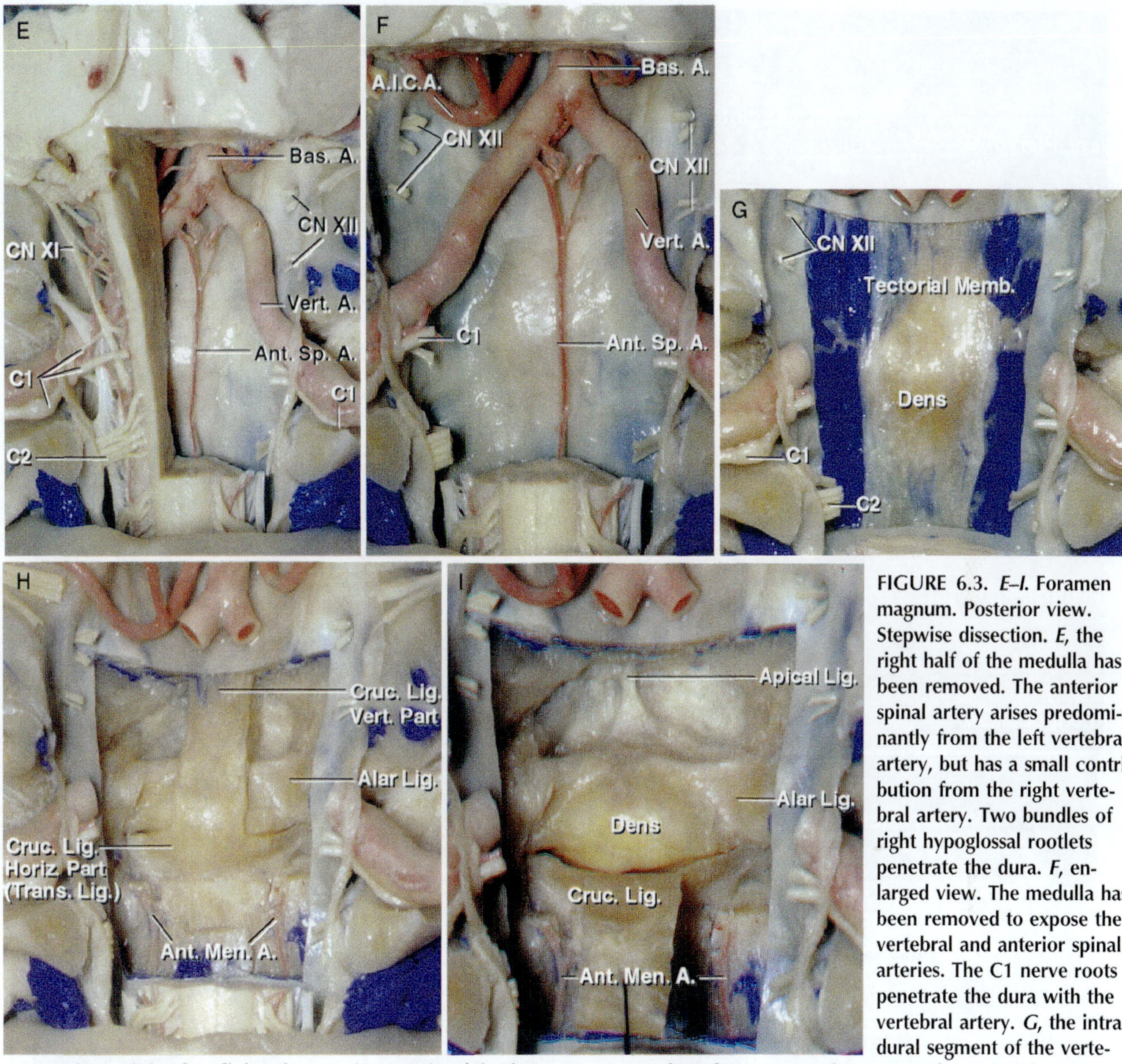

FIGURE 6.3. ***E–I.*** **Foramen magnum. Posterior view. Stepwise dissection.** ***E,*** **the right half of the medulla has been removed. The anterior spinal artery arises predominantly from the left vertebral artery, but has a small contribution from the right vertebral artery. Two bundles of right hypoglossal rootlets penetrate the dura.** ***F,*** **enlarged view. The medulla has been removed to expose the vertebral and anterior spinal arteries. The C1 nerve roots penetrate the dura with the vertebral artery.** ***G,*** **the intradural segment of the vertebral arteries and the dura lining the anterior margin of the foramen magnum have been removed to expose the tectorial membrane, a rostral extension of the posterior longitudinal ligament, and the vertebral venous plexus, which courses just outside the dura.** ***H,*** **the tectorial membrane has been removed to expose the cruciform and alar ligaments. The horizontal portion of the cruciform ligament, called the transverse ligament of the atlas, extends laterally to be attached to the medial edges of the lateral masses of the atlas, and the vertical portion ascends to attach to the anterior margin of the foramen magnum deep to the tectorial membrane. The alar ligaments pass upward and laterally and attach to the lateral edges of the foramen magnum. Anterior meningeal arteries pass along the dura and ligamentous structures in the anterior spinal canal.** ***I,*** **the vertical portion of the cruciform ligament has been folded downward to expose the synovial joint between the anterior surface of the cruciform ligament and the posterior surface of the dens. There is also another synovial joint between the anterior surface of the dens and the posterior surface of the anterior atlantal arch. The apical ligament of the dens extends upward to be attached to the margin of the foramen magnum.**

upper edges of the laminae of the axis. This membrane is pierced laterally by the second cervical nerve.

The atlanto-occipital joints

The atlas and the occipital bone are united by the articular capsules surrounding the atlanto-occipital joints and by the anterior and posterior atlanto-occipital membranes (*Figs. 6.2-6.4*). The articular capsules of the atlanto-occipital joints are sometimes deficient medially where the synovial cavities may communicate with the synovial bursa between the dens and the transverse ligament of the atlas. The anterior atlanto-occipital membrane is attached superiorly to the anterior edge

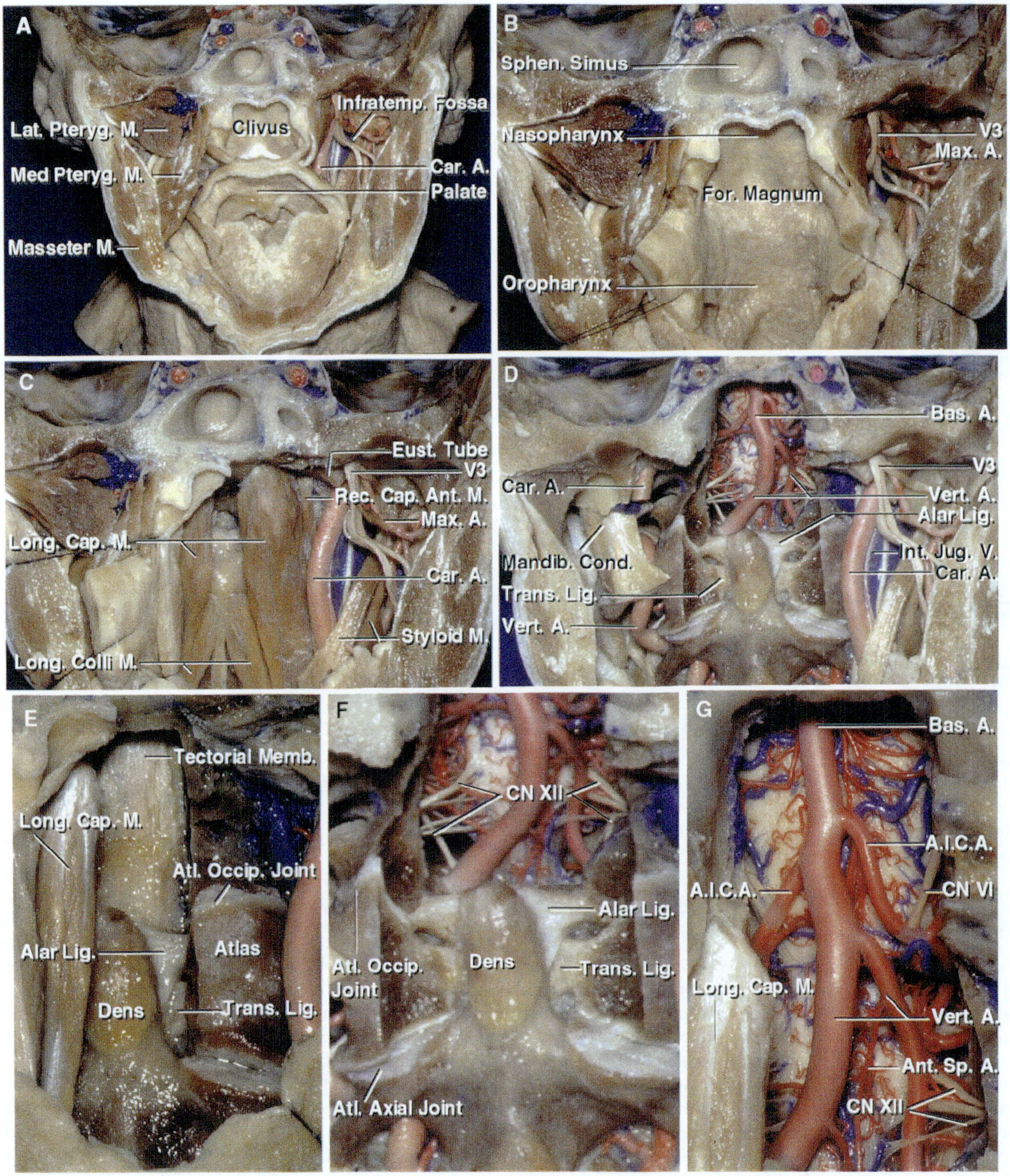

FIGURE 6.4. Anterior view. Stepwise dissection of a cross section showing the relationship of the foramen magnum and clivus to the nasal and oral cavities, pharynx, and infratemporal fossa. *A*, the soft palate, which has been preserved, is located at the level of the foramen magnum. The infratemporal fossa, located below the greater sphenoid wing and middle cranial fossa, contains the pterygoid muscles, maxillary artery, mandibular nerve branches, and the pterygoid venous plexus and opens posteriorly into the area around the carotid sheath, as shown on the left side. *B*, enlarged view. The soft palate has been divided in the midline and the leaves reflected laterally. The atlanto-occipital joints and the foramen magnum are located at approximately the level of the hard palate. The anterior arch of C1 and the dens are located behind the oropharynx, and the clivus is located behind the nasopharynx and sphenoid sinus. The prominence over the longus capitis and the

of the foramen magnum, inferiorly to the superior edge of the anterior arch of the atlas, and laterally to the capsule of the atlanto-occipital joints.

The posterior atlanto-occipital membrane is a thin sheet connected above to the posterior margin of the foramen magnum and below to the upper border of the posterior arch of the atlas. The lateral border of the membrane is free and arches behind the vertebral artery and the first cervical nerve root. The lateral edge of this membrane may be ossified in the area where it arches over the posterior aspect of the vertebral artery, thus creating a partial or complete osseous ring around the artery on the medial side of the atlanto-occipital joint.

Axis and occipital bone

Four fibrous bands, the tectorial membrane, the paired alar ligaments, and the apical ligament, connect the axis and the occipital bone (*Figs.* *6.3* and *6.4*). The tectorial membrane is a cephalic extension of the posterior longitudinal ligament that covers the dens and cruciform ligament. It is attached below to the posterior surface of the body of the axis, above to the upper surface of the occipital bone in front of the foramen magnum, and laterally to the medial sides of the atlanto-occipital joints. The alar ligaments are two strong bands that arise on each side of the upper part of the dens and extend obliquely superolateral to attach to the medial surfaces of the occipital condyles. The apical ligament of the odontoid process extends from the tip of the dens to the anterior margin of the foramen magnum and is situated between the anterior atlanto-occipital membrane and the superior prolongation of the cruciform ligament.

Muscular relationships

The foramen magnum is surrounded by the muscles attached to the occipital bone and upper cervical vertebrae (*Figs.* *6.4* and *6.5*). The trapezius covers the back of the head and neck. It extends from the medial half of the superior nuchal line, the external occipital protuberance, and the spinous processes of the cervical and thoracic vertebrae and converges on the shoulder to attach to the scapula and the lateral third of the clavicle. The sternocleidomastoid passes obliquely downward across the side of the neck from the lateral half of the superior nuchal line and mastoid process to the upper part of the sternum and the adjacent part of the clavicle. This muscle divides the side of the neck into an anterior triangle and a posterior triangle. The anterior triangle is bounded posteriorly by the anterior border of the sternocleidomastoid, above by the mandible, and anteriorly by the median line of the neck; the posterior triangle is bounded in front by the posterior border of the sternocleidomastoid, below by the middle third of the clavicle, and behind by the anterior margin of the trapezius. The splenius capitis, situated deep to and partially covered by the trapezius and sternocleidomastoid, extends from the bone below the lateral third of the superior nuchal line to the spinous processes of the lower cervical and upper thoracic vertebrae. Two muscles, both of which are situated deep to the splenius capitis and sternocleidomastoid and attach below to the upper thoracic and lower cervical vertebrae, are the semispinalis capitis, which attaches above in the area between the superior and inferior nuchal lines beginning medially at the external occipital crest and extending laterally to the occipitomastoid junction, and the longissimus capitis muscle, which attaches above to the posterior margin of the mastoid process.

The suboccipital muscles, located in the next layer, are a group of muscles situated deep to the splenius, semispinalis, and longissimus capitis in the suboccipital area. This group includes the superior oblique, which extends from the area lateral to the semispinalis capitis between the superior and inferior nuchal lines to the transverse process of the atlas; the inferior oblique, which extends from the spinous process and lamina of the axis to the transverse process of the atlas; the rectus capitis posterior major, which extends from and below the lateral part of the inferior nuchal line to the spine of the axis; and the rectus capitis posterior minor, which is situated medial to and is partially covered by the rectus capitis posterior major, extends

anterior arch of C1 are seen through the pharyngeal mucosa. *C,* the mucosa lining the posterior pharyngeal wall has been reflected to the right, exposing the longus capitis that attaches to the clivus and the part of the longus colli that attaches to the anterior arch of C1. The eustachian tube has been divided. The rectus capitis anterior extends from the transverse process of C1, posterolateral to the longus capitis, to attach to the occipital bone in front of the occipital condyle. *D,* the clivus and anterior arch of C1 have been removed. The dura has been opened to expose the vertebral and basilar artery. The dens has been preserved. The structures in the right infratemporal fossa and part of the right carotid artery and mandible have been removed to expose the right vertebral artery ascending between the C2 and C1 transverse processes. *E,* enlarged view of the step between *C* and *D.* The anterior arch of C1 has been removed to expose the odontoid process and the lower part of the clivus. The left longus coli and longus capitis have been reflected out of the exposure. The atlanto-occipital joint is exposed at the level of the odontoid apex. The transverse part of the cruciform ligament, also called the transverse ligament, extends across the back of the dens and attaches to a tubercle on the medial side of each lateral mass of the axis. The tectorial membrane, a cephalic extension of the posterior longitudinal ligament, lines the posterior clival surface. The alar ligaments attach to the lateral edges of the foramen magnum. *F,* enlarged view of the exposure shown in *D. G,* exposure after opening of the clivus. Both vertebral and anteroinferior cerebellar arteries (AICAs) and the anterior spinal artery are exposed. *A.,* artery; *A.I.C.A.,* anteroinferior cerebellar artery; *Ant.,* anterior; *Atl.,* atlanto-; *Cap.,* capitis; *Car.,* carotid; *CN,* cranial nerve; *Eust.,* eustachian; *For.,* foramen; *Infratemp.,* infratemporal; *Int.,* internal; *Jug.,* jugular; *Lat.,* lateral; *Lig.,* ligament; *Long.,* longus; *M.,* muscle; *Mandib.,* mandibular; *Max.,* maxillary; *Med.,* medial; *Memb.,* membrane; *Occip.,* occipital; *Pteryg.,* pterygoid; *Rec.,* rectus; *Sp.,* spinal; *Sphen.,* sphenoid; *Trans.,* transverse; *Vert.,* vertebral.

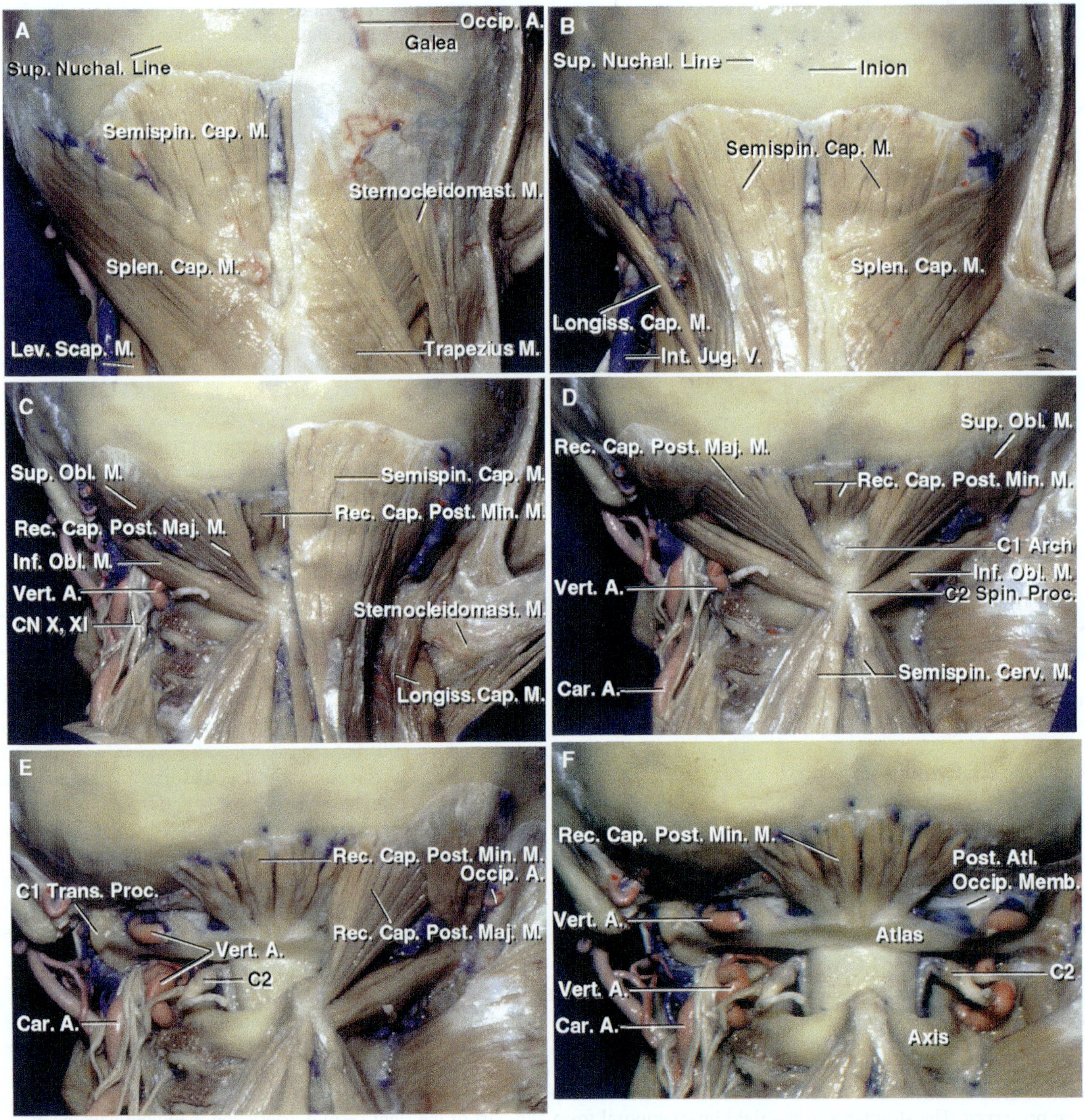

FIGURE 6.5. Suboccipital muscles. Stepwise dissection. *A*, the right trapezius and sternocleidomastoid have been preserved. The left trapezius and sternocleidomastoid have been reflected along with the galea aponeurotica to expose the underlying semispinalis capitis, splenius capitis, and levator scapulae. *B*, the right sternocleidomastoid and trapezius have been reflected to expose the splenius capitis. The left splenius capitis has been removed to expose the underlying semispinalis and longissimus capitis. *C*, the right splenius capitis has been removed to expose the semispinalis and longissimus capitis. The left semispinalis and longissimus capitis have been removed to expose the suboccipital triangle formed by the superior oblique, which passes from the C1 transverse process to the occipital bone, the inferior oblique, which extends from the transverse process of C1 to the spinous process of C2, and the rectus capitis posterior major, which extends from the occipital bone below the inferior nuchal line to the spinous process of C2. The vertebral artery courses in the depths of the suboccipital triangle as it passes behind the superior facet of C1 and across the upper edge of the posterior atlantal arch. *D*, both semispinalis capitis muscles have been reflected laterally to expose the suboccipital triangles bilaterally. *E*, the muscles forming the left suboccipital triangle have been removed. The vertebral artery ascends slightly lateral from the transverse process of C2 to reach the

from the medial part and below the inferior nuchal line to the tubercle on the posterior arch of the atlas.

The suboccipital triangle is a region bounded above and medially by the rectus capitis posterior major, above and laterally by the superior oblique, and below and laterally by the inferior oblique (*Fig. 6.5*). It is covered by the semispinalis capitis medially and by the splenius capitis laterally. The floor of the triangle is formed by the posterior atlanto-occipital membrane and the posterior arch of the atlas. The structures in the triangle are the terminal extradural segment of the vertebral artery and the first cervical nerve.

The platysma is a broad sheet extending downward from the lower part of the face and across the clavicle to the fascia covering the pectoralis major and deltoid. The anterior vertebral muscles insert on the clival part of the occipital bone anterior to the foramen magnum. This group includes the longus colli, which attach to the anterior surface of the vertebral column between the atlas and the third thoracic vertebra; the longus capitis, which extends from the clivus in front of the foramen magnum to the transverse processes of the third through the sixth cervical vertebrae; the rectus capitis anterior, which is situated behind the upper part of the longus capitis and extends from the occipital bone in front of the occipital condyle to the anterior surface of the lateral mass and transverse process of the atlas; and the rectus capitis lateralis, which extends from the jugular process of the occipital bone to the transverse process of the atlas.

The muscles described above are embedded in the cervical fascia. This fascia is divided into superficial and deep layers. The superficial layer is a lamina of loose connective tissue below the dermis, which invests the platysma. The deep layer lies internal to the platysma, invests the muscles, and condenses into fibrous sheaths that bind the arteries and accompanying veins together. The superficial lamina of the deep fascia attaches in the posterior midline to the ligamentum nuchae, thinly invests the trapezius, continues forward covering the posterior triangle of the neck, divides at the posterior border of the sternocleidomastoid to enclose the muscle, and at its anterior margin again forms a lamina that covers the anterior triangle of the neck and reaches the median plane, to be continuous with the corresponding lamina from the opposite side. The carotid sheath is a condensation of the cervical fascia, which invests the common and internal carotid arteries, the internal jugular vein, and the vagus nerve. The prevertebral lamina of the cervical fascia covers the prevertebral muscles, extends laterally to connect with the carotid sheath, and covers the scalene muscles to form a fascial floor for the posterior triangle of the neck. Superiorly it is attached to the base of the skull, and inferiorly it continues downward behind the pharynx and in front of the longus colli into the superior mediastinum. The deep fascia is fused above to the superior nuchal line, mastoid process, zygomatic arch, styloid process, and mandible, and below to the scapula, clavicle, and sternum.

Neural relationships

The neural structures situated in the region of the foramen magnum are the caudal part of the brainstem, cerebellum and fourth ventricle, the rostral part of the spinal cord, and the lower cranial and upper cervical nerves (*Figs. 6.3* and *6.6*) (5, 19).

Spinal cord

The spinal cord blends indistinguishably into the medulla at a level arbitrarily set to be at the upper limit of the dorsal and ventral rootlets forming the first cervical nerve (*Figs. 6.3* and *6.6*). It is easier to differentiate this level on the ventral than on the dorsal surface because the ventral rootlets of the first cervical nerve are always present, whereas the dorsal rootlets are absent in many cases. The fact that the junction of the spinal cord and medulla is situated at the rostral margin of the first cervical root means that the medulla, and not the spinal cord, occupies the foramen magnum.

The spinal cord immediately below the level of the foramen magnum is round, and it is divided by one fissure and several sulci. The anteromedian fissure and the posteromedian sulcus divide the spinal cord into symmetrical halves. The anteromedian fissure reaches a depth of several millimeters. The posteromedian sulcus is much shallower, and from it the posteromedian septum penetrates the spinal cord, almost reaching the central canal. The posterior lateral sulcus is situated along the line where the dorsal roots enter the spinal cord. The posterior funiculus is situated between the posteromedian and posterior lateral sulci. At the upper cervical level, the surface of each posterior funiculus is divided by another shallow longitudinal furrow, the posterior intermediate sulcus, into the fasciculus gracilis medially and the fasciculus cuneatus laterally. The region of the spinal cord between the posterior lateral sulcus and the anteromedian fissure is divided into anterior and lateral funiculi by the exiting ventral rootlets of the spinal nerves. The anterior funiculus includes the zone of emergence of the ventral roots. The lateral funiculus lies between the ventral roots and the posterior lateral sulcus. In the upper

transverse process of C1 and turns medially behind the superior facet of C1 to reach the upper surface of the posterior arch of C1. The C2 ganglion is located between the posterior arch of C1 and the lamina of C2. The dorsal ramus of C2 produces a medial branch that forms the majority of the greater occipital nerve. *F*, the muscles forming both suboccipital triangles have been removed. The rectus capitis posterior minor, which extends from the posterior arch of C1 to the occipital bone below the inferior nuchal line, has been preserved. The vertebral arteries cross the posterior arch of the atlas and penetrate the posterior atlanto-occipital membrane to reach the dura. *A.*, artery; *Atl.*, atlanto-; *Cap.*, capitis; *Car.*, carotid; *CN*, cranial nerve; *Inf.*, inferior; *Int.*, internal; *Jug.*, jugular; *Lev.*, levator; *Longiss.*, longissimus; *M.*, muscle; *Maj.*, major; *Memb.*, membrane; *Min.*, minor; *Obl.*, oblique; *Occip.*, occipital; *Post.*, posterior; *Proc.*, process; *Rec.*, rectus; *Scap.*, scapulae; *Semispin.*, semispinalis; *Spin.*, spinalis; *Splen.*, splenius; *Sternocleidomast.*, sternocleidomastoid; *Sup.*, superior; *Trans.*, transverse; *V.*, vein; *Vert.*, vertebral.

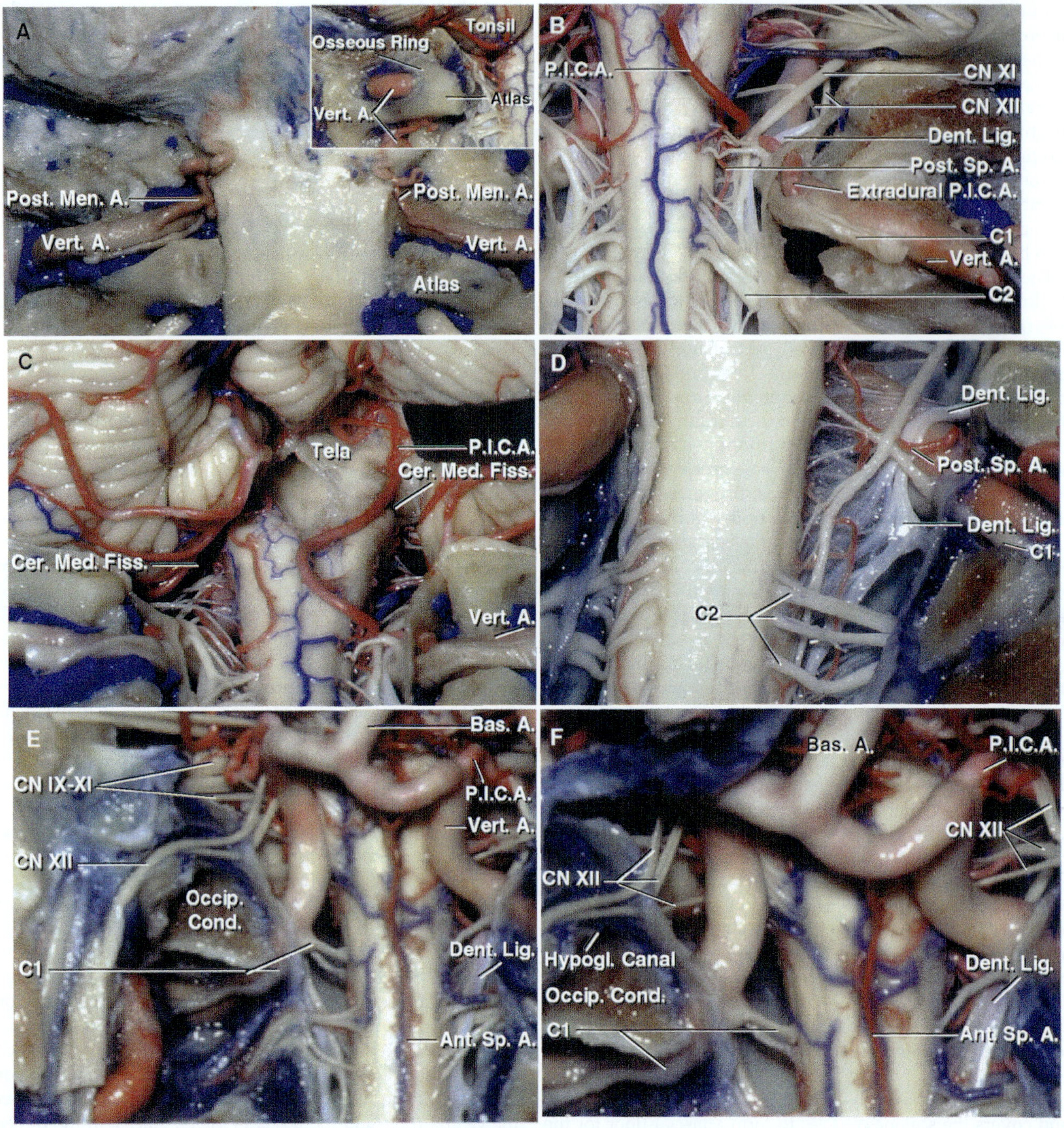

FIGURE 6.6. Foramen magnum. *A–D,* posterior views; *E* and *F,* anterior views. *A,* a suboccipital craniectomy and upper cervical laminectomy exposes the dura. The vertebral arteries pass medially across the upper surface of the atlas where they give off the posterior meningeal arteries that ascend to supply the dura on the posterior aspect of the foramen magnum and posterior fossa. *Insert, upper right.* The upper margin of the left half of the arch of the atlas forms an osseous ring around the vertebral artery just proximal to where it enters the dura. *B,* enlarged view of another foramen magnum after opening the dura. The right PICA arises outside the dura and penetrates the dura with the vertebral artery. The rostral end of the dentate ligament passes between the vertebral artery and the PICA to insert into the dura along the lateral margin of the foramen magnum. The accessory nerve ascends posterior to both the PICA and the vertebral artery. The vertebral artery gives rise to a posterior spinal artery that passes along the posterolateral aspect of the spinal cord and medulla. The hypoglossal rootlets are stretched over the posterior aspect of the vertebral artery. *C,* the right tonsil has been retracted to expose the caudal end of the fourth ventricle, which is located above the foramen magnum. The right PICA ascends through the foramen magnum and

cervical region, the rootlets that unite to form the spinal part of the accessory nerve emerge through the lateral funiculus.

Dentate ligament

The dentate ligament is considered with the spinal cord because it is attached to it (*Figs. 6.3* and *6.6*). This ligament is a white fibrous sheet that is attached to the spinal cord medially and to the dura mater laterally. The medial border of the dentate ligament, which is attached to the pia mater between the dorsal and ventral rootlets along the length of each side of the spinal cord, presents a series of triangular toothlike processes on each side that are attached at intervals to the dura mater. At the craniocervical junction, the dentate ligament is located between the vertebral artery and the ventral roots of C1 anteriorly and the branches of the posterior spinal artery and the spinal accessory nerve posteriorly; in addition, it is often incorporated into the dural cuff around the vertebral artery at the site of dural penetration. The most rostral attachment of the dentate ligament is located at the level of the foramen magnum, above where the vertebral artery pierces the dura. The ligament courses behind the accessory nerve at that level, although the dentate ligament is located anterior to the accessory nerve at lower levels. The second triangular process is attached to the dura below the site at which the vertebral artery and the roots of C1 pierce the dura. Sectioning the upper two triangular processes will increase access anterior to the spinal cord. The first cervical nerve courses along the posteroinferior surface of the vertebral artery as it pierces the dura. The ventral root is located anterior to the dentate ligament, and the dorsal root, which is infrequently present, passes posterior to the dentate ligament. There are frequently communications between the C1 nerve root and the spinal accessory nerve.

Brainstem

The lower medulla blends indistinguishably into the upper spinal cord at the level of the C1 nerve roots (*Figs. 6.3, 6.4,* and *6.6*). The anterior surface of the medulla is formed by the medullary pyramids, which face the clivus, the anterior edge of the foramen magnum, and the rostral part of the odontoid process. The lateral surface is formed predominantly by the inferior olives. The posterior surface of the medulla is divided into superior and inferior parts. The superior part is composed in the midline of the inferior half of the fourth ventricle, and laterally by the inferior cerebellar peduncles. The inferior part of the posterior surface is composed of the gracile fasciculus and tubercle medially, and the cuneate fasciculus and tubercle laterally.

Cerebellum

The suboccipital cerebellar surface rests above the posterior and lateral edge of the foramen magnum. Only the lower part of the hemispheres formed by the tonsils and the biventral lobules, and the lower part of the vermis formed by the nodule, uvula, and pyramid, are related to the foramen magnum. The biventral lobule sits above the lateral part of the foramen magnum, and the tonsils rest above the level of the posterior edge (*Figs. 6.3* and *6.6*). The cerebellar surface above the posterior part of the foramen magnum has a deep vertical depression, the posterior cerebellar incisura, which contains the falx cerebelli and extends inferiorly toward the foramen magnum. The tonsils, which sit above the posterior edge of the foramen magnum, are commonly involved in herniations through the foramen magnum. Each tonsil is an ovoid structure that is attached along its superolateral border to the remainder of the cerebellum. The cerebellomedullary fissure extends superiorly between the cerebellum and the medulla and is situated rostral to the posterior margin of the foramen magnum.

Cranial nerves

The accessory nerve is the only cranial nerve that passes through the foramen magnum (*Figs. 6.3* and *6.6*). It has a cranial part composed of the rootlets that arise from the medulla and join the vagus nerve, and a spinal portion formed by the union of a series of rootlets that arise from the lower medulla and upper spinal cord. In the posterior fossa, the accessory nerve is composed of one main trunk from the spinal cord and three to six small rootlets that emerge from the medulla. The most rostral medullary rootlets are functionally inferior vagal rootlets, since they arise from the vagal nuclei (25). The lower medullary rootlets join the spinal portion of the nerve. The upper medullary rootlets enter the jugular foramen without joining the spinal portion, but once inside the jugular foramen, they join either the vagus or accessory nerve. The spinal contribution arises from the cervical portion of the spinal cord as a series of rootlets situated midway between the ventral and dorsal rootlets. The lowest level of origin of the rootlets contributing to the accessory nerves was at the C7 root level in 2 of the 50 nerves examined,

along the posterior margin of the medulla to reach the cerebellomedullary fissure. *D*, another specimen. The rostral end of the dentate ligament passes between the posterior spinal artery and vertebral artery and attaches to the dura at the level of the foramen magnum. The accessory nerve ascends behind the posterior spinal artery. The C1 nerve root receives a contribution from the accessory nerve and passes through the dura with the vertebral artery and courses along the lower margin of the artery. The posterior spinal artery arises inside the dura and passes between the dentate ligament and accessory nerve and gives rise to ascending branches to the medulla and descending branches to the spinal cord. *E*, the anterior skull base has been removed. The vertebral arteries ascend in front of the brainstem and give rise to the anterior spinal artery. *F*, enlarged view. The C1 ventral roots penetrate the dura with the vertebral artery. The hypoglossal rootlets pass behind the vertebral arteries. *A.*, artery; *Bas.*, basilar; *Cer.Med.*, cerebellomedullary; *CN*, cranial nerve; *Cond.*, condyle; *Dent.*, dentate; *Fiss.*, fissure; *Hypogl.*, hypoglossal; *Lig.*, ligament; *Men.*, meningeal; *Occip.*, occipital; *P.I.C.A.*, posteroinferior cerebellar artery; *Post.*, posterior; *Sp.*, spinal; *Vert.*, vertebral.

C6 in 10, C5 in 13, C4 in 11, C3 in 7, C2 in 5, and Cl in 2 (5). These rootlets unite to form a trunk with a diameter of approximately 1.0 mm, which ascends through the foramen magnum between the dentate ligament and the dorsal spinal roots to enter the posterior cranial fossa behind the vertebral artery.

Of the 50 accessory nerves examined in our previous study, all had connections with the dorsal roots of the upper cervical nerves. The most common and largest anastomosis was with the dorsal root of the first cervical nerve (5, 22). Twenty-eight of the C1 dorsal roots arose solely from the accessory nerve without there being a contribution from the C1 level of the spinal cord. All of the 15 Cl dorsal roots that received rootlets arising from the spinal cord at the C1 level also had anastomotic fibers from the accessory nerve. Four of the 50 accessory nerves had an anastomotic connection with the C2 nerve root, 10 with the C3, 8 with the C4, and 2 with the C5.

The lower four cranial nerves are sufficiently close to the foramen magnum that they may be involved by lesions arising there (*Figs. 6.3* and *6.6*). Their intradural anatomy is described in the chapter of this issue on the cerebellopontine angle and posterior fossa cranial nerves.

Cervical nerve roots

Each dorsal and ventral root is composed of a series of six to eight rootlets that fan out to enter the posterolateral and anterolateral surfaces of the spinal cord, respectively (*Figs. 6.3* and *6.6*). The dorsal and ventral roots cross the subarachnoid space and transverse the dura mater separately, then unite close to the intervertebral foramen to form the spinal nerves. The rootlets in the region of the foramen magnum pass almost directly lateral to reach their dural foramina. The neurons of the dorsal roots collect to form ganglia located just proximal to the union of the dorsal and ventral root in the intervertebral foramina, however the first cervical dorsal root and associated ganglion may be absent. The C1, C2, and C3 nerves, distal to the ganglion, divide into dorsal and ventral rami. The dorsal rami divide into medial and lateral branches that supply the skin and muscles of the posterior region of the neck. The C1 nerve, termed the suboccipital nerve, leaves the vertebral canal between the occipital bone and atlas and has a dorsal ramus that is larger than the ventral ramus. The dorsal ramus courses between the posterior arch of the atlas and the vertebral artery to reach the suboccipital triangle, where it sends branches to the rectus capitis posterior major and minor, superior and inferior oblique, and the semispinalis capitis, and occasionally has a cutaneous branch that accompanies the occipital artery to the scalp. The C1 ventral ramus courses between the posterior arch of the atlas and the vertebral artery and passes forward, lateral to the lateral mass of the atlas and medial to the vertebral artery, and supplies the rectus capitis lateralis. The C2 nerve emerges between the posterior arch of the atlas and the lamina of the axis where the spinal ganglion is located extradurally, medial to the inferior facet of C1 and the vertebral artery. Distal to the ganglion, the nerve divides into a larger dorsal and a smaller ventral ramus. After passing below and supplying the inferior oblique muscle, the dorsal ramus divides into a large medial and a small lateral branch. It is the medial branch that is most intimately related to this suboccipital operative field and that forms the greater occipital nerve. It ascends obliquely between the inferior oblique and the semisplenius capitis, pierces the latter and the trapezius muscle near their attachments to the occipital bone, and is joined by a filament from the medial branch of C3. It supplies the semispinalis capitis muscle, ascends with the occipital artery, and supplies the scalp as far forward as the vertex, and occasionally the back of the ear. The lateral branch sends filaments that innervate the splenius, longissimus, and semisplenius capitis, and is often joined by the corresponding branch from the C3 nerve. The C2 ventral ramus courses between the vertebral arches and transverse processes of the atlas and axis and behind the vertebral artery to leave this operative field. Two branches of the C2 and C3 ventral rami, the lesser occipital and greater auricular nerves, curve around the posterior border and ascend on the sternocleidomastoid muscle to supply the skin behind the ear.

The first cervical nerve, located just below the foramen magnum, deserves special attention (*Figs. 6.3* and *6.6*). It differs from the other cervical nerves in the consistency and origin of the dorsal rootlets forming the nerve. The C1 ventral root is composed of four to eight rootlets that joined and coursed laterally. Before entering the dural foramina, the C1 ventral root, and the corresponding dorsal root if present, attaches to the posteroinferior surface of the initial intradural part of the vertebral artery, and both exit the dural sac through the funnel-shaped dural foramen around the vertebral artery. The ventral root joins the dorsal root in or external to the dural foramen.

The dorsal root of the first cervical nerve is more complicated than the ventral root because of the variations in its composition and its connections with the accessory nerve. In the 25 cervical spinal cords examined, in which one would expect to find 50 C1 dorsal roots arising from the posterior lateral sulcus, only 15 were found (5). The accessory nerve contributed a root to the C1 nerve in 28 of the 35 roots lacking a dorsal root arising from the spinal cord. In the remaining 7 cases, the C1 dorsal root was absent. Each of the 15 dorsal roots that arose from the spinal cord also had a contribution from the accessory nerve.

Arterial relationships

The major arteries related to the foramen magnum are the vertebral and posteroinferior cerebellar arteries (PICA), and the meningeal branches of the vertebral, and external and internal carotid arteries (*Figs. 6.3, 6.4,* and *6.6*) (16, 20, 21).

Vertebral artery

The paired vertebral arteries arise from the subclavian arteries, ascend through the transverse processes of the upper six cervical vertebrae, pass behind the lateral masses of the axis, enter the dura mater behind the occipital condyles, ascend through the foramen magnum to the front of the medulla, and join to form the basilar artery at the pontomedullary junction. Each artery is divided into intradural and extradural parts (*Figs. 6.3-6.6*).

The extradural part is divided into three segments. The first segment extends from the origin at the subclavian artery to the entrance into the lowest transverse foramen, usually at the C6 level. The second segment ascends through the transverse foramina of the upper six cervical vertebrae in front of the cervical nerve roots. This segment deviates laterally just above the axis to reach the laterally placed transverse foramen of the atlas. The third segment, the one most intimately related to the foramen magnum, extends from the foramen in the transverse process of the atlas to the site of passage through the dura mater. The artery, after passing through the transverse process of the atlas, is located on the medial side of the rectus capitis lateralis. The third segment passes medially behind the lateral mass of the atlas and atlanto-occipital joint and is pressed into the groove on the upper surface of the lateral part of the posterior arch of the atlas, where it courses along the floor of the suboccipital triangle. It enters the vertebral canal by passing anterior to the lateral border of the atlanto-occipital membrane. It is partially covered by the posterior atlanto-occipital membrane and semispinalis capitis, the rectus capitis posterior major, and the superior and inferior oblique muscles. It is surrounded by a venous plexus composed of anastomoses between the deep cervical and epidural veins. The C1 nerve root passes through the dura mater on the lower surface of the vertebral artery between the artery and the groove on the posterior arch of the atlas with the vertebral artery. This bony groove is frequently transformed into a bony canal that completely surrounds a short segment of the artery. Of the 50 arteries we examined, 24 (48%) were in a shallow groove, 12 (24%) were partially, but incompletely, surrounded by bone, and 14 (28%) coursed through a bony ring that completely surrounded the artery (*Fig. 6.6*) (5). The terminal extradural segment of the vertebral artery gives rise to the posterior meningeal and posterior spinal arteries, branches to the deep cervical musculature, and infrequently the PICA.

The intradural segment begins at the dural foramina just inferior to the lateral edge of the foramen magnum. The dura in this region is much thicker than in other areas, and it forms a funnel-shaped foramen around a 4- to 6-mm length of the artery. The first cervical nerve exits the spinal canal, and the posterior spinal artery enters the spinal canal through this dural foramen with the vertebral artery. These three structures are bound together at the foramen by fibrous dural bands. The initial intradural segment of the vertebral artery passes just superior to the dorsal and ventral roots of the first cervical nerve, and just anterior to the posterior spinal artery, the dentate ligament, and the spinal portion of the accessory nerve.

Once inside the dura mater, the artery ascends from the lower lateral to the upper anterior surface of the medulla. The intradural part of the artery is divided into lateral and anterior medullary segments (5, 16). The lateral medullary segment begins at the dural foramen and passes anterior and superior along the lateral medullary surface to terminate at the preolivary sulcus. The anterior medullary segment begins at the preolivary sulcus, courses in front of, or between, the hypoglossal rootlets, and crosses the pyramid to join with the other vertebral artery at or near the pontomedullary sulcus to form the basilar artery. In its ascending course, the anterior and lateral surfaces of the lateral medullary segments face the occipital condyles, the hypoglossal canals, and the jugular tubercles. The anterior medullary segment rests on the clivus. The branches arising from the vertebral artery in the region of the foramen magnum are the posterior spinal, anterior spinal, PICA, and anterior and posterior meningeal arteries.

Posterior spinal artery

The paired posterior spinal arteries usually arise from the posteromedial surface of the vertebral arteries, just outside the dura mater, but they may also arise from the initial intradural part of the vertebral arteries, or from the PICA (*Figs. 6.3* and *6.6*) (5, 16, 21). Care should be taken to preserve the posterior spinal artery during dural opening because it may be incorporated into the dural cuff around the vertebral artery. As each posterior spinal artery passes through the dura mater, it is surrounded by the same fibrous tunnel as the vertebral artery and the first cervical nerve root. In the subarachnoid space, it courses medially behind the rostral-most attachments of the dentate ligament, and on reaching the lower medulla, it divides into ascending and descending branches. The ascending branch courses through the foramen magnum and supplies the restiform body, the gracile and cuneate tubercles, the rootlets of the accessory nerve, and the choroid plexus near The foramen of Magendie, and may give rise to branches that anastomose with branches of the PICA. The descending branch passes downward between the dorsal rootlets and the dentate ligament on the posterolateral surface of the spinal cord, and supplies the superficial part of the dorsal half of the cervical spinal cord. It anastomoses with the posterior branches of the radicular arteries that enter the vertebral foramen at lower levels. The descending branch gives rise to collateral branches, each lower one being smaller and less constant than the last one, which course medially across the posterior surface of the spinal cord, and join to form an artery that courses in the midline, parallel to the posterior spinal arteries.

Posteroinferior cerebellar artery

The PICA is the largest branch of the vertebral artery (*Figs. 6.3* and *6.6*). It usually originates with the dura mater, but it may infrequently originate from the terminal extradural part of the vertebral artery. It may arise at, above, or below the level of the foramen magnum; of the 42 arteries found in 50 cerebellae examined, 35 arose above and 7 arose below the foramen (16). The tonsillomedullary PICA segment, which forms the caudal loop related to the lower part of the tonsil, is most intimately related to the foramen magnum. The lower end of the caudal loop was found to be above the edge of the foramen magnum in 37 of the 42 arteries examined, below the edge in 4, and at the level of the edge of the foramen in 1.

Anterior spinal artery

The anterior spinal artery is formed by the union of the paired anterior ventral spinal arteries, which originate from the anterior medullary segment of the vertebral arteries near the origin of the basilar artery (*Figs. 6.3, 6.4,* and *6.6*). The junction of the anteroventral spinal arteries was located above the level of the foramen magnum near the lower end of the olives in 84% of our specimens (5). In some cases, one of the anterior ventral spinal arteries continued inferiorly as the anterior spinal artery, and the other terminated on the anterior surface of the medulla or in a rudimentary channel connected the smaller anterior ventral spinal artery with a dominant one.

The anterior spinal artery descends through the foramen magnum on the anterior surface of the medulla and the spinal cord in or near the anteromedian fissure. On the medulla, it supplies the pyramids and their decussation, the medial lemniscus, the interolivary bundles, the hypoglossal nuclei and nerves, and the posterior longitudinal fasciculus (17). It anastomoses with the anterior branches of the radicular arteries entering the cervical foramina. There are few anastomoses with the anterior radicular branches if the descending channel is large, but it has frequent connections with the anterior radicular arteries if it is small.

Meningeal arteries

The dura mater around the foramen magnum is supplied by the anterior and posterior meningeal branches of the vertebral artery, and the meningeal branches of the ascending pharyngeal and occipital arteries (*Figs. 6.3* and *6.6*) (5, 20). These arteries, plus the dorsal meningeal branch of meningohypophyseal trunk that arises from the intracavernous segment of the internal carotid artery, supply all of the dura lining the posterior cranial fossa. Infrequently, the PICA, the posterior spinal artery, and the intradural part of the vertebral artery give rise to meningeal branches.

The anterior meningeal branch of the vertebral artery arises from the medial surfaces of the extradural part of the vertebral artery immediately above the transverse foramen of the third cervical vertebra (*Fig. 6.3*). The artery enters the spinal canal through the intervertebral foramen between the second and third cervical vertebrae, and ascends between the posterior longitudinal ligament and the dura mater. At the level of the apex of the dens, each artery courses medially to join its mate from the opposite side and forms an arch over the apex of the dens. Its branches supply the dura mater in the region of the clivus and the anterior part of the foramen magnum and upper spinal canal, and they anastomose with the branches of the ascending pharyngeal and dorsal meningeal arteries that supply the dura mater covering the anterior and anterolateral part of the posterior fossa. The anterior meningeal artery also gives rise to muscular and osseous branches that supply the body and odontoid process of the axis and the articulate plate of the atlanto-occipital and atlantoaxial joints.

The posterior meningeal artery arises from the posterosuperior surface of the vertebral artery as it courses around the lateral mass of the atlas, above the posterior arch or just before penetrating the dura; however, it may have an intradural origin, in which case, it penetrates the arachnoid to reach the dura (*Fig. 6.6*) (5). It pursues a tortuous ascending course and penetrates the dura before reaching the posterior edge of the foramen magnum. After passing through the foramen magnum, it ascends near the falx cerebelli and divides near the torcula into several branches that terminate in the posterior part of the tentorium and cerebral falx. It supplies the dura mater lining the posterolateral and posterior part of the posterior cranial fossa, and anastomoses with the meningeal branches of the ascending pharyngeal and occipital arteries.

The ascending pharyngeal branch of the external carotid artery usually sends two branches to the dura above the foramen magnum. One branch passes through the hypoglossal canal and the other enters through the jugular foramen (14). The branch passing through the hypoglossal canal divides into an ascending branch that passes upward in the dura covering the clivus and anastomoses with the branches of the dorsal meningeal artery, and a descending branch that courses inferomedially toward the anterior edge of the foramen magnum and anastomoses with branches of the arcade above the odontoid process formed by the anterior meningeal arteries. This anastomotic rete in the dura anterior to the foramen magnum and on the clivus gives osseous branches to the clivus. The branches that enter through the jugular foramen divide into branches that course posteriorly and posterosuperiorly to anastomose with the meningeal branches of the occipital and posterior meningeal arteries, and supply the dura mater in the posterior and posterolateral parts of the posterior cranial fossa.

The meningeal branch of the occipital artery is inconstant and, if present, it penetrates the cranium through the mastoid emissary foramen. It divides into one branch that courses posterosuperiorly to join the branches of the posterior meningeal artery that supplies the dura mater in the posterior part of the posterior fossa, and another branch that courses anterolaterally and joins the meningeal branches of the ascending pharyngeal artery.

Venous relationships

The venous structures in the region of the foramen magnum are divided into three groups: one composed of the extradural veins, another formed by the intradural (neural) veins, and a third constituted by the dural venous sinuses (13, 18). The three groups anastomose through bridging and emissary veins.

Extradural groups

Venous flow in this area empties into two systems: one drained by the internal jugular vein and another draining into the vertebral venous plexus. The internal jugular vein and its tributaries form the most important drainage system in the craniocervical area. The internal jugular vein originates at the jugular foramen by the confluence of the sigmoid and inferior petrosal sinuses (14, 18, 25). The venous plexus surrounding the vertebral artery in the suboccipital triangle is formed by numerous small channels that empty into the internal vertebral plexuses (between the dura and the vertebrae), which issue from the vertebral canal above the posterior arch of the atlas. This vertebral venous plexus and multiple small veins from the deep muscles communicate with the dense venous plexus, which accompanies the vertebral artery into the foramen in the transverse process of the atlas and descends through the transverse foramina of successive cervical vertebrae into the brachiocephalic vein. The posterior condylar emissary vein, which passes through the posterior condylar canal, forms a communication between the vertebral venous plexus and the sigmoid sinus. The venous plexus of the hypoglossal canal passes along the hypoglossal canal to connect the basilar venous plexus with the marginal sinus, which encircles the foramen magnum. Obliteration of a portion of the venous plexus exposes the upper extradural segment of the vertebral artery.

Dural venous sinuses

The venous channels in the dura mater surrounding the foramen magnum are the marginal, occipital, sigmoid, inferior petrosal, and basilar venous plexus. The marginal sinus is located between the layers of the dura in the rim of the foramen magnum. It communicates anteriorly, through a series of small sinuses, with the basilar sinus on the clivus, and posteriorly with the occipital sinus. It is usually connected to the sigmoid sinus or jugular bulb, by a sinus that passes across the intracranial surface of, and communicates with, the veins in the hypoglossal canal. These anastomoses provide an alternative route for venous drainage in the case of obstruction of the internal jugular vein. The occipital sinus courses in the cerebellar falx. Its lower end divides into paired limbs each of which courses anteriorly around the foramen magnum to join the sigmoid sinus or the jugular bulb and its upper end joins the torcula.

The basilar venous plexus is located between the layers of the dura mater on the upper clivus. It is formed by interconnecting venous channels that anastomose with the inferior petrosal sinuses laterally, the cavernous sinuses superiorly, and the marginal sinus and epidural venous plexus inferiorly. The inferior petrosal sinuses extend along the petroclival fissure and communicate above with the basilar sinus and below with the jugular bulb. The sigmoid sinus descends along the sigmoid groove and exits the cranium through the sigmoid part of the jugular foramen, and descends anterolateral to the occipital condyle, and anterior to the transverse process of the atlas.

Intradural (neural) veins

The intradural veins in the region of the foramen magnum drain the lower part of the cerebellum and brainstem, the upper part of the spinal cord, and the cerebellomedullary fissure. The veins of the medulla and spinal cord form longitudinal plexiform channels that anastomose at the foramen magnum. The median anterior spinal vein that courses in the anteromedian spinal fissure deep to the anterior spinal artery is continuous with the median anterior medullary vein that courses on the anteromedian sulcus of the medulla. The lateral anterior spinal vein courses longitudinally along the origin of the ventral roots and superiorly joins the lateral anterior medullary vein that courses longitudinally in the anterolateral medullary (preolivary) sulcus along the line of origin of the hypoglossal rootlets. The lateral posterior spinal vein, which courses along the line of origin of the dorsal roots in the posterior lateral spinal sulcus, is continuous above with the lateral medullary vein that courses along the retro-olivary sulcus, dorsal to the olive. The median posterior spinal vein, which courses along the posteromedian spinal sulcus, is continuous above with the main vein on the posterior surface of the medulla, the median posterior medullary vein that courses along the posteromedian medullary sulcus. The transverse medullary and transverse spinal veins cross the medulla and spinal cord at various levels, interconnecting the major longitudinal channels. Bridging veins may connect the neural veins with the dural sinus in the region of the foramen magnum.

DISCUSSION

Herniations

Herniation of cerebellar tissue into the foramen magnum may cause neural compression and even death. These herniations are commonly referred to as tonsillar herniations (8, 27), but the herniation usually involves the tonsils and biventral lobules, both of which are deeply grooved by the edge of the foramen magnum. The herniation may compress the medulla and be so severe that the herniated tissue undergoes necrosis. Patients with herniation at the foramen magnum may be asymptomatic; or may present with pain, signs of neural compression, increased intracranial pressure, and sudden unexpected death. Symptoms caused by dysfunction of the cerebellum, brainstem, and lower cranial and upper spinal nerves include pain in the neck and upper arms, dizziness, ataxia, disturbances of gait, diplopia, dysphagia, tinnitus, decreased hearing, nystagmus, weakness up to the degree of quadriparesis, and sensory deficit in the extremities. Coughing or sneezing may aggravate the symptoms and cause syncope. Some patients without previous symptoms who die suddenly are found to have herniations through the foramen magnum at autopsy. The occurrence of sudden death in these patients means that herniation at the foramen magnum is a precarious situation that can be aggravated by minor stresses (8). The common denominator in these cases with sudden death is herniation of the tonsils and adjacent part of the biventral lobule into the foramen magnum. The herniation may be bilateral and symmetrical, although more commonly it is not strictly symmetrical and may be unilateral. The herniated tonsils are tightly pressed against the medulla. Acute or chronic herniations may be seen with space-occupying lesions, such as cerebellar astrocytomas or cystic tumors. Chronic herniation is seen with the Arnold-Chiari malformation.

Tumors

Tumors arising in the region of the foramen magnum are divided by Cushing and Eisenhardt (4) into a craniospinal group that arises above and grows downward toward the foramen magnum, and a spinocranial group that arises below

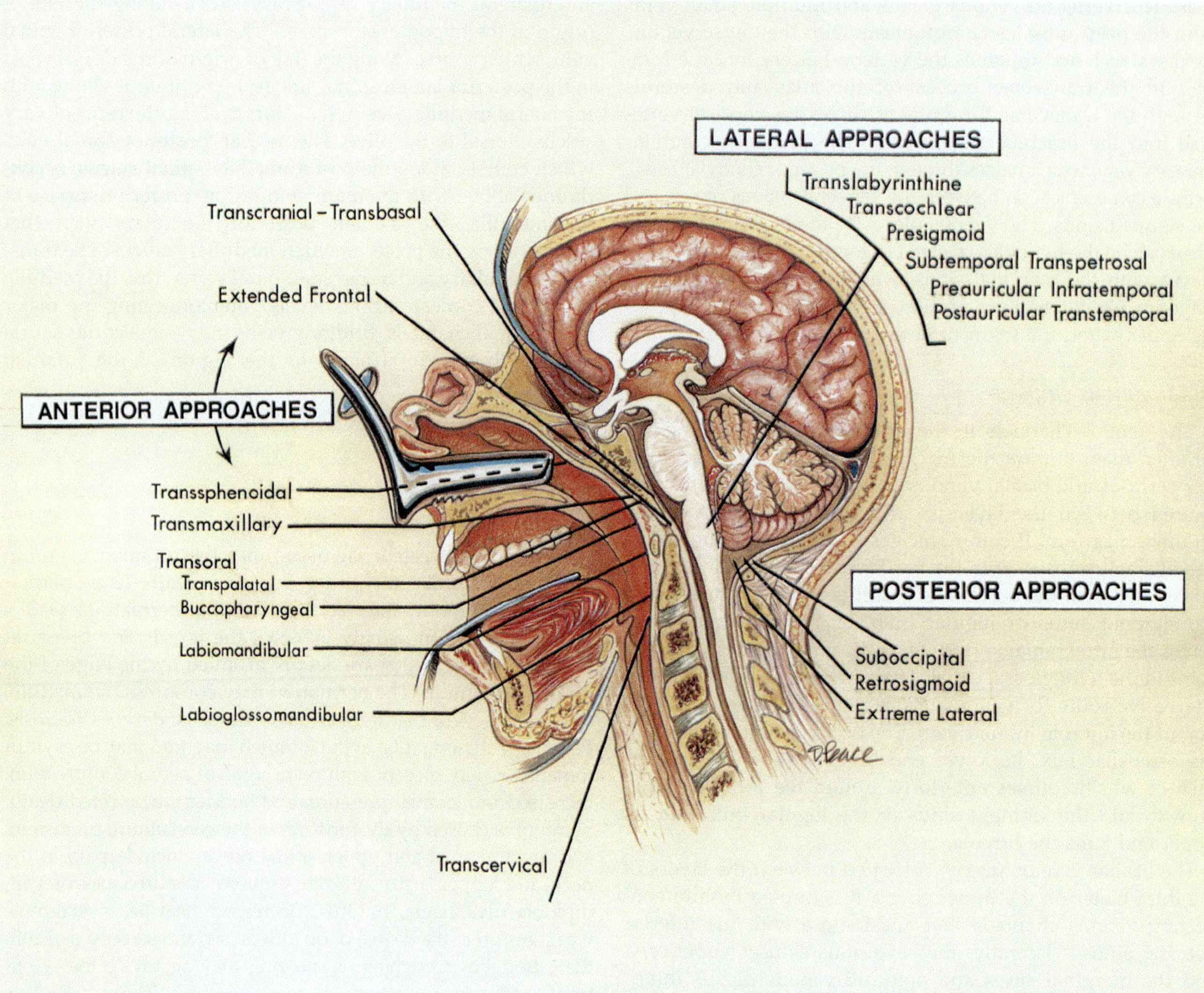

FIGURE 6.7. Surgical approaches to the foramen magnum. The posterior operative approach is commonly selected for intradural lesions. An anterior approach is frequently selected for extradural lesions situated anterior to the foramen magnum. A lateral approach may be selected for intradural lesions located lateral to and/or in front of the brainstem, especially if they involve or are contiguous with the temporal bone. The lateral approaches directed through the temporal bone are considered in a later section of this issue.

and grows upward toward the foramen magnum. The intradural extramedullary tumors in this region are usually benign, with meningiomas and schwannomas being the most frequent. The intramedullary tumors are represented mainly by astrocytomas and ependymomas. Cerebellar tumors, especially those originating in the fourth ventricle and those arising in the lower part of the cerebellar hemisphere or vermis, may extend into or through the foramen magnum into the upper spinal canal. Chordomas and metastases are the most common extradural tumors. The chordomas usually arise at the level of the clivus and may extend caudally into the foramen magnum.

Foramen magnum tumors have frequently eluded early diagnosis because they cause bizarre symptoms that simulate cervical, spondylosis, multiple sclerosis, or degenerative diseases (1, 23, 30). Symptoms or signs, common in other disorders that should also suggest the presence of a tumor in the region of the foramen magnum include neck stiffness and pain, involvement of the lower cranial nerves, especially the spinal accessory nerve, unilateral upper extremity weakness and atrophy, incoordination of the hands, gait disturbances, vague sensory disturbances or paresthesia in the extremities, objective sensory loss in a nonanatomic pattern, incoordination in the upper extremities, and pyramidal tract findings with spastic gait. Those tumors arising in the caudal part of the fourth ventricle or cerebellum may cause increased intracranial pressure by obstructing cerebrospinal fluid drainage at the level of the fourth ventricle.

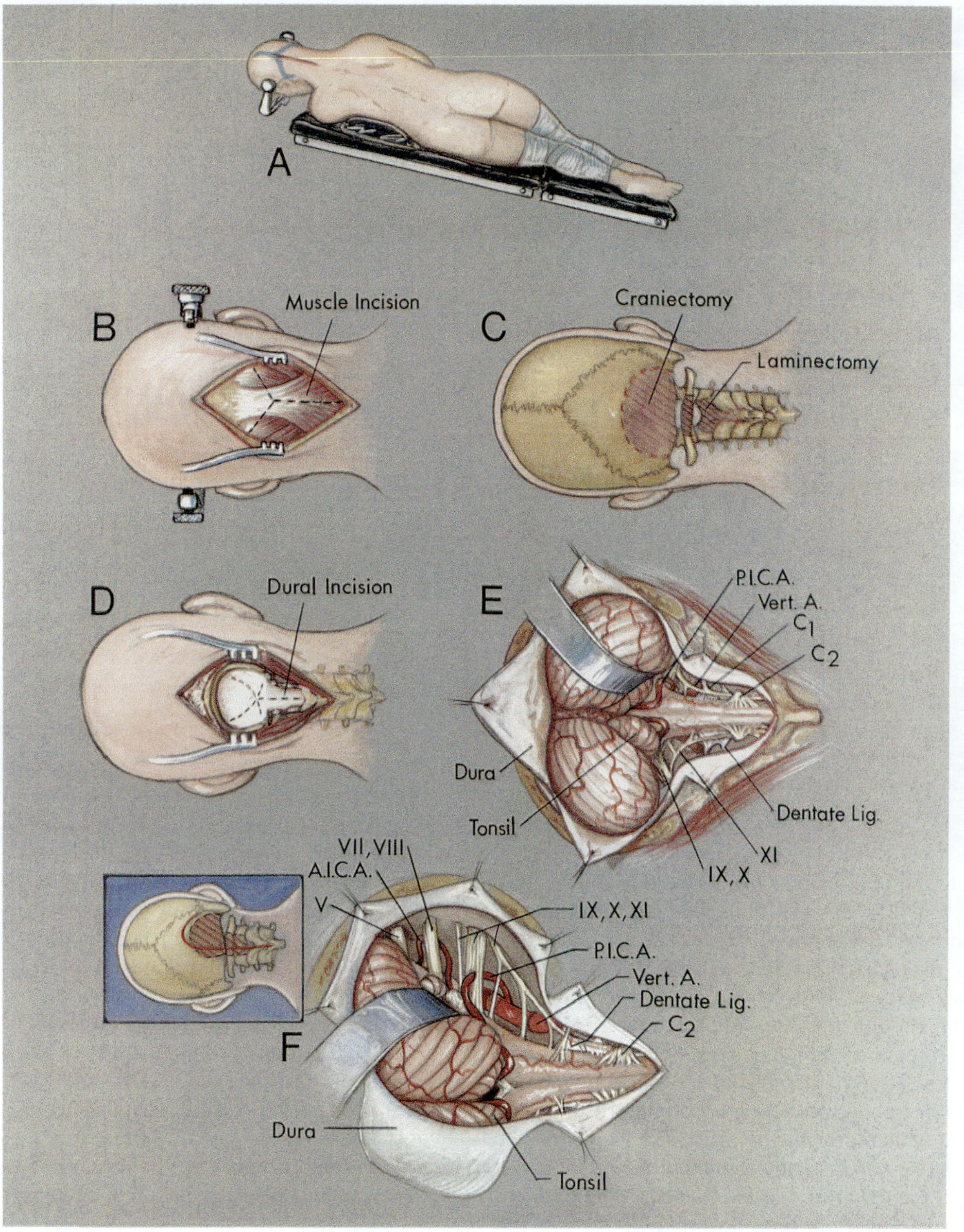

FIGURE 6.8. Suboccipital approaches. Either a vertical midline or hockey-stick incision is used, depending on the site of the lesion. *A*, the patient is most commonly placed in the three-quarter prone position. *B*, the vertical midline incision is selected for lesions situated in the upper spinal canal and for those located posteriorly or posterolaterally in the area above the foramen magnum. The subcutaneous tissues are separated from the underlying fascia near the inion to gain room for a Y-shaped incision in the muscles. The upper limbs of the "Y" begin at the level of the superior nuchal line and join below the inion. *C*, the incision is of sufficient length to complete a suboccipital craniectomy and a laminectomy of the axis and atlas (*oblique lines*). *D*, the dural incision is outlined (*interrupted lines*). *E*, intradural exposure. The major extracranial hazard is injury to the vertebral artery as it courses below the atlantoaxial joint and across the posterior arch of the atlas. The vertebral arteries and PICAs are in the lower part of the exposure. The accessory nerve ascends posterior to the dentate ligament. The glossopharyngeal, vagus, and accessory nerves pass toward the jugular foramen. *F, upper left.* Hockey-stick retrosigmoid exposure. Skin incision (*solid line*) and bone removal (*oblique lines*). *Lower right.* Intradural exposure. The hockey-stick incision extends superomedial from the mastoid process along the superior nuchal line to the inion and downward in the midline. This incision is selected if the lesion extends anterolateral or anterior to the brainstem toward the jugular foramen or cerebellopontine angle. This exposure permits the removal of the full posterior rim of the foramen magnum, the posterior elements of the atlas and axis, and, in addition, the ability to complete a unilateral suboccipital craniectomy of sufficient size to expose the anterolateral surface of the brainstem and the nerves in the cerebellopontine angle. Tumors in this area may extend upward through the cerebellomedullary fissure to be attached to the roof or floor of the fourth ventricle. Laterally situated tumors may be attached to the initial intradural segment of the vertebral artery and the thick dural cuff around the artery, which also incorporates the posterior spinal arteries and the C1 nerve root in fibrous tissue. As one moves superiorly along the lateral surface of the medulla, the origin of the PICA and the glossopharyngeal, vagus, accessory, facial, vestibulocochlear, and trigeminal nerves are encountered. The dura is closed with a dural substitute if closure of the patient's dura constricts the cerebellar tonsils or the cervicomedullary junction. *A.*, artery; *A.I.C.A.*, anteroinferior cerebellar artery; *Lig.*, ligament; *P.I.C.A.*, posteroinferior cerebellar artery; *Vert.*, vertebral.

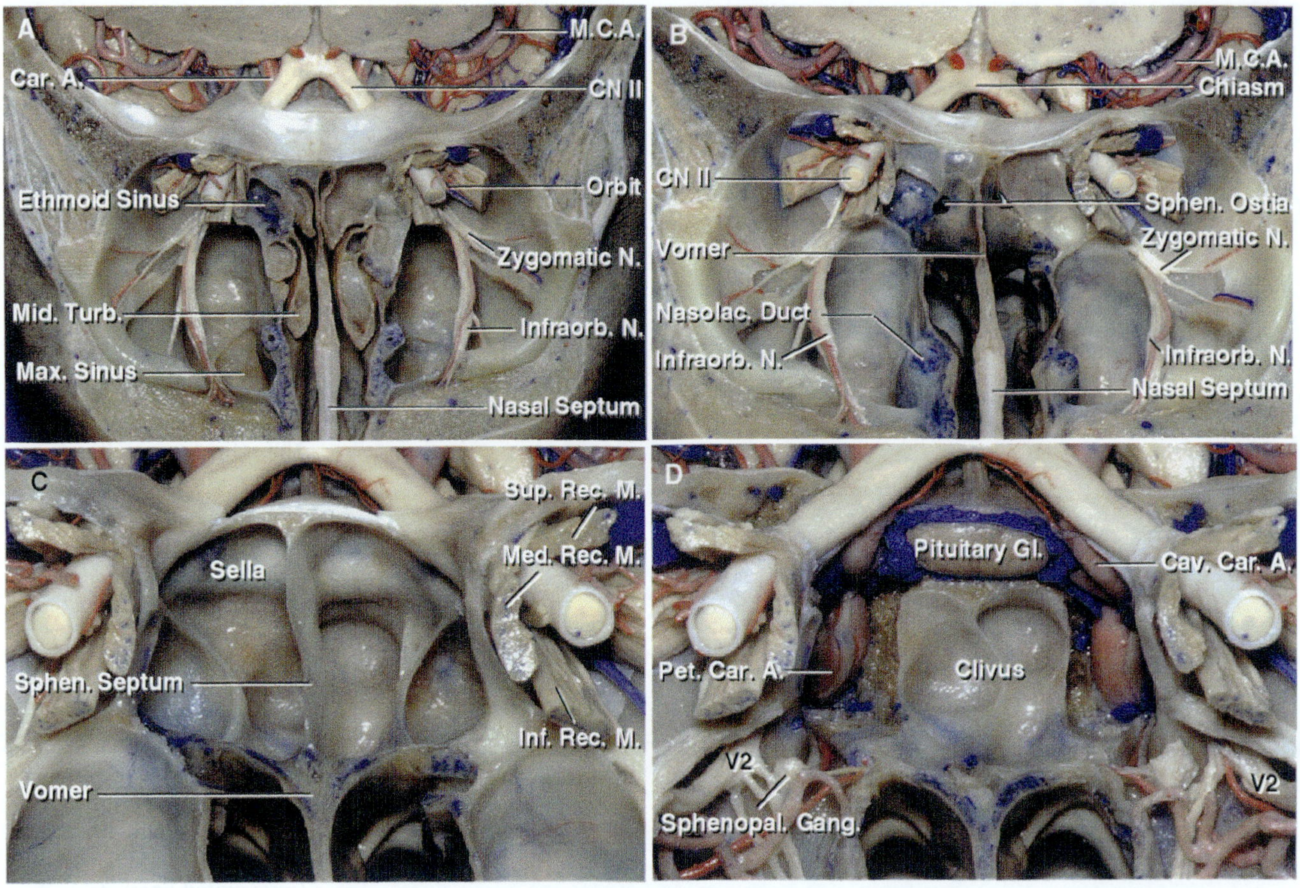

FIGURE 6.9. Transnasal route to the upper clivus. *A*, the section of the facial structures extends across the nasal cavity, superior and middle turbinates, maxillary sinuses, the orbits near the apex, and the ethmoid sinuses in front of the sphenoid sinus. The zygomatic and infraorbital nerves arise from the mandibular nerve in the pterygopalatine fossa, which is located behind the posterior wall of the maxillary sinus. *B*, the turbinates and posterior ethmoid air cells have been removed to expose the vomer and the anterior face of the sphenoid sinus. The nasolacrimal duct descends along the lateral wall of the nasal cavity and opens below the inferior turbinate into the inferior meatus. *C*, the anterior face of the sphenoid sinus has been removed to expose the multiseptated sphenoid sinus and the anterior wall of the sella. The bony prominences over the optic canals are situated in the superolateral margins of the sphenoid sinus. *D*, the anterior wall of the sella and the lateral walls of the sphenoid sinus have been removed to expose the petrous and cavernous carotid and the pituitary gland. The posterior wall of the sphenoid sinus, which forms the anterior surface of the upper clivus, has been preserved. *A.*, artery; *Car.*, carotid; *Cav.*, cavernous; *CN*, cranial nerve; *Gang.*, ganglion; *Gl.*, gland; *Inf.*, inferior; *Infraorb.*, infraorbital; *M.*, muscle; *Max.*, maxillary; *M.C.A.*, middle cerebral artery; *Med.*, medial; *Mid.*, middle; *N.*, nerve; *Nasolac.*, nasolacrimal; *Pet.*, petrous; *Rec.*, rectus; *Sphen.*, sphenoid; *Sup.*, superior; *Turb.*, turbinates.

Surgical approaches

The foramen magnum is most commonly approached from posteriorly or anteriorly, and less frequently from laterally (*Fig. 6.7*). The posterior operative approach is commonly selected for intradural lesions, and an anterior approach is frequently selected for extradural lesions situated anterior to the foramen magnum. A lateral approach may be selected for lesions located lateral to or in front of the brainstem, especially if they involve, or are located contiguous to the temporal bone and clivus. The lateral approaches directed through the temporal bone are reviewed in the chapter on the temporal bone.

Posterior approaches

The vertical midline incision is used for lesions situated in the upper spinal canal and posterior or posterolateral at the level of or above the foramen magnum (*Figs. 6.3, 6.6,* and *6.8*). The vertical midline skin incision is of sufficient length to complete a craniectomy above the foramen magnum and a laminectomy of the axis and atlas. The subcutaneous tissues are separated from the underlying fascia near the inion to gain room for a Y-shape muscle incision. The upper limbs of the "Y" begin at the level of the superior nuchal line, lateral to the external occipital protuberance, and join several centimeters below the inion, leaving a musculofascial flap along the su-

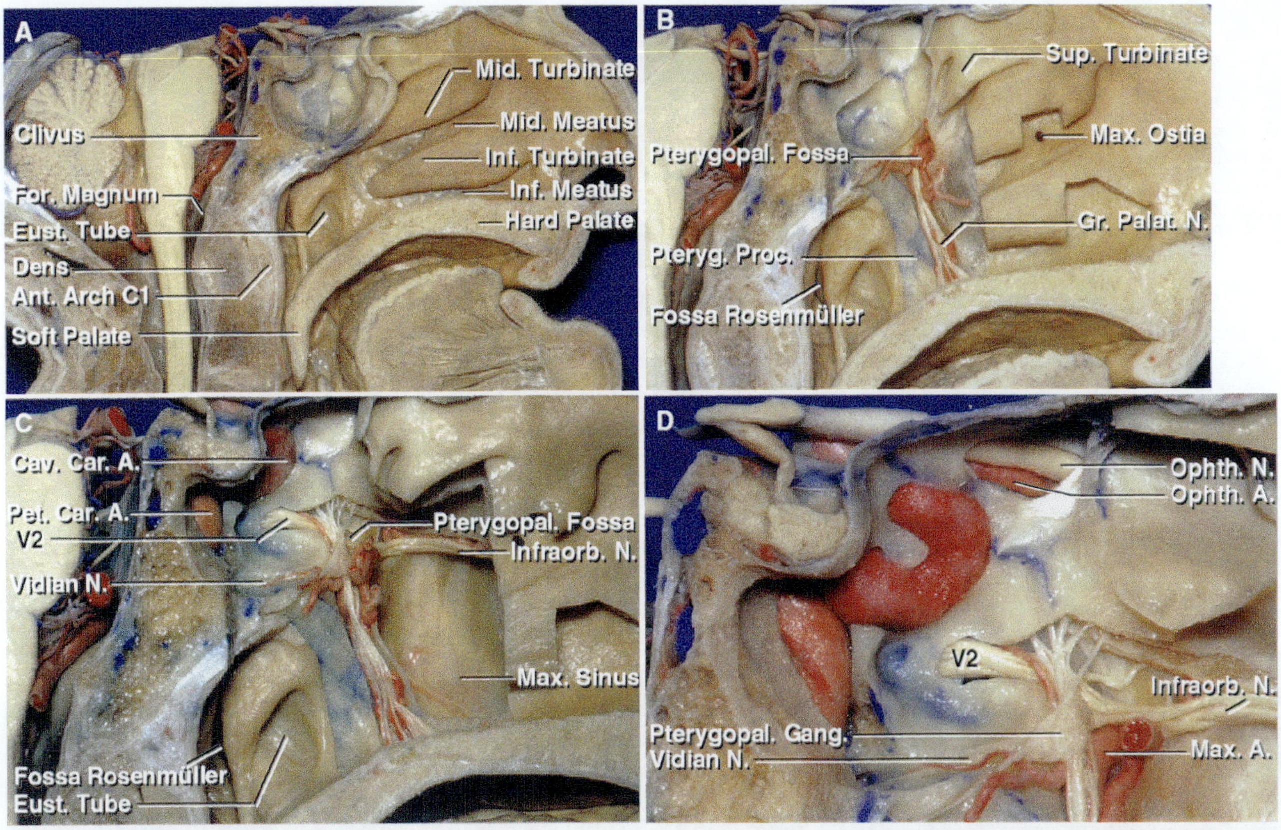

FIGURE 6.10. Nasal pathway to the clivus. Stepwise dissection showing the structures that form the lateral limit of the transnasal route to the clivus. *A*, the entire clivus is located above the level of the hard palate and, in most cases, can be accessed through the nasal cavity and nasopharynx. The nasal turbinates and meati and the eustachian tubes are in the lateral margin of the exposure. *B*, a portion of the superior, middle, and inferior turbinates has been removed and the area between the sphenoid pterygoid process and the posterior wall of the maxilla has been opened to expose the pterygopalatine fossa in the lateral wall of the nasal cavity. The ostia of the maxillary and frontal sinuses opens into the middle meatus located below the middle turbinate. The nasolacrimal duct opens below the lower turbinate into the inferior meatus. The eustachian tube, located in front the foramen magnum and lower edge of the clivus, opens into the nasopharynx at the posterior edge of the pterygoid process. Accessing the clivus plus the atlas and axis requires an approach that can be directed above and below the level of the palate. Rosenmuller's fossa is located behind the eustachian tube. *C*, the medial wall of the maxillary sinus has been opened to expose the infraorbital nerve, which arises in the pterygopalatine fossa and passes forward in the sinus roof. The maxillary nerve passes through the foramen rotundum to enter the pterygopalatine. The upper cervical carotid and eustachian tube form the lateral limit of the exposure of the lower clivus and the junction of the petrous and cavernous carotid limits the lateral exposure of the upper clivus. *D*, enlarged view. The bone and dura covering the optic canal in the superolateral part of the sphenoid sinus has been opened to expose the optic nerve and ophthalmic artery in the optic canal. The junction of the petrous and cavernous carotid limits the exposure below the level of the sella. The maxillary nerve exits the foramen rotundum and enters through the pterygopalatine fossa where it gives rise to the infraorbital, zygomatic, and greater palatine nerves, plus communicating rami to the pterygopalatine ganglion. Terminal branches of the maxillary artery intermingle with the neural structures in the pterygopalatine fossa. *A.*, artery; *Ant.*, anterior; *Car.*, carotid; *Cav.*, cavernous; *Eust.*, eustachian; *For.*, foramen; *Gang.*, ganglion; *Gr.*, greater; *Inf.*, inferior; *Infraorb.*, infraorbital; *Max.*, maxillary; *Mid.*, middle; *N.*, nerve; *Ophth.*, ophthalmic; *Palat.*, palatine; *Pet.*, petrosal; *Proc.*, process; *Pteryg.*, pterygoid; *Pterygopal.*, pterygopalatine; *Sup.*, superior.

perior nuchal line for closure. The inferior limb of the "Y" incision extends downward in the midline. The major extracranial hazard is injury to the vertebral artery as it courses along the lateral part of the posterior arch of the atlas. This artery is not encountered if the incision is strictly midline, but it is frequently encountered in the floor of the suboccipital triangle if the muscle incision deviates laterally, or when the muscles are stripped from the lateral part of the posterior arch of the atlas. The emissary veins and vertebral venous plexus should be obliterated quickly if they are opened.

The hockey-stick incision is selected if the lesion extends anterior or anterolateral to the brainstem toward the jugular foramen or the cerebellopontine angle. The skin incision extends from the mastoid process along the superior nuchal line to

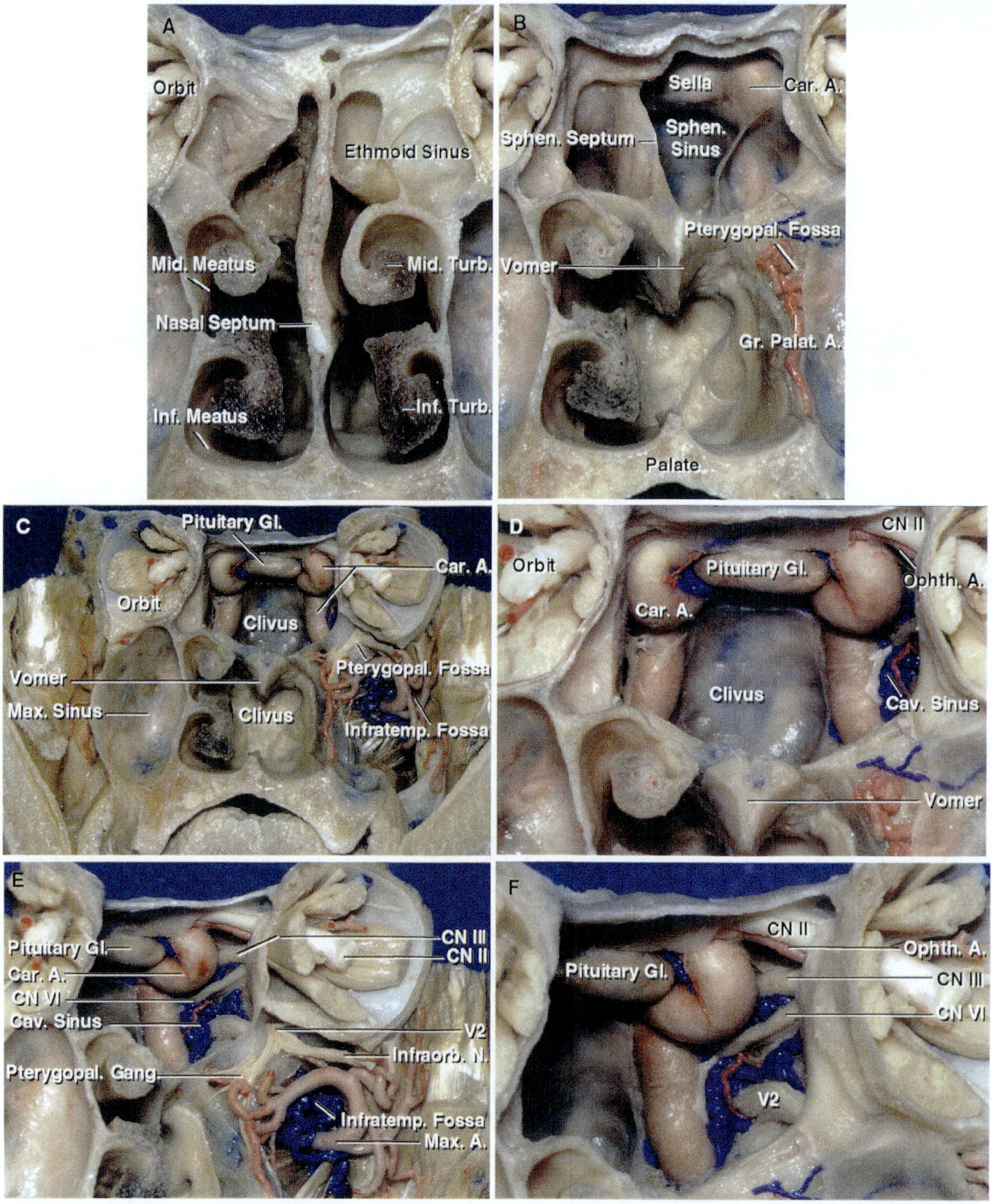

FIGURE 6.11. Nasal route to the clivus. *A*, this cross section extends through the nasal cavity, orbits, and maxillary and ethmoid sinuses. The ethmoid sinuses are situated in front of the sphenoid sinus. The middle and inferior turbinates have been preserved. *B*, the anterior wall of the sphenoid sinus has been opened to expose a multiseptated sinus and the anterior sellar wall. The left turbinates have been removed. Part of the posterior wall of the left maxillary sinus has been removed to expose the greater palatine artery which arises from the maxillary artery in the pterygopalatine fossa. The internal carotid arteries

the inion, and downward in the midline. A muscular cuff is left attached along the superior nuchal line to facilitate the closure. This incision permits removal of the full posterior rim of the foramen magnum, the posterior elements of the atlas and axis, and, in addition, to complete a unilateral suboccipital craniectomy of sufficient size to expose the anterolateral surface of the brainstem and the nerves in the cerebellopontine angle.

In opening the dura mater, using either the midline or hockey-stick approach, the marginal and occipital sinuses, along with the bridging veins passing from the neural surfaces to these and the sigmoid sinus, are encountered. Posterior intradural lesions may separate easily from the surface of the brain and spinal cord. On the other hand, they may be attached to the nerve roots and spinal cord, or they may extend upward through the cerebellomedullary fissure to be attached to the inferior medullary velum, choroid plexus, or the floor of the fourth ventricle. Opening the tela choroidea and inferior medullary velum may facilitate the exposure of tumors in this area. Care is required to avoid injury to the PICA as it courses around the tonsil and through the cleft between the superior pole of the tonsil and inferior medullary velum and tela choroidea.

Laterally situated tumors may be attached to the initial intradural segment of the vertebral artery and the thick dural cuff around the artery, which also incorporates the posterior meningeal and posterior spinal arteries, Cl nerve root, accessory nerve, and the dentate ligament. Dealing with these lesions may be facilitated by using a far-lateral approach, which is extended to include exposure of the atlanto-occipital joint, extradural vertebral artery, and transverse process of C1, combined with drilling of the occipital condyle, as described in detail in the chapter on the far lateral approach (29, 33). Dividing the attachments of the upper triangular processes of the dentate ligaments may facilitate the exposure of anteriorly situated lesions. Structures encountered in exposing superiorly along the lateral surface of the medulla include the PICA and the glossopharyngeal, vagus, accessory, and hypoglossal nerves. The vertebral artery may be followed upward to its junction with the basilar artery through the hockey-stick exposure. The most difficult lesions to remove are those situated anterior to the glossopharyngeal, vagus, and accessory nerves and the lateral medullary segment of the vertebral artery. Before sacrificing any rootlets of these nerves, an attempt should be made to gently separate the rootlets and to operate through the interval between the rootlets. Often, tumors expand and widen the interval between the rootlets, thus providing some access to medially placed lesions. Another route through which it may be easier to reach a lesion anterior to the medulla and pons is the interval between the lower margin of the vestibulocochlear and facial nerves and the upper margin of the glossopharyngeal nerve. It is uncommon to be able to work between the vagal rootlets; however, the lower cervical rootlets of the accessory nerve are very fine and are often separated by a wide interval. Consideration might be given to sacrificing a few of the lower accessory rootlets if it will make an otherwise incurable lesion curable. The intracapsular contents of the tumor are removed, and the remaining tumor capsule is separated from the surface of the brainstem and nerves rather than attempting to deliver the whole intact tumor through the limited exposure. Extreme care should be used when cutting into tumors situated anterolateral to the brainstem, since these tumors, especially meningiomas, may encase a segment of the vertebral artery or the PICA. The dura mater is closed with a dural substitute if closure of the patient's dura mater constricts the cerebellar tonsils or the cervicomedullary junction. A pseudomeningocele may form at the operative site if there is any tendency toward the development of hydrocephalus. Spinal drainage, repeated spinal punctures, or a shunting procedure may be required to decompress a postoperative pseudomeningocele.

Anterior operative approaches

The anterior approach was first used to reach lesions anterior to the spinal cord, and was subsequently used to expose lesions anterior to the brainstem (*Figs. 6.4, 6.5,* and *6.9-6.11*). The greatest advantage of the anterior approach is the direct route to the lesion, and the major disadvantages are the contaminated field and the frequency of cerebrospinal fluid fistula, pseudomeningocele, and meningitis after the exposure of intradural lesions by this approach. The depth of the operative field was once considered a disadvantage, but the use of the operating microscope has reduced the importance of that factor.

form serpiginous prominences in the lateral wall of the sphenoid sinus. *C*, the mucosa and bony wall of the sphenoid sinus have been removed to expose both the internal carotid arteries, which form the lateral limit of the transnasal exposure of the upper clivus. The pituitary gland has been exposed. Additional posterior wall of the left maxillary sinus has been removed to expose the infratemporal fossa, which contains the branches of the maxillary artery, the pterygoid muscles, pterygoid venous plexus, and branches of the mandibular nerve. The nasopharyngeal mucosa covering the longus capitis and the lower clivus is exposed in the interval between the palate and the vomer. *D*, enlarged view of the sphenoid sinus and sellar region. The anterior surface of the upper clivus is exposed below the pituitary gland. The lateral clival exposure is limited at this level by the internal carotid arteries. *E*, oblique view. The medial wall of the left cavernous sinus has been opened to expose the abducens and oculomotor nerves. The pterygopalatine fossa is located below the orbital apex. The maxillary nerve passes through the foramen rotundum and gives rise to the communicating rami to the pterygopalatine ganglion and the infraorbital nerve that courses along the floor of the orbit. *F*, enlarged view of the structures in the medial cavernous sinus. The ophthalmic artery courses below the optic nerve in the optic canal. *A.*, artery; *Car.*, carotid; *Cav.*, cavernous; *CN*, cranial nerve; *Gl.*, gland; *Gr.*, greater; *Inf.*, inferior; *Infratemp.*, infratemporal; *Max.*, maxillary; *Mid.*, middle; *Ophth.*, ophthalmic; *Palat.*, palatine; *Pterygopal.*, pterygopalatine; *Sphen.*, sphenoid; *Turb.*, turbinates.

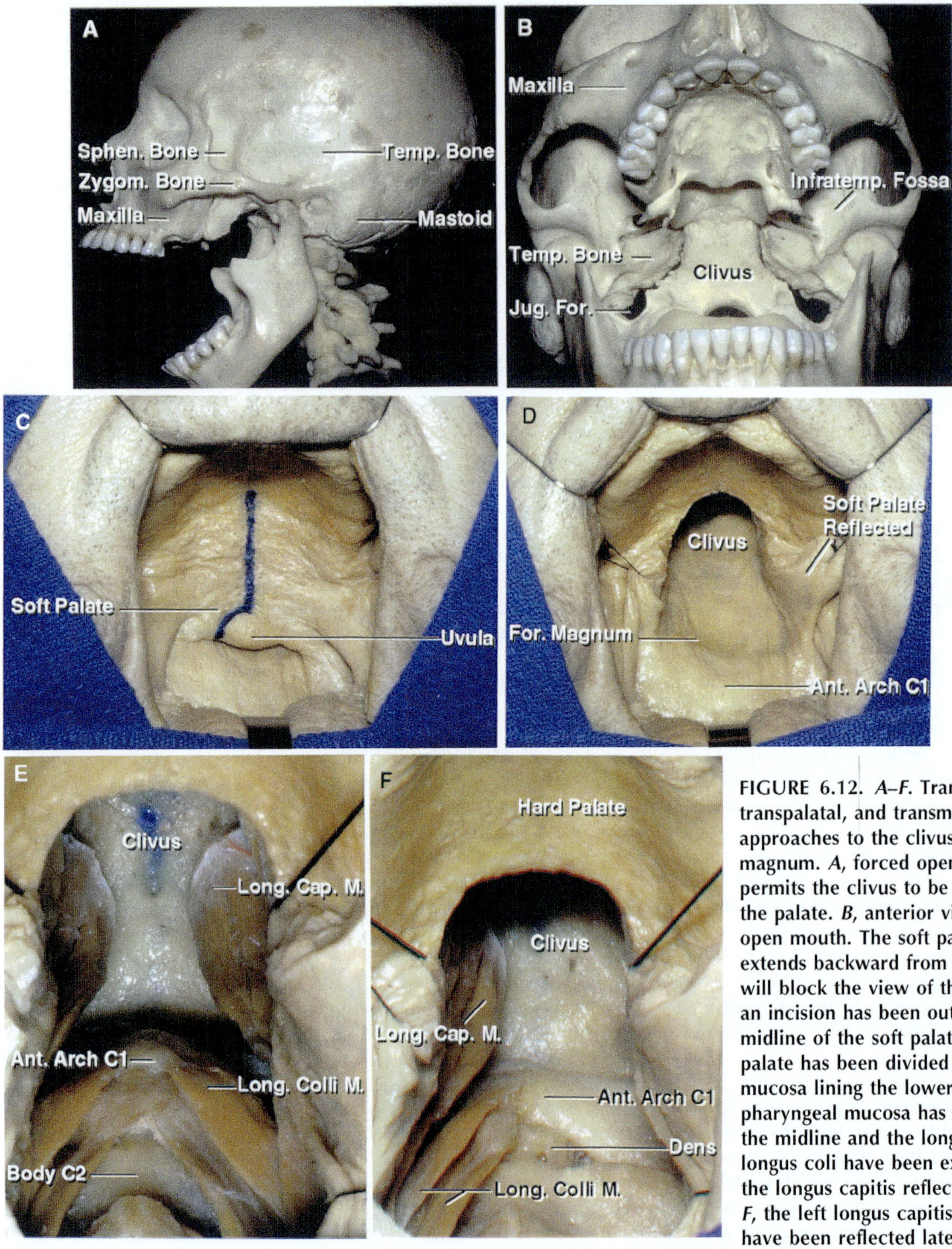

FIGURE 6.12. *A–F.* Transoral, transpalatal, and transmaxillary approaches to the clivus and foramen magnum. *A,* forced opening of the mouth permits the clivus to be exposed below the palate. *B,* anterior view through the open mouth. The soft palate, which extends backward from the hard palate, will block the view of the upper clivus. *C,* an incision has been outlined in the midline of the soft palate. *D,* the soft palate has been divided to expose the mucosa lining the lower clivus. *E,* the pharyngeal mucosa has been opened in the midline and the longus capitis and longus coli have been exposed and the longus capitis reflected laterally. *F,* the left longus capitis and longus coli have been reflected laterally. *A.,* artery; *A.I.C.A.,* anteroinferior cerebellar artery; *Ant.,* anterior; *Bas.,* basilar; *Cap.,* capitis; *CN,* cranial nerve; *For.,* foramen; *Gr.,* greater; *Infratemp.,* infratemporal; *Jug.,* jugular; *Long.,* longus; *M.,* muscle; *Max.,* maxillary; *N.,* nerve; *P.I.C.A.,* posteroinferior cerebellar artery; *Sp.,* spinal; *Sphen.,* sphenoid; *Temp.,* temporal; *Vert.,* vertebral; *Vert.,* vertebral; *Zygom.,* zygomatic.

Anterior approaches have been used to reach tumors of the atlas, axis, and clivus; for the resection and fixation of the odontoid process after ligamentous and osseous injury; for decompressing bony malformations of the craniovertebral junction, such as basilar invagination, which compress the medulla or spinal cord from anteriorly; and for approaching aneurysms of the lower third of the basilar artery, the vertebrobasilar junction, and the upper part of the vertebral arteries.

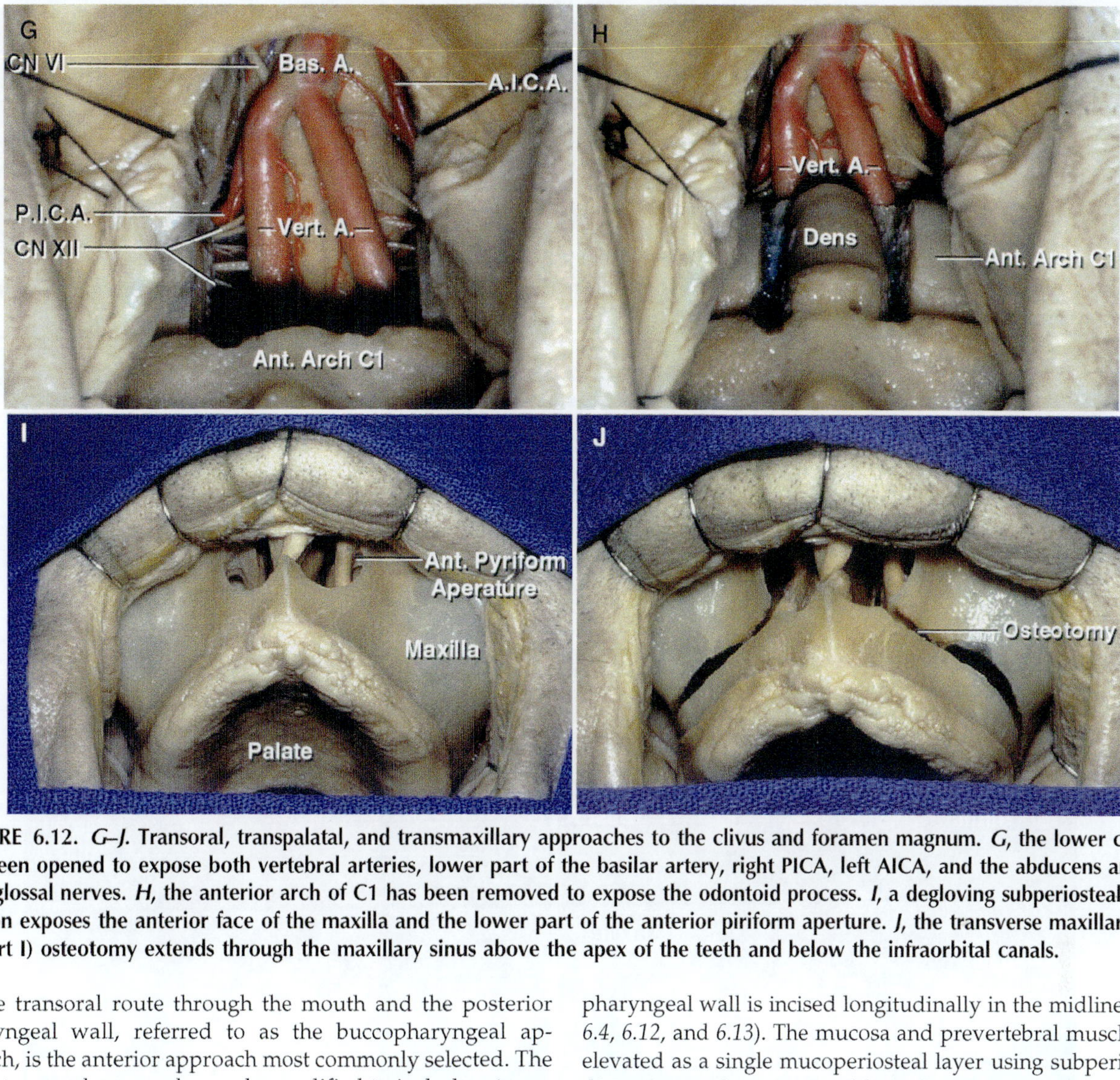

FIGURE 6.12. ***G–J.*** **Transoral, transpalatal, and transmaxillary approaches to the clivus and foramen magnum. *G,* the lower clivus has been opened to expose both vertebral arteries, lower part of the basilar artery, right PICA, left AICA, and the abducens and hypoglossal nerves. *H,* the anterior arch of C1 has been removed to expose the odontoid process. *I,* a degloving subperiosteal dissection exposes the anterior face of the maxilla and the lower part of the anterior piriform aperture. *J,* the transverse maxillary (LeFort I) osteotomy extends through the maxillary sinus above the apex of the teeth and below the infraorbital canals.**

The transoral route through the mouth and the posterior pharyngeal wall, referred to as the buccopharyngeal approach, is the anterior approach most commonly selected. The basic transoral approach may be modified to include a transpalatine approach in which the soft palate, or both the soft and hard palates, are opened, and a labiomandibular or labioglossomandibular approach in which the lip, mandible, and possibly the tongue and floor of the mouth are split to increase the exposure. Other types of anterior approaches are: the transcervical approach directed through the submandibular area along the anterior border of the sternocleidomastoid muscle (31); the transcranial-transbasal approach in which the clivus is reached through a bifrontal craniotomy after resection of the sphenoid and ethmoid sinuses (6); the extended frontal approach in which the bifrontal craniotomy is combined with an osteotomy of the orbital rims; and the transsphenoidal approach directed under the lip, along the nasal septum, and through the sphenoid sinus to the upper part of the clivus.

Transoral approaches

For the transoral approach, the soft palate is retracted to reach the anterior part of the atlas and axis, and the posterior pharyngeal wall is incised longitudinally in the midline (*Figs. 6.4, 6.12,* and *6.13*). The mucosa and prevertebral muscles are elevated as a single mucoperiosteal layer using subperiosteal dissection, and are retracted laterally. To expose the clivus, it is often necessary to split the soft palate in the midline. If added craniad exposure is needed, laterally based mucoperiosteal flaps may be elevated from the lower surface of the hard palate, and the posterior part of the hard palate may be removed. The mucosa covering the upper surface of the hard palate should be retracted and not opened. This permits the pharyngeal incision to be extended upward through the vault of the nasopharynx to the posterior border of the vomer. When elevating the mucoperiosteal layer from the clivus, the lateral margins slope dorsally into "gutter-like" depressions in which the tissue becomes thicker and more adherent. Depending on the lesion, the clivus, the anterior arch of the atlas, the dens, and bodies of C2 and C3 may be removed with a drill and rongeurs. The clival exposure between the occipital condyles is 2- to 2.5-cm wide and 2.5- to 3.0-cm long. Care must be taken to avoid the sixth through the twelve cranial nerves, the internal carotid arteries, the internal jugular veins, and the inferior petrosal sinuses that are on the periphery of

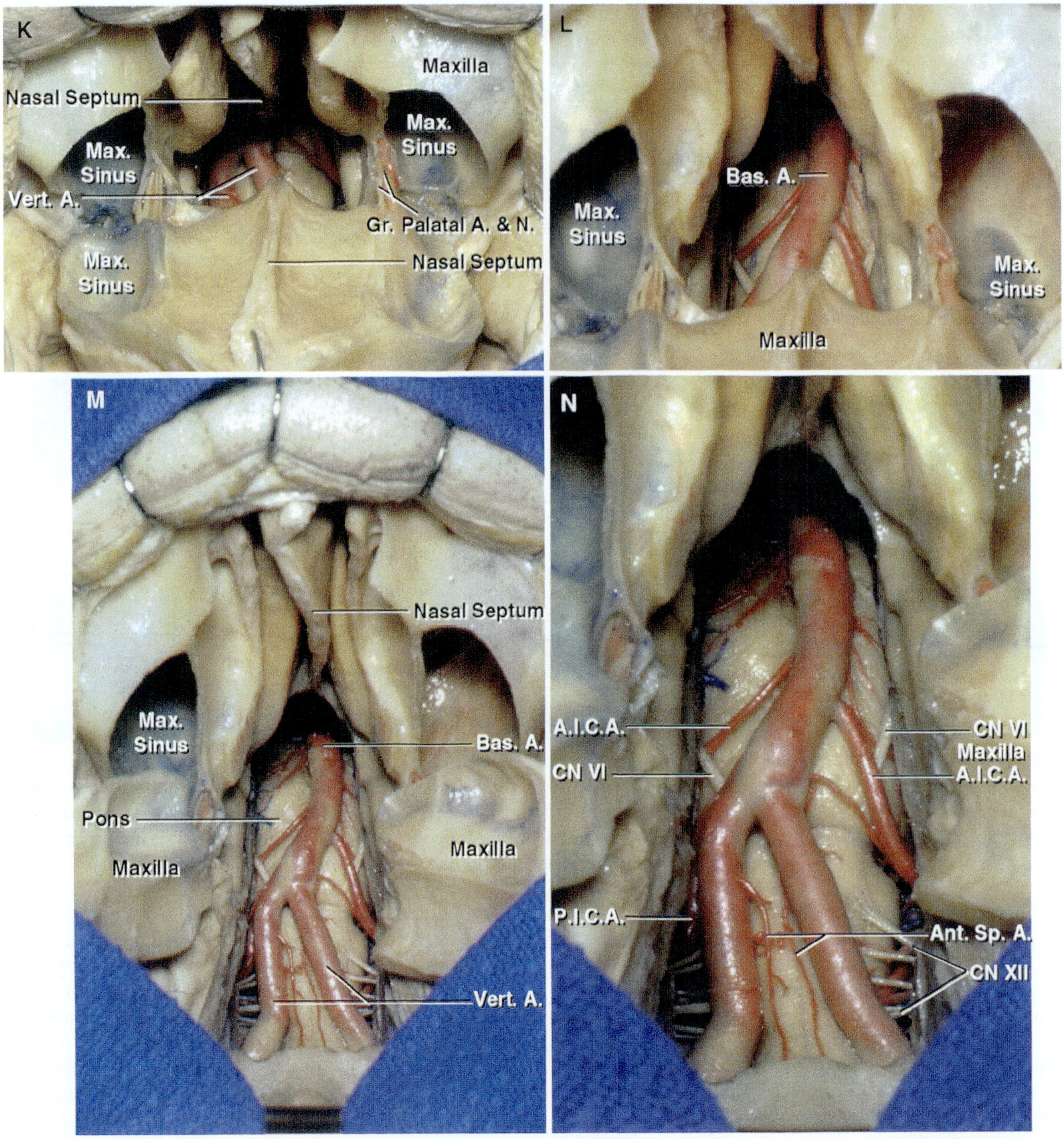

FIGURE 6.12. ***K–N.*** **Transoral, transpalatal, and transmaxillary approaches to the clivus and foramen magnum.** ***K,*** **the lower maxilla has been displaced downward. The clival window and vertebral arteries can be seen through the exposure.** ***L,*** **enlarged view of the clival opening.** ***M,*** **the maxilla has been split vertically in the midline and the halves reflected laterally, allowing the clival opening to be extended upward.** ***N,*** **enlarged view of the clival exposure. The right AICA passes behind the right abducens nerve and the left AICA passes in front of the left abducens nerve.**

the exposure. The most common lesions approached by this route are in an extradural location. Opening the dura mater will expose both vertebral arteries and the lower part of the basilar artery.

To increase the exposure and reduce the operative depth, the lip and chin may be incised vertically and a step-like mandibular osteotomy accomplished in the midline after removal of a central incisor tooth. Spreading the mandibular edges laterally, without splitting the tongue, permits the tongue to be depressed downward between the mandibular halves. If the exposure is still inadequate, the tongue and floor of the mouth may be split in the midline. Spreading the

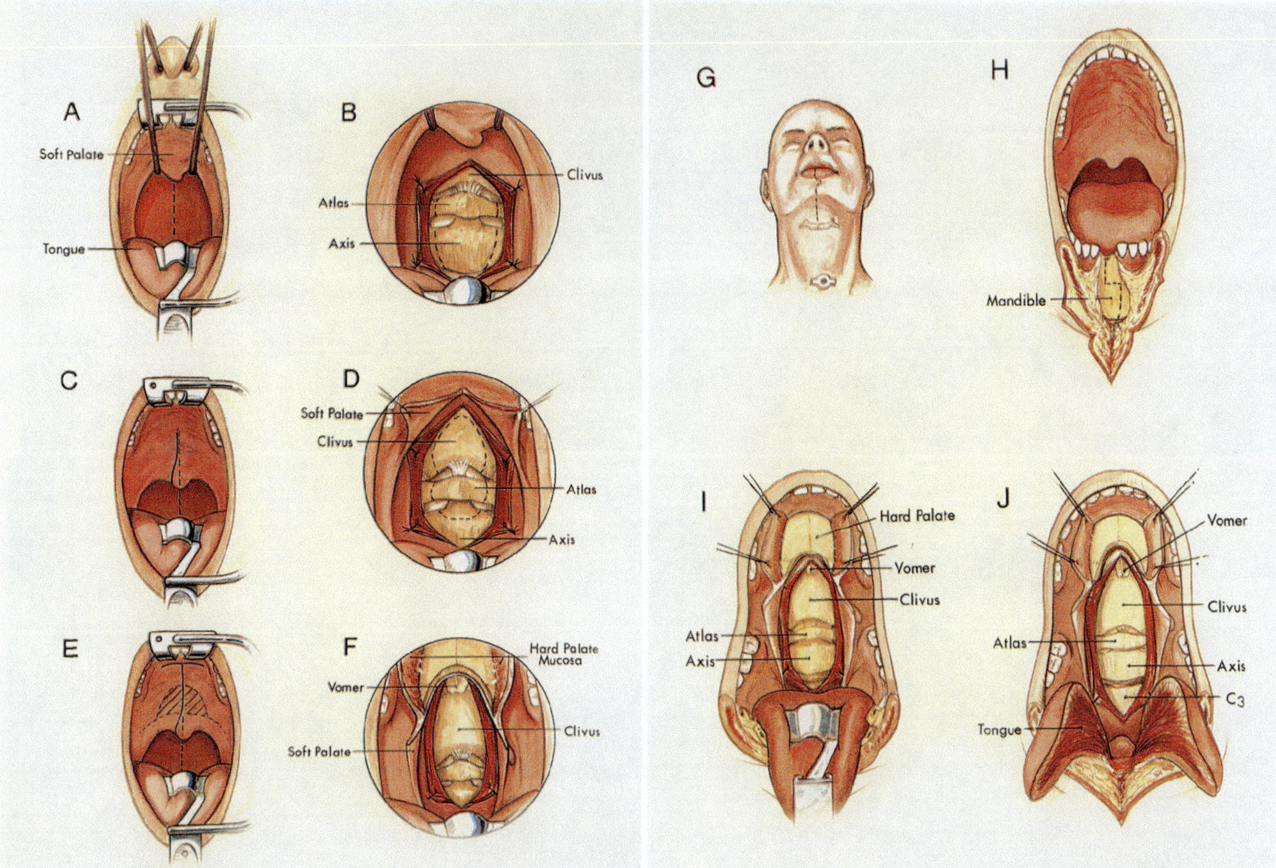

FIGURE 6.13. The transoral approach is the anterior approach most commonly selected. Variants of the transoral approach include the transpalatal variant in which the soft palate or both the soft and hard palates are opened, and the labiomandibular or labioglossomandibular variants in which the lip, chin, mandible, and possibly the tongue and floor of the mouth are split in the midline to increase the exposure. The transoral approach and its variants permit removal of the clivus, the anterior arch of the atlas, the odontoid process, and the bodies of C2 and C3. *A*, transoral approach. The patient is positioned with the head fixed so that lateral x-ray or image intensification is available to verify the location. A tracheostomy is commonly performed. Catheters inserted through the nasal passages and brought behind the soft palate and out the mouth or a silk suture brought through the base of the uvula and attached to a nasal catheter may be used to retract the soft palate. The posterior pharyngeal wall is incised longitudinally in the midline (*interrupted line*). *B*, the mucosa and muscles are retracted laterally as a single layer, using subperiosteal dissection to reach the atlas, axis, and lower clivus. The anterior arch of the atlas, the odontoid process, and the body of the atlas may be removed (*interrupted line*) to expose the dura. *C*, it may be necessary to split the soft palate in the midline to expose the clivus (palatal incision, *continuous line*; pharyngeal incision, *interrupted line*). *D*, the anterior surface of the clivus has been exposed through the transpalatal approach. The anterior arch of the atlas and the odontoid process may be removed and an opening made in the clivus (*interrupted line*). *E*, if further craniad exposure is needed, laterally based mucoperiosteal flaps may be elevated from the lower surface of the hard palate (*interrupted line*), and the soft palate split in the midline (*continuous line*). The posterior part of the hard palate may be removed (*oblique lines*). *F*, care is taken to retract rather than open the mucosa lining the upper surface of the hard palate. The pharyngeal incision is extended upward through the vault of the nasopharynx to the posterior border of the vomer. When elevating the mucoperiosteal layer from the clivus, the lateral margins slope dorsally into gutter-like depressions where the tissue becomes more adherent. The clivus, anterior arch of the atlas, dens, and bodies of C2 and C3 may be removed. The clival defect is packed with muscle or fat and may be reinforced with a bone graft. The prevertebral muscle and mucosal layers and the palatal openings are closed with absorbable sutures. *G*, the lower lip and mandible may be split (*interrupted line*) to increase the exposure and reduce the operative depth. *H*, a step-like mandibular osteotomy (*interrupted line*) is accomplished in the midline after removal of a central incisor tooth. *I*, spreading the mandibular halves laterally without splitting the tongue permits the tongue to be depressed downward between the mandibular halves. *J*, if the exposure is still inadequate, the tongue and floor of the mouth may be split in the midline. Spreading the mandibular-lingual halves exposes the pharynx down to the C3 level. The mucosa and musculature of the tongue and floor of the mouth are reapproximated; the mandibular osteotomy is closed with plates; and the lip, chin, and submandibular region are carefully closed after dealing with the lesion. (From, Rhoton AL Jr, de Oliveira E: Anatomical basis of surgical approaches to the region of the foramen magnum, in Dickman CA, Spetzler RF, Sonntag VKH (eds): *Surgery of the Craniovertebral Junction.* New York, Thieme, 1998, pp 13–57 [26].)

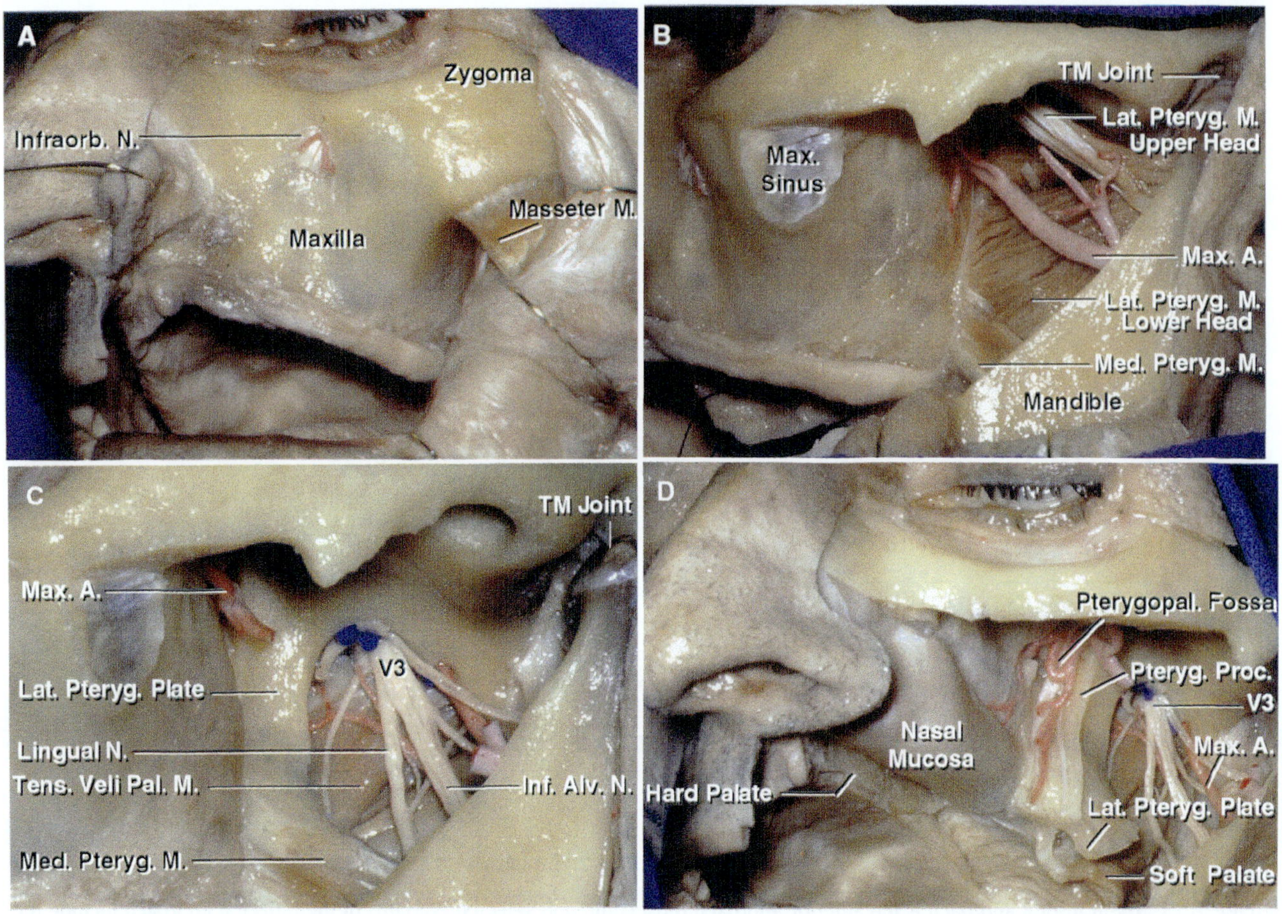

FIGURE 6.14. ***A–D.*** **Lower maxillotomy route to the clivus and foramen magnum.** ***A,*** **the approach can be made through a degloving incision inside the mouth; however, in this case, to more fully show the anatomy, a Weber-Fergusson paranasal incision with an infraorbital extension is used to expose the anterior face of the maxilla. The infraorbital nerve has been divided, although it can usually be preserved with the degloving incision. The masseter is attached along the lower margin of the zygoma.** ***B,*** **the mucosal lining the maxillary sinus is exposed below the zygomatic arch. The coronoid process of the mandible is removed or reflected with the temporalis muscle to expose the medial and lateral pterygoid muscles and the maxillary artery in the infratemporal fossa.** ***C,*** **the lateral pterygoid muscles and a segment of the maxillary artery have been removed. Removal of the lateral pterygoid exposes the mandibular nerve and its branches in the medial part of the infratemporal fossa.** ***D,*** **a lower maxillectomy has been completed. In this approach, the maxilla can be folded on a vascularized pedicle of soft palate into the floor of the mouth. The pterygoid process, which forms the posterior wall of the pterygopalatine fossa, has been preserved. The nasal mucosa remains intact. The maxillary artery exits the infratemporal fossa to enter the pterygopalatine fossa.** ***A.,*** **artery;** ***A.I.C.A.,*** **anteroinferior cerebellar artery;** ***Alv.,*** **alveolar;** ***Ant.,*** **anterior;** ***Bas.,*** **basilar;** ***Cap.,*** **capitis;** ***Car.,*** **carotid;** ***Cav.,*** **cavernous;** ***CN,*** **cranial nerve;** ***Eust.,*** **eustachian;** ***Gl.,*** **gland;** ***Inf.,*** **inferior;** ***Infraorb.,*** **infraorbital;** ***Int.,*** **internal;** ***Intercav.,*** **intercavernous;** ***Lat.,*** **lateral;** ***Long.,*** **longus;** ***M.,*** **muscle;** ***Max.,*** **maxillary;** ***Med.,*** **medial;** ***N.,*** **nerve;** ***Pal.,*** **palatini;** ***Pet.,*** **petrous;** ***Pteryg.,*** **pterygoid;** ***Pterygopal.,*** **pterygopalatine;** ***Tens.,*** **tensor;** ***TM.,*** **temporomandibular;** ***Vert.,*** **vertebral.**

mandibular-lingual halves exposes the pharyngeal wall down to the level of the arytenoid cartilages. After dealing with the lesion, the mucosa and musculature of the tongue and floor of the mouth are reapproximated, the mandibular osteotomy is repositioned with wire, and the lip, chin, and submandibular region are carefully closed.

Transmaxillary approach

Transmaxillary approaches have been advocated for pathology extending to the upper and middle third of the clivus, which is difficult to reach by the transoral approach (*Figs. 6.12* and *6.14-6.16*). Four different types of transmaxillary approaches have been used (2, 3). In one approach, a LeFort I osteotomy is completed, and the maxilla and hard palate are down-fractured into the oral cavity. In the second approach, called the extended maxillectomy, the LeFort osteotomy is combined with a midline incision of the hard and soft palate and the halves of the maxilla are swung laterally. In the third approach, the unilateral lower subtotal maxillotomy, half of the maxilla, and the hard palate are hinged on the soft palate

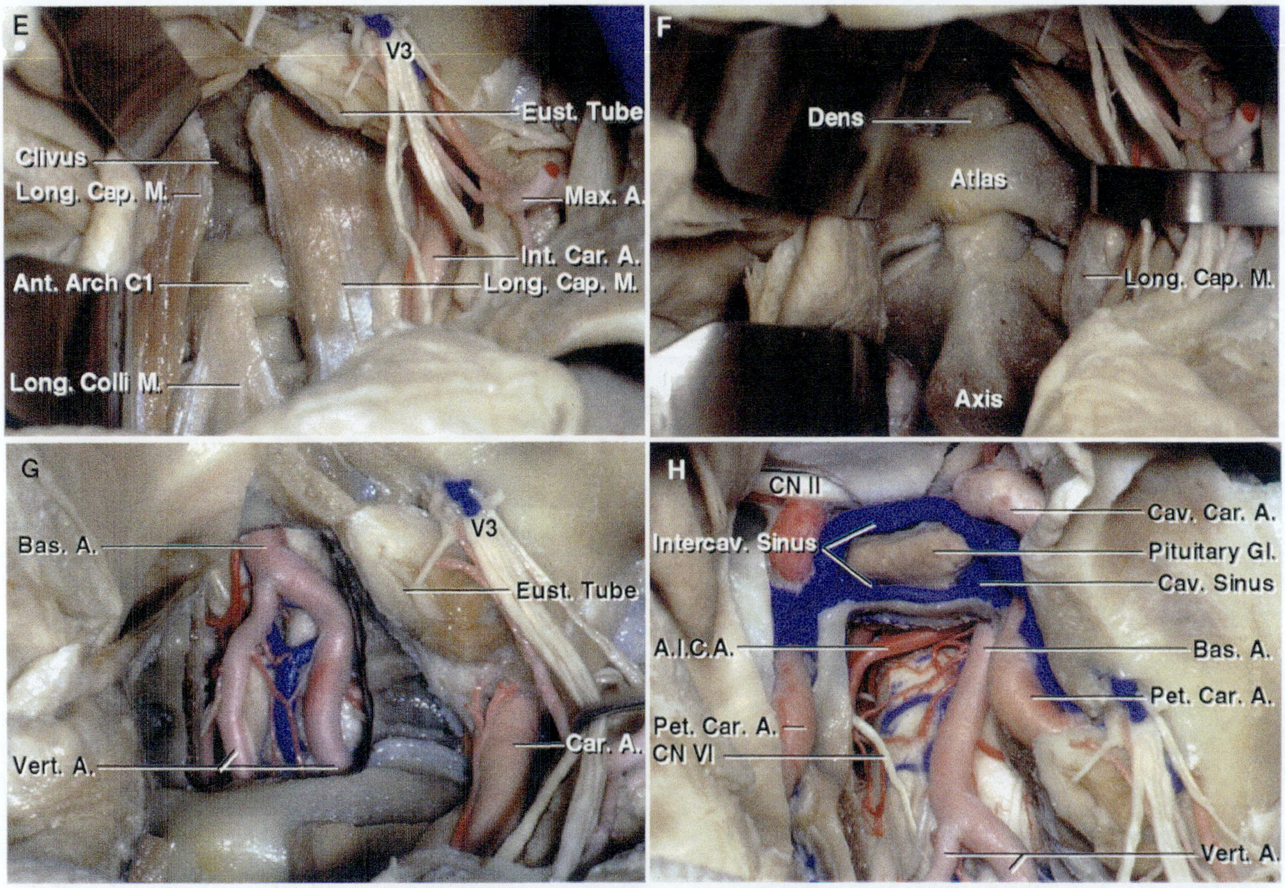

FIGURE 6.14. ***E–H.*** **Lower maxillotomy route to the clivus and foramen magnum.** ***E,*** **the nasal mucosa has been opened and the posterior pharyngeal wall reflected to the opposite side. The longus capitis attachments have been separated from the clivus.** ***F,*** **the longus capitis and longus coli have been reflected laterally to expose the anterior arch of the atlas and the dens and body of the axis.** ***G,*** **the clivus and the dura have been opened to expose the medulla and vertebral arteries.** ***H,*** **the exposure has been extended upward by removing the anterior wall of the sphenoid sinus and sella. The terminal part of the petrous carotids limits the lateral exposure at the level of the clivus, and the cavernous carotids limit the lateral exposure at the level of the sphenoid sinus. The intercavernous sinuses interconnect the paired cavernous sinuses.**

and folded downward into the floor of the mouth (6). The medial maxillotomy is a fourth and less extensive approach permitting exposure of the clivus. It involves removing the medial part of the anterior maxillary wall and the part of the maxilla bordering the anterior piriform aperture (*Fig. 6.15*). This provides an opening through the sinus and adjacent part of the nasal cavity that exposes the clivus above the level of the upper side of the hard palate. The sinus wall and the anterior piriform aperture can be reconstructed at the end of the procedure. It can commonly be performed through a degloving incision, although a lateral rhinotomy incision would be used if there is a need to extend the approach to the medial orbit (11, 12).

In the first approach, with a LeFort osteotomy, the upper lip is elevated and a mucosal incision is made along the upper alveolar margin, extending around the molars on both sides (*Fig. 6.16*). The mucosa is stripped off the anterior face of the maxilla below the infraorbital foramen. The saw cuts extend into the maxillary sinuses below the infraorbital foramen and high enough to avoid the dental roots, and extending into the nasal cavity leaving the branches of the internal maxillary artery and the nerves to the maxilla and palate intact. The mucosa on the nasal surface of the maxilla is dissected off, and the nasal septum is divided just above its attachment to the palate. The freed bone block includes, in one piece, the part of both maxilla and the maxillary teeth situated below the infraorbital foramen with their intact blood and nerve supply, which enters in the region of the infratemporal fossa and pterygoid plates. The fact that the soft palate is left intact reduces the incidence of speech and swallowing disorders. The intact maxillary block, however, blocks access to the craniovertebral junction, although it provides reasonable access to the upper and middle third of the clivus. In an effort to increase access to the craniovertebral junction, the LeFort osteotomy has been combined with a midline incision of the hard and soft palate, thus allowing the maxillary halves, with their attachment, to be reflected laterally (3). The disadvantage of the procedure is the difficulty obtaining good dental occlusion and proper functioning of the hard and soft palate.

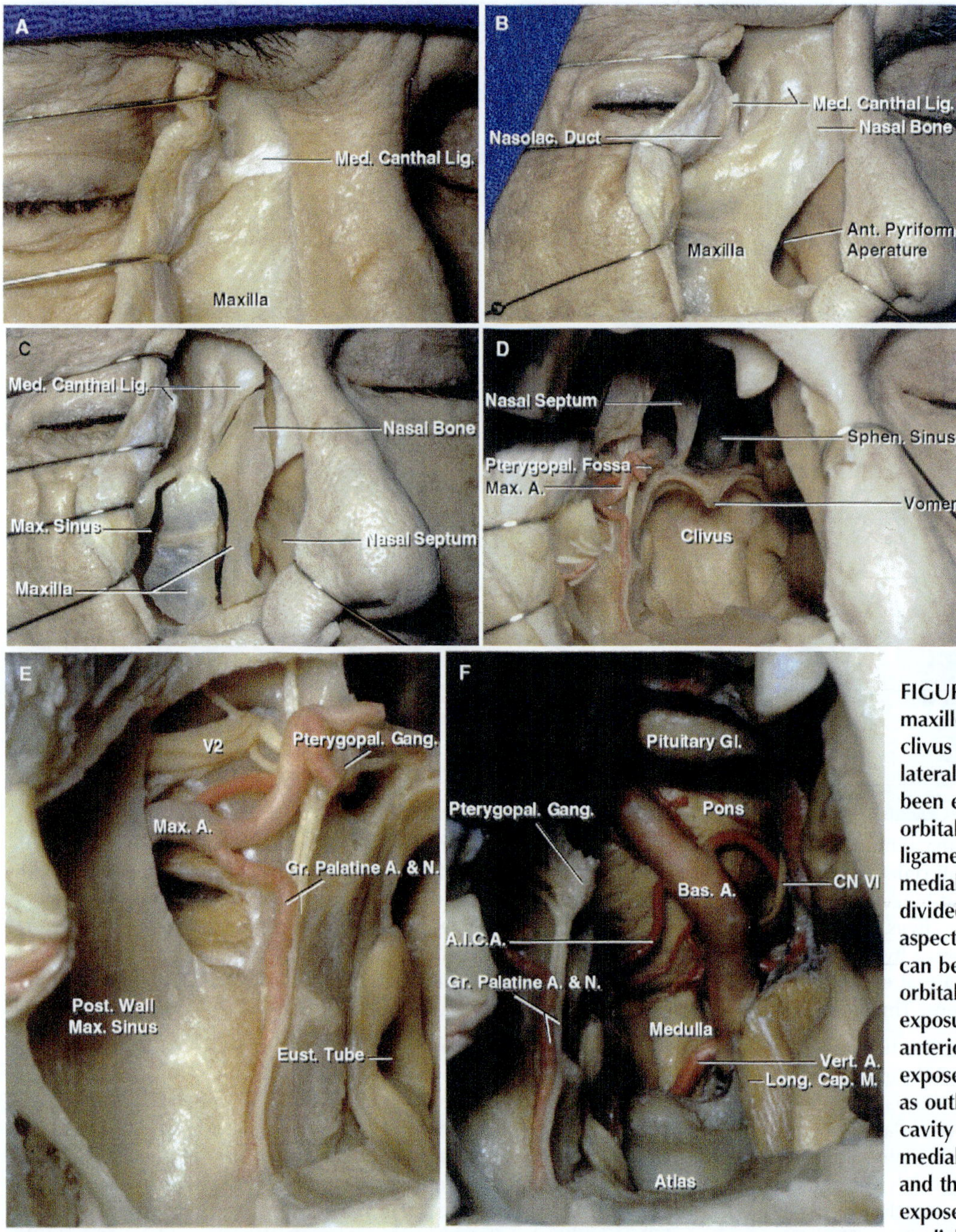

FIGURE 6.15. Medial maxillotomy approach to the clivus and foramen magnum. *A*, a lateral rhinotomy incision has been extended along the medial orbital rim. The medial canthal ligament has been exposed. *B*, the medial canthal ligament has been divided to expose the medial aspect of the orbit. The ligament can be preserved and the medial orbital wall left intact if orbital exposure is not needed. The anterior pyriform aperture is exposed. *C*, the osteotomies are as outlined to open the nasal cavity and medial maxilla. The medial one opens the nasal cavity and the lateral bone removal exposes the maxillary sinus. The medial maxillotomy aids in exposing the clivus. *D*, the exposure has been directed to the posterior nasopharyngeal wall behind which the clivus sits. The anterior wall of the sphenoid sinus has been removed, exposing the sphenoid septum. The posterior part of the nasal septum has been removed to expose the clivus below the sphenoid sinus. Removal of the medial part of the posterior wall of the maxillary sinus exposes the maxillary artery in the pterygopalatine fossa. *E*, enlarged view of the pterygopalatine fossa exposed by removing the medial part of the posterior wall of the maxillary sinus. The maxillary nerve and artery enter the pterygopalatine fossa. The maxillary artery is the major source of bleeding during surgery in this area. The maxillary artery enters the pterygopalatine fossa by passing through the pterygomaxillary fissure. The maxillary nerve enters the fossa by passing through the foramen rotundum and gives off communicating rami to the pterygopalatine ganglion. *F*, the pharyngeal mucosa has been opened, the longus capitis reflected laterally, and the clivus and dura opened to expose the basilar artery ascending in front of the pons. The pituitary gland is at the upper margin of the exposure. *A.*, artery; *A.I.C.A.*, anteroinferior cerebellar artery; *Ant.*, anterior; *Bas.*, basilar; *Cap.*, capitis; *CN*, cranial nerve; *Eust.*, eustachian; *Gang.*, ganglion; *Gl.*, gland; *Gr.*, greater; *Lig.*, ligament; *Long.*, longus; *M.*, muscle; *Max.*, maxillary; *Med.*, medial; *N.*, nerve; *Nasolac.*, nasolacrimal; *Post.*, posterior; *Pterygopal.*, pterygopalatine; *Sphen.*, sphenoid; *Vert.*, vertebral.

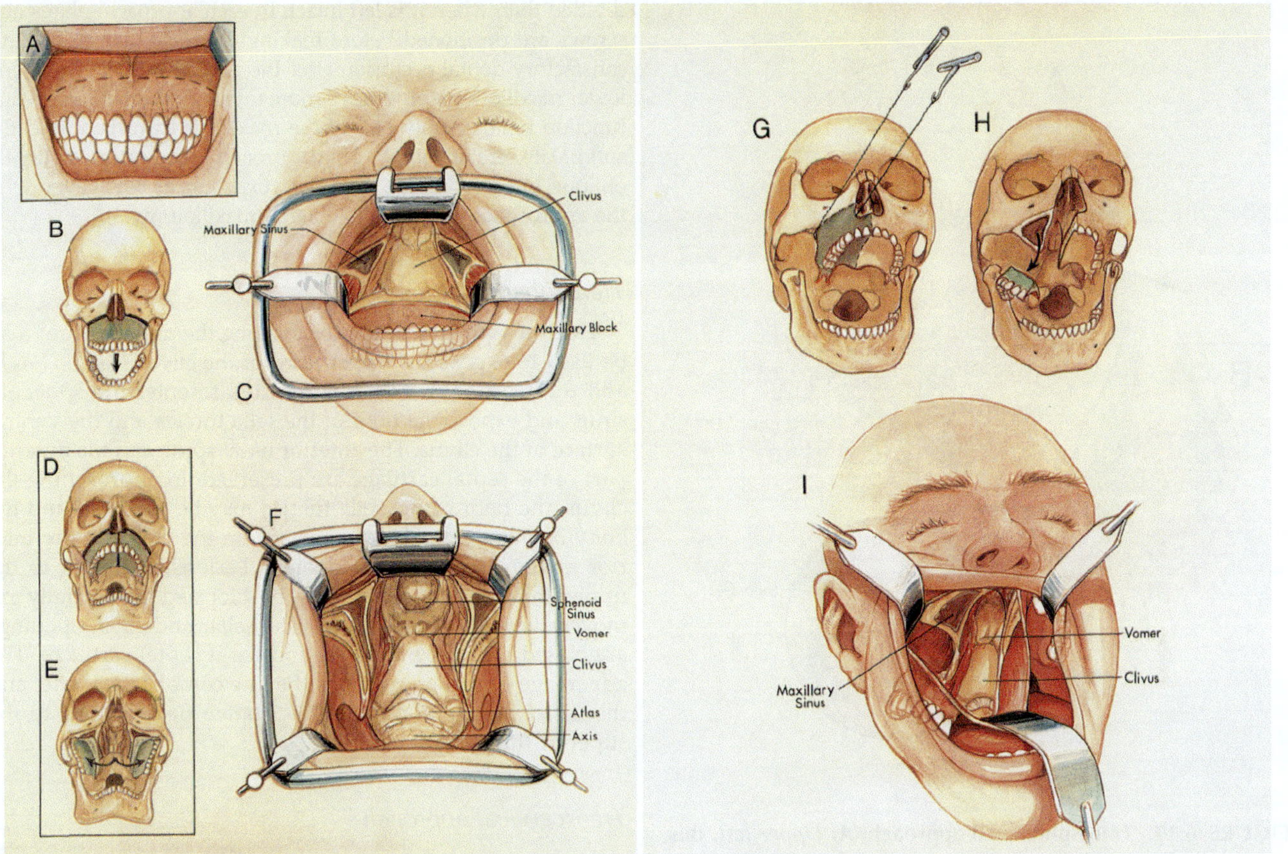

FIGURE 6.16. Transmaxillary approaches. Three variants of the transmaxillary approaches are shown. All three can be completed through an intraoral incision with degloving. Another type of incision extending onto the face, such as a Weber-Fergusson incision, might be considered. *A*, the upper lip is elevated and the mucosa is incised along the upper alveolar margin around the molars. The mucosa is elevated from the anterior face of the maxilla below the infraorbital foramen, but high enough to avoid the dental roots. The mucosa is elevated from the nasal surface of the maxilla, and the nasal septum is divided above its attachment to the palate. *B*, the saw cuts (*solid line*) extend into the maxillary sinus on both sides. The free block of maxilla is moved downward (*arrow*) to give access to the clivus. *C*, the intraoral retractor has been placed. Displacing the maxilla downward gives wide access to the clivus. *D*, a modified technique, called the extended maxillectomy, includes the LeForte I osteotomy with a midline incision of the hard and soft palate (*solid lines*). *E*, this allows the halves of the maxilla, which are attached to the muscles and vessels in the infratemporal fossa, to be reflected laterally, providing wider exposure to the clivus and upper cervical spine. *F*, retractors have been placed to expose the clivus and upper cervical area. The approach can be extended upward into the sphenoid and ethmoid sinuses and downward to C2 or C3. *G–I*. Unilateral maxillotomy. *G*, in this approach, half of the maxilla is mobilized by a bone cut, which extends back to the infratemporal fossa in the area just below the infraorbital foramen, and the maxilla is divided in the midline. A mucosal incision is made along the low surface of the hard palate parallel to the midline on the side opposite the saw cut through the hard palate, and the anterior face of the maxilla is degloved on one side. The soft palate is left intact. *H*, the unilateral block of maxilla, which is still attached to the structures in the infratemporal fossa along the pterygoid plates and to the soft palate, which is not interrupted, is folded downward into the floor of the mouth. *I*, the anterior part of the nasal septum is left undisturbed, but the posterior part is removed along with some of the turbinates and wall of the sinuses to provide a wide exposure of the clivus. This exposure can be enlarged to include the walls of the sphenoid and ethmoid sinuses. (From, Rhoton AL Jr: Anatomical basis of surgical approaches to the region of the foramen magnum, in Dickman CA, Spetzler RF, Sonntag VKH (eds): *Surgery of the Craniovertebral Junction.* New York, Thieme Medical Publishers, Inc., 1998, pp 13–57 [24].)

In the lower subtotal maxillotomy approach, the part of half of the maxilla, located below the orbital floor and infraorbital canal, is folded into the floor of the mouth on a hinge of vascularized tissue, including the internal maxillary artery and leaving the soft palate intact (*Fig. 6.14*) (2, 11). The hard palate is divided in the midline, care being taken to preserve the soft palate. This opens a route through the nasal and oral cavities to the clivus, foramen magnum, and upper cervical area.

In each of the approaches, the posterior part of the nasal septum and turbinates may be removed to expose the posterior pharyngeal wall and provide access to the clivus and upper cervical vertebrae. These approaches also provide ac-

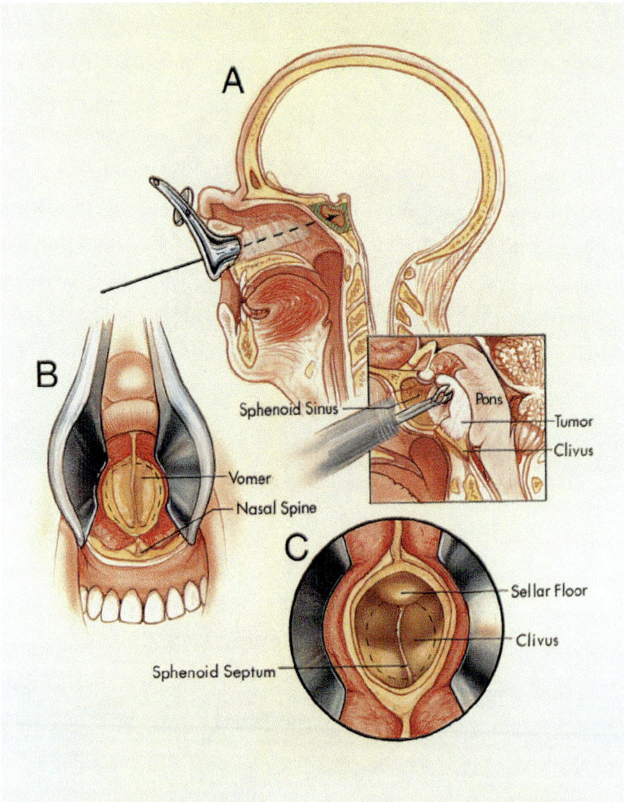

FIGURE 6.17. Transsphenoidal approach. *A, Upper left,* this approach, directed beneath the upper lip, along the nasal septum, and through the sphenoid sinus, may be used to expose the upper third of the clivus. The resectable area (*oblique lines*) includes the floor and anterior wall of the sella, the vomer, and the upper third of the clivus. This approach is suitable for biopsying some tumors that extend upward from the foramen magnum. *Lower right,* a cup forceps biopsies a clival tumor. *B,* view through nasal speculum. The anterior nasal spine is preserved and the anterior part of the septal cartilage remains attached to the septal mucosa on one side. The nasal speculum is inserted between the left side of the nasal septum and its mucosa. The nasal septum and the mucosa on the right side of the septum are pushed to the right by the speculum, and the mucosa on the left side of the septum is pushed to the left. The keel on the vomer is exposed. *C,* magnified view. The vomer has been removed to open the sphenoid sinus. The sellar floor is above the midline septum. In approaching the clivus, the floor of the sella is removed, and the opening in the bone is extended downward on the clivus (*interrupted lines*) to the inferior margin of the sphenoid sinus.

cess to the sphenoid and ethmoid sinuses and the sella, and the medial part of the floor of the anterior fossa. The posterior part of the mucosa on both sides of the nasal septum may be prepared to provide flaps that can be folded into the clival defect for closure. In addition, planning will allow for a temporalis muscle graft to be folded into the clival defect for closure. The incidence of swallowing and speech difficulties is significantly greater with those approaches in which the soft palate is divided than when it is left intact. In each approach, plates and screws are positioned before making the bone cuts to achieve satisfactory dental occlusion after the procedure. The unilateral lower maxillotomy provides a more rapid recovery of oropalatal function because only half of the maxilla is disturbed, and the soft palate remains intact. That approach to the clivus is slightly oblique, but can provide as wide an exposure as is achieved with the approaches involving a bilateral maxillotomy.

Transsphenoidal approach

The transsphenoidal approach along the nasal septum may be used to expose the upper third of the clivus (*Figs. 6.9-6.11* and *6.17*) (10). The vomer is resected to enter the sphenoid sinus and expose the floor of the sella turcica and the ventral surface of the clivus. The anterior nasal spine and the anterior part of the septal cartilage are preserved. In approaching the clivus, the floor of the sella turcica may be removed and the bony opening extended downward on the clivus to the inferior margin of the sphenoid sinus. Lesions extending to the upper third of the clivus may be biopsied or partially removed through this approach. The sellar and clival openings are closed with fat or muscle and nasal septal cartilage. The advantage of this approach is the low complication rate, and the disadvantage is the small operative field limited to the superior third of the clivus.

Transcervical approach

The transcervical approach, as performed by Stevenson et al., is directed through the fascial planes of the neck to the region of the foramen magnum (*Fig. 6.18*) (31). It avoids opening the oropharyngeal mucosa, but is selected infrequently because of the depth of the exposure and because it is not a direct midline exposure. A tracheostomy, which allows the jaws to be closed tightly, facilitates the exposure. The T-shaped skin incision includes a submandibular incision from the mastoid tip to the symphysis menti and an inferior extension carried from the midpoint of the submandibular incision across the sternocleidomastoid muscle. The fascial plane between the pharynx and the prevertebral muscles is reached through an exposure directed along the anterior border of the sternocleidomastoid muscle and between the carotid sheath laterally and the esophagus and trachea medially. The prevertebral fascia and muscles are retracted laterally to expose the ventral aspect of the clivus, atlas, and axis. Structures that may be divided from below to above to increase the exposure include the ascending pharyngeal and superior thyroid arteries, external laryngeal nerve, ansa hypoglossi, internal laryngeal nerve, lingual artery, hypoglossal nerve, stylohyoid muscle, anterior belly of the digastric muscle, stylohyoid ligament, glossopharyngeal nerve, and the stylopharyngeus and styloglossus muscles. The anterior arch of the atlas and the odontoid process, and a 2 cm width of clivus extending from the foramen magnum to the sphenooccipital synchondrosis may be removed. Deviation laterally may damage the internal jugular vein, internal carotid artery, eustachian tube, and the ninth through the twelfth cranial nerves.

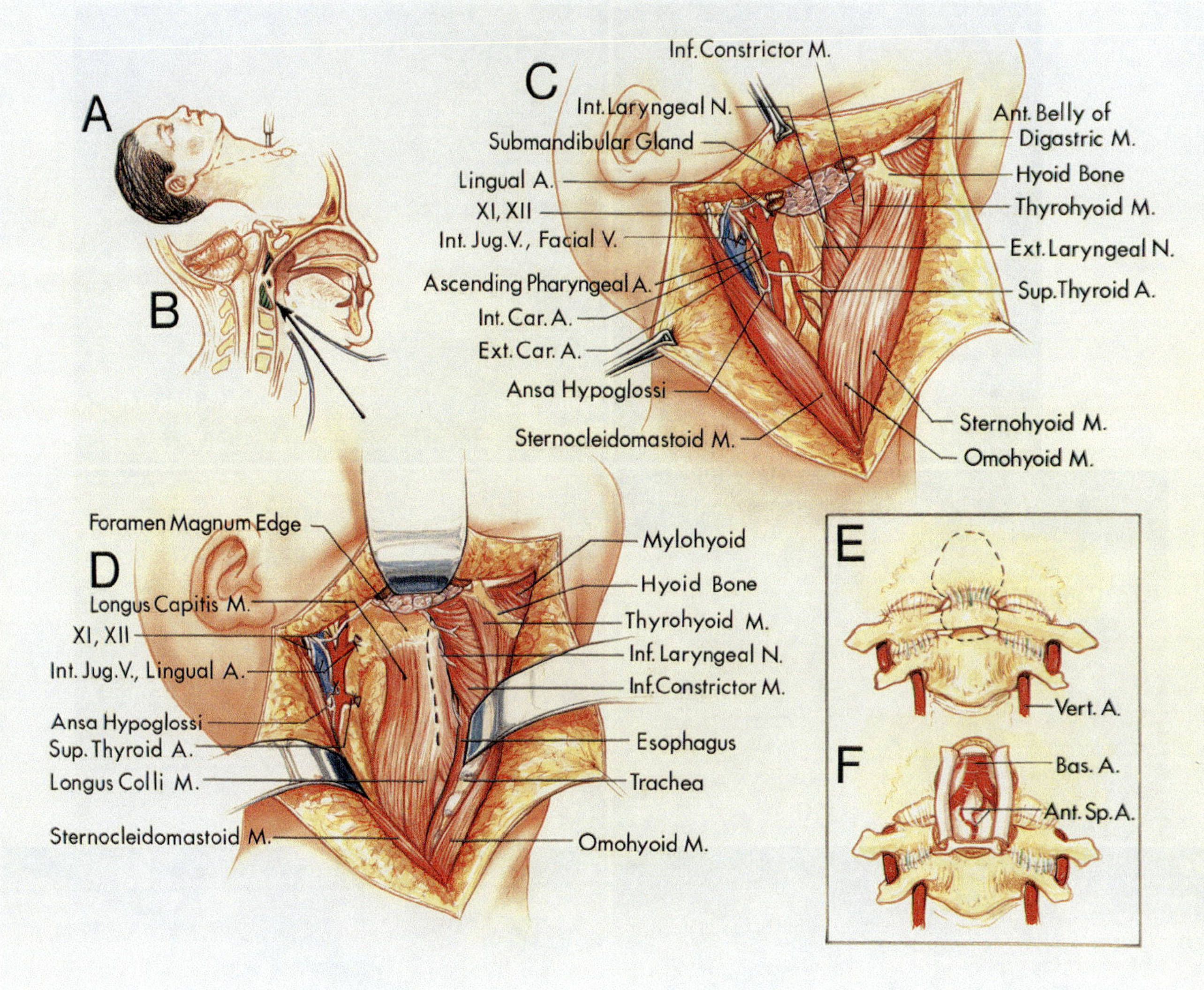

FIGURE 6.18. *A*, transcervical approach. A tracheostomy allows the jaws to be closed tightly. The T-shaped skin incision (***interrupted lines***) includes a submandibular incision extending from the mastoid tip to the symphysis menti and an inferior extension carried downward across the sternocleidomastoid muscle. *B*, the resectable area (***oblique lines***) includes the clivus, anterior arch of the axis, and the body of the odontoid process of the axis. *C*, the exposure is directed along the anterior border of the sternocleidomastoid and between the external and internal carotid arteries and internal jugular vein laterally, and the esophagus, hypopharynx, and trachea medially. Structures that may be divided to increase the exposure include the ascending pharyngeal and superior thyroid arteries, the external laryngeal nerve, ansa hypoglossi, internal laryngeal nerve, lingual artery, hypoglossal nerve, stylohyoid muscle, anterior belly of the digastric, stylohyoid ligament, glossopharyngeal nerve, and the stylopharyngeus and styloglossus. The accessory nerve passes behind the sternocleidomastoid. *D*, the prevertebral fascia and longus capitis and longus colli are separated in the midline from the clivus to C3 and are retracted laterally using subperiosteal dissection to expose the ventral aspect of the clivus, atlas, and axis. *E* and *F*, the anterior arch of the atlas and the odontoid process, and a 2.5-mm width of clivus extending from the foramen magnum to the spheno-occipital synchondrosis may be removed. The basilar, vertebral, and anterior spinal arteries are exposed in the dural opening. After dealing with the pathology, the dura is closed, muscle and fat are placed in the clival window, and the prevertebral and fascia are sutured in the midline. (From, Rhoton AL Jr: Anatomical basis of surgical approaches to the region of the foramen magnum, in Dickman CA, Spetzler RF, Sonntag VKH (eds): *Surgery of the Craniovertebral Junction*. New York, Thieme Medical Publishers, Inc., 1998, pp 13–57 [24].) *A.*, artery; *Ant.*, anterior; *Bas.*, basilar; *Car.*, carotid; *Ext.*, external; *Inf.*, inferior; *Int.*, internal; *Jug.*, jugular; *M.*, muscle; *Sp.*, spinal; *Sup.*, superior; *V.*, vein; *Vert.*, vertebral.

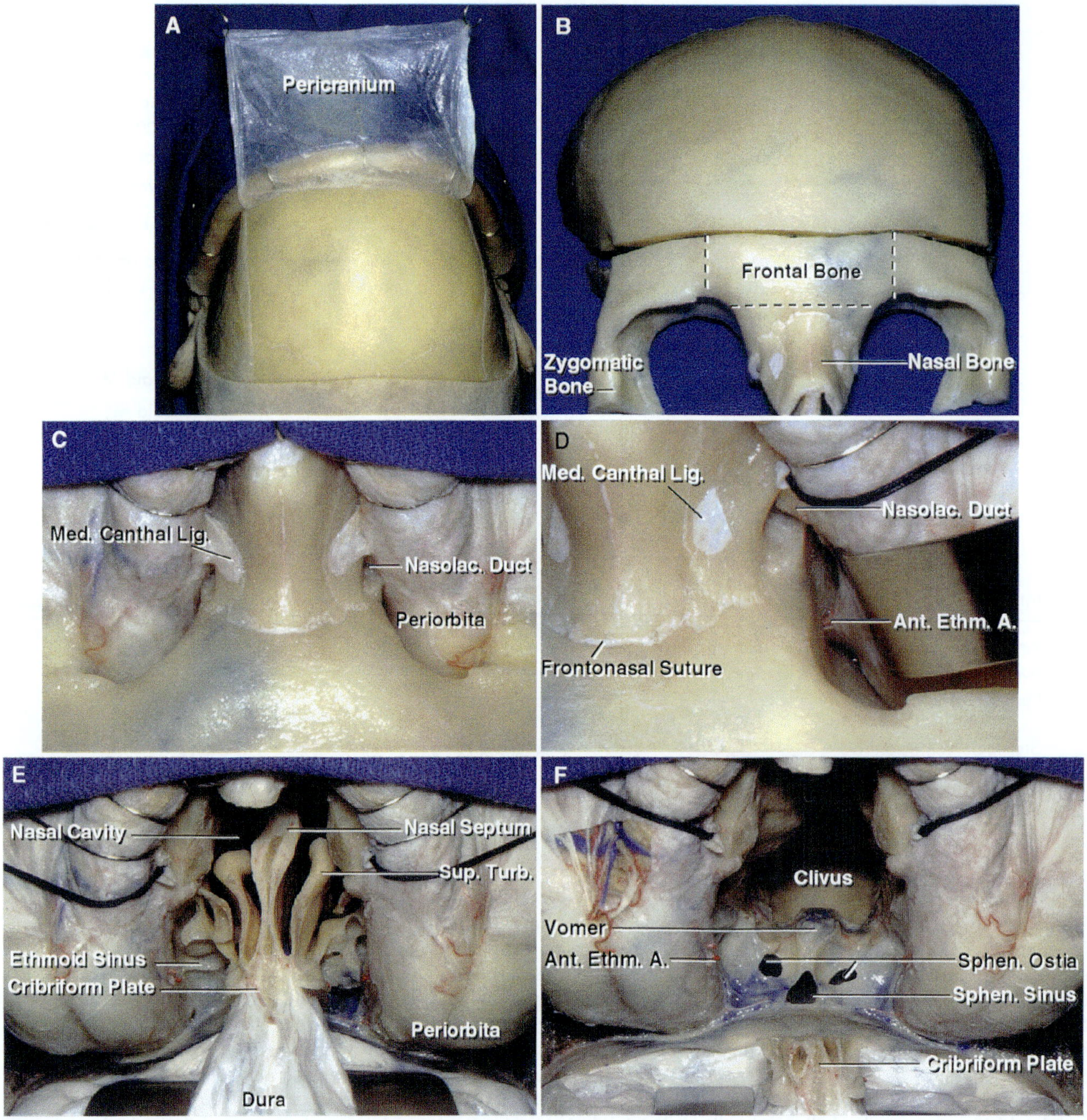

FIGURE 6.19. *A–F.* Relationships in the transbasal and extended frontal approaches. *A,* a bicoronal scalp flap has been reflected forward. The pericranium is commonly reflected as a separate layer for later use in closing the floor of the anterior cranial fossa. *B,* bone flap and osteotomy. The transcranial-transbasal approach uses only a bifrontal craniotomy bordering the floor of the anterior cranial fossae without the osteotomy. A large bifrontal craniotomy and a fronto-orbitozygomatic osteotomy have been completed. The osteotomized segment may extend through the nasal bone and lateral orbital rim, but for most clival lesions a more limited bone flap and osteotomy (*dotted lines*) will usually suffice and can be tailored as needed to deal with involvement of the nasal cavity, paranasal sinuses, or orbit. *C,* the periorbita has been separated from the walls of the orbit in preparation for the osteotomies. Division of the medial canthal ligament is not necessary for most lesions, but may be required for lesions extending into the lower nasal cavity or orbit. The ligaments should be re-approximated at the end of the procedure. *D,* the right medial canthal ligament has been divided and the orbital contents retracted laterally to expose the nasolacrimal duct and the anterior ethmoidal branch of the ophthalmic artery at the anterior ethmoidal foramen. *E,* the osteotomies have been completed and the frontal dura elevated. The dura remains attached at the cribriform plate. The upper part of both orbits are exposed. *F,* an osteotomy around the cribriform plate leaves it attached to the dura and olfactory bulbs, a maneuver

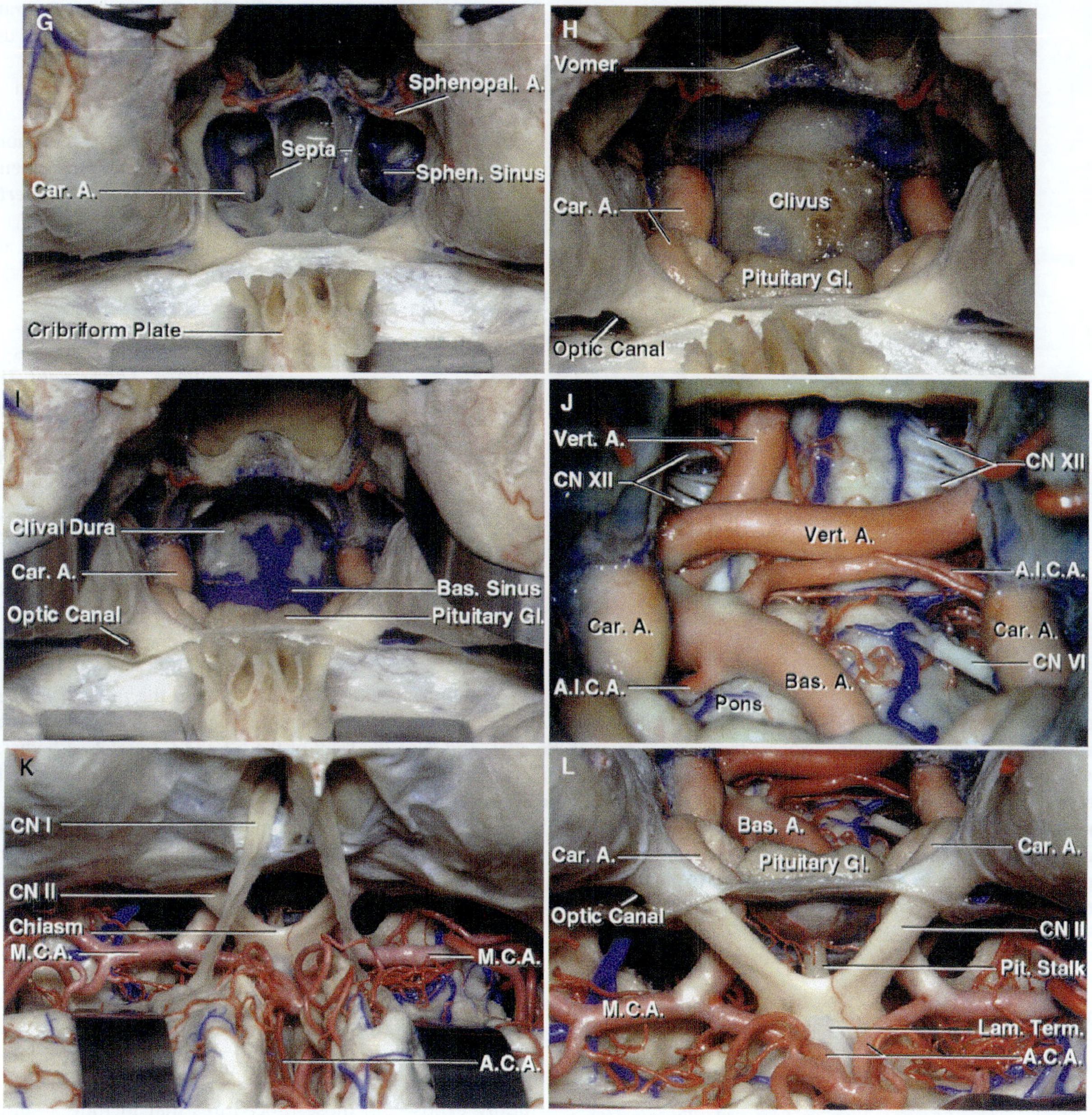

FIGURE 6.19. *G–L.* Relationships in the transbasal and extended frontal approaches. *G,* the sphenoid sinus has been opened to expose the septa within the sinus. The sphenopalatine arteries cross the anterior face of the sphenoid. *H,* the septa within the sphenoid sinus, the sellar floor, and the lateral sinus wall have been removed to expose the cavernous carotid arteries, pituitary gland, and optic canals. *I,* the clivus has been opened to expose the dura facing the brainstem. The basilar sinus, which interconnects the posterior parts of the cavernous sinus, is situated between the layers of dura on the upper clivus. *J,* the clivus has been opened to expose the tortuous vertebral arteries, which join to form the basilar artery at the left lateral margin of the clival opening. Both AICA origins are exposed. A vein splits the right abducens nerve into two bundles adjacent to the brainstem. *K,* the frontal dura has been opened and the frontal lobes elevated to expose the olfactory and optic nerves, the internal carotid, and the anterior and middle cerebral arteries. *L,* enlarged view. The subfrontal and clival openings are separated by the sella and pituitary gland. The lateral limit of the clival exposure is defined by the internal carotid arteries and optic nerves. The lamina terminalis is exposed above the optic chiasm.

that has been attempted to preserve olfaction, but is infrequently successful. The anterior face of the sphenoid sinus and both sphenoid ostia are exposed between the orbits. *A.,* artery; *A.C.A.,* anterior cerebellar artery; *A.I.C.A.,* anteroinferior cerebellar artery; *Ant.,* anterior; *Bas.,* basilar; *Car.,* carotid; *CN,* cranial nerve; *Ethm.,* ethmoidal; *Gl.,* gland; *Lam.,* lamina; *Lig.,* ligament; *M.C.A.,* middle cerebral artery; *Med.,* medial; *Nasolac.,* nasolacrimal; *Pit.,* pituitary; *Sphen.,* sphenoid; *Sphenopal.,* sphenopalatine; *Sup.,* superior; *Term.,* terminalis; *Turb.,* turbinates; *Vert.,* vertebral.

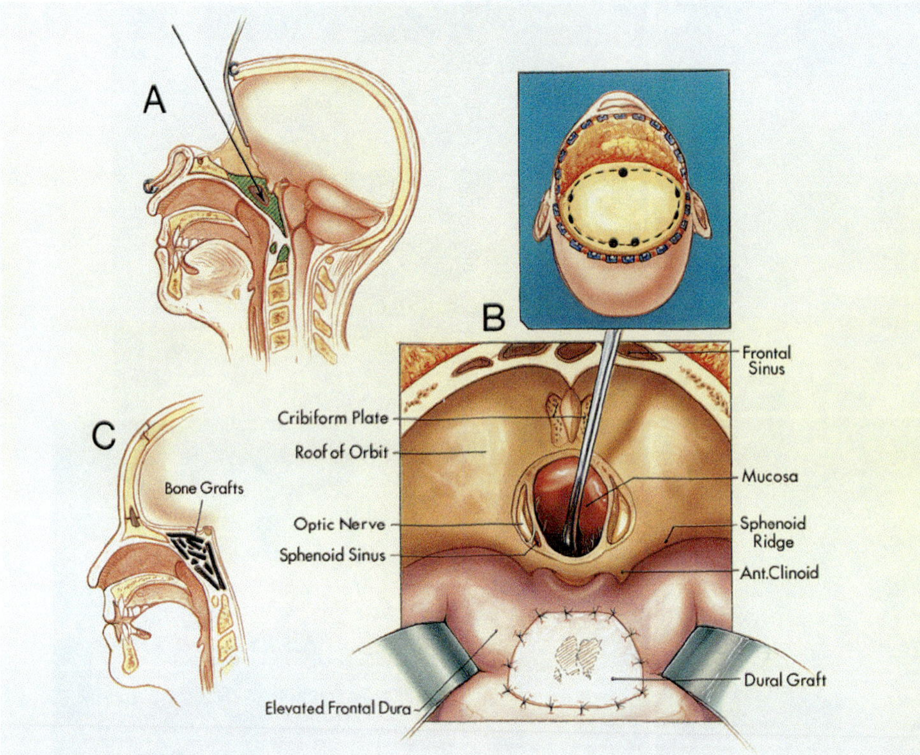

FIGURE 6.20. ***A,*** **the transcranial-transbasal approach may be used to approach tumors of the anterior edge of the foramen magnum if the tumor also involves and requires resection of part of the ethmoid and sphenoid bones (*oblique lines*). *B, insert.* The souttar scalp incision is situated behind the hairline, and the bifrontal craniotomy (*interrupted lines*) is placed strictly supraorbital without regard for the frontal sinuses (*oblique lines*). *Lower right.* The subfrontal dura is separated from the orbital roofs and the extradural dissection is carried to the lesser wings of the sphenoid bone, the tuberculum sellae, and the base of the anterior clinoid processes. The clivus is reached after resecting the posterior part of the floor of the anterior cranial fossa, the upper part of the walls of the ethmoid and sphenoid sinuses, and the floor of the sella. Proceeding downward, the clivus is removed to open the anterior margin of the foramen magnum. Separation of the pharyngeal mucosa from the front of the spine exposes the anterior arch of the atlas, and even the front of the C2 and C3 vertebral bodies. The nasal and pharyngeal mucosa should not be opened. Dural defects are closed with a leak-proof dural graft after dealing with the lesion. *C,* the orbital roof and the remainder of the cranial base are reconstructed using bone grafts. If the clivus has been removed, the graft above the ethmosphenoidal space is fitted into the edge of a vertical graft extending from the anterior margin of the foramen magnum or the anterior arch of the atlas to the floor of the sella. (From, Rhoton AL Jr: Anatomical basis of surgical approaches to the region of the foramen magnum, in Dickman CA, Spetzler RF, Sonntag VKH (eds): *Surgery of the Craniovertebral Junction.* New York, Thieme Medical Publishers, Inc., 1998, pp 13–57 [24].)**

Transcranial-transbasal approach

The subfrontal-transbasal approach may be used to approach tumors of the anterior side of the foramen magnum if the tumor also involves and requires resection of part of the ethmoid and sphenoid bones, and the clivus (*Figs. 6.19* and *6.20*). The transbasal approach, as performed by Derome (6), is made through a bicoronal scalp incision placed behind the hairline and a bifrontal free bone flap situated strictly supraorbital without regard for the frontal sinuses. The subfrontal dura mater is separated from the orbital roofs, the olfactory nerves are divided at the cribriform plates, and the extradural dissection is carried posteriorly to the lesser wings of the sphenoid bone, the tuberculum sellae, and the base of the anterior clinoid processes. Attempts have been made to leave the olfactory bulbs attached to the cribriform plate, but this has usually not prevented the loss of the sense of smell seen commonly after these procedures. The clivus is reached after resecting the posterior part of the floor of the anterior cranial fossa, the upper part of the walls of the ethmoid and sphenoid sinuses, and the floor of the sella turcica. Proceeding downward from the sellar floor, the clivus is removed to open the anterior margin of the foramen magnum. Separation of the pharyngeal mucosa from the front of the spine permits exposure of the anterior arch of the atlas, and even the C2 and C3 vertebral bodies. The nasal and pharyngeal mucosa are not opened in the transcranial transbasal approach, but are commonly exposed in those procedures that include a supraorbital osteotomy in addition to a bifrontal flap. Dural defects are closed with a leak-proof dural substitute, more than twice the size of the defect, which is sutured to the dura mater at the most remote margins of the exposure. The orbital roofs and the remainder of the cranial base are reconstructed using autogenous bone grafts. If the clivus has been removed, the graft above the ethmosphenoidal space is fitted into the edge of a vertical graft extending from the anterior margin of the foramen magnum or the anterior arch of the atlas to the floor of the sella. The advantages of the transbasal approach are that a tighter closure of the dura mater is possible than can be achieved through the transoral approaches, the subcranial mucosal planes can be preserved, and it can be combined with another intradural approach without the high risk of infection associated with the transoral approaches. The transbasal ap-

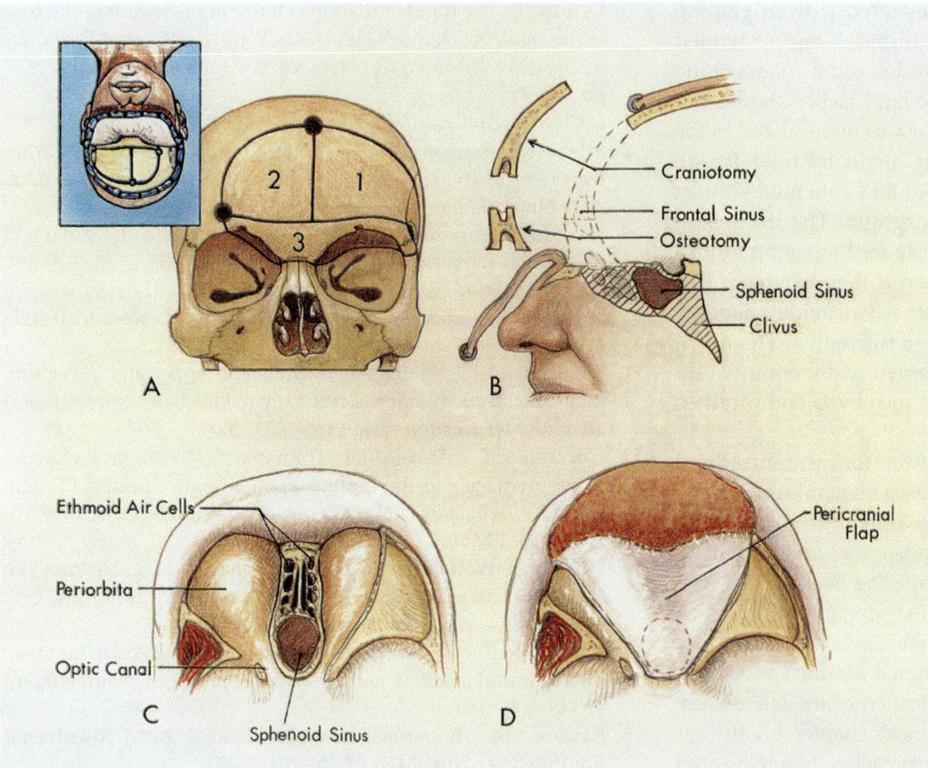

FIGURE 6.21. Extended frontal approach. ***A***, **the *upper left insert* shows the scalp flap and the order of the removal of the cranial bones (*1, 2, 3*). The third step, the orbitofrontoethmoidal osteotomy, includes both supraorbital ridges, the anterior part of the roof of the orbits, the frontal sinus, cribriform plate, and part of the ethmoid air cells in one block.** ***B***, **sagittal view. The oblique lines along the skull base show the possible extent of the bone removal. The foramen magnum is reached after removing the posterior part of the floor of the anterior fossa, the ethmoid air cells, walls of the sphenoid sinus, and the clivus.** ***C***, **the periorbita is exposed along both orbital roofs. The bone removal has been extended into the ethmoid air cells and the sphenoid sinus. The exposure can be extended along the clivus down to the foramen magnum.** ***D***, **use of pericranial flap for reconstruction. A fat graft is placed in the ethmoid and sphenoid sinuses before reflecting the pericranial flap over them. In addition, a fat graft may also be applied to the inner side of the pericranial flap. (From, Rhoton AL Jr: Anatomical basis of surgical approaches to the region of the foramen magnum, in Dickman CA, Spetzler RF, Sonntag VKH (eds):** ***Surgery of the Craniovertebral Junction.*** **New York, Thieme Medical Publishers, Inc., 1998, pp 13–57 [24].)**

proach may be combined with a transbasal-transsphenoidal route to gain access to the sella turcica. In the transbasal approach the clivus and sphenoid bone can be resected more extensively than by the transsphenoidal approach, but the subsellar area is hidden by the bulging dura in the transbasal approach. Both approaches may be combined to permit removal of all of the clivus below the level of the dorsum sellae. Anosmia is the only certain side effect. The most frequent complications are cerebrospinal fluid leaks, meningitis, and pseudomeningoceles.

Extended frontal approach

The extended frontal approach is similar to the transcranial-transbasal approach, except that it includes an orbitofrontoethmoidal osteotomy (*Figs. 6.19* and *6.21*) (28). It may also be used to approach tumors of the anterior side of the foramen magnum, especially if the tumor requires resection of part of the ethmoid and sphenoid bones as well as the clivus. The approach uses a souttar scalp incision, bifrontal bone flaps, and an orbitofronto-ethmoidal osteotomy in which the supraorbital ridges, and part of the orbital roofs and possibly the upper nasion, the roof of the ethmoid sinuses, and the cribriform plate are removed in a single block. The resection of the lesion may involve an extradural or combined intradural-extradural approach. The clivus and foramen magnum are reached after resecting the posterior part of the floor of the anterior cranial fossa, the upper walls of the ethmoid and sphenoid sinuses, and the floor of the sella. If needed, the supraorbital osteotomy can even be tailored in size and site to include the lateral orbital rims.

Selection of operative approach

Anterior extradural lesions of the clivus or upper cervical vertebrae are best reached by one of the anterior approaches. The transoral approach is selected for most anterior extradural lesions involving the foramen magnum because it provides a midline exposure and is the most direct route to the pathology. For more extensive lesions, a transmaxillary approach may be considered. Before selecting an anterior approach that would require that the dura mater be opened through the oropharynx, one should consider choosing a posterior approach since the incidence of cerebrospinal fluid leak, meningitis, and pseudomeningocele is high if the dura mater is opened through the oropharynx. The transcervical approach has the advantage of reaching the foramen magnum through the deep fascial planes of the neck rather than through the oropharynx; however, the depth of the exposure, the length of the time required to complete the dissection, and the fact that the foramen magnum is not approached from the midline have prevented it from gaining common usage. The transcranial-transbasal and extended frontal approaches offer another anterior route for reaching the foramen magnum, however these approaches should not be considered for approaching a tumor strictly localized in the region of the foramen magnum, but might be used for an extensive lesion involving the ethmoid and sphenoid sinuses as well as the clivus and foramen magnum. The transsphenoidal approach provides an easy route for biopsying lesions in the region of the foramen magnum if they extend to the upper third of the clivus, but it does not provide adequate exposure for removing larger lesions of the region. The transsphenoidal approach may be combined with another approach in removing lesions involving the clivus and foramen magnum.

The posterior approaches are preferred for most intradural lesions. The vertical midline incision, and a bilateral suboccipital craniectomy and upper cervical laminectomy is used for lesions situated in the upper spinal canal and posterior or posterolateral in the area above the foramen magnum. The hockey-stick incision and a unilateral suboccipital craniectomy and upper cervical laminectomy is selected if the lesion extends anterolateral or anterior to the brainstem toward the jugular foramen or cerebellopontine angle. The far-lateral modification of the lateral suboccipital approach, described in the next chapter on the far lateral approach, gives a more direct approach to lesions ventral to the brainstem and along the anterior rim of the foramen magnum, while reducing the need for retraction of neural structures (32, 33). The foramen magnum can also be reached through the approaches directed through the temporal bone, the subject of the chapter on the temporal bone; however, for reaching the foramen magnum and clivus, these approaches may require repositioning of the carotid artery or facial nerve, and possibly resection of the auditory and vestibular labyrinth.

Reprint requests: Albert L. Rhoton, Jr., M.D., Department of Neurological Surgery, University of Florida Brain Institute, P.O. Box 100265, 100 South Newell Drive, Building 59, L2-100, Gainesville, FL 32610-0265.

REFERENCES

1. Abbott KH: Foramen magnum and high cervical cord lesions stimulating degenerative disease of the nervous system. **Ohio State Med J** 46:645–651, 1950.
2. Cocke EW Jr, Robertson JH, Robertson JT, Crook JP Jr: The extended maxillotomy and subtotal maxillectomy for excision of skull base tumors. **Arch Otolaryngol Head Neck Surg** 116:92–104, 1990.
3. Crockard HA: The transmaxillary approach to the clivus, in Sekhar LN, Janecka IP (eds): *Surgery of Cranial Base Tumors*. New York, Raven Press, 1993, pp 169–180.
4. Cushing H, Eisenhardt L: *Meningiomas*. Springfield, Charles C Thomas, 1938, pp 169–180.
5. de Oliveira E, Rhoton AL Jr, Peace DA: Microsurgical anatomy of the region of the foramen magnum. **Surg Neurol** 24:293–352, 1985.
6. Derome P: The transbasal approach to tumors invading the base of the skull, in Schmidek HH, Sweet WH (eds): *Current Techniques in Operative Neurosurgery*. New York, Grune and Stratton, 1977, pp 223–245.
7. DiChiro G, Anderson WB: The clivus. **Clin Radiol** 16:211–223, 1965.
8. Friede RL, Roessmann U: Chronic tonsillar herniation: An attempt at classifying chronic herniations at the foramen magnum. **Acta Neuropathol (Berl)** 34:219–235, 1976.
9. Haas LL: The posterior condylar fossa, foramen, and canal and the jugular foramen. **Radiology** 69:546–552, 1957.
10. Hardy J, Grisoli F, Leclercq TA, Marino R: Trans-sphenoidal approach to tumors of the clivus [in French]. **Neurochirurgie** 23:287–297, 1977.
11. Hitotsumatsu T, Rhoton AL Jr: Unilateral upper and lower subtotal maxillectomy approaches to the skull base: Microsurgical anatomy. **Neurosurgery** 46:1416–1453, 2000.
12. Hitotsumatsu T, Matsushima T, Rhoton AL Jr: Surgical anatomy of the midface and the midline skull base, in Spetzler RF (ed): *Operative Techniques in Neurosurgery*. W.B. Saunders Co., 1999, vol 2, pp 160–180.
13. Huang YP, Wolf BS: Veins of the posterior fossa, in Newton TH, Potts DG (eds): *Radiology of the Skull and Brain*. St. Louis, C.V. Mosby, 1974, vol 2, book 3, pp 2155–2219.
14. Katsuta T, Rhoton AL Jr, Matsushima T: The jugular foramen: Microsurgical anatomy and operative approaches. **Neurosurgery** 41:149–202, 1997.
15. Kirdani MA: The normal hypoglossal canal. **Am J Roentgenol Radium Ther Nucl Med** 99:700–704, 1967.
16. Lister JR, Rhoton AL Jr, Matsushima T, Peace DA: Microsurgical anatomy of the posterior inferior cerebellar artery. **Neurosurgery** 10:170–199, 1982.
17. Margaretten I: Syndromes of the anterior spinal artery. **J Nerv Ment Dis** 58:127–133, 1923.
18. Matsushima T, Rhoton AL Jr, de Oliveira E, Peace DA: Microsurgical anatomy of the veins of the posterior fossa. **J Neurosurg** 59:63–105, 1983.
19. Matsushima T, Rhoton AL Jr, Lenkey C: Microsurgery of the fourth ventricle: Part 1—Microsurgical anatomy. **Neurosurgery** 11:631–667, 1982.
20. Newton TH: The anterior and posterior meningeal branches of the vertebral artery. **Radiology** 91:271–279, 1968.
21. Newton TH, Mani RL: The vertebral artery, in Newton TH, Pons DG (eds): *Radiology of the Skull and Brain*. St. Louis, C.V. Mosby, 1974, vol 2, book 2, pp 1659–1709.
22. Ouaknine G, Nathan H: Anastomotic connections between the eleventh nerve and the posterior root of the first cervical nerve in humans. **J Neurosurg** 38:189–197, 1973.
23. Piehl MR, Reese HH, Steelman HF: The diagnostic problem of tumors at the foramen magnum. **Dis Nerv Syst** 11:67–76, 1950.
24. Rhoton AL Jr: Anatomical basis of surgical approaches to the region of the foramen magnum, in Dickman CA, Spetzler RF, Sonntag VKH (eds): *Surgery of the Craniovertebral Junction*. New York, Thieme Medical Publishers, Inc., 1998, pp 13–57.
25. Rhoton AL Jr, Buza R: Microsurgical anatomy of the jugular foramen. **J Neurosurg** 42:541–550, 1975.
26. Rhoton AL Jr, de Oliveira E: Suboccipital and retrosigmoid approaches to the craniovertebral junction, in Dickman CA, Spetzler RF, Sonntag VKH (eds): *Surgery of the Craniovertebral Junction*. New York, Thieme Medical Publishers, Inc., 1998, pp 659–681.
27. Russell DS, Rubinstein LJ: *Pathology of Tumors of the Nervous System*. Baltimore, Williams & Wilkins, 1977, ed 4, p 368.

28. Sekhar LN, Nanda A, Sen CN, Snyderman CN, Janecka IP: The extended frontal approach to tumors of the anterior, middle and posterior skull base. J **Neurosurg** 76:198–206, 1992.
29. Sen CN, Sekhar LN: An extreme lateral approach to intradural lesions of the cervical spine and foramen magnum. **Neurosurgery** 27:197–204, 1990.
30. Stein BM, Leeds NE, Taveras JM, Pool JL: Meningiomas of the foramen magnum. **J Neurosurg** 20:740–751, 1963.
31. Stevenson GC, Stoney RJ, Perkins RK, Adams JE: A transcervical transclival approach to the ventral surface of the brainstem for removal of a clivus chordoma. **J Neurosurg** 24:544–551, 1966.
32. Tedeschi H, Rhoton AL Jr: Lateral approaches to the petroclival region. **Surg Neurol** 41:180–216, 1994.
33. Wen HT, Rhoton AL Jr, Katsuta T, de Oliveira E: Microsurgical anatomy of the transcondylar, supracondylar, and paracondylar extensions of the far-lateral approach. **J Neurosurg** 87:555–585, 1997.

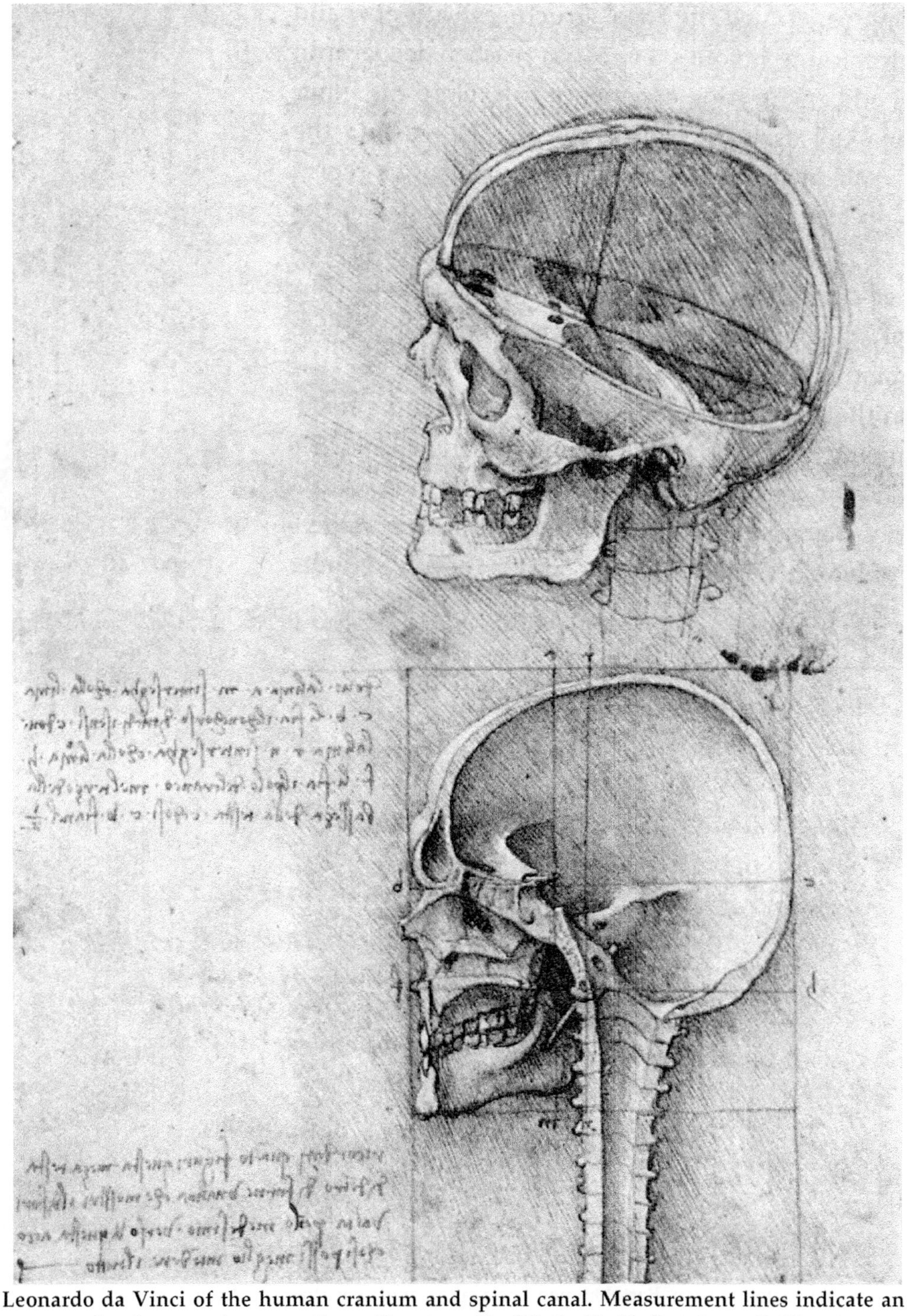

Drawings by Leonardo da Vinci of the human cranium and spinal canal. Measurement lines indicate an interest in the study of anatomic proportions. Courtesy, Dr. Edwin Todd, Pasadena, California.

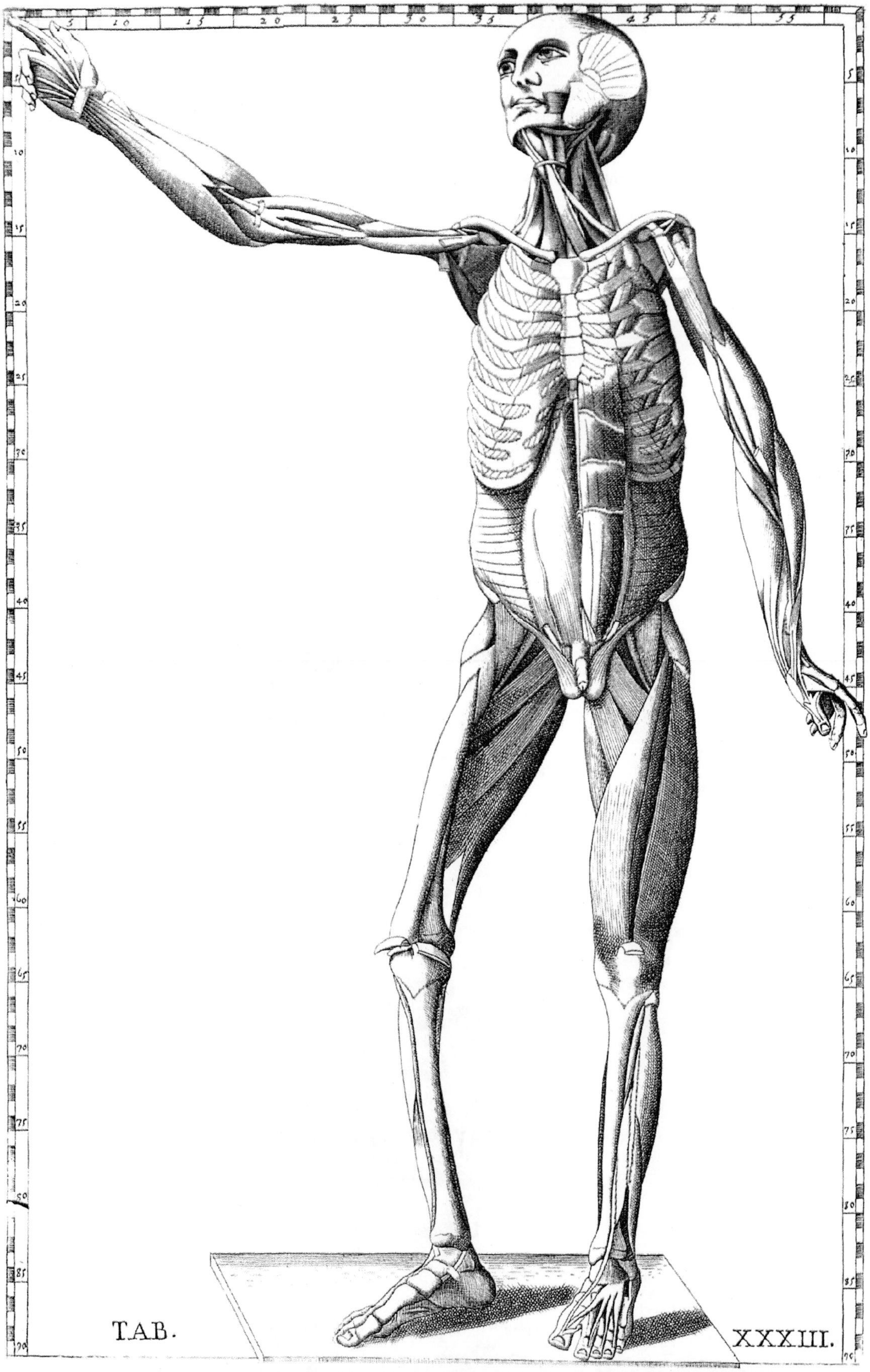

Anterior musculoskeletal anatomy, from, Bartolommeo Eustachio, *Tabulae anatomicae*. Rome, Sumptibus Laurentii & Thomae Pagliarini, 1728. Courtesy, Rare Book Room, Norris Medical Library, Keck School of Medicine, Los Angeles, California.

CHAPTER 7

The Far-lateral Approach and Its Transcondylar, Supracondylar, and Paracondylar Extensions

Albert L. Rhoton, Jr., M.D.

Department of Neurological Surgery, University of Florida, Gainesville, Florida

Key words: Cranial base, Cranial nerve, Craniocervical junction, Foramen magnum, Microsurgical anatomy, Occipital bone, Occipital condyle, Skull base, Surgical approach, Temporal bone, Vertebral artery

The basic far-lateral exposure is carried up to but does not include removal of the posterior part of the occipital condyle. It includes 1) dissection of the muscles along the posterolateral aspect of the craniocervical junction to permit an adequate exposure of the C1 transverse process and the suboccipital triangle; 2) early identification of the vertebral artery either above the posterior arch of the atlas or in its ascending course between the transverse processes of the atlas and axis; and 3) a suboccipital craniectomy or craniotomy with removal of at least half of the posterior arch of the atlas (5, 19, 20). It provides access for the following three approaches: the transcondylar approach directed through the occipital condyle or the atlanto-occipital joint and adjoining parts of the condyle; the supracondylar approach directed through the area above the occipital condyle; and the paracondylar exposure directed through the area lateral to the occipital condyle (*Fig. 7.1*). The transcondylar extension accompanied by drilling the condyles allows a more lateral approach and provides access to the lower clivus and premedullary area. The supracondylar approach provides access to the region of and medial to the hypoglossal canal and jugular tubercle. The paracondylar approach, which includes drilling of the jugular process of the occipital bone in the area lateral to the occipital condyle, accesses the posterior part of the jugular foramen, and the posterior aspect of the facial nerve and mastoid on the lateral side of the jugular foramen. In the standard posterior and posterolateral approaches, an understanding of the individual suboccipital muscles is not essential. However, these muscles provide important landmarks for the far-lateral approach and its modifications. Important considerations include the relationship of the occipital condyle to the foramen magnum, hypoglossal canal, jugular tubercle, the jugular process of the occipital bone, the mastoid, and the facial canal (1–3, 6, 7, 10, 12, 15–17).

STAGES OF APPROACH

The approach is divided into three anatomic stages (*Fig. 7.2*). The first stage, the muscular dissection, includes the skin incision, reflection of muscles, including those forming the suboccipital triangle, and examination of the relationship of the muscles to the occipital and vertebral arteries, the vertebral venous plexus, the transverse process of the atlas, and the upper cervical nerves. The second stage, the extradural dissection, examines landmarks for the suboccipital craniectomy, the extent of occipital condyle removal, and the exposure and identification of the hypoglossal canal, jugular process, jugular tubercle, and facial nerve. The final stage, the intradural exposure, reviews the relationships of the intradural segment of the vertebral artery and its branches, including the posteroinferior cerebellar artery (PICA), the lower cranial and upper cervical nerves, and the dentate ligament.

Muscular stage

For our study of the region, the exposure was done using a horseshoe scalp flap because it provided a better display of the muscular layers and their relationships to the neural and vascular structures (*Fig. 7.2A*). The incision began in the midline, approximately 5 cm below the external occipital protuberance, and was directed upward to just above the external occipital protuberance, turned laterally just above the superior nuchal line, reached the mastoid, and turned downward in front of the posterior border of the sternocleidomastoid muscle onto the lateral aspect of the neck to approximately 5 cm below the mastoid tip and below where the transverse process of the atlas can be palpated through the skin. The skin flap was reflected downward and medially to expose the most superficial layer of muscles formed by the sternocleidomastoid and splenius capitis muscles laterally and the trapezius and the semispinalis capitis muscles medially. In this description, the muscles are reflected separately but at an operation, the scalp and muscles superficial to the suboccipital triangle are reflected from the suboccipital area in a single layer, leaving a musculofascial cuff attached along the superior nuchal line for closure.

Muscular dissection

The sternocleidomastoid and trapezius are in the first layer encountered (*Fig. 7.2, B--H*). Dividing the sternocleidomastoid

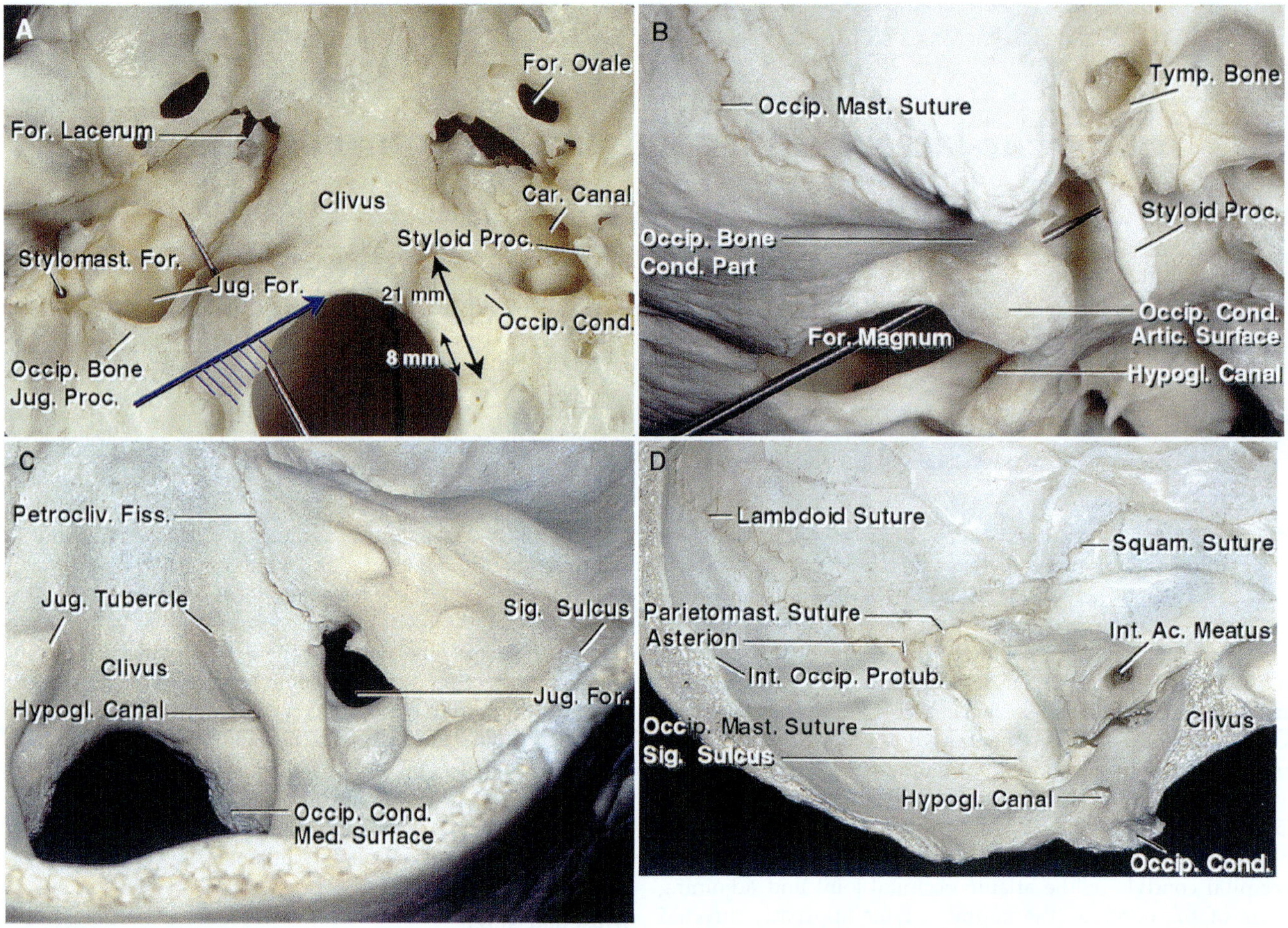

FIGURE 7.1. Osseous relationships. *A*, inferior view of the occipital condyles and foramen magnum. The occipital condyles are ovoid structures located along the lateral margin of the anterior half of the foramen magnum. Their articular surfaces are convex, face downward and laterally, and articulate with the superior facet of C1. A probe inserted through the hypoglossal canal passes forward approximately 45 degrees from the midsagittal plane in an anterolateral direction. The hypoglossal canal is located above the middle third of the occipital condyle and is directed from posterior to anterior and from medial to lateral. The intracranial end of the hypoglossal canal (*small oval*) is located approximately 5 mm above the junction of the posterior and middle third of the occipital condyle and approximately 8 mm from the posterior edge of the condyle. The extracranial end of the canal is located approximately 5 mm above the junction of the anterior and middle third of the condyle. The average length of the longest axis of the condyle is 21 mm. The *large arrow* shows the direction of the transcondylar approach and the *cross-hatched area* shows the portion of the occipital condyle that can be removed without exposing the hypoglossal nerve in the hypoglossal canal. The condylar fossa is frequently the site of a canal, the condylar canal, which transmits the posterior condylar emissary vein that connects the vertebral venous plexus with the sigmoid sinus just proximal to the jugular bulb. The condylar canal passes above and usually does not communicate with the hypoglossal canal. The jugular process of the occipital bone extends laterally from the posterior half of the occipital condyle to form the posterior margin of the jugular foramen. The portion of the jugular process located immediately behind the jugular foramen serves as the site of attachment for the rectus capitis lateralis muscle. The stylomastoid foramen is situated lateral to the jugular foramen. The styloid process is located anterior and slightly medial to the stylomastoid foramen. *B*, inferolateral view. A probe has been passed through the hypoglossal canal, which passes above occipital condyle. From its intracranial to its extracranial end it is directed forward, lateral, and slightly upward. *C*, superior view. The occipital condyle projects downward from the lateral margin of the anterior half of the foramen magnum. The intracranial entrance of the hypoglossal canal is located above the condyle. The jugular tubercles are located above and anterior to the hypoglossal canals. The jugular process of the occipital bone extends laterally from the condyles to form the posterior margin of the jugular foramen. The sigmoid sinus crosses the occipitomastoid suture and turns in a hooklike groove on the upper surface of the jugular process to reach the jugular foramen. Drilling the occipital condyle increases access to the anterolateral margin of the foramen magnum. Drilling in a supracondylar location below the hypoglossal canal accesses the lateral edge of the clivus. Drilling in the supracondylar location above the hypoglossal canal accesses the jugular tubercle, which projects upward and often blocks visualization of the junction of the middle and lower clivus and the region of the pontomedullary junction during the far-lateral approach. Drilling the jugular process in a

just below and with preservation of its upper attachment for closure and reflecting it laterally exposes the upper extension of the splenius capitis. Detaching the trapezius and splenius capitis muscles, while preserving a cuff of their upper attachments for closure, and reflecting them medially exposes the longissimus capitis muscle. Reflecting the longissimus capitis downward exposes the semispinalis capitis and the superior and inferior oblique muscles as well as the transverse process of the atlas, which has a prominent apex palpable through the skin between the mastoid process and mandibular angle. The semispinalis capitis is reflected medially to expose the suboccipital triangle, which is limited by three muscles; above and medially by the rectus capitis posterior major, above and laterally by the superior oblique, and below and laterally by the inferior oblique (*Fig. 7.2G*).

The triangle deep to these muscles is covered by a layer of dense fibrofatty tissue. The floor in the depth of the triangle is formed by the posterior atlanto-occipital membrane and the posterior arch of the atlas (*Fig. 7.2H*). The structures in the triangle are the vertebral artery and the C1 nerve, both of which lie in a groove on the upper surface of the lateral part of the posterior arch of the atlas. The suboccipital triangle is opened by reflecting the rectus capitis posterior major inferiorly and medially, the superior oblique laterally, and the inferior oblique medially. Opening the triangle exposes the portion of the vertebral venous plexus that surrounds the vertebral artery as it passes behind the atlanto-occipital joint and across the upper edge of the posterior arch of the atlas (*Fig. 7.2I*). Reflecting the superior oblique muscle, as described earlier, exposes the rectus capitis lateralis, a short, flat muscle that is an important landmark in identifying the jugular foramen (*Figs. 7.2, K* and *L*, and *7.3*). It arises from the upper surface of the transverse process of the atlas and attaches above to the rough, lower surface of the jugular process of the occipital bone behind the jugular foramen. The jugular process is a plate of occipital bone extending laterally from the posterior half of the occipital condyle. It is indented in front at the site of the jugular notch, which forms the posterior edge of the jugular foramen (*Fig. 7.1*). The rectus capitis lateralis, because it is attached to the jugular process at the posterior edge of the jugular foramen, provides a landmark for estimating the position of the jugular foramen and the facial nerve, which exits the stylomastoid foramen just lateral to the jugular foramen.

Vascular structures

Reflecting the muscles forming the suboccipital triangle, as described earlier, exposes the vertebral artery, which is surrounded by a rich venous plexus that must be obliterated and partially removed if the vertebral artery is to be exposed or transposed (*Fig. 7.2, H* and *I*).

The vertebral artery, above the transverse foramen of the axis, veers laterally to reach the transverse foramen of the atlas, which is situated further lateral than the transverse foramen of the axis. The artery, after ascending through the transverse process of the atlas, is located on the medial side of the rectus capitis lateralis muscle. From here it turns medially behind the lateral mass of the atlas and the atlanto-occipital joint and is pressed into the groove on the upper surface of the posterior arch of the atlas, where it courses in the floor of the suboccipital triangle and is covered behind the triangle by the semispinalis capitis muscle. The first cervical nerve courses on the lower surface of the artery between the artery and the posterior arch of the atlas (*Fig. 7.2, K–M*). After passing medially above the lateral part of the posterior arch of the atlas, the artery enters the vertebral canal by passing below the lower, arched border of the posterior atlanto-occipital membrane, which transforms the sulcus in which the artery courses on the upper edge of the posterior arch of the atlas into an osseofibrous casing that may ossify, transforming it into a complete or incomplete bony canal surrounding the artery (*Fig. 7.2H*) (5).

The third segment of the vertebral artery, the segment located between the C1 transverse process and the dural entrance, gives rise to muscular branches and the posterior meningeal arteries. The muscular branches arise as the artery exits the transverse foramen of C1 and courses around the lateral mass of the atlas to supply the deep muscles and anastomose with the occipital and ascending and deep cervical arteries (*Fig. 7.2I*). Some of the muscular branches may need to be divided to mobilize and transpose the vertebral artery. The posterior meningeal artery arises from the posterior surface of the vertebral artery as it passes behind the lateral mass or above the posterior arch of the atlas or just before penetrating the dura in the region of the foramen magnum, but it may also have an intradural origin from the

paracondylar location accesses the posterior margin of the jugular bulb, which is situated in the sigmoid portion of the jugular foramen. *D*, medial aspect of the occipital condyle and supracondylar region. The inner surface of the mastoid portion of the temporal bone is grooved by the sulcus of the sigmoid sinus. The asterion, the site of the junction of the lambdoid, parietomastoid, and the occipitomastoid sutures, is an important landmark used to define the transition between the transverse and sigmoid sinuses. The sigmoid sulcus crosses the occipitomastoid suture just behind the jugular foramen. The intracranial end of the hypoglossal canal is located above the junction of the posterior and middle thirds of the occipital condyle. The external occipital protuberance is located an average of 2 cm below the apex of the internal occipital protuberance and 1 cm below the lower margin of the torcular herophili. The parietal notch, located at the junction of the squamosal and parietomastoid sutures, defines the upper limit of the petrous portion of the temporal bone and the floor of the posterior portion of the middle fossa. The midportion of the parietomastoid suture approximates the anterior edge of the junction of the transverse and sigmoid sinuses. *Ac.*, acoustic; *Artic.*, articular; *Car.*, carotid; *Cond.*, condyle; *Fiss.*, fissure; *For.*, foramen; *Hypogl.*, hypoglossal; *Int.*, internal; *Jug.*, jugular; *Mast.*, mastoid; *Med.*, medial; *Occip.*, occipital; *Parietomast.*, parietomastoid; *Petrocliv.*, petroclival; *Proc.*, process; *Protub.*, protuberance; *Sig.*, sigmoid; *Squam.*, squamosal; *Stylomast.*, stylomastoid; *Tymp.*, tympanic.

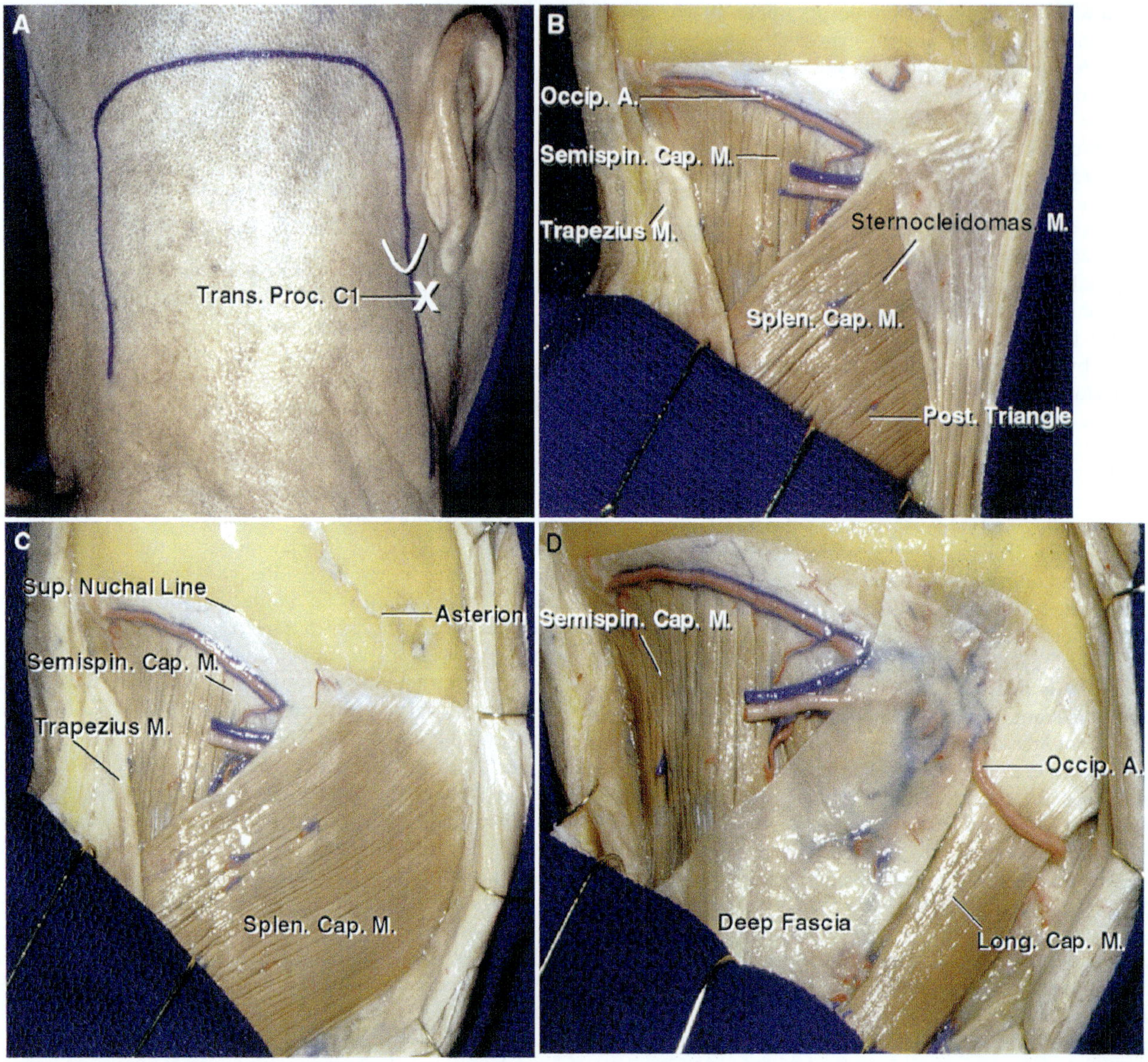

FIGURE 7.2. *A–D.* Far-lateral and transcondylar approach. *A*, a suboccipital scalp flap is commonly selected for the far-lateral exposure. The medial limb extends downward in the midline so that a wide upper cervical laminectomy can be completed if needed. The lateral limb extends below the C1 transverse process, which can be palpated between the mastoid tip and the angle of the jaw to access the vertebral artery as it ascends through the C1 transverse process. In this dissection, the muscles are reflected separately to show their anatomy; however, at an operation, the muscles superficial to the suboccipital triangle can be reflected from the suboccipital area in a single layer with the scalp flap, leaving a cuff of suboccipital muscle and fascia attached along the superior nuchal line to aid in closure. *B*, the scalp flap has been reflected to expose the sternocleidomastoid and trapezius, the edges of which form the margins of the posterior triangle of the neck. The splenius and semispinalis capitis are in the floor of the triangle. *C*, the sternocleidomastoid has been detached from the lateral part of the superior nuchal line and reflected laterally to expose the splenius capitis, which is attached just below the line. The asterion, located at the junction of the lambdoid, occipitomastoid, and parietomastoid sutures, most commonly overlies the lower half of the junction of the transverse and sigmoid sinuses. *D*, the splenius capitis has been reflected to expose the longissimus capitis and deep cervical fascia. The occipital artery may pass superficial or deep to the longissimus capitis. *A.*, artery; *Atl.*, atlanto; *Br.*, branch; *Cap.*, capitis; *CN*, cranial nerve; *Dent.*, dentate; *Digast.*, digastric; *Dors.*, dorsal; *Gang.*, ganglion; *Hypogl.*, hypoglossal; *Inf.*, inferior; *Lat.*, lateralis; *Lev.*, levator; *Lig.*, ligament; *Long.*, longissimus; *M.*, muscle; *Maj.*, major; *Mas.*, mastoid; *Memb.*, membrane; *Men.*, meningeal; *Min.*, minor; *Musc.*, muscular; *Obl.*, oblique; *Occip.*, occipital; *P.I.C.A.*, posteroinferior cerebellar artery; *Plex.*, plexus; *Post.*, posterior; *Proc.*, process; *Rec.*, rectus; *Scap.*, scapula; *Semispin.*, semispinalis; *Splen.*, splenius; *Suboccip.*, suboccipital; *Sup.*, superior; *Trans.*, transverse; *Vent.*, ventral; *Vert.*, vertebral.

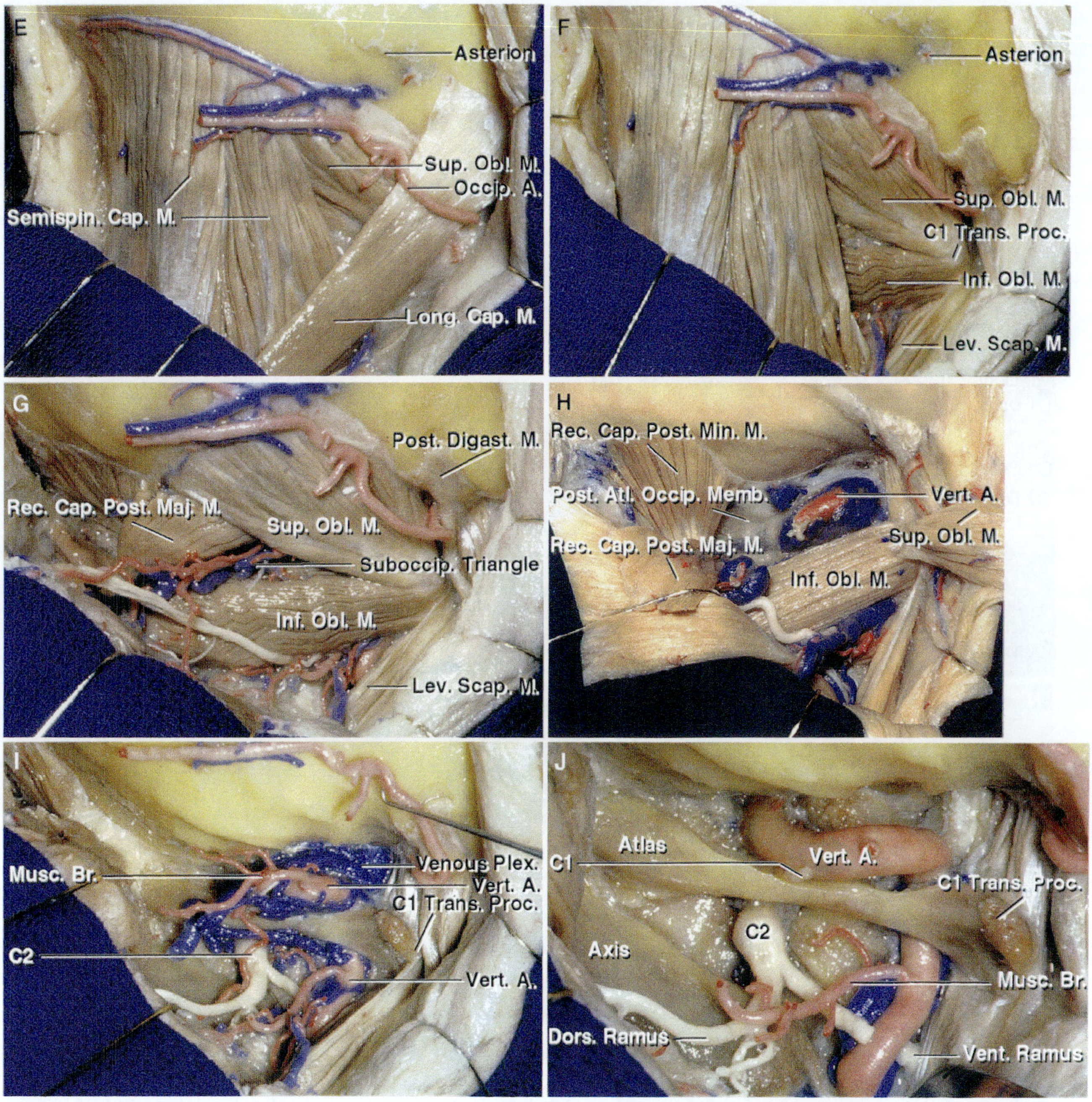

FIGURE 7.2. *E–J.* Far-lateral and transcondylar approach. *E*, the fascia has been removed to expose the occipital artery passing behind the superior oblique and semispinalis. *F*, the longissimus capitis has been reflected to expose the attachment of the superior and inferior oblique muscles to the C1 transverse process. *G*, the suboccipital triangle, in the depths of which the vertebral artery courses behind the atlanto-occipital joint and across the posterior arch of C1, is situated in the depths of the area between the superior and inferior oblique and the rectus capitis posterior major. *H*, the superior oblique muscle has been reflected laterally and the rectus capitis posterior major muscle inferomedially. The floor of the suboccipital triangle is formed by the posterior atlanto-occipital membrane and the posterior arch of the atlas. The vertebral artery and the C1 nerve root, which are surrounded by the vertebral venous plexus, course along the upper surface of the posterior arch of the atlas. *I*, the muscles forming the margins of the suboccipital triangle have been reflected to expose the vertebral artery ascending through the C1 transverse process and behind the atlanto-occipital joint and the surrounding venous plexus. *J*, the venous plexus around the vertebral artery has been removed. The vertebral artery gives off muscular branches, passes medially behind the atlanto-occipital joint and above the posterior arch of C1, and turns upward and anterior to penetrate the dura.

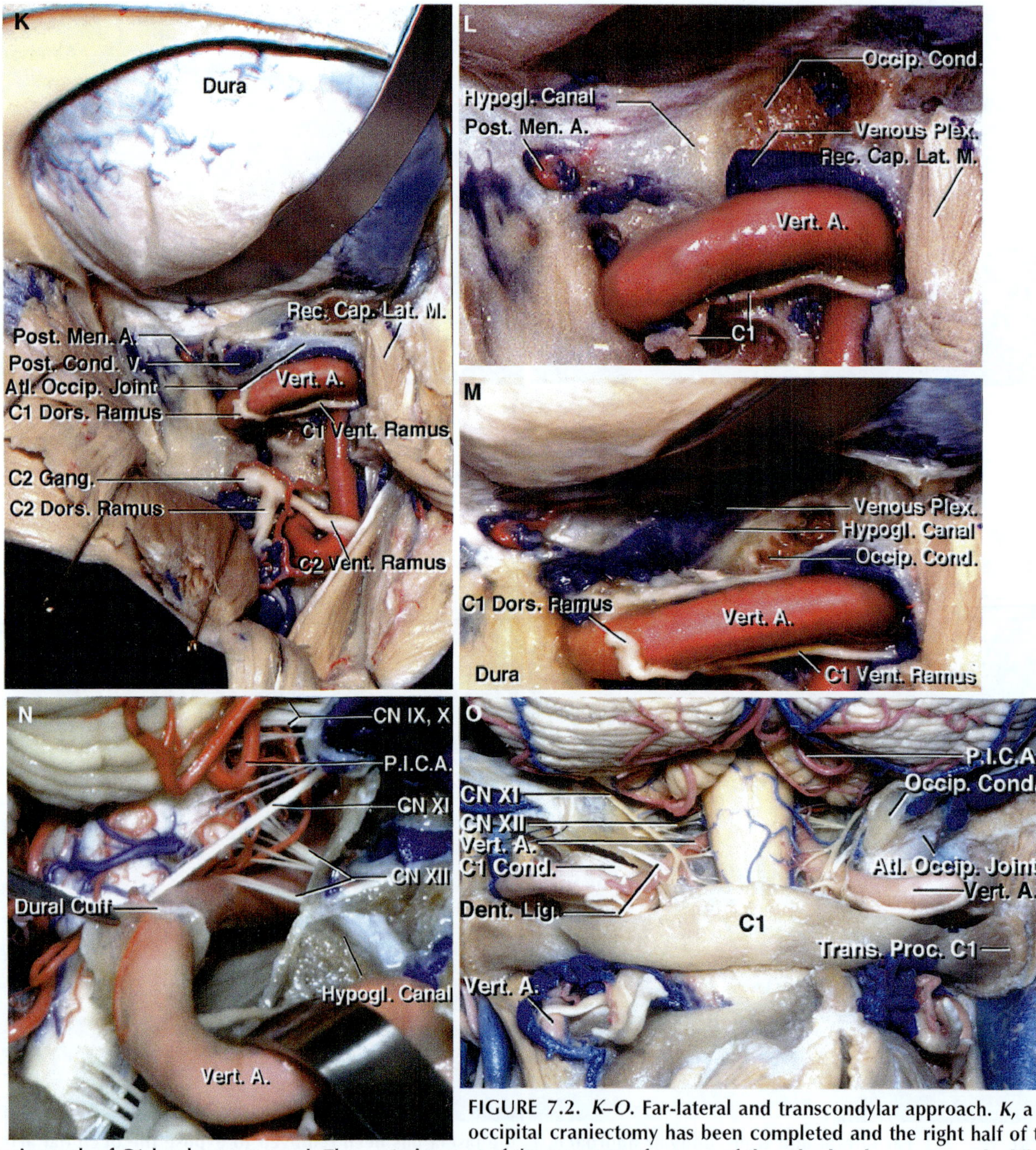

FIGURE 7.2. *K–O.* Far-lateral and transcondylar approach. *K*, a suboccipital craniectomy has been completed and the right half of the posterior arch of C1 has been removed. The posterior root of the transverse foramen of the atlas has been removed while preserving the portion of the tip of the transverse process of the atlas to which the rectus capitis lateralis, levator scapulae, and the superior oblique attach. The atlanto-occipital joint and the posterior condylar emissary vein are exposed. The ventral rami of the C1 and C2 nerve roots pass behind the vertebral artery. The dorsal ramus of C2 gives rise to the greater occipital nerve, which passes through the semispinalis capitis to reach the posterior scalp. *L*, the area above the occipital condyle has been drilled to the depth of the cortical bone surrounding the hypoglossal canal. The change from cancellous to cortical bone indicates that the hypoglossal canal has been reached. *M*, the hypoglossal canal has been opened to expose the venous plexus, which surrounds the hypoglossal nerve in the canal and connects the basilar venous plexus with the marginal sinus, which encircles the foramen magnum. The dorsal ramus of the C1 nerve root, also termed the suboccipital nerve, passes backward between the posterior arch of the atlas and the vertebral artery, supplies the muscles bordering the suboccipital triangle, and sends fibers to the rectus capitis posterior minor and the semispinalis capitis muscles. *N*, an upper cervical laminectomy has been completed and the dura opened. The dural incision completely encircles the vertebral artery, leaving a narrow dural cuff on the artery so that the

vertebral artery, in which case it pierces the arachnoid over the cisterna magna to reach the dura (*Fig. 7.2L*) (20).

The occipital artery is also exposed as the superficial and deep muscles in the region are reflected (*Fig. 7.2, C--G*). It originates from the posterior wall of the external carotid artery at the level of the angle of the mandible, ascends parallel and medial to the external carotid artery and lateral to the internal jugular vein to reach the area posteromedial to the styloid process. At that point, it changes its course to posterior and lateral, passing first between the rectus capitis lateralis and the posterior belly of the digastric and then between the superior oblique and the posterior belly of the digastric where it courses in the occipital groove medial to the mastoid notch, in which the posterior belly of the digastric muscle arises. After exiting the area between the superior oblique muscle and the posterior belly of the digastric, it courses medially, being related to the longissimus capitis and semispinalis capitis. If the occipital groove is present, the occipital artery will course deep to the longissimus capitis muscle, but if the groove is absent, the artery will course superficial to the longissimus capitis muscle (*Fig. 7.2E*). It courses medially behind the semispinalis capitis just below the superior nuchal line in the upper part of the posterior triangle to pass between the upper attachment of trapezius and the semispinalis capitis, where it pierces the attachment of the trapezius muscle to the superior nuchal line and ascends in the superficial fascia of the posterior scalp.

Osseous structures

The transverse process of the atlas, an important landmark in these approaches, projects further lateral than the transverse processes on the adjacent cervical vertebrae and has an apex that can be felt through the skin in the area between the mastoid process and angle of the mandible (*Fig. 7.2A*). Several muscles important in completing the exposure attach to the transverse process of the atlas (*Fig. 7.2G*). The rectus capitis lateralis arises from the anterior portion, and the superior oblique arises from the posterior portion of the upper surface of the transverse process. The inferior oblique muscle inserts on the lateral tip of the transverse process. The levator scapulae, splenius cervicis, and the scalenus medius attach to the inferior and lateral surface of the transverse process. The levator scapulae is also attached by tendinous slips to the posterior tubercles of the transverse processes of C2 to C4 (*Fig. 7.2, F* and *G*).

Neural structures

The neural structures encountered during the muscle dissection arise predominantly from the C1 and C2, and to a lesser extent from the C3 spinal nerves that are formed by the united dorsal and ventral roots and are described in the chapter on the foramen magnum (*Fig. 7.2, J–M*).

Extradural stage

The extradural stage begins with a suboccipital craniectomy or craniotomy, identification of the occipital condyle, and removal of at least half of the posterior arch of the atlas and possibly the posterior root of the transverse foramen, if mobilization of the vertebral artery is needed (*Fig. 7.2K*). Two osseous landmarks important in planning the suboccipital craniotomy are the asterion located along the lower half of the groove on the inner table of the cranium near the point where the transverse sinus empties into the sigmoid sinus, and the inion (external occipital protuberance) located an average of 1 cm below the apex of the internal occipital protuberance and the inferior margin of the confluence of the sagittal and transverse sinuses. In completing the removal of the posterior arch of the atlas, the tip of the transverse process is preserved along with the attachment of the superior oblique, which is reflected laterally while preserving the attachment of the rectus capitis lateralis.

At this stage, the segment of the vertebral artery extending from the transverse foramen of C2 to its entrance to the dura is exposed. Removal of the posterior root of the transverse foramen will permit the artery to be displaced downward and medially away from the atlanto-occipital joint to expose the occipital condyle (*Fig. 7.2, L--N*). The occipital condyles project downward along the lateral edges of the anterior half of the foramen magnum (*Figs. 7.1* and *7.3*). The articular surfaces, which are ovoid with the long axis in the AP direction, are located on the lower-lateral margin of the condyles. They face downward and laterally to articulate with the superior facets of the atlas, which face upward and medially.

The intracranial end of the hypoglossal canal is located approximately 5 mm above the junction of the posterior and middle third of the occipital condyle and appropriately 5 mm below the jugular tubercle (*Fig. 7.1*). The canal is directed forward and laterally at a 45-degree angle with the sagittal plane. The extracranial end of the hypoglossal canal is located immediately above the junction of the anterior and middle third of the occipital condyle and medial to the jugular foramen. The average length of the longest axis of the condyle is

artery can be mobilized. The drilling in the supracondylar area exposes the hypoglossal nerve in the hypoglossal canal, and can be extended extradurally to the level of the jugular tubercle to increase access to the front of the brainstem. *O*, comparison of the exposure with the far-lateral and transcondylar approaches. On the right side, the far-lateral exposure has been extended to the posterior margins of the atlantal and occipital condyles and the atlanto-occipital joint. The prominence of the condyles limits the exposure along the anterolateral margin of the foramen magnum. On the left side, a transcondylar exposure has been completed by removing the posterior part of the condyles. The dura can be reflected further laterally with the transcondylar approach than with the far-lateral approach. The condylar drilling provides an increased angle of view and room for exposure and dissection. The dentate ligament and accessory nerve ascend from the region of the foramen magnum.

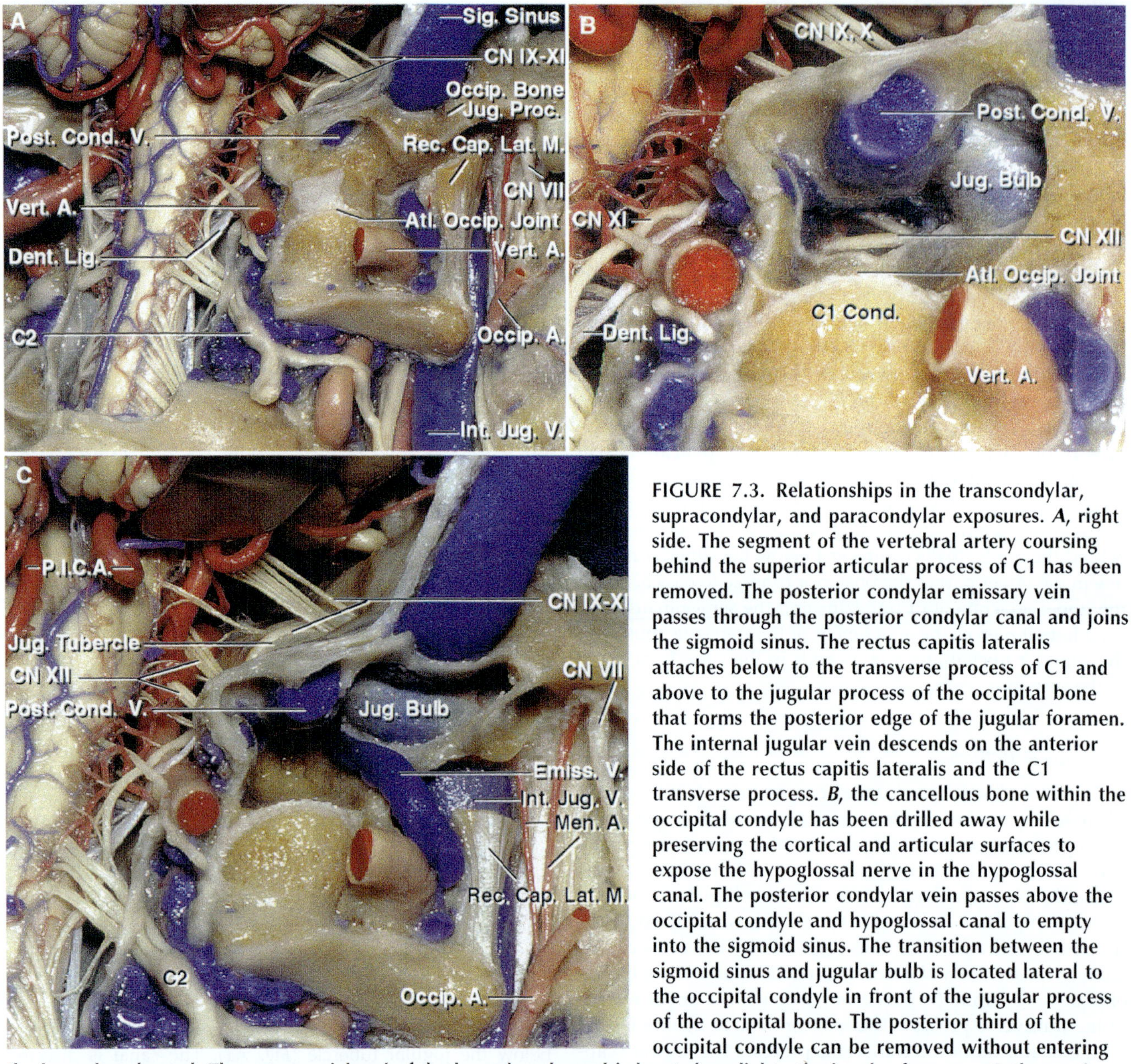

FIGURE 7.3. Relationships in the transcondylar, supracondylar, and paracondylar exposures. *A*, right side. The segment of the vertebral artery coursing behind the superior articular process of C1 has been removed. The posterior condylar emissary vein passes through the posterior condylar canal and joins the sigmoid sinus. The rectus capitis lateralis attaches below to the transverse process of C1 and above to the jugular process of the occipital bone that forms the posterior edge of the jugular foramen. The internal jugular vein descends on the anterior side of the rectus capitis lateralis and the C1 transverse process. *B*, the cancellous bone within the occipital condyle has been drilled away while preserving the cortical and articular surfaces to expose the hypoglossal nerve in the hypoglossal canal. The posterior condylar vein passes above the occipital condyle and hypoglossal canal to empty into the sigmoid sinus. The transition between the sigmoid sinus and jugular bulb is located lateral to the occipital condyle in front of the jugular process of the occipital bone. The posterior third of the occipital condyle can be removed without entering the hypoglossal canal. The extracranial end of the hypoglossal canal is located medial to the jugular foramen. *C*, the portion of the rectus capitis lateralis that attaches to the jugular process of the occipital bone has been removed to expose the internal jugular vein, and the jugular process of the occipital bone has been removed to expose the jugular bulb. The facial nerve is exposed laterally at the stylomastoid foramen. Several meningeal branches of the occipital artery ascend to pass through the jugular foramen. An emissary vein passes from the jugular bulb to the vertebral venous plexus. *A.*, artery; *Atl.*, atlanto; *Cap.*, capitis; *CN*, cranial nerve; *Cond.*, condyle; *Dent.*, dentate; *Emiss.*, emissary; *Int.*, internal; *Jug.*, jugular; *Lat.*, lateralis; *Lig.*, ligament; *M.*, muscle; *Men.*, meningeal; *Occip.*, occipital; *P.I.C.A.*, posteroinferior cerebellar artery; *Post.*, posterior; *Proc.*, process; *Rec.*, rectus; *Sig.*, sigmoid; *V.*, vein; *Vert.*, vertebral.

21 mm (range, 18–24 mm) and the average distance between the posterior edge of the occipital condyle and the posterior border of the intracranial end of the hypoglossal canal is 8.4 mm (range, 6–10 mm) (20). The hypoglossal canal is surrounded by cortical bone. The contents of the hypoglossal canal are the hypoglossal nerve, a meningeal branch of the ascending pharyngeal artery, and the venous plexus of the hypoglossal canal, which communicates the basilar venous plexus with the marginal sinus that encircles the foramen magnum (*Figs. 7.2M, 7.3B,* and *7.4, C* and *D*). Posterior to the occipital condyle, a depression, the condylar fossa, may be pierced by the condylar canal, which transmits the posterior condylar emissary vein, a communication between the vertebral venous plexus and the sigmoid sinus (*Fig. 7.3*). The canal

is directed slightly upward as it proceeds anteriorly to join the sigmoid sinus at the hook-like turn immediately proximal to where the sinus empties into the jugular bulb. The condylar canal does not communicate with the hypoglossal canal.

The jugular process of the occipital bone serves as a bridge between the condylar and squamosal parts of the occipital bone and forms the posterior margin of the jugular foramen (*Fig. 7.1*). It extends laterally from the posterior half of the condyle. The jugular process also serves as the site of attachment of the rectus capitis lateralis muscle behind the jugular foramen. The stylomastoid foramen, which transmits the facial nerve, is situated lateral to the jugular foramen at the anterior end of the mastoid notch (*Figs. 7.3C* and *7.4C*). The styloid process is located anterior to the stylomastoid foramen and anterolateral to the jugular foramen.

After removing the superficial layer of cortical bone covering the occipital condyle, soft cancellous bone will be encountered. Further drilling of the cancellous bone in and above the posterior third of the condyle exposes the second layer of hard, cortical bone that surrounds the hypoglossal canal (*Figs. 7.2N* and *7.3–7.6*). Subsequent drilling of this cortical bone exposes the venous plexus of the hypoglossal canal. The lateral aspect of the intracranial end of the hypoglossal canal is reached with removal of approximately the posterior third of the occipital condyle (8.4 mm of 21 mm) (*Fig. 7.1*) (20). Further drilling of the occipital condyle can be done after reaching the lateral aspect of the intracranial end of the hypoglossal canal, as the canal is directed anteriorly and laterally, permitting the lateral part of the posterior two-thirds of the condyle to be removed without entering the hypoglossal canal. The distance between the upper surface of the hypoglossal nerve and the roof of the hypoglossal canal averages 4.4 mm. Extensive drilling around the canal may allow the nerve to be transposed from its normal course (*Fig. 7.6*).

After exposing the hypoglossal canal above the occipital condyle, the bone of the jugular tubercle situated above the hypoglossal canal can be removed extradurally to gain additional exposure (1–3, 9, 10, 13). The jugular tubercle is a rounded prominence located at the junction of the basilar and condylar parts of the occipital bone (*Figs. 7.1, 7.4, C* and *D*, and *7.5, A–C*). It is situated above the hypoglossal canal and medial to the lower half of the intracranial end of the jugular foramen. The average distance from the posterior edge of the jugular tubercle (the site of the groove in which the lower cranial nerves course) to the upper border of the hypoglossal canal is 4.5 mm (20). The glossopharyngeal, vagus, and accessory nerves cross the posterior portion of the jugular tubercle in passing from the brainstem to the jugular foramen, sometimes coursing in a shallow groove on the surface of the tubercle (*Figs. 7.4* and *7.5*).

The prominence of the jugular tubercle blocks access to the basal cisterns and clivus anterior to the lower cranial nerves. As the jugular tubercle is removed extradurally the cranial nerves, which course along the back margin of the tubercle and are intradural, will not be visualized. As the drilling proceeds, bone will be removed from below the cisternal segment of the accessory and the vagus nerves that course above the tubercle just inside the dura. Caution is required in removing the jugular tubercle to avoid damaging the lower cranial nerves, either by direct trauma, by stretching the dura, or by the heat generated by the drilling (*Fig. 7.5, A–C*). The lateral margin of the jugular tubercle is situated just medial to and below the medial edge of the jugular bulb. If a more lateral exposure is needed, or the jugular foramen is to be opened from posteriorly, the jugular process of the occipital bone, which extends laterally from the occipital condyle, can be removed after detaching the rectus capitis lateralis muscle from its lower surface (*Figs. 7.3* and *7.4*). Removing the jugular process, which forms the posterior margin of the jugular foramen, will expose the transition between the sigmoid sinus, jugular bulb, and internal jugular vein. Care is required to avoid damaging the vertebral artery, because it passes upward through the transverse process of the atlas and turns medially in the area directly below the jugular process. For an even more lateral exposure, the posterior belly of the digastric muscle can be separated from the mastoid notch to expose the facial nerve just distal to the stylomastoid foramen (*Figs. 7.3C, 7.4, B* and *C*, and *7.6*). A partial mastoidectomy can be performed to expose the mastoid segment of the facial nerve in the facial canal at this stage.

Intradural stage

The dural incision begins behind the sigmoid sinus and extends behind the vertebral artery into the upper cervical area. The upper extent of the dural opening depends on how much of the cerebellopontine angle is to be exposed. Possible sources of bleeding during the dural opening are the marginal sinus that encircles the foramen magnum and the posterior meningeal artery, which usually originates from the vertebral artery extradurally, but may infrequently originate intradurally, in which case it crosses the lateral medullary cistern and pierces the arachnoid to reach the dura. Opening the dura exposes the intradural segment of the vertebral artery. As the artery pierces the dura, it is encased in a fibrous tunnel that binds the posterior spinal artery, dentate ligament, first cervical nerve, and the spinal accessory nerve to the vertebral artery (*Figs. 7.2, N* and *O, 7.3*) (14). Care should be taken to preserve the posterior spinal artery during the dural opening and mobilization of the vertebral artery because it may be incorporated into the dural cuff around the vertebral artery.

At the craniocervical junction, the dentate ligament is located between the vertebral artery and ventral roots of C1 anteriorly and the branches of the posterior spinal artery and spinal accessory nerve posteriorly, and is often incorporated into the dural cuff around the vertebral artery (*Figs. 7.2O, 7.3,* and *7.5*). The most rostral attachment of the dentate ligament is located at the level of the foramen magnum above where the vertebral artery pierces the dura and behind the accessory nerve, although the dentate ligament is located anterior to the accessory nerve at lower levels. Section of the upper two triangular processes will increase access anterior to the spinal cord. The first cervical nerve courses along the posteroinferior surface of the vertebral artery as it pierces the dura. The ventral root is located anterior to the dentate ligament, and the dorsal root, which is infrequently present, passes posterior

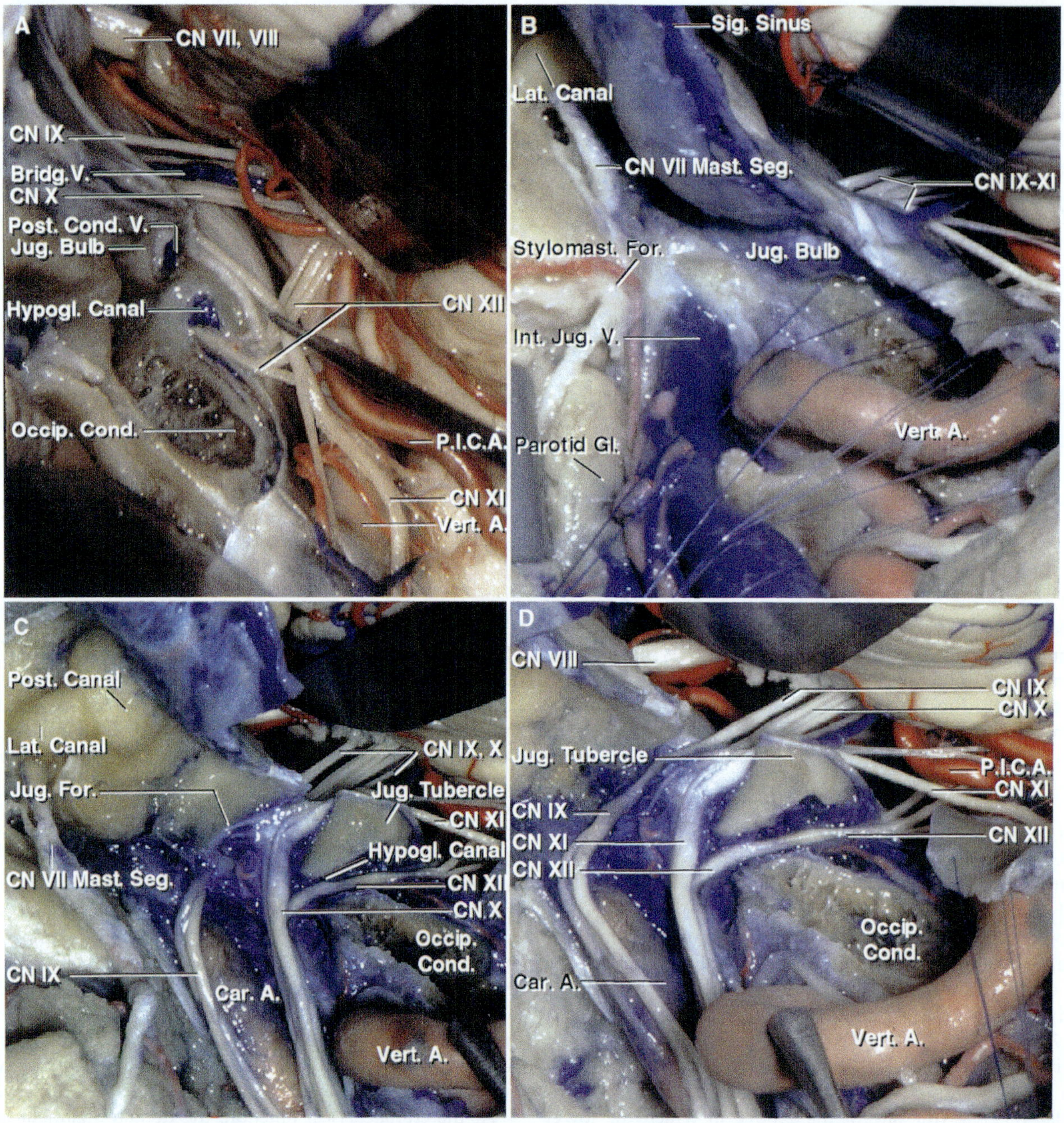

FIGURE 7.4. Relationships in the transcondylar, supracondylar, and paracondylar exposures. *A*, a left suboccipital craniectomy has been completed and the dura opened. The nerves entering the jugular foramen have been exposed. Bone has been removed above the occipital condyle to expose the hypoglossal nerve entering the hypoglossal canal. A bridging vein passes from the lateral aspect of the medulla to the jugular bulb. *B*, the rectus capitis lateralis has been detached from the cranial base and the jugular process of the occipital bone, which forms the posterior margin of the jugular foramen, has been removed to expose the jugular bulb. The posterior belly of the digastric muscle has been reflected forward and a mastoidectomy completed to expose the mastoid segment of the facial nerve. *C*, the jugular bulb and adjoining segment of the internal jugular vein have been removed to expose the glossopharyngeal, vagus, and accessory nerves passing through the jugular foramen and descending behind the internal carotid artery. The cortical bone lining the hypoglossal canal has been removed to expose the hypoglossal nerve and the venous plexus in the canal. The hypoglossal nerve joins the nerves exiting the jugular foramen to descend in the carotid sheath. A mastoidectomy has been completed to expose the bony capsule of the semicircular canals and the mastoid segment of the facial nerve. *D*, enlarged view of the nerves passing through the hypoglossal canal and jugular foramen in the supracondylar and paracondylar areas. *A.*, artery; *Bridg.*, bridging; *Car.*, carotid; *CN*, cranial nerve; *Cond.*, condyle; *For.*, foramen; *Gl.*, gland; *Hypogl.*, hypoglossal; *Int.*, internal; *Jug.*, jugular; *Lat.*, lateral, lateralis; *Occip.*, occipital; *P.I.C.A.*, posteroinferior cerebellar artery; *Post.*, posterior; *Seg.*, segment; *Sig.*, sigmoid; *Stylomast.*, stylomastoid; *Vert.*, vertebral.

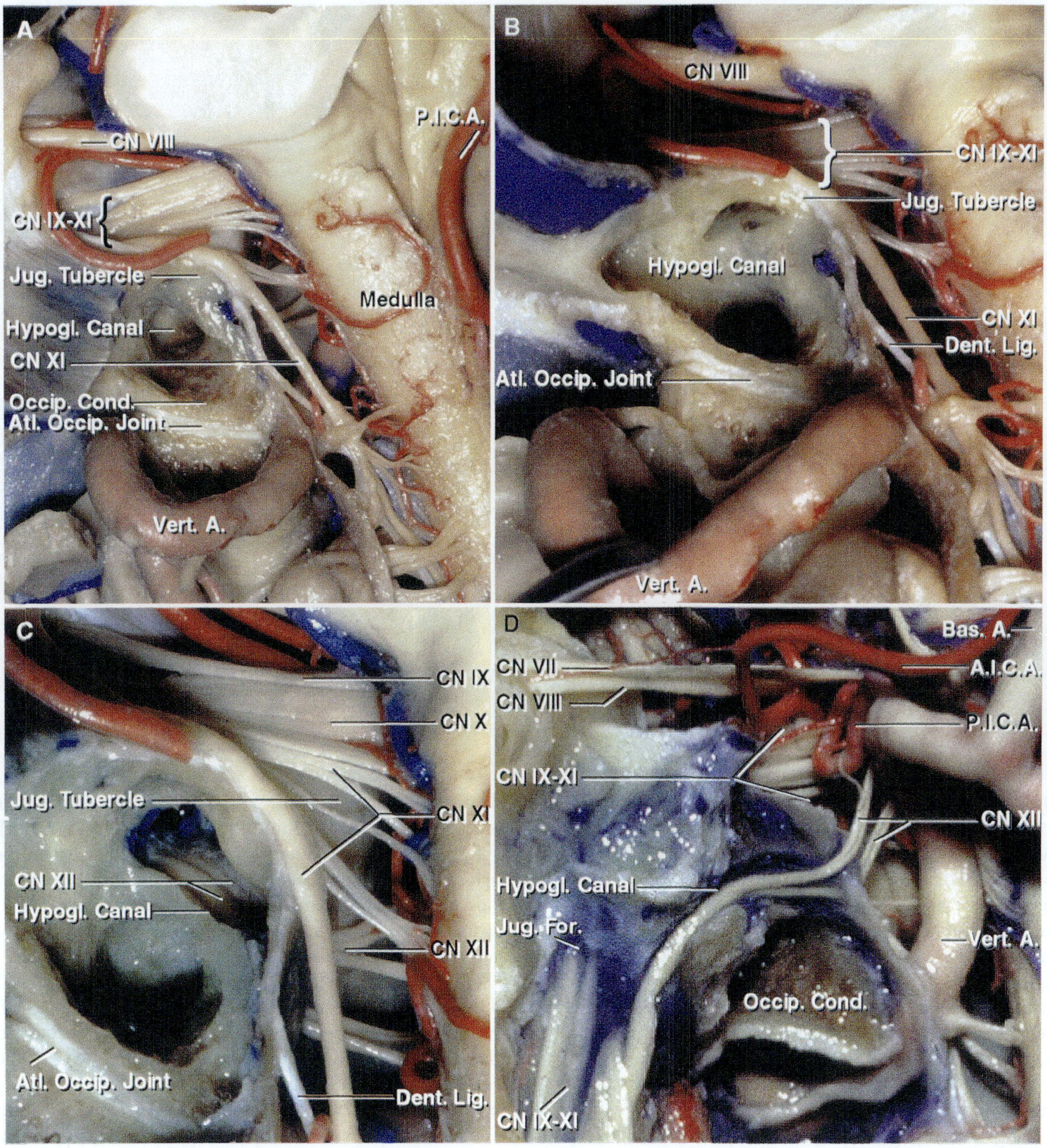

FIGURE 7.5. Posterior view of the left cerebellopontine angle. *A*, the glossopharyngeal, vagus, accessory, and hypoglossal nerves arise from the medulla. The hypoglossal canal has been exposed by drilling the cancellous bone above the occipital condyle. The posterior root of the transverse process of C1 has been removed. The accessory nerve crosses the jugular tubercle, the latter acting as a trochlea around which the accessory nerve courses to reach the jugular foramen. *B*, enlarged view. The area above the occipital condyle has been drilled to further expose the cortical bone around the hypoglossal canal. The atlanto-occipital joint has been preserved. *C*, the cortical bone lining the hypoglossal canal has been opened to expose the hypoglossal nerve and the hypoglossal venous plexus in the canal. *D*, anterior view. The anterior surface of the posterior fossa and the anterior wall of the hypoglossal canal have been removed to expose the hypoglossal nerve in its canal. The rootlets of the hypoglossal nerve originate ventral to the inferior olive and join before exiting the hypoglossal canal. The glossopharyngeal, vagus, and accessory nerves penetrate the dura on the medial side of the jugular bulb. The hypoglossal nerve exits the hypoglossal canal on the medial side of the jugular foramen. *A.*, artery; *A.I.C.A.*, anteroinferior cerebellar artery; *Atl.*, atlanto; *Bas.*, basilar; *CN*, cranial nerve; *Cond.*, condyle; *Dent.*, dentate; *For.*, foramen; *Hypogl.*, hypoglossal; *Jug.*, jugular; *Lig.*, ligament; *Occip.*, occipital; *P.I.C.A.*, posteroinferior cerebellar artery; *Vert.*, vertebral.

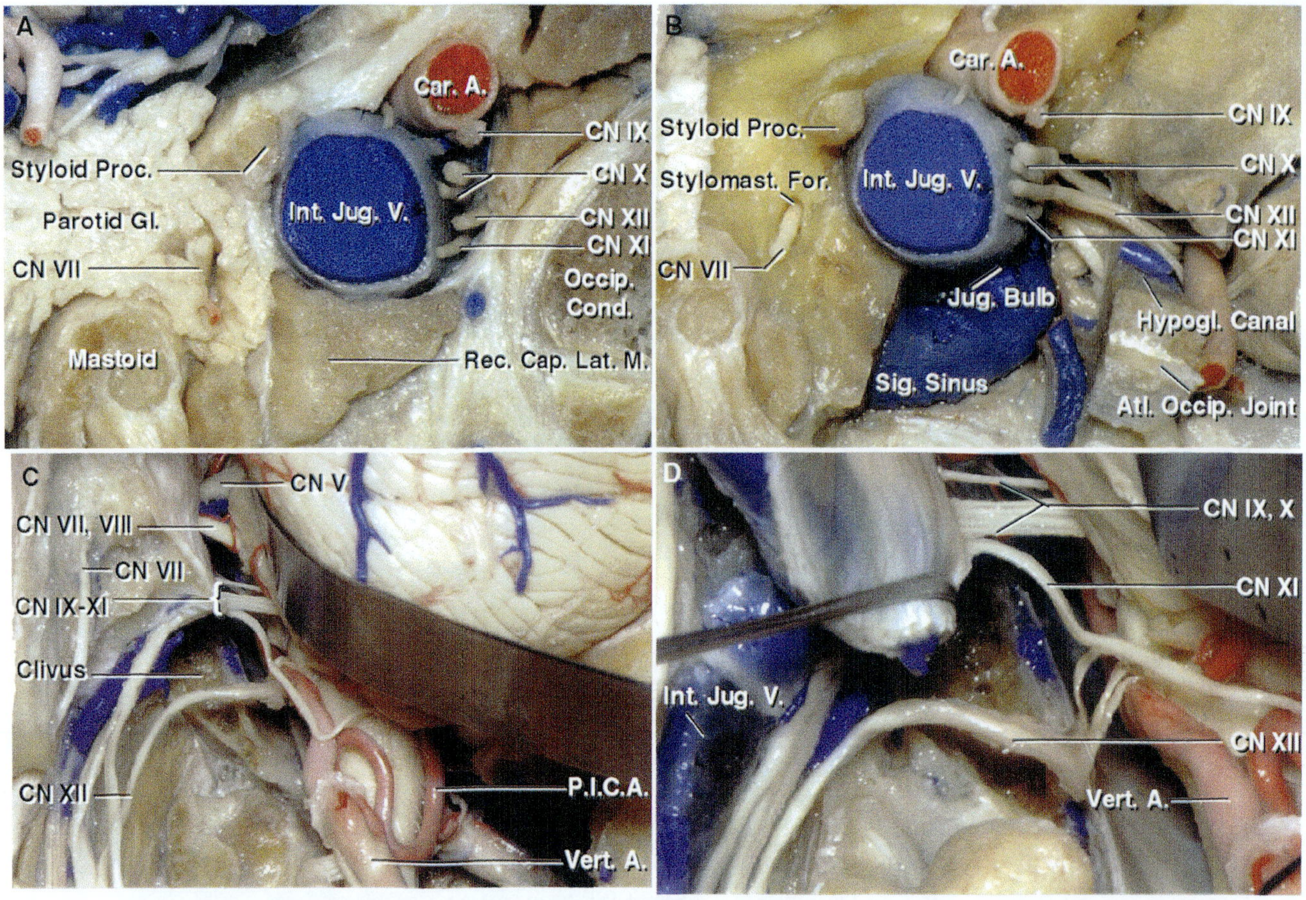

FIGURE 7.6. *A*, axial section extending through the occipital condyle and internal jugular vein below the right jugular foramen. The internal jugular vein descends just in front of the rectus capitis lateralis and behind the carotid artery. The occipital condyle is located on the medial side of the jugular foramen, and the styloid process, facial nerve, and parotid gland are on the lateral side. The nerves passing through the jugular foramen and hypoglossal canal collect together on the medial side of the internal jugular vein in an area just below the jugular foramen. *B*, the parotid gland has been removed. The facial nerve exits the stylomastoid foramen on the lateral side of the internal jugular vein. The styloid process is located along the anterolateral margin of the internal jugular vein. The central third of the occipital condyle has been removed to expose the hypoglossal nerve as it passes through the hypoglossal canal and joins the nerves exiting the jugular foramen on the medial side of the internal jugular vein. The rectus capitis lateralis and some of the jugular process of the occipital bone have been removed to expose the terminal part of the sigmoid sinus. *C–D*. Transposition of the hypoglossal nerve. *C*, the vertebral artery has been displaced medially. The occipital condyle, jugular tubercle, and the bone around and in front of the hypoglossal canal have been removed to expose the edge of the lower clivus. The dura ostium of the hypoglossal nerve has been opened so that the nerve can be mobilized. *D*, enlarged view of the mobilized hypoglossal nerve. *A.*, artery; *Atl.*, atlanto; *Cap.*, capitis; *Car.*, carotid; *CN*, cranial nerve; *Cond.*, condyle; *For.*, foramen; *Gl.*, gland; *Hypogl.*, hypoglossal; *Int.*, internal; *Jug.*, jugular; *Lat.*, lateralis; *M.*, muscle; *Occip.*, occipital; *P.I.C.A.*, posteroinferior cerebellar artery; *Proc.*, process; *Rec.*, rectus; *Sig.*, sigmoid; *Stylomast.*, stylomastoid; *V.*, vein; *Vert.*, vertebral.

to the dentate ligament. The rootlets forming the spinal portion of the accessory nerve, which arise from the cervical portion of the spinal cord midway between the dorsal and ventral rootlets as far caudally as C5, unite to form a trunk that ascends through the foramen magnum between the dentate ligament and the dorsal roots and enters the posterior fossa behind the vertebral artery (5).

The intradural segment of the vertebral artery, after emerging from the fibrous dural tunnel, ascends in front of the rootlets of the hypoglossal nerve to reach the front of the medulla oblongata where it unites near the junction of pons and medulla with its mate to form the basilar artery (*Fig. 7.2, N* and *O*). Before reaching the lower border of pons, the vertebral artery gives off the PICA, which courses backward around the lateral surface of the medulla and between the rootlets of glossopharyngeal, vagus, and accessory nerves. The anterior, lateral, and tonsillomedullary PICA segments and the intradural segment of the glossopharyngeal, vagus, and accessory nerves, which may be exposed in this approach, are described in greater detail in this issue in the chapters on the cerebellar arteries and cerebellopontine angle (*Figs. 7.2, N* and *O*, and *7.3-7.5*) (11).

DISCUSSION

The basic far-lateral approach without drilling of the occipital condyle may be all that is required to reach some lesions located along the anterolateral margin of the foramen magnum. However, it also provides a route through which the transcondylar, supracondylar, and paracondylar approaches and several modifications of these approaches can be completed. The transcondylar exposures can be categorized into several variants. An atlanto-occipital transarticular approach, in which the adjacent posterior parts of the occipital condyle and the superior articular facet of C1 are removed to facilitate completion of a circular dural incision, permitting the vertebral artery with the surrounding cuff of dura to be mobilized. A more extensive removal of the articular surfaces and condyles can be done to gain access to extradural lesions situated along the anterior and lateral margins of the foramen magnum. Another variant, the occipital transcondylar variant, is directed above the atlanto-occipital joint through the occipital condyle and below the hypoglossal canal to access the lower clivus and the area in front of the medulla. The supracondylar approach directed above the occipital condyle can also be varied, depending on the pathology to be exposed. The supracondylar exposure can be directed above the occipital condyle to the hypoglossal canal or both above and below the hypoglossal canal to the lateral side of the clivus. In the transtubercular variant of the supracondylar approach, the prominence of the jugular tubercle that blocks access to the area in front of the glossopharyngeal, vagus, and accessory nerves is removed extradurally to increase visualization of the area in front of the brainstem and to expose the origin of a PICA that arises from the distal part of the vertebral artery near the midline. The paracondylar approach also has several variants. In the transjugular variant, the exposure is directed lateral to the condyle through the jugular process of the occipital bone to the posterior surface of the jugular bulb. The approach can also be extended lateral to the jugular foramen into the posterior aspect of the mastoid to access the mastoid segment of the facial nerve and the stylomastoid foramen.

Many suboccipital operations are completed without requiring that each individual muscle be identified. However, identification of selective muscles is an essential part of completing the transcondylar, supracondylar, and paracondylar approaches. Muscles that are especially significant in identifying the neural, vascular, and osseous structures involved in these exposures are the three muscles forming the suboccipital triangle and the levator scapulae, rectus capitis lateralis, and the posterior belly of the digastric. Identification of the individual muscles is also helpful in exposing and preserving the occipital artery if it is needed for a bypass procedure and in preserving the peripheral branches of the upper cervical nerves. The levator scapulae muscle provides an excellent landmark for localizing the vertebral artery as it ascends between the transverse foramina of the atlas and axis where the artery is located medial to the upper attachments of the muscle. The main risk in this area is related to a tortuous vertebral artery that loops posteriorly as it ascends between the transverse processes of the axis and atlas, making it vulnerable to injury when one expects the artery to be passing straight upward from the lower to the upper transverse foramen. The artery is also susceptible to damage as it passes behind the superior articular facet of the atlas. The artery normally hugs the posterior surface of the superior articular facet of the atlas, extending upward only to the level of the atlanto-occipital joint. However, if the artery elongates and becomes tortuous it can loop upward behind the occipital condyle, even resting against the occipital bone behind the condyle. It also can loop backward and bulge posteriorly between the lips of the suboccipital triangle, which it can damage if one expects it to be found in the depth of the suboccipital triangle.

In obliterating and coagulating the venous plexus around the vertebral artery, there is the risk that some of the branches of the vertebral artery, which arise in an extradural location or even a hypoplastic vertebral artery, might be occluded or divided. The posterior spinal artery, and uncommonly the PICA, may arise extradurally in the region of the portion of the vertebral venous plexus, which may need to be partially excised or obliterated to gain access to the vertebral artery.

The far-lateral approach, in which the exposure is carried up to, but does not include, the posterior margin of the occipital condyle, may be selected for lesions located along the lateral or anterolateral aspect of the foramen magnum. It is frequently necessary to remove a small portion of both the occipital condyle and the superior articular facet of the atlas if there is a need to complete a circumferential dural incision around the site where the artery penetrates the dura, so that the artery can be displaced for access to lesions located ventral to the artery and in front of the cervicomedullary junction. For lesions requiring a greater anterior and superior exposure, the posterior third of the occipital condyle can be removed without entering the hypoglossal canal. It is possible to drill the cancellous bone of the occipital condyle to expose the lateral clivus and hypoglossal canal while preserving some of the cortical bone of the condyle and the articular surface so that the joint is not disrupted (*Figs. 7.3* and *7.5*). The cortical surface around the hypoglossal canal can be preserved if there is no need to expose the nerve within the canal.

Another key aspect of this approach is the condyle drilling, which requires an understanding of the relationship of the hypoglossal canal to the occipital condyle (*Figs. 7.3–7.6*). The maximum extent of the upper portion of occipital condyle that could be drilled without exposing the hypoglossal canal is the posterior third of its long axis. The occipital condyle sometimes can be covered by a hypertrophic superior articular facet of C1 that protrudes into the foramen magnum, making it easy to overlook the upper medial portion of the occipital condyle. In exposing lesions located along the anterior portion of the cervical cord, the inferior portion of the occipital condyle and the superior facet of C1 can be removed after retracting the vertebral artery inferior and medially. In drilling the upper posterior portion of the condyle, the posterior condylar vein may be a source of bleeding, which could be mistaken for bleeding from the venous plexus in the hypoglossal canal. After exposing the hypoglossal canal, the jugular tubercle, which is located just above and anterior to the canal, is identified. The drilling can be extended to a supracondylar location above the hypoglossal canal for removal of all or part of the jugular tubercle, so that the dura covering the tubercle can be pushed forward to gain access to the front of the medulla and the pontomedullary junction. Removal of the jugular tubercle may yield better visualization of the intradural segment of vertebral artery and the origin of the PICA, especially if the PICA originates from the upper part of the vertebral artery. The supracondylar approach, in which the jugular tubercle is removed and the hypoglossal canal is exposed or opened, provides a route for reaching extradural lesions located in the lower lateral part of the clivus in front of the hypoglossal canal. The extradural removal of the jugular tubercle should be performed with caution because of the risk of injuring the glossopharyngeal, vagus, and the accessory nerves that hug and often course in a shallow groove at the site where they cross the tubercle.

The paracondylar exposure, which accesses the posterior margin of the jugular foramen and the jugular bulb, can be completed without drilling the occipital condyle (8, 20). An excellent landmark for identifying the jugular process is the rectus capitis lateralis, which extends upward from the transverse process of the atlas to attach to the jugular process just behind the jugular bulb. The muscle is located medial to the site where the occipital artery enters the retromastoid area by passing between the rectus capitis lateralis and posterior belly of the digastric. The jugular foramen and jugular bulb is accessed by drilling the jugular process at the posterior margin of the foramen. Drilling lateral to the jugular bulb from this posterior exposure risks damaging the facial nerve in the facial canal at and just above the stylomastoid foramen. The posterior belly of the digastric muscle, which attaches along the digastric groove just posterior to the stylomastoid foramen, provides a useful landmark for identifying the facial nerve. A limited or more extensive mastoidectomy may be completed, depending on the length of the mastoid segment of the facial nerve to be exposed and the extent to which the bone on the lateral aspect of the jugular bulb must be removed. A wider exposure of the jugular foramen is obtained by a retrolabyrinthine transtemporal approach, in which a more extensive mastoidectomy is completed and the mastoid and the tympanic segments of the facial nerve are exposed so that the facial nerve can be transposed forward to provide access to both the lateral and the posterior margin of the jugular foramen.

Several controversies concern the positioning of the patient and the type of skin incision (20). The modified park bench position that we use offers the main advantage of avoiding air embolism (2, 3, 10, 14). The sitting position recommended by others is associated with a less distended venous plexus, but the rich net of veins around the cervical muscles, vertebral artery, and bone in the region offers the risk of air embolism (4, 13). A straight scalp incision has been recommended as being easier to open and close (10, 13). However, the thick cervical muscular mass and need for extensive retraction create a deep surgical field and the lateral position of the incision makes it difficult to complete a wide removal of the posterior C1 arch and C2 lamina, which is especially important if the lesion extends through the foramen magnum. We prefer an inverted horseshoe incision, with the medial limb extended so that a wide C1 to C2 laminectomy can be completed, and a lateral limb extended below the C1 transverse process so that the muscles attaching to the transverse processes are visualized (2, 5, 17, 18, 20). A musculofascial cuff is left attached along the superior nuchal line for closure. The flap on the upper part of the occipital squama can be reflected as a single layer, however it is helpful to identify the muscles forming the suboccipital triangle as an aid to exposing the vertebral artery. Anatomically, muscle dissection layer by layer offers the best preservation of the muscular landmarks. However, reflection of the superficial muscles individually carries a greater risk of flap dehiscence. Elevating the muscles attached to the upper part of the occipital squama with the scalp minimizes this problem and allows identification of important deep muscular landmarks, such as the suboccipital triangle and levator scapulae for localizing the vertebral artery and the rectus capitis lateralis for localizing the posterior portion of the jugular bulb.

Reprint requests: Albert L. Rhoton, Jr., M.D., Department of Neurological Surgery, University of Florida Brain Institute, P.O. Box 100265, 100 South Newell Drive, Building 59, L2-100, Gainesville, FL 32610-0265.

REFERENCES

1. Arnold H, Sepehrnia A: Extreme lateral transcondylar approach. **J Neurosurg** 82:313, 1995 (letter).
2. Babu RP, Sekhar LN, Wright DC: Extreme lateral transcondylar approach: Technical improvements and lessons learned. **J Neurosurg** 81:49–59, 1994.
3. Baldwin HZ, Miller CG, van Loveren HR, Keller JT, Daspit CP, Spetzler RF: The far lateral/combined supra- and infratentorial approach: A human cadaveric prosection model for routes of access to the petroclival region and ventral brainstem. **J Neurosurg** 81:60–68, 1994.
4. Bertalanffy H, Seeger W: The dorsolateral, suboccipital, transcondylar approach to the lower clivus and anterior portion of the craniocervical junction. **Neurosurgery** 29:815–821, 1991.
5. de Oliveira E, Rhoton AL Jr, Peace D: Microsurgical anatomy of the region of the foramen magnum. **Surg Neurol** 24:293–352, 1985.
6. Hakuba A, Tsujimoto T: Transcondyle approach for foramen magnum meningiomas, in Sekhar LN, Janecka IP (eds): *Surgery of Cranial Base Tumors*. New York, Raven Press, 1993, pp 671–678.
7. Heros RC: Inferolateral suboccipital approach for vertebral and vertebrobasilar aneurysms, in Wilkins RH, Rengachary SS (eds): *Neurosurgery Update: Vascular, Spinal, Pediatric, and Functional Neurosurgery*. New York, McGraw-Hill, 1991, vol II, pp 106–109.
8. Katsuta T, Rhoton AL Jr, Matsushima T: The jugular foramen: Microsurgical anatomy and operative approaches. **Neurosurgery** 41:149–202, 1997.
9. Kratimenos GP, Crockard HA: The far lateral approach for ventrally placed foramen magnum and upper cervical spine tumors. **Br J Neurosurg** 7:129–140, 1993.
10. Lang DA, Neil-Dwyer G, Iannotti F: The suboccipital transcondylar approach to the clivus and cranio-cervical junction for ventrally placed pathology at and above the foramen magnum. **Acta Neurochir (Wien)** 125:132–137, 1993.
11. Lister JR, Rhoton AL Jr, Matsushima T, Peace D: Microsurgical anatomy of the posterior inferior cerebellar artery. **Neurosurgery** 10:170–199, 1982.

12. Matsushima T, Ikezaki K, Nagata S, Inoue T, Natori Y, Fukui M, Rhoton AL Jr: Microsurgical anatomy for lateral approaches to the foramen magnum: With special reference to the far lateral approach and the transcondylar approach, in Nakagawa H (ed): *Surgical Anatomy for Microneurosurgery: Anatomy and Approaches to the Craniocervical Junction and Spinal Column* [in Japanese]. Tokyo, SciMed, 1994, vol VII, pp 81–89.
13. Perneczky A: The posterolateral approach to the foramen magnum, in Samii M (ed): *Surgery in and around the Brainstem and the Third Ventricle*. Berlin, Springer-Verlag, 1986, pp 460–466.
14. Rhoton AL Jr: Meningiomas of the cerebellopontine angle and foramen magnum. **Neurosurg Clin N Am** 52:349–377, 1994.
15. Sen CN, Sekhar LN: An extreme lateral approach to intradural lesions of the cervical spine and foramen magnum. **Neurosurgery** 27:197–204, 1990.
16. Sen CN, Sekhar LN: Surgical management of anteriorly placed lesions at the cranio-cervical junction: An alternative approach. **Acta Neurochir (Wien)** 108:70–77, 1991.
17. Sen C, Sekhar LN: Extreme lateral transcondylar and transjugular approaches, in Sekhar LN, Janecka IP (eds): *Surgery of Cranial Base Tumors*. New York, Raven Press, 1993, pp 389–411.
18. Spetzler RF, Grahm TW: The far-lateral approach to the inferior clivus and the upper cervical region: Technical note. **BNI Q** 6:35–38, 1990.
19. Tedeschi H, Rhoton AL Jr: Lateral approaches to the petroclival region. **Surg Neurol** 41:180–216, 1994.
20. Wen HT, Rhoton AL Jr, Katsuta T, de Oliveira E: Microsurgical anatomy of the transcondylar, supracondylar, and paracondylar extensions of the far-lateral approach. **J Neurosurg** 87:555–585, 1997.

DE HVMANI CORPORIS FABRICA LIBER VII.

DVODECIMA SEPTIMI LIBRI

FIGVRA.

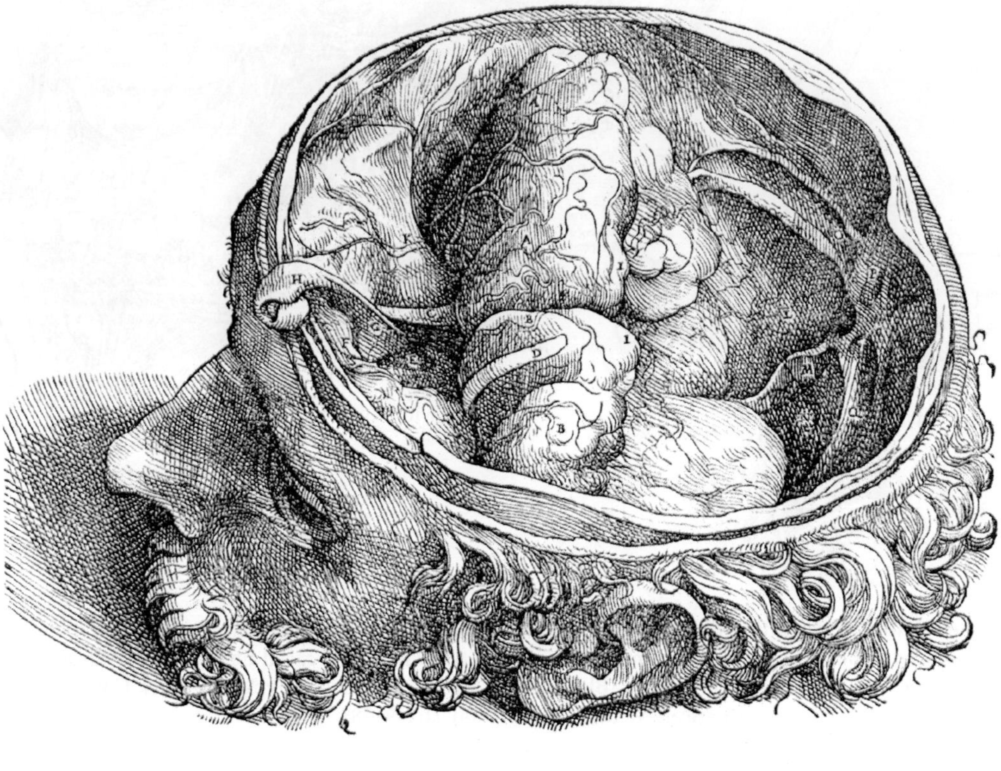

DVODECIMAE FIGVRAE, EIVSDEMQVE CHA-

racterum Index.

Cranium showing various anatomical structures. Vesalius was so confident that his work would be studied and plagiarized that he obtained the sponsorship and copyright protection of the Emperor, the King of France, and the Grand Council of Venice, the three great powers of his day. From, Andreas Vesalius, *De Humani Corporis Fabrica*. Basel, Ex officina Ioannis Oporini, 1543. Courtesy, Rare Book Room, Norris Medical Library, Keck School of Medicine, Los Angeles, California.

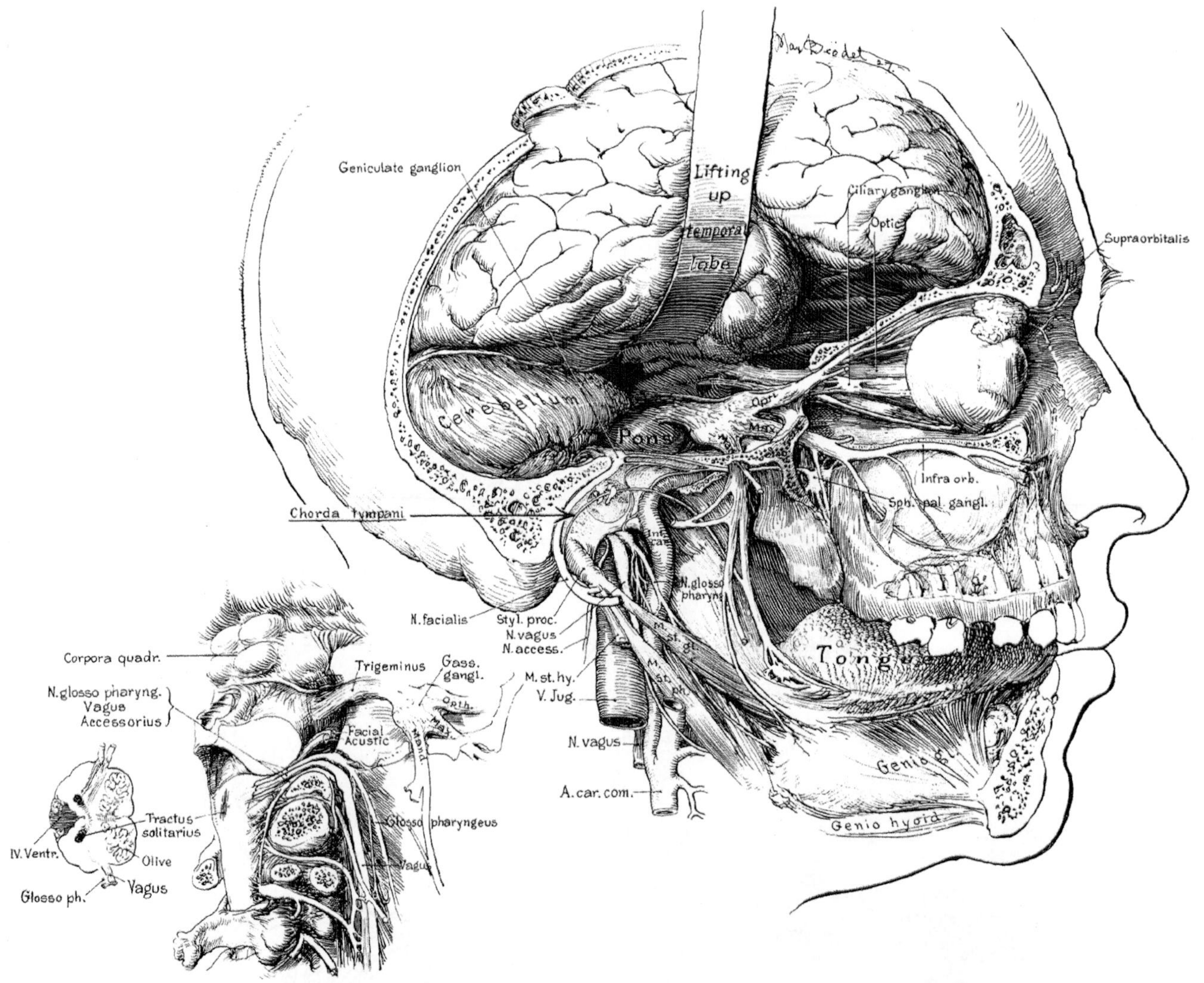

The course of the nerve fibers transmitting the sensation of taste. Dean Lewis and Walter Dandy described the course of taste fibers, which they believed to be from the tongue through the chorda tympani to the facial nerve, directly through the geniculate ganglion and the nervous intermedius into the pons. Black ink on Ross scratchboard by Max Brödel. Courtesy, Journal of the American Medical Association 21:249–288, 1930.

CHAPTER 8

The Temporal Bone and Transtemporal Approaches

Albert L. Rhoton, Jr., M.D.

Department of Neurological Surgery, University of Florida, Gainesville, Florida

Key words: Cranial base, Cranial nerves, Facial nerve, Internal carotid artery, Microsurgical anatomy, Skull base, Skull base neoplasm, Surgical approach, Temporal bone

The temporal bone is divided into squamosal, petrous, mastoid, tympanic, and styloid parts (*Figs. 8.1* and *8.2*). The squamosal part helps enclose the brain. The mastoid part is trabeculated and pneumatized to a variable degree and contains the mastoid antrum. The petrous part is compact and encloses the cochlea, the vestibule, and the semicircular, facial, and carotid canals (*Fig. 8.3*). The tympanic part forms part of the wall of the tympanic cavity and the external acoustic meatus. The styloid projects downward and serves as the site of attachment of several muscles. This section examines these parts in greater detail and defines the anatomic basis of the approaches directed through the temporal bone to the posterior fossa and petroclival region. The approaches examined are the middle fossa, translabyrinthine, transcochlear, combined supra- and infratentorial presigmoid, subtemporal anterior transpetrosal, subtemporal preauricular infratemporal, and the postauricular transtemporal approaches.

The approaches directed through the surface of the temporal bone forming the middle fossa floor include 1) the very limited middle fossa exposure of the internal acoustic meatus; 2) the anterior petrosectomy approach directed medial to the internal acoustic meatus through the petrous apex to access the upper anterior part of the posterior fossa and clivus; 3) the extended middle fossa approach, which may include not only resection of the roof of the internal acoustic meatus and petrous apex, but is extended lateral to the internal acoustic meatus to include resection, as needed, of the semicircular canals, vestibule, roof of the mastoid antrum and tympanic cavity, and the posterior face of the temporal bone; and 4) the subtemporal preauricular infratemporal fossa approach in which the middle fossa exposure is combined with exposure of the infratemporal fossa and, if needed, the petrous carotid, petrous apex, pterygopalatine fossae, and orbit.

The approaches directed through the mastoid in front of the sigmoid sinus vary in the amount of temporal bone resected. They include 1) the minimal mastoidectomy variant in which only enough presigmoid dura is exposed to open the dura in front of the sigmoid without exposing the labyrinth; 2) the retrolabyrinthine approach, which exposes the bony capsule of the labyrinth; 3) the partial labyrinthectomy, which includes removal of one or more of the semicircular canals; 4) the translabyrinthine approach, which includes resection of the semicircular canals and vestibule; and 5) the transcochlear modification, which includes removal of all the labyrinth, including the cochlear and possibly the petrous apex. These variants of the transmastoid approaches can all be combined, as needed, with the supra- and infratentorial presigmoid approaches to the middle and posterior fossa.

The final approach to be reviewed is the postauricular transtemporal approach, which allows lesions involving the mastoid, tympanic cavity, petrous apex, and jugular foramen to be followed backward to the areas exposed by the retrosigmoid and far-lateral approaches and forward to the infratemporal, pterygopalatine and middle fossae, lateral maxilla, and orbit. Selecting an approach directed through the temporal bone requires an understanding of its complex anatomy and its relationship to the petroclival region, the infratemporal fossa, and parapharyngeal space. Protecting and preserving the facial nerve, the petrous carotid artery, and the sensory organs of the inner ear that are contained within the temporal bone are important elements in operative approaches directed through the lateral aspect of the cranial base.

THE TEMPORAL BONE AND TRANSTEMPORAL APPROACHES

Lateral surface

When the skull and temporal bone are viewed from a lateral perspective, some landmarks useful in performing approaches directed around and through the temporal bone can be identified (*Fig. 8.2*). The posterior end of the superior temporal line continues inferiorly as the supramastoid crest and blends into the upper edge of the zygomatic arch. The supramastoid crest is located at the level of the floor of the middle fossa. The junction of the supramastoid crest with the squamous suture is located at the lateral end of the petrous ridge. The meeting point of the parietomastoid and squamous sutures is located a few millimeters below the lateral end of the petrous ridge. The anterior edge of the junction of the sigmoid and transverse sinuses is located at the junction of the squamous and parietomastoid suture.

The mastoid antrum, a pneumatized space opening into the tympanic cavity, is located about 1.5 cm deep to the su-

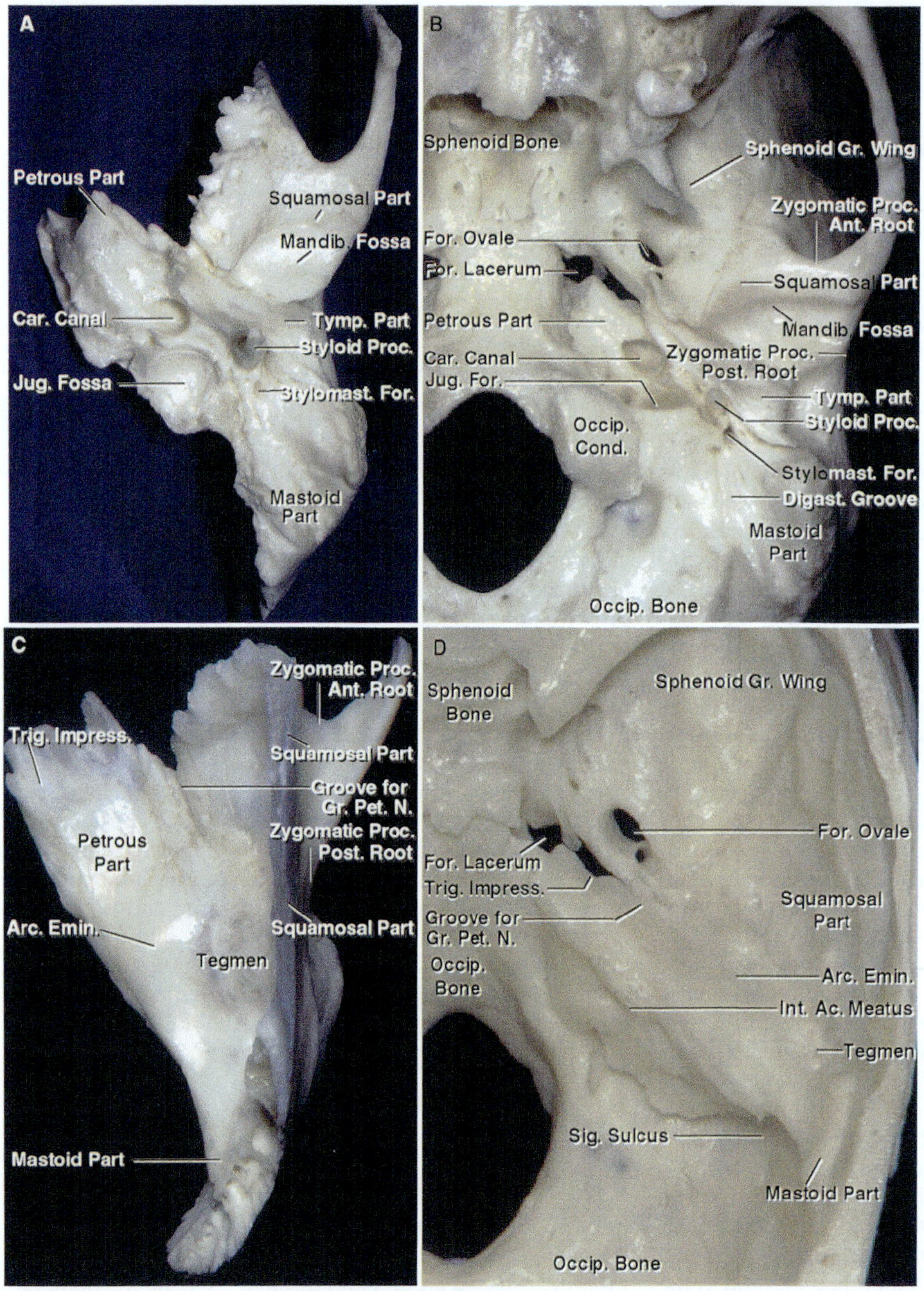

FIGURE 8.1. Temporal bone. *A* and *B*, inferior views. *A*, the temporal bone has a squamosal part, which forms some of the floor and lateral wall of the middle cranial fossa. It is also the site of the mandibular fossa in which the mandibular condyle sits. The tympanic part forms the anterior, lower, and part of the posterior wall of the external canal, part of the wall of the tympanic cavity, the osseous portion of the eustachian tube, and the posterior wall of the mandibular fossa. The mastoid portion contains the mastoid air cells and mastoid antrum. The petrous part is the site of the auditory and vestibular labyrinth, the carotid canal, the internal acoustic meatus, and the facial canal. The petrous part also forms the anterior wall and the dome of the jugular fossa. The styloid part projects downward and serves as the site of attachment of three muscles. *B*, inferior view of the temporal and surrounding bones. The squamosal and petrous parts articulate anteriorly with the greater wing of the sphenoid. The petrous apex faces the foramen lacerum and is separated from the clival part of the occipital bone by the petroclival fissure. The occipital bone joins with the petrous part of the temporal bone to form the jugular foramen. The mandibular fossa is located between the anterior and posterior roots of the zygomatic process. *C* and *D*, superior views. *C*, the medial part of the upper surface is the site of the trigeminal impression in which Meckel's cave sits. Farther laterally is the prominence of the arcuate eminence overlying the superior semicircular canal. Anterolateral to the arcuate eminences is the tegmen, a thin plate of bone overlying the mastoid antrum and epitympanic area. The temporal bone articulates anteriorly with the sphenoid bone, above with the parietal bone, and posteriorly with the occipital bone. The zygomatic process of the squamosal part has an anterior and a posterior root between which, on the lower surface, is located the mandibular canal. *D*, temporal and surrounding bones. The squamosal part of the temporal bone joins anteriorly with the sphenoid bone to form the floor of the middle cranial fossa. Posteriorly, it articulates with the occipital bone to form a portion of the anterior wall of the posterior fossa. Medially, it articulates with the clival portion of the occipital bone at the petroclival fissure. The sigmoid sulcus descends along the posterior surface of the mastoid portion and turns forward to enter the jugular foramen. The foramen lacerum is located at the junction of the temporal, sphenoid, and occipital bones. The porus of the internal acoustic meatus is located in the central part of the posterior surface. *Ac.*, acoustic; *Ant.*, anterior; *Arc.*, arcuate; *Car.*, carotid; *Cond.*, condyle; *Digast.*, digastric; *Emin.*, eminence; *For.*, foramen; *Gr.*, greater; *Impress.*, impression; *Int.*, internal; *Jug.*, jugular; *Mandib.*, mandibular; *N.*, nerve; *Occip.*, occipital; *Pet.*, petrosal; *Post.*, posterior; *Proc.*, process; *Sig.*, sigmoid; *Stylomast.*, stylomastoid; *Trig.*, trigeminal; *Tymp.*, tympanic.

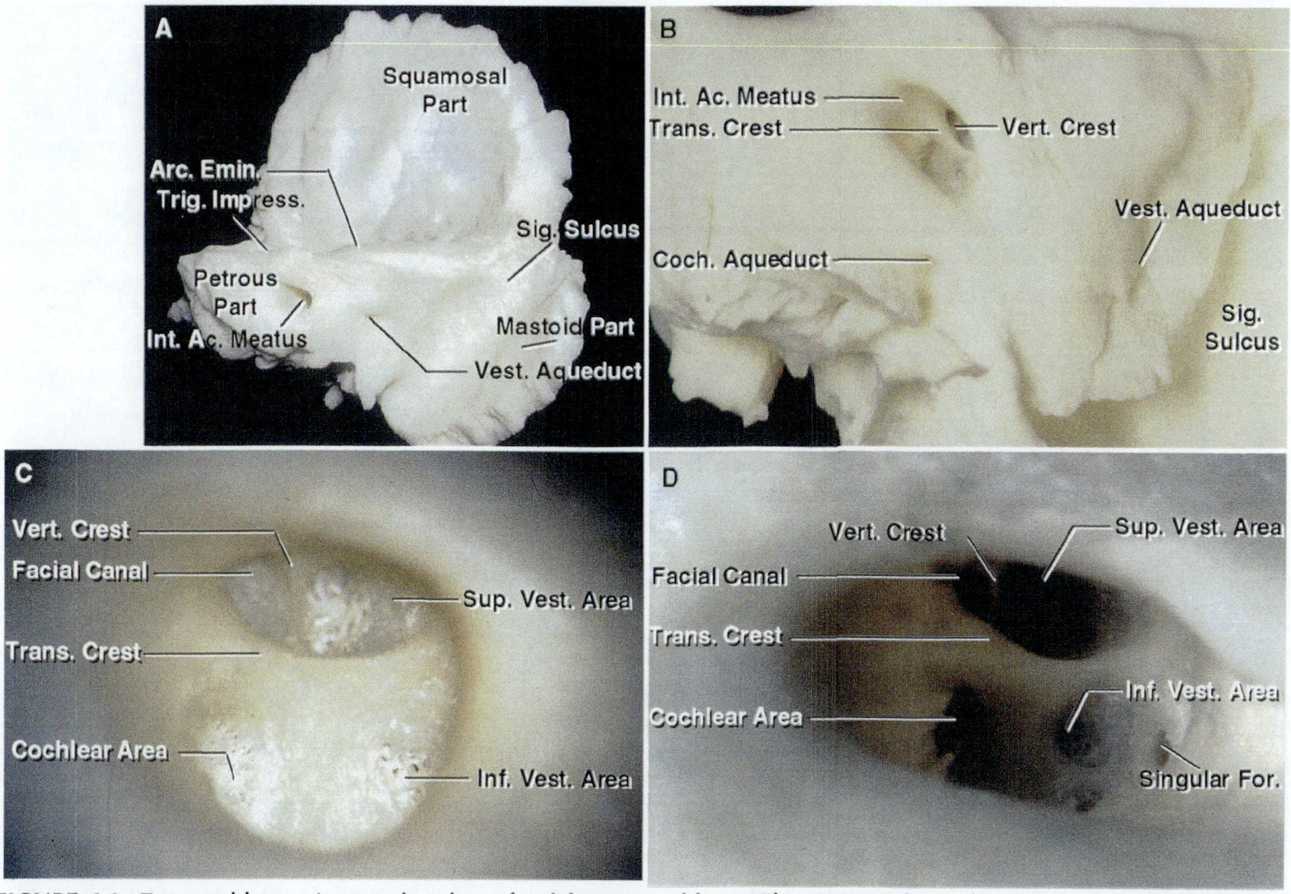

FIGURE 8.2. Temporal bone. ***A*****, posterior view of a right temporal bone. The squamosal part forms part of the floor and lateral wall of the middle fossa. The sigmoid sulcus descends along the posterior surface of the mastoid portion. The internal acoustic meatus enters the central portion of the petrous part of the bone. The trigeminal impression and arcuate eminence are located on the upper surface of the petrous part. The vestibular aqueduct connects the vestibule in the petrous part with the endolymphatic sac, which sits on the posterior petrous surface inferolateral to the internal acoustic meatus.** ***B*****, enlarged view. The transverse crest separates the meatal fundus into a superior part where the facial canal and superior vestibular areas are situated, and an inferior part where the cochlear and inferior vestibular areas are located. The vertical crest separates the facial and superior vestibular areas.** ***C*****, enlarged view of another internal acoustic meatus. The transverse crest divides the meatal fundus into superior and inferior parts. The anterior part above the transverse crest is the site of the facial canal and the posterior part is the site of the superior vestibular area. Below the transverse crest, the cochlear area is anterior and the inferior vestibular area is posterior.** ***D*****, another internal acoustic meatus. The view is directed to expose the singular foramen, for the singular branch of the inferior vestibular nerve that innervates the posterior ampullae. The inferior vestibular nerve also has a saccular and, occasionally, a utricular branch.** ***Ac.*****, acoustic;** ***Arc.*****, arcuate;** ***CN*****, cranial nerve;** ***Coch.*****, cochlear;** ***Emin.*****, eminence;** ***Ext.*****, external;** ***For.*****, foramen;** ***Impress.*****, impression;** ***Inf.*****, inferior;** ***Int.*****, internal;** ***Mandib.*****, mandibular;** ***Occipitomast.*****, occipitomastoid;** ***Parietomast.*****, parietomastoid;** ***Proc.*****, process;** ***Sig.*****, sigmoid;** ***Sp.*****, spine;** ***Sup.*****, superior;** ***Supramast.*****, supramastoid;** ***Trans.*****, transverse;** ***Trig.*****, trigeminal;** ***Vert.*****, vertebral;** ***Vest.*****, vestibular.**

prameatal triangle, a depression in the mastoid surface located between the posterosuperior edge of the external meatus, the supramastoid crest, and the vertical tangent along the posterior edge of the meatus. The suprameatal spine of Henle is located at the outer end of the posterosuperior edge of the external canal along the anterior edge of the suprameatal triangle and corresponds to the level of the lateral semicircular canal and tympanic segment of the facial nerve at a depth of approximately 1.5 cm. Several landmarks are also helpful in identifying the location of the junction of the transverse and sigmoid sinuses at the posterior aspect of the mastoid. The asterion located at the junction of the lambdoid, occipitomastoid, and parietomastoid sutures is usually located over the junction of the lower part of the transverse and sigmoid sinuses. A burr-hole placed at this site will usually expose the lower edge of this junction. A burr-hole located at the junction of the supramastoid crest and the squamosal suture will be located at the posterior part of the middle fossa floor just above and anterior to the upper edge of the junction of the transverse and sigmoid sinuses.

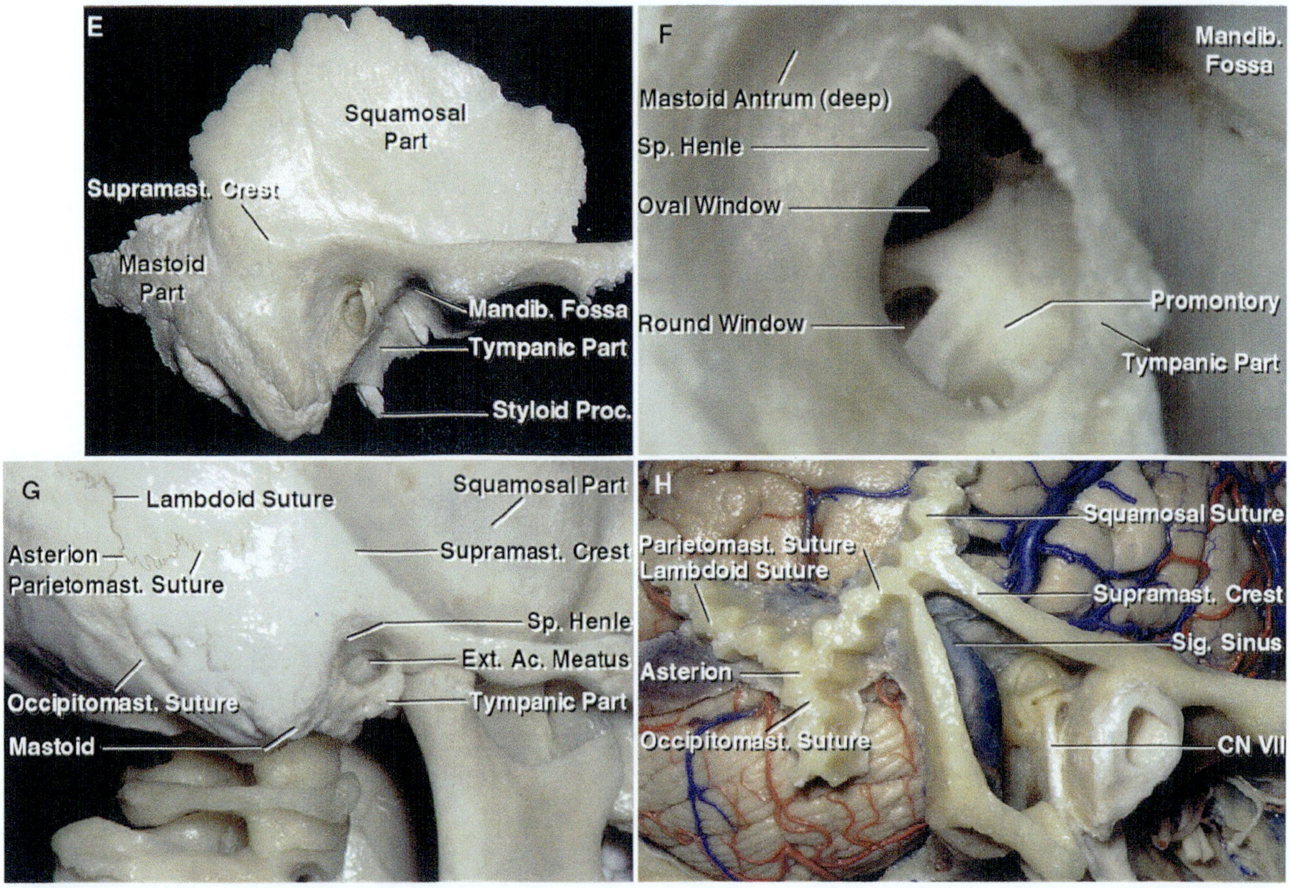

FIGURE 8.2. *E*, lateral view of the temporal bone. The squamosal part forms part of the lateral wall of the middle fossa, the posterior part of the zygomatic arch, and the upper part of the mandibular fossa. The tympanic part forms the posterior wall of the mandibular fossa and almost all of the wall of the external canal. The styloid process is ensheathed at its base by the tympanic part and projects downward, serving as the attachment of several muscles. The mastoid part is located posteriorly and contains the mastoid air cells that coalesce at the mastoid antrum. *F*, enlarged view of the external auditory canal. The spine of Henley, an excellent landmark for locating the deep site of the lateral canal and tympanic segment of the facial nerve, is located along the posterosuperior margin of the external canal. The mastoid antrum is located deep to the depressed area, called the suprameatal triangle, located behind the spine of Henley. The view into the canal exposes the tympanic cavity, which has the promontory overlying the basal turn of the cochlea and the oval and round windows in its medial wall. *G*, lateral surface of the temporal bone in the intact skull. The tympanic part forms the anterior and lower and part of the posterior wall of the external canal. The mandibular fossa is formed above and anteriorly by the squamosal part and behind by the tympanic part. The mastoid antrum is located posterosuperior to the spine of Henley, between the spine of Henley and the anterior part of the supramastoid crest. The asterion, the junction of the lambdoid, parietomastoid, and occipital mastoid sutures, is usually located over the lower half of the junction of the sigmoid and transverse sinuses. The midpoint of the parietal mastoid suture is usually located at the anterior margin of the junction of the transverse and sigmoid sinuses, and the lateral edge of the petrous ridge is located at the junction of the squamosal suture and the supramastoid crest. *H*, the supra- and infratentorial areas have been exposed while preserving the bone at the site of the sutures. The asterion, located at the junction of the lambdoid, occipitomastoid, and parietomastoid sutures, overlies the lower half of the junction of the transverse and sigmoid sinuses. The junction of the supramastoid crest and the squamosal suture is located at the posterior edge of the middle fossa and slightly anterior and above the junction of the transverse and sigmoid sinuses.

The tympanic part

The tympanic part of the temporal bone is a curved plate anterior to the mastoid process (*Figs. 8.1, 8.2,* and *8.4*). Its concave posterior surface forms the anterior wall, floor, and part of the posterior wall of the external acoustic meatus. The roof and upper posterior wall are formed by the squamosal part. Its surface contains a portion of the tympanic sulcus for attachment of the tympanic membrane, which closes the medial end of the external canal. The anterior surface, which is concave, forms the posterior wall of the mandibular fossa. Its lateral border forms most of the margin of the external acoustic meatus. Medially, it joins the petrous part at the petrotympanic fissure through which the chorda tympani passes. The carotid canal and the jugular foramen are located medial to the tympanic part.

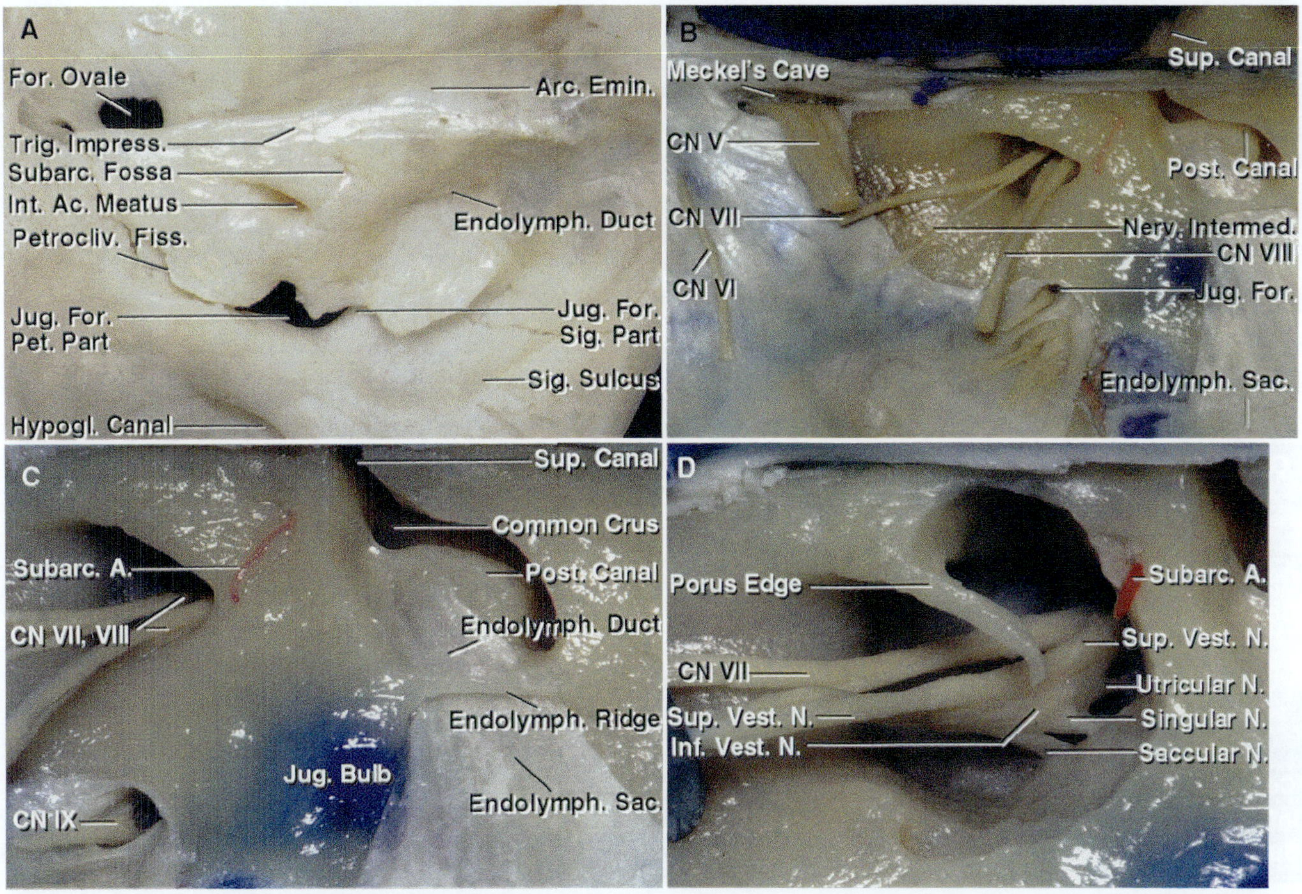

FIGURE 8.3. ***A–D.*** **Posterior surface of the temporal bone. *A*, the internal meatus is located near the center and the jugular foramen at the lower edge of the posterior surface. The sigmoid sinus descends along the posterior surface of the mastoid and turns forward on the occipital bone to pass through the sigmoid part of the jugular foramen. The inferior petrosal sinus descends along the petroclival fissure and passes through the petrosal part of the jugular foramen. The subarcuate fossa is located superolateral and the ostium for the vestibular aqueduct lateral to the internal acoustic meatus. The trigeminal impression is a shallow trough on the upper surface of the temporal bone behind the foramen ovale. The arcuate eminence overlies the superior semicircular canals. *B*, temporal bone with the nerves preserved. The abducens nerve ascends to enter Dorello's canal. The trigeminal nerve passes above the petrous apex to enter the porus of Meckel's cave. The facial and vestibulocochlear nerves enter the internal acoustic meatus, and the glossopharyngeal, vagus, and accessory nerves enter the jugular foramen. The posterior and superior semicircular canals have been exposed. *C*, enlarged view. The upper end of the posterior canal and the posterior end of the superior canal share the common crus. The endolymphatic duct extends downward from the vestibule and opens into the endolymphatic sac located beneath the dura inferolateral to the meatus. The endolymphatic ridge, the bridge of bone forming the posterior lip of the vestibular aqueduct, has been preserved. The jugular bulb can be seen through the thin bone below the internal meatus. *D*, enlarged view of the fundus of the meatus after removal of the posterior wall. The upper edge of the porus has been preserved. The subarcuate artery enters the subarcuate fossa. The inferior vestibular nerve gives rise to the singular branch to the posterior ampullae, plus utricular and saccular branches. The superior vestibular nerve innervates the ampullae of the superior and lateral semicircular canals and commonly gives rise to a utricular branch. *A.*, artery; *Ac.*, acoustic; *Arc.*, arcuate; *Car.*, carotid; *CN*, cranial nerve; *Coch.*, cochlear; *Emin.*, eminence; *Endolymph.*, endolymphatic; *Fiss.*, fissure; *For.*, foramen; *Hypogl.*, hypoglossal; *Impress.*, impression; *Inf.*, inferior; *Int.*, internal; *Intermed.*, intermedius; *Jug.*, jugular; *Lat.*, lateral; *N.*, nerve; *Nerv.*, nervus; *Pet.*, petrosal, petrous; *Petrocliv.*, petroclival; *Post.*, posterior; *Semicirc.*, semicircular; *Sig.*, sigmoid; *Subarc.*, subarcuate; *Sup.*, superior; *Trig.*, trigeminal; *Vest.*, vestibular.**

The styloid process, a slender spicule ensheathed by the inferior border of the tympanic bone, projects into the infratemporal fossa and is the site of attachment for the styloglossus, stylopharyngeus, and stylohyoid muscles (*Fig. 8.5*). It is located immediately anterior to the emergence of the facial nerve from the stylomastoid foramen and is covered laterally by the parotid gland. The stylomastoid foramen, the external end of the facial canal, opens between the styloid and mastoid

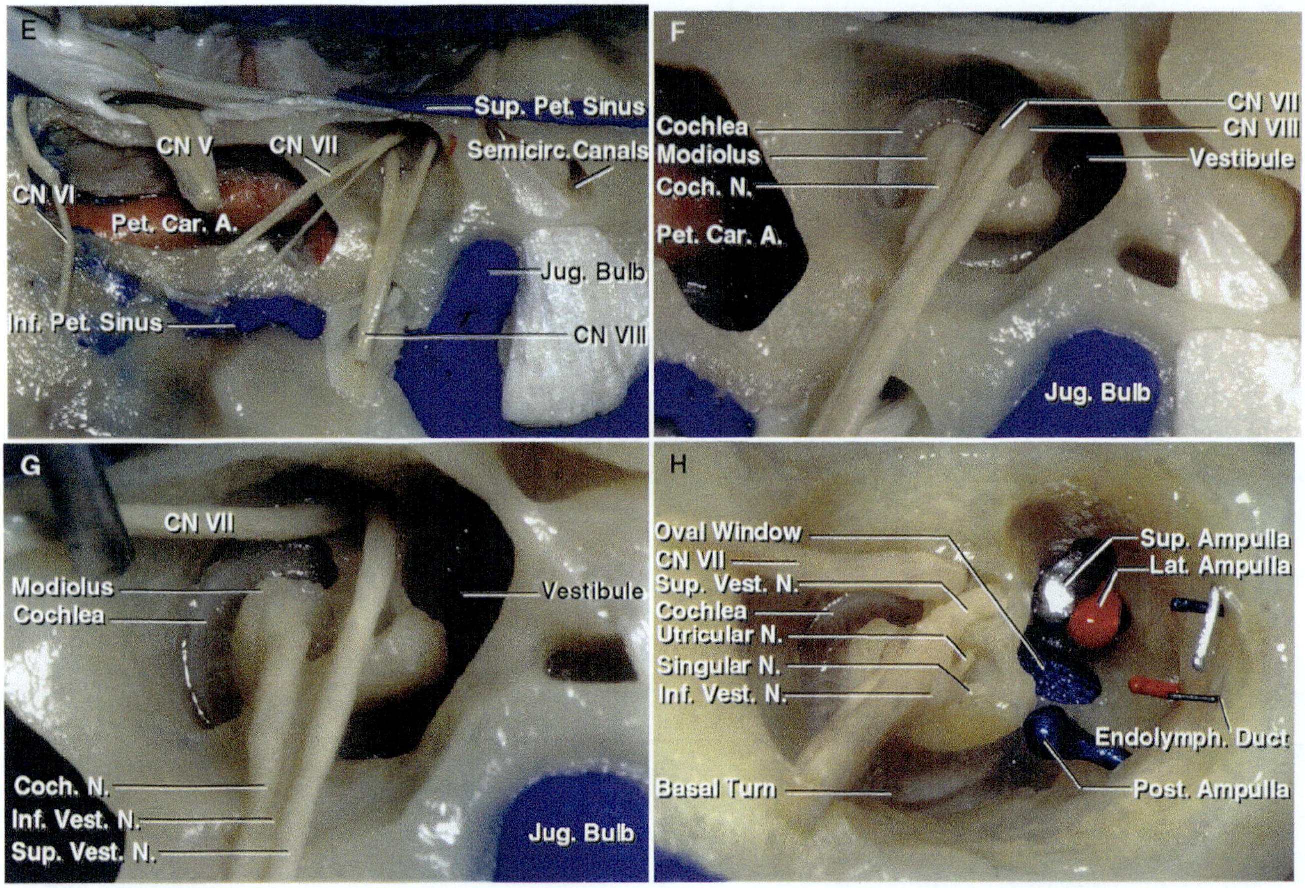

FIGURE 8.3. ***E–H.*** **Posterior surface of the temporal bone.** ***E,*** **the petrous apex medial to the internal acoustic meatus has been removed to expose the petrous carotid. The lateral genu of the petrous carotid, located at the junction of the vertical and horizontal segments of the petrous carotid, is situated below and medial to the cochlea. The jugular bulb extends upward toward the vestibule and semicircular canals adjacent to the posterior meatal wall. The inferior petrosal sinus courses along the petroclival fissure and enters the petrosal part of the jugular foramen, and the sigmoid sinus descends in the sigmoid groove and enters the sigmoid part of the foramen. The glossopharyngeal, vagus, and accessory nerves pass through the central or intrajugular part of the foramen between the sigmoid and petrosal parts.** ***F,*** **bone has been removed along the anterior margin of the meatal fundus to open the cochlea, and along the posterior margin to expose the vestibule. The jugular bulb extends upward toward the semicircular canals and vestibule.** ***G,*** **enlarged view. The cochlear nerve penetrates the modiolus of the cochlea where its fibers are distributed to the turns of the cochlear duct. The basal turn of the cochlea communicates below the modiolus with the vestibule.** ***H,*** **enlarged view of the vestibule and cochlea. The stapes has been removed from the oval window. The promontory in the medial wall of the tympanic cavity is located lateral to the basal turn of the cochlea. A** ***silver fiber*** **has been introduced into the superior canal, a** ***red fiber*** **into the lateral canal, and a** ***blue fiber*** **into the posterior canal. The ampullated ends are located at the bulbous ends of the three fibers. The common crus of the superior and posterior canals is located at the site where the tips of the blue and silver fibers overlap. The superior vestibular nerve passes to the ampullae of the superior and lateral canals. The singular branch of the inferior vestibular nerve innervates the posterior ampullae. A small** ***black fiber*** **has been introduced into the opening of the endolymphatic duct into the vestibule.**

processes. The facial nerve crosses the lateral surface of the styloid process, and the external carotid artery crosses the tip. Resecting the styloid process and reflecting the attached muscles downward exposes the internal jugular vein as it exits the jugular foramen and the carotid artery as it enters the carotid canal medial to the tympanic bone.

The squamous part

The externally convex surface of the squamosal part gives attachment to the temporalis muscle (*Figs. 8.1, 8.2,* and *8.5*). The supramastoid crest extends backward across its posterior part, giving attachment to the temporalis muscle and fascia. The suprameatal triangle, a depressed area, located below the anterior part of the crest and behind the posterosuperior margin of the external meatus, marks the deep location of the mastoid antrum. The cerebral surface of the squamosal part is concave, accommodating the temporal lobe and joining the greater wing of the sphenoid anteriorly. The zygomatic process of the squamosal part projects forward and with the zygomatic bone completes the zygomatic arch. The attachment of the zygomatic process to the squama is wide giving it anterior and posterior edges, referred to as the anterior and posterior roots. The temporalis fascia attaches to the superior border of the arch and the masseter attaches to the lower border. The posterior root of the zygomatic process blends posteriorly into the suprameatal crest. The anterior root is located at the anterior margin of the temporomandibular joint, with the joint forming a rounded fossa on the lower margin of the zygomatic process between the anterior and posterior roots. The upper margin of the zygomatic process between the two roots gives attachment to the posterior part of the temporalis muscle. The mandibular fossa, located on the lower margin of the process between the two roots, is delimited in front by the articular tubercle and posteriorly by the postglenoid tubercle adjacent to its junction with the tympanic bone. The squamotympanic fissure is located between the medial part of the squamosal part of the mandibular fossa and the medial part of the tympanic bone. The petrotympanic fissure is situated between the tympanic plate and the petrosal part and leads into the tympanic cavity; it contains the anterior ligament of the malleus and the anterior tympanic branch of the maxillary artery. The anterior canaliculus for the chorda tympani exits the tympanic cavity in the petrotympanic fissure. The rootlets of the temporal branch of the facial nerve cross the lateral aspect of the zygomatic arch and course through the subcutaneous tissues on the superficial layer of the temporal fascia. During resection of the zygomatic arch, the superficial temporalis fascia should be carefully dissected from the underlying deep fascia, starting as close as possible to the tragal cartilage, and carried forward, reflecting the superficial fascia anteriorly to avoid damage to the filaments of the temporal branch to the frontalis muscle.

The mastoid part

The mastoid is the posterior part of the temporal bone (*Figs. 8.1, 8.2,* and *8.4*). It projects downward to form the process that is the site of attachment, from superficial to deep, of the sternocleidomastoid, splenius capitis and longissimus capitis muscles, and the posterior belly of the digastric muscle (*Fig. 8.5*). The lower surface medial to the mastoid process is grooved by the mastoid notch to which the posterior belly of the digastric attaches. Medial to the notch, the occipital groove gives passage to the occipital artery. The fascia covering the anterior margin of the posterior belly of the digastric is continuous anteriorly with the connective tissue surrounding the emergence of the mastoid segment of the facial nerve from the stylomastoid foramen and can be used as a landmark for identifying the initial extracranial segment of the nerve. After exiting the stylomastoid foramen, the nerve divides in the substance of the parotid gland into temporal, zygomatic, buccal, marginal mandibular, and cervical branches (*Fig. 8.5*). The temporal and zygomatic branches cross the zygomatic arch and the superficial fascia of the temporalis muscle. Keeping the connective tissue surrounding the nerve at the stylomastoid foramen intact during mobilization of the facial nerve will reduce the risk of facial nerve damage. The posterior border of the mastoid process is perforated by one or more foramina through which an emissary vein to the sigmoid sinus and a dural branch from the occipital artery pass.

The medial aspect of the mastoid process is grooved by the sigmoid sinus (*Figs. 8.1-8.4*). The sinus represents the posterior limit of the mastoid cavity. The sinus meets the roof of the cavity at the level of the petrous ridge. The angle between the superior petrosal and sigmoid sinuses and the middle fossa dura delimits a dural space called the sinodural angle. The sinodural angle is an important landmark when exposing the contents of the mastoid. Inferiorly, the sigmoid sinus curves medially and forward, crossing the occipital bone to enter the jugular foramen. The superior aspect of the jugular foramen corresponds to the apex of the jugular bulb and constitutes the inferior limit of the mastoid cavity.

The medial limit of the mastoid cavity is formed by the block of solid bone, the otic capsule, containing the bony labyrinth (*Figs. 8.4* and *8.6*). The area of posterior fossa dura mater that can be exposed through the mastoid cavity between the sigmoid and superior petrosal sinuses, the otic capsule, and the jugular bulb is called Trautman's triangle. The size of this dural triangle is important in surgical procedures in which the dura delimited by the triangle must be opened medial to the sigmoid sinus. The distance from the anterior margin of the sigmoid sinus to the otic capsule at the level of the posterior semicircular canal averages 8 mm (range, 6–9 mm) on the right side, and 7 mm (range, 4–9 mm) on the left (44).

The distance between the apex of the jugular bulb and the superior petrosal sinus is also an important determinate of the size of exposure that can be achieved by opening Trautman's triangle. This distance is reduced if there is a high jugular bulb. The jugular bulb usually lies inferior to the ampulla of the posterior semicircular canal, but it can project superiorly as far as the level of the lateral semicircular canal (27). The average distance from the jugular bulb to the superior petrosal sinus is 14 mm (range, 10–19 mm) on the right side, and 16 mm (range, 11–21 mm) on the left (44).

The mastoid interior is composed of trabeculated bone, which coalesces to form a cavity, the mastoid antrum, that communicates through an opening, the aditus, that leads forward to the epitympanic part of in the tympanic cavity (*Figs. 8.4* and *8.6*). The lateral semicircular canal is medial to the epitympanic recess. The medial wall of the antrum faces the posterior semicircular canal. The roof is formed by the tegmen in the floor of the middle cranial fossa. The mastoid segment of the facial canal courses adjacent to the anteroinferior margin of the antrum. The lateral wall of the mastoid antrum, through which it is usually approached surgically, is formed by the postmeatal part of the squamous temporal bone. The lateral wall of the antrum is located deep to the suprameatal triangle, which is demarcated superiorly by the suprameatal crest, located at the level of the floor of the middle fossa; anteroinferior by the posterosuperior margin of the acoustic meatus, which indicates approximately the position of the descending or mastoid part of the facial canal; and posteriorly by a posterior vertical tangent to the posterior margin of the external meatus. The air cells in the mastoid may extend behind the sigmoid sinus and into the squamosal

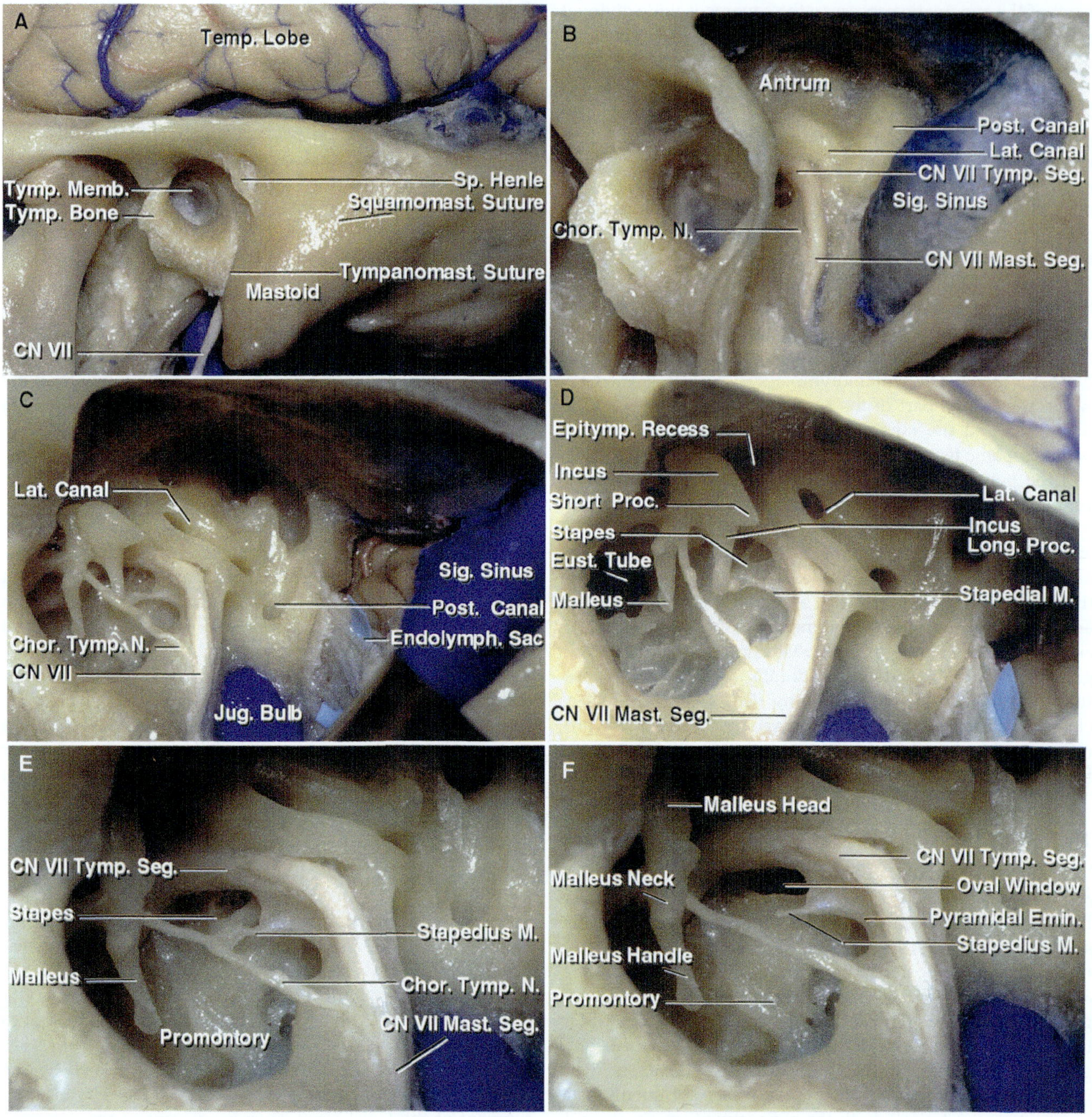

FIGURE 8.4. Tympanic cavity and mastoid antrum. *A*, the tympanic bone forms the anterior, lower, and part of the posterior wall of the external canal. The facial nerve exits the skull through the stylomastoid foramen, which is located medial to the tympanomastoid suture. The spine of Henley approximates the deep site of the tympanic facial segment and the lateral canal. The mastoid antrum is located between the posterosuperior wall of the external canal and middle fossa floor deep to the depression behind the spine of Henle. *B*, a mastoidectomy has been completed to expose the capsule of the posterior and lateral canals and the tympanic and mastoid facial segments. *C*, the posterior and superior wall of the external canal and the tympanic membrane have been removed while preserving the malleus and chorda tympani. The mastoid segment of the facial nerve descends through the facial canal and gives rise to the chorda tympani, which passes upward and forward across the tympanic membrane and malleus neck. *D*, enlarged view. The head of the incus articulates with the head of the malleus, the short process of the incus points backward toward the facial nerve, and the long process attaches to the stapes, which sits in the oval window. The stapedial muscle passes forward below the tympanic segment of the facial nerve and attaches to the neck of the stapes. *E*, the incus has been removed to expose the stapes sitting in the oval window. The chorda tympani

part of the temporal bone, the posterior root of the zygomatic process, the osseous roof of the external acoustic meatus, the floor of the tympanic cavity near the jugular bulb, and the petrous apex surrounding the carotid canal, eustachian tube, and labyrinth.

The tympanic cavity is a narrow air-filled space between the tympanic membrane laterally and the promontory containing the auditory and vestibular labyrinth medially (*Figs. 8.4, 8.6,* and *8.7*). It communicates posteriorly with the mastoid antrum and anteriorly through the eustachian tube with the nasopharynx. It contains the malleus, incus, and stapes. The tympanic cavity opens upward into the epitympanic recess, which contains the heads of the malleus and the incus. The roof of the tympanic cavity is formed by a thin plate, the tegmen tympani, which separates the middle fossa and tympanic cavities, and also roofs the mastoid antrum and the tensor tympani. The thin floor of the tympanic cavity separates the cavity from the jugular bulb. The medial part of the floor is perforated by an opening for the tympanic branch of the glossopharyngeal nerve. The lateral wall is formed by the tympanic membrane and the osseous ring to which the membrane attaches. The ring is deficient above near the openings of the anterior and posterior canaliculi for the chorda tympani (*Figs. 8.4* and *8.6*). The posterior canaliculus for the chorda tympani arises from the facial canal a few millimeters above the mastoid foramen and ascends in front of the facial canal to open into the tympanic cavity at the level of the upper part of the handle of the malleus. The chorda tympani passes in close relation to the tympanic membrane and the medial aspect of the neck of the malleus and forward to enter its anterior canaliculus at the medial aspect of the petrotympanic fissure, and descends vertically medial to the sphenoid spine and lateral pterygoid muscle to join the lingual nerve.

The medial wall of the tympanic cavity, which forms the lateral boundary of the inner ear and the petrosal part of the temporal bone, is the site of the promontory, the oval and round windows, and the prominence over the facial nerve (*Figs. 8.2* and *8.4*). The tympanic nerve plexus grooves the promontory overlying the lateral bulge of the basal turn of the cochlea. The apex of the cochlea lies near the medial wall of the cavity anterior to the promontory. The oval window is posterosuperior to the promontory and connects the tympanic cavity to the vestibule, and is occupied by the footplate of the stapes. The round window is posteroinferior to the oval window and opens under the overhanging edge of the promontory. The prominence of the facial canal is located above the oval window. The posterior wall of the tympanic cavity is mainly the site of the aditus, the opening of the tympanic cavity, into the mastoid antrum. The medial wall of the aditus has a round prominence overlying the lateral semicircular canal. The pyramidal eminence, which houses the stapedial muscle, is located just behind the oval window and anterior to the mastoid part of the facial canal. The stapedius extends forward from the eminence to attach to the neck of the stapes. The fossa incudis is a small depression low and posterior in the epitympanic recess; it contains the short process of the incus, which is fixed to the fossa by ligamentous fibers.

The anterior wall of the tympanic cavity narrows and leads into the eustachian tube, which communicates the nasopharynx with the tympanic cavity (*Figs. 8.4, 8.7,* and *8.8*). It has bony and cartilaginous parts. The bony part begins in the anterior part of the tympanic cavity and is directed anteriorly and medially. It joins the cartilaginous part at the junction of the squamous and petrous parts of the temporal bone. The cartilaginous part of the tube is attached to the lower margin of the sphenopetrosal groove, which is situated between the petrous bone and the greater wing of the sphenoid bone, and its base lies directly under the mucous membrane of the lateral wall of the nasaopharynx. Both the petrous carotid and eustachian tube are directed anteromedially, with the eustachian tube being located along the anterior margin of the carotid canal (*Figs. 8.7* and *8.8*). The tensor tympani muscle and its bony semicanal are located above the eustachian tube, parallel to the horizontal segment of the petrous carotid. The canals for the tensor tympani superiorly and the osseous part of the eustachian tube inferiorly open into the upper part of the anterior wall of the tympanic cavity. These canals are inclined downward, anteriorly, and medially; they open into the angle between the squamous and petrous parts of the temporal bone and are separated by a thin, bony septum. The canal for the tensor tympani extends posterolaterally on the medial wall of the tympanic cavity, to end above the oval window where the posterior end of the canal curves laterally to form a pulley, the trochleariform process, around which the tensor tympani tendon turns laterally to attach to the handle of the malleus.

crosses the neck of the malleus. The promontory is located superficial to the basal turn of the cochlea. The labyrinth and fundus of the internal meatus are located medial to the tympanic cavity. A line directed medially through the skull along the long axis of the external meatus will also approximate the site of the long axis of the internal meatus on the medial side of the promontory and acousticovestibular labyrinth. *F*, the stapes has been removed from the oval window. The handle of the malleus attaches to the tympanic membrane, the neck is crossed by the chorda tympani, and the head articulates with the incus, which has been removed. The tendon of the tensor tympani attaches to the upper part of the handle of the malleus. The stapedial muscle is housed within the pyramidal eminence and its tendon inserts on the stapedial neck. *Chor.*, chorda; *CN*, cranial nerve; *Emin.*, eminence; *Endolymph.*, endolymphatic; *Epitymp.*, epitympanic; *Eust.*, eustachian; *Jug.*, jugular; *Lat.*, lateral; *Long.*, longus; *M.*, muscle; *Mast.*, mastoid; *Memb.*, membrane; *N.*, nerve; *Post.*, posterior; *Proc.*, process; *Seg.*, segment; *Sig.*, sigmoid; *Sp.*, spine; *Squamomast.*, squamomastoid; *Temp.*, temporal; *Tymp.*, tympani, tympanic; *Tympanomast.*, tympanomastoid.

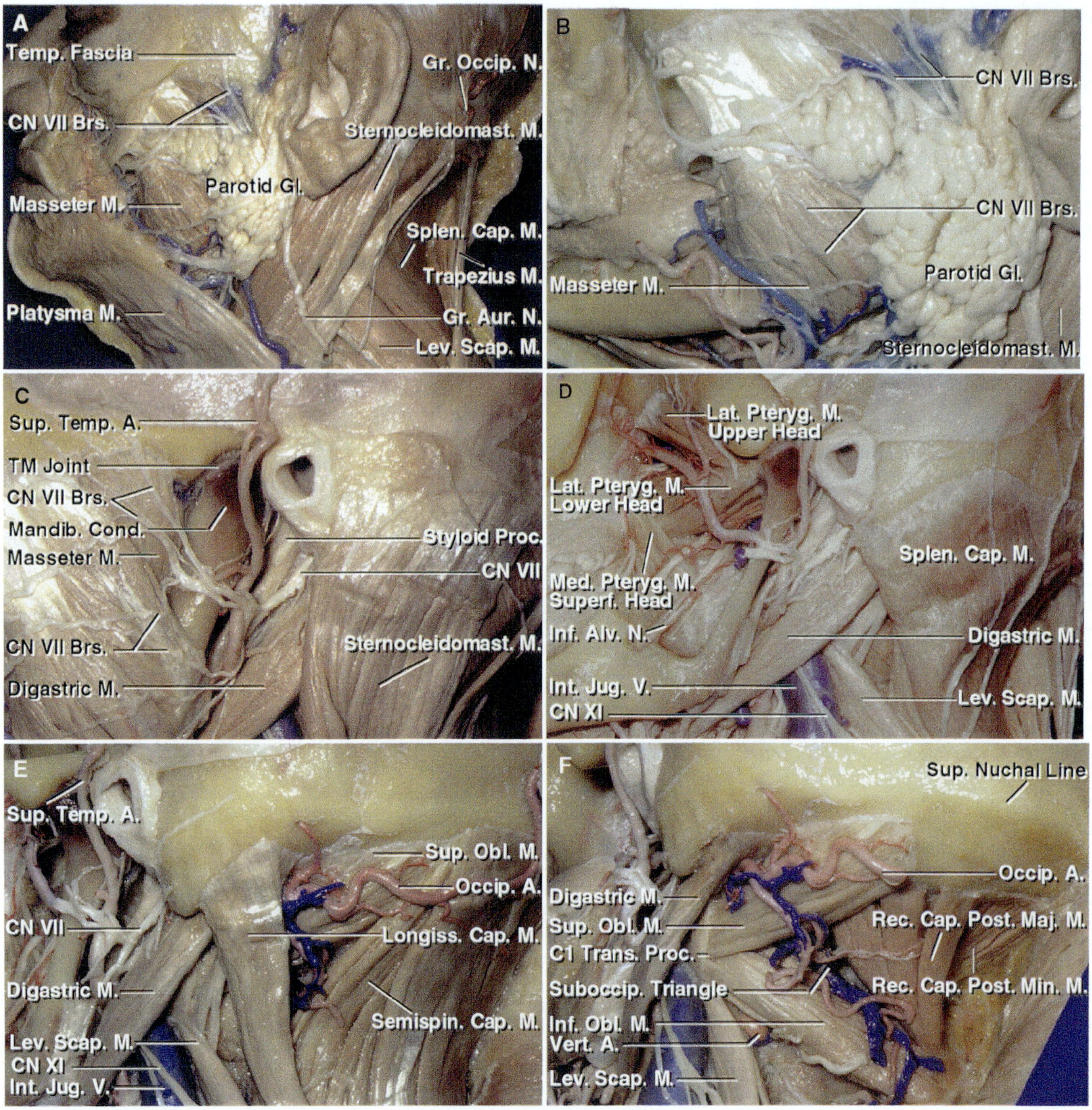

FIGURE 8.5. *A–F.* Muscular and osseous relationships. *A*, the skin and subcutaneous tissues have been removed to expose the parotid gland and the facial nerve branches that course deep to the parotid gland on their way to the facial muscles. The masseter muscle has two heads: a more superficial anterior head, which passes downward to the lateral surface of the angle of the jaw, and a deeper posterior head, which arises from the medial surface of the zygomatic arch and passes to the mandibular body. The sternocleidomastoid attaches to the lateral part of the superior nuchal line and mastoid process, descends in an anterior direction, and is crossed by the greater auricular nerve. The temporalis fascia attaches to the upper surface of the zygomatic arch. The trapezius muscle attaches to the medial part of the superior nuchal line. The posterior triangle of the neck, located between the sternocleidomastoid and trapezius, has the semispinalis capitis, splenius capitis, and levator scapulae in its floor. The terminal branches of the occipital artery and the greater occipital nerve reach the subcutaneous tissues by passing between the attachment of the trapezius and sternocleidomastoid muscles to the superior nuchal line. *B*, enlarged view. The facial nerve branches are exposed along the anterior edge of the parotid gland. *C*, the parotid gland has been removed to expose the facial nerve and its branches distal to the stylomastoid foramen. The nerve passes lateral to the styloid

The petrous part

The petrous part of the temporal bone is wedged between the sphenoid and occipital bones (*Figs. 8.1* and *8.3*). It contains the acoustic and vestibular labyrinth and is the site of the jugular fossa and the facial and carotid canals (*Figs. 8.3, 8.4,* and *8.7*). It has a base, apex, three surfaces and margins. The apex is located in the angle between the greater wing of the sphenoid and the occipital bone and is the site of the carotid canals medial opening. It forms the posterolateral limit of the foramen lacerum. The anterior surface faces the floor of the middle cranial fossa and its surface is grooved by the trigeminal impression for the trigeminal ganglion; anterolateral to this, it forms the roof of the carotid canal (*Figs. 8.1* and *8.7*). Lateral to the trigeminal impression is a shallow depression, which partially roofs the internal acoustic meatus and is limited laterally by the arcuate eminence, which overlies the superior semicircular canal. The posterior slope of the arcuate eminence overlies the posterior and lateral semicircular canals. Farther laterally, the roof covers the vestibule and part of the facial canal. The tegmen extends laterally from here and roofs the mastoid antrum and tympanic cavities and the canal for the tensor tympani. Opening the tegmen from above exposes the heads of the malleus, incus, the tympanic segment of the facial nerve, and the superior and lateral semicircular canals (*Fig. 8.7*). The tympanic segment of the facial nerve begins at the geniculate ganglion and ends at the level of the stapes, where the nerve turns downward below the lateral semicircular canal. The tegmen anteriorly is grooved by the greater petrosal nerve extending anterior and medial from the area in front of the arcuate imminence and crossing the floor of the middle fossa toward the foramen lacerum (*Figs. 8.7* and *8.8*). The greater petrosal nerve can be identified medial to the arcuate eminence as it leaves the geniculate ganglion by passing through the facial hiatus to reach the middle fossa floor. It runs beneath the dura of the middle fossa in the sphenopetrosal groove formed by the junction of the petrous and sphenoid bones, immediately superior and anterolateral to the horizontal segment of the petrous carotid. In a previous study, we found that bone of the middle cranial fossa was absent over the geniculate ganglion in 16% of the specimens, thus exposing the facial nerve and geniculate ganglion to the danger of injury during elevation of the dura from the floor of the middle fossa (31). Facial nerve injury can also result from damaging the branch of the middle meningeal artery, which passes through the facial hiatus to supply the nerve, or from traction applied to the ganglion when manipulating the greater petrosal nerve (30).

The lesser petrosal nerve from the tympanic plexus passes through the tympanic canaliculus, which is located anterior to the facial hiatus and courses in an anteromedial direction parallel to the greater petrosal nerve (*Fig. 8.8*). The cochlea lies below the floor of the middle fossa in the angle between the labyrinthine segment of the facial nerve and the greater petrosal nerve, just medial to the geniculate ganglion, anterior to the fundus of the internal acoustic meatus, and posterosuperior to the lateral genu of the petrous carotid artery. The cochlea is separated from the petrous carotid by a 2.1 mm (range, 0.6–10.0 mm) thickness of bone and can be injured during exposure of the petrous carotid. The middle meningeal artery, an important landmark when approaching the structures of the middle fossa, enters the cranial cavity through the foramen spinosum of the sphenoid bone. The foramen spino-

process, the external carotid artery, and mandibular neck. The superficial and deep heads of the masseter muscle are exposed. This lower end of the sternocleidomastoid muscle has been reflected posteriorly by dividing its attachment to the clavicle and sternum. The superficial temporal artery ascends in front of the ear. *D*, the upper part of the mandibular ramus and the lower part of the temporalis muscle and its attachment to the coronoid process have been removed while preserving the inferior alveolar nerve. The infratemporal fossa is located medial to the mandible and on the deep side of the temporalis muscle. The upper and lower heads of the lateral pterygoid, which insert along the temporomandibular joint, and the superficial head of the medial pterygoid, which extends from the lateral pterygoid plate to the angle of the jaw, have been exposed. The structures in the infratemporal fossa include the pterygoid muscles, branches of the mandibular nerve, the maxillary artery, and the pterygoid venous plexus. The sternocleidomastoid muscle has been reflected out of the exposure to expose the splenius capitis muscle. *E*, posterolateral view. The splenius capitis has been reflected downward to expose the longissimus capitis, superior oblique, and semispinalis capitis. The occipital artery passes along the occipital groove on the medial side of the digastric groove. *F*, the longissimus capitis has been reflected downward to expose the rectus capitis posterior minor and major, which descend from the occipital bone to attach to the spinous process of C1 and C2, respectively; the superior oblique, which passes from the occipital bone to the transverse process of C1; and the inferior oblique, which extends from the spinous process of C2 to the transverse process of C1. The vertebral artery, in its ascent from C2 to C1, is exposed medial to the attachment of the levator scapulae to the C1 transverse process. The C1 transverse process is situated immediately behind the internal jugular vein and a short distance below and behind the jugular foramen. *A.*, artery; *Alv.*, alveolar; *Ant.*, anterior; *Aur.*, auricular; *Brs.*, branches; *Cap.*, capitis; *Car.*, carotid; *CN*, cranial nerve; *Cond.*, condyle; *Constr.*, constrictor; *Eust.*, eustachian; *Ext.*, external; *Gl.*, gland; *Gr.*, greater; *Inf.*, inferior; *Int.*, internal; *Jug.*, jugular; *Lat.*, lateral; *Lev.*, levator; *Long.*, longus; *Longiss.*, longissimus; *M.*, muscle; *Maj.*, major; *Mandib.*, mandibular; *Max.*, maxillary; *Med.*, medial; *Memb.*, membrane; *Min.*, minor; *N.*, nerve; *Obl.*, oblique; *Occip.*, occipital; *Pal.*, palatini; *Parapharyng.*, parapharyngeal; *Pet.*, petrosal; *Post.*, posterior; *Proc.*, process; *Pteryg.*, pterygoid; *Pterygopal.*, pterygopalatine; *Rec.*, rectus; *Scap.*, scapula; *Semispin.*, semispinalis; *Splen.*, splenius; *Sternocleidomast.*, sternocleidomastoid; *Suboccip.*, suboccipital; *Sup.*, superior; *Superf.*, superficial; *Temp.*, temporal, temporalis; *Tens.*, tensor; *TM.*, temporomandibular; *Trans.*, transverse; *Tymp.*, tympanic; *V.*, vein; *Veli./Vel.*, veli; *Vert.*, vertebral.

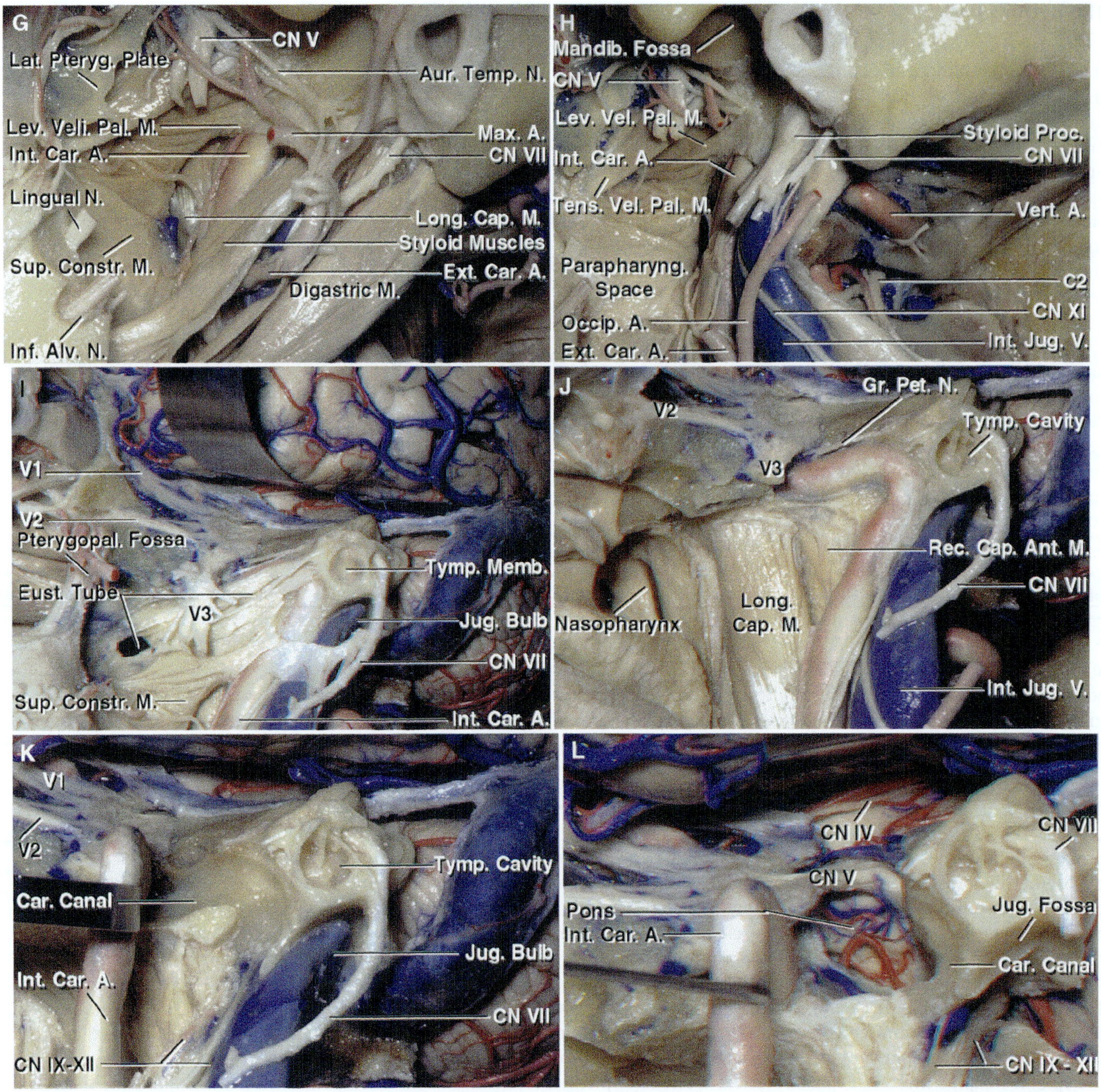

FIGURE 8.5. *G–L.* Muscular and osseous relationships. *G*, the mandibular condyle and ramus have been removed to expose the styloid process and attached muscles. The pterygoid muscles and some branches of the mandibular nerve have been removed to expose the auriculotemporal nerve, which splits into two roots that surround the middle meningeal artery. The levator veli palatini, which attaches the lower margin of the eustachian tube, is in the medial part of the exposure. The longus capitis is exposed medial to the internal carotid artery in the retropharyngeal area. *H*, the muscles that attach to the styloid process have been divided at their origin. The facial nerve crosses the lateral surface of the styloid process. The attachment of the tensor veli palatine to the skull base extends between the foramen ovale and the eustachian tube. *I*, the external auditory canal has been removed, but the tympanic membrane and cavity have been preserved. The levator veli palatine and part of the tensor veli palatine have been removed and the membranous part of the eustachian tube opened. The eustachian tube crosses anterior to and is separated from the petrous carotid by a thin shell of bone. The jugular bulb and lateral bend of the petrous carotid are located below the osseous labyrinth. The pterygopalatine fossa is exposed anteriorly. *J*, the eustachian tube has been resected and the mandibular nerve divided at the foramen ovale to expose the petrous carotid. This exposes the longus capitis and rectus capitis anterior, both of which are located behind the posterior pharyngeal wall. *K*, the petrous carotid has been reflected forward out of the carotid canal to expose the petrous apex medial to the carotid canal. *L*, the petrous apex and upper clivus have been drilled and the dura opened to expose the anterolateral aspect of the pons below the trigeminal nerve. The sigmoid sinus and the jugular bulb have been removed to expose the nerves exiting the jugular foramen.

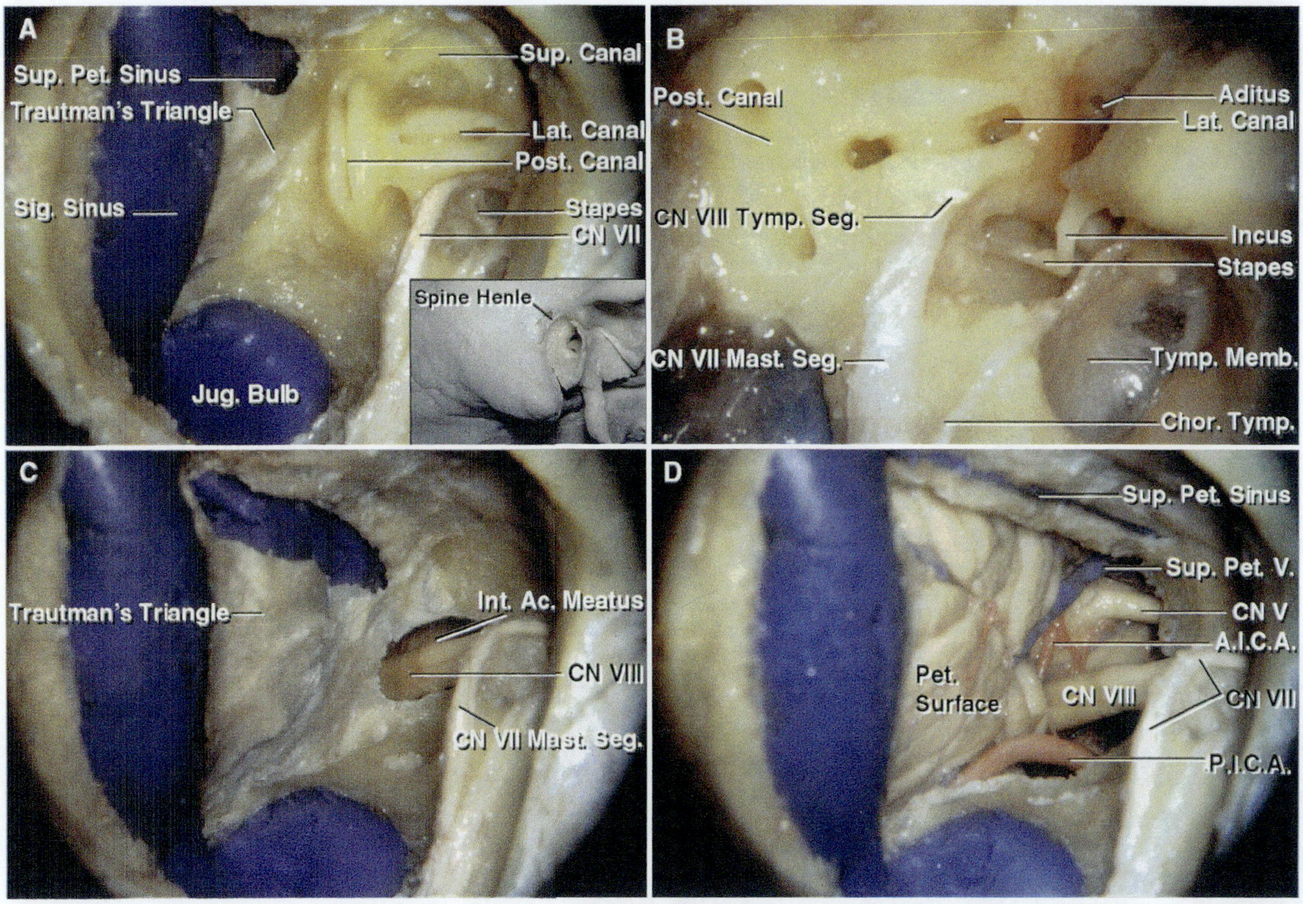

FIGURE 8.6. *A–D*. Translabyrinthine exposure. *A*, the *insert* shows the site of the exposure directed through the mastoid. The spine of Henley at the posterosuperior margin of the external meatus is a superficial landmark that approximates the deep site of the lateral semicircular canal and the tympanic segment of the facial nerve. The mastoidectomy has been completed. The superior petrosal and sigmoid sinuses, the jugular bulb, and the facial nerve are usually skeletonized in the approach, leaving a thin layer of bone over them. The semicircular canals, which are located in the cortical bone medial to the cancellous mastoid and the mastoid antrum, have been exposed. The dura between the sigmoid and superior petrosal sinuses, the jugular bulb, and the labyrinth, which faces the cerebellopontine angle, is referred to as Trautman's triangle. *B*, the mastoid antrum opens through the aditus into the epitympanic part of the tympanic cavity, which contains the upper part of the malleus and incus. The tympanic segment of the facial nerve passes between the lateral canal and the stapes in the oval window and then turns downward as the mastoid segment. The chorda tympani arises from the mastoid segment of the facial nerve and passes upward and forward along the deep surface of the tympanic membrane crossing the neck of the malleus. The incus, the head of which is located in the epitympanic area, has a long process that attaches to the stapes. *C*, the semicircular canals and vestibule have been removed and the dura lining the internal acoustic meatus has been opened to expose the vestibulocochlear nerve. *D*, the dura has been opened to expose the petrosal cerebellar surface and the structures in the cerebellopontine angle. Anatomic variants that limit the exposure include an anterior position of the sigmoid sinus, a high jugular bulb, or a low middle fossa plate. The jugular bulb may extend upward into the posterior wall of the internal acoustic meatus and be encountered as the posterior meatal wall is being removed by either the translabyrinthine or retrosigmoid approaches. *Ac.*, acoustic; *A.I.C.A.*, anteroinferior cerebellar artery; *Chor.*, chorda; *CN*, cranial nerve; *Coch.*, cochlear; *Inf.*, inferior; *Int.*, internal; *Intermed.*, intermedius; *Jug.*, jugular; *Laby.*, labyrinthine; *Lat.*, lateral; *Mast.*, mastoid; *N.*, nerve; *Nerv.*, nervus; *Pet.*, petrosal; *P.I.C.A.*, posteroinferior cerebellar artery; *Post.*, posterior; *Seg.*, segment; *Sig.*, sigmoid; *Sup.*, superior; *Tymp.*, tympani, tympanic; *V.*, vein; *Vest.*, vestibular.

sum is an average of 4.5 mm (range, 3–6 mm) anterolateral to the carotid canal and 14.0 mm (range, 11.0–17.0 mm) anterolateral to the geniculate ganglion (44).

The posterior surface of the petrosal part faces the posterior cranial fossa and cerebellopontine angle and is continuous with the mastoid surface (*Figs. 8.1-8.3*). The opening for the internal auditory meatus is situated midway between the base and the apex on the posterior surface. The lateral end of the meatus is divided into superior and inferior halves by the transverse crest. The area above the transverse crest is further

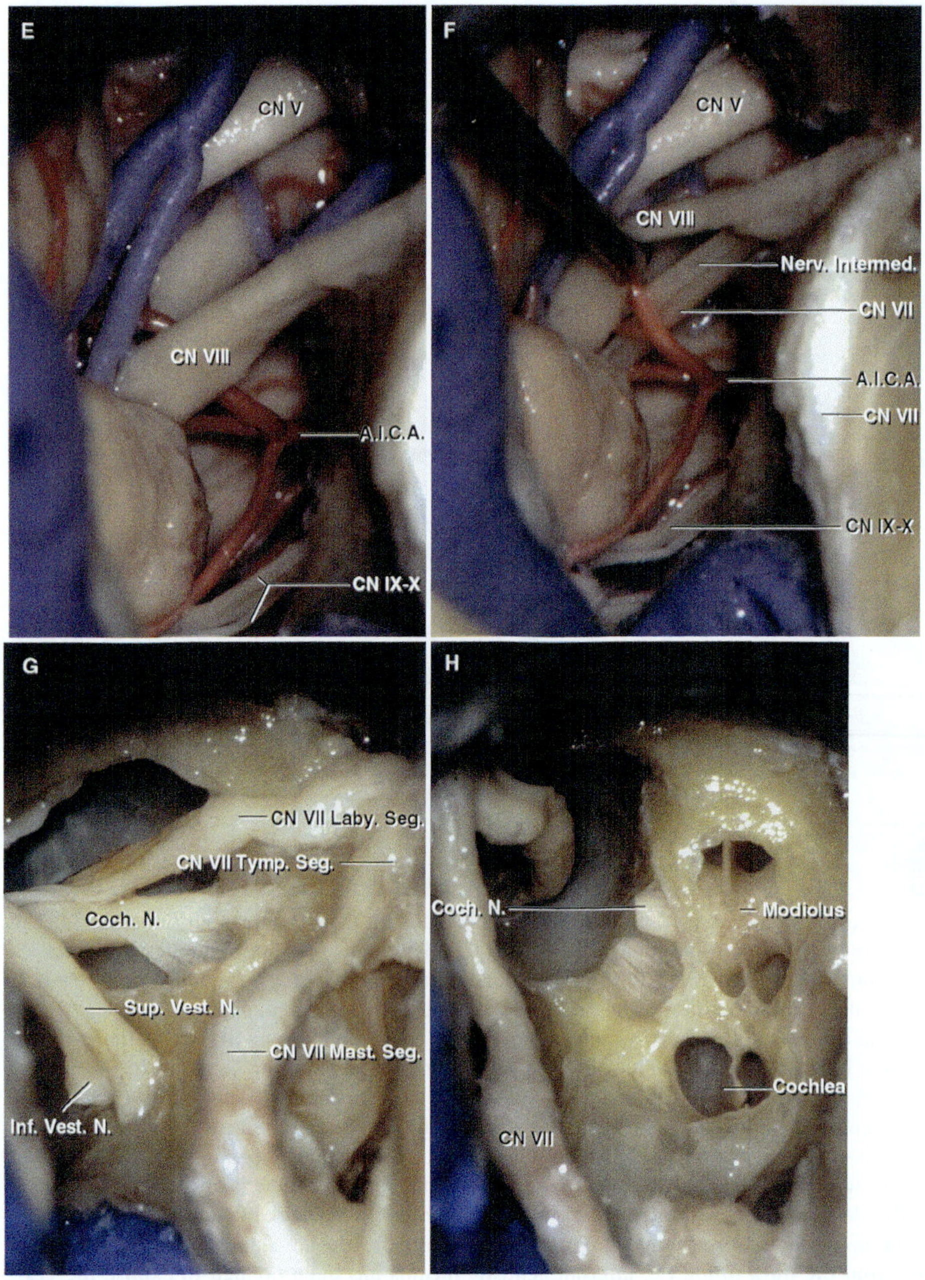

FIGURE 8.6. *E–H.* **Translabyrinthine exposure.** ***E*****, enlarged view of the exposure in the cerebellopontine angle. In this case, the glossopharyngeal and vagus nerves can be seen, although, in the translabyrinthine exposure, the jugular bulb often obstructs the view of the nerves entering the jugular foramen.** ***F*****, the vestibulocochlear nerve has been elevated to expose the facial nerve.** ***G*****, the labyrinthine, tympanic, and mastoid segments of the facial nerve have been exposed in preparation for transposition of the nerve for a transcochlear approach.** ***H*****, the facial nerve has been transposed backward and the bone anterior to the meatal fundus has been removed to expose the cochlea for a transcochlear approach in which the cochlea is removed to gain access to the side of the clivus and front of the brainstem. The cochlear nerve has been divided. The cochlear fibers innervating the cochlear duct pass through the modiolus.**

divided by the vertical crest, also called Bill's bar, which separates the anteriorly located facial canal from the posteriorly located superior vestibular area (29). The cochlea and inferior vestibular nerves penetrate the lateral end of the meatus below the transverse crest, with the cochlear nerve being located anteriorly. The posterior wall of the meatus, lateral to the porus is the site of a small bony opening, the subarcuate fossa, which gives passage to the subarcuate artery, a branch of the anteroinferior cerebellar artery (AICA), which usually ends blindly in the region of the superior semicircular canal. Inferolateral to the porus of the meatus is the opening for the vestibular aqueduct, which transmits the endolymphatic duct that opens below into the endolymphatic sac located between the dural layers. The opening of the cochlear aqueduct, also called the cochlear canaliculus and occupied by the perilymphatic duct, is situated inferior to the porus of the internal meatus at the anteromedial edge of the jugular foramen, just superior and lateral to where the glossopharyngeal nerve enters the intrajugular part of the jugular foramen.

The inferior surface is very irregular. The apex is connected medially to the clivus by fibrocartilage and gives attachment to the levator veli palatini and the cartilaginous portion of the eustachian tube (*Figs. 8.1* and *8.9*). Behind this is the opening of the carotid canal, behind which is the jugular fossa that contains the jugular bulb. The small foramen for the tympanic

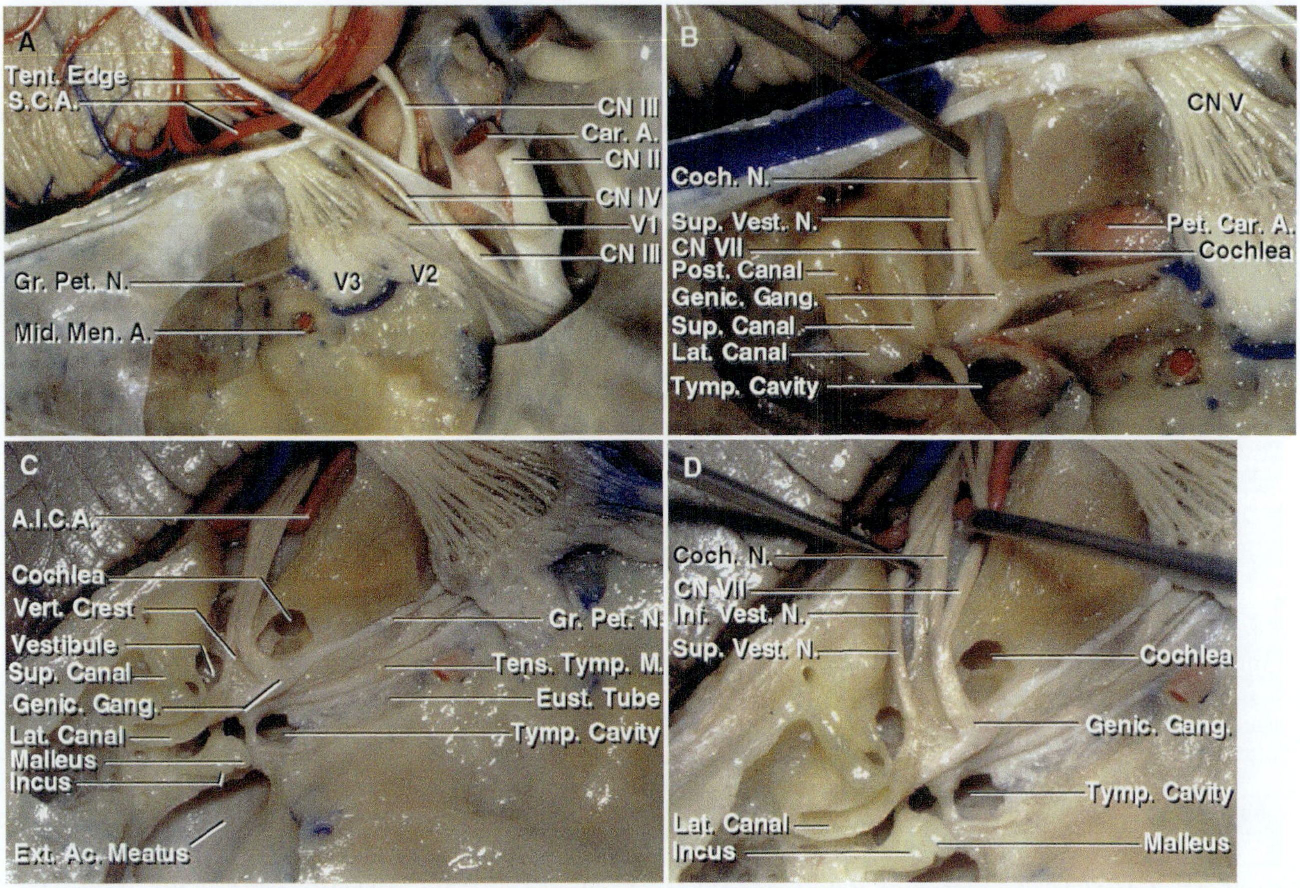

FIGURE 8.7. *A–D.* **Middle fossa exposure of the temporal bone.** *A*, **superolateral view. The tentorium, except the edge, has been removed. The dura has been removed from the middle fossa floor and cavernous sinus wall to expose the greater petrosal nerve, middle meningeal artery, and the nerves in the sinus wall.** *B*, **the middle fossa floor has been opened to expose the cochlea, semicircular canals, petrous carotid artery, and the facial, cochlear, and superior vestibular nerves in the meatus. The superior canal bulges upward into the middle fossa below the arcuate eminence. The cochlear nerve passes below the facial nerve to enter the cochlea, which is located above the lateral genu of the petrous carotid in the angle between the pregeniculate facial and greater petrosal nerves.** *C*, **another temporal bone drilled to expose the internal acoustic meatus, cochlea, vestibule, semicircular canals, tympanic cavity, and external meatus. The vestibule is located posterolateral and the cochlea is anteromedial to the fundus of the internal meatus. The vestibule communicates below the meatal fundus with the cochlea. The tensor tympani muscle and eustachian tube are layered along, but are separated from, the anterior surface of the petrous carotid by a thin layer of bone. The tegmen has been opened to expose the head of the incus and malleus in the epitympanic area. The internal acoustic meatus lies directly medial to, but is separated from, the external meatus by the tympanic cavity and the labyrinth.** *D*, **the nerves in the meatus have been separated to expose the superior and inferior vestibular, facial, and cochlear nerves.** *A.*, artery; *Ac.*, acoustic; *A.I.C.A.*, anteroinferior cerebellar artery; *Car.*, carotid; *CN*, cranial nerve; *Coch.*, cochlear; *Eust.*, eustachian; *Ext.*, external; *Gang.*, ganglion; *Genic.*, geniculate; *Gr.*, greater; *Inf.*, inferior; *Lat.*, lateral; *M.*, muscle; *Men.*, meningeal; *Mid.*, middle; *N.*, nerve; *Pet.*, petrosal, petrous; *Post.*, posterior; *S.C.A.*, superior cerebellar artery; *Sup.*, superior; *Tens.*, tensor; *Tent.*, tentorial; *Tymp.*, tympani, tympanic; *Vert.*, vertebral; *Vest.*, vestibular.

branch of the glossopharyngeal nerve is located on the ridge between the carotid canal and jugular foramen (*Fig. 9.2*). On the lateral wall of the jugular bulb is the mastoid canaliculus for the auricular branch of the vagus nerve. The superior border, located along the petrous ridge, is grooved by the superior petrosal sinus and serves as the attachment of the tentorium cerebelli, except medially where it is crossed by the posterior trigeminal root. The lower posterior border, located along the petroclival fissure, is the site of a groove in which resides the inferior petrosal sinus that connects the cavernous sinus and the medial wall of the jugular bulb. Behind this, the jugular fossa of the temporal bone joins with the jugular notch on the jugular process of the occipital bone to form the margins of the jugular foramen.

The jugular foramen is located at the lower end of the petro-occipital fissure and is divided into a larger lateral opening, the sigmoid part, that receives the drainage of the sigmoid sinus, and a small medial part, the petrosal part, that

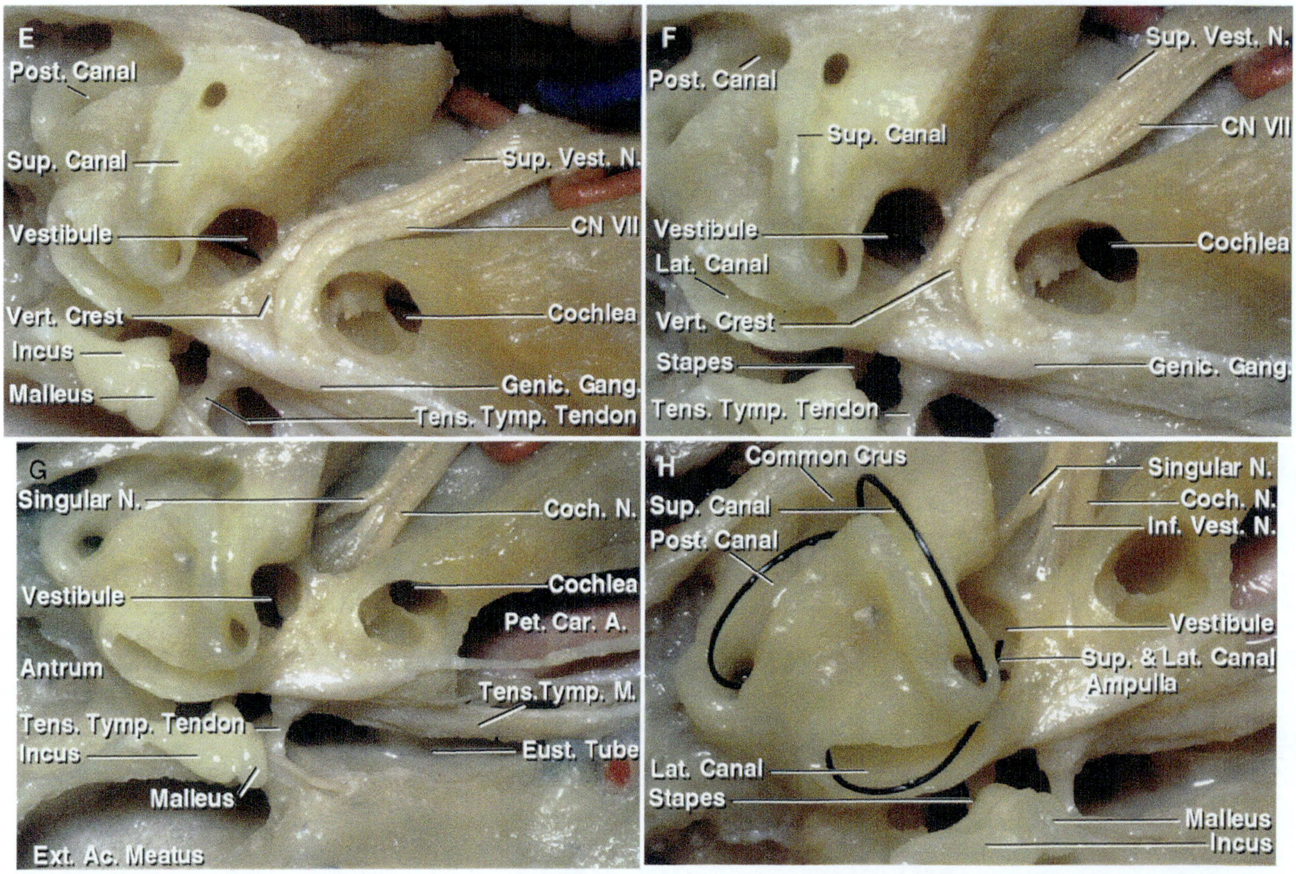

FIGURE 8.7. ***E–H.*** **Middle fossa exposure of the temporal bone. *E*, enlarged view. The vestibule, into which the semicircular canals open, communicates below the meatal fundus with the cochlea. The vertical crest, often called Bill's bar, separates the superior vestibular and facial nerves at the meatal fundus. The tendon of the tensor tympani makes a right-angle turn around the trochleariform process in the medial margin of the tympanic cavity to insert on the malleus. *F*, enlarged view. The superior canal projects upward in the floor of the middle fossa. The lateral canal is situated above the tympanic segment of the facial nerve in the posteromedial part of the epitympanic area, and the posterior canal is located lateral to the posterior wall of the internal acoustic meatus. *G*, bone has been removed below the greater petrosal nerve to expose the petrous carotid. The tensor tympani muscle above and the eustachian tube below are layered along the anterior surface of the petrous carotid. *H*, enlarged view. Suture has been placed in the three semicircular canals. The anterior end of the superior and lateral canals and the lower end of the posterior canal are the site of the ampullae. The posterior end of the superior canal and the upper end of the posterior canal join to form a common crus. The facial and superior vestibular nerves have been removed to expose the cochlear and inferior vestibular nerves. The singular branch of the inferior vestibular nerve innervates the posterior ampullae. The superior vestibular nerve innervates the superior and lateral ampullae.**

transmits the inferior petrosal sinus (*Fig. 9.1*). The intrajugular part, located between the sigmoid and petrosal parts, transmits the glossopharyngeal, vagus, and accessory nerves. The anterior border is joined laterally to the temporal squama at the petrosquamosal suture and medially articulates with the sphenoid's greater wing.

The bony labyrinth consists of three parts: the vestibule, the semicircular canals, and the cochlea. The vestibule, located in the central part of the bony labyrinth, is a small cavity at the confluence of the ampullate and nonampullated ends of the semicircular canals. It is situated lateral to the meatal fundus, medial to the tympanic cavity, posterior to the cochlea, and superior to the apex of the jugular bulb (*Figs. 8.3, 8.4,* and *8.7*).

The floor of the vestibule is separated from the apex of the jugular bulb by a thickness of bone that averages 6 mm (range, 4–8 mm) on the right side and 8 mm (range, 4–10 mm) on the left side (44). This distance is particularly important during translabyrinthine approaches since the height of the jugular bulb is a major determinant of the size of the exposure of the cerebellopontine angle that can be achieved with this approach. A high-placed jugular bulb may be the source of troublesome bleeding and air emboli if it is opened during exposure of the labyrinth or internal acoustic meatus.

The semicircular canals are situated posterosuperior to the vestibule (*Figs. 8.3, 8.4,* and *8.7*). The anterior part of the lateral semicircular canal is situated above the tympanic segment of

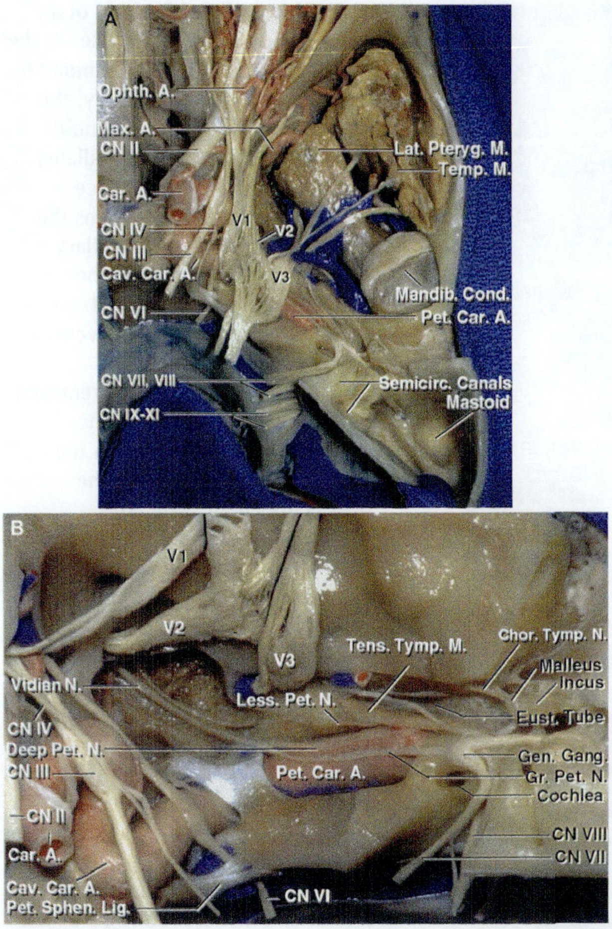

FIGURE 8.8 ***A*, superior view of the temporal bone and infratemporal fossa and orbit. The floor of the middle fossa has been removed to expose the temporalis muscle in the temporal fossa and the pterygoid muscles and branches of the third trigeminal division in the infratemporal fossa. The posterior part of the middle fossa forming the upper surface of the temporomandibular joint has been removed to expose the mandibular condyle. The internal acoustic meatus extends laterally from the posterior surface of the temporal bone. The mastoid is located behind the external canal and lateral to the semicircular canals and vestibule. *B*, enlarged view. The trigeminal nerve has been reflected forward and bone has been removed over the eustachian tube, tensor tympani muscle, petrous carotid, and internal acoustic meatus. Dura has been removed from the lateral wall of the cavernous sinus to expose the trochlear, trigeminal, and oculomotor nerves in the sinus wall and the abducens nerve passing below the petrosphenoid ligament and through Dorello's canal. The greater petrosal nerve is joined by the deep petrosal branches of the carotid sympathetic plexus to form the vidian nerve, which passes forward in the vidian canal, which has been unroofed. The lesser petrosal nerve arises from the tympanic branch of the glossopharyngeal nerve, which passes across the promontory in the tympanic nerve plexus and regroups to cross the floor of the middle fossa, exiting the skull to provide parasympathetic innervation through the otic ganglion to the parotid gland. The tensor tympani muscle and eustachian are layered along, but are separated from, the anterior surface of the petrous carotid by a thin layer of bone. *A.*, artery; *Car.*, carotid; *Cav.*, cavernous; *Chor.*, chorda; *CN*, cranial nerve; *Cond.*, condyle; *Eust.*, eustachian; *Gang.*, ganglion; *Gen.*, geniculate; *Gr.*, greater; *Lat.*, lateral; *Less.*, lesser; *Lig.*, ligament; *M.*, muscle; *Mandib.*, mandibular; *Max.*, maxillary; *N.*, nerve; *Ophth.*, ophthalmic; *Pet.*, petrosal, petrous; *Pteryg.*, pterygoid; *Semicirc.*, semicircular; *Sphen.*, sphenoid; *Temp.*, temporal; *Tens.*, tensor; *Tymp.*, tympani, tympanic.***

the facial nerve and can be used as a guide to locating that segment of the nerve. The posterior semicircular canal lies parallel to and in close proximity with the posterior surface of the petrous bone in the area just behind and lateral to the lateral end of the internal acoustic meatus. The superior semicircular canal projects toward the floor of the middle fossa, usually in close relation to the arcuate eminence. Each canal has an ampullated and a nonampullated end that opens into the vestibule. The anterior end of the lateral and superior canals and the inferior end of the posterior canal are the site of the ampullae, which are innervated by the vestibular nerves. The posterior ends of the superior and posterior canals, the ends opposite the ampullae, join to form a common crus that opens into the vestibule. The superior vestibular nerve innervates the ampullae of the superior and lateral canals, and the singular branch of the inferior vestibular nerve innervates the posterior ampulla. The vestibular nerves also have branches to the utricle and saccule located within the vestibule. The internal auditory meatus can be found medial to the arcuate eminence at an angle of about 60 degrees medial from the long axis of the superior semicircular canal. The superior canal is the most susceptible to damage in completing the middle fossa approach to the internal acoustic meatus. The posterior canal may be damaged in removing the posterior wall to expose the meatal contents by the retrosigmoid approach (*Fig. 8.3*).

During surgical approaches to the cerebellopontine angle in which the posterior meatal lip is removed, care should be taken to avoid opening the vestibular aqueduct, vestibule, posterior semicircular canal, or the common crus (*Figs. 8.2* and *8.3*). In our studies, we observed that there is a constant set of relationships among the structures around the posterior meatal lip. The common crus of the posterior and superior semicircular canals is located lateral to the entrance of the subarcuate artery into the subarcuate fossa. The vestibular aqueduct has an oblique orientation. It leaves the vestibule and runs in a posterior direction to open beneath the dura mater at a level corresponding to that of the posterior semicircular canal. The average distance between the posterior semicircular canal, at the level with the junction of the common crus, and the lateral edge of the porus was 7 mm (range, 5–9 mm) (44).

The carotid artery, at the point where it enters the carotid canal, is surrounded by a strong layer of connective tissue that makes it difficult to mobilize the artery at this point (*Figs. 8.9*

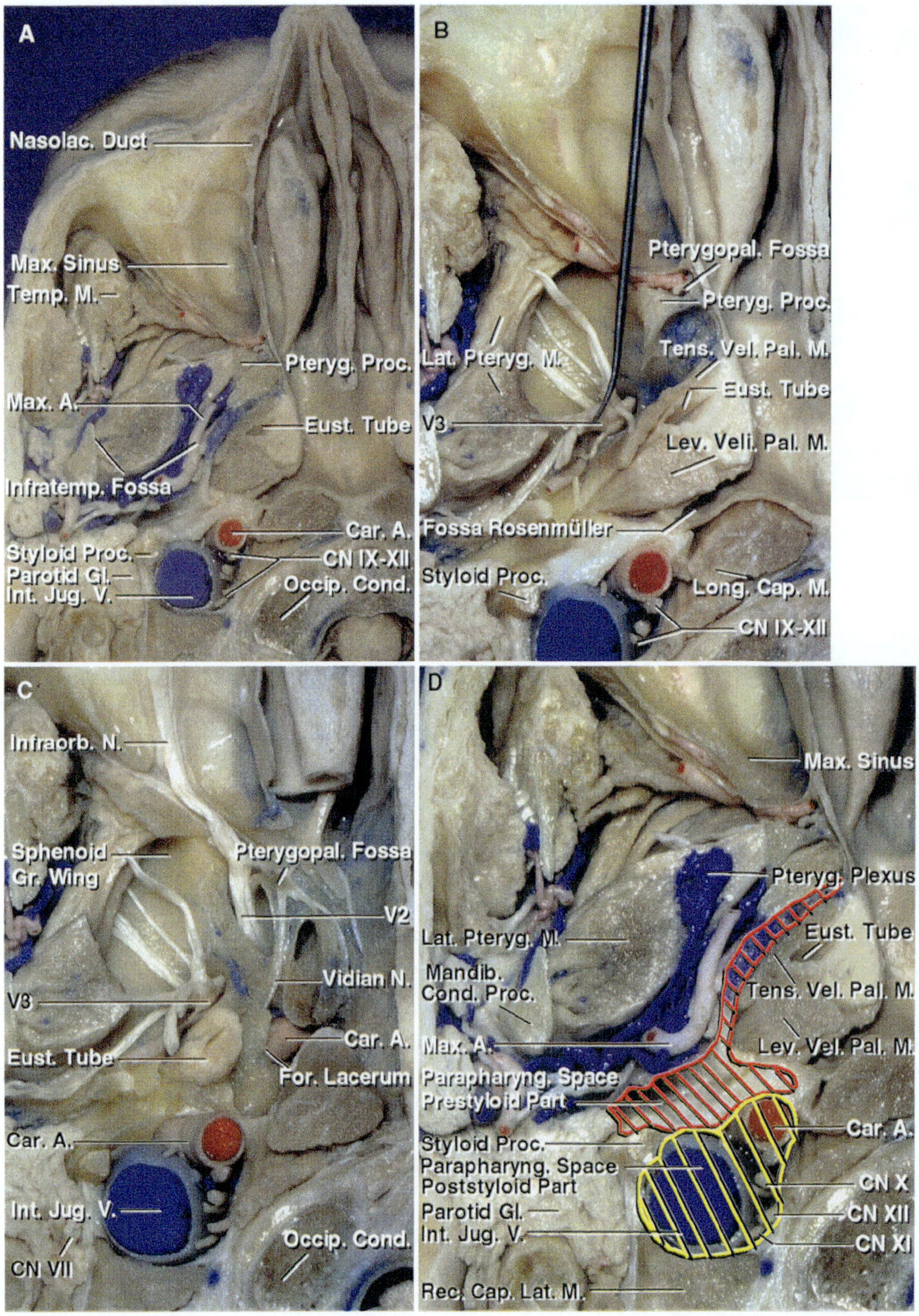

FIGURE 8.9. Inferior views of an axial section of the skull base. *A*, the infratemporal fossa is surrounded by the maxillary sinus anteriorly, the mandible laterally, the sphenoid pterygoid process anteromedially, and the parapharyngeal space posteromedially, and contains the mandibular nerve and maxillary artery and their branches, the medial and lateral pterygoid muscles, and the pterygoid venous plexus. *B*, part of the lateral pterygoid muscle has been removed to expose the branches of the trigeminal nerve coursing in the infratemporal fossa below the greater sphenoid wing. The pterygopalatine fossa is located between the posterior maxillary wall anteriorly, the sphenoid pterygoid process posteriorly, the nasal cavity medially, and the infratemporal fossa laterally. The pharyngeal recess (fossa of Rosenmüller) projects laterally from the posterolateral corner of the nasopharynx with its lateral apex facing the internal carotid artery laterally and the foramen lacerum above. The posterior nasopharyngeal wall is separated from the lower clivus and the upper cervical vertebra by the longus capitis, and the nasopharyngeal roof rests against the upper clivus and the posterior part of the sphenoid sinus floor. *C*, the sphenoid pterygoid process has been removed to expose the maxillary nerve passing through the foramen rotundum to enter the pterygopalatine fossa where it gives rise to the infraorbital nerve, which courses in the roof of the maxillary sinus. The maxillary nerve within the pterygopalatine fossa gives off communicating rami to the pterygopalatine ganglion. The vidian nerve, formed by the union of the deep petrosal nerve from the carotid sympathetic plexus and the greater petrosal nerve, courses forward through the vidian canal to join the pterygopalatine ganglion. The terminal part of the petrous carotid is exposed above the foramen lacerum. *D*, enlarged view with highlighting of the pre- (*red*) and poststyloid (*yellow*) compartments of the parapharyngeal space. The styloid diaphragm, formed by the anterior part of the carotid sheath, separates the parapharyngeal space into pre- and poststyloid parts. The prestyloid compartment, a narrow fat-containing space between the medial pterygoid and tensor veli palatini, separates the infratemporal fossa from the medially located lateral nasopharyngeal region containing the tensor and levator veli palatini and the eustachian tube. The poststyloid compartment, located behind the prestyloid part, contains the internal carotid artery, internal jugular vein, and the cranial nerves IX through XII. *A.*, artery; *Cap.*, capitis; *Car.*, carotid; *CN*, cranial nerve; Cond., condyle; *Eust.*, eustachian; *For.*, foramen; *Gl.*, gland; *Gr.*, greater; *Infraorb.*, infraorbital; *Infratemp.*, infratemporal; *Int.*, internal; *Jug.*, jugular; *Lat.*, lateral, lateralis; *Lev.*, levator; *Long.*, longus; *M.*, muscle; *Mandib.*, mandibular; *Max.*, maxillary; *N.*, nerve; *Nasolac.*, nasolacrimal; *Occip.*, occipital; *Pal.*, palatini; *Parapharyng.*, parapharyngeal; *Proc.*, process; *Pteryg.*, pterygoid; *Pterygopal.*, pterygopalatine; *Rec.*, rectus; *Tens.*, tensor; *V.*, vein; *Vel.*, veli.

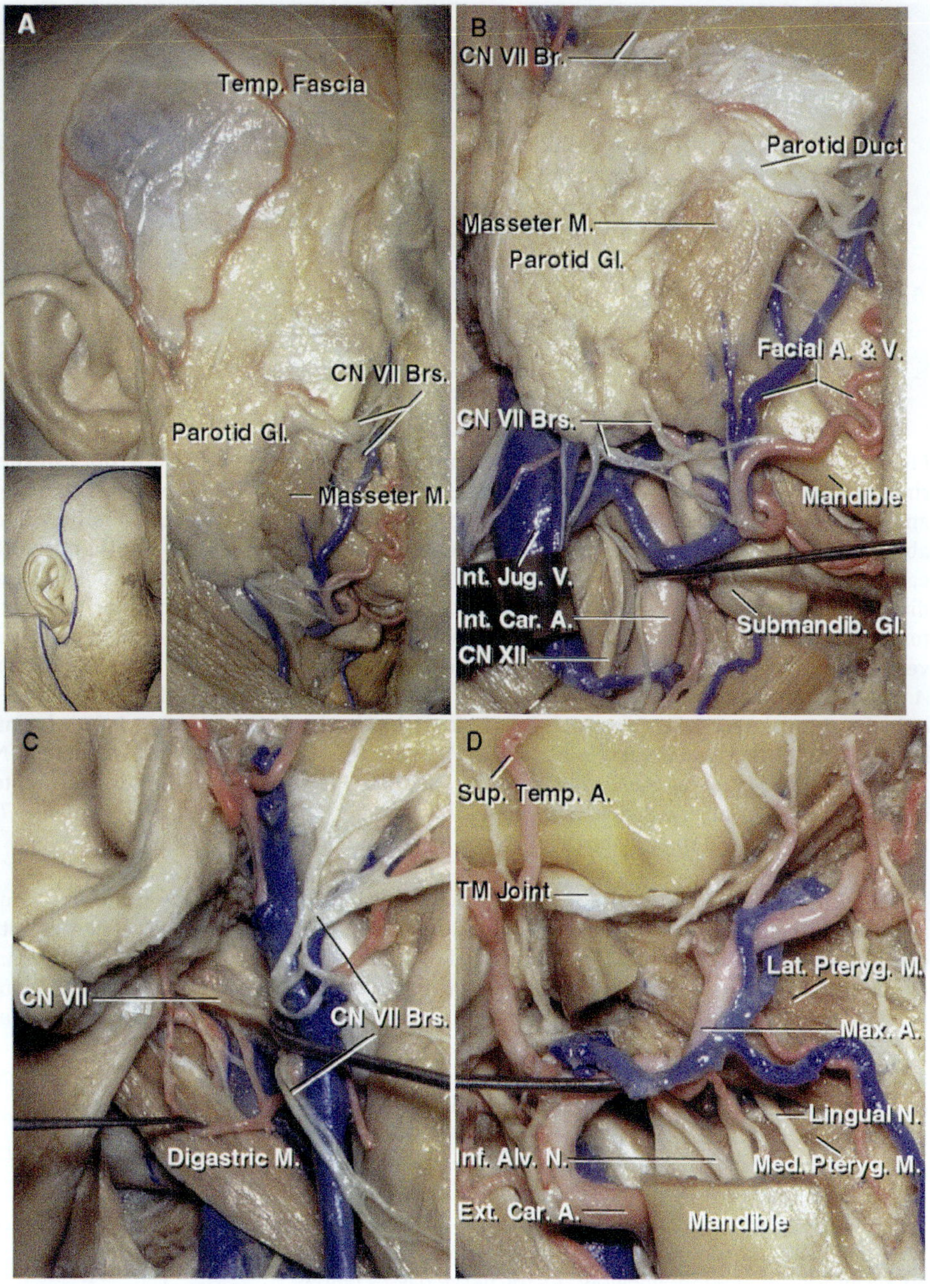

FIGURE 8.10. *A–D.* **Preauricular subtemporal-infratemporal fossa approach.** *A,* **the scalp flap has been reflected forward. The flap is positioned so that a neck dissection as well as a frontotemporal craniotomy can be completed. The scalp flap has been reflected forward while protecting the facial nerve and its branches. The neck dissection has been completed below the parotid gland. The facial nerve branches passing deep to the parotid have been preserved.** *B,* **the dissection has been carried around the parotid gland to expose the branches of the facial nerve. The internal jugular vein and internal carotid artery are exposed below the gland.** *C,* **the parotid gland has been removed to expose the branches of the facial nerve distal to the stylomastoid foramen.** *D,* **a segment of the mandibular ramus has been removed, leaving the mandibular condyle in the mandibular fossa, to expose the maxillary artery and pterygoid muscles in the infratemporal fossa. Branches of the third trigeminal division pass between the lateral and medial pterygoid muscles. The inferior alveolar nerve descends to enter the inferior alveolar foramen and canal.**

and *8.10*) (38, 39). The vertical segment of the artery passes upward in the canal toward the genu, where it curves anteromedially to form the horizontal segment. The eustachian tube and the tensor tympani muscle are located parallel to and along the anterior margin of the horizontal segment, where they are separated from the artery by a thin layer of bone.

The trigeminal ganglion and the adjacent part of the posterior root and their surrounding dural and arachnoidal cavern, called Meckel's cave, sit in an impression on the upper surface of the petrous apex above the medial part of the petrous carotid (*Figs. 8.1, 8.7,* and *8.8*). The length of the horizontal segment of the petrous carotid that can be exposed by removing bone lateral to the trigeminal ganglion averages 8.1 mm (range, 4.0–11.0 mm) (44). The length that can be exposed can be increased if the mandibular branch of the trigeminal nerve is retracted or divided, after which the average length that can be exposed increases to 20.1 mm (range, 17.5–28.0 mm) (*Figs. 8.7* and *8.8*) (10, 17). Gaining this added exposure can be particularly helpful during surgical procedures that are directed through the petrous apex to complete a vascular anastomosis, to occlude the artery for control of bleeding, and to allow for mobilization of the vertical and horizontal segments of the artery (40). A venous plexus of variable size, an extension of the cavernous sinus within the periosteal covering of the distal part of the canal, surrounds the artery.

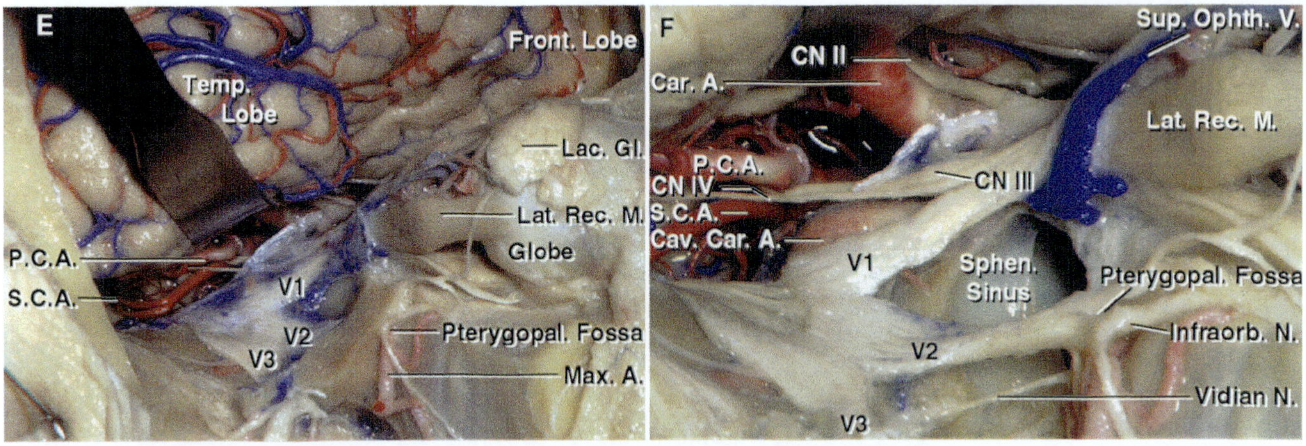

FIGURE 8.10. ***E***, **a frontotemporal craniotomy has been completed and the dura of the lateral wall of the cavernous sinus has been elevated. In addition, the lateral orbital wall has been removed to expose the globe, extraocular muscles, and lacrimal gland.** ***F***, **enlarged view of the region of the cavernous sinus. The PCA and SCA have been exposed coursing above and below the oculomotor and trochlear nerves, respectively. The optic nerve is exposed above the internal carotid artery. An opening has been made into the lateral wall of the sphenoid sinus between the first and second divisions. The maxillary nerve passes forward to join the terminal branches of the maxillary artery in the pterygopalatine fossa. The maxillary nerve continues forward along the floor of the orbit as the infraorbital nerve. The superior ophthalmic vein descends across the origin of the lateral rectus muscle and enters the anterior portion of the cavernous sinus.** ***A.***, **artery;** ***A.I.C.A.***, **anteroinferior cerebellar artery;** ***Alv.***, **alveolar;** ***Bas.***, **basilar;** ***Brs.***, **branches;** ***Cap.***, **capitis;** ***Car.***, **carotid;** ***Cav.***, **cavernous;** ***CN***, **cranial nerve;** ***Ext.***, **external;** ***Front.***, **frontal;** ***Gl.***, **gland;** ***Inf.***, **inferior;** ***Infraorb.***, **infraorbital;** ***Int.***, **internal;** ***Jug.***, **jugular;** ***Lac.***, **lacrimal;** ***Lat.***, **lateral;** ***Long.***, **longus;** ***M.***, **muscle;** ***Max.***, **maxillary;** ***Med.***, **medial;** ***N.***, **nerve;** ***Ophth.***, **ophthalmic;** ***P.C.A.***, **posterior cerebral artery;** ***Pet.***, **petrosal, petrous;** ***Pteryg.***, **pterygoid;** ***Pterygopal.***, **pterygopalatine;** ***Rec.***, **rectus;** ***S.C.A.***, **superior cerebellar artery; Sphen., sphenoid;** ***Submandib.***, **submandibular;** ***Sup.***, **superior;** ***Temp.***, **temporal;** ***Tens.***, **tensor;** ***TM.***, **temporomandibular;** ***Tymp.***, **tympani;** ***V.***, **vein;** ***Vert.***, **vertebral.**

The facial nerve in the temporal bone, which often blocks access to lesions within and deep to the temporal bone, is divided into three segments (*Figs. 8.4, 8.5,* and *8.7*). The first, or labyrinthine segment, which is located in the petrous part, extends from the meatal fundus to the geniculate ganglion and is situated between the cochlea anteromedially and the semicircular canals posterolaterally. The labyrinthine segment ends at the site at which the greater superficial petrosal nerve arises from the facial nerve at the level of the geniculate ganglion. From there, the nerve turns laterally and posteriorly along the medial surface of the tympanic cavity, thus giving the name tympanic segment to that part of the nerve. The tympanic segment runs between the lateral semicircular canal above and the oval window below. As the nerve passes below the midpoint of the lateral semicircular canal, it turns vertically downward and courses through the petrous part adjacent to the mastoid part of the temporal bone; thus the third segment, which ends at the stylomastoid foramen, is called the mastoid or vertical segment.

Petroclival region

These transtemporal operative approaches are often directed to the petroclival region located where the posterior surface of the petrous temporal bone meets the clival part of the occipital bone along the petroclival fissure. The junction of the two bones forms a line that extends from the jugular foramen to the petrous apex (*Fig. 8.1*). From a surgical standpoint, the intradural compartments of the petroclival region are divided along this petroclival line into 1) an inferior space related to the medulla and to the structures around the region of the foramen magnum; 2) a middle space related to the pons and to the structures in the prepontine and cerebellopontine angle; and 3) a superior space related to the contents of the interpeduncular cistern, and to the sellar and parasellar regions.

The inferior petroclival space

The inferior petroclival space corresponds to the anterior surface of the medulla and adjacent part of the clivus and anterior margin of the foramen magnum (4). The neurovascular structures in this region are those contained in the premedullary cistern. The superior limit is the junction of the pons and medulla. The inferior limit is the rostral margin of the first cervical nerve root, the site of the junction of the spinal cord and the medulla. The inferior petroclival space includes the lower four cranial nerves, lower part of the cerebellum, the vertebral artery and its branches, and the structures around the occipital condyle.

The middle petroclival space

The middle petroclival space corresponds to the anterolateral surface of the pons and cerebellum. Its superior limit is at the pontomesencephalic sulcus and the lower limit is at the pontomedullary sulcus. The lateral limits are formed by the posterior surface of the petrous bone and by the contents of

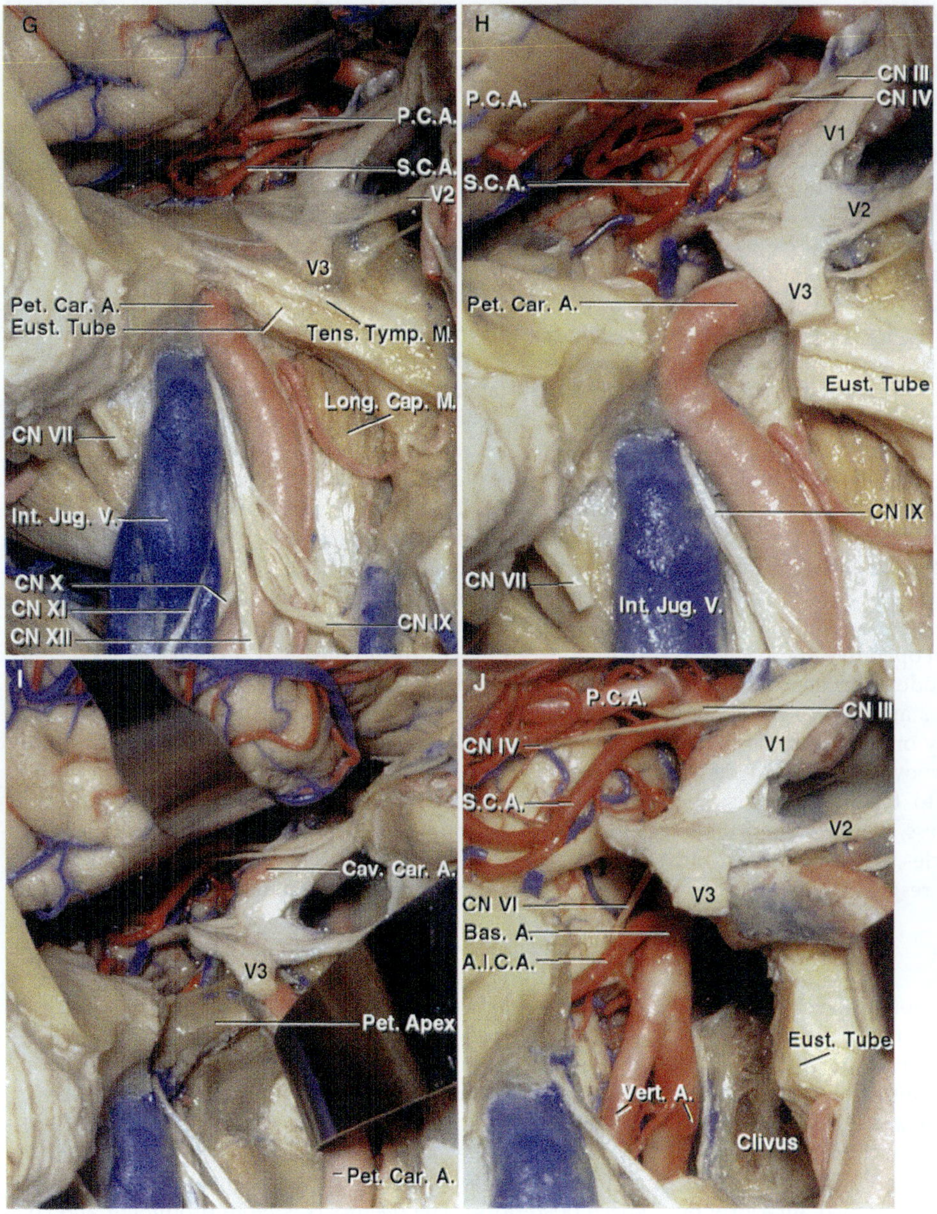

FIGURE 8.10. *G–J.* Preauricular subtemporal-infratemporal fossa approach. *G*, the floor of the middle fossa has been resected back to the level of the tensor tympani muscle and eustachian tube, and the petrous carotid artery. The nerves exiting the jugular foramen and hypoglossal canal pass laterally between the internal carotid artery and internal jugular vein to reach their end organs. *H*, the eustachian tube and tensor tympani have been resected and the bone lateral to the foramen ovale removed. This exposes the full length of the petrous carotid. *I*, the petrous carotid has been reflected forward out of the carotid canal to expose the petrous apex medial to the jugular foramen and lateral wall of the clivus. *J*, the petrous apex and adjacent part of the clivus medial to the jugular foramen and cochlea have been removed and the dura opened to expose the junction of the vertebral and basilar arteries and the origin of the AICA.

the cerebellopontine angle including the trigeminal, abducens, facial, and vestibulocochlear nerves, the basilar artery, and the AICA and the superior petrosal veins.

The superior petroclival space

The superior petroclival space is located anterior to the midbrain and corresponds to the anterior part of the tentorial incisura. It extends anteriorly and laterally to the sellar and parasellar regions. Its roof is formed by the diencephalic structures forming the floor of the third ventricle. The posterior limit is formed by the cerebral peduncles and the posterior perforated substance. The inferior limit is situated above the origin of the trigeminal nerve at the pontomesencephalic sulcus. It includes the intradural segment of the oculomotor and trochlear nerves, the basilar artery and its branching into the posterior cerebral artery (PCA) and superior cerebellar artery (SCA), and the cavernous carotid and its intracavernous branches to the dura of the upper clivus. The medial edge of the tentorium divides the superior petroclival space into infra- and supratentorial compartments.

Adjacent structures

The structures important in accessing the temporal bone from posteriorly and laterally have already been reviewed. This section reviews the structures located in front of the temporal bone that are important in reaching lesions that involve the bone or involve both the bone and areas anterior to it. They include several muscles, like the temporalis and masseter, the infratemporal fossa, and the parapharyngeal spaces.

The temporalis muscle, along with the deep temporal vessels, passes between the gap formed by the zygomatic arch and the floor of the temporal fossa (*Fig. 8.5*). The muscle attaches to the coronoid process of the mandible. The superficial and the deep temporalis fasciae attach, respectively, to the lateral and medial aspects of the upper border of the zygomatic arch. Inferiorly, the parotid fascia invests the parotid gland and the masseter muscle and attaches to the lower border of the zygomatic arch. The masseter muscle has two superimposed layers. A superficial layer which attaches to the zygomatic process of the maxilla and anterior part of the lower border of the zygomatic arch and a deep layer which attaches to the medial aspect of the whole zygomatic arch. Inferiorly it inserts onto the angle and ramus of the mandible.

The parotid gland, the parotid duct, and the branches of the facial nerve are located superficial to the masseter muscle (*Figs. 8.5, 8.9,* and *8.10*). In surgical procedures in which the mandibular condyle is resected or displaced inferiorly, the parotid gland, along with the branches of the facial nerve, can be dissected from the underlying masseter to avoid excessive traction on the facial nerve and to reduce the risk of facial palsy (33).

Muscles commonly encountered in operative approaches to the region of the temporal bone include the posterior belly of the digastric muscle and the muscles attached to the styloid process. The posterior digastric belly originates in the digastric groove, lateral to the occipital groove in which the occipital artery courses, and inserts onto the hyoid bone. The muscles attached to the styloid process, the stylohyoid, styloglossus, and stylopharyngeus muscles, extend to the hyoid bone, tongue, and pharyngeal wall, respectively.

Infratemporal fossa

The infratemporal fossa, a route through which some temporal bone lesions can be reached, is a not uncommon site of involvement by lesions that also involve the temporal bone (11). The osseous boundaries of the infratemporal fossa are the posterolateral maxillary surface anteriorly, the lateral pterygoid plate anteromedially, the mandibular ramus laterally, and the tympanic part of the temporal bone and the styloid process posteriorly. The fossa is domed anteriorly by the infratemporal surface of the greater sphenoid wing, the site of the foramina ovale and spinosum, and posteriorly by the squamous part of the temporal bone (*Figs. 8.8-8.10*). The inferior, posteromedial, and superolateral aspects are open without bony walls.

The structures located in the infratemporal fossa are the pterygoid muscles and venous plexus and the branches of the maxillary artery and mandibular nerve. The lateral pterygoid muscle crosses the upper part of the infratemporal fossa, originating from the upper and lower heads; the upper head arises from the infratemporal surface of the greater sphenoid wing, and the lower head originates from the lateral pterygoid plate (*Figs. 8.8-8.10*). Both heads pass posterolaterally and insert on the neck of the mandibular condylar process and the articular disc of the temporomandibular joint. The medial pterygoid muscle crosses the lower part of the infratemporal fossa and arises with superficial and deep heads; the superficial head arises from the lateral aspect of the palatine pyramidal process and the maxillary tuberosity and passes superficial to the lower head of the lateral pterygoid; and the deep head originates from the medial surface of the lateral pterygoid plate and the pterygoid fossa between the two pterygoid plates and passes deep to the lower head of the lateral pterygoid. Both heads descend backward and laterally to attach to the medial surface of the mandibular ramus below the mandibular foramen. The sphenomandibular ligament, located medial to the mandibular condylar process, descends from the sphenoid spine to attach to the lingula of the mandibular foramen. The structures located or passing between the sphenomandibular ligament and the mandible are the lateral pterygoid and the auriculotemporal nerve superiorly, and the inferior alveolar nerve, the parotid gland, the maxillary artery and its inferior alveolar branch inferiorly.

The maxillary artery is divided into three segments: mandibular, pterygoid, and pterygopalatine (*Figs. 8.8-8.10*). The mandibular segment arises from the external carotid artery near the posterior border of the condylar process, passes between the process and the sphenomandibular ligament, along the inferior border of the lower head of the lateral pterygoid, and gives rise to the deep auricular, anterior tympanic, middle and accessory meningeal, and the inferior alveolar arteries. The middle meningeal ascends medial to the lateral pterygoid to enter the foramen spinosum, the accessory meningeal arises from the maxillary or middle meningeal to enter the foramen ovale, and the inferior alveolar descends to enter the mandibular foramen. The pterygoid segment usually courses lateral to, but occasionally medial to, the lower head of the lateral pterygoid and gives rise to the deep temporal, pterygoid, masseteric, and buccal arteries. The pterygopalatine segment courses between the two heads of the lateral pterygoid and enters the pterygopalatine fossa by passing through the pterygomaxillary fissure. Its branching will be described with the pterygopalatine fossa.

The pterygoid venous plexus is located in the infratemporal fossa and has two parts: a superficial part located between the temporalis and lateral pterygoid; and a deep part situated between the lateral and medial pterygoids anteriorly, and between the lateral pterygoid and the parapharyngeal space posteriorly. The deep part is more prominent and connects with the cavernous sinus by emissary veins passing through the foramina ovale and spinosum, and occasionally through the sphenoidal emissary foramen (foramen of Vesalius). The main drainage of the pterygoid plexus is through the maxillary vein to the internal jugular vein.

The mandibular nerve enters the infratemporal fossa by passing through the foramen ovale on the lateral side of the parapharyngeal space, where it gives rise to several smaller branches, and then divides into a smaller anterior trunk and a larger posterior trunk (*Figs. 8.8-8.10*). The anterior trunk gives rise to the deep temporal and masseteric nerves, which supply the temporalis and the masseter, respectively, and the nerve to the lateral pterygoid. The buccal nerve, which conveys sensory fibers, passes anterolaterally between the two heads of the lateral pterygoid, and descends lateral to the lower head to reach the buccinator and the buccal mucosa. The posterior trunk gives off the lingual, inferior alveolar, and auriculotemporal nerves, which descend medial to the lateral pterygoid. The lingual and inferior alveolar nerves, the former coursing anterior to the latter, pass between the lateral and medial pterygoids. The auriculotemporal nerve usually splits to encircle the middle meningeal artery and passes posterolaterally between the mandibular ramus and the sphenomandibular ligament. The chorda tympani nerve, which contains the taste fibers from the anterior two-thirds of the tongue and the parasympathetic secretomotor fibers to the submandibular and sublingual salivary glands, enters the infratemporal fossa through the petrotympanic fissure, descends medial to the auriculotemporal and inferior alveolar nerves, and joins the lingual nerve. The otic ganglion is situated immediately below the foramen ovale on the medial side of the mandibular nerve. The ganglion receives the lesser petrosal nerve, which crosses the floor of the middle fossa anterolateral to the greater petrosal nerve to exit through the foramen ovale or the more posteriorly situated canaliculus innominatus and conveys parasympathetic secretomotor fibers to the parotid gland via the auriculotemporal nerve. The medial pterygoid nerve arises from the medial aspect of the mandibular nerve close to the otic ganglion and descends to supply the medial pterygoid and tensor veli palatini. The nervus spinosus, a meningeal branch, also arises near the otic ganglion and ascends through the foramen spinosum to innervate the middle fossa dura.

Parapharyngeal space

The parapharyngeal space is located in the lateral pharyngeal wall and is shaped like an inverted pyramid, with its base on the skull base superiorly and its apex at the hyoid bone inferiorly. The parapharyngeal space is subdivided into prestyloid and poststyloid compartments by the styloid diaphragm, a fibrous sheet that also constitutes the anterior part of the carotid sheath (*Figs. 8.5* and *8.9*). The prestyloid part, situated anteriorly between the fascia covering the opposing surfaces of the medial pterygoid and tensor veli palatini, is a thin fat-filled compartment separating the structures in the infratemporal fossa from the eustachian tube and the tensor and levator veli palatini muscles in the lateral nasopharyngeal wall. The upper portion of the prestyloid part is situated between two fascial sheets, which are oriented in a sagittal plane. The lateral sheet arises from the medial surface of the medial pterygoid, passes upward, backward, and medial to the mandibular nerve and the middle meningeal artery, incorporating the sphenomandibular ligament posteriorly, and reaching the retromandibular deep lobe of the parotid gland. The medial sheet is formed by the fascia overlying the lateral surface of the tensor veli palatini and is continuous inferiorly with the fascia over the superior pharyngeal constrictor and posteriorly with the thick styloid diaphragm, which envelopes the stylopharyngeus, styloglossus, and stylohyoid and blends into the carotid sheath. The superior border is located where the two fascial sheets fuse together and insert in the skull base along a line extending backward from the pterygoid process lateral to the origin of the tensor veli palatini, medial to the foramina ovale and spinosum to the sphenoid spine and the posterior margin of the glenoid fossa. The sharply angled inferior boundary is situated at the junction of the posterior digastric belly and the greater hyoid cornu. The poststyloid part, which contains the internal carotid artery, internal jugular vein, and the initial extracranial segment of cranial nerves IX through XII, is separated from the infratemporal fossa by the posterolateral portion of the prestyloid part. The glossopharyngeal nerve exits the skull through the intrajugular part of the jugular foramen, anterior to the vagus and accessory nerves, and passes forward, medial to the styloid process in close relationship to the lateral surface of the carotid artery as the artery enters the carotid canal (*Fig. 8.9*). Care is required to avoid injury to the glossopharyngeal nerve if the artery is to be mobilized at the carotid canal. The vagus nerve leaves the skull through the anteromedial edge of the intrajugular part of the foramen and courses deep within the carotid sheath, between the internal carotid artery and the jugular vein. The accessory nerve exits the intrajugular part and runs backward, lateral to the jugular vein and medial to the styloid process and the posterior belly of the digastric muscle, to innervate the sternocleidomastoid muscle.

The hypoglossal nerve exits through the hypoglossal canal, deep to the jugular vein and to the nerves emerging from the jugular foramen, and runs downward, between the carotid artery and the jugular vein (*Figs. 8.9* and *8.10*). It becomes superficial at the level of the angle of the jaw where it crosses the internal and external carotid arteries, close to the level of the common carotid bifurcation, to innervate the tongue.

Pterygopalatine fossa

The pterygopalatine fossa, which opens laterally into the medial part of the infratemporal fossa, is bounded posteriorly by the sphenoid pterygoid process, medially by the palatine perpendicular plate, that bridges the interval between the maxilla and pterygoid process, and opens superiorly through the medial part of the inferior orbital fissure into the orbital apex (*Figs. 8.5, 8.9,* and *8.10*) (11). The fossa contains the maxillary nerve, pterygopalatine ganglion, maxillary artery, and their branches, all embedded in fat tissue. Its lateral boundary, the pterygomaxillary fissure, opens into the infratemporal fossa and allows passage of the maxillary artery from the infratemporal into the pterygopalatine fossa, where the artery gives rise to its terminal branches. The lower part of the fossa is funnel-shaped, with its inferior apex opening into the greater and lesser palatine canals, which transmit the greater and lesser palatine nerves and vessels, and communicate with the oral cavity. The sphenopalatine foramen, located in the upper part of the fossa's medial wall, conveys the sphenopalatine nerve and vessels, and opens into the superior nasal meatus just above the root of the middle nasal concha. The foramen rotundum opens just below the superior orbital fissure through the superior part of the posterior wall of the fossa. The pterygoid canal opens through the sphenoid pterygoid process inferomedial to the foramen rotundum and conveys the vidian nerve carrying autonomic fibers to the pterygopalatine ganglion. The maxillary nerve, after entering the fossa, gives off ganglionic branches to the pterygopalatine ganglion. It then deviates laterally just beneath the inferior orbital fissure, giving rise to, in order, the zygomatic and posterosuperior alveolar nerves outside of the periorbita. It then turns medially as the infraorbital nerve, passing through the inferior orbital fissure to enter the infraorbital groove, where the anterior and middle superior alveolar nerves arise. Finally, it exits the infraorbital foramen to terminate on the cheek. The pterygopalatine ganglion, located in front of the pterygoid canal and inferomedial to the maxillary nerve, receives communicating rami from the maxillary nerve and gives rise to the greater and lesser palatine nerves from the lower surface of the ganglion, the sphenopalatine nerve and pharyngeal branch from the medial surface, and the orbital branch from the superior surface. The vidian nerve is formed by the union of the greater petrosal nerve, which conveys parasympathetic fibers arising from the facial nerve at the level of the geniculate ganglion, and the deep petrosal nerve, which conveys sympathetic fibers from the carotid plexus, to reach the lacrimal gland and nasal mucosa. The parasympathetic fibers synapse in the pterygopalatine ganglion, whereas the sympathetic fibers do not. The sympathetic fibers synapse in the superior cervical sympathetic ganglion.

The third or pterygopalatine segment of the maxillary artery enters the pterygopalatine fossa by passing through the pterygomaxillary fissure. This segment courses in an anterior, medial, and superior direction and gives rise to the infraorbital artery, which passes through the inferior orbital fissure and courses with the infraorbital nerve; the posterosuperior alveolar artery, which descends to pierce the posterolateral wall of the maxilla; the recurrent meningeal branches, which pass through the foramen rotundum; and the greater and lesser palatine arteries, which descend through the greater and lesser palatine canals; the vidian artery to the pterygoid canal; the pharyngeal branch to the palatovaginal canal; and finally the sphenopalatine artery, which passes through the sphenopalatine foramen to reach the nasal cavity and is considered to be the terminal branch of the maxillary artery because of its large diameter. The arterial structures in the pterygopalatine fossa are located anterior to the neural structures.

Arterial relationships

The arteries that may be involved in pathological abnormalities involving the temporal bone include the upper cervical and petrous portions of the internal carotid artery, the posteriorly directed branches of the external carotid artery, and the upper portion of the vertebral artery.

Common carotid artery

The common carotid artery bifurcates into the internal and external carotid arteries at the level of the upper border of the thyroid cartilage. The internal carotid artery initially ascends relatively superficial in the carotid triangle of the neck, but assumes a much deeper position after passing medial to the posterior belly of the digastric (*Figs. 8.9* and *8.10*). Below the digastric, it is crossed by the hypoglossal nerve and the ansa cervicalis, and by the lingual and facial veins. Medial to the digastric, it is crossed by the stylohyoid muscle and the occipital and posterior auricular arteries. Superior to the digastric, the internal carotid artery is separated from the external carotid artery by the styloid process and the muscles attached to it. At the entrance into the carotid canal, the artery is involved by a dense sheath of connective tissue and is separated from the internal jugular vein by the hypoglossal nerve and by the nerves exiting from the jugular foramen.

The internal carotid artery passes, almost straightly upward, posterior to the external carotid artery and anteromedial to the internal jugular vein to reach the carotid canal. At the level of the skull base, the internal jugular vein courses just posterior to the internal carotid artery, being separated from it by the carotid ridge. Between them, the glossopharyngeal nerve is located laterally and the vagus, accessory, and hypoglossal nerves medially.

After the internal carotid artery enters the carotid canal with the carotid sympathetic nerves and surrounding venous plexus, it ascends a short distance (the vertical segment), reaching the area below and slightly behind the cochlea, where it turns anteromedially at a right angle (the site of the lateral bend) and courses horizontally (the horizontal segment) toward the petrous apex (*Figs. 8.8-8.10*). At the medial edge of the foramen lacerum, it turns sharply upward at the site of the medial bend to enter the posterior part of the cavernous sinus.

External carotid artery

The external carotid artery ascends anterior to the internal carotid artery on the posteromedial margin of the parotid gland and medial to the digastric and stylohyoid muscles. Proximal to its terminal bifurcation into the maxillary and the superficial temporal arteries, it gives rise to six branches that can be divided into anterior and posterior groups according to their directions. The latter group is related to the region of the temporal bone.

The ascending pharyngeal artery, the first branch of the posterior group, often provides the most prominent supply to the meninges around the jugular foramen (18). It arises either at the bifurcation or from the lowest part of the external or internal carotid arteries. Rarely, it arises from the origin of the occipital artery. It courses upward between the internal and the external carotid arteries, giving rise to numerous branches to neighboring muscles, nerves, and lymph nodes. Its meningeal branches pass through the foramen lacerum to be distributed to the dura lining the middle fossa and through the jugular foramen or the hypoglossal canal to supply the surrounding dura of the posterior cranial fossa. The ascending pharyngeal artery also gives rise to the inferior tympanic artery, which reaches the tympanic cavity by way of the tympanic canaliculus along with the tympanic branch of the glossopharyngeal nerve.

The occipital artery, the second and largest branch of the posterior group, arises from the posterior surface of the external carotid artery and courses obliquely upward between the posterior belly of the digastric muscle and the internal jugular vein, and then medial to the mastoid process and either superficial or deep to the longissimus capitis muscle (*Fig. 8.5*). It courses deep to the latter muscle if it courses in the occipital groove of the mastoid bone, which is located medial to the digastric groove. After passing the longissimus capitis muscle, the occipital artery courses deep to the splenius capitis muscle, finally reaching a subcutaneous location by piercing the fascia between the attachment of the sternocleidomastoid and the trapezius muscles to the superior nuchal line. The occipital artery gives rise to several muscular and meningeal branches, anastomoses with other branches of the external carotid including the ascending pharyngeal and also with branches of the vertebral artery. Its meningeal branches, which enter the posterior fossa through the jugular foramen or the condylar canal, may make a significant contribution to tumors of the jugular foramen.

The posterior auricular artery, the last branch in the posterior group, arises above the posterior belly of the digastric muscle and travels between the parotid gland and the styloid process. At the anterior margin of the mastoid process, it divides into auricular and occipital branches, which are distributed to the postauricular and the occipital regions, respectively. The stylomastoid branch, which arises below the stylomastoid foramen, enters the stylomastoid foramen to supply the facial nerve. Its loss can lead to a facial palsy, even though it anastomoses with the petrosal branch of the middle meningeal artery. The posterior auricular branch may share a common trunk with the occipital artery, or sometimes it is absent, in which case, the occipital artery gives rise to the stylomastoid artery. Members of the anterior group, whose origins may be visualized in exposing lesions in the region, include the superior thyroid, lingual, and facial arteries.

The superficial temporal artery arises from the external carotid artery in the substance of the parotid gland behind the neck of the mandible where it is crossed by the temporal and zygomatic branches of the facial nerve (*Fig. 8.5*). It ascends over the posterior root of the zygoma and divides into anterior and posterior branches that run with the superficial temporal vein and the auriculotemporal nerve over the superficial temporalis fascia.

Vertebral artery

The vertebral artery and its meningeal, posterior spinal, and posteroinferior cerebellar branches, which may be exposed in approaches directed through the temporal bone, are detailed in the chapter on the foramen magnum (4, 20, 24).

Venous relationships

The venous drainage of the structures of the skull base is through the internal jugular veins, the sinuses in the dura mater, and a series of emissary veins communicating the intra- and extracranial compartments (25). The superior petrosal sinus sits on the petrous ridge and connects the cavernous and transverse sinuses. It receives tributaries from the inferior surface of the temporal lobe and from the petrosal veins that drain the cerebellum and brainstem. The inferior petrosal sinus courses along the petro-occipital fissure and drains the clival area. It consists of one or more channels that, at its lower end, course rostral or caudal to or between the nerves passing through the jugular foramen. It enters the medial wall of the jugular bulb just anterior to where the cranial nerves descend in the anteromedial wall of the jugular bulb (18). It joins the cavernous sinus at its upper margin. The transverse sinus begins at the level of the internal occipital protuberance and passes laterally and forward to the posterolateral part of the temporal bone where it joins the superior petrosal sinus and continues as the sigmoid sinus. It receives drainage from the tentorial surface of the cerebellum through the tentorial sinuses and from the temporal lobe through the vein of Labbé. The basilar venous plexus consists of multiple interconnecting channels situated between the layers of dura mater on the clivus. It forms the largest communication between the paired cavernous sinus and communicates through the inferior petrosal sinuses with the sinuses in the region of the foramen magnum (10).

SURGICAL APPROACHES

The suboccipital retrosigmoid approach, the traditional neurosurgical route to intradural pathologies arising in the region of the cerebellopontine angle, lower clivus, and foramen magnum, is reviewed in the chapter on the cerebellopontine angle. The approaches reviewed here are those directed through the temporal bone.

Middle fossa approach

This section focuses on the middle fossa approach to the internal acoustic meatus rather than on the more extensive approaches directed through the petrous apex to the petroclival region or the more extended approaches directed through the temporal bone lateral to the internal acoustic meatus. The middle fossa approach to the internal acoustic meatus is usually selected for small tumors that are located predominantly within the internal acoustic meatus in which there is an opportunity to preserve hearing. With this approach, the meatus is approached from above, through a temporal craniotomy located above the ear and zygoma (*Figs. 8.7* and *8.11*) (2). The dura under the temporal lobe is elevated from the floor of the middle cranial fossa until the arcuate eminence and the greater petrosal nerve are identified. The distance from the inner table of the skull to the facial hiatus, through which the greater petrosal nerve passes, ranges from 1.3 to 2.3 cm (average, 1.7 cm) (42). When separating the dura from the floor of the middle fossa, one should remember that bone may be absent over all or part of the geniculate ganglion. In our previous study of 100 temporal bones, all or part of the geniculate ganglion and the genu of the facial nerve were found to be exposed in the floor of the middle fossa in 15 bones (15%) (31). In 15 other specimens, the geniculate ganglion was completely covered, but no bone extended over the greater petrosal nerve. The greatest length of greater petrosal nerve covered by bone was 6.0 mm. More than 50% of the specimens had less than 2.5 mm of greater petrosal nerve covered. It also is important to remember that the petrous segment of the carotid artery may be exposed without a covering of bone in the floor of the middle fossa deep to the greater petrosal nerve (17) In a

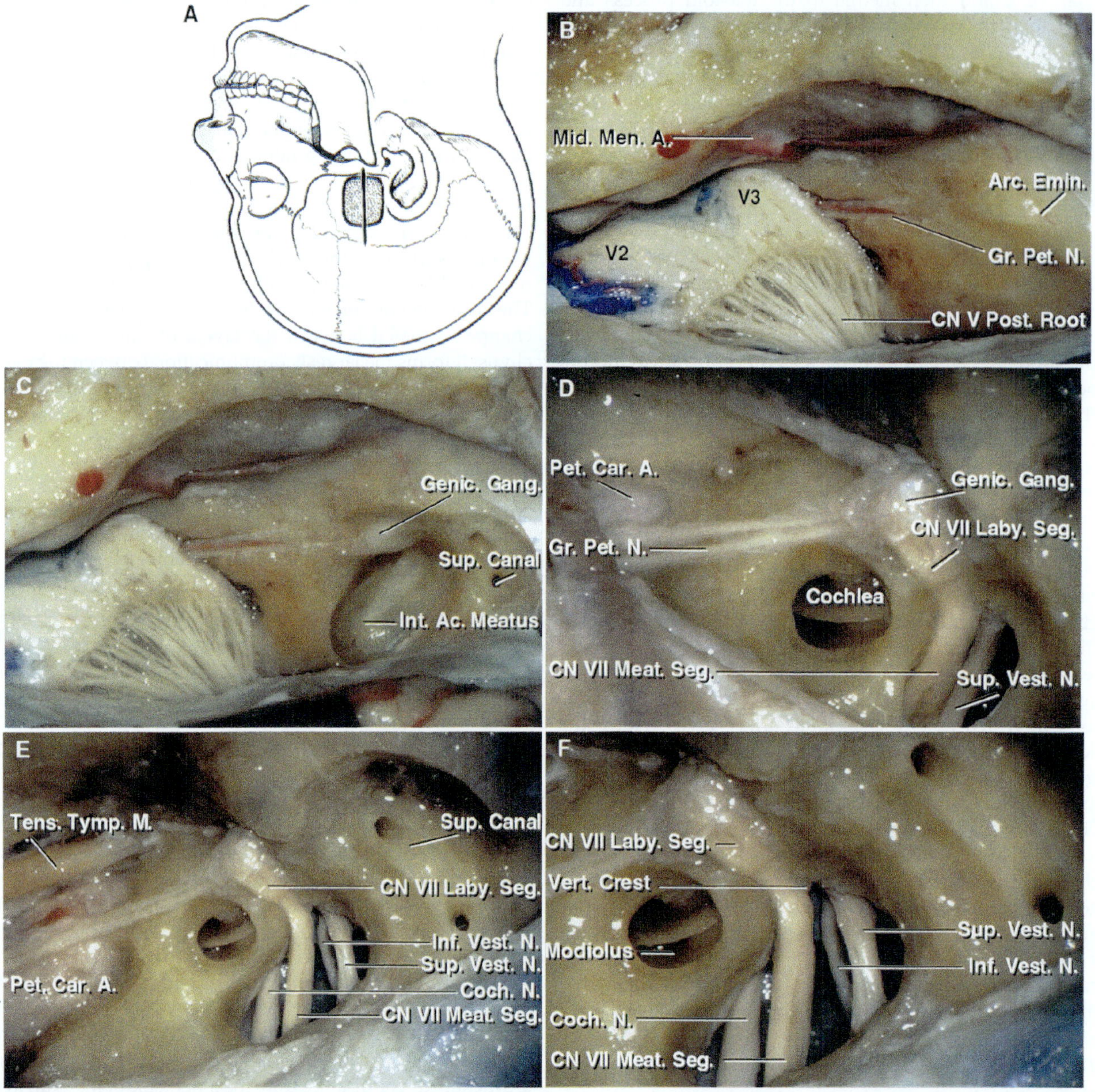

FIGURE 8.11. Middle fossa approach to the internal acoustic meatus. *A*, the vertical line shows the site of the scalp incision and the *stippled area* outlines the bone flap bordering the middle fossa floor. *B*, the dura has been elevated to expose the middle meningeal artery, the greater petrosal nerve, and the arcuate eminence. *C*, bone has been removed to expose the junction of the greater petrosal nerve and the geniculate ganglion. A portion of the upper wall of the internal meatus has been removed. The upper surface of the arcuate eminence has been drilled to expose the superior semicircular canal. In the middle fossa approach, for an acoustic neuroma, the cochlea and semicircular canal are not opened, as seen in this dissection illustrating some of the important structures that are to be avoided in opening the meatus. *D*, enlarged view. The cochlea, located below the middle fossa floor in the angle between the facial and greater petrosal nerves, has been opened in the area anteromedial to the meatal fundus. The roof of the meatus has been opened to expose the superior vestibular nerve, which innervates the ampullae of the superior and lateral canals and the meatal segment of the facial nerve. *E*, the vestibule and semicircular canals are located posterolateral and the cochlea is located anteromedial to the meatal fundus. The tensor tympani is layered along the anterior edge and the greater petrosal nerve above the petrous carotid. *F*, enlarged view. The vertical crest (Bill's bar) separates the facial and superior vestibular nerves at the meatal fundus. The superior and inferior vestibular nerves are located posteriorly and the facial and cochlear nerves anteriorly in the meatus, with the cochlear nerve passing below the facial nerve to enter the modiolus. The labyrinthine segment of the facial nerve courses superolateral to the cochlea. *A.*, artery; *Ac.*, acoustic; *Arc.*, arcuate; *Car.*, carotid; *CN*, cranial nerve; *Coch.*, cochlear; *Emin.*, eminence; *Gang.*, ganglion; *Genic.*, geniculate; *Gr.*, greater; *Inf.*, inferior; *Int.*, internal; *Laby.*, labyrinthine; *M.*, muscle; *Meat.*, meatal; *Men.*, meningeal; *Mid.*, middle; *N.*, nerve; *Pet.*, petrosal, petrous; *Post.*, posterior; *Seg.*, segment; *Sup.*, superior; Tens., tensor; Tymp., tympani; *Vert.*, vertebral; *Vest.*, vestibular.

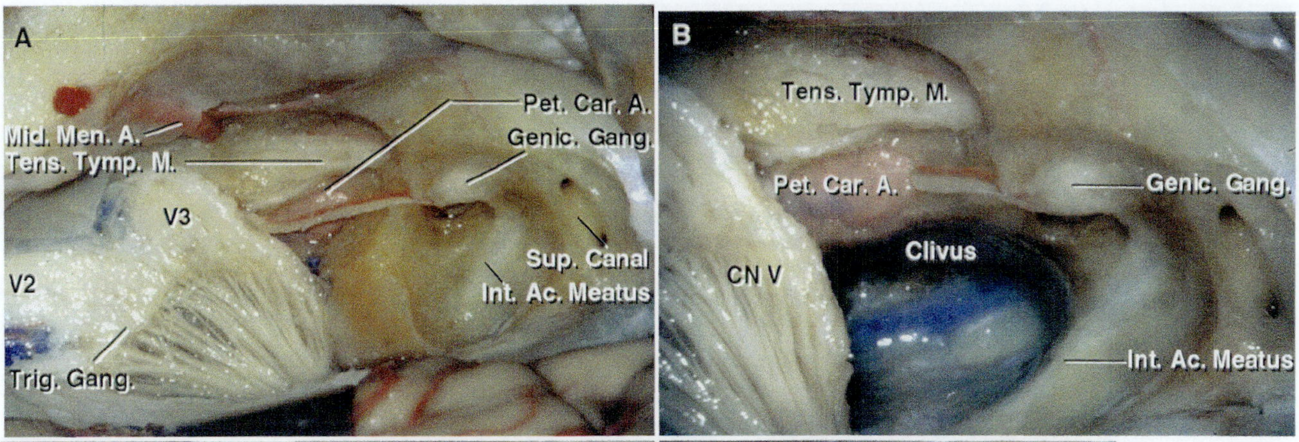

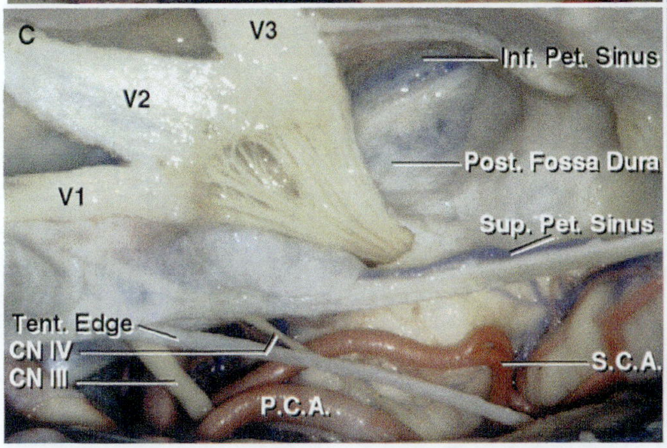

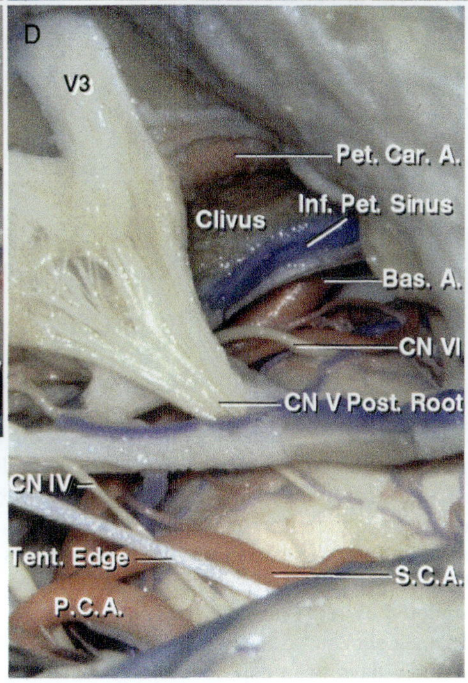

FIGURE 8.12. *A–D.* Anterior petrosectomy and extended middle fossa approach. *A*, the site of the bone flap is the same as shown in *Figure 8.11A*. The dura has been elevated from the floor of the middle fossa. Bone has been removed to expose the geniculate ganglion, the dura lining the internal acoustic meatus, the tensor tympani, some of the petrous carotid, and the superior semicircular canal. *B*, the bone of the petrous apex between the trigeminal nerve and the internal acoustic meatus has been removed to expose the side of the clivus. *C*, the exposure under the trigeminal nerve extends to the edge of the inferior petrosal sinus. *D*, the posterior fossa dura has been opened to expose the prepontine cistern, basilar artery, and abducens nerve. *A.*, artery; *Ac.*, acoustic; *A.I.C.A.*, anteroinferior cerebellar artery; *Bas.*, basilar; *Car.*, carotid; *Cav.*, cavernous; *Chor.*, chorda; *CN*, cranial nerve; *Ext.*, external; *Gang.*, ganglion; *Gen.*, geniculate; *Genic.*, geniculate; *Inf.*, inferior; *Int.*, internal; *Laby.*, labyrinthine; *Lat.*, lateral; *M.*, muscle; *Mast.*, mastoid; *Men.*, meningeal; *Mid.*, middle; *N.*, nerve; *P.C.A.*, posterior cerebral artery; *Pet.*, petrosal, petrous; *P.I.C.A.*, posteroinferior cerebellar artery; *Post.*, posterior; *S.C.A.*, superior cerebellar artery; *Seg.*, segment; *Sup.*, superior; *Tens.*, tensor; *Tymp.*, tympani; *Tent.*, tentorial; *Trig.*, trigeminal; *Tymp.*, tympani, tympanic.

previous study, we found that a 7-mm length of petrous carotid artery may be exposed without a bony covering in the area below where the greater petrosal nerve passes below the lateral margin of the trigeminal ganglion to reach the vidian canal at the anterior margin of the anterior margin of the foramen lacerum (30, 31). The foramen spinosum and middle meningeal artery and the foramen ovale and third trigeminal division are situated at the anterior margin of the extradural exposure. The extradural exposure can usually be completed without obliterating the middle meningeal artery at the foramen spinosum.

Two different methods are used for exposing the internal acoustic meatus. One is to remove bone over the greater petrosal nerve and to follow it to the geniculate ganglion and the genu of the facial nerve. From here, the labyrinthine portion of the facial nerve is followed to the lateral end of the internal auditory canal, after which the canal is unroofed. The other method is begun by drilling just in front of the petrous ridge in the area medial to the arcuate eminence. The angle between the long axis of the superior semicircular canal or the greater petrosal nerve and the long axis of the internal acous-

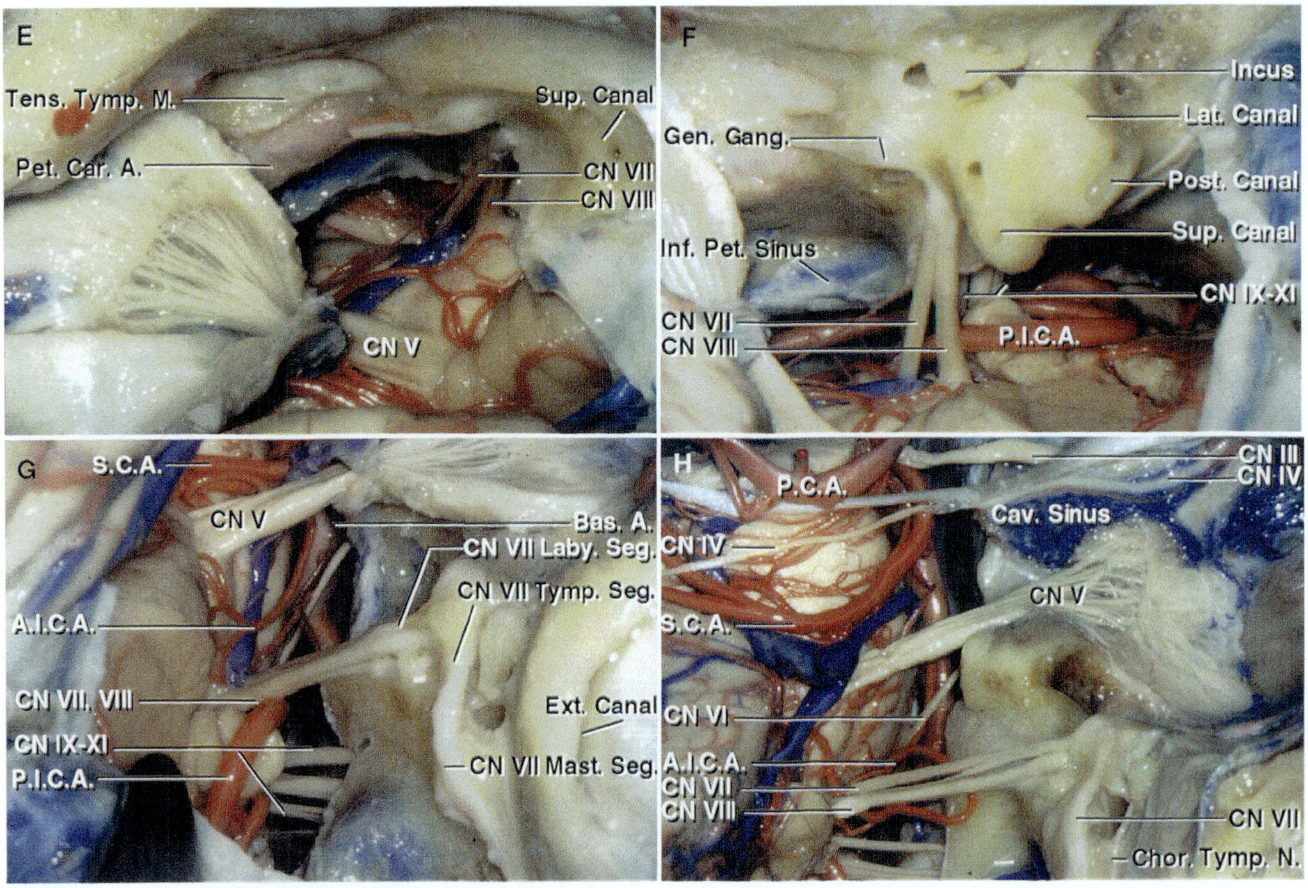

FIGURE 8.12. ***E–H.*** **Anterior petrosectomy and extended middle fossa approach. *E*, additional bone has been removed around the internal acoustic meatus and the dura opened to expose the facial and vestibulocochlear nerves. *F*, the exposure has been extended lateral to the internal acoustic meatus. The tegmen has been opened to expose the head of the incus in the epitympanic area. The osseous capsule of the labyrinth has been opened to expose the semicircular canals. The presigmoid dura behind the labyrinth has been exposed and opened. *G*, a translabyrinthine approach directed through the middle fossa has been completed by removing the semicircular canals and vestibule. The dura has been opened to give an exposure through the middle fossa similar to that seen with the presigmoid approach. The labyrinthine, tympanic, and mastoid segments of the facial nerve have been exposed. *H*, this extended middle fossa exposure extends from the lateral wall of the cavernous sinus, across the trigeminal nerve to the area lateral to the internal acoustic meatus, and provides wide access to the anterior part of the posterior fossa.**

tic meatus is helpful in selecting the site for drilling. The long axis of the central part of the internal acoustic meatus is located an average of 61 degrees behind the long axis of the greater petrosal nerve and an average of 37 degrees medial to the long axis of the arcuate eminence and superior semicircular canal. The drilling is directed anterolateral to the meatal fundus where the vertical crest is identified.

The lateral part of the bone removal near the meatal fundus is limited posteriorly by the superior semicircular canal, which is located a few millimeters behind and oriented parallel to the labyrinthine segment of the facial nerve (*Figs. 8.7* and *8.11*). The anteromedial edge of the exposure is limited by the cochlea, which sits only a few millimeters anterior to the site of bone removal, in the angle between the labyrinthine portion of the facial nerve and the greater petrosal nerve. The cochlea and the semicircular canals should be avoided in this approach if hearing is to be preserved. The vertical crest, which is identified at the upper edge of the meatal fundus, provides a valuable landmark for identifying the facial nerve. In the final stage of bone removal, the upper wall of the internal auditory canal is removed to expose the dura lining the entire superior surface of the internal auditory canal from the vertical crest to the porus. The dura is opened to expose the pathology.

The extended middle fossa approach used for the removal of larger acoustic neuromas includes wider opening of the posterior part of the petrous pyramid (21, 28, 42, 43). This approach combines different degrees of resection of the bony labyrinth with the subtemporal transtentorial routes (*Fig. 8.12*). Extending the resection of the petrous bone posteriorly over the mastoid and the bony labyrinth exposes the whole intrapetrous course of the facial nerve, and provides access to

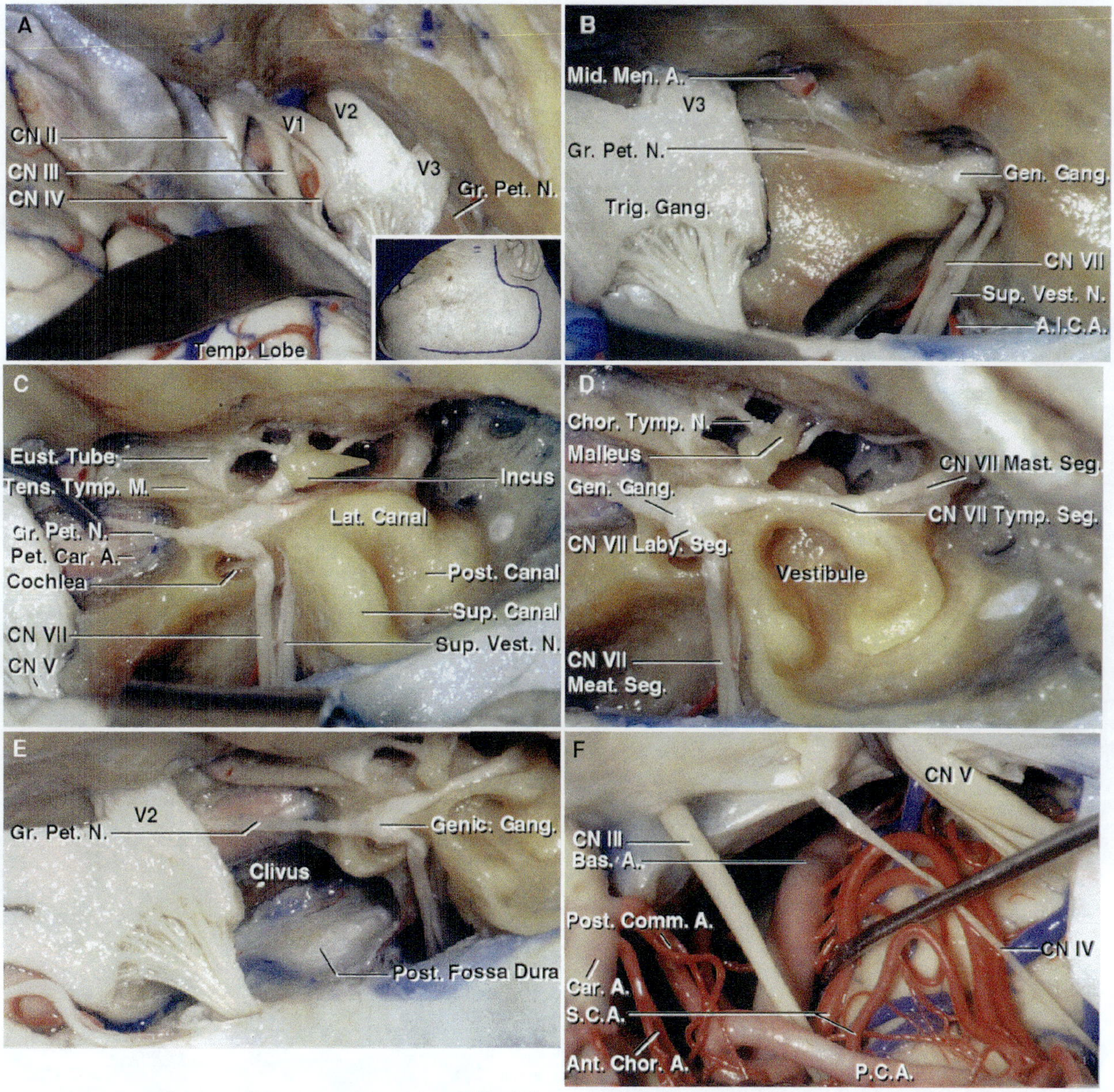

FIGURE 8.13. *A–F.* Subtemporal exposure of the right middle, infratemporal, and posterior fossae. *A,* the *insert* shows the side of the scalp incision. A frontotemporal craniotomy has been completed and the dura has been elevated from the middle fossa floor and lateral wall of the cavernous sinus. *B,* enlarged view. The bony roof over the geniculate ganglion and internal meatus has been removed and the dura lining the meatus opened to expose the facial and superior vestibular nerves. *C,* additional middle fossa floor has been removed to expose the petrous carotid, the cochlea in the angle between the greater petrosal nerve and pregeniculate part of the facial nerve, the semicircular canals and tympanic cavity. The tensor tympani muscle and eustachian tube are exposed in front of the petrous carotid artery. *D,* the bone between the superior and posterior canals has been removed to expose the vestibule with which both ends of the semicircular canals communicate. The vestibule contains the utricle and saccule and communicates below the fundus of the meatus with the cochlea. The meatal segment of the facial nerve courses in the internal acoustic meatus, the labyrinthine segment between the semicircular canals and the cochlea, the tympanic segment between the anterior margin of the lateral canal and the oval window on the medial side of the tympanic cavity, and the mastoid segment descends to exit the stylomastoid foramen. *E,* the petrous apex, medial to the cochlea and extending under the trigeminal nerve, has been removed to expose the lateral edge of the clivus and the posterior fossa dura. *F,* the medial tentorial edge has been divided behind the petrous ridge to expose the oculomotor, trochlear, and trigeminal nerves and the basilar artery. *A.,* artery; *A.I.C.A.,* anteroinferior cerebellar artery; Alv., alveolar; *Ant.,* anterior; *Bas.,* basilar; *Car.,* carotid; *Chor.,* chorda, choroidal; *CN,* cranial nerve; *Comm.,* communicating; *Eust.,* eustachian; *Gang.,* ganglion; *Gen.,* geniculate; *Genic.,* geniculate; *Gr.,* greater; *Inf.,* inferior; *Int.,* internal; *Jug.,* jugular; *Laby.,* labyrinthine; *Lat.,* lateral; *M.,* muscle; *Mandib.,* mandibular; *Mast.,* mastoid; *Max.,* maxillary; Meat., meatal; *Men.,* meningeal; *Mid.,* middle; *N.,* nerve; *P.C.A.,* posterior cerebral artery; *Pet.,* petrosal, petrous; *Post.,* posterior; *S.C.A.,* superior cerebellar artery; *Seg.,* segment; *Sup.,* superior; *Temp.,* temporal; *Tens.,* tensor; *Trig.,* trigeminal; *Tymp.,* tympani, tympanic; *V.,* vein; *Vert.,* vertebral; *Vest.,* vestibular.

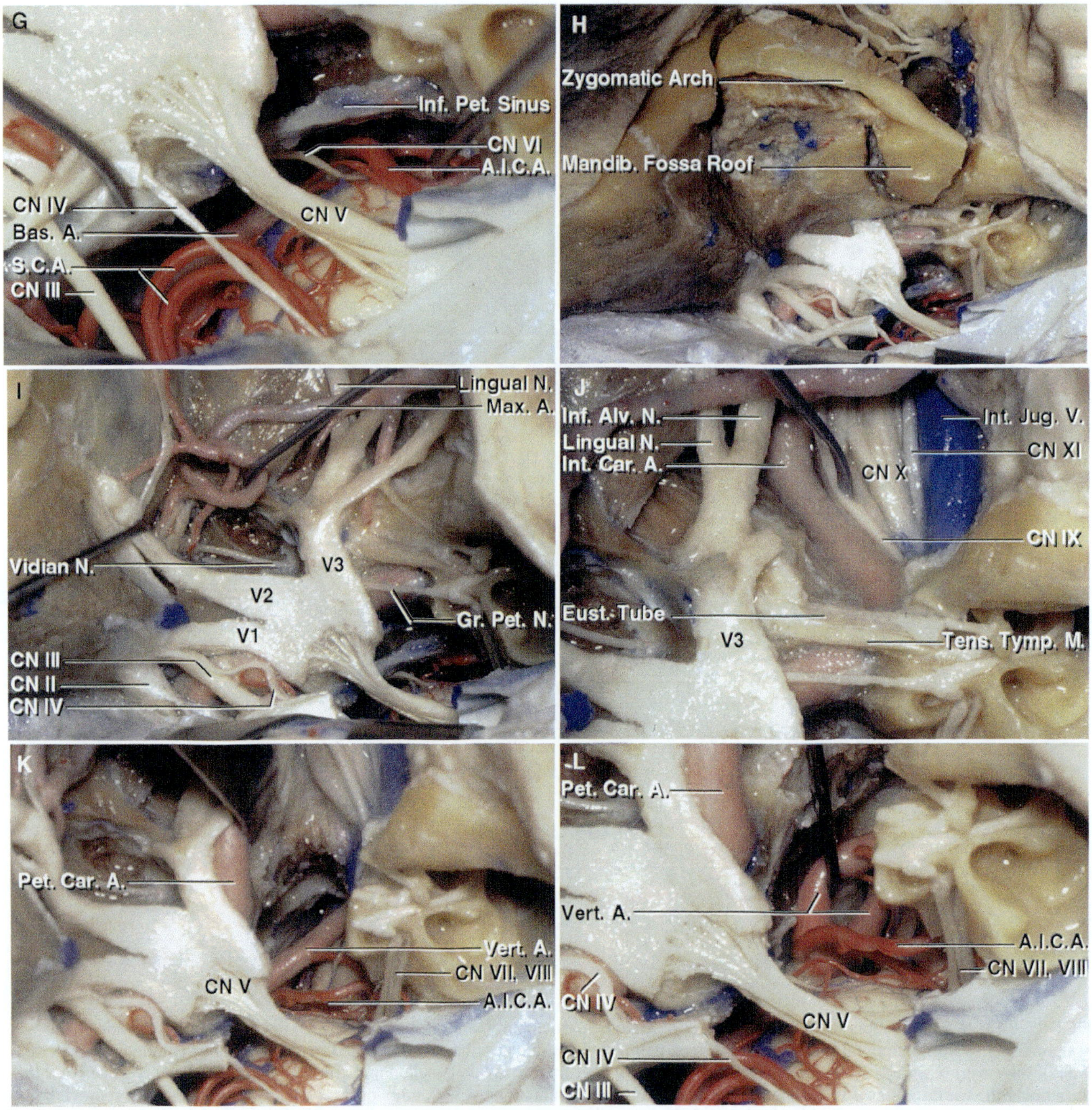

FIGURE 8.13. *G–L.* Subtemporal exposure of the right middle, infratemporal, and posterior fossae. *G,* the dural opening has been extended downward to expose the lateral edge of the clivus and the inferior petrosal sinus coursing along the petroclival fissure. The abducens nerve and the AICA are in the lower margin of the exposure. *H,* an osteotomy of the zygomatic arch and the floor of the middle fossa surrounding the mandibular fossa has been completed to aid in exposing the infratemporal fossa. *I,* the mandibular fossa and floor of the middle fossa, extending medially to the level of the foramen ovale, have been removed. Branches of the mandibular nerve and maxillary artery are exposed in the infratemporal fossa. The greater petrosal nerve joins the deep petrosal nerve from the carotid sympathetic plexus to form the vidian nerve, which passes forward in the vidian canal to reach the pterygopalatine fossa. *J,* the upper portion of the cervical carotid is exposed medial to the jugular foramen. The petrous carotid crosses behind the eustachian tube and tensor tympani. *K,* the eustachian tube and tensor tympani have been resected, the petrous carotid reflected forward out of the carotid canal, the petrous apex removed, and the posterior fossa dura opened to expose the vertebral artery and the AICA. *L,* enlarged view. The right vertebral artery has been displaced forward to expose the left vertebral artery. The AICA passes toward the nerves entering the internal acoustic meatus.

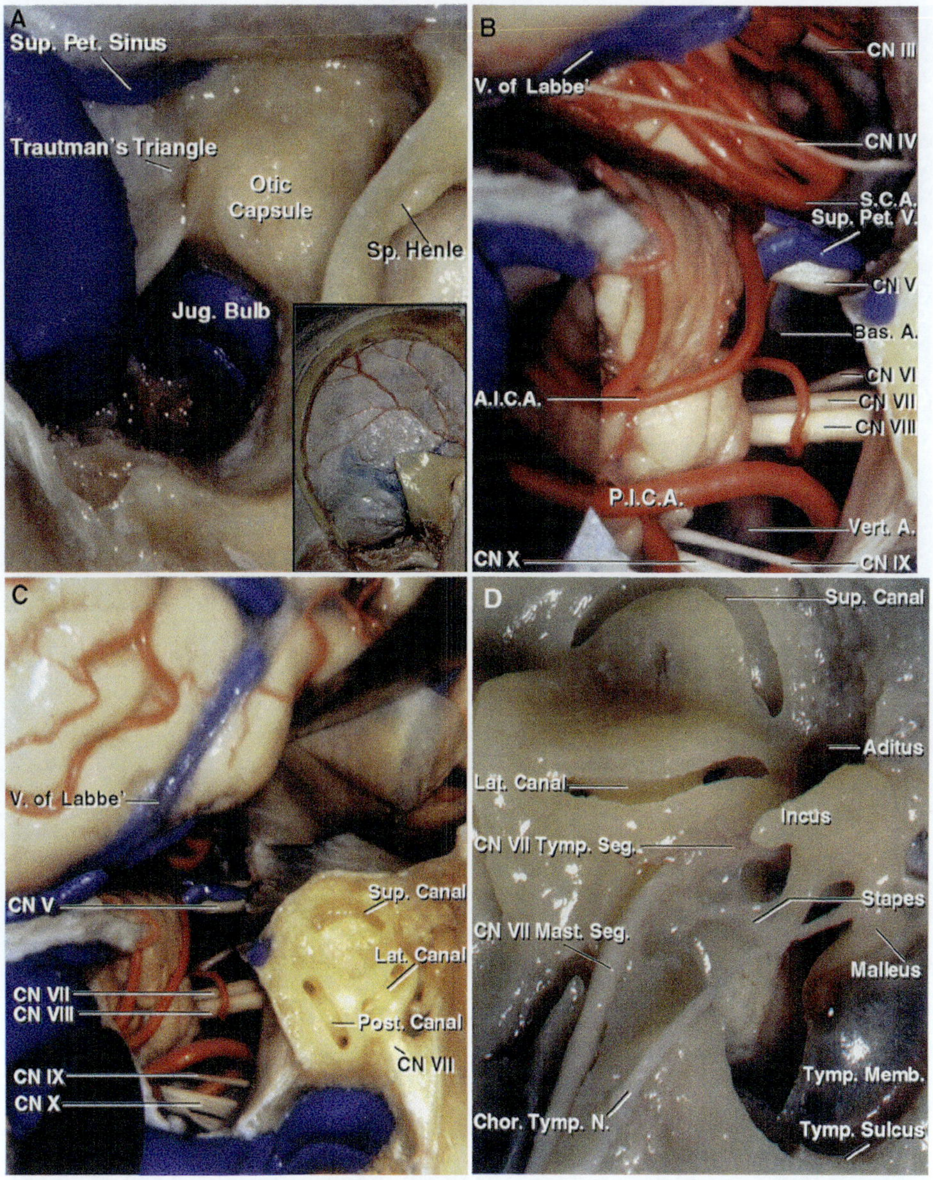

FIGURE 8.14. ***A–D.*** **Presigmoid approach.** ***A,*** **the** ***insert*** **shows the temporo-occipital craniotomy and the mastoid exposure. The mastoidectomy has been completed and the dense cortical bone around the labyrinth has been exposed. The tympanic segment of the facial nerve and the lateral canal are situated deep to the spine of Henley. Trautman's triangle, the patch of dura in front of the sigmoid sinus, faces the cerebellopontine angle.** ***B,*** **the presigmoid dura has been opened and the superior petrosal sinus and tentorium divided, taking care to preserve the vein of Labbé that joins the transverse sinus, and the trochlear nerve that enters the anterior edge of the tentorium. The abducens and facial nerves are exposed medial to the vestibulocochlear nerve. The posteroinferior cerebellar artery courses in the lower margin of the exposure with the glossopharyngeal and vagus nerves. The SCA passes below the oculomotor and trochlear nerves and above the trigeminal nerve.** ***C,*** **the semicircular canals have been opened. The superior canal is located under the middle fossa's arcuate eminence and the posterior canal is located immediately lateral to the posterior wall of the internal acoustic meatus.** ***D,*** **labyrinthine exposure in another specimen. The tympanic segment of the facial nerve courses below the lateral canal and turns downward as the mastoid segment where it gives origin to the chorda tympani, seen ascending along the inner surface of the tympanic membrane and neck of the malleus. The head of the malleus and incus are located in the epitympanic area above the level of the tympanic membrane. The mastoid antrum communicates through the aditus with the epitympanic area and tympanic cavity.** ***A.,*** **artery;** ***Ac.,*** **acoustic;** ***A.I.C.A.,*** **anteroinferior cerebellar artery;** ***Bas.,*** **basilar;** ***Br.,*** **branch;** ***Chor.,*** **chorda;** ***Cist.,*** **cisternal;** ***CN,*** **cranial nerve;** ***Coch.,*** **cochlear;** ***Gang.,*** **ganglion;** ***Genic.,*** **geniculate;** ***Inf.,*** **inferior;** ***Int.,*** **internal;** ***Jug.,*** **jugular;** ***Laby.,*** **labyrinthine;** ***Lat.,*** **lateral;** ***Marg.,*** **margin;** ***Mast.,*** **mastoid;** ***Meat.,*** **meatal;** ***Memb.,*** **membrane;** ***N.,*** **nerve;** ***Pet.,*** **petrosal;** ***P.I.C.A.,*** **posteroinferior cerebellar artery;** ***Post.,*** **posterior;** ***S.C.A.,*** **superior cerebellar artery;** ***Seg.,*** **segment;** ***Sp.,*** **spine;** ***Sup.,*** **superior;** ***Tymp.,*** **tympani, tympanic;** ***V.,*** **vein;** ***Vert.,*** **vertebral;** ***Vest.,*** **vestibular.**

the cerebellopontine angle by a combination of subtemporal, translabyrinthine, and presigmoid routes, all directed through the posterior part of the floor of the middle fossa.

Subtemporal anterior transpetrosal approach

This approach is made through a temporal craniotomy that extends down to the floor of the middle fossa (*Figs. 8.12* and *8.13*) (19). The dura is carefully elevated from the floor of the middle fossa to expose the middle meningeal artery, which may be obliterated and divided at the foramen spinosum. Further elevation of the dura toward the petrous ridge will expose the arcuate eminence and greater petrosal nerve posteriorly. The cochlea, which is to be preserved, and the anterior wall of the internal auditory canal constitute the lateral

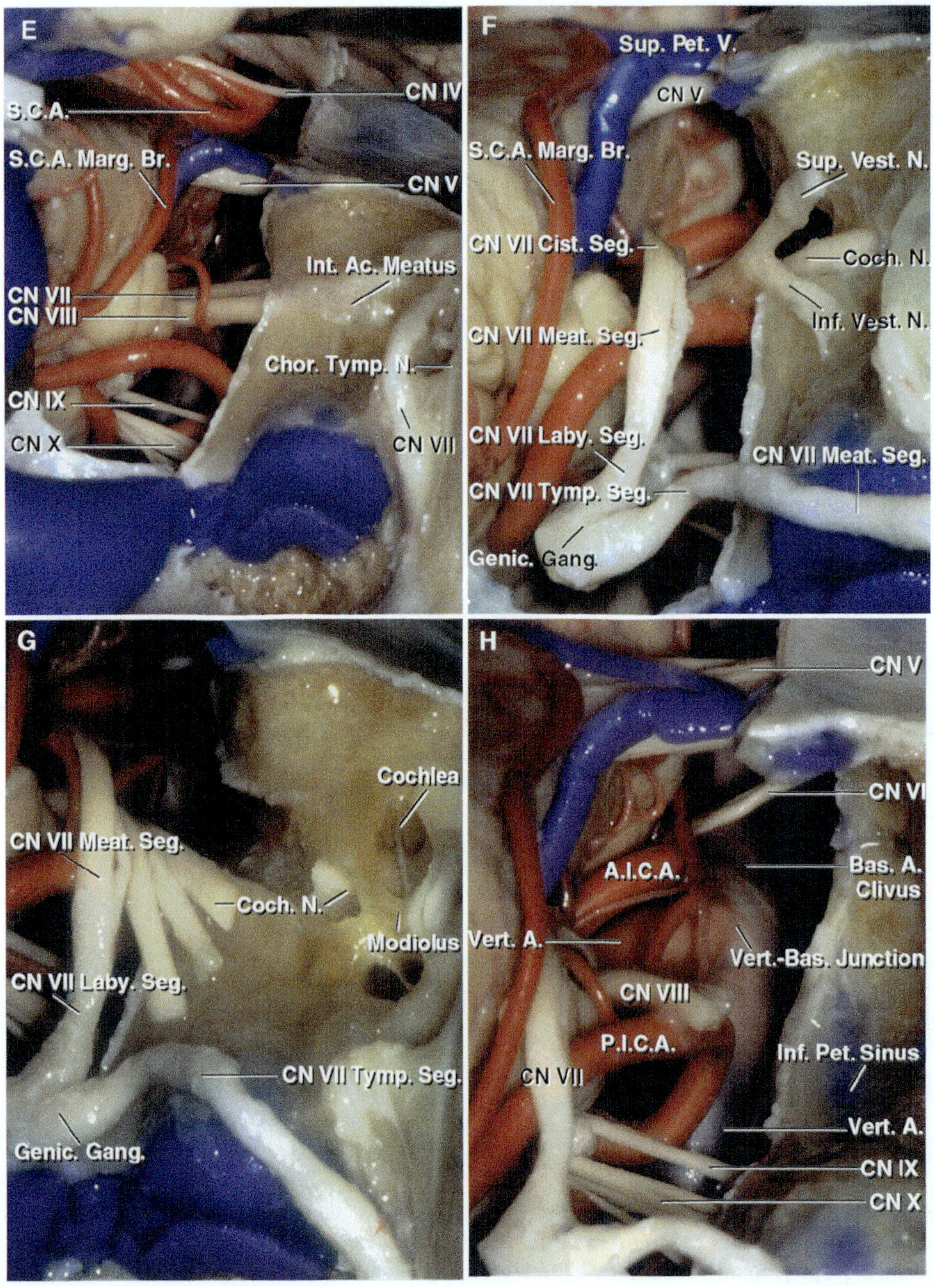

FIGURE 8.14. ***E–H.*** **Presigmoid approach.** ***E,*** **the labyrinthectomy has been completed to expose the internal acoustic meatus.** ***F,*** **the dura lining the meatus has been opened and the facial nerve has been transposed posteriorly. The facial segments are the cisternal segment located in the cistern medial to the meatal porus, the meatal segment that extends laterally from the porus to the meatal fundus, the labyrinthine segment that is located between the fundus and the geniculate ganglion, the tympanic segment that arises at the ganglion and the sharp turn, the genu, and passes between the lateral semicircular canal and the oval window, and the mastoid segment that descends to exit the stylomastoid foramen. The labyrinthine segment courses between the semicircular canals and vestibule on its posterolateral side and the cochlea on its anteromedial margin. The superior and inferior vestibular nerves have lost their end organs with the drilling of the semicircular canals and vestibule. The cochlear nerve passes laterally to enter the cochlea, which is still preserved in the bone anteromedial to the fundus of the meatus.** ***G,*** **the cochlear nerve has been divided and reflected and bone removed to expose the cochlea.** ***H,*** **the transcochlear exposure, completed by removing the cochlea and surrounding petrous apex, provides access to the front of the brainstem and vertebrobasilar junction, but at the cost of loss of hearing due to the labyrinthectomy and almost certain temporary or permanent facial weakness associated with the posterior transposition of the facial nerve.**

limit of the exposure through the petrous apex. The bone layer over the superior wall of the internal auditory canal, which averages 5 mm (range, 3–7 mm) in thickness, can be removed with a drill to improve the exposure (44). The petrous carotid forms the anterior limit of the exposure. The limit above the medial part of the bone resection is the trigeminal nerve in Meckel's cave. Drilling is directed behind the petrous carotid, through the petrous apex medial to the cochlea and under the trigeminal nerve. The petrous apex is removed and the bone removal is extended to the lateral side of the clivus, exposing the inferior petrosal sinus at the lateral edge of the clivus. Care is required to prevent damage to the abducens nerve as it passes through Dorello's canal located at the upper edge of the petroclival fissure. The width of the bone resection from the trigeminal impression to the posterior wall of the internal auditory canal averages 13 mm (range, 9–14 mm) (44). The depth of the exposure, from the trigeminal ganglion to the petroclival fissure, averages 13 mm (range, 9–17 mm). The cochlea lies below the floor of the middle fossa near the apex of the angle formed by the greater petrosal nerve anteriorly and the internal acoustic

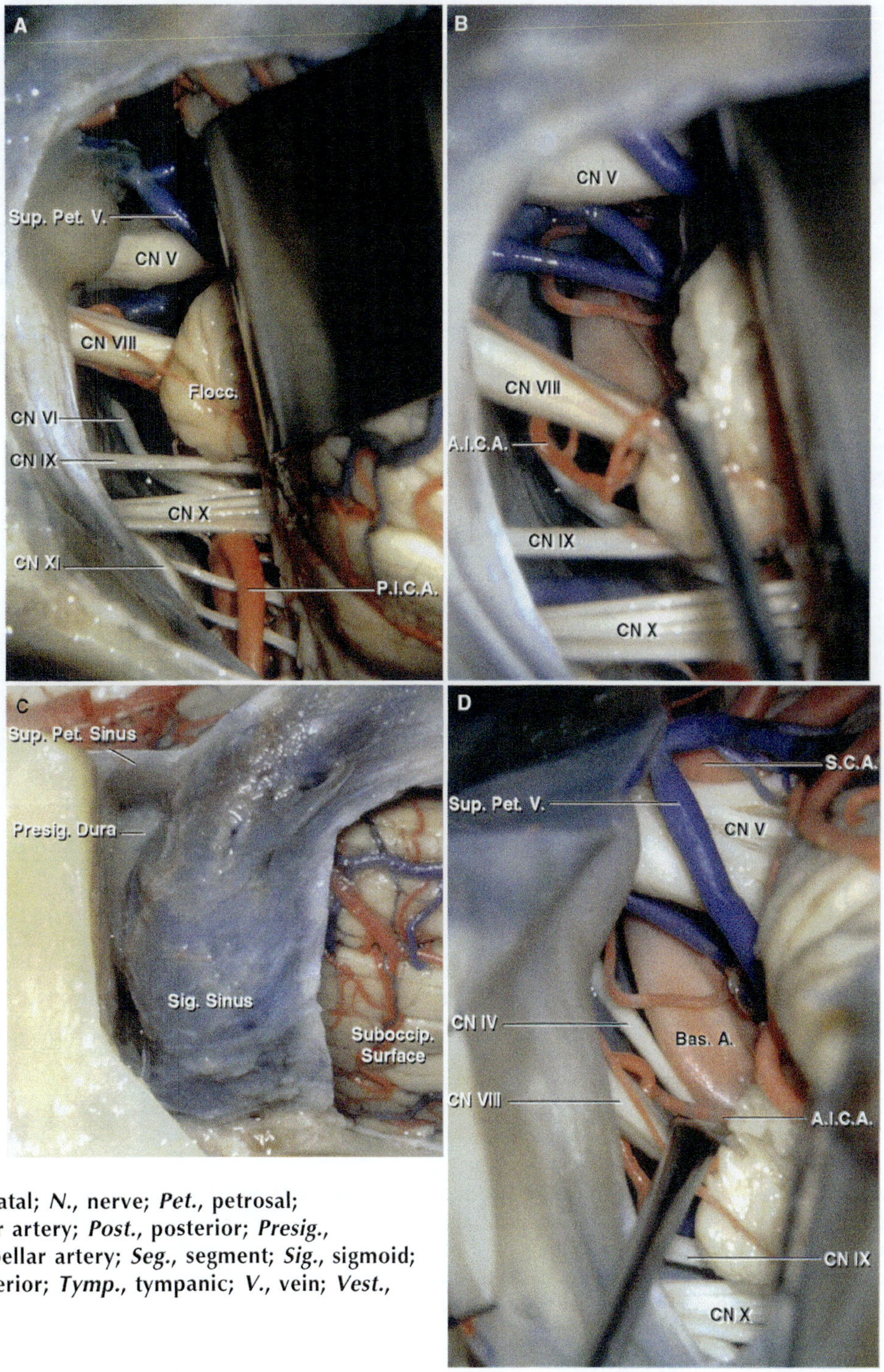

FIGURE 8.15. *A–D.* Comparison of the retrosigmoid approach and the minimal mastoidectomy, retrolabyrinthine, translabyrinthine, and transcochlear approach modifications of the presigmoid approach. *A,* retrosigmoid approach. The left cerebellum has been elevated to expose the cranial nerves V through XI in the cerebellopontine angle. The illustrations from each step are to be compared with the views from the other modifications of the approach. *B,* the facial and vestibulocochlear nerves and the flocculus have been retracted to expose the side of the basilar artery. *C,* for the minimal mastoidectomy, only enough bone is removed in front of the sigmoid sinus to open the presigmoid dura and divide the superior petrosal sinus and tentorium. *D,* the presigmoid dura has been opened and the sigmoid sinus has been retracted posteriorly. The view is approximately the same as that seen with the retrosigmoid exposure. The retrosigmoid approach provides a better view of the nerves entering the jugular foramen. *A.,* artery; *A.I.C.A.,* anteroinferior cerebellar artery; *Bas.,* basilar; *Cist.,* cisternal; *CN,* cranial nerve; *Coch.,* cochlear; *Flocc.,* flocculus; *Inf.,* inferior; *Laby.,* labyrinthine; *Lat.,* lateral; *Mast.,* mastoid; *Meat.,* meatal; *N.,* nerve; *Pet.,* petrosal; *P.I.C.A.,* posteroinferior cerebellar artery; *Post.,* posterior; *Presig.,* presigmoid; *S.C.A.,* superior cerebellar artery; *Seg.,* segment; *Sig.,* sigmoid; *Suboccip.,* suboccipital; *Sup.,* superior; *Tymp.,* tympanic; *V.,* vein; *Vest.,* vestibular.

meatus posteriorly. The cochlea is to be avoided if hearing is to be preserved.

After the bone removal is completed, the superior petrosal sinus is obliterated and divided in the area just lateral to the trigeminal nerve, and the dural incision is extended across the tentorium. The dural leaflets of the tentorium are retracted with sutures and the dural incision is carried downward to the lower margin of the opening through the petrous apex. The approach is then directed between the lower margin of the trigeminal nerve above, and the internal acoustic meatus inferiorly and laterally (20).

The exposure is small, as described above, and may require significant temporal lobe retraction, especially if the goal is to reach the lower aspect of the brainstem. To reach the anterior

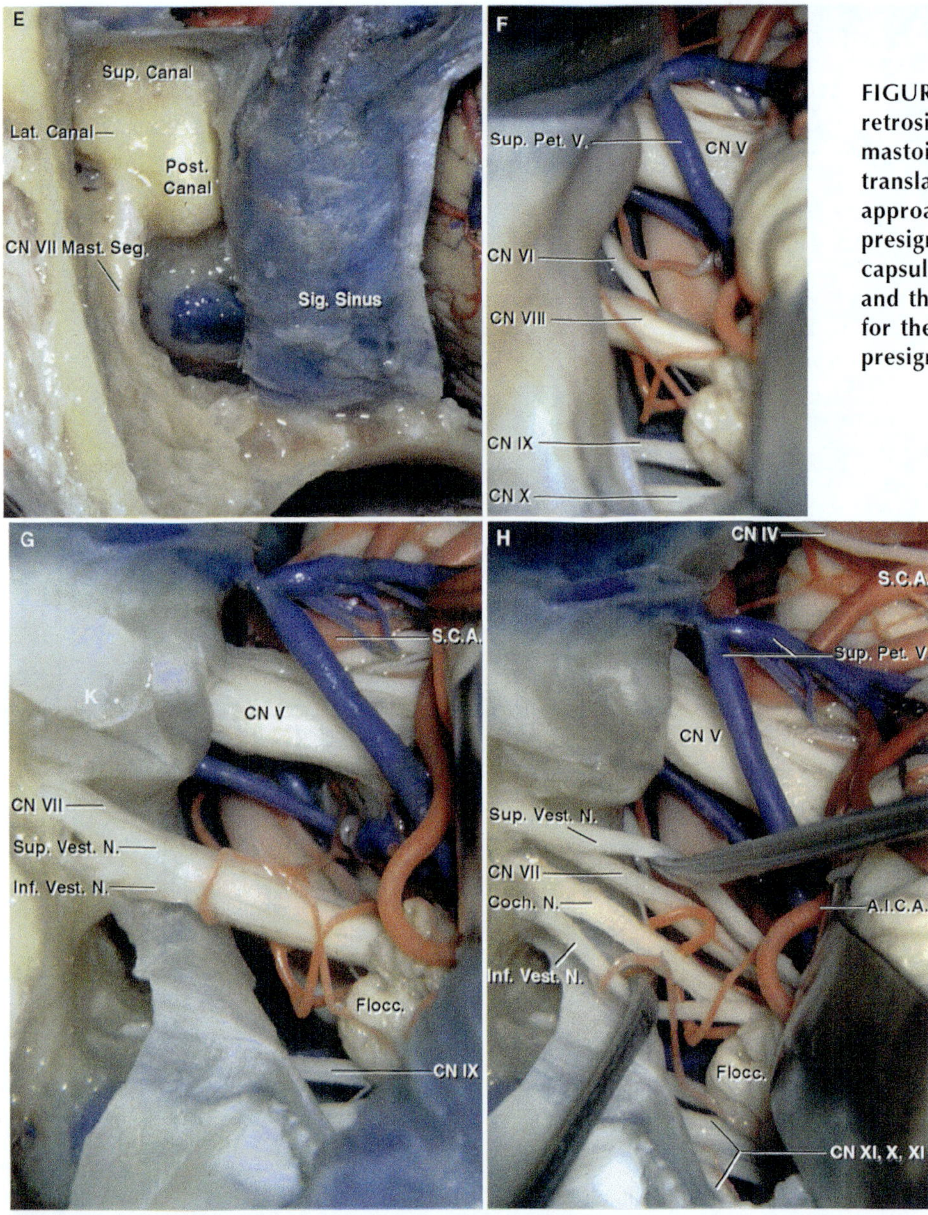

FIGURE 8.15. *E–H.* Comparison of the retrosigmoid approach and the minimal mastoidectomy, retrolabyrinthine, translabyrinthine, and transcochlear approach modifications of the presigmoid approach. *E*, the bony capsule around the semicircular canals and the facial nerve have been exposed for the retrolabyrinthine variant of the presigmoid approach. *F*, the exposure with the retrolabyrinthine version does not differ significantly from that achieved with the minimal mastoidectomy. *G*, the semicircular canals and vestibule have been removed and the dura lining the internal acoustic meatus has been opened to complete the translabyrinthine exposure. This yields an exposure of the internal acoustic meatus but provides only minimal improvement in the exposure of the structures medial to the porus of the meatus. *H*, the nerves have been separated beginning laterally at the fundus of the meatus and extending the cleavage plane medially toward the brainstem. The superior vestibular nerve is behind the facial nerve and the inferior vestibular nerve is behind the cochlear nerve.

aspect of the pons, the view must be directed from lateral to medial above the internal auditory canal. The angles of view through the area of the petrousectomy can be increased if the cranium is approached at a higher level through a frontotemporal craniotomy combined with zygomatic arch resection.

Translabyrinthine approach

In the translabyrinthine approach, the internal acoustic meatus and cerebellopontine angle are approached through a mastoidectomy and labyrinthectomy (*Fig. 8.6*) (16, 29, 38) There are two goals of bone removal in this approach. The first is to expose the dura of Trautman's triangle on the posterior surface of the temporal bone facing the cerebellopontine angle. The second is to remove enough bone to be able to identify the nerves lateral to the tumor as they course through the internal auditory canal and by the transverse and vertical crests. The approach may also be combined with a retrosigmoid or a supra- and infratentorial presigmoid approach.

A retroauricular incision starts above the pinna and extends inferiorly to the mastoid tip (3). A flap of periosteum and soft tissues overlying the mastoid and retromastoid areas is elevated. The cortical bone over the mastoid is drilled away and the mastoid air cells are removed, exposing the mastoid antrum, the cortical bone around the labyrinth, and the digastric ridge leading anteriorly to the mastoid segment of the facial nerve as it exits the stylomastoid foramen and the sinodural angle. Drilling is continued to expose the semicircular canals and to skeletonize the sigmoid sinus, middle fossa dura, mastoid segment of the facial nerve, and the upper surface of the jugular bulb, leaving only a thin shell of bone over these

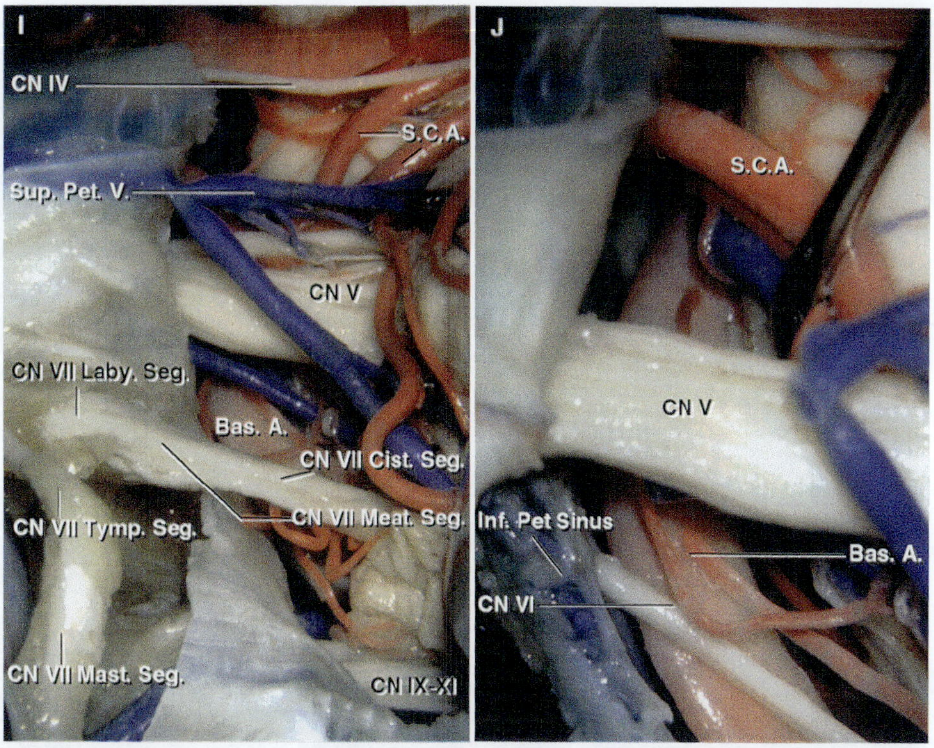

FIGURE 8.15. ***I* and *J*. Comparison of the retrosigmoid approach and the minimal mastoidectomy, retrolabyrinthine, translabyrinthine, and transcochlear approach modifications of the presigmoid approach. *I*, the labyrinthine, tympanic, and mastoid segments of the facial nerve have been exposed in preparation for the posterior transposition of the nerve needed to complete the transcochlear exposure. *J*, the facial nerve has been transposed and the cochlea and petrous apex removed to complete the transcochlear exposure of the anterior aspect of the brainstem and the basilar artery.**

structures. The lateral semicircular canal is the most laterally projecting canal and is the first one encountered by this approach. It provides a valuable landmark in identifying the tympanic segment of the facial nerve and the other canals. The nerve is found below the lateral canal. The retrofacial air cells are removed and the dome of the jugular bulb is identified inferiorly. In removing bone behind the internal acoustic meatus, it is important to remember that the jugular bulb may bulge upward behind the posterior semicircular canal or internal auditory meatus. The vestibular aqueduct and the endolymphatic sac may be opened and removed during the bone removal between the meatus and the jugular bulb. The cochlear canaliculus will be seen deep to the vestibular aqueduct as bone is removed in the area between the meatus and the jugular bulb. The lower end of the cochlear canaliculus is situated just above the area where the glossopharyngeal nerve enters the medial half of the jugular foramen. The labyrinthectomy portion of the procedure involves removing the semicircular canals and the vestibule to expose the dura lining the internal auditory canal. The lateral and posterior semicircular canals are drilled away. As the bone removal proceeds medially, the ampullae of the lateral and superior semicircular canals are exposed. At this point some bleeding can occur as the subarcuate artery is encountered in the bone near the center of the superior semicircular canal. The vestibule is an oval-shaped cavity located immediately lateral to the internal acoustic meatus, which forms the communication between the semicircular canals and the cochlea. Bone is removed medial and posterior to the vestibule, completely exposing it anterior and inferior to the facial nerve. Care is required to avoid injury to the facial nerve as it courses below the lateral canal and the ampullae of the posterior canal and around the superolateral margin of the vestibule.

The internal auditory canal is located medial and anterior to the tympanic segment of the facial nerve. The dura lining the internal canal is exposed by drilling away the semicircular canals and vestibule and the bone around the superior, posterior, and inferior margins of the internal canal. Further bone removal at the lateral end of the meatus exposes the transverse and vertical crests (*Fig. 8.2*). The intrameatal portion of the facial nerve is separated from the superior vestibular nerve at the lateral end of the canal by the vertical crest, also called Bill's bar, that can be used to positively identify the facial nerve (13, 16). The initial part of labyrinthine segment of the facial nerve, which lies just in front of the vertical crest, is exposed at the meatal fundus. After identifying the facial nerve, the dura lining the meatus is opened. The dural incision in Trautman's triangle is V-shaped with the apex of the "V" extending to the incision along the meatal dura. One limb of the "V" extends below the superior petrosal sinus and the other limb extends above the jugular bulb. The dural flap is then reflected posteriorly to expose the structures in the meatus and the cerebellopontine angle. The subarcuate artery, or the AICA, may be encountered in the dura of Trautman's triangle. Usually, the subarcuate artery arises from the AICA and passes through the dura on the upper posterior wall of the meatus as a fine stem. Occasionally, however, the subarcuate artery, along with its origin from the AICA, may be incorporated into the dura on the posterior face of the temporal bone. The approach may include transection of the external canal and obliteration of the middle ear with packing of the eustachian tube at closure.

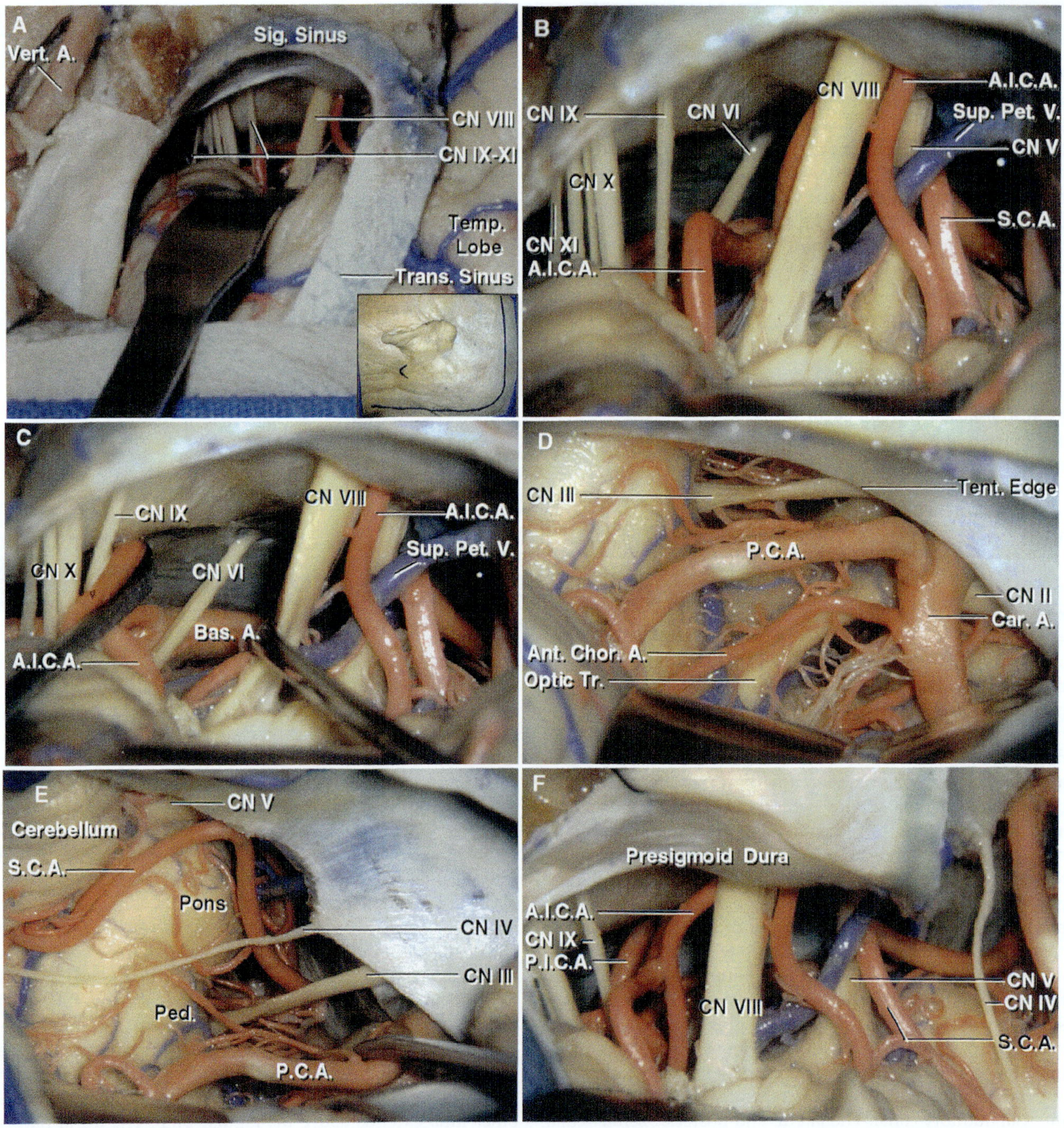

FIGURE 8.16. *A–F.* Comparison of the retrosigmoid and the various modifications of the presigmoid exposure. The modifications of the presigmoid approach include the minimal mastoidectomy, retrolabyrinthine, partial labyrinthine, translabyrinthine, modified transcochlear, and the full transcochlear approach with facial nerve transposition. *A*, the scalp incision (*insert*) is positioned for a supra- and infratentorial exposure through a temporo-occipital craniotomy. A temporo-occipital craniotomy has been completed and the dura opened to expose the temporal lobe and the retrosigmoid area. The transverse and sigmoid sinuses have been preserved. The cerebellum has been retracted to expose the nerves in the cerebellopontine angle. *B*, enlarged view of the retrosigmoid exposure to compare with the exposure obtained with the various modification of the presigmoid approach. *C*, in the retrosigmoid exposure the vestibulocochlear nerve has been elevated and the glossopharyngeal nerve depressed to expose the basilar artery at the origin of the AICA. *D*, subtemporal exposure. The temporal lobe has been elevated to expose the optic tract and oculomotor nerve and the PCA, internal carotid, and anterior choroidal arteries. *E*, the tentorium has been opened while preserving the trochlear nerve. The SCA courses below and the PCA above the

Transcochlear approach

The transcochlear approach is primarily an anteromedial extension of the translabyrinthine approach (*Fig. 8.6*) (3, 15, 16). It usually includes division and closure of the external canal, resection of at least the posterior part of the osseous external canal, and the tympanic membrane and ossicles, and obliteration of the eustachian tube. After exposing the dura lining the internal auditory canal, as described for the translabyrinthine approach, the incus is removed and the facial nerve is exposed from the geniculate ganglion to the stylomastoid foramen. The greater superficial petrosal nerve is transected and the facial nerve is transposed posteriorly. In the final stage, the bone removal is carried through the facial canal, after nerve transposition, and the cochlea and adjacent part of the petrous apex are drilled away (*Fig. 8.6*).

Medially, the bone removal extends to the edge of the clivus, exposing the inferior petrosal sinus from the jugular bulb below to the superior petrosal sinus above. The ascending portion of the petrous carotid is exposed at the anterior limit of the dissection. The bone removal, which now extends to the lateral edge of the clivus, could easily be carried medially into the clivus. Extending the dural opening in this area permits visualization of the abducent nerve medial to the internal acoustic meatus, the lower margin of the trigeminal nerve, the nerves entering the jugular foramen, a segment of the basilar artery, and the origin and initial segment of the AICA.

An alternative to transposing the facial nerve is to complete an extensive bone removal in the hypotympanic and retrofacial areas extending forward to the carotid canal, thus skeletonizing the mastoid segment of the facial nerve and leaving it suspended in a shell of bone, as described by Gantz and Fisch (7). In this approach, the external auditory canal is closed as a blind sac and the tympanic membrane, incus, and body of the malleus are removed (7). A mastoidectomy is performed, including the removal of the retrofacial, retrolabyrinthine, and supralabyrinthine compartments. The facial nerve is identified at its tympanic segment and at the stylomastoid foramen. The inferior part of the tympanic bone is removed to expose the infralabyrinthine compartment, the jugular bulb, and the intrapetrous carotid artery. The retrofacial dissection is carried medially and superiorly, removing the semicircular canals and vestibule. The dissection of the posterior fossa dura is carried inferiorly around the internal auditory canal and under the facial canal. The cochlea is drilled away by working inferior and anterior to the facial canal. The facial canal is then left as a bridge over the operative field and the dura is exposed between the carotid artery and the jugular bulb.

Combined supra- and infratentorial presigmoid approach

The presigmoid approach combines the supra- and infratentorial craniotomy centered on the mastoid and varying degrees of mastoid and labyrinthine resection (*Fig. 8.14*). The minimal degree of mastoid resection, which we refer to as a minimal mastoidectomy, exposes only enough of the presigmoid dura to open the dura in front of the sigmoid sinus for exposure of the cerebellopontine angle (*Figs. 8.15* and *8.16*). The next more extensive degree of mastoid resection, the retrolabyrinthine modification, is a more complete mastoidectomy exposing the bony capsule of the semicircular canals and skeletonizing at least a portion of the facial nerve. In the partial labyrinthectomy, one or two of the semicircular canals, commonly the superior and/or posterior canals, are resected with preservation of the lateral canal. Removal of these canals may, but not always, be associated with the loss of hearing (37). The posterior canal may be removed to increase access to the posterior fossa, and removing the superior canal alone gives a more direct access to the petrous apex along the middle fossa. The next more extensive modification is the translabyrinthine approach, in which the semicircular canals and vestibule are resected uniformly, resulting in the loss of hearing. The translabyrinthine approach provides excellent access to the internal auditory canal. The next more extensive modification is the transcochlear approach, in which the cochlea located anteromedial to the fundus of the meatus is removed, thus providing access to the medial part of the petrous apex and the side of the clivus. Another modification, which we call the extended translabyrinthine approach, and is similar to the transcochlear approach, involves drilling bone both anterior and posterior to the facial nerve, leaving the facial nerve skeletonized in a column of bone and working both anterior and posterior to the facial nerve to remove the cochlea and access the side of the clivus. Gaining access for drilling the cochlea anterior to the facial nerve commonly requires that at least part of the posterior part of the external canal be removed, that the tympanic cavity be obliterated, and that the internal carotid artery be exposed below the promontory.

In evaluating these approaches in our laboratory, we have found that the minimal mastoidectomy gives approximately

oculomotor and trochlear nerves. *F*, minimal mastoidectomy modification of the presigmoid approach. The minimal mastoidectomy approach is completed by removing only enough bone in the front of the sigmoid sinus so that the presigmoid dura can be opened to expose the posterior cranial fossa. The bony capsule of the labyrinth is not exposed in the minimal mastoidectomy as it is in the retrolabyrinthine approach. The exposure shown with the minimal mastoidectomy in this figure is to be compared with the retrosigmoid exposure shown in *B*. *A.*, artery; *Ac.*, acoustic; *A.I.C.A.*, anteroinferior cerebellar artery; *Ant.*, anterior; *Bas.*, basilar; *Car.*, carotid; *Chor.*, choroidal; *CN*, cranial nerve; *Comm.*, communicating; *Inf.*, inferior; *Int.*, internal; *Lat.*, lateral; *Mast.*, mastoid; *P.C.A.*, posterior cerebral artery; *Ped.*, peduncle; *Pet.*, petrosal; *P.I.C.A.*, posteroinferior cerebellar artery; *Post.*, posterior; *S.C.A.*, superior cerebellar artery; *Seg.*, segment; *Sig.*, sigmoid; *Sup.*, superior; *Temp.*, temporal; *Tent.*, tentorial; *Tr.*, trunk; *Trans.*, transverse; *V.*, vein; *Vert.*, vertebral.

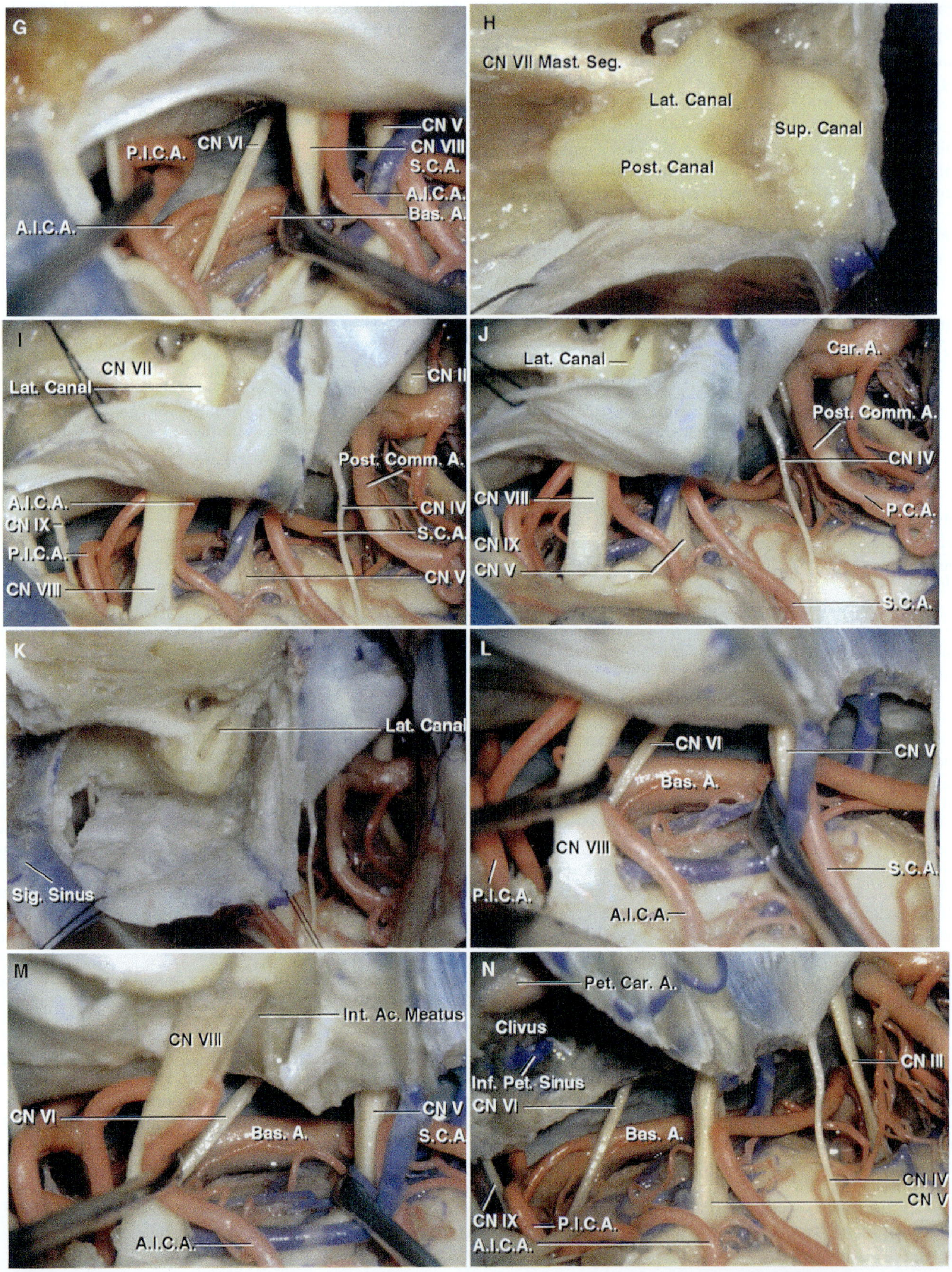
G
CN V
P.I.C.A.
CN VI
CN VIII
S.C.A.
A.I.C.A.
Bas. A.
A.I.C.A.
H
CN VII Mast. Seg.
Lat. Canal
Sup. Canal
Post. Canal
I
CN VII
Lat. Canal
CN II
Post. Comm. A.
A.I.C.A.
CN IV
CN IX
S.C.A.
P.I.C.A.
CN V
CN VIII
J
Lat. Canal
Car. A.
Post. Comm. A.
CN IV
CN VIII
P.C.A.
CN IX
CN V
S.C.A.
K
Lat. Canal
Sig. Sinus
L
CN VI
CN V
Bas. A.
CN VIII
S.C.A.
P.I.C.A.
A.I.C.A.
M
Int. Ac. Meatus
CN VIII
CN VI
CN V
Bas. A.
S.C.A.
A.I.C.A.
N
Pet. Car. A.
Clivus
CN III
Inf. Pet. Sinus
CN VI
Bas. A.
CN IV
CN V
CN IX
P.I.C.A.
A.I.C.A.

the same exposure as the retrolabyrinthine approach, but is done at reduced risk since the semicircular canals and facial nerve are not skeletonized (*Figs. 8.14* and *8.15*). Removing the posterior canal increases access to the posterior fossa, but access is only slightly increased over that achieved with the retrolabyrinthine approach. Removing the superior canal increases access to the middle fossa and petrous apex and reduces the needed retraction of the temporal lobe. The translabyrinthine approach does not significantly increase the access to the area medial to the porus of the internal acoustic meatus over that achieved with the minimal mastoidectomy or retrolabyrinthine approach, but does provide access to the internal auditory canal. The transcochlear modification, in which bone is removed up to the edge of the clivus, does significantly increase access to the front of the brainstem and clivus over that achieved with the lesser degrees of bony resection. The retrosigmoid, the presigmoid minimal mastoidectomy, and the retrolabyrinthine approaches were compared and yielded nearly the same exposure of the cerebellopontine angle, but the retrosigmoid approach did not provide the additional exposure of the middle fossa and petrous apex that could be achieved in the combined supra- and infratentorial presigmoid approach.

The skin incision is started in the temporal region above the zygoma, and extends above the ear and downward in the suboccipital area medial to the mastoid process (*Figs. 8.14, 8.15,* and *8.17*). The skin flap is reflected forward to the level of the external auditory canal. The temporal muscle is elevated and reflected anteriorly, and the muscles over the mastoid and suboccipital areas are swept inferiorly. A temporo-occipital craniotomy is performed and the transverse sinus is exposed. After the bone flap is elevated, a mastoidectomy is carried out without entering the labyrinth. The sigmoid sinus is skeletonized from the sinodural angle to the jugular bulb. Bone is removed superiorly to expose the floor of the middle fossa and the superior petrosal sinus. Trautman's triangle is exposed in the area lateral to the otic capsule.

The dura mater is then incised along the base of the temporal craniotomy, while preserving the junction of the vein of Labbé with the transverse sinus. The posterior fossa dura is opened anterior to the sigmoid sinus in Trautman's triangle. The dural incision is extended across the superior petrosal sinus to join the dural incision in the temporal dura. After division of the superior petrosal sinus, the tentorium is incised parallel to and just behind the petrous ridge and superior petrosal sinus. This dural incision is extended from the site of division of the superior petrosal sinus through the medial edge of the tentorium to the incisura behind where the trochlear nerve enters the tentorial edge. Care is taken to avoid injury to the IVth cranial nerve in its course near the tentorial margin. The posterior portion of the temporal lobe is elevated and the sigmoid sinus is displaced posteriorly along with the cerebellar hemisphere while preserving the junction of the vein of Labbé with the sigmoid sinus. The sigmoid sinus limits the ability for superior retraction of the temporal lobe and can be ligated to improve the exposure if bilateral venous angiography show adequate communication through the torcular to the opposite side (24). The petroclival region can be exposed from the middle fossa and tentorial incisura to near the foramen magnum, although access to the lower petroclival region may be limited by the jugular bulb. The presigmoid exposure provides a shorter working distance to the petroclival area and provides multiple angles for dissection. The major arteries in the posterior fossa are easily accessible. The exposure can also be combined with a far-lateral approach (*Fig. 8.17*).

Subtemporal preauricular infratemporal fossa approach

The subtemporal preauricular infratemporal approach is directed through the infratemporal and middle fossae to the part of the anterior surface of the petrous bone located medial to the cochlea and to the petroclival region (*Figs. 8.10, 8.13,* and *8.18*). This description outlines the full extent of the anatomic exposure available through this approach, but it can often be tailored to a smaller, more limited, approach. A curvilinear incision starting in the frontal region turns downward in front of the ear into the cervical region. The incision

FIGURE 8.16. *G–N.* Comparison of the retrosigmoid and the various modifications of the presigmoid exposure. *G,* deep exposure with the minimal mastoidectomy with retraction of the vestibulocochlear and glossopharyngeal nerves, to be compared with the retrosigmoid approach shown in *C.* The exposure is similar to that obtained with the retrosigmoid approach. *H,* retrolabyrinthine approach in which more extensive drilling of the mastoid has been completed to expose the osseous capsule of the semicircular canals. *I,* the dura has been folded forward after completing the retrolabyrinthine exposure. The exposure differs little from that obtained with the minimal mastoidectomy exposure shown in *F* and *G. J,* the exposure with the posterior canal partial labyrinthectomy is similar to that achieved with the minimal mastoidectomy. *K,* the partial labyrinthectomy has been extended by removing the superior canal in addition to removal of the posterior canal. *L,* the infratentorial exposure does not differ significantly from that achieved with the minimal mastoidectomy, as shown in *F* and *G.* Removal of the superior canal reduces the required temporal lobe retraction and aids in the exposure along the middle fossa floor and petrous apex. *M,* translabyrinthine exposure in which the semicircular canals and the vestibule have been removed. This adds the internal auditory canal to the exposure, but does not improve the exposure of the structures medial to the meatus, as compared with the minimal mastoidectomy or even the retrosigmoid approach. *N,* the facial nerve has been transposed posteriorly out of the field and the cochlea has been removed to complete the transcochlear approach. This approach greatly improves access to the front of the brainstem, clivus, and basilar artery, but is done at the cost of a temporary or permanent facial paralysis and loss of hearing.

may be extended downward only to the area just below the tragus if only the petrous apex and upper part of the infratemporal fossa are to be exposed, but it can be extended onto the upper neck if a neck dissection is needed. The skin flap is separated from the underlying tissues and reflected forward. The facial nerve and its major branches are identified distal to the stylomastoid foramen and followed to the parotid gland. The parotid gland is separated from the masseteric fascia to avoid excessive stretching of the facial nerve at the stylomastoid foramen (33, 38, 39). The superficial temporalis fascia in which the upper facial branches course is separated from the temporalis muscle and is reflected forward to prevent damage to the branch of the facial nerve to the frontalis muscle as the zygomatic arch is exposed. The zygomatic arch is divided at its anterior and posterior ends, and the temporalis muscle, with the overlying segment of the zygomatic arch, is reflected downward. The mandibular condyle and the capsule of the temporomandibular joint are either dislocated downward or excised. The temporomandibular joint can be removed in a single piece for later replacement by dividing the mandibular neck below the condyle and osteotomizing the middle fossa floor around the mandibular fossa (*Fig. 8.18*). The internal carotid artery, the internal jugular vein, and the vagus, accessory, and hypoglossal nerves may be exposed in the neck if needed. The posterior belly of the digastric muscle may be divided and the styloid process resected.

A frontotemporal craniotomy is then performed. The dura is elevated from the floor of the middle fossa to expose and obliterate the middle meningeal artery at the foramen spinosum and to expose the arcuate eminence, the third trigeminal division at the foramen ovale, and the greater petrosal nerve. The greater petrosal nerve is transected if necessary to avoid traction on the facial nerve. The floor of the middle fossa, including the lateral and inferior aspects of the superior orbital fissure, and the lateral margin of the foramina ovale may be removed to expose the structures in the infratemporal fossa.

If needed, bone can be removed medial to the mandibular fossa to expose the eustachian tube and the tensor tympani muscle, both of which may be resected (*Figs. 8.10*, *8.13*, and *8.18*). The bone removal is continued inferiorly, exposing the ascending portion of the petrous carotid. In this segment, the carotid artery is surrounded by a periosteal sheath, which encloses a periarterial venous plexus that is an extension of the cavernous sinus. At the entrance of the carotid canal, a dense fibrocartilaginous ring encircles the artery. If mobilization of the artery is required, care must be taken when dividing the ring not to damage the IXth cranial nerve that is in close proximity to the carotid canal as it exits the jugular foramen. After mobilizing the carotid artery and displacing it forward, the petrous apex and the clival region to the level of the foramen magnum can be approached medial to and behind the artery. During drilling, the very hard cortical bone along the petrous apex gives place to a crumbly cancellous bone in the region of the clivus, as the dura of the anterior and lateral aspects of the posterior fossa is being exposed. The area exposed is limited by Meckel's cave superiorly, by the cochlea and internal auditory canal laterally, by the abducens nerve in its course through the Dorello's canal medially, and by the hypoglossal canal inferiorly. If the dura is opened, the structures along the lateral and anterior aspects of the upper medulla and lower two-thirds of the pons will be exposed (41). The tentorium can be divided to give access to the upper clival region.

Dividing the third trigeminal division above the foramen ovale will permit exposure of the junction of the petrous and cavernous carotid along with the structures in the inferolateral portion of the cavernous sinus (17, 39). The pterygopalatine fossa, parapharyngeal space, lateral maxilla, and orbit can be exposed farther anteriorly. The lateral aspect of the sphenoid bone and the sphenoid sinus can also be approached by removing bone medial to the maxillary nerve at the root of the pterygoid process.

Postauricular transtemporal approach

The postauricular transtemporal approach is most commonly selected for lesions that involve the mastoid and tympanic cavities and track along the nerves and arteries to reach the middle and infratemporal fossa (*Figs. 8.19* and *8.20*). It can, however, be tailored at its posterior margin to include a retrosigmoid, far-lateral, or presigmoid exposure of the posterior fossa or, at its anterior limits, to include exposure of the pterygopalatine fossa and lateral parts of the maxillary orbit or anterior cranial fossa.

A question mark incision is started behind the hairline in the temporal region, extending behind the ear over the mastoid process and continuing inferiorly in front of the sternocleidomastoid muscle onto the neck. The skin flap is then reflected forward and the external auditory canal is divided at the bone-cartilage junction and closed as a blind sac. The sternocleidomastoid muscle is detached from the mastoid process and reflected inferiorly. The periosteum and posterior portion of the temporalis muscle are reflected anteriorly, thus exposing the temporal, mastoid, and retromastoid areas. The posterior belly of the digastric muscle is divided and reflected inferiorly. At this point, the facial nerve is identified distal to the stylomastoid foramen and is followed, along with its major branches, into the substance of the parotid gland (5). The internal jugular vein, the carotid bifurcation, and the glossopharyngeal, vagus, accessory, and hypoglossal nerves are exposed and isolated in the neck. This allows for proximal control of the internal carotid artery and ligation of the main feeding vessels from the external carotid artery to a neoplasm early in the procedure.

After this, temporal and/or retromastoid craniotomies may be performed with a simple mastoidectomy. The remaining skin of the external auditory canal, the tympanic membrane, the malleus, incus, and stapes arch (leaving the footplate) are removed. The facial nerve is completely skeletonized from the geniculate ganglion to the stylomastoid foramen.

If exposure of the jugular foramen and lower clival region is desired, a new facial canal is created by drilling a groove in the bone of the anterior attic wall, between the geniculate ganglion and the root of the zygoma. The facial nerve is carefully freed at the stylomastoid foramen, while leaving some of the surrounding connective tissue attached to the

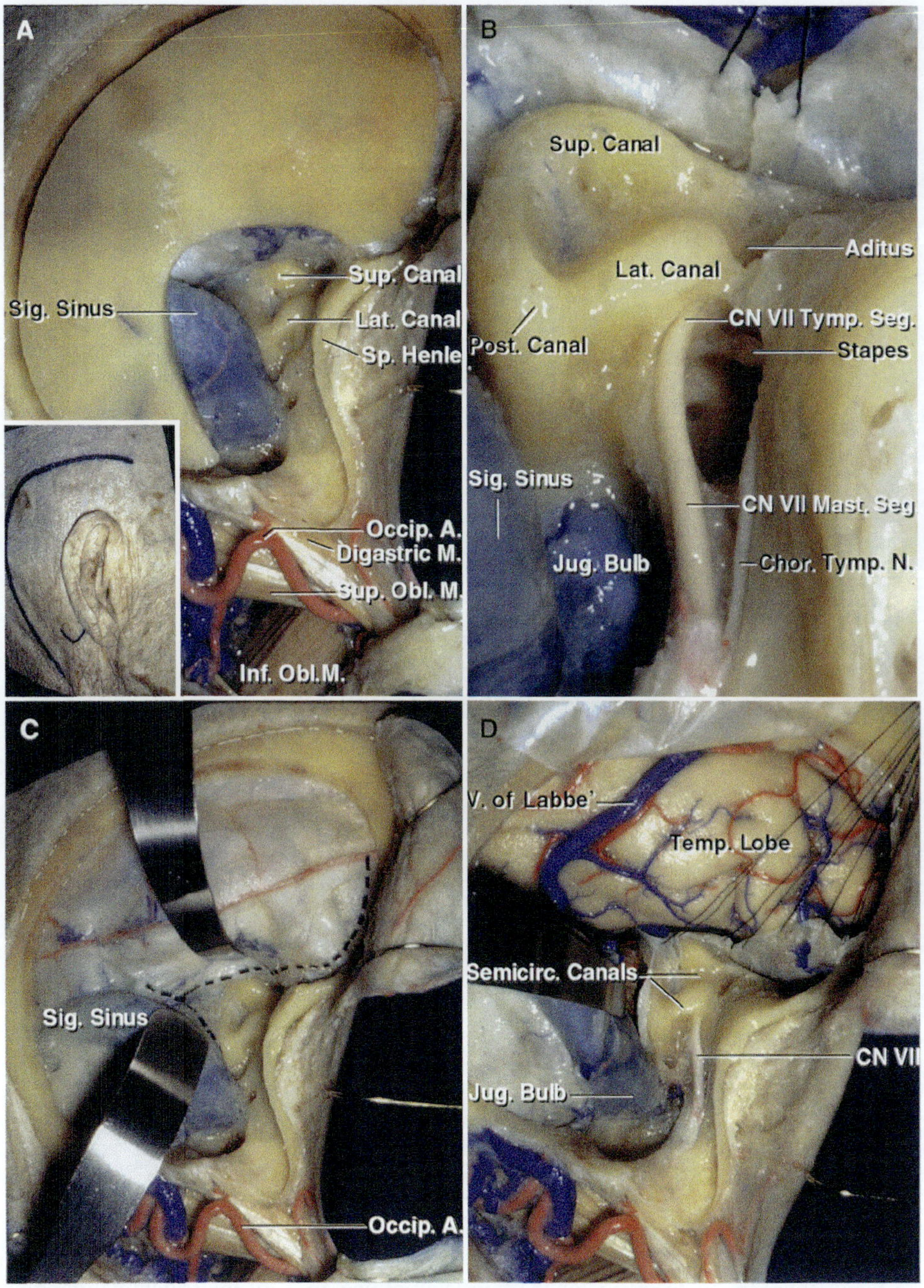

FIGURE 8.17. *A–D.* Combined presigmoid and far-lateral approach. *A*, the *insert* shows the site of the scalp incision and mastoid tip. The scalp flap has been reflected forward. The mastoidectomy exposes the dense cortical bone housing the semicircular canals. The bone flap is *outlined.* The occipital artery courses backward between the digastric and superior oblique. *B*, enlarged view. The tympanic segment of the facial nerve courses below the lateral canal. The chorda tympani arises from the mastoid segment of the facial nerve. The mastoid antrum, which has been drilled away, opens through the aditus into the epitympanic part of the tympanic cavity. *C*, the presigmoid and temporal dural incisions have been *outlined. D*, the temporal and presigmoid dura has been opened. One goal of the procedure is to preserve the vein of Labbé, which empties into the transverse sinus. *A.*, artery; *A.I.C.A.*, anteroinferior cerebellar artery; *Atl-Occip.*, atlanto-occipital; *Cap.*, capitis; *Car.*, carotid; *Chor.*, chorda; *Cist.*, cisternal; *CN*, cranial nerve; *Epitymp.*, epitympanic; *For.*, foramen; *Gang.*, ganglion; *Genic.*, geniculate; *Hypogl.*, hypoglossal; *Inf.*, inferior; *Jug.*, jugular; *Laby.*, labyrinthine; *Lat.*, lateral; *Lev.*, levator; *M.*, muscle; *Meat.*, meatal; *Memb.*, membrane; *Men.*, meningeal; *N.*, nerve; *Obl.*, oblique; *Occip.*, occipital; *P.C.A.*, posterior cerebral artery; *P.I.C.A.*, posteroinferior cerebellar artery; *Plex.*, plexus; *Post.*, posterior; *Rec.*, rectus; *S.C.A.*, superior cerebellar artery; *Scap.*, scapula; *Seg.*, segment; *Semicirc.*, semicircular; *Sig.*, sigmoid; *Sp.*, spine; *Suboccip.*, suboccipital; *Sup.*, superior; *Temp.*, temporal; *Trans.*, transverse; *Tymp.*, tympani, tympanic; *V.*, vein; *Vert.*, vertebral; *Vest.*, vestibular.

nerve, and the nerve is transposed anteriorly into the new bony groove of the epitympanum and imbedded for its protection into the parotid tissue (5).

The dura of the middle fossa and the sigmoid sinus from the sinodural angle to the jugular bulb is skeletonized. Then the sigmoid sinus and the jugular vein are ligated in this sequence, and the sigmoid sinus divided. Part of the wall of the sinus, bulb, and/or vein may be excised to increase the exposure. This allows for dissection of the lower cranial nerves at the jugular foramen, as well as for their mobilization and posterior displacement if necessary. The posterior mobilization of the lower cranial nerves allows for a direct exposure of the structures along the lateral and anterior aspects of the medulla and lower pons without the necessity for brain retraction. Dissection in the area of the jugular foramen has proven to be extremely difficult, as the lower cranial nerves are particularly fragile and difficult to isolate from the surrounding tissues.

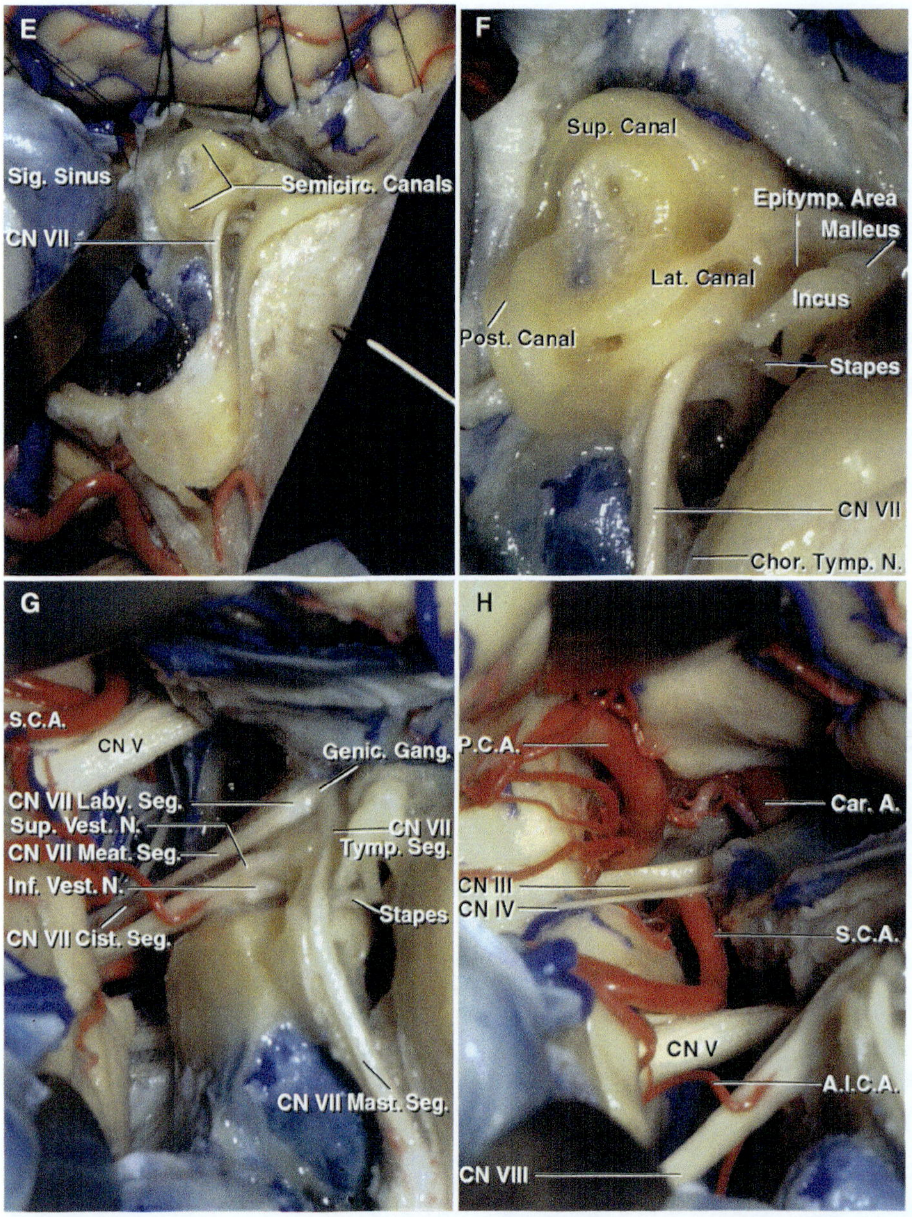

FIGURE 8.17. *E–H.* **Combined presigmoid and far-lateral approach.** *E,* **the dural incision has been extended through Trautman's triangle and across the superior petrosal sinus and tentorium, taking care to preserve the vein of Labbé and the trochlear nerve. The semicircular canals have been opened.** *F,* **enlarged view. The posterior canal faces the posterior fossa lateral to the internal acoustic meatus. The superior canal projects upward, below the arcuate eminence, toward the floor of the middle fossa. The lateral canal is a useful landmark for identifying the tympanic segment of the facial nerve, which courses between the canal and the stapes sitting in the oval window. The epitympanic area opens through the aditus into the mastoid antrum.** *G,* **the labyrinthectomy has been completed and the dura lining the meatus opened to expose the cisternal, meatal, labyrinthine, tympanic, and mastoid segments of the facial nerve. The SCA courses above the trigeminal nerve.** *H,* **enlarged view along the opened tentorial incisura. The oculomotor and trochlear nerves course between the PCA and SCA. The SCA rests against the upper surface of the trigeminal nerve.**

Exposure of the middle clival structures requires removal of the bony labyrinth, as described for the translabyrinthine approach. The internal auditory canal is exposed, the facial nerve identified, and the cochlear and vestibular nerves divided. The greater superficial petrosal nerve is sectioned at its origin from the geniculate ganglion. The facial nerve is freed from all its attachments in the temporal bone and reflected posteriorly. The bony portion of the external auditory canal and the tympanic bone are drilled away, exposing the ascending portion of the intrapetrous carotid artery medial to the eustachian tube.

The dissection is continued by drilling away the cochlea, starting at its basal turn, to expose part of the horizontal segment of the petrous carotid artery. Anterior displacement of the carotid artery and removal of the cochlea provides a wide exposure of the lateral and anterior portions of the pons and medulla. This exposure extends from the inferior aspect of the trigeminal ganglion to the foramen magnum. The exposure may be carried medially into the clivus and retropharyngeal space and anteriorly to expose the mucosa of the sphenoid sinus.

If the approach is to be extended to the parasellar and parasphenoidal areas, the zygomatic arch is divided and reflected inferiorly with the masseter muscle. The temporalis muscle is separated from its attachment to the coronoid process of the mandible and reflected anteriorly and superiorly. A temporal craniotomy is then performed, and extensive bone is removed along the whole lateral aspect of the middle cranial fossa. The ascending ramus of the mandible is either displaced anteriorly or resected, and the petrous carotid is exposed distally to the proximal portion of the intracavernous

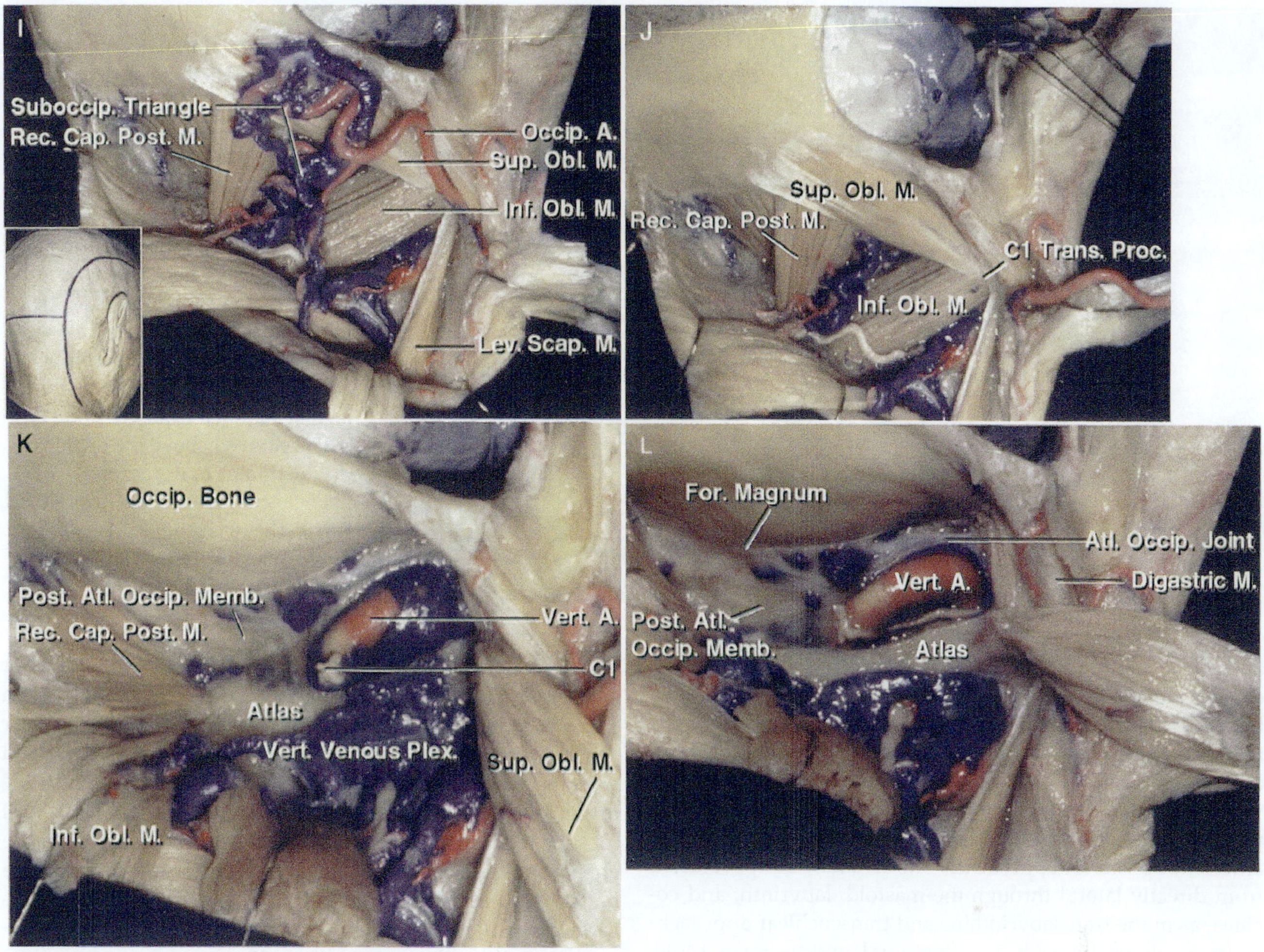

FIGURE 8.17. ***I–L.*** **Combined presigmoid and far-lateral approach.** ***I,*** **the** ***insert*** **shows the site of the additional skin incision needed to add a retrosigmoid craniotomy and far-lateral approach. The scalp flap has been reflected to expose the suboccipital triangle located between the superior and inferior oblique and the rectus capitis posterior major and in the depths of which the vertebral artery courses with a dense venous plexus.** ***J,*** **the venous plexus has been removed to expose the margins of the suboccipital triangle.** ***K,*** **the rectus capitis posterior major and the inferior oblique have been reflected medially and the superior oblique laterally to expose the vertebral artery and surrounding venous plexus behind the atlanto-occipital joint.** ***L,*** **the venous plexus has been removed to expose the vertebral artery coursing with the C1 nerve behind the atlanto-occipital joint and across the upper edge of the posterior atlantal arch.**

segment after removing the cartilaginous portion of the eustachian tube. The cavernous sinus can be approached and the intracavernous carotid artery exposed by dividing the mandibular segment of the trigeminal nerve. The approach can also be extended to the retrosigmoid area and down the vertebral artery to the C1 to C2 level, or to the suboccipital triangle for a far-lateral or transcondylar exposure. The lateral orbit and pterygopalatine fossa can be accessed at the anterior limit of the exposure.

DISCUSSION

Pathologies can arise anywhere within the petroclival region and frequently are not restricted to a single anatomic compartment of the cranial base. Involvement of multiple cranial nerves and arteries occurs because cranial base tumors tend to achieve considerable size before producing clinical manifestation (32). The distinction between the benign or malignant tumors in this area is not rigid because many benign tumors can have a very invasive characteristic. The selection of the best surgical approach depends on the location, extension, size, and nature of the pathology.

An advantage of these approaches directed through the temporal bone to the petroclival area is that they reach the area through tissue planes outside the oropharynx. They provide another route by which anterior intradural lesions situated medial to the nerves entering the internal acoustic meatus and jugular foramen can be approached without entering the nasopharynx. They also provide an avenue of exposure for lesions that involve the temporal and sphenoid bones in addition to the clivus. One or a combination of the lateral

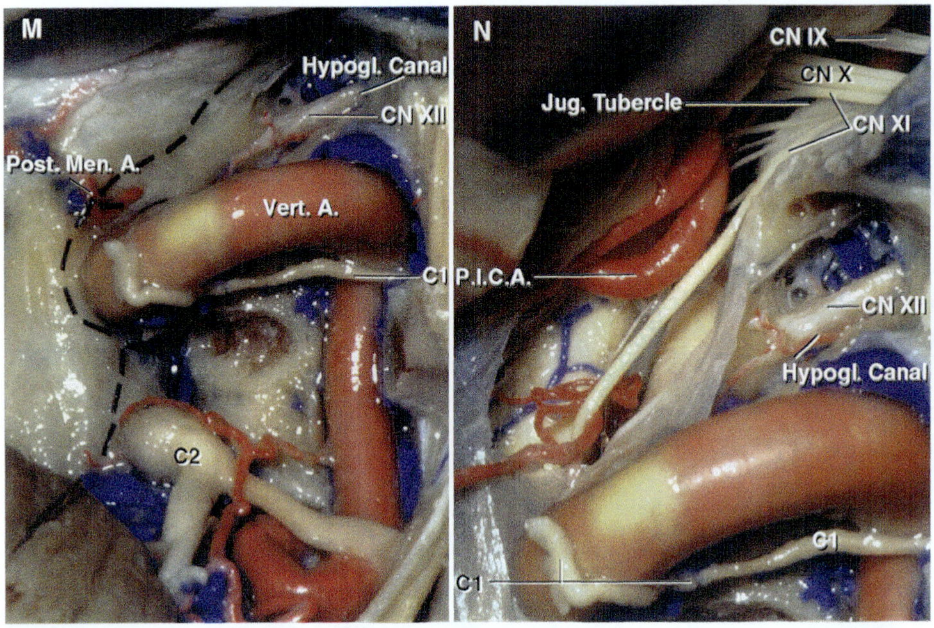

FIGURE 8.17. *M* **and** *N***, combined presigmoid and far-lateral approach.** *M***, a suboccipital craniotomy has been completed, the posterior arch and posterior ramus of the transverse process of the atlas removed, and the dural incision has been** *outlined***. The posterior meningeal artery arises before the vertebral artery penetrates the dura. The C1 nerve root adheres to the lower margin of the vertebral artery.** *N***, the dura has been opened and the nerves passing toward the jugular foramen exposed. Bone has been removed above the atlanto-occipital joint to expose the hypoglossal nerve in the hypoglossal canal. The accessory rootlets cross the jugular tubercle on their way to the jugular foramen.**

approaches is frequently used to expose intra- or extradural clival lesions that also involve the temporal and sphenoid bones. They also provide access to the anterior aspect of the midbrain, pons, and medulla and to the cerebellopontine angle and nerves in the posterior fossa. They may also provide better access to the temporal bone, jugular foramen, and petrous segment of the internal carotid artery than the other anterior or posterior approaches. The area may be approached from directly lateral through the mastoid, labyrinth, and cochlea, as in the translabyrinthine and transcochlear approaches; from above through a subtemporal middle fossa route; from behind in the retrosigmoid suboccipital approach; or from multiple directions using such combined supra- and infratentorial approaches as the presigmoid approach, to which a translabyrinthine or transcochlear approach may be added. Alternative or extended approaches, most of which include some route through the mastoid and petrous parts, include the anterior transpetrosal, the subtemporal preauricular infratemporal, and the far-lateral transcondylar approach.

The retrosigmoid suboccipital approach, described in the chapter on the cerebellopontine angle, offers a wide view of the cerebellopontine angle and of the intradural structures behind the ipsilateral lower clivus, but the dural surface of the petrous apex, upper clivus, and tentorial incisura are not well seen from this exposure (26, 35, 36, 46) (*Figs. 8.15* and *8.16*). Removal of posterior wall of the internal auditory canal through the retrosigmoid provides access to the contents of the meatus as far lateral as the vertical and transverse crests. The vestibule can be opened if needed to remove a tumor extending into the labyrinth. Care is required to avoid injury to the posterior semicircular canal and common crus if there is the possibility of preserving hearing (29). The retrosigmoid approach provides easy access to the intradural part of cranial nerves V, VII, VIII, and IX through XII. It also provides access to the nerve-related segments of the arteries of the posterior circulation. The vertebrobasilar junction can be exposed in some cases, although the lower cranial nerves and the jugular tubercle are frequent obstacles. Retraction of the pons and working between the cranial nerves is necessary to reach the origin of the AICA from the basilar artery. The far lateral modification of the retrosigmoid approach, described in the chapter on the far lateral approach, was devised to provide a better exposure of the lateral and anterior aspects of the cervicomedullary junction (45).

The presigmoid approach (1, 8, 32) combines a supra- and infratentorial exposure with various degrees of petrousectomy, while preserving the junction of the vein of Labbé with the transverse sinus (*Figs. 8.14-8.17*). The amount of resection of the petrous bone can vary from a retrolabyrinthine minimal mastoidectomy exposure to a translabyrinthine or transcochlear exposure with posterior displacement of the facial nerve. In selected cases, where angiography shows patency of the communication between the two transverse sinuses across the midline, the sigmoid sinus can be ligated to improve the exposure (24). Preservation of the drainage of the vein of Labbé and avoidance of excessive temporal lobe retraction are major goals of this approach to the upper clival region. Approaching the structures in the inferior petroclival space may be restricted by the jugular bulb, which could be overcome by division of the sigmoid sinus or by working posterior to it (36). The major advantages of this approach are the shorter working distance to clival lesions and the various angles for dissection that are provided. The approach provides access to the ipsilateral cranial nerves III through XII and to the major arteries in the posterior circulation. A major drawback to this exposure is provided by the anatomic variants, described below, that limit the size of the exposure through Trautman's triangle and the labyrinth.

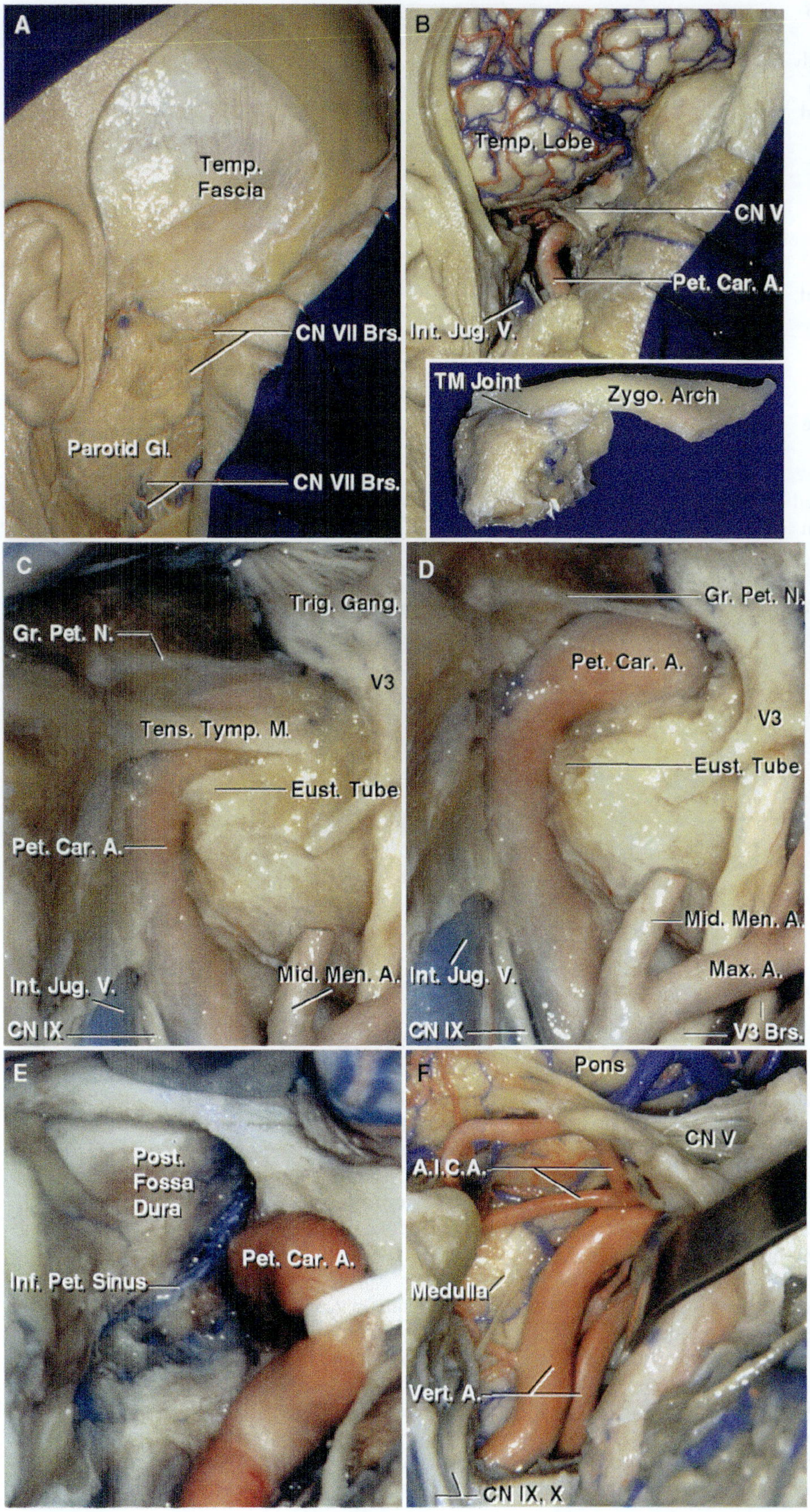

FIGURE 8.18. Preauricular subtemporal-infratemporal fossa approach. *A*, the scalp incision is positioned so that a frontotemporal craniotomy can be completed. The operation is often completed with an incision that extends downward only to the level of the tragus. However, it can be extended if a neck dissection is needed. The scalp flap has been reflected forward, taking care to protect the branches of the facial nerve. *B*, the temporalis muscle has been refracted forward and the craniotomy completed. The mandibular condyle and fossa and a portion of the zygomatic arch were removed in a single piece, as shown in the *insert,* and the middle fossa floor removed. *C*, exposure after removal of the middle fossa floor lateral to the foramen ovale and before resection of the tensor tympani muscle. The lower orifice of the carotid canal is located in front of the jugular foramen. The eustachian tube, which passes across the front of the petrous carotid, has been opened. *D*, the tensor tympani and eustachian tube have been resected to expose the horizontal segment of the petrous carotid. *E*, the internal carotid artery has been reflected forward and the petrous apex drilled to expose the posterior fossa dura and the inferior petrosal sinus coursing along the petroclival fissure. *F*, the dura facing the petrous apex has been opened and the vertebral arteries and AICA exposed. This exposure is directed through the petrous apex medial to the cochlea and jugular foramen and does not risk loss of facial nerve function or hearing, as do the approaches directed through the petrous apex that require facial nerve transposition and resection of the labyrinth. *A.*, artery; *A.I.C.A.*, anteroinferior cerebellar artery; *Brs.*, branches; *Car.*, carotid; *CN*, cranial nerve; *Eust.*, eustachian; *Gang.*, ganglion; *Gl.*, gland; *Gr.*, greater; *Inf.*, inferior; *Int.*, internal; *Jug.*, jugular; *M.*, muscle; *Max.*, maxillary; *Men.*, meningeal; *Mid.*, middle; *N.*, nerve; *Pet.*, petrosal, petrous; *Post.*, posterior; *Temp.*, temporal; *Tens.*, tensor; *TM.*, temporomandibular; *Trig.*, trigeminal; *Tymp.*, tympani; *V.*, vein; *Vert.*, vertebral; *Zygo.*, zygomatic.

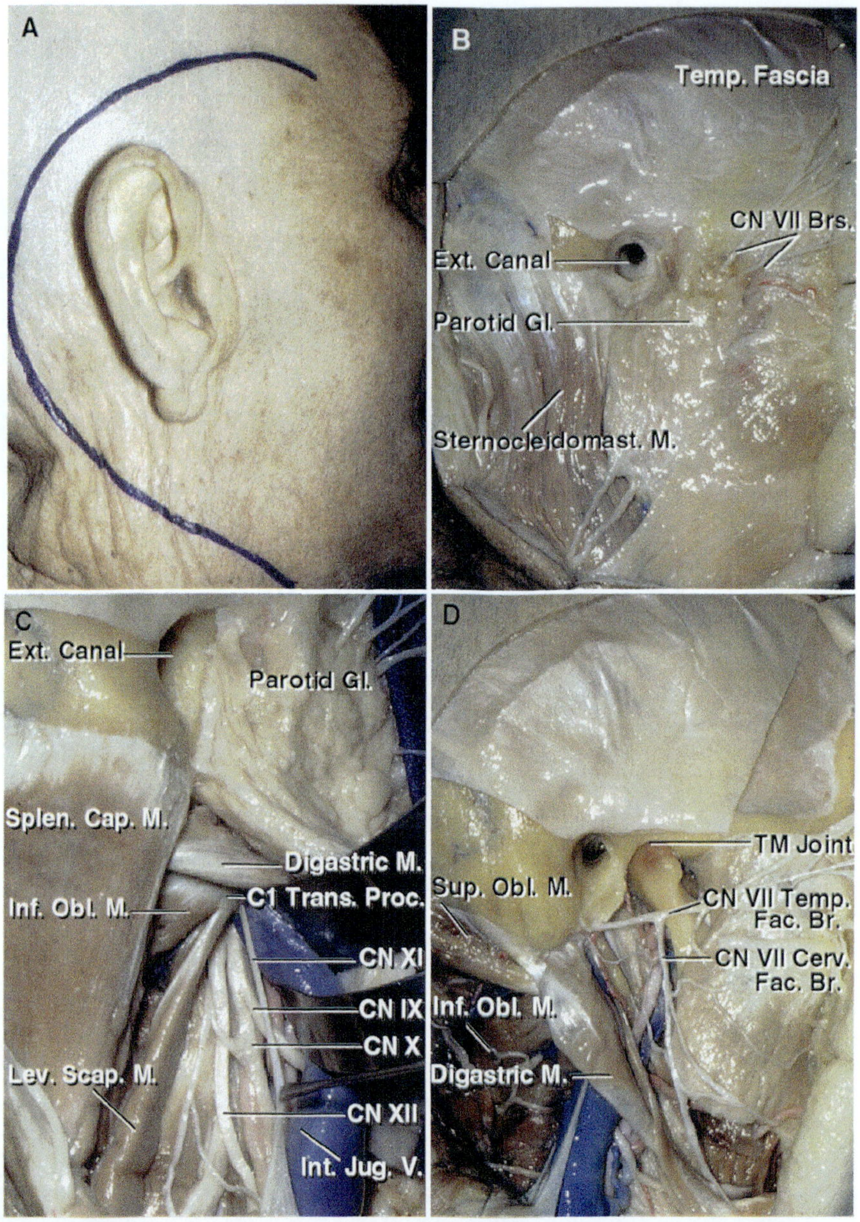

FIGURE 8.19. *A–D.* Anatomic basis of the postauricular transtemporal approach. *A*, the incision sweeps widely around the posterior margin of the ear so that a retrosigmoid, presigmoid, and far-lateral exposure can be obtained behind the ear, and a subtemporal, infratemporal, pterygopalatine, and orbital exposure can be obtained in front of the ear. *B*, the scalp flap has been reflected forward, the external canal transected, and the parotid gland and superficial branches of the facial nerve exposed. *C*, the sternocleidomastoid muscle has been reflected. The neck dissection exposes the internal jugular vein, C1 transverse process, and the glossopharyngeal, vagus, accessory, and hypoglossal nerves. The accessory nerve is retracted forward. *D*, the parotid gland has been removed to expose the temporofacial and cervicofacial trunks of the facial nerve and the temporomandibular joint. The splenius capitis muscle has been reflected downward to expose the superior and inferior oblique muscles, which insert on the transverse process of C1 and border the suboccipital triangle in which the vertebral artery courses. *A.*, artery; *Alv.*, alveolar; *Aur.*, auricular; *Br.*, branch; *Brs.*, branches; *Cap.*, capitis; *Car.*, carotid; *Cerv.*, cervical; *Chor.*, chorda, choroid; *CN*, cranial nerve; *Coch.*, cochlear; *Cond.*, condyle; *Endolymph.*, endolymphatic; *Eust.*, eustachian; *Ext.*, external; *Fac.*, facial; *Gang.*, ganglion; *Genic.*, geniculate; *Gl.*, gland; *Gr.*, greater; *Hypogl.*, hypoglossal; *Inf.*, inferior; *Infraorb.*, infraorbital; *Infratemp.*, infratemporal; *Int.*, internal; *Jug.*, jugular; *Laby.*, labyrinthine; *Lat.*, lateral; *Lev.*, levator; *M.*, muscle; *Mandib.*, mandibular; *Mast.*, mastoid; *Max.*, maxillary; *Med.*, medial; *N.*, nerve; *Obl.*, oblique; *Occip.*, occipital; *Pal.*, palatini; *P.C.A.*, posterior cerebral artery; *Ped.*, peduncle; *Pet.*, petrosal, petrous; *P.I.C.A.*, posteroinferior cerebellar artery; *Plex.*, plexus; *Post.*, posterior; *Proc.*, process; *Pteryg.*, pterygoid; *Pterygopal.*, pterygopalatine; *Rec.*, rectus; *S.C.A.*, superior cerebellar artery; Scap., scapula; *Seg.*, segment; *Semicirc.*, semicircular; *Sig.*, sigmoid; *Sphen.*, sphenoid; *Splen.*, splenus; *Sternocleidomast.*, sternocleidomastoid; *Sup.*, superior; Superf., superficial; *Symp.*, sympathetic; *Temp.*, temporal; *Tens.*, tensor; *TM.*, temporomandibular; *Trans.*, transverse; *Tymp.*, tympani, tympanic; *V.*, vein; *Vel.*, veli; *Vert.*, vertebral; *Vest.*, vestibular.

The translabyrinthine approach provides access to the facial nerve from its origin at the brainstem to the stylomastoid foramen, and exposure of the contents of the internal auditory meatus (*Fig. 8.6*) (12, 14). The lateral surface of the pons, the inferior aspect of the origin of the trigeminal nerve, and the facial and vestibulocochlear nerve complexes are well visualized, but exposure of the region inferior to the jugular bulb, above the trigeminal nerve, and anterior to the internal acoustic meatus is usually poor. The extent of exposure achieved with the translabyrinthine approach is dependent on several anatomic factors. A high jugular bulb, an anteriorly placed or large sigmoid sinus, or a low middle fossa plate may severely restrict the exposure (22, 27).

The transcochlear approach shares similar limitations with the translabyrinthine exposure, although the posterior transposition of the facial nerve in the transcochlear approach

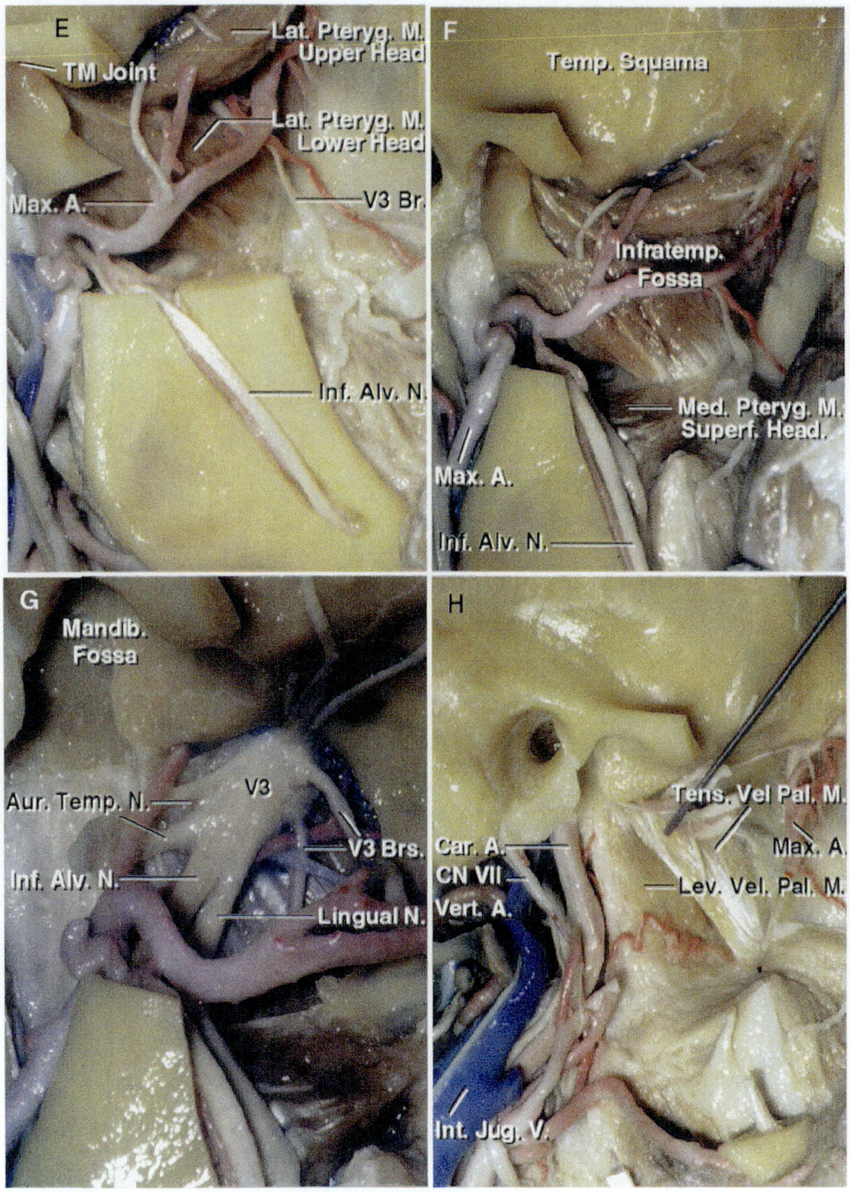

FIGURE 8.19. ***E–H.*** **Anatomic basis of the postauricular transtemporal approach.** ***E,*** **a segment of the mandibular ramus has been removed to expose the upper and lower head of the lateral pterygoid and the maxillary artery in the infratemporal fossa. The inferior alveolar canal and nerve have been exposed.** ***F,*** **the mandibular ramus, in front of the inferior alveolar canal, has been removed to provide a wider exposure of the inferotemporal fossa. The upper head of the lateral pterygoid muscle passes backward from the inferotemporal surface of the greater sphenoid wing and the lower head passes upward from the lateral pterygoid plate. Both heads insert on the mandibular neck and the joint capsule. The superficial head of the medial pterygoid muscle passes from the maxillary tuberosity and pterygoid plate to the mandibular angle. The deep head of the medial pterygoid arises from the pterygoid fossa between the pterygoid plates.** ***G,*** **enlarged view of the infratemporal area after removal of the mandibular condyle and lateral pterygoid muscles. The branches of the mandibular nerve are exposed below the foramen ovale. The largest branches are the lingual and superior alveolar nerves, which are predominantly sensory. The auriculotemporal nerve arises as two roots, which often pass around the middle meningeal artery before joining.** ***H,*** **the pterygoid muscles, a segment of the maxillary artery, and the mandibular and facial nerve branches have been reflected or removed to expose the internal jugular vein exiting the jugular foramen on the medial side of the stylomastoid foramen, the internal carotid artery ascending to enter the carotid canal, the tensor and levator veli palatini descending from their origin bordering the eustachian tube, and the terminal segment of the maxillary artery entering the pterygopalatine fossa.**

allows better visualization of the structures anterior to the internal auditory canal (15, 16). The area of exposure is very narrow and restricted by the maintenance of the bony external auditory canal, but can be increased by resecting the posterior part of the canal. Transposition of the facial nerve may be followed by a transient or permanent facial palsy.

The subtemporal anterior transpetrosal approach uses extradural resection of the anterior petrous pyramid via a temporal craniotomy (*Figs. 8.12* and *8.13*). It may be combined with zygomatic resection to increase access to the floor of the middle fossa (20). The area of the petrous apex removal extends from just medial to the internal auditory canal and cochlea to the petrous apex and petroclival junction, and from the petrous ridge posteriorly to the carotid canal anteriorly. A significant degree of temporal lobe retraction may be required. This may be reduced by using a frontotemporal craniotomy with zygomatic resection. Although only a small window in the petrous bone is provided, exposure can be expanded by dividing the adjacent part of the tentorium. The lateral and anterior surfaces of the pons and the upper clivus and adjacent part of the cavernous sinus can be approached through this route (*Fig. 8.13*). The facial, vestibulocochlear, trigeminal, and abducens nerves can be identified. The petrous carotid may limit the surgeon's line of vision and restrict

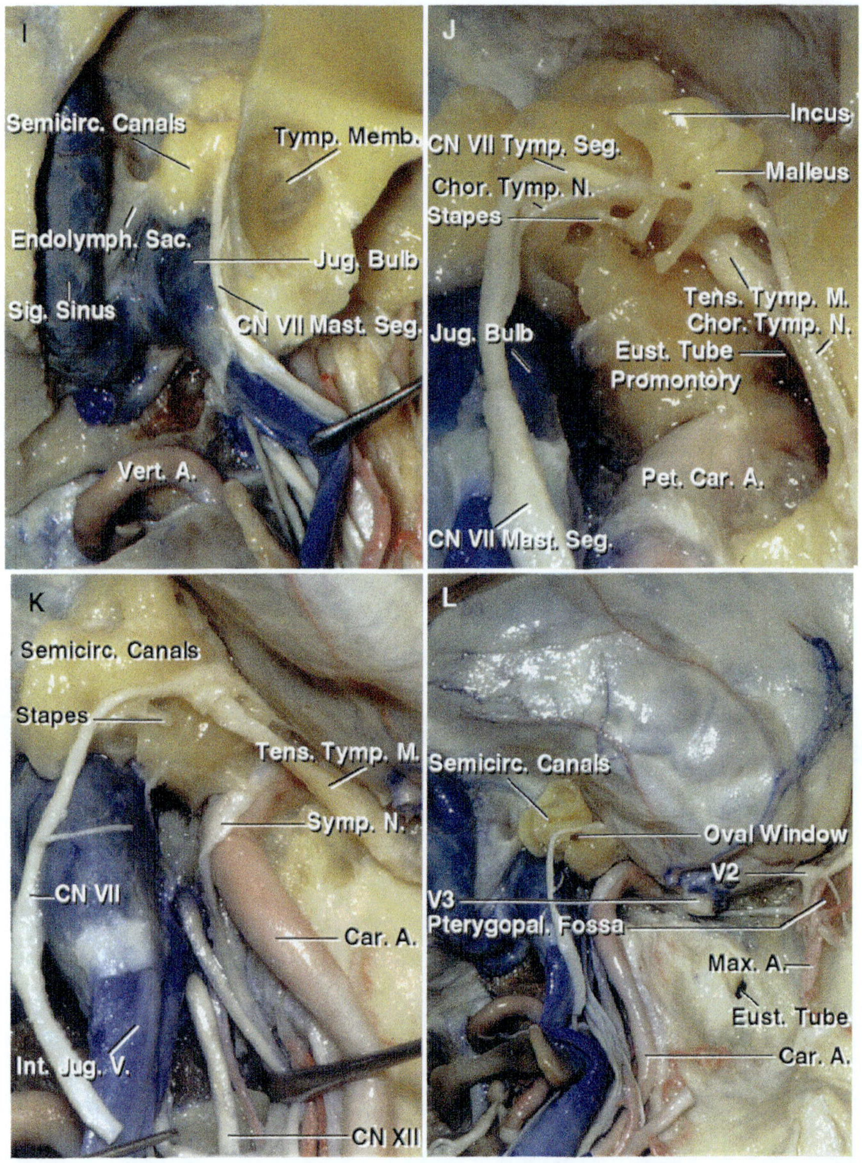

FIGURE 8.19. *I–L.* Anatomic basis of the postauricular transtemporal approach. *I*, a mastoidectomy has been completed to expose the semicircular canals and the mastoid segment of the facial canal. The endolymphatic sac sits under the presigmoid dura. *J*, the external canal has been resected to expose the structures in the tympanic cavity. The tympanic segment of the facial nerve courses between the lateral semicircular canal and the stapes sitting in the oval window. The chorda tympani arises from the mastoid segment of the facial nerve, passes forward along the inner surface of the tympanic membrane and the neck of the malleus to enter its anterior canaliculus, exits the skull along the petrotympanic suture, and joins the lingual nerve in the infratemporal fossa. The promontory overlies the basal turn of the cochlea. The tendon of the tensor tympani muscle makes a right-angle turn around the trochleiform process to insert on the malleus. *K*, the incus and malleus have been removed while preserving the stapes and the tensor tympani muscle. The petrous carotid has been exposed. The nerves exiting the jugular foramen have been retracted forward to expose the hypoglossal nerve exiting the hypoglossal canal. *L*, a frontotemporal craniotomy has been completed and the floor of the middle cranial fossa removed. The semicircular canals have been exposed above the jugular bulb and the stapes has been removed from the oval window. The maxillary nerve has been exposed in the pterygopalatine fossa. The membranous wall of the eustachian tube has been opened to expose the tube's opening into the nasopharynx.

access to the inferior part of the petroclival region, but this restriction may be overcome with anterior mobilization of the artery (39, 41). The approach provides access to the anterior aspect of the brainstem and basilar artery in the area between the trigeminal nerve above and the facial and vestibulocochlear nerves below. In approaching the basilar artery through this route, the size and location of the lesion in relation to the petrous ridge is critical. The trigeminal nerve can be mobilized to improve the exposure, although this may result in postoperative facial hypesthesia (19, 20). The anterior transpetrosal approach can be used alone for extradural pathologies restricted to the petrous apex or as a surgical step to approaching intradural pathologies in the petroclival region. It provides a route for resecting extradural lesions that extend from the level of the trigeminal nerve to the foramen magnum.

Removal of the posterior part of the petrous pyramid has been used for acoustic neuroma removal as part of extended approaches directed through the middle fossa (21, 28, 42, 43) (*Fig. 8.12*). The extended approaches combine different degrees of resection of the bony labyrinth with the subtemporal transtentorial routes. Extending the resection of the petrous bone posteriorly over the mastoid and the bony labyrinth exposes the whole intrapetrous course of the facial nerve, and provides access to the cerebellopontine angle by a combination of subtemporal, translabyrinthine, and presigmoid routes (*Figs. 8.12* and *8.13*) (9).

The subtemporal preauricular infratemporal approach reaches the skull base from an anterolateral direction (*Figs. 8.10*, *8.13*, and *8.18*). Division of the zygomatic arch, resection or displacement of the mandibular condyle, and extensive

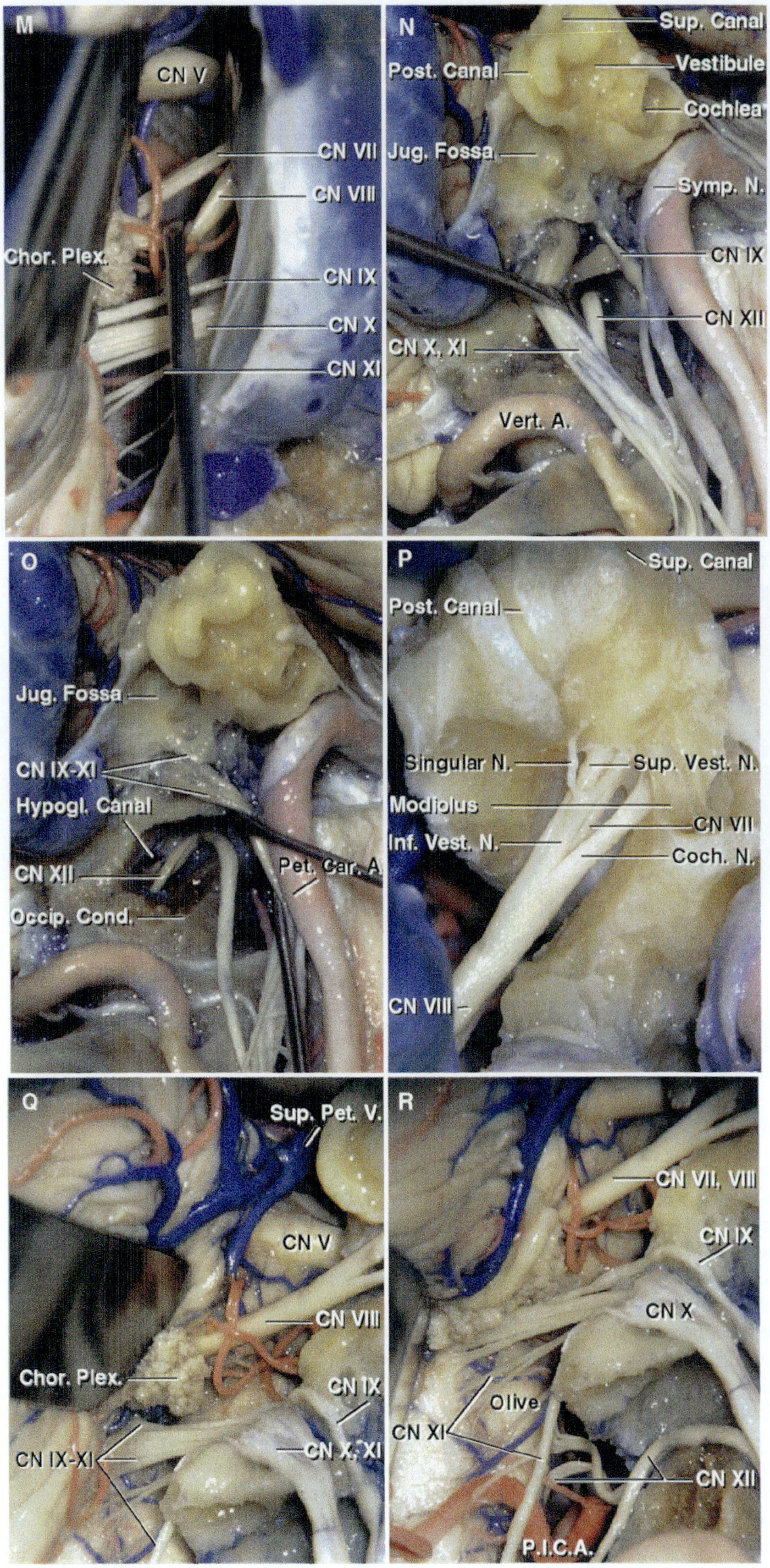

FIGURE 8.19. *M–R.* Anatomic basis of the postauricular transtemporal approach. *M,* a retrosigmoid craniotomy has been completed and the nerves in the cerebellopontine angle exposed. The vestibulocochlear nerve has been depressed to expose the facial nerve. *N,* the facial nerve has been reflected forward out of the facial canal. The promontory has been drilled to expose the cochlea and the vestibule. Both ends of the semicircular canals open into the vestibule, as does the basal turn of the cochlea. The jugular bulb has been removed to expose the jugular fossa in which the bulb resides. The jugular bulb is located below the vestibule. The nerves exiting the jugular foramen have been reflected backward to expose the hypoglossal nerve exiting the hypoglossal canal. The nerves passing through the jugular foramen and hypoglossal canal exit the skull on the medial side of the internal jugular vein and descend between the internal carotid artery and internal jugular vein. *O,* the bone above the occipital condyle has been drilled to expose the hypoglossal nerve in the hypoglossal canal. *P,* the posterior wall of the internal acoustic meatus has been removed to provide this presigmoid inferolateral view of the nerves in the internal meatus. The cochlear nerve separates off the main bundle of the vestibulocochlear nerve and penetrates the modiolus. The inferior vestibular nerve divides into the singular nerve to the posterior ampullae and a branch to the saccule. The superior vestibular nerve innervates the superior and lateral ampullae and sends a branch to the utricle. *Q,* the medial wall of the jugular fossa has been removed and the nerves passing through the jugular foramen have been exposed. The glossopharyngeal nerve passes through the foramen anterior to the vagus and accessory nerves. A large superior petrosal vein ascends to the superior petrosal sinus. *R,* the glossopharyngeal, vagus, and accessory rootlets arise behind and the hypoglossal rootlets arise anterior to the inferior olive.

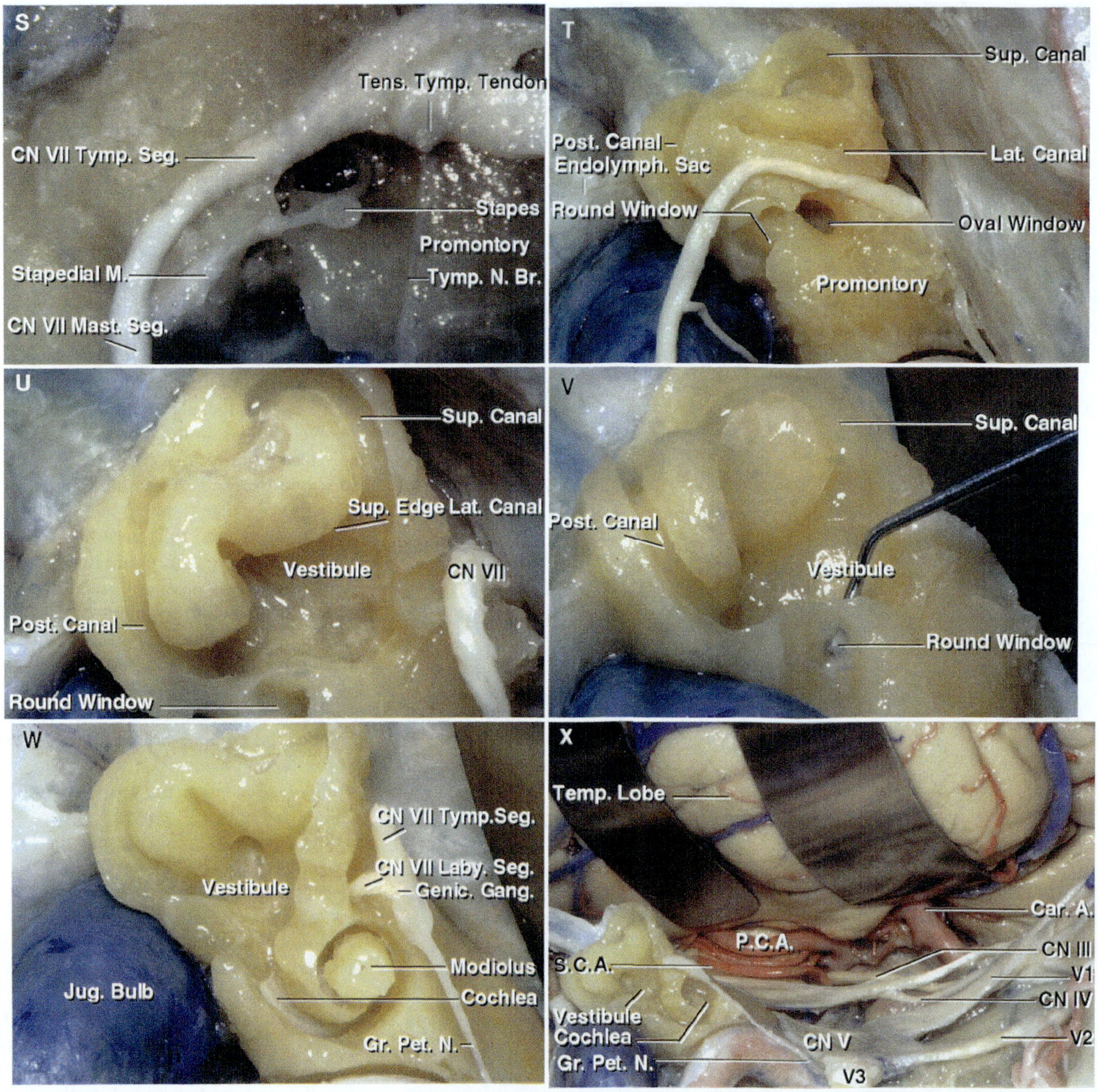

FIGURE 8.19. *S–X.* Anatomic basis of the postauricular transtemporal approach. *S,* enlarged view of the medial wall of the tympanic cavity before mobilizing the facial nerve. The stapedial muscle passes forward from the pyramidal eminence below the facial nerve and attaches on the neck of the stapes. The tensor tympani muscle passes backward and laterally, giving rise to a narrow tendon that makes a sharp turn around the trochleariform process at the lateral end of its semicanal to insert on the handle of the malleus. The basal turn of the cochlea is located deep to the promontory. The tympanic segment of the facial nerve courses above the stapes. *T,* enlarged view of the labyrinth. The semicircular canals have been unroofed and the stapes has been removed from the oval window. The round window is located below and behind the oval window. *U,* the facial nerve has been reflected forward out of the facial canal and the vestibule has been opened. The ampullae of the superior and the lateral canal open into the vestibule anteriorly and are innervated by the superior vestibular nerve. Only the upper edge of the superior canal was preserved in opening the vestibule. The ampullae of the posterior canal is located at its lower end and is innervated by the singular branch of the inferior vestibular nerve. *V,* a probe is directed through the vestibule to the inner surface of the membrane covering the round window, which is located behind and below the oval window. *W,* enlarged view of the labyrinth after opening the promontory to expose the cochlea. The jugular bulb is located below the vestibule and semicircular canals and the lateral genu of the internal carotid artery in position below the cochlea. The cochlea wraps around the modiolus through which the branches of the cochlear nerve are distributed to the cochlear duct. *X,* the temporal lobe has been elevated to expose the internal carotid, PCA, and SCA in the basal cisterns. The dura has been elevated from the lateral wall of the cavernous sinus.

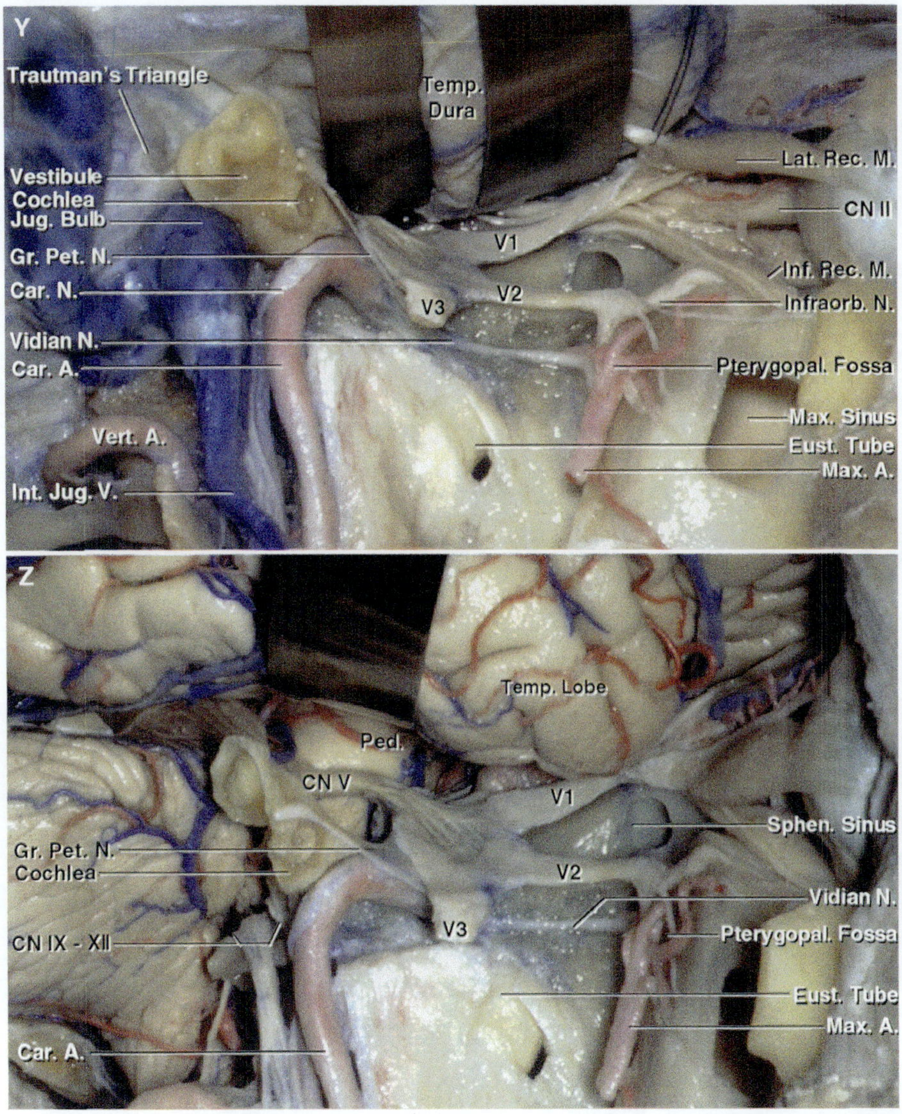

FIGURE 8.19. ***Y*** **and** ***Z*****, anatomic basis of the postauricular transtemporal approach.** ***Y*****, overview before opening the dura. The postauricular approach offers the potential for providing retrosigmoid, presigmoid, and far-lateral exposures and can be used to access the infratemporal and pterygopalatine fossae, the orbit, and the subtemporal areas. In this case, the exposure extends from the retrosigmoid area forward to the orbit. The maxillary sinus has been opened below the orbital floor.** ***Z*****, overview of exposure after opening the dura.**

resection of the lateral part of the middle fossa floor exposes the infratemporal fossa, the nasopharynx, the para- and retropharyngeal areas, and the ethmoid, sphenoid, and maxillary sinuses. The approach also provides access to the upper cervical and petrous carotid. The cavernous sinus also can be approached through its lateral and basal aspects. Anterior displacement of the petrous carotid allows direct access to the clivus and for extensive resection of the petrous bone medial to the cochlea. This exposes the extradural clival region from the level of the trigeminal nerve to the foramen magnum (33, 36, 38, 39). The approach can also provide access to the intradural space ventral to the brainstem (41). The exposure of the cerebellopontine angle and foramen magnum is limited because the approach is carried anterior and medial to cranial nerves VII through XII and the cochlea is not resected (36). Anterior transposition of the petrous carotid artery allows unhindered exposure of the origin of the AICA and the vertebrobasilar junction. The approach could be used as an alternative lateral route to vascular lesions of the midbasilar artery or at the vertebrobasilar junction, when these lesions cannot be exposed through either the retromastoid or subtemporal transtentorial approaches.

The postauricular transtemporal approach, which combines a transcochlear exposure with an infratemporal approach, may be used as an alternative to the preauricular infratemporal approach when the pathology involves the mastoid and the infratemporal fossa and extends to the facial recess, hypotympanic area, and jugular bulb (5, 6, 34) (*Figs. 8.19* and *8.20*). The structures of the lower and middle clivus can be exposed without the need for brain retraction. The facial nerve is displaced anterosuperiorly and the sigmoid sinus ligated and divided. Displacement of the facial nerve from its bony canal seriously interferes with its vascular supply and temporary or permanent loss of function is to be expected (33). Resection of the jugular bulb allows for exposure of the lower cranial nerves in the jugular foramen. Mobilization of the nerves in the medial part of the jugular foramen is extremely difficult and nerve damage is likely to occur if it is attempted. The lateral and anterior surfaces of the lower pons, medulla, and cervicomedullary junction are well exposed. The extent of exposure of the major arteries is dependent on the different anatomic variants and direction of displacement of the vessels. Exposure of the structures of the middle clivus requires posterior facial nerve displacement and drilling of the labyrinth with consequent destruction of any residual hearing. The lateral and part of the anterior surfaces of the pons can be exposed up to the point of emergence of the trigeminal nerve. Exposure of the superior petroclival space requires that the transtemporal exposure be combined with a subtemporal exposure. The transtemporal approach can

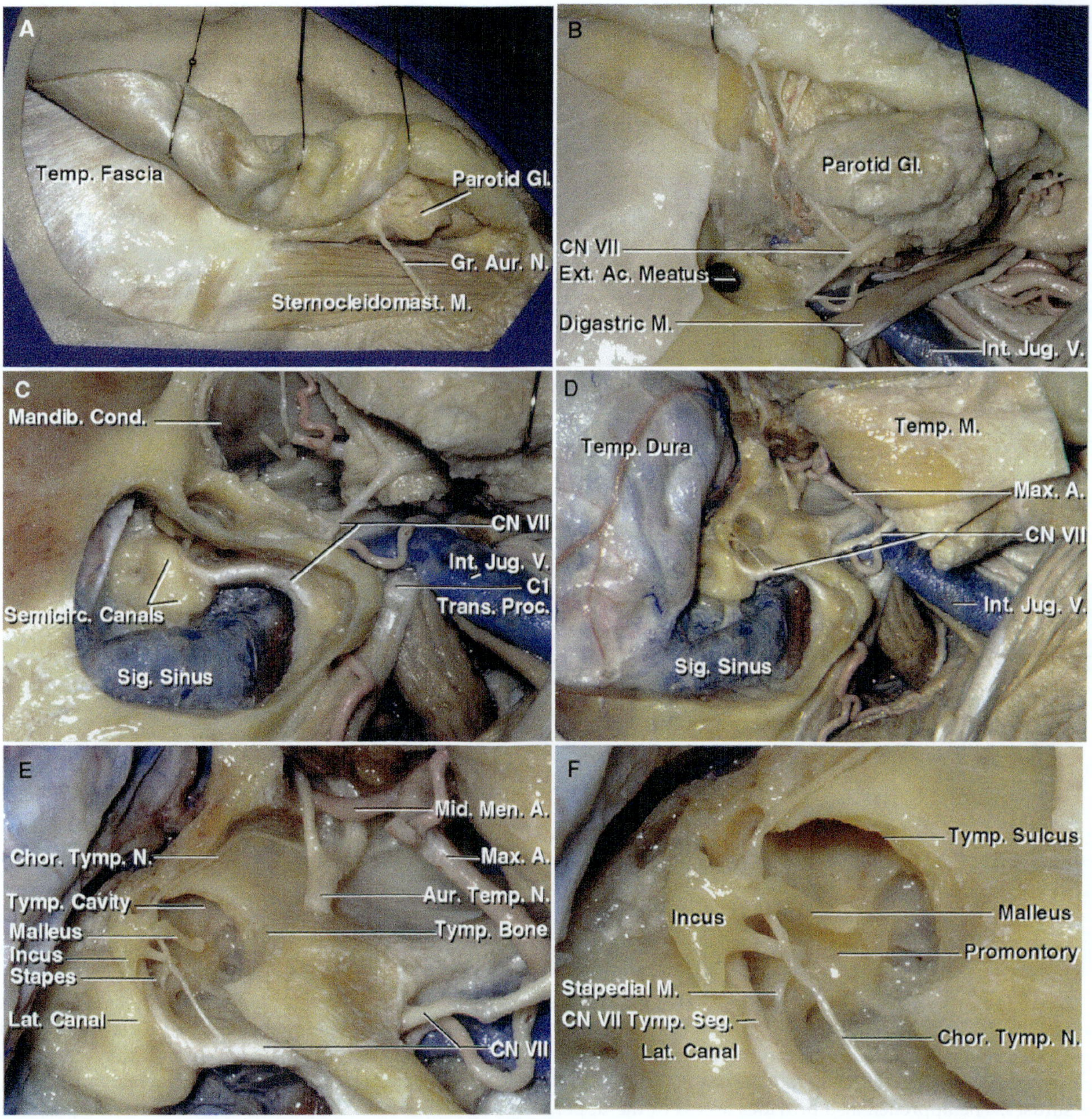

FIGURE 8.20. *A–F.* Postauricular transtemporal approach. This exposure includes the transtemporal and infratemporal approaches in combination with a craniotomy. *A*, the scalp flap has been reflected forward to expose the sternocleidomastoid, parotid gland, and the greater auricular nerve. *B*, the external canal has been divided to reflect the flap forward for a parotid and neck dissection that exposes the facial nerve and its trunks, the posterior digastric belly, and the internal jugular vein. *C*, the mastoidectomy has been completed to expose the presigmoid dura, the sigmoid sinus, and the semicircular canals. The mandibular condyle has been resected to provide access to the infratemporal fossa. *D*, a temporo-occipital craniotomy has been completed, the zygomatic arch opened, and the temporalis muscle reflected to expose the maxillary artery and pterygoid muscles in the infratemporal fossa. *E*, enlarged view of the temporal and infratemporal exposures. The posterior wall of the external canal has been removed. The auriculotemporal branch of the mandibular nerve is often split into two rootlets by the middle meningeal artery. *F*, enlarged view of the tympanic cavity. The anterior part of the lateral semicircular canal is located above the tympanic segment of the facial nerve. The promontory overlies the basal cochlear turn. *A.*, artery; *Ac.*, acoustic; *Aur.*, auricular; *Bas.*, basilar; *Car.*, carotid; *Chor.*, chorda; *CN*, cranial nerve; *Cond.*, condyle; *Ext.*, external; *Gl.*, gland; *Gr.*, greater; *Inf.*, inferior; *Int.*, internal; *Jug.*, jugular; *Lat.*, lateral; *M.*, muscle; *Mandib.*, mandibular; *Mast.*, mastoid; *Max.*, maxillary; *Mid.*, middle; *Men.*, meningeal; *N.*, nerve; *Pet.*, petrosal, petrous; *Proc.*, process; *Seg.*, segment; *Semicirc.*, semicircular; *Sig.*, sigmoid; *Sternocleidomast.*, sternocleidomastoid; *Sup.*, superior; *Temp.*, temporal; *Trans.*, transverse; *Tymp.*, tympani, tympanic; *V.*, vein; *Vert.*, vertebral.

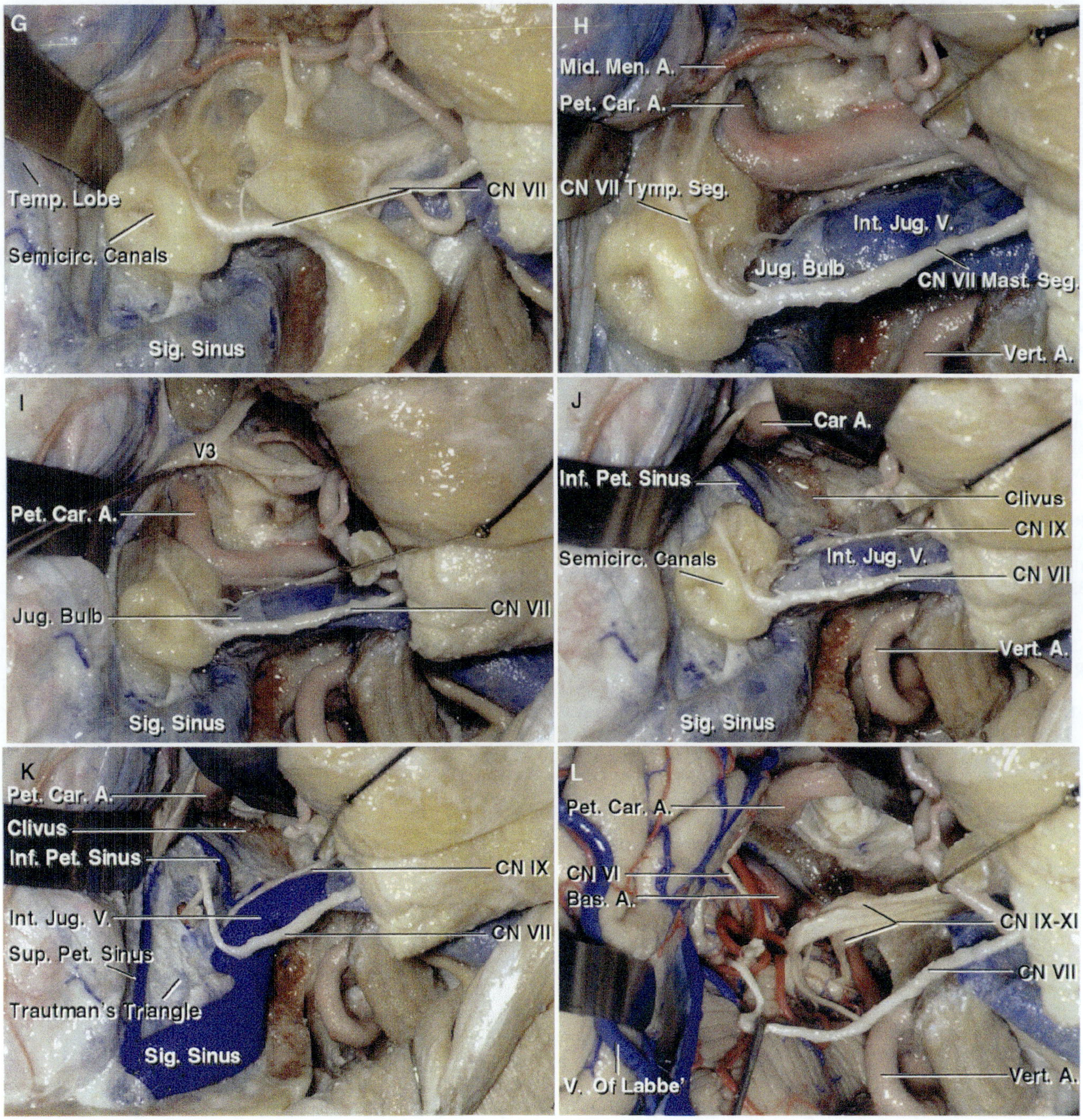

FIGURE 8.20. *G–L.* Postauricular transtemporal approach. *G,* the external canal has been resected in preparation for exposing the petrous carotid. *H,* the junction of the cervical and petrous carotid has been exposed in the area below the promontory. The lateral margin of the stylomastoid and jugular foramina have been removed to expose the jugular bulb below the semicircular canals. *I,* the mandibular nerve has been exposed below the foramen ovale. A more extensive exposure of the petrous carotid has been completed so that the artery can be reflected forward out of the carotid canal to provide access for drilling of the petrous apex. *J,* the petrous carotid has been reflected forward and the petrous apex removed to expose the clivus and inferior petrosal sinus. *K,* the facial nerve has been moved out of the facial canal, and a total labyrinth and petrous apicectomy have been completed. *L,* a segment of the sigmoid sinus and the jugular bulb have been removed to expose the nerves passing through the jugular foramen. The dura has been opened and the facial nerve displaced posteriorly. The temporal lobe has been elevated to expose the subtemporal area while preserving the vein of Labbé.

easily be extended to the infratemporal fossa, and the same exposure provided by the preauricular approach can be achieved. When this approach is combined with an infratemporal fossa exposure and anterior displacement of the intrapetrous carotid artery, the petrous part of the temporal bone can be completely removed, providing the widest possible exposure of the petroclival region (*Figs. 8.19* and *8.20*). The retrosigmoid, far-lateral, and transcondylar exposures can be obtained at the posterior margin of the exposure, and the anterior limit can be extended to include the pterygopalatine fossa and lateral part of the maxilla, orbit, and anterior cranial fossa.

Extensive removal of lesions involving the skull base frequently require reconstruction of the resultant bony, neural, and dural defects. The presence of cerebrospinal fluid leaks and the close proximity to contaminated spaces of the oro- or nasopharynx increases the risks of meningitis. Opened sinuses should be obliterated, dural incisions and openings should be sutured and sealed, nerves should be reanastomosed or grafted, and devascularized grafts of bone or dura should be covered with vascularized tissue whenever possible.

Reprint requests: Albert L. Rhoton, Jr., M.D., Department of Neurological Surgery, University of Florida Brain Institute, P.O. Box 100265, 100 South Newell Drive, Building 59, L2-100, Gainesville, FL 32610-0265.

REFERENCES

1. Al-Mefty O, Fox JL, Smith RR: Petrosal approach for petroclival meningiomas. **Neurosurgery** 22:510–517, 1988.
2. Brackmann DE: The middle fossa approach, in Sekhar LN, Janecka IP (eds): *Surgery of Cranial Base Tumors*. New York, Raven Press, 1993, pp 367–377.
3. Brackmann DE: Translabyrinthine/transcochlear approaches, in Sekhar LN, Janecka IP (eds): *Surgery of Cranial Base Tumors*. New York, Raven Press, 1993, pp 351–365.
4. de Oliveira E, Rhoton AL Jr, Peace D: Microsurgical anatomy of the region of the foramen magnum. **Surg Neurol** 24:293–352, 1985.
5. Fisch U, Pillsbury HC: Infratemporal fossa approach to lesions in the temporal bone and base of the skull. **Arch Otolaryngol** 105: 99–107, 1979.
6. Fisch U, Fagan P, Valavanis A: The infratemporal fossa approach for the lateral skull base. **Otolaryngol Clin North Am** 7:513–552, 1984.
7. Gantz BJ, Fisch U: Modified transotic approach to the cerebellopontine angle. **Arch Otolaryngol** 109:252–256, 1983.
8. Hakuba A, Nishimura S, Inoue Y: Transpetrosal-transtentorial approach and its application in the therapy of retrochiasmatic craniopharyngiomas. **Surg Neurol** 24:405–415, 1985.
9. Hakuba A, Nishimura S, Jang BJ: A combined retroauricular and preauricular transpetrosal-transtentorial approach to clivus meningiomas. **Surg Neurol** 30:108–116, 1988.
10. Harris FS, Rhoton AL Jr: Anatomy of the cavernous sinus: A microsurgical study. **J Neurosurg** 45:169–180, 1976.
11. Hitotsumatsu T, Rhoton AL Jr: Unilateral upper and lower subtotal maxillectomy approaches to the skull base: Microsurgical anatomy. **Neurosurgery** 46:1416–1453, 2000.
12. Hitselberger WE, House WF: Surgical approaches to acoustic tumors. **Arch Otolaryngol** 84:286–291, 1966.
13. House WF: Middle cranial fossa approach to the petrous pyramid. **Arch Otolaryngol** 78:460–469, 1963.
14. House WF: Evolution of transtemporal bone removal of acoustic tumors. **Arch Otolaryngol** 80:731–742, 1964.
15. House WF, Hitselberger WE: The transcochlear approach to the skull base. **Arch Otolaryngol** 102:334–342, 1976.
16. House WF, De la Cruz A, Hitselberger WE: Surgery of the skull base: Transcochlear approach to the petrous apex and clivus. **Otolaryngology** 86:770–779, 1978.
17. Inoue T, Rhoton AL Jr, Theele D, Barry ME: Surgical approaches to the cavernous sinus: A microsurgical study. **Neurosurgery** 26:903–932, 1990.
18. Katsuta T, Rhoton AL Jr, Matsushima T: The jugular foramen: Microsurgical anatomy and operative approaches. **Neurosurgery** 41:149–202, 1997.
19. Kawase T, Shiobara R, Toya S: Anterior transpetrosal-transtentorial approach for sphenopetroclival meningiomas: Surgical method and results in 10 patients. **Neurosurgery** 28:869–876, 1991.
20. Kawase T, Toya S, Shiobara R, Mine T: Transpetrosal approach for aneurysms of the lower basilar artery. **J Neurosurg** 63:857–861, 1985.
21. King TT, Morrison AW: Translabyrinthine and transtentorial removal of acoustic nerve tumors: Results in 150 cases. **J Neurosurg** 52:210–216, 1980.
22. King TT, Morrison AW: Translabyrinthine operation for the removal of acoustic nerve tumors, in Schmidek HH, Sweet WH (eds): *Operative Neurosurgical Techniques*. New York, W.B. Saunders Co., 1988, vol 1, pp 685–704.
23. Lister JR, Rhoton AL Jr, Matsushima T, Peace D: Microsurgical anatomy of the posterior inferior cerebellar artery. **Neurosurgery** 10:170–199, 1982.
24. Malis LI: Surgical resection of tumors of the skull base, in Wilkins RH, Rengachary SS (eds): *Neurosurgery*. New York, McGraw-Hill, 1985, vol 1, pp 1011–1021.
25. Matsushima T, Rhoton AL Jr, de Oliveira E, Peace D: Microsurgical anatomy of the veins of the posterior fossa. **J Neurosurg** 59:63–105, 1983.
26. Mayberg MR, Symon L: Meningiomas of the clivus and apical petrous bone: Report of 35 cases. **J Neurosurg** 65:160–167, 1986.
27. McElveen JT: The translabyrinthine approach to the cerebellopontine angle tumors, in Wilkins RH, Rengachary SS (eds): *Neurosurgery Update I: Diagnosis, Operative Technique, and Neuro-oncology*. New York, McGraw-Hill, 1990, pp 415–423.
28. Morrison AW, King TT: Experiences with a translabyrinthine-transtentorial approach to the cerebellopontine angle. **J Neurosurg** 38:382–390, 1973.
29. Pait TG, Harris FS, Paullus WS, Rhoton AL Jr: Microsurgical anatomy and dissection of the temporal bone. **Surg Neurol** 8:363–391, 1977.
30. Paullus WS, Pait TG, Rhoton AL Jr: Microsurgical exposure of the petrous portion of the carotid artery. **J Neurosurg** 47:713–726, 1977.
31. Rhoton AL Jr, Pulec JL, Hall GM, Boyd AS Jr: Absence of bone over the geniculate ganglion. **J Neurosurg** 28:48–53, 1968.
32. Samii M, Ammirati M, Mahran A, Bini W, Sepehrnia A: Surgery of petroclival meningiomas: Report of 24 cases. **Neurosurgery** 24:12–17, 1989.
33. Schramm VL Jr: Infratemporal fossa surgery, in Sekhar LN, Schramm VL Jr (eds): *Tumors of the Cranial Base: Diagnosis and Treatment*. Mount Kisco, Futura Pub. Co., 1987, pp 421–437.
34. Sekhar LN, Estonillo R: Transtemporal approach to the skull base: An anatomical study. **Neurosurgery** 19:799–808, 1986.
35. Sekhar LN, Jannetta PJ: Cerebellopontine angle meningiomas: Microsurgical excision and follow up results. **J Neurosurg** 60:500–505, 1984.

36. Sekhar LN, Jannetta PJ, Burkhart LE, Janosky JE: Meningiomas involving the clivus: A six-year experience with 41 patients. **Neurosurgery** 27:764–781, 1990.
37. Sekhar LN, Schessel DA, Bucur SD, Raso JL, Wright DC: Partial labyrinthectomy petrous apicectomy approach to neoplastic and vascular lesions of the petroclival area. **Neurosurgery** 44:537–550, 1999.
38. Sekhar LN, Schramm VL Jr, Jones NF: Operative management of large neoplasms of the lateral and posterior cranial base, in Sekhar LN, Schramm VL Jr (eds): *Tumors of the Cranial Base: Diagnosis and Treatment*. Mount Kisco, Futura Publishing Co, 1987, pp 655–682.
39. Sekhar LN, Schramm VL Jr, Jones NF: Subtemporal-preauricular infratemporal fossa approach to large lateral and posterior cranial base neoplasms. **J Neurosurg** 67:488–499, 1987.
40. Sekhar LN, Schramm VL Jr, Jones NF, Yonas H, Horton J, Latchaw RE, Curtain H: Operative exposure and management of the petrous and upper cervical internal carotid artery. **Neurosurgery** 19:967–982, 1986.
41. Sen CN, Sekhar LN: The subtemporal and preauricular infratemporal approach to intradural structures ventral to the brain stem. **J Neurosurg** 73:345–354, 1990.
42. Shiobara R, Ohira T, Kanzaki J, Toya S: A modified extended middle cranial fossa approach for acoustic nerve tumors. **J Neurosurg** 68:358–365, 1988.
43. Tator CH, Nedzelski JM: Facial nerve preservation in patients with large acoustic neuromas treated by a combined middle fossa transtentorial translabyrinthine approach. **J Neurosurg** 57:1–7, 1982.
44. Tedeschi H, Rhoton AL Jr: Lateral approaches to the petroclival region. **Surg Neurol** 41:180–216, 1994.
45. Wen HT, Rhoton AL Jr, Katsuta T, de Oliveira E: Microsurgical anatomy of the transcondylar, supracondylar, and paracondylar extensions of the far-lateral approach. **J Neurosurg** 87:555–585, 1997.
46. Yasargil MG, Mortara RW, Curcic M: Meningiomas of basal posterior cranial fossa, in Krayenbühl H (ed): *Advances and Technical Standards in Neurosurgery*. Wien, Springer-Verlag, 1980, vol 17, pp 3–115.

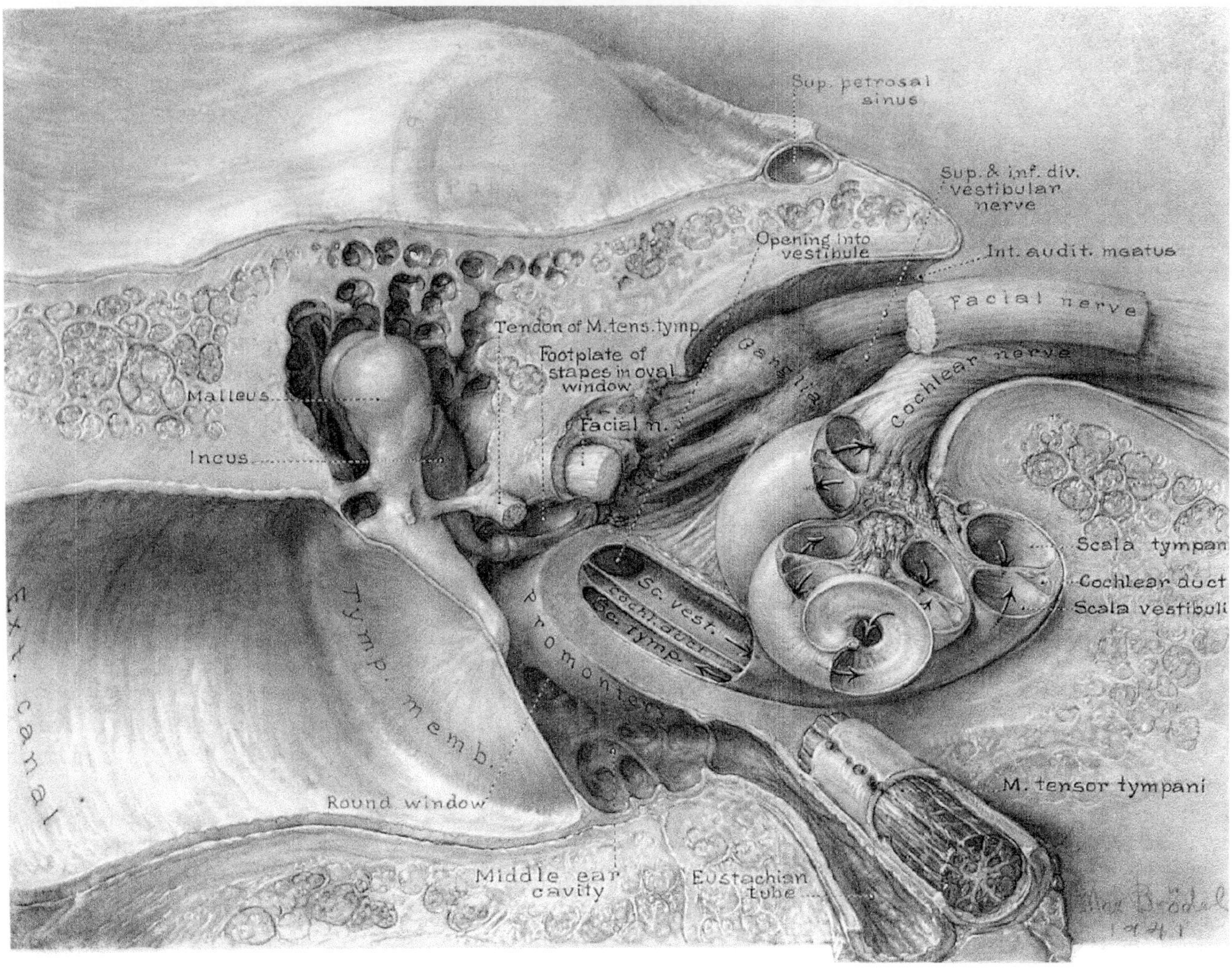

Anatomy of the human ear, a drawing by Max Brödel using Wolff's carbon pencil and dust on Ross stippleboard. Courtesy, W.B. Saunders Co.

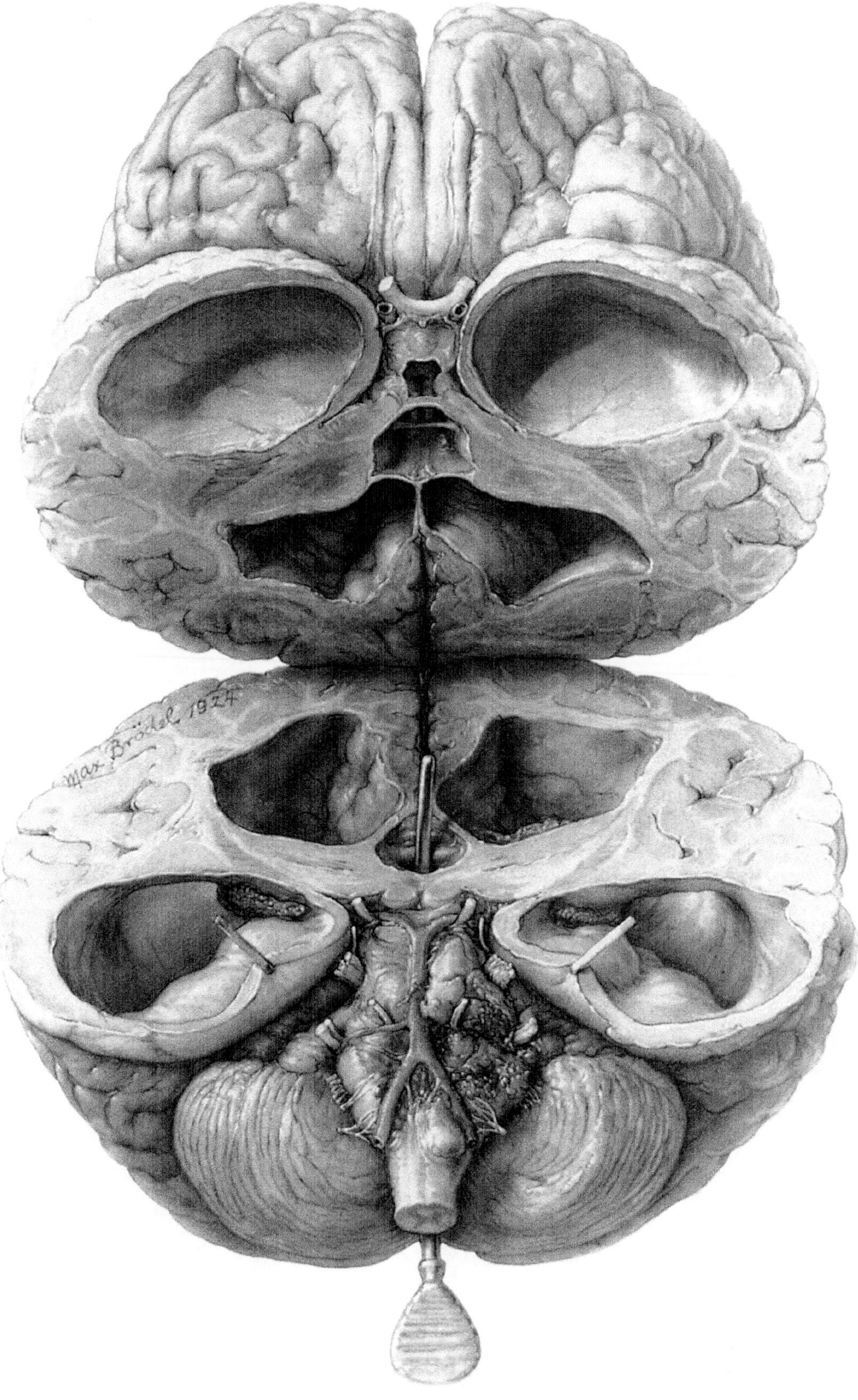

Max Brödel's drawing showing intracranial tumors and abscesses causing communicating hydrocephalus. In another article by Walter Dandy, Brödel shows the tumor spreading over the brain stem in the foreground. Courtesy, Annals of Surgery 81, 1925.

CHAPTER 9

Jugular Foramen

Albert L. Rhoton, Jr., M.D.

Department of Neurological Surgery, University of Florida, Gainesville, Florida

Key words: Cranial base, Cranial nerves, Jugular foramen, Microsurgical anatomy, Occipital bone, Skull base, Temporal bone, Venous sinuses

The jugular foramen is difficult to understand and to access surgically (3, 11, 15, 19, 24, 28). It is difficult to conceptualize because it varies in size and shape in different crania, from side to side in the same cranium, and from its intracranial to extracranial end in the same foramen, and because of its complex irregular shape, its curved course, its formation by two bones, and the numerous nerves and venous channels that pass through it (*Fig. 9.1*). The difficulties in exposing this foramen are created by its deep location and the surrounding structures, such as the carotid artery anteriorly, the facial nerve laterally, the hypoglossal nerve medially, and the vertebral artery inferiorly, all of which block access to the foramen and require careful management.

The jugular foramen is divided into three compartments: two venous and a neural or intrajugular compartment. The venous compartments consist of a larger posterolateral venous channel, the sigmoid part, which receives the flow of the sigmoid sinus, and a smaller anteromedial venous channel, the petrosal part, which receives the drainage of the inferior petrosal sinus. The petrosal part forms a characteristic venous confluens by also receiving tributaries from the hypoglossal canal, petroclival fissure, and vertebral venous plexus. The petrosal part empties into the sigmoid part through an opening in the medial wall of the jugular bulb between the glossopharyngeal nerve anteriorly and the vagus and accessory nerves posteriorly. The intrajugular or neural part, through which the glossopharyngeal, vagus, and accessory nerves course, is located between the sigmoid and petrosal parts at the site of the intrajugular processes of the temporal and occipital bones, which are joined by a fibrous or osseous bridge. The glossopharyngeal, vagus, and accessory nerves penetrate the dura on the medial margin of the intrajugular process of the temporal bone to reach the medial wall of the internal jugular vein. The operative approaches that access various aspects of the foramen and adjacent areas are the postauricular transtemporal, retrosigmoid, extreme lateral transcondylar, and preauricular subtemporal-infratemporal approaches.

OSSEOUS RELATIONSHIPS

The jugular foramen is located between the temporal bone and the occipital bone (*Figs. 9.1* and *9.2*). The right foramen is usually larger than the left. In a previous study, we observed that the right foramen was larger than the left in 68% of the cases, equal to the left in 12%, and smaller than the left in 20% (24). The foramen is configured around the sigmoid and inferior petrosal sinuses. It can be regarded as a hiatus between the temporal and the occipital bones. The structures that traverse the jugular foramen are the sigmoid sinus and jugular bulb, the inferior petrosal sinus, meningeal branches of the ascending pharyngeal and occipital arteries, the glossopharyngeal, vagus, and accessory nerves with their ganglia, the tympanic branch of the glossopharyngeal nerve (Jacobson's nerve), the auricular branch of the vagus nerve (Arnold's nerve), and the cochlear aqueduct.

The foramen is situated so that its long axis is directed from posterolateral to anteromedial, giving it an anterolateral margin formed by the temporal bone and a posteromedial margin formed by the occipital bone. From the intracranial end, it is directed forward, medially, and downward. One cannot see through the foramen when viewing the skull from directly above or below because of its roof, formed by the lower surface of the petrous part of the temporal bone. The foramen, when viewed from the intracranial side in a posterior to anterior direction, has a large oval lateral component, referred to as the sigmoid part, because it receives the drainage of the sigmoid sinus, and a small medial part, called the petrosal part, because it receives the drainage of the inferior petrosal sinus. The view through the foramen from directly below reveals the part of the temporal bone forming the dome of the jugular bulb, rather than a clear opening.

The junction of the sigmoid and petrosal parts is the site of bony prominences on the opposing surfaces of the temporal and occipital bones, called the intrajugular processes, which are joined by a fibrous, or less commonly, and osseous bridge, the intrajugular septum, separating the sigmoid and petrosal part of the foramen.

Although the margins of the jugular foramen are formed by the petrosal part of the temporal bone and the condylar part of the occipital bone, the other parts of these bones also have important relationships to the jugular foramen. The petroclival fissure, the fissure between the lateral edge of the clival part of the occipital bone and the petrous part of the temporal bone, intersects the anteromedial edge of the foramen, and the occipitomastoid suture, the suture between the mastoid por-

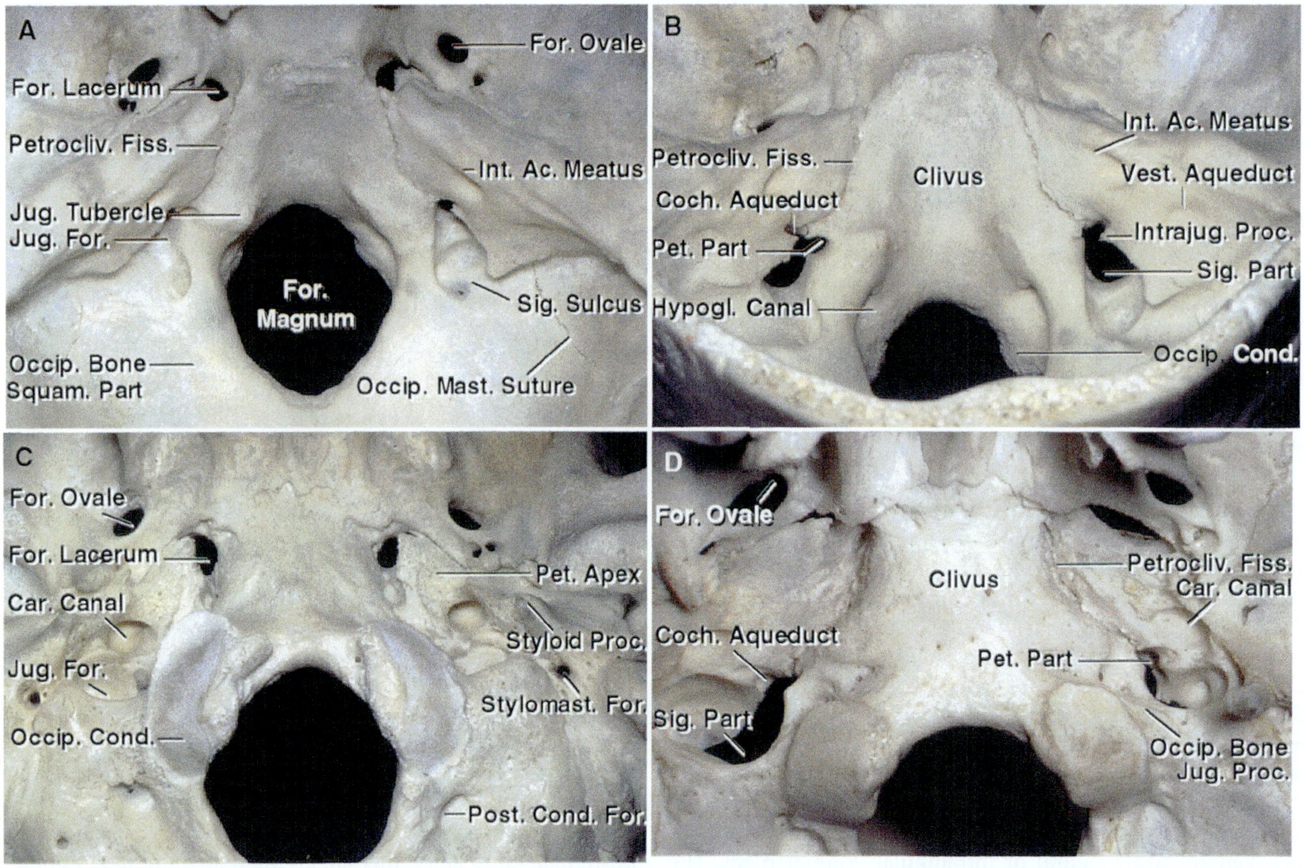

FIGURE 9.1. *A–D.* Osseous relationships. *A,* the jugular foramen is located between the temporal and occipital bones. One cannot see directly through the foramen from above, as shown, because it is directed forward under the temporal bone. The sigmoid groove descends along the mastoid and crosses the occipitomastoid suture where it turns forward on the upper surface of the jugular process of the occipital bone and enters the foramen by passing under the posterior part of the petrous temporal bone. *B,* the view directed from posterior and superior shows the shape of the foramen, which is not seen on the direct superior view. The foramen has a larger lateral sigmoid part through which the sigmoid sinus empties and a smaller anteromedial petrosal part through which the inferior petrosal sinus empties. The two parts are separated by the intrajugular processes of the occipital and temporal bones. The glossopharyngeal, vagus, and accessory nerves pass through the intrajugular portion of the foramen located between the sigmoid and petrosal parts. The foramen is asymmetric from side to side with the right side often being larger as shown. The cochlear aqueduct opens just above the anterior edge of the petrosal part. The vestibular aqueduct opens into the endolymphatic sac, which sits on the back of the temporal bone superolateral to the sigmoid part of the jugular foramen. *C,* jugular foramen viewed from directly below. One cannot see directly through the foramen from below because the foramen is covered above by the part of the petrous temporal bone forming the jugular fossa, which houses the jugular bulb. The entrance into the carotid canal is located directly in front of the medial half of the jugular foramen. The stylomastoid foramen is located lateral and the anterior half of the occipital condyle medial to the jugular foramen. The posterior condylar foramen is transversed by an emissary vein, which joins the sigmoid sinus. The hypoglossal canal passes above the middle third of the occipital condyle and opens laterally into the interval between the jugular foramen and carotid canal. *D,* the view directed from anterior and backward reveals the shape of the jugular foramen. The roof over the foramen formed by the jugular fossa of the temporal bone is shaped to accommodate the jugular bulb. The posterior margin of the foramen is formed by the jugular process of the occipital bone, which connects the basal (clival) part of the occipital bone to the squamosal part. The petroclival fissure intersects the anteromedial margin of the petrosal part of the foramen. *Ac.,* acoustic; *Car.,* carotid; *Coch.,* cochlear; *Cond.,* condyle; *Fiss.,* fissure; *For.,* foramen; *Hypogl.,* hypoglossal; *Int.,* internal; *Intrajug.,* intrajugular; *Jug.,* jugular; *Mast.,* mastoid; *Occip.,* occipital; *Pet.,* petrous; *Petrocliv.,* petroclival; *Post.,* posterior; *Proc.,* process; *Sig.,* sigmoid; *Squam.,* squamosal; *Stylomast.,* stylomastoid; *Temp.,* temporal; *Vest.,* vestibular.

tion of the temporal bone and the condylar part of the occipital bone, intersects its posterolateral edge.

The intrajugular processes of the temporal and occipital bones divide the anterior and posterior edges of the foramen between the sigmoid and petrosal parts. The intrajugular process of the temporal bone protrudes farther into the jugular foramen than the opposite process from the occipital bone, and may infrequently reach the smaller intrajugular process

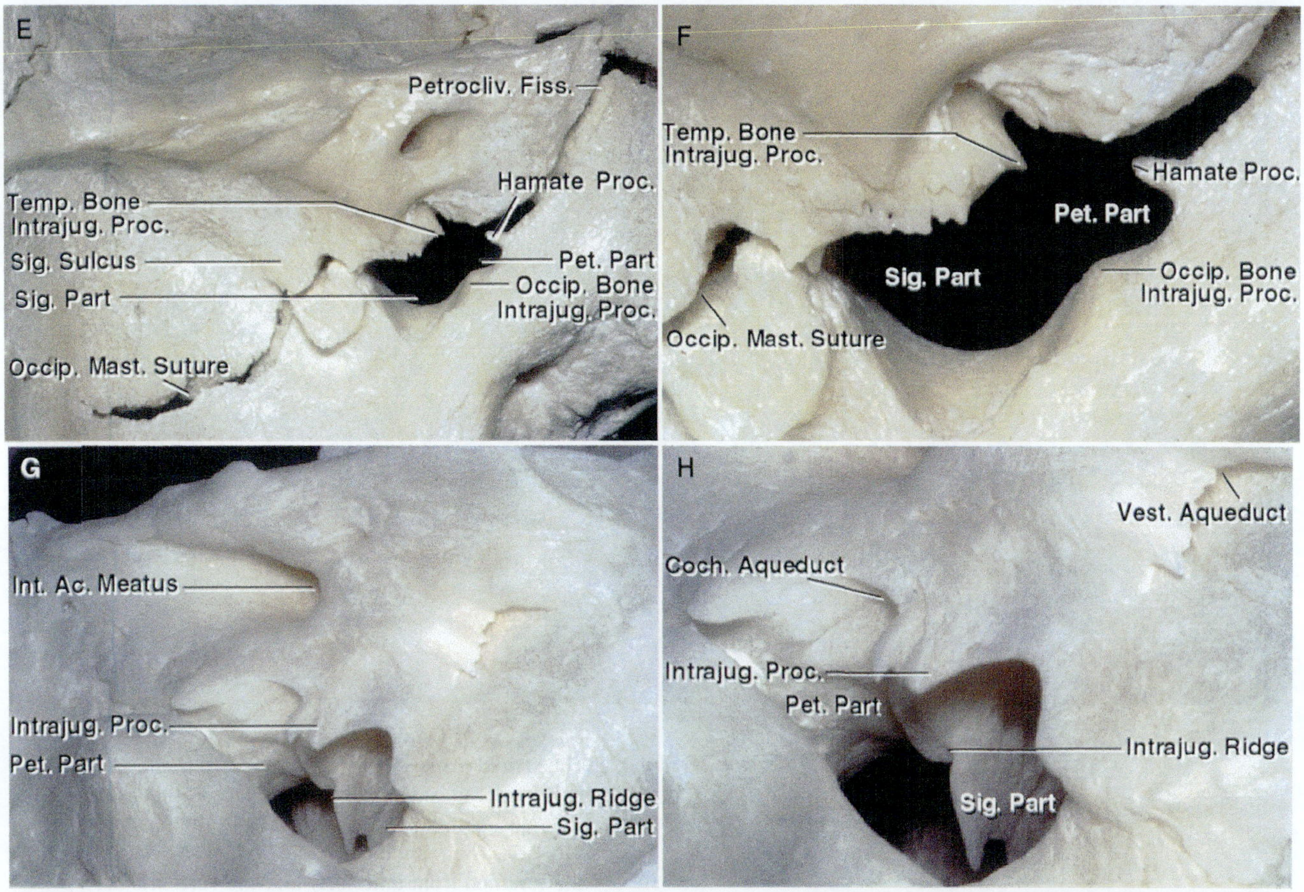

FIGURE 9.1. *E–H. E* and *F,* another jugular foramen. *Left side*: *E,* the sutures have been forced open to show the relationship of the foramen to the petroclival and occipitomastoid sutures. The jugular foramen has a larger lateral part, the sigmoid part, which receives the drainage of the sigmoid sinus, and a smaller medial part, the petrosal part, which receives the drainage of the inferior petrosal sinus. The intrajugular process of the occipital bone is somewhat more prominent than shown in *C* and projects forward toward the intrajugular process of the temporal bone. The hamate process normally extends along the medial edge of the petrosal part of the foramen to the adjacent part of the temporal bone, but in this case the sutures were forced open, leaving an interval between the hamate process and the temporal bone. *F,* enlarged view. *G* and *H,* another jugular foramen. *G,* the intrajugular process of the temporal bone projects into the interval between the sigmoid and petrosal parts of the foramen. A ridge, the intrajugular ridge, extends forward from the intrajugular process along the medial side of the jugular bulb. The glossopharyngeal nerve passes forward along the medial side of the intrajugular process and ridge. The vagus and accessory nerves enter the dura on the medial side of the process, but quickly descend and do not pass forward along the medial edge of the ridge as does the glossopharyngeal nerve. The jugular process of the occipital bone often has a small prominence on its surface that projects toward the intrajugular process of the temporal bone, and in some foramina, the intrajugular processes of the two bones are joined by an osseous bridge that converts the foramen into two osseous foramina. In this case, the intrajugular process of the occipital bone is absent. *H,* enlarged view. The cochlear aqueduct opens above the petrosal part of the foramen and the site where the glossopharyngeal nerve enters the intrajugular part of the foramen on the medial side of the intrajugular process. The vestibular aqueduct opens onto the posterior surface of the temporal bone superolateral to the jugular foramen.

of the occipital bone, dividing the jugular foramen into two bony foramina. A ridge, the intrajugular ridge, extends forward from the intrajugular process of the temporal bone along the medial edge of the jugular bulb (*Fig. 9.1*). The glossopharyngeal nerve courses along its medial edge. Occasionally, the edge of this ridge extends medially toward the adjacent part of the temporal bone to create a deep groove in which the nerve courses or it may reach the temporal bone to form a canal, which surrounds the glossopharyngeal nerve as it passes through the jugular foramen.

The drainage of the sigmoid sinus is directed forward into the sigmoid portion of the foramen, where a high domed recess, the jugular fossa, forms a roof over the top of the jugular bulb (*Figs. 9.1* and *9.3*). This recess, which has its summit slightly lateral to the entrance of the sigmoid sinus, is usually larger on the right side of the skull, reflecting the larger sigmoid sinus on

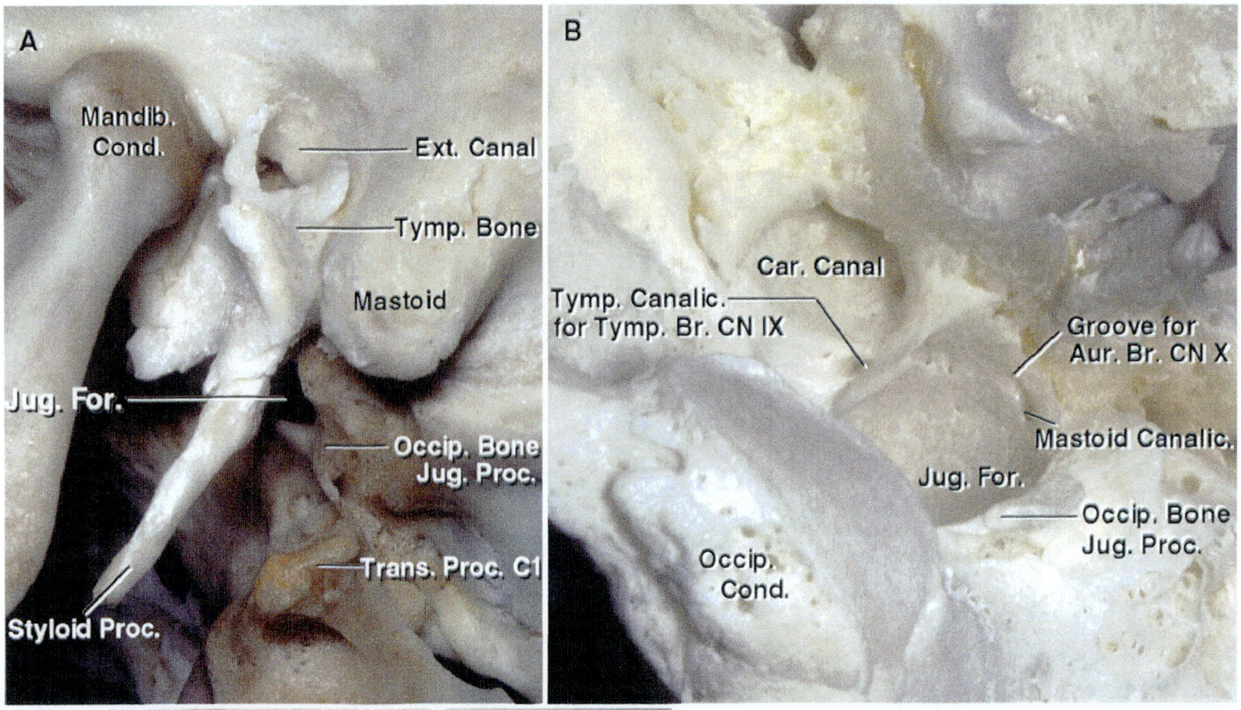

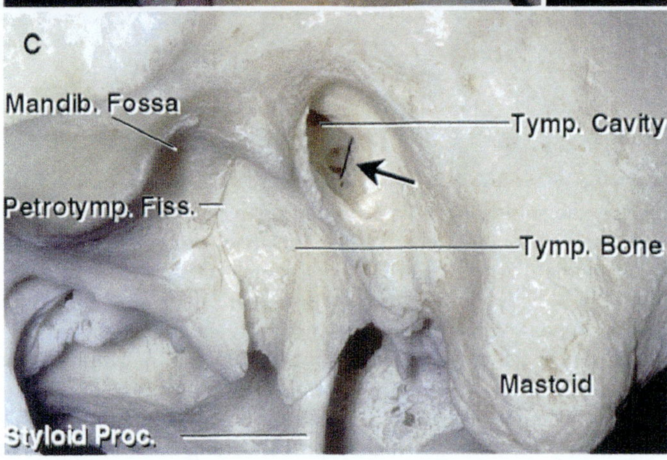

FIGURE 9.2. Osseous relationships. ***A,*** **lateral view. The styloid process projects downward and the facial nerve exits the stylomastoid foramen on the lateral side, and both block lateral access to the jugular foramen. The mandibular condyle blocks access to the foramen from anteriorly and the vertebral artery ascending through the C1 transverse process limits access from behind. The transverse process of C1 sits behind and often indents the posterior wall of the internal jugular vein.** ***B,*** **inferior view of the jugular foramen. The jugular foramen is located lateral to the anterior half of the occipital condyle. The temporal bone forms the dome over the jugular bulb. The jugular process of the occipital bone forms the posterior margin of the jugular foramen. The jugular foramen and carotid canal are separated by a narrow bony ridge, which is penetrated medially by the tympanic canaliculus through which passes the tympanic branch of the glossopharyngeal nerve (Jacobson's nerve). This branch of the nerve passes forward across the promontory in the medial part of the tympanic cavity, then crosses the floor of the middle fossa as the lesser petrosal nerve, and eventually reaches the otic ganglion, providing parasympathetic innervation to the parotid gland. The anterior wall of the sigmoid part of the foramen is the site of a shallow groove across which the auricular branch of the vagus nerve (Arnold's nerve) passes to enter the mastoid canaliculus. It exits the mastoid through the tympanomastoid suture.** ***C,*** **lateral view of the left temporal bone. A small fiber (*arrow*) placed in the tympanic canaliculus, shown in B, exits the canaliculus in the middle ear where the fibers of the tympanic branch of the glossopharyngeal nerve cross the promontory, and then regroup to cross the floor of the middle fossa as the lesser petrosal nerve. The styloid process projects downward lateral to the jugular foramen.** ***Aur.,*** **auricular;** ***Br.,*** **branch;** ***Canalic.,*** **canaliculus;** ***Car.,*** **carotid;** ***CN,*** **cranial nerve;** ***Cond.,*** **condyle;** ***Ext.,*** **external;** ***Fiss.,*** **fissure;** ***For.,*** **foramen;** ***Jug.,*** **jugular;** ***Mandib.,*** **mandibular;** ***Occip.,*** **occipital;** ***Petrotymp.,*** **petrotympanic;** ***Proc.,*** **process;** ***Trans.,*** **transverse;** ***Tymp.,*** **tympanic.**

that side. The dome of the recess is usually smooth as it conforms to the jugular bulb, but the summit may also be ridged and irregular. A small triangular recess, the pyramidal fossa, extends forward on the medial side of the intrajugular process of the temporal bone along the anterior wall of the petrosal part of the foramen. The external aperture of the cochlear canaliculus, which houses the perilymphatic duct and a tubular prolongation of the dura mater, opens into the anterior apex of the pyramidal fossa. The glossopharyngeal nerve enters this fossa below the point at which the cochlear aqueduct joins its apex.

The jugular process of the condylar portion of the occipital bone, which extends behind the jugular foramen and connects the clival and squamosal parts of the occipital bone, forms the posteromedial wall of the foramen. This process extends laterally from the area above the posterior half of the occipital condyle and is penetrated by the hypoglossal canal. The upper surface of the jugular process of the occipital bone in the area superomedial to the foramen presents an oval prominence, the jugular tubercle, which is located above the hypoglossal canal. The jugular tubercle often has a shallow furrow marking the site of passage of the glossopharyngeal, vagus, and accessory nerves across its surface. The terminal end of the sigmoid sinus courses forward on the superior surface of the jugular process in a deep hook-like groove, the sigmoid sulcus, which is directed medially into the sigmoid portion of the jugular foramen.

On the lateral wall of the jugular foramen, a few millimeters inside the external edge, just behind the point at which the occipitomastoid suture crosses the lateral edge of the foramen, is a small foramen, the mastoid canaliculus, and a shallow groove leading from medial to lateral across the anterior wall of the sigmoid part to the mastoid canaliculus (*Figs. 9.2* and *9.3*). The auricular branch of the vagus nerve (Arnold's nerve) courses along the groove and enters the canaliculus. The nerve passes through the mastoid and exits the bone in the inferolateral part of the tympanomastoid suture. At the site where the intrajugular ridge of the temporal bone meets the carotid ridge, a small canal, the tympanic canaliculus, is directed upward, leading the tympanic branch arising from the inferior glossopharyngeal ganglion (Jacobson's nerve) to the tympanic cavity (*Figs. 9.2*). Looking from below at the extracranial orifice of the jugular foramen, it can be recognized that the glossopharyngeal nerve courses along the medial side of the intrajugular process and ridge to reach the area below the tympanic canaliculus.

ADJACENT BONY STRUCTURES

On the intracranial side, the petrosal part of the foramen is located approximately 5 mm below the porus of the internal canal and 5 mm above the intracranial orifice of the hypoglossal canal (*Figs. 9.2* and *9.4*). The lateral edge of the foramen is located below and in approximately the sagittal plane through the lateral end of the internal acoustic meatus. The jugular tubercle, a rounded prominence located at the junction of the basal and condylar parts of the occipital bone, is situated approximately 8 mm medial to the medial edge of the jugular foramen. The otic capsule, which is situated in the petrous part of the temporal bone and which contains the semicircular canals and cochlea, is located superior to the dome of the jugular bulb.

The occipital condyle is located along the lateral margin of the anterior half of the foramen magnum in the area below and medial to the jugular foramen.

The hypoglossal canals, which pass through the condylar part of the occipital bone in the area above the occipital condyles, are located medial to the jugular foramina (*Figs. 9.1* and *9.3*). The intracranial end of the hypoglossal canal is situated below the jugular tubercle approximately 5 mm inferomedial to the petrosal part of the jugular foramen and several millimeters below the lower part of the petroclival fissure. A more detailed review is included in the chapter on the far-lateral approach.

The anterior margin of the jugular foramen, when viewed extracranially, is formed by the narrow ridge of temporal bone, the carotid ridge, which separates the foramen and the carotid canal (*Figs. 9.1* and *9.2*). The tympanic canaliculus opens on or near the medial part of the carotid ridge. The styloid process and the stylomastoid foramen are located lateral to the outer orifice of the jugular foramen, with the styloid process being located slightly anteromedial to the stylomastoid foramen. The facial nerve exits the stylomastoid foramen approximately 5 mm lateral to the lateral edge of the jugular foramen. The anterior margin of the jugular foramen is located just behind the part of the tympanic bone that forms the posterior wall of the temporomandibular joint and the anterior and inferior wall of the external auditory canal. The vaginal process of the tympanic bone, which separates both the carotid canal and sigmoid part of the foramen from the glenoid fossa, is the site of attachment of the styloid process to the skull base. The styloid process projects downward from the vaginal process of the tympanic bone, lateral to the foramen. The digastric groove is directed posteriorly from the styloid process along the medial margin of the mastoid process. Access to the jugular foramen is blocked laterally by mastoid and styloid processes, the transverse process of the atlas, and the mandibular ramus (*Figs. 9.3* and *9.4*).

The tympanic cavity, which is located medial to the tympanic membrane, is situated above and lateral to the jugular bulb and the sharp right-angled curve, called the lateral bend, at the junction of the vertical and horizontal segments of the petrous carotid artery (*Fig. 9.4*). Several structures that may be exposed during surgery for lesions in the jugular foramen are the vertical and horizontal segments of the petrous portion of the internal carotid artery, the eustachian tube, and the tensor tympani muscle. Both the cochlea and semicircular canals are located in the petrous part of the temporal bone above the dome of the jugular bulb (*Fig. 9.4*). The facial nerve in the temporal bone, which often blocks access to lesions in the jugular foramen, descends through the mastoid lateral to the jugular bulb. The endolymphatic sac is situated on the posterior surface of the petrous bone between the two layers of the dura in the corner at which the sigmoid sinus changes its course from a vertical direction to a horizontal one (*Figs. 9.3* and *9.5*).

Dural architecture

At the intracranial orifice, the jugular foramen is divided into three compartments by the dura mater: the petrosal compartment situated anteromedially, the sigmoid compartment situated posterolaterally, and the intrajugular or neural compartment situated between the petrosal and sigmoid parts at the site of the intrajugular processes of the temporal and occipital bones, the intrajugular septum, and the glossopharyngeal, vagus, and accessory nerves (*Figs. 9.3* and *9.5*). The dura over the intrajugular part of the foramen, which is located anteromedial to the sigmoid part, has two characteristic perforations, a glossopharyngeal meatus, through which the glossopharyngeal nerve passes, and a vagal meatus, through which the vagus and accessory nerves pass (*Figs. 9.5*

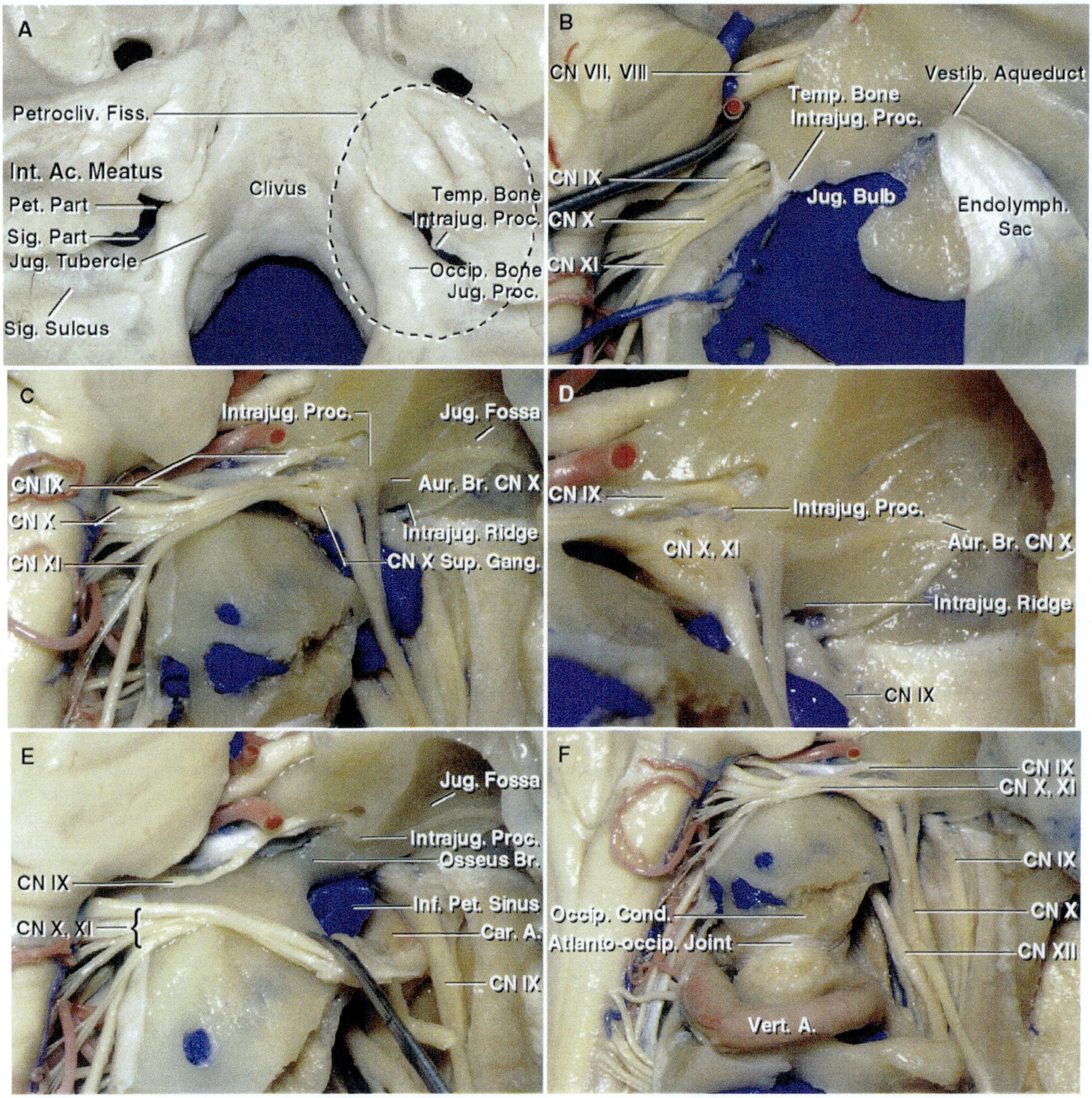

FIGURE 9.3. *A*, posterior superior view of the jugular foramen. The sigmoid sulcus makes a sharp turn just before emptying into the sigmoid portion of the jugular foramen. The inferior petrosal sinus extends along the petroclival fissure and enters the petrosal part of the foramen. The nerves enter the intrajugular part of the foramen located between the sigmoid and petrosal parts. The outlined area shows the approximate site from which *B* to *F* were taken. *B*, the sigmoid sinus descends in the sigmoid sulcus and makes a sharp anterior turn to enter the jugular foramen. The jugular bulb extends upward under the petrous temporal bone toward the internal acoustic meatus. The endolymphatic sac is located above the lower portion of the sigmoid sinus on the back of the temporal bone and opens above through the vestibular aqueduct into the vestibule. The glossopharyngeal, vagus and accessory nerves penetrate the dura on the medial side of the intrajugular process. *C*, the dura covering the jugular foramen and the jugular bulb have been removed. The nerves penetrate the dura on the medial side of the intrajugular process of the temporal bone. The intrajugular ridge extends forward along the medial side of the jugular bulb. *D*, enlarged view. The glossopharyngeal nerve passes forward along the medial side of the intrajugular ridge, but the vagus and accessory nerves, although entering the dura on the medial side of the intrajugular process, almost immediately turn downward and do not course along the medial edge of the intrajugular ridge in the medial wall of the jugular bulb, as

and *9.6*) (24). Both meatus are located on the medial side of the intrajugular processes and septum. The glossopharyngeal and vagal meatus are consistently separated by a dural septum ranging in width from 0.5 to 4.9 mm (13). The only intradural site at which the glossopharyngeal nerve is consistently distinguishable from the vagus nerve is just proximal to this dural septum. The close origins of the glossopharyngeal and vagus nerves at the brainstem, and the arachnoidal adhesions between the two in their course through the subarachnoid space may make separation difficult except in the area just proximal to the dural septum. The superior glossopharyngeal ganglion is easily visible intracranially in about one-third of nerves. The superior ganglion of the vagus can be seen intracranially in only one-sixth of nerves. Although the cranial and spinal portions of the accessory nerve most frequently enter the vagal meatus together, a dural septum may separate them.

The upper and lateral margins of the intrajugular part of the foramen are the site of a characteristic thick dural fold that forms a roof or lip that projects inferiorly and medially to partially cover the glossopharyngeal and vagal meatus (*Figs. 9.5* and *9.6*). This structure, called the jugular dural fold, was ossified on both sides in one specimen (13, 16, 17, 24, 31). The lip projects most prominently over the glossopharyngeal meatus and is comparable to, but smaller than, the posterior lip of the internal acoustic meatus. It is either predominantly bony or fibrous and may project a maximum of 2.5 mm over the margin of the glossopharyngeal meatus. The vagal lip is less prominent, projecting a maximum of 1 mm over the lateral margin of the vagal meatus.

Neural relationships

The glossopharyngeal, vagus, and accessory nerves arise from the medulla as a line of rootlets situated along the posterior edge of the inferior olive in the postolivary sulcus (*Figs. 9.3* and *9.5*). The hypoglossal nerve arises as a line of rootlets that exit the brainstem along the anterior margin of the lower two-thirds of the olive in the preolivary sulcus, a groove between the olive and medullary pyramid.

The glossopharyngeal nerve, at the point at which it penetrates the dural glossopharyngeal meatus, turns abruptly forward and then downward and courses through the jugular foramen in the groove leading from the pyramidal fossa below the opening of the cochlear aqueduct and along the medial side of the intrajugular ridge. After the nerve exits the jugular foramen, it turns forward, crossing the lateral surface of the internal carotid artery deep to the styloid process. As the nerve transverses the jugular foramen, it expands at the site of its superior and inferior ganglia (*Fig. 9.5*). At the external orifice of the jugular foramen, it gives rise to the tympanic branch (Jacobson's nerve), which traverses the tympanic canaliculus to enter the tympanic cavity where it gives rise to the tympanic plexus, the fibers of which course in shallow grooves on the promontory and regroup to form the lesser petrosal nerve, providing parasympathetic innervation by way of the otic ganglion to the parotid gland.

The vagal rootlets enter the dural subcompartment, called the vagal meatus, inferior to the glossopharyngeal meatus from which it is separated by a dural septum (*Figs. 9.5* and *9.6*). It is joined by the accessory nerve as it enters the dura. After its rootlets gather in the intracranial orifice of the foramen, the vagus nerve expands at the superior ganglion, which is about 2.5 mm in length, and ends below the extracranial orifice of the foramen. It sits on the dura, covering the jugular foramen, and there, along the medial side of the intrajugular process of the temporal bone, it turns downward. At the superior ganglion, the vagus nerve communicates with the accessory nerve, a portion of which blends into the ganglion. The auricular branch (Arnold's nerve) arises at the level of the superior vagal ganglion and is joined by a branch from the inferior glossopharyngeal ganglion (*Fig. 9.3*). The auricular branch passes laterally in a shallow groove on the anterior wall of the jugular bulb to reach the lateral wall of the jugular fossa, where it enters the mastoid canaliculus and ascends toward the vertical (mastoid) segment of the facial canal, giving off an ascending branch to the facial nerve as it crosses lateral to it before turning downward to exit the temporal bone through the tympanomastoid fissure.

The main trunk of the vagus nerve (or, more accurately, the superior ganglion) courses anterior and inferior as it crosses below the midportion of the intrajugular process of the temporal bone (*Figs. 9.3* and *9.5*). At the intracranial orifice of the foramen, the intrajugular process of the temporal bone separates the ganglion from the sigmoid sinus. In most cases, in the area immediately below the dura at the level of the intrajugular processes, there are no fibrous bands between the glossopharyngeal nerve and the vagal ganglion.

does the glossopharyngeal nerve. The auricular branch of the vagus nerve (Arnold's Nerve) arises from the vagus nerve, passes along the groove in the anterior wall of the jugular fossa, and penetrates the mastoid canaliculus in the lateral wall of the fossa. *E,* the nerves entering the jugular foramen have been displaced downward. The intrajugular process of the temporal bone projects backward to join the intrajugular process of the occipital bone, thus forming an osseous bridge that divides the foramen into two parts. The vagus and accessory nerves pass lateral to the osseous bridge and the inferior petrosal sinus descends below the bridge to open into the internal jugular vein. *F,* the hypoglossal nerve has been exposed on the lateral side of the occipital condyle. It exits the hypoglossal canal and joins the glossopharyngeal, vagus, and accessory nerves below the jugular foramen in the interval between the internal carotid artery and internal jugular vein. *A.,* artery; *Ac.,* acoustic; *Aur.,* auricular; *Br.,* branch; *Car.,* carotid; *CN,* cranial nerve; *Cond.,* condyle; *Endolymph.,* endolymphatic; *Gang.,* ganglion; *Inf.,* inferior; *Intrajug.,* intrajugular; *Jug.,* jugular; *Occip.,* occipital; *Pet.,* petrosal, petrous; *Petrocliv.,* petroclival; *Proc.,* process; *Sig.,* sigmoid; *Sup.,* superior; *Temp.,* temporal; *Vert.,* vertebral; *Vestib.,* vestibular.

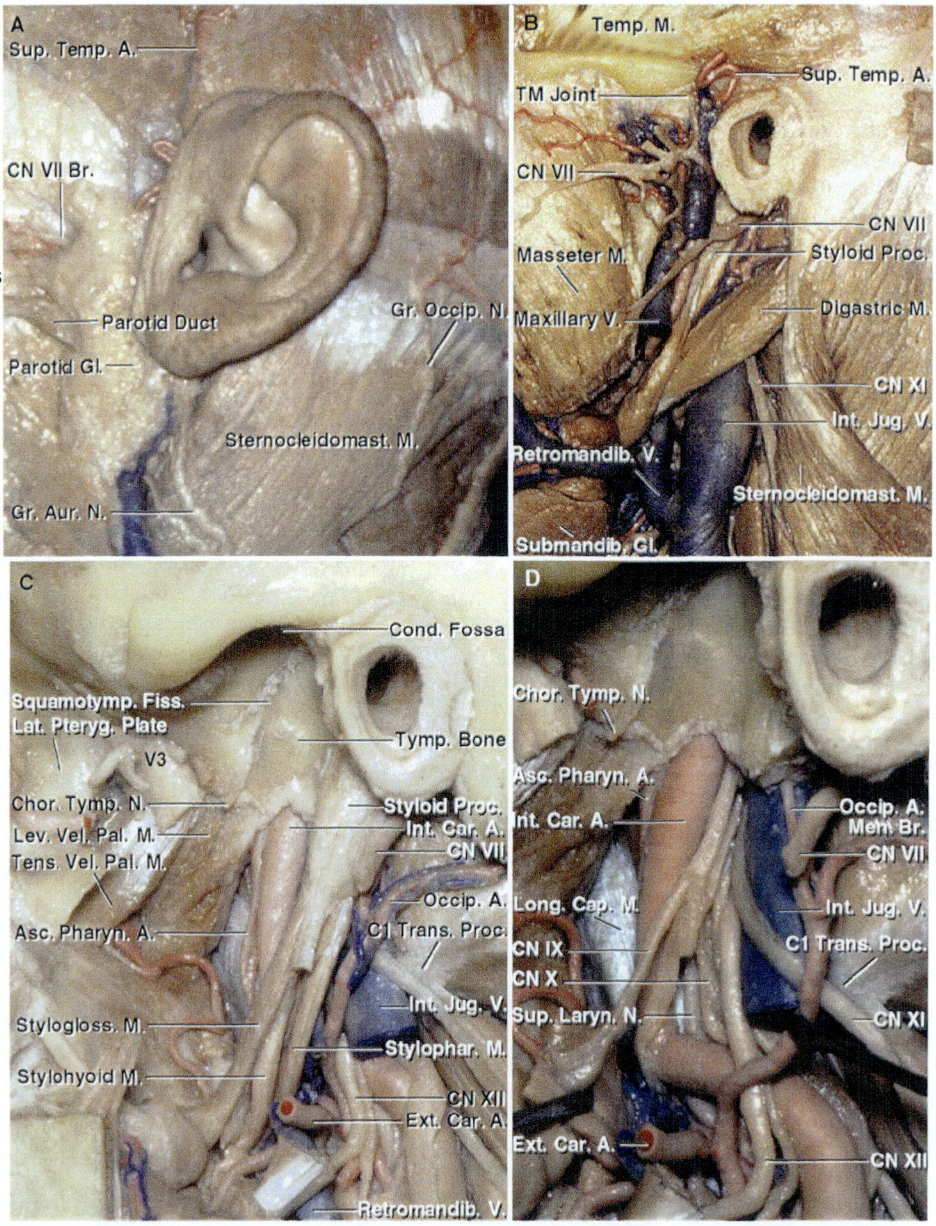

FIGURE 9.4. *A–D.* Stepwise dissection of the structures superficial to and surrounding the jugular foramen. *A,* the skin and scalp around the ear have been reflected to expose the area lateral to the jugular foramen. The sternocleidomastoid is exposed behind and the parotid gland in front of the ear. The greater occipital nerve and occipital artery reach the subcutaneous tissues by passing between the attachment of the trapezius and sternocleidomastoid muscles to the superior nuchal line. The external acoustic meatus is located a little forward of the deep site of the jugular bulb. *B,* removal of the superficial muscles and parotid gland exposes the facial nerve, temporalis and masseter muscles, posterior belly of the digastric, and the internal jugular vein. The sternocleidomastoid muscle has been reflected backward to expose the accessory nerve entering its deep surface. *C,* the mandibular ramus and condyle, medial and lateral pterygoid muscles, and posterior belly of the digastric have been removed to expose the styloid process, which is located lateral to the jugular foramen. The internal carotid artery ascends to enter the carotid canal in front of the jugular foramen. Both the jugular foramen and carotid canal are situated behind the tympanic part of the temporal bone, which forms the posterior wall of the condylar fossa. The tensor and levator vela palatini muscles are attached to the eustachian tube in the area below the horizontal segment of the petrous carotid. The infratemporal fossa is located below the greater wing of the sphenoid. The mandibular nerve passes through the foramen ovale to enter the upper part of the infratemporal fossa. Branches of the ascending pharyngeal artery pass through the jugular foramen to supply the surrounding dura. The hypoglossal nerve passes forward across the external and internal carotid artery. *D,* the styloid process has been removed to expose the glossopharyngeal, vagus, accessory, and hypoglossal nerves descending between the internal carotid artery and the internal jugular vein in the area immediately below the jugular foramen. The glossopharyngeal nerve descends along the lateral side of the internal carotid artery. The accessory nerve passes backward across the lateral surface of the internal jugular vein. The hypoglossal nerve passes through the hypoglossal canal, which is located below and medial to the jugular foramen, and descends with the nerves exiting the jugular foramen. The occipital artery gives rise to a meningeal branch, which passes through the jugular foramen to supply the surrounding dura, and to the stylomastoid artery, which passes through the stylomastoid foramen with the facial nerve. *A.*, artery; *Asc.*, ascending; *Aur.*, auricular; *Br.*, branch; *Cap.*, capitis; *Car.*, carotid; *Chor. Tymp.*, chorda tympani; *CN,* cranial nerve; *Cond.*, condylar; *Dors.*, dorsal; *Eust.*, eustachian; *Ext.*, external; *Fiss.*, fissure; *Gl.*, gland; *Gr.*, greater; *Inf.*, inferior; *Int.*, internal; *Jug.*, jugular; *Laryn.*, laryngeal; *Lat.*, lateral, lateralis; *Lev.*, levator; *Long.*, longus; *M.*, muscle; *Mast.*, mastoid; *Men.*, meningeal; *N.*, nerve; *Obl.*, oblique; *Occip.*, occipital; *Pal.*, palatini; *Pet.*, petrosal, petrous; *Pharyn.*, pharyngeal; *Post.*, posterior; *Proc.*, process; *Pteryg.*, pterygoid; *Rec.*, rectus; *Retromandib.*, retromandibular; *Scap.*, scapulae; *Seg.*, segment; *Semicirc.*, semicircular; *Sig.*, sigmoid; *Squamotymp.*, squamotympanic; *Sternocleidomast.*, sternocleidomastoid; *Stylogloss.*, styloglossus; *Stylomast.*, stylomastoid; *Stylophar.*, stylopharyngeus; *Submandib.*, submandibular; *Sup.*, superior; *Temp.*, temporal; *Tens.*, tensor; *TM.*, temporomandibular; *Trans.*, transverse; *Tymp.*, tympanic, tympany; *V.*, vein; *Vel.*, veli; *Vent.*, ventral; *Vert.*, vertebral.

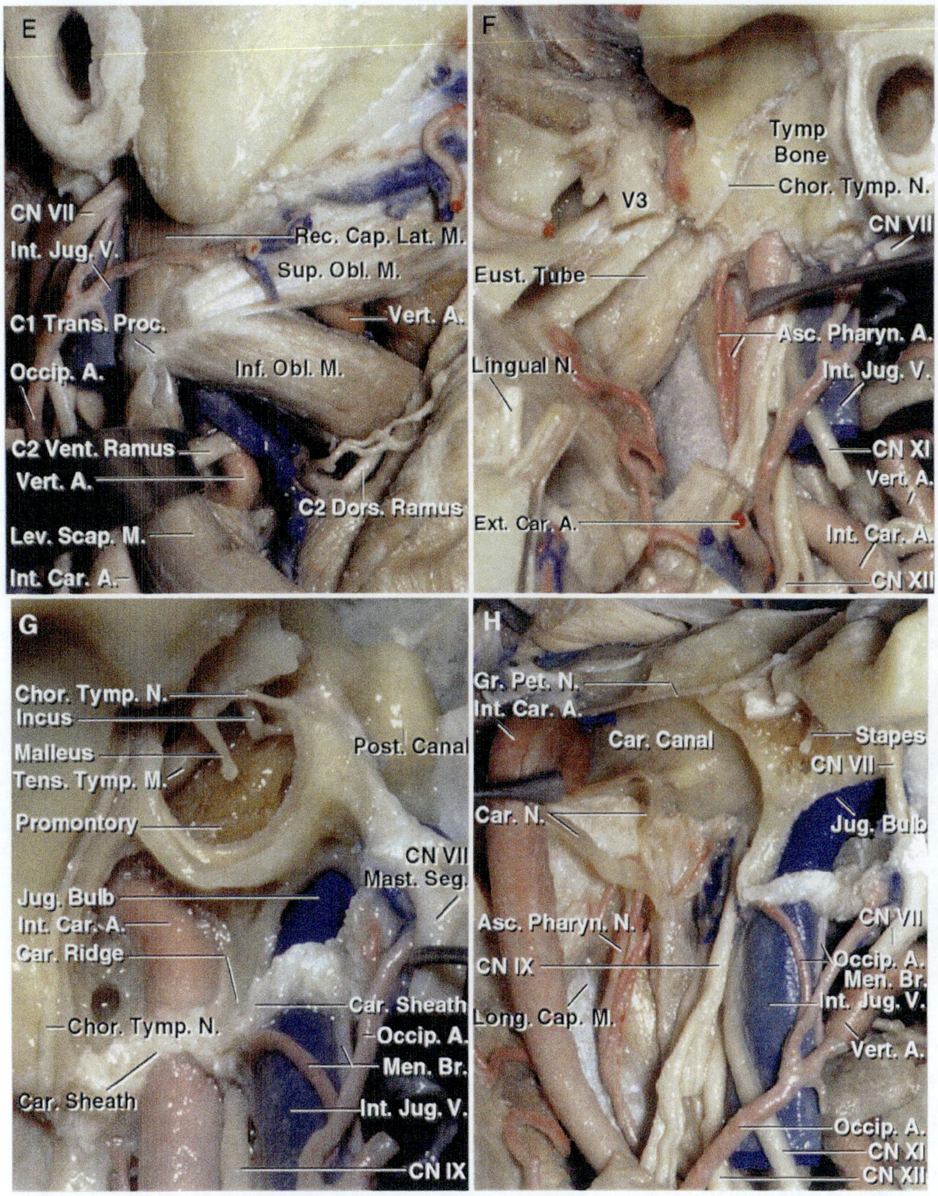

FIGURE 9.4. ***E–H. E,*** **the superior and inferior oblique have been exposed by reflecting the more superficial muscles. The C1 transverse process and rectus capitis lateralis rest against the posterior surface of the internal jugular vein. The rectus capitis lateralis attaches to the jugular process of the occipital bone at the posterior margin of the jugular foramen. Retracting the levator scapulae exposes the segment of the vertebral artery ascending through the C2 transverse foramen in front of the ventral ramus of the C2 nerve root. The vertebral artery, as it passes medially along the upper surface of the posterior arch of the atlas, is situated in the floor of the suboccipital triangle located between the superior and inferior oblique and rectus capitis posterior major.** ***F,*** **the internal carotid artery has been displaced posteriorly to expose the branches of the ascending pharyngeal, which pass through the foramen lacerum, jugular foramen, and hypoglossal canal to supply the surrounding dura. The chorda tympani exits the skull in the medial part of the condylar fossa by first passing through the petrotympanic and then along the squamotympanic sutures.** ***G,*** **the tympanic bone forming the lower and anterior margin of the external meatus has been removed, but the tympanic sulcus to which the tympanic membrane attaches has been preserved. The surface of the temporal and occipital bones surrounding the jugular foramen and carotid canal have an irregular surface that serves as the attachment of the upper end of the carotid sheath. The mastoid segment of the facial nerve and the stylomastoid foramen are situated lateral to the jugular bulb. The chorda tympani arises from the mastoid segment of the facial nerve and courses along the deep side of the tympanic membrane crossing the neck of the malleus. It exits the skull by passing through the petrotympanic and squamotympanic sutures and joins the lingual branch of the mandibular nerve distally. The carotid ridge separates the carotid canal and jugular foramen. Meningeal branches of the ascending pharyngeal and occipital arteries enter the jugular foramen. The glossopharyngeal, vagus, and accessory nerves pass through the jugular foramen on the medial side of the jugular bulb.** ***H,*** **the tympanic ring and bone lateral to the tympanic cavity have been removed. The internal carotid artery has been displaced forward out of the carotid canal to expose the carotid sympathetic nerves that ascend with the artery. The glossopharyngeal, vagus, accessory, and hypoglossal nerves exit the skull on the medial side of the internal carotid artery and jugular vein. The glossopharyngeal and hypoglossal nerves pass forward along the lateral surface of the internal carotid artery, and the accessory nerve descends posteriorly across the lateral surface of the internal jugular vein. The vagus nerve descends in the carotid sheath.**

The vagus nerve exits the jugular foramen vertically, retaining an intimate relationship to the accessory nerve (*Figs. 9.3–9.5*). At the level the two nerves exit the jugular foramen, they are located behind the glossopharyngeal nerve on the posteromedial wall of the internal jugular vein. As the vagus nerve passes lateral to the outer orifice of the hypoglossal canal, it is joined by the hypoglossal nerve medially. The vagus nerve begins to expand at the site of the inferior vagal

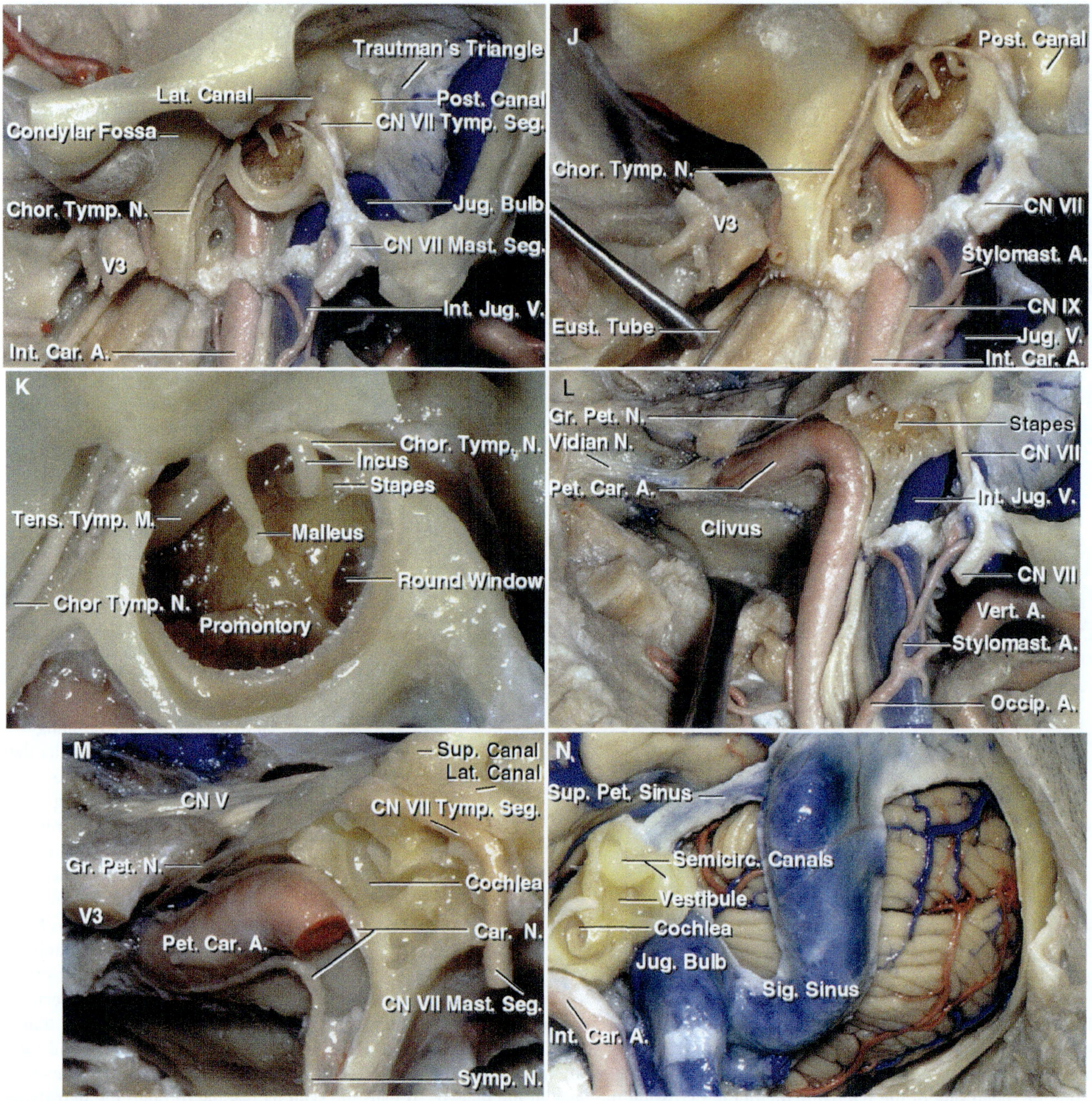

FIGURE 9.4. *I–N. I,* lateral view of mastoid and tympanic cavity before removing the tympanic ring. The tympanic segment of the facial nerve passes below the lateral semicircular canal and turns downward as the mastoid segment to exit the stylomastoid foramen. The stylomastoid foramen and the mastoid segment are located lateral to the jugular bulb. The semicircular canals are located above the jugular bulb. *J,* a probe has been placed in the eustachian tube, which passes downward, forward, and medially from the tympanic cavity and across the front of the petrous carotid. The third trigeminal division passes through the foramen ovale on the lateral side of the eustachian tube. *K,* enlarged view of the tympanic ring with the tympanic membrane removed. The tensor tympany muscle passes backward above the eustachian tube and gives rise to a tendon that turns sharply lateral around the trochleiform process to attach to the malleus. The chorda tympani crosses the inner surface of the tympanic membrane and neck of the malleus. The round window opens into the vestibule. The stapes sit in the oval window. The promontory is located lateral to the basal turn of the cochlea. *L,* the floor of the middle fossa and the tympanic sulcus have been removed to expose the jugular bulb and petrous carotid. The greater petrosal nerve courses along the floor of the middle fossa on the upper surface of the petrous carotid. The deep petrosal nerve arises from the sympathetic bundles on the internal carotid artery. The deep and greater petrosal nerves join to form the vidian nerve, which passes forward through the vidian canal to join the maxillary nerve and pterygopalatine ganglion in the pterygopalatine fossa. The pharyngobasilar fascia and upper part of the

ganglion just below the foramen and is approximately 2.5 cm in length.

Accessory nerve

Although the cranial and spinal portions of the accessory nerve most frequently enter the vagal meatus together, they may infrequently be separated by a dural septum. The spinal portion ascends toward the foramen magnum by crawling along the surface of the dura and may even be buried in the dura below the foramen magnum (*Figs. 9.3, 9.5*, and *9.6*). At the dural orifice of the jugular foramen, the nerve is often indistinguishable from the vagus nerve. The accessory nerve usually enters the same dural subcompartment as the vagus nerve and often adheres and blends into the vagus nerve at the level of the superior vagal ganglion. The accessory nerve departs the vagal ganglion after it exits the jugular foramen and descends obliquely laterally between the internal carotid artery and internal jugular vein and then backward across the lateral surface of the vein to reach its muscles. Approximately 30% of nerves descend along the medial, rather than the lateral, surface of the internal jugular vein (8).

Hypoglossal nerve

The hypoglossal nerve does not traverse the jugular foramen (*Figs. 9.3–9.5*). However, it joins the nerves exiting the jugular foramen just below the skull and runs with them in the carotid sheath. The nerve exits the inferolateral part of the hypoglossal canal and passes adjacent to the vagus nerve, descends between the internal carotid artery and the internal jugular vein to the level of the transverse process of the atlas, where it turns abruptly forward along the lateral surface of the internal carotid artery toward the tongue, leaving only the ansa cervicalis to descend with the major vessels.

ARTERIAL RELATIONSHIPS

The arteries that may be involved in pathological abnormalities at the jugular foramen include the upper cervical and petrous portions of the internal carotid artery, the posteriorly directed branches of the external carotid artery, and the upper portion of the vertebral artery (*Fig. 9.4*).

Internal carotid artery

The internal carotid artery passes, almost straightly upward, posterior to the external carotid artery and anteromedial to the internal jugular vein, to reach the carotid canal (*Fig. 9.4*). At the level of the skull base, the internal jugular vein courses just posterior to the internal carotid artery, being separated from it by the carotid ridge. Between them, the glossopharyngeal nerve is located laterally and the vagus, accessory, and hypoglossal nerves medially.

After the internal carotid artery enters the carotid canal with the carotid sympathetic nerves and surrounding venous plexus, it ascends a short distance (the vertical segment), reaching the area below and slightly behind the cochlea, where it turns anteromedially at a right angle (the site of the lateral bend) and courses horizontally (the horizontal segment) toward the petrous apex (*Fig. 9.4*). At the medial edge of the foramen lacerum, it turns sharply upward at the site of the medial bend to enter the posterior part of the cavernous sinus.

External carotid artery

The external carotid artery ascends anterior to the internal carotid artery. Proximal to its terminal bifurcation into the maxillary and the superficial temporal arteries, it gives rise to six branches, which can be divided into anterior and posterior groups according to their directions. The latter group is related to the jugular foramen.

The ascending pharyngeal artery, the first branch of the posterior group, often provides the most prominent supply to the meninges around the jugular foramen (*Fig. 9.4*) (18). It arises either at the bifurcation or from the lowest part of the external or internal carotid arteries. Rarely it arises from the origin of the occipital artery. It courses upward between the internal and the external carotid arteries, giving rise to numerous branches to neighboring muscles, nerves, and lymph nodes. Its meningeal branches pass through the foramen lacerum to be distributed to the dura lining the middle fossa and through the jugular foramen or the hypoglossal canal to supply the surrounding dura of the posterior cranial fossa. The ascending pharyngeal artery also gives rise to the inferior tympanic artery, which reaches the tympanic cavity by way of the tympanic canaliculus along with the tympanic branch of the glossopharyngeal nerve.

The occipital artery, the second and largest branch of the posterior group, arises from the posterior surface of the external carotid artery and courses obliquely upward between the posterior belly of the digastric muscle and the internal jugular vein (*Fig. 9.4*). Its meningeal branches, which enter the posterior fossa through the jugular foramen or the condylar canal, may make a significant contribution to tumors of the jugular foramen.

The posterior auricular artery, the last branch in the posterior group, arises above the posterior belly of the digastric muscle and travels between the parotid gland and the styloid process. At the anterior margin of the mastoid process, it divides into auricular and occipital branches, which are dis-

longus capitis have been reflected downward to expose the lower margin of the clivus. *M*, the jugular bulb has been removed from the jugular fossa located below the vestibule and semicircular canals. The vertical segment of the petrous carotid has been removed. The cochlea, which has been opened, is located above the lateral genu of the petrous carotid. The tympanic segment of the facial nerve passes posteriorly below the lateral semicircular canal. *N*, the retrosigmoid and presigmoid dura have been opened. The lateral wall of the vestibule and cochlea have been removed. The vestibule, semicircular canals, and cochlea are exposed above the jugular bulb and lateral genu of the petrous carotid.

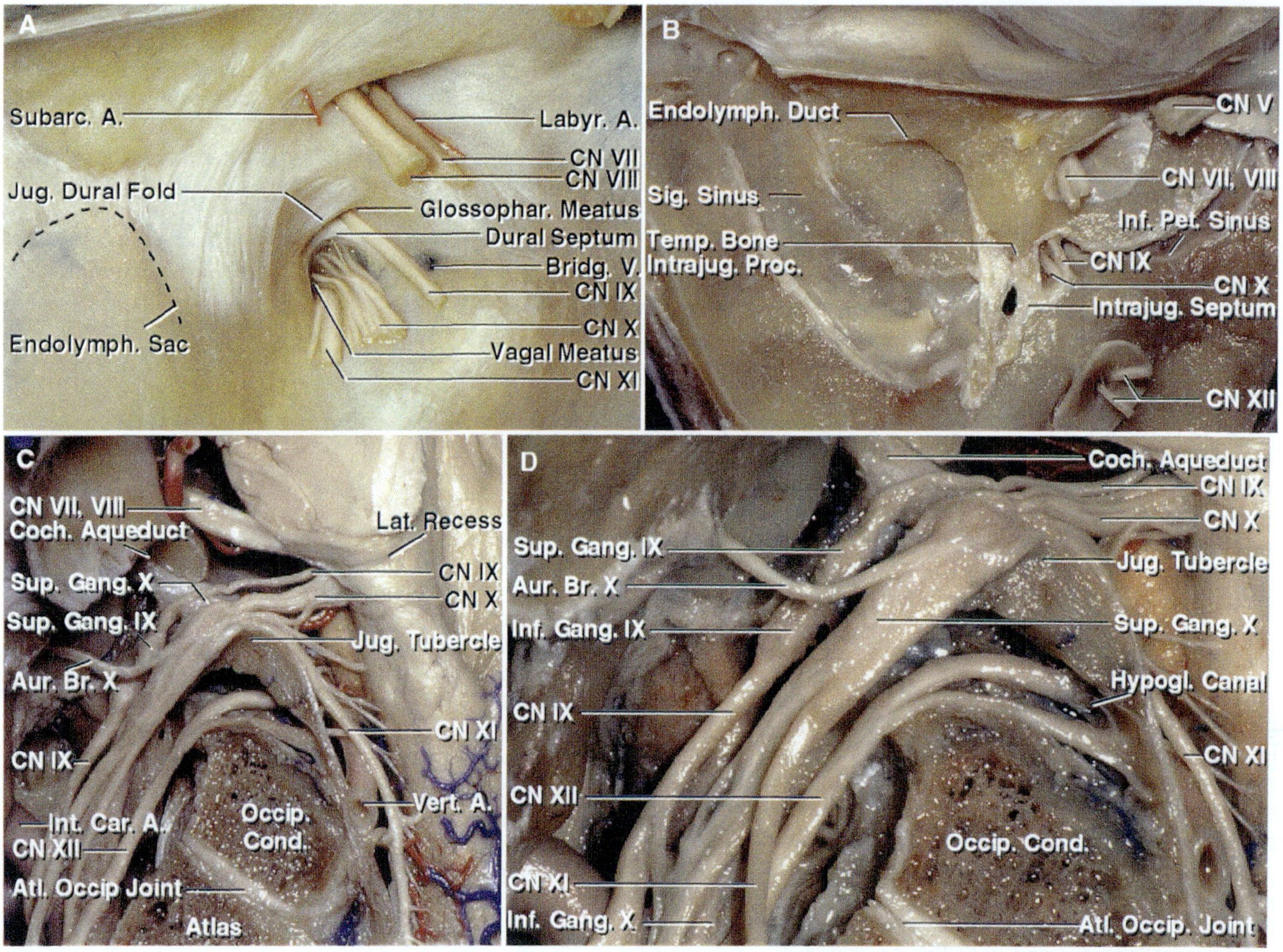

FIGURE 9.5. *A,* posterior view of the intracranial aspect of the left jugular foramen. The glossopharyngeal, vagus, and accessory nerves pierce the dural roof of the jugular foramen. The glossopharyngeal nerve is separated from the vagus nerve by a narrow dural septum. The jugular dural fold projects downward and medially from the lateral and upper margin of the jugular foramen over the site at which the nerves enter the dura roof of the foramen. The facial and vestibulocochlear nerves and labyrinthine artery enter the internal acoustic meatus. The subarcuate branch of the anteroinferior cerebellar artery enters the subarcuate fossa. The endolymphatic sac is located between the dural layers lateral to the jugular foramen. A bridging vein from the medulla joins the inferior petrosal sinus on the medial side of the jugular bulb. *B,* the dura has been removed from the posterior surface of the temporal bone. The intrajugular processes of the temporal and occipital bones, which are connected by a fibrous bridge, the intrajugular septum, separates the sigmoid and petrosal parts of the foramen. The glossopharyngeal, vagus, and accessory nerves enter the intrajugular part of the foramen by penetrating the dura on the medial side of the intrajugular process of the temporal bone. *C,* the glossopharyngeal nerve enters the jugular foramen below the cochlear aqueduct. The vagus nerve enters the jugular foramen behind the glossopharyngeal nerve. The auricular branch of the vagus nerve (Arnold's nerve) arises at the level of the superior ganglion and passes around the anterior wall of the jugular bulb. The accessory nerve is formed by multiple rootlets, which arise from the medulla and spinal cord. The accessory rootlets collect together to form a bundle that blends into the lower margin of the vagus nerve at the level of the jugular foramen. The lower vagal and accessory roots pass across the surface of the jugular tubercle. *D,* enlarged view. The glossopharyngeal nerve expands at the site of the superior and inferior ganglia. The superior ganglion of the vagus nerve is located at the level of or just below the dural roof of the foramen, and the inferior ganglion is located below the foramen at the level of the atlanto-occipital joint. *A.,* artery; *Atl.,* atlanto-; *Aur.,* auricular; *Br.,* branch; *Bridg.,* bridging; *Car.,* carotid; *CN,* cranial nerve; *Coch.,* cochlear; *Cond.,* condyle; *Endolymph.,* endolymphatic; *Gang.,* ganglion; *Glossophar.,* glossopharyngeal; *Hypogl.,* hypoglossal; *Inf.,* inferior; *Int.,* internal; *Intrajug.,* intrajugular; *Jug.,* jugular; *Labyr.,* labyrinthine; *Lat.,* lateral; *Occip.,* occipital; *Pet.,* petrosal; *Proc.,* process; *Sig.,* sigmoid; *Subarc.,* subarcuate; *Sup.,* superior; *Temp.,* temporal; *Vert.,* vertebral.

tributed to the postauricular and the occipital regions respectively. The stylomastoid branch, which arises below the stylomastoid foramen, enters the stylomastoid foramen to supply the facial nerve. Its loss can lead to a facial palsy even though it anastomoses with the petrosal branch of the middle meningeal artery. The posterior auricular branch may share a common trunk with the occipital artery, or sometimes it is absent, in which case, the occipital artery gives rise to the

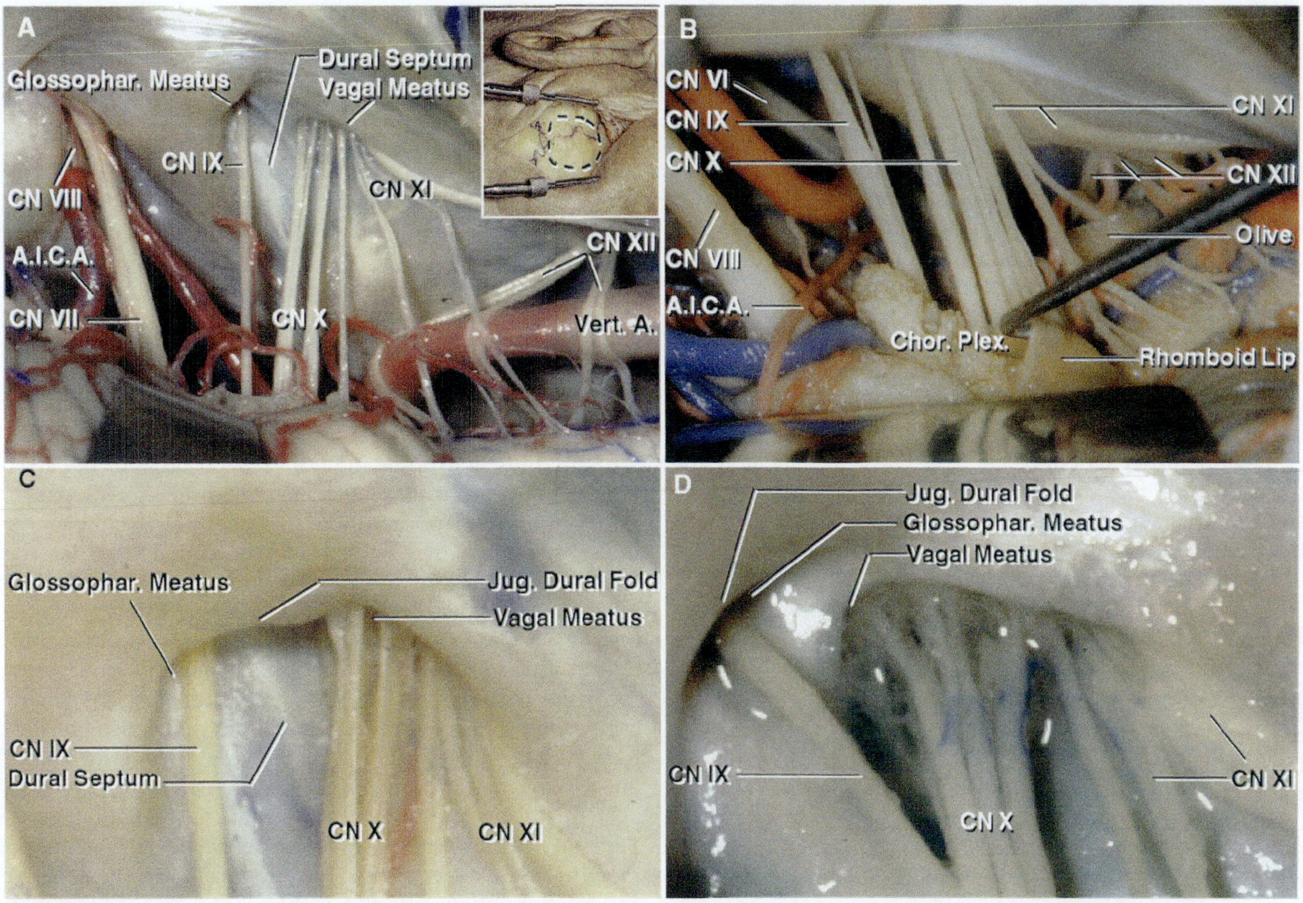

FIGURE 9.6. Retrosigmoid approach to jugular foramen. *A,* the detail shows the site of the vertical scalp incision and right retrosigmoid craniotomy. The cerebellum has been elevated to expose the nerves in the right cerebellopontine angle. The glossopharyngeal and vagal nerves are separated by the dural septum at the level of the dural roof of the jugular foramen. The glossopharyngeal nerve enters the glossopharyngeal meatus and the vagus nerve enters the vagal meatus with the branches of the accessory nerve. Both meatus are very shallow compared with the internal acoustic meatus. The superior and lateral margins of both meatus project downward and medially over the nerves entering the meatus. The vertebral artery displaces the hypoglossal rootlets of Cranial Nerve XII posteriorly so that they intermingle with the rootlets of the accessory nerve. *B,* another specimen showing the relationship of the rhomboid lip and choroid plexus protruding from the foramen of Luschka to the glossopharyngeal and vagus nerves. The choroid plexus protrudes laterally behind the glossopharyngeal nerves. The rhomboid lip is a thin layer of neural tissue that forms the ventral margin of the foramen of Luschka at the outer end of the lateral recess. *C* and *D,* enlarged view of two jugular foramina. The glossopharyngeal and vagus nerves are consistently separated by a dural septum at the level of the roof over the jugular foramen. The jugular dural fold projects downward and medially over the lateral edge of the glossopharyngeal and vagal meatus and over the site at which the nerves penetrate the dura. *A.,* artery; *A.I.C.A.,* anteroinferior cerebellar artery; Chor., choroid; *CN,* cranial nerve; *Glossophar.,* glossopharyngeal; *Jug.,* jugular; *Plex.,* plexus; *Vert.,* vertebral.

stylomastoid artery. Members of the anterior group, whose origins may be visualized in exposing lesions of the jugular foramen, include the superior thyroid, lingual, and facial arteries.

Vertebral artery

The vertebral artery, as it ascends to reach and pass through the transverse foramen of the atlas, is located below and behind the jugular foramen (*Fig. 9.4*). Branches encountered in approaches to lesions of the jugular foramen include the meningeal, posterior spinal, and posteroinferior cerebellar artery.

VENOUS RELATIONSHIPS

The jugular bulb and adjacent part of the internal jugular vein receives drainage from both intracranial and extracranial sources, which include the sigmoid and inferior petrosal sinuses, the vertebral venous plexus, the venous plexus of the hypoglossal canal, the posterior condylar emissary vein, and the vein coursing along the inferior aspect of the petroclival fissure (*Figs. 9.4* and *9.5*).

Sigmoid sinus and jugular bulb

The sigmoid sinus is the largest channel emptying into the jugular foramen (*Figs. 9.1* and *9.3–9.5*). After coursing down the sigmoid sulcus, the sinus turns anteriorly toward the jugular foramen, crossing the occipitomastoid suture immediately proximal to the foramen. From there, the sinus is directed forward below the petrous temporal bone at the site of the jugular bulb. The upward bulging of the superior margin of the jugular bulb creates a rounded fossa in the lower surface of the temporal bone below the internal auditory canal. The dome of the jugular bulb may extend upward in the posterior wall of the internal auditory canal to the level of the upper margin of the canal. The bulb is usually larger on the right side, reflecting the larger diameter of the sigmoid sinus on that side. From the level of the jugular bulb, flow is directed downward behind the tympanic bone and the carotid canal into the internal jugular vein.

Inferior petrosal sinus and venous confluens

The foramen also receives the inflow from the inferior petrosal sinus and the venous confluens in the petrosal part of the foramen. The inferior petrosal sinus, which courses on the intracranial surface of the petroclival fissure, communicates the cavernous sinus and basilar venous plexus at its upper end and with the jugular bulb at its lower end (*Figs. 9.3* and *9.5*). The inferior petrosal sinus, as it enters the petrosal part of the jugular foramen, forms a plexiform confluens with the venous plexus of the hypoglossal canal, the inferior petroclival vein, and tributaries from the vertebral venous plexus and posterior condylar emissary vein. This confluens, which fills the petrosal part of the foramen, usually consists of a main channel, 2 to 3 mm in diameter, and several smaller channels, less than 1 mm in diameter. It empties into the medial aspect of the jugular bulb through one or two openings in the venous walls between the glossopharyngeal and vagus nerves or into the internal jugular vein below the extracranial orifice.

The inferior petroclival vein courses along the extracranial surface of the petroclival fissure and is a mirror image of the inferior petrosal sinus, which courses along the intracranial surface of the fissure (*Fig. 9.5*). It empties into the venous confluens at the lower end of the inferior petrosal sinus at or just below the extracranial orifice of the jugular foramen or even above it, through bony clefts between the temporal and occipital bones.

Bridging veins

A bridging vein, which courses posterior to the glossopharyngeal, vagus, and accessory nerves from the dorsolateral medulla to the lower end of the sigmoid sinus, is present in about one-third of cerebellopontine angles (*Fig. 9.5*, also see *Fig. 3.12*). Infrequently, a bridging vein extends from the ventral medulla to the lower margin of the inferior petrosal sinus in front of the nerves.

MUSCULAR RELATIONSHIPS

Several muscles that are encountered in the surgical approaches to the jugular foramen and that provide important landmarks in the approach are reviewed in detail in the chapters on the foramen magnum and temporal bone (*Fig. 9.4*). These include the sternocleidomastoid, situated superficially in the lateral neck, and the splenius capitis, longissimus capitis, levator scapulae, and scalenus medius muscles in a deeper muscular layer.

More anteriorly is the posterior belly of the digastric muscle, which arises in the digastric groove located medial to the mastoid process and the longissimus capitis. The styloid process and its attached muscles appear in the triangular zone bounded by the posterior belly of the digastric, the external auditory canal, and the mandibular ramus. Reflecting the digastric muscle exposes the transverse process of the atlas, which is covered by the attachments of numerous muscles, including the superior and inferior obliques, which form the upper and lower margin of the suboccipital triangle. The rectus capitis lateralis muscle is the muscle most intimately related to the jugular foramen. It extends vertically behind the internal jugular vein from the transverse process of the atlas to the jugular process of the occipital bone.

On the posterior neck are the trapezius muscle, splenius capitis, and semispinalis capitis. Beneath the semispinalis capitis muscle, three muscles arise between the inferior nuchal line and the margin of the foramen magnum: the rectus capitis posterior major and minor and the superior oblique muscle. The suboccipital triangle, an area defined by the opposing margins of the rectus capitis posterior major and the superior and inferior oblique muscles, is the site at which the vertebral artery courses along the upper posterior surface of the atlas.

SURGICAL APPROACHES

Postauricular transtemporal approach

The postauricular transtemporal approach accesses the region from laterally, through the mastoid, and from below, through the neck (*Fig. 9.7*) (2, 4, 5). A C-shaped postauricular skin incision provides the exposure for a mastoidectomy and the neck dissection. The external auditory canal is either preserved or transected, depending on the anterior extent of the pathological abnormality. The neck dissection is completed initially to gain control of the major vessels and the branches supplying the tumor. The internal carotid artery, branches of the external carotid artery, internal jugular vein, and lower cranial nerves are exposed in the carotid sheath. A mastoidectomy with extensive drilling of the infralabyrinthine region accesses the jugular bulb. A limited mastoidectomy confined to the area behind the stylomastoid foramen and mastoid segment of the facial nerve, combined with removal of the adjacent part of the jugular process of the temporal bone, will provide access to the posterior and posterolateral aspect of the jugular foramen. Three obstacles to exposure of the full lateral half of the jugular foramen, the facial nerve, styloid process, and rectus capitis lateralis muscle are dealt with by transposing the facial nerve, removing the styloid process, and divid-

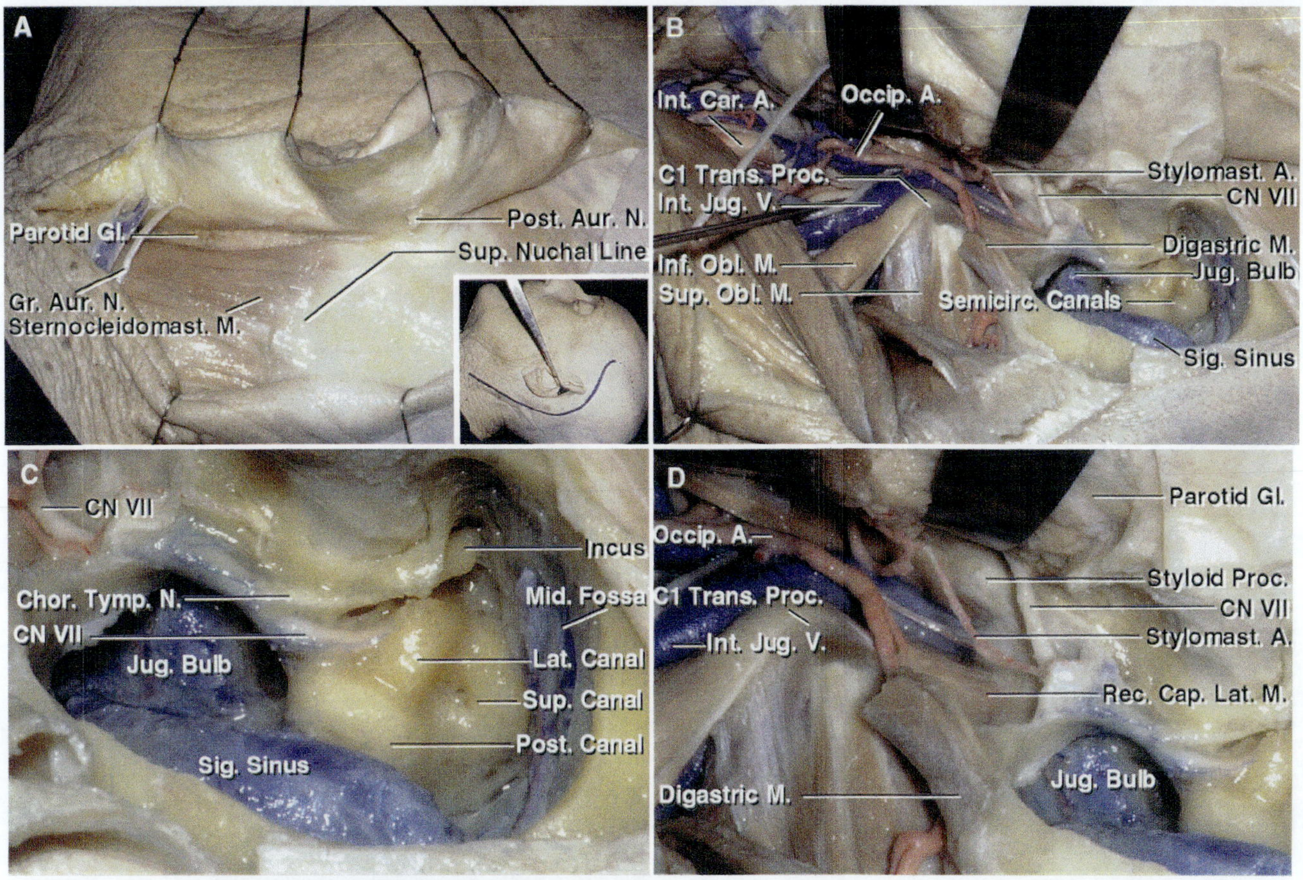

FIGURE 9.7. ***A–D.*** **Postauricular exposure of the jugular foramen.** ***A,*** **the detail shows the site of the scalp incision. The C-shaped retroauricular incision provides access for the mastoidectomy, neck dissection, and parotid gland displacement. The scalp flap has been reflected forward to expose the sternocleidomastoid and the posterior part of the parotid gland.** ***B,*** **the more superficial muscles and the posterior belly of the digastric have been reflected to expose the internal jugular vein and the attachment of the superior and inferior oblique to the transverse process of C1. A mastoidectomy has been completed to expose the facial nerve, sigmoid sinus, and capsule of the semicircular canals.** ***C,*** **enlarged view of the mastoidectomy. The jugular bulb is exposed below the semicircular canals. The chorda tympani arises from the mastoid segment of the facial nerve and passes upward and forward. The tympanic segment of the facial nerve courses below the lateral canal.** ***D,*** **enlarged view of the caudal part of the exposure shown in** ***C.*** **The facial nerve and styloid process cover the extracranial orifice of the jugular foramen. The facial nerve crosses the lateral surface of the styloid process. The stylomastoid artery arises from the postauricular artery. The rectus capitis lateralis attaches to the jugular process of the occipital bone behind the jugular foramen.** ***A.,*** **artery;** ***Aur.,*** **auricular;** ***Cap.,*** **capitis;** ***Car.,*** **carotid;** ***Chor. Tymp.,*** **chorda tympani;** ***CN,*** **cranial nerve;** ***Coch.,*** **cochlear;** ***Gl.,*** **gland;** ***Gr.,*** **greater;** ***Inf.,*** **inferior;** ***Int.,*** **internal;** ***Intrajug.,*** **intrajugular;** ***Jug.,*** **jugular;** ***Laryn.,*** **laryngeal;** ***Lat.,*** **lateral, lateralis;** ***M.,*** **muscle;** ***Med.,*** **medial;** ***Mid.,*** **middle;** ***N.,*** **nerve;** ***Obl.,*** **oblique;** ***Occip.,*** **occipital;** ***Pet.,*** **petrosal, petrous;** ***Post.,*** **posterior;** ***Proc.,*** **process;** ***Rec.,*** **rectus;** ***Semicirc.,*** **semicircular;** ***Sig.,*** **sigmoid;** ***Sternocleidomast.,*** **sternocleidomastoid;** ***Stylomast.,*** **stylomastoid;** ***Sup.,*** **superior;** ***Symp.,*** **sympathetic;** ***Tr.,*** **trunk;** ***Trans.,*** **transverse;** ***V.,*** **vein.**

ing the rectus capitis lateralis muscle. Anterior extensions of the pathological abnormality are reached by sacrificing the external and the middle ear structures. Sensorineural hearing can be preserved by maintaining the foot plate of the stapes in the oval window to avoid opening the labyrinth. Intracranial extensions of the lesion are reached by the retrosigmoid or presigmoid approaches after adding a suboccipital craniectomy. The lesion can be removed by a transtemporal infralabyrinthine approach directed through the temporal bone below the labyrinth without the neck dissection, if the extracranial extension of the lesion is not prominent. The exposure can be extended by opening the otic capsule (translabyrinthine approach).

Retrosigmoid approach

A pathological abnormality located predominantly intradurally can be resected by the retrosigmoid approach (*Fig. 9.6*). A lateral suboccipital craniectomy exposes the dura behind the sigmoid sinus. The dura is opened, and the cerebellum is gently elevated away from the posterior surface of the temporal bone to expose the cisterns in the cerebellopontine

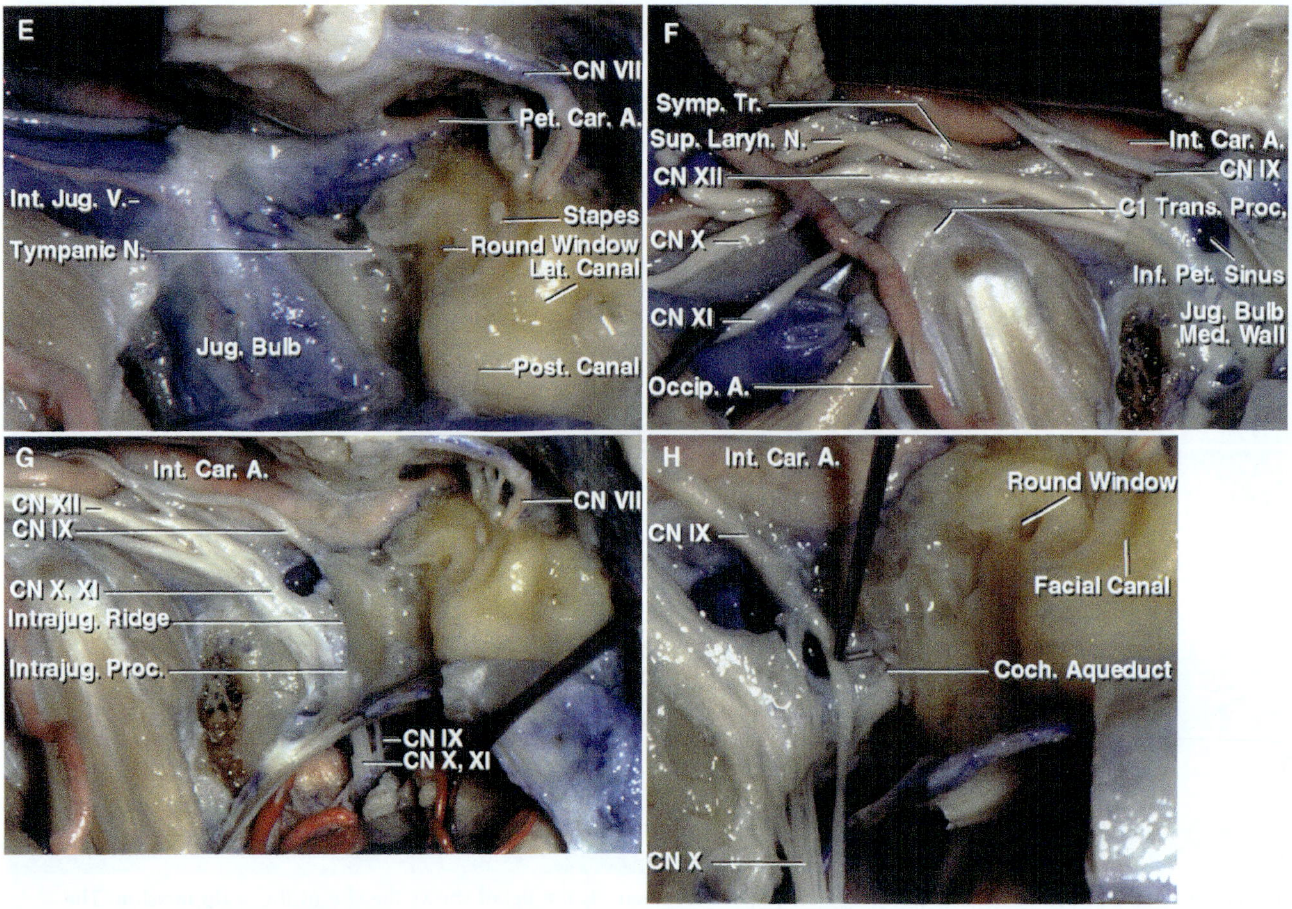

FIGURE 9.7. *E–H. E,* the external auditory canal has been transected and the middle ear structures have been removed, except the stapes, which has been left in the oval window. The lateral edge of the jugular foramen has been exposed by completing the mastoidectomy, transposing the facial nerve anteriorly, and fracturing the styloid process across its base and reflecting it caudally. The rectus capitis lateralis has been detached from the jugular process of the occipital bone. The petrous carotid is surrounded in the carotid canal by a venous plexus. *F,* a segment of the sigmoid sinus, jugular bulb, and internal jugular vein have been removed. The lateral wall of the jugular bulb has been removed while preserving the medial wall and exposing the opening of the inferior petrosal sinus into the jugular bulb. Removing the venous wall exposes the glossopharyngeal, vagus, accessory, and hypoglossal nerves, which are hidden deep to the vein. The main inflow from the petrosal confluens is directed between the glossopharyngeal and vagus nerves. *G,* the medial venous wall of the jugular bulb has been removed. The intrajugular ridge extends forward from the intrajugular process, which divides the jugular foramen between the sigmoid and petrosal parts. The glossopharyngeal, vagus, and accessory nerves enter the dura on the medial side of the intrajugular process, but only the glossopharyngeal nerve courses through the foramen entirely on the medial side of the intrajugular ridge. The vagus nerve also enters the dura on the medial side of the intrajugular process, but does not course along the medial side of the intrajugular ridge. *H,* the intrajugular process and ridge have been removed to expose the passage of the glossopharyngeal, vagus, and accessory nerves through the jugular foramen. The tip of a right-angle probe identifies the junction of the cochlear aqueduct with the pyramidal fossa, just above where the glossopharyngeal nerve penetrates the dura.

angle and the intracranial aspect of the cranial nerves entering the jugular foramen, hypoglossal canal, and internal acoustic meatus.

Far-lateral approach

An extended modification of the retrosigmoid approach, the far-lateral approach, the subject of another chapter in this issue, may be selected if the tumor extends down to the foramen magnum in front of or lateral to the lower brainstem (10, 30, 32, 33). In this approach, the jugular foramen is opened from behind. The dura is opened and the cerebellum elevated to expose the intracranial extension of the pathological abnormality at the lower clivus and at the foramen magnum. Several variations, depending on the location and extent of the pathological abnormality, include drilling the jugular tubercle extradurally and removing bone above without disturbing the condyle (21, 33). The extradural reduction of the jugular tubercle aids in minimizing the retraction of the brainstem needed to reach the area anterior to the medulla and pontomedullary junction.

Preauricular subtemporal-infratemporal approach

The preauricular subtemporal-infratemporal approach, reviewed in detail in the chapter on the temporal bone (see *Figs. 8.10* and *8.18*), exposes the jugular foramen anteriorly. It may be selected for tumors that extend along the petrous portion of the internal carotid artery, through the eustachian tube, or through the cancellous portion of the petrous apex (29). A preauricular hemicoronal scalp incision is extended down to at least the level of the tragus and possibly into the cervical region, depending on the extent of the pathological finding and whether a neck dissection is needed. The zygomatic arch is removed or reflected downward with the temporalis muscle, taking care to preserve the frontal branch of the facial nerve. A frontotemporal bone flap, which may include the superior or lateral orbital rim, is elevated, and the glenoid fossa and the mandibular condyle with the joint capsule are either dislocated inferiorly or removed. The dura is elevated, and the bone of the middle fossa medial to the glenoid fossa is removed until the carotid canal is opened. The eustachian tube and the tensor tympani muscle, which course anterior to the carotid canal, are sacrificed during this procedure, taking care to protect the lower cranial nerves as they exit the jugular foramen. The styloid process is divided at its base, and the internal carotid artery is reflected anteriorly to gain access to the clivus and anterior aspect of the jugular foramen. Drilling can be extended to the posterior fossa through Kawase's triangle or through the clivus to the contralateral internal carotid artery (14).

DISCUSSION

Pathologies

Tumors are the most common lesions to affect the jugular foramen; the majority are chemodectomas (glomus jugulare tumor), neurinomas, and meningiomas, with a small percentage of other tumors, such as chondrosarcomas and chordomas (12, 25). The glomus jugulare tumor arises either in the adventitia of the jugular dome or from the intumescences along the tympanic branch of the glossopharyngeal nerve or the auricular branch of the vagus nerve in the jugular foramen (9). Tumors of the same nature that arise in the tympanic cavity or in the mastoid on branches of these nerves are referred to as glomus tympanicum tumors. Small glomus jugulare tumors remain confined within the jugular foramen. However, the tumor can extend as follows: 1) along the eustachian tube into the nasopharynx and through the foramina at the base of the skull, 2) along the carotid artery to the middle fossa, 3) through the intracranial orifice of the jugular foramen or along the hypoglossal canal to the posterior fossa, 4) through the tegmen tympani to the floor of the middle fossa, 5) through the round window and the internal acoustic meatus to the cerebellopontine angle, and 6) through the extracranial orifice of the jugular foramen to the upper cervical region.

Neuromas arise either from the glossopharyngeal, vagus, or the accessory nerves, and meningiomas from arachnoid granulations in the jugular bulb or venous sinuses. Although each tumor has characteristic patterns of invasion and destruction, the basic anatomic environment is similar to that of the glomus jugulare tumor.

Selection of surgical approach

The approaches to the jugular foramen can be categorized into three groups: 1) a lateral group directed through the mastoid bone, 2) a posterior group directed through the posterior cranial fossa, and 3) an anterior group directed through the tympanic bone. This categorization is based on the anatomic fact that the block of the temporal bone, excluding the squamous part, is regarded as an irregular pyramid, having its base on the mastoid surface. In addition, the middle fossa approaches could be categorized as in the "superior group" and the neck dissection upward to the jugular foramen as in the "inferior group." However, the latter approaches are usually not suitable when used alone for pathological abnormalities of the jugular foramen.

Lateral approach

The lateral approach directed through a mastoidectomy, used alone or in combination with other approaches, is the route most commonly selected for lesions extending through the jugular foramen (7, 12, 22). Because the jugular foramen is situated under the otic capsule, the approach basic to this group is called the infralabyrinthine approach. The facial nerve is frequently transposed anteriorly to drill the bone inferior to the labyrinth. Avoiding injury to the facial nerve is one of the key points in the lateral approaches (1). Even with special care, some degree of transient facial palsy is common, possibly because of disturbance to the nerve's vasculature. The surgical field can be widened anteriorly by sacrificing the external auditory canal and middle ear structures or medially by drilling away the otic capsule (translabyrinthine approach) or cochlea (transcochlear approach).

The postauricular transtemporal approach, when combined with a neck dissection, provides satisfactory exposure of the jugular foramen, mastoid air cells, tympanic cavity, and the extracranial structures in and around the carotid sheath. Removal of the styloid process along with transposition of the facial nerve facilitates wide opening of the extracranial orifice of the jugular foramen and provides access to the lower part of the petrous portion of the internal carotid artery. A wider exposure for the extracranial tumor can be obtained by removing the transverse process of the atlas or dislocating or resecting the mandibular condyle. The intracranial extension of the tumor is approached either retrosigmoidally or presigmoidally after adding a lateral suboccipital craniectomy or craniotomy (4, 6, 10, 26, 27).

Posterior approach

This group includes the retrosigmoid approach and its more extensive far-lateral and transcondylar variants. These approaches are suited to the intracranial portion of the tumors. The conventional retrosigmoid approach provides access to the cerebellopontine angle and the intracranial orifice of the jugular foramen. However, extensions of the tumor through the foramen magnum or medially into the clivus are beyond the reach of this approach. The far-lateral and transcondylar modifications access these areas, providing an upward view from below by opening the posterolateral quarter of the foramen magnum and removing the posterior part of the occipital condyle. The posterior and posterolateral margin of the jugular foramen can be accessed by removing the part of the jugular process of the occipital bone located behind the jugular foramen and the portion of the mastoid located behind the mastoid segment of the facial nerve and stylomastoid foramen. A flatter view toward the midline clivus is obtained by additional extradural drilling of the jugular tubercle, although drilling in front of these nerves risks damaging the nerves as they cross the jugular tubercle (21, 23).

Anterior approach

The preauricular subtemporal-infratemporal approach is a major variant of this group of approaches. It uses the pathway anterior to the external auditory canal and through the tympanic bone, which are exposed by removal or displacement of the glenoid fossa and the temporomandibular joint. The approach alone can access the anterior part of the jugular foramen after reflecting the petrous portion of the internal carotid artery anteriorly. Further extensive drilling will expose the middle to upper clivus anteriorly. However, this approach is most often combined with a lateral approach to access an anterior extension of the pathology (22). Fisch et al. call this combined approach the infratemporal fossa approach, Type B or C according to the anterior extension of the exposure (4).

The selection of the optimal approach requires an understanding of the nature and the extension of the lesion. The combination of two or three approaches may be needed either in stages or in combination in one operative procedure (4, 25). Preoperative embolization will often reduce the blood loss with a vascular tumor. Intraoperative electrophysiological monitoring is of great help in avoiding nerve injury, in locating the neural trajectory in and around the tumor, or in predicting postoperative neural function (3, 20). Carefully planned reconstruction is required to reduce postoperative complications, especially leakage of cerebrospinal fluid, and to achieve a satisfactory cosmetic result.

Reprint requests: Albert L. Rhoton, Jr., M.D., Department of Neurological Surgery, University of Florida Brain Institute, P.O. Box 100265, 100 S. Newell Drive, Building 59, L2–100, Gainesville, FL 32610-0265.

REFERENCES

1. Brackmann DE: The facial nerve in the infratemporal approach. **Otolaryngol Head Neck Surg** 97:15–17, 1987.
2. Brackmann DE, Arriaga MA: Surgery for glomus tumors, in Brackmann DE (ed): *Otologic Surgery*. Philadelphia, W.B. Saunders Co., 1994, pp 579–593.
3. DiChiro G, Fischer RL, Nelson KB: The jugular foramen. **J Neurosurg** 21:447–460, 1964.
4. Fisch U, Fagan P, Valavanis A: The infratemporal fossa approach for the lateral skull base. **Otolaryngol Clin N Am** 17:513–552, 1984.
5. Gardner G, Cocke EW, Robertson JT, Trumbull ML, Palmer RE: Combined approach surgery for removal of glomus jugulare tumors. **Laryngoscope** 87:665–688, 1977.
6. Gardner G, Robertson JT, Robertson JH, Cocke EW, Clark WC: Glomus jugulare tumors: Skull base surgery, in Schmidek HH, Sweet WH (eds): *Operative Neurological Techniques*. Philadelphia, W.B. Saunders Co., 1988, ed 2, pp 739–752.
7. Goldenberg RA, Gardner G: Tumors of the jugular foramen: Surgical preservation of neural function. **Otolaryngol Head Neck Surg** 104:129, 1991.
8. Grant JCB: *An Atlas of Anatomy*. Baltimore, Williams & Wilkins, 1951.
9. Guild SR: Glomus jugulare in man. **Ann Otol Rhinol Laryngol** 62:1045–1071, 1953.
10. Hakuba A, Hashi K, Fujitani K, Ikuno H, Nakamura T, Inoue Y: Jugular foramen neurinomas. **Surg Neurol** 11:83–94, 1979.
11. Hovelacque A: *Osteologie*. Paris, G Doin and Cie, 1967, vol 2, pp 155–156.
12. Jackson CG, Cueva RA, Thedinger BA, Glasscock ME III: Cranial nerve preservation in lesions of the jugular fossa. **Otolaryngol Head Neck Surg** 105:687–693, 1991.
13. Katsuta T, Rhoton AL Jr, Matsushima T: The jugular foramen: Microsurgical anatomy and operative approaches. **Neurosurgery** 41:149–202, 1997.
14. Kawase T, Toya S, Shiobara R, Mine S: Transpetrosal approach for aneurysms of the lower basilar artery. **J Neurosurg** 63:857–867, 1985.
15. Kveton JF, Cooper MH: Microsurgical anatomy of the jugular foramen region. **Am J Otol** 9:109–112, 1988.
16. Lang J: Anatomy in and on the jugular foramen, in Frowein RA, Brock M, Klinger M (eds): *Advances in Neurosurgery*. Berlin, Springer-Verlag, 1989, vol 17, pp 125–132.
17. Lang J: *Clinical Anatomy of the Posterior Cranial Fossa and its Foramina*. New York, Thieme Medical Publishers, 1991, pp 92–95.
18. Lang J: Anatomy of the posterior cranial fossa, in Sekhar LN, Janecka IP (eds): *Surgery of Cranial Base Tumors*. New York, Raven Press, 1993, pp 131–146.
19. Lang J, Weigel M: Nerve-vessel relations in the region of the jugular foramen. **Anat Clin** 5:41–56, 1983.
20. Leonetti JP, Brackmann DE, Prass RL: Improved preservation of facial nerve function in the infratemporal approach to the skull base. **Otolaryngol Head Neck Surg** 101:74–78, 1989.
21. Matsushima, T, Ikezaki K, Nagata S, Inoue T, Natori Y, Fukui M, Rhoton AL Jr: Microsurgical anatomy for lateral approaches to the foramen magnum: With special reference to the far-lateral approach and the transcondylar approach, in Nakagawa H (ed): *Surgical Anatomy for Microneurosurgery VII*. Tokyo, SciMed Publications, 1995, pp 81–89.
22. Patel SJ, Sekhar LN, Cass SP, Hirsch BE: Combined approaches for resection of extensive glomus jugulare tumors: A review of 12 cases. **J Neurosurg** 80:1026–1038, 1994.
23. Perneczky A: The posterolateral approach to the foramen magnum, in Samii M (ed): *Surgery in and around the Brain Stem and the Third Ventricle*. Berlin, Springer-Verlag, 1986, pp 460–466.
24. Rhoton AL Jr, Buza R: Microsurgical anatomy of the jugular foramen. **J Neurosurg** 42:541–550, 1975.
25. Samii M, Bini W: Surgical strategy for jugular foramen tumors, in Sekhar LN, Janecka IP (eds): *Surgery of Cranial Base Tumors*. New York, Raven Press, 1993, pp 379–387.
26. Samii M, Draf W: Surgery of the middle skull base, in Samii M, Dwarf W (eds): *Surgery of the Skull Base: An Interdisciplinary Approach*. New York, Springer-Verlag, 1989, pp 234–359.

27. Samii M, Babu RP, Tatagiba M, Sepehrnia A: Surgical treatment of jugular foramen schwannomas. **J Neurosurg** 82:924–932, 1995.
28. Schwaber MK, Netterville JL, Maciunas R: Microsurgical anatomy of the skull base: A morphometric analysis. **Am J Otol** 11:401–405, 1990.
29. Sekhar LN, Schramm VL Jr, Jones NF: Subtemporal-preauricular infratemporal fossa approach to large lateral and posterior cranial base neoplasms. **J Neurosurg** 67:488–499, 1987.
30. Sen CN, Sekhar LN: An extreme lateral approach to intradural lesions of the cervical spine and foramen magnum. **Neurosurgery** 27:197–204, 1990.
31. Silverstein H, Willcox TO, Rosenberg SI, Seidman MD: The jugular dural fold: A helpful base landmark to the cranial nerves. **Skull Base Surg** 5:57–61, 1995.
32. Spetzler RF, Grahm TW: The far-lateral approach to the inferior clivus and the upper cervical region: Technical note. **Barrow Neurol Inst Q** 6:35–38, 1990.
33. Wen HT, Rhoton AL Jr, Katsuta T, de Oliveira E: Microsurgical anatomy of the transcondylar, supracondylar, and paracondylar extensions of the far-lateral approach. **J Neurosurg** 87:555–585, 1997.

ANDREAE VESALII BRVXELLENSIS

DECIMA TERTIA SEPTIMI LIBRI

FIGVRA.

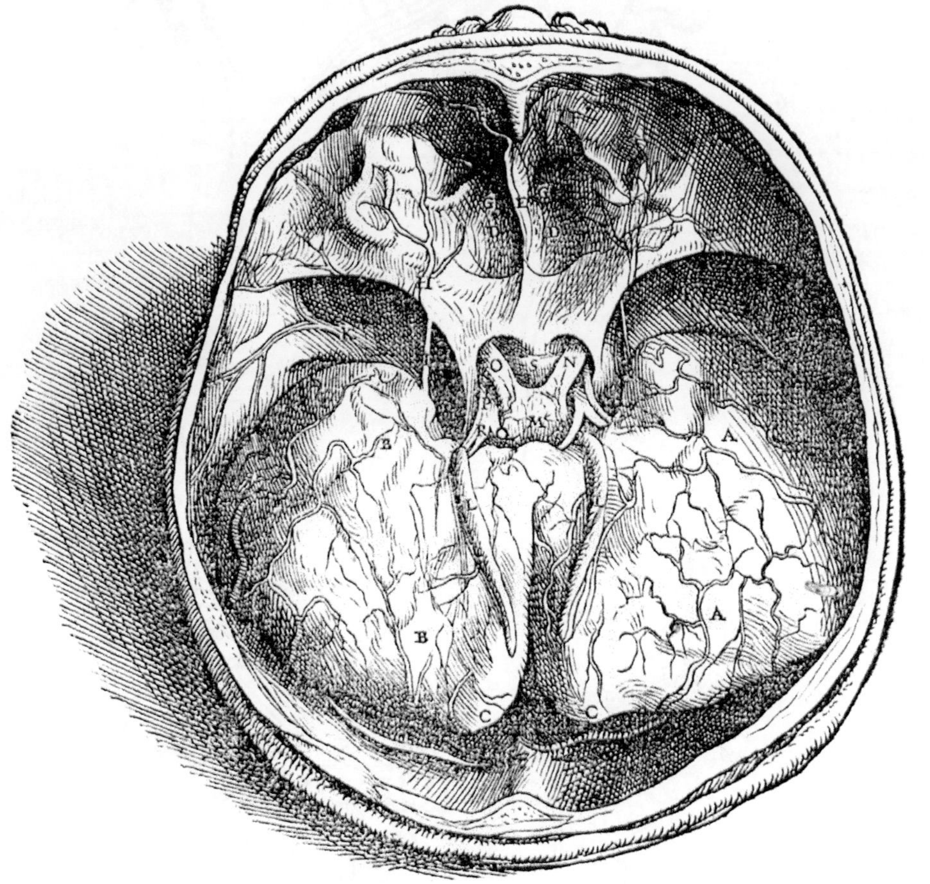

DECIMAE TERTIAE FIGVRAE, EIVSDEMQVE

characterum Index.

Cranial cavity with posterior fossa structures, including cerebellum and cranial nerves, from, Andreas Vesalius, *De Humani Corporis Fabrica*. Basel, Ex officina Ioannis Oporini, 1543. Courtesy, Rare Book Room, Norris Medical Library, Keck School of Medicine, Los Angeles, California.

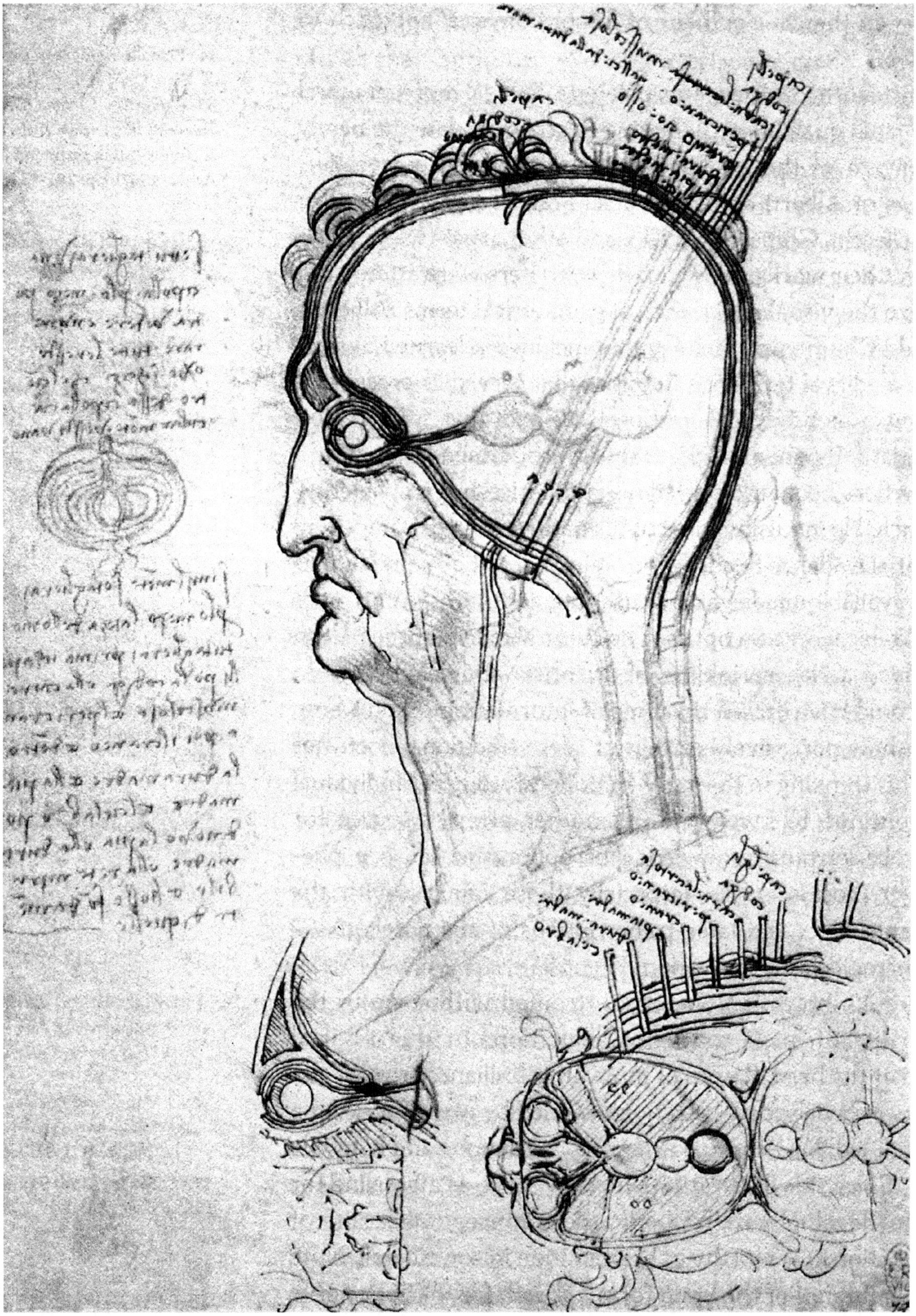

Sagittal transection of the head by Leonardo da Vinci showing his conception of the anatomy of the eye and the mechanisms of sight. Membranes of the brain form a sheath for the optic nerve, which in turn forms the layers of the eyeball to surround the vitreous humor. In the center is the crystalline humor, a fictitious counterpart of the lens.
Courtesy, Dr. Edwin Todd, Pasadena, California.

CHAPTER 10

The Posterior Fossa Cisterns

Albert L. Rhoton, Jr., M.D.

Department of Neurological Surgery, University of Florida, Gainesville, Florida

Key words: Brainstem, Cerebellum, Cranial nerve, Posterior cranial fossa, Subarachnoid cistern

The subarachnoid space, situated between the pia mater and the outer arachnoid membrane, expands at the base of the brain, around the brainstem, and in the tentorial incisura to form compartments filled with cerebrospinal fluid. Numerous trabeculae, septa, and membranes cross the space between the pia mater and the outer arachnoid membrane to divide the subarachnoid space into smaller compartments called cisterns. All of the cranial nerves and major intracranial arteries and veins pass through the cisterns. The cisterns provide a natural pathway through which most operations for intracranial aneurysms, extraaxial brain tumors, and disorders of the cranial nerves are directed. Some cisterns have sheet-like membranes, whereas others have indistinct porous trabeculated walls with openings of various sizes.

The arachnoid membrane that separates the posterior fossa cisterns includes Liliequist's membrane, which separates the chiasmatic and interpeduncular cisterns; the anterior pontine membrane, which separates the prepontine and cerebellopontine cisterns; the lateral pontomesencephalic membrane, which separates the ambient and cerebellopontine cisterns; the medial pontomedullary membrane, which separates the premedullary and prepontine cisterns; and the lateral pontomedullary membrane, which separates the cerebellopontine and cerebellomedullary cisterns. The three cisterns in which the arachnoid trabeculae and membranes are the most dense and present the greatest obstacle at operation are the interpeduncular and quadrigeminal cisterns and the cisterna magna. Numerous arachnoid membranes were found to intersect the oculomotor nerves.

The subarachnoid cisterns are divided into supratentorial and infratentorial groups. The cisterns located in the posterior cranial fossa or that communicate through the tentorial incisura are described here (*Fig. 10.1*) (15). They include paired and unpaired cisterns.

I. Posterior fossa cisterns
   A. Unpaired cisterns
      1. Interpeduncular cistern
      2. Prepontine cistern
      3. Premedullary cistern
      4. Quadrigeminal cistern
      5. Cisterna magna
   B. Paired cisterns
      1. Cerebellopontine cistern
      2. Cerebellomedullary cistern

INTERPEDUNCULAR CISTERN AND LILIEQUIST'S MEMBRANE

The interpeduncular cistern straddles the anterior portion of the tentorial incisura (*Figs. 10.1* and *10.2*). It is situated between the cerebral peduncles and the leaves of Liliequist's membrane at the confluence of the supra- and infratentorial parts of the subarachnoid space. The posterior wall of the cistern is formed by the posterior perforated substance. Its upper border is situated at the posterior edge of the mamillary bodies. Its lower border is situated at the junction of midbrain and pons. It is also bordered rostrally and caudally by Liliequist's membrane.

Liliequist's membrane arises from the outer arachnoid membrane covering the posterior clinoid processes and dorsum sellae (11, 12). As this membrane spreads upward from the dorsum and across the interval between the oculomotor nerves, it gives rise to two separate arachnoidal sheets (*Fig. 10.3*). One sheet, the diencephalic membrane, extends upward and attaches to the diencephalon at the posterior edge of the mamillary bodies and separates the chiasmatic and interpeduncular cisterns. The other sheet, called the mesencephalic membrane, extends backward and attaches along the junction of the midbrain and pons to separate the interpeduncular and prepontine cisterns. The lateral edge of the diencephalic and mesencephalic membranes attaches to the arachnoidal sheath surrounding the oculomotor nerves. The diencephalic membrane is the thicker of the two and is more frequently without perforations so that it acts as a barrier to the passage of air or other substances through the subarachnoid space. The mesencephalic membrane is thinner, more frequently incomplete, and contains an opening through which the basilar artery ascends to reach the interpeduncular fossa. The mesencephalic membrane may form a tight cuff around the basilar artery, but it more commonly has a large opening through which the basilar artery ascends. Many arachnoid trabeculae fan out from the superior edge of the diencephalic membrane to attach to the stalk of the pituitary gland, the mamillary

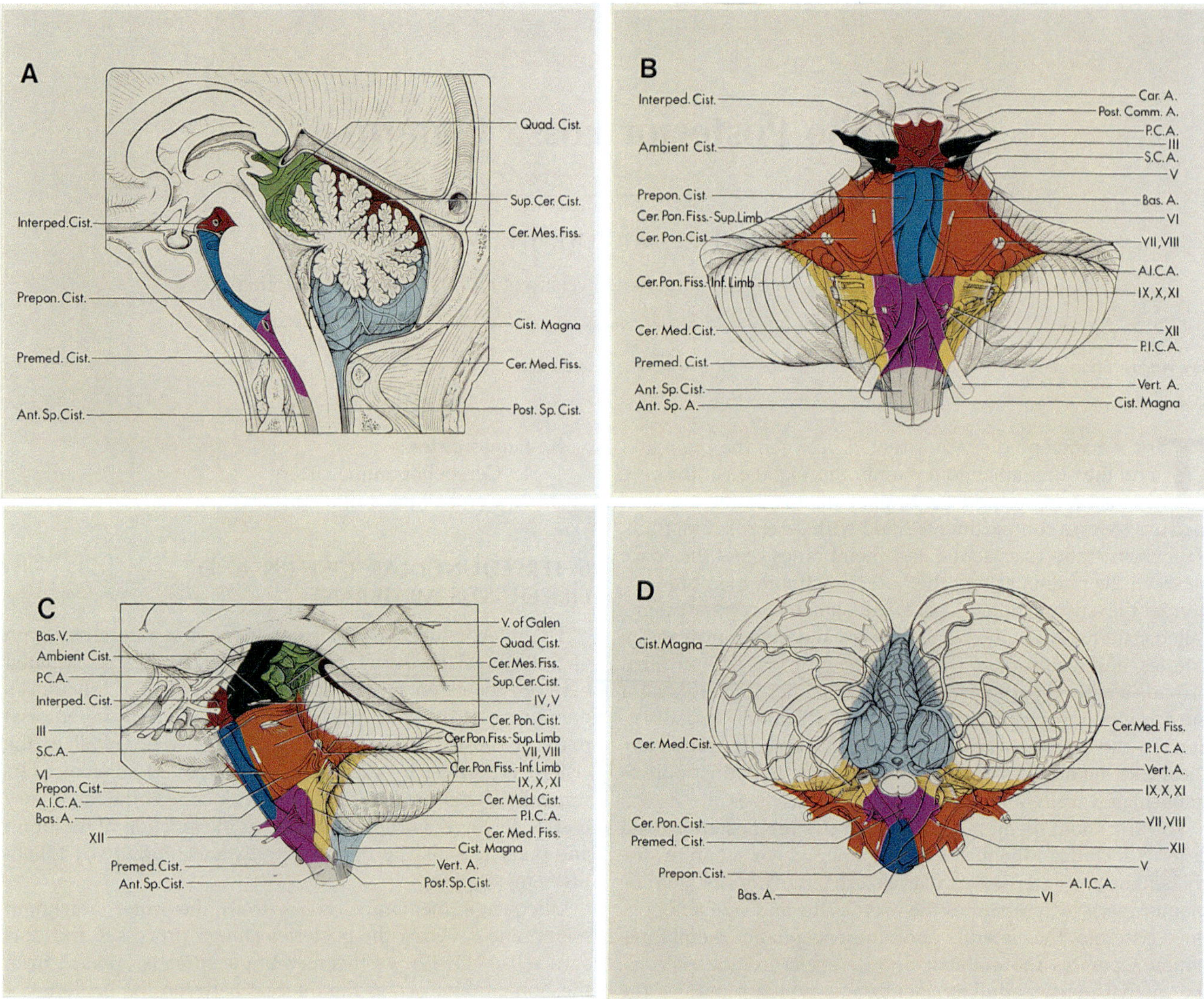

FIGURE 10.1. A–D. Posterior fossa cisterns. *A*, midsagittal section; *B*, anterior view; *C*, lateral view; *D*, inferior view. The cisterns in the posterior fossa are the interpeduncular (*red*), the prepontine (*dark blue*), the cerebellopontine (*orange*), the premedullary (*purple*), the cerebellomedullary (*yellow*), the quadrigeminal (*light green*), the superior cerebellar (*brown*), and the cisterna magna (*light blue*). The anterior spinal (*light gray*) and posterior spinal (*dark gray*) cisterns communicate through the foramen magnum with the posterior fossa cisterns. The ambient cistern (*dark green*) is a supratentorial cistern. The quadrigeminal cistern opens inferiorly into the cerebellomesencephalic fissure. The cerebellopontine cistern extends laterally to the cerebellopontine fissure. The latter fissure has superior and inferior limbs. The cisterna magna opens into the cerebellomedullary fissure. The apex of the basilar artery, the origin of the PCA, and the oculomotor nerves are situated in the interpeduncular cistern. The SCAs arise at the junction of the interpeduncular and prepontine cisterns. The trigeminal, abducens, facial, and vestibulocochlear nerves arise in the cerebellopontine cisterns. The basilar artery gives off the AICAs in the prepontine cistern. The SCAs and AICAs pass through the cerebellopontine cisterns. The vertebral arteries give rise to the PICAs and anterior spinal arteries in the premedullary cistern. The hypoglossal nerves pass through the premedullary cistern. The glossopharyngeal, vagus, and spinal accessory nerves arise in the cerebellomedullary cisterns. The PICAs pass through the cerebellomedullary cisterns and the cisterna magna. The basal vein empties into the vein of Galen in the quadrigeminal cistern. The carotid and posterior communicating arteries are in the supratentorial cisterns. *A.*, artery; *A.I.C.A.*, anteroinferior cerebellar artery; *Ant.*, anterior; *Bas.*, basilar; *Car.*, carotid; *Cer.*, cerebellar; *Cer. Med.*, cerebellomedullary; *Cer. Mes.*, cerebellomesencephalic; *Cer. Pon.*, cerebellopontine; *Cist.*, cistern, cisterna; *Comm.*, communicating; *Fiss.*, fissure; *Inf.*, inferior; *Interped.*, interpeduncular; *P.C.A.*, posterior cerebral artery; *P.I.C.A.*, posteroinferior cerebellar artery; *Post.*, posterior; *Premed.*, premedullary; *Prepon.*, prepontine; *Quad.*, quadrigeminal; *S.C.A.*, superior cerebellar artery; *Sp.*, spinal; *Sup.*, superior; *V.*, vein; *Vert.*, vertebral.

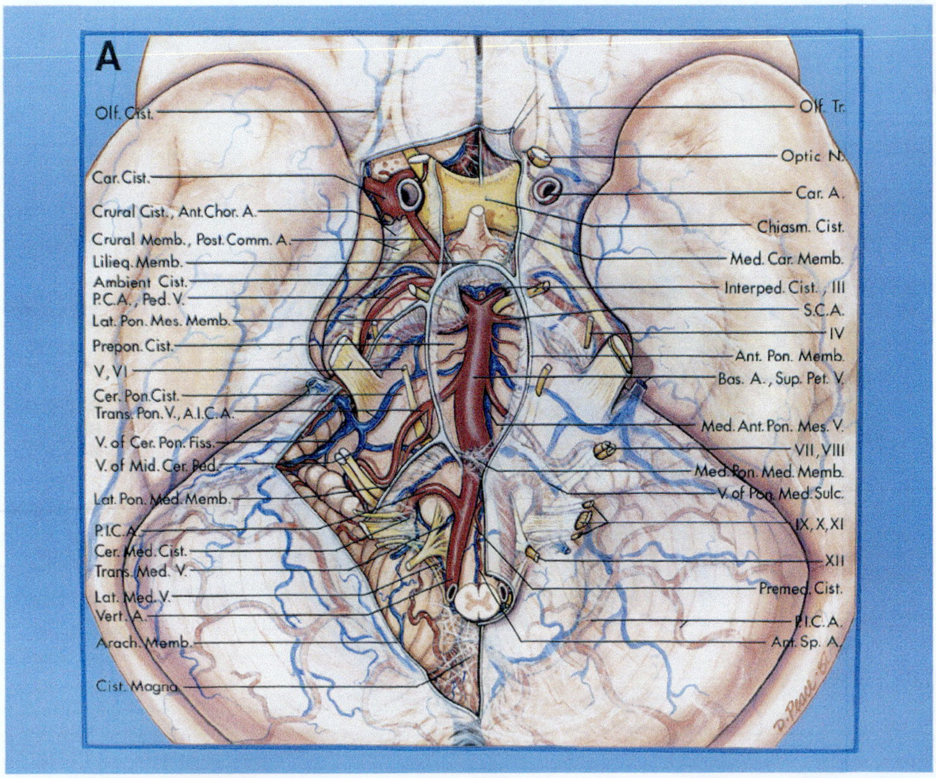

FIGURE 10.2. ***A.*** **Anterior view. The arachnoid membrane has been removed to expose the following cisterns: olfactory, carotid, chiasmatic, ambient, crural, interpeduncular, prepontine, premedullary, cerebellopontine, and cerebellomedullary and the cisterna magna. The oculomotor nerves course in an arachnoidal intersection situated in the junction of the walls of the carotid, chiasmatic, prepontine, interpeduncular, and cerebellopontine cisterns. The medial carotid membrane separates the carotid and chiasmatic cisterns. The crural membrane separates the crural and ambient cisterns. The anterior pontine membrane separates the prepontine and cerebellopontine cisterns. The lateral pontomesencephalic membrane separates the ambient and cerebellopontine cisterns. The medial pontomedullary membrane separates the prepontine and premedullary cisterns, and the lateral pontomedullary membrane separates the cerebellopontine and cerebellomedullary cisterns. The interpeduncular cistern is situated between the diencephalic and mesencephalic leaves of Liliequist's membrane. The bifurcation of the basilar artery is in the interpeduncular cistern. The carotid and posterior communicating arteries course within the carotid cisterns. The anterior choroidal artery arises in the carotid cistern and courses through the crural cistern. The optic nerves and chiasm and the stalk of the pituitary gland are situated in the chiasmatic cistern. The olfactory cisterns enclose the olfactory tracts. The SCAs arise at the junction of the interpeduncular and prepontine cisterns. The PCAs and trochlear nerves course through the ambient cisterns. The AICAs arise in the prepontine cistern. The premedullary cistern contains the hypoglossal nerves and vertebral arteries and the origin of the PICAs and anterior spinal arteries. The abducens, trigeminal, facial, and vestibulocochlear nerves and a segment of the SCA and AICA pass through the cerebellopontine cisterns. The cerebellomedullary cisterns contain the glossopharyngeal, vagus, and accessory nerves and a segment of the PICAs. The veins that course through the cisterns include the peduncular, transverse pontine, transverse medullary, lateral medullary, and median anterior pontomesencephalic veins and the veins of the pontomedullary sulcus, cerebellopontine fissure, and middle cerebellar peduncle. The veins in the cerebellopontine or cerebellomedullary cisterns join to form the superior petrosal veins.** ***A.,*** **artery;** ***A.C.A.,*** **anterior cerebral artery;** ***Ant.,*** **anterior;** ***Arach.,*** **arachnoid;** ***Bas.,*** **basilar;** ***Car.,*** **carotid;** ***Cer.,*** **cerebellar;** ***Cer. Med.,*** **cerebellomedullary;** ***Cer. Pon.,*** **cerebellopontine;** ***Chiasm.,*** **chiasmatic;** ***Chor.,*** **choroid;** ***Cist.,*** **cistern, cisterna;** ***Comm.,*** **communicating;** ***Fiss.,*** **fissure;** ***Front.,*** **frontal;** ***Interped.,*** **interpeduncular;** ***Lat.,*** **lateral;** ***Lilieq.,*** **Liliequist's;** ***M.C.A.,*** **middle cerebral artery;** ***Med.,*** **medial, medullary;** ***Memb.,*** **membrane;** ***Mid.,*** **middle;** ***N.,*** **nerve;** ***Olf.,*** **olfactory;** ***P.C.A.,*** **posterior cerebral artery;** ***Ped.,*** **peduncular;** ***Pet.,*** **petrosal;** ***P.I.C.A.,*** **posteroinferior cerebellar artery;** ***Pon.,*** **pontine;** ***Pon. Med.,*** **pontomedullary;** ***Pon. Mes.,*** **pontomesencephalic;** ***Premed.,*** **premedullary;** ***Prepon.,*** **prepontine;** ***S.C.A.,*** **superior cerebellar artery;** ***Sig.,*** **sigmoid;** ***Sp.,*** **spinal;** ***Sulc.,*** **sulcus;** ***Temp.,*** **temporal;** ***Tent.,*** **tentorium;** ***Tr.,*** **trunk;** ***Trans.,*** **transverse;** ***V.,*** **vein;** ***Vert.,*** **vertebral.**

bodies, and the posterior cerebral and posterior communicating arteries. The interpeduncular cistern communicates with the crural and ambient cisterns, which are situated in the tentorial area between the temporal lobe and midbrain.

The oculomotor nerves course in the lateral wall of the interpeduncular cistern and form the pillars to which the leaves of Liliequist's membrane attach. In addition, the oculomotor nerves are the site of attachment of other arachnoid membranes that separate the cisterns of the junction of the supra- and infratentorial areas (*Figs. 10.2* and *10.3*). The membranes that converge on and form a sleeve around the nerves are the mesencephalic membrane, which separates the interpeduncular and prepontine cisterns; the diencephalic membrane, which separates the interpeduncular and chiasmatic cisterns; the anterior pontine membrane, which separates the cerebellopontine and prepontine cisterns; the lateral pontomesencephalic membrane, which separates the ambient and cerebellopontine cisterns; the medial carotid membrane, which separates the chiasmatic and carotid cisterns; and the lateral carotid membrane, which forms the lateral wall of the carotid cistern.

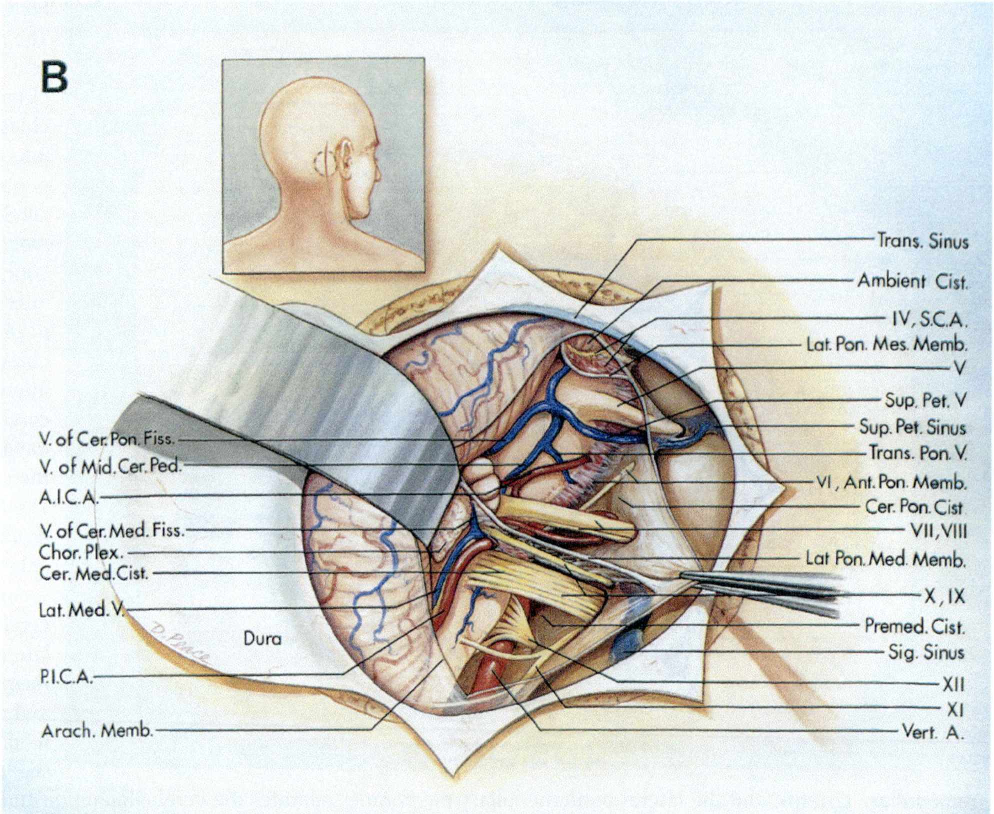

FIGURE 10.2. ***B.*** **Cisterns exposed through a unilateral suboccipital craniectomy. The insert (*upper left*) shows the site of the skin incision (*solid line*) and craniectomy (*interrupted line*). The arachnoid membrane forming the posterior wall of the cerebellopontine and cerebellomedullary cisterns has been opened. The anterior pontine membrane is medial to the abducens nerve. The lateral pontomedullary membrane separates the cerebellopontine and cerebellomedullary cisterns. The flocculus and choroid plexus protrude into the junction of the cerebellomedullary and cerebellopontine cisterns near the foramen of Luschka.**

The interpeduncular cistern contains the posterior thalamoperforating arteries, the bifurcation of the basilar artery, the origins of the posterior cerebral artery (PCA), superior cerebellar artery (SCA), and medial posterior choroidal arteries, the peduncular, posterior communicating, and median anterior pontomesencephalic veins, and the vein of the pontomesencephalic sulcus (3–5, 16, 24).

PREPONTINE CISTERN

The prepontine cistern lies between the arachnoid membrane resting on the clivus and the anterior surface of the pons (*Figs. 10.1–10.4*). The upper end of the cistern is wider than the lower. The prepontine cistern is separated from the interpeduncular cistern by the mesencephalic leaf of Liliequist's membrane. The lower boundary of the cistern is situated at the level of the pontomedullary sulcus, the site of a less well-defined membrane called the medial pontomedullary membrane. This membrane is formed by the thick trabeculae that surround the junction of the vertebral and the basilar arteries. The lateral edges of the prepontine cistern are separated from the cerebellopontine cisterns by the paired anterior pontine membranes. These membranes cross the interval between the pons and the outer arachnoid membrane that rests on the clivus. The anterior pontine membranes intersect the oculomotor nerves superiorly and extend downward along the medial side of the abducens nerves. The anterior pontine membranes become progressively thinner as they extend caudally and may disappear on the lower pons. No cranial nerves were found in the prepontine cistern. The basilar artery courses through and gives rise to the anteroinferior cerebellar artery (AICA) within this cistern (14).

CEREBELLOPONTINE CISTERN

The cerebellopontine cistern lies between the anterolateral surface of the pons and cerebellum and the arachnoidal membrane that rests on the posterior surface of the petrous bone (*Figs. 10.1–10.4*). Superiorly, at the level of the tentorium, this cistern is separated from the ambient cistern by the lateral pontomesencephalic membrane. This membrane is attached to the brainstem at the junction of the midbrain and pons and to the outer arachnoidal membrane near the free edge of the tentorium. Anteriorly, it intersects the oculomotor nerve. This membrane spans the interval between the PCA and SCA. Inferiorly, the cerebellopontine cistern is separated from the cerebellomedullary cistern by the lateral pontomedullary membrane, which crosses the subarachnoid space between the vestibulocochlear and glossopharyngeal nerves. The latter membrane stretches from the junction of the pons and medulla to the outer arachnoidal membrane. Medially, the cerebellopontine cistern is separated from the prepontine cistern by the anterior pontine membrane. Laterally, the cerebellopontine cistern extends to the edge of the cerebellar surface that wraps around the pons to form the cerebellopontine fissure.

The trigeminal nerve arises from the midpons and courses through the superolateral portion of the cistern. The abducens

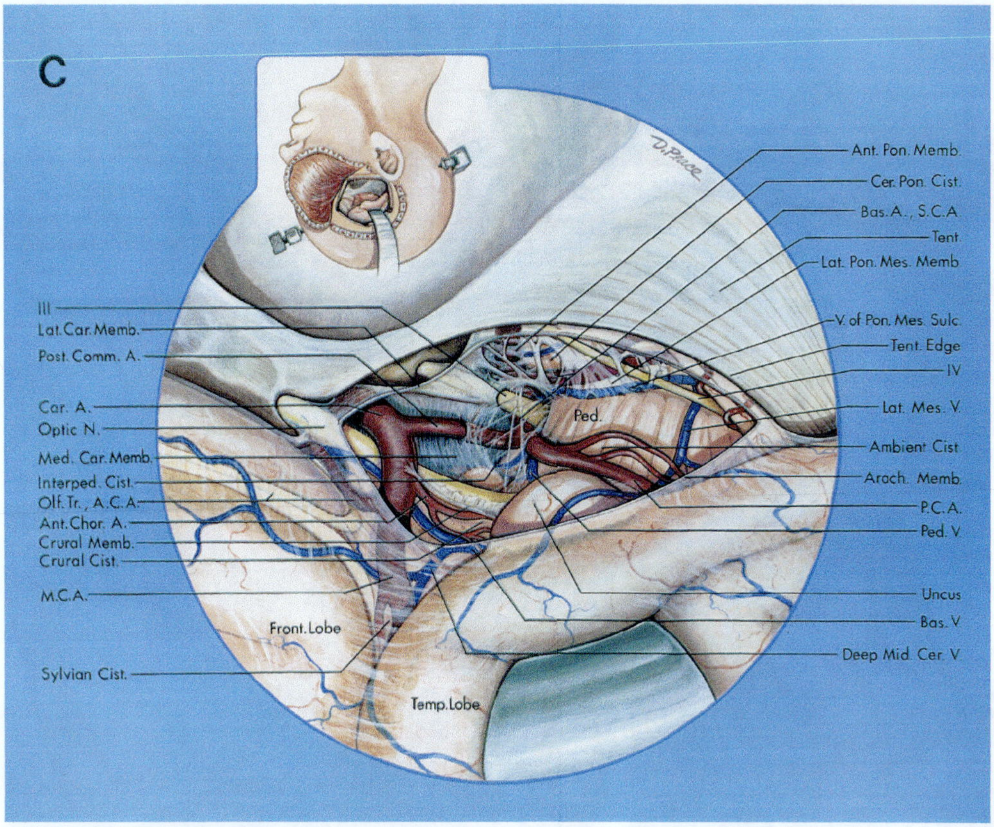

FIGURE 10.2. *C.* **Cisterns in the tentorial incisura. View through a right frontotemporal craniotomy. The insert shows the direction of view. The inferior surface of the temporal lobe has been elevated. The arachnoid membrane medial to the free edge of the tentorium has been opened to expose the carotid, ambient, crural, cerebellopontine, interpeduncular, and sylvian cisterns. The lateral carotid membrane is on the lateral side of the carotid artery, and the medial carotid membrane separates the carotid and chiasmatic cisterns. The crural membrane extends from the optic tract to the uncus and between the origins of the posterior communicating and anterior choroidal arteries.**

nerve arises at the level of the pontomedullary sulcus and ascends just lateral to the anterior pontine membrane. The facial and vestibulocochlear nerves arise in the inferior part of the cerebellopontine cistern just above the lateral pontomedullary membrane. The outer arachnoid membrane extends into the internal auditory canal and surrounds the intracanalicular segment of the facial and vestibulocochlear nerves. The flocculus projects into the cerebellopontine cistern behind the facial and vestibulocochlear nerves.

The SCA and AICA course through the cerebellopontine cistern (5, 14). The SCA enters the cerebellopontine cistern by passing through the junction of the anterior pontine membrane and the oculomotor nerve. It courses below the trochlear nerve and the lateral pontomesencephalic membrane, and above the trigeminal nerve in its passage through this cistern. The bifurcation of the SCA into rostral and caudal trunks may be situated in either the prepontine or the cerebellopontine cisterns. The AICA enters the lower part of the cerebellopontine cisterns by passing through or below the anterior pontine membrane. It commonly bifurcates into its rostral and caudal trunks within this cistern. The veins in this cistern converge on the area around the trigeminal nerve, where they unite to form the superior petrosal veins, which empty into the superior petrosal sinus (16).

PREMEDULLARY CISTERN

The premedullary cistern lies between the anterior surface of the medulla and the arachnoid membrane covering the lower part of the clivus (*Figs. 10.1, 10.2,* and *10.4*) (2). Its upper border is located at the junction of the pons and medulla. It is separated from the prepontine cistern by the medial pontomedullary membrane. Laterally, its border with the cerebellomedullary cistern is located at the dorsal margin of the inferior olive in front of the glossopharyngeal, vagus, and accessory nerves, at the site where the density of the arachnoid trabeculae crossing the subarachnoid space increases (1). Inferiorly, the premedullary cistern is continuous (without obstruction) with the anterior spinal cistern. The rootlets forming the hypoglossal nerves arise in the posterior wall of this cistern between the medullary pyramids and the inferior olives.

The vertebral arteries enter this cistern by ascending through the foramen magnum. They ascend obliquely through this cistern and join at the junction of the premedullary and prepontine cisterns. The paired anterior spinal arteries arise from the vertebral arteries and join to form a single trunk that courses in the midline on the anterior surface of spinal cord.

CEREBELLOMEDULLARY CISTERN

The cerebellomedullary cistern lies caudal to the junction of the pons and medulla (*Figs. 10.1, 10.2,* and *10.4*). It is separated from the cerebellopontine cistern by the lateral pontomedullary membrane and from the premedullary cistern by the trabeculae in front of the glossopharyngeal, vagus, and accessory nerves. Its inferior border is located at the level of the foramen magnum. The cistern extends backward from the

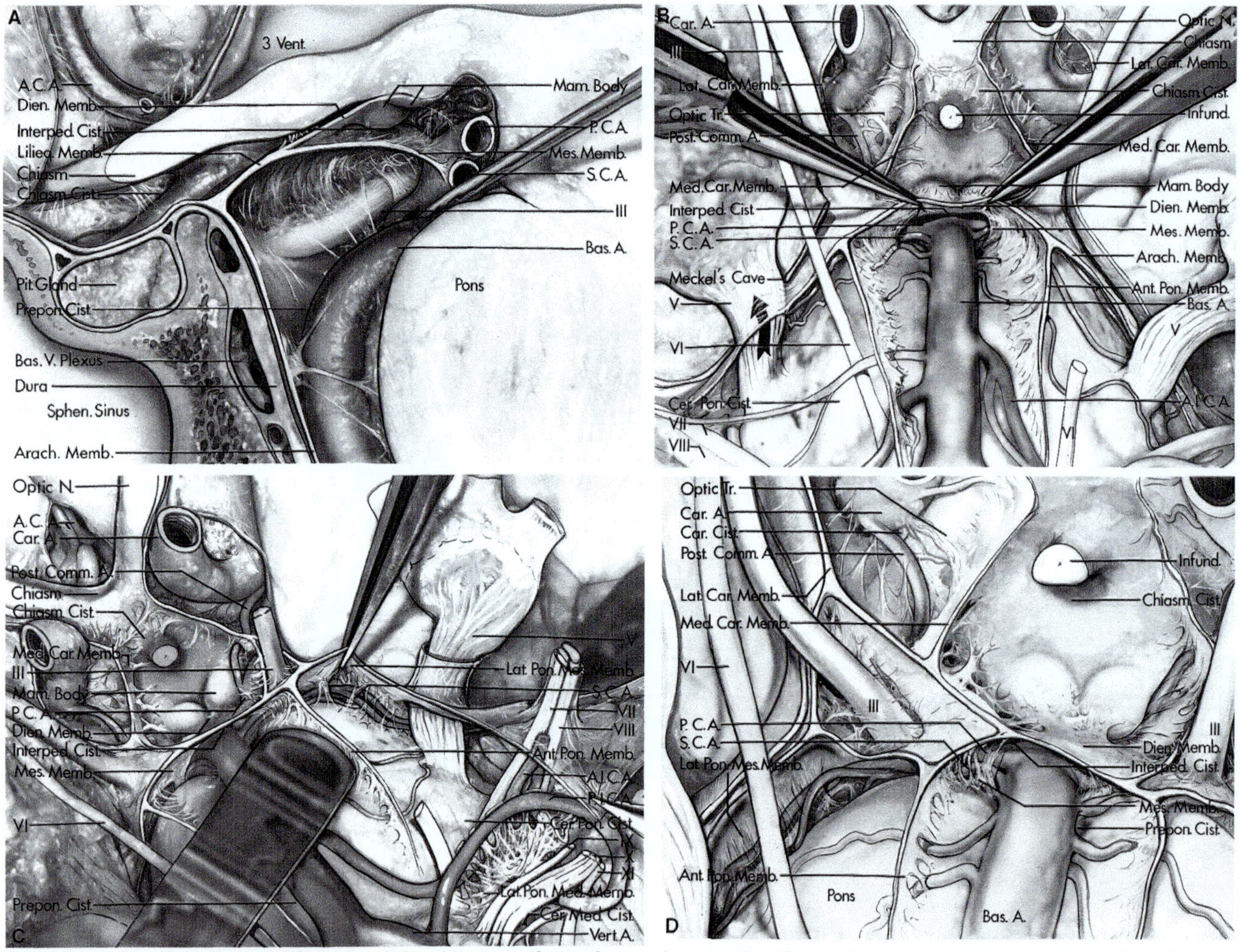

FIGURE 10.3. Liliequist's membrane and the cisterns and membranes intersecting the oculomotor nerve. *A*, parasagittal section to the left of the midline. Liliequist's membrane arises from the part of the outer arachnoid membrane that rests against the dorsum sellae and splits into the diencephalic and mesencephalic membranes. The diencephalic membrane is a complete membrane that attaches to the maxillary bodies and separates the chiasmatic and interpeduncular cisterns. The mesencephalic membrane, which attaches along the junction of the midbrain and pons, forms an incomplete wall between the interpeduncular and prepontine cisterns with an opening through which the basilar artery ascends. *B–D*, cisterns and membranes intersecting the oculomotor nerves. *B*, the ventral arachnoidal wall of the chiasmatic, carotid, interpeduncular, prepontine, and cerebellopontine cisterns has been removed. The lateral carotid membrane forms the lateral wall of the carotid cistern. The medial carotid membrane separates the carotid and the chiasmatic cisterns. The interpeduncular cistern is situated behind the mamillary bodies and the diencephalic membrane. The cerebellopontine cistern opens into Meckel's cave (*arrow*). The anterior pontine membrane separates the prepontine and cerebellopontine cisterns. *C*, the arachnoid membrane covering the cerebellopontine cistern has been stretched laterally to show the lateral pontomesencephalic membrane. The lateral pontomedullary membrane separates the cerebellomedullary and cerebellopontine cisterns. *D*, the arachnoidal cuff around the right oculomotor nerve has been opened. The medial and lateral carotid, mesencephalic, diencephalic, lateral pontomesencephalic, and anterior pontine membranes converge on and form a cuff around the oculomotor nerve. *A.*, artery; *A.C.A.*, anterior cerebral artery; *Ant.*, anterior; *Arach.*, arachnoid; *Bas.*, basilar; *Car.*, carotid; *Cer. Med.*, cerebellomedullary; *Cer. Pon.*, cerebellopontine; *Cist.*, cistern; *Comm.*, communicating; *Dien.*, diencephalic; *Infund.*, infundibulum; *Interped.*, interpeduncular; *Lat.*, lateral; *Mam.*, mamillary; *Med.*, medial; *Memb.*, membrane; *Mes.*, mesencephalic; *N.*, nerve; *P.C.A.*, posterior cerebral artery; *P.I.C.A.*, posteroinferior cerebellar artery; *Pit.*, pituitary; *Pon.*, pontine; *Post.*, posterior; *Prepon.*, prepontine; *S.C.A.*, superior cerebellar artery; *Sphen.*, sphenoid; *Tr.*, trunk; *V.*, vein, venous; *Vent.*, ventricle.

dorsal margin of the inferior olive around the dorsolateral medulla to the biventral lobule of the cerebellum.

The glossopharyngeal and vagus nerves and the medullary portion of the accessory nerve arise within and course through this cistern to reach the jugular foramen. The spinal portion of the accessory nerve ascends from the posterior spinal cistern to reach the cerebellomedullary cistern. The lateral recess of the fourth ventricle communicates with this cistern through the foramen of Luschka. The choroid plexus that projects from the foramen of Luschka sits on the posterior surface of the glossopharyngeal and vagus nerves.

The vertebral artery enters the dura mater at the lower border of this cistern and immediately leaves it to enter the premedullary cistern. The posteroinferior cerebellar artery (PICA) enters this cistern by reaching the anterior surface of the rootlets of the glossopharyngeal, vagus, and accessory nerves (13). From here, the artery passes dorsally between the rootlets of these nerves and pursues a posterior course around the medulla to enter the cisterna magna.

CISTERNA MAGNA

The cisterna magna lies dorsal to the medulla and cerebellar vermis (*Fig. 10.1*). Its posterior wall is formed by the arachnoid membrane that conforms to the inner surface of the occipital bone above the foramen magnum. A characteristic feature of the cisterna magna is the dense, mesh-like trabeculated arachnoid that extends from the cerebellar tonsils to the medulla and the margin of the foramen of Magendie.

The lower part of the cisterna magna is situated behind the medulla (17). Superiorly, the cisterna magna projects both anterior and posterior to the cerebellar vermis. Anteriorly, it opens into the cerebellomedullary fissure. The cisterna magna also opens behind the vermis into the posterior cerebellar incisura. The arachnoid membrane covering the incisura is reflected around the falx cerebelli. The upper limit of the extension behind the vermis is the tentorium. If the falx cerebelli is absent or small, the upper part of the cistern may be quite large. A median sheet of arachnoid may extend from the dorsal surface of the medulla to the outer arachnoid membrane to divide the cistern into sagittal halves. Inferiorly, the cisterna magna communicates without obstruction with the posterior spinal cistern.

The PICAs pass posteriorly around the medulla. They enter the cisterna magna near the point where they commonly divide into a lateral trunk, which supplies the hemisphere and tonsil, and a medial trunk, which supplies the vermis (3, 13).

QUADRIGEMINAL CISTERN

The quadrigeminal cistern encloses a space that corresponds to the pineal region (*Fig. 10.1*) (18, 19, 22, 26). The quadrigeminal plate is located at the center of the anterior wall of the cistern. In the midline, the anterior wall rostral to the colliculi is formed by the pineal gland. The suprapineal recess of the third ventricle bulges into the cistern above the gland. Laterally, the anterior wall is formed by the part of the pulvinar that lies medial to where the crus of the fornix wraps around the pulvinar. The fornix crosses the pulvinar midway between the medial and lateral edges of the pulvinar. The medial half of the pulvinar forms the anterior wall of the cistern and the lateral half of the pulvinar forms the anterior wall of the atrium of the lateral ventricle.

Each lateral wall of the cistern has an anterior and a posterior part. The anterior part is formed by the segment of the crus of the fornix that wraps around the pulvinar. The posterior part is formed by the part of the occipital cortex located below the splenium. Below the colliculi, the cistern extends into the cerebellomesencephalic fissure.

The roof of the cistern is formed by the lower surface of the splenium and the broad membranous envelope that surrounds the great vein and its tributaries. This envelope is applied to the lower surface of the splenium and is continuous anteriorly with the tela choroidea surrounding the velum interpositum. It is within this envelope in the superomedial part of the cistern that the intracisternal venous structures are found in the greatest density (16). The superomedial location of the veins contrasts with the location of the arteries, which are found in the greatest density in the inferolateral part of the cistern.

The quadrigeminal cistern communicates with the posterior pericallosal cistern, which extends around the splenium. It opens inferolaterally below the pulvinars into the ambient cisterns, which are located between the midbrain and the temporal lobes. It may communicate with the velum interpositum. The trochlear nerves arise in the quadrigeminal cistern just below the inferior colliculi and course forward around the midbrain and below the pulvinars to enter the ambient cisterns.

The trunks and branches of the PCA and SCA enter the lower-anterior part of the cistern and course below and lateral to the arachnoidal envelope around the vein of Galen and its tributaries (5, 16, 29). The PCAs commonly bifurcate into their calcarine and parieto-occipital branches within the cistern. Some of the lateral posterior choroidal arteries arise from the PCAs within this cistern (4). The medial posterior choroidal arteries arise from the PCAs in front of the midbrain and encircle the brainstem to enter the quadrigeminal cistern, where they turn forward beside the pineal body to reach the velum interpositum. The SCAs course through the part of the cistern that extends into the cerebellomesencephalic fissure. The perforating branches of the PCAs supply the walls of the cistern situated above the shallow groove separating the superior and inferior colliculi, and the SCAs supply the walls of the cistern below this groove.

The venous relationships in the cistern are the most complex in the cranium because the cistern is the site of convergence of the internal cerebral and basal veins and multiple other tributaries of the vein of Galen (18, 19). The internal cerebral veins exit the velum interpositum and the basal veins exit the ambient cisterns to reach the quadrigeminal cistern, where they join the vein of Galen. The latter vein passes below the splenium to enter the straight sinus at the tentorial apex. The veins that converge on the cistern to empty into the great, basal, or internal cerebral veins include the posterior pericallosal veins, which course around the splenium; the atrial veins, which drain the walls of the atria; the internal occipital veins, which originate on or near the calcarine and parieto-occipital sulci; and the vein of the cerebellomesencephalic fissure, which originates on the superior cerebellar peduncles and terminates with the superior vermian vein in the great vein.

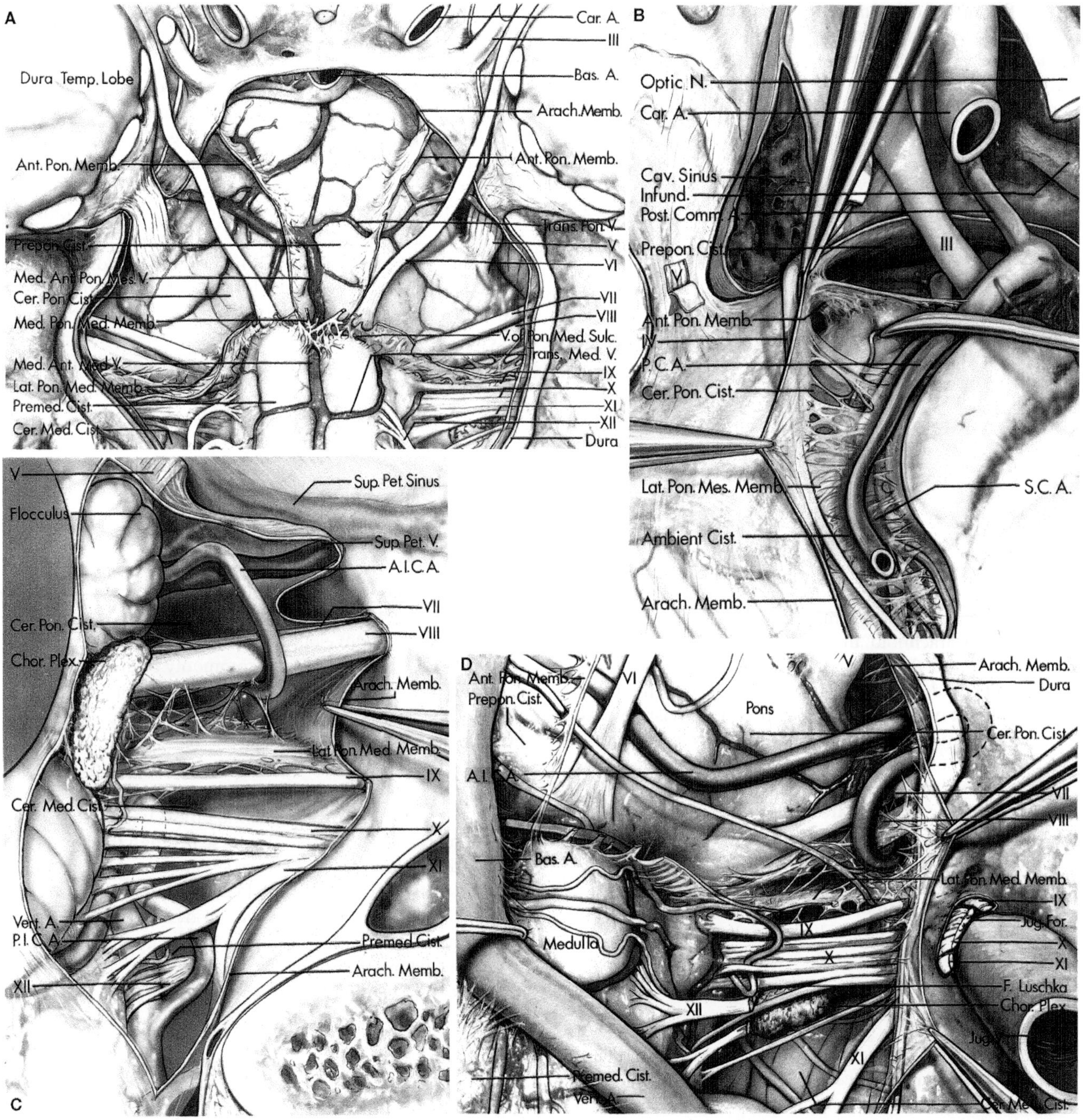

FIGURE 10.4. *A,* prepontine, cerebellopontine, cerebellomedullary, and premedullary cisterns. The arachnoid membrane that forms the anterior wall of the cerebellopontine, cerebellomedullary, prepontine, and premedullary cisterns has been removed. The lateral pontomedullary membrane separates the cerebellopontine and cerebellomedullary cisterns. The thick arachnoid trabeculae around the junction of the vertebral arteries form the median pontomedullary membrane that separates the premedullary and prepontine cisterns. The anterior pontine membrane separates the prepontine and cerebellopontine cisterns. The premedullary cistern extends backward to the anterior surface of the glossopharyngeal, vagus, and accessory nerves. *B,* the anterior pontine membrane, which separates the prepontine and cerebellopontine cisterns, passes forward from the pons to the clivus. The lateral pontomesencephalic membrane, which forms the floor of the ambient cistern and the roof of the cerebellopontine cistern, stretches across the interval between the PCA and SCA. A small flap of dura has been elevated to expose the trigeminal nerve in Meckel's cave. *C,* posterior view. The arachnoid membrane forming the posterior wall of the cerebellopontine and cerebellomedullary cisterns has been opened. The lateral pontomedullary membrane separates the cerebellopontine and

SUPERIOR CEREBELLAR CISTERN

This cistern is situated between the superior part of the vermis and the arachnoid membrane that rests against the lower border of the straight sinus. Anteriorly, it opens into the quadrigeminal cistern (*Fig. 10.1*). Posteriorly, it communicates below the torcular with the cisterna magna. Laterally, it blends into the subarachnoid space over the cerebellar hemispheres. The cistern contains the median and paramedian branches of the SCAs and the superior vermian vein.

DISCUSSION

Key and Retzius's excellent illustrations in 1875 accurately display the anterior pontine, medial and lateral pontomedullary, and lateral pontomesencephalic membranes and the membrane now called Liliequist's membrane (9). Liliequist noted that the membrane bearing his name, in pneumograms, is often seen as a fine line with a forward convexity extending from the dorsum sellae to the mamillary bodies (11, 12). In our study, this membrane was found to have two leaves: an upper leaf, called the diencephalic membrane, which attaches to the posterior edge of the mamillary bodies, and a caudal leaf, called the mesencephalic membrane, which attaches to the junction of the pons and the midbrain. The completeness and position of the diencephalic membrane favor its definition after lumbar subarachnoid injections of air, whereas a membrane like the mesencephalic membrane would not be seen on air studies because the large perforation in it, through which the basilar artery ascends, does not block the passage of air.

The oculomotor nerve is the site of intersection of multiple arachnoidal membranes (9). Six arachnoid membranes converge on the oculomotor nerve: the diencephalic, mesencephalic, anterior pontine, lateral pontomesencephalic, and medial and lateral carotid membranes. The medial carotid membrane separates the chiasmatic and carotid cisterns. The lateral carotid membrane, which is situated lateral to the carotid artery, extends from the optic to the oculomotor nerve (10, 25).

The three sites in the posterior fossa where the normal arachnoidal trabeculae and membranes present the greatest obstacle at operation are the interpeduncular and quadrigeminal and the cisterna magna. The multiple membranes that converge on the walls of the interpeduncular cistern make the operative exposure of lesions in this cistern more difficult. The tendency for the arachnoidal membranes and the nerves and arteries to which they attach to retract away from the site of an arachnoidal incision can be utilized to aid in exposing lesions in the interpeduncular cistern and also at other sites. If the arachnoid membrane is opened below the oculomotor nerve, the intact arachnoid membrane above the nerve will draw the nerve upward. After opening the arachnoid membrane below the oculomotor nerve, elevating the temporal lobe will elevate the oculomotor nerve and aid in exposing the structures below the nerve because the arachnoid above the oculomotor nerve is tethered to the temporal lobe. Opening the arachnoid above the nerve will allow the nerve to retract inferiorly and facilitate the exposure of structures above the nerve.

The second site at which the arachnoid trabeculae are especially dense is in the superomedial part of the quadrigeminal cistern, where the dense arachnoidal envelope surrounding the vein of Galen and its tributaries blends with the tela choroidea forming the walls of the velum interpositum. The part of the cistern situated below the vein of Galen that contains the PCA and SCA is less densely trabeculated.

The third site where the arachnoidal web is especially dense is in the cisterna magna, where the trabeculae bind the medulla and cerebellar tonsils to the branches of the PICA. It is commonly necessary to divide numerous trabeculae to remove a cerebellar tonsil and to expose and mobilize the infratonsillar loop of the PICA.

Opening a cisternal wall, with the resultant escape of cerebrospinal fluid, facilitates the approach to lesions in front of the brainstem and cerebellum. Allowing cerebrospinal fluid to escape from the cisterna magna during posterior fossa operations facilitates the exposure of lesions in the cerebellopontine, cerebellomedullary, prepontine, and premedullary cisterns. In some operations in which excessive retraction would be necessary to reach a cistern, opening the arachnoid over several surface folia and applying suction through a cottonoid laid over the arachnoidal opening will remove enough cerebrospinal fluid to relax the cerebellum and allow the operation to proceed.

Pathological processes in the subarachnoid space may conform to cisternal boundaries. The arachnoid septa and trabeculae separating the cisterns may prevent the spread of blood to adjacent cisterns after aneurysm rupture. The resulting location of the blood, as seen on computed tomographic scans and magnetic resonance imaging, often provides information pinpointing the site of a ruptured aneurysm. The thickening and staining of the arachnoid membranes that follow subarachnoid hemorrhage may make the approach to an aneurysm more difficult. Yasargil notes that aneurysms may become invested with the arachnoidal walls of the cisterns and that tension on the arachnoid membranes may be transmitted to the fundus of the aneurysm, even when dissection is being

cerebellomedullary cisterns. The PICA and hypoglossal nerves arise in the premedullary cistern. Choroid plexus protrudes into the junction of the cerebellomedullary and cerebellopontine cisterns. *D,* anterior view. The lateral pontomedullary membrane separates the cerebellopontine and cerebellomedullary cisterns. The anterior pontine membrane separates the prepontine and cerebellopontine cisterns. *A.,* artery; *A.I.C.A.,* anteroinferior cerebellar artery; *Ant.,* anterior; *Arach.,* arachnoid; *Bas.,* basilar; *Car.,* carotid; *Cav.,* cavernous; *Cer. Med.,* cerebellomedullary; *Cer. Pon.,* cerebellopontine; *Chor. Plex.,* choroid plexus; *Cist.,* cistern; *Comm.,* communicating; *F.,* foramen; *For.,* foramen; *Infund.,* infundibulum; *Jug.,* jugular; *Lat.,* lateral; *Med.,* medial, medullary; *Memb.,* membrane; *N.,* nerve; *P.C.A.,* posterior cerebral artery; *Pet.,* petrosal; P.I.C.A., posteroinferior cerebellar artery; Pon., pontine; *Pon. Mes.,* pontomesencephalic; *Post.,* posterior; *Premed.,* premedullary; *Prepon.,* prepontine; *S.C.A.,* superior cerebellar artery; *Sulc.,* sulcus; *Temp.,* temporal; *Trans.,* transverse; *V.,* vein; *Vert.,* vertebral.

carried out some distance away (27, 28). In dissecting an aneurysm, it is helpful to know which membranes may be attached to the aneurysm. Aneurysms arising at the basilar apex and at the origin of the SCA may project into the leaves of Liliequist's membrane; aneurysms arising at the origin of the AICA may have the anterior pontine membrane stretched around their surface; aneurysms arising at the origin of the PICA from the vertebral artery may project upward into the lateral pontomedullary membrane; and aneurysms arising at the junction of the vertebral with the basilar arteries may be enmeshed in the thick trabeculae that form the medial pontomedullary membrane (21).

An understanding of the arachnoidal membranes is especially important in dealing with aneurysms pointing in the direction of the oculomotor nerves. Traction on any of the membranes converging on the oculomotor nerve may rupture these aneurysms. The outer surface of the arachnoidal membranes that are adherent to an aneurysm may provide a plane of dissection that allows easier separation of the aneurysm from adjacent structures. It may be necessary to leave some of the arachnoid membrane attached to the fundus and wall of the aneurysm to prevent rupture of the aneurysm before a clip is applied.

A knowledge of the anatomy of the cistern will aid in dissecting some tumors. The arachnoidal walls of a cistern containing a tumor may protect the neural and vascular structures in adjacent cisterns from operative injury. Tumors may be classified into five categories on the basis of their relationship to the cisterns. These are: 1) growth within a single cistern; 2) growth within one cistern with compression of adjacent cisterns; 3) growth within multiple cisterns; 4) growth in adjacent structures with extension into the cisterns; and 5) growth in adjacent structures with compression of, but not extension into, the adjacent cisterns. A small pinealoma or acoustic neurinoma will be situated entirely within a single cistern. As it enlarges, it will stretch the arachnoidal walls of the cistern around its borders. Epidermoid tumors grow within multiple cisterns. These tumors, when situated in the posterior fossa, commonly involve the cerebellopontine, cerebellomedullary, and prepontine cisterns, and they may spread into the premedullary, interpeduncular, ambient, and quadrigeminal cisterns. Choroid plexus papillomas and ependymomas of the fourth ventricle may extend through the foramen of Magendie into the cisterna magna or through the foramen of Luschka into the cerebellomedullary cistern. Some gliomas of the cerebellum and brainstem may develop exophytic extensions into the cisterns. Meningiomas commonly arise external to and compress the cisterns without extending directly into them.

Acoustic neurinomas may stretch the anterior pontine, lateral pontomedullary, and lateral pontomesencephalic membranes around their borders (23). Preserving the arachnoid membrane that lies posterior to the tumor and extends into the internal acoustic meatus during removal of the posterior meatal wall with a drill will prevent bone dust from entering the subarachnoid space. A large tumor will displace the abducens nerve and anterior pontine membrane toward the midline. The lateral pontomedullary membrane crosses the interval between the tumor and the glossopharyngeal and vagus nerves and provides some protection for these nerves during tumor removal. Meningiomas may be removed without opening the outer arachnoid membrane. These tumors frequently displace the arachnoid membrane around their inner surface. The arachnoid membrane provides a barrier to injury of adjacent arteries and nerves during the removal of these tumors.

The arachnoid membranes surrounding the cerebellopontine and cerebellomedullary cisterns are best seen in decompression operations on the cranial nerves (6–8, 20). During these operations, the membranes are commonly found to be displaced by tortuous arteries. When one exposes the trigeminal nerve by the retrosigmoid route, the trochlear nerve is usually seen just above the trigeminal nerve. Placing the arachnoidal incision to expose the trigeminal nerve below the caudal edge of the trochlear nerve will allow the arachnoidal trabeculae inserting on the upper edge of the trochlear nerve to draw it upward, away from the operative site. After the outer arachnoidal membrane beside the trigeminal nerve is opened, the lateral pontomesencephalic membrane will come into view in the interval above the SCA. To complete a decompression operation on the trigeminal nerve, one rarely must expose the SCA as far medial as the point where it penetrates the anterior pontine membrane.

In completing an operation at the junction of the cerebellopontine and cerebellomedullary cisterns for hemifacial spasm, one sees the lateral pontomedullary membrane in the interval between the glossopharyngeal nerve and the nerves entering the internal acoustic meatus. One of the more common findings in hemifacial spasm is that the PICA has looped upward to compress the caudal surface of the facial nerve. This loop commonly pushes the lateral pontomedullary membrane ahead of it.

Reprint requests: Albert L. Rhoton, Jr., M.D., Department of Neurological Surgery, University of Florida Brain Institute, P.O. Box 100265, 100 S. Newell Drive, Building 59, L2–100, Gainesville, FL 32610-0265.

REFERENCES

1. Amundsen P, Newton TH: Subarachnoid cisterns, in Newton TH, Potts DG (eds): *Radiology of the Skull and Brain*. St. Louis, CV Mosby, 1974, vol 4, pp 3588–3711.
2. de Oliveira E, Rhoton AL Jr, Peace DA: Microsurgical anatomy of the region of the foramen magnum. **Surg Neurol** 24:293–352, 1985.
3. Fujii K, Lenkey C, Rhoton AL Jr: Microsurgical anatomy of the choroidal arteries: Fourth ventricle and cerebellopontine angles. **J Neurosurg** 52:504–524, 1980.
4. Fujii K, Lenkey C, Rhoton AL Jr: Microsurgical anatomy of the choroidal arteries: Lateral and third ventricles. **J Neurosurg** 52: 165–188, 1980.
5. Hardy DG, Peace DA, Rhoton AL Jr: Microsurgical anatomy of the superior cerebellar artery. **Neurosurgery** 6:10–28, 1980.
6. Jannetta PJ: Microsurgical approach to the trigeminal nerve for tic douloureux, in Krayenbühl H, Maspes PE, Sweet WH (eds): *Progress of Neurological Surgery*. Basel, Karger, 1976, vol 7, pp 180–200.
7. Jannetta PJ: Cranial nerve vascular compression syndromes (other than tic doulourex and hemifacial spasm), in Carmel PW (ed): *Clinical Neurosurgery*. Baltimore, Williams & Wilkins, 1981, vol 28, pp 445–456.

8. Jannetta PJ, Abbasy M, Maroon JC, Ramos FM, Albin MS: Etiology and definitive microsurgical treatment of hemifacial spasm. Operative techniques and results in 47 patients. **J Neurosurg** 47:321–328, 1977.
9. Key A, Retzius G: *Studien in der Anatomie des Nervensystems und des Bindegewebes*. Stockholm, Norstad 1875, vol 1, pp 111–123.
10. Lewtas NA, Jefferson AA: The carotid cistern: A source of diagnostic difficulties with suprasellar extensions of pituitary adenoma. **Acta Radiol Diagn (Stockh)** 5:675–690, 1966.
11. Liliequist B: The anatomy of the subarachnoid cisterns. **Acta Radiol** 46:61–71, 1956.
12. Liliequist B: The subarachnoid cisterns: An anatomic and roentgenologic study. **Acta Radiol** 185:1–108, 1959.
13. Lister JR, Rhoton AL Jr, Matsushima T, Peace DA: Microsurgical anatomy of the posterior inferior cerebellar artery. **Neurosurgery** 10:170–199, 1982.
14. Martin RG, Grant JL, Peace DA, Theiss C, Rhoton AL Jr: Microsurgical relationships of the anterior inferior cerebellar artery and the facial-vestibulocochlear nerve complex. **Neurosurgery** 6:483–507, 1980.
15. Matsuno H, Rhoton AL Jr, Peace DA: Microsurgical anatomy of the posterior fossa cisterns. **Neurosurgery** 23:58–80, 1988.
16. Matsushima T, Rhoton AL Jr, de Oliveira E, Peace DA: Microsurgical anatomy of the veins of the posterior fossa. **J Neurosurg** 59:63–105, 1983.
17. Matsushima T, Rhoton AL Jr, Lenkey C: Microsurgery of the fourth ventricle: Part 1—Microsurgical anatomy. **Neurosurgery** 11:631–667, 1982.
18. Ono M, Ono M, Rhoton AL Jr, Barry M: Microsurgical anatomy of the region of the tentorial incisura. **J Neurosurg** 60:365–399, 1984.
19. Ono M, Rhoton AL Jr, Peace DA, Rodriguez RJ: Microsurgical anatomy of the deep venous system of the brain. **Neurosurgery** 15:621–657, 1984.
20. Rhoton AL Jr: Microsurgical anatomy of the posterior fossa cranial nerves. **Clin Neurosurg** 26:398–462, 1979.
21. Rhoton AL Jr: Anatomy of saccular aneurysms. **Surg Neurol** 14:59–66, 1980.
22. Rhoton AL Jr: Microsurgical anatomy of the third ventricle: Part 2—Operative approaches. **Neurosurgery** 8:357–373, 1981.
23. Rhoton AL Jr: Microsurgical anatomy of the brain stem surface facing an acoustic neuroma. **Surg Neurol** 25:326–339, 1986.
24. Saeki N, Rhoton AL Jr: Microsurgical anatomy of the upper basilar artery and the posterior circle of Willis. **J Neurosurg** 46:563–578, 1977.
25. Wackenheim A, Braun JP, Babin E, Megret M: The carotid cistern. **Neuroradiology** 5:82–84, 1973.
26. Yamamoto I, Rhoton AL Jr, Peace DA: Microsurgical anatomy of the third ventricle: Part 1—Microsurgical anatomy. **Neurosurgery** 8:334–356, 1981.
27. Yasargil MG: *Microneurosurgery*. New York, Thieme-Stratton, 1984, vol 1, pp 5–53.
28. Yasargil MG, Kasdaglis K, Jain KK, Weber HP: Anatomical observations of the subarachnoid cisterns of the brain during surgery. **J Neurosurg** 44:298–302, 1976.
29. Zeal AA, Rhoton AL Jr: Microsurgical anatomy of the posterior cerebral artery. **J Neurosurg** 48:534–559, 1978.

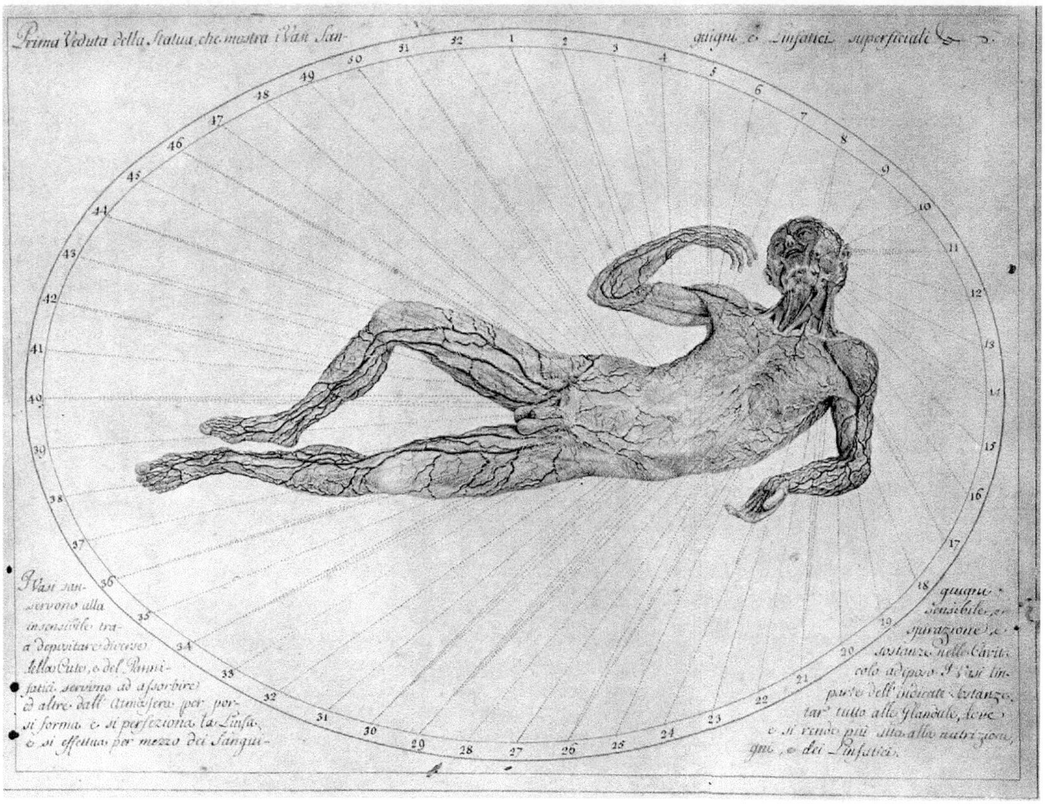

Key to various anatomic structures for an 18th century wax model in the Ceroplastica Laboratory of La Specola, Florence, Italy. The anatomic model reached its peak expression during this period. Courtesy, Ceroplastica Laboratory, La Specola, Florence, Italy.

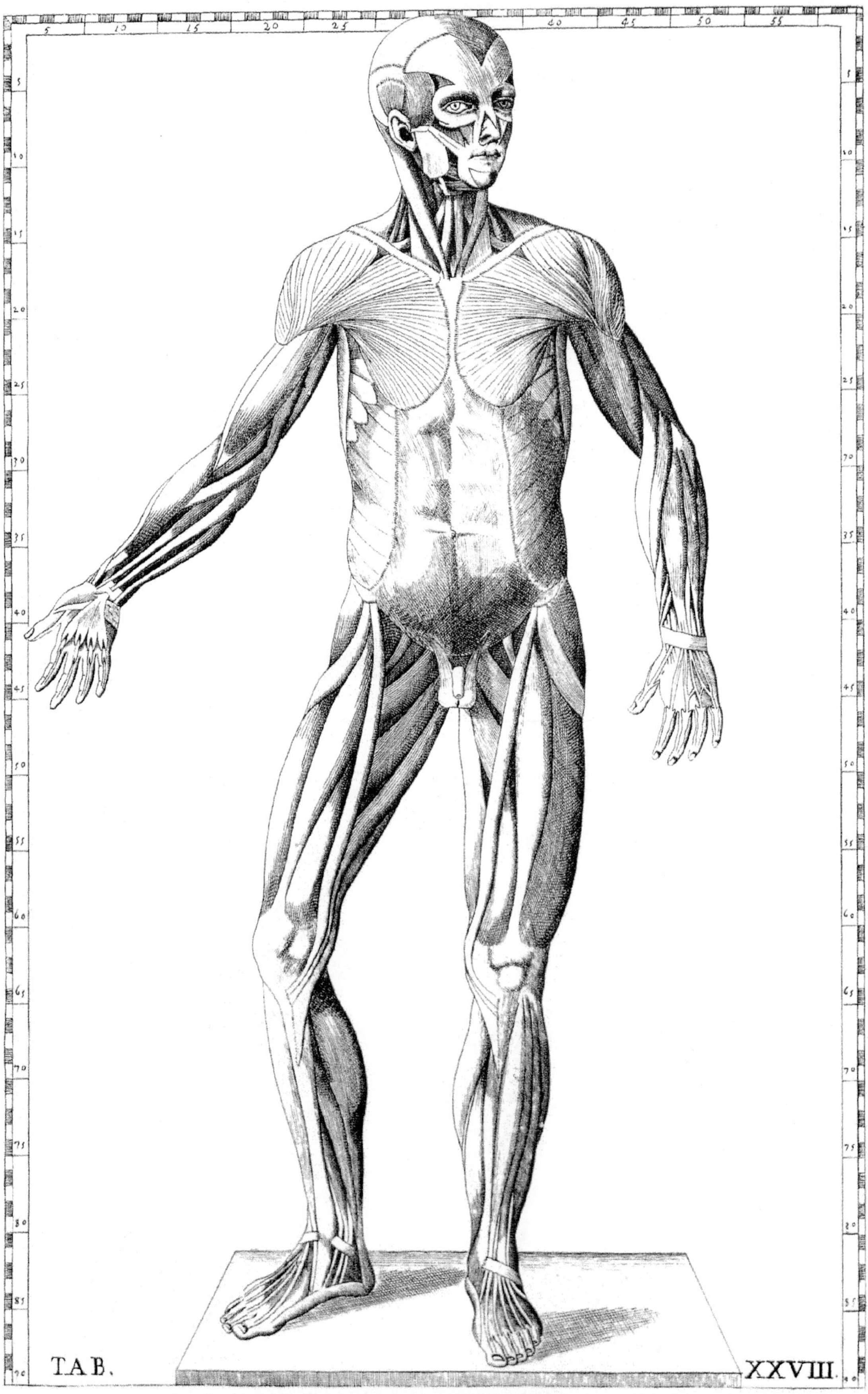

Superficial dissection showing anterior musculature, from, Bartolommeo Eustachio, *Tabulae anatomicae*. Rome, Sumptibus Laurentii & Thomae Pagliarini, 1728. Courtesy, Rare Book Room, Norris Medical Library, Keck School of Medicine, Los Angeles, California.

SUBJECT INDEX

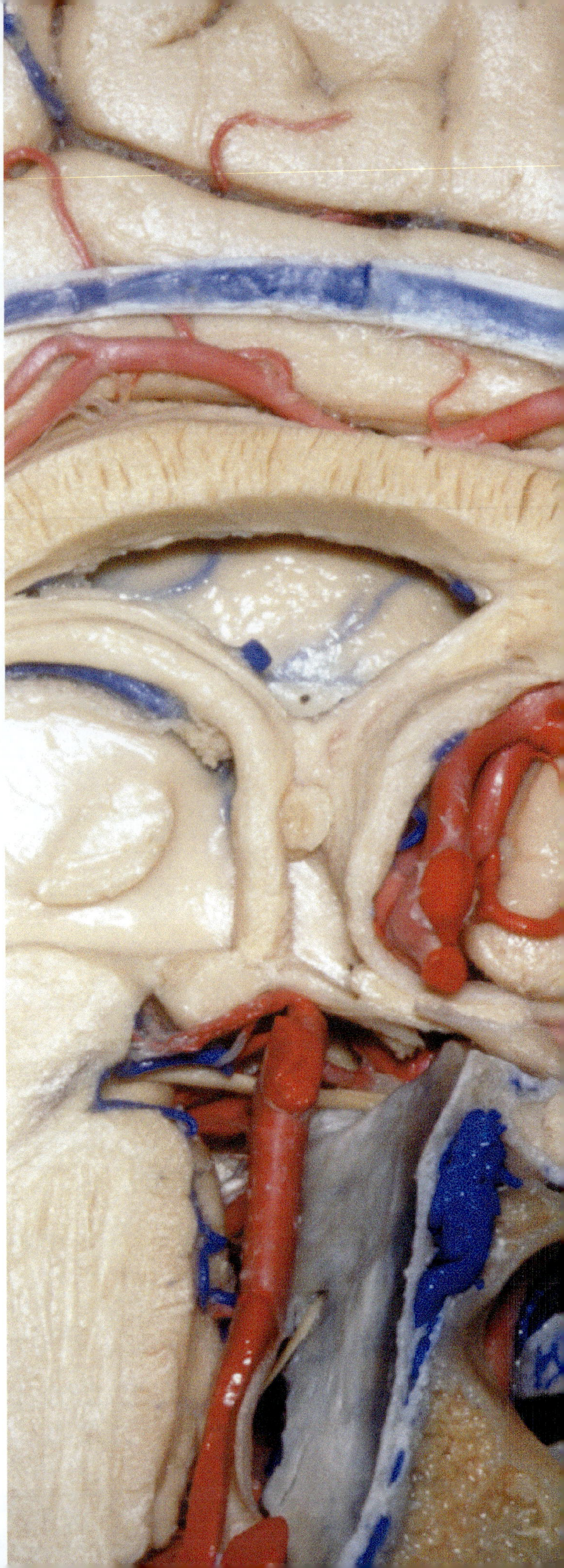

Rhoton's Anatomy

Note: Page numbers in italics have been used to indicate material found in illustrations and legends.

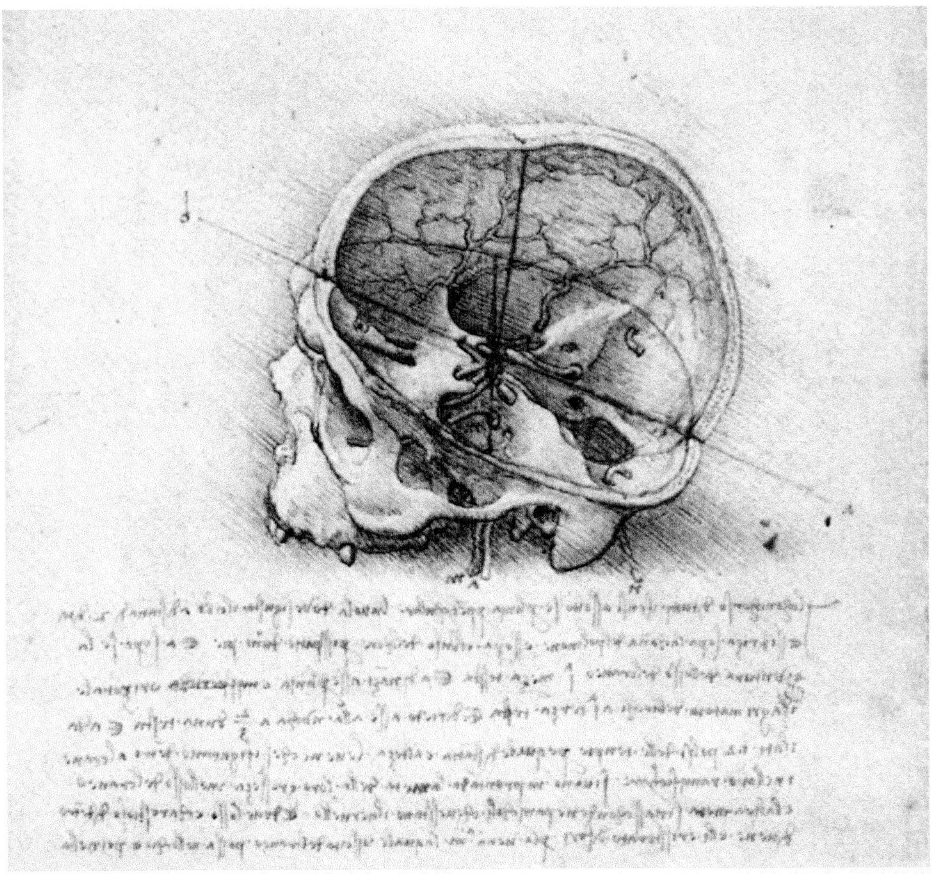

Cranial cavity drawing by Leonardo da Vinci captures the growing sense of a science of proporations for Renaissance artists. In addition to serving as anatomical specimens, his drawings remain consummate examples of draftsmanship. Courtesy, Dr. Edwin Todd, Pasadena, California.